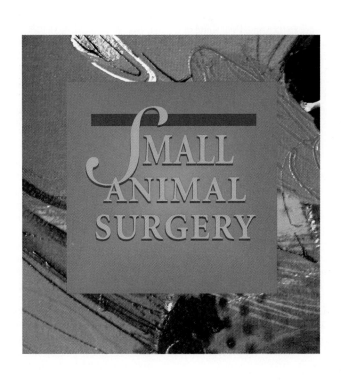

SMALL ANIMAL SURGERY

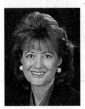

Theresa Welch Fossum, DVM, MS, PhD, Diplomate ACVS, Associate Professor and Chief of Surgery, Department of Small Animal Medicine and Surgery, College of Veterinary Medicine, Texas A&M University. Dr. Fossum is recognized as an outstanding veterinarian and an excellent teacher. She has received several awards for teaching excellence, including the Wiley Distinguished Teaching Professorship in Veterinary Medicine at Texas A&M University, 1994 to 1997. She frequently lectures and conducts laboratory sessions across the United States and in Europe and Japan. She has acted as principal investigator in a great number of funded research activities and received the American Kennel Club and American Veterinary Medical Foundation "Excellence in Canine Research" award in 1997 for her research of chylothorax. In addition, she has authored an impressive number of refereed publications and book chapters and acts as a reviewer for the leading veterinary journals.

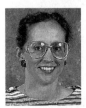

Cheryl S. Hedlund, DVM, MS, Diplomate ACVS, Professor of Surgery and Chief, Companion Animal Surgery and Anesthesia, School of Veterinary Medicine, Louisiana State University. Dr. Hedlund has been working in veterinary medicine since she was a child helping out in her father's rural veterinary practice. She is well respected in the field of veterinary medicine, particularly for her expertise in upper respiratory surgery. Dr. Hedlund frequently contributes articles to refereed publications and has authored many book chapters. She is a member of the Editorial Review Boards for *Veterinary Surgery* and *Journal of the American Animal Hospital Association* and acts as an ad hoc reviewer for other journals. Dr. Hedlund has served on the ACVS's Credentials Committee and is a member of the AVMA and AAHA, among other professional organizations.

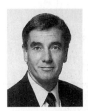

Donald A. Hulse, DVM, Diplomate ACVS, Professor, Department of Small Animal Medicine and Surgery, College of Veterinary Medicine, Texas A&M University. Dr. Hulse is well recognized for his accomplishments in teaching and in small animal orthopedics. He served as Section Chief of Small Animal Surgery from 1992 through 1996. He served on the ACVS's Examination Committee from 1992 to 1995. Dr. Hulse sat on the Board of Directors of the Veterinary Orthopedic Society from 1984 to 1987. He is also a member of the AVMA. Dr. Hulse's research in small animal orthopedics is extensive, including countless funded projects. His articles on orthopedics have been widely published, and he is a frequent contributor to veterinary books.

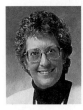

Ann L. Johnson, DVM, MS, Diplomate ACVS. Professor, Department of Veterinary Medicine, University of Illinois. Dr. Johnson is an internationally recognized veterinary orthopedic surgeon and educator. She has received the University of Illinois Award for Excellence in Graduate and Professional Teaching and the Purdue Outstanding Alumna Award in recognition of Distinguished Performance in Teaching, Research, and Organized Veterinary Medicine. She has been invited to lecture and conduct courses throughout the United States and Europe. Her research is significant and she has had countless journal articles and book chapters published. Dr. Johnson has been an active member of numerous committees in the ACVS since 1985 and was elected President of the ACVS in 1996. She is also a member of the AVMA, AO-Vet, and the Veterinary Orthopedic Society.

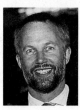

Howard B. Seim III, DVM, Diplomate ACVS, Associate Professor and Chief of Small Animal Surgery, Department of Clinical Sciences, Colorado State University. Dr. Seim has garnered accolades for his teaching ability. He was corecipient of the 1993 Merck AGVET Award for Creative Teaching and was awarded the 1995 Provosts' N. Preston Davis Award for Instructional Innovation. Dr. Seim has been teaching for 19 years, has been an active student advisor, and has participated in the AVMA's Mentor Program. Dr. Seim is also well recognized for his knowledge of and experience in the field of neurosurgery. He has presented innumerable scientific papers in this field, and has authored or coauthored many book chapters. Dr. Seim has obtained funding for a variety of research projects in the area of neurology. He has been a member of the Editorial Review Board of the *Journal of the AVMA* and of *Veterinary Surgery*. Dr. Seim served on the ACVS's Examination Committee from 1991 to 1995, and was Committee Chairman in 1993. He is also a member of AAHA.

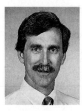

MEDICAL CONSULTANT–Michael D. Willard, DVM, MS, Diplomate ACVIM, Professor, Department of Small Animal Medicine and Surgery, College of Veterinary Medicine, Texas A&M University. Dr. Willard has been receiving awards for teaching excellence since 1987, among them the 1994 National Norden Award. In addition, he has numerous clinical presentations and has conducted some research in gastroenteric problems. Dr. Willard is also a member of the AVMA, AAHA, and the Comparative Gastroenterology Society. He serves as a reviewer for several veterinary journals. He has contributed numerous journal articles and several monographs and book chapters. Dr. Willard was responsible for reviewing most of the chapters in *Small Animal Surgery*, verifying the medical management of surgical diseases from an internist's perspective.

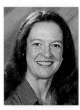

ANESTHESIA CONSULTANT – Gwendolyn L. Carroll, MS, DVM, Diplomate ACVA. Assistant Professor, Anesthesiology, Department of Small Animal Medicine and Surgery, College of Veterinary Medicine, Texas A&M University. Her primary interest is perioperative analgesia. Dr. Carroll is a member of the AVMA and the Veterinary Emergency and Critical Care Society, among other organizations. She was responsible for reviewing and verifying all anesthetic regimens and dosages included throughout *Small Animal Surgery*.

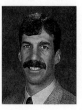

CONTRIBUTOR–Christopher E. Orton, DVM, MS, PhD, Diplomate ACVS, Professor, Department of Clinical Sciences, Colorado State University. Dr. Orton is a member of the American Physiological Society, the American Association of Veterinary Clinicians, and the AVMA. Dr. Orton's area of specialization is cardiothoracic surgery. He contributed Chapter 24, Surgery of the Cardiovascular System, to *Small Animal Surgery*.

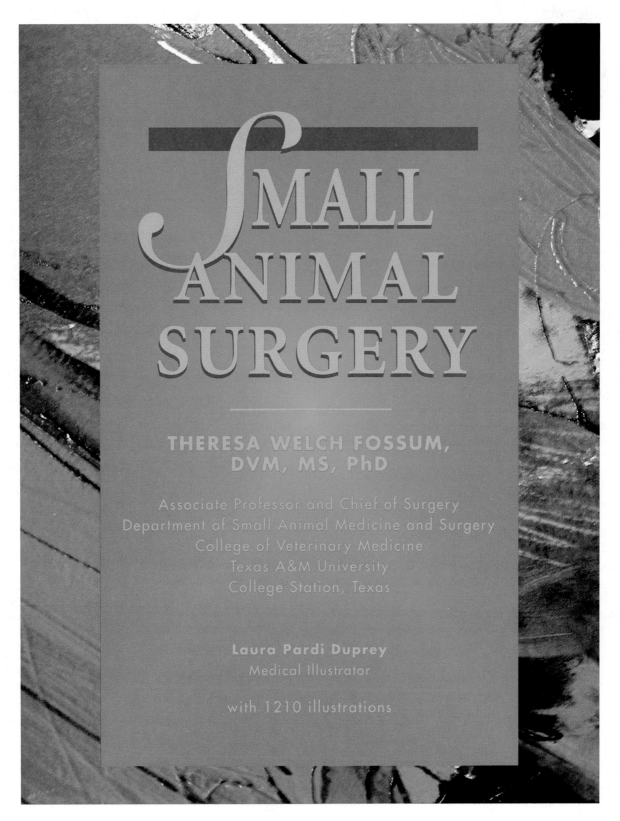

SMALL ANIMAL SURGERY

**THERESA WELCH FOSSUM,
DVM, MS, PhD**

Associate Professor and Chief of Surgery
Department of Small Animal Medicine and Surgery
College of Veterinary Medicine
Texas A&M University
College Station, Texas

Laura Pardi Duprey
Medical Illustrator

with 1210 illustrations

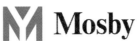 **Mosby**

St. Louis Baltimore Boston Carlsbad Chicago Naples New York Philadelphia Portland
London Madrid Mexico City Singapore Sydney Tokyo Toronto Wiesbaden

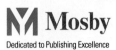
Mosby
Dedicated to Publishing Excellence

A Times Mirror
Company

Publisher: Don Ladig
Editor: Linda Duncan
Managing Editor: Penny Rudolph
Editorial Assistant: Angela Reiner
Project Manager: Mark Spann
Production Editor: Holly Roseman
Book Design Manager: Judi Lang
Book and Cover Designer: Jeanne Wolfgeher
Manufacturing Supervisor: Karen Boehme

NOTICE
Every effort has been made to ensure that the drug dosage schedules and current therapy contained herein are accurate and in accord with the standards accepted at the time of publication. However, as new research and experience broaden our knowledge, changes in treatment and drug therapy occur. Therefore, the reader is advised to check the product information sheet included in the package of each drug he/she plans to administer to be certain that changes have not been made in the recommended dose or in the contraindication. This is of particular importance in regard to new or infrequently used drugs.

Printed in the United States of America

Composition by GTS Graphics, Inc.
Printing/binding by Von Hoffman Press, Inc.

Mosby-Year Book, Inc.
11830 Westline Industrial Drive
St. Louis, Missouri 63146

ISBN 0-8151-3238-7

98 99 00 01 / 9 8 7 6 5 4 3

This book is dedicated to my husband (Matt Miller)
and sons, Chase and Kobe,
who made a personal sacrifice
while it was being written,
and to my students.

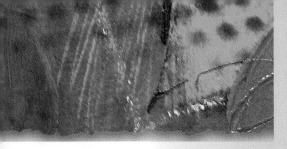

Preface

It takes only a quick glance to notice that Small Animal Surgery is vastly different from other veterinary surgical textbooks. When we initially conceptualized this book we agreed that our main objective would be to create an excellent reference for practitioners and students of veterinary surgery. Although the term user friendly is overused, we determined that this book should be not only well organized and informative but a pleasure to read. We agreed that the best way to achieve these goals was to break away from the typical mold used for veterinary textbooks. Most importantly we decided that we would have (1) a limited number of contributors, (2) an excellent and consistent artwork program, and (3) a precise and consistent format that varied minimally between chapters.

The bulk of this book was written by five surgeons. Dr. Howard Seim and myself were responsible for Part I, General Surgical Principles, while Dr. Cheryl Hedlund and myself contributed Part II, Soft Tissue Surgery, exclusive of the cardiovascular surgery chapter provided by Dr. Chris Orton. Drs. Don Hulse and Ann Johnson provided the material encompassed in Part III, Orthopedic Surgery. Lastly, Dr. Seim contributed Part IV, the Neurosurgery section. Because we wanted to provide the most up-to-date information on the medical management of surgical diseases, we enlisted the aid of an internist, Dr. Mike Willard. Mike reviewed most of the chapters, verifying information and providing his perspective to the case management detailed throughout this book.

SPECIAL FEATURES
Art Program

The artwork in this book is exceptional. Surgery is indeed a visual field and this book is a visual masterpiece. Most of the illustrations in this book are original drawings provided by a professional medical illustrator, Laura Duprey. To have had the opportunity to work with such a skilled medical illustrator was truly a privilege. If we could conceive of an illustration, Laura could make it reality. This detailed artwork, combined with the use of color photographs, makes understanding difficult surgical techniques much less formidable.

Consistent Chapter Format

Even with the limited number of authors, use of color, and exceptional illustrations, lack of a consistent format would limit the usefulness of this book. For this reason, we have used a single consistent format for all of the disease chapters of this book. Because we know veterinary practitioners are busy and it takes time to look up details such as drug dosages and formulas, we have used tables throughout the book to provide this information. Whenever a drug is mentioned in the text, the dose is included in a nearby table. Other innovations in this book are the use of notes to emphasize key points or concepts and the use of color text to highlight descriptions of surgical techniques. Surgical techniques are found throughout the text in the present tense. We have attempted to describe the techniques with great detail and in a readily understandable fashion. To achieve a consistent format required that there be some duplication of material. To prevent excessive duplication we have in some instances referred readers to other pages; however, where we felt that it would be beneficial to have the information duplicated (e.g., tables with drug dosages or formulas) we have done so.

OVERALL ORGANIZATION OF THE BOOK
General Format

This book comprises 37 chapters and is organized into four parts. The first 10 chapters of Part I, General Surgical Principles, were written with veterinary medical students in mind. The information contained within these chapters is the information we teach our students in their introductory surgery courses. Found within these chapters is detailed information on the basics of sterile technique, surgical instrumentation, suturing, preoperative care, and rational antibiotic use. The color photographs illustrating hand ties, pack preparation, and surgical instruments should be particularly useful. Chapter 11 contains information on postoperative care, including nutrition, for surgical patients. Because nutrition affects many body systems and is an important adjunct to case management, we have included detailed information on techniques for hyperalimentation in this chapter. Chapter 12 is a concise description of practical information on analgesics for surgical patients.

Parts II, III, and IV contain information on soft tissue surgery, orthopedic surgery, and neurosurgery, respectively. These chapters are divided into a section detailing general

General chapter format

I. General principles and techniques
    A. Definitions
    B. Preoperative concerns
    C. Anesthetic considerations
    D. Antibiotics
    E. Surgical anatomy
    F. Techniques
    G. Wound healing
    H. Suture materials/special instruments
    I. Postoperative care and assessment
    J. Complications
    K. Special age considerations
II. Specific diseases
    A. Definitions
    B. Synonyms
    C. General considerations and clinically relevant pathophysiology
    D. Diagnosis
        1. Clinical presentation
            a. Signalment
            b. History
        2. Physical examination findings
        3. Radiography/Ultrasonography
        4. Laboratory findings
    E. Differential diagnosis
    F. Medical management
    G. Surgical treatment
        1. Preoperative management
        2. Anesthesia
        3. Surgical anatomy
        4. Positioning
    H. Surgical technique
    I. Suture materials/special instruments
    J. Postoperative care and assessment
    K. Complications
    L. Prognosis

principles and techniques and a section on specific diseases. The General Principles and Techniques portion begins with definitions of procedures and terms relevant to the organ system detailed. Next are sections detailing information on preoperative concerns and anesthetic considerations. This is followed by a discussion on antibiotic use (including recommendations for antibiotic prophylaxis) and a brief description of pertinent surgical anatomy. Anatomy is too often neglected in surgical textbooks, or, because of formatting, is not well correlated with the techniques in a given chapter. We have circumvented this problem by including it as a separate and consistent heading under General Principles and Techniques. Surgical techniques that are broadly applicable to a number of diseases are also detailed in this section. However,

if a surgical procedure is specific to a particular disease, the description of the technique will be found instead with the specific disease description. Brief discussions on healing of the specific organ or tissue as well as suture materials and special instruments follow the surgical techniques descriptions. Information on wound healing is inconsistently found in most surgical textbooks, and decisions on choice of suture material are often neglected. The final headings in the General Principles and Techniques section are Postoperative Care and Assessment, Complications, and Special Age Considerations.

The Specific Diseases portion of each chapter begins with definitions, usually of the disease. Where relevant, synonyms for the diseases or relevant techniques are given. Next, general considerations and clinically relevant pathophysiology are detailed. This information is meant to provide practical material for case management rather than be a supplemental text for pathophysiology. The diagnosis discussions in this book are detailed and include information on signalment and history, physical examination findings, radiography and ultrasonography, and pertinent laboratory abnormalities. Sections on differential diagnoses and medical management of affected animals are consistently provided. These are followed by a detailed description of the relevant surgical techniques. We have attempted to detail most commonly used techniques, although we may have noted our preferences for particular methods. Information on positioning patients for a given procedure is often neglected in surgical textbooks; to avoid this we have provided this information as a separate heading. The remainder of the Specific Diseases section deals with postoperative care of the surgical patient, potential complications, and prognosis.

Anesthesia Protocols

In most surgery textbooks anesthesia is either totally neglected or is included in separate chapters near the end of the book. Busy practitioners often find it difficult to access this information and correlate it with the cases they are operating. Therefore, recommendations for anesthetizing animals with a particular disease or disorder are found in the Specific Diseases section of each chapter. We asked Dr. Gwendolyn Carroll to serve as our anesthesia consultant. Gwen was responsible for reviewing the general anesthetic information for each organ system included in the General Principles and Techniques sections. Also included in this book are numerous suggested anesthetic protocols, including drug dosages. Although we recognize that many veterinarians have established protocols that they prefer and with which they are comfortable, the protocols provided should prove to be a handy resource.

References

Rather than provide a long list of available references, we have chosen to give selected references under the heading Suggested Reading. Where a specific study or finding is indicated in the text, the reference has been noted by author name and year of publication and the reference included in a separate heading termed References. It was our feeling that with the ready availability of computerized bibliographic information, laundry lists of references are no longer necessary or preferable.

Product Appendix

To help readers find product information mentioned throughout the text, we have provided a product appendix at the end of the book. The product appendix contains trade names of products as well as a manufacturer source. These are not intended to be all-inclusive lists of suppliers of given products, but are instead meant to be a supplemental reference to assist veterinarians in locating particular products.

Index

We felt that an extensive index was mandatory. The index of *Small Animal Surgery* is thorough and exhaustive. Additionally, we have avoided cross-referencing readers to separate entries in the index. Rather, we have opted to duplicate the page source each time a topic is listed.

ACKNOWLEDGMENTS

A number of people have worked hard to make sure that this book is a quality reference. Special thanks to Linda Duncan, Penny Rudolph, Holly Roseman, Angela Reiner, and all the others at Mosby who worked on this project. We thank them for their dedication and care, but most of all for their vision. They believed that this could be a great addition to the available literature, and because of their faith, it moved from idea to reality.

We would also like to thank our mentors and colleagues, who have instilled in us a love of surgery and a dedication to our profession, and our students, who make it all worthwhile.

I would like to thank my fellow contributors who worked extremely hard to complete this task. It was an immense undertaking, and I will be forever grateful for their dedication and for the quality of the material they provided.

Finally, I would like to acknowledge the support and encouragement of my wonderful family: my husband, Matt Miller, and my sons, Chase and Kobe.

Theresa W. Fossum

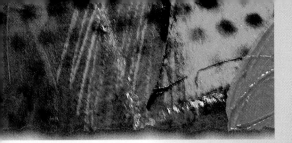

Contents

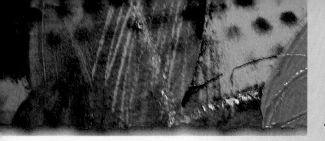

Detailed Contents

PART 1

CHAPTER 1

Principles of Surgical Asepsis

Whenever dermal integrity is disrupted, such as during surgery, microorganisms have access to inner tissues. Bacteria contaminating surgical wounds generally originate from the patient's endogenous flora, operating room personnel, and environment. To prevent wound contamination, rules of aseptic technique must be followed. These rules are not simply guidelines, but are laws of the operating room, and breaking them subjects patients to risk of infection or disease.

Aseptic technique is defined as methods and practices that prevent cross contamination in surgery. It involves proper preparation of the facilities and environment (Chapters 3 and 4), surgical site (Chapter 6), surgical team (Chapter 7), and surgical equipment (Chapters 2 and 8).

Introduction of microorganisms into the surgical wound is necessary for the development of infection. Microorganisms may gain entrance from exogenous (i.e., air, surgical instruments, surgical team, patient) or endogenous (i.e., organisms originating from within the patient's body) sources. It is impossible to eliminate all microorganisms from the surgical wound and sterile field; however, aseptic technique limits the patient's exposure to an amount of microorganisms that is not detrimental. Rules of aseptic technique and reasons to follow them are listed in Table 1-1.

PREPARATION OF SURGICAL PACKS

Regardless of the technique used for sterilization, instruments and linens (e.g., towels, gowns, and drapes) must be cleaned of gross contamination. Instruments should be cleaned manually or with ultrasonic cleaning equipment and appropriate disinfectants as soon after surgery as possible (see Chapter 8) and linens should be laundered. Items sterilized by pressurized steam or alternate methods (e.g., ethylene oxide, plasma) must be wrapped in a specific manner (see p. 3). The procedure for wrapping items is based on enhancing the ease of sterilization and preserving sterility of the item, not convenience or personal preference.

Before packing, instruments are separated and placed in order of their intended use. If steam or gas sterilization is used, the selected wrap should be penetrable by steam/gas, impermeable to microbes, durable, and flexible. Packing materials available, advantages and disadvantages of each, and the sterilization techniques with which each is compatible are listed in Table 1-2.

To allow maximal penetration specific guidelines should be followed when preparing packs for steam and gas sterilization. Presterilization wraps for steam sterilization comprise two thicknesses of two-layer muslin or nonwoven (i.e., paper) barrier materials. The poststerilization wrap (i.e., after sterilization and proper cool down period) consists of a waterproof, heat-sealable plastic dust cover; this wrap is not necessary if the item is to be used within 24 hours of sterilization. Small items may be wrapped, sterilized, and stored in heat-sealable paper/plastic peel pouches. Wrapping materials commonly used are listed in Table 1-2. Items to be gas sterilized are wrapped in heat-sealable plastic peel pouches or tubing or muslin wrap. When using plasma sterilization, items should be wrapped in heat-sealable Tyvek/Mylar pouches or polypropylene wraps. Time, temperature, and humidity recommendations for steam, ethylene oxide, and plasma sterilization are given in Chapter 2.

For steam and gas sterilization, instruments should be organized on a lint-free (huck) towel placed on the bottom of a perforated metal instrument tray. Instruments with box locks should be autoclaved while open. A 3- to 5-mm space between instruments is recommended for proper steam/gas circulation. Complex instruments should be disassembled when possible, and power equipment should be lubricated before sterilization. Items with a lumen should have a small amount of water flushed through them immediately before steam sterilization because water vaporizes and forces air out of the lumen; conversely, moisture left in tubing placed in a

TABLE 1-1

Rules of Aseptic Technique

Rule of Aseptic Technique	Reason for Rule
Surgical team members remain within the sterile area.	Movement out of the sterile area may encourage cross contamination.
Talking is kept to a minimum.	Talking releases moisture droplets laden with bacteria.
Movement in the operating room (OR) by all personnel is kept to a minimum; only necessary personnel should enter the operating room.	Movement in the OR may encourage turbulent air flow and result in cross contamination.
Nonscrubbed personnel do not reach over sterile fields.	Dust, lint, or other vehicles of bacterial contamination may fall on the sterile field.
Scrubbed team members face each other and the sterile field at all times.	A team member's back is not considered sterile even if wearing a wrap-around gown.
Equipment used during surgery must be sterilized.	Unsterile instruments may be a source of cross contamination.
Scrubbed personnel handle only sterile items; nonscrubbed personnel handle only nonsterile items.	Nonscrubbed personnel and nonsterile items may be a source of cross contamination.
If the sterility of an item is questioned, it is considered contaminated.	Nonsterile, contaminated equipment may be a source of cross contamination.
Sterile tables are only sterile at table height.	Items hanging over the table edge are considered nonsterile because they are out of the surgeon's vision.
Gowns are sterile from mid chest to waist and from gloved hand to 2 inches above the elbow.	The back of the gown is not considered sterile even if it is a wrap-around gown.
Drapes covering instrument tables or the patient should be moisture proof.	Moisture carries bacteria from a nonsterile surface to a sterile surface (strike-through contamination).
If a sterile object touches the sealing edge of the pouch that holds it during opening, it is considered contaminated.	Once opened, sealed edges of pouches are not sterile.
Sterile items within a damaged or wet wrapper are considered contaminated.	Contamination can occur from perforated wrappers or from strike-through from moisture transport.
Do not fold hands into the axillary region; rather clasp hands in front of the body above the waist.	The axillary region of the gown is not considered sterile.
If the surgical team begins the surgery sitting, they should remain seated until the surgery is completed.	The surgical field is sterile only from table height to the chest; movement from sitting to standing during surgery may increase cross contamination.

TABLE 1-2

Wrapping Materials for Pack Preparation

Material	Advantages	Disadvantages	Sterilization Method
Cotton muslin; 140 or 270 thread counts	Durable, flexible, reusable, easily handled	Requires double layer/double wrap, generates lint, not moisture resistant	Steam, ethylene oxide
Nonwoven barrier material (i.e., paper)	Inexpensive, single or double layer	Single-use, memory, not as durable, not moisture resistant, requires double wrap	Steam, ethylene oxide
Nonwoven polypropylene fabric*	Flexible, durable, excellent bacterial barrier, puncture resistant, lint free	Single-use, requires double wrap	Steam, ethylene oxide, plasma
Paper/plastic pouches† (heat sealed)	Convenient, long shelf life, water resistant	Instruments may puncture the pouch	Steam, ethylene oxide
Plastic pouches‡ (heat sealed)	Convenient, long shelf life, waterproof, puncture	Instruments may puncture the pouch	Plasma, ethylene oxide

*Spunguard.
†Paper and Mylar.
‡Mylar and Tyvek.

gas sterilizer may decrease the action of the gas below the lethal point. Containers (e.g., saline bowl) should be placed with the open end facing up or horizontal; containers with lids should have the lid slightly ajar. Multiple basins should be stacked with a towel between each. A standard count of radiopaque surgical sponges should be included in each pack. A sterilization indicator (see p. 9) should be placed in the center of each pack before wrapping. Solutions should be steam sterilized separately from instruments using the slow exhaust phase (see Table 2-2 on p. 8).

Linens may be steam sterilized. The maximum size and weight of linen packs that can be effectively steam sterilized is 12 × 12 × 20 inches and 6 kg, respectively. Closely woven table drapes should be packed separately. Layers of linen are alternated in their orientation to permit steam penetration. A sterilization indicator (see p. 9) should be placed in the center of each pack.

Wrapping Instrument Packs

Instrument packs should be wrapped so that they can be easily unwrapped without breaking sterile technique (Fig. 1-1).

Folding and Wrapping Gowns

Gowns must be folded so that they can be easily donned without breaking sterile technique (Fig. 1-2).

Folding and Wrapping Drapes

Drapes should be folded so that the fenestration can be properly positioned over the surgical site without contaminating the drape (Fig. 1-3).

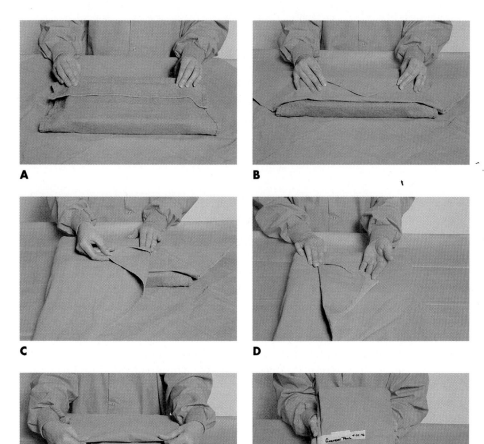

A

B

C

D

E

F

FIG. 1-1
Wrapping an instrument pack. **A,** Wrap the instrument pack in a clean huck towel. Place a large unfolded wrap in front of you and position the instrument tray in the center of the wrap so that an imaginary line drawn from one corner of the wrap to the opposite corner is perpendicular to the long axis of the instrument tray. **B,** Fold the corner of the wrap that is closest to you over the instrument tray and to its far edge. Fold the tip of the wrap over so that it is exposed for easy unwrapping. **C,** Fold the right corner over the pack, then, **D,** fold the left corner similarly. **E,** Turn the pack around and fold the final corner of the wrap over the tray, tucking it tightly under the previous two folds. **F,** Wrap the pack in a second layer of cloth or paper in a similar manner. Secure the last corner of the outer wrap with masking tape and a piece of heat-sensitive indicator tape.

FIG. 1-2
Folding and wrapping surgical gowns. **A,** Place the gown on a clean flat surface with the front of the gown facing up. Fold the sleeves neatly toward the center of the gown with the cuffs of the sleeves facing the bottom hem. **B,** Fold the sides to the center so that the side seams are aligned with the sleeve seams. **C,** Then fold the gown in half longitudinally (sleeves will be inside the gown). **D,** Starting with the bottom hem of the gown, fanfold it toward the neck. **E,** Fold a hand towel in half horizontally and fanfold it into about four folds. Place it on top of the folded gown, leaving one corner turned back to allow it to be easily grasped. **F,** Wrap the gown and towel in two layers of paper or cloth wrap as described in Fig. 1-1.

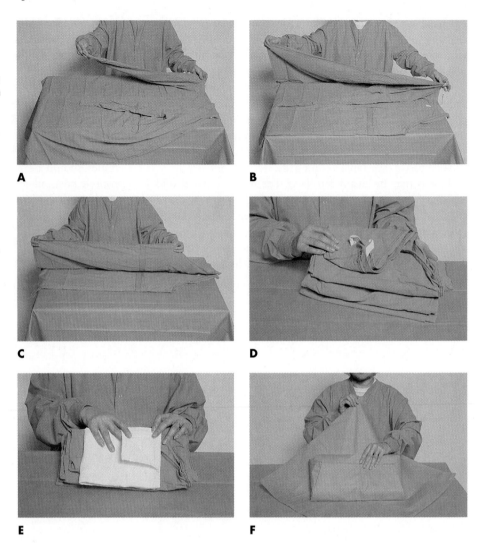

HANDLING AND STORAGE OF STERILIZED INSTRUMENTS/EQUIPMENT

Packs are allowed to cool and dry individually on racks when removed from the autoclave; instrument packs placed on top of each other during cooling may promote condensation of moisture, resulting in contamination via strike-through. When sterile packs are completely dry they should be stored in waterproof dust covers in closed cabinets (as opposed to uncovered on open shelves) to protect them from moisture or exposure to particulate matter (i.e., dust-borne bacteria). Excessive handling of sterile supplies should be discouraged, especially if items are pointed or have sharp edges. Sterile items should be handled gently; they should be protected from bending, crushing, or compression forces that could break a seal or puncture the package. Sterile packs should be stored away from ventilation ducts, sprinklers, and heat-producing light. Ideal environmental conditions include low humidity, low air turbulence, and constant controllable room temperature.

Sterile Shelf Life

Published expiration dates for sterilized items wrapped in various types of wrappers (Table 1-3) have become controversial. The reason for disputing time-related expiration is that events, not time, contaminate products. It has recently been shown that if items are packaged, sterilized, and handled properly, they remain sterile unless the package is opened, wet, torn, has a broken seal, or is damaged in some other way (i.e., event-related expiration). To use an event-related expiration system, appropriate protocols for sterilizing and handling items must be adopted.

Handling Sterilized Items

Sterile packs will not have an expiration date in the future; they will have the date on which the item was sterilized and a control lot number to trace an unsterile item. Heat-sealed waterproof dust covers will be placed on items not routinely used. All packages will state "sterility guaranteed until the package is damaged or opened." These items must be stored

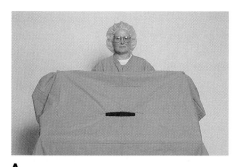

A

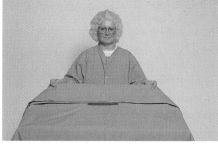

B

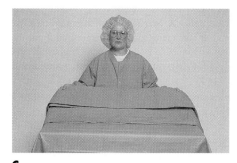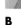

C

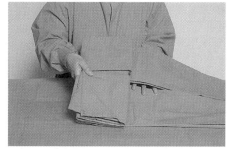

D

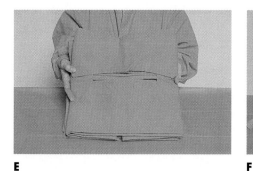

E

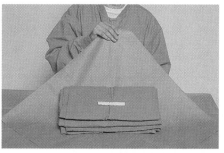

F

FIG. 1-3
Folding and wrapping drapes. **A,** Lay the drape out flat with the ends of the fenestration perpendicular to you and the sides of the fenestration parallel to you. **B,** Grasp the edges of the drape nearest you and fanfold the drape to the center. The edge of the drape should be exposed (dorsal) to allow it to be easily grasped during unfolding. **C,** Turn the drape around and fanfold the other half, similarly. **D,** Next, fanfold one end of the drape to the center (the fingers are through the fenestration); repeat with the other end. **E,** Note that when the drape is properly folded, the fenestration is on the ventral outermost aspect of the drape. **F,** Fold the drape in half and wrap it in two layers of paper or cloth wrap as described in Fig. 1-1.

in a manner that does not compromise packaging and sterility and should be rotated in such a way that the first processed item is used first.

If a sterile pack is damaged it should not be used. Damage to the sterile pack is defined as wraps that have moisture present, packs that have been placed in a dusty environment or stored near an air current source, items that have been dropped, bent, crushed, compressed, torn, or punctured, or packs that have a broken seal. Surgery personnel training must include how to protect sterile items from events that cause loss of sterility. They should carefully inspect the integrity of sterilized items to identify damaged goods. Plastic dust covers must be removed or wiped clean before reaching the surgical area.

Unwrapping/Opening Sterile Items

Sterile items are wrapped to allow operating room personnel to unwrap the item without contaminating it (see above). There are three popular methods of distributing sterile items.

TABLE 1-3

Recommended Storage Times for Sterilized Packs

Wrapper	Shelf Life
Double-wrapped, two-layer muslin	4 weeks
Double-wrapped, two-layer muslin, heat sealed in dust covers after sterilization	6 months
Double-wrapped, two-layer muslin, tape sealed in dust covers after sterilization	2 months
Double-wrapped nonwoven barrier materials (i.e., paper)	6 months
Paper/plastic peel pouches, heat sealed	1 year
Plastic peel pouches, heat sealed	1 year

Sterilized items from hospitals adopting event-related sterility assurance have an indefinite shelf life (see p. 4).

Unwrapping large sterile linen/paper/polypropylene packs that cannot be held during distribution. If the pack is too large, cumbersome, or heavy to be held during distribution, it may be opened onto a Mayo stand or back table. Place the pack on the center of the Mayo stand or back table and open each folded layer by pulling it toward you. This prevents your hand and arm from extending over the sterile area. Handle only the edge and underside of the wrap. Follow the same procedure for each fold. When the pack is opened, have a sterile team member place it on the sterile table.

Controversy exists concerning the correct way to open double-wrapped sterile packs: the outer layer only or both layers. There is evidence to support both techniques. The rationale for opening the outer layer only is that the risk of microbial shedding from the circulating nurse's hands and arms onto the sterile package contents is eliminated. The rationale for opening both wrappers is that when the outer surface of the inner wrapper is opened, it may become contaminated via dust particles and debris from the outer wrapper; if this wrapper is opened by the circulating nurse, the possibility of contamination is decreased. This decision should be made taking into consideration technical expertise of personnel and barrier quality.

Unwrapping sterile linen/paper packages that can be held during distribution. These packs may be opened and placed on a sterile table as described in Fig. 1-4 or, after opening, they may be grasped by a sterile team member.

Unwrapping sterile items in paper/plastic or plastic peel-back pouches. Identify the edges of the peel-back wrapper and carefully separate them. Peel the edges of the wrapper back slowly and symmetrically to ensure the sterile item does not contact the torn edge of the wrapper (the torn edge of a peel-back wrapper is nonsterile). If the item is small place it on the sterile area as described above, being careful not to lean across the sterile table. If the item is long or cumbersome have a sterile team member grasp it and gently pull it from the peel-back wrapper, taking care to not brush the item against the peeled edge of the wrapper. Scalpel blades and suture are opened similarly.

Pouring Solutions into Basins

Solutions (i.e., sterile saline, antiseptics) are poured into basins. The basin should be held away from the surgical table by a sterile team member to prevent the nonsterile assistant's hand and arm from extending over the sterile area. The solution is poured without splashing and with care to prevent it from dripping down the container onto the sterile person's hand. The solution container should not touch the sterile basin.

Suggested Reading

Donovan A, Turner DW, Smith A: Successful, documented studies favoring indefinite shelf life, *J Healthcare Material Management* 9:34, 1991.

Hooker R: Successfully eliminating outdates, *J Healthcare Material Management* 7:60, 1989.

Knecht CD et al: *Fundamental techniques in veterinary surgery,* ed 3, Philadelphia, 1987, WB Saunders.

Mayworm D: Sterile shelf life and expiration dating, *Journal HSPD* 2:32, 1984.

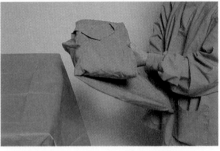

A

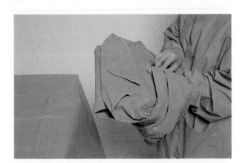

B

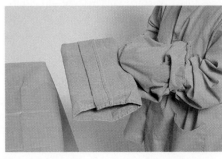

C

FIG. 1-4
A, To unwrap a sterile linen pack that can be held during distribution, hold the pack in your left hand if you are right-handed (and vice versa). **B,** Using your right hand, unfold one corner of the wrap at a time, being careful to secure each corner in the palm of your left hand to keep them from recoiling and contaminating the contents. **C,** Hold the final corner with your right hand; your hand should be completely covered by the wrap. When the pack is fully exposed and all corners of the wrap secured, gently set it onto the sterile field, being careful to not allow your hand and arm to reach across or over the sterile field.

CHAPTER 2

Sterilization and Disinfection

Sterilization refers to the destruction of all microorganisms (bacteria, viruses, spores) on something. It usually refers to objects that come in contact with sterile tissue or enter the vascular system (e.g., instruments, drapes, catheters, needles). Disinfection is the destruction of most pathogenic microorganisms on *inanimate* (i.e., nonliving) objects, while antisepsis is the destruction of most pathogenic microorganisms on *animate* (i.e., living) objects. Antiseptics are used to kill microorganisms during patient skin preparation and surgical scrubbing (see Chapters 6 and 7); however, the skin is not sterilized.

DISINFECTION

Disinfection usually involves liquid disinfectants. Selection of the appropriate disinfectant is based on the desired result. Some disinfectants are effective in destroying limited numbers of microorganisms; others are effective in killing all organisms, including spores. Common disinfectants, their usefulness, and necessary precautions are listed in Table 2-1.

STERILIZATION

Because the inner tissues of the body are sterile, any equipment or supplies that come in contact with these tissues must also be sterile. Methods of sterilizing surgical instruments or other equipment include steam, chemicals, plasma, and ionizing radiation.

Steam Sterilization

Pressurized steam is the most common method of sterilization used in hospitals. Steam destroys microbes via coagulation and cellular protein denaturation. To destroy all living microorganisms, the correct relationship between temperature, pressure, and exposure time is critical. If steam is contained in a closed compartment and pressure is increased, temperature increases, provided the volume of the compartment remains the same. If items are exposed long enough to steam at a specified temperature and pressure, they will become sterile. The unit used to create this high-temperature, pressurized steam is called an autoclave.

Failure to sterilize packs can occur if the packs are wrapped too tightly or are improperly loaded in the autoclave or gas sterilizer container. Instrument packs should be positioned vertically (i.e., on edge) and longitudinally in an autoclave. Heavy packs should be placed at the periphery where steam enters the chamber. Allow a small amount of air space between each pack to facilitate steam flow (1 to 2 inches between each pack and surrounding walls). Load linen packs so the fabric layers are oriented vertically (i.e., on edge). Do not stack linen packs because the increased thickness decreases steam penetration. Close supervision and exact standards for preparing, packaging, and loading of supplies are necessary for effective steam and gas sterilization.

Types of Steam Sterilizers

Gravity Displacement Sterilizer. The most commonly used steam sterilizer in veterinary practice is the gravity (or "downward") displacement sterilizer (Fig. 2-1). This

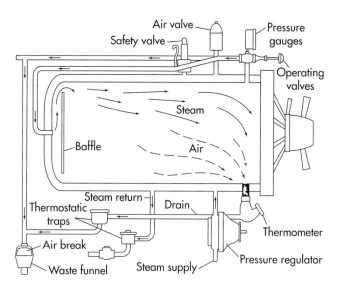

FIG. 2-1
Gravity displacement autoclave. (Modified from Slatter D: Textbook of small animal surgery, ed 2, Philadelphia, 1993, Saunders.)

TABLE 2-1

Common Disinfectants Used in Veterinary Practice

Agent	Practical Use	Disinfectant Properties	Antiseptic Properties	Mechanisms of Action	Precautions
Alcohol: isopropyl alcohol (50%-70%); ethyl alcohol (70%)	Spot cleaning; injection site preparation	Good	Very good	Protein denaturation, metabolic interruption, and cell lysis	Corrosive to stainless steel; volatile
Chlorine compounds: hypochlorite	Cleaning floors and countertops	Good	Fair	Release of free chlorine and oxygen	Inactivated by organic debris; corrosive to metal
Iodine compounds: iodophors (7.5%) scrub solution	Cleaning dark colored floors and countertops	Good	Good	Iodination and oxidation of essential molecules	Stains fabric and tissue
Glutaraldehyde: 2% alkaline solution	Disinfection of lenses and delicate instruments	Good; sterilizes	None	Protein and nucleic acid alkylation	Tissue reaction; odor (rinse instruments well before using)

sterilizer works on the principle that air is heavier than steam. Supplies to be sterilized are loaded into the inner chamber. A narrow, outer "jacket-type" chamber surrounds the inner chamber. Pressurized steam from the narrow, outer chamber enters the inner chamber to surround the supplies. Air in the inner chamber is pulled downward by gravity to the floor and exits through a temperature-sensitive valve. As steam accumulates and the temperature increases, the steam-release valve closes. Because function of this sterilizer is based on the ability of air to move to the bottom of the autoclave, careful wrapping (see p. 1) and loading of supplies are critical (see above). The minimum temperature/time standard for a gravity displacement sterilizer is 10 to 25 minutes at 270° to 275° F (132° to 135° C) or 15 to 30 minutes at 250° F (121° C). Table 2-2 contains recommended sterilization times for commonly sterilized items.

Prevacuum sterilizer. The prevacuum sterilizer relies on air being actively pulled out of the inner chamber, thereby creating a vacuum. Steam is injected into the chamber to replace the air. This method of sterilization provides greater steam penetration in a shorter time than the gravity displacement sterilizer. The minimum temperature/time standard for a prevacuum sterilizer is 3 to 4 minutes at 270° to 275° F (132° to 135° C).

Flash sterilizer. Emergency or "flash" sterilization is performed when an unwrapped, nonsterile item needs to be sterilized quickly. A gravity sterilizer is used. The item is placed unwrapped in a perforated metal tray and sterilized according to the manufacturer's time and temperature recommendations. With detachable handles, sterilized items are transported to the operating room in the metal tray. It is difficult to deliver flash-sterilized devices aseptically; the tray is hot, wet, and unwrapped and collects dust, debris, and microorganisms more readily than dry, cool trays with biobar-

TABLE 2-2

Exposure Periods for Sterilization in Gravity Displacement Sterilizers

Item	Minimum Time Required 250°-254° F (121°-123° C)
Scrub brushes (in dispensers, cans, individually wrapped)	30
Dressings (wrapped in muslin or paper)	30
Glassware (empty, inverted)	15
Instruments (wrapped in double-thickness muslin)	30
Instruments combined with suture, tubing, porous materials (wrapped in muslin or paper)	30
Metal instruments only (unwrapped)	15
Linen—maximum size 12 × 12 × 20 inches (6 kg wrapped)	30
Needles (individually packaged in glass vials or paper, lumens moist)	30
Needles (unwrapped, lumens moist)	15
Rubber catheters, drains, tubing (wrapped in muslin or paper; lumens moist)	30
Rubber catheters, drains, tubing (unwrapped; lumens moist)	20
Utensils (wrapped in muslin or paper, on edge)	20
Utensils (unwrapped, on edge)	15
Syringes (unassembled, individually packaged in muslin or paper)	30
Syringes (unassembled, unwrapped)	15
Suture—silk, cotton, nylon (wrapped in paper or muslin)	30
Solutions: 75-250 ml	20 (slow exhaust)
500-1000 ml	30 (slow exhaust)
1500-2000 ml	40 (slow exhaust)

rier protection. This type of sterilization should be used only in emergency situations when no other alternative is available. The minimum temperature/time standard for a gravity flash sterilizer is 4 minutes at 270° to 275° F (132° to 135° C).

Chemical (Gas) Sterilization

Ethylene oxide. Ethylene oxide is a flammable, explosive liquid that becomes an effective sterilizing agent when mixed with carbon dioxide or freon. Equipment that cannot withstand the extreme temperature and pressures of steam sterilization (i.e., endoscopes, cameras, plastics, power cables) can safely be sterilized with ethylene oxide, which kills microorganisms and their spores by alkylation. The process is enhanced by heat and moisture; the optimum temperature ranging from 120° to 140° F (49° to 60° C) and humidity from 20% to 40%. Length of time required for sterilization depends on concentration of ethylene oxide, humidity, temperature, and density and type of materials to be sterilized. Manufacturers' recommendations for ethylene oxide exposure time must be followed. It is critical for the safety of the patient and hospital personnel that all materials sterilized with ethylene oxide be aerated in a well-ventilated area for a minimum of 7 days, or 12 to 18 hours in an aerator.

Items should be clean and dry before ethylene oxide sterilization; moisture and organic material bonds with ethylene oxide and leaves a toxic residue. If an item cannot be disassembled and all surfaces cleaned, it cannot be sterilized. Items are packed and loaded loosely to allow gas circulation. Complex items (e.g., power equipment) are disassembled before processing (see p. 5). Items that cannot be ethylene oxide sterilized include acrylics, some pharmaceutical items, and solutions.

Environmental and safety hazards associated with ethylene oxide are numerous and severe. Recommended guidelines associated with equipment use should be followed carefully to prevent injury to the patient or hospital personnel. Ethylene oxide causes cutaneous burns (i.e., vesicant), nausea, vomiting, headaches, weakness, upper and lower respiratory irritation, and destruction of red blood cells (i.e., when improperly aerated items come in contact with the circulatory system). A category I carcinogen, it causes birth defects. Because ethylene oxide sterilization requires use of the hazardous and environmentally unsound chlorofluorocarbon 12, its use may soon be prohibited. The Environmental Protection Agency (EPA) has declared that the United States will cease using chlorofluorocarbon 12 by the year 2000.

Plasma Sterilization

Plasma sterilization is a method of low-temperature sterilization. This process uses reactive ions, electrons, and neutral atomic particles to sterilize items. Vapor phase hydrogen peroxide sterilization is a form of plasma sterilization that uses hydrogen peroxide to process instruments quickly and efficiently. Instruments can be sterilized in 75 minutes and are immediately available because aeration is not required. Items for sterilization must be wrapped in polypropylene, nonwo-

ven fabric (Table 1-2 on p. 2). Items that can be sterilized using this process are stainless steel, aluminum, brass, silicone, Teflon, latex, ethyl vinyl acetate, polycarbonate, polyethylene, polypropylene, polyvinyl chloride, and polymethylmethacrylate. Items that cannot be sterilized safely include linen, gauze sponges, wood products (including paper), some plastics, liquids, items that cannot be disassembled, items with copper or silver solder or using disphenole A epoxy, tubes and catheters greater than 12 inches, and tubes and catheters less than 3mm in diameter.

Ionizing Radiation

Most equipment available prepackaged from the manufacturer has been sterilized by ionizing radiation (i.e., cobalt 60). This process is restricted to commercial use because of expense. Items commonly used in the operating room that are sterilized with ionizing radiation include suture material, sponges, disposable items (i.e., gowns, drapes, table covers), powders, and petroleum goods. Prepackaged, sterilized items that have been opened but not used may not be able to be resterilized by other means because this could damage the item and be a health hazard.

Cold Chemical Sterilization

Chemicals used for sterilization must be noncorrosive to the items being sterilized. Glutaraldehyde is noncorrosive and provides a safe means for sterilizing delicate lensed instruments (i.e., endoscopes, cystoscopes, bronchoscopes). Most equipment that is safe for immersion in water is safe for immersion in 2% glutaraldehyde. Items for sterilization should be clean and dry; organic matter (e.g., blood, saliva) may prevent penetration of crevices or joints. Residual water causes chemical dilution. Complex instruments should be disassembled before immersion. Immersion times suggested by the manufacturer (e.g., 2% glutaraldehyde: 10 hours at 20° to 25° C for sterilization; 10 minutes at 20° to 25° C for disinfection) should be closely adhered to. After appropriate immersion time instruments should be rinsed thoroughly with sterile water and dried with sterile towels to avoid damaging the patients' tissues.

STERILIZATION INDICATORS

Simply placing an item in a sterilizer and initiating the process do not ensure sterility. Failure to achieve sterility may be caused by improper cleaning (if an item cannot be disassembled and all surfaces cleaned it cannot be sterilized), mechanical failure of the system used, improper use of equipment, improper wrapping, poor loading technique, and/or failure to understand concepts behind sterilization processes.

Sterilization indicators allow one to monitor the effectiveness of sterilization. Indicators undergo either a chemical or biologic change in response to some combination of time and temperature. Chemical indicators are generally paper strips or tape impregnated with a material that changes color

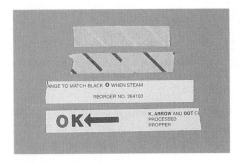

FIG. 2-2
Tape and indicator strips for steam sterilization. Diagonal stripes on the tape (top) turn from tan to black. The "K," arrow, and dot on the indicator strips (bottom) turn from white to black to match "O."

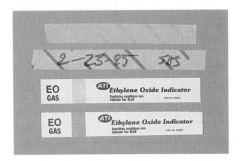

FIG. 2-3
Tape and indicator strips for ethylene oxide sterilization (before⇒after): tape, yellow⇒red; strips, yellow⇒blue.

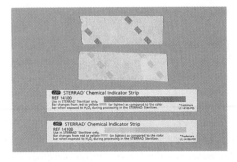

FIG. 2-4
Tape and indicator strips for plasma sterilization (before⇒after): tape, red⇒yellow; strips, red⇒yellow.

when a certain temperature is reached (Figs. 2-2 through 2-4). The chemical responds to conditions such as extreme heat, pressure, or humidity but does not take into consideration the duration of exposure that is critical to the sterilization process. Therefore it is important to remember that chemical indicators do not indicate sterility—only that certain conditions for sterility have been met. Chemical indicators are available for steam, gas, and plasma sterilization and are placed in the center of each pack and on the outside of the item to be sterilized. Some autoclaves have a temperature-time graph on the control panel. This indicator method is reliable at measuring the temperature reached and the duration that each load is exposed to that temperature. A written record can be kept of each processed load.

The surest way to determine sterility is with the use of a biologic indicator. A strain of highly resistant, nonpathogenic, spore-forming bacteria (i.e., *Bacillus stearothemophilus* for steam; *Bacillus subtilis* for gas) contained in a glass vial or a strip of paper is placed in the load of goods to be sterilized. After the sterilization cycle is complete, the vial or strip is recovered and cultured; growth of the organism documents inadequate sterilization. Biologic indicators should be used at least weekly to test the effectiveness of the sterilization process.

Sterilization indicators should not be heavily relied on because of the problems mentioned above. There is no substitution for close supervision of personnel, a general understanding of sterilization processes, and maintaining high standards for preparing, packing, and loading supplies.

Suggested Reading

Harris MH: Flash sterilization, *AORN Journal* 55:1547, 1992.
Lemarie RJ, Hosgood G: Antiseptics and disinfectants in small animal practice, *Comp Cont Educ Pract Vet* 17:1339, 1995.
Moss R: Clinical issues, *AORN Journal* 61:869, 1995.

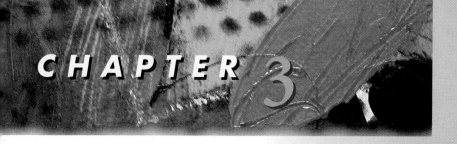

CHAPTER 3

Surgical Facilities, Equipment, and Personnel

A variety of physical layouts are suitable for modern operating rooms and surgical areas; the goals of all designs are patient safety and work efficiency. The surgical area should be located close to anesthesia and surgical preparation areas, critical care, radiology, and central supply. However, it should be isolated from general traffic flow (i.e., examination rooms, offices, reception area, wards). In large facilities (i.e., universities, surgical referral centers) the surgical area should be a separate working unit isolated from general hospital traffic.

STRUCTURE AND DESIGN OF THE SURGICAL AREA

Because of the constant danger of contamination to surgical patients, the surgical area is divided to clearly delineate "clean," "mixed," and "contaminated" areas. Clean areas include operating rooms, scrub sink areas, and sterile supply rooms. Mixed areas include hallways between operating rooms and nurses' stations, instrument and supply processing areas, storage areas, and utility rooms. Contaminated areas include anesthesia preparation rooms, dressing rooms, lounges, and offices.

A common floor plan used in most surgical areas is one in which the surgical suites are arranged around a central operating room nurses' work station. Easy access to each operating room from the work station ensures efficient traffic flow, reducing cross contamination between areas. Clean areas should be restricted to clean traffic and contaminated areas to contaminated traffic. Persons entering a clean area from a contaminated area must don proper surgical attire (see Chapter 7); the ideal location for moving from a contaminated to a clean area (or vice versa) is through a locker room. Surgical personnel leaving a clean area and entering a contaminated area must cover their clothing before leaving and discard these items when returning to the clean area. Doors between clean and contaminated areas should be kept closed at all times. Food and drink is permitted only in contaminated areas. Movement of clean and sterile supplies and equipment should be separated as much as possible from contaminated supplies and equipment by space, time, and/or traffic patterns. Soiled linen and trash should be kept in a contaminated area. Patients should be clipped and vacuumed in a contaminated area before transport to a clean area (e.g., operating room).

☞ **N O T E ·** To avoid contaminating the surgical suite, clip the patient and perform an initial surgical preparation in a separate area.

DESCRIPTION AND FUNCTION OF ROOMS IN THE SURGICAL AREA
Dressing Room

Dressing rooms are used by surgical personnel to change into proper surgical attire. The dressing room should have closed cabinets for storing scrub suits, shoe covers, masks, and caps and a separate area for hanging street clothes. A hamper for dirty laundry should be available to minimize carrying contaminated linen throughout the hospital.

Anesthesia and Surgical Preparation Room

The anesthesia induction and surgical preparation room should be located adjacent to the surgical area yet out of major hospital traffic patterns. This area should be supplied with equipment or medications that may be necessary in the event of an emergency (i.e., defibrillator, laryngoscopes, endotracheal tubes, suction, oxygen, crash cart). Anesthetic equipment (i.e., machines, drugs), laryngoscopes, clippers (i.e., mounted on the wall or hanging from the ceiling), vacuums (i.e., large canister or central), skin preparation materials (i.e., antiseptic soaps, alcohol, sterile gauze sponges), sharps containers, needles and syringes, and monitoring equipment should be readily available to ensure efficient anesthesia and preoperative patient preparation.

☞ **N O T E** • Drugs and equipment needed in the event of an emergency can be stored in a mobile "crash cart" that facilitates movement from the anesthesia preparation room to the operating room and to recovery.

Preparation counters and surfaces should be impervious and easily cleaned and disinfected. Stainless steel preparation tables with built-in sinks are ideal. Gas-scavenger systems should be present at each anesthesia preparation table. General lighting is achieved by main overhead fluorescent lights, supplemented by a spotlight directed at each preparation table. A sink designated for cleaning anesthetic hoses, endotracheal tubes, and rebreathing bags, plus a plastic rack for draining and drying rebreathing bags and hoses, should be available. An erasable anesthesia/surgery scheduling board, easily visible to anesthesia and surgical personnel, should have a list of the day's procedures.

Room temperature should be kept between 62° and 68° F and humidity at 50% or less to reduce microbial growth. Gurney surfaces should be padded, and circulating water heating blankets should be used to prevent hypothermia. Well-constructed gurneys should be available for patient transportation. They should be made from stainless steel, have relatively large wheels with bearings that can be readily lubricated, and have rubber bumpers mounted on the corners to prevent damage to doors and walls. An adhesive microfilm dust pad should be placed at the doorway between the anesthesia preparation room and surgical area to collect dust, hair, and other particulates on gurney rollers, shoes, and anesthetic equipment.

Anesthesia Supply Room

The anesthesia supply room should be adjacent to the anesthesia and surgical preparation room. Equipment necessary to keep anesthesia machines working properly, extra endotracheal tubes, anesthetic monitoring equipment, oxygen "E" tanks, hoses, catheters, and airway connectors are stored here. It may also contain a cabinet for storing nongaseous anesthetic agents. This may be a convenient location to store large oxygen tanks that supply oxygen to each anesthesia preparation table and operating room.

Nurses' Work Station

The nurses' work station should be centrally located within the surgical area (i.e., clean area). An autoclave (for flash sterilization), incubator/blanket warmer (e.g., irrigation fluids and towels to wrap patients postoperatively), refrigerator (e.g., medications, solutions), and formalin containers are kept in this area. Daily surgery log, operating room protocols, and a telephone are also located here. Soiled instruments may be sent to a central supply or decontaminated, washed, lubricated, and wrapped or packaged for resterilization here. If this area is used for decontaminating and wrapping instruments, it should be divided into two separate areas to prevent cross contamination of clean supplies.

Sterile Instrument Room

The sterile instrument room is a clean area that houses all sterilized and packaged instruments and supplies. It is generally located near the nurses' work station (see above discussion). Surgery personnel assemble items needed for a particular case from supplies located in this room. Items should be logically arranged on shelves (e.g., alphabetical order) and routinely checked for "outdates" (i.e., "time related" expiration; see p. 4) and package integrity (i.e., "event related" expiration; see p. 4).

Equipment Room

Large pieces of equipment such as anesthetic machines, lasers, monitoring equipment, operating microscopes, and portable surgery lights can be stored in an equipment room. Equipment should be kept free of dust and cleaned routinely using the protocol described for operating room disinfection (see p. 15). The equipment room is a valuable area because it prevents the storage of large and expensive equipment in hallways where it could be a hazard or become damaged.

Housekeeping Supply Room

Supplies used to decontaminate and clean surgical suites may be stored in the supply room or closet. Cleanup equipment and supplies stored here must be restricted to use within the operating room to prevent cross contamination from other hospital areas.

Scrub Sink Area

Scrub sink areas should be centrally located to the operating room suites. Antiseptic soap in an appropriate dispenser (i.e., foot activated), scrub brushes (i.e., sterilized reusable brushes or disposable polyurethane brush/sponge combination), and fingernail cleaners should be located within easy reach at each scrubbing station. Deep stainless steel sinks equipped with knee-, elbow-, or foot-operated water activators are ideal. If reusable brushes are utilized, the dispensing container and clean brushes must be detached and autoclaved regularly. The scrub sink area must be located away from wrapped sterile supplies because of possible contamination by water droplets and spray from the sinks. Scrub sinks should never be used to clean equipment or instruments or dispose of body fluids.

Gowning and Gloving Area

Gowning and gloving can commence outside or inside the operating room. Controversy exists as to which location results in the least amount of cross contamination; there is no evidence to suggest one location over another.

☞ **N O T E** • If the operating room is small or if several people are "scrubbing in," gowning and gloving in a separate area may help prevent contamination of personnel, sterile supplies, or the prepped surgical site.

Operating Room

Operating rooms are the individual rooms where surgeries are performed. Room size should be large enough to allow personnel to move around sterile equipment without contamination, and to accommodate large pieces of equipment needed for various procedures. Room design should be uncluttered and simple so there are no areas that trap dust or are difficult to clean. Floors, ceilings, and other surfaces should be smooth, nonporous, and constructed of fireproof materials. Smooth surfaces allow thorough cleaning and disinfection and prevent trapping biologic material that could cross contaminate. Surface materials should be able to withstand frequent washing and cleaning with strong disinfectants.

Ventilation systems for surgical suites should be designed to provide positive air pressures within the operating room and lower air pressures within adjoining corridors. The ideal ventilation system should deliver a minimum of 15 to 20 air exchanges per hour. Positive pressures inside the operating room decrease the likelihood of contaminated air from adjacent corridors mixing with operating room air. Scavenging systems that pull anesthetic gases out of operating room air should be installed in each operating room. The operating room environment should be kept at a constant humidity and temperature. Humidity is controlled to minimize static electricity and microbial growth; ideal humidity is 50% or less. Air temperature is maintained at 62° to 68° F.

General lighting in the operating room is achieved by use of main overhead fluorescent lights supplemented by the use of one, or preferably two, halogen spotlights. Halogen lamps are preferred because of the pale, bluish cast emitted, which results in less eye fatigue, and their low heat production. Fiberoptic headlamps worn by surgeons are now available in comfortable, lightweight models; headlamps virtually eliminate shadowing of the surgical site. Surgical spotlights are mounted in the ceiling directly over the operating table and should have maximum maneuverability. Track lighting is undesirable because dust and bacteria may become trapped in their tracks.

Stainless steel operating tables should be fully adjustable for height (hydraulic mechanism) and degree of tilt. Tabletops should be either a flat, one-piece surface or have V-trough capabilities. Portable V-troughs and insulating table pads should be available. The patient's body temperature must be maintained during surgery, especially if they weigh less than 10 kg or the surgical procedure is longer than 2 hours. Maintaining body temperature is usually accomplished by placing the patient on a circulating water blanket. Special tabletop attachments to allow visualization of the patient's head by the anesthesiologist should also be provided so that the patient can be monitored without contaminating the surgical field.

An instrument table (i.e., Mayo stand) or back table should be available; the table selected should be large enough to accommodate all instrumentation required for the surgical procedure. Instrument tables should be made of stainless steel and should be adjustable in height. A kick bucket is used by surgical team members to discard soiled sponges during surgery. The bucket frame should have wheels so it can be easily moved (i.e., kicked) about the operating room. Plastic bag liners for kick bucket containers facilitate clean-up.

Suction (portable or piped in) should be available in each operating room. Suction units with disposable containers are easily cleaned and are reliable and cost-efficient. Suction hoses should not be reused unless they are sterilized because they are a common source of surgical wound contamination. Other accessory equipment such as physiologic monitors, the anesthesia supply cart, intravenous stands, and sitting stools should be available. Each operating room should be provided with a radiographic view box, preferably flush mounted to facilitate cleaning. Portable imaging devices are optimal for evaluating orthopedic implant placement but may be cost prohibitive. The operating room should have a wall clock to determine elapsed time; particularly when vascular occlusion is necessary.

Supply cabinets with tight-fitting doors (to minimize dust accumulation) should be located in each room to store suture material, dressings, sponges, scalpel blades, and frequently used instruments. Operating room doors should be kept closed to decrease mixing of operating room air with corridor air.

Postoperative Recovery Area

The postoperative recovery area should be adjacent to the surgical area yet separate from other hospitalized patients. Patients should be placed in individual, heated cages and carefully monitored until complete recovery. Patients requiring intensive care should be taken directly to the critical care facility. The temperature of recovery rooms should be warmer than operating rooms (i.e., 70° to 77° F). Warming cabinets with a supply of warm fluids and blankets should be available. Analgesic medications should be available, as well as any equipment or medications that may be necessary in the event of an emergency (i.e., defibrillator, laryngoscopes, endotracheal tubes, suction, oxygen, crash cart).

Minor Procedures Surgery Room

A separate room adjacent to the anesthesia preparation area should be designated for minor, contaminated surgical procedures (i.e., lacerations, biopsies, wound management, dental procedures, endoscopy). The room should be equipped with an operating table, spotlight, gas and suction lines for anesthesia equipment, suture, antiseptic preparation materials, and minor surgical instrument packs. Because of the nature of surgical procedures performed in this room, it should be properly cleaned and disinfected after each surgical procedure and at the end of each surgery day (see Chapter 4).

PERSONNEL

Responsibilities and functions of every member of the surgical team should be clearly defined in writing. This is done to clarify the job description and to establish accountability of each employee. These policies must be carefully followed and strictly enforced to ensure safe and efficient operation of the surgical area. Periodic evaluations should be made of all staff members. Provisions for training programs, educational self-improvement, and information dissemination should be made available, as well as current books, periodicals, and audiovisual tapes of new procedures and techniques.

The surgeon's role is to guide the flow and scope of what happens in the operating room during surgery. Surgical assistance is often provided by the veterinary technician. Surgical assistants carry out functions that assist the surgeon in performing a safe operation, including developing a working knowledge of the procedure being performed, providing retraction and hemostasis, and manipulating instrumentation and tissues into proper position to complete the surgical task. A knowledgeable surgical assistant is invaluable.

An anesthesiologist is responsible for the meticulous monitoring and adjustment of the patient's physiologic status during surgery. He or she is trained to render immediate care in the event of a physiologic crisis. Occasionally the surgeon and anesthesiologist must work together to carefully time surgical maneuvers (i.e., cardiothoracic surgery). A properly trained anesthesiologist allows the surgeon to concentrate on the surgical procedure.

Operating Room Supervisor/Surgical Technician

In large facilities the operating room supervisor oversees technicians working in the surgical area. It is his or her responsibility to organize work schedules, train new staff, set policies for the surgical area, implement and enforce policies, and develop educational programs and seminars. He or she actively takes part in day-to-day technical aspects of running a surgical area (i.e., circulates, opens surgical packs, retrieves special instruments). In a small facility (i.e., one operating room) the operating room supervisor assumes all of the surgical technician's tasks mentioned above. He or she may also have other technical tasks to perform as a veterinary technician (i.e., anesthesia, restraint, receptionist). Qualifications for a well-educated technician include graduation from an approved veterinary technician program and 1 or 2 years of basic training in a veterinary practice or veterinary teaching hospital.

Suggested Reading

Fuller JR: *Surgical technology: principles and practice,* ed 3, Philadelphia, 1994, WB Saunders Co.
Moss R: Operating room ventilation, *AORN* 36:455, 1996.

CHAPTER 4

Care and Maintenance of the Surgical Environment

Surgery puts a patient at risk for nosocomial (hospital acquired) infections unless strict environmental, equipment care, and maintenance standards are established and followed. Because most surgical infections develop from bacteria that enter the incision site during surgery, proper preparation of the surgical environment is crucial to reduce the likelihood of infection.

The operating room is considered a clean area (see Chapter 3); appropriate attire must be worn by all personnel entering or leaving it (see Chapter 7). To render the surgical environment as microorganism-free as possible, routine cleaning/disinfection should be performed. The term *cleaning* refers to removal of soil (i.e., blood, serum, urine, pus); *disinfection* refers to treatment of surfaces, materials, and equipment with disinfectants to reduce bacterial numbers. Cleaning and disinfection are usually performed simultaneously, unless large amounts of organic material or other body fluids are present.

DAILY CLEANING ROUTINES
Operating Room

At the beginning of each surgery day all horizontal surfaces, lights, operating room equipment, and furniture should be damp dusted with a lint-free cloth and hospital grade disinfectant (Table 4-1). After each surgical procedure, areas contaminated by organic debris (e.g., floors, doors, counters, equipment, operating table) should be cleaned/disinfected. If biohazards (i.e., infectious diseases, chemotherapeutic agents) were encountered during surgery, special precautions should be taken during cleaning and disinfection (i.e., specific disinfectant, cleaning time, disinfectant contact time).

At the close of each day, operating tables, counters, lights, equipment, floors, windows, cabinets, and doors should be cleaned/disinfected in preparation for the following day's activities. Linen and waste bags should be collected, linen laundered, and waste disposed of properly. Kick buckets should

---

TABLE 4-1

Daily Care and Maintenance of the Operating Room

At the Beginning of Each Day
- Wipe flat surfaces of furnishings and lights with a cloth dampened with a disinfectant solution.

After Each Surgical Procedure
- Collect used instruments and place them in a cool water and detergent or enzymatic solution.
- Collect waste materials and soiled linens and place in proper containers.
- Wipe instrument and surgical tables, stands, kick buckets, and heating pads with a disinfectant.
- If necessary, clean the floor (move the surgical table and clean under it if body fluids have collected there).

After the Last Surgical Procedure of the Day
- Clean and disinfect kick buckets.
- Check ceilings, walls, cabinet doors, counter surfaces, and all furniture and clean as necessary.
- Clean/care for individual items (i.e., monitoring devices, anesthesia equipment, surgical lights) according to the manufacturer's instructions.
- Wipe counter surfaces and cabinet doors with a disinfectant solution.
- Wipe instrument and surgical tables, stands, heating pads, and light fixtures with a disinfectant solution. Disassemble the surgical table if necessary to thoroughly clean it.
- Check supplies and restock as necessary.
- Roll wheeled equipment (e.g., surgical table, monitoring devices) through a small amount of disinfectant solution placed on the floor.
- Wet vacuum or damp mop the floor.

be disinfected and plastic bags replaced. Surgical lights, monitoring equipment, and anesthesia equipment are cleaned/disinfected following manufacturers' specific guidelines. Wheels and coasters of all movable equipment and gurneys are cleaned/disinfected. The operating room should be restocked with commonly used instruments, suture, gauze sponges, needles, and syringes, and the floor should be wet vacuumed or damp mopped. Wet vacuuming is preferred over mopping because mops are a major source of infection. If mops are used, mop heads should be laundered and dried daily. They should be rinsed between uses and soaked in disinfectants.

Scrub Sinks

Scrub sink areas need special attention during the day because water (a vehicle for bacterial contamination) is frequently splashed on floors and walls, and blood and other organic debris can be tracked from the scrub sink area to the surgical suite (Table 4-2). This area should be cleaned as needed throughout the day (i.e., floors mopped, used scrub brushes and fingernail cleaners removed, soap dispensers cleaned, sinks and walls washed) and disinfected at the end of the day.

Anesthesia and Surgical Preparation Rooms

Sinks, vacuum canisters, trash buckets, gurneys, and anesthesia preparation tables should be kept clean of organic debris and disinfected as needed throughout the day (Table 4-3). Hair removed during patient preparation should be vacuumed from surgical tables and floors. Blood, urine, feces, tissue, serum, and purulent material should be contained and discarded. Needles and other sharp instruments should be disposed of in appropriate containers. Discarded biohazards should be disposed of in color-coded bags or be clearly marked as biohazard materials.

Plumbing fixtures, floors, cabinets, anesthesia equipment, utility rooms, furniture, and other equipment should be cleaned and disinfected daily. At the end of the day the sink should be disinfected and a cup of disinfectant solution poured down the drain. The inner surface of garbage containers should be disinfected. Portable vacuums should have the bag and filter removed and replaced as needed; the outside surfaces of the vacuum (including hose and nozzle) should be wiped clean and disinfected. Clippers should be cleaned according to manufacturer's instructions. Floors should be wet vacuumed or damp mopped and supplies restocked. If a mop is used the mop bucket should be emptied and cleaned, and all cleaning equipment and supplies should be returned to a designated storage closet.

Recovery Room

Cages, sinks, trash buckets, and gurneys should be cleaned of organic debris and disinfected as needed throughout the day. Plumbing fixtures, floors, cabinets, anesthesia equipment, utility rooms, furniture, and other equipment should be cleaned and disinfected daily, as described in the discussion on care of anesthesia and surgical preparation rooms.

When a surgical patient has vacated a cage in the recovery room, the cage must be carefully disinfected before use by the next patient. Before cage disinfection, padding, paper, and organic matter should be removed. Disinfectant should be sprayed on all cage surfaces, including the door. Dry organic matter should be scrubbed with a brush until it is released. Lastly, the area in front of the cage should be cleaned and disinfected. Before reuse, linen (i.e., pads, blankets, heating blanket covers) should be laundered. Plastic circulating water heating blankets should be cleaned and disinfected.

TABLE 4-2

Daily Care and Maintenance of the Scrub Room/Sinks

Between Scrubbing Sessions
- Dispose of wrappings from packs.
- Dispose of debris in sinks.

After the Last Surgical Procedure of the Day
- Remove waste and clean waste receptacles with a disinfectant. Line waste receptacles with a plastic bag.
- Check supplies and restock.
- Clean and refill soap dispensers.
- Wipe counter surfaces, cabinet doors, walls adjacent to sink, and switch plates.
- Scrub and disinfect sinks.
- Wet vacuum or damp mop the floor.

TABLE 4-3

Daily Care and Maintenance of the Patient Preparation Area

Between Patient Preparations
- Discard waste material (e.g., feces).
- Properly dispose of urine and clean the sink.
- Remove hair from clipper blades and lubricate according to manufacturer's instructions.
- Check walls, counters, and cabinet doors and clean with a disinfectant if necessary.
- Vacuum and clean the floor as necessary to remove hair clippings.

At the End of the Day
- Remove waste and clean waste receptacles with a disinfectant. Line waste receptacles with a plastic bag.
- Wipe light fixtures and supply lines with a disinfectant.
- Clean clippers according to manufacturer's instructions.
- Vacuum the floor to remove hair clippings. Change filter in vacuum. Wipe outside of vacuum, hose, and nozzle with a disinfectant.
- Check walls and ceiling and clean as necessary.
- Check supplies and restock.
- Wipe counter surfaces, cabinet doors, walls adjacent to sink, and switch plates with a disinfectant.
- Scrub and disinfect sinks.
- Wet vacuum or damp mop the floor.

This protocol helps maintain a consistently low level of microbes in the surgical recovery area to reduce nosocomial surgical site infections; however, special precautions are necessary for some infectious diseases (e.g., parvovirus).

WEEKLY AND MONTHLY CLEANING ROUTINES

Surgical suites should be emptied of moveable equipment and thoroughly cleaned once a week. Shelves of supply cabinets, walls, windows, windowsills, ceilings, light fixtures, surgical tables, utility and supply carts and castors, utility rooms, equipment storage areas, and infrequently used equipment should be cleaned and disinfected. At least once a week operating room floors should be wet vacuumed and ventilation duct grills should be vacuumed. Once a month the walls, floors, and ceilings should be mopped and wheels and other moveable parts of equipment and gurneys should be lubricated.

Suggested Reading

Allen G, Josephson A: Meeting infection control standards in the operating room, *AORN* 62: 595, 1995.

Tracy DL: *Small animal surgical nursing,* ed 2, St Louis, 1994, Mosby.

CHAPTER 5

Preoperative Assessment of the Surgical Patient

Surgical patient selection and preparation require attention to a number of details. The patient should always receive a complete physical examination, followed by appropriate laboratory workup. A thorough history helps determine the extent of physical and laboratory examinations. Preoperative information also allows comparison of the animal's status before and after surgery (e.g., ability to micturate before and after spinal surgery). General assessment and stabilization of the surgical patient are discussed here, while preoperative considerations for specific diseases are provided throughout the text.

HISTORY TAKING

A thorough history from the owner/caregiver aids evaluation of the underlying disease process and identification of other abnormalities that might affect outcome. Although an abbreviated history is often necessary in emergencies, a thorough history should eventually be obtained. The history should include the presenting complaint, signalment, diet, exercise, environment, past medical problems, and present treatment. It is particularly important to detect acute or chronic corticosteroid or antimicrobial therapy, as well as evidence of infection elsewhere in the patient's body.

Questions should be framed to avoid vague responses and obtain specific information (e.g., "When was your dog last vaccinated?" vs. "Is your dog current on his vaccinations?"). Vomiting, diarrhea, altered appetite, exposure to toxins/foreign bodies, coughing, exercise intolerance, and other abnormalities should be noted. Animals with a history of seizures must be identified to avoid drugs that precipitate seizures (e.g., acepromazine). Severity, duration, and progression of the specific disease or presenting complaint should be ascertained.

PHYSICAL EXAMINATION

The animal should be systematically evaluated during the physical examination, and all body systems should be included. The animal's general condition (body condition, attitude/mental status) should be noted. Traumatized animals should have neurologic (see Chapter 33) and orthopedic (see Chapter 28) examinations, in addition to respiratory, gastrointestinal, cardiovascular, and urinary system evaluations. Emergencies may allow only a cursory examination until the animal has been stabilized. Evaluation of preanesthetic physical status (Table 5-1) is one of the best determinants of the likelihood of cardiopulmonary emergencies during or after surgery; the more deteriorated the physical status, the higher the risk of anesthetic and surgical complications.

LABORATORY DATA

The animal's physical status and the procedure being performed dictate the extensiveness of the laboratory workup. Hematocrit, total protein (TP), and urine specific gravity may suffice in young healthy animals undergoing elective procedures (e.g., ovariohysterectomy, declawing) and in healthy animals with localized disease (e.g., patellar luxation). If the animal is older than 5 to 7 years of age, or if anticipated surgical time exceeds 1 to 2 hours, animals with physical status of I or II (see Table 5-1) should have a CBC, serum biochemistry panel, and urinalysis. Animals with systemic signs (e.g., dyspnea, heart murmur, anemia, ruptured bladder, gastric dilatation-volvulus, shock, hemorrhage) should also have a complete CBC, serum biochemistry profile, and urinalysis done.

Additional laboratory data are dictated by the animal's presenting signs and underlying disease (Table 5-2). Identification of associated or underlying disease influences preop-

TABLE 5-1

Physical Status in Surgical Patients

Physical Status	Animal Condition	Examples
I	Healthy with no discernable disease	Elective procedure being performed (e.g., ovariohysterectomy, declaw, castration)
II	Healthy with localized disease or mild systemic disease	Patellar luxation, skin tumor, cleft palate without aspiration pneumonia
III	Severe systemic disease	Pneumonia, fever, dehydration, heart murmur, anemia
IV	Severe systemic disease that is life threatening	Heart failure, renal failure, hepatic failure, severe hypovolemia, severe hemorrhage
V	Moribund; patient is not expected to live longer than 24 hours with or without surgery	Endotoxic shock, multiorgan failure, severe trauma

erative management, surgical procedure performed, prognosis, and postoperative care. Animals with neoplasia should be evaluated for metastasis (e.g., thoracic radiographs, lymphadenopathy). Those with cardiac disease should have thoracic radiographs, cardiac ultrasound, and/or electrocardiograms (see Chapter 24). Heartworm status should be checked before surgery in endemic areas. Traumatized animals should have thoracic radiographs to evaluate the diaphragm, pleural space, and lungs (e.g., pulmonary contusions, pneumothorax, diaphragmatic hernia). Although economic considerations are important, thorough preoperative evaluation of surgical patients is cost-effective because it often prevents or predicts costly complications.

DETERMINATION OF SURGICAL RISK

Once a complete history, physical examination, and laboratory data have been obtained, the surgical risk can be determined and a prognosis given. An *excellent* prognosis should be given if there is minimal potential for complications and a high probability that the patient will return to normal after surgery. If there is a high probability for a good outcome but there is some potential for complications, a *good* prognosis is warranted. If serious complications are possible but uncommon, recovery may be prolonged, or the animal may not return to its presurgical function, a *fair* prognosis is warranted. When the underlying disease or surgical procedure is associated with many and/or severe complications, recovery is expected to be prolonged, likelihood of death during or after the procedure is high, or the animal is unlikely to return to its presurgical function, a *guarded* prognosis should be given.

Occasionally the risk of the surgical procedure may outweigh its potential benefits. For example, removal of an apparently benign skin mass may not be warranted in an animal with hepatic or renal dysfunction. Likewise, patients with thoracic metastases may not benefit from removal of the primary tumor (e.g., limb amputation for osteosarcoma). Quality of life must be considered in veterinary patients; those with severe, debilitating, untreatable disease may not benefit from surgery. However, in some patients, surgery may improve the animal's quality of life even if length of life is limited.

CLIENT COMMUNICATION

Client communication is extremely important to ensure owner satisfaction after surgery. Owners should be informed before surgery of the diagnosis, surgical or nonsurgical options, potential complications, postoperative care, and cost. Although cost cannot always be predicted because of unanticipated complications, owners should be kept apprised of the animal's status and procedures that may affect the initial cost estimate. If the disease is hereditary, neutering should be recommended.

PATIENT STABILIZATION

Patients should be stabilized as thoroughly as possible before surgery. Occasionally, stabilization is impossible and surgical intervention must be rapid; however, replacing fluid deficits and correcting acid-base and electrolyte abnormalities before anesthetic induction are usually justified. Intravenous fluids are indicated in all animals undergoing general anesthesia and surgery, including elective procedures in healthy animals. The need for perioperative antibiotics is dictated by the animal's disease and the procedure being performed. Recommendations for antibiotic prophylaxis and therapy are given with discussions of specific diseases throughout this text. Perioperative antibiotic use is discussed in Chapter 10.

Patient history, clinical signs, physical examination findings, and total CO_2 are helpful in identifying significant acid-base abnormalities. Blood pH, PaO_2, $PaCO_2$, and bicarbonate concentrations may be measured to determine the extent of such abnormalities. Sodium bicarbonate therapy should be considered in patients that are markedly acidemic (pH less than 7.2). The amount of bicarbonate to be given can be calculated using the formula in Table 5-3.

The nutritional state is often critical in chronically diseased animals. Preoperative parenteral or enteral hyperalimentation (see Chapter 11) is sometimes recommended to improve nutritional status before surgery. For example, cleaning particulate matter from the nasal cavity, appropriate antibiotics, and enteral hyperalimentation for several weeks before surgery may decrease infection and improve wound healing in patients with cleft palate.

Traumatized patients must be evaluated swiftly to detect life-threatening abnormalities. Fluid therapy should be initiated if hemorrhage or shock is suspected. Normal blood volume of dogs and cats is approximately 90 and 70 ml/kg, re-

TABLE 5-2

Brief Considerations for Selected Clinical Pathologic Findings

Laboratory Abnormality	Comments	Major Differential Diagnoses
High blood urea nitrogen (BUN)	Obtain urine specific gravity before initiating fluid therapy.	Prerenal azotemia, primary renal disease, postrenal azotemia
Low BUN		Hepatic insufficiency (e.g., portosystemic shunt, cirrhosis), severe polyuria/polydipsia, low protein diet
High alanine aminotransferase (ALT)	ALT may be normal in some animals with severe hepatic disease.	Hepatic disease
Low albumin	Substantial inconsistencies between laboratories	Hepatic disease, loss from urine or gastrointestinal tract, severe exudative cutaneous lesion (e.g., burn)
High serum alkaline phosphatase	Source of elevation (e.g., liver, bone) can be determined by isoenzyme analysis; commonly elevated in young growing animals or caused by steroids or anticonvulsants; falsely elevated with severe lipemia or severe bilirubinemia (>8 g/dl).	Hepatic disease, steroid therapy, extrahepatic biliary obstruction, some neoplasms
High bilirubin	Exposure to fluorescent light may degrade bilirubin.	Hepatocellular disease, extrahepatic biliary obstruction, intrahepatic cholestasis, hemolytic anemia
High calcium		Paraneoplastic syndrome (lymphosarcoma, anal sac adenocarcinoma), primary hyperparathyroidism, calciferol-containing rodenticides, hypervitaminosis D, hypoadrenocorticism, granulomatous disease, renal disease
Low calcium	Artificially low in animals with low albumin	Renal disease (especially acute), pregnancy (eclampsia), hypovitaminosis D, hypoparathyroidism
High creatinine	Emaciated animals will have falsely decreased serum creatinine.	Renal disease, uroabdomen, muscle trauma (minor elevations)
High glucose	Stress may increase glucose to 200-400 mg/dl in cats.	Diabetes mellitus
Low glucose	Delayed separation of red blood cells (RBCs) will falsely lower glucose.	Hepatic disease, insulinoma, hypoadrenocorticism, extrahepatic neoplasms, septicemia/toxemia, starvation of neonates
High sodium	Primarily caused by loss of free water	Vomiting, diarrhea, renal failure, diabetes insipidus, inappropriate fluid therapy
Low sodium	Primarily caused by failure to excrete free water, occasionally due to loss of sodium	Vomiting, diarrhea, hypoadrenocorticism, diuretic therapy, inappropriate fluid therapy
High potassium	Thrombocytosis may falsely elevate potassium; hemolysis will increase potassium in selected breeds.	Hypoadrenocorticism, renal failure, uroabdomen, drug therapy
Low potassium		Vomiting, diarrhea, diuretic therapy, chronic renal failure (especially in cats), inappropriate fluid therapy
High eosinophils		Parasitism (heartworm, gastrointestinal), eosinophilic diseases, mast cell tumor, hypersensitivities
High basophils		Parasitism (heartworm), mast cell tumors

TABLE 5-2

Brief Considerations for Selected Clinical Pathologic Findings—cont'd

Laboratory Abnormality	Comments	Major Differential Diagnoses
High lymphocytes		±lymphosarcoma, ±FeLV
Low lymphocytes		Severe stress, lymphangiectasia, chylothorax, acute viral diseases
High RBCs		Dehydration, polycythemia, hypoxia (right to left shunts)

TABLE 5-3

Calculation of Volumes Needed for Blood Transfusion or Bicarbonate Therapy

Blood Transfusions

$$\text{Blood needed (ml)} = \text{recipient's weight (kg)} \times \frac{\text{desired PCV} - \text{recipient's PCV}}{\text{donor's PCV}} \times 70 \text{ [cat] or } 90 \text{ [dog]*}$$

Note: A rough estimate is that 2.2 ml of blood/kg of body weight increases the recipient's PCV by 1%.

Bicarbonate Therapy

Bicarbonate needed (mEq) = 0.3 × base deficit[†] (mEq) × body weight (kg) (Give one half IV over 10-15 minutes and reevaluate. Give the remainder over 4 to 6 hours if necessary), or give 1-2 mEq/kg IV; repeat only if indicated based on assessment of acid-base balance and potassium concentration.

Note: Because CO_2 is an end product of bicarbonate administration, adequate ventilation should be assured.
*Total blood volume is estimated at 90 ml/kg for dogs and 70 ml/kg for cats.
[†]Some calculate the base deficit as the difference between the desired bicarbonate and the actual bicarbonate (vs. normal bicarbonate and actual bicarbonate). Animals that are acidotic enough to require bicarbonate therapy need repeated monitoring.

spectively. Treatment of acute hypovolemia seeks to establish a circulating blood volume that allows adequate tissue perfusion. Generally, the patient in shock can be given 60 to 90 ml/kg of polyionic isotonic fluid intravenously in the first hour without adverse effects; however, patients with pulmonary, cardiovascular, or renal disease may be less tolerant of rapid fluid administration. If hemodilution is not a concern, balanced electrolyte solutions (i.e., lactated Ringer's solution, Normosol-R) may be given. Hypertonic saline solutions are beneficial in reducing total fluid requirements, limiting edema, and increasing cardiac output (see Table 23-24 on p. 556). Transfusions (i.e., whole blood, packed red cells) may be necessary in anemic patients. Animals with preoperative packed cell volumes (PCVs) of less than or equal to 20% usually benefit from blood transfusions. The major preoperative concern in anemic patients is maintaining oxygen-carrying capacity, and this requires blood transfusion. The amount of donor blood needed can be estimated by the formula given in Table 5-3.

Needle thoracentesis should be performed in severely dyspneic animals with suspected pleural cavity disease (i.e., pneumothorax, pleural effusion). Tube thoracostomy (see p. 678) and/or oxygen supplementation via oxygen cage,

nasal insufflation (see p. 618), or mask may be necessary. Thoracic radiographs should be taken after severely dyspneic patients have been stabilized. Abdominal abnormalities (i.e., hemorrhage, uroabdomen, bile peritonitis, mesenteric avulsion) are common in traumatized animals. The animal's ability to void and urine characteristics should be noted. Uroabdomen should be identified (i.e., abdominal pain, peritoneal effusion, and/or postrenal azotemia) and treated appropriately (see p. 496). Early recognition of peritonitis is important to reduce patient morbidity and improve survival. Diagnostic peritoneal lavage may be useful in such patients (see p. 198).

Suggested Reading

Krotje LJ: Cyanosis: physiology and pathogenesis, *Compend Contin Educ Pract Vet* 9:271, 1987.

Morgan RV: Respiratory emergencies. I. *Compend Contin Educ Pract Vet* 5:228, 1983.

Morgan RV: Respiratory emergencies. II. *Compend Contin Educ Pract Vet* 5:305, 1983.

Murtaugh RJ, Ross JN: Cardiovascular resuscitation following traumatic injury, *Compend Contin Educ Pract Vet* 9:369, 1987.

CHAPTER 6

Preparation of the Operative Site

Endogenous microbial flora (particularly *Staphylococcus aureus* and *Streptococcus* spp.) are the most common source of surgical wound contaminants. Normal or resident organisms live in the skin's superficial cornified layers and outer hair follicles. Resident canine flora include *Staphylococcus epidermidis*, *Corynebacterium* spp., and *Pityrosporon* spp. while *S. aureus*, *Staphylococcus intermedius*, *Escherichia coli*, *Streptococcus* spp., *Enterobacter* spp., and *Clostridium* spp. are transient pathogens. Eliminating exposure to this flora is extremely important during surgery. Although it is impossible to sterilize skin without impairing its natural protective function and interfering with wound healing, preoperative preparation reduces infection.

DIETARY RESTRICTIONS

Food intake is generally restricted 6 to 12 hours before anesthesia to avoid intra- or postoperative emesis and aspiration pneumonia. Access to water is generally not curtailed. Operations of the large intestine often require specialized preparations (i.e., dietary restriction for 48 hours) and/or enteric antibiotics (i.e., oral kanamycin, neomycin, or penicillin G). Food should not be withheld for long periods in young animals because hypoglycemia could occur.

EXCRETIONS

The animal should be allowed to defecate and urinate shortly before anesthesia. Colonic surgery may require enemas. An empty urinary bladder often facilitates abdominal procedures. If urine is not evacuated naturally, the bladder may be manually expressed under general anesthesia or a sterile urethral catheter passed into the urinary bladder.

TREATMENT OF HAIR

Before preparing the patient for surgery, the patient's identity, the surgical procedure being performed, and the surgical site should be verified. It is useful to bathe the animal the day before the surgical procedure to remove loose hair, debris, and external parasites. Hair should be liberally clipped around the proposed incision site so that the incision can be extended within a sterile field (Fig. 6-1). A general guideline

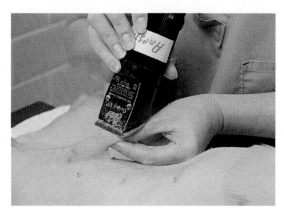

FIG. 6-1
Liberally clip hair around the proposed incision site so that the incision can be extended within a sterile field. In male dogs be sure to clip the prepuce.

is to clip at least 20 cm on each side of the incision. The hair can be removed most effectively with an electric clipper and a No. 40 clipper blade. Patients with dense hair coats may be clipped first with a coarser blade (No. 10). The higher the blade number, the shorter the remaining hair. Clippers should be held using a "pencil grip" and initial clipping should be done with the hair growth pattern. Subsequent clipping should be against the pattern of hair growth to obtain a closer clip. Depilatory creams are less traumatic than other hair removal methods but induce a mild dermal lymphocytic reaction. They are most useful in irregular areas where adequate hair removal is difficult. Razors are occasionally used for hair removal (e.g., around the eye), but cause microlacerations in skin that may increase irritation and promote infection.

After hair removal is completed, loose hair is removed with a vacuum. For limb procedures, if exposure of the paw is unnecessary, the paw can be excluded from the surgical area by placing a latex glove over the distal extremity and securing it to the limb with tape (Fig. 6-2). The glove should be covered with tape or Vetrap. The foot is then "draped-out" of

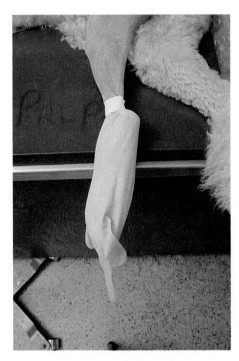

FIG. 6-2
For limb procedures where exposure of the paw is not required, exclude the paw from the surgical area by placing a glove over the distal extremity and securing it to the limb with tape. Wrap the glove with tape or Vetrap.

the sterile field (see below). To enhance manipulation of limbs during surgery a "hanging-leg" preparation may be done. This requires that the limb be circumferentially clipped; the limb is hung from an IV pole during prepping to allow all sides to be scrubbed.

Before transporting the animal to the surgical suite, the incision site is given a general cleansing scrub and ophthalmic antibiotic ointments or lubricants are placed on the cornea and conjunctiva. In male dogs undergoing abdominal procedures, the prepuce should be flushed with an antiseptic solution (Fig. 6-3). The skin is scrubbed with germicidal

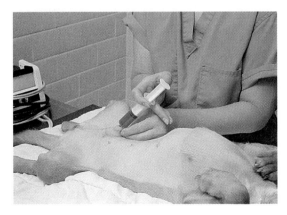

FIG. 6-3
Flush the prepuce of male dogs with antiseptic solution before performing the sterile preparation.

soaps to remove debris and reduce bacterial populations. The area is lathered well until all dirt and oils are removed. This is a generous scrub that often encompasses the hair surrounding the operation site to remove unattached hair and dander that may be disturbed during draping.

Commonly used scrubbing solutions are iodophors, chlorhexidine, alcohols, hexachlorophene, and quaternary ammonium salts. Alcohol is not effective against spores but produces a fast kill of bacteria and acts as a defatting agent. Using alcohol by itself is not recommended, but it is commonly used in conjunction with povidone-iodine (see below). Hexachlorophene and quaternary ammonium salts are less effective than other available agents.

POSITIONING

Before the sterile application of the epidermal germicide, the animal is moved to the operating room, positioned so that the operative site is accessible to the surgeon, and secured with ropes, sandbags, troughs, tape, or vacuum-activated positioning devices. Avoid interfering with respiratory function and peripheral circulation as well as the musculature and its innervation. Monitoring devices should be connected or the connections rechecked after positioning. The animal is generally placed on a water circulating heating pad and if electrocautery is being used, the ground plate should be positioned under the patient. If a hanging-leg preparation is being done, the limb should be carefully suspended with tape from an IV pole.

STERILE SKIN PREPARATION

Sterile preparation begins after the animal has been transported and positioned in the surgical suite. Gauze sponges are sterilized in a pack along with bowls into which the germicides can be poured. Sponges are handled with sterile sponge forceps or a gloved hand using aseptic technique. The dominant hand should be used to perform the sterile preparation, while the less dominant hand is used to retrieve sponges from the preparation bowl. Transferring the sterile sponges to the dominant hand before scrubbing the animal helps ensure that the hand picking up the sponges remains sterile during the procedure.

Scrubbing is started at the incision site, usually near the center of the clipped area. A circular scrubbing motion is used, moving from the center to the periphery. Sponges should not be returned from the periphery to the center because bacteria could be transferred onto the incision site; sponges are discarded after reaching the periphery. Frequently, when using povidone-iodine and alcohol, the site is scrubbed alternatively with each solution three times to allow for 5 minutes of contact time. However, using alcohol between the povidone-iodine scrubs decreases contact time of povidone-iodine with skin and may decrease its efficacy. Excess solution on the table or in body "pockets" should be blotted with a sterile towel or sponges. When the final povidone-iodine scrub is completed, a 10% povidone-iodine solution should be sprayed or painted on the site (Fig. 6-4). If chlorhexidine is the preparation solution, it remains in

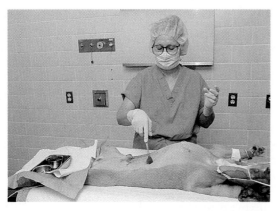

FIG. 6-4
If using povidone-iodine, spray or paint a 10% povidone-iodine solution on the site after the preparation is completed.

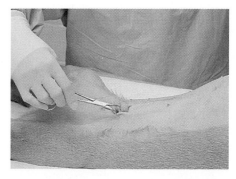

FIG. 6-5
If an abdominal incision extends to the pubis in male dogs, clamp the prepuce to one side with a sterile towel clamp.

contact with the skin at the end of the preparation procedure or may be rinsed with saline. Because chlorhexidine binds to keratin, contact time is less critical than with povidone-iodine. Two 30-second applications have been advocated as being adequate for antimicrobial activity.

Use of a 1-minute alcohol cleansing and application of an antimicrobial film provides equivalent bactericidal activity to a 5-minute iodophor scrub and paint (Geelhoed, Sharp, Simon, 1983). Comparison of three skin preparations (povidone-iodine or 4% chlorhexidine gluconate with either saline or 70% isopropyl alcohol rinse) showed no significant differences in percentages of bacterial reduction for surgical times up to 8 hours in dogs (Osuna, DeYoung, Walker, 1990); however, significantly more skin reactions occurred with povidone-iodine than with chlorhexidine. Approximately 50% of dogs prepared with iodophors in this study developed erythema, edema, papules, wheals, and/or weeping of serum from the skin. The authors concluded that povidone-iodine and chlorhexidine with a saline rinse were equally effective under clinical conditions; however, 4% chlorhexidine with a 70% isopropyl alcohol rinse was inferior because it resulted in fewer negative cultures after surgery.

DRAPING

Once the animal has been positioned and the skin prepared, the animal is ready to be draped. If electrocautery is being used, sufficient time should elapse between the skin preparation and application of drapes to permit complete evaporation of flammable substances (e.g., alcohol, defatting agents) from the skin. If an abdominal incision extends to the pubis in male dogs, the prepuce should be clamped to one side with a sterile towel clamp (Fig. 6-5). The purpose of drapes is to create and maintain a sterile field around the operative site. Draping is performed by a gowned and gloved surgical team member and begins with placement of field drapes (quarter drapes) to isolate the unprepared portion of the animal. These towels should be placed one at a time at the periphery of the prepared area. Field drapes may be huck towels or disposable nonabsorbent towels. Drapes should not be

flipped, fanned, or shaken because rapid movement of drapes creates air currents on which dust, lint, and droplet nuclei can migrate. Drapes, supplies, and equipment extending over or dropping below table level should be considered unsterile because they are not within the surgeon's visual field and their sterility cannot be verified.

Once the towels are placed they should not be readjusted toward the incision site because this carries bacteria onto the prepared skin. Towels are secured at the corners with Bachhaus towel clamps (Fig. 6-6). The tips of the towel clamps, once placed through the skin, are considered nonsterile and should be handled appropriately. Generally, field towels do not cover the edges of the table; do not brush a sterile gown against this unsterile field. When the animal and incision site are protected by field drapes, final draping can be performed (Fig. 6-7). A large drape is placed over the animal and the entire surgical table to provide a continuous sterile field. Cloth drapes should have an appropriately sized and positioned opening that can be placed over the incision site while the drape covers the remaining surfaces.

To drape a limb, field drapes should be placed and secured as described above to isolate the surgical site or the proximal aspect of the limb if the leg is hung (Fig. 6-8). The

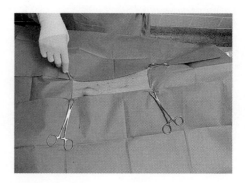

FIG. 6-6
Secure field drapes at the corners with sterile Bachhaus towel clamps. The tips of the towel clamps, once placed through the skin, are considered nonsterile and should be handled appropriately.

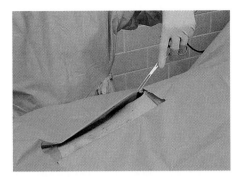

FIG. 6-7
If the drape does not have a fenestration, cut an appropriately sized one. The edges of the drape can be secured to the field drapes with Allis tissue forceps (not towel clamps). Do not put holes through the outer drape.

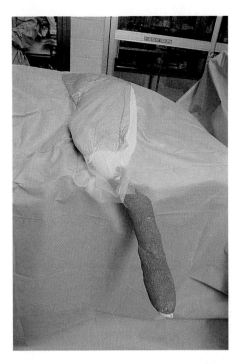

FIG. 6-9
The limb is placed through a fenestration of a lap or fanfold drape and the drape is secured. A plastic adhesive drape has been applied to the skin and surrounding drapes.

nonprepared area of the limb is held by a nonsterile member of the surgical team and the tape holding the elevated limb is cut. The limb is presented to the sterile surgical member so that it may be taken with a hand in a sterile stockinette or towel. The limb should not be turned loose until it is securely held by the sterile surgical team member. If a stockinette is used, it should be carefully unrolled down the limb and secured with towel clamps. If a sterile towel is used, the limb should be carefully wrapped with the towel before securing it to skin with a towel clamp. Water-impermeable (disposable) towels (plus the towel clamp) should then be covered with sterile Kling. If a cloth towel is used, it (and the towel clamp) should be covered with sterile Vetrap. The limb is now ready to be placed through a fenestration of a lap or fanfold drape and the drape secured (Fig. 6-9). The end of the stockinette is wrapped with sterile Vetrap.

To reduce skin exposure and subsequent contamination during the surgery, additional skin draping, or "toweling-in," can be performed after the skin incision is made. Alternatively, plastic adhesive drapes can be applied to the skin and surrounding drapes for the same purpose. When the animal and nearby unsterile surfaces are covered with sterile drapes, the instrument tray can be arranged, and surgery can commence.

References

Geelhoed GW, Sharpe K, Simon GL: A comparative study of surgical skin preparation methods, *Surg Gynecol Obstet* 157:265, 1983.

Osuna DJ, DeYoung DJ, Walker RL: Comparison of three skin preparation techniques in the dog. I: experimental trial, *Vet Surg* 19:14, 1990.

Osuna DJ, DeYoung DJ, Walker RL: Comparison of three skin preparation techniques. II: clinical trial in 100 dogs, *Vet Surg* 19:20, 1990.

Suggested Reading

Bilbrey SA, Dulisch ML, Stallings B: Chemical burns caused by benzalkonium chloride in eight surgical cases, *J Am Anim Hosp Assoc* 25:31, 1989.

Thompson JP, et al: Neurotoxicosis associated with the use of hexachlorophene in a cat, *J Am Vet Med Assoc* 190:1311, 1987.

Trim CM, Simpson ST: Complication following ethylene oxide sterilization: a case report, *J Am Anim Hosp Assoc* 18:507, 1982.

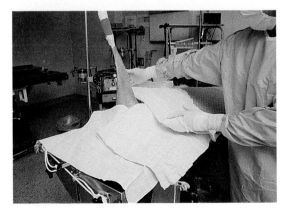

FIG. 6-8
When performing a hanging-leg preparation place field drapes around the limb and secure them with towel clamps.

CHAPTER 7

Preparation of the Surgical Team

Surgical personnel are a major cause of microbial contamination during surgery. Careful preparation of the surgical team and nonsterile personnel reduces bacterial numbers in the surgical suite but does not eliminate them. A correlation has been noted between the number of people, their movements, and the number of airborne bacteria in a surgical suite (Fuller JR, 1994). To minimize contamination during surgery, strict guidelines should be followed regarding surgical attire of all surgical room personnel (including observers). If possible, surgical room personnel should be reduced to only those essential for anesthesia or surgical support.

SURGICAL ATTIRE

All persons entering the operating room suite, regardless of whether a surgery is in progress or not, should be appropriately clothed. To minimize microbial contamination from operating room personnel, scrub clothes rather than street clothes should be worn in the operating suite. With two-piece pant suits, loose fitting tops should be tucked into the trousers. Tunic tops that fit close to the body may be worn outside the trousers. The sleeves of the top should be short enough to allow the hands and arms to be scrubbed. Pants should have an elastic waist or drawstring closure. Non-scrubbed personnel should wear long-sleeved jackets over their scrub clothes. Jackets should be buttoned or snapped closed during use to minimize the risk of the edges inadvertently contaminating sterile surfaces. Scrub clothes should be laundered between wearings and changed if they are visibly soiled or wet to prevent transfer of microorganisms to the surgical environment. Wearing scrub clothes outside the surgical environment increases microbial contamination. If a scrub suit must be worn outside the surgery room, a lab coat or single-use gown should be used to cover it.

Other surgical attire includes hair coverings, masks, shoe covers, gowns, and gloves. Hair is a significant carrier of bacteria; when left uncovered it acts as a filter and collects bacteria. Because shedding from hair has been shown to affect surgical wound infection rates, complete coverage is necessary. Even when surgery is not in progress, caps and masks should be worn in the surgical suite. Caps should completely cover all head and face hair, and masks should cover the mouth and nostrils. Sideburns and/or beards necessitate hoods (Fig. 7-1) for complete coverage. Skullcaps that fail to cover the side hair above the ears and hair at the nape of the neck should not be worn.

Any footwear that is comfortable can be worn in the surgery area. Shoe covers should be donned when first entering the surgical area and should be worn when leaving it to keep shoes clean. New shoe covers are donned upon returning to the surgical area. Shoe covers are generally made of reusable or disposable materials that are water-repellant and that resist tearing.

Masks constructed from lint-free material containing a hydrophilic filter web sandwiched between two outer layers

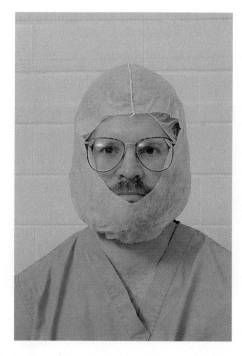

FIG. 7-1
Facial hair and sideburns should be covered with a hood.

should be worn whenever entering a sterile area. Their major function is to filter and contain droplets of microorganisms expelled from the mouth and nasopharynx during talking, sneezing, and coughing. Masks must be fitted over the mouth and nose and be secured in a manner that prevents venting. The dorsal aspect of the mask is secured by shaping the reinforcing top edge tightly around the nose.

Surgical gowns may be reusable and made of woven materials (usually cotton), or they may be disposable. Disposable (single-use) gowns are nonwoven and are made directly from fibers, rather than yarn. Loosely woven, all-cotton fabric, type 140 muslin is commonly used for reusable gowns. This fabric is instantly permeable to bacteria when it becomes wet. 270 pima cloth that has been treated to produce a durable, water-repellant finish is more expensive but provides a better bacterial barrier. Fifty/fifty polyester/cotton blend cloth is available as a tightly woven fabric that resists bacterial penetration. Laundering woven gowns widens the fabric pores, decreasing their effectiveness as microbial barriers. Nonwoven gown materials include olefins and polyesters. The number of microorganisms isolated from the surgical environment is lower when disposable (single-use), nonwoven materials are used.

SURGICAL SCRUB

Surgical scrubs are used to clean the hands and forearms to reduce bacterial numbers that come in contact with the wound via scrubbed personnel during surgery. All sterile surgical team members perform a hand and arm scrub before entering the surgical suite. Objectives of a surgical scrub include mechanical removal of dirt and oil, reduction of the transient bacterial population (i.e., bacteria deposited from the environment), and residual depression of the skin's resident bacterial population (i.e., bacteria persistently isolated from the skin) during the procedure. Relying on gloves alone (without a surgical scrub) to prevent microbial contamination is not recommended; up to 50% of surgical gloves contain holes at the completion of surgery. This number may increase with long or difficult surgeries.

Antimicrobial soaps or detergents used for scrubbing should be rapid-acting, broad-spectrum, and nonirritating, and should inhibit rapid rebound microbial growth. They should not depend on cumulation for activity. The most commonly used surgical scrub solutions are chlorhexidine gluconate, povidone-iodine, and hexachlorophene (Table 7-1).

Surgical scrubs physically separate microbes from skin and inactivate them via contact with the antimicrobial

TABLE 7-1

Common Antimicrobial Soaps Available for Surgical Scrubs

Antimicrobial Soap	Mechanism of Action	Properties
Chlorhexidine gluconate	Disruption of cell wall and precipitation of cell proteins	• Broad spectrum (more effective against gram-positive than gram-negative bacteria or fungi) • Good virucide • Residual activity because it binds to keratin • Not inactivated by organic material • May be less irritating to skin than iodophors
Hexachlorophene	Disruption of cell wall and precipitation of cell proteins	• Bacteriostatic for gram-positive cocci • Minimal activity against gram-negative bacteria, fungi, or viruses • Not inactivated by organic material • Cumulative (nullified by alcohol) • May be neurotoxic
Iodophors	Cell wall penetration, oxidation, replaces microbial contents with free iodine	• Broad spectrum (gram-negative and gram-positive bacteria, fungi, and viruses) • Some activity against spores • Inactivated by organic material • Requires minimum of 2 minutes of skin contact
Parachloromethaxylenol (PCMX)	Disruption of cell wall and enzyme inactivation	• Broad spectrum (more effective against gram-positive than gram-negative bacteria, fungi, or viruses) • Slow onset of action
Triclosan	Disruption of cell wall	• Broad spectrum (ineffective against many *Pseudomonas* spp.) • Minimally affected by organic material

solution. Two accepted methods of performing a surgical scrub are the anatomic timed scrub (i.e., 5-minute scrub) and counted brush stroke methods (strokes per surface area of skin). Each method is described in Table 7-2 (Fig. 7-2). Recommendations regarding the number of times one should lather and rinse during the scrub, number of strokes per surface area, and time spent on each surface area vary; however, both methods ensure sufficient exposure of all skin surfaces to friction and antimicrobial solutions. If the hands and arms are grossly soiled, scrub time should be lengthened or brush counts increased; however, skin irritation or abrasion should be avoided because this causes bacteria residing in deeper tissues (e.g., around base of hair follicles) to become more superficial, increasing the number of potentially infective organisms on the skin surface. Contact time between the antimicrobial soap or detergent should be based on documentation of product efficacy in the scientific literature. An initial 5- to 7-minute scrub for the first case of the day, followed by a 2- to 3-minute scrub between additional surgical operations, is generally adequate.

Before scrubbing, all jewelry (including watches) should be removed from the hands and forearms because they are reservoirs for bacteria. Fingernails should be free of polish and trimmed short, and cuticles should be in good condition. Artificial nails (e.g., bondings, tips, wrappings, tapes) should never be worn. A higher number of gram-negative microorganisms has been cultured from the fingertips of personnel wearing artificial nails than from personnel with natural nails, both before and after hand washing. Fungal growth between artificial nails and the natural nail has also been reported and can contaminate the surgical wound. Hands and forearms should be free of open lesions and breaks in skin integrity because such skin infections may contaminate surgical wounds.

Once the scrub has been started nonsterile items cannot be handled. If the hands or arms are inadvertently touched by a nonsterile object (including surgical personnel), the scrub should be repeated. During and after scrubbing procedures the hands should be kept higher than the elbows. This allows water and soap to flow from the cleanest area (hands) to a less clean area (elbow). A single scrub brush can generally be used for the entire procedure. No difference has been documented in the effectiveness of a sterilized reusable brush and disposable polyurethane brush/sponge combination.

TABLE   7-2

Surgical Scrub Procedure

- Locate scrub brushes, antibacterial soap, nail cleaners.
- Remove watches and rings.
- Wet hands and forearms thoroughly.
- Apply 2-3 pumps of antimicrobial soap to hands and wash hands and forearms.
- Clean nails and subungual areas with a nail cleaner under running water.
- Rinse arms and forearms.
- Apply 2-3 pumps of antimicrobial soap to hand and forearm.
- Apply 2-3 pumps of antimicrobial soap to the sterile scrub brush.

Anatomic Timed Method	**Counted Brush Stroke Method**
Note starting time; scrub each side of each finger, between fingers, and back and front of the hand for two minutes.	Apply 30 strokes (one stroke consists of up and down or back and forth motion) to the very tips of your fingers and thumb.
Proceed to scrub the arms, keeping the hand higher than the arm.	Divide each finger and thumb into four parts and apply 20 strokes to each of the four surfaces, including the finger webs (see Fig. 7-2, *A*).
Scrub each side of the arm to 3 inches above the elbow for 1 minute.	Scrub from the tip of the finger to the wrist when scrubbing the thumb, index, and small fingers.
Total scrub time is 2 to 3 minutes per hand and arm.	Divide your forearms into four planes and apply 20 strokes to each surface (see Fig. 7-2, *B*).

- Rinse the scrub brush well under running water and transfer the brush to your scrubbed hand. Do not rinse the scrubbed hand and arm at this time.
- Repeat the process on your other hand and arm.
- When both hands and arms have been scrubbed, drop the scrub brush in the sink.
- Starting with the fingertips of one hand, rinse under water by moving your fingertips up and out of the water stream and allowing the rest of your arm to be rinsed off on the way out of the stream.
- Always allow the water to run from your fingertips to your elbows (see Fig. 7-2, *C*).
- Never allow your fingertips to come below the level of your elbows.
- Never shake your hands to get rid of excess water; allow the water to drip from your elbows.
- Rinse off your other hand similarly.
- Hold your hands upright and in front of you so that they can be seen, and proceed to the gowning and gloving area.

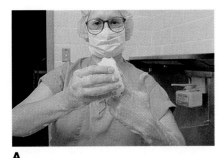

A

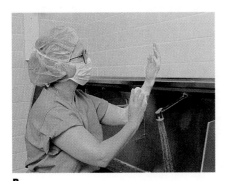

B

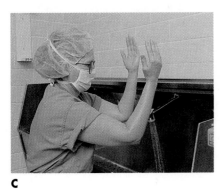

C

FIG. 7-2
A, Divide each finger and thumb into four parts and scrub each of the four surfaces, including the finger webs. **B,** Divide your forearm into four planes and scrub each surface. **C,** When rinsing always allow the water to run from your fingertips to your elbows.

When the scrub has been completed, the hand and arms should be dried with a sterile towel. Pick up the sterile towel from the table taking care not to drip water on the gown beneath it and step back from the sterile table. Hold the towel lengthwise and dry one hand and arm working from hand to elbow with one end of the towel; use a blotting motion (Fig. 7-3). Bend over at the waist when drying the arms so the end of the towel will not brush against your scrub suit. Once the hand and arm are dry bring the dry hand to the opposite end of the towel. Dry the other hand and arm in a similar manner. Drop the towel into the proper receptacle or on the floor if a receptacle is not provided. Do not lower your hands below waist level.

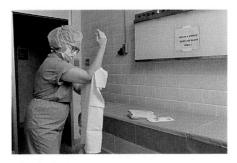

FIG. 7-3
When drying your hands and arms, use one end of the towel to dry one hand and arm (work from hand to elbow). Then bring the dry hand to the opposite end of the towel and dry the other hand and arm in a similar manner.

GOWNING

Gowns are a barrier between the skin of the surgical team member and the patient. They should be constructed of a material that eliminates the passage of microorganisms between sterile and nonsterile areas (see p. 27). They should be resistant to fluid, linting, stretch, pressure, and friction (especially at the forearms, elbow, and abdominal areas) and should be comfortable, economical, and fire resistant. Gowns are available as disposable (single-use) or reusable.

The technique of gowning is described below and illustrated in Fig. 7-4. Gowning and gloving should be done from a surface separate from other sterile supplies (the surgical table) or the surgical patient to avoid dripping water onto the sterile field and contaminating it. Gowns are folded so that the inside of the gown faces outward. Grasp the gown firmly and gently lift it away from the table. Step back from the sterile table to allow room for gowning. Hold the gown at the shoulders and allow it to gently unfold. Do not shake the gown because this increases the risk of contamination. Once the gown is opened identify the armholes and guide each arm through the sleeves. Keep your hands within the cuffs of the gown. Have an assistant pull the gown up over your shoulders and secure it by closing the neck fasteners (see Fig. 7-4, *A*) and tying the inside waist tie. If a sterile-back gown is used, do not secure the front tie until you have donned sterile gloves (see Fig. 7-4, *B*).

GLOVING

Latex rubber gloves are barriers between the surgical team member and the patient; however, they are not a substitute for proper scrubbing methods. If the glove of a properly scrubbed hand is perforated during a surgical procedure, bacteria are rarely cultured from the punctured glove. Lubricating agents for latex gloves such as magnesium silicate (talcum) or low cross-linked cornstarch allow gloves to slide more easily onto the hand. These agents cause considerable irritation to various tissues, even if

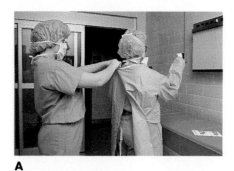

A

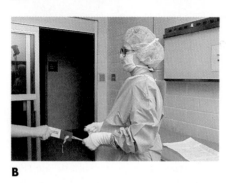

B

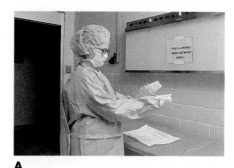

A

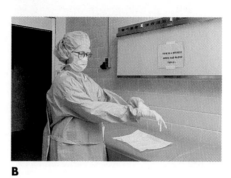

B

FIG. 7-4
A, Have an assistant pull the gown up and over your shoulders and secure it by closing the neck fasteners and tying the inside waist tie. **B,** If a sterile-back gown is used, do not secure the front tie until you have donned sterile gloves.

FIG. 7-5
Closed gloving. **A,** Working through the gown sleeve, pick up one glove from the wrapper. Lay the glove palm down over the cuff of the gown with the thumb and fingers of the glove facing toward your elbow. **B,** Grasp the cuff of the glove with your index finger and thumb. With the index finger and thumb of the other hand (within the cuff), take hold of the opposite side of the edge of the glove. Lift the cuff on the glove up and over the gown cuff and hand. Turn loose and come to the palm side of the glove and take hold of the gown and glove, pulling them toward the elbow while pushing the hand through the cuff and into the glove. Proceed with the opposite hand using the same technique.

gloves are vigorously rinsed in sterile saline before surgery. Therefore the surgeon should use gloves in which the inner surfaces are lubricated with an adherent coating of hydrogel.

Gloving can be performed by three separate methods: (1) gloving yourself using a closed method; (2) gloving yourself using an open method; and (3) assisted gloving.

Closed Gloving

The closed method of gloving ensures that the hand never comes in contact with the outside of the gown or glove (Fig. 7-5).

Open Gloving

The open method of gloving is used when only the hands need to be covered (e.g., urinary catheterization, bone marrow biopsy, sterile patient preparation) or during surgery when one glove becomes contaminated and must be changed. It should not be used routinely for gowning and gloving (Fig. 7-6).

Fig. 7-7 illustrates what to do if both gloves are being donned.

Assisted Gloving

The steps involved in assisted gloving are illustrated in Fig. 7-8.

Removing Gloves Aseptically

This procedure is described in Fig. 7-9.

MAINTAINING STERILITY OF SURGICAL PERSONNEL

The techniques described in this chapter for gowning and gloving minimize the risk of the operative team contaminating the surgical field. However, vigilance is necessary to prevent contamination of gowns or gloves. Once gowned, the surgical team should always face the sterile field. An unsterile area should not be leaned over or touched. Arms and hands should remain above the waist and below the shoulders. The arms should not be folded; they should be clasped in front of the body, above the waist. Scrubbed persons should avoid changing levels and should be seated only when the entire surgical procedure will be performed at this level.

The front of the gown should be considered sterile from the chest to the level of the sterile field; the back of the gown is not considered sterile (even if a sterile-back or wrap-

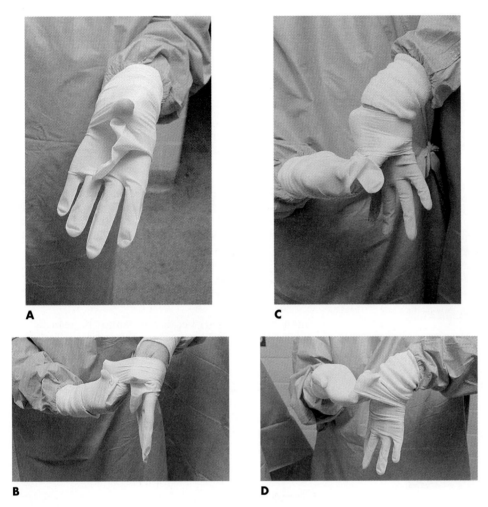

FIG. 7-6
Open gloving when one hand is sterile. **A,** Open the glove wrapper and pick up the correct glove at the folded edge with your sterile hand. Gently put your hand into the glove until your fingers are in the fingers of the glove. Place your thumb inside or near the thumb of the glove and hook the cuff of the glove over your thumb. Let go of the glove. **B,** Place the finger of your sterile hand under the cuff at the palm of the glove and **C,** bend the wrist of the hand being gloved 90 degrees. **D,** Gently walk your fingers around the cuff until they are at the front of the cuff and at the same time pull the cuff up and over

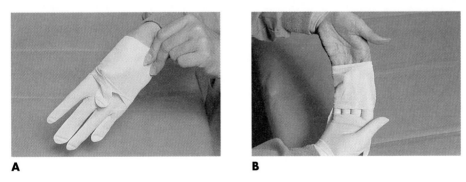

FIG. 7-7
Open gloving when neither hand is sterile. **A,** Pick up one glove by its inner cuff with the opposite hand. Slide the glove onto the opposite hand; leave the cuff down. **B,** Using the partially gloved hand, slide your fingers into the outer side of the opposite glove cuff. Slide your hand into the glove and unfold the cuff; do not touch your bare arm as the cuff is unfolded. With the gloved hand, slide your fingers under the outside edge of the opposite cuff and unfold it.

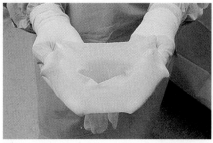

A

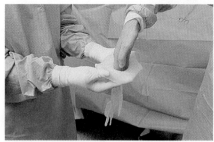

B

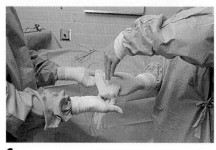

C

FIG. 7-8

Assisted gloving. **A,** Have the assistant pick up one glove and place his or her fingers and thumb under the cuff of the glove. **B,** With the thumb of the glove facing you, slip your hand into the glove. Then, have the assistant bring the cuff of the glove up and over the cuff of your gown and gently let it go. **C,** Have the assistant pick up the other glove. Assist by holding the cuff of the glove open with the fingers of your sterile hand, while putting your ungloved hand into the open glove. The assistant keeps his or her thumbs under the cuff while you thrust your hand into it.

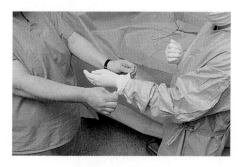

FIG. 7-9

To remove gloves aseptically, the nonsterile assistant grasps the glove near the cuff (being careful not to touch the gown) and pulls it gently from the fingertips. Regloving should be performed using the assisted gloving technique described in Fig. 7-8.

around gown is used) because it cannot be seen by the scrubbed person. The sleeves should be considered sterile from 2 inches above the elbow to the stockinette cuff. Because the stockinette cuff collects moisture (making it an ineffective microbial barrier), it is considered unsterile and should be covered by sterile gloves at all times. The neckline, shoulders, and area under the arms should also be considered unsterile because they may be contaminated by perspiration or by collar and shoulder surfaces rubbing together during head and neck movements.

Reference

Fuller JR: *Surgical technology: principles and practice,* ed 3, Philadelphia, 1994, WB Saunders.

Suggested Reading

Paulson DS: Comparative evaluation of five surgical hand scrub preparations, *AORN Journal* 6:246, 1994.

CHAPTER 8

Surgical Instrumentation

INSTRUMENT CATEGORIES

Each type of surgical instrument is designed for a particular use and should be used only for that purpose. Use of instruments for procedures for which they are not designed (e.g., using Metzenbaum scissors to cut suture, tissue forceps to hold bone) may break or dull the instrument.

Scalpels

Scalpels are the primary cutting instrument used to incise tissue (Fig. 8-1). Reusable scalpel handles (No. 3 and 4) with detachable blades are most commonly used in veterinary medicine; however, disposable handles and blades are available. Blades are available in various sizes and shapes, de-

pending on the task for which they are used. A No. 10 blade is most commonly used in small animal surgery.

Scalpels are usually used in a "slide cutting" fashion where the direction of pressure applied to the knife blade is at a right angle to the direction of scalpel pressure. When incising skin, the scalpel blade should be kept perpendicular to the skin surface. Scalpels can be held using a pencil grip, fingertip grip, or palmed grip. The pencil grip allows shorter, finer, and more precise incisions, because the scalpel is at a 30 to 40 degree greater angle to the tissues than with the other grips (Fig. 8-2). This angle reduces cutting edge contact, making it less useful for long incisions. The fingertip position offers the most accuracy and stability in making long incisions.

Scissors

Scissors come in a variety of shapes, sizes, and weights and are generally classified according to the type of point (e.g., blunt-blunt, sharp-sharp, sharp-blunt), blade shape (e.g., straight, curved), or by the cutting edge (plain, serrated) (Fig. 8-3). Curved scissors offer greater maneuverability and

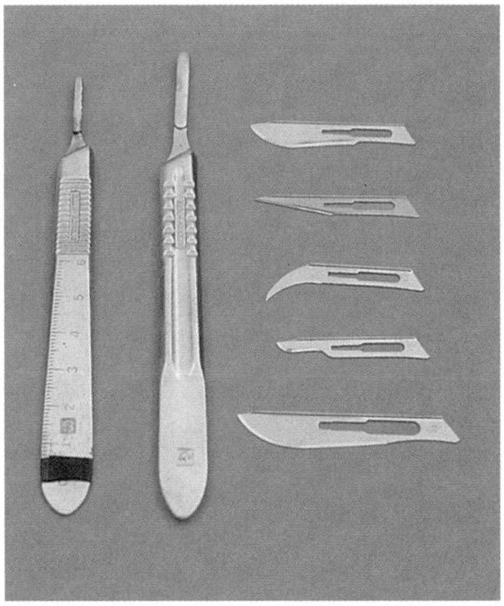

FIG. 8-1
Scalpel handles (No. 3, left; No. 4, right) and blades (top to bottom): No. 10, 11, 12, 15, and 20.

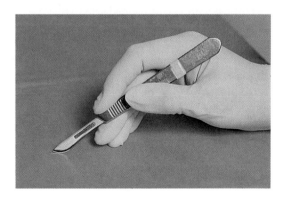

FIG. 8-2
Scalpels are generally held using a pencil grip because it allows short, fine, and precise incisions.

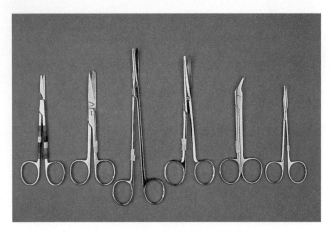

FIG. 8-3
Scissors (left to right): stitch (suture removal), sharp/blunt, Metzenbaum, Mayo, wire, tenotomy.

visibility, while straight scissors provide the greatest mechanical advantage when cutting tough or thick tissue. Metzenbaum or Mayo scissors are most commonly used in surgery; the former scissors are more delicate and should be reserved for fine, thin tissues. Mayo scissors are used for cutting heavy tissues (i.e., fascia). Suture scissors, not tissue scissors, should be used to cut suture. Suture scissors used in the operating room are different from suture removal scissors. The latter have a concavity on one blade that prevents the suture from being lifted excessively during removal. Delicate scissors (e.g., tenotomy, iris) are often used in ophthalmic procedures and other surgeries where fine, precise cuts are necessary. Bandage scissors have a blunt tip that, when introduced under the bandage, reduces the risk of cutting skin.

Scissors may be used for sharp cutting or blunt dissection. They are held with the tips of the thumb and ring finger through the finger rings and with the index finger resting on the shanks near the fulcrum. The ring finger or thumb should not be allowed to "fall through" the handle; the rings should be kept near the distal finger joint. Most scissors are designed for use with a right-handed grip so that the natural pushing of the thumb and pulling of the fingers in a gripping motion applies maximal shear and torque to the blades. When used in the left hand, the thumb blade is positioned such that a grasping motion that pushes with the thumb causes loss of shear and torque forces. It takes considerable practice for a left-handed surgeon to use right-handed scissors. Left-handed instruments are manufactured by most instrument companies.

Direction, control, and accuracy in cutting depend on the stability of the tissue between the scissor blades and the stability of the scissors within the operator's grip. The more obtuse the angle between the blades when cutting, the less the scissors stabilize the tissue and the less accurate the cut. Using the end of the blade stabilizes the tissue more securely and results in a more precise cut. Scissors should not be

completely closed if the incision is to be continued or a ragged incision results; they should be nearly closed, advanced, and nearly closed again. Blunt dissection (i.e., separation of tissue by inserting the points and opening the handles) may be used to separate muscles and fat. Blunt dissection should not be used in tougher tissues or where precise cuts are possible.

Needle Holders

Needle holders are used to grasp and manipulate curved needles (Fig. 8-4). Choice of size and type of needle holder is determined by the characteristics of the needle to be held and location of the tissue being sutured. Heavier, larger needles require wider, heavier jawed needle holders. If needle holders are used to hold suture, the jaws should be finely serrated or smooth to prevent damaging (i.e., fraying, cutting) the suture. Long needle holders facilitate working in deep wounds. High-quality needle holders are made of noncorrosive high-strength alloy and have a glare-free finish. The tips are hardened by coating with a diamond surface or fusing tungsten carbide to the face. Tungsten carbide inserts may be replaced when they become damaged or fail to hold suture adequately.

Most needle holders have a ratchet lock just distal to the thumb (e.g., Mayo-Hegar, Olsen-Hegar), but some (e.g., Castroviejo) have a spring and latch mechanism for locking. Mayo-Hegar needle holders are commonly used in veterinary medicine when medium to coarse needles are being manipulated. Olsen-Hegar needle holders are used similarly but have scissor blades allowing suture to be tied and cut with the same instrument. The disadvantage of Olsen-Hegar needle holders is that expertise is required to prevent unintentionally cutting the suture during tying. Mathieu needle holders have a ratchet lock at the proximal end of the handles of the holder, which permits locking and unlocking simply by a progressive squeezing together of the needle holder handles.

Needles should generally be placed perpendicular to the needle holder because this allows the greatest maneuverabil-

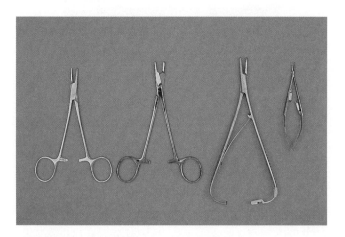

FIG. 8-4
Needle holders (left to right): Mayo-Hegar, Olsen-Hegar, Mathieu, Castroviejo.

ity. Needles placed at an angle require that the handles move through a wide arc during suturing. Needles are generally grasped near their center because this allows the needle to be advanced through tissue with greater force and less risk of needle breakage. When the needle is grasped near the eye or swage, maximum needle length is available for suturing and there is less risk of needle slippage; however, unless delicate tissue is being sutured, the needle is more likely to bend or break. Conversely, holding the needle near the pointed end allows the greatest driving force when suturing tough tissue, but grasping the needle for extraction is difficult.

Needle holders may be held using a palmed grip (no fingers are placed in the rings; upper ring rests against the ball of the thumb [Fig. 8-5]), thenar grip (i.e., upper ring rests on the ball of the thumb, ring finger is inserted through the lower ring [Fig. 8-6]), thumb-ring finger grip (thumb is placed through the upper ring and ring finger through the lower ring [Fig. 8-7]), or pencil grip (i.e., used with Castroviejo needle holders; index finger and thumb rest on the shafts of the needle holders [Fig. 8-8]). The palmed grip is most advantageous when tough tissue is being sutured that requires a strong needle-driving force; however, the needle cannot be released and regrasped after a stitch without read-

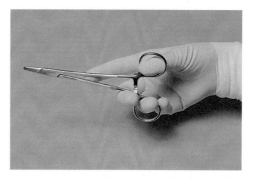

FIG. 8-7
The thumb-ring finger grip allows for the most precision of all grips and is preferable when suturing delicate tissues.

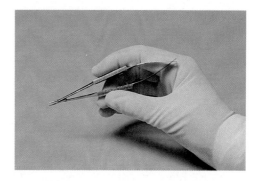

FIG. 8-8
A pencil grip is used with Castroviejo needle holders.

justing to another grip, making suturing less precise. Left-handed surgeons cannot palm right-handed instruments because the boxlock closes rather than opens with pressure. The thenar grip allows the needle to be released and regrasped for extraction without changing grips. Although it allows mobility, releasing the needle holder by exerting pressure on the upper ring with the ball of the thumb causes the handles of the needle holder to "pop" apart. Some movement of the needle occurs during this procedure. The greatest advantage of a thumb-ring finger grip is that it allows precision when releasing a needle. Although it may be slower than the palmed or thenar grips, it is preferred when tissue is delicate or when precise suturing is required.

Tissue Forceps

Tissue (thumb) forceps are tweezerlike, nonlocking instruments that are used to grasp tissue (Fig. 8-9). The proximal ends are bonded together to allow the grasping ends to spring open or be squeezed shut. They are available in a variety of shapes and sizes; tips (grasping ends) may be pointed, flattened, rounded, smooth, serrated, or have small or large teeth. Tissue forceps with large teeth should not be used to handle tissue that is easily traumatized; smooth tips are recommended with delicate tissue (e.g., blood vessels). The most commonly used tissue forceps (e.g., Brown-Adson) have small serrations on the tips that cause minimal trauma but facilitate holding tissue securely.

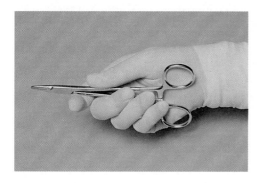

FIG. 8-5
A palmed grip provides a strong driving force but less precision.

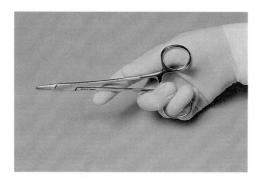

FIG. 8-6
A thenar grip provides good mobility, but releasing the needle holder by applying pressure with the ball of the thumb to the upper ring causes the handles to "pop" apart. This causes some movement of the needle within the tissue being sutured.

Tissue forceps are generally used in the nondominant hand. They should be held so that one blade functions as an extension of the thumb and the other blade functions as an extension of the opposing fingers (i.e., pencil position [Fig. 8-10]). Holding the shanks in the palm greatly limits maneuverability. When they are not in use they can be palmed and held with the ring and little fingers, leaving the index and middle fingers free.

Tissue forceps are used to stabilize tissue and/or expose tissue layers during suturing. During suturing, tissue forceps are used on the far side of the wound to grasp the layer above the one being sutured. This layer is retracted upward and outward with the forceps, exposing the layer to be sutured. The needle point can then be placed at the desired level. Before the needle is driven completely through the tissue, the forceps should be moved from the superficial layer to grasp the layer being sutured. This layer can then be lifted to expose the needle's exit as it is passed through the tissue. On the near side the tissue layer being sutured is grasped and lifted to expose the desired needle entrance site. After the needle point is placed at the desired site, the tissue forceps are moved and are used to retract the more superficial layer, thereby exposing the exit site. When needles are grasped during suturing they should be grasped perpendicular to the shaft.

Hemostatic Forceps

Hemostatic forceps are crushing instruments used to clamp blood vessels (Fig. 8-11). They are available with straight or curved tips and vary in size from smaller (3-inch) mosquito hemostats with transverse jaw serrations to larger (9-inch) angiotribes. Serrations on the jaws of larger hemostatic forceps may be transverse, longitudinal, diagonal, or a combination of these. Longitudinal serrations are generally gentler to tissue than cross serrations. Serrations usually extend from the tips of the jaws to the boxlocks, but in Kelly forceps transverse (i.e., horizontal) serrations extend only over the distal portion of the jaws. Similarly sized Crile forceps have transverse serrations that extend the entire jaw length. Kelly and Crile forceps are used on larger vessels. Rochester-Carmalt forceps are

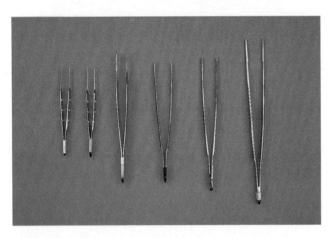

FIG. 8-9
Tissue forceps (left to right): Bishop-Harmon (smooth tip), Bishop-Harmon (toothed), Brown-Adson, 1×2 tissue, serrated, DeBakey.

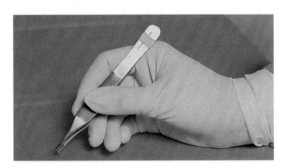

FIG. 8-10
Holding tissue forceps using a pencil grip provides greater maneuverability than other grips.

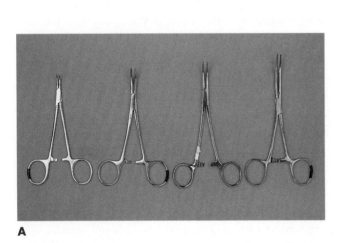

A

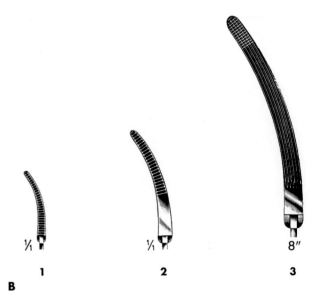

B

¹⁄₁	¹⁄₁	8″
1	**2**	**3**

FIG. 8-11
A, Hemostatic forceps (left to right): mosquito hemostats. **B,** Jaw detail of hemostatic forceps: (1) Mosquito, (2) Kelly, and (3) Rochester-Carmalt.

larger crushing forceps, often used to control large tissue bundles (e.g., during ovariohysterectomy). They have longitudinal grooves with cross grooves at the tip ends to prevent tissue slippage. Specialized cardiovascular forceps (e.g., Satinsky) are available that allow occlusion of only a portion of the vessel. The serrations of cardiovascular clamps provide tissue compression without cutting delicate vessel walls. Large teeth located at the tip ends of some forceps (i.e., Oschner) help prevent tissue slippage within the forceps.

Curved hemostats should be placed on tissue with the curve facing up. As little tissue as possible should be grasped to minimize trauma, and the smallest hemostatic forceps that will accomplish the job should be used. To avoid having fingers momentarily trapped within the rings of hemostats, fingertips should be placed on the finger rings or fingers should be inserted into the rings only as far as the first joint.

Retractors

Hand-held (Fig. 8-12) and self-retaining retractors (Fig. 8-13) are used to retract tissue and improve exposure. The ends of handheld retractors may be hooked, curved, spatula-shaped, or toothed. Some handheld retractors may be bent (i.e., malleable) to conform to the structure or area of the body being retracted. Senn (rake) retractors are double-ended retractors. One end has three fingerlike, curved prongs; the other end is a flat, curved blade. Self-retaining retractors maintain tension on tissues and are held open with a boxlock (e.g., Gelpi, Weitlaner) or other device (e.g., setscrew). Examples of the latter are Balfour and Finochietto retractors (Fig. 8-14). Balfour retractors are generally used to retract the abdominal wall, while Finochietto retractors are commonly used during thoracotomies.

Miscellaneous Instruments

Instruments are available to suction fluid (Fig. 8-15), clamp drapes or tissues (Fig. 8-16), cut and remove pieces of bones (rongeurs [Figs. 8-17 and 8-18]), hold bones during fracture repair (Fig. 8-19), scrape surfaces of dense tissue (curettes), remove periosteum (periosteal elevators [Fig. 8-20]), cut or

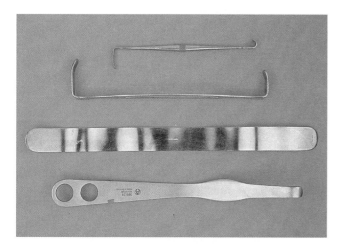

FIG. 8-12
Handheld retractors (top to bottom): Senn, Army-Navy, malleable, Hohmann.

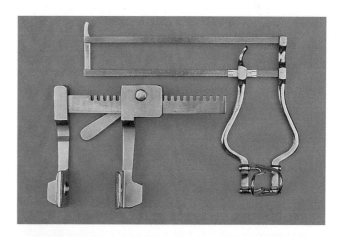

FIG. 8-14
Self-retaining retractors: Finochietto (left), Balfour (right).

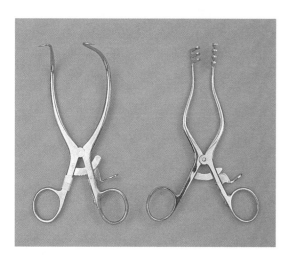

FIG. 8-13
Self-retaining retractors: Gelpi (left), Weitlaner (right).

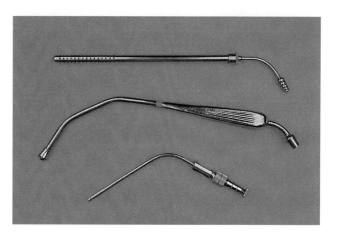

FIG. 8-15
Suction tips (top to bottom): Poole, Yankauer, Frazier.

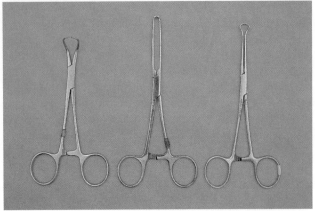

FIG. 8-16
Clamps and forceps (left to right): Backhaus towel clamp, Allis tissue forceps, Babcock forceps.

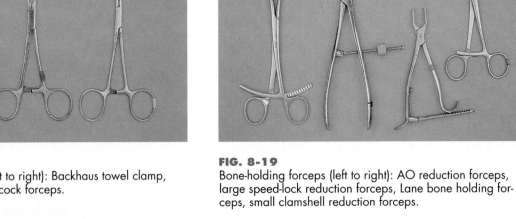

FIG. 8-19
Bone-holding forceps (left to right): AO reduction forceps, large speed-lock reduction forceps, Lane bone holding forceps, small clamshell reduction forceps.

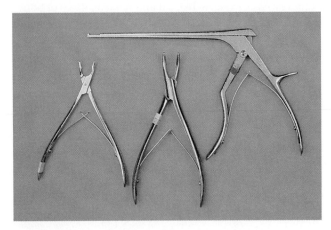

FIG. 8-17
Rongeurs (left to right): Lempert, Ruskin, Kerrison.

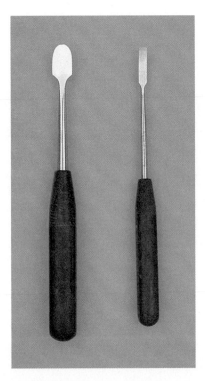

FIG. 8-20
Periosteal elevators: AO—round edge (left), AO—curved blade, straight edge (right).

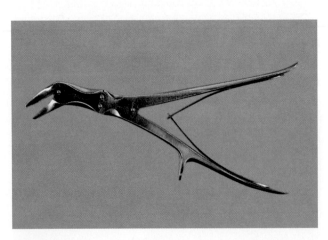

FIG. 8-18
Duck-bill double-action rongeurs.

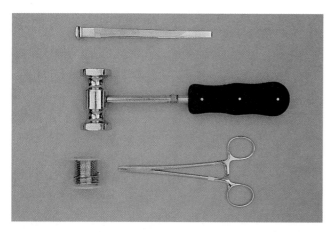

FIG. 8-21
Orthopedic equipment (top to bottom): chisel, mallet, orthopedic wire, and wire twisters.

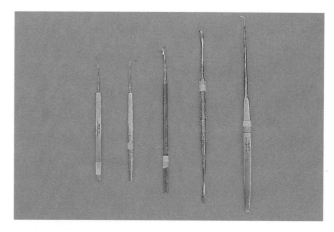

FIG. 8-24
Neurosurgery equipment (left to right): lens loop; small, nerve-root retractor; tartar scraper; Freer dissector; large, right-angle, nerve-root retractor.

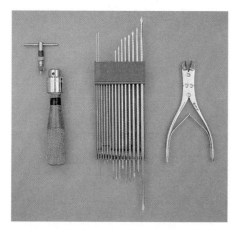

FIG. 8-22
Orthopedic equipment (left to right): Jacob's chuck and key, Steinmann pins and Kirschner wires (pin caddy), pin cutter.

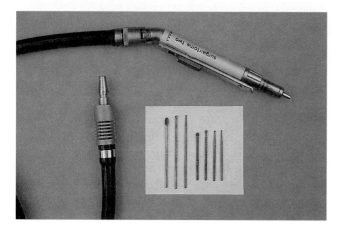

FIG. 8-23
Hall air drill and assorted bits.

shape bone and cartilage (osteotomes and chisels [Fig. 8-21]), and bore holes in bone (trephines). Numerous other specialized instruments have been developed to facilitate specific surgical procedures. Some instruments used in orthopedic and neurologic procedures are illustrated in Figs. 8-22 through 8-24. Other orthopedic instruments are described in Chapter 28.

INSTRUMENT CARE AND MAINTENANCE

Good surgical instruments are valuable investments. They must be used properly and receive routine care and maintenance to prevent corrosion, pitting, and/or discoloration (Table 8-1). Instruments should be rinsed in cool water immediately after the surgical procedure to prevent blood, tissue, saline, or other foreign matter from drying on them. Many manufacturers recommend that instruments be rinsed, cleaned, and sterilized in distilled or deionized water because tap water contains minerals that may discolor and stain. If tap water is used for rinsing, instruments should be dried thoroughly to avoid staining. Instruments with multiple components should be disassembled before cleaning. Delicate instruments should be cleaned and sterilized separately.

Cleaning

Ultrasonic and enzymatic cleaning are effective and efficient. Before putting soiled instruments in an ultrasonic cleaner, they should be washed in cleaning solution to remove all visible debris. Dissimilar metals (e.g., chrome and stainless steel) should not be mixed in the same cycle. All instruments should be placed in the ultrasonic cleaner with the ratchets and boxlocks open. Instruments should not be piled on top of each other because delicate instruments could become damaged. They should be removed from the cleaner and rinsed and dried at the completion of the cycle. If an ultrasonic cleaner is not available, instruments should be cleaned as thoroughly as possible, paying particular attention to boxlocks, serrations, and hinges. Nylon brushes and cool

8-1

Causes of Instrument Corrosion, Pitting, or Discoloration

Type/Cause of Damage	Solution
Corrosion	
• Excessive moisture left on the surface of the instrument or within the instrument pack	• Preheat the autoclave; allow to cool slowly; check autoclave valves for leaks
• Rinsing with tap water; deposition of alkali earth deposits on walls of autoclave, which deposit on instruments	• Use distilled or deionized water during sterilization; clean autoclave with acetic acid periodically
• Prolonged exposure to enzymatic cleaning solutions	• Do not expose carbon steel instruments to enzymatic cleaners for longer than 5 minutes
Pitting	
• Exposing instruments to saline or foreign materials	• Rinse instruments with distilled water immediately after the procedure
• Detergent residue on instruments during autoclaving	• Avoid detergents with chloride bases, which form hydrochloric acid when combined with steam
• Use of alkaline detergents that remove the chromium oxide coat	• Use detergents that have a pH near 7
• Simultaneously cleaning metals of dissimilar composition in an ultrasound cleaner	• Separate instruments made from dissimilar metals during cleaning
Rust deposition	
• Deposition of iron on instrument from tap water	• Use distilled or deionized water during cleaning, rinsing, and sterilization
• Deposition and oxidation of carbon particles on stainless steel instruments when they are sterilized with chrome-plated instruments that have exposed metal	• Separate the two types of steel during sterilization; replace plated instruments that are peeling or imperfect
Spotting	
• Condensation and slow evaporation of water droplets containing sodium, calcium and/or magnesium on instruments	• Follow instructions for autoclave use; open door after steam has been exhausted; check valves or gaskets; use distilled or deionized water
Staining	
Purplish-black	
• Exposure to ammonia	• Avoid detergents with ammonia; rinse instruments thoroughly
• Use of amine chemicals to clean lime deposits in steam lines	• Use distilled or deionized water in autoclaves to prevent lime deposits
Bluish-gray	
• Prolonged use of cold-sterilization solutions	• Use distilled water and rust inhibitors in cold sterilization solutions
Brownish	
• Deposition of copper on instruments during sterilization; formation of a chromic oxide film when the instrument is heated	• Use a dishwashing compound that does not contain polyphosphates, which can solubilize copper components of the sterilizer

cleaning solution may be used for most instruments. Rasps and serrated areas may require a wire brush. A cleaning solution with a neutral pH should be used to avoid staining. Cleaning solutions should be prepared and used per the manufacturer's instructions. Enzymatic solutions remove proteinaceous materials from general surgical instruments and endoscopic equipment.

Lubricating and Autoclaving

Autoclaving is not a substitute for proper instrument cleaning. Before autoclaving, instruments with boxlocks and hinges, and power equipment should be lubricated with in-

strument milk or surgical lubricants. Industrial oils interfere with steam sterilization and should not be used. Instruments are generally grouped into packs or kits (Tables 8-2 and 8-3) according to their use. Before autoclaving, instruments should be wrapped in cloth or placed on a cloth inside a fenestrated pan to absorb moisture. Instruments should be sterilized with the boxlocks or hinges open. The chamber should not be overloaded and stacking of instruments should be avoided to prevent damaging delicate instruments. Kits should be double wrapped (see p. 5) and sealed with tape (e.g., Auto Clave Tape), and a monitor (e.g., OK sterilization indicators, Sterrad chemical indicator strip) should be added before autoclaving (see p. 5). To prevent condensation avoid rapid cooling of instruments. Additional information regarding autoclaving and other methods of sterilization is given in Chapter 2.

Cold Sterilization

Cold sterilization is used for some instruments but does not guarantee sterility. Instruments that cannot be autoclaved are best sterilized using alternate means (e.g., ethylene oxide, plasma sterilization; see p. 9). Solutions that contain benzyl ammonium chloride (BAC) should not be used with instruments that have tungsten carbide inserts because BAC dissolves the tungsten.

TABLE 8-2

Suggestions for Basic Soft Tissue Pack (i.e., spay, laparotomy, wound repair)

Instrument	Quantity
Halsted-mosquito hemostats, curved, 5-inch	2
Halsted-mosquito hemostats, straight, 5-inch	2
Kelly hemostats, curved, 5.5-inch	2
Crile forceps, straight, 5.5-inch	2
Rochester-Carmalt hemostats, curved, 7.25-inch	4
Mayo-Hegar or Olsen-Hegar needle holders, 7-inch	1
Brown-Adson tissue forceps	1
Allis tissue forceps, 5×6 teeth, 6-inch	4
Backhaus towel clamps, 5.25-inch	4
Metzenbaum scissors, curved, 8-inch	1
Mayo scissors, curved, 8-inch	1
Suture scissors, sharp/blunt, straight, 5-inch	1
Instrument tray	1
Senn retractors	2
Blade handle, No. 3	1
Ovariohysterectomy "spay" hook	1
Saline bowl	1
Radiopaque sponges (4×4)	20

TABLE 8-3

Suggestions for Basic Orthopedic Pack (augmented with a general pack described in Table 8-2)

Instrument	Quantity
Jacobs chuck and key	1
Spoon Hohmann retractor	2
Army-Navy retractor	2
Periosteal elevator	1
Wire twister	1
Medium pin cutter	1
Kern or Lane bone-holding forceps	2
Reduction forceps	1
Orthopedic wire (18, 20, and 22 gauge)	1 each size
Kirschner wires	2 each size
Intramedullary pins	2 each size

DRAPING AND ORGANIZING THE INSTRUMENT TABLE

Instrument tables should be height adjustable to allow them to be positioned within reach of surgical personnel. The instrument table should not be opened until the animal has been positioned on the surgical table and draped. Large, water-impermeable table drapes should cover the entire instrument table. To open these drapes, the drape and outer wrap are positioned on the instrument table. The exposed underneath surface of the drape is gently grasped and the ends and then the sides are unfolded. Once the drape has been opened, nonsterile personnel should not reach over it. Mayo stands are often used in procedures that require additional instruments (e.g., bone plating); specially designed stand covers are available to cover these tables. When the instrument pack has been opened (see p. 6), instruments should be positioned so that they can be readily retrieved. Layout is generally determined by surgeon's preference, but grouping similar instruments (i.e., scissors, retractors) facilitates their use. Whenever a body cavity is opened, sponges should be counted at the beginning of the procedure (before making the incision) and again before closure to ensure that none have been inadvertently left in the body cavity. Contaminated instruments or soiled sponges should not be placed back on the instrument table.

CHAPTER 9

Biomaterials, Suturing, and Hemostasis

SUTURES AND SUTURE SELECTION
Suture Characteristics

An ideal suture is easy to handle; reacts minimally in tissue; inhibits bacterial growth; holds securely when knotted; resists shrinking in tissues; is noncapillary, nonallergenic, noncarcinogenic, and nonferromagnetic; and absorbs with minimal reaction after the tissue has healed. Such an ideal suture does not exist; therefore surgeons must choose a suture that most closely approximates the ideal for a given procedure and tissue to be sutured. A wide choice of suture and needle combinations are available.

Suture size. The smallest diameter suture that will adequately hold the mending wounded tissue should be used, to minimize trauma as the suture is passed through the tissue and to decrease the amount of foreign material left in the wound. A suture need be no stronger than the sutured tissue. Suture volumes in relationship to sizes are given in Table 9-1. The most commonly used standard for suture size is the USP (United States Pharmacopeia), which denotes dimensions from fine to coarse, according to a numerical scale; 10-0 is the smallest and 7 is the largest. The USP uses different standards for surgical gut and for other materials (Table 9-2). The smaller the suture size, the less its tensile strength. Stainless steel wire is usually sized according to the metric or USP scale or by the Brown and Sharpe (B and S) wire gauge.

Flexibility. The flexibility of suture is determined by its torsional stiffness and diameter, which influence its handling and use. Flexible sutures are indicated when ligating vessels or performing continuous suture patterns. Less flexible sutures (e.g., wire) cannot be used to ligate small bleeders. Nylon and surgical gut are relatively stiff compared with silk suture; braided polyester sutures have intermediate stiffness.

Surface characteristics and coating. The surface characteristics of a suture influence the ease with which it is pulled through tissues ("drag") and the amount of trauma doing so causes. Rough sutures cause more injury than smooth sutures. Smooth surfaces are particularly important in delicate tissues such as the eye. However, the disadvantages of sutures with smooth surfaces include that they require increased tension to ensure good apposition of tissues, and they have reduced knot security (see below). Braided materials have more friction or drag than do monofilament sutures. Braided materials are often coated to decrease capillarity (see below) and yield a smooth surface. Substances used for coating include Teflon, silicone, wax, paraffin-wax, and calcium stearate.

Capillarity. Capillarity is the process by which fluid and bacteria are carried into the interstices of multifilament fibers. Because neutrophils and macrophages are too large to enter the interstices of the fiber, such infection may persist (particularly in nonabsorbable sutures). All braided materials (e.g., silk) are capillary; monofilament sutures are less capillary. Capillarity of some sutures is reduced by coating. Capillary suture materials should not be used in contaminated or infected sites.

TABLE 9-1

Percentage Volumetric Reduction with Decreased Suture Size

USP	EP	Percentage
3	6	
2	5	28
1	4	33
0	3.5	31
2-0	3	27
3-0	2	51
4-0	1.5	40
5-0	1	49
6-0	0.7	54
7-0	0.5	50
8-0	0.4	44
9-0	0.3	40
10-0	0.2	50

From Zederfeldt BH, Hunt TK: *Wound closure: materials and techniques*, Wayne, NJ, 1990, Davis & Geck.

TABLE 9-2

Suture Sizes

Actual Size (mm)	Metric Gauge	Synthetic Suture Materials (USP)	Surgical Gut (USP)	Brown and Sharpe Wire Gauge
0.02	0.2	10-0		
0.03	0.3	9-0		
0.04	0.4	8-0		
0.05	0.5	7-0	8-0	41
0.07	0.7	6-0	7-0	38-40
0.1	1	5-0	6-0	35
0.15	1.5	4-0	5-0	32-34
0.2	2	3-0	4-0	30
0.3	3	2-0	3-0	28
0.35	3.5	0	2-0	26
0.4	4	1	0	25
0.5	5	2	1	24
0.6	6	3,4	2	22
0.7	7	5	3	20
0.8	8	6	4	19
0.9	9	7		18

Knot tensile strength. Knot tensile strength is measured by the force (in pounds) that the suture strand can withstand before it breaks when knotted. Sutures should be as strong as the normal tissue through which they are being placed; however, the tensile strength of the suture should not greatly exceed the tensile strength of the tissue.

Relative knot security. Relative knot security is the holding capacity of a suture expressed as a percent of its tensile strength. The knot-holding capacity of a suture material is the strength required to untie or break a defined knot by loading the part of the suture that forms the loop, whereas the suture material's tensile strength is the strength required to break an untied fiber with a force applied in the direction of its length.

Specific Suturing Materials

Suture materials may be classified according to their behavior in tissue (absorbable or nonabsorbable), structure (monofilament or multifilament), or their origin (synthetic, organic, or metallic). Monofilament sutures are made of a single strand of material. They have less tissue drag than multifilament suture material and do not have interstices that may harbor bacteria. Care should be used in handling monofilament sutures because nicking or damaging them with forceps or needle holders weakens them and predisposes to breakage. Multifilament sutures consist of several strands of suture that are twisted or braided together. Multifilament sutures are generally more pliable and flexible than monofilament sutures. They may be coated to decrease tissue drag and enhance handling characteristics (see above).

Absorbable suture materials. Absorbable suture materials (e.g., surgical gut, polyglycolic acid, polyglactin 910, polydioxanone, and polyglyconate) lose most of their tensile strength within 60 days and eventually disappear from the tissue implantation site because they are phagocytized or hydrolyzed (Table 9-3). The time for loss of strength and the time for complete absorption vary between sutures.

Catgut (surgical gut). The word *catgut* is derived from the term *kitgut* or *kitstring* (the string used on a kit or fiddle). Misinterpretation of the word *kit* as referring to a young cat led to the use of the term *catgut*. Surgical gut is actually made from the submucosa of sheep intestine or the serosa of bovine intestine and is approximately 90% collagen. It is broken down by phagocytosis and elicits a marked inflammatory reaction, compared with other sutures. Plain surgical gut loses strength rapidly after tissue implantation. "Tanning" (crosslinking of collagen fibers), by exposure with chrome or aldehyde, slows absorption. Surgical gut is available as plain, medium chromic, or chromic; increased tanning generally implies prolonged strength and reduced tissue reaction. Surgical gut is rapidly removed from infected sites or areas where it is exposed to digestive enzymes and is quickly degraded in catabolic patients. The knots may loosen when wet.

Synthetic absorbable materials. Synthetic absorbable materials (e.g., polyglycolic acid, polyglactin 910, polydioxanone, polyglyconate) are generally broken down by hydrolysis. Polyglycolic acid (Dexon) is braided from filaments extracted from glycolic acid. It loses 35% of its tensile strength by 14 days and 65% by 21 days. Polyglycolic acid is available in both coated and uncoated forms. Polyglactin 910 (Vicryl) is a multifilament suture made of a copolymer of lactide and glycolide with polyglactin 370. It is coated with calcium stearate. Its rate of tensile strength loss is similar to polyglycolic acid. Polydioxanone (PDS II) and polyglyconate (Maxon) sutures are monofilament sutures that retain tensile strength longer than polyglycolic acid or polyglactin 910. Polydioxanone suture has a 14% loss of tensile strength in 14 days, 31% in 42 days, and complete absorption in 6 months. Calcinosis circumscripta has been associated with polydioxanone suture in

TABLE 9-3

Characteristics of Suture Materials Commonly Used in Veterinary Medicine

Generic Name	Trade Name	Manufacturer	Suture Characteristics	Reduction in Tensile Strength*	Complete Absorption (Days)	Relative Knot Security[†]	Tissue Reaction[‡]
Chromic surgical gut (catgut)	—	—	Absorbable Multifilament	33% at 7 days 67% at 28 days	60	− wet + dry	+++
Polyglactin 910	Vicryl	Ethicon	Absorbable Multifilament	35% at 14 days 60% at 21 days	60	++	+
Polyglycolic acid	Dexon "S" (uncoated) Dexon II (coated)	Davis & Geck	Absorbable Multifilament	35% at 14 days 65% at 21 days	60–90	++	+
Polydioxanone	PDS II	Ethicon	Absorbable Monofilament	14% at 14 days 31% at 42 days	180	++	+
Polyglyconate	Maxon	Davis & Geck	Absorbable Monofilament	30% at 14 days 45% at 21 days	180	++	+
Silk	Perma-Hand	Ethicon Davis & Geck	Nonabsorbable Multifilament	30% at 14 days 50% at 1 year	>2 years	−	+++
Polyester	Mersiline (uncoated) Ethibond (coated) Dacron (uncoated) Ti•cron (coated)	Ethicon Ethicon Davis & Geck Davis & Geck	Nonabsorbable Multifilament			−	++
Polyamide (Nylon)	Ethilon (monofilament) Nurolon (multifilament) Dermalon (monofilament) Surgilon (multifilament)	Ethicon Ethicon Davis & Geck Davis & Geck	Nonabsorbable Monofilament Multifilament	30% at 2 years (mo)) 75% at 180 days (mu)		+	−
Polypropylene	Prolene Surgilene Fluorofil	Ethicon Davis & Geck Mallinckrodt Veterinary	Nonabsorbable Monofilament			+++	−
Polybutester	Novafil	Davis & Geck	Nonabsorbable Monofilament			++	−
Polymerized caprolactum	Supramid Braunamid Vetcassette II	S. Jackson B. Braun Melsungen Ag Mallinckrodt Veterinary	Nonabsorbable Multifilament			++	++ (if coating breaks)
Stainless steel wire	Flexon (multifilament)	Davis & Geck Ethicon	Nonabsorbable Monofilament Multifilament			+++	−

*Values given are approximate. Actual loss of tensile strength may vary depending on suture and tissue.
[†](−) = poor (<60%); (+) = fair (60% to 70%); (++) = good (70% to 85%); (+++) = excellent (>85%).
[‡](−) = minimal to none; (+) = mild; (++) = moderate; (+++) = severe.

dogs. Polyglactin 910 and polyglycolic acid are more rapidly hydrolyzed in alkaline environments, but are relatively stable in contaminated wounds. Polyglycolic acid may be rapidly degraded in infected urine. There is minimal tissue reaction to synthetic absorbable suture materials, and time for loss of strength and absorption is fairly constant in different tissues. Infection or exposure to digestive enzymes does not significantly influence the rates of absorption of synthetic absorbable sutures.

Nonabsorbable suture materials

Organic nonabsorbable materials. Silk is the most common organic nonabsorbable suture material used. It is a braided multifilament suture made by a special type of silkworm and is marketed as uncoated or coated. Silk has excellent handling characteristics and is often used in cardiovascular procedures; however, it does not maintain significant tensile strength after 6 months and is therefore contraindicated for use with vascular grafts. It should also be avoided in contaminated sites; one silk suture may decrease the number of bacteria required to induce infection in a wound from 10^6 to 10^3.

Synthetic nonabsorbable materials. Synthetic nonabsorbable suture materials (see Table 9-3) are marketed as braided multifilament (e.g., polyester or coated caprolactum) or monofilament (e.g., polypropylene, polyamide, polyolefins, or polybutester) threads. They are typically strong and induce minimal tissue reaction. Nonabsorbable suture materials, which consist of an inner core and an outer sheath (e.g., Supramid), should not be buried in tissues because they may predispose to infection and fistulation. The outer sheath is frequently broken, allowing bacteria to reside under it.

Metallic sutures. Stainless steel is the metallic suture most commonly used. It is available as a monofilament or multifilament twisted wire. The reaction to stainless steel is generally minimal; however, the knot ends evoke an inflammatory reaction. Stainless steel has a tendency to cut tissue and may fragment and migrate. It is stable in contaminated wounds and is the standard for judging knot security and tissue reaction to suture materials.

Surgical Needles

A variety of needle shapes and sizes are available; selection of a needle depends on the type of tissue to be sutured (e.g., penetrability, density, elasticity, and thickness), topography of the wound (e.g., deep or narrow), and characteristics of the needle (i.e., type of eye, length, and diameter). Needle strength, ductility, and sharpness are important factors in determining the handling characteristics and use of a needle. The amount of angular deformation a needle can withstand before becoming permanently deformed is called *surgical yield*. *Ductility* is the needle's resistance to breaking under a specified amount of bending. The sharpness of a needle is related to the angle of the point (see below) and the taper ratio of the needle. The sharpest needles have a long, thin, tapered point with smooth cutting edges. Most surgical needles are made from stainless steel wire because it is strong, corrosion free, and does not harbor bacteria.

The three basic components of a needle are the attachment end (i.e., swaged or eyed), body, and point (Fig. 9-1, *A*). Eyed needles must be threaded and, because a double-strand of suture is pulled through the tissue, a larger hole is created than when swaged suture material is used. Eyed needles may be closed (i.e., round, oblong, or square) or French (i.e., with a slit from the inside of the eye to the end of the needle for ease of threading) (Fig. 9-1, *B*). Eyed needles are threaded from the inside curvature. With swaged sutures the needle and suture are a continuous unit, minimizing tissue trauma and increasing ease of use.

The needle body comes in a variety of shapes (Fig. 9-1, *C*); tissue type and depth and size of the wound determine the appropriate needle shape. Straight (Keith) needles are generally used in accessible places where the needle can be manipulated directly with the fingers (e.g., placement of purse-string sutures in the anus). Curved needles are manipulated with needle holders. The depth and diameter of a wound are important when selecting the most appropriate curved needle. One-fourth (¼) circle needles are primarily used in ophthalmic procedures. Three-eighths (⅜) and one-half (½) circle needles are the most commonly used surgical needles in veterinary medicine (e.g., abdominal closure). Three-eighths circle needles are more easily manipulated than one-half cir-

cle needles because they require less pronation and supination of the wrist. However, because of the larger arc of manipulation required, they are awkward to use in deep or inaccessible locations. A one-half circle or five-eighths (⅝) circle needle (despite requiring more pronation and supination of the wrist) is easier to use in confined locations.

The needle point (i.e., cutting, taper, reverse cutting, or side-cutting; Fig. 9-1, *D*) affects the sharpness of a needle and type of tissue in which the needle is used. Cutting needles generally have two or three opposing cutting edges. They are designed to be used in tissues that are difficult to penetrate (e.g., skin). With conventional cutting needles the third cutting edge is on the inside (i.e., concave) curvature of the needle. The location of the inside cutting edge may promote "cut-out" of tissue because it cuts toward the edges of the wound or incision. Reverse cutting needles have a third cutting edge located on the outer (i.e., convex) curvature of the needle. This makes them stronger than similarly sized conventional cutting needles and reduces the risk of tissue cutout. Side-cutting needles (i.e., spatula needles) are flat on the top and bottom. They are generally used in ophthalmic procedures. Taper needles (i.e., round needles) have a sharp tip that pierces and spreads tissues, without cutting them. They are generally used in easily penetrated tissues (e.g., intestine, subcutaneous tissues, or fascia). Taper-cut needles are a combination of a reverse cutting edge tip and a taper point body and are generally used for suturing dense, tough fibrous tissue (e.g., tendon) and for some cardiovascular procedures (e.g., vascular grafts). Blunt-point needles have a rounded, blunt point that can dissect through friable tissue without cutting. They are occasionally used for suturing soft, parenchymal organs (e.g., liver or kidney).

Suture Selection for Different Tissue Types

Considerations for suture selection include how long the suture will be required to help strengthen the wound or tissue, risk of infection, effect of the suture material on wound healing, and the dimension and strength of suture required.

Abdominal closure. Monofilament sutures should be used in skin to prevent wicking or capillary transport of bacteria to deeper tissues. Synthetic monofilament nonabsorbable sutures (e.g., Prolene, Novafil, and Fluorofil) generally have good relative knot security and are relatively noncapillary. Polymerized caprolactam (Supramid, Vetafil) is preferred for skin sutures by some surgeons because of its superior handling characteristics; however, this suture should not be buried in deeper tissues. Absorbable sutures (e.g., PDS or Maxon) may be used in skin, but they should be removed because absorption requires contact with body fluids. Subcutaneous sutures are used to obliterate dead space and decrease tension on skin edges; absorbable suture material (e.g., PDS or Maxon) is preferred. The rectus fascia may be closed with either an interrupted or continuous suture pattern. For the former, numerous suture materials are adequate; however, suture that is rapidly removed (e.g., surgical gut) should be avoided in catabolic patients. When a continuous suture pattern is used, strong monofilament suture

FIG. 9-1
A, Basic components of a needle. **B,** Types of eyed needles. **C** and **D,** Needle body shapes and sizes.

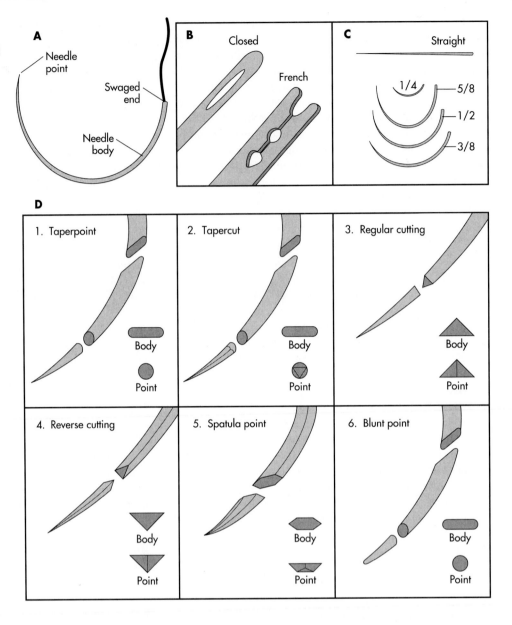

with good knot security should be used (e.g., PDS, Maxon, Prolene, or Novafil). One size larger suture than would normally be used is preferred when performing a continuous suture pattern. The knots should be tied carefully, and three or four square knots (six or eight throws) should be placed. Absorbable suture (e.g., PDS or Maxon) may be preferable, to prevent large amounts of foreign material from remaining permanently within the incision.

Muscle and tendon. Muscle has poor holding power and is difficult to suture. Absorbable or nonabsorbable suture material may be used. Sutures placed parallel to the muscle fibers are likely to pull out. Suture material used for tendon repair should be strong, nonabsorbable, and minimally reactive. Suture with a taper or Taper-cut needle is generally less traumatic. The largest suture that will pass without trauma through the tendon should be used.

Parenchymal organs and vessels. Parenchymal organs (e.g., liver, spleen, and kidney) are generally sutured

with absorbable, monofilament sutures (e.g., PDS or Maxon). Multifilament sutures should be avoided in areas of contamination, and sutures with increased drag (e.g., Dexon or Vicryl) may tend to cut through tissues. Nonabsorbable suture (e.g., Prolene) should be used for vascular grafts. A special manufacturing process tapers the end of Prolene suture, allowing it to be swaged to a needle of similar diameter, which is advantageous for vascular anastomoses.

Hollow viscus organs. Absorbable sutures are generally recommended in hollow viscus organs (e.g., trachea, gastrointestinal tract, or bladder) to prevent tissue retention of foreign material once the wound is healed. Additionally, nonabsorbable suture may be calculogenic when placed in the urinary bladder or gallbladder. Dexon suture was found to rapidly dissolve when incubated in sterile (6 days) or infected (3 days) urine (Sebeseri et al, 1975).

Infected or contaminated wounds. If possible, sutures should be avoided in highly contaminated or infected wounds because even the least-reactive nonabsorbable sutures elicit some degree of infection in tissues contaminated with either *E. coli* or *S. aureus*. Multifilament nonabsorbable sutures (e.g., silk or polyester) should not used in infected tissues because they potentiate infection and may fistulate. Absorbable suture material is preferred; however, surgical gut should be avoided because its absorption in infected tissue is unpredictable. In one study, synthetic monofilament nylon and polypropylene sutures elicited less infection in contaminated tissue than did metallic sutures (Edlich et al, 1973).

OTHER BIOMATERIALS
Tissue Adhesives

Cyanoacrylates (e.g., n-butyl and isobutyl-2-cyanoacrylate) are commonly used for tissue adhesion during some procedures (e.g., declaws, tail docking, and ear cropping). Products advocated for use in veterinary patients include Tissueglue, Vetbond, and Nexabond. These adhesives rapidly polymerize in the presence of moisture and produce a strong, flexible bond. Adhesion of the contact tissues generally takes less than a minute (0 to 15 seconds), but may be prolonged if there is excessive hemorrhage. Persistence of the glue in the dermis may result in granuloma formation or dehiscence, and placement in an infected site may be associated with fistulation. When Nexabond and Vetbond were compared for wound closure after feline onychectomy, no differences were found (Martinez et al, 1993). A major indication in humans is life-threatening bleeding that cannot be stopped by conventional means. CNS indications include embolization of abnormal vessels (e.g., arteriovenous fistulae) or highly vascular tumors before surgical resection. Nexabond and Vetbond have been combined with sutures for tendon repair.

Adhesive Surgical Membranes

Adhesive surgical membranes or tapes designed for wound closure are available; however, there have been few reports of their use in veterinary patients. One study of the use of an adhesive polyurethane membrane for skin closure in cats found that it was quicker and easier to apply than sutures (Court et al, 1989). It adhered strongly to skin and provided adequate support. Histologically, wounds closed with the polyurethane membrane were characterized by milder inflammatory reactions and greater vascular infiltration than were sutured wounds.

Staples and Ligating Clips

Clips (e.g., Hemoclips or Ligaclips) may be used for vessel ligation. They are particularly useful when the vessel is difficult to reach or when multiple vessels must be ligated. Use of ligating clips on vessels greater than 11 mm in diameter is not recommended. The vessel should be dissected free of surrounding tissue before the clip is applied, and 2 to 3 mm of vessel should extend beyond the clip to prevent slippage. The vessel should be one third to two thirds of the size of the clip. Staples (e.g., Michel clips, Proximate plus skin staples) are used to appose wound edges or attach drapes to skin.

When using staples for skin closure, the staple must be appropriately bent so that it cannot be easily removed by the animal. A special staple-remover facilitates clip removal after healing. Approximation of linea alba incisions with stainless steel fascial staples compares favorably with closure with a simple continuous pattern of polypropylene suture material, with regard to breaking strength and clinical, histologic, and morphometric appearance (Kirpensteijn et al, 1993). Stainless steel staples are commonly used in thoracic (e.g., pulmonary resection, or right atrial tumor resection) and gastrointestinal anastomoses (see p. 298).

Autologous Fibrin Glue

Autologous fibrin glue is a biologic adhesive made of fibrinogen, factor XIII, fibronectin, thrombin, apoprotinin, and calcium chloride. It is made from the patient's blood before surgery. In humans, uses of the glue include fixation of skin grafts (i.e., without sutures) and stabilization of gastrointestinal and nerve anastomoses. It has also been used as a preclot material on vascular grafts and as a seal for sutured vascular anastomoses. There is limited experience with the use of fibrin glue in small animals.

Surgical Mesh

Surgical mesh may be used to repair hernias (e.g., perineal hernias) or reinforce traumatized or devitalized tissues (abdominal hernias). Occasionally it is used to replace excised traumatized or neoplastic tissues (see p. 672). Surgical mesh is available in nonabsorbable (e.g., Mersilene [polyester] fiber mesh and Prolene [polypropylene] mesh) or absorbable (e.g., Vicryl [polyglactin 910] and Dexon [polyglycolic acid]) forms. Although surgical mesh is generally elastic, it does not stretch significantly as the patient grows and thus should be used cautiously in immature patients. Fibrous tissue grows through the mesh interstices. Nonabsorbable mesh placed in contaminated wounds may extrude or fistulate and should be removed when the tissue has healed and the mesh is no longer required for support.

COMMON SUTURE TECHNIQUES
Suture Patterns

Suture patterns may be classified as interrupted or continuous, by how they appose tissues (e.g., appositional, everting, or inverting), or by which tissues they primarily appose (e.g., subcutaneous or subcuticular). Appositional sutures (e.g., simple interrupted sutures) bring the tissue in close approximation; everting sutures (e.g., continuous mattress suture) turn the tissue edges outward, away from the patient and toward the surgeon. Inverting sutures (e.g., Lembert, Connell, Cushing) turn tissue away from the surgeon, or toward the lumen of a hollow viscus organ.

Subcutaneous sutures. Subcutaneous sutures are placed to eliminate dead space and provide some apposition of skin so that less tension is placed on skin sutures (Fig. 9-2, *A*). Subcutaneous sutures are generally placed in a simple continuous manner; however, in some instances (e.g., where drainage might be necessary), simple interrupted sutures are preferable. Subcuticular closure may be used in place of skin sutures to reduce scarring or eliminate the need for suture removal (e.g., fractious animals or castrations). The suture is begun by burying the knot (see below) in the dermis. Suture is advanced in the subcuticular tissue, but in contrast to a continuous subcutaneous line, bites are parallel to the long axis of the incision. The suture line is completed with a buried knot (Fig. 9-2, *B*). Absorbable suture material is preferred for subcuticular suture patterns.

Interrupted Suture Patterns

Simple interrupted. A simple interrupted suture is made by inserting the needle through tissue on one side of an incision or wound, passing it to the opposite side, and tying (Fig. 9-3, *A*). The knot is offset so that it does not rest on the incision, and the ends of the suture are cut (for skin sutures, the ends are left long enough to allow them to be grasped during removal). The sutures should be placed approximately 2 to 3 mm away from the skin edge. Right-handed surgeons place sutures from right to left in a horizontal fashion; left-handed surgeons do the opposite.

Simple interrupted sutures are easy and quick to place. They are appositional unless excessive tension is applied; then inversion may occur. Inversion of skin causes poor healing; care should therefore be used to ensure that skin sutures are loose and the edges are apposed. The primary advantage of simple interrupted sutures is that disruption of a single suture does not cause the entire suture line to fail. However, simple interrupted sutures take more time than continuous patterns and result in more foreign material (knots) in the wound.

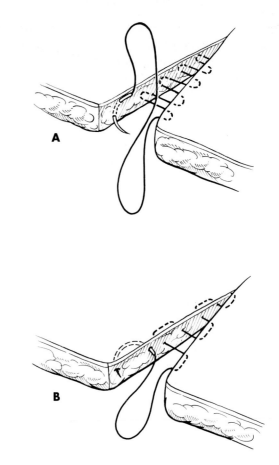

FIG. 9-2
Suture patterns: **A,** subcutaneous, and **B,** subcuticular.

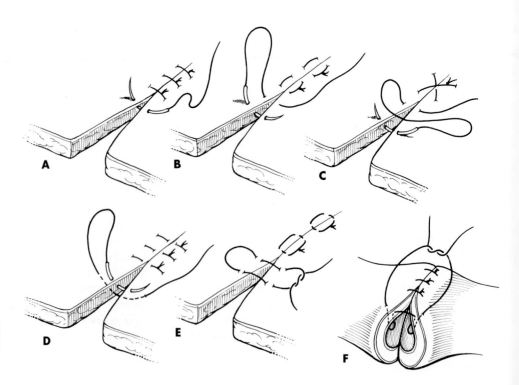

FIG. 9-3
Interrupted suture patterns: **A,** simple interrupted, **B,** horizontal mattress, **C,** cruciate, **D,** vertical mattress, **E,** Halsted, and **F,** Gambee.

Horizontal mattress sutures. Horizontal mattress sutures are placed by inserting the needle on the far side of the incision, passing it across the incision, and exiting it on the near side, as described for a simple interrupted suture (Fig. 9-3, *B*). The needle is then advanced 6 to 8 mm along the incision and reintroduced through the skin on the near side. It then crosses the incision, exiting from the skin on the far side, and the knot is tied. Horizontal mattress sutures are generally separated by 4 to 5 mm. They are primarily used in areas of tension and can be rapidly applied; however, they often cause tissue eversion. Care should be exercised to appose, rather than evert, tissue margins, and the suture should be angled through the tissue so that it passes just below the dermis. Mattress sutures can be modified to form a cross over or under the incision (cruciate) (Fig. 9-3, *C*).

Vertical mattress. To place a vertical mattress suture, the needle is introduced approximately 8 to 10 mm from the incision edge on one side, passed across the incision line, and exited at an equal distance on the opposite side of the incision (Fig. 9-3, *D*). The needle is reversed and inserted through skin on the same side, approximately 4 mm from the skin edge, and the knot tied. Vertical mattress sutures are stronger than horizontal mattress sutures, when used in areas of tension. Placement of vertical mattress sutures is relatively time-consuming; however, eversion of skin margins is less a problem than with horizontal mattress sutures. When two vertical mattress sutures are placed in a parallel fashion before tieing, the pattern is known as a Halsted suture (Fig. 9-3, *E*).

Gambee. Gambee sutures are used in intestinal surgery to reduce mucosal eversion. The suture is introduced as for a simple interrupted suture from the serosa through muscularis and mucosa to the lumen (Fig. 9-3, *F*). It is then returned from the lumen through the mucosa to muscularis, before it crosses the incision. After crossing the incision it is introduced in the muscularis and is continued through the mucosa to the lumen. The needle is then reintroduced through the mucosa and muscularis, to exit from the serosal surface, and the suture tied. Gambee sutures reduce mucosal eversion and may reduce wicking of material from the intestinal lumen to the exterior.

Continuous Suture Patterns

Simple continuous. A simple continuous suture consists of a series of simple interrupted sutures, with a knot on either end; the suture is continuous between the knots (Fig. 9-4, *A*). To begin a simple continuous suture line, a simple interrupted suture is placed and knotted, but only the end that is not attached to the needle is cut. The needle is directed through skin, perpendicular to the incision. The resulting suture line has a suture perpendicular to the incision line below the tissue and advances forward above it. If both the deep and superficial portions of the suture line advance, the suture is termed a *running suture* (Fig. 9-4, *B*). To end a continuous suture, the needle end of the suture is tied to the last loop of suture that is exterior to the tissues. If an eyed needle is used, the needle is advanced through the tissue, and the short end of the suture is grasped. A loop of suture is pulled

through with the needle, and this loop is tied to the single end on the contralateral side.

Simple continuous suture lines provide maximal tissue apposition and are relatively airtight and fluidtight, when compared with a series of simple interrupted sutures. They are frequently used to close the linea alba and subcutaneous tissues. Care should be used when placing continuous suture lines in areas where tightening of the suture may cause a purse-string–like effect (e.g., intestinal anastomosis).

Ford interlocking. Ford interlocking sutures are modifications of a simple continuous pattern, in which each passage through the tissue is partially locked, as illustrated in Fig. 9-4, *C*. To terminate this suture pattern, the needle is introduced in the opposite direction from that used previously (near to far) and the end held on that side. The loop of suture formed on the opposite side is tied to the single end. Locked suture patterns are rapid to place and may appose tissues better than a simple interrupted pattern. The disadvantages are that they use a large amount of suture and may be difficult to remove.

Lembert. A Lembert pattern is a variation of a vertical mattress pattern, applied in a continuous fashion. It is an inverting pattern that is often used to close hollow viscera. The needle penetrates serosa and muscularis approximately 8 to 10 mm from the incision edge and exits near the wound margin on the same side. After passing over the incision, the needle penetrates approximately 3 to 4 mm from the wound margin and exits 8 to 10 mm away from the incision. This pattern is repeated along the length of the incision (Fig. 9-4, *D*).

Connell and Cushing. These patterns are frequently used to close hollow organs because they cause tissue inversion and provide a watertight seal. Connell and Cushing patterns are similar, except that a Connell pattern enters the lumen, whereas a Cushing pattern extends only to the submucosal area (Fig. 9-4, *E* and *F*). The suture line is begun with a simple interrupted or vertical mattress suture. The needle is advanced parallel to the incision and introduced into the serosa, passing through the muscular and mucosal surfaces. From the deep surface (lumen with a Connell), the needle is advanced parallel along the incision and returned through the tissues to the serosal surface. Once outside the viscera, the needle and suture are passed across the incision and introduced at a point that corresponds to the exit point on the contralateral side. The suture is then repeated. The suture should cross the incision perpendicularly. When the suture is tightened, the incision inverts. A Parker-Kerr suture is a modification of Cushing and Lembert patterns that has been advocated for closing the stump of hollow viscera (Fig. 9-4, *G*). It is seldom used because it causes excessive tissue inversion.

Tendon Sutures

Sutures may be used to approximate severed ends of a tendon or to secure one end of a tendon to bone or muscle.

Three-loop pulley suture. The three-loop pulley pattern is made with three loops oriented approximately 120 degrees to each other. The initial loop is placed perpendicular to the long axis of the tendon ends, in a near-far fashion Fig. 9-5). The second loop is placed in a plane 120 degrees

FIG. 9-4
Continuous suture patterns: **A,** simple continuous, **B,** running configuration, **C,** Ford interlocking (**C2** and **C3** illustrate how to end the suture line), **D,** Lembert, **E,** Connell, **F,** Cushing, and, **G,** Parker-Kerr.

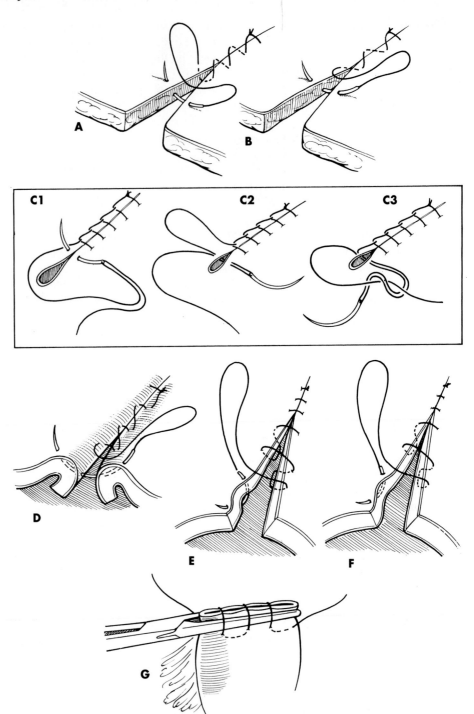

from the first, at a point midway between the near and far positions. The final loop is placed in a far-near pattern, 120 degrees from the first two sutures.

Bunnell's suture. A modified Bunnell's suture pattern may be used to appose severed tendons. The needle is passed from one side of the proximal end of the severed tendon and crossed diagonally across the tendon to the opposite side, where it exits (see Fig. 9-5). The suture is reintroduced approximately 1 mm distal to the exit site and crossed diagonally to the other side of the tendon, where it exits from the severed end. It is introduced into the distal portion of the

severed tendon from the cut end, and two cruciate sutures are placed. The suture exits at the severed end of the distal portion of the tendon and is reintroduced into the proximal tendon. The pattern is repeated in this portion of the tendon, with the suture exiting near the original entrance site. The tendon ends are apposed and the suture tightened.

This pattern is used less frequently than in the past because it is difficult to place and may damage the tendon's microcirculation. Ischemia resulting from the suture may cause the suture to pull out or may result in death of the tendon ends. The resultant gap must then be filled with fibrous tissue.

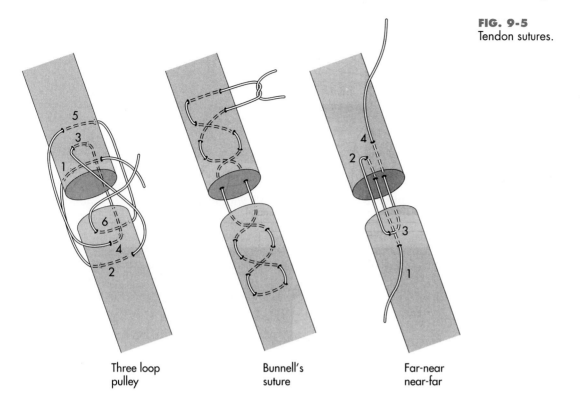

FIG. 9-5
Tendon sutures.

Three loop
pulley

Bunnell's
suture

Far-near
near-far

Far-near-near-far. A far-near-near-far suture may be used in flat tendons. The needle is passed through the tendon, perpendicular to, and 5 mm from, the severed tendon end (see Fig. 9-5). The needle then enters the distal section of the severed tendon in the same vertical plane, 2 mm from the tendon edge. It is looped back to the proximal section of tendon, where it enters 2 mm from the severed edge. The suture is again looped back to the distal section of tendon, to enter 5 mm from the severed tendon edge. Suture ends are pulled taut and tied using a surgeon's knot. This pattern minimally disrupts blood flow and provides good resistance to tension because all suture passes are in the same vertical plane.

Knot Tieing

The knot is the weakest point of a suture. A knot consists of at least two throws laid on top of each other and tightened. The throws can be joined parallel, as in a square knot (Fig. 9-6), or crosswise, as in a granny knot (see Fig. 9-6). Correct knot-tieing technique is important because incorrectly tied knots (e.g., tumbled knots or half hitches [see Fig. 9-6] or granny knots) may lead to dehiscence. Factors that influence knot security are the material coefficient, length of the cut ends, and structure configuration of the knot. The most reliable configuration for a knot is superimposition of squared knots. A surgeon's knot (see Fig. 9-6) cannot be tightened and stands only slight strain on the suture loop. Although it is often used in areas of tension, it is generally not recommended for use with coated or monofilament materials and should be avoided unless tissue tension is such that use of the standard square knot would result in poor tissue apposition. It should never be used to ligate vessels. Multifilament sutures generally have better knot-holding properties than do monofilament materials; however, coating the suture to decrease drag decreases knot security. To avoid strangulating tissues excessive tension should be avoided when tieing knots (except when ligatures are being applied for hemostasis). Excessively tight skin sutures cause patient discomfort and increase the likelihood that the animal will prematurely remove the sutures.

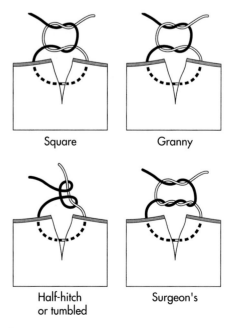

Square

Granny

Half-hitch
or tumbled

Surgeon's

FIG. 9-6
Types of knots.

Instrument ties. In veterinary medicine, instrument ties (Fig. 9-7, *A-D*) are more commonly used than hand ties because there is less waste of suture. The first loop is made as illustrated in Fig. 9-7, after which the suture should not be lifted or have uneven pressure applied to either end, or the throw will loosen. If one end is pulled with greater tension than the other, a half hitch will form (see Fig. 9-6). Opposing suture ends should be pulled perpendicular to the long axis of the incision. Lifting one hand will cause the suture to tumble, forming a sliding two half hitch knot. Failure to correctly cross the hands results in a granny knot.

Hand ties. Hand ties are particularly useful in confined or hard to reach areas or when sutures have been preplaced, as in a thoracotomy closure. Hand ties generally require that suture ends be left longer than is required for an instrument tie. A one-handed or two-handed technique may be used. The two-handed technique generally allows improved control and accuracy; however, the one-handed technique is more useful in confined areas. Techniques for tieing one-handed and two-handed knots are shown in Fig. 9-8, *A-I* and Fig. 9-9, *A-L*.

Burying the knot. The knots of subcutaneous and subcuticular suture patterns are often buried to reduce irritation caused by the knots against more superficial tissues. Refer to Fig. 9-10 for a detailed description of this procedure.

Suture Removal

Skin sutures should generally be removed once healing is sufficiently complete, to prevent dehiscence; they are usually removed after 10 to 14 days. However, prolonged healing (i.e., extremely debilitated animals) may require that sutures be left in place for a longer period. Additionally, if fibrosis is desired (e.g., aural hematoma), delayed suture removal may be considered.

HEMOSTATIC TECHNIQUES AND MATERIALS

Hemostasis is a complex process that involves platelet activation and circulating clotting factors. Numerous diseases or conditions may interfere with clotting in surgical patients. The reader is referred to a medicine text for an in-depth discussion of normal clotting and alterations of clotting caused by diseased states. Obtaining hemostasis allows appropriate tissue visualization during the procedure and prevents life-threatening hemorrhage. Low-pressure hemorrhage from small vessels can be controlled by applying pressure to the bleeding points with gauze sponges. Once a thrombus has formed, the sponge should be gently removed to avoid disrupting clots.

Large vessels must be ligated. Double ligatures are recommended for larger vessels, particularly arteries. Transfixation ligatures may be indicated for larger vessels to prevent the ligature from slipping off the vessel end (Fig. 9-11). Using the smallest suture possible for vessel ligation improves knot security. A surgeon's throw should not be used during vessel ligation (see above).

Electrocoagulation

Electrocoagulation, or vascular coagulation, is widely used for hemostasis. It is generally used in vessels less than 1.5 to 2 mm in diameter; larger vessels should be ligated (see above). The term *electrocautery* is often erroneously used to mean *electrocoagulation*. With electrocautery, the needle tip or scalpel is heated before it is applied to the tissue; whereas with electrocoagulation, heat is generated in the tissue as a high-frequency current is passed through it. Excessive use of electrocautery or electrocoagulation retards healing. Electrocoagulation may be with monopolar or bipolar devices.

FIG. 9-7
A, An instrument tie is made by placing the tips of the needle holders between the two strands of suture. Wrap the strand nearest you (white or long end) around the needle holders to form a loop and grasp the end of the far piece of suture (black; short end) in your needle holders. **B,** Bring it toward you (through the loop) by reversing your hands, and tighten the suture gently. **C,** For the second throw wrap the strand farthest from you (white; long end) over the needle holders to form a loop, grasp the end of the suture nearest you (black; short end) and, **D,** pull it through the loop, snugging it down gently to avoid tightening the suture excessively. Keep your hands low and parallel when tightening the suture to avoid causing the knot to tumble.

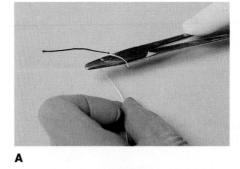

A

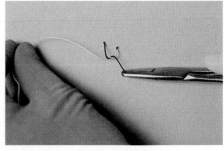

B

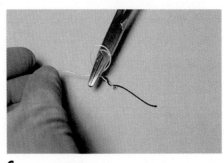

C

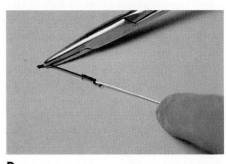

D

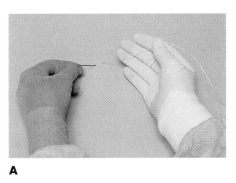

A

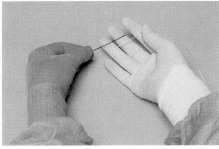

B

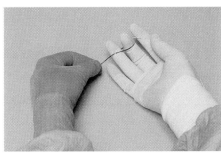

C

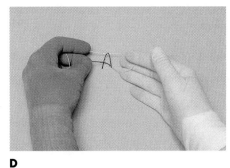

D

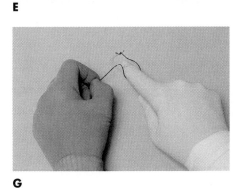

E

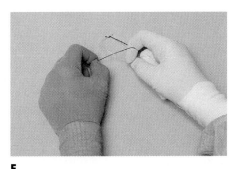

F

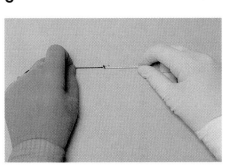

G

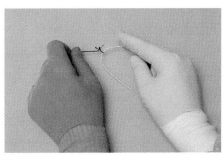

H

I

FIG. 9-8
One-handed square knot (right-handed). **A,** Reflect the right suture (*white*) between the three fingers of your right hand (*white glove*) and hold it between your index finger and thumb. **B,** Hold the left suture (*black*) in your left hand (*dark glove*) and pass it between the index finger and second finger of your right hand. **C,** Flex the distal phalanx of the second finger of your right hand and draw the left strand to the right of the right strand. Extend the tip of the second finger so that the white strand is drawn with it through the loop. **D,** Pull the right strand through the loop by the tips of the second and third fingers on your right hand. **E,** Cross your hands and apply even tension to the two strands. **F,** Place the index finger of your right hand between the right (*black*) and left (*white*) strands so that the left-hand strand forms a loop with the right. Flex the distal phalanx of your right index finger and, **G,** then extend it to draw the right hand strand through the loop. **H,** Pull the right strand through the loop and, **I,** apply even tension to complete the square knot. (Modified from Knecht CD et al: *Fundamental techniques in veterinary surgery,* ed 2, Philadelphia, 1981, WB Saunders.)

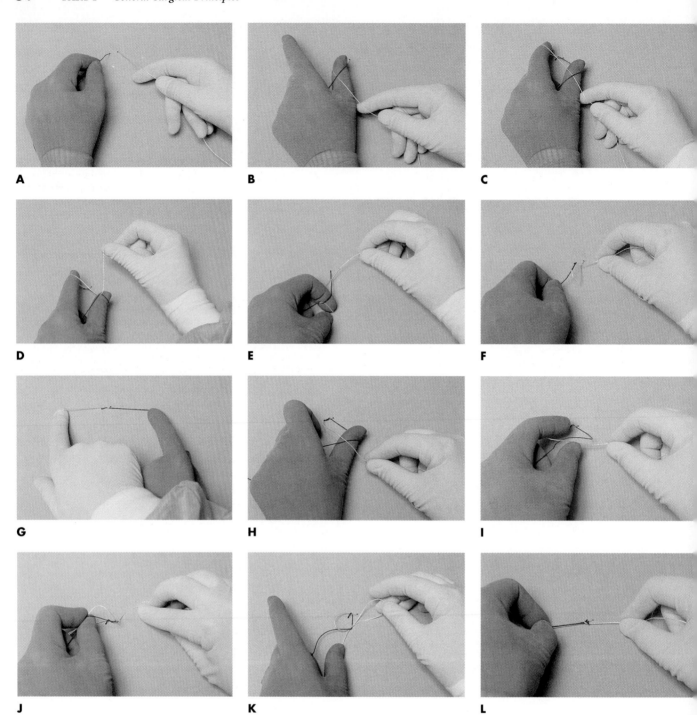

FIG. 9-9

Two-handed square knot (right-handed). **A,** Extend the index finger of your right hand (*white glove*) as a bridge and place the right (*white*) strand over it. Hold the left (*black*) strand in the palm of your left hand (*dark glove*). **B,** Pass your left thumb below and around the right strand and then to the left of the left strand. **C,** Introduce your left index finger between the crossed strands (with your left thumb). **D,** Carry the right strand to your left index finger and thumb, and, **E,** then (using your left index finger and thumb) carry it through the loop. **F,** Return the suture to your right hand, **G,** cross your hands, and apply even tension to the suture ends. **H,** Place your left thumb between the two strands and make a loop with your right hand. **I,** Place your left index finger through the loop and use it and your left thumb to grasp the left (*white*) strand and, **J,** pull or push it through the loop. **K,** Pass the left strand from your left hand to your right thumb and index finger after passing it through the loop and, **L,** apply even tension to the suture strands to tighten the square knot. (Modified from: Knecht CD et al: *Fundamental techniques in veterinary surgery,* ed 2, Philadelphia, 1981, WB Saunders.)

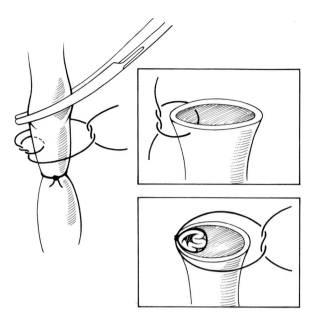

FIG. 9-11
To place a transfixation ligature on a vessel, introduce the needle through the previously ligated tissue. Place a single throw in the suture on the near side and then tie the suture on the opposite side of the vessel.

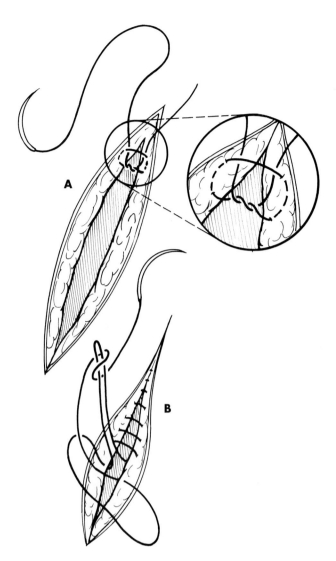

FIG. 9-10
A, To bury a simple interrupted suture introduce the needle deep in the far subcutaneous tissue and pass it toward the dermis. Then pass it across the incision line and reintroduce it in the near subcutaneous tissues at the dermis, exiting deep in the incision line. **B,** To bury a knot at the end of a continuous suture line lift a loop of suture from the incision line. Introduce the needle from the deep surface to superficial on one side, pass it across the incision, and insert it from superficial to deep in the tissue near the loop.

Monopolar coagulation. Monopolar coagulation is the most commonly used method. It involves the flow of current from an active electrode (handpiece), through the patient, to a ground plate. The small surface area of the handpiece concentrates the current density, increasing the temperature of the contact tissue, and causing coagulation. The larger surface area of the ground plate decreases the current density so that minimal tissue heating occurs. Good contact of the ground plate to the patient is essential to prevent thermoelectric burns; conduction gel is usually placed on the ground plate to enhance contact. The tip of the handpiece is generally touched to a hemostat that has been ap-

plied to the bleeding vessel. Direct application of the handpiece tip to tissue is usually avoided. Fulguration may be indicated in some procedures (i.e., perianal fistulae). Fulguration is the destruction of living tissue by electric sparks generated by high-frequency current. The electrode is held near the tissue, but not in direct contact with it, so that a spark of current arcs from the electrode to the patient. When using monopolar coagulation, the field must be relatively dry and the electrode kept clean and free of debris.

Bipolar coagulation. Bipolar coagulation involves the use of a forcepslike handpiece. Current passes from one tip, through the tissue being held between the forceps, to the opposite tip. The tips must be held approximately 1 mm apart for a current to be generated. Bipolar coagulation is used when precise coagulation is necessary to avoid damaging adjacent structures (e.g., thyroidectomy or ophthalmic procedures).

Hemostatic Agents

Substances available to control hemorrhage during surgery include bone wax and hemostatic materials made of gelatin or cellulose. Bone wax is a sterile mixture of semisynthetic beeswax and a softening agent (i.e., isopropyl palmitate). It may be pressed into cavities in bone (e.g., mandibular foramen) or applied to the bone surface to inhibit bleeding. It is poorly resorbed and should be used sparingly because it may act as a physical barrier to healing and promote infection.

Surgicel is made of oxidized regenerated cellulose. When saturated with blood it becomes a gelatinous mass that provides a substrate for clot formation. It can be cut to the desired size and placed on an area of hemorrhage. Surgicel is absorbed by the body; however, removal is recommended because it may inhibit callus formation and promote infection. It is not activated by tissue fluids other than blood, and thus should only be used at sites of hemorrhage. Gelfoam is an absorbable gelatin sponge that may be used in a similar fashion to Surgicel. When applied to an area of hemorrhage, it swells and exerts pressure on the wound. Absorption occurs over a 4- to 6-week period. It may cause granuloma formation and should not be left in infected sites, the brain, or areas with a high risk of infection.

References

Court MH, Bellenger CR: Comparison of adhesive polyurethane membrane and polypropylene sutures for closure of skin incisions in cats, *Vet Surg* 18:211, 1989.

Edlich RF et al: Physical and chemical configuration of sutures in the development of surgical infection, *Ann Surg* 177:679, 1973.

Kirpensteijn J et al: Comparison of stainless steel fascial staples and polypropylene suture material for closure of the linea alba in dogs, *Vet Surg* 22:464, 1993.

Martinez SA, Hauptman, J, Walshaw R: Comparing two techniques for onychectomy in cats and two adhesives for wound closure, *Vet Med* 88:516, 1993.

Sebeseri O et al: The physical properties of polyglycolic acid sutures (Dexon) in sterile and infected urine, *Invest Urology* 12:490, 1975.

Suggested Reading

Barton B, Moore EE, Pearce WH: Fibrin glue as a biologic vascular patch: a comparative study, *J Surg Res* 40:510, 1986.

Bellenger CR: Sutures: the purpose of sutures and available suture materials, *Comp Cont Educ Pract Vet* 4:507, 1982.

Coyne BE, Bednarski RM, Bilbrey SA: Thermoelectric burns from improper grounding of electrocautery units: two case reports, *J Am Anim Hosp Assoc* 29:7, 1993.

Crowe DT Jr: Closure of abdominal incisions using a continuous polypropylene suture: clinical experience in 550 dogs and cats, *Vet Surg* 7:74, 1978.

Dinsmore RC: Understanding surgical knot security: a proposal to standardize the literature, *J Am Coll Surgeons* 180:689, 1995.

Fucci V, Elkins AD: Electrosurgery: principles and guidelines in veterinary medicine, *Compend Contin Educ Pract Vet* 13:407, 1991.

Goldenberg IS: Catgut, silk, and silver—the story of surgical sutures, *Surgery* 46:908, 1959.

Hampel NL, Johnson RG, Pijanowski GJ: Effects of isobutyl-2-cyanoacrylate on skin healing, *Compend Contin Educ Pract Vet* 13:80, 1991.

Heath MM: Needle selection in veterinary surgery, *Comp Cont Educ Vet Pract* 4:45, 1983.

Kirby BM et al: Calcinosis circumscripta associated with polydioxanone suture in two young dogs, *Vet Surg* 18:216, 1989.

Matsumoto T: Vienna international symposium-tissue adhesives in surgery, *Arch Surg* 96:226, 1968.

Ota K et al: Experimental and clinical use of adhesive on parenchymatous organs, *Arch Surg* 96:231, 1968.

Rosin E: Single layer, simple continuous suture pattern for closure of abdominal incisions, *J Am Anim Hosp Assoc* 21:751, 1985.

Rosin E: Knot security of suture materials, *Vet Surg* 18:269, 1989.

Smeak DD, Wendelberg KL: Choosing suture materials for use in contaminated or infected wounds, *Compend Contin Educ Pract Vet* 11:467, 1989.

Trier WC: Considerations in the choice of surgical needles, *Surg Gynecol Obstet* 149:84, 1979.

Vinters HV et al: The histotoxicity of cyanoacrylates: a selective review, *Neuroradiology* 27:279, 1985.

CHAPTER 10

Surgical Infections and Antibiotic Selection

The golden age of modern antibiotic therapy began with the discovery and mass production of penicillin in 1941. Since then, many potentially fatal infections have been prevented through the use of antibiotics; however, they are commonly misused. The widespread use of prophylactic antibiotics in surgical patients has resulted in deemphasis of surgical asepsis and the development of antibiotic-resistant bacteria. The accumulation of resistant bacteria in hospitals and the associated increase in bacterial infections have been accentuated by prolonged, extensive surgical procedures, increased invasiveness of supportive measures, lengthy hospital stays, increased survival of geriatric and debilitated patients, and use of immunosuppressive drugs.

Antibiotic selection is often based on preconceived bias and tradition, rather than on identified or expected bacterial flora. Antibiotic therapy may be prophylactic or therapeutic. *Prophylactic* antibiotic therapy should be used only when indicated by likelihood of infection or when infection would be catastrophic; selection should be based on expected bacterial flora in the targeted tissue. *Therapeutic* antibiotic selection should ideally be based on culture and sensitivity results. This is often not possible, and initial selection is based on expected flora, with antibiotics changed according to culture and sensitivity results. Inappropriate use of antibiotics may cause them to be ineffective or cause serious morbidity and mortality as a result of toxicity or development of resistant microbes.

Bacterial survival in a host depends on the virulence of the bacteria, bacterial numbers, host immunocompetence, and wound factors that deactivate host defenses (i.e., presence of blood clots, ischemic tissue, pockets of fluid, or foreign material). Successful antibiotic therapy requires reduction of bacterial numbers such that host defenses are effective. Competent host defenses allow bacteriostatic agents that slow protein synthesis or prevent bacterial replication to be adequate (see below). However, compromised host defenses (directly or by the presence of negative wound factors) may necessitate bactericidal antibiotics. In addition to using appropriate antibiotics, wound factors may need to be corrected through wound debridement, drainage, or removal of foreign material, to achieve a successful outcome.

MECHANISMS OF ANTIBIOTIC ACTION

Antibiotics that inhibit bacterial growth are termed *bacteriostatic;* those that kill bacteria are termed *bactericidal.* The distinction between bactericidal and bacteriostatic classifications of antibiotics is relative and depends on the ratio between MBC (minimum bactericidal concentration) and MIC (minimum inhibitory concentration). The MIC (generally expressed in μg/ml) is the lowest concentration that inhibits visible bacterial growth. MIC represents the concentration necessary for bacterial inhibition in the patient's plasma or tissues; MBC is the lowest concentration that kills 99.9% of bacteria in plasma or tissues. Antibiotics with a small MBC/MIC ratio (i.e., less than 4) are classified as bactericidal, because plasma and tissue levels that kill 99.9% of the bacteria are typically achieved. Conversely, if the ratio between MBC and MIC is large, it may be difficult to achieve plasma or tissue levels that kill bacteria, and we consider these to be bacteriostatic drugs.

The antibiotic dose used must kill bacteria without harming the host. When the dose required to kill bacteria is greater than that tolerated by the host or greater than that which can be achieved, the bacteria are "resistant" to that drug. Because distribution of antibiotics in body tissues is variable, culture and sensitivity results may be misleading. For example, a urinary tract infection that is "marginally sensitive" to a particular antibiotic, based on sensitivity testing, may be successfully treated if the antibiotic is concentrated in urine. Conversely, if the infection involves the central nervous system and the particular antibiotic does not penetrate the blood-brain barrier, treatment is unlikely to succeed. An effective antibiotic is one that reaches the target tissue and then inhibits or kills the microorganism.

Antibiotics are typically classified according to their mechanism of action. They may destroy or alter the bacterial cell wall or inhibit its synthesis, or inhibit protein or DNA synthesis.

Destruction of Bacterial Cell Walls

One group of antibiotics inhibits synthesis of or promotes destruction of bacterial cell walls. Included in this group are the β-lactam ring antibiotics (e.g., penicillins, cephalosporins, carbapenems, and monobactams), vancomycin, bacitracin, polymixin, nystatin, amphotericin B, and the imidazole antifungal agents. β-Lactams function by binding to the cell wall, decreasing strength and rigidity, and affecting cell division and growth. β-Lactam antibiotics tend to be bactericidal. Penicillins are effective against gram-positive aerobes and gram-positive and gram-negative anaerobes, but some are inactivated by bacterial penicillinases (a type of β-lactamase), and some bacteria are impermeable to them (e.g., methicillin-resistant staphylococci). Penicillinase inhibitors (e.g., clavulanic acid) may be combined with penicillins (e.g., amoxicillin or ticarcillin plus clavulanic acid) to enhance their activity.

Cephalosporins are more effective than penicillins against gram-negative rods (e.g., Enterobacteriaceae), but may be inactivated by cephalosporinases (a type of β-lactamase). Most are poorly effective against anaerobes (cefoxitin is an exception). First-generation cephalosporins are effective against most gram-positive and some gram-negative organisms. Second-generation cephalosporins have greater activity against gram-negative bacteria and anaerobes, but have no additional efficacy against gram-positive organisms. Third-generation cephalosporins are highly effective against more than 90% of gram-negative bacteria, but are often less active against gram-positive organisms than first-generation cephalosporins. Some third-generation cephalosporins have specific gram-negative spectra.

Imipenem and aztreonam are newer β-lactam antibiotics that are highly resistant to β-lactamases. They are as effective against gram-negative organisms as aminoglycosides, but are not nephrotoxic. Imipenem (a carbapenem) has the broadest antibacterial spectrum of any systemic antimicrobial, and is effective against virtually all clinically relevant bacterial species, including gram-negative and gram-positive anaerobes and aerobes. Imipenem should only be used in severely ill patients who fail to respond to other antibiotics. Its broad spectrum of activity is likely to encourage abuse, resulting in emergence of resistant bacteria. Aztreonam, a synthetic monobactam, is unaffected by bacterial β-lactamase. It is highly effective against many gram-negative aerobes, but has little activity against anaerobes. It has no activity against gram-positive bacteria and must be used in combination to achieve broad-spectrum activity.

Inhibition of Protein Synthesis

Chloramphenicol, tetracycline, erythromycin, and clindamycin bind to bacterial ribosomes, causing reversible inhibition of protein synthesis. Chloramphenicol has broad-spectrum activity against streptococci, staphylococci,

Brucella, Pasteurella, and anaerobes; activity against *Pseudomonas* is poor. Chloramphenicol is highly lipophilic and readily enters cells, the central nervous system, and the eye. It may be poorly absorbed in fasted cats because their inactive gastrointestinal tracts do not release the parent drug from its ester group. Chloramphenicol may cause idiosyncratic, fatal anemia in humans, but dogs and cats usually only experience mild, transient anemia (if even that).

Tetracyclines are effective against many gram-positive and gram-negative bacteria, *Chlamydia, Rickettsia,* spirochetes, *Mycoplasma,* bacterial L-forms, and some protozoa. They are usually ineffective against staphylococci, enterococci, *Pseudomonas,* and Enterobacteriaceae. Tetracyclines are distributed well to most tissues (not central nervous system). They achieve good intracellular concentrations. Calcium-containing products chelate tetracyclines and interfere with oral absorption. Binding of calcium can be a problem in young or pregnant animals, and tooth discoloration and inhibited bone growth can occur.

Erythromycin is readily absorbed from the upper gastrointestinal system and diffuses well throughout most tissues. Serum concentrations decline rapidly 4 to 6 hours after administration. Erythromycin is readily concentrated by the liver and eliminated by bile. It is very effective against gram-positive bacteria, but has relatively little effect against gram-negative organisms. It is effective against *Streptococcus* spp., *Staphylococcus* spp., *Bacillus anthracis,* P. *multocida,* *Helicobacter* spp., and clostridia. In one retrospective study, erythromycin caused vomiting in 57% of animals to which it was administered orally, probably because it stimulates gastric motility via motilin receptors. Clarithromycin and azithromycin have recently become available. Azithromycin achieves extremely high tissue concentrations and only needs to be given once daily.

Clindamycin is a semisynthetic derivative of lincomycin, and has a limited spectrum of activity compared with erythromycin. Clindamycin is active against gram-positive pathogens, including *Staphylococcus, Streptococcus, Clostridium,* several *Actinomyces,* and some *Nocardia,* and is extremely effective against many anaerobic bacteria. Clindamycin is often used when treating infections that are resistant to penicillins and erythromycin, or in patients that cannot tolerate these drugs. It is effective against staphyloccocal osteomyelitis, but ineffective against gram-negative bacteria.

Aminoglycosides (e.g., amikacin, gentamicin, and tobramycin) also disrupt protein synthesis, but bind irreversibily to bacterial ribosomes and are bactericidal. They are effective against gram-negative and gram-positive bacteria, including Enterobacteriaceae and pseudomonads, and have a synergistic effect with β-lactam antibiotics. Their activity is reduced in necrotic tissue because of free nucleic acid material. Anaerobes are resistant to aminoglycosides because they lack the receptor necessary for transport into the bacterial cell. Aminoglycosides are polar and thus lipid-insoluble, resulting in limited distribution in extracellular fluid and cerebrospinal fluid. Distribution into pleural fluid, bone, joints, and peritoneal cavity is good. None of the aminoglycosides is well-absorbed orally. They are considered to be "concentration-dependent," as opposed to "time-dependent," indicating that they can be given at higher doses at longer intervals (e.g., once daily), which maintains effectiveness but decreases renal toxicity. Dehydration, electrolyte loss, and preexisting renal disease increase aminoglycoside nephrotoxicity. Ototoxicosis and neuromuscular blockade are other potential adverse effects.

Inhibition of DNA Synthesis

Fluoroquinolones (e.g., enrofloxacin, norfloxacin, ciprofloxacin, ofloxacin) and potentiated sulfas (e.g., trimethoprim sulfa) inhibit DNA synthesis. Fluoroquinolones inactivate DNA gyrase, preventing uncoiling of the DNA molecule during DNA replication and transcription to mRNA. They are rapidly bactericidal and are effective for soft tissue infections, pneumonia, osteomyelitis, and urinary tract infections caused by gram-negative organisms and staphylococci. They are also effective against *R. rickettsiae* and possibly L-forms, but are variably effective against streptococci and ineffective against most anaerobes. They have excellent activity against Enterobacteriaceae, including some that are resistant to aminoglycosides and cephalosporins. An additional reported advantage is activity against *P. aeruginosa;* however, recent reports suggest that higher-than-recommended doses are required. Although development of resistance to fluoroquinolones was initially considered unlikely, some *Pseudomonas, Escherichia coli, Enterococcus* spp., and *Staphylococcus* spp. have become resistant. In one hospital, 80% of methicillin-resistant staphylococci developed resistance to ciprofloxacin within 1 year of its introduction in human patients. Indiscriminate use will likely continue the development of resistant strains. Potential side effects include vomiting, central nervous system effects in animals of all ages, and cartilage lesions in developing animals.

Trimethoprim-sulfonamide combinations are effective for the treatment of osteomyelitis, prostatitis, pneumonia, tracheobronchitis, pyoderma, and urinary tract infections. When used in combination, they are bactericidal and function by inhibiting sequential steps in folate synthesis. Combination therapy is less likely to cause development of resistant strains. Trimethoprim-sulfonamide combinations have a broad spectrum of activity, including most streptococci, many staphylococci, and *Nocardia*. They have relatively little activity against anaerobes, and none against *Pseudomonas*. Potential side effects include keratoconjunctivitis sicca, thrombocytopenia, anemia, vomiting, hypersensitivity (i.e., vasculitis or arthritis), and hepatic disease. Some breeds (e.g., Doberman pinschers and rottweilers) and some families of dogs seem more likely to have side effects.

CAUSES OF ANTIBIOTIC FAILURE AND MECHANISMS OF ANTIBIOTIC RESISTANCE

Successful antibiotic drug therapy relies on administering appropriate doses so that bacteria at the site of infection are killed or suppressed sufficiently to allow the patient's im-

mune system to control the infection. Factors that contribute to antibiotic failure include inappropriate dose (i.e., excessive or suboptimal), frequency, or route of administration; length of treatment; inappropriate antibiotic selection (i.e., not based on culture and sensitivity); inability of the antibiotic to reach the cause of infection (i.e., foreign body or implant); inability of the antibiotic to reach the target tissue in sufficient dosages (e.g., cross blood-brain barrier); antibiotic resistance by bacteria (see below); depressed host immunity (i.e., concurrent severe or debilitating illness); pharmacokinetics of the drug; drug reactions; antibiotic antagonism; and incorrect diagnoses (i.e., viral diseases or foreign bodies).

Antibiotic resistance may be the result of enzymatic destruction of the antibiotic (e.g., some bacteria produce β-lactamases, which inhibit β-lactam drugs), alteration of bacterial permeability to the antibiotic (e.g., streptococci have a natural permeability barrier to aminoglycosides, which may be overcome if a cell wall–active drug is simultaneously used), alteration of the structural target for the antibiotic (e.g., resistance to aminoglycosides can be gained by alteration of the protein composition of the bacterial ribosome that serves as the receptor in susceptible organisms), or development of alternative metabolic pathways that bypass the reaction antagonized by the particular antibiotic.

SURGICAL INFECTION
Classification of Surgical Wounds

Surgical wounds are classified by degree of contamination, to help predict the likelihood of developing infection. Bacterial infection is defined as having greater than 10^5 bacteria per gram of tissue. The classification scheme was developed by the National Research Council to allow a basis for comparison between types of wounds and between institutions. Although this scheme is helpful, there is some overlap and inconsistency between and within groups. The overall infection rate for all types of surgical wounds is approximately 5%. Further classification of surgical wounds by degree of contamination results in significant differences in infection rates.

Clean wounds are nontraumatic wounds without inflammation or infection, in which breaks in aseptic technique do not occur (or are not identified) and luminal organs are not entered. The published infection rates for these surgical wounds range from 0% to 3.5%. Within this category, wounds associated with severe trauma with multiple fractures, traumatic procedures (i.e., carpal arthrodesis), and fractures of the distal radius or tibia requiring plating are most likely to result in postoperative infection. Antibiotic prophylaxis has not reduced the infection rate except when surgery is performed by students or when surgery duration exceeds 90 minutes. Thus antibiotic prophylaxis is not indicated for clean wounds unless a prolonged procedure is anticipated or when inexperienced personnel are performing the surgery.

Clean-contaminated wounds are identified when nonsterile luminal organs are entered without significant spillage of contents. Included in this category are procedures during which the gastrointestinal or respiratory tracts, oropharynx, or vagina are entered, the urinary or biliary tracts are entered in the absence of infected urine or bile, or when there is a minor break in aseptic technique (e.g., perforation of a surgical glove). The published infection rate in this type of surgical wound is 4.5%, with clean-contaminated fractures of the pelvis and long bones most frequently becoming infected. Antimicrobial prophylaxis is indicated in clean-contaminated wounds; antibiotic selection is based on anticipated flora.

Contaminated wounds involve a major break in surgical technique, gross spillage of gastrointestinal contents, fresh traumatic wounds, or entrance of the urinary or biliary tract when gross infection is present. Published infection rates vary from 5.8% to 14.6%, with contaminated fractures of long bones and pelvis and contaminated urogenital procedures most frequently becoming infected. For contaminated wounds, antibiotic prophylaxis is indicated; drug selection is initially based on anticipated bacterial flora and modified based on culture and sensitivity results. These wounds are not infected initially, but have the potential to become so. The fate of contaminated wounds can be markedly altered by early management. Delicate debridement, copious lavage, and antibiotic therapy can convert these wounds to "clean" ones, whereas inadequate therapy often results in a dirty, infected wound.

Dirty wounds are those in which gross infection is present (e.g., traumatic wounds with retained devitalized tissue, foreign bodies, or fecal contamination) at the time of surgical intervention. Management of this type of wound requires antibiotic therapy (initial selection based on anticipated flora, later modified by bacterial culture and sensitivity), copious lavage, debridement, drainage, and potentially wet-to-dry bandages (to further debride the wound during the early postoperative period).

Classifications of Surgical Infections

Infections can plague surgical patients in four major settings: (1) primary surgical disease (e.g., osteomyelitis secondary to an open fracture, pyometra, peritonitis secondary to gastrointestinal perforation, or prostatic abscessation), (2) a complication of a surgical procedure not commonly associated with infection, (3) a complication of support procedures, and (4) associated with prosthetic implants. Bacteria causing infections associated with primary surgical diseases are characteristic of the nonsterile source (e.g., skin, urinary tract, or gastrointestinal tract). These infections are subject only to surgical treatment and not surgical prevention. Initial antibiotic selection is based on expected bacterial flora and later modified by culture and sensitivity results.

Sites of surgical procedures that are not normally associated with infection become infected when bacteria are introduced from nonsterile surfaces (e.g., skin, gastrointestinal tract, or urinary tract) to sterile tissues. All surgical procedures result in some bacterial contamination. Development of infection depends on the number and virulence of bacteria, competence of host defenses, and amount of tissue damage and dead space occurring from the procedure. Infections can be minimized through meticulous surgical technique,

copious wound lavage, closure of dead space, and appropriate antibiotic prophylaxis.

Infection may be a complication of support procedures, particularly when extensive support procedures are performed in debilitated, traumatized, or immunocompromised patients. Intravenous catheters may be associated with sepsis that persists until catheter removal. Patients with prolonged intravenous catheterization should be monitored carefully for infection. Cephalic catheters should be changed every 48 to 72 hours, although jugular catheters often last for 7 to 10 days, if managed properly. Urinary catheters are a common source of infection in perioperative patients. Patients with indwelling urinary catheters are not protected from infection by systemic antibiotics. Indwelling urinary catheters should be connected to closed drainage systems to help prevent ascending infection. Prolonged endotracheal intubation supports the development of infection through the presence of a foreign body, disruption of the mucociliary apparatus, and disruption of an effective cough reflex.

Prosthetic implants are foreign substances used to support, rebuild, or in some fashion mimic the function of an anatomic structure (i.e., total hip, polypropylene mesh, nonabsorbable suture, vascular prostheses, metallic implants, or methylmethacrylate bone cement). The presence of foreign material in contaminated or infected wounds significantly increases the chance for chronic infection and implant rejection. Antibiotic treatment is seldom successful until the implant is removed because implants inhibit medications and defense mechanisms from reaching bacteria. However, if sterile biocompatible implants are placed using appropriate aseptic surgical technique and antibiotic prophylaxis, infection and subsequent implant rejection are rare. Transient bacteremia (e.g., ultrasonic dental prophylaxis) may seed porous implants (i.e., methyl methacrylate) with bacteria and produce an infection. Therefore patients with surgical implants requiring such procedures should be treated with prophylactic antibiotics before the procedure.

Prevention of Surgical Infection

Preventing surgical wound infection is the primary objective of aseptic surgery. Factors that may determine whether microbial contamination occurs on a surgical wound include host factors (i.e., age, physical condition, nutritional status, diagnostic procedures, concurrent metabolic disorders, and nature of the wound), operating room practice, and characteristics of bacterial contaminants. Patients older than 10 years may be predisposed to infection because of an inability to mount an appropriate immune response, or they may have concurrent debilitating disorders (i.e., hyperadrenocorticism, diabetes mellitus, protein-losing enteropathy). Patients younger than 1 year may be predisposed because of an underdeveloped immune system. Patients with protein-calorie malnutrition (see Chapter 11) are at increased risk, especially if malnutrition is causing hypoproteinemia. Diagnostic procedures (i.e., urethral catheterization, thoracocentesis and abdominocentesis, intravenous catheterization), immunosuppressive therapy (i.e., corticosteroids or cancer chemotherapy), long periods of hospitalization, previous antibiotic therapy, remote infections, and wound or body cavity drains may also predispose to infection. Local conditions at the surgical site (i.e., presence of necrotic tissue, hematoma, serum pockets, local infection, foreign bodies, dead space) may also influence patient susceptibility to infection because they allow bacterial proliferation, yet inhibit normal host response.

Operating room practice (i.e., principles of aseptic technique, sterilization and disinfection, preparation of the surgical environment, gowning and gloving, and preparation of the surgical patient, operative site, and surgical team) are important in preventing surgical infection and are discussed in Chapters 1 through 7. Considerable evidence supports the assumption that endogenous bacteria (i.e., bacteria from the patient) account for the majority of wound infections. Also important in preventing surgical infection is proper atraumatic tissue handling and instrument usage. Traumatized tissue supports bacterial growth, but has impaired host defenses. Traumatized or necrotic tissue also has reduced oxygen content, which permits anaerobic bacterial growth. Phagocytosis and humoral immunity are significantly decreased when tissue integrity is interrupted during surgery. Inexperienced surgeons cause more tissue trauma than experienced surgeons, producing greater susceptibility to infection. The overall surgical infection rate for all classifications of wounds in a university setting (i.e., students, interns, residents, and staff surgeons) was approximately 5%, while in a specialty referral center (i.e., staff surgeons only) it was 3.5%.

Characteristics of bacterial contaminants may influence surgically acquired infection. The agents most likely to cause surgical wound infection are environmentally resistant bacteria. These infections are generally acquired during hospitalization and are referred to as *nosocomial* infections. Surgical wounds are a common site for nosocomial infections. Overuse of antibiotics, indwelling catheters (i.e., intravenous or urinary), diagnostic procedures (i.e., transtracheal wash, thoracocentesis and abdominocentesis, bone marrow biopsy), advanced age (i.e., older than 10 years), and chronic debilitating disease are risk factors for nosocomial infections. Prevention of nosocomial infections requires control of endogenous flora (i.e., patient preparation [see Chapter 6]), decreased bacterial transmission (i.e., hand washing, gloves, disinfection, and sterilization [see Chapters 2, 7, and 8]), control of the hospital environment (i.e., maintaining proper cleaning, disinfection, and hospital sterilization protocols [see Chapter 4]), and rational antibiotic use (i.e., based on patient need and culture and sensitivity results).

THERAPEUTIC AND PROPHYLACTIC ANTIBIOTIC USE
Prophylactic Antibiotics

Prophylactic antibiotics must be present at the surgical site during the time of potential contamination to prevent growth of contaminating pathogens. Surgical procedures that may warrant use of prophylactic antibiotics are listed in Table 10-1. Antibiotics are not a substitute for proper aseptic technique, meticulous and atraumatic tissue handling, careful hemostasis, judicious use of sutures, preservation of blood supply, elimination of dead space, and anatomic apposition of tissues.

Rational selection of antibiotics for antimicrobial prophylaxis requires that the most likely contaminating microorganism(s) is identified and that the microorganism is susceptible to the drug used. Empirical selection of drugs is necessary for antimicrobial prophylaxis. Antibiotic selection should be based on clinical experience plus published studies of the microbiology of small animal infection. Empirical selection of an antibiotic to prevent or treat infection requires a drug that is at least 80% effective against the probable pathogen(s). The pathogens usually responsible for postoperative wound infection in small animal surgical patients are *Staphylococcus* spp. (especially *aureus*), *E. coli*, *Pasteurella* spp. (especially in cats), and *Bacteroides fragilis* (anaerobic).

TABLE 10-1

Examples of Surgical Procedures That May Warrant Prophylactic Antibiotic Administration

General Indications	Gastrointestinal Procedures
• Surgery time longer than 90 minutes	• Colonic anastomosis or colectomy
• Prosthesis implantation (e.g., mesh, pacemaker, vascular prosthesis, bone cement)	• Strangulation/obstruction
	• Pancreatic abscess
• Patients with a preexisting prosthesis (e.g., total hip, pacemaker, bone cement) undergoing surgical procedures (e.g., dental prophylaxis, traumatic wounds, colorectal surgery)	• Gastric resection for gastric dilatation-volvulus
	• Anal and rectal surgery
	• Esophageal surgery
• Severely infected or traumatized wounds	• Perineal herniorrhaphy
	• Hepatobiliary surgery with infection
Orthopedic Procedures	
• Total hip replacement	**Urogenital Procedures**
• Open fracture repair	• Renal, ureteral, bladder, or urethral surgery with infected urine
• Extensive fracture repair	
Respiratory Procedures	
• Resection of infected lung lobe(s)	
• Closure of esophagobronchial fistula	

TABLE 10-2

Organisms Most Commonly Isolated from Various Body Systems

Specific Procedure	Likely Pathogens
Thoracic surgeries (pulmonary and cardiovascular procedures)	*Staphylococcus* spp. Gram-negative bacilli
Orthopedic surgeries (e.g., total hip replacement, prolonged internal fixation)	*Staphylococcus* spp.
Gastric and upper intestinal surgeries (high-risk patients)	Gram-positive cocci Enteric gram-negative bacilli
Biliary tract surgeries (high-risk patients)	Enteric gram-negative bacilli Anaerobes (esp. *Streptococcus* spp., *Clostridium* spp.)
Colorectal surgeries	Enteric gram-negative bacilli Anaerobes (esp. *Bacteroides* spp., *Streptococcus* spp.)
Urogenital (e.g., pyometra, endometritis)	*E. coli*, *Streptococcus* spp., anaerobes
Deep, penetrating wounds (e.g., wounds less than 6 hours old [wounds older than 6 hours require therapeutic antibiotics], bite wounds)	Anaerobes Facultative bacteria
Dentistry (patients with valvular heart disease)	*Staphylococcus* spp., *Streptococcus* spp., facultative bacteria, anaerobes

The most likely organisms associated with surgical procedures are listed in Table 10-2 according to body system. Special considerations used in the selection and administration of prophylactic antibiotics are provided in Table 10-3.

Therapeutic Antibiotics

Therapeutic use of antibiotics is based on clinical judgment, knowledge of the antibiotic's mechanism of action (see above), and microbiologic factors. When an antibiotic is in-dicated, the goal is to choose a drug that is selectively active for the most likely infecting microorganism(s), has the least toxicity, kills bacteria at the site of infection, and does not negatively influence the host's immune system. Therapeutic antibiotics are indicated in surgical patients with over-whelming systemic infection (i.e., septicemia or bacteremia), infection present at the surgical site or in a body cavity (i.e., wound infection, pyothorax, or abdominal abscess), or any contaminated or dirty surgical procedure listed in Table 10-1. Generally, antibiotic therapy is instituted before surgery and continued for at least 2 to 3 days after resolution of all clinical signs; maximum duration of therapy depends on drug toxicity and the disease being treated.

Special considerations in the selection and administration of therapeutic antibiotics are listed in Table 10-4. Success of antibiotic therapy is initially determined by observing the patient's response for a minimum of 3 days. If the animal's condition has not improved by then, determination should be made whether the original diagnosis is correct; the culture and sensitivity are accurate; the pathogen is susceptible to the antibiotic; the proper dose, route, and frequency are being used; a foreign body or undrained focus of infection is present; a new infection is superimposed on the original infection; and/or the host defense mechanism is severely compromised. In most surgical infections, antibiotic therapy needs adjunctive therapy (i.e., drainage of accumulations of serum, pus, or blood from surgical wounds or body cavities, concurrent debridement of necrotic tissue, continued lavage of infected wounds, removal of foreign bodies or infected implants, removal of urinary calculi, removal of pus from abdominal abscess, debridement of chronic osteomyelitis, drainage of suppurative arthritis) to be effective.

TABLE 10-3

Considerations for Selection and Administration of Prophylactic Antibiotics

Considerations/Action

Antibiotic Selection

- Determine system involved and most likely organism (see Table 10-2)
- Cefazolin attains appropriate concentrations to prevent bacterial growth of the most common contaminants

Timing of Antibiotic Administration

Beginning of surgery (at anesthetic induction)

Cefazolin dose

20 mg/kg

Routes of Antibiotic Administration

Intravenously at induction; may repeat in 2-3 hours depending on length of surgery

Duration of Antibiotic Administration

Discontinue immediately after surgical wound closure

TABLE 10-4

Considerations for Selection and Administration of Therapeutic Antibiotics

Considerations/Action

Antibiotic Selection

- Determine system involved and most likely pathogen, to establish primary therapy (see Table 10-2)
- Obtain representative samples for Gram's stain, cytology, and culture and susceptibility testing (e.g., fluid, tissue, implants, necrotic debris)
- Ensure antibiotic reaches target tissue
- If several antibiotics are effective, select the one that is least expensive, least toxic, and most convenient to administer

Timing of Antibiotic Administration

As soon as samples have been obtained, begin empirical antibiotic therapy

Dose

Follow recommended doses carefully

Routes of Antibiotic Administration

Treat for a minimum of 3 days; assess animal's condition; if improving, continue therapy; if no improvement, reevaluate

Duration of Antibiotic Administration

Duration depends on effect of antibiotic, toxicity, and disorder being treated; give for at least 2 to 3 days after resolution of all signs

Suggested Reading

Dorfman M, Barsanti J, Budsberg SC: Enrofloxacin concentrations in dogs with normal prostates and dogs with chronic bacterial prostatitis, *Am J Vet Res* 56:386, 1995.

Hardie EM: Life-threatening bacterial infection, *Comp Cont Educ Pract Vet* 17:763, 1995.

Hirsh DC, Spencer SJ: Antimicrobial susceptibility of selected infectious bacterial agents obtained from dogs, *J Am Anim Hosp Assoc* 3:487, 1994.

Neer TM: Clinical pharmacologic features of fluoroquinolone antimicrobial drugs, *J Am Vet Med Assoc* 193:577, 1988.

Papich MG: Antimicrobial drugs. In Ettinger SJ, Feldman EC, eds: *Textbook of veterinary internal medicine*, ed 4, Philadelphia, 1995, WB Saunders.

Petersen SW, Rosin E: Cephalothin and cefazolin in vitro antibacterial activity and pharmacokinetics in dogs, *Vet Surg* 24:347, 1995.

Richardson DC et al: Pharmacokinetic disposition of cefazolin in serum and tissue during canine total hip replacement, *Vet Surg* 21:1, 1992.

Rosin E et al: Cefazolin antibacterial activity and concentrations in serum and surgical wound in dogs, *Am J Vet Res* 534:1317, 1993.

Vasseur PB et al: Surgical wound infection rates in dogs and cats: data from a teaching hospital, *Vet Surg* 17:60, 1988.

Wilkens B et al: Effects of cephalothin, cefazolin, and cefmetazole on the hemostatic mechanism in normal dogs: implications for the surgical patient, *Vet Surg* 24:25, 1995.

CHAPTER 11

Postoperative Care of the Surgical Patient

Care of the surgical patient does not end when the procedure is finished. Postoperative care of surgical patients often determines the ultimate outcome; with critical patients it may determine whether they survive. Postoperative care involves normalization of homeostasis, control of pain (see Chapter 12), and early recognition of complications. Early recognition of potentially catastrophic conditions facilitates treatment and, ultimately, recovery. Recommendations for postoperative care are included with information regarding treatment of specific diseases throughout this text; general recommendations for animals undergoing surgery are included in this chapter.

After surgery, patients should be moved to a quiet recovery room where they can be observed. Geriatric patients, ill or debilitated patients (e.g., renal dysfunction, hepatic disease, vomiting, diarrhea), and patients undergoing long surgeries should be maintained on intravenous fluids until they are able to eat and drink. Close attention to fluid rate and urinary losses is necessary to prevent volume depletion, severe electrolyte imbalances, and/or acid-base disorders. Temperature, pulse, and respiration should be monitored at least every hour (more frequently in critical patients) until the temperature is normal and the animal is alert. Hypothermic animals may need to be actively rewarmed with heated cages, hot water bottles or gloves, or warmed blankets. Recumbent animals should be alternated between left and right lateral recumbency or placed in sternal recumbency until they are able to sit or stand without assistance. Evaluation of hematocrit, blood gases, blood pressure, and/or oxygen saturation may be necessary. Oxygen supplementation via an oxygen cage, nasal insufflation (see p. 618), or mask should be considered for hypoxemic (P_aO_2 less than 60 mm Hg) animals. Patients unable to urinate without assistance (e.g., patients with intervertebral disk disease) require special care; treatment of animals with neurologic disease is discussed in Chapters 33 to 37.

Anesthesia, toxic/metabolic disorders, primary brain stem disease, and increased intracranial pressure may cause central nervous system (CNS) depression. Patients with delayed recovery from anesthetic episodes should be evaluated for increased intracranial pressure, particularly if there was preexisting CNS disease or trauma. Seizures are paroxysms of abnormal brain function and may occur postoperatively as a result of anesthetic drugs (i.e., ketamine), diagnostic procedures (i.e., myelography), primary intracranial disease secondary to intracranial surgery, and/or secondary effects of other disease processes on brain function (e.g., portosystemic shunts, hypocalcemia following thyroid or parathyroid surgeries, hypoglycemia associated with insulinomas). Most seizures are short-lived and cease before treatment can be instituted; however, patients in status epilepticus or with cluster seizures should be treated immediately, even if the primary cause is not ascertained.

Mechanical ventilation may be necessary after surgery in some animals (i.e., severe hypoxemia [P_aO_2 less than 50 to 60 mm Hg], severe hypercarbia [P_aCO_2 greater than 50 to 60 mm Hg], increased intracranial pressure). Volume-cycled or pressure-cycled ventilators may be used. Respiratory rate and tidal volume should be adjusted to maintain P_aCO_2 between 30 to 40 mm Hg and P_aO_2 levels greater than 60 mm Hg. Excessive airway pressures should be avoided. P_aO_2 is generally five times that of the F_IO_2 (fractional concentration of inspired oxygen); values less than this may suggest gas exchange impairment (e.g., if a patient is breathing in 40% O_2, the expected P_aO_2 level is 200 mm Hg). Depending on the degree of impairment, additional treatment (e.g., positive end expiratory pressure [PEEP]) may be necessary. PEEP increases functional residual capacity and volume for gas exchange, lessening alveolar collapse. PEEP can be provided with sophisticated equipment or by placing the expiratory limb of the breathing circuit under water. The pressure against which the patient breathes (usually 2 to 5 cm H_2O) depends on the depth the expiratory limb extends under water.

Hemorrhage may be a result of surgery or the underlying disease. Severe hemorrhage decreases circulating blood volume and oxygen-carrying capacity, resulting in eventual cardiovascular collapse. Clinical signs of severe hemorrhage may be obvious; however, occult hemorrhage into a body cavity may be hard to recognize. Pale mucous membranes, slow capillary refill time, weak pulses, and a high heart rate are nonspecific signs of hemorrhage, but these parameters should be monitored closely after surgery. The hematocrit should be evaluated frequently if bleeding is a concern; however, acute blood loss frequently occurs without changes in the hematocrit. Although normal animals can lose approximately 10% of their blood volume without severe consequences, many postoperative patients are unable to tolerate this much hemorrhage. Ongoing hemorrhage should be eliminated and blood volume replaced. The choice of replacement product is dictated by the onset of the deficit, clinical signs, and potential for complications. If hemodilution is not a concern, balanced electrolyte solutions (i.e., Normosol) may be given. Two to three times the volume of blood lost may be given rapidly (not to exceed 60 to 90 ml/kg). Central venous pressures may be monitored to assess volume replacement. Evaluating packed cell volume (PCV) and total solids at frequent intervals following resuscitation is indicated. The optimal PCV in critical patients is 25% to 35%. A slightly lower than normal PCV decreases blood viscosity, effectively decreasing afterload and improving cardiac output. If the PCV is less than or equal to 20% or if hemodilution or ongoing hemorrhage is likely to cause the PCV to fall below this level, blood products should be administered (see Table 5-3, p. 21). Fresh, whole blood replaces red cell mass, plasma proteins, platelets, and clotting factors. If the animal is not hypoproteinemic, packed red blood cells may be given. All blood products should be administered through a filtered administration set. Calcium-containing fluids should not be used to dilute or flush these lines because they may cause clotting within the tubing. Patients that are hypoproteinemic but not anemic may be given plasma or other colloidal solutions (e.g., hetastarch, dextrans) to increase plasma oncotic pressure (see p. 197).

NUTRITIONAL MANAGEMENT OF THE SURGICAL PATIENT

An important component of postoperative care is nutritional support of debilitated or anorexic patients. Malnutrition is defined as the progressive loss of lean body mass and adipose tissue because of inadequate intake of or increased protein and caloric demand. Possible consequences of protein-calorie malnutrition include organ and muscle atrophy, impaired immunocompetence, ineffective wound healing, anemia, hypoproteinemia, decreased resistance to infection, and death. Thus patients with protein-calorie malnutrition require nutrient supplementation during treatment of their underlying disorder.

A variety of disorders may cause protein-calorie malnutrition (e.g., starvation, anorexia, malabsorption, severe trauma, surgical stress, sepsis, large surface area burns, various types of malignancies). In addition, surgery, postoperative complications, and surgically-induced anorexia create an increased metabolic demand for protein and calories. There is no age, sex, or breed predisposition for patients with

malnutrition; it is common in animals with severe illness (i.e., 25% to 65% incidence in veterinary practice).

Diagnosis of protein-calorie malnutrition is possible if three or more of the criteria listed in Table 11-1 are present. Physical examination may reveal poor hair coat, pressure sores or nonhealing wounds, tissue wasting, skeletal muscle atrophy, and/or emaciation. Additional physical findings vary depending on the cause of malnutrition. Thoracic and abdominal radiographs of malnourished patients are generally nonspecific. Imaging techniques occasionally reveal an underlying cause for the patient's hyporexia, anorexia, or emaciation (i.e., intestinal obstruction, abdominal mass, thoracic mass). Biochemical changes in patients with protein-calorie malnutrition may include hypoproteinemia/hypoalbuminemia, anemia, hypoglycemia, hyperglycemia, and/or hyperlipidemia. Other changes may be related to the specific underlying disease.

Prevention and Treatment of Malnutrition

Nutritional supplementation plus identification and appropriate treatment of the underlying disease are goals for treating malnourished patients. Hyperalimentation is the administration of adequate nutrients to malnourished patients or those at risk. Enteral hyperalimentation provides nutrients to a functional gastrointestinal tract (i.e., nasoesophageal, pharyngostomy, esophagostomy, gastrostomy, or enterostomy tube), while parenteral hyperalimentation provides nutrients intravenously.

Predicting malnutrition (e.g., prolonged postoperative anorexia, early stages of a potentially chronic disorder) and supplementing nutrients before depletion occurs help prevent malnutrition in hospitalized patients. Specific treatment depends on the patient's calculated energy needs, the diet chosen, and the route of administration (i.e., enteral vs. parenteral). Basal energy requirement (BER) is based on body weight; maintenance energy requirement (MER) is determined from BER and the number and severity of clinical problems (i.e., cage rest, postsurgical stress, trauma, cancer, sepsis, or major burn). These calculations are based on specific patient data and are applied to the formulas in Fig. 11-1.

TABLE 11-1

Diagnosis of Protein-Calorie Malnutrition

- Weight loss of more than 10% normal body weight
- Anorexia or hyporexia (i.e., suboptimal intake of nutrients) for more than 5 days or an expected decrease in nutrient intake of more than 5 days
- Increased nutrient loss (i.e., vomiting, diarrhea, severe wounds/burns)
- Increased nutrient needs (i.e., trauma, surgery, infection, burns, fever)
- History of chronic illness
- Serum albumin concentration less than or equal to 2.5 g/dl

Calculate basal energy requirement (BER)

Animals less than 2 kg body weight: $70 \times \left(\boxed{}^{0.75} \right) = \boxed{\boxed{}}$

body weight (kg)   BER (kcal/day)

Animals more than 2 kg body weight: $30 \times \boxed{} + 70 = \boxed{\boxed{}}$

body weight (kg)   BER (kcal/day)

Calculate maintenance energy requirement (MER)

Associated clinical problems	Factor
Cage rest	1.00 - 1.25
Postsurgical stress	1.25 - 1.35
Trauma or cancer	1.35 - 1.50
Sepsis	1.50 - 1.70
Major burns	1.70 - 2.00

$\boxed{} \times \boxed{} = \boxed{\boxed{}}$

factor   BER   MER
chosen   (kcal/day)   (kcal/day)

Calculate volume of formula required (See Tables 11-2 and 11-3 for formula composition.)

$\boxed{} \quad \boxed{} \div \boxed{} = \boxed{\boxed{}}$

name of formula chosen   MER   kcal/ml   mls of formula
    (kcal/day)   per day

Calculate protein requirement

Species	Maintenance	Hepatic or renal failure
Canine:	5.0 - 7.5 g/100 kcal	< 3.0 g/100 kcal
Feline:	6.0 - 9.0 g/100 kcal	< 4.0 g/100 kcal

$\boxed{} \times \boxed{} = \boxed{\boxed{}}$

protein   MER   protein
requirement   (100 kcal/day)   requirement
chosen   (g/day)
g/100 kcal

Calculate needed protein supplementation if required

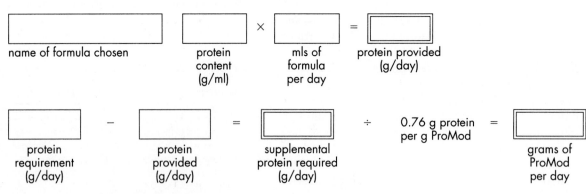

$\boxed{} \quad \boxed{} \times \boxed{} = \boxed{\boxed{}}$

name of formula chosen   protein   mls of   protein provided
    content   formula   (g/day)
    (g/ml)   per day

$\boxed{} - \boxed{} = \boxed{} \div \begin{matrix} 0.76 \text{ g protein} \\ \text{per g ProMod} \end{matrix} = \boxed{\boxed{}}$

protein   protein   supplemental   grams of
requirement   provided   protein required   ProMod
(g/day)   (g/day)   (g/day)   per day

FIG. 11-1
Formulas used to calculate basal and maintenance energy requirements for dogs and cats.

Diets for enteral use. The ideal enteral diet should be well tolerated, readily digested and absorbed, contain essential nutrients, be readily available, inexpensive, have a long shelf life, and be easy to use. Generally, diets should be isotonic (i.e., approximately 300 mOsm/L), have a caloric density of approximately 1.0 kcal/ml, include fiber at 1.0 to 1.5 g/100 kcal, and provide approximately 16% of total calories as protein (i.e., protein content of at least 4.0 g/100 kcal) and approximately 30% of calories as fat. Diets for enteral use are generally divided into monomeric and polymeric categories. Monomeric diets are usually composed of crystalline amino acids as the protein source, glucose and oligosaccharides as the carbohydrate source, and safflower oil as the essential fatty acid source. They generally have twice normal osmolality, can be used in patients with primary gastrointestinal disorders (e.g., short bowel syndrome, inflammatory bowel disease, pancreatic exocrine insufficiency), and are expensive. The most commonly used commercially available monomeric diet is Vivonex HN; its composition is listed in Table 11-2.

Polymeric diets contain large molecular weight proteins, carbohydrates, and fats, approach isotonic osmolality, require normal gastrointestinal digestive processes, contain about 1 kcal/ml, and are more economical. These diets include blenderized diets and commercially available liquid diets (Tables 11-2 and 11-3). Commercial polymeric diets are available in a variety of osmolalities, caloric densities, and compositions. Examples of commonly used commercial polymeric diets and their compositions are listed in Table 11-2. These diet formulas are indicated for malnourished patients with intact digestive and absorptive function or suspected food allergy and should be used in patients that must be fed through small diameter tubes (i.e., nasoesophageal, gastroduodenostomy, and enterostomy tubes).

The most cost-effective, well-balanced diets for enteral administration are those blenderized from prescription pet food or homemade diets. Caloric density and protein content vary with the diet chosen. Examples of blenderized diets and their compositions are given in Table 11-3. Blenderized diets can be administered through size 8 French diameter or larger tubes; a commercially available liquid diet is recommended when feeding through smaller diameter tubes (i.e., 5 French).

Diets for total parenteral nutrition. Diets available for total parenteral nutrition (TPN) should be customized to meet an animal's protein, carbohydrate, and fat requirements; caloric needs are calculated as described in Fig. 11-1. 8.5% amino acids with electrolytes (protein source), 10% to 20% lipids (fat source), and 50% dextrose (carbohydrate source) are generally used. B-complex vitamins are added at 1 to 2 ml per liter. TPN can achieve nitrogen balance, accelerate wound healing, and improve patient recovery from severe protein-calorie malnutrition. However, potential problems include catheter management (i.e., sterile placement, maintaining sterility of catheter entrance, routine changing of infusion sets), expensive equipment (i.e., infusion pump), expensive feeding formulas, technical problems (i.e., constant patient monitoring during administration, diet preparation and storage), and/or sepsis. Additionally, if the gastrointestinal tract is not adequately stimulated by luminal nutrients and hormonal or neurovascular mechanisms, the intestines and pancreas may atrophy. Intestinal mucosal compromise predisposes the intestinal wall to bacterial translocation into the portal circulation and possible sepsis. These problems make total parenteral hyperalimentation less desirable than enteral hyperalimentation.

Oral feeding is preferable if adequate nutrients can be consumed to meet protein and calorie requirements. Several techniques have been used to successfully coax an animal to eat. If the owners can manage the patient at home, it may eat better there. Petting and vocal reassurance are also helpful, albeit time consuming. Highly palatable foods or food

TABLE 11-2					
Commercially Available Diets and Their Composition*					
Product	**Caloric Content (kcal/ml)**	**Protein Content (g/100 kcal)**	**(g/ml)**	**Fat Content (g/100 kcal)**	**Osmolality (mOsm/kg)**
Polymeric Diets					
Jevity	1.06	4.20	0.045	3.48	310
Osmolite HN	1.06	4.44	0.047	3.68	310
Impact	1.00	5.50	0.055	2.80	375
Vital HN	1.00	4.17	0.042	1.08	460
Clinicare feline	0.92	7.00	0.064	4.60	368
Clinicare canine	0.99	5.00	0.050	6.10	340
ProMod	1.48	N/A	0.76 g protein per g ProMod	N/A	N/A
Monomeric Diets					
Vivonex HN	1.00	4.60		0.90	810

*These figures should be used for energy requirement calculations in Fig. 11-1.

TABLE 11-3

Blenderized Diets for Dogs and Cats

Homemade diets

Liquid diet for dogs and cats

Ingredients
1 jar baby food
1 cooked egg
15 ml corn oil
15 ml corn syrup
100 ml water

Nutrient availability
1.0 kcal/ml

Liquid diets for cats

Ingredients
Equal parts egg yolk, strained baby food, and water

3 oz egg yolk
3 oz strained baby food
3 oz water
1 tsp cooking oil
1 T corn syrup

Nutrient availability
1.1 kcal/ml

1.5 kcal/ml

Prescription diets

Product	Amount of Diet	Amount of Water	Caloric Content (kcal/ml)	Protein Content (g/100 kcal)	(g/ml)	Fat Content (g/100 kcal)
Feline a/d	1 can*	none	1.20	8.75	0.105	5.50
	1 can*	1 can‡	0.60	4.38	0.053	2.75
Feline p/d	1/2 can†	3/4 cup§	0.80	9.29	0.074	6.22
Feline k/d	1/2 can†	1-1/4 cup‖	0.90	4.36	0.039	7.54
Feline c/d	1/2 can†	1-1/4 cup‖	0.62	8.87	0.055	5.96
Canine a/d	1 can	none	1.20	8.75	0.105	5.50
	1 can	1 can‡	0.60	4.38	0.053	2.75
Canine k/d	1/2 can	1-1/4 cup‖	0.62	3.06	0.019	5.29
Canine u/d	1/2 can	1-1/4 cup‖	0.66	1.94	0.013	5.13
Canine i/d	1/2 can	1-1/4 cup‖	0.57	5.86	0.033	3.41

*1 can is equal to 156 g
†1/2 can is equal to 224 g
‡1 can is equal to 156 ml
§3/4 cup is equal to 170 ml
‖1-1/4 cup is equal to 284 ml

Preparation technique

Ingredients
Mix the appropriate quantity of each ingredient (see chart above).

Preparation
Blend at high speed for 60 sec.
Strain twice through kitchen strainer (1-mm mesh).

Advantages
Provides all required nutrients, low cost, protein content, branched chain amino acid content, normal stool consistency, manageable viscosity for 8 French catheter or larger.

Disadvantages
Cannot be used if feeding tube has a smaller than 8 French lumen diameter.

coverings (e.g., gravy) may stimulate the appetite. Warming foods (i.e., microwave oven) increases aroma and palatability. Supplementing potassium (i.e., 1 to 2 mEq/kg orally), vitamin B-complex (in maintenance fluids), and/or zinc may increase appetite. Drugs that may stimulate appetite, and their recommended dosages, are given in Table 11-4. These drugs are rarely adequate in stimulating a severely anorexic animal to eat sufficiently, but they may stimulate partially anorexic patients to resume eating.

Methods of Providing Hyperalimentation

Total parenteral nutrition. Total parenteral nutrition is indicated when the intestines cannot adequately absorb nutrients (e.g., massive, small-bowel resection; impaired,

TABLE 11-4

Drugs Used as Appetite Stimulants

Cyproheptadine (Periactin)
Cats - 2 mg/cat PO

Diazepam (Valium)
Cats* - 2-5 mg/cat PO or 0.2 mg/kg IV
Dogs - 0.2 mg/kg IV

Oxazepam (Serax)
Cats - 2.5 mg/cat PO
*Rarely causes hepatic necrosis in cats.

small-intestine motility; severe malabsorption). Severe, prolonged pancreatitis and severe malnutrition are also potential indications. To place TPN catheters, patients should be tranquilized or anesthetized. A 16-gauge, 18-cm, single-lumen, silicone elastomer catheter is inserted in the right or left external jugular vein. The catheter tip should be positioned in the cranial vena cava, and a subcutaneous tunnel created such that the catheter hub emerges on the dorsum of the neck. The catheter is anchored to the vein, subcutaneous tissue along the tunnel, and skin at the exit point with 4-0 to 5-0 nonabsorbable monofilament suture. An extension set is attached to the catheter hub and the catheter is bandaged in place with sterile gauze, cast padding, and self-adherent wrap. The catheter should be flushed with heparinized saline (0.9% sterile saline with 1 IU/ml heparin) after each use.

The predetermined nutrient formulation (based on calculations described above and in Fig. 11-1 and Table 11-2) should be administered using an infusion pump. Generally, 50% of the calculated nutrient requirements should be administered the first day and 100% the second day. Serum electrolytes, glucose, total protein, serum lipids, PCV, and blood urea nitrogen (BUN) should be evaluated daily, and body weight and temperature should be measured twice daily. Every 2 days the neck bandage should be removed, the catheter entrance site cleaned with povidone-iodine solution, extension and administration sets changed, and a new bandage applied. Complications associated with TPN include catheter kinking and displacement, phlebitis, thrombosis, sepsis, hyperglycemia, hyperlipidemia, azotemia, and electrolyte imbalances.

Enteral hyperalimentation. Enteral hyperalimentation is practical, safe, easy, economical, physiologic, well-tolerated, and has minimal morbidity in patients with a functional gastrointestinal tract. Enteral hyperalimentation is indicated in any such animal with overt or impending protein-calorie malnutrition. Examples include hypermetabolic patients (e.g., patients with severe burns, sepsis, postsurgical stress, trauma, cancer) and patients with chronic anorexia/malnutrition (e.g., evidenced by greater than 10% loss of normal body weight and hypoalbuminemia). Enteral

hyperalimentation can also be used whenever 5 to 7 days of anorexia is anticipated (e.g., after oral, pharyngeal, esophagogastric, duodenal, pancreatic, or biliary tract surgery), during postoperative management of cancer patients (particularly if chemotherapy is instituted), and in patients with a mental status preventing self-feeding (e.g., patients with head trauma, brain surgery).

Although enteral hyperalimentation is desirable in most patients with actual or pending protein-calorie malnutrition, infusion of nutrients into the intestines may stimulate exocrine pancreatic function, precluding the use of enteral nutrients in the management of pancreatitis. Patients with adynamic ileus, small-bowel obstruction, and/or severe, intrinsic small-bowel disease (e.g., malabsorption as a result of inflammatory bowel disease or lymphosarcoma) should have nutrients delivered parenterally.

Generally, oral administration of food is more efficient, easier, safer, and allows greater flexibility in formula composition. However, the further aboral materials are delivered, the less efficient the assimilation and digestion of nutrients and the greater care needed when choosing formula composition. Route of administration also dictates feeding tube diameter (Table 11-5), which dictates usable feeding formulas. Various formulas have different viscosities and particulate matter size (see above). The most common routes of administration for enteral hyperalimentation include oral, nasoesophageal, pharyngostomy, esophagostomy, gastrostomy, gastroduodenostomy, and enterostomy. Each route has its indications, contraindications, advantages, disadvantages, and complications.

Nasoesophageal intubation. Nasoesophageal intubation is easy, effective, and efficient. Availability of small-bore, soft polyvinyl and Silastic feeding tubes (i.e., 5 French), low-viscosity; nutritionally complete, liquid diet formulations (see Table 11-2); and patient tolerance of tube placement makes nasoesophageal tube placement popular. Nasoesophageal tube placement is indicated in patients with protein-calorie malnutrition that will not undergo oral, pharyngeal, esophageal, gastric, or biliary tract surgery. These tubes can be left in place for several weeks, are well tolerated, and can be easily removed. The patient can drink and

TABLE 11-5

Tube Diameter Based on Route of Administration of Enteral Diets

5 French diameter tubes
- Nasoesophageal
- Enterostomy (jejunostomy)

8 French or larger diameter tubes
- Pharyngostomy
- Esophagostomy
- Gastrostomy

swallow around the tube, thus eliminating the need for repeated orogastric intubation.

Light general anesthesia may be needed when placing nasoesophageal tubes; however, topical anesthetics or light sedation usually suffices. Proparacaine hydrochloride (0.5 to 1 ml; 0.5%) is instilled into the nasal cavity and the head is elevated to encourage the local anesthetic to coat the nasal mucosa. Repeat application of local anesthetic ensures adequate anesthesia of the nasal mucous membrane. If the patient will not tolerate nasal intubation, heavy sedation plus topical lidocaine (e.g., 1 to 2 ml of 2% lidocaine) or light general anesthesia may be required.

An appropriate sized feeding tube should be selected (Table 11-6). Length of tube to be placed in the esophagus can be estimated by placing the tube from the nasal planum, along the side of the patient, to the seventh or eighth intercostal space. A tape marker is placed on the tube once the appropriate measurement has been taken. The feeding tube should not pass through the lower esophageal sphincter because this may cause sphincteric incompetence, esophageal reflux of hydrochloric acid, and esophagitis. The tip of the tube should be lubricated with 5% lidocaine viscous before passage, and the patient's head should be held in a normal functional position (i.e., avoid hyperflexion or hyperextension). The tube is placed in the ventrolateral aspect of the external nares and passed in a caudoventral and medial direction into the nasal cavity. After the prominent alar fold is identified, the tube is directed from a ventrolateral location in the external nares to a caudoventral and medial direction as it enters the nasal cavity (Fig. 11-2). When the tube is introduced 2 to 3 cm inside the nostril, contact with the median septum at the floor of the nasal cavity can be felt. Pushing the external nares dorsally facilitates opening the ventral meatus. The proximal end of the tube is elevated and the tube advanced into the oropharynx and esophagus. It will generally "drop" into the oropharynx and stimulate a swallowing reflex.

Esophageal placement is confirmed by injecting 3 to 5 ml of sterile saline through the tube and seeing if a cough is elicited, or by injecting 6 to 12 ml of air and auscultating for borborygmus at the xiphoid. Placement can also be confirmed by radiographing the chest. If the patient requires general anesthesia, correct tube placement can be visually confirmed. Once satisfied that the tube is properly placed, it should be sutured to the nose and head to prevent removal

by the patient. It is important that the tube not contact the whiskers of cats. The tube should be positioned directly over the dorsal aspect of the nose and forehead (Fig. 11-3) and secured with a Chinese finger-trap suture (Fig. 11-4). In dogs the tube is secured to the lateral aspect of the nose and dorsal nasal midline with a Chinese finger-trap suture or cyanoacrylate glue (Fig. 11-5). An Elizabethan collar should be used immediately postoperatively until it is determined whether the patient will tolerate the tube. A column of water should be placed in the tube before capping it to prevent air intake, reflux of esophageal contents, and/or tube occlusion by diet.

Esophagostomy tube. Esophagostomy tube feeding is indicated in anorexic patients with disorders of the oral cavity or pharynx and in anorexic patients with a functional gastrointestinal tract distal to the esophagus. They are contraindicated in patients with primary or secondary esophageal dysfunction (e.g., esophageal stricture, after esophageal foreign body removal or esophageal surgery, esophagitis, megaesophagus). Advantages of esophagostomy tubes include ease of placement, acceptance by patients,

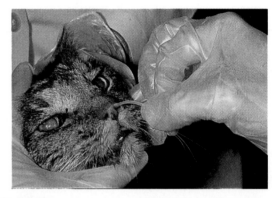

FIG. 11-2
Direct the nasoesophageal tube from ventrolaterally in the external nares to caudoventrally and medially as it enters the nasal cavity.

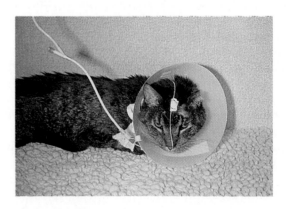

FIG. 11-3
Secure nasoesophageal feeding tubes to the dorsal nasal midline and forehead of cats.

TABLE 11-6
Recommended Tube Sizes for Nasoesophageal Placement
Cats, dogs smaller than 15 kg—5 Fr × 91 cm Dogs larger than 15 kg—8 Fr × 91 cm

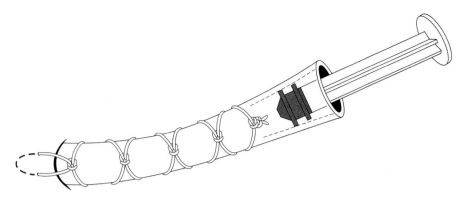

FIG. 11-4
Use a Chinese finger-trap friction suture to secure feeding tubes to skin.

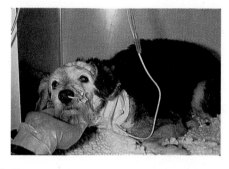

FIG. 11-5
Secure nasoesophageal feeding tubes to the lateral aspect of the nose in dogs.

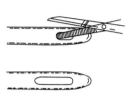

FIG. 11-6
For esophagostomy tubes, enlarge the lateral openings of the tubes to 3 to 4 mm to encourage smooth flow of blended diets. (From Devitt CM, Seim HB III: Clinical evaluation of tube esophagostomy in small animals, *J Am Anim Hosp Assoc* 33:55, 1997.)

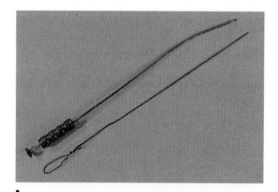

A

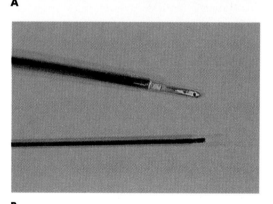

B

FIG. 11-7
A, Eld feeding tube placement device. **B,** Activated spring-loaded blade. (From Devitt CM, Seim HB III: Clinical evaluation of tube esophagostomy in small animals, *J Am Anim Hosp Assoc* 33:55, 1997.)

large-bore tubes that allow blenderized diets, ease of tube care and feeding, ability for patients to eat and drink around the tube, and flexibility to perform tube removal anytime after placement. Esophageal tube placement eliminates coughing, laryngospasm, and/or aspiration occasionally associated with pharyngostomy tubes. The major disadvantage of esophagostomy tubes is the need for general anesthesia for tube placement.

The animal should be anesthetized and placed in right lateral recumbency with the left side uppermost. The tube can be placed on either the right or left side of the midcervical region; however, the esophagus lies left of the midline, making left-sided placement more desirable. The midcervical area from the angle of the mandible to the thoracic inlet is prepared for aseptic surgery. A speculum is placed to hold the mouth open, and a 20 to 24 French polyvinyl chloride feeding tube is premeasured from its insertion point to the level of the seventh and eighth intercostal space and marked (ensuring mid-esophageal to caudal-esophageal placement). The two lateral openings of the feeding tube should be enlarged to encourage smoother flow of blended diet (Fig. 11-6). An Eld feeding tube placement device (Fig. 11-7) is used. The oblique tip of the instrument shaft is placed into the oral cavity to the level of the mid cervical region (i.e., equal distance between the angle of the mandible and thoracic inlet). The tip should be palpated as it bulges through the cervical skin. A small skin incision is made over the device tip and the spring-loaded instrument blade is activated until it is visible through the skin incision (Figs. 11-8, *A* and *B*). With the tip of the scalpel blade the incision is carefully enlarged in the subcutaneous tissues, cervical musculature, and esophageal wall to allow penetration of the instrument shaft (see Fig. 11-8, *B*). A 2-0 nonabsorbable suture is placed through the side holes of the feeding tube and the

hole in the instrument blade. The suture is tightened until the tip of the instrument blade and feeding tube tip are in close apposition (Fig. 11-8, *C*). The instrument blade is retracted into the instrument shaft so the feeding tube tip enters the instrument shaft (i.e., deactivating the instrument blade), and lubricant is placed on the tube and instrument shaft. The instrument is retracted and the feeding tube pulled into the oral cavity to its predetermined measurement (Fig. 11-9, *A*). The suture is removed to free the feeding tube from the instrument blade and a stylet is placed through one

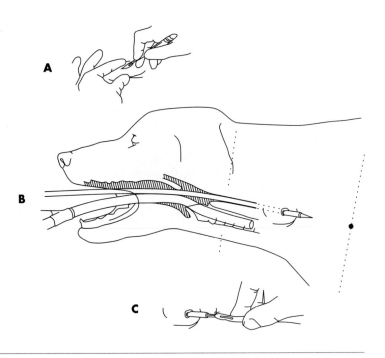

FIG. 11-8
A, For esophageal tube placement, place the instrument shaft in the oral cavity and palpate the tip as it bulges the cervical skin; make an incision over the device tip. **B,** Activate the instrument blade until it is visible through the skin incision; enlarge the incision to allow penetration of the instrument shaft. **C,** Use 2-0 nonabsorbable suture (e.g., nylon) to secure the tip of the feeding tube to the tip of the blade; retract the blade so the feeding tube tip contacts the instrument shaft. (From Devitt CM, Seim HB III: Clinical evaluation of tube esophagostomy in small animals, *J Am Anim Hosp Assoc* 33:55, 1997.)

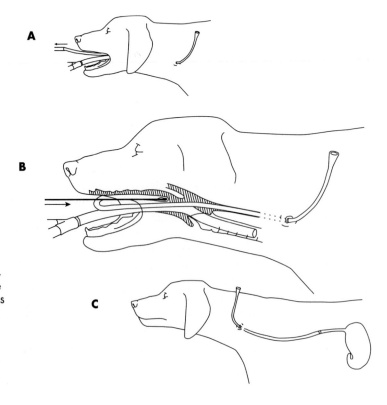

FIG. 11-9
Esophageal tube placement (cont'd from Fig. 11-8). **A,** Retract the instrument and pull the feeding tube into the oral cavity. **B,** Place a stylet into one of the lateral holes of the feeding tube and against its tip; advance the tube into the esophagus. **C,** The esophageal tube should lie in the mid-esophageal region. (From Devitt CM, Seim HB III: Clinical evaluation of tube esophagostomy in small animals, *J Am Anim Hosp Assoc* 33:55, 1997.)

of the side holes of the feeding tube and against its tip (Fig. 11-9, *B*). The tube is lubricated and advanced into the esophagus until the entire oral portion of the feeding tube disappears (Fig. 11-9, *C*) and the tube passes down the esophagus without twisting or bending. The stylet is retracted from the oral cavity, with care to ensure its release from the tube. The tube is secured to the cervical skin with a Chinese finger-trap suture of No. 1 nonabsorbable suture (see Fig. 11-4). The exit point of the tube can be left exposed or loosely bandaged. A column of water is placed in the tube and the exposed end is capped with a 3-cc syringe.

Most patients tolerate esophagostomy tubes, and Elizabethan collars are not needed. Esophagostomy tubes can be safely removed immediately after placement or left in place for several weeks or months. Care of the tube exit site may require periodic cleansing with an antiseptic solution. Tube removal is performed by cutting the finger-trap suture and gently pulling the tube. No further exit wound care is necessary; the hole seals in one or two days and is healed by 7 to 10 days.

Complications associated with esophagostomy tube placement include early removal by the patient, or vomiting the tube and chewing off the end. No significant long-term complications have been reported (e.g., esophagitis, esophageal stricture, esophageal diverticulum, subcutaneous cervical cellulitis). Reflux esophagitis can occur from improper tube placement (i.e., through the lower esophageal sphincter) or esophageal irritation can be caused by the tube itself. Mid-esophageal placement of polyvinyl chloride rubber tubes markedly reduces the incidence of esophageal injury and reflux esophagitis.

Pharyngostomy tubes. Whenever it is necessary to provide nutritional supplementation to an anorexic patient (i.e., patients suffering protein-calorie malnutrition) or to patients that are unable or reluctant to ingest food orally (i.e., patients with cleft palate, mandibular or maxillary fractures, oral neoplasia), a pharyngostomy tube may be considered. Pharyngostomy tubes should not be used for nutritional management of patients with esophageal disorders (i.e., esophagitis, esophageal stricture, recent esophageal surgery or esophageal foreign body removal, esophageal neoplasia). The major advantage of a pharyngostomy tube over a nasoesophageal tube is tube diameter. Pharyngostomy tubes are generally 20 to 24 French, thus accommodating a wider variety of diets. Pharyngostomy tubes are placed into the mid esophagus; they should never be placed through the lower esophageal sphincter. Esophagostomy tubes (see above) are easier to maintain in dogs and cats than pharyngostomy tubes.

For tube placement the patient is anesthetized and positioned in lateral recumbency with the incision site uppermost. A 4-cm-square area just caudal to the angle of the mandible is aseptically prepared. The mouth is held open with a mouth speculum. A 24 French, polyvinyl chloride feeding tube is premeasured from the insertion point to the level of the seventh or eighth intercostal space and marked, ensuring mid-esophageal placement. An index finger is positioned into the pharynx, near the base of the tongue (Fig. 11-10), and the epiglottis, arytenoid cartilages, and hyoid apparatus are palpated. The orally located index finger is flexed toward the lateral aspect of the neck to identify the junction of the intrapharyngeal ostium and laryngopharynx (this is the proper location for pharyngostomy tube exit). Enough pressure should be applied to the lateral pharyngeal wall to create an externally visible bulge. Large, curved forceps (e.g., curved Rochester-Carmalt forceps) can be substituted for the index finger to maintain the bulge. A 1- to 2-cm skin incision is made over the bulge, and curved forceps are used to bluntly dissect subcutaneous tissue, pharyngeal muscle, and pharyngeal mucosa until the index finger or forceps becomes

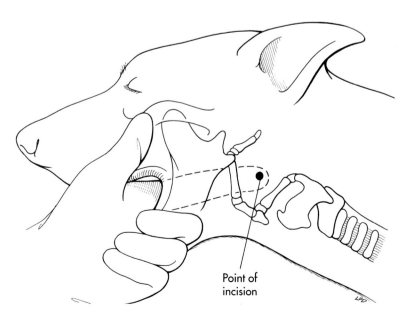

Point of incision

FIG. 11-10
Proper location of pharyngostomy tube exit relative to the hyoid apparatus.

visible. If the index finger rather than forceps is being used to maintain the bulge, it is replaced with curved forceps, and the tip of the pharyngostomy tube is grasped and pulled through the incision, into the oral cavity, and out of the mouth (Fig. 11-11, *A*). The tip of the tube is reinserted into the mouth and passed into the mid esophagus (i.e., pre-marked location on the feeding tube) (Fig. 11-11, *B*). The tube is secured at its exit point with a Chinese finger-trap suture (see Fig. 11-4) and to the patient's neck to encourage the tube to remain dorsally. A column of water is placed in the tube and it is capped with a 3-cc syringe. When the tube is no longer required, the Chinese finger-trap suture can be cut, the tube pulled, and the pharyngeal wound allowed to heal by contraction and epithelialization.

If the pharyngostomy tube is placed ventral and medial to the intrapharyngeal ostium and laryngopharynx, partial airway obstruction, coughing, and gagging may result. If the tube is placed through the lower esophageal sphincter, reflux esophagitis may occur. Vomiting up the tube has also been reported.

Gastrostomy tubes. Gastrostomy tubes are indicated in anorexic patients with a functional gastrointestinal tract distal to the stomach or in patients undergoing operations of the oral cavity, larynx, pharynx, or esophagus. These tubes are contraindicated in patients with primary gastric disease (e.g., gastritis, gastric ulceration, gastric neoplasia). Advantages of gastrostomy tubes include ease of placement, patient tolerance, availability of large-bore feeding tubes, easy tube care and feeding, and the fact that oral feeding can commence while the tube is in place. Disadvantages include needing specialized equipment (e.g., endoscope) and general anesthesia, waiting 12 to 24 hours after tube placement before initiating feeding, and the fact that, depending upon placement technique, tubes cannot be removed for at least 10 to 12 days (i.e., to encourage adhesion formation between the stomach and the abdominal wall).

Gastrostomy tubes can be placed percutaneously without the aid of an endoscope, percutaneously with the aid of an endoscope, or via laparotomy. Tubes placed percutaneously without the aid of an endoscope can be performed with or without gastropexy.

Percutaneous Placement of a Gastrostomy Tube with Gastropexy. Advantages of this technique include ease of tube placement, ease of finding the stomach in an anorectic patient, quick placement, no need for special equipment (i.e., endoscope, feeding tube placement device),

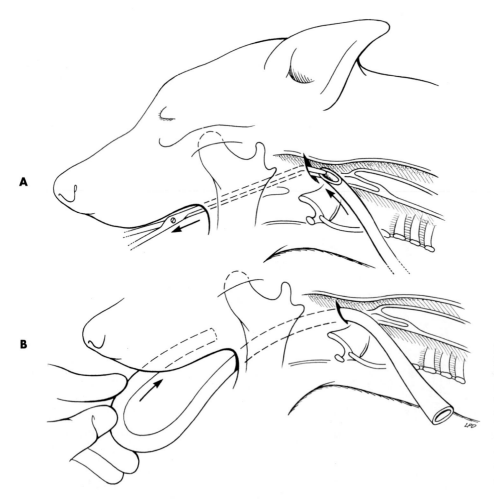

FIG. 11-11
A, To place a pharyngostomy tube, pass a long forceps in the mouth to the point of tube entrance; incise over the instrument tip, grasp the tip of the tube, and pull the tube out through the mouth. **B,** Reinsert the tip of the tube into the mouth and pass the tube to its premarked mid-esophageal location.

surgical gastropexy ensures an immediate seal between the stomach wall and body wall, and confirmation of proper tube placement is performed during placement. Feeding tubes can be safely removed at any time after placement.

General anesthesia and standard skin preparation of the left paralumbar fossa is performed. The left flank area is prepared for aseptic surgery and the area is draped. An unsterile assistant passes a large-bore, stiff, plastic tube into the stomach. The sterile surgeon palpates the left flank area until the end of the stomach tube can be palpated and grasped (Fig. 11-12, *A*). The tube is held stable as a skin incision is made over the end of the stomach tube. The subcutaneous tissues and abdominal muscles are bluntly dissected to expose the wall of the stomach over the tube; care is taken not to enter the lumen of the stomach (Fig. 11-12, *B*). A pursestring suture is placed in the stomach wall around the tube (Fig. 11-12, *C*). A No. 11 scalpel blade is used to puncture the stomach wall by punching the blade into the lumen of the tube. A 20-24 French Foley catheter is placed into the lumen of the stomach and into the tube (Fig. 11-13, *A*). Traction is placed on the pursestring suture as the stomach tube is slowly withdrawn. Once the Foley catheter is out of the lumen of the stomach tube, the bulb is inflated and gentle traction is placed on the catheter to bring it against the stomach wall (Fig. 11-13, *B*). The pursestring suture is tied snugly around the Foley catheter. Three to four simple interrupted sutures of 2-0 absorbable suture (i.e., PDS, Maxon) are placed from the stomach wall to the body wall to firmly pexy the stomach in place. Subcutaneous tissues and skin are closed around the existing Foley catheter and the tube is secured to skin with a Chinese finger-trap suture of No. 1 nonabsorbable suture (Fig. 11-13, *C*).

Percutaneous Gastrostomy Tube Placement Without Gastropexy. Advantages of this technique are that no special instrumentation is required for placement and it is easy to perform. Its disadvantages are that the stomach is not pexied to the body wall (i.e., early removal by the patient could result in peritonitis) and confirmation of tube placement can only be performed endoscopically or radiographically.

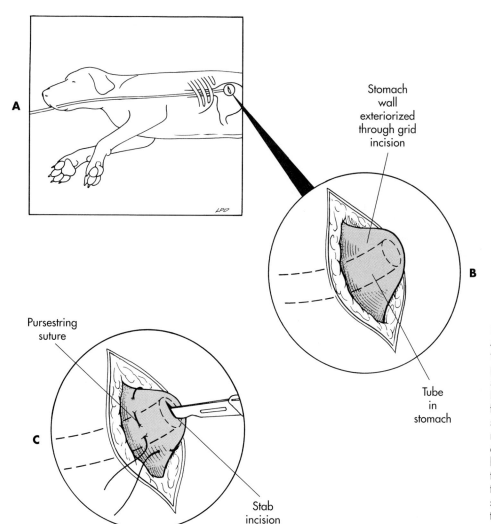

FIG. 11-12
A, For percutaneous gastrostomy tube placement with gastropexy, pass a large bore stiff plastic stomach tube into the stomach. Palpate the end of the tube at the flank. **B,** Grasp the tube and secure it with thumb and finger, make an incision through skin and subcutaneous tissue, and bluntly dissect abdominal muscles to expose the gastric wall over the tube. **C,** Place a pursestring suture in the gastric wall around the tube and puncture the wall with a scalpel blade.

Stomach wall exteriorized through grid incision

Tube in stomach

Pursestring suture

Stab incision

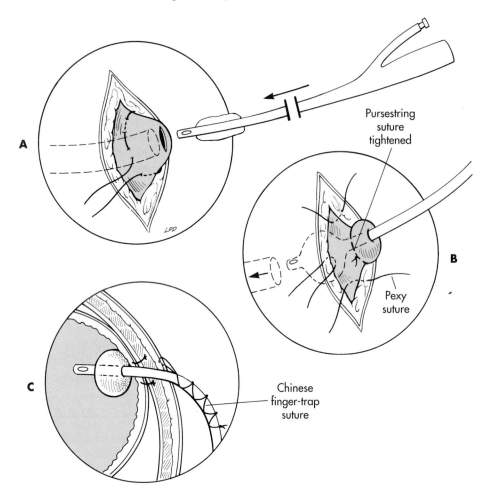

FIG. 11-13
A, Percutaneous gastrostomy tube placement with pexy (cont'd from Fig. 11-12). Place the Foley or Pezzer catheter into the lumen of the stomach and into the tube. **B,** Tighten the pursestring suture, remove the stomach tube, inflate the Foley catheter bulb, and suture the gastric wall to the abdominal wall. **C,** Notice proper tube placement of the inflated Foley catheter, gastropexy, and Chinese finger-trap suture to secure the tube in place.

The patient is positioned and prepared as described above. A 20 French Pezzer urinary catheter is prepared as follows. Cut off and discard the dilated proximal end of the tube. Cut off 1.5 cm of the remaining tube and set aside for use as an external flange. Cut the remaining proximal end of the tube at a sharp angle. A strand of No. 1 Braunamid is cut to the length of the prepared feeding tube. A stiff, large-bore stomach tube or feeding tube placement device (Fig. 11-14, *A*) is passed into the stomach until it can be palpated bulging against the left body wall 1 to 2 cm caudal to the last rib and 2 to 3 cm distal to the transverse spinous processes of lumbar vertebrae two or three. If a stomach tube is being used, an 18-gauge hypodermic needle is passed through skin and into the lumen of the stomach tube. A strand of No. 1 suture is placed through the needle, into the stomach tube, and out through the mouth. The stomach tube is removed. If a feeding tube placement device is being used (see esophagostomy tube placement above), the device is activated and the No. 1 suture is threaded through the hole in the instrument blade (Fig. 11-14, *B*). The blade is retracted into the instrument shaft and the instrument is withdrawn out through the mouth (Fig. 11-14, *C*). In each case the No. 1 suture enters the stomach through the left flank and exits through the oral cavity. The end of the suture exiting the oral cavity is threaded through the narrow end of an 18-gauge sovereign catheter and is tied to the proximal end of the prepared Pezzer urinary catheter (i.e., feeding tube) (Fig. 11-14, *D*). The Pezzer catheter is pulled tightly into the flange of the catheter and is lubricated. The No. 1 suture exiting the left flank is pulled until the catheter tip exits the skin (Fig. 11-14, *E*). The skin incision is enlarged to 3 to 4 mm, allowing easy delivery of the catheter. The catheter is pulled until the mushroom tip is snugly against the body wall, ensuring a seal between the stomach wall and body wall. The catheter is secured to the skin with a Chinese finger-trap suture using No. 1 nonabsorbable suture (e.g., Novafil).

Percutaneous Endoscopic Gastrostomy Tube Placement. The advantage of endoscopic placement is direct visualization of the tube throughout placement. The disadvantages are the inability to perform surgical gastropexy to ensure an early and permanent seal between the stomach wall and body wall, and the 10- to 12-day wait to remove the tube after placement.

Percutaneous endoscopic tube placement without gastropexy is performed as described for percutaneous placement without gastropexy with the exception that the No. 1

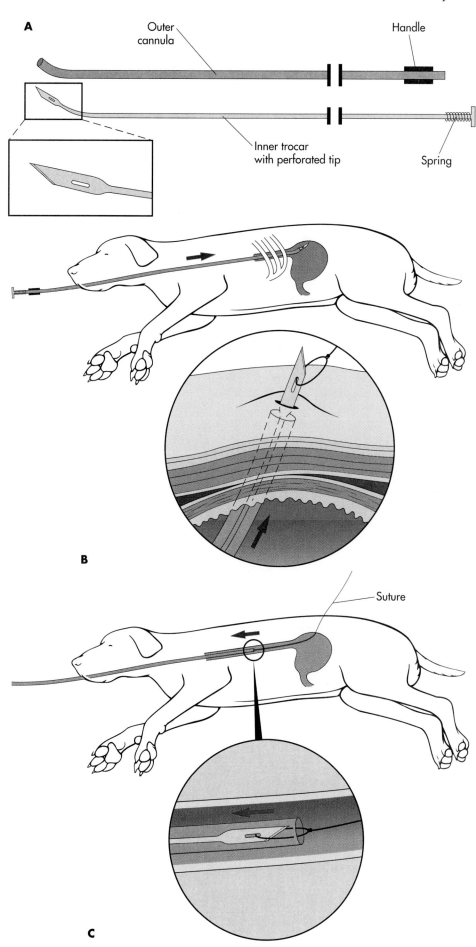

A, Outer cannula

Handle

Inner trocar with perforated tip

Spring

B

C

Suture

FIG. 11-14
A, Schematic view of a device designed to place gastrostomy tubes without endoscopy. The trocar (lower) is placed through the cannula (upper). The cutting tip (detailed insert) is not extended until the device is properly placed. **B,** Schematic view showing how the device is placed in an animal receiving a gastrostomy tube. Note that the tip of the device ultimately arrives at a point behind the last rib. Push the trocar tip through the cannula so that the blade tip extends through the skin (see insert) and tie a suture to the tip. **C,** Retract the entire device (cannula and trocar) out through the mouth, bringing the suture with it.
Continued

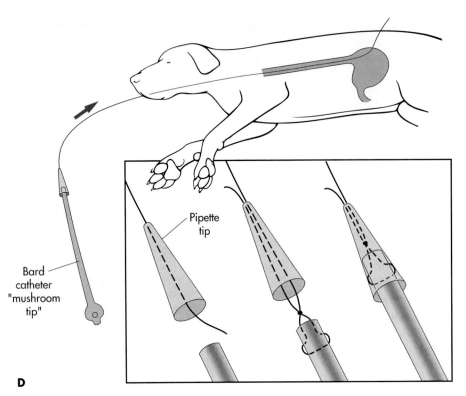

Pipette tip

Bard catheter "mushroom tip"

D

E

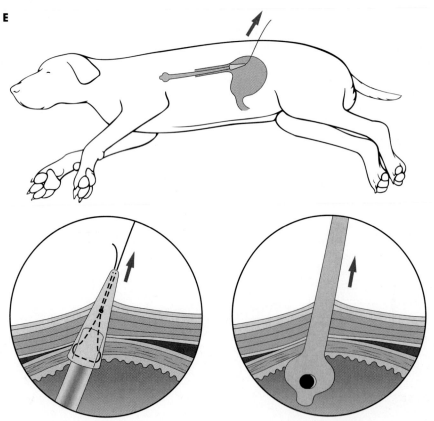

FIG. 11-14, CONT'D
D, Fasten the end of the suture that is brought out of the mouth to the tip of a mushroom tip catheter. Note how a pipette tip is placed where the suture attaches to the tip of the catheter.
E, Pull the suture through the skin, pulling the mushroom catheter into the stomach. The pipette tip facilitates passage of the catheter through the abdominal wall. Withdraw the catheter until the mushroom tip is against the gastric mucosa and the stomach is pulled snugly against the abdominal wall.

suture is placed from the left flank out through the oral cavity with the aid of an endoscope. The endoscope is passed into the stomach and its lumen is insufflated with air. A 1-mm skin incision is made in the left flank 1 to 2 cm caudal to the last rib and 2 to 3 cm distal to the transverse spinous processes of lumbar vertebrae two or three. An 18-gauge needle is thrust through the skin incision and into the stomach lumen. The strand of No. 1 suture is passed through the needle, into the stomach, retrieved endoscopically, and brought out through the mouth. Once the strand of suture is entering the left flank and exiting the oral cavity, placement of the feeding tube is as described for percutaneous surgical placement without gastropexy.

Gastrostomy Tube Placement via Laparotomy. This procedure is generally performed when tube placement is ancillary to another abdominal procedure (i.e., biopsy, mass removal). The distal end of a 20 French Foley or Pezzer catheter (i.e., bulb or mushroom tip) is placed into the abdominal cavity through a stab incision in the left body wall. The ventral surface of the stomach is exteriorized and a pursestring suture is placed in the ventrolateral body wall. A stab incision is made in the center of the pursestring suture with a No. 11 scalpel blade and the distal end of the feeding catheter is placed in the lumen of the stomach. The pursestring suture is tightened around the catheter and the bulb of the catheter (i.e., Foley) is inflated with saline. Gentle traction is placed on the catheter to bring the body of the stomach in close apposition to the left body wall. The stomach wall is pexied to the abdominal wall with four 2-0 synthetic absorbable sutures. The feeding tube is secured to the skin with a Chinese finger-trap suture of No. 1 nonabsorbable suture (e.g., Novafil). Abdominal closure is routine.

The most severe complication of gastrostomy tube placement is early removal with leakage of gastric contents into the abdominal cavity and subsequent generalized peritonitis. This complication can be prevented by choosing a technique that results in a sutured pexy of stomach to body wall (i.e., percutaneous surgical placement with gastropexy or via laparotomy). Pezzer catheters last longer (weeks to months) in the stomach than Foley catheters because the balloons of Foley catheters disintegrate. Other complications include vomiting and peristomal infection.

Enterostomy tube. Enterostomy feeding tubes are indicated in patients with gastric, intestinal, or pancreatic disease and in patients having biliary tract surgery in which the intestinal tract distal to the disease or surgical site is functional. Immediate feeding of a highly digestible, low-bulk diet in patients undergoing colonic surgery can be accomplished using an enterostomy tube. Patients with preexisting protein-calorie malnutrition that must undergo major abdominal surgery are candidates for early enteral hyperalimentation via enterostomy.

Celiotomy is required for placement of an enterostomy feeding tube. A 5 French, 36-inch, infant feeding tube is recommended. The distal tip of the feeding tube is brought into the abdominal cavity through a 2- to 3-mm stab incision on the right or left body wall using a No. 11 scalpel blade or 10-gauge hypodermic needle (Fig. 11-15). A segment of proximal jejunum is selected and the normal direction of flow of ingesta is identified (i.e., aboral and oral end). The selected intestine must be easily mobilized to the feeding tube entrance location on the body wall. A 1- to 1.5-cm linear incision is made in the seromuscular layers of the antimesenteric border of the selected jejunal segment (Fig. 11-16, *A*). A No. 11 scalpel blade is used to enter the lumen of the jejunum at the most aboral end of the incision. The distal end of the feeding tube is inserted through the incision and 10 to 12 inches of the tube are passed in an aboral direction into the jejunal lumen. The exiting portion of the tube is positioned in the 1- to 1.5-cm seromuscular incision and sutured in this "tunnel" by inverting the seromuscular layer over the tube with three or four Cushing sutures of 4-0 absorbable suture material (i.e., Maxon, PDS) (Figs. 11-16, *B* and *C*). The jejunal tube exit site is pexied to the exit site at the body wall with four to five simple interrupted sutures of 4-0 absorbable suture, and the feeding tube is secured to skin using a Chinese finger-trap suture of 2-0 nonabsorbable material (e.g., Novafil).

Alternatively, from a laparotomy approach, a 10-gauge needle may be passed through the abdominal wall from peritoneum to skin (see Fig. 11-15). The feeding tube is introduced into the abdominal cavity through the needle and the needle is removed, leaving the feeding tube with its hub outside the abdominal cavity (Fig. 11-17). Then the needle is

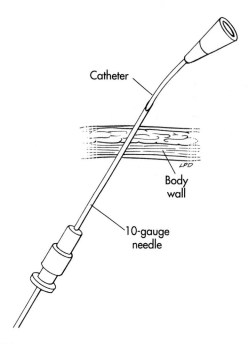

FIG. 11-15
During placement of an enterostomy tube, a 10-gauge hypodermic needle facilitates transabdominal placement of a 5 French feeding tube.

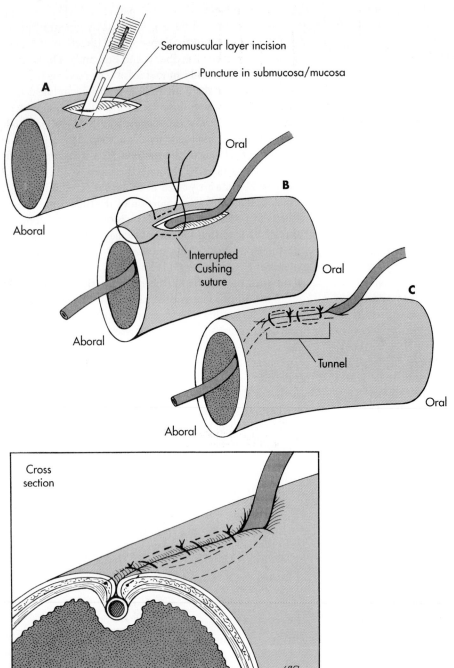

Seromuscular layer incision

Puncture in submucosa/mucosa

A

Oral

Aboral

B

Interrupted Cushing suture

Oral

Aboral

C

Tunnel

Oral

Aboral

Cross section

LPD

FIG. 11-16
A, For enterostomy tube placement, make a 1- to 1.5-cm linear incision in the seromuscular layers of the antimesenteric border of the selected jejunal segment; use the tip of the blade to puncture a hole in the aboral aspect of the seromuscular incision. **B** and **C,** Place the distal end of the feeding tube through the incision; lay the exiting portion of the tube in the 1- to 1.5-cm seromuscular incision and construct a "tunnel" by inverting the seromuscular layer over the tube with three or four Cushing sutures of 4-0 absorbable material.

introduced at an acute angle into the jejunal lumen and exited at an oblique angle, creating a seromuscular tunnel. The catheter is advanced into the beveled end of the needle and the needle is removed, leaving the catheter in the jejunal lumen. The catheter is threaded into the jejunal lumen and jejunum is sutured to the body wall and secured to skin with a Chinese finger-trap friction suture (see Fig. 11-4). If the seromuscular tunnel is inadequate, a 1.5- to 2-cm serosal tunnel may be created using one to two Cushing sutures before pexy (Fig. 11-18).

In medium to large dogs (the thin bowel wall may make this technique difficult in small dogs and cats), a 10-gauge needle may be introduced into the antimesenteric border of the jejunal wall and the needle inserted between the seromuscular and submucosal layers of the jejunal wall for a distance of 1.5 to 2 cm (Figs. 11-19, *A* and *B*). Once a 3- to 4-cm tunnel is created, the needle is directed into the lumen and a 5 French, 36-inch Silastic or polyurethane catheter is passed through the needle. The needle is removed, leaving a 3- to 4-cm seromuscular tunnel. The catheter is exteriorized

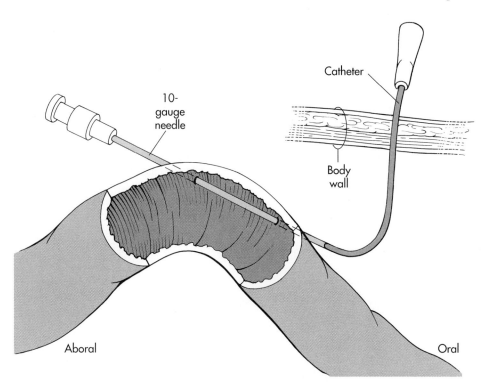

FIG. 11-17
Introduce the needle at an acute angle into the lumen of the jejunum and exit at an oblique angle, creating a seromuscular tunnel.

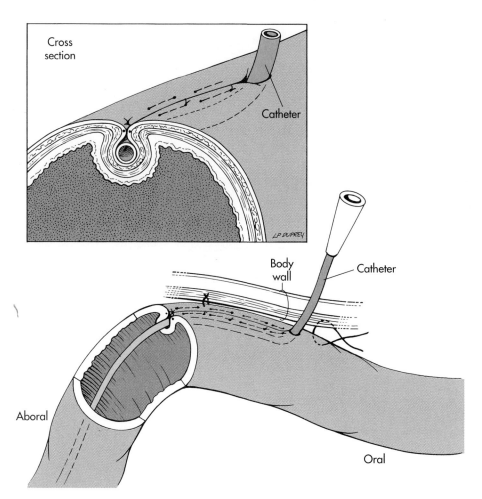

FIG. 11-18
If the seromuscular tunnel is inadequate, create a 1.5- to 2-cm serosal tunnel using one or two Cushing sutures; pexy sutures are used to secure the jejunum to the body wall.

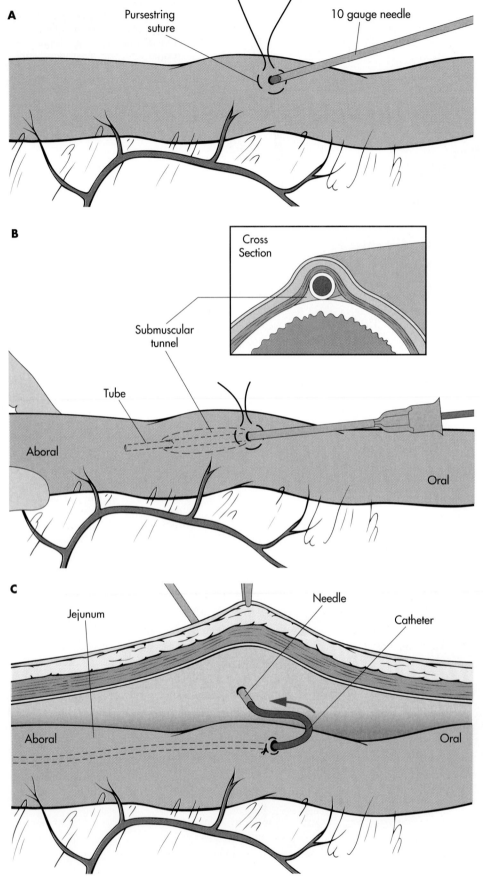

A

Pursestring
suture

10 gauge needle

B

Cross
Section

Submuscular
tunnel

Tube

Aboral

Oral

C

Jejunum

Needle

Catheter

Aboral

Oral

FIG. 11-19
A, A pursestring suture is placed at the antimesenteric border of the jejunum at the site of catheter entrance. **B,** A 10-gauge needle is introduced into the antimesenteric border of the jejunal wall, between the seromuscular and submucosal layers, for a distance of 3 to 4 cm. **C,** The catheter is exteriorized through a separate stab incision in the body wall.

Continued

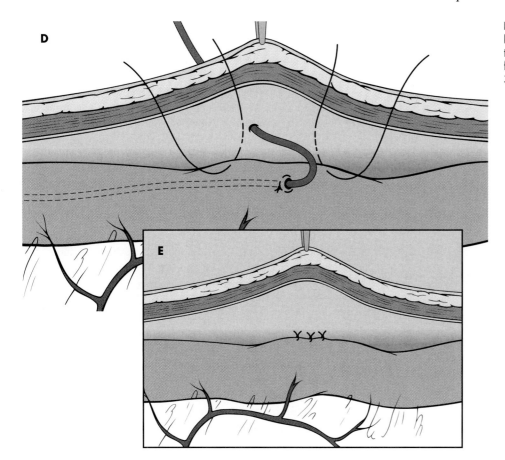

through a separate stab incision in the body wall (Fig. 11-19, *C*) and secured to skin with a Chinese finger-trap suture (see Fig. 11-4). The jejunum is attached to the body wall with three to four simple interrupted sutures of 3-0 or 4-0 absorbable suture material (e.g., Maxon, PDS) (Figs. 11-19, *D* and *E*). Omentum may be interposed between the jejunum and body wall.

Patients with enterostomy feeding tubes can be fed immediately postoperatively. The feeding tube exit point should be incorporated into a body bandage to prevent premature removal by the patient, technical staff, or client. A column of water should be kept in the tube between uses. Possible complications include premature removal, tube-induced jejunal perforation, peritoneal leakage, and subcutaneous leakage. Subcutaneous leakage is prevented by securely fixing the tube to skin, and peritoneal leakage is prevented by paying close attention to include a 360 degree jejunal-abdominal wall pexy.

Calculation of Rate and Volume of Feeding

Once the number of calories needed to meet the patient's total caloric requirement has been calculated, rate and volume of feeding are determined based on route of administration (e.g., oral, nasoesophageal, esophagostomy, pharyngostomy,

gastrostomy, or enterostomy). When feeding into the stomach (i.e., oral, nasoesophageal, esophagostomy, pharyngostomy, and gastrostomy tubes), the quantity of diet fed is determined by the patient's stomach capacity. Normal canine and feline gastric capacity is approximately 80 ml of fluid/kg of body weight. However, anorexic patients can accommodate only 30 to 40 cc of fluid/kg of body weight when feeding begins. A gradual increase in volume over a 2- to 3-day period allows the stomach to accommodate progressively larger volumes. A minimum of three feedings daily should be used; however, if vomiting and abdominal distention occur, the volume should be reduced and number of feedings per day increased.

When feeding into the small intestine (i.e., enterostomy tubes), rate and volume of diet must be carefully regulated to avoid overdistention. Each patient is unique in the amount of fluid the small intestine will accommodate; a guideline for feeding via enterostomy tube is outlined in Table 11-7. These are guidelines only; some patients require a longer adjustment time (5 to 7 days), while others allow total volume feeding in 2 to 3 days. Signs of overfeeding include vomiting, diarrhea, abdominal distention, and/or cramping. Diluting diet concentration and decreasing the rate and volume of administration generally resolve these complications.

TABLE 11-7

Guidelines for Feeding Via an Enterostomy Tube

- Calculate total caloric requirement.
- Give 1/4 of the calculated volume during the first 24 hours; a minimum of four to five feedings/day is recommended.*
- Give 1/2 of the calculated volume during the second 24 hours in four to five feedings.*
- Give 3/4 of the calculated volume during the third 24 hours in four to five feedings.*
- Give the entire calculated volume during the fourth 24 hours in four to five feedings.*

*Continuous feeding via infusion pump is preferred.

Complications

Three types of complications can occur during enteral hyperalimentation: mechanical, gastrointestinal, and metabolic. In most instances complications can be prevented by proper tube placement technique, use of appropriate-diameter, soft-rubber feeding tubes, use of proper diets, carefully calculated feeding schedules, and proper tube management during and between feedings.

Mechanical complications. Mechanical complications include inadvertent tube placement in the trachea (i.e., nasoesophageal, esophagostomy, pharyngostomy) or peritoneal cavity (i.e., gastrostomy, enterostomy), gut perforation by the feeding tube (i.e., enterostomy), regurgitating or vomiting the tube (i.e., nasoesophageal, esophagostomy, pharyngostomy), esophageal irritation (i.e., nasoesophageal, esophagostomy, pharyngostomy), infection at the tube exit site, tube occlusion, or tube removal by the patient. Inadvertent placement of feeding tubes in the trachea or peritoneal cavity can be prevented by careful attention during tube placement. A small amount of sterile aqueous contrast material should be injected through the feeding tube and a radiograph taken if there is any question of tube location. Gut perforation has been virtually eliminated by use of small-bore, Silastic or soft-rubber enterostomy feeding tubes. Premature tube removal by the patient can be prevented by adequate mechanical restraint devices (e.g., bandaging and Elizabethan collar) and secure attachment of the tube to its exit site (i.e., Chinese finger-trap suture). Patient tolerance has been enhanced by the use of small-bore, soft-rubber feeding tubes. Esophagitis secondary to nasoesophageal, esophagostomy, and pharyngostomy tube placement has been reported; however, the use of Silastic or soft rubber (i.e., polyvinyl) feeding tubes has decreased esophageal irritation. Also, mid-esophageal placement effectively eliminates reflux esophagitis.

Infection at the tube site can be minimized by proper tube management. The area should be kept clean and covered with a bandage. Care should be taken when feeding the patient to keep diet formula from contaminating the exit site. Rhinitis secondary to nasoesophageal tube placement has been reported, but use of small-bore, soft-rubber tubes has minimized this.

Small-bore feeding tubes (3 to 5 French) can become occluded with diet. This is best prevented by using commercial liquid diets instead of blenderized diet. Taking care to flush material out of the tube when feeding is complete and capping the tube to maintain a column of water also help prevent occlusion caused by gastrointestinal reflux. Large-bore feeding tubes accept blenderized diets, but similar precautions should be used to prevent occlusion. If a tube becomes occluded a carbonated liquid (i.e., sparkling water, cola) can be infused into the tube; effervescence of the liquid may encourage removal of clogged material. If this is unsuccessful, tube replacement may be necessary.

Gastrointestinal complications. Common gastrointestinal complications of enteral nutritional therapy include vomiting, cramping, abdominal distention, and/or diarrhea. The most common causes are feeding too rapidly, feeding too large a volume, and feeding diets with high osmolality. Treatment is aimed at decreasing the rate and volume fed or diluting the diet.

Metabolic complications. The most common metabolic complication of enteral nutritional therapy is hyperglycemia secondary to rapid absorption of glucose. Insulin may be used to control the hyperglycemia. Dosage rates are 0.5 to 1 IU/kg neutral protamine Hagedorn (NPH) insulin subcutaneously in dogs and 0.25 IU/kg NPH insulin subcutaneously in cats. Observe for hypophosphatemia and hypo- or hyperkalemia, especially in emaciated animals.

Suggested Reading

Abood SK, Buffington CAT: Enteral feeding of dogs and cats: 51 cases, *J Am Vet Med Assoc* 201:619, 1992.

Abood SK, Buffington CAT: Improved nasogastric intubation technique for administration of nutritional support in dogs, *J Am Vet Med Assoc* 199:577, 1991.

Bright RM, Colin FB: Percutaneous endoscopic tube gastrostomy in dogs, *Am J Vet Res* 49:629, 1988.

Bright RM, DeNovo RC, Jones JB: Use of a low-profile gastrostomy device for administering nutrients in two dogs, *J Am Vet Med Assoc* 207:1184, 1995.

Burkholder WJ: Metabolic rates and nutrient requirements of sick dogs and cats, *J Am Vet Med Assoc* 205:614, 1995.

Crowe DT: Clinical use of an indwelling nasogastric tube for enteral nutrition and fluid therapy in the dog and cat, *J Am Anim Hosp Assoc* 22:675, 1986.

Crowe DT: Enteral nutrition for critically ill or injured patients. III. *Compend Contin Educ Pract Vet* 8:826, 1986.

Crowe DT, Downs MO: Pharyngostomy complications in dogs and cats and recommended technical modifications: experimental and clinical investigations, *J Am Anim Hosp Assoc* 22:493, 1986.

DeBowes LJ, Coyne B, Layton CE: Comparison of French-Pezzer and Malecot catheters for percutaneously placed gastrostomy tubes in cats, *J Am Vet Med Assoc* 202:1963, 1993.

Graham PA, Maskell IE, Nash AS: Canned high fiber diet and postprandial glycemia in dogs with naturally occurring diabetes mellitus, *J Nutr* 124:2712S, 1994.

Heyland D et al: Enteral nutrition in the critically ill patient: a prospective survey, *Crit Care Med* 23:1055, 1995.

Hill RC: A rapid method of estimating maintenance energy requirement for body surface area in inactive adult dogs and in cats, *J Am Vet Med Assoc* 202:1814, 1993.

Jacobs G et al: Treatment of idiopathic hepatic lipidosis in cats: 11 cases (1986-1987), *J Am Vet Med Assoc* 195:635, 1989.

Lippert AC et al: Total parenteral nutrition in clinically normal cats, *J Am Vet Med Assoc* 194:669, 1989.

Macy DW, Gasper PW: Diazepam-induced eating in anorexic cats, *J Am Anim Hosp Assoc* 21:17, 1985.

Mauterer JV et al: New techniques and management guidelines for percutaneous nonendoscopic tube gastrostomy, *J Am Vet Med Assoc* 205:574, 1994.

McCrackin MA et al: Endoscopic placement of a percutaneous gastroduodenostomy feeding tube in dogs, *J Am Vet Med Assoc* 203:792, 1993.

Moore EE, Moore FA: Immediate enteral nutrition following multisystem trauma: a decade perspective, *J Am Coll Nutr* 10:633, 1991.

Nelson RW et al: Effects of dietary fiber supplementation on glycemic control in dogs with alloxan-induced diabetes mellitus, *Am J Vet Res* 52:2060, 1991.

Rawlings, CA: Percutaneous placement of a midcervical esophagostomy tube: new technique and representative cases, *J Amer Anim Hosp Assoc* 29:526, 1993.

Ray PA, Thatcher CD, Swecker WS: Nutritional management of dogs and cats with cancer, *Vet Med* 12:1185, 1992.

Slater MR, Scarlett JM: Nutritional epidemiology in small animal practice, *J Am Vet Med Assoc* 207:571, 1995.

Tennant B, Willoughby K: The use of enteral nutrition in small animal medicine, *Compend Cont Educ Pract Vet* 15:1054, 1993.

Wills JM: Diagnosing and managing food sensitivity in cats, *Vet Med* 9:884, 1992.

Wolfe BM, Keltner RM, Kaminski DL: The effect of an intraduodenal elemental diet on pancreatic secretion, *Surg Gynecol Obstet* 140:241, 1975.

CHAPTER 12

Treatment of Perioperative Pain

There are real, undesirable consequences to unrelieved pain. Postoperative pain management influences the quality of patient care as well as surgical outcome. Evidence suggests that acute, unrelieved pain produces potentially life-threatening physiologic effects. Patients treated perioperatively for pain return to normal functions (e.g., grooming, eating, drinking) sooner than those who are untreated. Therefore analgesic requirements should be anticipated and incorporated into each patient's anesthetic management. Choice of analgesic is based on the drug's pharmacokinetics and pharmacodynamics. Response should be monitored and appropriate adjustments made.

PAIN ASSESSMENT

Assessment of pain is based on expectations, physiologic parameters, and behavioral responses. Expectations are influenced by clinical experiences. Procedures likely to be painful include amputations; thoracotomies (especially median sternotomy); ear resections; some abdominal procedures, such as nephrectomy, prostatectomy, and hepatic resection; and pelvic fracture repair. Most physiologic changes involve sympathetic nervous system activation. Changes in heart rate, peripheral circulation, and breathing patterns may indicate pain, distress, or discomfort. However, physiologic parameters should not be used exclusively for assessing pain because other variables (i.e., drug administration, hypovolemia) may alter them. Several recognized behavioral characteristics of pain may be used in conjunction with physiologic responses to evaluate postoperative patients. The most recognized behavioral manifestation of pain is vocalization (i.e., crying, howling, barking, growling, purring, moaning). However, not all patients in pain vocalize; many animals suffer quietly. Changes in posture or facial expression, guarding or protecting a limb, self-mutilation, dilated pupils, salivation, muscle rigidity or weakness, and changes in sleeping, eating, or elimination patterns also suggest pain. Activity level may change; patients may be either restless or reluctant to move. There may also be attitude alterations (e.g., a previously gentle dog may become aggressive; a previously social animal may become timid). Cats are particularly difficult to assess, but one of the most consistent (albeit not specific) indicators of pain in cats is cessation of grooming.

Although there is debate regarding pain perception and recognition in domestic animals, there is general agreement that it is reasonable to use changes in physiologic parameters in conjunction with behavioral characteristics to determine pain. Little time should be spent determining if a patient is in pain; you should treat if you are unsure. If analgesia produces undesirable side effects or does not promote clinical improvement, treatment may be discontinued. A common argument against providing analgesia is that a pain-free patient will injure the surgical site. However, comfortable patients are no more likely to injure a surgical site than patients in pain. Tranquilization, not pain, should be used to restrict movement.

PAIN MANAGEMENT

Environmental manipulations may facilitate patient comfort. Familiarizing the patient with the environment preoperatively and inducing and recovering the patient in a dry, warm, quiet environment helps. Avoiding sleeplessness and anxiety in the perioperative period enhances postoperative pain management. Tranquilizers or sedatives may reduce perioperative anxiety and make the experience less distressing. However, tranquilizers such as acepromazine or diazepam should not be used alone in patients with pain. Adequate intraoperative and postoperative padding and positioning lessen postoperative pain from areas that were not operated on but that may result from anesthesia (e.g., ischemia of the skin and underlying tissues, neural deficits). Corneal, oral, lingual, tracheal, and dental injuries should be avoided during induction and recovery. The bladder should be emptied before recovery to avoid postoperative discomfort. Other interventions involve analgesics or analgesic techniques, including local anesthetics.

Good postoperative pain management begins preoperatively. Systemic drugs may be administered on a schedule (e.g., every 4 hours), by continuous infusion (e.g., morphine, lidocaine), or by continuous absorption (e.g., transdermal fentanyl). Local and regional techniques with local anesthetics and opioids may also be used. Analgesics should be administered preemptively. To be most effective, nociception should be inhibited with analgesic therapy before the initiation of the painful stimulus. If a patient is in pain preoperatively, administration of an analgesic before induction facilitates handling and manipulation and improves patient comfort.

Opioids

If an opioid analgesic is used, it should be chosen before surgery. Using a single, opioid analgesic agent throughout the perioperative period is reasonable. Unless contraindicated, the analgesic agent to be used postoperatively should also be used pre- and intraoperatively. The two primary considerations for choosing opioids are efficacy and duration. Some opioids are indicated for mild to moderate pain (e.g., buprenorphine), while others are more beneficial for moderate to severe pain (e.g., oxymorphone). An analgesic should be administered based on its duration of activity rather than "as needed." Pharmacokinetic and pharmacodynamic information provides a rational defense against "as needed" medication. For opioids of short duration, ease and expense of redosing must be considered. In most cases, to avoid painful intramuscular injections intravenous injection is preferred when an intravenous port is available.

Opioid agonists and agonist-antagonists commonly employed perioperatively include morphine, oxymorphone, butorphanol, and buprenorphine. Morphine (Table 12-1) is the prototype opioid agonist and is indicated for moderate to severe pain. Onset of action and duration of action are about 15 to 30 minutes and 4 hours, respectively. Cardiovascular effects include vagally-induced bradycardia, direct depression of the sinoatrial node, and slowed atrioventricular (AV) conduction. Morphine does not sensitize the myocardium to catecholamines. Ventilation is directly depressed (dose-dependent) by inhibiting central respiratory centers. Morphine also alters the rhythm of breathing. Hypoventilation may cause increased intracranial pressure as a result of elevated P_aCO_2. Nausea and vomiting result from chemoreceptor trigger zone stimulation. Morphine may cause hypothermia and miosis in dogs and mydriasis and hyperthermia in cats. Histamine may be released when administered intravenously; slow intravenous administration minimizes this risk. Morphine is administered as continuous intravenous infusions in human pain management and is being used clinically in veterinary medicine. It is frequently used for epidural administration (see later in this section and Table 12-2).

Oxymorphone (see Table 12-1) is similar to morphine, but does not cause histamine release. It is appropriate for moderate to severe pain and is particularly useful in managing critically ill patients that require intraoperative analgesic supplementation to decrease the amount of inhalant required. Oxymorphone causes sedation, panting, and sometimes hypothermia.

Fentanyl and meperidine are effective analgesics but have short durations of action. Fentanyl (see Table 12-1), a synthetic opioid, has a more rapid onset of action than morphine. In veterinary medicine fentanyl is used for intraoperative management of critically ill patients in balanced anesthetic techniques but is not used extensively for pain management unless administered transdermally. Fentanyl may be administered intravenously, intramuscularly, epidurally (Table 12-2), transmucosally, and transdermally.

TABLE 12-1

Commonly Used Systemic Opioid Analgesics

Drugs	Sample Surgeries	Dosage (mg/kg)*†	Route	Duration*
Butorphanol	Elective reproductive surgery, caudal abdominal procedures, gall bladder surgery, bile peritonitis, distal limb fractures	0.2–0.4	IV, SC, IM	2–3 hours
Buprenorphine	Elective reproductive surgery, caudal abdominal procedures, distal limb fractures	0.005–0.015	IV, IM	4–6 hours
Fentanyl	Used as premedicant; too short acting for analgesia	0.005	IV, SC, IM	<1 hour
Morphine	Thoracotomies, amputations, pelvic fractures, ear ablations	0.1–0.4	IV‡, SC, IM	3–4 hours
Oxymorphone	Thoracotomies, amputations, pelvic fractures, ear ablations	0.05–0.1	IV, SC§, IM	3–4 hours

Modified from Carroll GL: How to manage perioperative pain, *Vet Med* 91:353, 1996.
*Dosages and duration are based on clinical experience and may need to be individualized for a given situation and patient. Higher dosages may be needed for recalcitrant pain.
† The lower dosages are used for intravenous routes and cats.
‡ Morphine may be associated with hypotension when administered intravenously; morphine may be associated with excitement in cats.
§ Subcutaneous administration may be less efficacious.

TABLE 12-2

Epidural Drugs in Dogs*

Drug	Uses	Dosage	Onset	Duration
Lidocaine 2%[†]	Motor and sensory block: abdominal and hindlimb procedures	1 ml/3.4 kg (T$_5$)[‡] 1 ml/4.5 kg (T$_{13}$–L$_1$)[‡]	10 min	1–1.5 hours
Bupivacaine 0.25% or 0.5%[†]	Motor and sensory block: abdominal and hindlimb procedures	1 ml/4.5 kg[‡]	20–30 min	4–6 hours
Fentanyl	Sensory block: abdominal and hindlimb procedures	0.001 mg/kg	4 to 10 min	6 hours
Morphine	Sensory block: thoracotomies, forelimb and hindlimb amputations, cranial and caudal abdominal procedures, hindlimb and pelvic fractures	0.1 mg/kg[§] (preservative free)	25 min	~20 hours
Buprenorphine	Sensory block: abdominal, and hindlimb procedures	0.003–0.005 mg/kg diluted with saline	—	12–18 hours
Oxymorphone	Sensory block: abdominal, pelvic, and hindlimb procedures	0.1 mg/kg	—	About 10 hours

Modified from Carroll GL: How to manage perioperative pain, *Vet Med* 91:353, 1996.
*Dosages, onset, and duration are based on clinical experience; each patient should be evaluated individually.
[†] Avoid head down position after epidural with local anesthetic.
[‡] A block to T$_1$ leads to intercostal nerve paralysis; a block to C$_7$–C$_5$ leads to phrenic nerve paralysis.
[§]The dose for epidural morphine in cats is 0.03 mg/kg.

Transcutaneous fentanyl administration avoids the problem of a short duration of action and is being increasingly used in dogs and cats. Fentanyl may cause bradycardia, ventilatory depression, and skeletal muscle rigidity. Meperidine administered intravenously can cause significant histamine release and should be avoided. Meperidine has little place in veterinary pain management because of its short duration of action.

Buprenorphine (see Table 12-1) is a partial opioid agonist. Its onset is about 30 minutes and its duration is 4 to 6 hours. Buprenorphine's affinity for mu receptors causes prolonged duration of action and difficulty associated with antagonism. It is used for mild to moderate pain in veterinary patients. Buprenorphine causes little sedation or dysphoria in dogs and cats. Its prolonged duration of action makes it useful if redosing is problematic.

Butorphanol (see Table 12-1) is a mixed agonist-antagonist. It has a low affinity for mu receptors (not a complete antagonist), a moderate affinity for kappa receptors (produces analgesia), and minimal affinity for sigma receptors (decreased incidence of dysphoria). Butorphanol has minimal effects on the biliary and gastrointestinal tracts and is particularly effective for visceral pain such as bile peritonitis and pancreatitis. The advantage of agonist-antagonists is analgesia with minimal ventilatory depression. There is a ceiling effect; additional doses do not produce additional depression. The ceiling effect on ventilation is accompanied by a modest ability to decrease anesthetic requirements. Mixed agonist-antagonists can attenuate the efficacy of subsequently administered agonists.

Ventilatory depression and sedation caused by opioids may be reversed with opioid antagonists. Opioids should be antagonized carefully in patients with pain because the antagonist also reverses analgesia. Patients in pain may breathe shallowly; they usually ventilate better when comfortable.

Patients who have had thoracotomies and/or high abdominal procedures may have small tidal volumes because they guard themselves from pain incurred during breathing. Although an opioid may depress ventilation, its analgesic effect is more likely to decrease splinting, allowing larger tidal volumes and improved ventilation. Antagonism of opioids with naloxone, an opioid antagonist, has been associated with catecholamine release, hypertension, dysrhythmias, and even fatal outcomes in people. Dilution of naloxone with saline and slow intravenous titration decreases the likelihood of untoward side effects. Agonist-antagonists such as nalbuphine or butorphanol are preferable because they are associated with fewer reversal side effects than complete antagonism with naloxone. Some analgesia may also be preserved. Titration of a 1:10 diluted solution of nalbuphine (5 mg/ml diluted to 0.5 mg/ml) appears to antagonize sedation and respiratory depression, maintain analgesia, and avoid the dangerous side effects associated with high dose naloxone reversal. Similarly, butorphanol may be used for antagonism of mu opioids (e.g., oxymorphone) in veterinary patients.

Local Anesthesia

Adjuncts to opioid administration generally involve local anesthetics. Lidocaine is commonly administered as a continuous intravenous infusion in humans to supplement opioid therapy for recalcitrant pain. Subantiarrhythmic doses of lidocaine (5 to 30 μg/kg/min, IV) can supplement opioid analgesia in dogs when opioid analgesia alone is insufficient. Generally, local anesthetics are used in regional techniques that tend to be more effective when performed before surgical stimulation. Local anesthesia decreases the intensity of postoperative pain beyond the expected duration of the local anesthetic, probably by suppressing the sustained hyperexcitable state ("windup") responsible for maintaining postoperative pain. Several local anesthetic techniques (i.e., epidurals, ring blocks, splash blocks, local infiltration, brachial plexus blocks, regional anesthesia, intercostal blocks, and interpleural blocks using local anesthetics) are effective in obtunding pain. These techniques decrease inhalant requirements, which facilitates intraoperative patient management. The two most commonly used local anesthetics in small animal practice are lidocaine and bupivacaine. Bupivacaine lasts longer than lidocaine but also has a longer onset of action. Do not exceed a total dose of 2 mg/kg bupivacaine in dogs. Lower doses of bupivacaine can be used in cats.

Epidurals

Epidurals are useful for intraoperative management of high risk patients, perioperative analgesia, cesarean section, caudal anesthesia/analgesia, thoracotomies, and forelimb amputations. Epidural anesthesia is easily accomplished and provides hours of relative comfort (see Table 12-2). Specific contraindications for epidurals include hemorrhagic diathesis and sepsis. Epidural administration of local anesthetics, but not opioids, is contraindicated in hypovolemia; pretreatment with fluids may improve response. The dose of anesthetic should be decreased in geriatric, pregnant, and obese patients plus those with space-occupying lesions. The dose should also be decreased by 50% if CSF fluid is encountered when performing an epidural.

Epidural complications include infection, hemorrhage, and failure to produce analgesia or anesthesia. Local anesthetic administration results in sensory and motor blockade, while opioid administration affects only sensory function. Local anesthetic administration results in no or mild sedation, minimal nausea and vomiting, and occasionally urinary retention. Opioid administration may cause marked sedation, nausea, vomiting, urinary retention, and/or pruritus. With respect to cardiopulmonary function, epidural administration of a local anesthetic may result in decreased heart rate, cardiac output, and blood pressure. Postural hypotension can be expected. Local administration at appropriate doses usually does not impair the respiratory system, but excessive doses can produce convulsions. Opioid administration at appropriate doses produces minimal change in heart rate, cardiac output, or blood pressure but may cause early and late respiratory depression. The respiratory depression can be antagonized.

Opioids may be combined with local anesthetics in selected cases. Some opioid epidurals (i.e., morphine) have extended duration of activity and craniad migration as a result of low lipid solubility. Morphine epidurals relieve thoracotomy pain in dogs, and may even provide analgesia for forelimb amputations and cranial abdominal procedures.

Intercostal and Interpleural Neural Blocks

Thoracotomy pain can be managed with intercostal neural blockade and/or interpleural analgesia plus systemic opioids. Postthoracotomy interpleural administration or intercostal bupivacaine hydrochloride nerve blocks have proven efficacious, especially when combined with systemic opioid administration. The intercostal nerves supplying the incision site, two nerves cranial to the site, and two nerves caudal to the thoracotomy incision are selectively blocked. Interpleural analgesia is an alternative to intercostal neural blockade and offers prolonged analgesia without multiple needle sticks. Bupivacaine is diluted with saline and instilled in the chest tube of the thoracotomy patient. The operated side is placed down and sufficient time (20 minutes for bupivacaine) allowed for absorption of the local anesthetic. If a chest tube is present additional bupivacaine can be placed postoperatively (e.g., after 6 hours). If intercostal and interpleural blocks are both employed, the bupivacaine dose should be adjusted to stay below 2 mg/kg total dose. Potential complications include pneumothorax, respiratory failure, and/or drug toxicity.

Regional Techniques

Regional local anesthetics often help recovery and allow the patient to adjust to the onset of discomfort. Sufficient time must be allowed for tissues to absorb local anesthetics. Wound perfusion/infiltration is the simplest technique for providing wound analgesia, but there is poor efficacy in infected wounds. Effective local infiltration is used for incisional pain, nerve pain (amputation), and ear ablation. Brachial plexus anesthesia alleviates pain distal to the elbow. Infiltration of nerve stumps after amputation or brachial plexus block before amputation provides postsurgical pain relief. When performing a splash block following an ear ablation, the local anesthetic should remain in contact with tissues for 15 to 20 minutes before being removed.

Nonsteroidal Antiinflammatory Drugs

Nonsteroidal antiinflammatory drugs (NSAIDs) have been used for treating chronic pain and are only now being investigated for acute pain. Most NSAIDs are marketed as oral preparations and have not been utilized in perioperative pain management. They can be associated with clotting problems, gastrointestinal ulceration, and potential renal damage, which limits their utility. Some NSAIDs are available as injectable preparations and may be effective analgesic adjuncts.

POSTOPERATIVE PATIENT EVALUATION

Heart rate, respiration, and mucous membrane color should be monitored in postoperative patients. Successful analgesic therapy will often cause these variables to normalize. Appropriate analgesia causes the patient to be sedate but arousable. It is appropriate for the patient to sleep. Postoperatively the patient should be monitored for normal behavior such as eating, drinking, urinating, and grooming, which indicate the patient is not in severe pain.

Reference

Carroll GL: How to manage perioperative pain, *Vet Med* 91:353, 1996.

Suggested Reading

Andree RA: Sudden death following naloxone administration,

Anesthesia and Analgesia 59:782, 1980.

Cousins MJ: Management of postoperative pain. *Proceedings of the International Anesthesia Research Society 60th Congress,* Las Vegas, 1986, International Anesthesia Research Society.

DesMarteau JK, Cassot AL: Acute pulmonary edema resulting from nalbuphine reversal of fentanyl-induced respiratory depression, *Anesthesiology* 65:237, 1986.

Edwards WT, Breed RJ: The treatment of acute postoperative pain in the postanesthesia care unit, *Anesthesiology Clinics of North America* 8:235, 1990.

Gregg R: Spinal analgesia, *Anesthesiology Clinics of North America* 7:79, 1989.

Hansen BD: Analgesic therapy, *Compend Cont Educ Pract Vet* 16:868, 1994.

Hansen B, Hardie E: Prescription and use of analgesics in dogs and cats in a veterinary teaching hospital: 258 cases (1983-1989), *J Am Vet Med Assoc* 202:1485, 1993.

Lee VC: Non-narcotic modalities for the management of acute pain, *Anesthesiology Clinics of North America* 7:101, 1989.

Levy JH: The allergic response. In Barash PG, Cullen BF, Stoelting RK, editors: *Clinical Anesthesia,* Philadelphia, 1989, JB Lippincott.

Light GS et al: Pain and anxiety behaviors of dogs during intra-venous catheterization after premedication with placebo, acepromazine or oxymorphone, *Applied Animal Behavior Science* 37:331, 1993.

McCrackin MA et al: Butorphanol tartrate for partial reversal of oxymorphone-induced postoperative respiratory depression in the dog, *Vet Surg* 23:67, 1994.

Moldenhauer CC et al: Nalbuphine antagonism of ventilatory depression following high-dose fentanyl anesthesia, *Anesthesiology* 62:647, 1985.

Morton DB, Griffiths PHM: Guidelines on the recognition of pain, distress and discomfort in experimental animals and an hypothesis for assessment, *Vet Record* 116:431, 1985.

Pascoe PJ, Dyson DH: Analgesia after lateral thoracotomy in dogs, *Vet Surg* 22:141, 1993.

Scherk-Nixon M: A study of the use of a transdermal fentanyl patch in cats, *J Am Anim Hosp Assoc* 32:19, 1996.

Schultheiss PJ, Morse BC, Baker WH: Evaluation of a transdermal fentanyl system in the dog, *Contemporary Topics* 34:75, 1995.

Thompson SE, Johnson JM: Analgesia in dogs after intercostal thoracotomy, *Vet Surg* 20:73, 1991.

Tverskoy M et al: Postoperative pain after inguinal herniorrhaphy with different types of anesthesia, *Anesth Analg* 70:29, 1990.

CHAPTER 13

Surgery of the Integumentary System

GENERAL PRINCIPLES AND TECHNIQUES

WOUND MANAGEMENT

SURGICAL ANATOMY

The skin is composed of epidermis, dermis, and associated adnexa. The outermost layer, the epidermis, is thin but protective; it is especially thin in areas with abundant hair and slightly thicker in areas without much hair. The thickest epidermis is on the nose and foot pads where it is keratinized. The epidermis is avascular, receiving nourishment from fluid that penetrates the deeper layers and from dermal capillaries. The thicker, vascular dermis lies deep to the epidermis and nourishes and supports it. It is composed of collagenous, reticular, and elastic fibers surrounded by a mucopolysaccharide ground substance. Fibroblasts, macrophages, plasma cells, and mast cells are found throughout this layer. The dermis contains blood and lymph vessels, nerves, hair follicles, glands, ducts, and smooth muscle fibers. The hypodermis or subcutis lies below the dermis.

Musculocutaneous vessels are the primary vessels supplying skin in human beings, apes, and swine; however, dogs and other loose-skinned animals lack musculocutaneous vessels. Musculocutaneous vessels run perpendicular to the skin surface, whereas the vessels supplying the skin of dogs and cats approach and travel parallel to the skin and are direct cutaneous vessels. Thus some human pedicle grafting techniques have limited application in dogs and cats. Terminal arteries and veins branch from the direct cutaneous vessels and form the subdermal (deep) plexus, cutaneous (middle) plexus, and the subpapillary (superficial) plexus. The subdermal plexus supplies hair bulbs and follicles, tubular glands, the deeper portion of the gland ducts, and arrectores pili muscles. The cutaneous plexus supplies sebaceous glands and reinforces the capillary network around hair follicles,

tubular gland ducts, and arrectores pili muscles. The subpapillary plexus lies on the outer layer of dermis and capillary loops from this plexus project into the epidermis and supply it. The capillary loop system is poorly developed in dogs and cats compared to human beings and swine, which is why canine skin does not usually blister with superficial burns.

The subdermal plexus is of major importance to skin viability. In areas where there is a panniculus muscle (cutaneous trunci, platysma, sphincter colli superficialis, sphincter colli profundus, preputialis, suprammarius muscles), the subdermal plexus lies both superficial and deep to it. Therefore you must undermine in the fascial plane beneath the cutaneous musculature to preserve the integrity of the subdermal plexus. Where the panniculus is absent, such as in the extremities, the subdermal plexus runs in the deep surface of the dermis, necessitating that you undermine well below the dermal surface.

WOUND HEALING

Wound healing is a preferred biological process. It is a combination of physical, chemical, and cellular events that restore wounded tissue or replace it with collagen. Wound healing begins immediately after injury or incision. The four phases of wound healing are inflammatory, debridement, repair, and maturation. Wound healing is dynamic; several phases occur simultaneously. The first 3 to 5 days are the *lag phase* of wound healing because inflammation and debridement predominate and wounds have not gained appreciable strength. Healing is influenced by host factors, wound characteristics, and other external factors.

Stages of Wound Healing

Inflammatory phase. Hemorrhage cleans and fills wounds immediately after injury. Blood vessels initially constrict (for 5 to 10 minutes) to limit hemorrhage, but then dilate and leak fibrinogen and clotting elements into wounds.

The extrinsic coagulation mechanism is activated by thromboplastin released from injured cells. Fibrin and plasma transudates fill wounds and plug lymphatics, localizing inflammation and "gluing" wound edges together. Blood clot formation stabilizes wound edges and provides limited wound strength. Scabs form when the blood clot dries. They protect wounds, prevent further hemorrhage, and allow healing to progress underneath their surface. Inflammatory mediators (i.e., histamine, serotonin, proteolytic enzymes, kinins, prostaglandins, complement, lysosomal enzymes, thromboxane, growth factors) cause inflammation that begins immediately after injury and lasts approximately 5 days. White blood cells leaking from blood vessels into wounds initiate the debridement phase.

Debridement phase. An exudate composed of white blood cells, dead tissue, and wound fluid forms on wounds during the debridement phase of wound healing. Neutrophils and monocytes appear in wounds (approximately 6 hours and 12 hours after injury, respectively) and initiate debridement. Neutrophil numbers increase for 2 to 3 days. They prevent infection and debride organisms and debris by phagocytosis. Degenerating neutrophils release enzymes, facilitating the breakdown of extracellular debris and necrotic material, and they stimulate monocytes. Monocytes become macrophages within wounds at 24 to 48 hours. These cells remove necrotic tissue, bacteria, and foreign material and they are chemotactic. Chemotactic factors (i.e., complement, collagen fragments, bacterial endotoxins, inflammatory cell products) direct macrophages to injured tissue. Macrophages also recruit mesenchymal cells, stimulate angiogenesis, and modulate matrix production within wounds. Platelets release growth factors important for fibroblastic activity. Lymphocytes appear later in the debridement phase than neutrophils and macrophages. Lymphocytes secrete soluble factors that may stimulate or inhibit migration and protein synthesis by other cells. However, they usually improve the rate and quality of tissue repair. Although healing is severely impaired when macrophage function is suppressed, neutropenia or lymphopenia does not adversely affect healing or development of wound-tensile strength in sterile wounds.

Repair phase. The repair phase usually begins 3 to 5 days after injury. Macrophages stimulate DNA and fibroblast proliferation. Tissue oxygen content of approximately 20 mm Hg and slight acidity also stimulate fibroblast proliferation and collagen synthesis. Fibroblasts originate from undifferentiated mesenchymal cells in surrounding connective tissue and migrate to wounds along fibrin strands in the fibrin clot. Fibroblasts migrate into wounds just ahead of new capillary buds as the inflammatory phase subsides (2 to 3 days). They invade wounds to synthesize and deposit collagen, elastin, and proteoglycans that mature into fibrous tissue. Orientation is initially haphazard, but after 5 days, tension on wounds causes fibroblasts, fibers, and capillaries to orient parallel to the incision or wound margin. Wound fibrin disappears as collagen is deposited. Collagen synthesis is associated with an early increase in wound-tensile strength.

The amount of collagen reaches a maximum within 2 to 3 weeks after wounding. As the collagen content of wounds increases, the number of fibroblasts and the rate of collagen synthesis decrease, marking the end of the repair stage. The fibroblastic phase of healing lasts 2 to 4 weeks depending on the nature of the wound. Fibroblast migration, proliferation, collagen production, and capillary ingrowth are delayed if macrophages are absent.

Capillaries invade wounds behind migrating fibroblasts. Capillary buds originate from existing blood vessels and unite with other capillary buds or disrupted vessels. New capillaries increase oxygen tension in wounds, which augments fibroplasia. Mitotic activity in adjacent mesenchymal cells increases as blood begins to flow in new capillaries. Lymphatic channels develop similarly to capillary buds; however, their development is slower. Lymphatic drainage of wounds is poor during early healing. The combination of new capillaries, fibroblasts, and fibrous tissue forms bright red, fleshy granulation tissue between 3 to 5 days after injury. Granulation tissue is formed at each wound edge at a rate of 0.4 to 1.0 mm/day. Unhealthy granulation tissue is white and has a high fibrous tissue content with few capillaries. Granulation tissue fills defects and protects wounds. It provides a barrier to infection, a surface for epithelial migration, and a source of special fibroblasts called *myofibroblasts*. Myofibroblasts have an important role in wound contraction. They are believed to contain proteins (actin and myosin) that contribute to wound contraction. Myofibroblasts are not found in normal tissues, incised and coapted wounds, or tissues surrounding a contracting wound.

☞ **N O T E ·** Healthy granulation tissue is highly resistant to infection.

Epithelium is an important barrier to external infection and internal fluid loss. Epithelial repair involves mobilization, migration, proliferation, and differentiation of epithelial cells. Epithelialization begins almost immediately (24 to 48 hours) in sutured wounds with good edge-to-edge apposition because there is no defect for granulation tissue to fill. In open wounds epithelialization begins when an adequate granulation bed has formed (usually 4 to 5 days). Chalone inhibits epithelial mitosis in normal tissue but is decreased in wounds allowing epithelial cells along wound margins to divide and migrate across the granulation tissue. Other growth factors secreted by platelets, macrophages, and fibroblasts may also be involved. Increased basal cell mitotic activity occurs as early as 24 to 48 hours. Epithelial migration is random but guided by collagen fibers. Migrating epithelial cells enlarge, flatten, and mobilize, losing their attachments to the basement membrane and other epithelial cells. Basal cells at wound edges develop microvilli and extend broad, thin pseudopodia over the exposed surface of collagen bundles. They develop intracytoplasmic microfilaments and selectively fix antiactin and antimyosin antibodies. Epithelial cells in the layers behind these altered cells migrate over them until they contact the wound surface. Cells continue to slide forward until the wound surface is covered. The migrating cells move under scabs and produce collagenase, which dissolves the base of the scab so it can be shed. Contact with other epithelial cells on all sides inhibits further cell migration (contact inhibition). Initially, new epithelium is only one cell layer thick and is fragile, but it gradually thickens as additional cell layers form. After a basement membrane is established epithelial cells become plump, develop mitoses, and proliferate, restoring the normal, stratified, squamous epithelium architecture. Some hair follicles and sweat glands may regenerate, depending on the depth of skin damage. Epithelial migration also occurs along suture tracts, which may lead to a foreign body reaction, sterile abscess, and/or scarring. Epithelialization of suture tracts can be minimized by early removal of sutures. New epithelium is usually visible 4 to 5 days after injury. Epithelialization occurs faster in a moist versus a dry environment. It will not occur over nonviable tissue. Epithelial migration is energy-dependent and related to oxygen tension. Anoxia prevents epithelial migration and mitosis; whereas, hyperbaric oxygen therapy may enhance migration. Wet-dry bandages (see p. 103) debride newly formed epithelium, delaying reepithelialization.

Wound contraction reduces the size of wounds subsequent to myofibroblast contraction in granulation tissue. Contraction occurs simultaneously with granulation and epithelialization but is independent of epithelialization. Centripetal, full-thickness skin edges are pulled inward by contraction and wounds may be noticeably smaller by 5 to 9 days after injury. Contraction progresses at a rate of approximately 0.6 to 0.7 mm/day. Wound contraction is limited if skin around wounds is fixed, inelastic, or under tension, and it is inhibited if myofibroblast development or function is impaired. Contraction can also be impaired by antiinflammatory steroids, antimicrotubular drugs, and local application of smooth muscle relaxants. Wound contraction stops when wound edges meet, tension is excessive, or myofibroblasts are inadequate.

Maturation phase. Wound strength increases to its maximum level because of changes in the scar during the maturation phase of wound healing. Wound maturation begins once collagen has been adequately deposited in wounds (17 to 20 days after injury) and may continue for several years. Collagen fibers remodel with alteration of their orientation and increased cross-linking, which improves wound strength. Fibers orient along lines of stress. Nonfunctionally oriented collagen fibers disappear and functionally oriented fibers become thicker. There is a gradual decrease of type III collagen and an increase in type I collagen. Normal tissue strength is never regained in wounds (80% of original strength). The number of capillaries in fibrous tissue decreases, causing the scar to become paler. Additionally, scars become less cellular, flatten, and soften during maturation. Collagen synthesis and lysis occur at the same rate in maturing scars.

Host Factors Affecting Wound Healing

Old animals tend to heal slowly, probably because of concurrent diseases or debilitation. Malnourished animals and those with serum protein concentrations less than 1.5 to 2 g/dl may have delayed wound healing and decreased wound strength. Hepatic disease may cause clotting factor deficiencies. Hyperadrenocorticism delays wound healing because of excess circulating glucocorticoids. Animals with diabetes mellitus have delayed wound healing and a predisposition to wound infections. Uremia occurring within 5 days of injury impairs healing by altering enzyme systems, biochemical pathways, and cellular metabolism.

Wound Characteristics Affecting Wound Healing

Foreign material in wounds, such as dirt, debris, sutures, and surgical implants, can cause an intense inflammatory reaction that interferes with normal wound healing. The release of enzymes designed to degrade foreign bodies destroys wound matrix, prolongs the inflammatory phase, and delays the fibroplastic phase of tissue repair. Soil may contain infection-potentiating factors that inhibit antibiotics, leukocytes, and antibodies. Exposure of the wound to antiseptics delays healing and may predispose to infection. Warmth (30° C or 86° F) allows wounds to heal more quickly and with greater tensile strength than if they are at room temperature. A moist wound promotes recruitment of vital host defenses and cells, encouraging wound healing. Bandages facilitate keeping wounds warm and moist. Wounds created with sharp surgical incisions heal more rapidly and with less necrosis at the wound margin than when scissors, electroscalpels, or lasers are used. Wound infection interferes with the repair phase of healing. Contaminated tissues become infected if invasive bacteria multiply to 10^5 organisms per gram of tissue. Development of wound infection depends on the degree of tissue trauma, the amount of foreign material present, the delay between injury and treatment, and the effectiveness of host defenses. Bacterial toxins and associated inflammatory infiltrates cause cell necrosis and vascular thrombosis. Wound exudates can separate tissue layers and further delay healing. Inflammation caused by infection further compromises vasculature causing additional necrosis.

Healing is dependent on blood supply, which delivers oxygen and metabolic substrates to cells. Impairment of blood supply by trauma, tight bandages, or wound movement slows healing. Macrophages resist hypoxia, but epithelialization and fibroblastic protein synthesis are oxygen dependent. Collagen synthesis requires 20 mm Hg PO_2. Hyperbaric oxygen therapy increases tissue oxygen and produces more rapid gains in wound strength. Accumulation of fluid in dead space delays healing because the hypoxic fluid environment of a seroma inhibits migration of reparative cells into wounds. Fluid mechanically prevents adhesion of flaps or grafts to the wound bed.

Recruitment, proliferation, and function of cells in wound healing are probably controlled by growth factors—

proteins that are synthesized and released by cells involved in wound healing. Numerous growth factors have been identified including platelet-derived growth factor, epidermal growth factor, fibroblast growth factor, and type β transforming growth factor. Platelet-derived growth factors are found in granules, while macrophages must be stimulated to synthesize and release growth factors.

Fibronectins are glycoproteins critical to wound healing. They stimulate cell attachment and migration and are found in soluble form in plasma and insoluble form in connective-tissue matrix. Macrophages, endothelium, fibroblasts, and epithelium can synthesize and release fibronectin. Fibronectin in the coagulum probably assists the initial migration of cellular elements (macrophages and epithelium) into wounds. It binds bacterial cell wall components, collagen, actin, thrombospondin, heparan sulfate, hyaluronic acid, fibrin, cell surface receptors, and other fibronectin molecules. Fibronectin may also be important in providing an early wound-healing matrix and interlinking cellular and matrix components during healing. Fibronectin in wounds decreases as healing nears completion. Proteoglycans are also important in all phases of wound healing. The matrix during cell migration contains elevated concentrations of nonsulfated glycosaminoglycans (i.e., hyaluronate). As wound maturation progresses, more sulfated glycosaminoglycans (i.e., chondroitin sulfate, heparan sulfate) appear.

External Factors Affecting Wound Healing

Some drugs and radiation therapy delay wound healing. Corticosteroids depress all phases of wound healing and increase the chance of infection. Vitamin A and anabolic steroids may reverse the effects of corticosteroids on wound healing. Antiinflammatory drugs suppress inflammation but have little effect on wound strength. Aspirin therapy may delay blood clotting. Some chemotherapeutic drugs (e.g., cyclophosphamide, methotrexate, doxorubicin) inhibit wound healing. Radiation therapy can have a profound adverse effect on wound healing, depending on dose and time of exposure relative to time of injury. It decreases the quantity of blood vessels and causes increasing dermal fibrosis. Therefore chemotherapeutics and radiation therapy should be avoided for 2 weeks following surgery. Vitamin A, vitamin E, and aloe vera may promote healing in irradiated wounds.

MANAGEMENT OF OPEN AND/OR SUPERFICIAL WOUNDS

Wounds should be covered with a clean, dry bandage immediately after injury or at presentation to prevent further contamination and hemorrhage. Life-threatening injuries should be treated and the animal stabilized before further wound management. When appropriate, bandages should be removed and the wound assessed and classified as either contaminated or infected, and as an abrasion, laceration, avulsion, puncture, crush, or burn wound. The "golden period" is the first 6 to 8 hours between wound contamination at injury and bacterial multiplication greater than 10^5 organisms per gram of tissue. A wound is classified as infected rather than contaminated when bacterial numbers exceed 10^5 organisms per gram of tissue. Infected wounds are often dirty and covered with a thick viscous exudate.

Abrasions are superficial and involve destruction of varying depths of skin by friction from blunt trauma or shearing forces. Abrasions are sensitive to pressure or touch and they bleed minimally. A laceration is created by tearing, which damages the skin and underlying tissues. They may be superficial or deep and have irregular edges. Avulsion wounds are characterized by tearing of tissues from their attachments and creation of skin flaps. Avulsion injuries on limbs with extensive skin loss are called "degloving injuries." A penetrating or puncture wound is created by a missile or sharp object, such as a knife, pellet, or tooth, that damages tissues. Wound depth and width vary depending on velocity and mass of the object creating the wound. The extent of tissue damage is directly proportional to the velocity of the missile. Pieces of hair, skin, and debris can be embedded in the wound. Crushing injuries can be a combination of other types of wounds with extensive damage and contusions to skin and deeper tissues. Burns may be partial or full-thickness skin injuries caused by heat or chemicals (see p. 132).

☞ **N O T E** • Most large "degloving injuries" of the limbs of dogs and cats heal well with appropriate wound management. Grafting is often unnecessary.

Wounds of less than 6 to 8 hours with minimal trauma and contamination are treated by lavage, debridement, and primary closure. Penetrating wounds should not be primarily apposed without surgical exploration. Severely traumatized and contaminated wounds, wounds older than 6 to 8 hours, or infected wounds should be treated as open wounds to allow debridement and reduction of bacterial numbers. Most wounds are surgically apposed after infection has been controlled; however, some wounds heal by contraction and epithelialization.

Anesthesia is often required for initial wound inspection and care. The objective of open wound care is to convert the open, contaminated wound into a surgically clean wound that can be closed. Aseptic technique, gentle tissue handling, and hemostasis are essential. After initial inspection severely contaminated or infected wounds should be cultured. The area surrounding the wound should be clipped and prepped. The wound may be protected from clipped hair and detergents by applying a sterile water-soluble lubricant (K-Y Jelly) or placing saline-soaked sponges in the wound. Alternatively, the wound may be temporarily closed with sutures, towel clamps, staples, or Michel clips. Hair may be clipped from the wound margin with scissors dipped in mineral oil to prevent hair from falling into the wound. Povidone-iodine or chlorhexidine gluconate skin scrubs can be used to prepare the clipped skin. Detergents in antiseptic scrubs cause irritation, toxicity, and pain to exposed tissues and may potentiate wound infection. Alcohol kills and fixes exposed tissues on contact and should be used only on intact skin.

☞ **NOTE** • Bite wounds are contaminated and should be treated as open wounds or closed with drainage.

Initial wound management begins with copious lavage using warm, sterile saline or tap water (500 to 1000 ml). Sterile isotonic saline or a balanced electrolyte solution are preferred lavage solutions. Tap water is effective and, although it causes some hypotonic tissue damage, it is less detrimental than distilled or sterile water. Wound lavage reduces bacterial numbers mechanically by loosening and flushing away bacteria and associated necrotic debris. Occasionally the addition of antibiotics or antiseptics such as chlorhexidine or povidone-iodine (see p. 97) to the lavage solution reduces bacterial numbers; however, these agents may damage tissue. Antiseptics have little effect on bacteria that have established infection. Lavaging is preferred to scrubbing the wound with sponges. Sponges inflict tissue damage that impairs the wound's ability to resist infection and allows residual bacteria to elicit an inflammatory response.

Bacteria are effectively removed from the wound surface by high-pressure lavage using a 35- or 60-ml syringe and 18-gauge needle, which generates approximately 7 to 8 psi of pressure. The syringe may be connected to a bag of fluid with a three-way stopcock and intravenous tubing to facilitate refilling. Higher pressure (70 psi), generated by pulsatile lavage instruments (Water pik, Teledyne, or Pulsavac Debridement System) is more effective in reducing bacterial numbers and removing foreign debris and necrotic tissue, but may drive bacteria and debris into loose tissue planes and damage underlying tissue. Bulb syringes do not generate enough pressure to adequately remove bacteria and debris.

Devitalized tissue may be removed by surgical excision, enzymes (see p. 96), or wet-dry bandages (see p. 103). The extent of devitalized tissue is usually obvious within 48 hours of injury. Devitalized tissue should be surgically excised in layers beginning at the surface and progressing to the depths of the wound. Bone, tendons, nerves, and vessels must be preserved, but bone sequestra should be removed because they may prevent complete granulation of the wound (especially with metacarpal and metatarsal degloving injuries) and predispose to infection. Muscle should be debrided until it bleeds and contracts following appropriate stimuli. Contaminated fat should be liberally excised because it is easily devascularized and harbors bacteria. Alternatively the entire wound can be excised en bloc if there is sufficient healthy tissue surrounding the wound and vital structures can be preserved. The danger of surgical debridement is removal of excessive amounts of potentially viable tissue. When dealing with penetrating wounds or punctures it may be necessary to enlarge the wound to assess the extent of injury and allow debridement. After surgical debridement wounds are often treated as open wounds with medications and wet-dry bandages. The wound should be closed when it appears healthy or when a bed of healthy granulation tissue has formed (unless wound closure by contraction and epithelialization is anticipated).

ANTIBIOTICS

Selective antibiotic use may be beneficial in preventing or controlling integument infections following injury or surgery. Minimally or moderately contaminated wounds within the first 6 to 8 hours of injury may be cleaned and closed or treated without the need for antibiotics. Severely contaminated, crushed, and/or infected wounds or wounds older than 6 to 8 hours may benefit from antibiotic therapy. Contaminated wounds and those with established infection should be cultured before initiating antibiotics, and antibiotic selection should be based on results of culture and sensitivity testing. Ideally, quantitative bacterial counts should be performed before grafts or flaps are placed over granulating wounds. Reconstruction should be delayed if bacterial counts are greater than 10^5 organisms/g of tissue.

Systemic antibiotics should be given if there is a high risk of bacteremia or disseminated infections. A broad-spectrum antibiotic should be administered while awaiting culture results. Antibiotic blood levels should be present at the time of surgery when antibiotics are used prophylactically for clean or clean-contaminated procedures. Prophylactic antibiotics should optimally be given intravenously at the time of anesthetic induction (see Chapter 10). Contamination that occurs during surgery is usually limited to the patient's skin flora. Thus drugs effective against gram-positive skin flora, especially *Staphylococcus* spp., should be selected (e.g., 20 mg/kg cefazolin intravenously).

TOPICAL WOUND MEDICATIONS
Topical Antibiotics

Topical antibiotics rather than systemic antibiotics are preferred for open wounds. Mildly or moderately contaminated wounds do not appear to benefit from combined topical and systemic antibiotic therapy; however, combined therapy is advantageous in heavily contaminated wounds. Antibiotics applied within 1 to 3 hours of contamination are often effective in preventing infection. The benefits of topical drugs should outweigh their cytotoxic effects. Antibiotics used effectively as topical ointments or added to lavage solutions are penicillin, ampicillin, carbenicillin, tetracycline, kanamycin, neomycin, bacitracin, polymyxin, and the cephalosporins. Once infection is established there is no beneficial effect of topical or systemic antibiotics in preventing suppuration of wounds undergoing closure. Wound coagulum prevents topical antibiotics from reaching effective levels in tissues deep within the wound and prevents systemic antibiotics from reaching superficial bacteria. These wounds must be debrided to allow antimicrobial access to bacteria.

Advantages of topical antibiotics over antiseptics in wound management include selective bacterial toxicity, efficacy in the presence of organic material, and combined efficacy with systemic antibiotics. Disadvantages include expense, reduced antimicrobial spectrum, potential for bacterial resistance, creation of "super infections," systemic or local toxicity, hypersensitivity, and increased nosocomial infections. Antibiotic solutions are preferred to ointments and powders. Ointments liberate antibiotics slowly and may be occlusive, promoting anaerobic bacterial growth. Powders act as foreign bodies and should not be used. Topical cefazolin (combined systemic and topical dose should not exceed 20 mg/kg) provides high levels of antibiotic in the wound fluid. The minimum inhibitory concentration is prolonged in wounds when applied topically compared with systemic administration (Matushek, Rosin, 1991). Topically administered cephazolin is 95% bioavailable and rapidly absorbed; thus systemic levels equal wound fluid levels within 1 hour (Matushek, Rosin, 1991).

Triple Antibiotic Ointment

Triple antibiotic ointment (bacitracin, neomycin, polymyxin) is effective against a broad spectrum of pathogenic bacteria commonly infecting superficial skin wounds. Its efficacy against *Pseudomonas* species is poor. The zinc-bacitracin component is responsible for enhancing reepithelialization of wounds. These drugs are poorly absorbed so systemic toxicosis (nephrotoxicity, ototoxicity, neurotoxicity) is rare. It is more effective for preventing infections than treating them.

Silver Sulfadiazine

Silver sulfadiazine in a 1.0% water-miscible cream (Silvadene) is effective against most gram-positive and gram-negative bacteria and most fungi. It has the ability to penetrate necrotic tissue and enhances wound epithelialization. It is the drug of choice to treat burn wounds.

Nitrofurazone

Nitrofurazone (Furacin) has broad-spectrum antibacterial and hydrophilic properties. The polyethylene base gives it hydrophilic properties, enabling it to draw body fluid from wound tissue, which helps dilute tenacious exudates so they can be absorbed into bandages. Nitrofurazone may delay wound epithelialization.

☞ **NOTE** · Use gloves when placing your hand in a jar of nitrofurazone to prevent contaminating the contents.

Gentamicin Sulfate

Gentamicin sulfate, available as a 1% ointment or powder (Garamycin), is especially effective in controlling gram-negative bacterial growth (*Pseudomonas* spp., *Escherichia coli*, *Proteus* organisms). It is often used before and after grafting and for wounds that have not responded to triple antibiotic ointment. Gentamicin in an oil-in-water cream base may initially inhibit wound contraction. However, gentamicin in an isotonic solution does not inhibit contraction; it promotes epithelialization (Lee et al, 1984).

Enzymatic Debriding Agents

Enzymatic debriding agents are used as an adjunct to wound lavage and surgical debridement. They are beneficial in patients that are poor anesthetic risks or when surgical debridement may damage healthy tissue needed for reconstruction. Enzymatic agents break down necrotic tissue and liquefy coagulum to allow better antibiotic contact with wounds and enhanced exposure for development of cellular and humoral immunity. They do not damage living tissue if used properly. Burned skin, necrotic bone, and connective tissue are not digested by available enzymes. Enzymes must remain in contact with the wound for an adequate time to produce the desired effect. Local tissue irritation may occur with enzyme use. Granulex-V is an enzymatic debriding agent containing trypsin, balsam of Peru, and castor oil. Trypsin debrides and liquefies protein but can cause local inflammation and pyrogenic reactions; balsam of Peru stimulates capillary beds to increase wound circulation; castor oil improves epithelialization by reducing epithelial desiccation and cornification. Elase is an enzymatic debriding agent containing deoxyribonuclease and fibrinolysin. Travase Ointment contains *Bacillus subtilis* protease as a debriding enzyme. Preparation-H is a hemorrhoid medication composed of a water-soluble extract of yeast (brewer's yeast *Saccharomyces cerevisiae*) sometimes used on granulating wounds. It stimulates oxygen consumption, angiogenesis, epithelialization, and collagen synthesis in wounds and has been called the *wound respiratory factor*.

☞ **NOTE** · Do not use enzymatic debriding agents on extensive burn wounds because they may cause pain and may be toxic if large amounts are absorbed.

Other Topical Agents

Aloe vera has been used on burns for its antibacterial activity against *Pseudomonas aeruginosa*. The antiprostaglandin and antithromboxane properties of aloe vera medications are beneficial in maintaining vascular patency and thus help avert dermal ischemia. Aloe vera medications may also stimulate fibroblastic replication and have antibacterial properties. Acemannan, a component of aloe vera extract gel, promotes wound healing. Allantoin, another component of aloe vera extract gel, stimulates tissue repair in suppurating wounds and resistant ulcers by promoting epithelial growth. Use on full-thickness wounds is discouraged because of its antiinflammatory effects. Hydrophilic agents cause diffusion of fluids through wound tissues to the surface or into the bandage. This dilutes the tenacious coagulum and debris on the wound surface and allows easier absorption. Copolymer flakes (Avalon Copolymer Flakes) and dextranomer (Debrisan) are hydrophilic agents that absorb tissue fluid with minimal tissue reaction. An organic acid combination of malic, benzoic, and salicylic acids (Derma-Clens) enhances fluid absorption by devitalized tissue to promote its separation from wounds. Underlying healthy tissue is not damaged by the acids and the 2.8 pH discourages microbial growth.

LAVAGE SOLUTIONS
Chlorhexidine Diacetate

A 0.05% solution of chlorhexidine diacetate is the preferred wound lavage and wetting solution because of its wide spectrum of antimicrobial activity and sustained residual activity. Additionally, it has antibacterial activity in the presence of blood and other organic debris, minimal systemic absorption and toxicity, and promotes rapid healing. A 0.05% solution is created by diluting one part of stock solution with 40 parts of sterile water. Saline should not be used for dilution because a precipitate will form. More potent solutions may slow granulation tissue formation with prolonged wound contact. Residual activity may last as long as 2 days and effectiveness increases with repeat application.

Povidone-Iodine

A 1% or 0.1% povidone-iodine solution (10% stock solution diluted 1:10 or 1:100 respectively) is frequently used as a wound lavage solution because of its wide spectrum of antimicrobial activity. Iodine compounds are active against vegetative and sporulated bacteria, fungi, viruses, protozoa, and yeast. Povidone-iodine is a water-soluble, strongly acidic (pH 3.2) iodophor produced by combining molecular iodine with polyvinylpyrrolidone. Frequent reapplication (every 4 to 6 hours) is required when it is used as a wetting solution because residual activity lasts only 4 to 8 hours and organic matter (i.e., blood, serous exudate) inactivates the free iodine in povidone-iodine. Iodine absorption through skin and mucous membranes may result in excess systemic iodine concentrations and cause transient thyroid dysfunction. The low pH of povidone-iodine can cause or intensify metabolic acidosis when absorbed. Scrubbing wounds with povidone-iodine detergents damages tissues and potentiates infection. In one study, contact hypersensitivities were reported in 50% of dogs scrubbed with povidone-iodine compounds (Osuna, DeYoung, Walker, 1990).

☞ **N O T E** • Dilute povidone-iodine appropriately (0.1% to 1%)! More concentrated solutions are not more effective because less free iodine is available.

Tris-EDTA

Tris-EDTA [disodium-calcium salt of ethylenediaminetetraacetic acid buffered with tris(hydroxymethyl) aminomethane] added to lavage solutions causes increased permeability of gram-negative bacteria to extracellular solutes and leakage of intracellular solutes. Treated bacteria are more susceptible to destruction by lysozymes, antiseptics, and antibiotics. Tris-EDTA in sterile water rapidly lyses *P. aeruginosa, E. coli,* and *Proteus vulgaris.* The addition of Tris-EDTA to a 0.01% chlorhexidine gluconate solution increases the antimicrobial effectiveness 1000-fold (Pearman, Bailey, Harper, 1988). Antimicrobial synergism against *E. coli* occurs between Tris-EDTA and penicillin, oxytetracycline, or chloramphenicol. Similarly, Tris-EDTA and gentamicin, oxytetracycline, polymyxin B, nalidixic acid, or triple sulfonamide have synergistic activity against *P. vulgaris.*

Acetic Acid

Acetic acid at 0.25% or 0.5% is occasionally used as a lavage solution. Its antibacterial effect is achieved by lowering the wound pH. Wound acidification is beneficial in wounds containing urea-splitting organisms such as *Pseudomonas* spp.; however, resistance to acetic acid may develop.

Miscellaneous Lavage Solutions

Lavage solutions that should be avoided include hydrogen peroxide and Dakin's solution. Hydrogen peroxide, even in low concentrations, damages tissues and is a poor antiseptic. It is an effective sporicide; therefore if clostridial spores are suspected it may be beneficial. It dislodges bacteria and debris from wounds by effervescent action. Dakin's solution is a 0.5% solution of sodium hypochlorite (1:10 dilution of laundry bleach). It releases free chlorine and oxygen into tissues, killing bacteria and liquefying necrotic tissue. Even at half or quarter strength Dakin's solution is detrimental to neutrophils, fibroblasts, and endothelial cells; therefore it should not be used as a wound lavage solution (Kozol, Gillies, Elgebaly, 1988).

ASSESSMENT OF SKIN VIABILITY

Skin circulation may deteriorate for 5 days after surgery because of edema and other factors. Skin viability is clinically assessed by color, warmth, pain sensation, and bleeding. Viability may also be assessed by dyes, transcutaneous oxygen or carbon dioxide, and laser-Doppler velocimetry. The appearance of nonviable skin is black, bluish-black, or white, and the area may be nonpliable, cool, and devoid of sensation. Normal skin is warm, pliable, and pink with normal capillary refill (difficult to assess) and pain sensation. Areas of questionable viability are often blue or purple and capillary refill and sensation are poor.

Intravenous injection of the vital stains fluorescein (10 mg/kg) or xylenol orange (90 mg/kg) have been used to assess vascular integrity of skin but have not been shown to be advantageous over visual observation (Bellah, Krahwinkel, 1985). Transcutaneous oxygen or carbon dioxide monitoring allows immediate evaluation for ischemia but requires prolonged, quiet recumbency (Rochat et al, 1993). Additionally, trancutaneous oxygen or carbon dioxide sensors left in place for more than 3 hours may cause superficial burns. Skin generally survives if transcutaneous PO_2 values of approximately 60 mm of Hg are maintained. Transcutaneous PO_2 values between 30 to 60 mm of Hg may be associated with partial or complete survival. Transcutaneous PCO_2 values are lower at the base (approximately 53 mm Hg) than at the apex (approximately 106 mm Hg) of skin flaps where ischemia is most apt to occur (Rochat et al, 1993). Laser-Doppler velocimetry is an indication of capillary blood flux that may give an accurate assessment of local circulation. Probes must be placed away from major vessels to monitor relative blood flow, volume, and velocity, factors that vary with species, site, and instrumentation (Manning et al, 1991).

PRINCIPLES OF INTEGUMENTARY SURGERY

Fundamental surgical principles for reconstructive surgery are listed in Table 13-1. Incisions made with scalpel blades cause less tissue trauma than those made with scissors, electrosurgery, or lasers. Skin edges should be manipulated atraumatically using skin hooks or fine-tooth forceps. The deep or subdermal plexus must be preserved during dissection and excision to ensure skin survival. It is important to undermine at the level of the subcutaneous fat to avoid transection of the subdermal plexus. To avoid transecting the direct cutaneous arteries that supply the subdermal plexus, dissection should be performed under the cutaneous muscles (i.e., panniculus, prepucialis, supramammaricus, platysma, sphincter colli) or in the distal extremities in the deep dermal layer.

Sutures

Suture acts as a foreign body in wounds. Buried suture greatly decreases the critical number of bacteria required to cause infection because suture causes direct irritation, harbors bacteria, and generates ischemic islands of tissue. The smallest size and fewest sutures possible should be used to close a wound. Approximating sutures should be used to bring tissue edges into anatomic apposition. A 3-0 or 4-0 absorbable suture (e.g., polyglyconate, polydioxanone, polyglactin 910) with a swaged taper-point needle should be used for closure of subcutaneous and subcuticular tissue. A 3-0 or 4-0 monofilament, nonabsorbable suture (e.g., nylon, polypropylene) with a reverse-cutting needle is preferred for most skin sutures. Cyanoacrylate tissue adhesives may be used in selected procedures to facilitate skin closure or secure drains.

Drains

Drains allow evacuation of potentially harmful fluids (e.g., blood, pus, serum) from wounds and help eliminate dead space. They are often necessary for treatment of bite wounds, lacerations, skin avulsions or separations, mastectomies, seromas, abscesses, and hygromas. Drains may also be used to help maintain contact between a flap or graft and its bed. Drains may be either passive or active. Passive drains (e.g., Penrose drains) depend on gravity for fluid evacuation whereas active drains require a vacuum. Penrose drains are used most commonly to drain subcutaneous spaces. Active drains increase drain efficiency and reduce drain-related infection. They are especially useful in draining deep wounds and after grafting. Active drains may be open with an air vent into the wound, or closed. Vented drains (e.g., sump) have the danger of retrograde contamination of particulate matter and bacteria passing through the air vent into the wound. Filtered vents reduce the risk of contamination. Many portable, closed suction systems are commercially available (e.g., Snyder Hemovac). An effective closed suction drain can be easily made using a butterfly catheter and an evacuated tube or syringe. The syringe adaptor is removed from the plastic tubing and the tube is fenestrated before placing the drain in the wound. After wound closure the needle is inserted into the evacuated tube (5 to 10 ml) to apply suction. Alternatively, the needle can be removed, the tube fenestrated, and the adaptor attached to a syringe with suction applied. The vacuum tube is replaced when it loses negative pressure or fills with fluid. The volume of fluid collected should be measured and recorded.

☞ **N O T E** • Fluid drains around Penrose drains rather than through them. Fenestrating Penrose drains decreases their surface area, decreasing drainage.

The major disadvantage of drains is that they serve as retrograde conduits for skin contaminants to gain entrance into the wound. The presence of drains also impairs tissue resistance to infection and may disrupt graft adherence. Thus the smallest diameter and fewest number of drains with the fewest number of exit holes should be used to avoid complications. Superficial, passive drains should be secured to the skin at the dorsal aspect of the wound by direct visualization or blind suture placement. They should be exited through a stab incision at least 1 cm from the primary incision and positioned such that they allow maximal flow by gravity. To avoid incisional dehiscence and herniation, drains should not exit from the primary incision. They should be secured to the skin so that they cannot be prematurely removed or allowed to retract into the wound. Drains should be protected with a bandage that is changed before "strike-through" occurs. Strike-through is the saturation of a bandage with fluid that wets both the inner and outer surfaces. An Elizabethan collar or bucket can prevent self-inflicted drain or bandage damage. The animal should be kept in a clean, dry environment and have limited exercise. Drain malfunction may be caused by tissue fragments, fibrin, or viscous exudates. Drains are foreign bodies and will cause drainage until removed. Removal should be performed when the discharge is serosanguineous and the volume has diminished. Most

---

TABLE 13-1

Fundamental Surgical Principles

- Use strict asepsis in preparation of surgical team, room, and instruments, and during surgery.
- Handle tissues gently.
- Preserve vascularity.
- Remove necrotic tissue.
- Maintain hemostasis.
- Approximate tissues anatomically without tension.
- Obliterate dead space.
- Use appropriate suture materials and implants.

wound drains can be removed after 2 to 5 days. Closed suction drains placed under grafts are usually removed after 48 to 72 hours when drainage has diminished. Care should be used when removing drains to avoid disruption of the skin-wound bed interface.

Tourniquets

Tourniquets are helpful in controlling hemorrhage of the distal extremities to improve visualization and reduce operating time. Pneumatic tourniquets with pressures less than 300 mm Hg for less than 3 hours should be used. The limb should be elevated for about 5 minutes or exsanguinated with a rubber bandage before tourniquet application. Application of pressure is more even if two to three layers of orthopedic padding are placed under the tourniquet. The tourniquet cuff should be applied at a point of maximal circumference where nerves and blood vessels are protected against direct compression. Complications of tourniquet use are ischemia, hypoxia, or acidosis of local tissue, neuropraxia, and muscle damage.

WOUND CLOSURE

Wounds may be closed immediately (primary wound closure), within 1 to 3 days after injury when they are free of infection but before granulation tissue has appeared (delayed primary wound closure), after the formation of granulation tissue (secondary closure), or they may be allowed to contract and epithelialize (second intention healing). Wounds closed in the presence of contamination, necrotic tissue, excessive tension, and/or dead space are apt to dehisce, often with the loss of additional tissue because of bacterial toxins and pressure necrosis. If there is any doubt as to whether a wound should be closed it is best to leave it open. Factors that affect the decision to close wounds include:

1. *Time lapse since injury.* Wounds older than 6 to 8 hours are initially treated with bandages.
2. *Degree of contamination.* Wounds obviously contaminated should be thoroughly cleansed and initially treated with bandages.
3. *Amount of tissue damage.* Wounds with substantial tissue damage have reduced host defenses and are more likely to become infected; therefore they should initially be treated with bandages.
4. *Completeness of debridement.* Wounds should remain open if the initial debridement was conservative and further debridement is needed.
5. *Blood supply.* A wound with questionable blood supply should be observed until the extent of nonviable tissue is determined.
6. *The animal's health.* Animals unable to tolerate prolonged anesthesia are best treated with bandages until their health has improved.
7. *Closure without tension or dead space.* Wounds should be managed with bandages if excessive tension or dead space is present in order to prevent dehiscence,

fluid accumulation, infection, and/or delayed wound healing.
8. *Location of the wound.* Large wounds in some areas (e.g., limbs) are not amenable to closure.

Delayed primary closure is indicated for mildly contaminated, minimally traumatized wounds that require some cleansing and debridement or when the wound is older than 6 to 8 hours. Wounds are first lavaged and debrided to control local contamination or infection. These wounds should be treated with bandages after injury and before closure. After lavage and debridement, wounds that are minimally contaminated with little tissue loss and that are less than 6 to 8 hours old (within the golden period) may be closed primarily. Traumatic wounds contaminated by feces, saliva, purulent exudate, or soil should not be closed primarily. Instead they should be thoroughly explored and lavaged with sterile saline to remove debris and reduce bacterial numbers. Transected tendons can be anastomosed in clean wounds (see p. 59). Large motor nerves that are transected sharply and cleanly can be primarily apposed; otherwise, nerve repair should be delayed for 2 to 3 weeks when the wound has healed. If there is excessive dead space surrounding a wound, Penrose or suction drains should be used. Subcutaneous tissues should be apposed with 3-0 or 4-0 buried interrupted or continuous approximating sutures (e.g., polydioxanone or polyglyconate). The skin edges may be brought into apposition with buried walking sutures (see p. 110) or subcuticular sutures (e.g., 3-0 or 4-0 polydioxanone, polyglyconate). Approximating sutures should be used in skin (e.g., 3-0 or 4-0 polypropylene or nylon).

Wounds with considerable tissue loss, contamination, or infection, or those that are older than 6 to 8 hours should be treated as open wounds. Initially they should be lavaged, explored, and debrided. Tendons, ligaments, and vessels may be damaged beyond repair. Identifiable tendon ends should be tagged. A wet-dry bandage (see p. 103) should be applied and the area immobilized to allow debridement and formation of a healthy granulation bed. The wounds will initially heal by contraction and epithelialization and may heal completely (second intention healing). Second intention healing is often less expensive and results in normal appearing skin if contraction is complete. Body wounds are more apt to completely close by second intention than are leg wounds. Disadvantages of second intention healing include contracture with disfigurement, incomplete healing, and fragile epithelial scars with large wounds. Alternatively, healthy wounds may be repaired by secondary closure or use of a flap or graft. Secondary closure occurs at least 3 to 5 days after injury when a healthy granulation bed has formed. The granulation tissue helps control infection in the wound and fills tissue defects. Secondary closure is called for when the wound is severely contaminated or traumatized, epithelialization and contraction will not completely close the wound, or second intention healing is undesirable. Secondary closure involves resecting the granulation bed and skin margins, lavaging the wound, and apposing skin edges. Secondary closure also can be accomplished by resecting skin margins, debriding the surface of the healthy granulation bed, and apposing skin edges over the granulation tissue. Excising the entire granulation bed gives a more cosmetic closure. If secondary closure is not possible a flap or graft can be applied over the defect. After wound closure an absorbent nonadherent bandage should be applied to support the wound and absorb exudate. Bandages should be changed once or twice daily if a drain is used; if little drainage is expected and drains are not used, once every 3 to 4 days may be adequate.

POSTOPERATIVE CARE AND ASSESSMENT

Postoperative wound care should optimize healing and be tailored to the type of wound. Wounds should be evaluated frequently for infection, tension, fluid accumulation, dehiscence, and necrosis. They should be protected with clean, dry bandages. Bandages act as a barrier against exogenous bacteria and support the wound during the first few days after surgery. Healing, sutured wounds become increasingly resistant to bacterial penetration. The patient and the patient's environment should be kept clean, and adequate nutrition should be provided. Analgesics (see Chapter 12) and antibiotics should be used postoperatively as needed.

☞ **NOTE** · Excessively tight sutures are painful. To reduce the risk of animals mutilating the surgical site or prematurely removing sutures, keep skin sutures loose.

Infection may be suspected if the patient has fever, leukocytosis, anorexia, and/or depression. Although these abnormalities can be a normal response to stress and surgery and do not diagnose infection, they are generally more exaggerated with infection than nonseptic inflammation. If infection is suspected samples should be collected for culture and Gram's stains. If a surgical wound becomes infected the sutures should be removed and the incision treated as an open wound with appropriate bandages (see p. 94). Topical or systemic antibiotics (see above) are used to control infection based on results of susceptibility testing. The wound may be closed after infection has resolved.

Sutures should be removed from wounds in 7 to 14 days, despite the fact the wound has regained only 20% to 30% of its original strength. Scarring and infection associated with sutures is greater when sutures are left for longer periods. Most complications are prevented by using good surgical and wound management techniques. Potential complications include inflammation, edema, seroma and hematoma formation, drainage, infection, dehiscence, necrosis, granulomas, contracture, and failure to heal. Seromas are caused by excessive dead space or motion. They are prevented by closing dead space, using drains, and applying bandages to immobilize and support the wound. Seromas are treated by immobilizing the area and applying a pressure bandage. Large seromas may be drained, although this increases the risk of infection. Dehiscence may occur if sutures are placed too close to the margin, tension exceeds suture strength, sutures absorb too quickly, or sutures strangulate and cut through tissue. Dehiscence may also occur secondary to self-trauma, infection, severe cough, hypoproteinemia, or hypovolemia. Wounds that dehisce may be allowed to heal by second intention or may be debrided and resutured. A granuloma is a chronic inflammatory process that may be caused by the presence of foreign material in a wound. Contracture or excess scar formation most commonly occurs at sites of motion (e.g., elbow, stifle) or body orifices. Contracture limits motion and may be disfiguring. Scar revision or excision is necessary when contracture interferes with activities. Wounds may fail to heal when the area is infected or has been irradiated, or when the animal has received chemotherapy or is severely debilitated or malnourished.

References

Bellah JR, Krahwinkel DJ: Xylenol orange as a vital stain to determine the viability of skin flaps in dogs, *Vet Surg* 13:111, 1984.

Kozol RA, Gillies C, Elgebaly SA: Effects of sodium hypochlorite (Dakin's solution) on cells of the wound module, *Arch Surg* 123:420, 1988.

Lee AH et al: Effects of gentamicin solution and cream on the healing of open wounds, *Am J Vet Res* 45:1487, 1984.

Matushek KJ, Rosin E: Pharmacokinetics of cephazolin applied topically to the surgical wound, *Arch Surg* 126:890, 1991.

Osuna DJ, DeYoung DJ, Walker RL: Comparison of three skin preparation techniques. II. Clinical trial in 100 dogs, *Vet Surg* 19:20, 1990.

Pearman JW, Bailey M, Harper WE: Comparison of the efficacy of "Trisdane" and kanamycin-colistin bladder instillations in reducing bacteriuria during intermittent catheterizations of patients with acute spinal cord trauma, *Br J Urol* 62:140, 1988.

Rochat MC et al: Evaluation of skin viability in dogs using transcutaneous carbon dioxide and sensor current monitoring, *Am J Vet Res* 54:476, 1993.

Suggested Reading

Blass CE, Moore RW: The tourniquet in surgery: a review, *Vet Surg* 13:111, 1984.

Burke JF: The effective period of preventative antibiotic action in experimental incisions and dermal lesions: role of antibiotics in wound lavage, *Surgery* 50:161, 1961.

Harari J: *Surgical complications and wound healing in the small animal practice*, ed 1, Philadelphia, 1993, WB Saunders.

Keller WG et al: Rapid tissue expansion for the development of rotational skin flaps in the distal portion of the hindlimb of dogs: experimental study, *Vet Surg* 23:31, 1994.

Lee AH et al: The effects of petrolatum, polyethylene glycol, nitrofurazone, and a hydroactive dressing on open wound healing, *J Am Anim Hosp Assoc* 22:443, 1986.

Manning TO et al: Cutaneous laser-Doppler velocimetry in nine animal species, *Am J Vet Res* 52:1960, 1991.

Pavletic MM: Plastic and reconstructive surgery, *Vet Clinics of N Am (Sm Anim)* 20, 1990.

Rochat MC et al: Transcutaneous oxygen monitoring for predicting skin viability in dogs, *Am J Vet Res* 54:468, 1993.

Swaim SF, Henderson RA: *Small animal wound management,* ed 1, Philadelphia, 1990, Lea & Febiger.

BANDAGES

Bandages provide wound cleanliness, control wound environment, reduce edema and hemorrhage, eliminate dead space, immobilize injured tissue, and minimize scar tissue. Additionally, they provide comfort, absorb and allow characterization of wound secretions, and provide an aesthetic appearance. Bandages keep wounds warm, which improves wound healing and facilitates oxygen dissociation. Covering wounds with a bandage promotes an acid environment at the wound surface by preventing carbon dioxide loss and absorbing ammonia produced by bacteria. An acid environment increases oxygen dissociation from hemoglobin and subsequently increases oxygen availability in wounds.

Bandages should be comfortable and clean. Uncomfortable bandages annoy patients, who may then mutilate the bandage and/or wound. Pressure should be applied over and distal to wounds rather than proximal to them, to minimize venous or lymphatic compromise. When the outer layer of bandages becomes wet, bacteria readily pass from the outer surface and colonize wounds. Most wounds are unbandaged, inspected, and treated daily; however, wounds with excessive tissue damage, exudate, or established infection may require twice daily bandage changes. Adherent bandages should be changed more frequently if the gauze is saturated with exudate and slides on the wound at bandage changes. Bandages applied over wounds with healthy granulation tissue and support bandages used to immobilize fractures may need changing only once every 2 to 4 days. Analgesia or anesthesia may be required for initial bandage changes.

WOUND DRESSING MATERIALS

Bandages have three basic layers including the contact (primary) layer, intermediate (secondary) layer, and outer (tertiary) layer.

Contact or Primary Layer

The contact layer touches the wound surface and should remain in contact with it during movement. It is used to debride tissue, deliver medication, transmit wound exudate, or form an occlusive seal over the wound. The contact layer should minimize pain and prevent excess loss of body fluids. It may be adherent or nonadherent and occlusive or semiocclusive. An adherent contact layer is used when wound debridement is required, whereas a nonadherent contact layer is selected when granulation tissue has formed. Semiocclusive bandages allow air to penetrate and exudate to escape from the wound surface. They are the most commonly used bandages in veterinary medicine. Occlusive bandages are impermeable to air and are used on nonexudative wounds to keep tissues moist.

Dry adherent. A dry adherent contact layer should be selected when the wound surface has loose necrotic tissue and foreign material or large quantities of low-viscosity exudate that does not aggregate. An absorbent wide-mesh gauze is used, without cotton filler. Dry gauze absorbs exudate and adheres to necrotic tissue and debris. The bandage should be removed after the primary layer has absorbed fluid and debris and dried. The disadvantages of a dry adherent contact layer are that it is painful to remove, viable cells may be removed with necrotic debris, and the wound may desiccate.

Wet adherent. A wet adherent contact layer should be used when the wound surface has necrotic tissue, foreign matter, or a viscous exudate. Sterile, wide-mesh gauze soaked with saline is applied to the wound. A 0.05% solution of chlorhexidine diacetate (Nolvasan solution) may also be used as a wetting solution. The fluid dilutes the exudate so that it can be absorbed by the intermediate layer of the bandage. Necrotic tissue and foreign material adhere to the gauze as it dries and are removed with the bandage. Wet bandages absorb faster than dry bandages and are more comfortable. Potential disadvantages of a wet adherent contact layer are pain and tissue damage during bandage change, bacterial proliferation, tissue maceration, and strike-through (see p. 98). Rewetting the dried dressing with warm saline facilitates removal and reduces pain during bandage changes.

Nonadherent. Nonadherent contact layers do not stick to the wound surface and most are semiocclusive. They may be used when wounds are in the repair phase of healing or if necrotic debris is absent. Nonadherent contact layers retain moisture to promote epithelialization and prevent wound dehydration. They allow excess fluid to drain to prevent tissue maceration. Wide-mesh gauze impregnated with petrolatum (Adaptic or Xeroform), polyethylene glycol (Furacin Dressing or Aquaphor), or petrolatum-based antibiotic ointment is used as the nonadherent contact layer when wounds have newly formed granulation tissue and some exudate but are not epithelialized. Petrolatum gauze slows epithelialization. Polyethylene glycol is a hydrophilic, water-soluble substance that serves as the base of some ointments and is used to prevent adherence and increase capillarity. Xeroform is a semi-occlusive dressing composed of a fine mesh gauze impregnated with 3% bismuth tribromophenate and petrolatum. It allows egress of fluid and bacteria from the wound through the mesh. Fibrin from the wound bed causes temporary bonding of the dressing to wounds as the dressing dries. It is inexpensive and associated with low infection rates but painful to remove. Epithelialization is rapid. Nonadherent dressing without petrolatum (a cotton nonadherent film dressing, such as Telfa Pads or a rayon/polyethylene dressing, such as Release) should be used once epithelialization begins. These dressings are removed with little pain because they do not adhere to the wound surface.

Another type of nonadherent contact layer is an occlusive dressing. Occlusive dressings are not permeable to air. They are used on healthy wounds with minimal exudation during the repair phase of healing. Occlusive dressings accelerate wound epithelialization and collagen synthesis. They require less frequent changes than other types of bandages. Some types of occlusive dressings have a hydrocolloid, adhesive layer dressing (Dermaheal or DuoDERM). The hydrocolloid adheres to skin around the wound, while the dressing over the wound interacts with the wound fluid to create a nonadherent occlusive hydrocolloid gel. These dressings are used on wounds with an established granulation tissue bed, advanced contraction, minimal fluid production, and initial epithelialization. The wound should first be lavaged and dried. Then the hydrocolloid dressing is warmed between the palms to make it soft and pliable. The dressing is cut to an appropriate size and shape to cover the wound and the protective film is removed. The dressing is applied with light pressure until it adheres to the skin. Adherence is a problem in dogs and cats but may be improved by clipping the hair adjacent to the wound. It may be necessary to apply a light intermediate and outer bandage layer to hold the hydrocolloid dressing in place over mobile areas. The dressing is removed after 2 to 3 days when the outer surface of the hydrocolloid feels like a fluid-filled blister or if leakage occurs. The gel is lavaged or wiped from the wound and a new dressing applied. Wounds dressed with hydrocolloid contact layers are less painful and epithelialize more rapidly than wounds covered by semiocclusive, nonadherent dressings; however, wound contraction is reduced. The dressings are not transparent so wound monitoring is difficult.

DuoDERM is an oxygen impermeable dressing used to treat dermal ulcers, burns, abrasions, and graft donor sites. Its outer layer is a polyurethane foam that is impermeable to oxygen and water; its inner layer is a hydrocolloid polymer complex that is occlusive and hydrophilic. Oxygen impermeability promotes the rate of epithelialization and collagen synthesis and decreases wound exudate pH, thereby potentially reducing bacterial counts. The dressing does not adhere to the wound bed and is comfortable. Fluid accumulates under the dressing. The dressing should be discontinued when epithelialization is complete.

Other occlusive nonadherent contact layers include polyurethane films, hydrogels and hydrophilic beads, flakes, powders, and pastes. Polyurethane films and hydrogels are transparent, expensive, and contraindicated on infected wounds. Polyurethane films are used on flat, granulating surfaces. Hydrophilic polymers rapidly absorb large amounts of wound fluid and are indicated for use in deep, granulating and/or infected wounds. Biobrane is an expensive, temporary wound dressing composed of an ultrathin, semipermeable, silicone membrane bonded to a flexible, knitted, nylon fabric with pores. The two layers are covalently bonded to porcine collagen peptides to increase wound adherence. Biobrane is flexible and stretches to conform to the area. It is incorporated into the wound and is therefore comfortable. The wound can be seen through the dressing and minimal fluid collects. The dressing is removed when epithelialization is complete or infection is detected. Biologic dressings may serve as contact layers on wounds with minimal exudate. Biologic dressings include grafts and amniotic membrane.

Intermediate or Secondary Layer

The intermediate layer of a bandage is an absorbent layer that removes and stores deleterious agents (e.g., blood, serum, exudate, debris, bacteria, enzymes) away from the wound surface. Bacterial growth is retarded if the bandage allows fluid evaporation and exudate becomes concentrated. The intermediate layer should have capillarity for absorption and should be thick enough to collect the fluid. The intermediate layer also serves to pad the wound from trauma, splint the wound to prevent movement, and hold the contact layer against the wound. Absorbent cotton, combine roll, or cast padding (Specialist cast padding or Kerlix Rolls) may be used. Enough pressure must be applied during application of this layer to avoid spaces between the wound and contact layer and between the contact layer and intermediate layer. Such spaces allow fluid to accumulate, which promotes tissue maceration; however, excessive compression impairs absorption and interferes with blood supply and wound contraction. The outer layers of the intermediate layer can be made nonabsorptive by applying petrolatum, which inhibits environmental fluid from reaching the wound.

Outer or Tertiary Layer

The tertiary layer holds the other bandage layers in place and protects them from external contamination. Roll gauze (Conform Stretch Bandages or Kling), stockinette (Specialist tubular stockinette), or surgical adhesive tape is used for the outer bandage layer. The latter is most commonly used. Porous tape allows fluid evaporation and promotes dryness but allows surface bacteria to contaminate the wound when it becomes wet. Conversely, wound bacteria can migrate through bandages and contaminate the environment. Waterproof tape protects the wound from environment fluids, but creates an occlusive bandage that may lead to tissue maceration. Elastic adhesive tapes (Elastikon porous adhesive tape or Vetrap) apply pressure, conform to the area, and immobilize it. Support rods or splints may be incorporated into the outer layer of the bandage if additional immobilization is required.

TYPES OF BANDAGES

When applying bandages appropriate materials of adequate width should be used to avoid a tourniquet effect. Porous materials allow air circulation and escape of moisture. All bandages should be applied as smoothly as possible to avoid ridges and lumps that may cause irritation and skin necrosis. Owners must be instructed on proper bandage care. Bandages should be evaluated frequently for signs of slippage or strike-through. The surface of all bandages should be kept clean and dry. Patients should be observed for discomfort, swelling, hypothermia, skin discoloration, dryness, and/or odor, which may indicate the area has been bandaged improperly. Bandages applied too tightly impair circulation and produce soft tissue damage. Digits should be exposed when extremity bandages are applied to allow sensation and circulation to be monitored. Loose bandages cause pressure sores, decubital ulcers, or slippage. Patients should be restrained from chewing at the bandage and should have exercise limited to short leash walks. Bandages should be protected from dirt and moisture by covering them with a plastic bag or other waterproof material when the patient is outside. The waterproof material should be removed within 30 minutes to prevent excess moisture accumulation under the bandage.

☞ **N O T E ·** To monitor bandaged extremities for swelling leave the distal phalanges exposed. Separation of the nails indicates swelling.

Absorbent Bandages

Absorbent bandages are indicated for open contaminated and infected wounds. Absorbed debris is removed from the wound surface to allow better healing. The contact layer is an absorbent pad (Kerlix) followed by an absorbent intermediate layer (Kerlix Rolls) to hold the pad in place. The thickness of the intermediate absorbent wrap varies with the amount of expected drainage. An elastic contouring wrap (Conform Stretch Bandages or Kling) is placed over the absorbent wrap to conform the bandage and apply slight pressure. Adhesive tape is the final covering. The bandage should be changed daily or more often if strike-through occurs.

Adherent Bandages

Adherent bandages include wet-dry, wet-wet, and dry-dry bandages.

Wet-dry. Wet-dry bandages are the most common type of adherent bandage used in veterinary medicine. Wet bandages assist debridement by liquefying coagulum and absorbing necrotic debris while leaving viable tissue intact. The principle of a wet saline bandage is that, as the sponges dry, wick action pulls debris and exudate into the sponge and away from the wound. Advantages of wet-dry bandages are: (1) antimicrobials can be used in the wetting solution, (2) a physiologic environment can be maintained, (3) comfort is maintained, and (4) exudate is removed. However, bacteria may flourish in a moist environment and tissue maceration may occur. Topical antibiotics used in conjunction with a wet bandage should be in a water-soluble form and placed in the solution used to wet the sponges. *Place several layers of sterile gauze sponges over the wound and soak them with saline or a 0.05% to 0.1% chlorhexidine solution. Cover the wet sponges with an absorbent bandage. Change the bandage daily or more often if strike-through occurs. To remove the primary layers of the bandage (dry gauze sponges), moisten the sponges with saline and lift them from the wound.* Removal of the primary bandage layer may cause bleeding or oozing.

Wet-wet. A wet-wet bandage is similar to a wet-dry bandage except the contact layer is expected to remain wet and is not allowed to dry before bandage removal. A wet-wet bandage is used to transport heat and enhance capillary movement of exudate from the wound. It creates a moist environment to help clean the wound but has little debriding

capacity. They are used on wounds with large amounts of viscous exudate and little debris or necrotic tissue. Disadvantages of wet-wet bandages include increased management time, tissue maceration that promotes infection, and environmental contamination of the wound by bacteria if fluid reaches the bandage surface.

Dry-dry. Dry-dry bandages are used on wounds with loose necrotic tissue and debris or large quantities of low-viscosity exudate. *Apply a dry, wide-mesh gauze to the wound, followed by an absorbent intermediate layer and tape. Leave the bandage in place until absorbed fluid and debris have dried in the intermediate layer.* Dry-dry bandages are painful to remove, viable cells may be dislodged with necrotic debris, and tissue may desiccate.

Nonadherent Bandages

Wet-dry, wet-wet, and dry-dry bandages should be replaced with nonadherent bandages when drainage becomes serosanguineous and granulation tissue forms on the wound. The contact layer is a nonadherent pad (Release or Telfa) followed by an intermediate absorbent wrap (Kerlix Rolls) to hold the pad in place. The thickness of the intermediate absorbent wrap varies with the amount of expected drainage. *Place an elastic contouring wrap (Conform Stretch Bandages or Kling) over the absorbent wrap to conform the bandage and apply slight pressure. Place adhesive tape as the final covering. Change the bandage every 1 to 3 days, or as needed.*

Occlusive Bandages

Occlusive bandages allow wound fluid and normal body moisture to accumulate and prevent external fluid contamination of the wound. Bandages become occlusive when the outer layer is waterproof adhesive tape, rubber, or plastic. Another type of occlusive bandage is a hydrocolloid material that serves as a nonadherent contact layer (Dermaheal or DuoDERM) (see discussion of wound dressing materials, p. 102). Occlusive dressings are beneficial in speeding the rate and quality of healing in comparison with dressings that allow wound desiccation. However, wound contraction is reduced when hydrocolloid dressings that adhere to the wound edges are used. Occlusive bandages are used to retain moisture over partial-thickness wounds without necrosis or infection.

Tie-Over Bandages

The contact and absorbent layers of a bandage can be held in place with a tie-over bandage when the wound is in an area inaccessible to standard bandaging techniques (e.g., hip, shoulder, axilla). *Place several sutures (e.g., 2-0 or 0 nylon or polypropylene) in the skin surrounding the wound, tieing them with a loose loop. Apply an adherent or nonadherent contact layer and an intermediate bandage layer on the wound. Hold these layers in place by lacing sterile gauze or umbilical tape through the loose skin sutures. Cover the area with an outer bandage layer, if possible.*

Stabilizing Bandages

Bandages help immobilize fractures to minimize further tissue damage during transport for definitive fracture fixation. These bandages are heavily padded and are frequently referred to as Robert Jones bandages (see p. 706 for application technique). After fracture fixation with splints, external fixators, or internal fixation, stabilizing bandages may be used to support injured tissues, reduce swelling, and treat open wounds. The type of bandage applied to the wound is determined by the type of wound and condition of the tissues.

Postoperative or Closed Wound Bandages

Bandages applied to areas devoid of an open wound may serve to absorb fluid from a drain or incision line, support the incision, compress dead space, apply pressure, and prevent trauma or contamination. These bandages improve patient comfort by supporting wounds. *Place a nonadherent, absorbent dressing over the incision line and several layers of wide-mesh, absorbent gauze over the drain. Determine the thickness of the intermediate layer based on the amount of drainage expected. Be sure to use adequate padding over the end of the drain to prevent strike-through. Assess the character and amount of drainage with each bandage change.*

Pressure Bandages

Pressure bandages are used to facilitate control of minor hemorrhage, edema, and excess granulation tissue. Direct application of a corticosteroid ointment to the wound may help control excess granulation tissue. The more convex the surface, the greater the pressure exerted by the dressing on the tissue. *Apply an absorbent nonadherent contact layer over the area of hemorrhage or excess granulation tissue. Use a thick absorbent intermediate layer and elastic adhesive tape for the outer bandage layer. Wrap the elastic tape carefully to avoid excess pressure, which can impair arterial, venous, and lymphatic circulation, and cause tissue necrosis or nerve damage. Observe for discomfort, swelling, hypothermia, dryness, or odor, which may indicate the area has been bandaged too tightly. Remove the bandage within 24 to 48 hours if it was applied to control hemorrhage.*

Pressure Relief Bandages

Bandages designed to prevent pressure over an area (usually a bony prominence) are used to treat or prevent pressure sores (see p. 137). Avoiding pressure encourages healing over bony prominences. Most pressure relief bandages use a doughnut-shaped bandage or pipe insulation (Fig. 13-1). The bandage should be sufficiently large and thick so that pressure over the bony prominence is avoided. The circular opening in the bandage is used to treat the wound without removing the bandage and distributes pressure around, rather than over, the wound. *Create a doughnut-shaped bandage by rolling a towel or cloth into a tight cylinder, securely taping it to maintain the roll, and forming it*

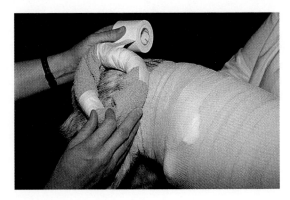

FIG. 13-1
A pressure relief bandage being applied over the greater trochanter in a dog. The bandage is made from a firmly rolled towel that is cut, taped, and applied over the bony prominence.

into an appropriately sized circle. Center the doughnut-shaped bandage over the lesion or bony prominence and secure it to the skin with tape so it will not slip. These bandages may be difficult to maintain in position. Taping directly to the skin may cause skin irritation. Pipe insulation bandages are usually used to protect the olecranon. *Create bandages from foam rubber pipe insulation tubes by splitting the tube and cutting a hole where the bony prominence will lie. If necessary, use two or three thicknesses of pipe. Stack and tape the pieces of pipe together. When using over the olecranon, first pad the cranial surface of the radial-humeral joint with cast padding to prevent joint flexion and keep the dog from lying in sternal recumbency. Then, tape the cast padding and pipe insulation in place. Use a spica type bandage (see discussion on bandaging extremities, p. 107), if necessary, to hold the bandage in position.*

BANDAGING TECHNIQUES
Bandaging the Thorax and Abdomen

The thorax and abdomen are often bandaged to cover wounds, surgical incisions, or drainage devices. These bandages should be applied firmly but without constricting the chest or abdomen. Abdominal pressure bandages are occasionally used when abdominal hemorrhage is suspected. Their effectiveness lasts only 1 to 2 hours and they should be removed within 4 hours. When placing an abdominal pressure bandage, bandage layers should be applied firmly. A rolled towel can be placed along the midline to reinforce the bandage before tape is applied.

Apply an adherent or nonadherent contact layer over the incision or wound. Place several layers of sterile gauze sponges over the end of Penrose drains. Hold the contact layer in position with combine rolls, cast padding, or cotton. Use padding, gauze, and tape rolls 3 to 6 inches in width. Wrap the padding circumferentially around the torso with slight pressure. Overlap each wrap by approxi-

mately one half to one third the width of the roll. Increase the thickness of the intermediate layer with increasing amounts of expected drainage. Reduce rostral or caudal slippage of the bandage by wrapping the intermediate and outer bandage layers between the legs and over the shoulders or hips in a criss-cross fashion. Encircle the torso with one wrap of bandage material, then direct the bandage from the right inguinal area (axillary area) to the left perineal area (shoulder area). Encircle the torso again and continue across the right perineal area (shoulder area), through the left inguinal area (axillary area), to the left flank (thorax). Repeat the criss-cross pattern several times. Also reduce slippage by adhering 0.5 to 1 inch of tape to the hair. Do not wrap the bandage so tightly that thoracic expansion is inhibited. Hold the intermediate layer in place with elastic gauze (Kling) or stockinette. Cut a length of stockinette (3 inches for cats and small dogs; 4 to 6 inches for medium and large dogs) slightly longer than the length of the body from head to rump. Cut small holes in the stockinette to accommodate the legs. Place the stockinette over the head and pull the front legs through the leg holes before rolling the stockinette caudally. Pull the hind legs through the leg holes. Secure the bandage with tape. In male dogs cut a hole in the bandage to accommodate the prepuce or divert urine with a catheter to keep the bandage dry. During bandaging manipulate the ends of tube drains so they can be easily accessed for aspiration or infusion.

Bandaging the Head

Most head bandages are placed to protect an ear that has been traumatized or has surgical incisions. Similar bandages can be used to cover the eye. Head bandages may interfere with breathing if they are applied too snugly or with neck flexion. A properly applied bandage should allow insertion of the fingers between the bandage and chin to allow room for neck flexion without airway obstruction. If the bandage is too tight an incision can be made partway across the bandage under the chin. Leaving one ear out of the bandage helps to keep the bandage from sliding. Extreme caution should be used when removing the bandage to prevent laceration or amputation of the pinna.

Apply 1-inch porous tape directly to the edge of the pinna to form a stirrup, fold the ear over an absorbent pad or gauze sponges onto the dorsum of the head, and wrap the tape around the head to secure the ear in position. Using a similar technique pad and place the opposite pinna over the first pinna if indicated. Place a nonadherent contact layer over an incision or gauze sponges over the end of a passive drain. Hold the pinna and contact layers in position with 2- to 3-inch cast padding or cotton roll. Encircle the head, passing the rolls of bandage material cranial and caudal to the opposite ear unless both ears are being immobilized. Starting under the chin, wrap loosely and overlap each wrap by approximately one-third the width of the roll. Cover this intermediate bandage layer with overlapping wraps of elastic gauze or a stockinette. To prevent

slippage secure the bandage in position with elastic tape attached to the skin and hair at the cranial and caudal edges of the bandage. During bandaging manipulate the ends of tube drains so they can be easily accessed for aspiration or infusion. If necessary to medicate the ear, cut holes in the bandaging over the external acoustic meatus.

Bandaging the Extremities

A soft-padded extremity bandage is used to cover abrasions, lacerations, or incisions and can be modified to accommodate splints for joint or bone immobilization. Modifications of the basic padded bandage may be necessary to allow immobilization, prevent slippage, or protect digits. Immobilization is accomplished by placing a spoon splint, molded thermoplastic splint, fiberglass splint, or aluminum rods between the intermediate and outer bandage layers. These materials may sometimes replace the outer layer. It is important to ensure adequate padding at the ends of the splint material to avoid skin irritation.

Begin by applying a 1-inch porous tape stirrup to the dorsal and ventral or medial and lateral surfaces of the paw (Fig. 13-2, A). Extend stirrups 3 to 8 inches beyond the digits to help prevent the bandage from slipping distally. If necessary, use a loose layer of elastic gauze to help secure the stirrups. Insert small pledgets of cotton or other absorbent material between the digits and the metatarsal/metacarpal pads and digital pads. Apply an appropriate contact layer over the wound (see p. 101). Snugly apply cast padding around the paw beginning at the level of the second and fifth digital pads. Wrap obliquely so the third and fourth digits protrude slightly beyond the bandage (Fig. 13-2, B). Overlap the cast padding (2- to 3-inch width) one half to two thirds of its width as it is advanced up the leg. Continue the bandage to the proximal radius and ulna (tibia and fibula) or above the elbow (stifle), depending on the site of the injury. Use enough padding to create the bulkiness necessary for protection. Snugly wrap elastic gauze (2- to 3-inch width) over the cast padding to conform the padding to the limb, overlapping each turn by one half the width of the material. Separate the tape stirrups and attach them to their respective sides of the bandage (Fig. 13-2, C). Apply an outer layer of elastic tape (2- to 3-inch width), overlapping one half the width with each turn (Fig. 13-2, D). Avoid over-stretching the tape to prevent compromising limb circulation. Check exposed digits three and four frequently for swelling, coolness, and discomfort; remove the bandage and evaluate the limb if these signs are observed.

☞ **N O T E** • Have the owners check the digits for swelling daily after the animal is released from the hospital.

Slippage can be prevented by extending the bandage to encircle the shoulder and thorax (hip and caudal abdomen), creating a spica bandage (Fig. 13-3). The spica bandage

FIG. 13-2
A, For a leg bandage apply a 1-inch porous tape stirrup to the dorsal and ventral or medial and lateral surfaces of the paw. Insert an absorbent material between the digits and metacarpal or metatarsal and digital pads. **B,** Apply cast padding or cotton over an appropriate contact layer, overlapping wraps by one half to two thirds the width of the roll. Keep the third and fourth digits exposed. Conform the padding to the limb by applying elastic gauze. Apply a splint for greater immobilization between the padding and elastic gauze (optional). **C,** Fold the tape stirrups over the gauze. **D,** Apply an outer layer of 2- to 3-inch wide elastic tape, overlapping one half of the width of the tape with each turn.

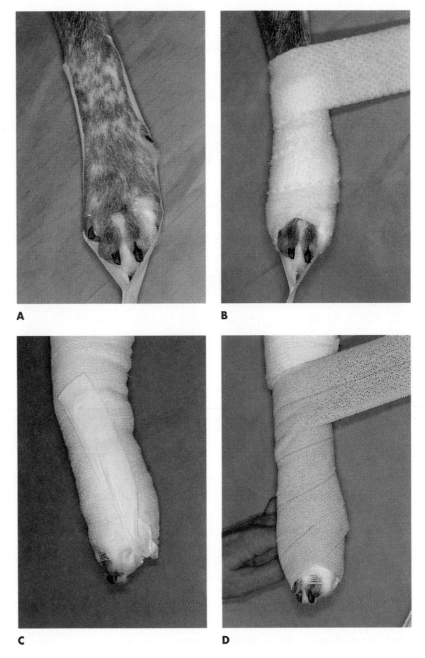

A

B

C

D

immobilizes the shoulder or hip in addition to the more distal joints and often incorporates splint material. The intermediate and outer bandage layers criss-cross cranial and caudal to the affected limb and caudal and cranial to the contralateral limb as described on p. 105 for abdominal and thoracic bandages. The bandage is reinforced with splint rod, fiberglass casting tape, or thermoplastic splint material if fractures are being temporarily stabilized or if additional wound immobilization is desired.

Temporary immobilization of injuries below the elbow or stifle can also be accomplished by applying a Robert Jones bandage or modified Robert Jones bandage. A Robert Jones bandage is a large bulky bandage that provides stabilization by applying compression to a thick cotton layer (see p. 706). A modified or light Robert Jones bandage is similar to a Robert Jones bandages but there is much less cotton padding, making it less bulky. Modified Robert Jones bandages are used to reduce limb edema postoperatively.

Onychectomy, digit amputation, or pad reconstruction may benefit from a bandage to protect the digits and reduce hemorrhage. In these cases stirrups should be applied laterally and the digits covered with gauze sponges or a nonadherent contact layer. *Reflect layers of 2-inch cast padding from dorsal to ventral and then ventral to dorsal over the*

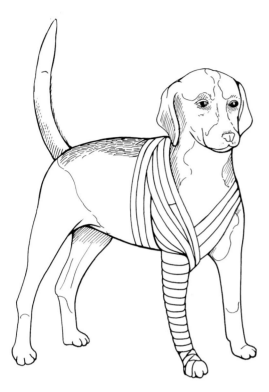

FIG. 13-3
For proximal extremity lesions continue the bandage up the leg, around the chest or abdomen, and between the legs to create a spica-type bandage.

end of the paw (Fig. 13-4, A). Extend the cast padding in a spiral pattern to the mid radius and ulna (tibia and fibula). Leave the proximal ends of the tape stirrup exposed to aid bandage removal. Cover the cast padding with elastic gauze. Fold the tape stirrups to their respective sides. Cover the bandage with tape from the distal extremity to the proximal hair (Fig. 13-4, B). Alternatively, Tubegauz, a thin, elastic stockinette, may be used to cover the contact layer and cast padding. It is applied with a "bale" or metal cage cylinder. *Insert the foot in the bale covered with Tubegauz, grasp the stockinette proximally, pull the bale to the end of the foot using a slight rotating motion and twist 180 to 360 degrees. Push the bale up and pull it down the limb to add additional layers of stockinette. Cover the stockinette with tape. Increase tension by increasing the rotation of the bale along the long axis of the leg. Avoid applying the stockinette too tightly. Remove the bandage by incising the proximal aspect to expose the proximal ends of the tape stirrups. Pull the tabs of the stirrup down the leg to loosen and remove the bandage.*

Suggested Reading

Swaim SF: Management and bandaging of soft tissue injuries of dog and cat feet, *J Am Anim Hosp Assoc* 21:329, 1985.
Swaim SF, Henderson RA: *Small animal wound management*, ed 1, Philadelphia, 1990, Lea & Febiger.

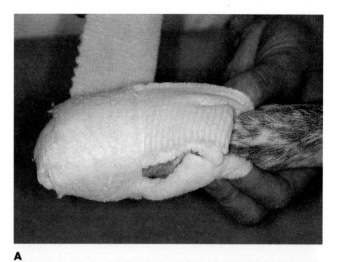

A

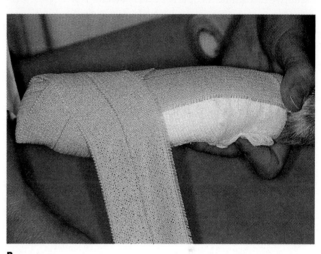

B

FIG. 13-4
A paw bandage is placed similar to a leg bandage, except the digits are covered. **A,** After placing stirrups and the contact layer, reflect cast padding over the digits from dorsal to ventral and then ventral to dorsal. Then wrap the padding around the distal limb. **B,** Conform the bandage to the limb with elastic gauze and secure the bandage with elastic tape in a similar fashion.

PRINCIPLES OF PLASTIC AND RECONSTRUCTIVE SURGERY

SKIN TENSION AND ELASTICITY

Reconstructive surgery is commonly performed to close defects occurring secondary to trauma, to correct or improve congenital abnormalities, or after removal of neoplasms. A variety of reconstructive procedures are available; selection of the appropriate technique(s) is important to prevent complications and avoid unnecessary cost. Although large lesions (particularly those on the trunk) will often heal by contraction and epithelialization (see pp. 92 and 93), wound closure may be preferred. Occasionally, large or irregular defects can be closed using relaxing incisions or "plasty" techniques (e.g., V-Y plasty, Z- plasty). Large defects or those on the extremities may require that tissue be mobilized from other sites. Pedicle flaps are tissues that are partially detached from the donor site and mobilized to cover a defect (see p. 116), and grafts involve the transfer of a segment of skin to a distant (recipient) site (see p. 128). Careful planning and meticulous, atraumatic surgical technique are necessary to prevent excessive tension, kinking, and circulatory compromise. The amount of skin available for transfer varies between sites on the same animal and between breeds. Little skin can be mobilized in the extremities, whereas large defects over the trunk can often be closed by advancing adjacent tissue. The character of the recipient bed influences the choice of reconstructive technique. Properly developed and transferred local flaps can survive on avascular beds, while grafts and distant flap transfers require vascular beds (i.e., healthy granulation tissue, muscle, periosteum, and paratenon).

Hirudiniasis, or the attachment of leeches to skin, can help in reconstructive and microvascular surgery. Leeches are only recommended for tissues with impaired venous circulation. The medicinal leech is *Hirudo medicinalis.* After a blood meal a leech can go for months without eating. Leeches produce a small bleeding wound that mimics venous outflow. The leech eats an average of 5 ml of blood, but blood oozes from the wound for 24 to 48 hours after the leech detaches because of anticoagulants and vasodilator substances introduced into the wound. There is a significant risk of infection with *Aeromonas hydrophila* when leeches are used.

TENSION LINES AND TENSION RELIEF

Location of the wound, elasticity of surrounding tissue, regional blood supply, and character of the wound bed should be considered when planning reconstructive surgery. Skin tension and elasticity are assessed by grasping and lifting the skin in the proposed flap/graft area and allowing it to spontaneously retract. Evaluating the amount of tension that can be tolerated by tissues is subjective. Apposing incision edges under too much tension causes incisional discomfort and pressure necrosis, resulting in sutures "cutting out" (see p. 110) and partial or complete incisional dehiscence. Methods to reduce tension include undermining wound edges, selecting appropriate suture patterns, using relief incisions, and tissue expansion. If these methods do not allow primary apposition, wounds may be allowed to heal by second intention or be reconstructed with flaps or grafts.

Tension Lines

Tension lines are formed by the predominant pull of fibrous tissue within the skin. General lines of tension have been mapped in animals, but variations occur depending on breed, conformation, sex, and age (Fig. 13-5). Tension causes incised skin edges to separate and it widens linear scars (Fig. 13-6). Incisions should be made parallel to tension lines. Incisions and wounds along tension lines heal better, faster, and

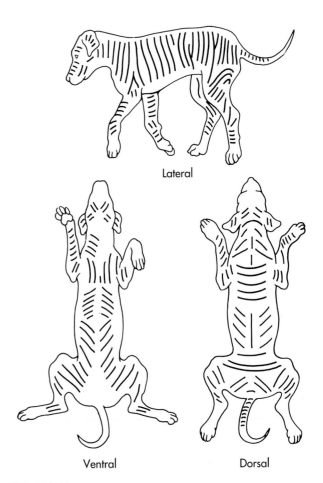

Lateral

Ventral   Dorsal

FIG. 13-5
Approximate skin tension lines in dogs. (Modified from Irwin DHG: Tension lines in the skin of the dog, *J Small Anim Pract* 7:595, 1966.)

with more aesthetic results, whereas those made across tension lines gape widely. Incisions made at an angle to tension lines take a curvilinear shape. Incisions made across tension lines require more sutures for closure and are more likely to dehisce than those made parallel to tension lines. Traumatic wounds should be closed in the direction that will avoid or minimize tension. Before closure the wound edges should be manipulated to determine which direction the suture line should run to have the least tension (Fig. 13-7). If there is minimal tension wounds should be closed in the direction of their long axis. The direction of closure should avoid or minimize the creation of "dog ears."

Tension Relief

Skin is undermined by using scissors to separate skin and/or panniculus muscle from underlying tissue. Undermining skin adjacent to a wound is the simplest tension-relieving procedure. It releases skin from underlying attachments so that its full elastic potential can be used as it is stretched over a wound. Skin should be undermined deep to the panniculus muscle layer to preserve the subdermal plexus and direct cutaneous vessels that run parallel to the skin surface (Fig.

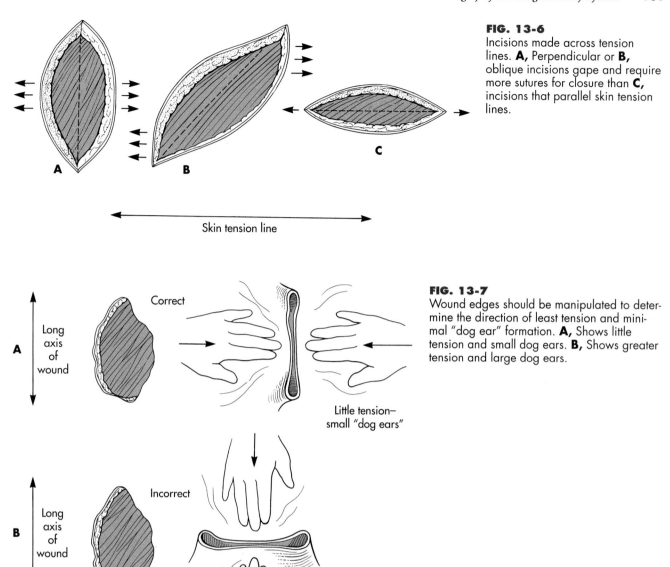

FIG. 13-6
Incisions made across tension lines. **A,** Perpendicular or **B,** oblique incisions gape and require more sutures for closure than **C,** incisions that parallel skin tension lines.

Skin tension line

FIG. 13-7
Wound edges should be manipulated to determine the direction of least tension and minimal "dog ear" formation. **A,** Shows little tension and small dog ears. **B,** Shows greater tension and large dog ears.

13-8). Where there is no panniculus, skin should be undermined in the loose areolar fascia deep to the dermis to preserve the subdermal plexus. Elevated skin should include a portion of the superficial fascia with the dermis to preserve the direct cutaneous arteries. Avoid injury to the subdermal plexus by using atraumatic surgical technique, including cutting skin with sharp scalpel blades instead of scissors and avoiding crushing instruments (e.g., Allis tissue forceps). Brown-Adson thumb forceps, skin hooks, or stay sutures should be used to manipulate skin. Tissue layers are separated by repeatedly inserting Metzenbaum scissors with the blades closed, opening the blades, and then withdrawing the scissors in an open position. Tissue is snipped with the scis-

sors as necessary. Alternatively, the partially opened scissors can be advanced along the cleavage plane without snipping. While undermining, determine if tension relief is adequate by periodically attempting to approximate the skin edges.

Bleeding is usually insignificant during undermining. Excessive bleeding may be controlled with electrocoagulation or ligation; however, skin tension and bandaging usually control hemorrhage and prevent seromas. Undermining areas with delayed wound closure requires that the epithelialized skin edge be separated from the granulation tissue. The skin should be excised with a scalpel blade at the junction of normal skin and new epithelium. The incision should be continued through the granulation tissue at the normal

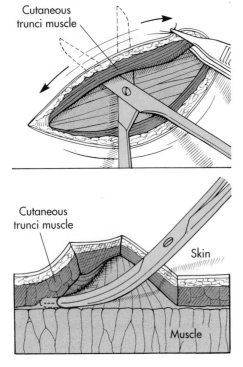

Cutaneous
trunci muscle

Cutaneous
trunci muscle

Skin

Muscle

FIG. 13-8
Before wound closure use scissors to undermine skin and subcutaneous tissue or skin and panniculus muscle and separate them from the underlying tissue.

cleavage line of subcutaneous fascia, deep to the subdermal plexus. Wound closure under excessive tension, rough surgical technique, and division of direct cutaneous arteries interfere with cutaneous circulation and may cause skin necrosis, wound dehiscence, or infection. Surgical manipulation of recently traumatized skin should be minimized until circulation improves. Resolution of contusions, edema, and infection indicates improved skin circulation.

Tissue Expansion

Tissue expanders are inflated in subcutaneous tissues to stretch the overlying skin, allowing creation of larger flaps for closing defects. They are beneficial in overcoming tissue shortage and obtaining skin with desirable qualities. Tissue expanders have an inflatable bag and reservoir made of silicone elastomer. Although expensive, they are available in various sizes and shapes (e.g., Intravent Intraoperative Tissue Expanders, Radovan Tissue Expander). Careful planning is required for optimum expansion and reconstruction. The base of the expander should approximate the size of the donor site. The incision for insertion of the expander should be made parallel to tension lines at the leading edge of the future flap or skin adjacent to the site will be inappropriately stretched. The device is placed subcutaneously and inflated with saline. Rapid expansion requires intermittent, intraoperative, short-term inflation of the expander. It involves inflating the expander for 2 to 3 minutes, deflating and letting the tissue rest for 3 to 4 minutes, and then repeating the cy-

cle two to three times before creating a flap. Gradual expansion involves injecting to a given pressure or volume at intervals spanning days to weeks (usually every 2 to 7 days). Inflation at injection is continued until the skin feels tense, looks blanched, or discomfort is perceived. When the tissue is sufficiently stretched to allow reconstruction, the device is removed and a skin flap created to close the defect. Complications of tissue expanders include pain, seroma formation, scar widening, infection, dehiscence, skin necrosis, and implant failure. Axial pattern flaps (see p. 120) are preferable to tissue expanders.

SUTURE PATTERNS
Subdermal Sutures

Subdermal fascia is strong and tolerates tension better than subcutaneous tissue or skin. Sutures placed in subdermal or subcuticular tissue reduce tension on skin sutures and bring skin edges into apposition. These sutures also reduce scarring. 3-0 or 4-0 polydioxanone or polyglyconate with a buried knot is used for subdermal/subcuticular sutures.

Walking Sutures

Walking sutures move skin across a defect, obliterate dead space, and distribute tension over the wound surface. Skin is advanced toward the center of the wound by placing rows of interrupted, subdermal sutures beginning at the depths of the wound. The suture (e.g., 3-0 polydioxanone or polyglyconate) should be placed through fascia of the body wall at a distance closer to the center of the wound than the bite through the subdermal fascia or deep dermis (Fig. 13-9). Walking sutures do not penetrate the skin surface. Tieing the suture advances skin toward the wound center. Successive rows of walking sutures further advance the skin toward the center of the wound. The number of walking sutures should be minimized to avoid creating subcutaneous loculi. Subdermal and skin sutures are used to complete wound closure.

External Tension Relieving Sutures

External tension relieving sutures help prevent sutures from cutting out, which occurs when pressure on skin within the suture loop exceeds the pressure that allows blood flow. Pressure is reduced by spreading it over a larger area of skin. Placing sutures further from the skin edge or using mattress or cruciate sutures helps to disperse pressure. Other suture patterns that help relieve tension include alternating wide and narrow bites using simple interrupted sutures, or placing far-near-near-far or far-far-near-near sutures. The standard tension relieving suture is the vertical mattress suture. A tension relieving row of vertical mattress sutures should be placed 1 to 2 cm away from the primary row of sutures apposing skin edges. The vertical mattress sutures (2-0 to 0 polypropylene or nylon) are placed while the skin is approximated with towel clamps or skin hooks before skin edge apposition with approximating sutures (e.g., 3-0 or 2-0 polypropylene or nylon). These tension relieving vertical mattress sutures can usually be removed by the third day after surgery when fibrin has stabilized the edges.

proximated. Undermining is begun at the edge of the defect at the point of maximum skin tension and continued until the edges can be apposed under tension. The wound is closed and a relaxing incision is made at the point where undermining stopped or where tension lines are observed (Fig. 13-11, *A*). The incision should begin at the point of maximum skin tension and extend as necessary to relieve excess tension. The relief incision may be made before skin closure, if necessary. A nonadherent pad is placed over the relief incisions and suture line, followed by a padded bandage. Initially the bandage should be changed every 1 or 2 days.

Multiple Punctate Relaxing Incisions

Multiple punctate relaxing incisions are small, parallel, staggered incisions made in skin adjacent to a wound to allow closure with reduced tension (Fig. 13-11, *B*). Skin around the wound is undermined and a continuous subdermal suture pattern placed. The suture is tightened starting at one end of the incision and working toward the other end. If skin edges do not appose in an area, small incisions approximately 1 cm long are made in adjacent skin on either side of the wound, approximately 1 cm from the wound. If excessive tension persists a second row of incisions may be made 0.5 cm lateral to the first row. The suture is tightened to appose wound edges; the procedure is continued along the length of the wound. Skin sutures are placed to appose the original wound. A nonadherent bandage should be placed. Bandages should be changed daily during the early stages of healing and less often as healing progresses. Tension relieving incisions heal by second intention. Multiple punctate relaxing incisions are more cosmetic than single relaxing incisions but provide less relaxation.

V-to-Y Plasty

V-to-Y plasty is a type of relaxing incision that provides an advancement flap to cover a wound. It is used to close chronic, inelastic wounds or wounds that would distort adjacent structures if closed under tension. A V-shaped incision is made adjacent to the wound (Fig. 13-11, *C*). The original wound is closed after undermining skin (Fig. 13-11, *D*). The V relief incision is closed in the shape of a Y. Closure is begun at the ends of the V until tension develops (Figure 13-11, *E*). The remainder of the relief incision is closed as the stem of the Y (Fig. 13-11, *F*).

Z Plasty

Z plasty is a technique that lengthens or relaxes an incision. The Z may be incorporated into the wound or a separate Z made adjacent to the wound to facilitate closure with less tension. The central limb of the Z is the wound or primary incision. The two arms of the Z are made the same length as the central limb (Fig. 13-11, *G*). The angles of the Z can vary between 30 and 90 degrees, but 60 degrees is advised. Larger angles give more length gain (45 degrees = 50% increase; 60 degrees = 75% increase). Length is gained along the original central limb of the Z when the flaps of the Z are transposed (Fig. 13-11, *H*). A Z-shaped incision is made with the central

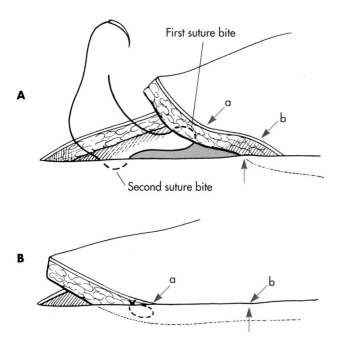

FIG. 13-9
Use walking sutures to advance skin toward the center of the wound. **A,** Place the suture through the fascia of the body wall at a distance closer to the center of the wound than the bite through the subdermal fascia or deep dermis. **B,** Note the distance from *a* to *b* increases because of skin stretching when the suture is tied.

PREVENTION OF "DOG EARS"

"Dog ears" or puckers may be prevented or corrected at the end of a suture line by unequal suture spacing or by resecting a small ellipse or triangle of skin. Placing sutures close together on the convex side of the defect and further apart on the concave side of the wound may prevent dog ears (Fig. 13-10, *A*). Dog ears may be corrected by outlining with an elliptical incision, removing redundant skin, and apposing the skin edges in a linear or curvilinear fashion (Fig. 13-10, *B*). Alternately, the dog ear may be incised in the center to form two triangles; one triangle should be excised and the other used to fill the resultant defect (Fig. 13-10, *C* and *D*), or both triangles may be excised and the edges apposed, creating a linear suture line (Fig. 13-10, *E*).

RELAXING INCISIONS

Relaxing incisions, or incisions made near a defect to allow apposition of skin edges, are beneficial in allowing skin closure around fibrotic wounds, over important structures, or before radiation therapy after extensive tumor excision. They are rarely indicated except on the legs or around the eye and anus.

Simple Relaxing Incisions

Relief incisions heal by contraction and epithelialization in 25 to 30 days. Some relaxing incisions surrounded by loose elastic tissue can be closed primarily after the wound is ap-

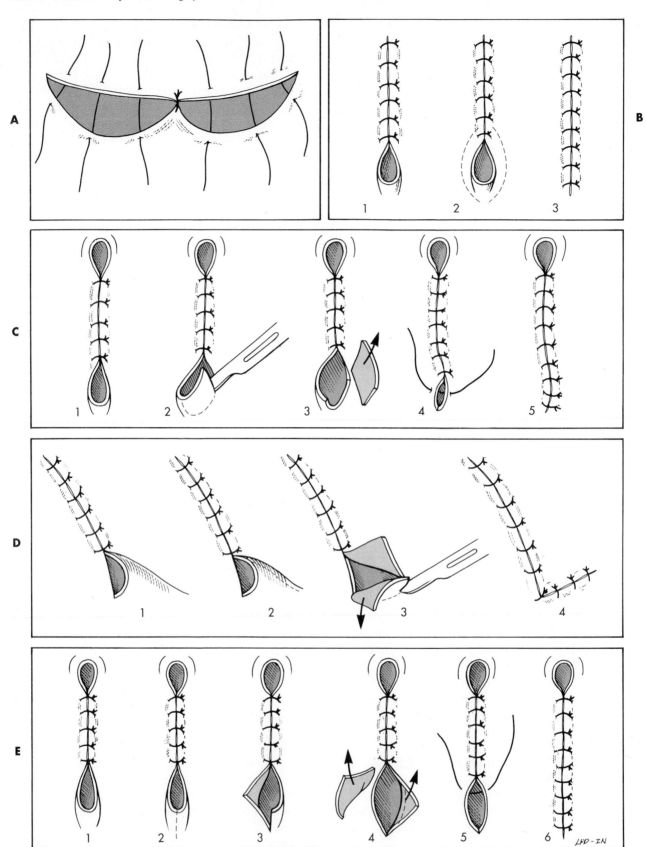

FIG. 13-10
Prevent or correct dog ears or puckers at the end of suture lines by **A,** unequal suture spacing or by **B,** resecting an elliptical segment of skin, **C,** and **D,** one large triangle, or **E,** two smaller triangles of skin.

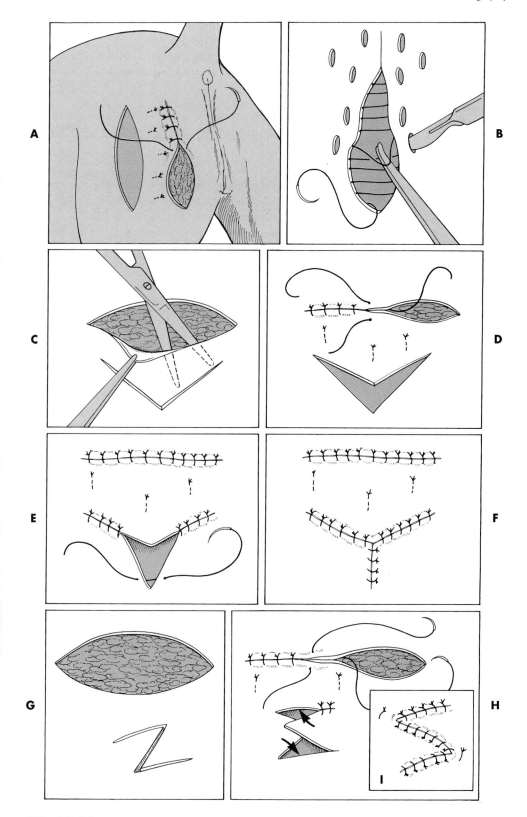

FIG. 13-11

Make relaxing incisions near the defect to allow skin apposition. **A,** Unilateral or bilateral simple relaxing incisions are made adjacent to the wound after undermining skin. **B,** Multiple punctate incisions are made parallel to the wound after preplacing a continuous subcuticular suture pattern. **C-F,** A V-Y plasty provides an advancement flap to cover the wound. **G-I,** A-Z plasty can be made adjacent to or involving the wound to allow wound closure.

arm of the Z parallel to the direction length is needed. The flaps are undermined prior to transposition and suturing (Fig. 13-11, *I*).

REMOVAL OF SKIN TUMORS

Prior to tumor removal, skin tension and elasticity should be assessed, but excessive tumor manipulation should be avoided. Direction of skin tension lines, shape of excision, and closure should be planned before surgery. A large area should be clipped and aseptically prepared for surgery, especially if there is a chance skin flaps may be necessary for closure. Excision of skin tumors should include the tumor, previous biopsy sites, and wide margins of normal tissue in three dimensions (i.e., length, width, depth). For benign tumors remove the tumor and 1 cm of normal tissue; for malignant tumors a margin of more than 2 to 3 cm may be necessary for complete local excision. Induration of the periphery of the lesion resulting from a fibroplastic host response may help identify the gross limits of the tumor. Margin width should be greater for aggressive, infiltrative tumors (i.e., mast cell tumors, melanomas, squamous cell carcinomas, soft tissue sarcomas, feline mammary adenocarcinomas, hemangiopericytomas, infiltrating lipomas). Tumor invasion is affected by the type of surrounding tissue. Tissue easily infiltrated by tumor cells (i.e., fat, subcutaneous tissue, muscle, parenchyma) should be resected with the tumor. Cartilage, tendon, ligaments, fascia, and other collagen-dense, vascular-poor tissue are resistant to neoplastic invasion; therefore these tissues are often spared during resection. Excision of infiltrative/aggressive tumors should extend at least one fascial layer below detectable tumor margins. Radical tumor excision (i.e., removal of an entire compartment or structure, amputation, lobectomy) is indicated for poorly localized tumors or those with high-grade malignancy.

All resections should be performed as atraumatically as possible and adjacent tissue protected to prevent tumor seeding. When removing multiple masses from the same animal, first remove lesions believed benign and change instruments and gloves (drapes if necessary) after removal of each mass to avoid spreading tumor cells from one site to another. Ligate the blood supply as early as possible to prevent systemic spread of tumor cells or substances (i.e., histamine, heparin). Irrigate the wound bed after tumor incision. Biopsy regional lymph nodes to stage the disease. Replace tumor contaminated (or potentially contaminated) instruments, drapes, and gloves prior to wound closure.

> ☞ **N O T E** · Submit all excised skin masses for histopathologic examination. Occasionally "benign appearing" tumors (e.g., lipomas) are actually malignant (e.g., mast cell tumors) tumors.

Tumor margins should be marked with sutures or dyes and all resected specimens submitted for histologic evaluation. Adequate fixation with 10% neutral, buffered formalin requires that specimens be not larger than 5 to 10 mm in width. The sample should be placed in approximately 10 parts of formalin to one part of tissue. Identification of tumor type is imperative in determining appropriate postoperative therapy and prognosis. The most common reason for local tumor recurrence is inadequate surgical margins.

REMOVAL OF IRREGULAR SKIN DEFECTS

Although it is advisable to remove skin lesions with an elliptical shaped skin incision to facilitate closure, some lesions result in irregular shaped defects because of their size or location. Skin elasticity and tension lines should be assessed prior to excision and closure.

Circular Defects

Circular excision of lesions saves the most normal skin when compared with other excision patterns. Skin tension lines may convert defects of other shapes into circular defects. Circular defects are difficult to close because dog ears (puckers) tend to develop. They may be closed using a variety of techniques. The linear, combined V, and bow tie techniques are preferred (Swaim, Lee, McGuire, 1984). Conversion of a circular defect by a fusiform or elliptical excision with 4:1 length to width ratios resects more skin than necessary (156%). The linear technique may be used for small defects when skin edges can be apposed without the formation of large dog ears. Sutures are placed parallel to the direction of skin tension lines, beginning at the center of the defect. Then the dog ears at each end of the suture line are excised and the remaining defects apposed (Fig. 13-12, *A*). The combined V technique is used when skin apposition results in dog ears and there is limited skin for reconstruction. This technique does not remove additional normal skin. Two equilateral triangles are designed on opposite sides of the circular defect with the central axis 45 degrees from the long axis (tension lines) of the defect. The sides of each triangle are incised so the vertex of the V is pointing to the longitudinal axis of the defect. The skin flaps are rotated and sutured to convert the circular defect into a smaller irregular fusiform defect. The edges of the converted defect are apposed with approximating sutures (Fig. 13-12, *B*). The bow tie technique is used when skin apposition results in large dog ears and there is abundant skin surrounding the defect. This technique removes 36% additional skin. Two equilateral triangles are removed from opposite sides of the circular defect, with the central axis of each triangle 30 degrees from the long axis of the skin tension lines. The flaps are transposed and sutured into their new positions to shorten the sides of the original circle and transform the shape of the defect (Fig. 13-12, *C*).

Triangular Defects

Triangular lesions may be closed by shifting local tissues or rotating flaps. A simple closure technique is to begin at each point of the triangle and suture toward the center of the defect to create a Y-shaped suture line (Fig. 13-13, *A*). A rotational flap is a semicircular or three-quarter–circular flap of

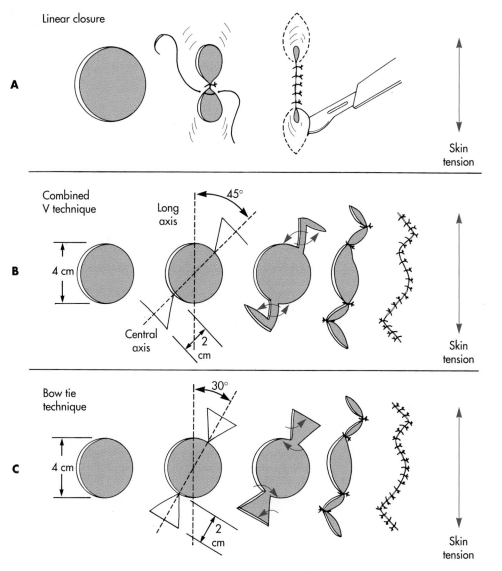

Linear closure

A

Combined V technique

B

4 cm

Long axis

45°

Central axis

2 cm

Skin tension

Bow tie technique

C

4 cm

30°

2 cm

Skin tension

FIG. 13-12
A, To close small circular defects use a linear closure if skin edges can be apposed without creating large dog ears. **B,** Use a combined V technique when there is limited skin for reconstruction and **C,** a bow-tie technique when there is abundant skin.

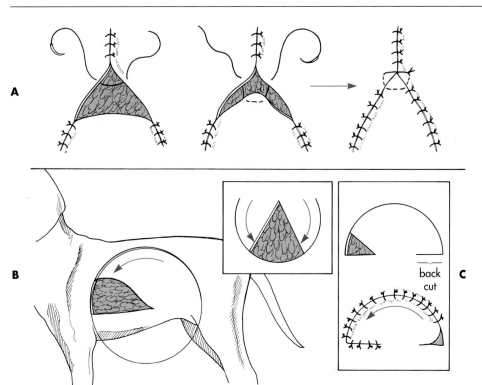

A

B

C

back cut

FIG. 13-13
A, To repair triangular defects close the defect as a Y by beginning at each point and suturing toward the center, **B,** or create one or two rotational flaps at the defect edge. **C,** A backcut or excision of Bürow's triangle may be needed to relieve tension at the flap base.

skin that is rotated about a pivot point into the defect (Fig. 13-13, *B*). Rotational flaps are used when there is skin available on only one side of the defect or when moving skin from one side of the defect results in distortion of adjacent structures (i.e., near eye or anus). Bilateral rotational flaps are used when there is little moveable skin but it is moveable on two sides of the defect. Flaps should be sufficiently large (about 4:1) to avoid tension on surrounding tissue. If tension is noted, a backcut into the base of the flap may ease tension and allow the flap to move by a combination of rotation and transposition (Fig. 13-13, *C*). Tension may also be relieved by removing a small triangle of skin (Bürow's triangle) at the end of the semicircle opposite the defect.

Square and Rectangular Defects

Square or rectangular defects may be closed using centripetal, unilateral, or bilateral advancement flaps, or rotational flaps. Centripetal closure begins with suture closure at each corner of the defect and advances toward the center to form an X suture line (Fig. 13-14, *A*). This technique should be used when skin is available on all four sides of the defect. A unilateral or single pedicle advancement flap should be used to close defects with mobile skin on only one side and in the same plane as the defect. Parallel incisions are made from two corners of the defect at least as long as the width of the defect. Skin is undermined and advanced over the defect (Fig. 13-14, *B*). If necessary, relaxing incisions are made at the base of the flap. An H-plasty or a double pedicle advancement flap is used to close large defects that have mobile skin available on two sides of the defect (Fig. 13-14, *C*). A rotational or transposition flap is used to cover defects that have mobile skin on only one side of the defect and available skin in a different plane than the defect (Fig. 13-14, *D*). These flaps become effectively shorter with increasing rotation. They should be longer than the size of the defect to achieve adequate coverage without tension. The width of the base of the flap should at least equal the width of the defect. The diagonal from the pivot point of the flap to the farthest corner of the defect should be equal to the diagonal from the flap's pivot point across the flap. A dog ear forms at the base of the flap opposite the pivot point.

Fusiform Defects

Fusiform or elliptical defects are closed by first placing a suture across the widest part of the defect. Continue to divide each remaining segment in half with subsequent sutures to achieve a linear closure without dog ears (Fig. 13-15).

☞ **N O T E** • Fusiform incisions are generally the easiest to close. Place the long axis of the incision parallel to skin tension lines.

Crescent Defects

Crescent-shaped defects have one side longer than the other. These defects are closed beginning at the midpoint. Each remaining segment is divided in half with subsequent sutures, while spacing sutures on the convex side closer together than sutures on the concave side. Dog ears are removed as needed (Fig. 13-16).

References

Swaim SF, Lee AH, McGuire JA: Techniques for reconstructing circular skin defects in dogs, *Vet Surg* 13:18, 1984.

Suggested Reading

Harari J: *Surgical complications and wound healing in the small animal practice,* Philadelphia, 1993, WB Saunders.
Pavletic MM: Plastic and reconstructive surgery, *Vet Clinics of N Am (Sm Anim)* 20: 67, 1990.
Swaim SF, Henderson RA: *Small animal wound management,* Philadelphia, 1990, Lea & Febiger.
Swaim SF, Henderson RA, Sutton HH: Correction of triangular and wedge shaped skin defects in dogs and cats, *J Am Anim Hosp Assoc* 16:225, 1980.

PEDICLE FLAPS

Pedicle flaps are "tongues" of epidermis and dermis that are partially detached from donor sites and used to cover defects. The base or pedicle of the flap contains the blood supply essential for flap survival. Pedicle flaps often allow immediate coverage of a wound bed and avoid prolonged healing, excessive scarring, and contracture associated with second intention healing. They can be classified in various ways based on location, blood supply, and tissue formation. A specific flap may be classified in more than one way. Most flaps are called *subdermal plexus flaps;* however, those with direct cutaneous vessels are termed *axial pattern flaps.* Flaps that remain attached to the donor bed by only the direct cutaneous vessels and subcutaneous tissues are *island flaps.* Flaps created adjacent to the defect in loose elastic skin are *local flaps.* Those created at a distance from the defect are *distant flaps* and usually require multiple stage reconstruction. Flaps that include tissue other than skin and subcutaneous tissue are termed *compound* or *composite flaps* and may include muscle (myocutaneous), cartilage, or bone.

Increasing the width of a pedicle flap does not increase the surviving length of the flap. However, narrowing the base of the pedicle by backcut techniques increases the possibility of necrosis. The base of flaps should be slightly wider than the width of the flap body. Multiple small flaps may be preferable to large flaps if circulation is questionable. Delaying flap transfer 18 to 21 days after initial creation may improve circulation and survival in ischemic flaps (delay phenomenon). Donor sites should have enough skin to permit primary closure and skin transfer to the recipient site. Donor sites with excessive motion and stress should be avoided. Reconstruction should be planned so that the color and direction of hair growth after transfer of flaps or grafts to the recipient site is similar to that of the donor site.

Hyperbaric oxygen treatment may improve flap or graft survival. Hyperbaric oxygen treatment consists of breathing

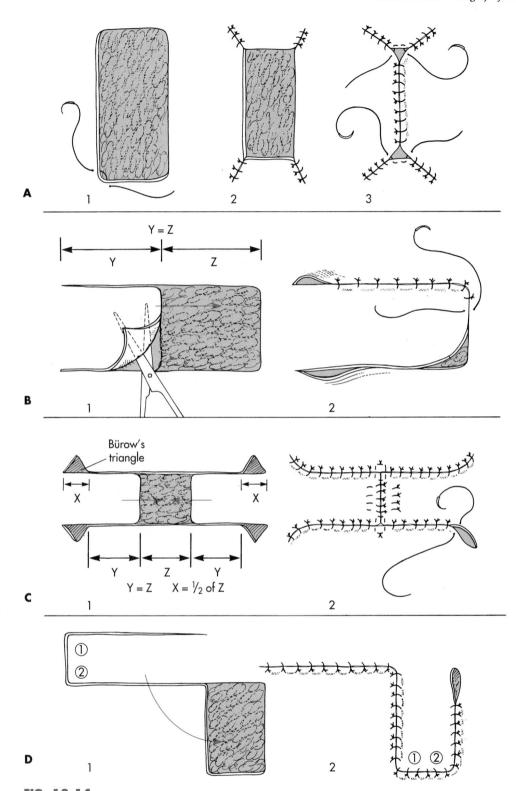

FIG. 13-14
A, To repair square or rectangular defects close from the corners and advance to the center to form an X suture line. **B,** Use a unilateral or **C,** bilateral advancement flap to close defects with mobile skin on only one or two sides of the defect. **D,** Use a rotational or transposition flap to cover defects with mobile skin in a different plane than the defect.

FIG. 13-15
Close fusiform defects (*1*) by placing the first suture across the widest part of the wound. Continue to divide each segment of the defect in half with subsequent sutures (*2* and *3*).

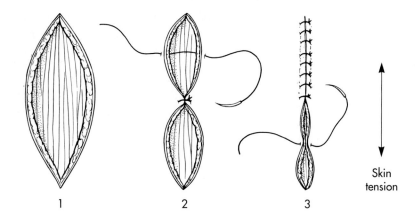

Skin tension

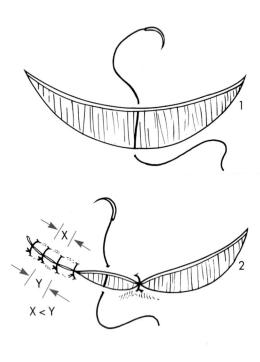

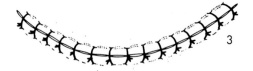

FIG. 13-16
Close crescent defects by (*1*) beginning at the midpoint and dividing each segment of the defect in half with subsequent sutures (*2* and *3*). Space sutures closer on the convex than the concave aspect of the defect.

100% oxygen in a chamber where pressure is maintained at greater than 1 atm absolute or greater than sea level pressure. Hyperbaric oxygen therapy hyperoxygenates hypoxic tissue, stimulates fibroblasts, and enhances tissue revascularization.

Venous congestion in a flap may be suspected if the flap becomes dusky or bluish in color, capillary return is quicker than normal, and rapid or dark bleeding occurs in response to a needle prick. Venous congestion may lead to failure of flaps and grafts.

ADVANCEMENT FLAPS

Advancement flaps are local subdermal plexus flaps. They include single pedicle, bipedicle, and V-Y advancement flaps (see Figs. 13-11, 13-13, and 13-14). Flaps are formed in adjacent, loose, elastic skin that can be slid over the defect. An advancement flap is developed parallel to lines of least tension to facilitate its forward stretch over a wound. Advancement flap stretching is opposed by retractive forces that may lead to dehiscence.

ROTATIONAL FLAPS

Rotational flaps are local flaps that are pivoted over a defect with which they share a common border. They are semicircular in shape and may be paired or single. They may be used to close triangular defects without creating a secondary defect. A curved incision is created and undermined in a stepwise fashion until it covers the defect without tension (see Fig. 13-13).

TRANSPOSITION FLAPS

Transposition flaps are rectangular, local flaps that bring additional skin when rotated into defects. A Z-plasty is a modified transposition flap (see Fig. 13-11, *G-I*). Ninety-degree transposition flaps are aligned parallel to the lines of greatest tension to obtain the bulk of the flap required to cover the defect. The donor site is easily closed because minimal tension lines are perpendicular to the suture line. The width of the flap equals the width of the defect (Fig. 13-14, *D*). Flap length is determined by measuring from the pivot point of the flap to the most distant point of the defect. Flap length decreases in length as the arc of rotation increases past 90 degrees because of kinking and skin folding. Dog ears occur but flatten with time.

POUCH AND HINGE FLAPS

Pouch flaps (bipedicle flaps) and hinge flaps (single pedicle flaps) are direct, distant flaps useful for reconstructing lower extremity skin defects. Reconstruction using the pouch or hinge flap requires three stages: (1) debridement and granulation, (2) flap creation and healing, and (3) flap release. After a healthy bed of granulation tissue has formed, the skin on the limb and ipsilateral thoracoabdominal area is prepared for aseptic surgery. The limb is positioned along the animal's side and two parallel dorsoventral incisions are made at locations that allow complete coverage of the defect (Fig. 13-17, *A*). If pad tissue is absent only a single cranial incision is necessary. The flap is undermined and the foot placed within the pouch. Skin at the wound edges is apposed with the edges of the flap using interrupted approximating sutures (e.g., 3-0 or 4-0 polypropylene or nylon). Three to four interrupted sutures are placed through the skin of the flap into the granulation tissue to immobilize the flap over the defect. The limb is bandaged against the body for 14 days and the bandage changed every 3 to 4 days. The limb is released from the pouch by making two horizontal incisions (dorsal and ventral) an appropriate distance from the paw to allow coverage of the palmar aspect of the defect (Fig.

13-17, *B*). The medial aspect of the paw is lavaged to remove exudate and is debrided if necessary. The ends of the skin flap are trimmed and sutured in place. The donor site is lavaged and closed with interrupted approximating sutures (e.g., 3-0 to 4-0 polypropylene or nylon) (Fig. 13-17, *C*). Although this technique is successful in covering distal extremity skin defects, some animals may not tolerate the limb being positioned against the body wall; plus it causes temporary joint stiffness.

TUBED PEDICLE FLAPS

A tubed pedicle flap uses a multistaged procedure to "walk" an indirect, distant flap to a recipient site. The tube is made wider and longer (2 to 3 cm) than the recipient bed because these tubes contract as a result of decreased elasticity and fibrosis before transfer. The tube is created by making two parallel incisions through the skin in an area where remaining skin can be reapposed without excess tension (Fig. 13-18, *A*). Skin is undermined between

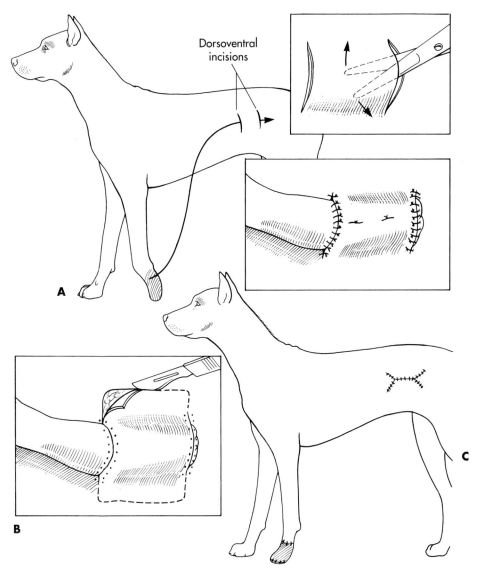

Dorsoventral incisions

A

B

C

FIG. 13-17
A, For a pouch flap make two parallel dorsoventral incisions and undermine skin to create a pouch. Position the limb inside the pouch and suture the edges of the defect to the flap. **B,** After 2 to 3 weeks, release the limb and cover the remainder of the defect. Make two horizontal incisions to free the flap, then suture it to the remaining edges of the defect. **C,** Close the donor site.

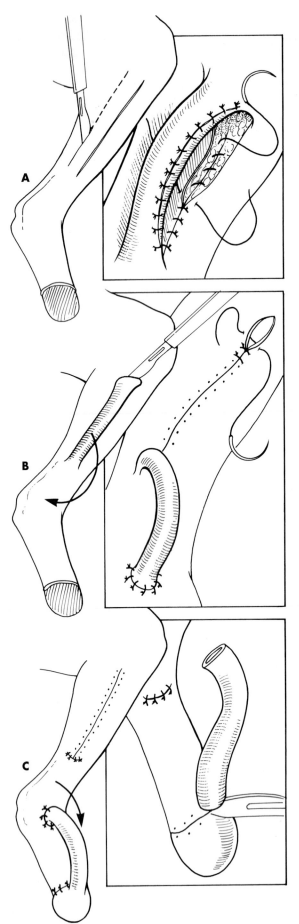

the two incisions. The incised edges of the flap are sutured together with approximating sutures (e.g., 3-0 or 4-0 polypropylene or nylon) creating a tube attached at both ends. Edges of the donor site are apposed with approximating sutures (e.g., 3-0 or 4-0 nylon or polypropylene). After 18 to 21 days one end of the tube is transected and transposed to the recipient bed. Alternatively, the end of the tube nearer the donor site may be transposed and after an additional 18 to 21 days the other end of the tube is transected and transposed over the defect (Fig. 13-18, *B*). The tube is incised and unrolled as needed to cover the defect and the edges of the tube are sutured to the edges of the defect (Fig. 13-18, *C*). Skin edges at the tube's origin are apposed. The remaining end of the tube is transected after 18 to 21 days to complete coverage of the defect if necessary. The disadvantage of this technique is the number of stages and time required to accomplish wound closure.

AXIAL PATTERN FLAPS

Axial pattern flaps are pedicle flaps that include a direct cutaneous artery and vein at their base. The terminal branches of these vessels supply the subdermal plexus. They have better perfusion than pedicle flaps whose circulation is from the subdermal plexus alone. Axial pattern flaps are elevated and transferred to cutaneous defects within their radius. They are usually rectangular or L-shaped flaps. Axial pattern flaps have been described using the caudal auricular artery branches, omocervical artery, thoracodorsal artery, superficial brachial artery, caudal superficial epigastric artery, deep circumflex iliac, genicular artery, and lateral caudal arteries as direct cutaneous arteries in dogs (Fig. 13-19). Although similar flaps can be created in cats, only the thoracodorsal and caudal superficial epigastric axial pattern flaps have been evaluated. Axial pattern flaps require careful planning, measuring, and mapping on the skin surface to minimize errors. Axial pattern flaps can be modified to create island arterial flaps by severing the cutaneous pedicle but preserving the direct cutaneous artery and vein. Island flaps have the potential for use as a free flap for transfer and microvascular anastomosis.

Axial pattern flaps are used most commonly to facilitate wound closure following tumor resection or trauma. Flap survival of axial pattern flaps is approximately twice the survival rate of subdermal plexus flaps of comparable size. Axial pattern flaps also provide durable, full-thickness skin that can be transposed primarily without the need for a vascular bed or postoperative immobilization. Complications include wound drainage, partial dehiscence, distal flap necrosis, infections, and seroma formation. Cosmetic results are good.

FIG. 13-18
A, For a tubed pedicle flap make two parallel incisions in mobile skin. Create a tube by suturing the edges together and appose the donor site. *Note:* The tube may need to be created more proximally on the limb than illustrated in order to have sufficiently mobile skin to close the donor site defect. **B,** Approximately 3 weeks later advance the tube toward the defect by severing one end of the tube and suturing it nearer the defect. **C,** After another 3 weeks sever the other end of the tube and use it to cover the defect or advance it closer to the defect.

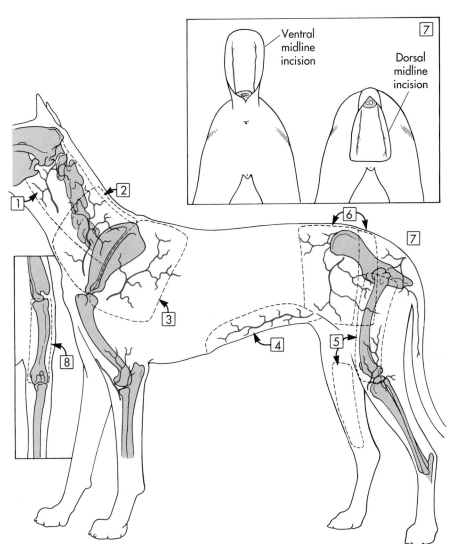

FIG. 13-19
Direct cutaneous vessels used in axial pattern flaps. *1*, Caudal auricular; *2*, omocervical; *3*, thoracodorsal; *4*, caudal superficial epigastric; *5*, medial genicular; *6*, deep circumflex iliac; *7*, superficial lateral caudal (*inset*); and *8*, superficial brachial (*inset*). *Dashed lines* outline anticipated flaps corresponding with each direct cutaneous vessel.

Caudal Auricular Axial Pattern Flap

The sternocleidomastoideus branches of the caudal auricular artery and vein may be used to reconstruct defects involving the head and neck. The sternocleidomastoideus branches are located between the lateral aspect of the wing of the atlas and the vertical ear canal and are directed caudodorsally. *Outline the flap with the base centered over the lateral aspect of the wing of the atlas (see Fig. 13-19). Draw a caudal incision line parallel to the base at a point rostral to the scapular spine. Then draw dorsal and ventral lines that connect the base and the caudal incision line at a width that allows donor site closure. Incise the dorsal, ventral, and caudal lines and elevate the flap deep to the platysma muscle until the sternocleidomastoideus branches of the caudal auricular artery are identified. Rotate the flap into the defect, place drains, and appose skin edges.*

Omocervical Axial Pattern Flap

Omocervical axial pattern flaps are used for defects involving the face, head, ear, shoulder, neck, and axilla. They incorporate the superficial cervical branch of the omocervical artery and associated vein. Vessels originate adjacent to the prescapular lymph node at a site corresponding to the cranial shoulder depression and course dorsally just cranial to the scapula. *Position the patient in lateral recumbency with the forelimb in relaxed extension perpendicular to the trunk. Draw a line over the scapular spine to identify the caudal incision. Draw the cranial incision line parallel to the scapular spine at a site equal to the distance between the scapular spine and the cranial shoulder depression at the cranial edge of the scapula. Extend the lines to and continue along the dorsal midline. Extend the flap to the contralateral scapulohumeral joint if necessary. Incise the outlined flap and undermine deep to the sphincter coli superficialis muscle. Transpose the flap. Eliminate dead space with Penrose or closed suction drains and close the defects.*

Thoracodorsal Axial Pattern Flap

Thoracodorsal axial pattern flaps are used to cover defects involving the shoulder, forelimb, elbow, axilla, and thorax (Fig. 13-20). In cats the thoracodorsal flap extends to the

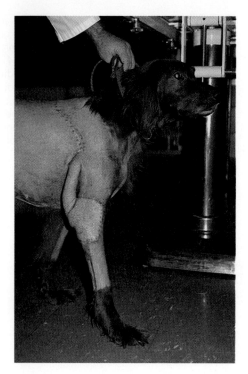

FIG. 13-20
A thoracodorsal axial pattern flap has been tubed and applied over an elbow wound.

carpus. It is based on a cutaneous branch of the thoracodorsal artery and associated vein located at the caudal shoulder depression at a level parallel to the dorsal border of the acromion. *Position the patient in lateral recumbency with the forelimb in relaxed extension perpendicular to the trunk. Outline the flap by drawing a line over the scapular spine to mark the cranial incision (see Fig. 13-19). Draw the caudal incision line parallel to the scapular spine at a site approximately twice the distance from the acromion to the caudal shoulder depression. Extend the lines to and continue along the dorsal midline. Flaps extended ventral to the contralateral scapulohumeral joint usually survive. Create an L flap for extended coverage by extending the dorsal incision line by about 50% and creating a parallel incision line beginning at the approximate midpoint of the caudal incision line. Incise the outlined flap and undermine deep to the cutaneous trunci muscle. Transpose the flap. Create a tube as needed for distant transposition. Eliminate dead space with Penrose or closed suction drains and close the defects.*

Superficial Brachial Axial Pattern Flaps

Superficial brachial axial pattern flaps are used to cover defects involving the antebrachium and elbow. These flaps depend on a small branch of the brachial artery located 3 cm proximal to the elbow (superficial brachial artery). *Position the patient in dorsal recumbency with the leg suspended in an elevated position. Outline the flap by drawing parallel to the humeral shaft two lines that extend dorsally and*

gradually converge at or below the greater tubercle. Center the base of the flap over the anterior third of the flexor surface of the elbow. Elevate the flap to the base, being especially careful to preserve the subdermal plexus, superficial brachial vessels, and cephalic vein. Rotate the flap into the defect, place drains, and appose skin edges.

Caudal Superficial Epigastric Axial Pattern Flap

The caudal superficial epigastric axial pattern flap is a versatile flap that is used to cover defects involving the caudal abdomen, flank, prepuce, perineum, thigh, and hind leg. In cats the flap extends over the metatarsal area. The flap includes the three to four caudal mammary glands and is supplied by the caudal superficial epigastric artery and associated vein that pass through the inguinal ring. *Position the patient in dorsal recumbency. Outline the flap with the ventral midline as the location of the medial incision. Incorporate the base of the prepuce in the male dog. Mark a parallel lateral incision at a distance equal the distance of the mammary teats to the midline. Determine the number of mammary glands to include in the flap based on the size of the defect. Create the flap by connecting the two parallel lines between the first and second or second and third glands with a crescent shaped incision. Undermine the flap at the level of the external abdominal oblique aponeurosis, deep to the supramammarius muscle. Make the flap wider as needed to cover the defect if there is abundant skin for closure. Transpose the flap, place drains, and appose skin edges.*

☞ **N O T E** • When used for limb defects, these flaps result in mammary tissue being transposed to the leg. The mammary tissue may remain functional.

Deep Circumflex Iliac Axial Pattern Flap

The dorsal branch of the deep circumflex iliac vessel is used in flaps to cover defects involving the caudal thorax, lateral abdominal wall, ipsilateral flank, lateral lumbar area, medial or lateral thigh, greater trochanter, and pelvic area. The dorsal and ventral branches of the deep circumflex iliac artery originate at a point cranioventral to the wing of the ilium. *Position the patient in lateral recumbency with the hind limb in relaxed extension perpendicular to the body. Outline the flap by first drawing a line midway between the cranial border of the wing of the ilium and the greater trochanter. For the cranial incision draw a second line parallel to the first line and equal to the distance between the iliac border and the caudal line. Extend the lines to the dorsal midline and create an L extension if needed to cover the defect (see Fig. 13-19). Elevate the flaps below the level of the cutaneous trunci muscle. Incise the outlined flap. Transpose the flap, place drains, and appose skin edges.*

The ventral branch of the deep circumflex iliac artery is used in flaps to cover defects of the lateral abdominal wall and as an island flap for pelvic and sacral defects. *Make the reference lines as for the previous flap. Draw the caudal in-*

cision line extending distally cranial to the border of the femoral shaft. Extend the cranial incision line down the flank/thigh region, parallel to the caudal flap border. Connect the two lines above the patella. Elevate the flaps below the level of the cutaneous trunci muscle. Incise the outlined flap. Transpose the flap, place drains, and appose skin edges.

Genicular Axial Pattern Flaps

Genicular axial pattern flaps are used to cover defects involving the lateral and medial tibia and potentially the tibiotarsal joint. These flaps are dependent on the short genicular branch of the saphenous artery and medial saphenous vein. *Position the patient in lateral recumbency. Mark a point 1 cm proximal to the patella and 1.5 cm distal to the tibial tuberosity (see Fig. 13-19). Extend these two points dorsally parallel to the femoral shaft ending at the base of the greater trochanter. Connect the parallel lines dorsally. Incise the outlined flap. Elevate the flap and rotate it to cover the defect. Place drains and appose skin edges.*

Reverse Saphenous Conduit Flaps

Reverse saphenous conduit flaps are used for defects at or below the tarsus. They are created by ligating and dividing the vascular connection between the femoral artery and vein and the saphenous artery and medial saphenous vein. Reverse blood flow occurs because of anastomoses between the cranial branch of the saphenous artery and the perforating metatarsal artery (via medial and lateral plantar arteries), cranial branch of the lateral saphenous vein, and other venous connections with the cranial and caudal branches of the medial saphenous veins distal to the tibiotarsal joint. Preoperative angiography ensures the presence and function of the saphenous artery, medial saphenous vein, and femoral artery and vein. *Position the patient in lateral recumbency with the affected limb down. Roughly outline the flap by marking a line across the central third of the inner thigh at or slightly above the level of the patella. Make parallel lines 0.5 to 1.0 cm cranial and caudal to the branches of the saphenous artery and medial saphenous vein. Make the transverse incision as marked to expose the saphenous vessels and nerve. Ligate and transect the saphenous artery and medial saphenous vein at their junction with the femoral artery and vein. Extend the incisions distally as marked in a slightly converging fashion. Undermine deep to the saphenous vessels by elevating a portion of the medial gastrocnemius muscle fascia with the flap. Ligate and divide the peroneal (fibular) artery and vein. Do not elevate the flap beyond the anastomosis between the cranial branch of the medial saphenous vein and the cranial branch of the lateral saphenous vein. Rotate or partially tube the pedicle transfer to the defect. Place drains and appose the defects.*

Lateral Caudal Axial Pattern Flap

The lateral caudal arteries of the tail may be used to reconstruct areas involving caudodorsal trunk defects. The tail skin may also be used as a tube flap to cover defects on the hind leg. The lateral caudal vessels are bilateral and located in the subcutaneous tissue of the tail. The lateral caudal arteries arise from the caudal gluteal arteries and have several anastomotic branches with the median caudal artery. Use of this flap requires tail amputation. *Make a dorsal midline incision along the length of the tail to cover dorsocaudal defects (see Fig. 13-19). Make a ventral midline skin incision to cover defects on the hind leg. Dissect the subcutaneous tissues from the deep caudal fascia, preserving the right and left lateral caudal arteries and veins. Amputate the tail at the third or fourth caudal intervertebral space (see p. 144). Transpose the skin flap over the defect, place drains, and appose skin edges.*

Suggested Reading

Harari J: *Surgical complications and wound healing in the small animal practice,* Philadelphia, 1993, WB Saunders.

Henney LHS, Pavletic MM: Axial pattern flap based on the superficial brachial artery in the dog, *Vet Surg* 17:311, 1988.

Kerwin SC et al: The effect of hyperbaric oxygen treatment on a compromised axial pattern flap in the cat, *Vet Surg* 22:31, 1993.

Kostolich M, Pavletic MM: Axial pattern flap based on the genicular branch of the saphenous artery in the dog, *Vet Surg* 16:217, 1987

Pavletic MM: Canine axial pattern flaps, using the omocervical, thoracodorsal, and deep circumflex iliac direct cutaneous arteries, *Am J Vet Res* 42:391, 1981.

Pavletic MM: Caudal superficial epigastric arterial pedicle grafts in dogs, *Vet Surg* 9:103, 1980.

Pavletic MM: Plastic and reconstructive surgery, *Vet Clinics of N Am (Sm Anim)* 20:105, 1990.

Pavletic MM et al: Reverse saphenous conduit flap in the dog, *J Am Vet Med Assoc* 182:380, 1983.

Remedios AM, Bauer MS, Bowen CV: Thoracodorsal and caudal superficial epigastric axial pattern skin flaps in cats, *Vet Surg* 18:380, 1989.

Smith MM et al: Direct cutaneous arterial supply to the tail in dogs, *Am J Vet Res* 53:145, 1992.

Smith MM et al: Axial pattern flap based on the caudal auricular artery in dogs, *Am J Vet Res* 52:922, 1991.

Swaim SF, Henderson RA: *Small animal wound management,* Philadelphia, 1990, Lea & Febiger.

Trevor PB et al: Clinical evaluation of axial pattern skin flaps in dogs and cats: 19 cases (1981-1990), *J Am Vet Med Assoc* 201:608, 1992.

MYOCUTANEOUS AND MUSCLE FLAPS

Muscle flaps with overlying skin (myocutaneous flaps) or without skin (muscle flaps) may be created to facilitate herniorrhaphy, cover soft tissue defects, contribute circulation to fractures, and combat infection. They should only be used when reconstruction with local flaps (see p. 116), axial pattern flaps (see p. 120), or free grafts (see p. 128) is not feasible. These flaps must be sufficiently large to cover the defect and have an easily accessible and constant dominant vascular supply. Donor sites should be easily closed. Muscles in dogs and cats that may be sacrificed without loss of function include cutaneous trunci, gracilis, trapezius, sternohyoideus, sternothyroideus, deep pectoral, anconeus, ulnaris lateralis, ulnar head of flexor carpi ulnaris, sartorius, semitendinosus, rectus femoris, cranial tibial, long digital extensor, and portions of the latissimus dorsi.

MYOCUTANEOUS FLAPS

Myocutaneous flaps described in the veterinary literature include latissimus dorsi, cutaneous trunci, gracilis, and trapezius muscles. These muscles are superficial, allowing easy access and elevation, and have direct cutaneous arteries exiting the muscle surface to supply overlying skin. A vascular pedicle sufficient to maintain circulation is required to facilitate flap rotation into defects. Increased rotation may impair circulation and require that the flap length be reduced. Distant transfer of gracilis and some trapezius flaps is possible with microvascular anastomosis.

Latissimus Dorsi Myocutaneous Flap

The latissimus dorsi muscle is a flat, triangular muscle overlying the dorsal half of the lateral thoracic wall. It originates from thoracolumbar fascia of the thoracic and lumbar spinous processes and from muscular attachments to the last two or three ribs. The aponeurosis of the latissimus dorsi inserts on the major teres tuberosity of the humerus. The muscle flexes the shoulder, drawing the limb caudally. The ventral portion of the muscle is supplied by branches of the thoracodorsal artery (dorsal and lateral thoracic arteries) that penetrate the muscle and supply the cutaneous trunci muscle and skin. Intercostal arteries supply segmental branches to the dorsal portion of the latissimus dorsi muscle and overlying cutaneous trunci muscle. Latissimus dorsi myocutaneous flaps are bulky because they contain the cutaneous trunci muscle and skin, subcutaneous fat, and latissimus dorsi muscle. They are best suited for thoracic defects, although they may be used for forelimb defects. Anatomic landmarks are the ventral border of the acromion, adjacent caudal border of the triceps muscle, head of the last rib, and distal third of the humerus that corresponds to the axillary skin fold (Fig. 13-21).

Plan and outline the flap with a marking pen with the patient in lateral recumbency and the forelimb placed in relaxed extension perpendicular to the trunk. Draw parallel lines caudodorsally and connect them to outline the flap. Incise skin and extend the incision through the underlying latissimus dorsi muscle. The muscle flap equals the size of the skin flap. Elevate the latissimus dorsi and skin as a unit. Isolate, ligate, and divide the lateral intercostal vessels deep to the latissimus muscle. Identify and preserve the thoracodorsal artery and vein. Transpose the flap to the desired location without occluding the thoracodorsal vessels. Place Penrose or closed suction drains at the donor site and beneath the flap at the recipient site. Secure the flap in position and close the donor site.

Cutaneous Trunci Myocutaneous Flap

The cutaneous trunci muscle arises from the pectoralis profundus and forms a thin leaf covering most of the dorsal, lateral, and ventral walls of the abdomen (see Fig. 13-21). It is more closely associated with skin than underlying structures. Blood supply is from small muscular branches and direct cutaneous arteries supplying the overlying skin. The cutaneous

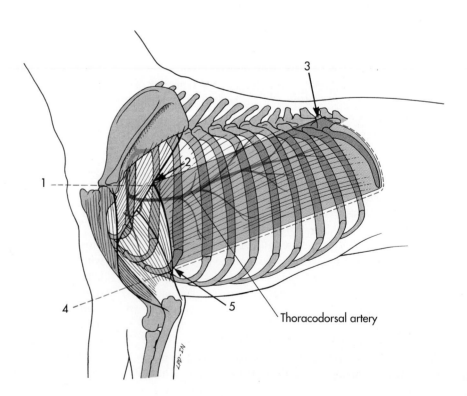

FIG. 13-21
Landmarks for the latissimus dorsi and cutaneous trunci myocutaneous flaps include: *1*, ventral border of the acromion; *2*, adjacent caudal border of the triceps muscle; *3*, vertebral attachment of last rib; *4*, distal third of the humerus; and *5*, axillary skin fold. Draw a line from *2* to *3* and a second, parallel line from *5*. Connect the two parallel lines dorsally.

Thoracodorsal artery

trunci overlying the latissimus dorsi muscle receives two to four short direct cutaneous branches of the thoracodorsal artery caudal to the border of the triceps muscle. Elevating the cutaneous trunci muscle with skin helps preserve the subdermal plexus. Cutaneous trunci myocutaneous flaps are more pliable and elastic than latissimus dorsi myocutaneous flaps and are preferred for forelimb flaps. *Plan and outline the flap the same as for a latissimus dorsi myocutaneous flap. Incise the skin as outlined but do not extend the incision beyond subcutaneous tissue between the cutaneous trunci and latissimus dorsi. Elevate the cutaneous trunci by dissecting the loose subcutaneous tissue. Ligate and divide branches of the proximal lateral intercostal direct cutaneous vessels. Transpose the flap to its desired location without occluding the thoracodorsal vessels. Place Penrose or closed suction drains beneath the flap at recipient and donor sites. Secure the flap in position and close the donor site.*

Trapezius Osteomyocutaneous Flap

Trapezius osteomyocutaneous flaps are generally used for defects in the neck, cranial thorax, or proximal thoracic limb; however, they may be transferred to distant sites with microvascular anastomosis. The trapezius is a thin, triangular muscle divided into cervical and thoracic parts. The cervical part of the trapezius is overlapped by the cleidocervicalis

muscle and the thoracic part by the latissimus dorsi muscle. The muscle originates from the median raphe of the neck and supraspinous ligament from the level of the third cervical vertebra to the ninth thoracic vertebra and inserts on the scapular spine. It acts to elevate and abduct the forelimb. Lameness and scapular fractures may occur when this flap is used. Only the scapular spine and not the scapular body remains viable. The bone in this flap is weak and should be used as a source of osteogenesis rather than support. Dorsal, caudal, and cranioventral borders of the flap are 2 cm ventral to the dorsal midline, 2 cm caudal to the scapular spine, and a line between the acromion and transverse process of the third cervical vertebra, respectively.

Make a triangular skin incision over the cervical part of the trapezius muscle (Fig. 13-22). Incise the origin of the cervical part of the trapezius on the dorsal midline. Dissect the incised trapezius from the cleidocervicalis and omotransversarius muscles, preserving the attachment to the scapular spine and the prescapular branch of the superficial cervical vascular pedicle. Dissect the caudal half of the supraspinatus muscle from its attachment on the scapular spine and body. Incise the deltoideus and thoracic part of the trapezius attachments to the scapular spine. Dissect the cranial half of the infraspinatus from the scapular spine

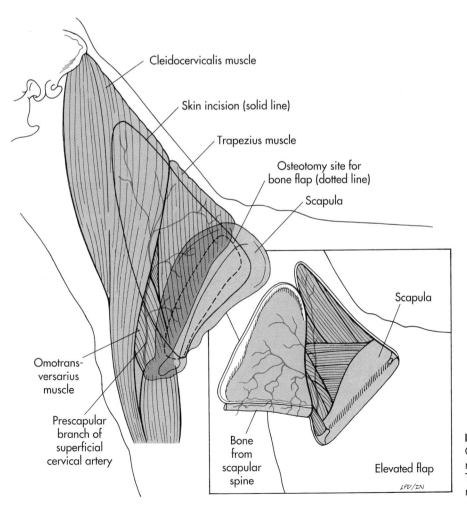

Cleidocervicalis muscle

Skin incision (solid line)

Trapezius muscle

Osteotomy site for bone flap (dotted line)

Scapula

Scapula

Omotransversarius muscle

Prescapular branch of superficial cervical artery

Bone from scapular spine

Elevated flap

LPD/IN

FIG. 13-22
Outlined trapezius osteomyocutaneous flap for regional reconstruction. The inset shows the flap ready for relocation.

and body. Create a bone flap using an air-powered burr or saw. Dissect the medial attachments of the subscapularis and serratus ventralis muscles from the bone flap. Elevate the osteomusculocutaneous flap and transfer it to the recipient site, preserving the prescapular branch of the superficial cervical vascular pedicle. Place a Penrose drain at the donor site and close the defect with approximating sutures (i.e., muscle—2-0 or 3-0 polydioxanone or polyglyconate; subcutaneous tissue—3-0 or 4-0 polydioxanone or polyglyconate; skin—3-0 or 4-0 nylon or polypropylene). Apply a bandage over the donor and recipient sites for support and fluid absorption.

MUSCLE FLAPS

Muscle flaps may be transposed beneath skin to fill defects, repair hernias, and treat paralysis. Many muscles have been used to facilitate adjacent visceral repair and to fill defects. Use of muscle in reconstruction is limited by availability and the surgeon's imagination. The latissimus dorsi may be used with or without a cutaneous flap to cover thoracic wall defects (see above). The muscle flap may be used with mesh or other implants to give support and is sutured to adjacent muscle or fascial planes. Diaphragmatic hernia repair has been facilitated by using the transversus abdominis muscle. The internal obturator, superficial gluteal, and semitendinosus muscles have been used in perineal hernia repair (see p. 353). Esophageal repair may be facilitated by use of intercostal, diaphragm, sternocephalicus, or sternothyroideus muscles (see p. 238). Biceps femoris or deep gluteal muscle flaps are sometimes used to cushion the femoral head and neck osteotomy site (see p. 948).

External Abdominal Oblique Muscle Flap

The external abdominal oblique muscle is elastic and mobile and may be used to facilitate repair of defects in the abdominal wall or caudal thoracic wall. This flap may be used to fill defects larger than 10 cm × 10 cm in medium-sized dogs. The external abdominal oblique muscle is a long, flat muscle covering the ventral half of the lateral thoracic wall and lateral abdominal wall. Its fibers are directed caudoventrally. It is divided into a costal part arising from the fifth to thirteenth ribs and a lumbar part arising from the last rib and the thoracolumbar fascia. It has a wide aponeurosis that inserts on the linea alba and cranial pubic ligament and contributes to the external rectus fascia, external inguinal ring, and prepubic tendon. The cranial branch of the cranial abdominal artery supplies the middle zone of the lateral abdominal wall and is accompanied by the cranial hypogastric nerve and satellite vein. The deep branch of the deep circumflex artery anastomoses with the cranial and caudal abdominal arteries and is the main supply to the caudodorsal fourth of the abdominal wall. It is accomplished by a satellite vein and joined by the lateral cutaneous femoral nerve.

Make a paracostal skin incision from the level of the epaxial muscles to the ventral midline, beginning 5 cm caudal to the thirteenth rib. Identify and divide the lumbar fascial edge of the external abdominal oblique muscle, leaving a 0.5-cm margin of fascia along the muscular edge (Fig. 13-23). Undermine the lumbar external abdominal oblique muscle. Identify and preserve the neurovascular

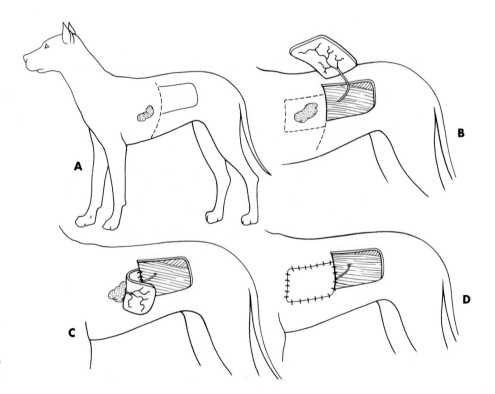

FIG. 13-23
Create an external abdominal oblique flap to reconstruct defects involving the caudal thorax or abdominal wall. **A,** Make a paracostal incision from the epaxial muscles toward the ventral midline, beginning 5 cm caudal to the 13th rib. **B,** Incise the lumbar fascial edge of the external abdominal oblique muscle and undermine it, preserving the neurovascular pedicle. **C** and **D,** Transpose and suture the muscle over an adjacent defect.

pedicle (branches of the cranial abdominal artery and cranial hypogastric nerve and satellite vein) in a craniodorsal location caudal to the thirteenth rib. Divide the dorsal fascial attachment and sever the lumbar external abdominal oblique muscle at the level of the thirteenth rib. Transpose the flap to an adjacent defect. Overlap the defect with the flap and suture the inner fascial surface with 2-0 polydioxanone or polyglyconate using a simple interrupted pattern. Place Penrose or closed suction drains and appose the defect edges.

Cranial Sartorius Muscle Flap

Cranial sartorius muscle flaps are used to repair prepubic tendon ruptures or femoral hernias when tissue trauma, retraction, and fibrosis preclude adequate anatomic reapposition. It may also be used to cover femoral trochanteric ulcers. The sartorius muscle consists of two long, flat, strap-like muscles on the craniomedial surface of the thigh. The origin of the cranial part of the sartorius is the crest of the ilium and the thoracolumbar fascia. The cranial sartorius inserts on the patella with the rectus femoris of the quadriceps. A single major vascular pedicle, branches of the femoral artery and vein, enters the proximal one third of the muscle caudally. The muscle acts to extend the stifle and flex the hip.

Incise skin over the cranial sartorius extending to the inguinal region and dissect subcutaneous tissues to expose the muscle (Fig. 13-24, A). Isolate the muscle by blunt and sharp dissection from the caudal sartorius and quadriceps femoris muscles and other tissues. Transect the muscle distally at its insertion on the tibia and elevate it to its vascular pedicle, which enters the proximal one third of the muscle caudally. Rotate the flap up to 180 degrees into adjacent defects. Alternately, create an island muscle flap by subperiosteal elevation of the muscle's ilial origin. Suture muscle borders to adjacent fascial planes to cover the defect with absorbable suture material (e.g., 2-0 or 3-0 polydioxanone or polyglyconate). Place Penrose or closed suction drains in the donor and recipient sites and close the defect(s).

Caudal Sartorius Muscle Flap

Caudal sartorius muscle flaps can be rotated distally to cover defects over the tibial or metatarsal area. These flaps may facilitate fracture repair when healing is impaired by osteomyelitis or poor circulation. Preoperative angiography ensures that the saphenous artery is not the primary source of circulation to the traumatized area and distal extremity. The caudal sartorius muscle originates from the cranial ventral iliac spine and adjacent ventral border of the ilium. It inserts on the cranial border of the tibia in common with the

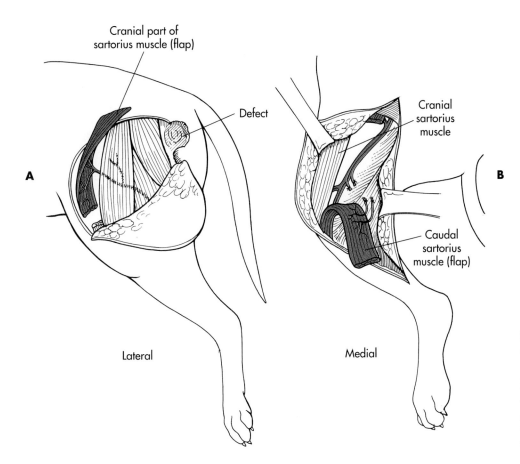

Cranial part of sartorius muscle (flap)

Defect

Cranial sartorius muscle

A

B

Caudal sartorius muscle (flap)

Lateral

Medial

FIG. 13-24
A, Use a cranial sartorius muscle flap to reconstruct prepubic tendon ruptures, femoral hernias, or femoral trochanteric ulcers. **B,** Elevate a caudal sartorius muscle flap to cover defects over the tibia or metatarsus.

gracilis. The caudal sartorius muscle has a segmental blood supply with a dominant vascular pedicle off the saphenous artery and medial saphenous vein at the distal third of the muscle belly. It acts to flex the hip and stifle.

Make a skin incision on the medial aspect of the thigh along the length of the caudal sartorius and dissect subcutaneous tissues to expose the muscle (Fig. 13-24, B). Transect the caudal sartorius muscle approximately 4 cm distal to its origin on the ilium. Double ligate and transect the saphenous artery and medial saphenous vein where they join the femoral artery and vein. Avoid traumatizing the saphenous vessels in the medial tibial region and along the caudal border of the muscle. Transect the caudal sartorius near the tibial crest for complete mobilization. This creates an island muscle flap dependent on the saphenous artery and medial saphenous vein. Extend the skin incision and further mobilize the vascular pedicle as needed. Transfer the flap to the desired location and secure. Place a Penrose or closed suction drain and close the defects at the donor recipient sites.

Temporalis Muscle Flap

Temporalis muscle flaps are used to close orbitonasal defects or improve cosmesis after orbital exenteration. The temporalis muscle is fan shaped and arises from the temporal fossa, inserting on the mandibular coronoid process. The temporal and masseter muscles fuse between the zygomatic arch and coronoid process. The temporal branches of the superficial temporal artery, cranial deep temporal artery, and caudal deep temporal artery supply the temporalis muscle. The blood supply enters the muscle near its narrow insertion on the mandible and runs in a ventral-dorsal direction, paralleling the muscle fibers. The muscle closes the mandible in conjunction with the masseter and medial pterygoid muscles.

Make a cranial to caudal incision centered over the orbit to expose the temporalis muscle (Fig. 13-25). Preserve the superficial temporal artery. Dissect and transect the temporalis fascia from the zygomatic arch. Incise and subperiosteally elevate the desired portion of temporalis muscle. Rotate the flap around its insertion to the recipient site, resecting the zygomatic arch and lateral orbital ligament as needed. Secure the flap over the defect with approximating sutures (e.g., 2-0 or 3-0 polydioxanone or polyglyconate). Obliterate dead space with Penrose or closed suction drains and close cutaneous defects routinely.

Suggested Reading

Alexander LG, Pavletic MM, Engler SJ: Abdominal wall reconstruction with a vascular external abdominal oblique myofascial flap, *Vet Surg* 20:379, 1991.

Chambers J et al: Identification and anatomic categorization of the vascular patterns of the pelvic limb muscles of dogs, *Am J Vet Res* 51:305, 1990.

Chambers J et al: Treatment of trochanteric ulcers with cranial sartorius and rectus femoris muscle flaps, *Vet Surg* 19:424, 1990.

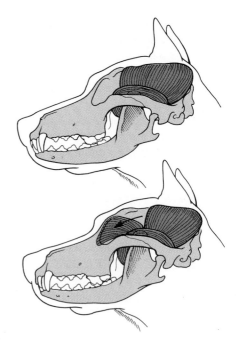

FIG. 13-25
Use a temporalis muscle flap to close orbitonasal defects.

Gregory CR et al: Definition of the gracilis musculocutaneous flap for distant transfer in cats, *Am J Vet Res* 53:153, 1992.

Pavletic MM: Plastic and reconstructive surgery, *Vet Clinics of N Am (Sm Anim)* 20:127, 1990.

Pavletic MM et al: A comparison of the cutaneous trunci myocutaneous flap and latissimus dorsi myocutaneous flap in the dog, *Vet Surg* 16:283, 1987.

Philbert D, Fowler JD: The trapezius osteomusculocutaneous flap in the dog, *Vet Surg* 22:444, 1993.

Philbert D, Fowler JD, Clapson JB: Free microvascular transplantation of the trapezius musculocutaneous flap in the dog, *Vet Surg* 21:435, 1992.

Purinton PT, Chambers J, Moore JL: Identification and categorization of the vascular patterns to muscles of the thoracic limb, thorax and neck of dogs, *Am J Vet Res* 53:1435, 1992.

Tomlinson J, Presnell KR: Use of the temporalis muscle flap in the dog, *Vet Surg* 10:77, 1981.

Weinstein MJ et al: Cranial sartorius muscle flap in the dog, *Vet Surg* 18:286, 1989.

Weinstein MJ, Pavletic MM, Boudrieau RJ: Caudal sartorius muscle flap in the dog, *Vet Surg* 17:203, 1988.

SKIN GRAFTS

Skin grafts are the transfer of a segment of free dermis and epidermis to a distant recipient site. They may be full thickness (epidermis and entire dermis) or partial thickness (epidermis and a variable portion of the dermis). They are used for defects that cannot be reconstructed by direct apposition or skin flaps (usually limb and large trunk defects). Skin graft survival depends upon absorption of tissue fluid and revascularization. Autografts (same animal) are most useful; however, allografts (same species) and xenografts (different species) that are eventually rejected may be used to temporarily cover and protect large burned or denuded areas. Making templates of the defect and graft and drawing reference lines on the skin are helpful in planning reconstruction.

Successful graft healing or graft "take" is dependent on establishment of arterial connections and adequate drainage. This must occur by the seventh or eighth postoperative day or the graft will die. The graft bed must supply adequate vasculature for the graft. Healthy granulation tissue or a fresh clean wound free of infection and debris may serve as the graft bed. Bone, cartilage, tendon, and nerve that are denuded of their overlying connective tissue do not support grafts. Poor graft take occurs over avascular fat, crushing injuries, infected tissue, irradiated tissue, old or hypertrophic granulation tissue, and chronic ulcers. Chronic granulation tissue should be excised to allow new granulation tissue to form before grafting (approximately 4 to 5 days). The surface of healthy granulation tissue may be debrided by excising a thin layer (0.5 to 2.0 mm) with a blade or rubbing with a gauze sponge before grafting. If bleeding persists hemorrhage may be controlled with pressure or pinpoint electrocoagulation. The graft bed should be covered with moistened sponges while preparing the graft. A graft adheres to its bed by fibrin contraction soon after being placed. Fibrous tissue forms after fibroblasts, leukocytes, and phagocytes invade the area. The strength of graft adherence increases as fibrous tissue forms; by the tenth postoperative day a firm union has occurred. Good graft contact with the graft bed is essential to adherence and graft take. To achieve good contact the graft bed must be free of debris and irregularities. Mobilizing the graft with sutures and bandages minimizes graft movement over the wound and facilitates adhesion.

Plasmatic imbibition initially nourishes the graft and keeps the graft vessels dilated until the graft revascularizes. Capillary action pulls the fibrinogen-free, serum-like fluid and cells from the graft bed into the dilated vessels of the graft. Absorption of hemoglobin products gives the graft a bluish-black color. The absorbed fluid diffuses into the interstitial tissue of the graft, producing edema; edema reaches its maximum at 48 to 72 hours after grafting. As venous and lymphatic drainage improves, fluid is taken away from the graft and the edema regresses. Anastomosis of graft vessels with graft bed vessels of similar sizes (inosculation) may begin within 1 day of grafting. Vascular buds from the graft bed follow the fibrin scaffold to meet pre-existing severed graft vessels. Vascular anastomoses form and blood flow to the graft begins. Initially blood flow is sluggish and disorganized but improves and approaches normal by the fifth or sixth day. Fluid accumulations (i.e., seroma, hematoma) inhibit inosculation. Grafts may also be revascularized by the ingrowth of new vessels from the bed into the graft. New vessels form by endothelial sprouting and anastomosis with another sprout or formed vessel. Vascular sprouts may be found within the lower layers of the graft in 48 to 72 hours. New vascular connections remodel, differentiate, and mature until a system of arterioles, venules, and capillaries forms. New lymphatic vessels develop in the graft and establish lymphatic drainage by the fourth or fifth postoperative day.

Fluid accumulation within or under the graft and movement of the graft prevent good vascular connections from developing between the graft and the bed. A bandage should be placed immediately after grafting and left undisturbed for 24 to 48 hours to facilitate graft immobilization, fluid absorption, and graft adhesion and to protect the graft from trauma. Frequency of bandage changes depends on the wound and varies from daily to every 3 to 4 days for at least 3 weeks. Grafts are pale when initially placed in a wound. They appear black and blue during the next 48 hours. The dark colors fade and a light reddish tinge appears by 72 to 96 hours. The entire graft should be red 7 to 8 days after surgery if graft survival is complete. Normal color gradually returns by the fourteenth day. Persistently pale areas are avascular and will undergo necrosis and slough. Black coloration indicates dry ischemic necrosis. Do not resect areas of questionable viability.

The most common causes of graft failure are separation from the graft bed, infection, and movement. They cause graft failure by disrupting the delicate fibrin bonds that bind the graft to the bed. Without adherence, revascularization and organization are impossible. Hematoma or seroma formation under the graft is a common cause of graft failure. Fluid mechanically separates the graft from its bed, impairing nutrition and revascularization. Meticulous hemostasis during graft bed preparation helps prevent hematomas and seromas. Nonexpanded mesh grafts and closed suction drainage are the best methods of facilitating drainage. Mesh grafts have the advantage of not requiring placement of a tube that may disrupt graft adhesion and healing. Initial bandage change is recommended 24 to 48 hours after grafting to detect and drain fluid accumulation under the graft. The danger of fluid accumulation is greater than the risk of moving the graft during bandage manipulations. Infection is detrimental to graft survival because bacteria may cause dissolution of fibrin attachments or produce sufficient exudate to lift a graft from the recipient bed. Plasminogen activators and proteolytic enzymes released by bacteria disrupt the fibrin seal. β-Hemolytic streptococci and *Pseudomonas* spp. produce large amounts of plasmin and proteolytic enzymes. *Pseudomonas* spp. also produce elastase, which breaks down elastin; elastin adheres to fibrin, facilitating graft adhesion.

Donor site skin should have hair of the same color, texture, length, and thickness as hair surrounding the recipient site. The donor site should have enough skin to allow closure without tension after graft removal. Hair follicles may be damaged during graft harvesting and preparation, or by poor graft revascularization. Removal of subcutaneous tissue may damage the base of hair follicles and reduce hair regrowth. Hair regrowth is usually noticed within 2 to 3 weeks after grafting; however, hair color may be altered after grafting. Split-thickness grafts result in sparse hair regrowth. Hair regrowth with strip, punch, and expanded mesh grafts is patchy. Full-thickness sheet grafts and nonexpanded mesh grafts result in the best hair regrowth and cosmetic appearance.

Reinnervation of grafts depends on the type and thickness of the graft, amount of scar tissue formation, and innervation of surrounding tissue. Return of sensation is greatest in flaps, less in full-thickness grafts, and least in split-thickness grafts. Reinnervation occurs from the margins of the graft. Pain is the first sensation to return, followed by touch, and lastly temperature discrimination.

FULL-THICKNESS SKIN GRAFTS

Full-thickness skin grafts include the epidermis and entire dermis. They are indicated to cover large defects on flexor surfaces thus preventing contracture and distal extremity defects (Fig. 13-26, *A* and *B*). After healing, full-thickness grafts resemble normal skin in hair growth, color, texture, and elasticity. They become pliable, movable, and durable. Full-thickness grafts take as well as split-thickness grafts. Disadvantages include planning, tedious removal of subcutaneous tissue, and areas of nonviability. Full-thickness grafting techniques include meshes, plugs, strips, and sheets of skin.

Sheet Grafts

Sheet grafts are indicated to prevent contracture of defects on the distal aspect of the limbs and over flexor surfaces. They should only be used over noninfected granulation beds and when minimal fluid production is expected because graft adhesion is prevented by fluid accumulation or drains. Sheet grafts are less flexible, less expansive, and less conforming than mesh grafts. They utilize as the donor site skin of the lateral thoracic wall, back, shoulder, or other areas with abundant skin. The lateral thoracic wall is the preferred donor site as the skin is relatively thin and well haired.

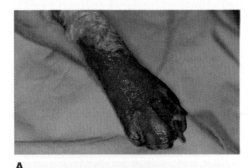

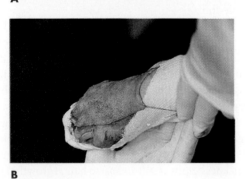

FIG. 13-26
A, Injuries involving the distal extremities commonly require grafting. Grafts should be applied over healthy granulation tissue. **B,** A full-thickness sheet graft has been applied over the wound.

Aseptically prepare the surgical sites. Debride, lavage, and control hemorrhage in the graft bed before placing the graft. Make a pattern of the defect using a sterile towel or paper template. Using the pattern of the defect as a guide, harvest a segment of skin from the donor site with the hair oriented in the proper direction. Excise all subcutaneous tissue from the graft with a scalpel blade during harvest or it will interfere with revascularization. Alternatively, excise the graft, stretch, and fix it to a piece of stiff cardboard and then remove subcutaneous tissues with scissors. Keep the donor site moist with saline-soaked sponges while the graft is being placed. Place the graft in the defect with the hair properly oriented. Tack the graft in position with interrupted sutures. Place a closed suction drain beneath the graft and appose the edges of the graft and wound with staples or simple interrupted or continuous sutures (e.g., 3-0 or 4-0 nylon or polyproplyene) placed 3 to 4 mm apart. Close the donor site by undermining and apposing wound edges or using a pedicle flap. Bandage the graft site with a nonadherent, absorbable bandage. Change the evacuation tube as needed. Change the bandage and evaluate the graft 24 to 48 hours after surgery. Continue rebandaging as needed for 21 days.

Plug, Punch, or Seed Grafts and Strip Grafts

Plug, punch, or seed grafts and strip grafts are placed in a prepared granulation tissue bed. They are indicated for limb wounds and wounds with low-grade infection or irregular surfaces. These grafts are difficult to immobilize after implantation. Wounds that are parallel to the long axis of the limb lend themselves to strip grafting. Plugs and strip grafting are easy to perform and require no special equipment. However, excessive bleeding from the graft bed may float plugs out of the recipient site or delay revascularization. Cosmetic appearance is poor because of epithelial scarring and sparse hair growth because the wounds heal by epithelialization from each graft and wound edge. *Prepare the graft bed by debriding and treating as an open wound for several days. Harvest plugs of skin from the donor site with a 5-mm biopsy punch or tent the skin and resect a small piece of tissue. Harvest 5-mm–wide strips of skin free-hand for strip grafting. Remove subcutaneous tissues from the dermis. For plugs make small slit-like pockets (2 to 4 mm deep, 5 to 7 mm apart) in the granulation tissue, almost parallel to the wound surface. Insert a plug in each pocket, holding it in position with gentle pressure for 1 to 2 minutes. Alternatively, cut holes in the granulation tissue with a 4-mm skin biopsy punch and insert the skin plugs into these holes. Make grooves 2 mm wide and 3 to 5 mm apart for strip grafting. After hemorrhage has been controlled lay a skin strip in each groove and anchor it with an interrupted suture at each end. Bandage and splint the graft site with nonadherent, absorbent materials. Excise and reappose the donor site or treat as an open wound with bandages. Change the graft bandage 3 to 4 days after surgery, being careful to avoid dislodging any of the grafts. Rebandage the area as needed until healing is complete.*

☞ **N O T E** • Expect minimal hair growth when using plug, punch, or seed grafts.

Mesh Grafts

Mesh grafts may be either full-thickness or split-thickness grafts in which parallel rows of staggered slits have been cut. Meshing a sheet graft allows drainage, flexibility, conformity, and expansion. The degree of expansion is directly related to the length of the slits; longer slits equal greater expansion. As the graft is expanded it shortens in the perpendicular plane. A sheet graft is meshed with a special meshing dermatome (Fig. 13-27) or free-hand (Fig. 13-28). Free-hand slits are made in a sheet graft when it is fixed to cardboard after subcutaneous tissue has been removed. Slits are made with a No. 11 scalpel blade and should be approximately 5 to 15 mm long and 2 to 6 mm apart and oriented in rows. Cosmesis is improved if slits are placed parallel to the skin tension lines.

A nonexpanded, full-thickness mesh graft is recommended for most grafts because it may be used under a wide range of circumstances, has a high success rate, and has good cosmetic appearance. Meshing allows a graft to conform and adhere to irregular surfaces and allows placement on graft beds with exudation or blood. Meshing allows drainage and thereby facilitates graft adherence. Cosmetic appearance equals that of sheet grafts (Fig. 13-29, *A* and *B*). Survival is 90% to 100% when grafts are applied on healthy granulation beds and managed properly. Expanded mesh grafts are indicated when donor sites are limited and defects are large. They should be cut longer than the defect to account for shortening with expansion. A diamond-shaped pattern with tufts of hair between epithelial scars results when a mesh graft is expanded. This may not be cosmetically acceptable.

SPLIT-THICKNESS SKIN GRAFTS

Split-thickness skin grafts are composed of epidermis and a variable thickness of dermis. Feline skin is too thin for split-thickness grafting. Graft take with split-thickness grafts is similar to that of full-thickness grafts. Split-thickness grafts are less durable and more subject to trauma than full-thick-

ness grafts, and hair growth may be absent or sparse. Finally, the graft may appear scaly. Hair regrowth at the donor site of thick split-thickness grafts may also be sparse if allowed to heal as an open wound, rather than being resected. Skin of the lateral thoracic wall, back, shoulder, or another area with abundant skin may be used as the donor site.

Aseptically prepare the surgical sites. Debride, lavage, and control hemorrhage in the graft bed before placing the

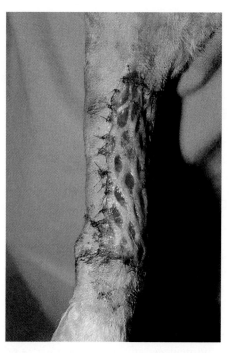

FIG. 13-28
Skin grafts may be meshed by making small, full-thickness incisions through the graft. The incisions are aligned in parallel rows.

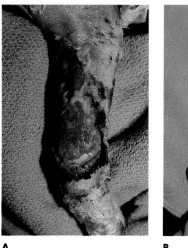

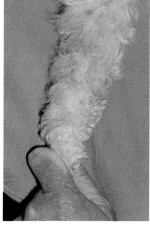

A   **B**

FIG. 13-29
A, Appearance of the skin graft in Fig. 13-28 at 6 days; note that there is partial graft loss. **B,** However, the cosmetic appearance after 100 days is good.

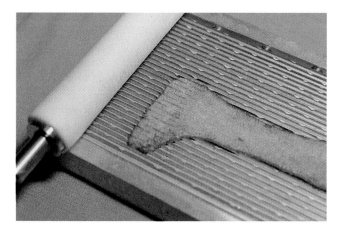

FIG. 13-27
A dermatome may be used to mesh skin grafts.

graft. Harvest the split-thickness graft with a dermatome or free-hand. Inject sterile saline subcutaneously under the donor site to elevate the skin. Lubricate the skin surface with sterile mineral oil or water-soluble gel if using a dermatome. Pull the skin in opposite directions over the donor site to make it taut. Harvest the graft. Using a scalpel, make a partial-thickness incision perpendicular to the skin surface. Then, holding a modified safety razor almost parallel to the skin surface, begin cutting. Place stay sutures in the cut edge of the graft to apply traction while cutting. Change blades as they become dull. Place the graft on the bed with hair growth oriented in the proper direction. Overlap the wound edges with the graft by 2 to 4 mm. Anchor the graft in place with interrupted sutures or skin staples. Irrigate under the graft with saline or thrombin. Apply a nonadherent absorbent bandage with a splint to immobilize the area. Use a tie-over bandage if necessary. Holes inadvertently perforating the graft will allow drainage and eventually heal. After harvest and grafting, excise the donor site and close it or manage it as an open wound with bandages. Increased pain is associated with the wound when it is managed as an open wound. Perform the first bandage change 24 to 48 hours after surgery. Drain the area if a seroma or hematoma has formed by making a small incision in the graft and aspirating. Expect the graft overlapping the skin to necrose. Rebandage the area and change the bandage only as needed as movement of the graft bed interferes with revascularization.

Stamp Grafts

Stamp grafts are square patches of split-thickness skin applied to a granulating wound. The graft bed and graft are prepared and managed in the same manner as other split-thickness grafts. The graft is cut into patches ranging from 5 mm^2 to 25 mm^2. Patches are spaced 1 to 10 mm apart in graft bed depressions. These grafts are particularly susceptible to movement and easily displaced by bandages.

Suggested Reading

Bauer MS, Pope ER: The effects of skin graft thickness on graft viability and change in original graft area in dogs, *Vet Surg* 15:321, 1986.

Bradley DM, Shealy PM, Swaim SF: Meshed skin graft and phalangeal fillet for paw salvage: a case report, *J Am Anim Hosp Assoc* 29:427, 1993.

Harari J: *Surgical complications and wound healing in the small animal practice*, Philadelphia, 1993, WB Saunders.

Pavletic MM: Plastic and reconstructive surgery, *Vet Clinics of N Am (Sm Anim)* 20:14, 1990.

Pope ER, Swaim SF: Wound drainage from under full-thickness skin grafts in dogs. I. Quantitative evaluation of four techniques, *Vet Surg* 15:65, 1986.

Pope ER, Swaim SF: Wound drainage from under full-thickness skin grafts in dogs. II. Effect on cosmetic appearance, *Vet Surg* 15:72, 1986.

Swaim SF, Henderson RA: *Small animal wound management*, Philadelphia, 1990, Lea & Febiger.

SURGICAL MANAGEMENT OF SPECIFIC SKIN DISORDERS

BURNS AND OTHER THERMAL INJURIES

Burns occur when heat energy is applied at a faster rate than tissue can absorb and dissipate it. Fires, electric heating pads, hair dryers, scalding water, steam, hot cooking oil, exhaust systems, and hot pipes are common sources of thermal burns in domestic animals. Extent of injury is influenced by temperature of the heat source, duration of contact, and tissue conductance. A transition zone separates completely devitalized tissue from uninjured tissue. The area in direct contact with the heat coagulates; cellular proteins denature and blood vessels coagulate. The transition zone is characterized by reduced blood flow, intravascular sludging, and potentially reversible tissue damage. Progressive dermal ischemia may occur in this area because of the release of vasoactive substances (e.g., thromboxane A_2, histamine, leukotrienes, prostaglandins, oxygen radicals), tissue edema, desiccation, and bacterial invasion. The transition zone is surrounded by an area of hyperemia where minimal damage occurs and healing is complete. It can be difficult to determine burn depth and area of involvement because the depth of injury is not uniform and the skin surface is often covered by dry coagulum and is leathery. An eschar is the residue of skin elements that have been coagulated by the heat. It is composed almost entirely of tough denatured collagen fibers. Scabs contain dead cells and flimsy fibrin and are not a strong protective covering like an eschar.

Superficial or first-degree burns affect only epidermis. The area is painful, thickened, erythematous, and desquamated. Healing occurs rapidly (within 3 to 6 days) by epithelialization from the stratum germinativum or adnexal structures of the dermis. Because canine skin does not act as an organ for heat dissemination as does human skin, dogs do not have the same rich superficial vascular plexus as humans. Therefore they show less erythema with superficial burns than humans. Superficial partial-thickness burns are moist, blanch with pressure, and are sensitive to pain. They usually heal within 3 weeks because of epithelialization from deeper portions of the skin appendages. Healing is usually complete and occurs without grafting. Deep, partial-thickness or second-degree burns cause marked destruction of the dermis. The only remaining adnexal epithelium is in the upper layers of the subcutaneous fat. Subcutaneous edema and marked inflammation occur and hair does not epilate easily. Progressive damage during the first 24 hours results from the heat of injury and the release of proteolytic enzymes, prostaglandins, and vasoactive substances. Although they frequently heal without grafting, healing takes months and scarring may be extensive. Healing occurs by reepithelialization from deep adnexa and wound margins. They must be protected against trauma and contamination while healing. Inappropriate therapy may allow a second-degree burn to progress to a third-degree burn, especially if bacterial infection occurs. Full-thickness or third-degree burns form a dark brown, insensitive, leathery eschar. All skin structures are destroyed and hair epilates easily. Third-degree burns are less painful than first- or second-degree burns because nerves have been destroyed. Superficial vascular thrombosis and deep vascular permeability cause subcutaneous edema and necrosis. Healing occurs by contraction and reepithelialization unless the wound is reconstructed. Some indication of injury depth may be obtained by elevating the eschar. First- and second-degree burn eschars split when elevated and bent to reveal underlying epidermis or dermis, whereas third-degree burns may not split or the split may extend to subcutaneous tissues.

Burn wounds are sterile or colonized only by superficial bacteria during the first 24 hours. The large volume of dead tissue provides an excellent medium for bacterial growth and occlusion of local blood supply impairs delivery of humeral and cellular defense mechanisms and systemic drugs to the wound. Superficial bacteria proliferate and invade the deeper tissues under the eschar within 4 to 5 days after injury. Initially most organisms are gram-positive cocci, but by 3 to 5 days the wound is colonized with gram-negative bacteria, typically *Pseudomonas* spp. Early eschar removal and topical antibiotics are needed to minimize progression of damage.

Burns frequently cause shock and multiple organ failure because of fluid loss, fluid shifts, electrolyte imbalances, protein losses, myocardial depression, increased peripheral vascular resistance, and increased blood viscosity. Cardiac abnormalities, immunosuppression, anemia, renal failure, liver failure, and disseminated intravascular coagulation occur in some animals. More severe systemic signs are associated with large burn surface areas. Respiratory distress may occur from smoke inhalation, thermal burns of the upper airway, and carbon monoxide poisoning. Smoke inhalation causes pulmonary edema with vascular congestion, interstitial edema, and atelectasis. Pneumonia often occurs several days after smoke inhalation.

Burns from contact, rather than fire, may not be immediately recognized. Moisture and flattening of the hair coat may be noted a few days after injury. This is rapidly followed by hair and skin loss, which makes demarcation of the burn area obvious. Burns may be avoided during surgery by using circulating warm water pads (less than or equal to 42° C) rather than electrical wire element pads. Thermal burns from hot, water-filled gloves or bottles may also occur. Anesthetized or hypothermic animals are particularly susceptible to burns from hot water bottles because of reduced circulation associated with vascular constriction. The longer the exposure, the greater the risk of burns. Burns may also be avoided by properly grounding patients when using electrosurgical units.

TREATMENT

The first priority in treating burns is to minimize tissue loss by administering first aid and preventing shock. Prevention of septic complications by good wound management is the next priority. Early wound debridement and reconstruction are important to minimize morbidity. Immediately after thermal injury (within 2 hours), cooling the affected areas may limit further extension of tissue destruction. The area should be lavaged with cold water or cold packs applied to the wound. Analgesics should be given as necessary to alleviate pain (e.g., buprenorphine; 0.005 to 0.015 mg/kg intravenously, intramuscularly, or subcutaneously every 4 to 6 hours). Vital signs, mental status, hematocrit, total protein, urine output, central venous pressure, electrolytes, blood gases, and daily body weight should be monitored.

The size of the burn area can be estimated by measuring the area of burned skin with a metric ruler, dividing that area by the total surface area of the animal (Table 13-2) and multiplying by 100. Alternately, a rough estimate can be

TABLE 13-2

Burns: Calculation of Total Body Surface Area

Conversion Chart
Body Weight (kg) to Total Body Surface Area (m^2)

kg	m^2	kg	m^2
1.0	0.10	26.0	0.88
2.0	0.15	27.0	0.90
3.0	0.20	28.0	0.92
4.0	0.25	29.0	0.94
5.0	0.29	30.0	0.96
6.0	0.33	31.0	0.99
7.0	0.36	32.0	1.01
8.0	0.40	33.0	1.03
9.0	0.43	34.0	1.05
10.0	0.46	35.0	1.07
11.0	0.49	36.0	1.09
12.0	0.52	37.0	1.11
13.0	0.55	38.0	1.13
14.0	0.58	39.0	1.15
15.0	0.60	40.0	1.17
16.0	0.63	41.0	1.19
17.0	0.66	42.0	1.21
18.0	0.69	43.0	1.23
19.0	0.71	44.0	1.25
20.0	0.74	45.0	1.26
21.0	0.76	46.0	1.28
22.0	0.78	47.0	1.30
23.0	0.81	48.0	1.32
24.0	0.83	49.0	1.34
25.0	0.85	50.0	1.36

Total body surface area = $weight^{0.425} \times height^{0.725} \times 0.007184$ ($m^2 = kg^{0.425} \times cm^{0.725} \times 0.007184$) or total body surface area = $0.1 \times weight (kg)^{2/3}$

From Swaim SF: *Surgery of traumatized skin: management and reconstruction in the dog and cat*, Philadelphia, 1980, WB Saunders.

gained using the rule-of-nine; each forelimb of the animal represents approximately 9% of the total body surface area (TBSA), each rear limb is 18% (two nines), and the dorsal and ventral thorax and abdomen are each 18%. Animals with partial-thickness burns involving less than 15% of the TBSA require minimal supportive therapy, while those with burns involving more than 15% TBSA require emergency supportive care. Euthanasia should be considered for those with burns involving more than 50% TBSA (Davis, 1980). Shock doses of lactated Ringer's solution or hypertonic saline solution should be administered to minimize and reverse signs of shock. The amount of isotonic fluid required during the first 24 hours may be estimated using the formula 3 to 4 ml/kg/percent of TBSA burned. Hypertonic saline solutions are beneficial in reducing total fluid requirements, limiting edema, and increasing cardiac output. Hypertonic saline (4 ml/kg bolus) plus lactated Ringer's solution (1 ml/kg/percent of TBSA of burn) may be administered. Serum sodium concentration should not exceed 160 mEq/L when giving hypertonic saline. Nonprotein colloid solutions (i.e., dextran 70, dextran 40, hetastarch) given in the early postburn period improve survival and reduce edema formation. Administration of protein colloids (i.e., fresh-frozen plasma or albumin) to hypoproteinemic patients should be delayed for 8 to 12 hours to allow stabilization of membrane permeability and increased lymph return that reduces protein loss. Protein colloids given within the first 8 to 12 hours are lost into the burn wound and worsen edema formation. Dogs with partial-thickness burns involving 20% TBSA may lose 28% of their plasma volume during the first 6 hours (Salzberg, Evans, 1950). Transfusions (i.e., whole blood, packed red blood cells) may be necessary in anemic patients.

Respiratory distress should be treated by giving oxygen (mask, nasal insufflation, tracheostomy tube) and bronchodilators. The half-life of carbon monoxide is reduced with oxygen therapy. Continuous positive pressure ventilation may be necessary in some animals. Tracheostomy (see p. 613) and mechanical ventilation are indicated in patients with upper airway swelling or severe tracheobronchial secretions. Trachea and bronchi should be suctioned if necessary. Systemic antibiotics should be administered if bronchopneumonia occurs.

Aggressive nutritional support counters the increased metabolic demand and protein losses that occur in burn patients (see Chapter 11). A high-protein, high-caloric diet should be fed to animals with moderate to severe wounds. Early enteral feeding is important in preventing gastroduodenal ulceration. Histamine H_2-receptor antagonists should be given if gastroduodenal ulceration is suspected (see p. 288).

BURN WOUND MANAGEMENT

Necrotic tissue may be debrided from burn wounds with enzymes or dissection (see p. 96). Enzymatic debridement spares viable tissue that may be removed by dissection or surgical excision, but results are variable; best results are obtained when applied to moist, pliable eschar. Loose and obviously devitalized tissue in partial-thickness burns may be removed with scissors, hydrotherapy, or gauze sponge abrasion. With full-thickness burns, sharp excision to muscle fascia is necessary. Early burn excision is recommended to minimize secondary infections and systemic effects (e.g., endotoxins, blood loss).

Small burn wounds can be excised and closed primarily. Closure is achieved by skin advancement or skin flaps. Larger wounds may be allowed to heal by contraction and epithelialization, or they may be grafted. Second intention healing may take months or be incomplete, and the resulting scar may be cosmetically unacceptable. Therefore many large burns are debrided, allowed to form a healthy granulation bed, and then reconstructed using rotating skin flaps, axial pattern flaps, tissue expansion, or grafts. Early wound closure decreases wound management, reduces secondary infection, and shortens hospitalization. Scars are fragile and may erode and bleed easily. Squamous cell carcinomas occasionally occur in burn scars.

Estimate the burn depth and calculate the size of the burn in relationship to the TBSA obtained from a weight-conversion chart (see above and Table 13-2). Clip the wound and surrounding hair before gently lavaging with an antiseptic solution (e.g., 0.05% chlorhexidine diacetate). Cover the wound with a topical aloe vera compound or silver sulfadiazine (see p. 96). If treatment is begun soon after the burn, use aloe vera or dipyridamole (thromboxane synthetase blocker) to help preserve patency of the dermal vasculature. After the first 24 hours apply water-soluble, 1% silver sulfadiazine cream (Silvadene cream) to the wound once or twice daily. Silver sulfadiazine is bactericidal with activity against gram-positive and gram-negative bacteria and Candida. Bandage the wound and aseptically manage it during daily bandage changes. Remove the proteinaceous gel from the surface of the wound during bandage changes and before reapplication of silver sulfadiazine. Use gentle hydrotherapy to remove debris and clean the wound.

References

Davis LE: Thermal burns. In Swaim SF, editor: *Surgery of traumatized skin: management and reconstruction in the dog and cat*, Philadelphia, 1980, WB Saunders.

Salzberg AM, Evans EI: Blood volumes in normal and burned dogs, *Ann Surg* 132:746, 1950.

Suggested Reading

Demling RH: Fluid replacement in burned patients, *Surg Clin North Am* 67:15, 1987.

ELECTRICAL INJURIES

Electrical burns occur when current touches one point on the body, with or without an exit point. Chewing on electrical cords is the most common cause of electrical injury in small animals. Resistance to electrical current flow is greatest in bone and least in nerves (bones > fat > tendon > skin > muscle > blood > nerve). Low-voltage electrical current follows the path of least resistance, which is usually along blood vessels. Tissue necrosis occurs from vascular thrombosis and release of vasoactive substances. Tissue damage may be massive because of deep extension of the generated heat. Immediate death can result from respiratory paralysis or ventricular fibrillation.

Animals are often found collapsed in a tonic state with an electrical cord in their mouth. The body stiffens from contraction of striated muscles while receiving the electric current. Generalized tonoclonic activity with vomiting and defecation can also occur. If the animal survives, the tonic state resolves when the cord is removed from the mouth, although the animal may be weak and ataxic for a short period. Burns primarily occur on the lips, gums, palate, or tongue. These areas may initially appear charred, pale gray, or tan. Edema develops after 1 to 2 days. Extent of injury may not be apparent for 2 to 3 weeks. Pulmonary edema frequently occurs, causing dyspnea and moist rales.

☞ **N O T E** · Suspect an electrical cord injury in an otherwise healthy puppy with an acute onset of respiratory distress.

TREATMENT

Affected patients should be examined frequently for pulmonary edema. Pulmonary edema may be treated with diuretics (i.e., furosemide 2.5 to 5.0 mg/kg intramuscularly or intravenously, once or twice a day) and aminophylline (10 mg/kg intravenously or intramuscularly three times a day). Morphine (1 mg/kg intramuscularly or subcutaneously) may be given to dogs to reduce anxiety. Ventilatory support is needed if there is no response to medication.

Repair of damaged tissue should be delayed until the full extent of the injury is known. Minor burns may be allowed to heal by second intention. Oronasal fistulae must be repaired (see p. 216). Large lip wounds should be repaired to prevent oral drying and improve cosmesis.

Suggested Reading

Swaim SF: *Surgery of traumatized skin: management and reconstruction in the dog and cat,* Philadelphia, 1980, WB Saunders.
Swaim SF, Henderson RA: *Small animal wound management,* Philadelphia, 1990, Lea & Febiger.

FROSTBITE

Severe or prolonged cold may cause necrosis of exposed tissues. Extremities (i.e., ear, tail, scrotum, mammary glands) are most commonly affected because of sparse hair coat and poor peripheral circulation. Frozen tissue is pale, hypoesthetic, and cool. Thawed viable tissue is hyperemic, painful,

and scaly. Nonviable tissue undergoes dry gangrene or mummification and sloughs. Superficial injuries involve skin and subcutaneous tissue while deep injuries extend beyond subcutaneous tissues. Ice crystals form in intracellular and extracellular spaces causing cell damage and death.

TREATMENT

Affected body parts should be rapidly rewarmed in warm water (i.e., 102° to 107.6° F or 39° to 42° C) for about 20 minutes to improve circulation. Affected areas become erythematous and edematous, form large vesicles, and are often painful, necessitating analgesics (see Chapter 12). Topical aloe vera or silver sulfadiazine should be applied to the affected areas. Bandages are used to prevent self-trauma. Conservative therapy should be continued until viable tissue can be distinguished from nonviable tissue (i.e., 3 to 6 weeks). Necrotic tissue should then be debrided and the area reconstructed if necessary. Healing may be complete beneath the mummified tissue.

Suggested Reading

Swaim SF, Henderson RA: *Small animal wound management,* Philadelphia, 1990, Lea & Febiger.

CHEMICAL INJURIES

Chemical burns from strong acids or alkalis destroy tissue by denaturing proteins or interfering with cell metabolism. Mechanisms of injury include oxidation, reduction, corrosion, dehydration, denaturation, and vesication. The severity depends on chemical type, strength, volume, contact time, penetration, and mechanism of action. Corrosives (i.e., sodium containing drain and oven cleaners, phenol disinfectants) cause protein denaturation resulting in erosion and ulceration. Dehydrating chemicals (i.e., sulfuric and hydrochloric acid) desiccate tissues, while oxidizing agents (i.e., chromic acid, hypochlorite, potassium permanganate) coagulate protein. Denaturing agents (i.e., picric acid, tannic acid, acetic acid, formic acid, hydrofluoric acid) fix or stabilize tissue by the formation of salts. Vesicants (i.e., dimethyl sulfoxide, cantharides, halogenated hydrocarbons, gasoline) liberate tissue amines (histamine, serotonin), causing blisters.

TREATMENT

Immediately after chemical exposure, resultant burns should be flushed with large volumes of water to remove the chemical and prevent further injury. This dilutes the chemical and dissipates the heat of chemical reactions. Hydrofluoric acid must be neutralized to stop penetration; apply aqueous benzalkonium chloride, which precipitates residual fluoride ion. Ten percent calcium gluconate should then be injected into and around the lesion (0.5 ml/cm²). The animal should be prevented from licking the wound to avoid chemical burns of the tongue, oropharynx, and/or esophagus. Antimicrobials should be applied as described for thermal burns (see p. 134). Early debridement may prevent further chemical penetration and tissue destruction; however, excessive tissue removal should be avoided.

Suggested Reading

Bilbrey SA, Dulisch ML, Stallings B: Chemical burns caused by benzalkonium chloride in eight surgical cases, *J Am Anim Hosp Assoc* 25:31, 1989.

Swaim SF, Henderson RA: *Small animal wound management*, Philadelphia, 1990, Lea & Febiger.

SNAKEBITES

Snakebites may cause severe local tissue damage and systemic effects. Venomous snakes in the United States include the Crotalidae (pit vipers) and Elapidae subfamilies. The Crotalidae subfamily includes the copperhead, cottonmouth water moccasin, and rattlesnake. Pit vipers have a triangular head with facial pits located between the nostrils and eyes and vertically elliptical pupils. Their fangs are hollow, retractable teeth near the rostral maxilla. Coral snakes are members of the Elapidae subfamily. They (along with many nonpoisonous snakes) have round heads, no pits, and round pupils. Coral snakes have small fangs fixed in the cranial maxilla. Their short fangs allow them to hang from animals they bite. Nonvenomous snakes have teeth, but no fangs.

Coral snake venom is primarily neurotoxic, causing moderate tissue reaction and pain at puncture sites. There is a delay of several hours before onset of systemic signs, which worsen gradually over 18 hours. Effects may last 7 to 10 days. Neurotoxicity caused by coral snake venom is characterized by central nervous system depression, vasomotor instability, and muscle paralysis. Coral snake envenomation may cause lethargy, tremors, ptosis, dysphonia, incoordination, and hematuria. Larger doses may cause vomiting, salivation, defecation, and generalized parasympathetic stimulation followed by paralysis and death. The primary cause of death is respiratory paralysis.

Crotalid venoms are primarily enzymatic in activity (i.e., phospholipase A, phosphatases, exopeptidase, hyaluronidase, L-amino-acid oxidase, proteases, endopeptidase). These venoms are hematotoxic, vasculotoxic, and necrogenic. They alter the resistance and integrity of blood vessels causing hypotension and bleeding, affect cardiac dynamics and nervous system function, and produce respiratory depression and myonecrosis. Bites most commonly occur on the face and legs. Signs of envenomation are variable and depend on the snake species, volume of venom, and size of the victim. The bite of a pit viper usually produces two puncture marks surrounded by edema. The fang marks may bleed. Erythema, edema, and pain are immediate local effects. Envenomation has not occurred if these signs are not seen within 20 minutes of the bite. Progressive swelling and sometimes local hemorrhage occur with moderate to severe envenomation. Tissue discoloration caused by petechiae and ecchymosis occurs, followed by local tissue necrosis. Tissue damage varies with the depth of bite and amount of venom injected. Systemic signs of envenomation are usually lethargy, vomiting, diarrhea, hypotension, and shock. Other signs may include anorexia, salivation, thirst, lymph node pain, weakness, bradycardia or tachycardia, generalized tremors, coma, tachypnea, pulmonary edema, urinary and fecal incontinence, paralysis, convulsions, and hemorrhage. Venom-induced coagulation defects may be severe.

TREATMENT

Treatment goals include neutralizing the venom, treating systemic effects and wounds, and reconstructing tissue defects. The bite wound should be immobilized and excitement or exertion avoided. The wound should be lavaged and cleaned with antiseptics or germicidal soaps. Tourniquets, incision, suction, or manipulation of the bitten area is rarely of benefit and must be performed immediately after the bite to have any beneficial effect. They can easily cause additional tissue damage. If a tourniquet is applied, it should be placed 10 cm proximal to the fang marks, be lightly constrictive, and should be released every 30 minutes for 60 to 90 seconds. Tourniquets can prevent dilution of the venom and decrease tissue perfusion, thereby promoting ischemia and tissue necrosis.

The site should be clipped to facilitate examination for fang marks. Hospitalization and observation for systemic signs are indicated. Results of hemograms, coagulation profiles, urinalysis, and serum biochemical analyses should be monitored every 6 hours. Persistent decreased platelet counts and prolonged clotting times suggest progressive venom activity. Myoglobinuria indicates rhabdomyolysis and hemoglobinuria indicates hemolysis. The electrocardiogram should be monitored. The circumference of the edematous area around the bite should be measured and recorded to monitor progression.

Antivenin (Antivenin Crotalidae Polyvalent or North American Coral Snake Antivenin) should be administered only if a snake bite is known to have occurred. It should be administered as soon as possible to limit tissue necrosis and prevent systemic reactions. Pretreating with antihistamines and skin testing the animal with antivenin prior to intravenous administration will decrease anaphylactic reactions. Recommended doses range from 1 to 5 vials. Although it is not known how long antivenin can be given after envenomation and still be effective, administration after 8 hours is of questionable value. The animal should be supported with intravenous fluids. Corticosteroids may help treat shock and reduce edema. Broad-spectrum antibiotics are used to inhibit wound infection. Additional supportive care may include analgesics, sedatives, transfusions, and oxygen.

Necrotic tissue should be treated as an open, infected wound (see p. 94). Wet-dry absorbent bandages (see p. 103) should be applied until healthy granulation tissue has formed. Then nonadherent absorbent bandages (see p. 103) should be used and the wound allowed to heal by second intention or reconstructed with flaps or grafts.

Suggested Reading

Mansfield PD: The management of snake venom poisoning in dogs, *Compend Contin Educ Pract Vet* 6:988, 1984.

Marks SL, Mannella C, Schaer M: Coral snake envenomation in the dog: report of four cases and review of the literature, *J Am Anim Hosp Assoc* 26:629, 1990.

Swaim SF, Henderson RA: *Small animal wound management,* Philadelphia, 1990, Lea & Febiger.

PRESSURE SORES

Pressure is exerted on bony prominences when animals lie down. The lateral humeral epicondyle, tuber calcanei, greater femoral trochanter, tuber coxae, and ischiatic tuberosity are most susceptible to pressure sores. The acromion of the scapula, lateral tibial condyle, lateral malleolus, olecranon, and sternum are less common sites. Soft tissues including skin, loose connective tissue, fat, deep fascia, and periosteum cover these prominences. All intervening tissues are compressed when pressure is exerted on a bony prominence. Typically, repeated trauma and inflammation are mild and protective callus develops. Prolonged or severe compression leads to soft tissue ischemia and cell death. Pressure sores form when animals are recumbent for long periods because of paralysis, fractures, injuries, or illness. Pressure sores may also develop under improperly fitted or padded casts and bandages. They are prevented by providing well-padded bedding (i.e., water mattress, air mattress, fleece), repositioning the animal frequently, and keeping the animal clean and dry. Bony prominences should be checked daily for signs of an impending ulcer (i.e., hyperemia, moisture, easily epilated hair).

As pressure sores begin developing, blood vessels dilate and inflammatory edema of skin and subcutaneous tissues occurs. If trauma persists, tissues break down causing a hematoma or an open sore. Untreated hematomas are not absorbed because surrounding tissues are damaged. The fluid is mucinous and yellow to red. Tissues thicken around the hematoma, forming a false bursa or hygroma. The wall of the hygroma or false bursa is thick and tough, composed of granulation tissue and collagen. The lining of this sac is pale and smooth, or rough with irregular villus-like projections extending into the lumen. Open sores may involve the epidermis and dermis, or extend through subcutaneous tissues and fascia to bone. Osteomyelitis or septic arthritis may develop.

TREATMENT

Early pressure sores are treated by padding bedding and bandaging the limb to eliminate pressure over the bony prominence. A well-padded doughnut-type bandage or pipe insulation bandage should be applied to prevent trauma (see p. 104). Treatment for open or chronic pressure sores is similar, but response is poorer. Open wounds should be treated with topical antibiotics (see p. 95) and wet-dry bandages (see p. 103) to encourage debridement and granulation. Dead space should be drained and infected tissues and bone surgically debrided when deep ulcers are present.

Small superficial wounds may heal by second intention. Secondary closure is performed after healthy granulation tissue has formed in large, deep wounds. Skin edges should be undermined and apposed if possible. Skin flaps (i.e., local advancement, transposition, axial pattern, or musculocutaneous [see pp. 116 to 128]) and grafts may be needed for a tension-free closure. Suture lines should not be positioned over bony prominences. A well-padded bandage and a soft-padded bed should be used to protect the site during healing. Ulcers may recur if the cause goes uncorrected.

Suggested Reading

Swaim SF, Henderson RA: *Small animal wound management,* Philadelphia, 1990, Lea & Febiger.

ELBOW HYGROMA

An elbow hygroma (elbow seroma, olecranon bursitis) is a fluid-filled cavity surrounded by dense fibrous connective tissue occurring over the lateral aspect of the olecranon (Fig. 13-30). Caused by chronic trauma, they often occur bilaterally as nonpainful swellings. Most elbow hygromas occur in young (i.e., 6 to 18 months old), large-breed dogs before a protective callus forms over the bony prominence; however, they may occur in older animals with neuromuscular disease. Elbow hygromas vary in size, becoming larger and thicker with repeated trauma. They are usually sterile initially, but bacteria may be introduced during aspiration. Infected hygromas are painful. Small, nonpainful hygromas are cosmetic problems that persist if not treated. Hygromas also occur over other bony prominences (i.e., tuber calcanei, greater trochanter, tuber coxae, tuber ischium, external occipital protuberance, thoracic vertebral dorsal spinous processes).

TREATMENT

The primary treatment for elbow hygromas is elimination of repeated elbow trauma (i.e., soft, padded bed and padded elbow bandage). A spica-type bandage may be needed to prevent slippage (see p. 107). Aspiration of the hygroma is of little benefit and may introduce bacteria. Although surgery should be avoided if possible, development of a fibrous

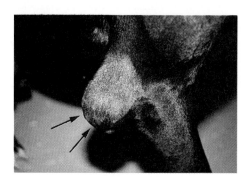

FIG. 13-30
Elbow hygroma in a dog. Note the fluid-filled swelling over the olecranon (*arrows*).

capsule or infection may necessitate it. Infection requires drainage and administration of appropriate antibiotics. Prolonged drainage may be obtained by placement of Penrose drains into the hygroma. The advantage of this technique is that the protective callus is preserved. Penrose drains should not be used on ulcerated hygromas. *For nonulcerated (infected or sterile) hygromas, prepare the limb for aseptic surgery and make several dorsal and ventral stab wounds into the hygroma cavity. Probe the cavity, breaking down fibrous septa, and lavage it. Place multiple Penrose drains into the hygroma cavity and secure them. Apply a nonadherent absorbent bandage (see p. 103) to absorb drainage and prevent trauma. Change the bandage daily. Remove drains when drainage becomes minimal and scar tissue adherence occurs (i.e., 2 to 3 weeks). Continue to bandage the elbow for at least one week after drain removal, or until healing is complete.*

Occasionally, hygromas are surgically excised when fibrous tissue, fistulae, or infection develops without a large fluid-filled cavity. The naturally protective callus is removed during excision and postoperative management is often complicated. Incisions may dehisce and ulcerate, bandages are difficult to maintain, and recurrence is common. Wounds that dehisce may not heal. Small hygromas can be excised and the defect closed by undermining and advancing local tissue until skin edges can be approximated with interrupted sutures. The cavity lining should be debrided and lavaged and Penrose drains placed before closure. Complete excision of fibrous tissue is unnecessary. Suture lines should be positioned medial or lateral to the olecranon if possible. It is difficult to excise large hygromas and close the wound without using skin flaps (i.e., axial pattern [see p. 120], pedicle [see p. 116], or myocutaneous [see p. 123]). The limb should be bandaged for a minimum of 4 weeks. An external coaptation splint (i.e., spica bandage; see p. 107) protects and pads the elbow.

Suggested Reading

Johnston DE: Hygroma of the elbow in dogs, *J Am Vet Med Assoc* 167:23, 1975.
Swaim SF, Henderson RA: *Small animal wound management,* Philadelphia, 1990, Lea & Febiger.

LICK GRANULOMA

Lick granulomas (acral lick dermatitis, acral pruritic nodule, acropruritic granuloma, psychogenic dermatoses, neurodermatitis) are self-induced by continuous licking or chewing. They are usually single and unilateral and may occur anywhere although the cranial aspect of the carpus/metacarpus and lateral aspect of the tarsus/metatarsus are most commonly affected. They usually occur in older, large-breed dogs. Although wounds, foreign bodies, infections, and musculoskeletal pain may be initiating factors, most are believed to be psychogenic and associated with boredom, inactivity, or environmental change. The lesion is sparsely haired, thick-

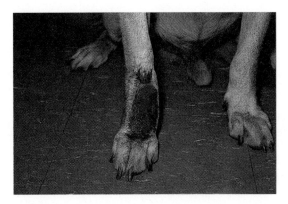

FIG. 13-31
Lick granulomas often occur in the carpal/metacarpal or tarsal/metatarsal area. They are sparsely haired, thickened, firm, ulcerated, erythematous, and surrounded by a hyperpigmented halo.

ened, firm, ulcerated, erythematous, and surrounded by a hyperpigmented halo (Fig. 13-31). Superficial tissues may erode and expose bone. Dermatologic examination, skin scraping, fungal culture, biopsy, radiographs, electrodiagnostics, allergy testing, and/or hypoallergenic diet trials may be needed. Radiographs may reveal periosteal proliferation secondary to soft tissue inflammation or associated arthritis, osteomyelitis, osteosarcoma, or foreign bodies. Biopsy to rule out neoplasia and deep cultures to determine bacterial involvement and antimicrobial sensitivity are recommended.

TREATMENT

Treatment should be initiated before the lesion becomes chronic and nonresponsive. If an underlying cause is identified, it should be treated or eliminated. Previously recommended treatments have included activity and/or environmental modification, bandaging, collars, muzzles, topical antichew agents, glucocorticoids, orgotein, radiation therapy, cryosurgery, surgical excision, behavior-modifying drugs, cobra venom, acupuncture, and other medications (i.e., fluocinoleone acetonide, flunixin meglumine, dimethylsulfoxide, proteolytic enzymes). Results have been inconsistent and recurrence is common. Although not commonly performed, surgical excision of a lick granuloma followed by reconstruction using direct apposition, flaps, or grafts is possible. The surgical site should be protected with a bandage until suture removal. However, the lesion usually recurs at the same or a different site unless the causative factor(s) is eliminated.

☞ **N O T E** • Warn owners that recurrence (at the same or another location) is common.

Suggested Reading

Rivers B, Walter PA, McKeever PJ: Treatment of canine acral lick dermatitis with radiation therapy: 17 cases (1979–1991), *J Am Anim Hosp Assoc* 29:541, 1993.

Swaim SF, Henderson RA: *Small animal wound management,* Philadelphia, 1990, Lea & Febiger.

DERMOID SINUS (PILONIDAL SINUS)

A dermoid sinus or cyst is a tubular skin indentation that extends ventrally as a blind sac from the dorsal midline. It is a neural tube defect caused by incomplete separation of skin and the neural tube during embryonic development. Sinus depth varies; some are superficial while others extend to the supraspinous ligament or dura mater. They are most common in Rhodesian ridgebacks, occurring along the dorsal midline cranial and caudal to their midline ridge, but have also been reported in a Shih Tzu and boxer. Multiple or single draining tracts may be identified, especially in the cervical region. Cervical sinuses are generally attached to the dorsal spinous process of the second cervical vertebra. Because the lesion is believed to be hereditary, affected animals should be neutered.

Lesions can be recognized at a young age as openings on the dorsal midline with protruding hair. A tube or cord is palpated in the subcutaneous tissue when a skin fold is elevated in the area of the sinus. The cord is 1 to 5 mm in diameter and courses toward the spine. Cystlike subcutaneous swellings may also be palpated. The lumen of the sinus is filled with inspissated sebum, exfoliated keratin debris, and hair. Sinus infection and abscessation may occur. Myelitis, meningomyelitis, or encephalitis can occur if the infected sinus extends to the spine.

Samples should be collected for cytology and microbial culture and sensitivity testing. Metrizamide fistulography and myelography may reveal spinal communications. Excised tissue should be submitted for histologic examination to rule out other causes of draining tracts. Differential diagnoses include foreign bodies, sebaceous cysts, abscesses, epidermal inclusion cysts, follicular retention cysts, and intracutaneous cornifying epitheliomas. Histology of the dermoid sinuses is consistent with normal skin plus adnexa.

TREATMENT

Dermoid sinuses may be resected if they are associated with drainage or neurologic signs. Strict asepsis is essential to avoid postoperative meningitis if the sinus extends to the dura. Incomplete excision may occur if the sinus attaches to the dura and causes a chronic draining lesion. The prognosis is guarded if neurologic signs occur before surgery. *Clip and aseptically prepare a large area around the sinus. Position the dog in ventral recumbency and make an elliptical incision around the sinus opening. Carefully dissect the sinus to its origin and free its attachment. Divide or split the nuchal ligament if necessary. Perform a laminectomy or hemilaminectomy (see p. 1055) if the sinus tract extends to the dura. Lavage thoroughly before closure. If the nuchal ligament has been transected, reappose it with a locking loop or modified Bunnel's suture pattern (see p. 50). Appose muscles and deep tissues with interrupted absorbable sutures to eliminate dead space (e.g., 3-0 or 4-0 polydioxanone or polyglyconate). If a large amount of dead space is still present, place a closed suction drain at the site. Appose subcutaneous tissues and skin routinely. Submit tissue samples for culture and sensitivity testing and histologic evaluation. Give analgesics, antibiotics, and bandage the site after surgery. Neuter affected animals.*

Suggested Reading

Angarano DW, Swaim SF: Congenital skin diseases. In Bojrab MJ, editor: *Disease mechanisms in small animal surgery,* ed 2, Philadelphia, 1993, Lea & Febiger.

INTERDIGITAL PYODERMA

Interdigital pyoderma (granuloma, acne, furunculosis) is a bacterial pododermatitis that may coexist with other conditions. Sometimes erroneously called an interdigital cyst, pododermatitis may be caused by parasites, allergies, mycoses, irritants, neoplasms, and metabolic, neurologic, or autoimmune disease. Bacterial infections are usually secondary to demodicosis, allergy, hypothyroidism, or hyperglucocorticoidism. Immunosuppression is suspected in some animals. The primary bacterial pathogen is *Staphylococcus intermedius.* Secondary opportunistic bacteria include *Proteus* spp., *P. aeruginosa,* and *E. coli.*

Varying degrees of pruritus, pain, paronychia, swelling, erythema, and hyperpigmentation are common. Papules, pustules or nodules, draining tracts, and ulcers may be present. Chronic infections may produce interdigital fibrosis and pyogranulomas. Antibiotic and steroid therapy may cause remission, but recurrence is common. The underlying cause should be identified and treated. Diagnostics include hematologic and serum biochemistry profiles, urinalysis, skin scraping, culture and sensitivity testing, cytology, and biopsy. Consider referring animals that do not respond to conservative treatment to a dermatologist.

TREATMENT

Conservative surgical treatment involves incision, exploration, and debridement of all fistulous tracts. Lesions should be medicated with antibacterial agents (e.g., chlorhexidine, povidone-iodine, nitrofurazone) and bandaged for 24 to 48 hours. Subsequently, they should be soaked with an antibacterial solution for 15 to 20 minutes twice daily. Oral antibiotics chosen based on sensitivity testing are continued for 6 to 8 weeks. Lesions failing to respond to this treatment may require fusion podoplasty (see p. 151).

Suggested Reading

Bellah JR: Intertriginous dermatitis. In Bojrab MJ, editor: *Disease mechanisms in small animal surgery,* ed 2, Philadelphia, 1993, Lea & Febiger.

Swaim SF, Henderson RA: *Small animal wound management,* Philadelphia, 1990, Lea & Febiger.

Swaim SF et al: Fusion podoplasty for the treatment of chronic fibrosing interdigital pyoderma in the dog, *J Am Anim Hosp Assoc* 27:264, 1991.

REDUNDANT SKIN FOLDS

Redundant skin is characteristic of some breeds and is exacerbated by obesity. Chronic skin overlap or apposition creates skin folds of varying depths. Pyoderma occurs in the skin fold recesses (intertriginous dermatitis) because it is a poorly ventilated, dark, warm, moist environment. Commonly involved organisms include *Staphylococcus, Streptococcus, E. coli, Pseudomonas, Proteus,* and *Candida* spp. Friction at contact points, retention of secretions, and bacterial proliferation cause skin maceration and superficial ulceration. Affected areas become painful and foul smelling, causing the animal to further traumatize the area by scooting, rubbing, licking, or scratching.

Skin fold resection is the most effective treatment for skin fold pyoderma (see below). First, medical therapy should reduce infection, inflammation, and secretions or exudates. Medical therapy consists of clipping hair from the folds and surrounding area, applying topical antibacterial solutions and medicated soaps, using antiseborrheic shampoos and astringents, and giving appropriate systemic antimicrobials. Culture and sensitivity testing is necessary to select appropriate antimicrobials. Corticosteroids are sometimes needed to reduce pruritus-induced self-trauma. Weight reduction is beneficial for obese animals. Continuous medical therapy is palliative, not curative. The surgical site must be kept clean and dry and protected from trauma. Continued antimicrobial therapy may be necessary. General complications of skin fold resection and reconstruction are self-trauma, infection, dehiscence, and pyoderma recurrence.

LIP FOLDS

Breeds with excessive mandibular labial tissue (large pendulous lips) (e.g., spaniels, St. Bernards, Newfoundlands, Labrador retrievers, golden retrievers, Irish setters) most commonly have lip fold dermatitis. It may also occur following partial maxillectomy or mandibulectomy. The fold usually occurs behind the mandibular canine tooth where food and saliva accumulate. Affected dogs rub and paw their faces, and the skin becomes inflamed and thickened. Halitosis and pruritus are the most common presenting complaints.

Lip Fold Resection (Cheiloplasty)

Position the anesthetized animal in dorsal recumbency to allow access to both lips. Clip and aseptically prepare the mandibular area (Fig. 13-32, A). Make an elliptical incision around the affected area, paralleling the horizontal ramus of the mandible (Fig. 13-32, B). The incision may involve the mucocutaneous junction. Elevate and remove the outlined skin segment, preserving underlying muscles. Control hemorrhage with ligation, electrocoagulation, and pressure. Assess the adequacy of resection and excise additional skin if necessary. Lavage the site and appose subcutaneous and subcuticular tissues with continuous or interrupted approximating sutures (e.g., 3-0 or 4-0 polydioxanone or polyglyconate). Place interrupted appositional sutures in the skin (e.g., 3-0 or 4-0 polypropylene or nylon) (Fig. 13-32, C). Use an Elizabethan collar or bucket to prevent self-inflicted trauma to the surgical site. Keep the area clean and dry, removing food and saliva as needed.

FIG. 13-32
A, Cheiloplasty for lip fold dermatitis. **B,** Make an elliptical incision and excise the infected skin. **C,** Appose healthy skin edges with approximating sutures.

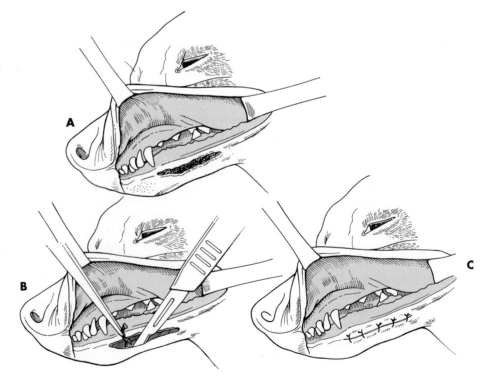

Antidrool Cheiloplasty

Antidrool cheiloplasty reduces the loss of food and saliva from the lateral vestibules of the oral cavity when there is excessive eversion or denervation of the lower lip. Oral function is usually normal after surgery, but inflammation and infection occasionally occur at the surgical site. Permanent flap adhesion and cheek scars are expected. *Position the anesthetized patient in lateral recumbency. Clip the lateral face, lavage the oral cavity, and aseptically prepare the skin for surgery. Grasp the lower lip 2 to 3 cm rostral to the commissure and elevate it dorsally until the lip is taut when the dog's mouth is completely opened (Fig. 13-33, A). The site of maximal tautness is usually near the level of the caudal root of the upper fourth premolar. Beginning near an imaginary line between the medial canthus of the eye and the commissure, make a 2.5- to 3-cm, horizontal, full-thickness incision through the maxillary skin at the site of tautness (Fig. 13-33, B). Control hemorrhage with ligation or electrocoagulation. The dorsal labial vein lies just dorsal to the proposed incision site. Use scissors to remove a 2-mm strip of mucosa adjacent to the mucocutaneous junction of the lower lip, beginning 2 cm rostral to the commissure and extending 2.5 cm (Fig. 13-33, C). Create 0.5- to 0.75-cm mucosal and skin flaps by undermining on each side of the in-*

cision (Fig. 13-33, D). Place stay sutures at the rostral and caudal aspects of the flaps. Evert the flaps through the cheek incision with the stay sutures (Fig. 13-33, E). Secure and bury the flap edges in the cheek skin incision with 3 to 4 preplaced vertical mattress sutures (e.g., 2-0 or 3-0 polypropylene or nylon) (Fig. 13-33, F and G). Add additional approximating skin sutures if necessary to achieve good skin apposition. Reposition the patient and repeat the procedure on the other side. Lavage the oral cavity with water after meals. Fit the dog with an Elizabethan collar or bucket to prevent self-inflicted trauma if necessary. Remove sutures at 21 days. Delay suture removal because constant lip movement may interfere with healing.

NASAL FOLDS

Brachycephalic breeds (i.e., English bulldogs, French bulldogs, Pekingese, Boston terriers, pugs, Persian cats) characteristically have facial or nasal skin folds across the bridge of the nose. Prominent folds cause pyoderma and a foul odor. Hair rubbing on the cornea is associated with keratitis, ulceration, epiphora, pain, and blepharospasm. Facial folds remain moist and become stained secondary to epiphora. Fold resection and ophthalmic medications are necessary. Excision of too much skin may cause ectropion or promote dehiscence.

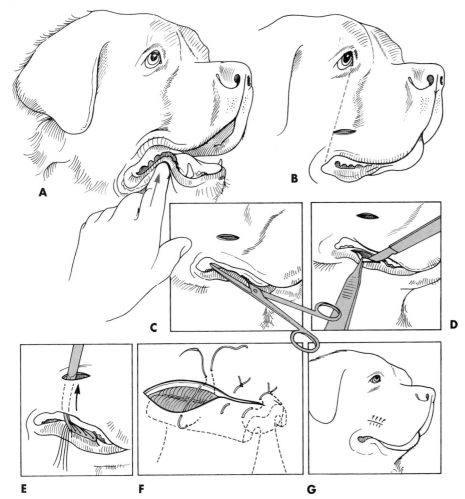

FIG. 13-33
A, For cheiloplasty in dogs that drool excessively, elevate the everted lip dorsally until it is taut when the dog's mouth is opened maximally. **B,** Make a 2.5- to 3-cm, horizontal, full-thickness incision through the maxillary skin at the site of tautness near the upper fourth premolar. **C,** Remove a 2-mm strip of mucosa 2.5 cm long from the mucocutaneous junction of the lower lip beginning 2 cm rostral to the commissure. **D,** Create 0.5- to 0.75-cm flaps. **E,** evert the flaps through the skin incision, **F** and **G,** and secure with vertical mattress sutures.

Nasal Skin Fold Resection

Position the patient in ventral recumbency. Protect the eyes with a petrolatum-based ophthalmic ointment. Clip and aseptically prepare the dorsum of the nose and lips. Estimate the amount of skin that must be resected to eliminate the skin folds without causing excess tension or ectropion. Make an elliptical incision around or through the skin folds in nonmacerated tissue. Keep the caudal incision approximately 1 cm away from the medial canthus. Undermine and remove the outlined skin segment. Avoid traumatizing the nasolabialis muscle and facial vessels during dissection. Control hemorrhage with ligatures, electrocoagulation, and pressure. Lavage the area with sterile saline. Bury three or four interrupted sutures in the subcutaneous and subcuticular tissues to align and appose the skin edges and assess the adequacy of resection. Resect more skin if skin recesses remain. If necessary, undermine the skin edges to allow apposition without tension. Place additional interrupted, subcuticular sutures (e.g., 4-0 polydioxanone or polyglyconate) with buried knots. Use approximating skin sutures (e.g., 4-0 nylon or polypropylene) and cut the ends short to prevent further corneal irritation. Place an Elizabethan collar or bucket to prevent self-trauma. Keep the site free of exudates and ocular discharge. Continue to medicate the eyes.

VULVAR FOLDS

Vulvar skin folds occur in obese females and those with infantile, recessed vulvas. Urine and vaginal secretions are trapped by the skin fold resulting in superficial perivulvar dermatitis. Clinical signs include perineal pain, odor, and urinary tract infections. Episioplasty is a vulvar reconstructive procedure that removes the skin fold (see p. 532 for a description of the technique). Skin fold pyoderma should be resolved medically before surgery. Complications include inflammation, swelling, infection, dehiscence, and recurrent perivulvar dermatitis. Excessive suture line tension may cause dehiscence. Perivulvar dermatitis will recur if inadequate skin is excised.

☞ **N O T E** • Weight reduction may be beneficial if the animal is obese.

TAIL FOLDS

Redundant skin often overlaps deformed terminal caudal vertebrae ("screwtails," "corkscrew" tails, ingrown tails). Tail fold pyoderma occurs most commonly in brachycephalic breeds but has also been reported in Schipperke dogs and Manx cats. The skin fold may be several inches deep with severe pyoderma. The depth of the folds varies with the animal's size, amount of fat, abundance of skin, and degree of vertebral deviation. Fecal contamination, licking, and scooting exacerbate the condition. Signs include perineal pruritus, pain, odor, ulcers, and fistulous tracts. Differential diagnoses should include perianal fistula, anal sacculitis, perianal tumors, trauma, and foreign bodies. Draining tracts should be probed or a fistulogram performed to determine their site of origin. To remove all skin recesses at the tailhead, complete caudectomy is necessary (see also p. 145).

Tail Fold Resection

Give perioperative antibiotics based on skin fold culture and sensitivity results. Scrub the skin folds separate from the remainder of the surgical field. Resect the tail and skin folds en bloc being careful during dissection to avoid penetrating the skin folds or traumatizing the rectum. Manipulate the tail with bone-holding forceps or towel clamps. Ankylosis or severe ventral deviation may make the vertebrae immobile. Transect the tail cranial to the deviated vertebrae with Gigli wire or a bone cutter if the intervertebral space cannot be located. Smooth sharp bone edges with rongeurs. Lavage thoroughly and insert Penrose drains before apposing the subcutaneous tissues with absorbable sutures (e.g., 3-0 or 4-0 polydioxanone or polyglyconate). Drains should exit ventral to the incision and lateral to the anus. Close skin with nonabsorbable sutures (e.g., 3-0 or 4-0 nylon or polypropylene). Keep the area clean and free of exudate and fecal contamination by applying warm moist compresses two to three times daily for 15 to 20 minutes. Remove drains in 3 to 5 days.

Suggested Reading

Harari J: *Surgical complications and wound healing in the small animal practice,* Philadelphia, 1993, WB Saunders.

Pavletic MM: Plastic and reconstructive surgery, Vet Clinics of N Am (Sm Anim) 20, Philadelphia, 1990, WB Saunders.

Smeak DD: Anti-drool cheilooplasty: clinical results in 6 dogs, *J Am Anim Hosp Assoc* 25:181, 1989.

Swaim SF, Henderson RA: *Small animal wound management,* Philadelphia, 1990, Lea & Febiger.

SURGERY OF THE TAIL

Caudectomy (i.e., amputation of a portion of the tail) is usually performed to comply with breed standards or tradition; however, therapeutic caudectomy is indicated for traumatic lesions, infection, neoplasia, and possibly perianal fistula. The tail should be amputated with 2 to 3 cm of normal tissue margins when resecting tumors or traumatic lesions. Amputation should be performed near the anus if the end of the tail chronically bleeds because of repeated abrasion or chewing. Amputation near the base is recommended for avulsed tails and if necessary for tail fold pyoderma and perianal fistula.

CAUDECTOMY IN PUPPIES

Cosmetic caudectomy (i.e., tail docking) in puppies is performed between 3 to 5 days of age and does not require anesthesia. The desired tail length should be determined by referring to breed standards and consulting with the owner (Table 13-3). Healing after caudectomy in puppies is usually

TABLE 13-3

Tail Docking Guidelines

Breed	Length at less than 1 week
Sporting Breeds	
Brittany Spaniel	Leave 1 in
Clumber Spaniel	Leave $\frac{1}{4}$ to $\frac{1}{3}$ of length
Cocker Spaniel	Leave $\frac{1}{3}$ of length (approximately $\frac{3}{4}$ in)
English Cocker Spaniel	Leave $\frac{1}{3}$ of length
English Springer Spaniel	Leave $\frac{1}{3}$ of length
Field Spaniel	Leave $\frac{1}{3}$ of length
German Shorthaired Pointer	Leave $\frac{2}{5}$ of length
German Wirehaired Pointer	Leave $\frac{2}{5}$ of length
Sussex Spaniel	Leave $\frac{1}{3}$ of length
Vizsla	Leave $\frac{2}{3}$ of length
Weimaraner	Leave $\frac{2}{3}$ of length (approximately $1\frac{1}{2}$ in)
Welsh Springer Spaniel	Leave $\frac{1}{3}$ to $\frac{1}{2}$ of length
Wirehaired Pointing Griffon	Leave $\frac{1}{3}$ of length
Working Breeds	
Bouvier des Flanders	Leave $\frac{1}{2}$ to $\frac{3}{4}$ in
Boxer	Leave $\frac{1}{2}$ to $\frac{3}{4}$ in (two vertebrae)
Doberman Pinscher	Leave $\frac{3}{4}$ in (two vertebrae)
Giant Schnauzer	Leave $1\frac{1}{4}$ in (three vertebrae)
Old English Sheepdog	Leave one vertebrae (close to body)
Rottweiler	Leave one vertebrae (close to body)
Standard Schnauzer	Leave 1 in (2 vertebrae)
Welsh Corgi (Pembroke)	Leave one vertebrae (close to body)
Terrier Breeds	
Airedale Terrier	Leave $\frac{2}{3}$ to $\frac{3}{4}$ of length*
Australian Terrier	Leave $\frac{2}{5}$ of length
Fox Terrier	Leave $\frac{2}{3}$ to $\frac{3}{4}$ of length*
Irish Terrier	Leave $\frac{3}{4}$ of length
Kerry Blue Terrier	Leave $\frac{1}{2}$ to $\frac{2}{3}$ of length
Lakeland Terrier	Leave $\frac{2}{3}$ to $\frac{3}{4}$ of length
Miniature Schnauzer	Leave $\frac{3}{4}$ in (less than 1 in)
Norwich Terrier	Leave $\frac{1}{4}$ to $\frac{1}{3}$ of length
Sealyham Terrier	Leave $\frac{1}{3}$ to $\frac{1}{2}$ of length
Soft Coated Wheaten Terrier	Leave $\frac{1}{2}$ to $\frac{2}{3}$ of length
Welsh Terrier	Leave $\frac{2}{3}$ to $\frac{3}{4}$ of length*
Toy Breeds	
Affenpinscher	Leave $\frac{1}{3}$ in (close to body)
Brussels Griffon	Leave $\frac{1}{4}$ to $\frac{1}{3}$ of length (approximately $\frac{1}{3}$ in)
English Toy Spaniel	Leave $\frac{1}{3}$ of length (approximately $1\frac{1}{2}$ in)
Miniature Pinscher	Leave $\frac{1}{2}$ in (two vertebrae)
Silky Terrier	Leave $\frac{1}{3}$ of length (approximately $\frac{1}{2}$ in)
Toy Poodle	Leave $\frac{1}{2}$ to $\frac{2}{3}$ (approximately 1 in)
Yorkshire Terrier	Leave $\frac{1}{3}$ of length (approximately $\frac{1}{2}$ in)
Nonsporting Breeds	
Miniature Poodle	Leave $\frac{1}{2}$ to $\frac{2}{3}$ of length (approximately $1\frac{1}{8}$ in)
Schipperke	Close to body
Standard Poodle	Leave $\frac{1}{2}$ to $\frac{2}{3}$ of length (approximately $1\frac{1}{2}$ in)
Miscellaneous Breeds	
Cavalier King Charles Spaniel (optional)	Leave $\frac{2}{3}$ of length with white tip
Spinoni Italiani	Leave $\frac{3}{5}$ of length

*Tip of docked tail should be approximately level with top of skull when puppy is in show position

uncomplicated. Puppies rarely irritate the surgical site, but bitches may lick sutures out within a few days. If caudectomy is not performed during the first week of life it should be delayed until the puppy is 8 to 12 weeks old and performed under a general anesthetic.

Have an assistant restrain the puppy. Clip and aseptically prepare the proposed site of resection. Retract the tail's skin toward the tailhead. Immobilize the tail between the thumb and index finger and apply pressure to help control hemorrhage. Palpate the desired transection site. Transect the tail between adjacent caudal vertebrae with Mayo scissors, nail trimmers, scalpel blade, or a tail docker/cutter (Tail Docker/Cutter). You may use scissors to assist with skin retraction. Place the ventral blade at the desired transection site. Position the dorsal blade more distally at an oblique angle. Rotate the blades into a perpendicular position while maintaining firm contact with the skin to push the skin cranially (Fig. 13-34, A). Maintaining the scissors in this position, transect through an intervertebral space (Fig. 13-34, B). Control hemorrhage with pressure or electrocautery. Extend the retracted skin over the remaining tail, assess the tail length, and resect more if necessary. Appose skin edges with two or three approximating sutures (e.g., 4-0 nylon or polypropylene) (Fig. 13-34, C).

CAUDECTOMY IN ADULTS

Caudectomy in dogs older than 1 week requires general or epidural anesthesia. The surgical site should be observed for swelling, draining, inflammation, and pain. Healing after caudectomy is uncomplicated if excess skin tension and self-trauma are avoided. The site should be protected with a bandage or restraining device if necessary. Complications include infection, dehiscence, scarring, fistula recurrence, and anal sphincter or rectal trauma. Incisions that dehisce after partial amputation may heal by second intention, which usually leaves a hairless scar. Reamputation may be necessary to relieve irritation and improve cosmesis.

Partial Amputation

Wrap the distal tail with gauze or insert it into an exam glove and secure the covering with tape. Clip a generous area near the amputation site and aseptically prepare it for surgery. Position the patient in a perineal position or lateral recumbency. Retract the skin toward the tailhead. Make a double V incision in the skin distal to the desired intervertebral transection site. Orient the V to create dorsal and ventral skin flaps that are longer than the desired tail length (Fig. 13-35, A). Identify and ligate the medial and lateral caudal arteries and veins slightly cranial to the transection site (Fig. 13-35, B). Incise soft tissues slightly distal to the desired intervertebral space and disarticulate the distal tail with a scalpel blade. If bleeding occurs place a circumferential ligature around the distal end of the remaining tail or religate the caudal vessels (Fig. 13-35, C). Appose subcutaneous tissue and muscle over the exposed vertebrae with interrupted approximating sutures (e.g., 3-0 polydioxanone or polyglyconate). Fold the dorsal skin flap over the caudal vertebrae (Fig. 13-35, D). Trim the ventral skin flap as needed to allow skin apposition without tension. Appose skin edges with approximating sutures (e.g., 3-0 or 4-0 nylon or polypropylene with a reverse cutting needle) (Fig. 13-35, D). Protect the surgical site with a bandage or by placing an Elizabethan collar or bucket over the animal's head.

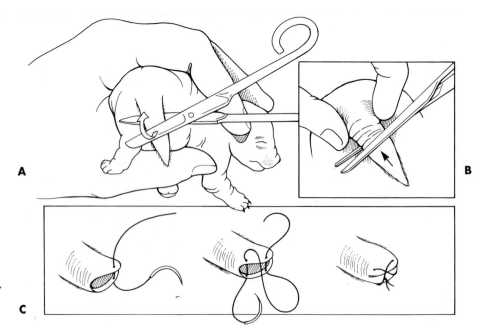

FIG. 13-34
A, For puppy caudectomy retract the tail's skin toward the tailhead and immobilize the tail between the thumb and index finger. **B,** Rotate the scissors toward the tailhead to push the skin toward the body. Transect the tail through the desired intervertebral space. **C,** Appose skin edges with approximating sutures.

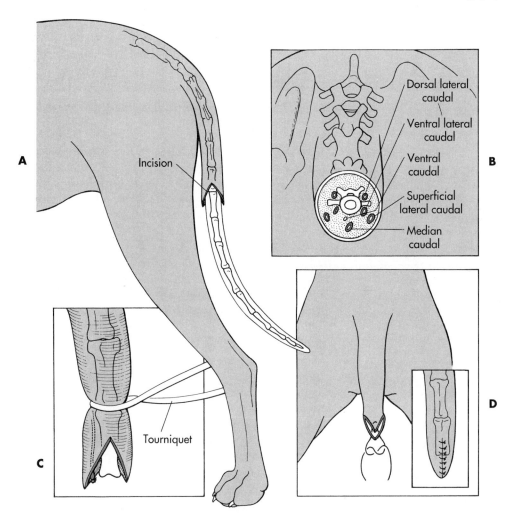

FIG. 13-35
A, For adult partial caudectomy retract the tail's skin toward the tailhead and make a double V incision in the skin distal to the desired transection site. **B,** Ligate the median and lateral caudal arteries and veins. **C,** Transect the soft tissues distal to the desired intervertebral space. Transect the tail through the desired intervertebral space. A proximally placed tourniquet assists hemostasis. **D,** Appose soft tissues and skin with approximating sutures.

Complete Caudectomy

Anesthetize the patient; clip and aseptically prepare the entire perineum and tailhead area. Position the animal in ventral recumbency. Make an elliptical incision around the tail base (Fig. 13-36, A). Incise subcutaneous tissues to expose the muscles. Separate the attachments of the levator ani, rectococcygeus, and coccygeus muscles to the caudal vertebra (Fig. 13-36, B). Ligate the medial and lateral caudal arteries and veins before or after transection. Transect the tail by disarticulation with a scalpel blade at the second or third caudal vertebra. Lavage the site after hemostasis is controlled. Appose the levator ani muscles and subcutaneous tissues with simple interrupted or continuous suture patterns (e.g., 3-0 or 4-0 polydioxanone or polyglyconate). Excise redundant skin if necessary and appose skin edges with approximating, nonabsorbable sutures (e.g., 3-0 or 4-0 nylon or polypropylene).

☞ **N O T E** • Use an Elizabethan collar or similar restraining device after caudectomy in adult animals to prevent self-mutilation.

Suggested Reading

Rigg DL, Schwink KL: Tail amputation in the dog, *Compendium Contin Educ Pract Vet* 5:719, 1983.

SURGERY OF THE DIGITS AND FOOTPADS

ONYCHECTOMY

Onychectomy (i.e., declawing) is removal of the third digital phalanx (P3) (Fig. 13-37, *A*). It is usually performed between 3 and 12 months of age to prevent cats from scratching furniture or people. Usually only the forelimb claws are removed. Although it is recommended that declawed cats be kept indoors because the procedure interferes with a cat's ability to protect itself, those with hindlimb claws can climb to escape some dangers. Alternatives to elective onychectomy are to glue a vinyl cap to each claw every 6 to 8 weeks (SoftPaws) or perform deep digital flexor tendonectomy (see below). Vinyl caps blunt the claws to render them less damaging.

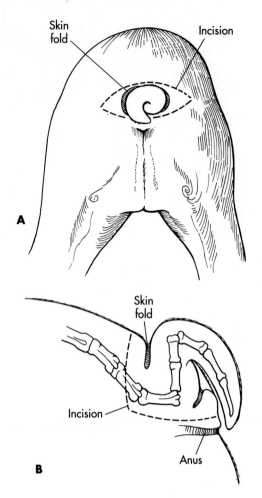

FIG. 13-36
A, Complete caudectomy with tail fold pyoderma requires an elliptical incision around diseased skin and **B,** deep dissection to locate the caudal vertebrae rostral to the vertebral deviation.

Onychectomy or more extensive digit amputation may remove infected nailbeds and neoplasms. The most common nailbed tumors are squamous cell carcinomas, melanomas, soft tissue sarcomas, and osteosarcomas. Complete excision may require that adjacent phalanges be removed with the affected claw. Onychomycosis, usually caused by *Tricophyton mentagrophytes*, produces dry, cracked, brittle, and deformed nails with inflamed alopecic nailbeds. Follicular infections with *Demodex* and *Staphylococcus* organisms produce similar lesions.

Dissection Onychectomy

In cats either a scalpel or guillotine-type nail clipper may be used to remove the third phalanx. The dissection technique is used for canine onychectomy. Onychectomy is performed with the patient under general anesthesia. Clipping hair from the paw and around the toes is advised in dogs and long-haired cats. Although most germinal cells are located in the ungual crest, the entire process must be removed to prevent claw regrowth.

Aseptically scrub the paw, digits, and nails for surgery. Position the animal in lateral recumbency and apply a tourniquet below the elbow to minimize blood loss and improve visualization. Tourniquet application above the elbow in cats may cause damage to the radial, median, or ulnar nerves because their arm muscles lack protective bulk. Alternatively, have an assistant compress the brachial artery with a thumb or index finger against the humeral shaft by applying pressure just cranial to the triceps muscle on the medial aspect of the brachium. Drape the feet. Extend the claw by grasping the tip with a towel clamp or by pushing up on the digital pad. Circumferentially incise the hairless, cuticle-like skin away from the claw near the articulation between the second and third phalanx (Fig. 13-37, B). Transect the common digital extensor tendon and dorsal ligaments with a No. 11 or No. 12 scalpel blade. Follow the contour of the proximal end of P3 to transect the deep digital flexor tendon and dissect the phalanx from the digital pad and other soft tissue attachments (i.e., joint capsule, collateral ligaments, other tendons). Avoid cutting the digital pad. Remove all 10 claws from the front paws for elective onychectomy. Appose skin edges with a bandage, single interrupted cruciate sutures, or cyanoacrylate tissue adhesive (e.g., Vetbond Tissue Adhesive). Do not place sutures through the digital pads. Apply tissue adhesives over the apposed surface of the skin and not between the cut edges. Apply a bandage from the paw to the distal antebrachium (see p. 107) and remove the tourniquet.

☞ **N O T E** · Be sure to count the excised claws prior to bandaging the foot to prevent inadvertently leaving a claw.

Nail Clipper Onychectomy

Prepare the paws for surgery as described in the section on dissection onychectomy. Trim the claws to facilitate positioning the nail trimmer in the interphalangeal space. Position a sharp guillotine-type nail clipper (Resco nail shears) around the claw (Fig. 13-37, C). Extend the claw by grasping the tip with a towel clamp. Position the blade dorsally at the joint space and transect the extensor tendon(s). Rotate the blade ventrally with continuous contact with the skin. Lift the claw dorsally to close the joint space and deviate the flexor process ventrally. After ensuring that the digital pad is proximal to the line of transection and the instrument is in the joint space, close the instrument to amputate the phalanx. Inspect the articular surfaces for complete excision of P3 (Fig. 13-37, D). If a small portion of the palmar aspect of P3 remains, grasp it with thumb forceps and carefully dissect if from the digital pad with a scalpel blade. Remove all 10 claws from the front paws for elective onychectomy. Appose skin edges with a single interrupted suture or tissue adhesive. Apply a bandage from the paw to the distal antebrachium (see p. 106) and remove the tourniquet.

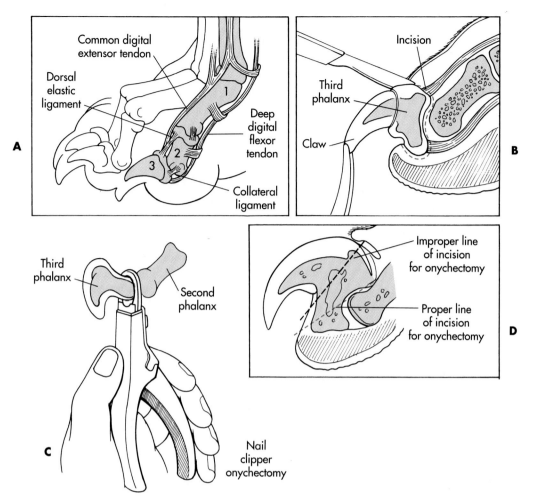

FIG. 13-37
A, Distal phalangeal anatomy for onychectomy. **B,** Dissection onychectomy disarticulates the third phalanx by transecting tendons, ligaments, and other soft tissue attachments. **C,** Nail clipper onychectomy should remove the entire ungual crest, but often leaves a portion of the ventral flexor process of P3. Proper and improper lines of transection are shown in **D.**

☞ **N O T E** · Use extreme care to avoid cutting the digital pads. When this occurs, the animal may be lame for a prolonged time. Skin edges may be left open—sutures or tissue adhesives are optional.

Postoperative Care and Complications

Mild bleeding should be expected when the bandage is removed after 12 to 24 hours; if bleeding persists the bandage should be reapplied for 2 to 3 days. Shredded paper, instead of litter, should be used for 2 weeks while the nailbeds heal. Sutures are usually removed by the cat within a week. Convalescence is more rapid in young growing cats than in older or obese cats. Complications (i.e., pain, hemorrhage, pad damage, lameness, swelling, infection, claw regrowth, second phalanx protrusion, and palmagrade stance) occur in 50% of patients. Cutting the digital pads prolongs postoperative pain and lameness. Early postoperative pain is more common after blade than nail clipper onychectomy (Tobias, 1994). Hemorrhage is most common in older animals and when wounds are not sutured. Late postoperative complications are more common when nail clippers are used (Tobias, 1994). Tissue adhesives may cause postoperative lameness (frequently non–weight-bearing) and infections and may be extruded from the wounds as a foreign body. Improper tourniquet use may cause neuropraxia, tissue necrosis, and lameness. The radial nerve is most often affected, but signs usually resolve in 6 to 8 weeks. Tight bandages can result in ischemic necrosis of the paw. Incomplete removal of the germinal cells in the dorsal aspect of the ungual crest allows claw regrowth. If only a small remnant of the flexor process remains, claw regrowth is not anticipated. Claw regrowth should be suspected if draining tracts develop. The regrown claw is usually deformed.

☞ **N O T E** · Warn owners that animals may be lame for several weeks after onychectomy.

DEEP DIGITAL FLEXOR TENDONECTOMY

The deep digital flexor tendon inserts on the flexor process of the third phalanx and is needed to flex the phalanx. Claws remain retracted after the deep digital flexor tendons are severed, which limits the cat's ability to scratch; however, the nails become thick and blunt and must be trimmed regularly. Hemorrhage, infection, and lameness may occur postoperatively. Tendonectomy of the superficial digital flexor (which inserts on the proximal aspect of P2) instead of the deep digital flexor results in an abnormal flat-footed stance. Problems may include interphalangeal joint immobility, fibrosis, pain, and claw ingrowth into the digital pads. Cats may require onychectomy to relieve clinical signs. Thus this technique is not routinely recommended.

☞ **N O T E** · After deep digital flexor tendonectomy the nails must be routinely clipped. Owners who are unlikely or unwilling to provide this aftercare should be advised against this procedure.

Anesthetize the cat and position it in dorsal or lateral recumbency. Clip and aseptically prepare the paws. Apply a tourniquet below the elbow to minimize hemorrhage. Make a 3- to 5-mm skin incision over the palmar surface of the second phalanx (P2), near the P2-P3 interphalangeal joint and digital pad (Fig. 13-38, A). The glistening, white tendon of the deep digital flexor lies directly beneath the skin. Dissect under the tendon with mosquito hemostats or small scissors (Fig. 13-38, B). Excise a 5-mm segment of tendon with a scalpel blade (Fig. 13-38, C). Appose the skin edges with an interrupted suture or tissue adhesive as for onychectomy. Repeat the procedure on each digit and trim each claw. Use torn paper rather than litter for 2 weeks. Limit activity and discourage jumping for 1 week.

DEWCLAW REMOVAL

The dewclaw is the first digit of the canine rear paws. The first and second phalanges of the digit are inconsistent. Dewclaws are absent in some dogs and double in others. Great Pyrenees and briard breeds must have double rear dewclaws to meet breed standards. In other breeds loosely attached dewclaws are removed to prevent trauma during hunting or grooming (Table 13-4). Often only the rear dewclaws are removed. Dewclaws should be removed at 3 to 5 days of age, at the same time as caudectomy. After 5 days of age, hemorrhage is more excessive and anesthetics are necessary. Complications include hemorrhage, pain, infection, and dehiscence. Premature suture removal may cause scarring. Bandages applied too tightly may cause swelling or ischemic necrosis.

Puppy Dewclaw Removal

Aseptically prepare the medial aspect of the paw. Have an assistant cup the puppy in his or her hands and immobilize the paw. Abduct the digit and transect the web of skin attaching the dewclaw to the paw with Mayo scissors (Fig. 13-39, A). Disarticulate the metatarsal(carpal)-phalangeal joint or transect the bone near the metatarsal or metacarpal bone with a scalpel blade or Mayo scissors. Control hemorrhage with pressure or electrocautery. Appose skin margins with a single approximating suture or allow second intention healing.

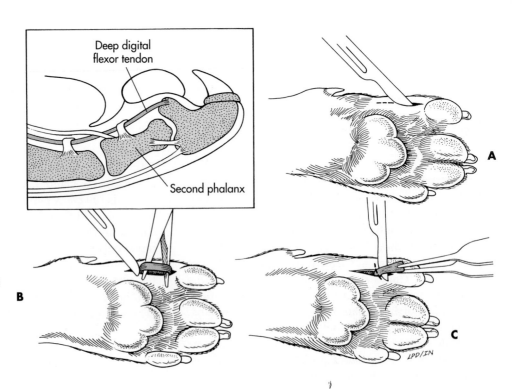

FIG. 13-38
A, For deep digital tendonectomy make a 3- to 5-mm incision over the palmar surface of the second phalanx. **B** and **C,** Elevate and excise a 5-mm segment of deep digital flexor tendon. The inset illustration shows the relationship of the deep digital flexor tendon to P1, P2, and P3.

Deep digital flexor tendon

Second phalanx

TABLE 13-4

Breeds Recommended for Dewclaw Removal

- Alaskan Malamute
- Basset Hound*
- Belgian Malinois
- Belgian Sheepdog
- Belgian Tervuren
- Bernese Mountain Dog
- Boxer
- Cardigan Welsh Corgi
- Chesapeake Bay Retriever
- Dalmatian
- Dandie Dinmont Terrier
- Kerry Blue Terrier
- Komondor
- Lakeland Terrier
- Norwegian Elkhound
- Papillon
- Puli*
- Rottweiler
- Shetland Sheepdog
- Siberian Husky
- Silky Terrier
- St. Bernard
- Vizsla
- Weimaraner

*Optional removal.

Adult Dewclaw Removal

If dewclaw removal is not performed within the first week of life, it should be delayed until after 3 months of age and performed under a general anesthetic. It is convenient to remove dewclaws at the time of neutering. *Position the patient in lateral recumbency. Clip and aseptically prepare the paws for surgery. Make an elliptical incision around the base of the digit where it articulates with the metatarsal or metacarpal bone (Fig. 13-39, B). Abduct the digit and dissect subcutaneous tissues to the metacarpophalangeal or metatarsophalangeal joint. If the first and second phalanges are firmly attached, free them with a No. 11 blade. Ligate the dorsal common and axial palmar digital arteries. Disarticulate the metacarpophalangeal or metatarsophalangeal joint with a scalpel blade. Results using bone cutters to transect the first phalanx near the metacarpophalangeal or metatarsophalangeal joint are less cosmetic. Appose subcutaneous tissues with 3-0 or 4-0 simple continuous or interrupted approximating sutures using absorbable suture material (i.e., polydioxanone, polyglyconate, polyglactin 910, or chromic catgut). Appose skin with interrupted approximating sutures (i.e., 3-0 or 4-0 nylon or polypropylene) (Fig. 13-39, C). Apply a soft, padded bandage to protect the surgical site for 3 to 5 days. Remove sutures at 7 to 10 days.*

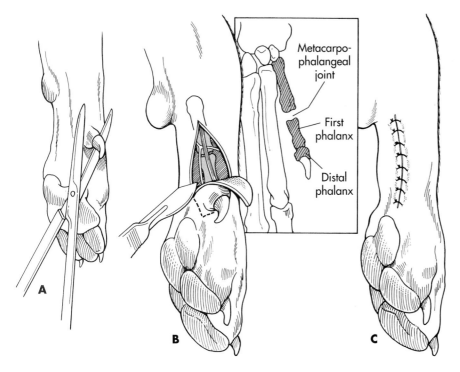

FIG. 13-39
A, For dewclaw removal in puppies, abduct and transect the dewclaw with scissors, disarticulating at the metatarsal(carpal)-phalangeal joint. **B,** In adults make an elliptical incision around the base of the dewclaw, dissect subcutaneous tissues, and ligate the dorsal common and axial palmar arteries. Then disarticulate the joint or transect P1 with bone cutters (*inset*). **C,** Appose subcutaneous tissues and skin with approximating sutures.

DIGIT AMPUTATION

Digit amputation is performed because of neoplasia, chronic bacterial or fungal infections, osteomyelitis, or severe trauma. Affected digits are swollen and painful with thickened, dystrophic, or absent claws. Occasionally a digit is amputated to facilitate salvage of a weight-bearing pad or portion of the paw. The primary weight-bearing digits are the third and fourth digits. The level of amputation is determined by the site of the lesion and disease process. General anesthesia is required. Complications include hemorrhage, infection, dehiscence, and recurrence. Tight bandages may cause swelling or ischemic necrosis. Lameness results if more than two digits or the third or fourth digits are removed.

Digital tumors occur in older dogs (mean, 10 years) and are often initially misdiagnosed as infections. Bone invasion is common. Squamous cell carcinomas, malignant melanomas, soft tissue sarcomas, and osteosarcomas are common digital tumors. Squamous cell carcinomas, mast cell tumors, and melanomas arising in the subungual epithelium are aggressive and sometimes metastatic. Black dogs are predisposed to subungual squamous cell carcinomas. One-year survival following digital amputation varies from 45% to 100%, depending on the tumor type.

Clip and aseptically prepare the paw for surgery. Position the dog in ventral or lateral recumbency with the leg suspended. Place a tourniquet and drape the area. Release the aseptically prepared paw into the sterile field. Begin a dorsal skin incision at the distal end of the appropriate metacarpal (metatarsal) or proximal end of the first phalanx. Make a transverse encircling incision at the appropriate interphalangeal joint (inverse Y incision) (Fig. 13-40, A and B). Preserve the digital pad if only the third phalanx is removed. Transect the flexor and extensor tendons, ligaments, and joint capsule. Ligate the digital arteries and veins with 3-0 or 4-0 absorbable suture. Disarticulate with a scalpel blade or transect the phalanx with bone cutters. Include the sesamoid bones with the excision. Suture the extensor tendon to the dorsal surface of the pad when it is preserved. Appose subcutaneous tissues over the end of the bone with interrupted absorbable sutures (e.g., 3-0 or 4-0 polydioxanone or polyglyconate). Appose skin with approximating sutures (e.g., 3-0 or 4-0 nylon or polypropylene) (Fig. 13-40, C). Apply a padded bandage and if necessary an Elizabethan collar or bucket. Keep the bandage clean and dry. Change the bandage in 2 to 3 days or as needed to evaluate the wound. Remove the bandage and sutures after 7 to 10 days.

FOOTPAD INJURIES

The footpad is the toughest area of the canine skin and is designed to absorb shock, standing, and abrasive forces. The stratum corneum is usually pigmented, thick, and keratinized, with a rough surface of conical papillae. Footpad injuries include laceration, degloving, abrasion, avulsion, burns, and tumors. Injuries may not heal well as a result of the weight-bearing forces and pad loss. Weight-bearing areas without pads may ulcerate.

Superficial Pad Loss

Wounds with superficial pad loss are allowed to heal by second intention and treated with nonadherent absorbent or semiabsorbent bandages and a spoon splint. A functional pad is maintained if epithelial tissue remains at the periphery and the wound is able to heal by contraction and epithelialization. Splinting the paw promotes healing because wound contractile forces are antagonized by weight bearing, which pushes the wound edges apart. Aloe vera extract gel has a positive effect on early stages of paw pad healing. Bandaging and splinting the paw should be continued until reepithelialization and some keratinization occur. Exercise should be

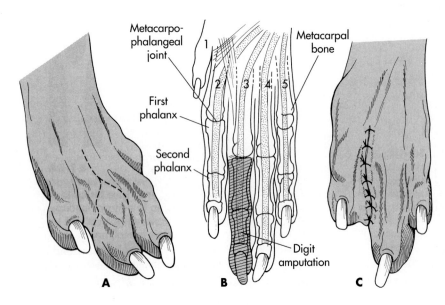

FIG. 13-40
A, For digit amputation begin the skin incision dorsally and extend it laterally on each side of the involved digit. **B,** Ligate digital vessels and transect the tendons, ligaments, and joint capsule to disarticulate the digit between P3-P2, P2-P1, or P1-metacarpal(tarsal). **C,** Appose subcutaneous tissues over the end of the bone and approximate skin edges.

restricted while the limb is bandaged. After bandage removal exercise may be gradually allowed on nonabrasive surfaces.

Lacerations

Improperly managed simple lacerations can become chronic nonhealing wounds because forces applied on the pads during standing or walking flatten and spread the pad, separating the lacerated edges. Proper management of lacerated pads includes lavage, suturing, and bandaging. Acute lacerations should be thoroughly lavaged and minimally debrided. Old, severely contaminated, or infected lacerations need wet-dry bandages for several days. The edges of chronic lacerations should be debrided to remove necrotic tissue and provide a bleeding edge for apposition. Deep layers of the pad should be apposed with buried simple interrupted absorbable sutures (e.g., 3-0 and 4-0 polydioxanone or polyglyconate). Epithelial edges are apposed with interrupted approximating sutures (e.g., 3-0 or 4-0 polypropylene or nylon), taking bites several millimeters from the cut edge. After closure the pad should be protected with a nonadherent, thick, absorbent bandage and a spoon splint (see p. 706). The bandage should be changed every 1 to 3 days depending on the amount of drainage. Sutures should be removed after 10 to 14 days and the splint/bandage reapplied for 3 to 4 days. The splint should then be removed but the paw rebandaged for an additional 3 to 6 days to allow the wound to strengthen. Alternatively, the pad may be protected with a commercial boot after suture removal (Dog Bootie). Exercise should be restricted while the limb is bandaged. Exercise on a nonabrasive surface after bandage removal may be gradually instituted.

Paw Salvage

Degloving or crushing injuries to the paw may cause a nonfunctional paw. Amputation or multiple surgical procedures are required to maintain paw function when injury is severe. Free grafts, axial pattern flaps, or thoracic wall pouch flaps may be used to replace skin. Indoor cats and small dogs that walk primarily on carpets may function well on grafted skin that does not contain pads; however, most dogs require salvage or replacement of the metacarpal/metatarsal pad. Replacement of metatarsal, metacarpal, or weight-bearing digital pads may be achieved by transposing adjacent pads, segmental digital pad grafts, or microneurovascular free digital pad transfer (Fig. 13-41, A and B). Tissue should not be transposed over a pad injury caused by tendon malfunction, bone malalignment, or nerve damage until the cause is corrected. A digital pad is transposed to replace a portion of the metatarsal or metacarpal pad. The phalanges of digit two or five are removed through a palmar incision. The digital pad is maintained on a pedicle of skin and is transposed to the metatarsal/metacarpal pad (Bradley, Shealy, Swaim, 1993). Alternatively, severe trauma to all digits may necessitate digital amputation and transposition of the metatarsal or metacarpal pad over the bone ends to provide a weight-bearing surface (Barclay, Fowler, Basher, 1987). Free segmental digital pad grafts (6 × 8 mm) sutured into recessed

recipient beds in granulation tissue allow pad reepithelialization with a tough keratinized and effective weight-bearing surface (Swaim et al, 1993). Microneurovascular pad transfer requires specialized instrumentation and training. The paw should be bandaged after surgery as described above for lacerations.

FUSION PODOPLASTY

Fusion podoplasty is a salvage procedure used to treat severed flexor tendons or chronic interdigital pyoderma. Fusion podoplasty is not recommended on all four paws during a single surgery because of the prolonged operative time and postoperative discomfort. *Clip and aseptically prepare the paw. Position the anesthetized patient in dorsal or lateral recumbency. Secure a tourniquet around the distal limb. Excise the interdigital web and skin between the digital and metacarpal/metatarsal pads. Preserve 2 to 3 mm of skin adjacent to the nail. Avoid damage to the digital vessels and nerves during dissection. Control hemorrhage with electrocoagulation, pressure, and ligation. Thoroughly lavage the wound. Suture the digital pads in apposition with simple interrupted sutures (e.g., 3-0 polypropylene or nylon). Approximate the digital and metacarpal/metatarsal pads with simple interrupted sutures; direct apposition of epithelial edges may not be possible. Before the last few pad sutures are inserted place a small Penrose drain across the paw deep to the sutures. Approximate adjacent skin edges dorsally with simple interrupted sutures (e.g., 3-0 polypropylene or nylon). Leave a gap between skin edges at the end of the digits to allow drainage. Repeat the procedure on the opposite paw if indicated. Remove the tourniquet. Apply an antibiotic ointment followed by a nonadherent, absorbent bandage and spoon splint extending from the paw to the elbow or hock. Change the bandage/splint daily until drainage diminishes, usually within 10 to 14 days. Remove the drain and extend the interval between bandage/splint changes to every 2 to 3 days. Soak the paw in an antiseptic solution before rebandaging if a Pseudomonas spp. infection is suspected. Remove sutures between 10 to 21 days after surgery but continue bandaging until granulation is complete. Additional debridement may be indicated if nonhealing wounds or draining tracts persist after surgery. When healing nears completion a lighter bandage or a paw bootie (Dog Bootie) allows transition between a heavy splinted bandage and full weight bearing.*

References

Barclay CG, Fowler JD, Basher AW: Use of the carpal pad to salvage the forelimb in a dog and cat: an alternative to total limb amputation, *J Am Anim Hosp Assoc* 23:527, 1987.

Bradley DM, Shealy PM, Swaim SF: Meshed skin graft and phalangeal fillet for paw salvage: a case report, *J Am Anim Hosp Assoc* 29:427, 1993.

Swaim SF et al: Free segmental paw pad grafts in dogs, *Am J Vet Res* 54:2161, 1993.

Tobias KS: Feline onychectomy at a teaching institution: a retrospective study of 163 cases, *Vet Surg* 23:274, 1994.

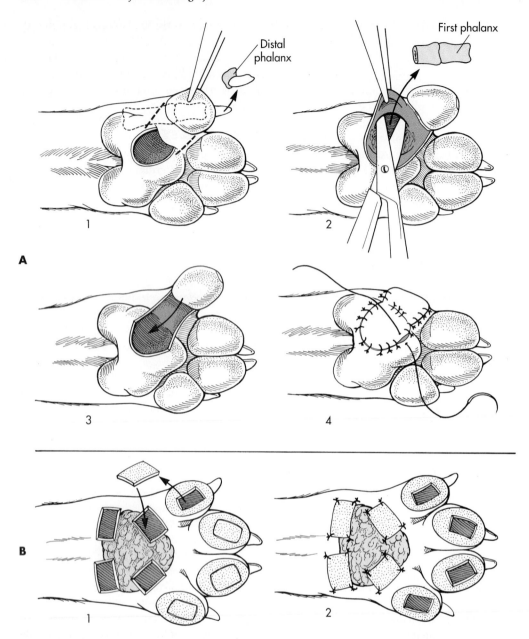

FIG. 13-41
Weight-bearing pads may be replaced or salvaged. **A,** Partially or completely replace a pad by removing P3 and P2 from digit two or five and transposing the pad and skin to the injured area (phalangeal fillet technique). **B,** The metacarpal or metatarsal pad may be salvaged by grafting from digital pads. Place the free segmental graft on a healthy granulation bed and across the skin-pad junction.

Suggested Reading

Brewer WG et al: Canine digital tumors: retrospective review of 63 cases (1980-1990), a veterinary comparative oncology group cooperative study—preliminary results, *Veterinary Cancer Society Newsletter* 17:7, 1993.

O'Brien MG, Berg J, Engler SJ: Treatment by digital amputation of subungual squamous cell carcinoma in dogs: 21 cases (1987-1988), *J Am Vet Med Assoc* 201:759, 1992.

Rife J: Deep digital flexor tendonectomy-an alternative to amputation onychectomy for declawing cats, *J Am Anim Hosp Assoc* 24:73, 1988.

Swaim SF: Management and bandaging of soft tissue injuries of dog and cat feet, *J Am Anim Hosp Assoc* 21:329, 1985.

Swaim SF, Henderson RA: *Small animal wound management,* Philadelphia, 1990, Lea & Febiger.

Swaim SF et al: Fusion podoplasty for the treatment of chronic fibrosing interdigital pyoderma in the dog, *J Am Anim Hosp Assoc* 27:264, 1991.

CHAPTER 14

Surgery of the Ear

GENERAL PRINCIPLES AND TECHNIQUES

DEFINITIONS

Otitis externa is inflammation of the vertical and/or horizontal ear canal(s), and **otitis media** is inflammation of the tympanic cavity and membrane.

PREOPERATIVE CONCERNS

To anticipate surgical complications it is imperative that the extent and severity of disease be determined in animals undergoing ear surgery. A head tilt may indicate severe pain or otitis media/interna (see p. 168). The latter should be suspected if the head tilt is associated with circling, nystagmus, and/or vestibular dysfunction (Table 14-1). Facial nerve function should be determined before surgery. Facial nerve deficits (i.e., poor palpebral reflex, lip droop, facial spasms) in patients with chronic otitis externa suggest concurrent middle ear disease. However, facial nerve paralysis may also occur as a result of intraoperative trauma. It is wise to perform a Schirmer's tear test in animals with ocular discharge to differentiate preoperative abnormalities in tear production (i.e., "dry eye") from surgically induced facial nerve trauma.

Otoscopic examination should determine if the tympanic membrane is intact and should define the severity of horizontal and vertical canal changes. Always inspect both ear canals, even if unilateral ear disease exists. Skull radiographs are used to determine if concurrent middle ear disease or neoplasia exists (see p. 176). Proliferation of cartilage or bone around the horizontal ear canal should be noted. After radiographs the ear should be cleaned, but using a solution greater than 0.2% chlorhexidine, iodine and iodophors, ethanol, or benzalkonium chloride should be avoided if the tympanic membrane is ruptured. Chlorhexidine may cause cochlear and vestibular dysfunction in cats when applied to the ear canal in combination with cetrimide. However, ototoxicity was not observed when dogs with surgically ruptured tympanic membranes were treated with 0.2% chlorhexidine (Merchant et al, 1993).

Owner's expectations must be considered; owners should be questioned as to their perception of the dog's hearing before surgery because total ear canal ablation may diminish hearing and be unacceptable. However, most owners do not report substantial alterations in their pets' hearing after this procedure, probably because marked hearing loss is frequently present before surgery. Similarly, brain stem–auditory evoked responses reveal that auditory function decreases minimally after total ear canal ablation in dogs with chronic otitis externa.

ANESTHETIC CONSIDERATIONS

Most animals undergoing ear surgery are healthy and a variety of anesthetic protocols can be used. Ear surgery, particularly total ear canal ablation, vertical canal resection, and lateral ear canal resection, is painful. Although butorphanol (0.2-0.4 mg/kg subcutaneously or intramuscularly) and buprenorphine (5-15 μg/kg intramuscularly) are

---

TABLE 14-1

Signs of Middle and Inner Ear Disease

- Head tilt
- Nystagmus
- Asymmetric ataxia
- Circling
- Stumbling
- Rolling
- Difficulty standing
- Nausea
- Vomiting
- Horner's syndrome
- Facial nerve paralysis
  - Diminished palpebral reflex
  - Widened palpebral fissure
  - Drooping of the ear and lip
  - Excessive drooling

common premedicants in dogs, oxymorphone (Table 14-2) appears to be a better analgesic for dogs undergoing ear surgery. Saturating the surgical site with bupivacaine hydrochloride (splash block; use a volume sufficient to cover the area but do not exceed 2 mg/kg) before closing the incision following resections or ablations may increase patient comfort in the early postoperative period. The area should not be flushed following a splash block for at least 20 minutes. A variety of anesthetic protocols (i.e., chamber induction with isoflurane, barbiturates, or a combination of ketamine and diazepam) can be used following premedication with butorphanol or buprenorphine to anesthetize cats for ear surgery (see Table 14-2). Ketamine should not be given to cats with neurologic dysfunction.

Postoperative analgesics should be given after ear surgery. If oxymorphone was used as a premedicant, it should be readministered 3 to 4 hours later (0.05-0.1 mg/kg intravenously, subcutaneously, or intramuscularly). If the animal appears dysphoric or anxious postoperatively, tranquilization may be necessary; however, tranquilizers should only be used in animals that have been given sufficient analgesics. If there are no contraindications to acepromazine administration (i.e., hypotension, seizures), low doses may be given (0.025-0.05 mg/kg subcutaneously, intramuscularly, or intravenously; not to exceed 1 mg).

TABLE 14-2

Selected Anesthetic Protocols for Ear Surgery

Dogs
Premedication

Give atropine (0.02-0.04 mg/kg SC or IM) or glycopyrrolate (0.005-0.011 mg/kg SC or IM) plus oxymorphone (0.05-0.1 mg/kg SC or IM; see text)

Induction

Thiopental sodium (10-12 mg/kg IV) or propofol (4-6 mg/kg IV)

Maintenance

Isoflurane or halothane

Cats
Premedication

Give atropine (0.02-0.04 mg/kg SC or IM) or glycopyrrolate (0.005-0.011 mg/kg SC or IM) plus butorphanol (0.2-0.4 mg/kg SC or IM) or buprenorphine (5-15 µg/kg IM)

Induction

Use chamber induction with isoflurane; or thiopental sodium or propofol at dose given above for dogs; or diazepam plus ketamine (see text) (0.27 mg/kg and 5.5 mg/kg, respectively) combined and administered IV to effect

Maintenance

Isoflurane or halothane

ANTIBIOTICS

Preoperative antibiotics are recommended in animals undergoing aural surgery. Bacterial cultures should be performed in those with purulent discharge and appropriate antibiotics initiated before surgery (Fig. 14-1). Severe infection should be treated for several weeks before surgery with systemic and/or topical antibiotics. In less severely affected animals, broad-spectrum antibiotics may be given before the surgical procedure, or during surgery but after intraoperative cultures have been taken. Cultures of deep tissues taken during surgery are often more useful than preoperative cultures. If possible, ototoxic antibiotics (i.e., gentamicin, kanamycin, neomycin, streptomycin, tobramycin, amikacin, polymyxin B) should be avoided; however, careful systemic use of aminoglycosides is necessary in some patients (e.g., *Pseudomonas* sp.). Initial ototoxicity caused by aminoglycosides is reversible by calcium administration, suggesting that these drugs interfere with maintenance of endolymph ion balance, which may impair electrical activity and nerve conduction.

SURGICAL ANATOMY

The ear is composed of three parts: (1) the inner ear, which consists of a membranous and a bony labyrinth and functions for hearing and balance, (2) the middle ear, which is formed by the tympanic cavity and connects to the pharynx via the auditory tube (eustachian tube), and (3) the external ear formed by the auditory meatus and a short canal (Fig. 14-2). The middle and external ears are separated by the tympanic membrane, and the opening of the horizontal canal into the middle ear is known as the external acoustic meatus. The three auditory ossicles (stapes, malleus, and incus) connect the tympanic membrane to the inner ear. The tympanic cavity is air filled and in dogs is composed of a small dorsal epitympanic recess and a large ventral tympanic bulla. The long axis of the tympanic cavity is about 15 mm long in medium-sized dogs. The auditory ossicles reside in the middle portion of the tympanic cavity. The feline tympanic cavity is divided into two compartments by a thin, bony septum that arises along

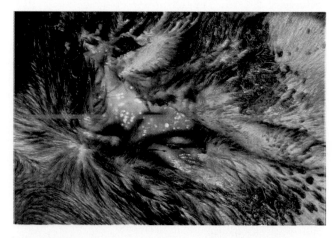

FIG. 14-1
Purulent discharge in a dog with chronic otitis externa.

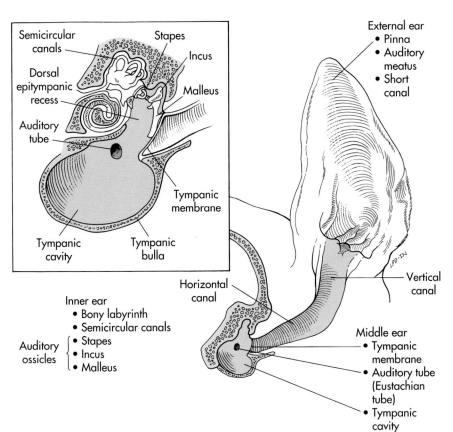

FIG. 14-2
Anatomy of the ear.

the cranial aspect of the bulla and curves to attach to the mid-point of the lateral wall (Fig. 14-3). The majority of the lateral wall of the smaller craniolateral compartment is formed by the tympanic membrane. These compartments communicate through a narrow fissure on the caudomedial aspect of the bony septum. Near this fissure the sympathetic nerves form a plexus on a structure known as the promontory. Because of their vulnerable location these nerves are often traumatized (i.e., Horner's syndrome; see p. 169) during surgical curettage of the feline middle ear. The tympanic membrane is normally thin and semitransparent but may become thickened or ruptured when diseased. The facial nerve exits the stylomastoid foramen caudal to the ear and courses ventral to the horizontal canal in close proximity to the middle ear.

The external ear varies in size and shape between dog breeds. The auricular cartilage determines the appearance of the canine pinna. The base of the ear is composed of a number of ridges that are important landmarks for ear surgery (Fig. 14-4). These include the tragus, lateral crus of helix, pretragic incisure, and intertragic incisure. The external opening of the vertical canal is known as the external auditory meatus. There are numerous muscles that attach to the cartilage of the ear and allow it to move to localize sound.

SURGICAL TECHNIQUES

Numerous surgical techniques have been described for the treatment of ear disease in dogs and cats. Only the more commonly performed techniques are described here.

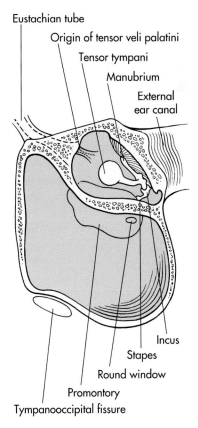

FIG. 14-3
The feline tympanic cavity.

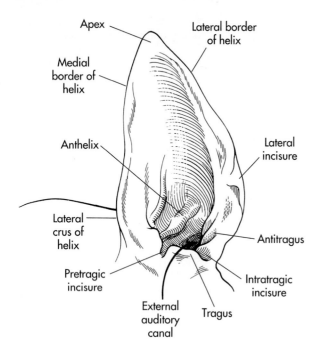

FIG. 14-4
Landmarks of the external ear.

☞ **NOTE** • When performing a lateral ear canal resection or vertical canal ablation be prepared to perform a total ear canal ablation if the opening of the horizontal canal is stenotic or too narrow to allow adequate drainage.

Lateral Ear Canal Resection

Lateral ear canal resection increases drainage and improves ventilation of the ear canal. It also facilitates placement of topical agents into the horizontal canal. Lateral ear canal resection is indicated in patients with minimal hyperplasia of the ear canal epithelium or small neoplastic lesions of the lateral aspect of the vertical canal. It should not be performed in animals with obstruction or stenosis of the horizontal ear canal, concurrent otitis media (unless performed in conjunction with ventral bulla osteotomy; see below), or in those with severe epithelial hyperplasia. Dogs with underlying disease (i.e., hypothyroidism or primary idiopathic seborrhea) often respond poorly to this surgery. In one study nearly 50% of dogs undergoing lateral ear canal resection for chronic otitis externa had a poor outcome (Gregory, Vasseur, 1983). It is important that owners understand that lateral ear canal resection is not a curative procedure and that medical management of the ear may be necessary for the remainder of the animal's life. A modification of the original technique for lateral ear resection described by Lacroix established a "drainboard" and is known as a Zepp procedure (Fig. 14-5).

☞ **NOTE** • The ventral flap in the Zepp procedure acts as a drainboard and restricts hair growth at the horizontal canal opening.

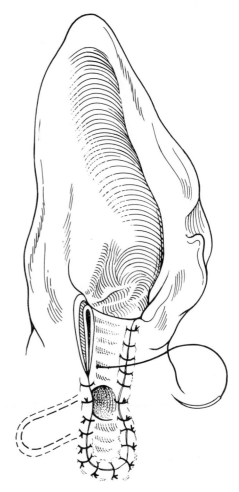

FIG. 14-5
Lateral ear resection (Zepp procedure).

Clip the entire side of the face and both sides of the pinna. Gently flush the ear and remove as much debris as possible. Position the animal in lateral recumbency with the head elevated on a towel and prepare the pinna and surrounding skin for aseptic surgery. Place quarter drapes around the ear with the entire pinna draped into the surgical site. Stand at the ventral aspect of the dog's head and position a forceps into the vertical ear canal to determine its ventral extent. Mark a site below the horizontal ear canal that is one half the length of the vertical ear canal (Fig. 14-6, A). Make two parallel incisions in the skin lateral to the vertical ear canal that extend from the tragus ventrally to the marked site (Fig. 14-6, B). These incisions should be one and one half times the length of the vertical ear canal. Connect the skin incisions ventrally and, using a combination of sharp and blunt dissection, reflect the skin flap dorsally exposing the lateral cartilaginous wall of the vertical ear canal. During dissection stay as close as possible to the cartilage of the ear canal to avoid inadvertently damaging the facial nerve. Note the parotid gland at the ventral extent of the incision and avoid damaging it. While standing at the dorsal aspect of

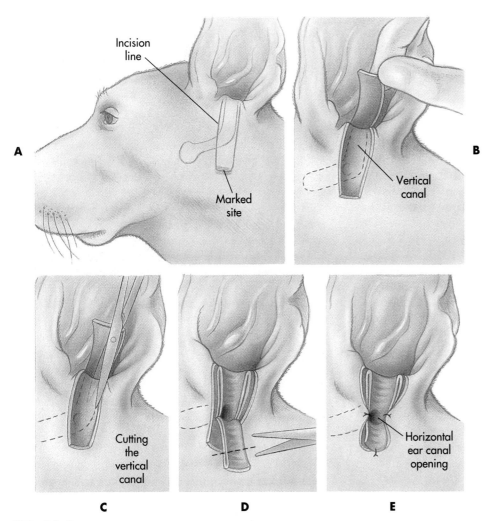

FIG. 14-6
A, For a lateral ear canal resection, mark a site that is one half the length of the vertical ear canal below the horizontal ear canal. **B,** Lateral to the vertical ear canal make two parallel incisions that extend from the tragus ventrally to the marked site. **C,** Connect the skin incisions ventrally and reflect the skin flap dorsally exposing the lateral cartilaginous wall of the vertical ear canal. Use Mayo scissors to cut the vertical canal. **D,** Reflect the cartilage flap distally and inspect the opening of the horizontal canal. Resect the distal one half of the cartilage flap to make the drainboard and remove the skin flap. **E,** Place sutures from the epithelial tissues to skin. Begin suturing at the opening of the horizontal canal, then suture the drainboard.

the animal's head, use Mayo scissors to cut the vertical canal (Fig. 14-6, C). Place one blade of the scissors within the canal at the pretragic or tragohelicine incisure at the cranial (medial) aspect of the external auditory meatus and incise the canal ventrally to the level of the horizontal canal. Repeat the process beginning at the intertragic incisure (caudal or lateral aspect of the external auditory meatus). Angle the scissors 30 degrees while making the cuts. Do not allow the incision to converge toward the lateral aspect of the canal or the drainboard will be too narrow. Be sure to extend the incisions as far distally as the beginning of the horizontal canal or the drainboard will not lie flat against the skin. Reflect the cartilage flap distally, inspect the opening of the horizontal canal, and if in-

dicated, obtain cultures (Fig. 14-6, D). Occasionally the opening can be widened by making two small cuts at the cranial and caudal aspect. Resect the distal one half of the cartilage flap to make the drainboard, and remove the skin flap. The ligament between the horizontal and vertical flaps usually acts as a hinge to allow the drainboard to lie flat, but in some cases scoring the cartilage on the ventral aspect of the drainboard will facilitate this. Place absorbable or nonabsorbable monofilament sutures (3-0 or 4-0) from the epithelial tissues to skin (Fig. 14-6, E). Begin suturing at the opening of the horizontal canal first, then suture the drainboard. Lastly, suture the cranial and caudal aspects of the medial wall of the vertical ear canal to skin (see Fig. 14-6, E).

☞ **N O T E** • Be sure that owners understand that medical management will continue to be necessary after lateral ear canal resection.

Vertical Ear Canal Ablation

Vertical canal ablation can be performed when the entire vertical canal is diseased but the horizontal canal is normal. It may be the technique of choice when neoplasia is confined to the vertical canal, or in some animals with chronic otitis externa. Total removal of the vertical canal may result in decreased postoperative exudation and pain. This technique may also provide a more cosmetic appearance of the ear than lateral ear canal resection when there is an abundance of hyperplastic tissue present in and around the vertical canal (Fig. 14-7).

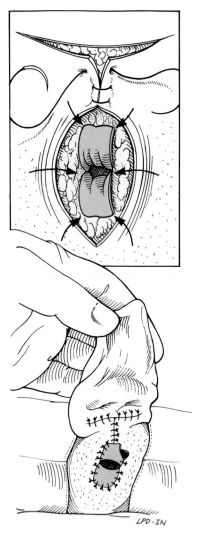

FIG. 14-7
Vertical ear canal resection can be performed when the entire vertical canal is diseased, but the horizontal canal is normal.

Position and prep the animal as for a lateral ear canal resection. Make a T-shaped incision with the horizontal component parallel and just below the upper edge of the tragus (Fig. 14-8, A). From the midpoint of the horizontal incision make a vertical incision that extends to the level of the horizontal canal. Retract the skin flaps, reflect loose connective tissue, and expose the lateral aspect of the vertical canal (Fig. 14-8, B). Continue the horizontal incision through the cartilage around the external auditory meatus with a scalpel blade. Remove as much of the diseased tissue on the medial surface of the pinna as possible but avoid damaging the major branches of the great auricular artery. Use curved Mayo scissors to dissect around the proximal and medial aspect of the vertical canal. During dissection stay as close as possible to the cartilage of the ear canal to avoid inadvertently damaging the facial nerve. Free the entire vertical canal from all muscular and fascial attachments (Fig. 14-8, C). Transect the vertical canal ventrally 1 to 2 cm dorsal to the horizontal canal and submit it for histologic examination (Fig. 14-8, D). Incise the remnant of the vertical canal cranially and caudally to create dorsal and ventral flaps (Fig. 14-8, E). Reflect the ventral flap downward and suture it to the skin for a drainboard using absorbable or nonabsorbable monofilament sutures (2-0 to 4-0). Suture the dorsal flap to the skin and close subcutaneous tissues with an absorbable suture material (2-0 or 3-0). Then close skin in a T shape (Fig. 14-8, F).

Total Ear Canal Ablation

Total ear canal ablation (Fig. 14-9) is indicated in animals with chronic otitis externa in which appropriate medical management has failed, when severe calcification/ossification of the ear cartilage is present, or when severe epithelial hyperplasia extends beyond the pinna or vertical ear canal. It is commonly performed in animals with lateral ear resections that have failed. Animals with severely stenotic ear canals may also benefit from this procedure. Occasionally, neoplasia of the horizontal canal can be treated by total ear canal ablation. Because of the potential for serious complications this surgery should not be performed in animals with mild disease or by surgeons unfamiliar with the anatomy of the ear. Associated skin disease (i.e., seborrhea, atopy, food or contact allergy dermatitis) should be treated. In many cases effective dermatologic therapy usually benefits the ears also. If the skin condition is unresponsive, total ear canal ablation is preferred over lateral ear resection (see p. 156) and should be performed in conjunction with either a lateral or ventral bulla osteotomy (see pp. 160-161).

☞ **N O T E** • Most animals with severe, chronic otitis externa have concurrent otitis media. Removing the avenue for exudative material to drain by performing a total ear canal ablation without treating the otitis media is disastrous. Therefore a bulla osteotomy should always be performed in conjunction with total ear canal ablation for otitis externa/media.

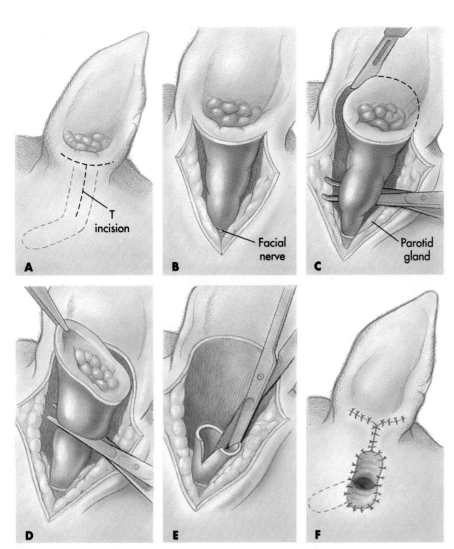

FIG. 14-8
A, For vertical ear canal resection, make a T-shaped incision with the horizontal component parallel and just below the upper edge of the tragus. From the midpoint of the horizontal incision, make a vertical incision which extends to the level of the horizontal canal. **B,** Retract the skin flaps, reflect loose connective tissue, and expose the lateral aspect of the vertical canal. **C,** Continue the horizontal incision through the cartilage around the external auditory meatus with a scalpel blade. Use curved Mayo scissors to dissect around the proximal and medial aspect of the vertical canal. Free the entire vertical canal from all muscular and fascial attachments. **D,** Transect the canal ventrally 1 to 2 cm dorsal to the horizontal canal and submit the canal for histologic examination. **E,** Incise the remnant of the vertical canal cranially and caudally to create dorsal and ventral flaps. **F,** Reflect the ventral flap downward and suture it to the skin for a drainboard. Suture the dorsal flap to the skin and close subcutaneous tissues. Then close skin in a T shape.

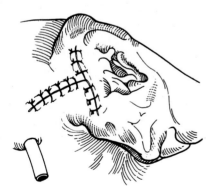

FIG. 14-9
Total ear canal ablation.

Position the animal in lateral recumbency with the head elevated with a towel and prepare the pinna and surrounding skin for aseptic surgery. Make a T-shaped incision with the horizontal component parallel and just below the upper edge of the tragus (Fig. 14-10, A). From the mid- *point of the horizontal incision make a vertical incision that extends to just past the level of the horizontal canal (see Fig. 14-10, A). Retract the skin flaps, reflect loose connective tissue, and expose the lateral aspect of the vertical canal. Continue the horizontal incision around the opening of the vertical ear canal with a scalpel blade (Fig. 14-10, B). Then use curved Mayo scissors to dissect around the proximal and medial aspect of the vertical canal (Fig. 14-10, C). During dissection stay as close as possible to the cartilage of the ear canal to avoid inadvertently damaging the facial nerve. Avoid damaging the major branches of the great auricular artery at the medial aspect of the vertical canal. Identify the facial nerve as it courses caudoventrally to the horizontal canal (gently retract it if necessary). If the facial nerve is entrapped within thickened and calcified horizontal canal tissue, carefully dissect the nerve from the horizontal canal. Continue the dissection to the level of the external acoustic meatus (Fig. 14-10, D). Excise the horizontal canal attachment to the external acoustic meatus with a scalpel blade, rongeur, or Mayo scissors but be careful to avoid damaging the facial nerve.*

FIG. 14-10

A, For total ear canal resection make a T-shaped incision with the horizontal component parallel and just below the upper edge of the tragus. From the midpoint of the horizontal incision, make a vertical incision that extends to just past the level of the horizontal canal. **B,** Retract the skin flaps, reflect loose connective tissue, and expose the lateral aspect of the vertical canal. Continue the horizontal incision around the opening of the vertical ear canal with a scalpel blade. **C,** Dissect around the proximal and medial aspect of the vertical canal. **D,** Continue the dissection to the level of the external acoustic meatus. **E,** Excise the horizontal canal attachment to the external acoustic meatus with a scalpel blade, rongeur, or Mayo scissors and use a curette to carefully remove secretory tissue that is adherent to the rim of the external acoustic meatus. **F,** If infection is considered likely, place an ingress-egress drain to allow the area to be flushed postoperatively. Close subcutaneous tissues and skin.

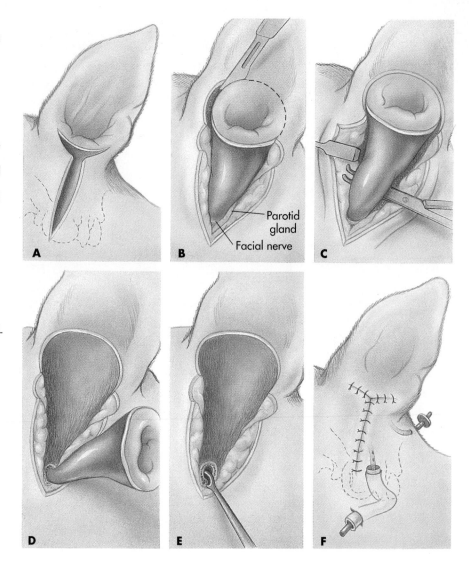

Remove the entire ear canal and obtain deep cultures around or just inside the external acoustic meatus. Submit the ear for histologic examination. Use a curette to carefully remove secretory tissue that is adherent to the rim of the external acoustic meatus (Fig. 14-10, E). Be sure to remove all epithelial tissues in this region or chronic fistulation will occur. Perform a lateral bulla osteotomy (see below). Flush the area with sterile saline solution before closure. If obvious infection remains or extensive drainage is likely, place an ingress-egress drain to allow the area to be flushed postoperatively. Otherwise use blunt dissection to exit a Penrose drain (¼ to ½ inch wide) or soft rubber tubing ventral to the incision in a dependent area (through a separate stab incision), or use closed suction drainage (e.g., butterfly catheter and Vacutainer tube). The end of the drain near the tympanic cavity may be secured with a single suture of chromic catgut (4-0 or 5-0). Secure the drain to the skin at the exit site. If an ingress-egress system is used

place the tube via a separate stab incision proximal to the surgical incision at the dorsal aspect of the head and exit it ventrally through a separate incision (Fig. 14-10, F). Close the subcutaneous tissues with an absorbable suture material (2-0 or 3-0) and close skin in a T shape (see Fig. 14-10, F).

Lateral Bulla Osteotomy

Lateral bulla osteotomy exposes the tympanic cavity so that exudate and secretory epithelium can be removed, which improves drainage. It should be performed in conjunction with total ear canal ablation in animals with chronic otitis externa and middle ear disease. Although a lateral bulla osteotomy affords less exposure to the tympanic cavity than a ventral osteotomy, it does not require that the animal be repositioned and is preferred when performed in conjunction with total ear canal ablation.

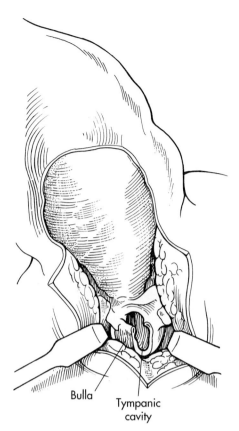

FIG. 14-11
Lateral bulla osteotomy.

Bluntly dissect the tissues from the lateral aspect of the bulla using a small periosteal elevator. Rongeur the lateral aspect of the bulla until the caudal aspect of the middle ear canal is exposed (Fig. 14-11). Extend the bony excision as needed to fully visualize contents of the tympanic cavity. Use a curette to remove infected materials but avoid curetting in the dorsal or dorsomedial area of the tympanic cavity so as to not damage the auditory ossicles or inner ear structures. Gently irrigate the cavity with saline in order to remove all remaining debris.

Ventral Bulla Osteotomy

Ventral bulla osteotomy allows increased exposure of the tympanic cavity and can be performed alone or in conjunction with lateral ear resection. It is the technique of choice for suspected middle ear neoplasia and nasopharyngeal polyps involving the feline middle ear. This technique provides better drainage of the bulla than does lateral bulla osteotomy and allows both bullae to be opened without repositioning the animal.

☞ **NOTE** • Ventral bulla osteotomy allows better visualization of the bulla than lateral bulla osteotomy but requires that the animal be repositioned when performing total ear canal ablation.

Place the patient in dorsal recumbency and prepare a generous area surrounding the angle of the mandible for aseptic surgery. Palpate the bulla immediately caudal and medial to the vertical ramus of the mandible. Draw an imaginary line connecting the mandibular rami and a second imaginary line along the long axis of the ventral aspect of the head (Fig. 14-12, A). Make a 7- to 10-cm incision parallel with the midline of the dog and centered 2 cm toward the affected side from where these imaginary lines intersect (see Fig. 14-12, A). Incise the platysma muscle, retract the linguofacial vein if necessary, and deepen the incision by bluntly dissecting the digastricus muscle (lateral) from the hyoglossus and styloglossus muscles (medial). Avoid damaging the hypoglossal nerve located on the lateral aspect of the hypoglossus muscle. Confirm the location of the bulla and use self-retaining retractors (i.e., Gelpi or Weitlander) to spread the digastricus and glossal muscles and retract them from the bulla (Fig. 14-12, B). Palpate the bulla craniomedial to the cornu process of the hyoid bone and caudomedial to the angle of the mandible. Bluntly dissect tissues from the ventral surface of the bulla and use a Steinmann pin to make a hole in its ventral aspect (Fig. 14-13). Enlarge the opening with small rongeurs (i.e., Lempert). Examine the interior of the bulla for inflammatory debris, neoplastic tissue, or foreign bodies and obtain samples for culture, sensitivity, and histopathologic examination. Be sure to examine both compartments of the bulla in cats (see the discussion on surgical anatomy on p. 154; see Fig. 14-13). Flush the cavity with warm saline and if there is evidence of infection, or if continued drainage is anticipated, place a small fenestrated drain tube within the cavity and exit it through a separate stab incision. Suture the fenestrated portion of the drain tube to the bulla with small (4-0 to 6-0) chromic gut suture. Depending on the amount of exudation, remove the drain in 3 to 7 days.

HEALING OF THE EAR

Hyperkeratinization of the epidermis and hyperplasia of the dermis and epidermis of the ear canals occur secondary to chronic infection or inflammation. Additionally, sebaceous glands become less numerous and active, while apocrine tubular glands distend and increase their secretions. Healing of the surgical techniques previously described is routine unless incisional infections develop that cause dehiscence. Such wounds are best left open to granulate, unless they are very large.

SUTURE MATERIALS/SPECIAL INSTRUMENTS

Electrocautery is useful for ear surgery because numerous vessels are encountered. Small curettes simplify removal of the epithelial tissues on the bony rim at the external acoustic meatus. Rongeurs are used to remove the lateral aspect of the bulla when performing a total ear canal resection. A Steinmann pin, hand chuck, and rongeurs are necessary for ventral bulla osteotomy (unless the bone has been eroded by infection or neoplasia). Self-retaining retractors are useful

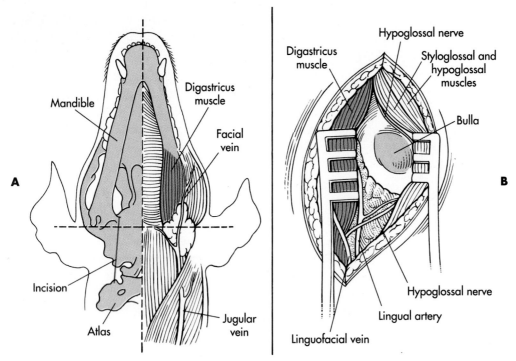

FIG. 14-12

A, For ventral bulla osteotomy, draw an imaginary line connecting the mandibular rami and a second imaginary line along the long axis of the ventral aspect of the head. Make a 7- to 10-cm incision parallel with the midline of the dog and centered 2 cm toward the affected side from where these imaginary lines intersect. **B,** Incise the platysma muscle, retract the linguofacial vein if necessary, and deepen the incision by bluntly dissecting the digastricus muscle (lateral) from the hypoglossal and styloglossal muscles (medial). Confirm the location of the bulla and use self-retaining retractors to spread the digastricus and glossal muscles and retract them from the bulla.

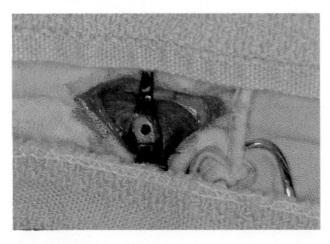

FIG. 14-13

During ventral bulla osteotomy in cats, be sure to examine both compartments of the bulla. The cat's nose is toward the left. (Courtesy H. Boothe, Texas A&M University.)

when performing a ventral bulla osteotomy to allow retraction of the muscles that are superficial to the bulla. Culture swabs (both aerobic and anaerobic) should be available whenever ear surgery is performed. Monofilament suture (i.e., polydioxanone, polyglyconate, polypropylene, nylon) should be used to suture the epithelial tissues of the canal to skin.

POSTOPERATIVE CARE AND ASSESSMENT

Postoperative analgesics should be given following ear canal resections or ablations (see the discussion on anesthetics on p. 153) and tranquilizers may be administered if the animal appears dysphoric or anxious (see p. 154). A bandage should be placed over the ear(s) and an Elizabethan collar or sidebar used to prevent bandage removal and/or ear mutilation. If swelling is excessive a hot pack can be applied to the side of the face several times a day for the first few days after surgery. The animal should be monitored postoperatively because bandages and/or excessive swelling (particularly after bilateral total ear canal ablation and lateral bulla osteotomy) may impair respiration. Antibiotics should be based on culture results and continued for 3 to 4 weeks. After total ear canal ablation in which ingress-egress drains have been placed, the drains should be flushed with sterile saline, dilute chlorhexidine (0.05%), or a Tris-ethylenediaminetetraacetic acid (EDTA) solution (Table 14-3), 2 to 3 times a day until the infection appears to be resolving (i.e., decreased bacterial numbers, nondegenerative neutrophils). Penrose drains can generally be removed in 3 to 7 days. Sutures can be removed in 10 to 14 days.

TABLE 14-3

Modified Tris-EDTA Solution*

1 liter of distilled water
1.2 g EDTA
6.05 g Tris
1 ml glacial acetic acid
Note: pH of solution should be approximately 8.
Modified from Neer TM, Howard PE: Otitis media, *Compend Contin Educ Pract Vet* 4:410, 1982.

*Add 1-3 ml with gentamicin otic drops 2-3 times a day to affected ear.

COMPLICATIONS

Complications other than inadequate drainage and continued otitis externa are uncommon after lateral ear resection or vertical ear canal ablation. Relief of clinical signs associated with otitis externa may not occur in dogs with underlying dermatologic disease that cannot be effectively managed. Making the opening of the horizontal canal insufficient for drainage and performing these techniques in animals with concurrent middle ear disease without treating the middle ear infection results in persistent or recurrent signs of otitis externa. Facial nerve palsy is a rare complication of vertical ear canal ablation. Complications of total ear canal ablation (i.e., superficial wound infections, facial nerve paralysis, vestibular dysfunction, deafness, chronic fistulation or abscessation, and avascular necrosis of the skin of the pinna) are potentially more serious than with the other techniques discussed in this chapter. Facial nerve paralysis usually resolves within a few weeks of surgery and is caused by stretching or retraction of the nerve; however, permanent damage occurs if the nerve is transected or severely stretched. Facial nerve damage may result in loss of the blink response and parasympathetic nerve innervation to the lacrimal glands. The eye should be kept moistened with artificial tears or an ophthalmic lubricant to prevent corneal ulceration. If normal lid function does not return within 4 to 6 weeks and/or ulceration of the eye occurs because of chronic drying, enucleation may be indicated; however, this is seldom necessary.

☞ **N O T E** · Facial nerve paralysis, vestibular dysfunction, and Horner's syndrome may all be caused by otitis media/interna or surgery. Preoperative presence of these abnormalities must be recognized to avoid having them considered as surgical complications.

Signs of middle and inner ear disease may persist after surgery, but if they worsen acutely an abscess of the tympanic cavity should be suspected. Superficial wound infections are common and are attributed to surgical manipulation of infected tissues, inadequate closure of dead space, inadequate drainage, and resistance to antibiotics. In cats

surgical curettage of the tympanic cavity may cause a transient Horner's syndrome, which usually resolves in 2 to 3 weeks (see discussion on surgical anatomy on p. 154). Facial nerve paralysis has also been reported after ventral bulla osteotomy in cats.

☞ **N O T E** · Warn owner that Horner's syndrome (usually temporary) is common in cats after ventral bulla osteotomy.

SPECIAL AGE CONSIDERATIONS

Young cats with middle or inner ear signs, or a previous history of respiratory disease should be examined for nasopharyngeal polyps (see p. 168).

References

Gregory CR, Vasseur PB: Clinical results of lateral ear resection in dogs, *J Am Vet Med Assoc* 182:1087, 1983.

Merchant SR et al: Otoxicity assessment of a chlorhexidine otic preparation in dogs, *Prog Vet Neurol* 4:72, 1993.

Suggested Reading

Beckman SL, Henry WB Jr., Cechner P: Total ear canal ablation combining bulla osteotomy and curettage in dogs with chronic otitis externa and media, *J Am Vet Med Assoc* 196:84, 1990.

Elkins AD: Surgery of the external ear canal, *Probl Vet Med* 3:239, 1991.

Lane JG, Little CJL: Surgery of the canine external auditory meatus: a review of failures, *J Small Anim Pract* 27:247, 1986.

Little CJL, Lane JG: The surgical anatomy of the feline bulla tympanica, *J Small Anim Pract* 27:371, 1986.

Matsuda H et al: The aerobic bacterial flora of the middle and external ears in normal dogs, *J Small Anim Pract* 25:269, 1984.

Matthiesen DT, Scavelli T: Total ear canal ablation and lateral bulla osteotomy in 38 dogs, *J Am Anim Hosp Assoc* 26:257, 1990.

McCarthy RJ, Caywood DD: Vertical ear canal resection for end-stage otitis externa in dogs, *J Am Anim Hosp Assoc* 28: 545, 1992.

Sharp NJH: Chronic otitis externa and otitis media treated by total ear canal ablation and ventral bulla osteotomy in thirteen dogs, *Vet Surg* 19:162, 1990.

Smeak DD, DeHoff WD: Total ear canal ablation, *Vet Surg* 15:161, 1986.

Stout-Graham M et al: Morphologic measurements of the external horizontal ear canal of dogs, *Am J Vet Res* 51:990, 1990.

SPECIFIC DISEASES

OTITIS EXTERNA

DEFINITIONS

Otitis externa is an inflammation of the epithelium of the horizontal and vertical ear canals and surrounding structures (i.e., external auditory meatus and pinna).

SYNONYMS

Swimmer's ear is a term used to describe otitis externa that occurs after swimming or bathing.

GENERAL CONSIDERATIONS AND CLINICALLY RELEVANT PATHOPHYSIOLOGY

Otitis externa is common in dogs (i.e., 3.9% to 20% of hospital admissions) and cats (i.e., 2% to 6.6% of hospital admissions). It may be associated with other dermatologic diseases, particularly allergic or immune-mediated skin disease (i.e., food allergy dermatitis, atopy, contact dermatitis) or systemic diseases (i.e., endocrinopathies such as hypothyroidism or Sertoli cell tumors). Bacterial infections, foreign bodies (i.e., foxtails), parasites (i.e., *Otodectes cynotis, Demodex canis, Sarcoptes scabiei, Notoedres cati,* ticks), fungi, yeasts (i.e., *Mallassezia pachydermis*), or neoplasia may also be the cause. *O. cynotis* is responsible for more than 50% of feline otitis externa.

Predisposing causes of otitis externa include excessive moisture or increased humidity in the canal, narrow ear canal conformation, or obstruction of the ear canal. The normal ear canal is inhabited by bacteria (i.e., *Staphylococcus* and *β-Streptococcus* spp.). High humidity and temperature promote moisture retention in the ear, which allows maceration of the epithelial lining and fosters secondary bacterial colonization. The most frequent bacteria isolated from ears of dogs with chronic otitis externa are *Corynebacterium* spp., *Escherichia coli, Proteus mirabilis, Pseudomonas aeruginosa,* and *Staphylococcus intermedius.* From the ears of cats: *Pasteurella multocida* and *Staphylococcus intermedius.* Chronic otitis externa causes secondary changes in the ear canal (i.e., epithelial hyperplasia and ossification of chronically inflamed tissue) that perpetuate the infection and make medical management difficult because of constriction of the external ear canal lumen. Additionally, ulceration and secondary infection with pyogenic bacteria, yeast, and/or fungi commonly occur. In chronic otitis externa the apocrine glands increase in size, number, and secretory activity, while the sebaceous glands decrease in number and become less active.

DIAGNOSIS

Clinical Presentation

Signalment. Dogs and cats of any breed or age may develop otitis externa, but some groups are at higher risk. Dogs with long, pendulous ears (e.g., spaniels, basset hounds) and those with abundant hair in the ear canal (e.g., poodles) are commonly affected. Of the erect-eared dogs, German shepherds are most frequently affected. Spaniel breeds, particularly cocker spaniels, may have abnormal keratinization and increased sebaceous gland secretion of the pinna and/or ear canal. Chronic bacterial infections and hyperplastic changes in the sebaceous glands and epithelial lining of the ear often lead to scarring and ear canal obstruction.

History. Animals with otitis externa may present for evaluation of acute or chronic signs. If a foreign body is lodged in the ear of an animal, head shaking and scratching at or near the ear are typical. Head shaking and ear scratching are also common among animals with parasitic infections and acute bacterial infections. A purulent, odoriferous discharge may be noted with chronic infections. The dog may constantly rub his head on objects and appear in pain when his head or ear is touched.

Physical Examination Findings

Palpation of the ear may suggest thickening or calcification of the ear canal. A thorough otoscopic examination should be performed even if it requires tranquilization. Examination of the ear canal is often difficult if hyperplasia or exudation is present; general anesthesia may be necessary to allow meticulous inspection. The extent of involvement of the vertical and horizontal ear canals and the status of the tympanic membrane should be determined. Purulent yellow or cream-colored exudates may be associated with gram-negative infections, particularly *Pseudomonas* and *Proteus* spp. Dark brown or black exudates are more commonly associated with yeast infections or those caused by *Staphylococcus* or *Streptococcus* spp. A bloody exudate may be suggestive of neoplasia. A definitive diagnosis requires examination of exudate collected during the procedure by placing sterile swabs into the canal through the otoscope cone. The exudate should be examined for parasites, bacteria, fungi, and/or yeast, and bacterial and fungal cultures performed if indicated. The ear should be flushed with a bulb syringe and/or soft catheter and alligator forceps should be available to remove foreign bodies and debris. Biopsy of the external ear canal may allow diagnosis of neoplasia and some allergic conditions. A complete dermatologic examination should be performed in all animals with otitis externa unless an obvious cause such as a foreign body is found.

Radiography

Skull radiographs should be performed to determine if concurrent otitis media exists (see p. 169). Calcification of the external auditory canal is common with chronic otitis externa (Fig. 14-14); this finding may influence the choice of surgical techniques. Occasionally, radiographic signs suggestive of neoplasia (i.e., bony lysis of the petrous temporal bone) are found.

Laboratory Findings

Specific laboratory abnormalities are not found. Thyroid function tests should be performed if hypothyroidism is suspected.

DIFFERENTIAL DIAGNOSIS

The diagnosis of otitis externa is usually simple; however, differentiation of the various causes may be difficult. It is important to identify treatable underlying causes of otitis externa before considering surgical intervention; optimal re-

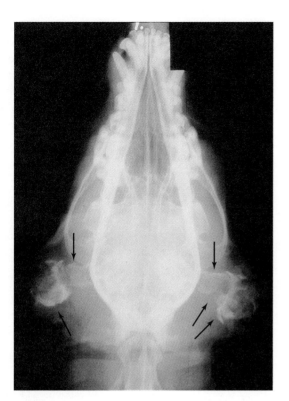

FIG. 14-14
Calcification of the external ear canals (*arrows*) in a dog with chronic otitis externa. (Courtesy L. Homco, Texas A&M University.)

sults require underlying diseases to be appropriately treated. In some cases surgery will be unnecessary if the underlying cause is treated. Concurrent otitis media should be identified in animals undergoing surgery for otitis externa.

☞ **NOTE** · Lateral ear canal resection and vertical canal ablation often fail if concurrent dermatologic or middle ear disease is not resolved.

MEDICAL MANAGEMENT

Treatment of otitis externa involves identifying the underlying or perpetuating causes, cleaning and drying the ear, and using appropriate topical and/or systemic medications. There are many topical agents available for treatment of otitis externa (Table 14-4). Most contain various combinations of antibiotics and parasiticidal, antiinflammatory, and/or antifungal agents. Refer to a medicine text for an in-depth discussion of the use of these various agents. Consideration of the ototoxicity of the various agents should be taken into account before their use, particularly if the tympanic membrane has been ruptured. Because ceruminous material decreases the ability of topical medications to reach the infection and may inactivate some drugs, the ears must be thoroughly cleaned before treatment. Persistence of clinical signs following treatment of otitis externa may suggest concurrent otitis media.

SURGICAL TREATMENT

Surgical therapy of otitis externa should be considered when medical management fails, or in cases where there are proliferative growths or stenotic canals. The surgical alternatives in animals with otitis externa that do not have middle ear involvement include a lateral ear canal resection (see p. 156), vertical ear canal ablation (see p. 158), or total ear canal resection (see p. 158). If otitis media exists a lateral ear canal resection in conjunction with a ventral bulla osteotomy (see p. 161) or an ear canal ablation with lateral bulla osteotomy (see p. 160) can be performed.

Preoperative Management

Preoperative antibiotic therapy is recommended. Bacterial cultures should be performed if purulent discharge is present, and appropriate antibiotics should be initiated before surgery. In other animals perioperative antibiotics (i.e., β-lactamase–resistant penicillins or cephalosporins) may be given intravenously immediately before the surgical procedure, or may be administered during surgery but after intraoperative cultures have been obtained.

Anesthesia

See p. 153 for anesthetic recommendations for animals with ear disease.

Surgical Anatomy

Refer to p. 154 for a description of the surgical anatomy of the ear canal.

Positioning

Refer to pp. 156–159 for positioning for the various surgical procedures.

SURGICAL TECHNIQUE

The choice of surgical techniques depends on the severity and extent of the disease. See p. 156–161 for a description of the surgical techniques used in animals with ear disease. A discussion of the indications and contraindications of each procedure is provided.

SUTURE MATERIALS/SPECIAL INSTRUMENTS

See p. 161 for a discussion of appropriate suture materials and instruments for surgery of the ear.

POSTOPERATIVE CARE AND ASSESSMENT

Postoperative pain is common in animals undergoing ear surgery. See p. 153 for a discussion of analgesic therapy in these patients. After administration of adequate analgesics, tranquilizers may be given if the animal appears dysphoric or anxious (see p. 154). The ear should be bandaged following surgery in order to minimize contamination and trauma to the surgical site. Animals will often shake their heads excessively after ear surgery and may try to paw or scratch at the

TABLE 14-4

Topical Otic Preparations

Product	Company	Active Ingredients					Vehicle
		Antibiotics	Antiinflammatory	Antiparasitic	Antiyeast	Other (e.g., Anesthetics, Astringents)	
Adams ear desiccant	Adams		aloe vera			colloidal sulfur, dioctyl sodium sulfosuccinate, urea peroxide, EDTA	propylene glycol
Adams ear mite lotion	Adams		aloe vera	pyrethrins			
Cerumite	Evsco			pyrethrins			squalene
Clear$_x$ treatment dryer	DVM		hydrocortisone			acetic acid, colloidal sulfur, dioctyl sodium sulfosuccinate, urea peroxide	
Conofite 1% lotion	Pitmann Moore				micronazole nitrate		polyethylene glycol
Cort/Astrin	Vedco		hydrocortisone			Burow's solution	water
Epi-Otic	Allerderm					lactic acid, salicylic acid	propylene glycol
Forte topical	Upjohn	procaine penicillin, neomycin, polymyxin	hydrocortisone				mineral oil
Gentocin otic	Schering	gentamicin	betamethasone				alcohol, glycerin, propylene glycol

Liquichlor	Evsco	chloramphenicol	prednisolone			tetracaine	mineral oil, squalene
Micropearls Coal Tar Spray	Evsco					coal tar	water
Mitiban	Upjohn				amitraz		water
Mitox	SmithKline-Beecham	neomycin			carbaryl	sulfactamide, tetracaine	mineral oil
Oti-Clens	SmithKline-Beecham					malic acid, benzoic acid, salicylic acid	propylene glycol
Otomax	Schering-Plough	gentamicin	betamethasone	clotrimazole			mineral oil
Otomite	Allerderm				0.05% pyrethrins		olive oil
Otomite Plus	Allerderm				0.15% pyrethrins		olive oil
Panalog ointment	Solvay	neomycin, thiostreptosin	triamcinolone acetonide	nystatin			polyethylene, mineral oil
Panodry	Solvay					boric acid, isopropyl alcohol	silicone fluid
Solvaprep	Solvay					surfactants	propylene glycol
Synotic	Syntex		fluocinolone, DMSO				propylene glycol
Tresaderm	MSD-Agvet	neomycin	dexamethasone	thiabendazole		alcohol, glycerin	propylene glycol

bandage. Close supervision in the early postoperative period and use of an Elizabethan collar or sidebar are recommended.

PROGNOSIS

Chronic otitis externa is a difficult disease to treat with medical therapy or surgery. A poor surgical outcome may be the result of technical failures (e.g., not making the horizontal canal opening large enough with lateral ear canal resection or vertical ear canal ablation), lack of owner compliance in continuing to treat the ear (with lateral ear canal resection or vertical ear canal ablation), unrealistic expectations on the part of the owner, unrecognized middle ear disease, faulty diagnoses (e.g., not recognizing neoplasia as the underlying cause), or failure to treat the underlying disease or perpetuating cause. Surgical procedures designed to increase drainage (i.e., lateral ear canal resection, vertical ear canal ablation) often fail in animals with untreated dermatologic disease or unrecognized middle ear disease. Clinical signs resolved in 41% of dogs undergoing lateral ear resection for the treatment of chronic otitis externa; whereas 47% of the dogs showed no improvement after surgery (Gregory, Vasseur, 1983). Of 36 dogs undergoing vertical ear canal ablation for chronic otitis, only 23% had complete resolution of clinical signs, but 95% were improved (i.e., decreased frequency of medical treatment required, increased ease of application of topical medication, and overall client satisfaction) (McCarthy, Caywood, 1992). Total ear canal ablation combined with bulla osteotomy reportedly resolved clinical signs in 97% of the surgically treated ears (Beckman, Henry, Cechner, 1990).

Partial or complete facial nerve paralysis has been reported to occur in 5% to 58% of cases treated with total ear canal ablation. Other complications include persistent infection (dissecting cellulitis, prolonged wound drainage, incisional dehiscence, periauricular abscess formation), nystagmus, head tilt, postural abnormalities, and loss of hearing (see p. 153).

References

Beckman SL, Henry WB Jr., Cechner P: Total ear canal ablation combining bulla osteotomy and curettage in dogs with chronic otitis externa and media, *J Am Vet Med Assoc* 196:84, 1990.

Gregory CR, Vasseur PB: Clinical results of lateral ear resection in dogs, *J Am Vet Med Assoc* 182:1087, 1983.

McCarthy RJ, Caywood DD: Vertical ear canal resection for end-stage otitis externa in dogs, *J Am Anim Hosp Assoc* 28:545, 1992.

Suggested Reading

August JR: Otitis externa, *Vet Clin North Am Small Anim Pract* 18:731, 1988.

Henderson JT, Radasch RM: Total ear canal ablation with lateral bulla osteotomy for the management of end-stage otitis in dogs, *Comp Cont Educ Pract Vet* 17:157, 1995.

Wooley RE et al: In vitro action of combinations of antimicrobial agents with edta-trimethamine of *Proteus vulgaris* of a canine origin, *Am J Vet Res* 45:1451, 1984.

OTITIS MEDIA AND INTERNA

DEFINITIONS

Otitis media is inflammation of the middle ear; **otitis interna** is inflammation of the inner ear. **Myringotomy** is a surgical puncture of the tympanic membrane to relieve pressure or obtain samples for analysis.

SYNONYMS

The auditory tube is also known as the **eustachian tube.** Inflammatory polyps found in the feline middle ear are referred to as **nasopharyngeal polyps.**

GENERAL CONSIDERATIONS AND CLINICALLY RELEVANT PATHOPHYSIOLOGY

Otitis media may be secondary to bacterial infections, yeast or fungal infections, neoplasia, trauma, or foreign bodies. Inflammatory or nasopharyngeal polyps are additional causes of feline otitis media. The most common cause of otitis media is bacterial infection; more than half of the animals with chronic end-stage otitis externa have documented evidence of otitis media at surgery. Consequently, pathogens cultured from the middle ear are similar to those cultured from the ears of animals with otitis externa (i.e., *Staphylococcus* spp., *Streptococcus* spp., *Pseudomonas* sp., *Escherichia coli*, and *Proteus mirabilis*). In addition to infections spreading to the middle ear across the tympanic membrane, they may also ascend from the pharynx via the auditory tube, or may reach the inner ear via the bloodstream. Bilateral otitis media is usually indicative of bacterial infection. Otitis media may lead to otitis interna (Table 14-5).

Inflammatory or nasopharyngeal polyps are benign masses that may be located in the nasopharynx, auditory tube, and/or tympanic cavity. Although rarely, they may rupture the tympanic membrane and protrude into the external ear canal. They often cause signs of unilateral otitis media when located in the tympanic cavity. These polyps may occur as a result of ascending infection from the pharynx or may arise as a result of chronic otitis media. Suspected congenital polyps have also been reported in kittens.

TABLE 14-5

Clinical Signs Associated with Otitis Interna (Vestibular Dysfunction)

- Head tilt to affected side
- Circling to affected side
- Falling to affected side
- Rolling to affected side
- Nystagmus (horizontal or rotary), with fast component away from affected side
- Asymmetric ataxia with strength preserved
- Positional or vestibular strabismus with the eyeball ipsilateral to the lesion deviated ventrally
- Postural reactions (except for the righting reflex)

Neoplasia originating in the middle ear is uncommon in both dogs and cats. Tumors originating in the external ear canal that secondarily extend into the tympanic cavity are more common than primary middle ear tumors in dogs. Benign tumors of the middle ear cavity of dogs (i.e., papillary adenomas, fibromas) have been more commonly reported than malignant tumors. Epidermoid cysts (cholesteatomas) occur in the canine middle ear. These cysts are often associated with chronic otitis media and must be differentiated from neoplastic lesions. Squamous cell carcinoma is the most common tumor of the feline middle and inner ear. Other tumors found in the middle ear of cats have included fibrosarcomas, anaplastic carcinomas, lymphoblastic lymphosarcoma, and ceruminous gland adenocarcinoma.

DIAGNOSIS
Clinical Presentation

Signalment. Most animals that develop otitis media secondary to otitis externa are middle-aged. Older animals more commonly develop neoplasia of the middle ear and young cats are more apt to have nasopharyngeal polyps. There is no known breed or sex predisposition in cats with nasopharyngeal polyps or animals with neoplastic middle ear disease. Canine breeds predisposed to otitis externa (see p. 164) also have a higher incidence of otitis media.

History. The history and clinical signs of animals with otitis media do not differ substantially from those with otitis externa alone (see p. 163). Affected animals commonly scratch or paw at their ears and they may shake their heads excessively. There may be an odor to the ear, and animals often appear in pain on manipulation or palpation of their ears or adjacent skull. A history of chronic, poorly responsive otitis externa is common. Some animals present for evaluation of vestibular signs caused by otitis interna (see Table 14-5). Pain during eating or when the mouth is opened may be noted, especially in cats with neoplastic middle ear disease. Ipsilateral facial nerve paralysis is also common in animals with middle ear neoplasia. Neoplastic lesions of the middle ear rarely extend into the nasopharynx causing gagging, retching, and/or dyspnea. Cats with nasopharyngeal polyps often have nasal discharge, sneezing, or stridor. If there is a concurrent pharyngeal polyp, dysphagia and/or dyspnea may be noted. Deafness may be reported with bilateral disease, but loss of hearing is seldom evident with unilateral lesions.

Physical Examination Findings

Discharge from the external auditory canal, hyperplasia, and ulceration of the aural epithelial tissues are often obvious upon physical examination in animals with otitis media and externa. Neurologic abnormalities referable to the inner ear or facial nerve paralysis (Table 14-6) are not present in most animals with otitis media. Horner's syndrome may occur as a result of damage of the sympathetic trunk as it courses through the middle ear. Clinical signs associated with the syndrome are ptosis, miosis, enophthalmus, and protrusion of the third eyelid.

TABLE 14-6

Clinical Signs Associated with Facial Nerve Paralysis

- Diminished palpebral reflex
- Widened palpebral fissure
- Drooping of the ear and lip
- Excessive drooling
- Blepharospasm
- Elevation and wrinkling of the lip
- Caudal displacement of the labial commissure
- Elevation of the ear on the affected side

Otoscopic examination of these patients often requires general anesthesia. The tympanic membrane may be ruptured or it may bulge outward because of purulent material, blood, or serum. An intact tympanic membrane does not exclude middle ear disease. Abundant mucus within the middle ear cavity has been associated with adenomatous lesions. The normal tympanic membrane appears shiny and is gray or white in color; it becomes opaque with infection. If the tympanic membrane is ruptured, samples for cytology and culture can be taken directly from the middle ear. Otherwise, samples can be obtained using a 20-gauge, 3½-inch spinal needle inserted through the ventral half of the tympanum (myringotomy). If the opening is too small it may be enlarged with a small cannula.

Inflammatory polyps usually appear as pedunculated, smooth, shiny, light-pink masses. The oral cavity of animals with inflammatory polyps or neoplastic masses should be carefully examined because extension into the pharynx may occur. Neoplastic lesions may be friable but they are often difficult to differentiate grossly from chronically infected tissue.

Radiography

The most valuable radiographic view for evaluating animals with suspected otitis media is the frontal open-mouth projection (also known as rostrocaudal open-mouth view) in which the animal is placed on its back with his head flexed 80 to 90 degrees to the film (Fig. 14-15). The mouth is held open with gauze strips hooked on the upper and lower canine teeth and the x-ray beam is centered on the temporomandibular joints. The tongue and endotracheal tube must be retracted from the field of view, using gauze secured to the lower mandible. The tympanic bullae and their contents are demonstrated with this view. The most common findings with middle ear disease are opacification of the air-filled tympanic cavities and thickening and sclerosis of the walls of the bullae (Fig. 14-16). Lateral oblique views (Fig. 14-17) with the head tilted 10 to 15 degrees show individual bullae, while ventrodorsal or dorsoventral views evaluate the external ear canals and architecture of the petrous temporal bones. Lysis or periosteal reaction of the bullae and petrous temporal bone should increase suspicion of neoplasia. Radiography is not sensitive for detecting middle ear disease; up to 25% of animals with middle ear disease do not have radiographic abnormalities. A soft-tissue mass within the pharyngeal region may be noted in cats with inflammatory polyps.

☞ **N O T E** • Some animals with middle ear disease have radiographically normal bullae.

Laboratory Findings

Specific laboratory abnormalities are uncommon.

DIFFERENTIAL DIAGNOSIS

Differential diagnoses for disease of the middle and inner ear cavity include bacterial infections, fungal or yeast infections, inflammatory polyps, neoplasms, foreign bodies, trauma, sebaceous gland and ceruminous gland hyperplasia, paraaural abscesses, and idiopathic vestibular disease. Otitis media is common in animals with otitis externa, but because clinical signs are similar, the former often goes unrecognized.

MEDICAL MANAGEMENT

The most important aspect of treating otitis media is to remove infected tissues or exudate, neoplasms, polyps, or foreign bodies from the tympanic cavity. The external ear canal should be cleaned and concurrent otitis externa must be treated (see p. 163). Medical management of animals with acute otitis media consists of myringotomy, cultures of middle ear contents, irrigation of the tympanic cavity, and topical (see Table 14-4) and systemic antibiotics. If there is no improvement within 3 to 4 weeks, ventral bulla osteotomy should be considered.

SURGICAL TREATMENT

Surgery is often necessary to distinguish between the various potential causes of middle ear disease. Surgical treatment of otitis media caused by infection includes bulla osteotomy, culture of affected tissues or exudate, drainage, and long-term antibiotics. If neurologic signs are present before surgery the owner should be warned that they are likely to persist after surgery. Benign neoplastic or inflammatory lesions can usually be removed via a bulla osteotomy; however, Horner's syndrome is a common, short-term complication of bulla osteotomy in cats (see p. 163). Neoplasia of the bulla warrants a poor prognosis.

☞ **N O T E** • Warn owners that neurologic signs may not resolve after surgery.

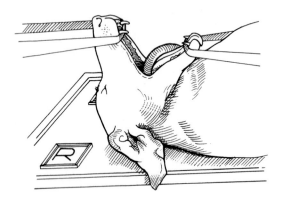

FIG. 14-15
Positioning for a frontal open-mouth projection.

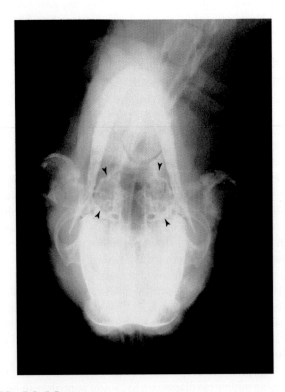

FIG. 14-16
Frontal open-mouth projection showing opacification, thickening, and sclerosis of the bullae (*arrows*). (Courtesy L. Homco, Texas A&M University.)

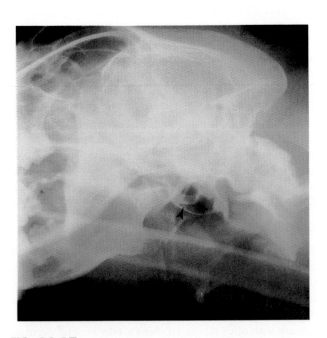

FIG. 14-17
Lateral oblique radiograph of a dog with unilateral otitis media. Note the thickened wall of the left bulla (*arrows*), compared with the normal, thin-walled, right bulla. (Courtesy L. Homco, Texas A&M University.)

Preoperative Management

Preoperative antibiotics may be given; however, intraoperative cultures are often performed in animals with middle ear disease. In such patients intravenous antibiotics should be given immediately after cultures have been obtained.

Anesthesia

Refer to p. 153 for anesthetic recommendations for animals with ear disease. Chamber or mask induction should not be used in dyspneic animals (i.e., some cats with nasopharyngeal polyps). Because nitrous oxide increases middle ear pressure, it may be wise to avoid its use in animals with middle ear disease.

Surgical Anatomy

The middle ear is composed of the tympanic cavity and its contents, and the auditory tube. Refer to p. 154 for a description of the surgical anatomy of the ear.

Positioning

The animal is positioned in lateral recumbency for a lateral bulla osteotomy and in dorsal recumbency for a ventral bulla osteotomy.

SURGICAL TECHNIQUE

Approach the middle ear via a lateral bulla osteotomy (see p. 160) in conjunction with a total ear canal ablation (see p. 158) or via a ventral bulla osteotomy (see p. 161).

SUTURE MATERIALS/SPECIAL INSTRUMENTS

Refer to p. 161 for a description of surgical supplies needed for bulla osteotomy.

POSTOPERATIVE CARE AND ASSESSMENT

Cats with concurrent upper airway disease (i.e., nasopharyngeal polyps) may have respiratory distress after extubation and may require supplementary oxygen. Oxygen may be given by mask or nasal insufflation in these animals.

PROGNOSIS

Animals with bacterial otitis media may have persistent neurologic signs despite surgical treatment. In one study, cats with otitis interna before surgery had permanent head tilts postoperatively (Trevor, Martin, 1993). However, these cats usually had a normal level of activity despite their neurologic dysfunction. The prognosis for benign tumors is good; however, surgical cures are rare with malignant tumors (because of their extensive nature at the time of diagnosis). Inflammatory polyps may recur if they are simply removed from the external ear using traction. Recurrence is less likely if traction plus bulla osteotomy is performed.

Reference

Trevor PB, Martin RA: Tympanic bulla osteotomy for treatment of middle ear disease in cats: 19 cases (1984-1991), *J Am Vet Med Assoc* 101:123, 1993.

Suggested Reading

Kapatkin AS et al: Results of surgical treatment for nasopharyngeal inflammatory polyps in 31 cats, *Vet Surg* 18:59, 1989.

Kapatkin AS et al: Results of surgery and long-term follow-up in 31 cats with nasopharyngeal polyps, *J Am Anim Hosp Assoc* 26:387, 1990.

Little CJL, Pearson GR, Lane JG: Neoplasia involving the middle ear cavity of dogs, *Vet Rec* 124:54, 1989.

Neer TM, Howard PE: Otitis media, *Compend Contin Educ Pract Vet* 4:410, 1982.

Remedios AM, Fowler JD, Pharr JW: A comparison of radiographic versus surgical diagnosis of otitis media, *J Am Anim Hosp Assoc* 27:183, 1991.

Rogers KS: Tumors of the ear canal, *Vet Clin North Am Small Anim Pract* 18:859, 1988.

AURAL HEMATOMAS AND TRAUMATIC LESIONS OF THE PINNA

DEFINITIONS

An **aural hematoma** is a collection of blood within the cartilage plate of the ear.

SYNONYMS

Auricular hematoma

GENERAL CONSIDERATIONS AND CLINICALLY RELEVANT PATHOPHYSIOLOGY

Aural hematomas may occur in dogs or cats and are usually characterized as fluctuant, fluid-filled swellings on the concave surface of the pinna. The entire portion of the concave surface of the pinna may be involved, or only a portion. The cause of aural hematomas is not well understood; however, it appears that head shaking or scratching at the ear caused by pain or irritation associated with otitis externa (i.e., usually bacterial otitis in dogs and *Otodectes cynotis* in cats) is responsible in many cases. Head shaking may cause sinusoidal wave motions to occur in the ear resulting in cartilage fracture. The hematoma appears to originate from branches of the great auricular artery within the fractured auricular cartilage, rather than between the skin and cartilage, as was initially postulated. Some animals that develop aural hematomas do not have evidence of concurrent ear disease; hematoma formation in some patients may be associated with increased capillary fragility (i.e., Cushing's disease).

Lacerations of the ear may occur as a result of fighting or other trauma. These wounds may be superficial, involving the skin on one surface of the ear only, or may perforate the cartilage and involve both skin surfaces. Depending on the severity of the wounds, some may be left to heal by second intention while others have a more cosmetic appearance if sutures are placed. Rarely a portion of the ear may be avulsed and cause an unacceptable cosmetic deformity.

DIAGNOSIS
Clinical Presentation

Signalment. Dogs and cats with otitis externa are at increased risk to develop aural hematomas.

History. A history of violent head shaking and/or acute or chronic otitis externa (see p. 163) may be noted; in some animals there may be no history of previous ear disease.

Physical Examination Findings

Hematomas initially appear fluid filled, soft, and fluctuant, but eventually may become firm and thickened as a result of fibrosis. The ear may then develop a "cauliflower" appearance.

Radiography

Skull radiographs may be indicated if underlying otitis externa/media has predisposed the animal to aural hematoma.

Laboratory Findings

Specific laboratory abnormalities are uncommon.

DIFFERENTIAL DIAGNOSIS

Aural hematoma is diagnosed at physical examination; however, the underlying ear disease must be diagnosed and treated to decrease the likelihood of recurrence.

MEDICAL MANAGEMENT

Underlying ear disease should be appropriately treated (see p. 165). Needle aspiration of aural hematomas has been attempted (with and without concurrent injection of corticosteroid); however, recurrence is common with this technique.

SURGICAL TREATMENT

Numerous techniques have been described for the surgical treatment of aural hematomas. The goals of surgery are to remove the hematoma, prevent recurrence, and retain the natural appearance of the ear (i.e., minimize thickening and scarring). The most commonly used procedure involves incising the tissues overlying the hematoma, evacuating blood clots and fibrin, and holding the cartilage in apposition with sutures until scar tissue can form. Alternately, drains or cannulas have been used to provide drainage for several weeks during the healing process. To prevent enlargement or fibrosis, hematomas should be treated soon after they occur (i.e., within several days).

Linear lacerations that involve only one skin surface may be left to heal by second intention or may be sutured. The laceration should be cleaned and the edges debrided if necrotic tissue is present. The skin margins can be apposed with simple interrupted sutures. If a flap of tissue has been elevated away from the cartilage it should be sutured. Sutures are placed through the skin at the margins of the wound; additionally, sutures should be placed through the skin and cartilage at the center of the flap to obliterate any dead space where fluid might collect. Full-thickness injuries through the ear margin should be sutured. The skin on both sides of the defect may be sutured with simple interrupted sutures, or alternately, a vertical mattress suture may be used to appose the skin and cartilage on one side of the ear and simple interrupted sutures used to appose the skin on the opposite side of the ear (Fig. 14-18).

Preoperative Management

Concurrent otitis externa (see p. 163) should be treated simultaneously. Appropriate cultures should be submitted and the ear canal cleaned and flushed.

Anesthesia

Animals with aural hematomas are usually healthy and a variety of anesthetic protocols can be used. Tranquilization may be necessary upon recovery from anesthesia once sufficient analgesics have been provided (see p. 154). Refer to p. 153 for the anesthetic management of animals with ear disease.

Surgical Anatomy

Structural support of the pinna is provided by cartilage interposed between the two skin surfaces. Branches of the great auricular arteries and veins supply the pinna. These main vessels are located along the convex surface of the ear and small branches penetrate the scapha to supply the concave surface. The sensory innervation to the ear is supplied by the second cervical nerve (convex surface) and the auriculotemporal branches of the trigeminal nerve (concave surface).

Positioning

Animals are generally placed in lateral recumbency for aural hematoma and laceration repair.

SURGICAL TECHNIQUES
Aural Hematomas

Make an S-shaped incision on the concave surface of the ear and expose the hematoma and its contents from end to end (Fig. 14-19). Remove the fibrin clot and irrigate the

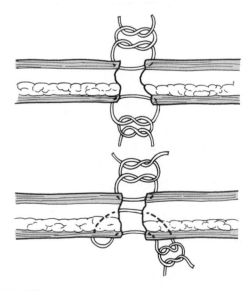

FIG. 14-18
Suture placement for repair of pinna lacerations.

cavity. Place ¾- to 1-cm long sutures through the skin on the concave surface of the ear and underlying cartilage. Place the sutures parallel to the major vessels (vertical rather than horizontal). They may be placed through the cartilage without incorporating the skin on the convex surface of the ear or they may be full-thickness. Place an ample number of sutures so that there are no pockets in which fluid can accumulate. Do not ligate the branches of the great auricular artery visible on the convex surface of the ear. Do not suture the incision closed; it should gap slightly to allow for continued drainage. Place a light protective bandage over the ear and support the ear over the animal's head (see p. 175 under Postoperative Care). Remove the bandage and sutures in 10 to 14 days.

If there is minimal fibrin present a teat cannula or drain can be placed in lieu of the above described procedure (Fig. 14-20, *A*). Trim half of the collar of the cannula to allow the tube to rest comfortably against the ear (Fig. 14-20, *B*). Aspirate the contents of the hematoma using a large needle (14 or 16 gauge) inserted into the hematoma

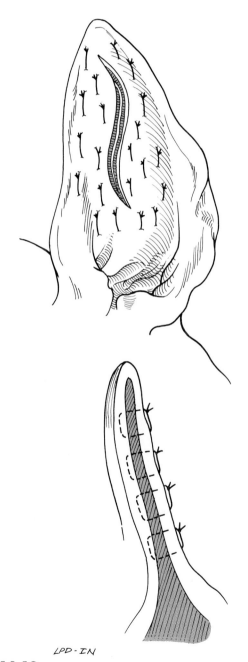

FIG. 14-19
Sutures should be placed vertically rather than horizontally for aural hematoma repair. They may be placed through the cartilage without incorporating the skin on the convex surface of the ear, or they may be full-thickness.

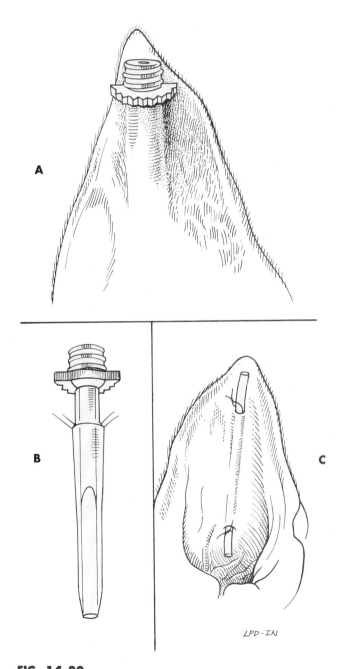

FIG. 14-20
A, If there is minimal fibrin present a teat cannula can be used for aural hematoma repair. **B,** Trim half of the collar of the cannula to allow the tube to rest comfortably against the ear.
C, Alternatively, a ¼-inch fenestrated latex drain can be used.

at its most distal margin. Insert the cannula through the needle hole and suture it to the ear. (The cannula is placed in the most distal aspect of the hematoma—even in erect-eared animals—to prevent drainage from entering the concha). Do not bandage or support the ear over the top of the head.

A ¼-inch fenestrated latex drain can be used instead of a teat cannula (Fig. 14-20, C). Make a stab incision in the proximal and distal limits of the hematoma. Empty the hematoma of fluid and fibrin and use a mosquito or alligator forceps to bring the drain into the hematoma cavity. Suture the ends of the drain to the skin where they protrude from the cavity. Place a light bandage over the ear (see p. 175 under Postoperative Care).

Avulsions of the Ear Margin

Small avulsions of the ear margin may be treated by resecting surrounding tissue to restore a normal ear contour. The skin edges are sutured over the cartilage using a continuous suture pattern. Larger defects of the ear may be repaired using a pedi-cle flap obtained from the side of the neck in dogs with pendulous ears or the dorsum of the head in dogs with erect ears.

☞ **N O T E ·** Defects of the ear margins can be repaired for cosmetic reasons, but repair should be delayed after excision of neoplasms until it has been determined that recurrence is unlikely.

Prepare the ear and donor site for aseptic surgery. Debride the margins of the ear defect. Place the ear on the donor site and incise the skin extending the limbs 0.5 to 1 cm longer than the defect (Fig. 14-21, A). Suture the flap to the skin on the convex surface of the ear (Fig. 14-21, B). Place a nonadherent dressing over the wound and leave the ear bandaged for 10 to 14 days. Then sever the flap from the donor site in the shape of the defect on the concave side of the ear (Fig. 14-21, C). Gently fold the flap over the ear margin and suture it to the skin (Fig. 14-21, D). Remove skin sutures in 10 to 14 days.

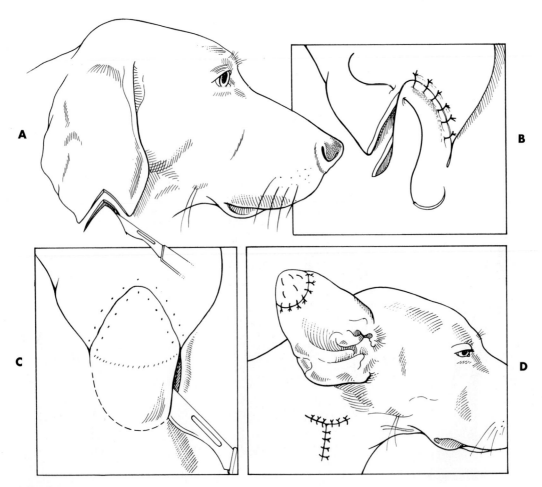

FIG. 14-21
A, To repair defects on the pinna place the ear on the donor site and incise the skin extending the limbs 0.5 to 1 cm longer than the defect. **B,** Suture the flap to the skin on the convex surface of the ear. **C,** After 10 to 14 days sever the flap from the donor site in the shape of the defect on the concave side of the ear. **D,** Gently fold the flap over the ear margin and suture it to skin.

SUTURE MATERIALS/SPECIAL INSTRUMENTS

Monofilament, nonabsorbable (i.e., polypropylene or nylon) or absorbable (i.e., polydioxanone or polyglyconate) suture material (3-0 or 4-0) should be used to suture the ear. Other materials that may be used in animals with aural hematomas are Dr. Larson's plastic teat tubes or Silastic medical grade tubing.

POSTOPERATIVE CARE AND ASSESSMENT

A bandage can be used to protect the ear from contamination and self-inflicted trauma after hematoma repair. Maintaining bandages on the head can be difficult. One method is to place short strips of tape on the rostral and caudal margin of the convex surface of the pinna (Fig. 14-22, *A*). The tape should extend beyond the ear border. Longer pieces of tape are placed on the concave surface of the pinna so that these tape pieces contact the tape on the convex surface (Fig. 14-22, *B*). The ear is placed over the top of the head (cotton can be placed between the ear and the top of the head to support the ear) and a nonadherent pad placed over the incision (Fig. 14-22, *C*). The long pieces of tape are applied to the skin. Cast padding and Kling are applied over the ear; the nonaffected ear on the other side is not incorporated in the bandage (Fig. 14-22, *D*). Vetrap or a stockinette (cut a hole for the nonaffected ear) can be placed as the external layer. The bandage can then be secured to the head cranially or caudally with Elastikon or 1-inch tape that is applied to both the hair and bandage.

☞ **N O T E** · Be sure to check head bandages periodically to ensure that they are not too tight and are not restricting breathing.

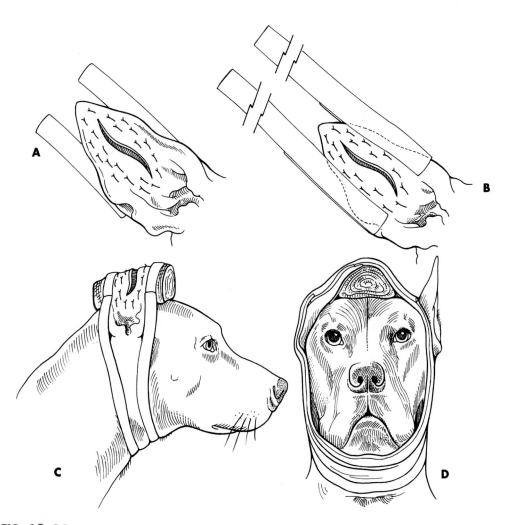

FIG. 14-22
A, To bandage the ear place short strips of tape on the rostral and caudal margin of the convex surface of the pinna. **B,** Use longer pieces of tape on the concave surface of the pinna so that these tape pieces contact the tape on the convex surface. **C,** Place the ear over the top of the head and place a nonadherent pad over the incision. **D,** Apply cast padding and Kling over the ear, then use Vetrap or a stockinette as an external layer.

PROGNOSIS

Aural hematomas seldom recur if they are properly treated and the underlying ear disease is appropriately treated.

Suggested Reading

Dubielzig RR, Wilson JW, Seireg AA: Pathogenesis of canine aural hematomas, *J Am Vet Med Assoc* 185:873, 1984.

Kagan KG: Treatment of canine aural hematoma with an indwelling drain, *J Am Vet Med Assoc* 183:972, 1983.

Kolata RJ: A simple method for treating canine aural hematomas, *Canine Practice* 11:47, 1984.

Wilson JW: Treatment of auricular hematoma, using a teat tube, *J Am Vet Med Assoc* 182:1081, 1983.

NEOPLASIA OF THE PINNA AND EXTERNAL EAR CANAL

DEFINITIONS

The **pinna** is that portion of the ear that projects outward from the skull.

GENERAL CONSIDERATIONS AND CLINICALLY RELEVANT PATHOPHYSIOLOGY

Neoplasms of the external ear canal are relatively uncommon in dogs and cats; however, they may arise from any structure that lines or supports the ear canal. The most common tumors of the external ear canal arise from the ceruminous glands (ceruminous gland adenomas or adenocarcinomas). Squamous cell carcinomas, basal cell tumors, and mast cell tumors may also be found. Although tumors of the external ear canal are more common than those arising within the internal or middle ear cavities, clinical signs of middle or inner ear disease may predominate if these tumors extend through the tympanic membrane (see p. 169). Neoplasms of the external ear are frequently associated with concurrent bacterial and yeast infections. It has been hypothesized that chronic otitis causes hyperplasia that may eventually induce dysplastic and neoplastic changes. The mere presence of a tumor in the ear canal often obstructs drainage, resulting in otitis externa. Most canine ceruminous gland tumors are benign; such tumors are usually malignant in cats.

Any tumor that affects the skin may arise on the pinna, but the most frequent tumor of the pinna in cats is squamous cell carcinoma. These tumors are most commonly diagnosed in older cats, particularly white cats. The association between a lack of protective pigmentation and the occurrence of these tumors suggests that solar radiation may be a causative factor. Although these tumors are highly invasive, metastasis is uncommon. If metastasis does occur it is usually to the regional lymph nodes and lungs. Tumors may also be noted on the nares and eyelids. Other tumors of the pinna of dogs and cats are melanoma, fibrosarcoma, basal cell tumor, fibroma, lymphoma, histiocytoma, papilloma, and mast cell tumor.

DIAGNOSIS

Clinical Presentation

Signalment. Most neoplastic lesions of the external ear are found in middle-aged to older animals. Older male cats may be at increased risk to develop ceruminous gland tumors of the ear canal. Squamous cell carcinoma of the ear pinna occurs almost exclusively in older white-eared cats or multi-colored cats with little pigmentation of their pinna.

History. The history of a patient with a tumor arising from the external ear canal usually differs minimally from those with primary bacterial otitis externa (see p. 163). The history of cats with squamous cell carcinoma is often insidious and begins with the owner intermittently noticing crusty eczematous lesions at the edge of the ear.

☞ **N O T E** • Presenting signs of ear tumors may mimic otitis externa.

Physical Examination Findings

Small, pedunculated masses of the external ear canal suggest ceruminous gland hyperplasia or adenomas, papillomas, or inflammatory polyps. Infiltrative masses suggest ceruminous gland adenocarcinoma (Fig. 14-23). Squamous cell carcinomas usually originate on the tips of the ears where there is little hair and may initially appear as hyperemic skin. As the lesions progress, erosion, ulceration, crusting, and thickening become noticeable (Fig. 14-24). The ear may bleed with mild trauma.

Radiography

Radiographic signs of neoplasia (i.e., bony lysis of the petrous temporal bone) may be noted on skull radiographs of animals with neoplasia of the external ear canal. Although metastasis usually occurs late in the course of disease, pulmonary metastasis may be noted with some ear tumors; therefore, thoracic radiographs are recommended.

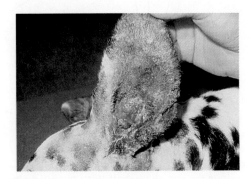

FIG. 14-23
Ceruminous gland adenocarcinoma on the ear pinna of a 6-year-old dog that presented for chronic otitis externa.

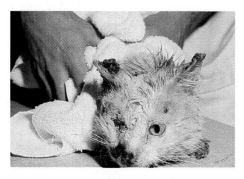

FIG. 14-24
Squamous cell carcinomas on the ear tips of a cat. Note the crusting and thickened appearance of the pinna.

Laboratory Findings

The diagnosis of ear neoplasia requires that the lesion be biopsied.

DIFFERENTIAL DIAGNOSIS

Neoplastic lesions of the ear pinna must be differentiated from nonneoplastic lesions (i.e., dermatitis caused by insect bites, immune-mediated lesions). Suspicious lesions should be biopsied to improve the chances of complete resection.

MEDICAL MANAGEMENT

Squamous cell carcinoma may be prevented or reduced by applying sunscreens to nonpigmented areas of the ear and/or preventing physical exposure to ultraviolet radiation. Cryotherapy and radiation are alternatives to surgical removal of the pinna. Cryotherapy may be curative in small, superficial tumors, but local recurrence is common. Radiation therapy is less disfiguring than surgical removal of the lesions and is a viable alternative for small, superficial tumors and preneoplastic lesions.

SURGICAL TREATMENT

For neoplasms of the external ear canal, vertical or total ear canal ablations are usually required (see p. 158). The aim of surgical treatment of squamous cell carcinoma is to remove the neoplasm with a wide margin of normal surrounding skin. This may require pinnectomy alone, or a vertical ear canal ablation plus removal of the pinna. The owner should be prepared for the resulting cosmetic deformity.

Preoperative Management

If concurrent otitis externa is present, perioperative antibiotics based on culture results should be given. Preoperative cytology will help determine the need for radical resection when neoplasia is suspected.

Anesthesia

See p. 153 for anesthetic recommendations for animals with ear disease.

Surgical Anatomy

Refer to pp. 154 for a description of the surgical anatomy of the ear canal and pinna.

Positioning

Positioning for ear surgery is described with the discussion on surgical techniques on pp. 156–159.

SURGICAL TECHNIQUE

The most important aspect of surgery of ear neoplasms is to achieve wide margins to prevent local recurrence. This may require that the entire pinna and ear canal be removed. If aggressive surgical therapy cannot provide clean margins, adjunctive therapy (i.e., radiation) should be considered. Refer to pp. 156–159 for a description of surgical techniques commonly used for diseased or neoplastic ears.

☞ **N O T E** · Malignant ear tumors must be excised with wide margins of normal tissue. The owner should be advised of the resulting cosmetic defect before surgery.

For pinnectomy, remove the affected portion of the ear and suture the remaining skin over the exposed cartilage.

For small tumors on the central portion of the convex surface of the pinna, resect the neoplasm and mobilize the skin around the defect by undermining between the cartilage and skin. Suture the skin margins or, if necessary, leave the defect open to heal by second intention under a light bandage. For small tumors on the concave surface of the ear, repair the skin defect by elevating a flap from surrounding skin and rotating it into the defect. Suture the flap to the wound margins. After a delay of 10 to 14 days, transect the flap and suture the edge to the defect. Close the donor site primarily.

SUTURE MATERIALS/SPECIAL INSTRUMENTS

See p. 161 for a discussion of suture materials and surgical instruments for ear surgery.

POSTOPERATIVE CARE AND ASSESSMENT

An Elizabethan collar or sidebar should be used to prevent the animal from mutilating the ear after surgery. Ear surgery is painful and postoperative analgesics (i.e., oxymorphone) should be provided (see p. 153). If the animal appears dysphoric or anxious, tranquilizers may be given once they have received adequate postoperative analgesics (see p. 154).

PROGNOSIS

For malignant ceruminous gland tumors of the external ear, ablation is seldom curative. Adjunctive therapy (radiation therapy) should be considered. Local recurrence of squamous cell carcinomas is common if wide margins are not obtained at surgery. The prognosis is poor with squamous cell carcinoma of the middle and inner ear; however, amputation of the pinna for squamous cell carcinoma of the ear margin may be curative.

Suggested Reading

Kirpensteijn J: Aural neoplasms, *Semin Vet Med Surg (Small Anim)* 8:17, 1993.

Legendre AM, Krahwinkel DJ: Feline ear tumors, *J Am Anim Hosp Assoc* 17:1035, 1981.

Little CJL, Pearson GR, Lane JG: Neoplasia involving the middle ear cavity of dogs, *Vet Rec* 124:54, 1989.

Rogers KS: Tumors of the ear canal, *Vet Clin North Am Small Anim Pract* 18:859, 1988.

Trevor PB, Martin RA: Tympanic bulla osteotomy for treatment of middle-ear disease in cats: 19 cases (1984-1991), *J Am Vet Med Assoc* 202:123, 1993.

CHAPTER 15

Surgery of the Abdominal Cavity

GENERAL PRINCIPLES AND TECHNIQUES

DEFINITIONS

Celiotomy is a surgical incision into the abdominal cavity; **laparotomy** is often used synonymously, although it technically refers to a flank incision.

PREOPERATIVE CONCERNS

Celiotomy is performed for a variety of reasons. Surgery may be indicated for diagnostic (e.g., obtaining biopsies) or therapeutic purposes. Many animals undergoing abdominal exploratory surgery have chronic disease, but abdominal surgery must be performed on an emergency basis in some patients with acute clinical signs. A sudden onset of clinical signs referable to the abdominal cavity (e.g., abdominal distention, pain, vomiting) is called an *acute abdomen*. Some conditions (e.g., gastric dilation-volvulus, colonic perforation, severe hemorrhage) are life threatening, and initiation of appropriate therapy must be prompt. Conditions that require surgery must be differentiated from those that can be managed medically. Although obviously unnecessary surgery must be avoided, surgery cannot always be delayed until it is certain the patient will benefit from it.

The decision to operate is based on historical and physical examination findings, radiographic/ultrasonographic studies, and/or laboratory analyses. Physical examination can be unreliable in predicting the severity of abdominal trauma. The inaccuracy associated with examining patients with acute abdominal disease (particularly that associated with trauma) may be attributed in part to the patient's condition at the time of examination and delayed development of clinical signs associated with some injuries. Depressed or lethargic animals may not exhibit pain during abdominal palpation. Clinical signs of hemorrhage often are not apparent immediately after trauma; delays of 3 to 4 hours between trauma and development of shock and collapse are common in patients with liver or spleen lacerations. Thus traumatized animals should be closely observed for at least 8 to 12 hours.

In most instances life-threatening hemorrhage will become apparent before this time. However, animals with traumatic bile peritonitis often are without clinical signs for several weeks. Likewise, traumatic mesenteric avulsion is seldom associated with clinical signs until subsequent peritonitis develops (usually several days after trauma occurs). Sensitive diagnostic tests such as diagnostic peritoneal lavage (see p. 198) may facilitate identification of patients with significant abdominal trauma, before the development of overt clinical signs.

☞ **N O T E ·** Paracentesis and diagnostic peritoneal lavage can be performed after abdominal trauma to help determine whether surgery is warranted. Evidence of gastrointestinal or urinary tract trauma is often made before the onset of obvious clinical signs when these techniques are used. Physical examination accurately predicts which traumatized animals require surgery in only about 50% of cases (see the discussion on peritonitis on p. 193).

Preoperative management of most animals undergoing exploratory laparotomy is dictated by their underlying abdominal disease. General observations include noting the animal's attitude and posture, temperature, respiratory rate and effort, and heart rate and rhythm. Additionally, auscultation, percussion, and palpation of the abdomen, plus a rectal examination, should be performed. Serial examinations are important to detect trends or deterioration in patient status. An intravenous catheter should be placed for fluid and drug administration, and blood samples should be drawn. Useful initial blood work in an animal with acute abdomen includes hematocrit, serum total protein, serum glucose concentrations, complete blood count (CBC), platelet count, and blood urea nitrogen. Other laboratory tests (i.e., serum biochemistry profile, clotting parameters) can be performed, depending on the animal's condition and suspected underlying disease. Urine may be collected via cystocentesis or catheterization for urinalysis. An indwelling urinary catheter may be used to quantitate urinary output if necessary. Abdominal radiographs may detect peritoneal fluid (i.e., uroabdomen, peritonitis) or abnormal accumulations of air. Surgery is warranted if free air is present in the abdominal cavity because this usually indicates rupture or perforation of the gastrointestinal tract. Animals with acute abdominal signs of uncertain cause should have diagnostic peritoneal lavage (see p. 198) performed if radiographs are nondiagnostic. Electrolyte and hydration abnormalities should be corrected before surgery.

☞ **NOTE ·** Do not delay celiotomy excessively in traumatized animals. It may be better to perform a negative exploratory than wait until overt signs of illness develop. Remember, clinical signs of hemorrhage may not be evident until several hours after trauma. Similarly, mesenteric avulsion may not cause obvious clinical signs for 5 to 7 days and biliary tract rupture may not be apparent for several weeks.

ANESTHETIC CONSIDERATIONS

The anesthetic management of animals with abdominal disease depends on their underlying disease. Young, healthy animals can be premedicated with an anticholinergic and opioid (i.e., oxymorphone, butorphanol, buprenorphine) and induced with thiopental, propofol, or a combination of diazepam and ketamine given intravenously to effect (Table 15-1). Refer to subsequent chapters for the anesthetic management of sick and/or debilitated animals.

ANTIBIOTICS

The appropriate use of antibiotics in patients undergoing abdominal surgery depends on the underlying disease, the animal's overall general health, and the length and type of surgical procedure being performed. Surgeries of less than 1.5 to 2 hours in which a contaminated, hollow viscus is not opened do not usually warrant prophylactic antibiotics (see Chapter 10).

TABLE 15-1

Selected Anesthetic Protocols

Premedication
Atropine (0.02-0.04 mg/kg SC or IM) or glycopyrrolate (0.005-0.011 mg/kg SC or IM) plus oxymorphone (0.05-0.1 mg/kg SC or IM) or butorphanol (0.2-0.4 mg/kg SC or IM) or buprenorphine (5-15 µg/kg IM)

Induction
Thiopental sodium (10-12 mg/kg IV) or propofol (4-6 mg/kg IV) or diazepam plus ketamine (0.27 mg/kg and 5.5 mg/kg, respectively) combined and administered IV to effect

Maintenance
Isoflurane or halothane

SURGICAL ANATOMY

The rectus sheath is composed of an external and internal leaf (Fig. 15-1). The external leaf is formed by the aponeurosis of the external abdominal oblique muscle and a portion of the aponeurosis of the internal abdominal oblique muscle. The aponeurosis of the transversus abdominis muscle joins the external leaf near the pubis (see Fig. 15-1). The internal leaf consists of a portion of the aponeurosis of the internal abdominal oblique muscle, aponeurosis of the transversus abdominis muscle, and transversalis fascia. The internal leaf disappears in the caudal third of the abdomen where the aponeurosis of the internal abdominal oblique muscle joins the external leaf, leaving the caudal rectus abdominis muscle covered only by a thin sheet of transversalis fascia and peritoneum (see Fig. 15-1).

☞ **NOTE ·** The linea is easier to find near the umbilicus because it becomes thinner near the pubis.

SURGICAL TECHNIQUES

The abdomen is generally explored via a ventral midline incision. In most animals the entire abdomen (including inguinal areas) and caudal thorax should be prepared for aseptic surgery to allow extension of the incision into the thoracic and/or pelvic cavities if necessary. Prepping too small an area is a common mistake, particularly when abdominal exploration is performed in trauma patients. To adequately visualize all abdominal structures, the incision must extend from the xiphoid process to the pubis. If only a specific abdominal structure is to be examined, the incision length can be shortened. A caudal abdominal incision that extends from the umbilicus to the pubis is adequate for bladder exploration; similarly a cranial abdominal incision (i.e., umbilicus to xiphoid process) allows evaluation of the liver and stomach. Occasionally, the midline incision is extended laterally at the xiphoid process (1 cm caudal to the last rib) to facilitate exposure of the liver, biliary system, and diaphragm. A paracostal (paralumbar) celiotomy can be used to expose the kidney and adrenal glands; it is most commonly used for unilateral adrenalectomy. Counting surgical sponges before surgery and before abdominal closure will help prevent inadvertently leaving them in the abdominal cavity.

Ventral Midline Celiotomy in Cats and Female Dogs

With the patient in dorsal recumbency make a ventral midline skin incision beginning near the xiphoid process and extending caudally to the pubis (Fig. 15-2, A). Sharply incise the subcutaneous tissues until the external fascia of the rectus abdominis muscle is exposed. Ligate or cauterize small subcutaneous bleeders and identify the linea alba. Tent the abdominal wall and make a sharp incision into the linea alba with a scalpel blade. Palpate the interior surface of the linea for adhesions. Use scissors to extend the incision cranially and/or caudally to near the extent of the skin

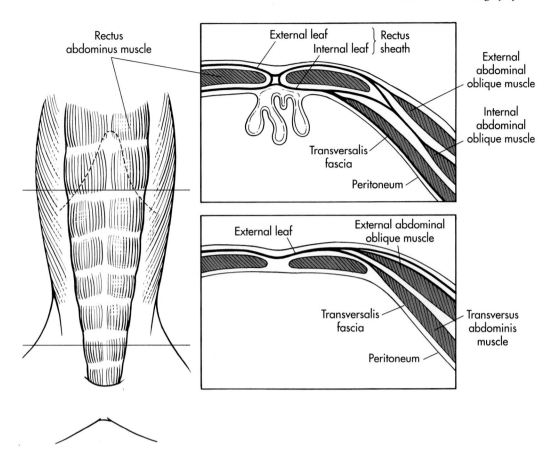

FIG. 15-1
Anatomy of the rectus sheath.

incision. Digitally break down the attachments of one side of the falciform ligament to the body wall or excise it and remove it entirely if it interferes with visualization of cranial abdominal structures. Clamp the cranial end of the falciform ligament and ligate or cauterize bleeders before removing it.

Ventral Midline Celiotomy in Male Dogs

With the dog positioned in dorsal recumbency, place a towel clamp on the prepuce and clamp it to the skin on one side of the body (Fig. 15-2, B). Drape the tip of the prepuce and clamp outside the surgical field. Make a ventral midline skin incision beginning at the xiphoid process and continuing caudally to the prepuce. Curve the incision to the left or right (the opposite side from where the prepuce is clamped) of the penis and prepuce and extend it to the level of the pubis (see Fig. 15-2, B). Incise subcutaneous tissues and fibers of the preputialis muscle to the level of rectus fascia in the same plane as the skin incision. Ligate or cauterize large branches of the caudal superficial epigastric vein at the cranial aspect of the prepuce. Retract incised skin and subcutaneous tissues laterally and locate the linea alba and external fascia of the rectus abdominis muscle. Do not attempt to locate the caudal linea alba until subcutaneous tissues have been incised and abdominal musculature fascia identified. Tent the abdominal wall and

make a sharp incision into the linea alba with a scalpel blade. Palpate the interior surface of the linea for adhesions. Use scissors to extend the incision cranially and/or caudally to near the extent of the skin incision.

Paracostal Celiotomy

Position the animal in lateral recumbency and place a rolled towel or sandbag between the animal and the operating table. Make a skin incision from the ventral vertebral column to near the ventral midline. Center the incision halfway between the wing of the ilium and the last rib. Extend the incision through the external abdominal oblique muscle with scissors. Separate internal abdominal oblique and transversus abdominis muscle fibers and expose peritoneal and transversalis fascia. Tent the peritoneum and sharply incise it with scissors.

Abdominal Exploration

Systematically explore the entire abdomen. Various techniques may be used; however, every surgeon should develop a consistent pattern to ensure that the entire abdominal cavity and all structures are visualized and/or palpated in each animal (Table 15-2). *Use moistened laparotomy sponges to protect tissues from drying during the procedure. If generalized infection is present or if diffuse intraoperative contamination has occurred, flush the*

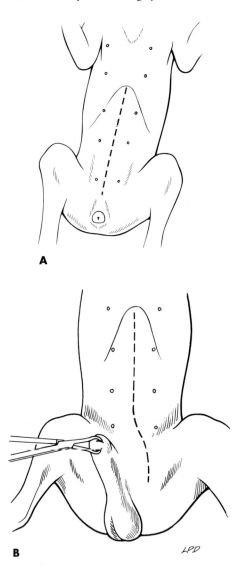

FIG. 15-2
Ventral midline celiotomy. **A,** In cats and female dogs. **B,** In male dogs.

TABLE 15-2
Systematic Exploration of the Abdominal Cavity

1) Explore the cranial quadrant
  • Examine the diaphragm (including esophageal hiatus) and entire liver (palpate the liver)
  • Inspect the gallbladder and biliary tree; express the gallbladder to determine patency
  • Examine the stomach, pylorus, proximal duodenum, and spleen
  • Examine both pancreatic limbs (palpate it gently!), portal vein, hepatic arteries, and caudal vena cava
2) Explore the caudal quadrant
  • Inspect the descending colon, urinary bladder, urethra, and prostate or uterine horns
  • Inspect the inguinal rings
3) Explore the intestinal tract
  • Palpate the intestinal tract from the duodenum to the descending colon and observe the mesenteric vasculature and nodes
4) Explore the gutters
  • Use the mesoduodenum to retract the intestine to the left and examine the right "gutter." Palpate the kidney and examine the adrenal gland, ureter, and ovary.

  • Use the descending colon to retract the abdominal contents to the right. Examine the left kidney, adrenal gland, ureter, and ovary.

abdomen with copious amounts of warmed, sterile saline solution. Historically, many different antiseptics (i.e., povidone-iodine, chlorhexidine) and antibiotics have been added to lavage fluids. Povidone-iodine is the most widely used antiseptic; however, it has not shown a beneficial effect in repeated experimental and clinical trials and may be detrimental in animals with established peritonitis because the carrier, polyvinylpyrrolidone, inhibits macrophage chemotaxis. Similarly, there is no substantial evidence that adding antibiotics to lavage fluid benefits patients treated with appropriate systemic antibiotics. *Remove lavage fluid and blood and inspect the abdominal cavity before abdominal closure to ensure that all foreign material and surgical equipment have been removed. Perform a sponge count and compare it with the preoperative count to ensure that surgical sponges have not been left in the abdominal cavity.*

Abdominal Wall Closure

Close the linea alba with simple interrupted sutures or a simple continuous suture pattern. A simple continuous suture pattern does not increase the risk of dehiscence when properly performed (i.e., secure knots, appropriate suture material), and it allows for rapid closure. Preferably strong, absorbable suture material (i.e., polydioxanone or polyglyconate) should be used for continuous suture patterns and six to eight knots placed at each end of the incision line. Monofilament, nonabsorbable suture material (i.e., nylon, polypropylene) has been associated with suture sinus formation in dogs and should be avoided. Surgical gut and stainless steel wire should not be used for continuous suture patterns. *On each side of the incision incorporate 4 to 10 mm of fascia in each suture. Place interrupted sutures 5 to 10 mm apart, depending on the animals' size. Tighten sutures sufficiently to appose, but not strangulate, tissue because the latter will adversely affect wound healing.*

Incorporate full-thickness bites of the abdominal wall in the sutures if the incision is midline (i.e., through the linea alba; Fig. 15-3). Do not incorporate the falciform ligament between the fascial edges. If the incision is lateral to the linea alba and muscular tissue is exposed (i.e., paramedian), close the external rectus sheath without including muscle in the sutures. Do not attempt to include peritoneum in the sutures. Close subcutaneous tissues with a simple continuous pattern of absorbable suture material and reappose preputialis muscle fibers. Use nonabsorbable (simple interrupted or continuous appositional patterns;

see Chapter 9) sutures or stainless steel staples to close skin. Place skin sutures without tension.

For paracostal celiotomy, close individual muscle layers with synthetic absorbable or nonabsorbable suture material in a continuous or interrupted pattern. Attempt to eliminate dead space between muscle layers. Appose subcutaneous tissue with absorbable suture in a continuous or interrupted pattern and close skin with nonabsorbable suture in a simple interrupted or continuous pattern.

HEALING OF THE ABDOMINAL WALL

The ability of tissues to hold sutures without tearing depends on the tissue's strength and orientation of collagen fibrils. Skin and fascia are strong, whereas muscle and fat are weak. Because the holding layer of abdominal incisions is fascia rather than muscle, dehiscence is common if rectus fascia is not incorporated in sutures. Peritoneum heals rapidly across the incision and does not contribute to wound strength; therefore closure of this layer is not beneficial. Experimental and clinical studies in dogs suggest that suturing peritoneum may increase the incidence of postoperative intraabdominal adhesions.

☞ **N O T E** · The holding layer of the abdominal wall is fascia, not muscle. Fascia must be incorporated into the suture line to prevent dehiscence.

SUTURE MATERIALS/SPECIAL INSTRUMENTS

Useful instruments for celiotomy include Balfour abdominal retractors, Poole or Yankauer suction tips, malleable retrac-

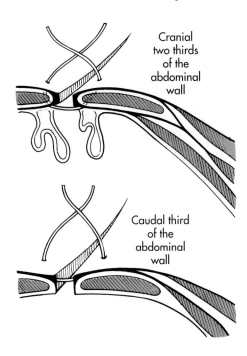

Cranial
two thirds
of the
abdominal
wall

Caudal third
of the
abdominal
wall

FIG. 15-3
To close a midline incision, incorporate full-thickness bites of the linea alba (or external sheath only) in the sutures.

tors, and Mixter (right-angle) forceps. Laparotomy pads and 4 × 4 sponges should have radiopaque markers. See the previous discussion on abdominal wall closure for choice of suture material.

POSTOPERATIVE CARE AND ASSESSMENT

The abdominal incision should be checked twice daily for evidence of redness, swelling, or discharge. If the animal licks or chews at the incision, an Elizabethan collar or sidebar should be used to prevent iatrogenic suture removal. Early signs of altered wound healing are inflammation and edema. Serosanguineous drainage from the incision and swelling are consistent signs of acute incisional dehiscence. Dehiscence usually occurs 3 to 5 days postoperatively when minimal healing has occurred and the sutures have weakened; however, it may occur earlier if knots were tied improperly or if fascia was not incorporated into the sutures. Evisceration usually results in sepsis and severe blood loss secondary to mutilation of exposed intestine and must be treated promptly. The abdomen should be bandaged, fluid therapy initiated, and broad-spectrum antibiotics given while the animal is prepared for surgery. If technical failure is suspected (i.e., poor knot tieing, improper suturing), the entire suture line should be removed and replaced. Debridement of the wound edges is not necessary and will delay wound healing. The intestine should be closely inspected for viability and damaged sections resected if appropriate (see p. 295). The abdominal cavity should be lavaged with copious amounts of warmed, sterile saline. Open abdominal drainage (see p. 198) should be considered in animals with generalized peritonitis. Wound disruption after 10 to 21 days usually results in hernia formation rather than evisceration. Hernial repair in these animals may require excision of fibrotic tissues. Subsequent closure requires that tissue layers be accurately apposed.

COMPLICATIONS

Dehiscence (incisional hernias) may occur if improper surgical technique is used (see the discussion above). The most common causes of wound dehiscence in the early postoperative period are suture breakage, knot slippage or untieing, or sutures cutting through tissue. An increased rate of dehiscence may occur in animals with wound infections, fluid or electrolyte imbalances, anemia, hypoproteinemia, metabolic disease, treatment with corticosteroids or chemotherapeutic agents or radiation, immunosuppression (i.e., feline immunodeficiency virus [FIV], feline leukemia virus), or abdominal distention. Suture sinus formation has been reported with nonabsorbable suture material. Surgical resection of affected tissues and removal of offending sutures are necessary in such cases.

☞ **N O T E** · Never use chromic gut suture in a continuous fashion in the linea alba.

SPECIAL AGE CONSIDERATIONS

Debilitated, very young or old, or hypoproteinemic animals may have delayed healing; chromic gut suture should be avoided for abdominal wall closure in these animals.

Suggested Reading

Freeman LJ et al: Tissue reaction to suture material in the feline linea alba, *Vet Surg* 16:440, 1987.

Hess JL et al: Comparison of stainless steel staples and synthetic suture material on skin wound healing, *J Am Anim Hosp Assoc* 15:501, 1979.

Hosgood G, Pechman RD, Casey HW: Suture sinus in the linea alba of two dogs, *J Small Anim Pract* 33:285, 1992.

Rosin E: Single layer, simple continuous suture pattern for closure of abdominal incisions, *J Am Anim Hosp Assoc* 21:751, 1985.

Wood DS, Collins JE, Walshaw R: Tissue reaction to nonabsorbable suture materials in the canine linea alba: a histological evaluation, *J Am Anim Hosp Assoc* 20:39, 1984.

SPECIFIC DISEASES

UMBILICAL AND ABDOMINAL HERNIAS

DEFINITIONS

External abdominal hernias are defects in the external wall of the abdomen that allow protrusion of abdominal contents, while **internal abdominal hernias** are those that occur through a ring of tissue confined within the abdomen or thorax (i.e., diaphragmatic hernia, hiatal hernia). External abdominal hernias may involve the abdominal wall anywhere other than the umbilicus, inguinal ring, femoral canal, or scrotum. **Umbilical hernias** occur through the umbilical ring. The contents of **true hernias** are generally enclosed within a peritoneal sac; however, because **false hernias** allow protrusion of organs outside of a normal abdominal opening, the contents are seldom contained within a peritoneal sac. **Omphaloceles** are large midline umbilical and skin defects.

SYNONYMS

Abdominal hernias may be defined depending on their location (i.e., ventral, prepubic, subcostal, hypochondral, paracostal, or lateral). The cranial pubic ligament was formally called the *prepubic tendon.*

GENERAL CONSIDERATIONS AND CLINICALLY RELEVANT PATHOPHYSIOLOGY

Abdominal hernias generally occur secondary to trauma (e.g., vehicular accidents, bite wounds); however, they have occasionally been reported as congenital lesions. Congenital cranial abdominal hernias (i.e., cranial to the umbilicus) have been reported in association with peritoneopericardial diaphragmatic hernias in dogs and cats. Abdominal hernias are false hernias because they do not contain a hernial sac. When

associated with blunt trauma, they arise as a result of rupture of the wall from within because intraabdominal pressure is increased while abdominal muscles are contracted. The most common sites for traumatic abdominal hernias are the prepubic region and flank. Cranial pubic ligament hernias often occur in association with pubic fractures (Fig. 15-4). Paracostal hernias may result in migration of abdominal contents along the thoracic wall (see Fig. 15-4). Rarely, abdominal contents will enter the chest through defects in the intercostal muscles.

Umbilical hernias are usually congenital, caused by flawed embryogenesis (see Fig. 15-4). Umbilical vessels, the vitelline duct, and the stalk of the allantois pass through the umbilical ring in the fetus, but this aperture closes at birth leaving an umbilical cicatrix. If the aperture fails to contract or is too large or improperly formed, a hernia results. The hernia is lined by a peritoneal sac and these hernias are considered true hernias. The cause of umbilical hernias is seldom known but most are thought to be inherited. Many male dogs with umbilical hernias are also cryptorchid. Omphaloceles allow abdominal organs to protrude externally (eviscerate). The abdominal contents are initially covered by amniotic tissue but this membrane covering is easily ruptured. Most affected neonates either die or are euthanized at birth.

DIAGNOSIS
Clinical Presentation

Signalment. A majority of animals with umbilical or abdominal hernias are young. Umbilical hernias are believed to be heritable in some breeds (i.e., Airedale, basenji, Pekingese). Cranial ventral abdominal hernias associated with peritoneopericardial diaphragmatic hernias may be inherited in weimaraners.

History. A history of trauma is common with abdominal hernias. The hernia may initially be overlooked while more obvious or life-threatening injuries are treated. Small umbilical hernias often are not noticed until the animal is examined for neutering. If strangulation or intestinal obstruction occurs the animal may present for vomiting, abdominal pain, anorexia, and/or depression.

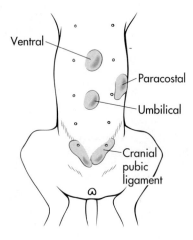

FIG. 15-4
Location of abdominal and umbilical hernias.

Physical Examination Findings

Abdominal structures (i.e., organs or omentum) in the subcutaneous space or between muscle layers usually cause asymmetry of the abdominal contour. The size of the swelling may not correspond to the hernia size, particularly if intestine has migrated into the hernia. The swelling should be carefully palpated to discern the contents of the hernia (i.e., intestine, bladder, spleen) and to locate the abdominal defect. These patients should be thoroughly examined to determine whether concurrent abdominal or thoracic injury or abnormality exists. Cranial pubic ligament rupture is often difficult to palpate because of subcutaneous swelling and pain.

☞ **N O T E** • Do not forget to examine the diaphragm and heart in animals with cranial abdominal hernias.

Umbilical hernias usually present as a soft ventral abdominal mass at the umbilical scar. Deep palpation of the swelling reveals umbilical ring size and helps characterize contents. The hernial ring is not palpable in some animals because the ring closes subsequent to falciform fat or omental herniation. Occasionally, intestine or other abdominal structures can be palpated; they can generally be reduced into the abdominal cavity. If the umbilical sac is warm or painful and the contents are irreducible, intestinal strangulation or obstruction should be suspected.

☞ **N O T E** • Evaluate dogs with congenital hernias for other defects (e.g., cryptorchidism with umbilical hernias).

Radiography/Ultrasonography

Radiographs should be taken in animals with abdominal hernias. Routine ventral dorsal and lateral views may show the presence of associated abdominal or thoracic injury (i.e., abdominal fluid, diaphragmatic hernia). Abdominal radiographs may help confirm the presence of a hernia (i.e., subcutaneous intestinal loops and loss of the ventral abdominal stripe) when the abdominal wall defect cannot be palpated because of swelling or pain. Radiographs are generally not indicated in small umbilical hernias. Ultrasound may also help define the contents of hernias.

Laboratory Findings

Laboratory abnormalities are uncommon with umbilical hernias unless strangulation or intestinal obstruction is present. Abnormalities associated with abdominal hernias vary depending on the severity of concurrent internal injuries.

DIFFERENTIAL DIAGNOSIS

Most hernias are diagnosed on physical examination. Differentials for abdominal swellings include abscesses, cellulitis, hematomas/seromas, and neoplasia.

MEDICAL MANAGEMENT

Initial treatment of animals with abdominal hernias is directed toward diagnosing and treating shock and concurrent life-threatening internal injuries.

SURGICAL TREATMENT

Most abdominal hernias can be repaired by suturing torn muscle edges or apposing the disrupted abdominal wall edge to pubis, ribs, or adjacent fascia. Rarely, synthetic mesh is needed to repair the defect. Some hernias (i.e., intestinal strangulation, urinary obstruction, concurrent organ trauma) require emergency surgical correction. However, the extent of devitalized muscle may not initially be apparent and delaying surgery until muscle damage can be accurately assessed will facilitate surgical correction in stable patients. The most common complications of surgery are hernia recurrence and wound infection. Abdominal hernias secondary to bite wounds are usually contaminated; wound infection and dehiscence of skin and/or hernial repair are common. Mesh should not be placed in these hernias, and the wounds should be drained. Treatment of infected wounds includes cultures, drainage, antibiotics, and/or flushing. Abdominal exploration should be performed at herniorrhaphy to diagnose concurrent abdominal organ injury (i.e., mesenteric avulsion, gastric or intestinal perforation, diaphragmatic herniation, bladder rupture).

☞ **N O T E** • Do not use nonabsorbable suture or mesh in infected wounds; it may fistulate.

Many umbilical hernias resolve spontaneously in young animals or are small and are not corrected until the animal is neutered. Spontaneous closure may occur as late as 6 months of age. Intestinal strangulation is most likely when the hernial defect is about the size of intestine and the hernial sac is large. Strangulation is unlikely in very small or large defects. If abdominal viscera contained within the hernia cannot be reduced, surgery should be performed as soon as possible.

Preoperative Management

Preoperative care depends on the animal's status and concurrent injuries. Hydration and electrolyte abnormalities should be corrected before surgery.

Anesthesia

If there are no concurrent abdominal injuries or disease, the animal can be anesthetized using a variety of anesthetic protocols (see Table 15-1). The underlying disease dictates anesthetic management of sick or debilitated patients. Refer to subsequent chapters for detailed information regarding the anesthetic management of these patients.

Surgical Anatomy

The abdominal wall is composed of four muscle layers (external and internal abdominal oblique muscles, rectus abdominis muscle, and transversus abdominis muscle). Abdominal hernias may occur at insertions or attachments of these muscles or through muscle bellies themselves. The cranial pubic ligament (prepubic tendon) is a band of transverse fibers that connects the iliopectineal eminence and pectineal muscle origin of one side with those on the other side. This ligament attaches the rectus abdominis muscle to the pelvis.

Positioning

For ventral hernias the animal is placed in dorsal recumbency and the area around the hernia prepared for aseptic surgery. Repair of cranial pubic ligament ruptures may be facilitated by placing the animal in dorsal recumbency with the rear limbs flexed and pulled cranially.

SURGICAL TECHNIQUE
Abdominal Hernias

For most abdominal hernias perform a ventral midline abdominal incision to allow the entire abdomen to be explored. Assess the extent of visceral herniation. Reduce herniated contents and amputate or excise necrotic or devitalized tissue around the hernia. Close muscle layers of the hernia with simple interrupted or simple continuous sutures. If a large area of devitalized tissue is removed, use synthetic mesh such as Marlex or Prolene to close the defect (do not place in infected sites). Fold the edges of the mesh over and suture folded edges to viable tissue using simple interrupted sutures. Cranial pubic ligament injuries can be difficult to repair. If necessary, drill holes in the pubic bone to anchor sutures.

Paracostal hernias. *Repair paracostal hernias via a midline incision or one made directly over the hernia. Explore the hernia and suture the torn edges of the transverse, internal, and external abdominal oblique muscles. Incorporate a rib in the suture if muscle has been avulsed from the costal arch.*

Cranial pubic ligament hernias. *With cranial pubic ligament injuries, make a ventral midline skin incision and identify the ruptured tendon and its pubic insertion. Evaluate inguinal rings and vascular lacuna; these hernias may extend into the femoral region as a result of inguinal ligament rupture. Reattach the free edge of the abdominal wall to the cranial pubic ligament with simple interrupted sutures. Alternately, suture the tendon remnant to muscle fascia and periosteum covering the pubis or anchor it to the pubis by drilling holes in the pubic bone through which sutures can be placed (Fig. 15-5). If the hernia extends into the femoral region, it may be necessary to suture body wall to the medial fascia of the adductor muscles. Take care when doing so to avoid damaging the femoral vessels or nerves.*

Umbilical Hernias

For umbilical hernias palpate the hernial ring, reduce abdominal contents if possible, and incise skin over the umbilicus. If the hernia contains only fat or omentum, ligate the hernial neck and excise the sac and its contents. Alternately, if adhesions are not present, invert the sac and its

contents into the abdominal cavity. Do not debride wound margins. Suture edges of the defect with monofilament, synthetic, absorbable suture (i.e., polydioxanone or polyglyconate) in a simple interrupted pattern. If hernial contents cannot be reduced make an elliptical incision around the swelling to prevent damaging the contents. Incise the hernial sac and replace contents into the abdominal cavity. If the contents are irreducible or strangulation or intestinal obstruction is present, extend the abdominal defect on the midline. Explore the abdomen before closing the defect and inspect the intestines for viability. Umbilical hernia repair seldom requires mesh implantation.

SUTURE MATERIALS/SPECIAL INSTRUMENTS

Strong absorbable (i.e., polydioxanone or polyglyconate) or nonabsorbable suture (i.e., polypropylene or nylon) should be used to repair abdominal or ventral hernias. Types of synthetic mesh used to repair some large defects include Marlex mesh and Prolene mesh.

POSTOPERATIVE CARE AND ASSESSMENT

Postoperative care of these patients is dictated by the presence of concurrent injuries or disease. They should be kept quiet and the wound should be observed frequently for infection or dehiscence. Vomiting, fever, and/or leukocytosis may indicate peritonitis (see p. 193).

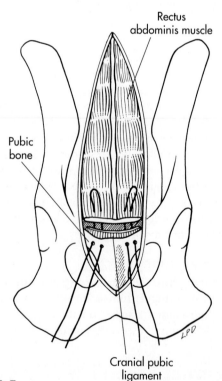

FIG. 15-5
To repair cranial pubic ligament injuries, it may be necessary to anchor the ligament to the pubis by drilling holes in the pubic bone through which sutures can be placed.

PROGNOSIS

The prognosis is generally good and recurrence is uncommon. In one study of 24 animals with abdominal hernias, recurrence was noted within 48 hours in two animals and at 32 days in one animal (Waldron, Hedlund, Pechman, 1986). Nineteen of 24 animals had excellent long-term results.

Reference

Waldron DR, Hedlund CS, Pechman R: Abdominal hernias in dogs and cats: a review of 24 cases, *J Am Anim Hosp Assoc* 22:817, 1986.

Suggested Reading

Mann FA et al: Cranial pubic ligament rupture in dogs and cats, *J Am Anim Hosp Assoc* 22:519, 1986.

Smeak DD: Management and prevention of surgical complications associated with small animal abdominal herniorrhaphy; gastrointestinal surgical complications, *Probl Vet Med* 1:254, 1989.

INGUINAL, SCROTAL, AND FEMORAL HERNIAS

DEFINITIONS

Inguinal hernias are protrusions of organs or tissues through the inguinal canal adjacent to the vaginal process. **Scrotal hernias** occur when inguinal ring defects allow abdominal contents to protrude into the vaginal process adjacent to the spermatic cord. **Femoral hernias** occur through a defect in the femoral canal.

GENERAL CONSIDERATIONS AND CLINICALLY RELEVANT PATHOPHYSIOLOGY

Inguinal hernias may arise as a result of a congenital inguinal ring abnormality or may occur following trauma (Fig. 15-6). The inguinal ring defect allows abdominal contents (e.g., intestine, bladder, uterus) to enter subcutaneous spaces. Congenital hernias may be associated with other abnormalities (e.g., umbilical hernias, perineal hernias, cryptorchidism). Whether inguinal hernias are heritable in most breeds is unknown; neutering is recommended in dogs with nontraumatic hernias until genetics of this condition are known.

The causes of inguinal herniation in small animals are poorly understood. Both neutered and intact male and female dogs may develop nontraumatic inguinal hernias. They may be unilateral or bilateral; unilateral inguinal hernias occur more commonly on the left side than right. Sex hormones have been incriminated in the formation of inguinal hernias in mice, but their role in dogs is unclear. Pregnancy and obesity may be associated with inguinal hernia formation. Traumatic inguinal hernias may occur as a result of a congenital musculature weakness or abnormality of the inguinal ring.

Scrotal hernias are rare, indirect hernias (see Fig. 15-6). They are usually unilateral and strangulation of abdominal contents is common. Little is known regarding cause and heritability. A congenital defect or trauma may predispose some dogs to hernia formation. An increased incidence of testicular tumors has been reported in conjunction with scrotal hernias.

Femoral hernias are rare in dogs and cats. They occur when abdominal contents or fat protrude through the femoral canal, caudomedial to the femoral vessels (see Fig. 15-6). They may be mistaken for inguinal hernias. Femoral hernias may occur following trauma and avulsion of the cranial pubic ligaments or they may be caused by transecting the origin of the pectineus muscle from the pubis during subtotal pectineal myectomy.

DIAGNOSIS
Clinical Presentation

Signalment. Nontraumatic inguinal hernias are most frequently reported in intact, middle-aged female dogs or young (less than 2 years of age) male dogs. Inguinal hernias presumably arise in young male dogs because late testicular descent causes delayed inguinal ring closure. Breeds that are predisposed include Pekingese, cairn terrier, basset, basenji, and West Highland white terrier. Older bitches may be predisposed to develop inguinal hernias because they have a relatively large diameter ring with a short canal. Herniation is most commonly associated with enlargement of the entrance to the vaginal process in these dogs. Inguinal hernias are rare in cats. Scrotal hernias have been reported most commonly in chondrodystrophic dogs, particularly shar-peis. No breed or sex predisposition has been reported for femoral hernias.

History. Animals with inguinal hernias may present for evaluation of a nonpainful swelling in the inguinal region, or for vomiting, lethargy, pain, and/or depression if the hernial contents are incarcerated. Small hernias often go unnoticed unless organ entrapment or incarceration occurs. Omentum is the most common organ present in canine

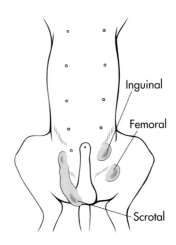

FIG. 15-6
Location of scrotal, inguinal, and femoral hernias.

inguinal hernias. Uterus is often located within the hernias of affected intact females. These hernias are often chronic and do not cause clinical signs until pregnancy or pyometra develops.

☞ **N O T E** · Recommend neutering dogs with inguinal hernias.

Animals with scrotal and femoral hernias usually present for evaluation of scrotal or medial thigh swelling, respectively, or for vomiting and pain if intestinal incarceration occurs.

Physical Examination Findings

The physical characteristics of the swelling vary depending on the hernial contents and the degree of associated vascular obstruction. Often a soft, nonpainful, unilateral or bilateral swelling is noted in the inguinal region. If intestinal strangulation has occurred, or a gravid uterus or urinary bladder is contained within the hernia, the swelling may be large, fluctuant, and painful. Finding nonviable small intestine is more common in young (less than 2 years) male dogs with nontraumatic hernias than in older animals. Associated vascular and/or lymphatic obstruction may cause testicular and spermatic cord edema. Concurrent abnormalities (e.g., perineal hernia, cryptorchidism) may be noted. Unilateral inguinal hernias are more common than bilateral hernias. Bilateral hernias occur more commonly in young dogs, and careful palpation of the contralateral inguinal region for occult hernias is recommended in all dogs.

Scrotal hernias usually appear as a firm, cordlike mass extending into the caudal aspect of the scrotum. Pain and bluish-black tissue discoloration may be noted if intestinal strangulation has occurred. Femoral hernias cause swelling on the medial aspect of the thigh that may extend into the inguinal region. The swelling is located caudal to the inguinal ligament and ventrolateral to the pelvic brim.

Radiography/Ultrasonography

Abdominal radiographs may help identify herniation of a gravid uterus, intestine, or bladder in an inguinal hernia. Loss of the caudal abdominal stripe may be noted in affected animals. Ultrasonography is useful with scrotal hernias to assess viability of testicular blood flow and whether spermatic cord torsion or hydrocele is present.

Laboratory Findings

Laboratory abnormalities are uncommon unless intestinal incarceration has occurred.

DIFFERENTIAL DIAGNOSIS

Differentiation of mammary tumors, lipomas, lymphadenopathy, hematomas, abscesses, and/or mammary cysts from inguinal hernias is facilitated by placing the animal on its back and attempting to reduce the contents of the swelling. Incarceration of intestine may prevent reduction

and make differentiation of these abnormalities difficult. Occasionally, older, obese cats will have abdominal fat deposits which may be confused with hernias on physical examination. Differentials for scrotal hernias include trauma, testicular or scrotal neoplasia, orchitis, and severe scrotal inflammation or swelling. Differentials for femoral hernias include neoplasia, abscesses, and lymphadenopathy. Femoral and inguinal hernias may be difficult to distinguish from each other before surgery.

☞ **N O T E** · Do not mistake the caudal abdominal fat pad in obese cats for a hernia.

MEDICAL MANAGEMENT

The animal should be stabilized before surgery.

SURGICAL TREATMENT

Prompt surgical correction is recommended to prevent complications associated with intestinal strangulation or pregnancy. Removal of nondescended testicles should be performed at inguinal hernia repair. Necrosis of ipsilateral descended testicles may occur secondary to vascular obstruction and necessitate orchiectomy. If a gravid uterus is contained within the inguinal hernia the animal can be spayed, or if the fetus is viable and pregnancy termination is not desired, an attempt can be made to reduce the uterus and close the inguinal ring. However, parturition or uterine enlargement may be associated with recurrence.

☞ **N O T E** · Warn owners of intact female dogs with inguinal hernias that the hernia may recur if the dog is bred or develops pyometra.

Preoperative Management

If intestinal incarceration or strangulation is suspected, antibiotics should be given before surgery.

Anesthesia

If the animal is healthy a variety of anesthetic protocols can be used safely (see Table 15-1). If nonviable intestine is present see p. 293 for anesthetic recommendations for animals undergoing intestinal surgery. Anesthetic protocols for pregnant animals are on p. 521.

Surgical Anatomy

The inguinal canal is a sagittal slit in the caudoventral abdominal wall through which the genital branch of the genitofemoral nerve, artery, and vein, the external pudendal vessel, and the spermatic cord (males) or round ligament (females) pass (Fig. 15-7). The vascular structures are located in the caudomedial aspect of the canal. The inguinal canal is bounded by the internal and external inguinal rings. The internal inguinal ring is formed by the caudal edge of the internal abdominal oblique muscle (cranial), rectus abdominis muscle (medial), and inguinal ligament (lateral and caudal),

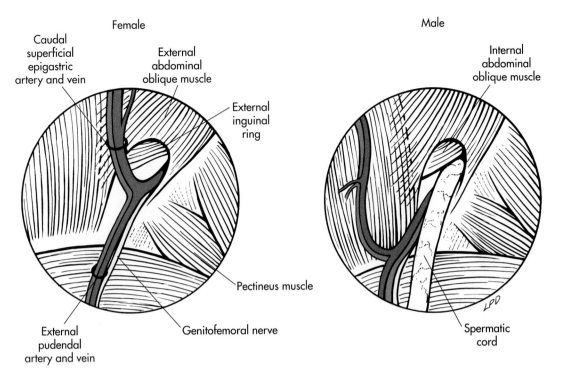

Female
Caudal superficial epigastric artery and vein
External abdominal oblique muscle
External inguinal ring
Pectineus muscle
External pudendal artery and vein
Genitofemoral nerve

Male
Internal abdominal oblique muscle
Spermatic cord

FIG. 15-7
Components of the inguinal canal.

while the external inguinal ring is a longitudinal slit in the aponeurosis of the external abdominal oblique muscle. Direct hernias occur when peritoneal evagination occurs as a separate outpocketing distinct and separate from the vaginal process, while indirect hernias are protrusions through the normal evagination of the vaginal process.

Positioning

The animal is positioned in dorsal recumbency and the caudal abdominal and inguinal areas prepared for aseptic surgery.

SURGICAL TECHNIQUE

The goal of surgery is to reduce the abdominal contents and close the external inguinal ring so that herniation of abdominal contents cannot recur. The approach for inguinal hernias depends on whether the hernia is unilateral or bilateral, whether the contents can be reduced, and whether intestinal strangulation or concurrent abdominal trauma is present. Although an incision can be made parallel to the flank fold directly over the lateral aspect of the swelling, a midline incision is usually preferred in female dogs because it allows palpation and closure of both inguinal rings through a single skin incision. Inguinal hernias can usually be closed without the use of prosthetic materials. Occasionally repair of recurrent or large traumatic defects requires synthetic mesh placement (see p. 47) or a cranial sartorius muscle flap (see p. 127). Bilateral orchiectomy is recommended with scrotal hernias to lessen recurrence.

☞ **N O T E •** Some surgeons prefer to incise directly over the inguinal rings, even with bilateral hernias.

Inguinal Hernias

Make a caudal abdominal midline skin incision in female dogs cranially from the brim of the pelvis (Fig. 15-8). Deepen the incision through subcutaneous tissues to the ventral rectus sheath. Expose the hernial sac by bluntly dissecting beneath mammary tissue and identify the hernial sac and ring (Fig. 15-9, A). Reduce abdominal contents by twisting the sac and milking contents through the ring, or if necessary incise the hernial sac and make an incision in the craniomedial aspect of the ring to enlarge it (Fig. 15-9, B). After reducing abdominal contents amputate the base of the hernial sac and close it with

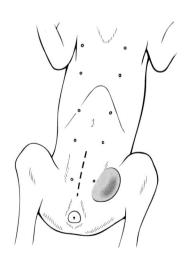

FIG. 15-8
Incision for inguinal hernia repair.

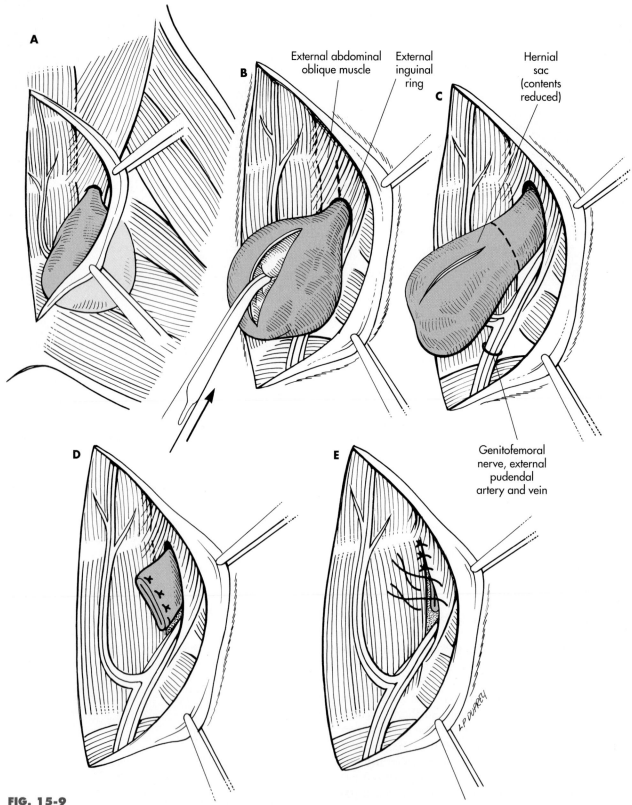

A, External abdominal oblique muscle, External inguinal ring

C, Hernial sac (contents reduced)

Genitofemoral nerve, external pudendal artery and vein

FIG. 15-9
A, For inguinal hernia repair, bluntly dissect beneath mammary tissue and identify the hernial sac and ring. **B,** If necessary, incise the hernial sac. **C,** Reduce the hernial contents, and amputate the base of the sac. **D,** Close the sac, **E,** and the inguinal ring.

horizontal mattress sutures (Fig. 15-9, C and D), a simple continuous suture pattern, or an inverting suture pattern (i.e., Cushing plus Lembert). Close the inguinal ring with simple interrupted sutures of absorbable or nonabsorbable synthetic suture material (Fig. 15-9, E). Avoid compromising the external pudendal vessels and genitofemoral nerve that exit from the caudomedial aspect of the ring (or the spermatic cord in intact male dogs). Palpate the contralateral ring and close it if necessary before skin closure.

If hernial contents cannot be reduced, perform a celiotomy and explore abdominal contents. Expose the inguinal ring as described above and reduce hernial contents (enlarge the inguinal ring if necessary). Resect nonviable intestine or perform an ovariohysterectomy and close the inguinal ring(s).

Scrotal Hernias

Incise the skin over or lateral to the inguinal ring and parallel to the flank fold (Fig. 15-10). Expose the hernial sac and reduce abdominal contents (incise the hernial sac if necessary). If hernial repair is performed in conjunction with orchiectomy (preferred), open the hernial sac and ligate the contents of the spermatic cord (Fig. 15-11, A). Remove the testicle after disrupting the ligament of the tail of the epididymis and ligate the hernial sac at the level of the internal inguinal ring (Fig. 15-11, B). If castration is not being performed, make an incision into the hernial sac (parietal vaginal tunic) and evaluate the hernial contents (Fig. 15-11, C). Reduce the herniated contents and place a transfixing ligature or several horizontal mattress sutures in the hernial sac to reduce the size of the vaginal orifice (Fig. 15-11, D). Partially close the external inguinal ring with interrupted sutures (Fig. 15-11, E). Do not compromise the spermatic cord or vascular structures at the caudomedial ring aspect.

If hernial contents cannot be reduced or if viscera are strangulated and necrotic, perform a midline celiotomy as described previously. After resecting intestine, expose the inguinal ring and repair the hernia. Perform a scrotal ablation if severe contamination of the vaginal process and scrotum has occurred.

Femoral Hernias

Incise skin parallel to the inguinal ligament and expose the hernial sac. Reduce sac contents and ligate the hernial sac as high in the femoral canal as possible. If the inguinal ligament is intact, close the femoral canal by placing sutures between the inguinal ligament and pectineal fascia. Do not damage or compromise neurovascular structures of the femoral canal (Fig. 15-12). Close subcutaneous tissues and skin. If strangulation of abdominal organs is present, perform a midline celiotomy. Reduce abdominal contents, then invert and ligate the sac. Dissect laterally from the skin incision to the femoral canal and close the femoral canal defect as described above.

SUTURE MATERIALS/SPECIAL INSTRUMENTS

Monofilament absorbable (polydioxanone or polyglyconate) or nonabsorbable (polypropylene or nylon) suture material should be used to close the hernial ring. Multifilament nonabsorbable suture may be associated with a higher incidence of wound infection. Mesh can be used as an overlay to reinforce the primary hernia repair (see p. 47).

POSTOPERATIVE CARE AND ASSESSMENT

Routine use of drains is not recommended; however, hernial sites should be assessed postoperatively for evidence of infection or hematoma/seroma formation. Prompt removal of skin sutures, drainage, and topical therapy is indicated if abscessation occurs to prevent dehiscence of the hernia repair. Exercise should be restricted to leash walks for several weeks. An Elizabethan collar may be necessary to prevent the animal from licking at the surgical site. Testicular swelling postoperatively may indicate compromise of testicular lymphatic and/or vascular drainage. With femoral hernias, hobbles may be necessary during healing to prevent limb abduction, and femoral nerve function should be assessed postoperatively. Nerve deficits or severe pain may indicate compromise of the femoral nerve during the repair; reoperation is warranted in such cases.

PROGNOSIS

The prognosis is excellent unless intestinal leakage and perforation occur. The overall complication rate in one study of 35 dogs with inguinal hernias was 17% with a mortality rate of 3% (Waters, Roy, Stone, 1993).

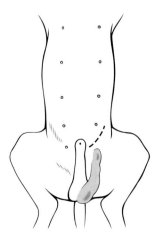

FIG. 15-10
Incision for scrotal hernia repair.

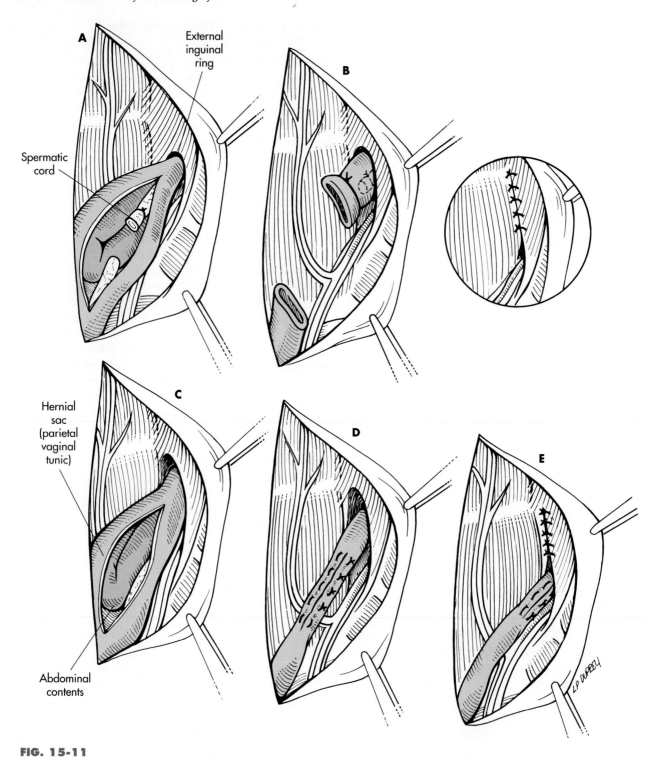

FIG. 15-11

If scrotal hernia repair is performed in conjunction with orchiectomy, **A,** open the hernial sac and ligate the contents of the spermatic cord. **B,** Remove the testicle and ligate the hernial sac at the level of the internal inguinal ring. If castration is not performed, **C,** make an incision into the hernial sac, **D,** reduce the contents, and decrease the size of the vaginal orifice. **E,** Partially close the external inguinal ring.

References

Waters DJ, Roy RG, Stone EA: A retrospective study of inguinal hernia in 35 dogs, *Vet Surg* 22:44, 1993.

Suggested Reading

Fry PD: Unilateral inguinal scrotal hernia in a castrated dog, *Vet Rec* 532, 1991.

Manderino D, Bucklan L: Complete small-bowel obstruction caused by scrotal hernia in a dog, *Mod Vet Pract* 3:365, 1987.

Mitchener KL et al: Use of ultrasonographic and nuclear imaging to diagnose scrotal hernia in a dog, *J Am Vet Med Assoc* 196:1834, 1990.

Penzhorn BL, Petrick SWT: Hydrocele associated with unilateral inguinal hernia in a young basset hound, *J Small Anim Pract* 27:81, 1986.

Pugh CR, Konde LJ: Sonographic evaluation of canine testicular and scrotal abnormalities: a review of 26 case histories, *Vet Radiol* 32:243, 1991.

Strande A: Inguinal hernia in dogs, *J Small Anim Pract* 30:520, 1989.

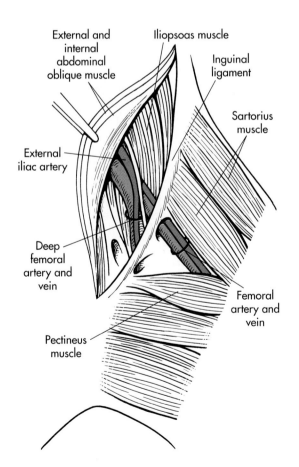

FIG. 15-12
Neurovascular structures of the femoral canal.

Labels: External and internal abdominal oblique muscle; Iliopsoas muscle; Inguinal ligament; Sartorius muscle; External iliac artery; Deep femoral artery and vein; Femoral artery and vein; Pectineus muscle

PERITONITIS

GENERAL CONSIDERATIONS AND CLINICALLY RELEVANT PATHOPHYSIOLOGY

Secondary generalized peritonitis is the predominant form of peritonitis in dogs and is usually caused by bacteria. Primary generalized peritonitis occurs in cats associated with feline infectious peritonitis. Generalized peritonitis may result from intestinal or gallbladder perforation, rupture, or necrosis (e.g., gastric or intestinal foreign bodies, intussusception, mesenteric avulsion, gastric dilatation-volvulus, necrotizing cholecystitis), pancreatic abscessation, prostatic abscesses, or foreign body penetration.

DIAGNOSIS
Clinical Presentation

Signalment. Any age, sex, or breed of dog or cat may develop peritonitis. It is particularly common in young animals that have perforating foreign bodies and in those that receive abdominal trauma (e.g., vehicular trauma or bite wounds).

History. The history of peritonitis in a patient is often nonspecific. The animal may not show signs of illness for several days after the traumatic episode. Mesenteric avulsions often do not cause clinical signs of peritonitis for 5 to 7 days after the injury. Animals with traumatic bile peritonitis may be asymptomatic for several weeks after the injury. Most animals are presented for lethargy, anorexia, vomiting, diarrhea, and/or abdominal pain.

☞ **N O T E ·** Early detection of peritonitis (before the onset of overt clinical signs) requires abdominocentesis or diagnostic peritoneal lavage.

Physical Examination Findings

Affected animals are usually in pain during abdominal palpation. The pain may be localized but generalized pain is more common and the animal will often tense or "splint" the abdomen during palpation. Vomiting and diarrhea may be noted. Abdominal distension may be noted if sufficient fluid has accumulated. Pale mucous membranes, prolonged capillary refill times, and tachycardia may indicate that the animal is in shock. Dehydration and arrhythmias may also occur.

Radiography/Ultrasonography

The classic radiographic finding in animals with peritonitis is loss of abdominal detail with a focal or generalized "ground-glass" appearance. The intestinal tract may be dilated with air and/or fluid. Free air in the abdomen may be noted with rupture of a hollow organ or sometimes occurs without gut rupture as a result of gas-producing anaerobes. A more localized peritonitis may occur secondary to pancreatitis and can cause the duodenum to appear fixed and elevated. Ultrasonography is useful to localize fluid accumulation and help determine etiology.

Laboratory Findings

The most common laboratory finding in animals with peritonitis is a marked leukocytosis. The predominant cell type is the neutrophil and a left shift is often apparent. Other abnormalities may include anemia, dehydration, and electrolyte and acid-base abnormalities.

Abdominocentesis should be performed (see p. 198) and fluid retrieved for analysis. See pp. 496 and 398 for fluid analysis of animals with uroabdomen and bile peritonitis, respectively. Inflammatory fluids should have an elevated number of neutrophils, which may appear degenerative. Significant numbers of leukocytes accumulate in the peritoneal cavity within 2 to 3 hours of contamination with blood, bile, urine, feces, or gastric or pancreatic secretions. Leukocyte counts in abdominal fluid of normal dogs are usually less than 500 cells/μl. Following peritoneal lavage (see p. 198) in dogs, white blood cell (WBC) counts of 1000 to 2000 cells/μl are indicative of mild to moderate irritation, while counts of greater than 2000 cells/μl indicate marked peritonitis (Hardie, 1995). The presence of degenerate leukocytes and bacteria in the lavage fluid also suggests intraabdominal infection. However, the presence and number of WBCs should be correlated with other clinical findings when considering abdominal exploration. Elevated leukocyte counts are found in most dogs following abdominal surgery. In animals that have undergone recent surgery, 7000 to 9000 cells/μl indicates mild to moderate peritonitis and greater than 9000 cells/μl indicates marked peritonitis (Hardie, 1995).

After abdominocentesis the amount of blood in the abdominal cavity can be estimated by observing the lavage sample. A red color reflects the presence of red blood cells (RBCs) and a deep red color usually indicates severe hemorrhage. If newsprint cannot be read through the plastic tubing, then hemorrhage is significant. If print can be seen through the tubing, only moderate or minimal hemorrhage is present. The amount of blood in the abdominal cavity can be estimated using the equation in Table 15-3. Surgical intervention is indicated when there is a substantial increase in the packed cell volume (PCV) of lavage samples taken within 5 to 20 minutes of each other, or if an animal in shock does not respond to aggressive fluid therapy.

TABLE 15-3

Estimation of the Amount of Blood in Abdominal Fluid

Formula:

$$X = \frac{L \times V}{P - L}$$

X = amount of blood in the abdominal cavity
L = the PCV of the returned lavage fluid
V = the volume of lavage fluid infused into the abdominal cavity
P = the PCV of the peripheral blood before the IV infusion of fluids

---

DIFFERENTIAL DIAGNOSIS

Advanced peritonitis with significant accumulation of abdominal fluid is not difficult to diagnose. The difficulty usually arises in determining the etiology of the effusion or infection. Early peritonitis, before the onset of overt clinical signs, is difficult to diagnose and may require diagnostic peritoneal lavage (see p. 198).

MEDICAL MANAGEMENT

The goals of management of animals with peritonitis are to treat the cause of the contamination, resolve the infection, and restore normal fluid and electrolyte balances. Food should be withheld if the animal is vomiting. Fluid replacement therapy should be initiated as soon as possible, particularly if the animal is dehydrated or appears to be in shock (up to 90 ml/kg intravenously, based on the animal's condition). Hypokalemia (Table 15-4) and hyponatremia may be present and require intravenous supplementation. Hypoglycemia is common if the animal has septic shock (systemic inflammatory response syndrome) and glucose may need to be added to the fluids (i.e., 2.5% to 5% dextrose). Standard shock therapy (i.e., fluid replacement, antibiotics, plus or minus soluble corticosteroids) should be initiated. If severe metabolic acidosis is present, bicarbonate therapy may be indicated (Table 15-5).

Broad-spectrum antibiotic therapy should be initiated as soon as the diagnosis is made. Ampicillin plus enrofloxacin (Table 15-6) is an effective combination against most bacteria responsible for peritonitis in dogs. However, amikacin sulfate plus clindamycin or amikacin sulfate plus metronidazole may be necessary if anaerobic infection is present (see Table 15-6). A second-generation cephalosporin such as cefoxitin sodium (see Table 15-6) may also be used if gram-negative plus anaerobic infection is suspected. If renal compromise is present in an animal with a resistant bacterial infection, imipenem may be considered (see Table 15-6). Initial antibiotic therapy should be altered based on results of aerobic and anaerobic culture results of lavage fluid or cultures obtained at surgery.

Low-dose heparin (Table 15-7) increases survival and significantly reduces abscess formation in experimental peritonitis. The inflammatory process in peritonitis is associated with an outpouring of fibrous exudate that causes intraabdominal loculation of bacteria. The loculated bacteria are protected from host defense mechanisms and antibiotics that may not be able to penetrate the fibrin clots. Although the exact mechanism of its beneficial effect is still unknown, there does not appear to be any doubt that heparin is indicated in patients with severe peritonitis. Heparin may also be incubated with plasma and given to animals with disseminated intravascular coagulation (DIC) (see Table 15-7).

Flunixin meglumine is beneficial in experimental peritonitis (see Table 15-7). Dogs treated with banamine in addition to gentamicin sulfate and fluids had higher blood pressures, less hemoconcentration, less metabolic acidosis, and higher survival rates than dogs treated with gentamicin sulfate and fluids alone (Hardie, Rawlings, Collins, 1985). Banamine blocks thromboxane and prostacyclin produc-

TABLE 15-4

Intravenous Potassium Supplementation Guidelines

Serum Potassium* (mEq/L)	mEq KCl/L of Fluid	Maximal Infusion Rate† (ml/kg/hr)
<2.0	80	6
2.1-2.5	60	8
2.6-3.0	40	12
3.1-3.5	28	16

*If serum potassium not available, add potassium to a total concentration of 20 mEq/L.
†Do not exceed 0.5 mEq/kg/hr

TABLE 15-5

Sodium Bicarbonate Therapy

1-2 mEq/kg, IV; repeat only if indicated based on assessment of acid-base balance and potassium concentration

or

$0.3 \times$ base deficit (mEq) $\times$ b.w. (kg) (Give half IV over 10 to 15 minutes and reevaluate. Give the remainder over 4 to 6 hours if necessary.)

TABLE 15-6

Antibiotic Therapy in Animals with Peritonitis

Ampicillin
22 mg/kg IV, TID or QID

Enrofloxacin (Baytril)
5-10 mg/kg IV, BID

Amikacin (Amiglyde-V)
30 mg/kg IV, SID

Clindamycin (Antirobe)
11 mg/kg IV, TID

Metronidazole (Flagyl)
10 mg/kg IV, TID

Cefoxitin (Mefoxin)
30 mg/kg IV, QID

Imipenem (Primaxin)
3-10 mg/kg IM, slow IV, TID or QID

TABLE 15-7

Adjunctive Therapy in Dogs with Peritonitis

Heparin
50-100 units/kg SC, BID

Heparin activated plasma
Incubate 5-10 units/kg heparin with 1 unit fresh plasma for 30 minutes; give 10 ml/kg IV

Flunixin meglumine (Banamine)
1 mg/kg IV, once or twice if in septic shock

tion. However, it must be used with caution in dogs because of the potential of gastrointestinal (GI) and renal toxicity.

SURGICAL TREATMENT

Abdominocentesis is the percutaneous removal of fluid from the abdominal cavity, usually for diagnostic purposes, although it may occasionally be therapeutic. Indications include shock without apparent cause, undiagnosed disease with signs involving the abdominal cavity, suspicion of postoperative GI dehiscence, blunt or penetrating abdominal injuries (i.e., gunshot wounds, dog bites, automobile accidents), and undiagnosed abdominal pain. A multifenestrated catheter should be used to enhance fluid collection. Physical and radiographic examinations should precede abdominocentesis to rule out instances where it may not be safe and to guide needle placement. Four-quadrant paracentesis may be performed if simple abdominocentesis is not successful in retrieving fluid. It is similar to simple abdominocentesis except that multiple abdominal sites are assessed by dividing the abdomen into four quadrants through the umbilicus and tapping each of these four areas. Diagnostic peritoneal lavage should be performed in animals with suspected peritonitis if the above methods are unsuccessful in obtaining fluid for analysis (see p. 198).

☞ **NOTE** • To enhance fluid collection during needle paracentesis use an over-the-needle catheter in which several side ports have been added.

Exploratory surgery is indicated when the cause of peritonitis cannot be determined or when bowel rupture, intestinal obstruction (e.g., bowel incarceration, neoplasia), or mesenteric avulsion is suspected. Serosal patching and plication are techniques that decrease the incidence of intestinal leakage, dehiscence, or repeated intussusception (see pp. 301 and 302). Animals requiring surgery and that have peritonitis secondary to intestinal trauma (disruption of mesenteric blood supply, bowel perforation, chronic intussusception, foreign body) are frequently hypoproteinemic. The role that protein levels play in healing intestinal incisions is not well understood. However, most surgeons are concerned that hypoproteinemic patients may not heal as quickly as patients with normal protein levels despite one study that showed similar complication rates among animals with normal protein levels and those that were hypoproteinemic and undergoing intestinal surgery (Harvey, 1990). Most experimental evidence has shown that retardation of wound healing is not seen with moderate protein depletion but only with severe deficiencies (less than 1.5 to 2 g/dl).

☞ **NOTE** • Choose your suture carefully in hypoproteinemic and debilitated patients. Do not use gut suture in these animals.

Although the practice of lavaging the abdominal cavity of animals with peritonitis is controversial, lavage is generally indicated with diffuse peritonitis. Lavage should be done with care in animals with localized peritonitis to prevent causing diffuse dissemination of infection. When lavage is performed, as much of the fluid as possible should be removed because fluid inhibits the body's ability to fight off infection, probably by inhibiting neutrophil function. Historically, many different agents have been added to lavage fluids, especially antiseptics and antibiotics. Povidone-iodine is the most widely added antiseptic; however, its use may be contraindicated in established peritonitis. Furthermore, no beneficial effect of this agent has been shown in repeated experimental and clinical trials. Although a great many antibiotics have been added to lavage fluids over the years, there is no substantial evidence that their addition is of any benefit to patients who are being treated with appropriate systemic antibiotics. Warmed sterile physiologic saline is the most appropriate lavage fluid.

Open abdominal drainage (OAD) is a useful technique for managing animals with peritonitis. Reported advantages include improvement in the patient's metabolic condition secondary to improved drainage, reduced abdominal adhesion and abscess formation, and access for repeated inspection and exploration of the abdomen. With this technique the abdomen is left open and sterile wraps are placed around the wound. The frequency of the wrap changes is dependent upon the amount of fluid being drained and the amount of external soiling. Experimentally, dogs with peritonitis treated by OAD recovered faster than those treated with closed abdomens. Peritoneal bacterial numbers were significantly less in OAD dogs when compared with control dogs, and at necropsy there were fewer abdominal adhesions and less peritoneal fluid in the former group. Complications of open abdominal drainage include persistent fluid loss, hypoalbuminemia, weight loss, adhesions of abdominal viscera to the bandage, and contamination of the peritoneal cavity with cutaneous organisms.

Preoperative Management

Animals with peritonitis should be stabilized before surgery if they are in shock. Preoperative management of peritonitis is similar to that described in the previous discussion on medical management. Nutritional management of animals with peritonitis is extremely important. If they are debilitated, vomiting, or likely to not resume eating for several days after surgery, enteral or parenteral hyperalimentation should be considered (see Chapter 11).

Anesthesia

Animals with peritonitis are often endotoxic and/or hypotensive. Small amounts of endotoxins are normally absorbed from the intestine and transported via the portal system to the liver, where they are removed and destroyed by hepatocytes. Hypotension in dogs is associated with intense portal vasoconstriction. This vasoconstriction causes break-down of the intestinal mucosal barrier, allowing increased endotoxin to be absorbed from the intestines. If hepatic function is impaired (common in septic animals), small doses of endotoxin that would normally be nonharmful may be lethal. Thus hypotension should be corrected before and prevented during and after surgery in animals with peritonitis. Animals with total protein less than 4.0 g/dl or albumin less than 1.5 g/dl may benefit from perioperative colloid administration. Colloids may be given preoperatively, intraoperatively, and/or postoperatively for a total dose of 20 ml/kg/day. If colloids are given during surgery (7 to 10 ml/kg), acute intraoperative hypotension should be treated with crystalloids.

Dobutamine or dopamine (Table 15-8) may be given during surgery for inotropic support. Dobutamine is less arrhythmogenic and chronotropic than dopamine and is preferred if the patient is hypotensive and anuric. If the patient is anuric and normotensive, low dose dopamine (0.5 to 1.5 μg/kg/min intravenously) plus furosemide (0.2 mg/kg intravenously) may be preferable. These patients should be monitored for arrhythmias or tachycardia.

Hepatic necrosis occurs during sepsis and causes reduced liver function. The pathogenesis of hepatic necrosis is uncertain but may be caused by hypotension and hypoxia. These animals may have reduced ability to metabolize drugs, and prolonged duration of action or altered function of drugs may result. Acepromazine should not be used in animals with peritonitis if severe hepatic dysfunction is suspected (see p. 367). Diazepam plus an opioid are useful premedicants in patients with hepatic dysfunction (see p. 368). Diazepam used alone may disinhibit some behaviors. It should be used with caution in hypoalbuminemic patients. Most opioids have little or no adverse effect on the liver; however, intravenous morphine should be avoided in dogs with hepatic dysfunction because it may cause hepatic congestion as a result of histamine release and hepatic vein spasm. Although some opioid analgesics may have prolonged action when hepatic function is reduced, their effects can be antagonized. Barbiturates (e.g., thiopental) should be used cautiously or avoided in patients with significant hepatic dysfunction. Selected anesthetic protocols for use in animals with peritonitis are provided in Table 15-9. An anticholinergic may be given if the animal is bradycardic (Table 15-10).

Surgical Anatomy

Surgical anatomy of the abdominal cavity is described on p. 180.

Positioning

For abdominocentesis and diagnostic lavage the abdomen should be clipped and prepared aseptically. These procedures may be performed with the animal in lateral recumbency or standing.

TABLE 15-8

Inotropic Support of Hypotensive Animals

Dobutamine
2-10 μg/kg/min IV

Dopamine
2-10 μg/kg/min IV

TABLE 15-9

Selected Anesthetic Protocols for Use in Animals with Peritonitis That Are Debilitated or in Shock

Dogs
Induction

Oxymorphone (0.1 mg/kg IV) plus diazepam (0.2 mg/kg IV). Give in incremental dosages. Intubate if possible. If necessary, give etomidate (0.5-1.5 mg/kg IV). Alternately, if there is no vomiting, use mask induction or give thiopental or propofol at reduced doses.

Maintenance

Isoflurane

Cats
Premedication

Butorphanol (0.2-0.4 mg/kg SC or IM) or buprenorphine (5-15 μg/kg IM) or oxymorphone (0.05 mg/kg SC or IM)

Induction

Diazepam (0.2 mg/kg IV) followed by etomidate (0.5-1.5 mg/kg IV). Alternately, if there is no vomiting, use mask or chamber induction or give thiopental or propofol at reduced dosages. If there are no contraindications to ketamine, reduced dosages of diazepam and ketamine may also be used.

Maintenance

Isoflurane

TABLE 15-10

Anticholinergics

Atropine
0.02-0.04 mg/kg IV, SC, or IM

Glycopyrrolate
0.005-0.011 mg/kg IV, SC, or IM

SURGICAL TECHNIQUES
Abdominocentesis

Insert an 18- or 20-gauge, $1\frac{1}{2}$-inch plastic over-the-needle catheter (with added side holes) into the abdominal cavity at the most dependent part of the abdomen. Do not attach a syringe; instead allow the fluid to drip from the needle and collect in a sterile tube. If sufficient fluid is obtained, place the fluid in a clot tube and an ethylenediamine-tetraacetic acid (EDTA) tube, submit samples for aerobic and anaerobic culture, and make four to six smears for analysis. If fluid is not obtained, apply gentle suction using a 3-ml syringe. It is difficult to puncture bowel by this method because mobile loops of bowel move away from the tip of the needle as it strikes them. Perforations created by a needle this size usually heal without complications. The major disadvantage of needle paracentesis is that it is insensitive to the presence of the small volumes of intraperitoneal fluid and thus a negative result can be meaningless. At least 5 to 6 ml of fluid/kg body weight must be present in the abdominal cavity of dogs to obtain positive results in a majority of cases using this technique.

Diagnostic Peritoneal Lavage

Make a 2-cm skin incision just caudal to the umbilicus and ligate any bleeders to avoid false positive results. Spread loose subcutaneous tissues and make a small incision in the linea alba. Hold the edges of the incision with forceps while the peritoneal lavage catheter (Stylocath) (without the trocar) is inserted into the abdominal cavity (Fig. 15-13). Direct the catheter caudally into the pelvis. With the catheter in place, apply gentle suction. If blood or fluid cannot be aspirated, connect the catheter to a bottle of warm sterile saline and infuse 20 ml/kg of fluid into the abdominal cavity. When the calculated volume of fluid has been delivered, roll the patient gently from side to side, place the bottle on the floor, vent it, and collect the fluid by gravity drainage. Do not be surprised if you do not retrieve all of the fluid, particularly in dehydrated animals.

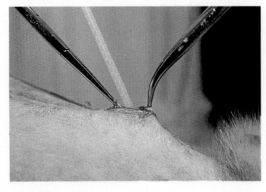

FIG. 15-13
Diagnostic peritoneal lavage.

Exploratory Laparotomy

Perform a ventral midline incision from the xiphoid process to the pubis (see pp. 180–181). Obtain a sample of fluid for culture and analysis. Explore and inspect the entire abdomen. Find the source of infection and correct it. Break down adhesions that may hinder drainage. Lavage the abdomen with copious amounts of warm sterile saline if the infection is generalized. Remove as much necrotic debris and fluid as possible. Close the abdomen routinely or perform open abdominal drainage.

Open Abdominal Drainage

After completing the abdominal procedure, leave a portion of the abdominal incision (usually the most dependent portion) open to drain. Generally, make the opening just large enough to allow a gloved hand to be inserted. Close the cranial and caudal aspects of the incision with monofilament suture using a continuous suture pattern. Place a sterile laparotomy pad over the opening, then place a sterile wrap over the laparotomy pad. Change the wrap at least twice daily initially with the animal standing; sedation is seldom necessary (use sterile bandage materials and wear sterile gloves). The volume of drainage dictates the number of wrap changes needed. Break down adhesions to the incision that may interfere with drainage. Abdominal lavage may be attempted but is seldom necessary. Place a diaper over the wrap to decrease contamination from urine. Assess the fluid daily for bacterial numbers and cell morphology. When bacterial numbers have decreased and normal neutrophil morphology is present (nondegenerative), close the incision (generally in 3 to 5 days). If the opening is small it may be left to heal by second intention.

SUTURE MATERIALS/SPECIAL INSTRUMENTS

Monofilament synthetic nonabsorbable (i.e., polypropylene or nylon) or slowly absorbable (i.e., polydioxanone or polyglyconate) suture should be used to close the abdomen in animals with peritonitis. Braided suture (i.e., dacron, silk, braided nylon) or suture that may be rapidly degraded (i.e., chromic gut) should not be used.

POSTOPERATIVE CARE AND ASSESSMENT

Fluid therapy should be continued postoperatively in most animals with peritonitis and is mandatory in those being managed with an open abdomen. Electrolytes, acid-base, and serum protein should be assessed in the postoperative period and corrected as necessary. Nasal oxygen may benefit animals that are septic. Assuring that patients with peritonitis have adequate caloric intake postoperatively is often difficult. The animal's energy requirement is much greater following injury or illness than at rest. Generally, the formula 30 $Wt_{kg}+70$ is used to calculate the resting animal's energy requirement. Postoperatively, the metabolic rate of dogs and cats increases 25% to 35% over resting levels. With mild trauma the increase in energy requirement is 35% to 50%, and with sepsis 50% to 70% more calories are required. The factor 1.5 has been used to estimate the energy requirement of ill or injured dogs and cats. Meeting these caloric requirements in dogs with intestinal disease is particularly difficult and may require enteral or parenteral nutritional support (see Chapter 11). If hypoproteinemia becomes severe, plasma transfusions should be considered.

PROGNOSIS

The prognosis for animals with generalized peritonitis is guarded; however, with proper and aggressive therapy, many survive. Some authors have suggested that the mortality rate is as high as 68% (Hosgood, Salisbury 1988). The mortality rates reported in animals with generalized peritonitis treated with open abdominal drainage have varied from 33% to 48%.

References

Hardie EM: Life-threatening bacterial infection, *Compend Contin Educ Pract Vet* 17:763, 1995.

Hardie EM, Rawlings CA, Collins LG: Canine *Escherichia coli* peritonitis: long term survival with fluid, gentamicin sulfate and flunixin meglumine treatment, *J Am Anim Hosp Assoc* 21:691, 1985.

Harvey HJ: Complications of small intestinal biopsy in hypoalbuminemic patients, *Vet Surg* 19:289, 1990.

Hosgood G, Salisbury SK: Generalized peritonitis in dogs: 50 cases (1975-1986), *J Am Vet Med Assoc* 193: 1488, 1988.

Suggested Reading

Crowe DT: Abdominocentesis and diagnostic peritoneal lavage in small animals, *Modern Veterinary Practice* 13:877, 1984.

Donner GS, Ellison GW: The use and misuse of abdominal drains in small animal surgery, *Comp Cont Educ Pract Vet* 10:705, 1986.

Hau T, Simmons RL: Heparin in the treatment of experimental peritonitis, *Ann Surg* 187:294, 1987.

Woolfson JM, Dulisch ML: Open abdominal drainage in the treatment of generalized peritonitis in 25 dogs and cats, *Vet Surg* 15:27, 1986.

CHAPTER 16

Surgery of the Digestive System

Surgery of the Oral Cavity and Oropharynx

GENERAL PRINCIPLES AND TECHNIQUES

DEFINITIONS

Maxillectomy is removal of a portion of the maxilla, while **mandibulectomy** is removal of a portion of the mandible. **Tonsillectomy** is excision of one or both tonsils. **Glossectomy** is excision of a portion of the tongue. **Cheiloplasty** is performed to alter the shape of the lip, generally to reduce drooling. **Mucoceles** are subcutaneous collections of saliva and/or mucus. **Ranulas** are collections of cystic fluid from the mandibular or sublingual salivary glands that occur beneath the tongue on either side of the frenulum.

PREOPERATIVE CONCERNS

Surgical diseases of the oral cavity and oropharynx are common in dogs and cats. They include congenital and traumatic abnormalities, foreign bodies, neoplasia, salivary gland disease, and dental disease. Patients with oral cavity or oropharyngeal disease may present for drooling, dysphagia, anorexia, bleeding from the mouth, and/or fetid breath. Some animals are asymptomatic until the lesions become large or are discovered on routine physical examination. Others present because of a mass, oral hemorrhage, oral pain, difficulty eating, nasal regurgitation, chronic rhinitis, and/or dyspnea. They may have a history of dental disease, weight loss, or trauma. Diagnosis is based on history, clinical signs, physical examination, cytology, radiographs, computed tomography (CT) scans, magnetic resonance imaging (MRI), and/or biopsy.

Before performing major surgery, a thorough physical examination, complete blood cell count (CBC), serum biochemical profile, and urinalysis should be performed; performing an electrocardiogram is optional. Animals undergoing maxillectomy or mandibulectomy and those predisposed to coagulopathies should have their coagulation system checked and blood cross-matching done before surgery. Doberman pinschers should be evaluated for the presence of von Willebrand's disease. Skull radiographs or CT scans can usually determine the extent of the lesion. Thoracic radiographs are indicated to evaluate for metastasis, cardiac size, and pulmonary disease. The teeth of animals with periodontal disease should be cleaned several days before major reconstructive surgery to improve tissue health and reduce oral bacterial numbers. Nutrition should be maintained by tube feeding if necessary (see Chapter 11). Animals with oronasal fistulae can be fed via feeding tubes to decrease rhinitis and inhalation pneumonia before surgery. Metabolic abnormalities should be corrected and mature animals fasted 12 to 18 hours (pediatric animals 4 to 8 hours) before anesthetic induction. After induction the mouth should be flushed with dilute betadine or chlorhexidine solution to reduce bacterial numbers.

ANESTHETIC CONSIDERATIONS

Oral cavity and oropharyngeal surgery can sometimes be hindered by an orally placed endotracheal tube. Therefore endotracheal intubation may be performed through a pharyngotomy or tracheotomy incision (see p. 209). It is important that the endotracheal tube and its cuff prevent blood and fluid from entering the lower airways. One or two gauze sponges can be placed in the oropharynx around the endotracheal tube to help absorb fluids. Postoperative swelling of oral mucous membranes can potentially obstruct the glottis; it can be minimized by corticosteroid pretreatment (e.g., dexamethasone, 1-2 mg/kg subcutaneously or intramuscularly before anesthetic induction or intravenously at induction). Most animals with oral disease are healthy and numerous anesthetic protocols can be used (Table 16-1). Blood and/or hypertonic saline should be available in the event that severe hemorrhage occurs. Placement of two cephalic catheters will allow simultaneous administration of blood and inotropes if necessary. Evaluation of arterial blood pressure during surgery is warranted, and ace-

TABLE 16-1

Selected Anesthetic Protocols for Use in Animals with Oral Disease

Premedication

Give atropine (0.02-0.04 mg/kg SC or IM) or glycopyrrolate (0.005-0.011 mg/kg SC or IM) plus oxymorphone* (0.05-0.1 mg/kg SC or IM) or butorphanol (0.2-0.4 mg/kg SC or IM), or buprenorphine (5-15 µg/kg IM)

Induction

Thiopental (10-12 mg/kg IV) or propofol (4-6 mg/kg IV) to effect or a combination of diazepam and ketamine (diazepam 0.27 mg/kg plus 5.5 mg/kg ketamine IV) titrated to effect

Maintenance

Isoflurane or halothane

*Use 0.05 mg/kg in cats.

TABLE 16-2

Prophylactic and Therapeutic Antibiotics for Oral Surgery

Cefazolin (Ancef, Kefzol)

20 mg/kg IV

Amoxicillin (Amoxi-Tabs, Amoxi-Drops, Amoxi-Inject)

22 mg/kg PO, IM or SC, BID to TID

Clindamycin (Antirobe)

11 mg/kg PO, BID

Metronidazole (Flagyl)

10 mg/kg PO, TID

TABLE 16-3

Principles of Oral Surgery

- Use atraumatic technique.
- Control hemorrhage using pressure and ligation.
- Avoid tension; make flaps 2 to 4 mm greater than the defect.
- Support flaps—do not suture over defects.
- Use appositional sutures (e.g., simple interrupted, simple continuous, cruciate, vertical mattress).

promazine should be avoided. Specific recommendations for anesthetizing animals with concurrent organ dysfunction (i.e., hepatic failure, renal failure) appear in the chapters discussing general techniques for the organ system of concern.

ANTIBIOTICS

The oral cavity and oropharynx are contaminated (aerobic, facultative, and anaerobic bacteria), but saliva is antimicrobial and the blood supply to this region is excellent; thus infections after oral surgery are rare. One dose of prophylactic antibiotic effective against gram-positive aerobes and anaerobes (e.g., amoxicillin) may be given at induction (Table 16-2). Therapeutic antibiotics (e.g., cefazolin plus metronidazole, or amoxicillin, or clindamycin; see Table 16-2) are indicated in debilitated and immunosuppressed patients and those with severe periodontal disease.

SURGICAL ANATOMY

The oral cavity is divided into the vestibule and oral cavity proper. The vestibule is the cavity lying outside the teeth and gums, but inside the lips and cheeks. The ducts of the parotid and zygomatic salivary glands open in the dorsocaudal part of the vestibule. The oral cavity proper is the area bounded by the hard palate and a small part of the soft palate dorsally, by the dental arches laterally and rostrally, and by the tongue and adjacent mucosa ventrally. The tongue is attached to the floor of the oral cavity by the lingual frenulum. The oropharynx extends from the level of the palatoglossal arches to the caudal border of the soft palate and base of the epiglottis. Dorsally the oropharynx is bounded by the soft palate and ventrally by the root of the tongue. The palatine tonsils are found in the lateral wall of the oropharynx.

The blood supply to this region originates from branches of the common carotid arteries. The paired major and minor palatine arteries are important (Fig. 16-1). Two or three vessels emerge from the major palatine foramen at the caudal edge of the fourth upper premolar and course rostrally, midway between the midline and dental arcade. The right and left major palatine arteries anastomose caudal to the incisors. The minor palatine arteries enter the palate caudal to the last molar and lateral to the major palatine artery, then course caudomedially to ramify in the caudal hard palate and soft palate. The major blood supply to the mandible is via the mandibular alveolar artery, which enters the mandibular canal on the medial surface of the mandible (see Fig. 16-1). The entry point is where an oblique line connecting the last molar tooth and angular (muscular) process (which is hidden beneath the pterygoid muscle) meet. The mandibular alveolar artery ends at the middle mental foramen where it branches to form the caudal, middle, and rostral mental arteries and exits via the mental foramina. The mandibular canal also transmits the mandibular vein and mandibular alveolar nerve.

☞ **NOTE** • The vascularity of the oral cavity promotes rapid healing and inhibits infection.

SURGICAL TECHNIQUES

Atraumatic surgical technique is important to reduce tissue damage and swelling and to encourage rapid healing (Table 16-3). Hemorrhage is expected and should be controlled with pressure and vessel ligation. Electrosurgery should be used sparingly because excessive use delays healing and may result in dehiscence. Electrocoagulation should be applied

FIG. 16-1
The major blood supply to the maxilla and mandible is via the major and minor palatine arteries and the mandibular alveolar artery respectively.

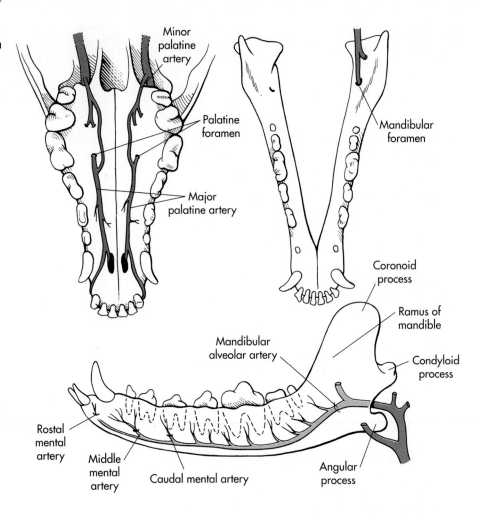

only to discrete, isolated areas. There is a potential to ignite flammable gases (i.e., oxygen) leaking around the endotracheal tube when electrosurgery or laser surgery is used.

Tension-free closure is imperative to prevent wound dehiscence and subsequent oronasal fistula. Flaps created during reconstructive procedures should be approximately 2 to 4 mm larger than the defect and major vessels entering these flaps must be preserved. Tension on these flaps should be minimized by adequate mobilization. Flaps should be manipulated with skin hooks or stay sutures to minimize trauma. Suture lines should be placed over connective tissue or bone, rather than the defect, to help support mucosal flaps. Cleanly incised edges of tissue should be apposed with a two-layer closure in an appositional suture pattern (simple interrupted, cruciate, or apposing vertical mattress). Monofilament suture material (i.e., 4-0 or 3-0 polydioxanone or polypropylene) minimizes wicking and tissue reaction. A temporary acrylic obturator can be cemented or wired to the teeth to protect healing tissues in the occasional case where tongue or pharyngeal muscle activity is apt to break down the suture line.

Biopsy Techniques

Impression smears or aspirates should be obtained from oral lesions before incisional or excisional biopsy. Cytology may allow a tentative diagnosis that is helpful in planning further diagnostics. When obtaining biopsies, areas of superficial necrosis should be avoided; deeper, viable tissues should be sampled. If the biopsy results do not correlate with the gross appearance of the mass, a second deeper and larger biopsy should be taken. An incisional biopsy using a needle or wedge biopsy technique should be performed if the definitive diagnosis will change the course of therapy. A Tru-Cut or Vim-Silverman needle can be used to obtain small cores from several areas of the mass, whereas wedge biopsies should be performed from nonnecrotic areas of the mass when larger pieces of tissue are needed. A loop or needle electrode of an electrosurgical unit is useful in obtaining oral biopsies. The specimen will be nondiagnostic if too much current is applied, especially to a small sample. Tissue coagulation can be prevented by keeping the power setting on the electrosurgical unit as low as possible. Diseased tissue is often friable and difficult to appose with sutures after a biopsy; however, pressure over the cut area is usually sufficient to control hemorrhage. If necessary, silver nitrate cautery can be used. An excisional biopsy (e.g., partial maxillectomy, mandibulectomy, tonsillectomy, glossectomy, or lip resection) should be performed and the area reconstructed if the definitive histologic diagnosis will not alter the course of therapy. All specimens should be submitted for histologic evaluation.

☞ **N O T E** · Submit all oral masses for histologic examination, regardless of whether they appear benign or not.

Temporary Carotid Artery Ligation

Some surgeons perform temporary carotid artery occlusion before maxillectomy to minimize blood loss. *To do so, place the animal in dorsal recumbency and prepare the ventral cervical area for surgery. Expose the trachea through a 5- to 8-cm ventral cervical midline incision. Palpate the carotid pulse and exteriorize the carotid sheath. Separate the common carotid artery from the vagosympathetic trunk and internal jugular vein. Temporarily occlude the carotid artery with a vascular clamp or tie. Repeat the procedure on the opposite carotid artery. Temporarily appose skin with a continuous suture pattern or staples during the maxillectomy procedure. After maxillectomy reopen the cervical wound and remove the vascular clamps or ties. Lavage the area thoroughly and appose the sternohyoid muscles, subcutaneous tissue, and skin in separate layers.* **This procedure may not be safe in cats.**

Partial Maxillectomy

The most common reason for maxillectomy is to resect an oral neoplasm (Fig. 16-2). Varying amounts of the maxilla and hard palate may be excised, depending on the gross and radiographic extent of the tumor or lesion (Fig. 16-3). Depending on the area being resected partial maxillectomies may be classified as hemimaxillectomies (rostral, central, or caudal) or premaxillectomies (bilateral rostral). Hemimaxillectomy, without a definition of site, usually refers to removal of one entire maxilla. Partial maxillectomy is limited by the surgeon's ability to reconstruct the oronasal defect; lesions that cross the midline of the palate are difficult to successfully reconstruct.

Clip and aseptically prepare the maxillary and nasal skin. Flush the mouth with antiseptic solution. Place the patient in dorsal recumbency for lesions of the premaxilla and open the mouth to its maximum extent by placing a mouth speculum or taping the mouth open. Place the patient in lateral or dorsal recumbency for lesions caudal to the premaxilla. Determine the extent of resection based on the size of the soft tissue lesion and radiographic degree of bony involvement. Generally, excise the mass and a minimum of 1 to 2 cm of normal soft tissue and bone on all borders (Fig. 16-4). Remove the mass en bloc by first making mucosal (buccal, gingival, and hard palate) incisions around the tissue to be resected. Avoid rectangular excision because

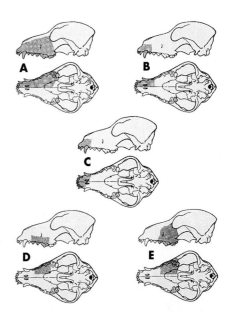

FIG. 16-3
Areas resected with partial maxillectomy techniques: **A,** hemimaxillectomy; **B,** rostral hemimaxillectomy; **C,** premaxillectomy (bilateral rostral hemimaxillectomy); **D,** central hemimaxillectomy; and **E,** caudal hemimaxillectomy. (From *Vet Surg* 15:17, 1986.)

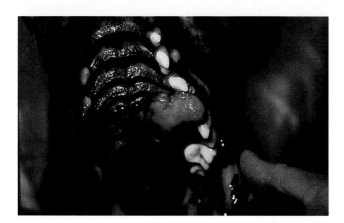

FIG. 16-2
An odontogenic tumor involving the maxillary dental arcade, palate, and maxilla.

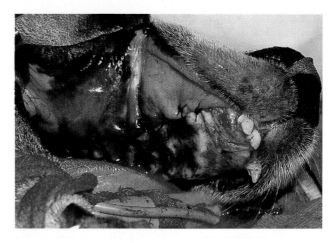

FIG. 16-4
Appearance of the oral cavity of a dog after a rostral hemimaxillectomy. A buccal flap has been advanced across the defect and secured with apposition sutures.

the corners are susceptible to dehiscence. Then using a periosteal elevator, undermine and reflect the gingival and palatal mucosa.

Use an oscillating saw or an osteotome and mallet to cut the maxilla, incisive bone, and/or palate. Resect all premolar and molar teeth for lesions extending to the third premolar because of the outward turn of the dental arch. When performing a caudal maxillectomy, remove a portion of the zygomatic arch and orbit if necessary to obtain clean borders. Elevate the tissue block and sever any remaining soft tissue attachments to complete the resection. The nasal cavity is exposed (Fig. 16-5). *Remove involved nasal turbinates with ronguers and hemostats if disease extends into the nasal cavity. Control hemorrhage by ligating identifiable vessels and applying pressure to other areas. Isolate and ligate the major palatine and infraorbital artery and vein if included in the resection site. Use bone wax or electrofulguration to help control bone hemorrhage.*

Lavage and inspect the defect to ensure all grossly diseased tissue has been excised. Close the defect by elevating a buccal mucosal flap from the adjacent cheek or lip (Fig. 16-6). Elevate enough buccal mucosa and submucosa to allow a tension-free approximation with the gingival and palatal mucosa. Place the first layer of simple interrupted sutures in the submucosa with the knot directed toward the nasal cavity. Place a second layer of interrupted approximating sutures (i.e., simple, cruciate, vertical) to accurately appose buccal mucosa to the palatal and gingival mucosa. A double-flap technique may be used to close premaxillectomy defects to provide mucosa on both the nasal and oral surfaces. However, an epithelial surface on the nasal aspect of the flap is not necessary because the connective tissue surface of the flap is covered with respiratory epithelium within 1 to 2 weeks. If carotid artery occlusion was performed, release the occlusion after the defect is closed.

☞ **N O T E** · Clipping and prepping the skin for maxillectomies is optional.

Partial Mandibulectomy

The most common reason for mandibulectomy is to resect an oral neoplasm. Occasionally mandibular fractures are also treated by partial mandibulectomy. Varying amounts of mandible may be excised depending on the extent of the tumor or lesion (Fig. 16-7). Depending on the extent of resection hemimandibulectomies may be classified as rostral, rostral-bilateral, central, caudal, or total (Fig. 16-8). These techniques may be combined when more extensive resection is necessary. Following mandibulectomy, cheiloplasty (commissuroplasty) may be performed to minimize excessive drooling and lateral protrusion of the tongue (Fig. 16-9). It is accomplished by removing the mucocutaneous junction of the upper and lower lip to the level of the second premolar or canine tooth. The commissure is advanced rostrally during

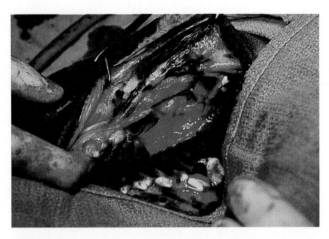

FIG. 16-5
A central hemimaxillectomy was used to remove the lesion shown in Fig. 16-2 and an additional 1 to 2 cm of normal tissue. Note that the nasal cavity is exposed.

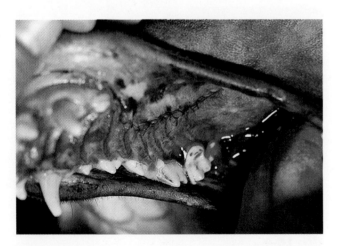

FIG. 16-6
A buccal mucosal flap was advanced over the defect evident in Fig. 16-5 and secured with approximating sutures.

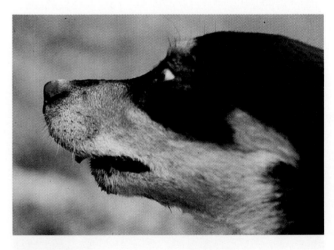

FIG. 16-7
Postoperative appearance after rostral mandibulectomy. Note that the tongue is barely apparent despite the short mandible.

closure. The upper and lower lip margins are apposed in three layers (oral mucosa, muscle and connective tissue, and skin) (Fig. 16-10). Opening the mouth fully during the first 2 weeks may cause dehiscence. Tension-relieving button sutures or a loose tape muzzle may be used to help prevent this. During rostral mandibulectomies, redundant skin and mucosa may be eliminated by excising and apposing V-shaped wedges. The base of the V is along the mucocutaneous junction (see Fig. 16-10).

Position the patient in lateral, sternal, or dorsal recumbency with the neck extended (Figs. 16-11, A and 16-12, A). Clip and aseptically prepare the skin of the lateral face and ventral mandible. Flush the mouth with antiseptic solution. Determine the amount to be resected based on size of the soft tissue lesion and radiographic degree of bony involvement. Generally, excise the mass and a minimum of 1 to 2 cm of normal soft tissue and bone on all borders. Retract the commissure and lip to give maximal exposure. If necessary, improve visualization by incising the commissure to the level of the mandibular angle (Fig. 16-12, B). Begin en bloc resection by first incising mucosa (buccal, gingival, and sublingual) around the diseased area (Figs. 16-11, B and 16-12, B). Using a periosteal elevator, undermine and reflect gingival mucosa to expose

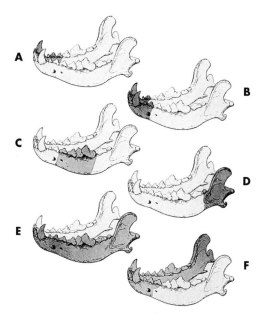

FIG. 16-8
Areas resected with partial mandibulectomy techniques: **A,** rostral hemimandibulectomy (unilateral rostral hemimandibulectomy); **B,** rostral mandibulectomy (bilateral rostral mandibulectomy); **C,** central hemimandibulectomy; **D,** caudal hemimandibulectomy; **E,** total hemimandibulectomy; and **F,** three quarter mandibulectomy. (From *J Am Anim Hosp Assoc* 24:287, 1988.)

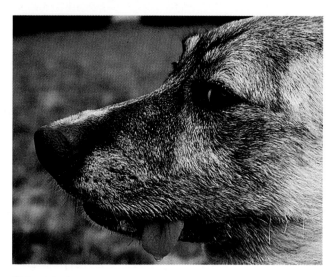

FIG. 16-9
Postoperative appearance after hemimandibulectomy in which a cheiloplasty was not performed. Although the tongue is moveable, it protrudes from the oral cavity.

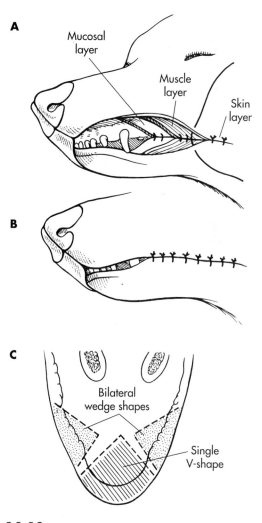

FIG. 16-10
To perform a cheiloplasty, **A,** excise lip margins to the level of the second premolar. **B,** Appose the incised lip margins in three layers (mucosa, muscle, skin). **C,** To improve cosmesis after rostral mandibulectomy, excise redundant skin from one or more of the indicated sites.

FIG. 16-11
For rostral mandibulectomy **A,** position the patient in dorsal recumbency. **B,** Incise mucosa 1 to 2 cm from the lesion, exposing the underlying muscles. Elevate the muscles. **C,** Appose the labial and sublingual mucosa following en bloc excision.

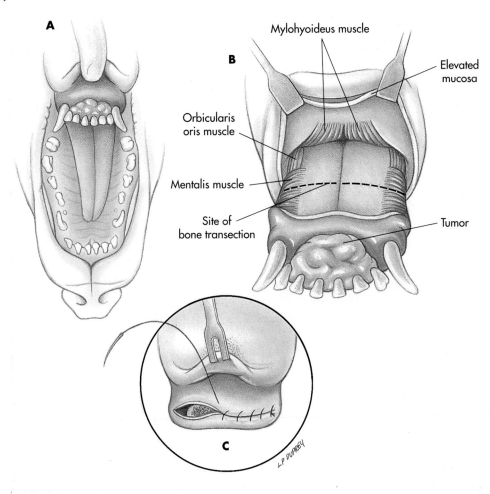

the lateral and ventral aspects of the ramus. Transect or elevate and retract muscles (mentalis, orbicularis oris, buccinator, mylohyoideus, geniohyoideus, genioglossus, masseter, digastricus, temporalis, and pterygoideus) attached to the portion of the mandible being resected (Figs. 16-11, B, 16-12, C, and 16-12, D). Use an oscillating saw or an osteotome and mallet to transect the ramus and separate the symphysis. Alternatively, use a Gigli wire to transect the ramus. Complete a total hemimandibulectomy by incising the joint capsule and disarticulating the temporomandibular joint (Fig. 16-12, C). Locate the temporomandibular joint by rotating the mandible and palpating the articulation. Ligate or cauterize the mandibular artery (see Fig. 16-12, D). Sever any remaining soft tissue attachments to complete the resection. Avoid traumatizing the lingual frenulum or sublingual and mandibular salivary ducts. Contour the ostectomy sites with bone rongeurs, removing sharp bone and tapering the edges to facilitate closure. Stabilizing the remaining mandible is not necessary. Close the defect by elevating a mucosal flap from the adjacent lip or cheek (Figs. 16-11, C and 16-12, E). Elevate enough mucosa and submucosa to allow a tension-free approximation with the gingival and sublingual mucosa. Place the first layer of simple interrupted sutures in the submucosa with the knots buried. Place a second layer of interrupted approximating sutures

(simple, cruciate, or vertical) to accurately appose the labial, sublingual, and gingival mucosa.

☞ **NOTE** • Alternatively, a single-layer simple continuous or interrupted closure may be used.

Tonsillectomy

When neoplasia of the palatine tonsils is suspected, they should be biopsied or removed. Squamous cell carcinoma and lymphosarcoma are the most common tumors of the tonsils. Enlarged tonsils are occasionally removed if they contribute to airway obstruction or dysphagia, and in cases of nonresponsive chronic tonsillitis.

Administer dexamethasone (1 to 2 mg/kg) at the time of induction to minimize postoperative swelling and edema. Position the animal in ventral recumbency with the maxilla suspended from an IV stand or similar device. Open the mouth maximally and secure it open with tape or gauze. Locate the tonsil in the tonsillar fossa or crypt on the dorsolateral wall of the oropharynx just caudal to the palatoglossal arch (Fig. 16-13). Retract the edge of the tonsillar crypt caudodorsally to expose the tonsil. Grasp the tonsil at its base with an Allis tissue forceps or hemostat and retract it from the crypt. Transect the hilar mucosa at the base of the

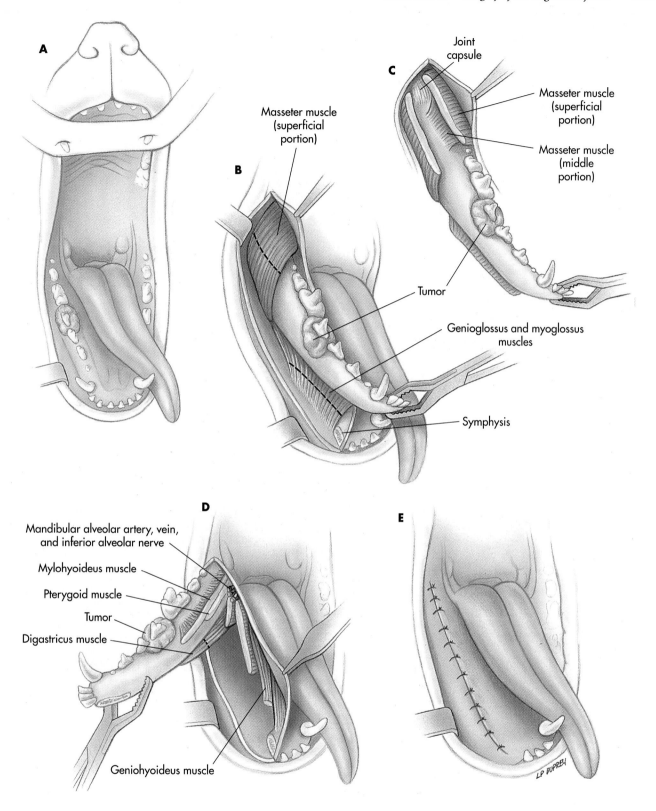

A

B

Masseter muscle
(superficial
portion)

C

Joint
capsule

Masseter muscle
(superficial
portion)

Masseter muscle
(middle
portion)

Tumor

Genioglossus and myoglossus
muscles

Symphysis

D

Mandibular alveolar artery, vein,
and inferior alveolar nerve

Mylohyoideus muscle

Pterygoid muscle

Tumor

Digastricus muscle

Geniohyoideus muscle

E

LP DUPREY

FIG. 16-12

For total hemimandibulectomy **A,** position the patient in ventral recumbency. **B,** Incise mucosa 1 to 2 cm from the lesion. Incise the commissure to allow better exposure of the caudal mandible. **C,** Separate the mandibular symphysis and identify the muscles. Dissect and transect the lateral mandibular muscles and expose the temporomandibular joint. **D,** Dissect and transect the medial muscles of the mandible and identify the mandibular artery entering the mandibular foramen. Ligate the mandibular vessels, disarticulate, and remove the mandible. **E,** Appose the buccal and sublingual mucosa with approximating sutures.

FIG. 16-13
A, The palatine tonsils are located in the dorsolateral pharynx. **B,** During tonsillectomy evert the tonsil from the crypt, begin transection along the base, and ligate tonsillar vessels. **C,** Close the crypt with a simple continuous pattern to help control hemorrhage.

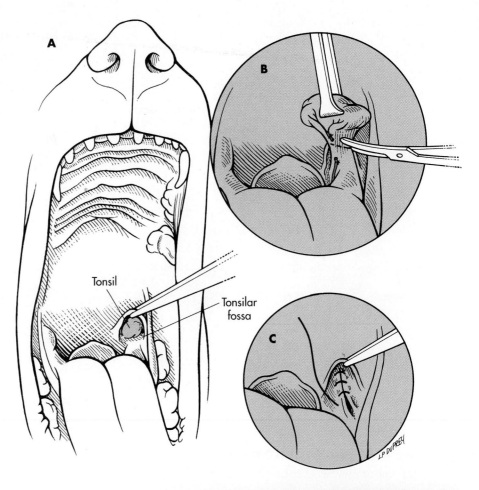

Tonsil

Tonsilar fossa

tonsil with Metzenbaum scissors or a tonsillectomy snare. Ligate the tonsillar artery as it enters the caudal aspect of the tonsil. (Some surgeons excise the tonsil using electrosurgery or laser surgery.) Appose the edges of the tonsillar crypt with a simple continuous suture pattern of 3-0 or 4-0 monofilament absorbable suture to minimize hemorrhage.

☞ **N O T E** · Submit the tonsil plus the regional lymph nodes for histologic examination.

Glossectomy

The primary reason for partial tongue amputation is neoplasia, which usually occurs on the margin or base of the tongue. The most common tongue tumor is squamous cell carcinoma (Fig. 16-14); others include malignant melanoma, granular cell myeloblastoma, and mast cell tumor. Amputation of 40% to 60% of the rostral tongue is usually well tolerated. Amputation at the base of the tongue makes eating and drinking difficult; however, intake can be accomplished by learning to suck in food and water or by tossing chunks of food to the base of the tongue. Most lacerations of the tongue are amenable to repair with a one- or two-layer closure rather than amputation. *When performing partial glossectomy, resect the diseased portion of tongue and a minimum of 2 cm of normal tissue after placing a noncrushing clamp across the base of the tongue. Wedge the*

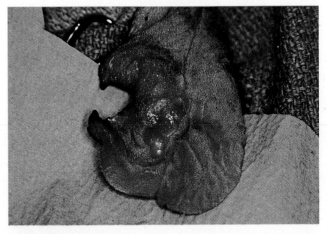

FIG. 16-14
Appearance of a tongue squamous cell carcinoma in a dog.

incision so slightly more tongue muscle than dorsal or ventral mucosa is excised. Control hemorrhage by ligation, pressure, or electrosurgery. Appose the epithelial edges with a simple continuous suture pattern using 3-0 or 4-0 monofilament absorbable suture (Fig. 16-15).

☞ **N O T E** · Dogs seem to adapt better than cats to tongue amputations.

Pharyngotomy

Pharyngotomy is performed to allow endotracheal intubation or tube feeding. *Position the patient in right lateral recumbency with the neck extended. Insert a gloved finger into the mouth and digitally identify the larynx and hyoid apparatus. Select a pharyngotomy site in the dorsal pharynx caudal to the epihyoid bone. Using the finger or a curved hemostat, tent the appropriate pharyngotomy site laterally (Fig. 16-16, A). Incise skin, platysma muscle, sphincter colli muscle, and pharyngeal mucosa at this site. Grasp the end of the tube with an orally placed hemostat and pull the tube into the oral cavity (Fig. 16-16, B). Direct the distal end of the tube into the trachea or the esophagus (Fig. 16-16, C). Secure the tube to the skin. After tube removal allow the pharyngotomy site to heal by second intention.*

Salivary Gland Excision

The most common reasons to remove salivary glands are to treat salivary mucoceles or neoplasia. The mandibular and sublingual salivary glands are most commonly removed as treatment for cervical, sublingual, and pharyngeal salivary mucoceles. Neoplasms (usually adenocarcinomas or carcinomas) occur most frequently in the parotid and mandibular salivary glands. Salivary gland excision is described on pp. 229 to 231.

HEALING OF THE ORAL CAVITY AND OROPHARYNX

Oral cavity and oropharyngeal mucosa heal more rapidly than skin because phagocytic activity (primarily monocytes rather than polymorphonuclear leukocytes) and epithelialization are greater and occur earlier in mucosa. Excellent mucosal blood supply, warmer temperatures, higher metabolic activity, and a higher mitotic rate contribute to rapid healing of mucosa. Apposed wounds reepithelialize within a few days, while defects heal by second intention.

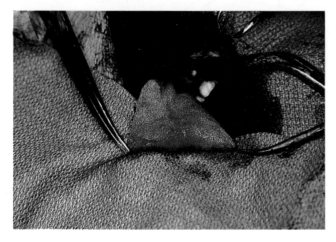

FIG. 16-15
Postoperative appearance of the tongue in Fig. 16-14 after partial glossectomy. The glossectomy was completed by apposing epithelial edges with a simple continuous suture pattern.

SUTURE MATERIALS/ SPECIAL INSTRUMENTS

Special instruments that may facilitate surgical procedures of the oral cavity include periosteal elevators, an oscillating saw or osteotome and mallet, Gigli wire, rongeurs or bone cutters, vascular bulldog clamps, vascular ties, tissue hooks, Metzenbaum scissors, noncrushing clamps (Doyen intestinal forceps), and Penrose drains. Although many suture materials may be used successfully in the oral cavity and oropharynx, 3-0 or 4-0 polydioxanone or polyglyconate (monofilament absorbable) and 3-0 or 4-0 polypropylene or nylon (monofilament nonabsorbable) are preferred.

POSTOPERATIVE CARE AND ASSESSMENT

After oral surgery gauze sponges should be removed from the caudal pharynx, and the nasopharynx should be suctioned. Extubation should be delayed until a well-developed swallowing reflex is present. Patients should be recovered in a slightly head down position and the tube removed with the cuff slightly inflated to encourage blood clots to be expelled through the mouth, rather than being aspirated or swallowed. These patients should be monitored for signs of airway obstruction or pain, and analgesics should be provided as needed (Table 16-4). Elizabethan collars or similar restraining devices should be used in some animals to prevent disruption of the surgical site. Occasionally an acrylic oral splint is used to protect the surgical site.

☞ **N O T E** • Remember to suction the oral cavity and oropharynx before extubation, extubate with the cuff partially inflated, and monitor for airway obstruction during recovery.

Oral intake should not be allowed for the first 8 to 12 hours after surgery (except in pediatric patients who are at risk for hypoglycemia); hydration should be maintained with intravenous fluids. Water should be offered after 12 hours and the animal observed for signs of dysphagia, pain, and/or regurgitation. If no serious problems are identified, soft food may be offered between 12 to 24 hours after surgery. Gruel is not necessary and may seep between sutures and inhibit healing. Feeding through a gastrostomy, pharyngostomy,

TABLE 16-4

Postoperative Analgesics after Digestive Surgery

Oxymorphone (Numorphan)
0.05-0.1 mg/kg IV or IM every 4 hours (as needed)

Butorphanol (Torbutrol, Torbugesic)
0.2-0.4 mg/kg IV, IM, or SC every 2 to 4 hours (as needed)

Buprenorphine (Buprenex)
5-15 μg/kg IV, IM every 6 hours (as needed)

FIG. 16-16
For placement of a pharyngostomy (feeding) tube **A,** make an incision caudal to the epihyoid bone in the dorsal pharynx. **B,** Push an orally placed forceps through the incision, grasp the tube, pull it into the mouth, and then direct it down the esophagus. **C,** Place esophageal tubes dorsal to the glottis to prevent airway obstruction or interference with epiglottic movement.

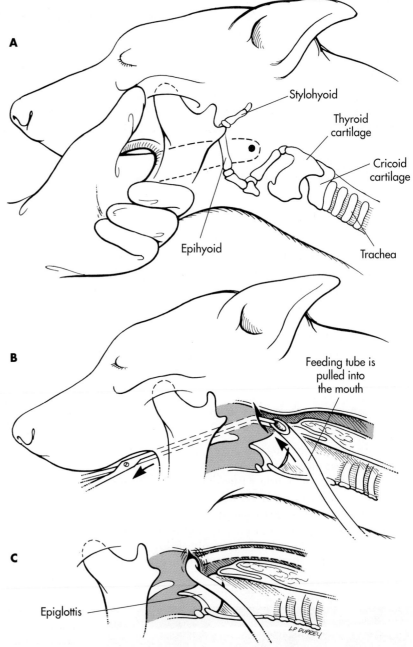

or esophagostomy tube is occasionally necessary for animals with severe wounds or those unwilling to eat within 3 days after surgery (see Chapter 11). Soft food should be fed until the wound is healed, and the animal should be prevented from chewing on sticks, toys, or other hard surfaces. Healing should be evaluated at 3 to 5 days, 2 weeks, and 4 weeks after surgery. Additional reconstruction may be necessary if areas of partial dehiscence do not heal by second intention or an oronasal fistula remains after 4 to 6 weeks. Animals with neoplasia should be evaluated every 3 to 6 months for signs of tumor recurrence.

After maxillectomy, epistaxis, serous to mucoid nasal discharge, and pain are expected. Crusting of the nares and epiphora may occur when the nasolacrimal duct is transected. Subcutaneous emphysema occasionally occurs when a large portion of the nasal cavity is exposed. Emphysema, crusting, and nasal discharge are short-term sequelae, usually resolving in days to weeks. Cosmesis is usually good with a slight facial concavity and lip elevation after lateral maxillectomy. Removal of a canine tooth results in more noticeable concavity. Premaxillectomies involving all incisors and one or both canine teeth result in ventral drooping of the nose and displacement of the maxillary lip caudal to the mandibular canine teeth. Extensive premaxillectomies (caudal to the first premolar) shorten the nose and may result in an obvious prognathic appearance (protrusion of the lower jaw).

☞ **NOTE** • Respiration may cause lateral deviation of the skin adjacent to the maxillectomy site for a few days. This resolves as fibrosis occurs.

Cosmesis and function after partial mandibulectomy are good (see Fig. 16-7). Mandibular "drift" and instability occur more often when the osteotomy is caudal to the second premolar. The remaining hemimandible may deviate medially, resulting in malocclusion, clicking of the teeth, and/or trauma to the palatal or gingival mucosa. Most animals adapt, and serious problems seldom occur. If erosion or ulceration develops, the involved canine tooth may be pulled or shortened. Rostral mandibulectomy (bilateral) caudal to the third or fourth premolar may cause difficulty with prehension and is less cosmetic. Tongue protrusion may occur, but most patients are able to keep the tongue retracted. Cheiloplasty may decrease drooling and lateral tongue protrusion in animals after partial maxillectomies.

☞ **NOTE** • Dogs do better with hemimandibulectomies than cats. Warn owners that some cats refuse to eat after this procedure.

COMPLICATIONS

Minor swelling of the skin and mucous membranes should be expected after partial maxillectomy or mandibulectomy but should resolve within 2 to 3 days. Infection is a potential complication because the oral cavity is contaminated. However, infection is rarely seen if the blood supply is maintained and good surgical technique is used. Partial dehiscence may occur 3 to 5 days after surgery if tissue is severely traumatized, blood supply is inadequate, or excessive motion or tension affects any area of the repair (Table 16-5). The most common postoperative complication after tonsillectomy is hemorrhage. Regrowth of tonsillar tissue may occur if excision is incomplete. After pharyngotomy complications of airway obstruction and aspiration pneumonia may be seen if the pharyngostomy tube is located cranial or ventral to the epihyoid bone.

SPECIAL AGE CONSIDERATIONS

Pediatric patients with congenital cleft palate should be fed with a tube until they are 8 to 12 weeks old and may be more safely anesthetized. Pediatric patients are at higher risk of hypothermia and hypoglycemia, thus they should not be

TABLE 16-5

Common Errors in Oral Surgery

- Failing to diagnose and treat before secondary problems develop
- Failing to accurately appose healthy tissue margins
- Causing dehiscence to occur by disrupting blood supply or applying excessive tension when suturing
- Failing to resect all diseased tissue

fasted for more than 4 to 8 hours. Neoplasia is more common in geriatric patients; before surgery they should be thoroughly evaluated for concurrent disease and evidence of metastasis.

Suggested Reading

Carpenter LG et al: Squamous cell carcinoma of the tongue in 10 dogs, *J Am Anim Hosp Assoc* 29:17, 1993.

Salisbury SK: Problems and complications associated with maxillectomy, mandibulectomy and oronasal fistula repair, *Problems in Veterinary Medicine: Head & Neck Surgery* 3:53, 1991.

Salisbury SK, Lantz GC: Long-term results of partial mandibulectomy for treatment of oral tumors in 30 dogs, *J Am Anim Hosp Assoc* 24:285, 1988.

Salisbury SK, Richardson DC, Lantz GC: Partial maxillectomy and premaxillectomy in the treatment of oral neoplasia in the dog and cat, *Vet Surg* 15:16, 1986.

Smith MM: Surgery of the canine salivary system, *Compend Contin Educ Pract Vet* 7:457, 1985.

Withrow SJ, Holmberg DL: Mandibulectomy in the treatment of oral cancer, *J Am Anim Hosp Assoc* 19:273, 1983.

SPECIFIC DISEASES

CONGENITAL ORONASAL FISTULA (CLEFT PALATE)

DEFINITIONS

A **congenital oronasal fistula** is an abnormal communication between the oral and nasal cavities involving the soft palate, hard palate, premaxilla, and/or lip. The **primary palate** consists of the lip and premaxilla. Incomplete closure of the primary palate is a **primary cleft** or **cleft lip (harelip).** The **secondary palate** consists of the hard and soft palates. Incomplete closure of either of these structures is a **secondary cleft** or **cleft palate.**

SYNONYMS

Cleft palate, secondary cleft, cleft lip, harelip, primary cleft, cheiloalveoloschisis, lateral cleft of the soft palate

GENERAL CONSIDERATIONS AND CLINICALLY RELEVANT PATHOPHYSIOLOGY

Congenital palatal defects result when the two palatine shelves fail to fuse during fetal development (Fig. 16-17). The most critical time for development and closure of the fetal palate appears to be 25 to 28 days of gestation in dogs. Incomplete closure of either the primary or secondary palate is attributed to inherited (recessive or irregular dominant, polygenic traits), nutritional, hormonal (steroids), mechanical (in utero trauma), and toxic (including viral) factors. Primary cleft palate alone is rare; however, secondary cleft palate may occur alone or in combination with primary clefts. Some affected neonates are unable to nurse effectively

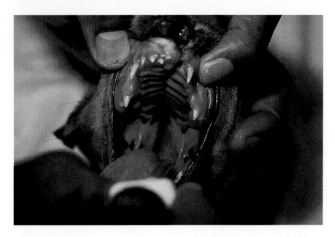

FIG. 16-17
A puppy with a cleft extending through the primary and secondary palate.

and die soon after birth. Others contaminate their nasal cavity with saliva and food. Signs of rhinitis and other respiratory infections are common.

DIAGNOSIS
Clinical Presentation

Signalment. Dogs, particularly brachycephalic breeds, are more commonly affected with cleft palate than cats. Purebred dogs have a higher incidence than mixed breeds. Breeds at high risk for cleft palate include Boston terrier, Pekingese, bulldog, miniature schnauzer, beagle, cocker spaniel, and dachshund. Siamese cats have a higher incidence than other cat breeds. The cleft is present at birth, although it is not always recognized immediately.

History. A history of difficulty nursing, nasal regurgitation, nasal discharge, and failure to thrive are common problems. Signs related to incomplete separation of the oral and nasal cavity include drainage of milk from the nares during or after nursing; gagging, coughing, and/or sneezing while eating; poor growth; and respiratory infection (i.e., rhinitis, aspiration pneumonia).

Physical Examination Findings

All puppies and kittens should be checked on initial presentation for evidence of a cleft palate. Diagnosis of congenital oronasal fistula is made by visual examination. Incomplete closure of the lip is easily recognized when the patient is first examined; however, a thorough oral exam is required to identify incomplete closure of the premaxilla, hard palate, and/or soft palate. Anesthesia may be necessary to thoroughly assess the soft palate. A secondary cleft may occur without a primary cleft. Patients may be thin and stunted. Abnormal respiratory sounds are auscultated if aspiration pneumonia is present. Affected neonates should be carefully evaluated for concurrent congenital anomalies.

☞ **N O T E** · Always evaluate animals with cleft palates for other congenital anomalies.

TABLE 16-6
Antibiotic Treatment of Aspiration Pneumonia

Chloramphenicol (Chloromycetin)
Dogs—50 mg/kg PO, TID to QID
Cats—50 mg/kg PO, BID

Trimethoprim-sulfadiazine (Tribrissen)
Dogs—15 mg/kg PO or IM, BID
Cats—15 mg/kg PO, BID

Ampicillin
22 mg/kg PO, IV, IM, or SC, TID to QID

Clindamycin (Antirobe, Cleocin)
11 mg/kg PO or IV, BID

Radiography/Ultrasonography

Radiographic examination of the skull is not necessary; however, thoracic radiographs are useful in evaluating for aspiration pneumonia.

Laboratory Findings

Laboratory abnormalities are not present unless the animal has aspiration pneumonia or is cachectic.

DIFFERENTIAL DIAGNOSIS

Traumatic or acquired clefts, rhinitis, nasal foreign body, and aspiration pneumonia are potential differential or concurrent diagnoses.

MEDICAL MANAGEMENT

Affected patients should be tube fed to maintain an adequate nutritional status and to decrease the incidence of aspiration pneumonia until they are old enough for surgery. Aspiration pneumonia may be treated with antibiotics, fluids, oxygen, bronchodilators, and/or expectorants. Use of corticosteroids is controversial for acute aspiration and of no benefit for chronic aspiration. A tracheal wash with culture and sensitivity should be performed if aspiration pneumonia is severe. Broad-spectrum antibiotics with efficacy against anaerobes (Table 16-6) are indicated for severe aspiration or purulent rhinitis. Animals with severe rhinitis may benefit from having the nasal infection treated before surgical closure of the defect. With the animal under general anesthesia, cultures should be obtained from the nasal cavity, and the nose and oral cavity should be flushed of debris and exudate. To prevent recontamination of the nasal cavity with food, the animal should be given nothing per os for 10 to 14 days. Nutrition can be provided via tube feeding (e.g., tube gastrostomy; see p. 74) during this time.

SURGICAL TREATMENT

Most animals with defects of the primary and secondary palate are euthanized or die. Surgical treatment is generally delayed until the patient is at least 8 to 12 weeks of age in order to allow growth and easier access to the palate. Older patients seem to have less friable tissue that holds suture better. Rarely, repairing clefts before 25 weeks results in a narrower maxilla and occlusal problems. The primary goal of repairing a cleft palate is to reconstruct the nasal floor. Multiple procedures may be necessary before the entire cleft is permanently reconstructed. Affected patients should be neutered because this is considered to be a hereditary defect.

Preoperative Management

Pediatric patients should not be fasted more than 4 to 8 hours. After anesthetic induction, oral intubation, and cuff inflation, the nasal and oral cavities should be flushed with saline and a dilute antiseptic solution. If the animal is not on antibiotics, perioperative antibiotics may be given intravenously at induction. Feed poorly nourished animals through a gastrostomy or esophagostomy tube for several days before surgery.

Anesthesia

After 8 weeks of age puppies and kittens are better able to metabolize drugs and are better anesthetic risks. Special precautions should be taken to prevent hypothermia and hypoglycemia in young patients. Intubation through a pharyngotomy (see p. 209) or tracheotomy incision (see p. 613) may facilitate repair of secondary clefts. The former is generally preferred if it will allow adequate visualization of the defect. General anesthetic recommendations for animals undergoing oral surgery are provided on p. 200. Guarded tracheostomy tubes should be used to prevent kinking during the procedure. Care should be taken to prevent and recognize dislodgement of the anesthetic tubing from the endotracheal tube during oral manipulations.

Surgical Anatomy

The major palatine arteries emerge from the major palatine foramen midway between the midline and caudal edge of the upper fourth premolar (see Fig. 16-1). The main artery courses rostrally equidistant between the lingual border of the teeth and palatal midline to anastomose with the major palatine artery of the contralateral side caudal to the incisors. The minor palatine arteries enter the palate at the level of the last molar, caudal and slightly lateral to the major palatine foramen. The minor palatine arteries course caudomedially and ramify in the caudal hard palate and soft palate. The soft palate is also supplied by branches of the ascending pharyngeal artery.

Positioning

Animals should be positioned in dorsal recumbency with the mouth maximally opened to facilitate repair of a secondary palate. They may be positioned in ventral or dorsal recumbency to repair a primary palate.

SURGICAL TECHNIQUE

The first step in the repair of combined primary and secondary clefts is to separate the oral and nasal cavities by reconstructing the nasal floor. Following successful separation

the lip defect is reconstructed. Areas where flaps were harvested for closure of primary or secondary clefts are allowed to heal by second intention. Granulation and epithelialization are usually complete within 2 to 3 weeks.

Closure of Hard Palate Defects

The two most frequently used procedures to repair secondary clefts are sliding bipedicle flaps and overlapping flap techniques. Sliding bipedicle flaps are created to close hard palate defects. The disadvantage of this technique is that the repair is unsupported and directly over the defect. *Incise the margins of the defect and make bilateral releasing incisions along the margins of the dental arcade (Fig. 16-18, A). Elevate the mucoperiosteal layer on both sides of the defect with a periosteal elevator (Fig. 16-18, B). Avoid damaging the major palatine arteries. Control hemorrhage with pressure and suction. Appose the nasal mucosal edges or periosteum at the margin of the defect with buried interrupted sutures (knots within the nasal cavity), if possible. Slide the elevated mucoperiosteal flaps across the defect and appose with simple interrupted sutures (Fig. 16-18, C and D). Allow the denuded hard palate near the dental arcades to heal by second intention.*

An alternate technique for repair of hard palate defects is the overlapping "sandwich" technique (Figs. 16-19 and 16-20). This technique is advantageous because it does not place the repair over the palate defect. *Incise one margin of the defect separating the oral and nasal mucosa (see Fig. 16-20, A). Elevate the mucoperiosteum at this edge approximately 5 mm. At the opposite side of the defect create a mucoperiosteal rotational flap large enough to cover the defect with its base hinged at the margin of the palatal defect (see Fig. 16-20, B). Begin the incision near and parallel to the dental arcade creating a flap 2 to 4 mm larger than the defect. Make perpendicular incisions at the rostral and caudal end of the incision extending to the cleft. Elevate this mucoperiosteal flap being careful not to disrupt the margin of the defect (see Fig. 16-20, B). Dissect carefully around the palatine artery to release it from fibrous tissue. Rotate the flap across the defect (see Fig. 16-20, C). Place the edge of the flap under the mucoperiosteal flap on the opposite side. Preplace and then tie a series of horizontal mattress sutures to secure the flaps in position (see Fig. 16-20, D).*

☞ **N O T E** • Warn owners that multiple surgeries may be needed to completely close large, hard palate defects.

Closure of Soft Palate Defects

Close soft palate clefts by first incising the margins of the cleft to separate the oral and nasal mucosa. Continue incisions made in the margins of hard palate clefts caudally into the soft palate (see Fig. 16-20, D). Isolate the nasal mucosa, palatal muscles, and oral mucosa. Appose the palatal edges in three layers beginning caudally and working rostrally to a point adjacent to the caudal or midpoint of the

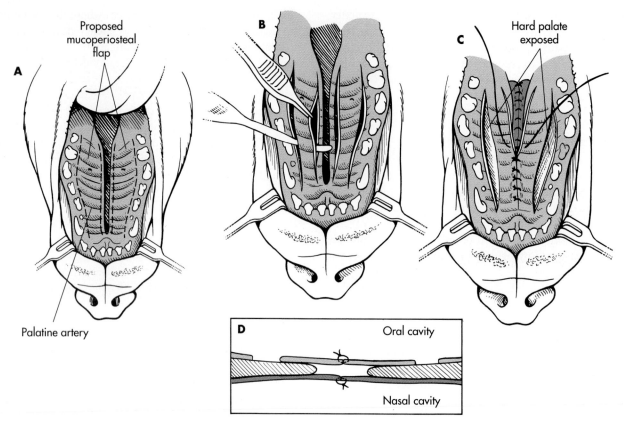

FIG. 16-18
A sliding bipedicle flap repair may be used to repair a congenital oronasal fistula. **A,** The dotted lines represent the mucoperiosteal incisions necessary to create two sliding flaps. **B,** Mucoperiosteum is elevated from the hard palate with the major palatine artery. **C,** Nasal mucosa and mucoperiosteum are apposed in two layers over the defect in the hard palate. **D,** Cross-sectional view of the repair.

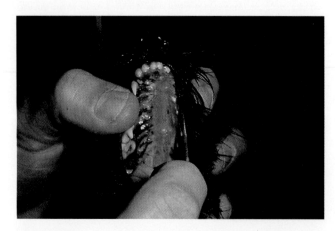

FIG. 16-19
The secondary palate of the puppy in Fig. 16-17 was repaired with an overlapping flap technique. The defect over the hard palate was allowed to heal by second intention.

tonsil. First appose the nasal mucosa using a series of simple interrupted sutures with nasally oriented knots or use a simple continuous pattern. Then appose the palatal muscle and connective tissue mucosa with a simple continuous su-

ture pattern. Lastly, appose the oral mucosa with a simple continuous or interrupted suture pattern. Make tension-relieving incisions in the oral mucosa from the lingual aspect of the last molar to near the tip of the soft palate. An overlapping flap technique, rotational flaps from the hard or soft palate, or nasopharyngeal mucosal flaps can also be used to repair soft palate defects.

☞ **NOTE ·** Some surgeons fracture the pterygoid hamulus (where the palatal muscles attach) with an osteotome to decrease tension on the soft palate.

Closure of Primary Clefts

Cosmetic repair of primary clefts can be very complicated, requiring elaborate planning to achieve a successful outcome (Fig. 16-21, *A*). *Create a mucosal flap to separate the nasal from the oral cavity (Fig. 16-21, B). If the cleft extends into the premaxilla, evaluate the position of the deciduous incisors and pull them if necessary. Suture the buccal or gingival mucosal flap to the nasal mucosa. Use a free hand modified Z-plasty for reconstruction of the lip defect (Fig. 16-21, C). Close the lip defect so the distance from the ven-*

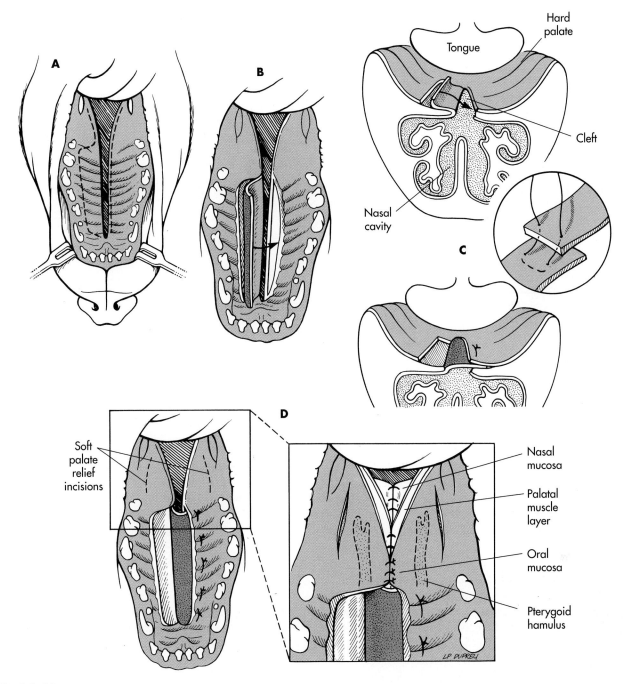

FIG. 16-20
Repair of a congenital oronasal fistula may be done using an overlapping flap technique.
A, The dotted lines represent the incisions necessary to allow soft tissue closure. **B,** Elevate the mucoperiosteal flap and rotate it medially to cover the hard palate defect. **C,** Insert the edge of this flap between the hard palate and the mucoperiosteum on the opposite side of the defect. Secure the flaps in position with horizontal mattress sutures. **D,** Complete the repair by apposing the incised edges of the cleft soft palate in three layers. Make lateral relief incisions to reduce tension on the repair.

tral nostril to the free ventral edge of the lip is the same on both sides. Make multiple small flaps if necessary for a cosmetic closure. Place a layer of sutures in the fibromuscular layer (orbicularis oris muscle and connective tissue) before skin closure.

POSTOPERATIVE CARE AND ASSESSMENT

Soft food should be fed for a minimum of 2 weeks after surgery, and chewing on hard objects (e.g., bones, sticks, chew toys) should be prevented. Gastrostomy or esophagostomy

FIG. 16-21

A, Schematic drawing of a repair of a primary cleft palate involving the lip, premaxilla, and nostril. **B,** First create a flap from the nasal wall and suture it to a labial mucosal flap to separate the nasal and oral cavity. **C,** Repair the cleft lip with one or a series of Z-plasties: (1) Make incisions from *A* to *B* and *a* to *c*. (2) Place a suture between *A* and *a* and *B* and *b* to transpose the flaps. (3) Place additional sutures as needed.

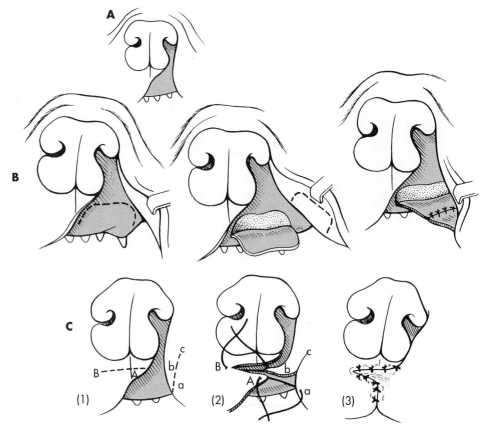

feeding for 7 to 14 days may facilitate healing. Reevaluation at 2 weeks may require anesthesia to identify small defects.

COMPLICATIONS

Dehiscence and subsequent incomplete healing of oronasal fistulae are the most common complications. Dehiscence usually occurs within 3 to 5 days of surgery but may occur later. Early dehiscence may occur if tension is excessive, blood supply is poor, or the tissue is traumatized. Motion of the tongue against the repair and particulate matter in the surgical site can also lead to dehiscence. Early dehiscence of the lip occurs if the orbicularis oris muscle has not been apposed. Contraction of the unapposed muscle during lip movement causes excess tension on the suture line. Tissues are friable after dehiscence; thus repair of early dehiscence should be delayed for 4 to 6 weeks to allow tissues to revascularize and regain strength. Late dehiscence is a result of growth-induced stress on the repair and is best treated after the patient matures.

PROGNOSIS

The prognosis is good for animals with successful cleft palate repair; however, multiple surgeries may be required. Chronic rhinitis and aspiration pneumonia persist if large defects are not repaired. Untreated patients with small clefts may have few clinical signs.

References

Kirby BM: Oral flaps: principles, problems, and complications of flaps for reconstruction of the oral cavity, *Problems in Veterinary Medicine: Reconstructive Surgery* 2:494, 1990.

Waldron DR, Martin RA: Cleft palate repair, *Problems in Veterinary Medicine: Head & Neck Surgery* 3:142, 1991.

Wijdeveld MGMM et al: Maxillary arch dimensions after palatal surgery at different ages in beagles, *J Dent Res* 68:1105, 1989.

ACQUIRED ORONASAL FISTULAE

DEFINITIONS

Acquired oronasal fistulae are abnormal communications between the nasal and oral cavity caused by trauma or disease.

SYNONYMS

Traumatic cleft palate, palatal defect

GENERAL CONSIDERATIONS AND CLINICALLY RELEVANT PATHOPHYSIOLOGY

Acquired palatal defects are most frequently caused by dental disease (Fig. 16-22). An oronasal fistula results when a deep maxillary periodontal pocket progresses to the apex of the tooth, lysing bone between the apex of the alveolus and the nasal cavity or maxillary sinus. They may also result from trauma (i.e., bite wounds, gunshot wounds, blunt trauma to the head, electrical burns) or be a complication of surgery (e.g., mass excision or ventral rhinotomy), radiation, or hyperthermic treatment of oral lesions. Foreign bodies lodged between the dental arcades may cause pressure necrosis of the hard palate and subsequent oronasal fistula (Fig. 16-23).

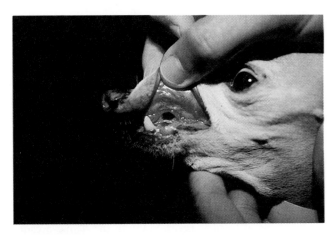

FIG. 16-22
An oronasal fistula that occurred from loss of the canine tooth.

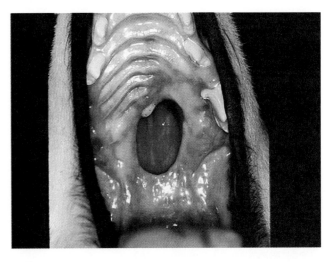

FIG. 16-23
An acquired oronasal fistula caused by a foreign body that lodged between the dental arcades.

Ingested food that passes through the fistula into the nasal cavity may be expelled from the nostril by sneezing. Chronic rhinitis is common.

DIAGNOSIS
Clinical Presentation

Signalment. Any breed or sex may acquire an oronasal fistula. Oronasal fistulae secondary to dental disease or tumors are seen more often in middle-aged to older animals. Oronasal fistulae secondary to trauma may occur at any age.

History. Oronasal fistula should be suspected in patients with chronic rhinitis and a history of dental disease, trauma, or previously treated oral tumors. Common clinical signs are sneezing and chronic unilateral serous or mucopurulent nasal discharge.

Physical Examination Findings

Diagnosis can be made by identifying an abnormal communication between the oral and nasal cavities (see Figs. 16-22 and 16-23). Small fistulae associated with periodontal disease are not easily identified unless the area around the involved tooth is explored with a narrow dental probe. If passing the probe into the gingival pocket causes epistaxis, a fistula is present. The palatal aspect of the maxillary canine tooth is a common site for an oronasal fistula. Anesthesia is generally required to probe periodontal pockets.

Radiography/Ultrasonography

Skull radiographs may identify underlying causes of fistulae, such as periapical abscesses, advanced periodontal disease, maxillary neoplasia (see p. 222), or broken and retained tooth roots. Lysis around tooth roots is indicative of periapical abscesses.

Laboratory Findings

Inflammatory changes on a complete blood cell count (CBC) may be secondary to rhinitis or aspiration pneumonia.

DIFFERENTIAL DIAGNOSIS

Differential diagnoses include any disease that causes chronic rhinitis (e.g., fungal disease, foreign body, congenital oronasal fistula, invasive oral neoplasia). These conditions can generally be differentiated based on physical examination and/or histopathology. Histopathology should be performed to distinguish fistulae secondary to neoplasia from those associated with infection or trauma.

☞ **N O T E** • Always biopsy to rule out neoplasia.

MEDICAL MANAGEMENT

Broad-spectrum antibiotics effective against anaerobes (i.e., chloramphenicol, trimethoprim-sulfadiazine, ampicillin, clindamycin) should be given if severe purulent rhinitis is present in a patient (see Table 16-6). Such animals may benefit from having the nasal infection treated before closure of the defect. With the patient under general anesthesia, cultures should be obtained from the nasal cavity, and the nose and oral cavity should be flushed of debris and exudate. To prevent recontamination of the nasal cavity with food, the animal should be given nothing per os for 10 to 14 days. Nutrition can be provided via tube feeding (e.g., tube gastrostomy; see p. 74) during this time.

SURGICAL TREATMENT

Most oronasal fistulae require surgical reconstruction, although small or traumatic fistulae occasionally heal spontaneously. A variety of surgical techniques have been described for repair, including simple suturing of the fistula edges, mucosal flaps, mucoperiosteal flaps, double reposition flaps, and two-staged tongue flaps. Successful repair of oronasal fistulae requires a well-supported, airtight, tension-free closure. Flap techniques are more successful than direct apposition of the fistula edges because there is less tension and increased support for the repair. Teeth involved in the fistula should be extracted several weeks before reconstruction of the defect. Central lesions may require that normal teeth be extracted to allow creation of adequate mucosal flaps. If the fistula is of dental origin it may be necessary to perform a limited maxillectomy (at least 5 mm from each margin), to remove necrotic or diseased bone. Traumatic oronasal fistulae may require stabilization of the maxilla and hard palate with small pins or wire. Interdental wiring (see p. 769) using the carnassial teeth and/or the canine teeth can be used to help bring bone edges into apposition. Areas where flaps were harvested heal by second intention in 2 to 3 weeks. Use of acrylic, Silastic, or metal obturators fitted over the defect has also been described (Lantz, 1984).

Preoperative Management

Pediatric patients should not be fasted for longer than 4 to 8 hours. After anesthetic induction the nasal and oral cavities should be flushed with saline-diluted antiseptic solution. Aggressive management of rhinitis (see Medical Management on p. 217) may decrease infection and improve suture holding capability of tissues.

Anesthesia

General anesthetic recommendations for animals undergoing oral surgery are provided on p. 200. Intubation through a pharyngotomy (see p. 209) or tracheotomy incision (see p.

613) may facilitate repair of large or centrally located oronasal fistulae. The former is generally preferred if it will allow adequate visualization of the defect. Guarded tracheostomy tubes should be used to prevent kinking during the procedure. Care should be taken to prevent and recognize dislodgement of the anesthetic tubing from the endotracheal tube during oral manipulations.

Surgical Anatomy

Surgical anatomy of the hard palate is discussed on p. 201.

Positioning

The patient should be positioned in lateral recumbency to repair oronasal fistulae associated with the dental arcade. Dorsal recumbency with the mouth opened maximally facilitates repair of more centrally located fistulae involving the secondary palate.

SURGICAL TECHNIQUE
Direct Apposition

Direct apposition of the fistula should be performed only if the fistula is very small. *Debride the fistula to healthy, bleeding mucosal edges (Figs.16-24, A and B). Incise or debride the margin of the fistula and elevate the edges enough to allow approximation without excess tension. Appose mucosa with interrupted appositional sutures (i.e., simple, cruciate, or vertical mattress) (Fig.16-24, C).*

FIG. 16-24
Small fistulae may be repaired using a direct appositional technique. **A,** Incise mucosa around the fistula, **B,** elevate the gingival flaps, and debride the edges of the fistula. **C,** Appose mucosa over the defect.

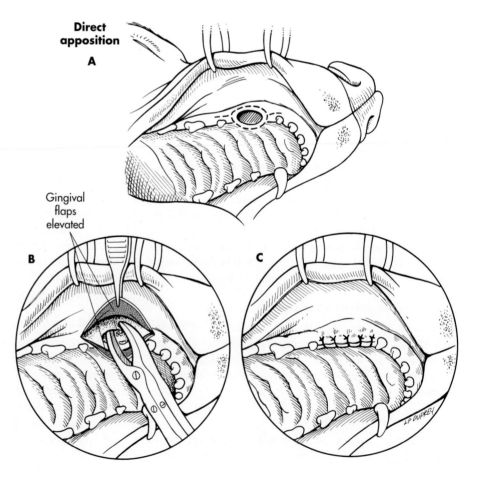

Direct apposition
A

Gingival flaps elevated

B

C

Single-Layer Flap Repair

Debride the epithelial margin of the fistula (Fig. 16-25, A). Incise the gingival and buccal mucosa to outline a flap 2 to 4 mm larger than the debrided fistula (Fig. 16-25, B). Make these incisions perpendicular to the dental arcade. Elevate the gingival mucosa with a periosteal elevator. Then undermine the buccal mucosa until the flap can be advanced across the defect without tension (Fig. 16-25,

C). Using a rongeur, remove infected alveolar and maxillary bone. Expose approximately 1 to 2 mm of the hard palate at the medial aspect of the fistula by excising 1 to 2 mm of mucoperiosteum. Lavage the surgical site with saline. Suture the gingival-buccal flap to the mucoperiosteum of the hard palate using interrupted approximating (i.e., simple, cruciate, or vertical mattress) monofilament, absorbable sutures.

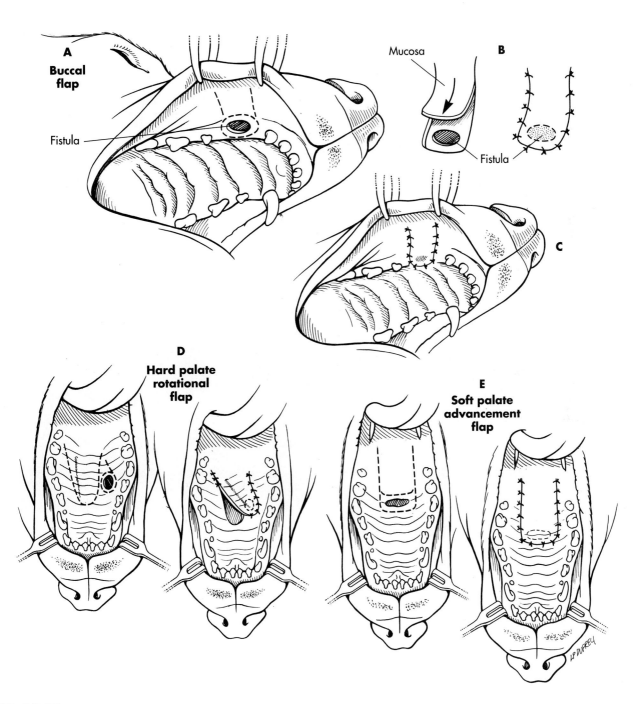

FIG. 16-25
For a single flap technique for fistula repair, **A,** debride the fistula **B** and **C,** and advance a buccal flap over the defect. **D,** Create a hard palate rotational flap by debriding the fistula and rotating a mucoperiosteal hard palate flap over the defect. **E,** To repair lesions at the junction of the hard and soft palate, debride and close the defect with a soft palate advancement flap.

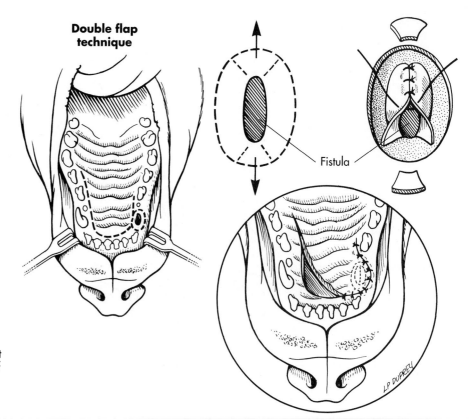

FIG. 16-26
A double-layer flap technique may be performed using tissue surrounding the fistula and a flap from the mucoperiosteum of the hard palate. Create the first flap by rotating the gingival margins of the fistula medially and apposing with sutures. Cover this flap with a rotational mucoperiosteal hard palate flap.

Rotational Flap Repair

A rotational or advancement flap may be created from the hard palate or soft palate (Figs. 16-25, *D* and *E*), or an overlapping technique similar to that described for repair of congenital oronasal fistulae (see p. 213) may be used. *Do not debride the palatal epithelial margin during debridement of the fistula because this edge serves as the base of the mucoperiosteal flap and must remain continuous with the nasal mucosa to be effective. Create a flap in the mucoperiosteum 2 to 4 mm larger than the debrided fistula (Figs. 16-26 and 16-27). Elevate the flap without disrupting the palatal margin of the fistula. Fold the flap over the defect and suture it to the gingival mucosa with interrupted, approximating, monofilament, absorbable sutures.* Granulation tissue fills the defect over the hard palate and the area reepithelializes within a few weeks.

Double-Flap Repair

Double-flap techniques may be used with large dental fistulae and fistulae located in more central areas of the palate. Double-flap techniques provide a mucosal surface on both the oral and nasal sides of the fistula. If buccal flaps are planned to close large central defects, teeth extraction may be necessary. The extraction sites should be allowed to heal before reconstruction. *Create one or two mucoperiosteal flaps, 2 to 4 mm larger than the defect (Fig. 16-28, A). To ensure a good blood supply, incorporate the major palatine artery in palatal flaps. Transpose and suture the flap in place for the first layer of the closure (Fig. 16-28, B). This flap provides "nasal" mucosa. Cover this layer with a mu-*

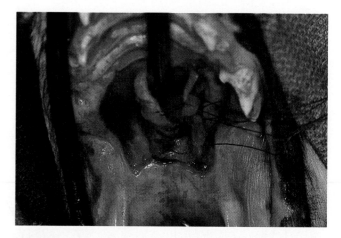

FIG. 16-27
Intraoperative photograph showing repair of an oronasal fistula using a double-layer flap technique. The margins of the fistula have been elevated and rotated medially to cover the defect. This flap was covered with a buccal mucosa flap.

cosal flap (gingival and buccal) to provide the "oral" mucosal layer of the closure (Figs. 16-28, C and D). Allow the denuded hard palate to heal by second intention.

POSTOPERATIVE CARE AND ASSESSMENT

Intravenous fluids should be provided until the animal begins eating and drinking (usually within 24 hours of surgery). Soft food should be fed for 2 to 3 weeks, and chew-

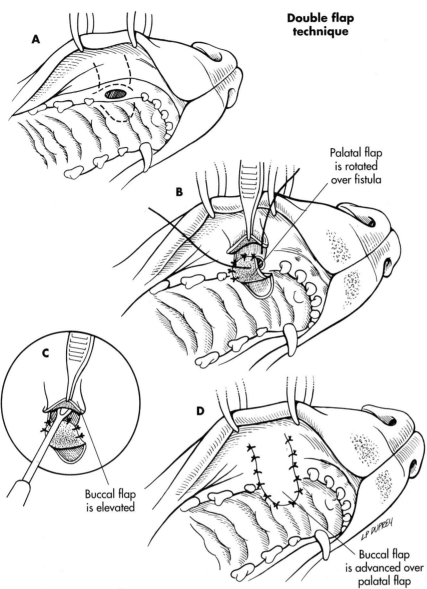

Double flap technique

FIG. 16-28
A double-layer flap technique for fistula repair may be performed using a mucoperiosteal hard palate flap and a buccal flap. **A** and **B,** Create a flap from the mucoperiosteum of the hard palate, **C** and **D,** cover it with a second flap advanced from the buccal mucosa.

Palatal flap is rotated over fistula

Buccal flap is elevated

Buccal flap is advanced over palatal flap

ing on hard objects (i.e., toys, sticks) must be prevented to avoid dehiscence or perforation of the flap separating the oral and nasal cavities. If the animal paws at the mouth, an Elizabethan collar should be used. Severe rhinitis should be treated with antibiotics (see Table 16-6). Healing should be evaluated 2 and 4 weeks postoperatively.

COMPLICATIONS

Most oronasal fistulae are successfully repaired if flaps can be apposed without tension and with a good blood supply. Dehiscence and recurrence of the oronasal fistula are expected if conditions for healing are not ideal. Motion of the tongue against the repair and particulate matter in the surgical site can also lead to dehiscence. Tension, poor blood supply, infection, lack of flap support, and traumatic technique may inhibit healing. Additional attempts to repair recurring fistulae should be delayed 4 to 6 weeks to allow sites of previous flap harvesting to heal, revascularize, and mature before additional flaps are created. Rhinitis should resolve after suc-

cessful fistula healing if irreversible mucosal changes have not occurred.

PROGNOSIS

Traumatic clefts may heal spontaneously in 2 to 4 weeks. Signs of rhinitis caused by regurgitation of food into the nasal cavity may be controlled with chronic antibiotic therapy. The long-term prognosis for most patients with nontraumatic fistulae is poor when surgical correction is not possible because fistulae do not heal without surgical reconstruction.

References

Ellison GW: A double reposition flap technique for repair of recurrent oronasal fistulas in dogs, *J Am Anim Hosp Assoc* 22:803, 1986.
Kirby BM: Oral flaps: principles, problems, and complications of flaps for reconstruction of the oral cavity, *Problems in Veterinary Medicine: Reconstructive Surgery* 2:494, 1990.

Lantz GC: Maxillary splint rod for repair of selected facial fractures, *J Am Anim Hosp Assoc* 20:905, 1984.

Salisbury SK: Problems and complications associated with maxillectomy, mandibulectomy and oronasal fistula repair, *Problems in Veterinary Medicine: Head & Neck Surgery* 3:153, 1991.

ORAL TUMORS

DEFINITIONS

Oral tumors encompass those neoplasms that arise from gingiva, buccal mucosa, labial mucosa, tongue, tonsil, or dental elements.

SYNONYMS

For malignant melanoma–**melanosarcoma;** for ameloblastoma–**adamantinoma**

GENERAL CONSIDERATIONS AND CLINICALLY RELEVANT PATHOPHYSIOLOGY

The oral cavity is the fourth most common site of neoplasia in dogs and cats; oral tumors account for 5% (dogs) to 7% (cats) of all malignant tumors in these species. Oral tumors originate from mucosa, tongue, periodontium, odontogenic tissue, mandible, maxilla, tonsils, and lips and spread by direct extension or invade adjacent bone and cartilaginous tissue. Metastatic spread is by lymphatics or blood to the regional lymph nodes and lungs. All tumors should be clinically staged according to the TNM classification system (primary tumor, regional lymph nodes, and metastasis) described by the World Health Organization (Table 16-7).

The most common malignant canine tumors are malignant melanoma, squamous cell carcinoma, and fibrosarcoma, whereas squamous cell carcinoma is the most common malignant oral feline tumor. Other malignancies are listed in Table 16-8. Benign oral tumors are rare in cats. The most common benign oral neoplasms in dogs are epulides; other benign oral lesions are listed in Table 16-8.

Malignant melanomas are the most frequently occurring malignant oral tumor in dogs; they rarely occur in cats (Table 16-9). Melanomas are rapidly growing tumors that appear white-gray to brown-black and are firm and vascular. They usually occur on the gingiva and are characterized by early, local invasion. Some types are easily mistaken on histopathology for fibrosarcoma. Metastasis to regional lymph nodes and lung occurs in 80% of the cases. Wide surgical excision using partial maxillectomy, mandibulectomy, tonsillectomy, or glossectomy is recommended. Radiation therapy may be used but there is a high rate of recurrence. Response to radiotherapy is better if concurrent hyperthermia is used. Chemotherapy and immunotherapy have been of little or no benefit in the treatment of malignant melanomas.

Squamous cell carcinomas (SCC) are the most common malignant oral tumors of cats and the second most common malignant oral tumor in dogs (Table 16-10). They occur on the gingiva, lip, tongue, or tonsil. The masses are red, friable, vascular, and sometimes ulcerated. Most tumors in the rostral oropharynx are locally invasive and have a low metastatic potential, whereas those located in the caudal oropharynx tend to be more infiltrative and metastasize more rapidly. Canine gingival SCC tend to be highly invasive and osteolytic but have a low rate of metastasis. Feline gingival SCC have a poorer prognosis than canine SCC. Wide resection is recommended for gingival tumors. They are radiosensitive and combining radiotherapy with hyperthermia has been effective. Tonsillar SCC grow rapidly and are associated with early local invasion and a high rate of lymph node and lung metastasis. Tonsillar carcinoma has not been reported in cats. They occur more commonly in male, urban dogs. The prognosis for tonsillar SCC is guarded. Squamous cell carcinomas may also occur on the tongue.

Fibrosarcomas are primarily found in dogs (Table 16-11). They most commonly occur on the maxillary gingiva and hard palate and appear as pink-red, firm, smooth, multilobulated masses that are often attached to underlying tissue. Local infiltration with bony involvement is common, but distant metastasis is uncommon. Although local recurrence is high with any treatment, wide surgical resection is recommended. Most fibrosarcomas are poorly responsive to chemotherapy. Fibrosarcomas are generally radioresistant, although median tumor control time with radiation alone has been reported to be 12 months (McChesney et al, 1989). Cryotherapy is believed to stimulate recurrence.

Osteosarcomas comprise approximately 10% of canine mandibular and maxillary tumors. They are locally aggressive and have a high metastatic potential. Response to conventional therapies (i.e., surgery, radiation, chemotherapy) is poor.

The epulides are the most common class of benign oral neoplasms, accounting for 30% of all canine oral neoplasms (Table 16-12). They are rarely seen in cats. They are firm, gingival masses that arise from the periodontal ligament. There are three types of epulides: fibromatous, ossifying, and acanthomatous. Fibromatous epulides are noninvasive, firm, smooth, pink masses that originate at the gingival sulcus and may be single or multiple and pedunculated or sessile (Fig. 16-29). They contain periodontal ligament stroma as the primary cell type. Ossifying epulides are similar to fibromatous epulides except that they contain large amounts of osteoid matrix within the stroma of the periodontal ligament. They are firm and difficult to cut. Malignant transformation to osteosarcoma has been reported. Acanthomatous epulides are classified as benign masses but they are often locally aggressive and are sometimes difficult to differentiate from squamous cell carcinoma histologically. They are the most frequent type of epulis and frequently infiltrate bone, causing lysis. Acanthomatous epulides occur most frequently rostral to the mandibular canine teeth. They are composed primarily of epithelial cells arranged in sheets and cords intimately associated with the underlying stroma and invading bone. Wide surgical excision is recommended, although they are

TABLE 16-7

Clinical Stage Classification System for Canine/Feline Tumors of the Oral Cavity*

The following are the minimum requirements for assessing the T, N, and M categories (if these cannot be met, the symbols TX, NX, and MX should be used).

- T categories: clinical and surgical examination
- N categories: clinical and surgical examination
- M categories: clinical and surgical examination, radiography of thorax

T: Primary Tumor

Tis—preinvasive carcinoma (carcinoma in situ)
T0—no evidence of tumor
T1—tumor less than 2 cm maximum diameter
    T1a—without bone invasion
    T1b—with bone invasion
T2—tumor 2 to 4 cm maximum diameter
    T2a—without bone invasion
    T2b—with bone invasion
T3—tumor greater than 4 cm maximum diameter
    T3a—without bone invasion
    T3b—with bone invasion
The symbol *m* added to the appropriate T category indicates multiple tumors.

N: Regional Lymph Nodes (RLN)†

N0—no evidence of regional lymph node involvement
N1—movable ipsilateral nodes
    N1a—nodes not considered to contain growth‡
    N1b—nodes considered to contain growth‡
N2—movable contralateral or bilateral nodes
    N2a—nodes not considered to contain growth‡
    N2b—nodes considered to contain growth‡
N3—fixed nodes

M: Distant Metastasis

M0—no evidence of metastasis
M1—distant metastasis (including distant nodes) detected—specify site(s) _____

Stage grouping

	T	N	M
I	T1	N0, N1a or N2a	M0
II	T2	N0, N1a or N2a	M0
III‡	T3	N0, N1a or N2a	M0
	Any T	N1b	
IV	Any T	Any N2b or N3	M0
	Any T	Any N	M1

*The regional lymph nodes are the cervical, submandibular, and parotid nodes.
†(−)=histologically negative, (+)=histologically positive.
‡Any bone involvement.
From document VPH/CMO/80.20, World Health Organization; reproduced with permission.

radiosensitive. They will recur locally if not treated adequately. Ameloblastomas (adamantinoma) are benign tumors that arise from the dental lamina. They usually occur in younger dogs and involve the rostral mandible.

Oral papillomas are benign tumors that are caused by a papillomavirus or papovavirus in young dogs. They occur primarily on the buccal and gingival mucosa, appearing as multiple gray-white pedunculated lesions. Papillomas spontaneously regress within 2 months in most dogs as immunity to the viral agent develops. Surgical resection is necessary only to confirm the diagnosis or in dogs that are dys-

phagic as a result of many large papillomas. Some animals have been treated with autogenous vaccines.

DIAGNOSIS
Clinical Presentation

Signalment. Breeds that appear to be predisposed to oral tumors include boxers, German shepherds, golden retrievers, cocker spaniels, German shorthaired pointers, collies, Old English sheepdogs, and weimaraners. Oral tumors are generally observed in middle-aged and older animals (older than 7 to 10 years). Exceptions to this include oral

TABLE 16-8
Oral Tumor Types

Malignant
- Malignant melanoma
- Squamous cell carcinoma
- Fibrosarcoma
- Osteosarcoma
- Lymphosarcoma
- Mast cell tumor
- Gingival hemangiosarcoma
- Neurofibrosarcoma
- Anaplastic sarcoma
- Chondrosarcoma
- Myxosarcoma
- Invasive nasal tumors
- Transmissible venereal tumor
- Histiocytic neoplasia

Benign
- Epulides
- Viral papillomatosis
- Odontogenic tumors (adamantinoma* or ameloblastoma)
- Fibroma
- Peripheral giant cell granuloma
- Chondroma
- Lipoma
- Hemangioma
- Plasma cell tumor

*Biologic behavior is unpredictable.

TABLE 16-9
Characteristics of Oral Malignant Melanomas

- Most common malignant oral tumor in dogs (~20%)
- Rare in cats
- Most common on gingiva
- More common in male dogs
- Mean age of affected animals is 9 to 11 years (10.3)
- Breeds with pigmented oral mucosa, cocker spaniels, and German shepherds may be predisposed
- Metastasis is common
- Prognosis is poor; median survival is 8 to 9 months

TABLE 16-10
Characteristics of Oral Squamous Cell Carcinomas

- Most common tumor in cats (~70%)
- Second most common tumor in dogs (with fibrosarcoma) (~15%)
- Occur on gingiva, lip, tongue, or tonsil
- Biological behavior varies with location and species; regional lymph node involvement common with tongue and tonsillar SCC

TABLE 16-11
Characteristics of Oral Fibrosarcomas

- Second most common malignant oral tumor in dogs (with squamous cell carcinoma)
- Occur most commonly on gingiva and hard palate
- More common in large breeds (i.e., > 20 kg), male dogs
- Younger dogs may be affected (mean age < 7 years)
- Locally invasive; high metastatic potential in dogs < 2 years of age

TABLE 16-12
Characteristics of Epulides

- Most common oral tumor in dogs (~30%)
- Mean age ~8.2 years
- More common in large breed (i.e., > 20 kg) dogs
- Do not metastasize
- Acanthomatous epulis most common form

papillomatosis, which occurs in dogs 1 year old or less, and fibrosarcoma, which has a mean age of occurrence of approximately 5 years.

☞ **NOTE** · Remember, some melanomas are not pigmented (amelanotic).

Melanomas are more common in males (reported male:female ratio as high as 4:1) with an average onset age of 9 to 11 years. Breeds with pigmented oral mucosa and cocker spaniels and German shepherds appear to have an increased incidence. Squamous cell carcinomas are common in cats of either sex that are older than 10 years. Nontonsillar squamous cell carcinomas are most common in small breed dogs of either sex between 8 to 10 years of age. Fibrosarcomas occur more commonly in large breed dogs, particularly Dobermans and golden retrievers. Males are affected more frequently than females (2:1). For fibrosarcomas age of onset is younger (4 to 5 years) in large breed dogs (more than 25 kg) than smaller dogs (more than 8 years). Fibromatous epulides are common in boxers.

History. Oral tumors are often large when recognized by an owner; however, some are found during yearly examinations or routine dentistry. Neoplasia should be suspected during dentistry if teeth are excessively mobile. Affected animals frequently present for evaluation of a visible mass, oral bleeding, difficulty eating, and/or halitosis. Anorexia, weight loss, loose or displaced teeth, salivation, facial deformity, and/or nasal discharge may also be noted. A history of recent tooth extraction may precede rapid growth of a mass at the extraction site. Clinical signs in dogs with tonsillar SCC may be related to oropharyngeal obstruction (i.e., dyspnea, anorexia, cough, and/or drooling), and a large ventral cervical swelling may be found associated with lymph node metastasis.

Physical Examination Findings

Oral tumors arising from the rostral portion of the oral cavity are generally easily visualized; however, seeing tonsillar or caudal oropharyngeal tumors may require sedation or anes-

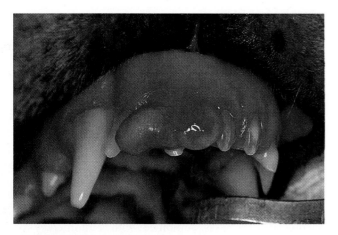

FIG. 16-29
Appearance of a fibromatous epulis surrounding the maxillary incisors in a dog.

thesia. General anesthesia is often necessary to define the extent of disease. The surface of growing neoplasms may appear ulcerated, infected, and necrotic. Regional lymph nodes should be evaluated for evidence of enlargement, nodularity, and adherence to surrounding tissue.

> ☞ **N O T E ·** When you first observe the tumor, measure it and record its location (particularly if treatment is delayed).

Radiography/Ultrasonography

Thoracic radiographs should be performed to look for pulmonary metastasis and concurrent pulmonary or cardiovascular disease. Both lateral radiographic views should be taken because tumors may be missed on a single lateral view. Further therapy may not be indicated if metastasis is noted. Skull radiographs are performed under general anesthesia and are used to assess the extent of the lesion and bony involvement. Malignant tumors show a tendency for irregular, destructive, or aggressive bone loss, whereas bone production predominates in benign tumors.

Laboratory Findings

Laboratory examination of animals with oral tumors should include a CBC, chemistry profile, urinalysis, bleeding time, and electrocardiogram. Abnormalities related to the tumor (other than anemia of chronic blood loss) are uncommon.

DIFFERENTIAL DIAGNOSIS

Granulation tissue (secondary to foreign body, trauma, or infection), eosinophilic granuloma complex, and gingival hyperplasia are the primary differentials. Fluctuant swellings in the sublingual and pharyngeal area may be salivary mucoceles (see p. 227) or congenital cysts. Other differential diagnoses include nasopharyngeal polyp, osteomyelitis, and feline plasma cell gingivitis-pharyngitis. Cytologic or histologic analysis of masses may be necessary to differentiate neoplastic from some nonneoplastic oral lesions.

> ☞ **N O T E ·** Always biopsy oral masses to rule out neoplasia.

MEDICAL MANAGEMENT

Cytologic analysis of the tumor and draining lymph nodes is indicated before surgery. Excisional or incisional biopsy (see p. 202) is usually necessary to determine prognosis and treatment. Treatment modalities (other than surgery) that have been used alone or in combination for oral tumors include radiotherapy, hyperthermia, chemotherapy, cryosurgery, immunotherapy, and photodynamic therapy. Squamous cell carcinomas are radiosensitive and are successfully treated by this modality. Fibrosarcomas are radioresistant. Melanomas may be sensitive to radiotherapy but distant metastasis frequently renders it ineffective. Radiation-induced tumors occur in up to 20% of the irradiated sites. The prognosis following treatment with chemotherapy, immunotherapy, hyperthermia, and photodynamic therapy needs further investigation. Refer to a medicine text for additional information regarding these techniques.

SURGICAL TREATMENT

Treatment protocols must be based on the tumor type, site, extent, stage, age and health of the patient, and treatment limitations. Early, aggressive therapy offers the best chance of success in treating oral malignancies. Aggressive surgical excision (e.g., mandibulectomy, maxillectomy) may be curative for gingival tumors if resection is complete and metastasis has not occurred. Because most gingival tumors invade bone, mandibulectomy or maxillectomy is usually necessary. Shaving the tumor down to bone will generally result in recurrence. Caudal tumors and those crossing the midline may be nonresectable or it may be difficult to successfully reconstruct the area with flaps. Excision of the middle and caudal maxilla is limited by the size of mucosal flap that can be created. Mandibulectomy is limited by the medial and caudal extent of the tumor (see p. 204). Tumors invading into the sublingual musculature and caudal pharynx may not be resectable. Tumor extension into the lip necessitates full-thickness lip resection with partial maxillectomy (see p. 203) or mandibulectomy. Owners are often more receptive to major oral resections if they see pictures of animals having had procedures similar to what you are recommending for their pet.

Preoperative Management

Perioperative antibiotics are indicated for oral tumors, which often have focal areas of necrosis and infection (see p. 201). Debilitated animals require intravenous fluids and enteral or parenteral hyperalimentation before surgery.

Anesthesia

General anesthetic protocols for animals undergoing oral surgery are on p. 200. Sedation or general anesthesia may be required for fine-needle aspiration depending on tumor location and the animal's disposition. General anesthesia is generally recommended for biopsy because of subsequent bleeding. Surgical excision of tumors requires general anesthesia with inhalant anesthetics. Because most affected animals are old, isoflurane is the inhalant anesthetic of choice. Cuffed endotracheal tubes, preferably tubes that are guarded to prevent kinking, should be used. Intubation may be accomplished through a pharyngotomy (see p. 209) or tracheotomy (see p. 613) if necessary to facilitate surgery. Sterile sponges should be placed in the caudal oropharynx to prevent aspiration of blood.

☞ **N O T E** · Use guarded endotracheal tubes.

Surgical Anatomy

Surgical anatomy of the oropharynx is given on p. 201.

Positioning

Mandibular lesions are usually resected with the patient in lateral recumbency. Maxillary lesions may be resected with the patient in lateral or ventral recumbency.

SURGICAL TECHNIQUE

Identify the soft tissue and/or bone to be resected and remove them according to the techniques for maxillectomy, mandibulectomy, glossectomy, and tonsillectomy described on pp. 203 to 208. After mandibulectomy or maxillectomy but before closure you may radiograph the excised segment to help determine whether adequate bone was removed; however, tumor growth up the mandibular foramen may necessitate wider margins than radiographic evaluation of bone destruction might predict. If available, intraoperative cytology is often more beneficial in determining the adequacy of resection. *Submit excised tissues for histologic analysis. If additional bone is excised mark the caudal border to allow determination of whether additional resection is needed (i.e., if this margin contains tumor).*

POSTOPERATIVE CARE AND ASSESSMENT

Sponges should be removed from the caudal oropharynx, and the oral cavity and nasopharynx should be suctioned before anesthetic recovery. Analgesics (i.e., oxymorphone, butorphanol, or buprenorphine; see Table 16-4) should be provided postoperatively. Soft food and water may be offered the day after surgery. Intravenous fluids may be discontinued when the animal maintains hydration by drinking. Dogs are seldom reluctant to eat after surgery; however, cats may require 2 to 3 days to adapt. Reevaluation should be performed 1 and 2 weeks following surgery to assess healing. Sutures are usually extruded or sloughed 2 to 4 weeks postoperatively. Facial swelling usually resolves within 3 to 7 days following surgery. Thoracic radiographs may be taken at 3, 6, and 12 months postoperatively to evaluate for metastases, and oral examinations should be performed regularly to look for tumor recurrence. Following partial maxillectomy or mandibulectomy, excessive dental tartar may accumulate on the teeth of the opposite dental arch.

COMPLICATIONS

Tumor recurrence and dehiscence are the most common complications following major oral reconstruction. Overall, tumor recurrence following resection with tumor-free margins is less than 40% (Salisbury, Lantz, 1988; White, 1991). Recurrence in these cases is due to the presence of a multifocal tumor, development of a new tumor, or inadequate pathologic assessment. Dehiscence occurs in less than one third of cases with major reconstruction (Kosovsky et al, 1991; Salisbury, Lantz, 1988). Suture line tension, excessive electrocautery use, ischemic necrosis of a mucosal flap, excessive flap movement, infection, and tumor recurrence are major causes of dehiscence. Dehiscence occurs more frequently if surgery is combined with radiotherapy or chemotherapy because these adjuvant therapies may inhibit wound healing.

PROGNOSIS

The prognosis for oral tumors depends on the tumor type, biologic behavior, and stage of disease. The prognosis is good for benign oral tumors, whereas the prognosis for malignant oral tumors is poor. The best chance for cure or control of malignant or benign oral tumors is surgical resection and reconstruction. Elimination of local disease is essential. Overall, the 1-year survival rate is 46% with a median survival time of 8 months for dogs with malignant maxillary tumors (White, 1991; Wallace, 1992). For malignant mandibular tumors the overall 1-year survival rate is 45% with a median survival time of 11 months (White, 1991; Salisbury, Lantz, 1988). Dogs with tumors rostral to the maxillary canine or the first mandibular premolar teeth have a better prognosis. This may be because of earlier recognition, altered tumor behavior based on location, or prevalence of tumor type.

☞ **N O T E** · Warn owners that partial mandibulectomy and maxillectomy alleviate most clinical signs but may not cure the disease.

Squamous cell carcinomas respond best to surgery because they are localized and usually have not metastasized. In dogs more than 50% of SCCs are controlled locally for a year or more, and mean survival is approximately 13 to 19 months. Reports of 1-year survival rates vary from 50% to 91%. Fibrosarcomas are localized but locally aggressive and are often difficult to completely resect. Recurrence of up to 80% within the first year following resection has been reported. Mean survival varies from 10 to 14 months and 1-year survival rates vary from 21% to 50% after excision of fibrosarcomas. Melanomas have the poorest prognosis because they metastasize early. Less than 20% of affected animals are disease free 1 year after surgery, and mean survival is 9 months. Reported median survival times vary from 8 to 10 months. Tumors arising from the tongue have a poor prognosis. They are controlled locally in only 25% of animals 1 year after resection or radiation therapy.

References

Kosovsky JK et al: Results of partial mandibulectomy for the treatment of oral tumors in 142 dogs, *Vet Surg* 21:397, 1991.

McChesney SL et al: Radiotherapy of soft tissue sarcomas in dogs, *J Am Vet Med Assoc* 194:60, 1989.

Salisbury SK, Lantz GC: Long-term results of partial mandibulectomy for treatment of oral tumors in 30 dogs, *J Am Anim Hosp Assoc* 24:285, 1988.

Wallace J, Matthiesen DT, Patnaik AK: Hemimaxillectomy for the treatment of oral tumors in 69 dogs, *Vet Surg* 21:337, 1992.

White RAS: Mandibulectomy and maxillectomy in the dog: long term survival in 100 cases, *J Small Anim Pract* 32:69, 1991.

Suggested Reading

Oakes MG et al: Canine oral neoplasia, *Compend Contin Educ Pract Vet* 15:15, 1993.

Schwarz PD et al: Mandibular resection as a treatment for oral cancer in 81 dogs, *J Am Anim Hosp Assoc* 27:601, 1991.

Schwarz PD et al: Partial maxillary resection as a treatment for oral cancer in 61 dogs, *J Am Anim Hosp Assoc* 27:617, 1991.

SALIVARY MUCOCELES

DEFINITIONS

A **salivary mucocele** is a collection of saliva that has leaked from a damaged salivary gland or duct and is surrounded by granulation tissue. A **cervical mucocele** is a collection of saliva in the deeper structures of the intermandibular space, the angle of the jaw, or the upper cervical region. A **sublingual mucocele** or **ranula** is a collection of saliva in the sublingual tissue caudal to the openings of the sublingual and mandibular ducts, while a **pharyngeal mucocele** is a collection of saliva in the tissues adjacent to the pharynx. A **zygomatic mucocele** is a collection of saliva ventral to the globe. **Complex mucoceles,** consisting of two or more types, occur in some animals. **Marsupialization** is the process of incising a mucocele and suturing the edges to the mucosa. The interior of the mucocele suppurates and gradually closes by granulation.

SYNONYMS

Sialocele, ranula, salivary cyst, honey cyst

GENERAL CONSIDERATIONS AND CLINICALLY RELEVANT PATHOPHYSIOLOGY

Tearing of a salivary gland or duct results in leakage of saliva into the surrounding tissue. Salivary mucoceles are not cysts. Cysts are cavities that are lined by epithelium, whereas the granulation tissue lining of a mucocele is produced secondary to inflammation caused by free saliva in the tissues. The cause of salivary mucoceles is rarely identified, although blunt trauma (choke chains), foreign bodies, and sialoliths have been suggested. The sublingual salivary gland is most commonly involved. Saliva takes the path of least resistance, most commonly accumulating in the cranial cervical or inter-

mandibular area (Fig. 16-30), sublingual area (Fig. 16-31), or pharyngeal tissues (Fig. 16-32). Saliva irritates the tissue and causes inflammation. During this initial phase the swelling may be firm and painful but the animal is usually asymptomatic. Granulation tissue forms in response to the inflammation and prevents saliva from migrating further. The diagnosis of salivary mucocele is primarily based on history, clinical signs, and pathologic findings. Radiographs may determine which gland is involved and histopathology is diagnostic.

DIAGNOSIS
Clinical Presentation

Signalment. Dogs are more frequently affected than cats. All breeds are susceptible, but some reports indicate that poodles, German shepherds, dachshunds, and Australian silky terriers are more commonly affected. There is a slight predisposition for males to be affected. Any age animal may present with a mucocele.

History. Clinical signs depend on the location of the mucocoele. Most dogs have cervical or intermandibular mucocoeles and are usually asymptomatic. These animals are usually

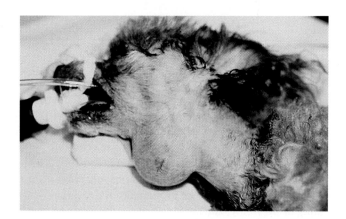

FIG. 16-30
Cervical mucocele in a dog.

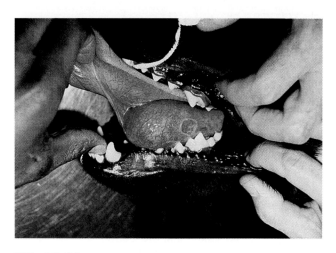

FIG. 16-31
Intraoperative appearance of a mucocele (ranula) located lateral to the tongue in the sublingual tissue.

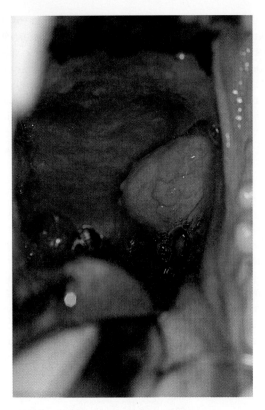

FIG. 16-32
Pharyngeal mucocele in a dog.

presented with a history of a gradually developing, fluctuant, nonpainful mass. Patients with a sublingual mucocele (i.e., ranula) may present with abnormal prehension and oral bleeding; bleeding is caused by trauma during chewing. Respiratory distress and dysphagia are common in patients with pharyngeal mucoceles. Swelling in the oropharyngeal area may cause abnormal tongue movements and interfere with eating or breathing, and swelling in the orbital area with zygomatic mucoceles may cause exophthalmos and divergent strabismus.

☞ **NOTE ·** Clients should be asked where they first noticed the swelling because this may help determine the affected side.

Physical Examination Findings

The parotid and mandibular glands are easily palpated. The sublingual gland is occasionally palpable in the cooperative or sedated patient. Palpation of the glands is expected to be normal and without discomfort. Most mucoceles are soft and fluctuant, while tumors and abscesses are generally firm. Mucoceles are nonpainful except during the acute phase of swelling. It is sometimes difficult to identify the affected side when mucoceles are located on the ventral midline or intermandibular space. Examining these animals in dorsal recumbency often allows the mucocele to gravitate to the affected side. Palpation of some cervical mucoceles will cause the sublingual tissues to bulge on the affected side. Concur-

rent sublingual and cervical mucoceles originate from the side where the sublingual mucocele is found. Blood-tinged saliva may occur in patients with sublingual mucoceles because teeth often traumatize the mucocele. Periorbital facial swelling, exophthalmos, and periocular pain are signs of a zygomatic mucocele. Optic neuropathy secondary to pressure may occur with zygomatic mucoceles.

☞ **NOTE ·** Animals with pharyngeal mucoceles often present in acute respiratory distress. Appropriate therapy must be rapidly instituted or many of these patients will die.

Radiography/Ultrasonography

Plain radiographs rarely help except in cases with sialoliths, foreign bodies, or neoplasia. Thoracic radiographs are indicated to evaluate for metastasis if neoplasia is suspected. Sialography, the injection of an iodinated water-soluble contrast agent into a salivary duct, is difficult and usually unnecessary to confirm the diagnosis or determine the site of origin.

Laboratory Findings

Laboratory abnormalities are seldom present in affected animals. Salivary gland function and duct patency can be evaluated by placing a drop of topical ophthalmic atropine solution on the tongue to stimulate saliva to flow. However, it may be difficult to distinguish flow from individual ducts. Paracentesis should be performed under aseptic conditions to prevent infection of the mucocele. Aspiration of a clear, yellowish, or blood-tinged, ropey, mucoid fluid with a low cell count is consistent with saliva. Staining a smear with a mucus-specific stain such as periodic acid-Schiff (PAS) confirms the presence of saliva. An elevated white blood cell count may indicate concurrent sialoadenitis.

DIFFERENTIAL DIAGNOSIS

Sialoadenitis, salivary neoplasia, sialolith (calcium phosphate or carbonate), cervical abscess, foreign body, hematoma, cystic or neoplastic lymph nodes, thyroglossal cyst, cystic Rathke's pouch, and branchial cysts may cause swellings in the same region as mucoceles. Occasionally mucoceles may be difficult to distinguish from cysts or tumors. Histopathology is necessary to diagnose a salivary gland tumor and to differentiate a congenital cyst from a mucocele. Congenital cysts have an epithelial lining, while mucoceles are lined by granulation tissue.

MEDICAL MANAGEMENT

Repeated drainage or injection of cauterizing or antiinflammatory agents will not eliminate mucoceles but will complicate subsequent surgery by leading to abscessation or fibrosis.

SURGICAL TREATMENT

Complete excision of the involved gland-duct complex and drainage of the mucocele are curative. The side of mucocele origin may be determined by oral examination, palpation, sialography, and/or exploration of the mucocele.

☞ **N O T E** · If you are having trouble identifying the affected side in an animal with a cervical mucocele, place the animal in dorsal recumbency. The mucocele will often gravitate to the side of the lesion.

Preoperative Management

Animals with pharyngeal mucoceles may present in acute respiratory distress and rapid intubation may be necessary. Intubation may not be possible through the mouth and a temporary tracheostomy may be required. Once these animals are intubated they are generally stable and surgical excision of the mucocele can be delayed while further diagnostics are performed if necessary. Intravenous antibiotics may be given at induction but are not essential.

Anesthesia

Most animals undergoing salivary gland excision for mucoceles are healthy, and a variety of anesthetic protocols can be used. General anesthetic recommendations for animals undergoing oral surgery (i.e., for ranulas or pharyngeal mucoceles) are listed on p. 200. Oral intubation may be difficult in patients with large pharyngeal mucoceles (see above), and placement of the endotracheal tube via tracheostomy is often necessary to allow adequate visualization of the lesion.

Surgical Anatomy

Dogs and cats have four major pairs of salivary glands of surgical significance (Fig. 16-33). They include the parotid, mandibular, sublingual, and zygomatic glands. The parotid gland is a triangular shaped serous gland located ventral to the horizontal ear canal. Numerous arteries, veins, and nerves are closely associated with the medial aspect of the

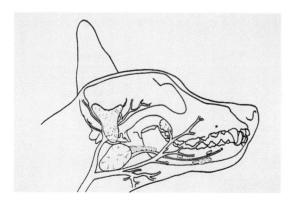

FIG. 16-33
Surgical anatomy of the salivary glands. The parotid gland lies ventral to the ear canal. The mandibular gland is ventral to the parotid gland, lying between the maxillary and linguofacial veins. The sublingual gland follows the rostral course of the mandibular duct toward the oral cavity. The zygomatic gland is protected by the zygomatic arch.

gland. The parotid duct papilla is located on the mucosal surface of the cheek at the level of the upper carnassial tooth (fourth premolar). The mandibular gland is large, ovoid, and lies within a fibrous capsule caudal and ventral to the parotid gland. It is located between the linguofacial and maxillary veins as they merge to join the external jugular vein. The mandibular duct runs with the sublingual gland toward the floor of the mouth and opens on a small papilla lateral to the rostral border of the frenulum (Table 16-13). The sublingual gland is divided into a monostomatic and polystomatic portion. The monostomatic portion of the sublingual gland originates on the rostroventral border of the mandibular gland. The ducts from this portion of the sublingual gland course with the mandibular duct but often open on separate papillae. The polystomatic portion of the sublingual gland is divided into several loosely connected lobules that surround the mandibular duct and lie immediately beneath the oral mucosa, secreting directly into the oral cavity. The zygomatic gland, an irregularly ovoid gland, is located on the floor of the orbit ventrocaudal to the eye and medial to the zygomatic arch. The zygomatic gland has several ducts that run ventrally and open on a fold of mucosa lateral to the last upper molar tooth. The major zygomatic duct can usually be identified at this location about 1 cm caudal to the parotid papilla.

Positioning

Salivary gland excision is performed with the animal in lateral recumbency. Ventral recumbency and maximal opening of the mouth facilitates marsupialization of pharyngeal mucoceles and ranulas.

SURGICAL TECHNIQUE
Mandibular and Sublingual Salivary Gland Excision

The mandibular and sublingual salivary glands are excised together because the sublingual gland is intimately associated with the mandibular salivary gland duct; removal of one would traumatize the other. Removal of glands on the involved side is all that is necessary for mucocele resolution; however, both pairs of mandibular and sublingual glands may be resected without risk of xerostomia. If it is not clear

TABLE 16-13

Oral Openings of the Salivary Gland Ducts

Parotid Duct
- Labial mucosa at level of upper carnassial tooth

Mandibular Duct
- Papilla lateral to the rostral border of the frenulum

Sublingual Duct
- Opens with the mandibular duct near the lingual frenulum

Zygomatic Gland
- Lateral to the last upper molar tooth

from which side the mucocele originated, make a stab incision in the mucocele and digitally palpate the lumen. The unaffected side is rounded and smooth. The affected side has a tract or tunnel toward the site of leakage. *Position the patient in lateral recumbency. Place a pad under the neck to rotate the ventral aspect dorsally and fix the neck in an extended position. Locate the mandibular salivary gland between the linguofacial and maxillary veins as they join the external jugular vein (Fig. 16-34, A). Incise skin, subcutaneous tissue, and platysma muscle from the angle of the mandible caudally to the external jugular vein to expose the fibrous capsule of the mandibular gland (Fig. 16-34, B). Avoiding the branch of the second cervical nerve that crosses the capsule, incise the capsule and dissect it away from the mandibular and monostomatic sublingual salivary glands. Ligate the artery (branch of the great auricular artery) and vein as they are encountered on the dorsomedial aspect of the gland. Continue dissecting cranially, following the mandibular duct, sublingual duct, and polystomatic sublingual glands toward the mouth (see Fig. 16-34, B). Incise the fascia between the masseter and digastricus muscles. Expose the entire mandibular and sublingual salivary gland complex by retracting the digastricus muscle and applying caudal traction on the mandibular gland. If necessary, perform digastricus muscle myotomy or tunnel the caudal sublingual gland duct complex under the digastricus muscle to improve visualization. Dissect (digital and sharp) rostrally until the lingual branch of the trigeminal nerve is identified and only ducts remain in the com-*

plex. Avoid traumatizing the lingual or hypoglossal nerves. Try to identify the gland-duct defect causing the mucocele because failure to identify this defect may indicate the mucocele originated from the contralateral gland-duct complex. Ligate and transect the mandibular sublingual gland-duct complex just caudal to the lingual nerve. Traction on the gland-duct complex may cause the ducts to tear. If this occurs near the point of proposed transection or on the oral aspect of the gland-duct defect, no further dissection is needed. However, if the tear occurs before the gland-duct defect or when the defect is not identified and glandular tissue is identified oral to the tear, further resection of glandular tissue is recommended to prevent recurrence. Lavage the surgical site before closure. Appose the digastric muscle if it has been incised with horizontal mattress or cruciate sutures. Close the dead space with a few sutures in the capsule and deep tissue. Routinely appose superficial muscles, subcutaneous tissue, and skin. Following excision, submit the glands and ducts to rule out neoplasia, and submit a portion of the mucocele wall to rule out congenital cysts.

Drain cervical mucoceles by making a stab incision at the most dependent point; place a Penrose drain if desired. Protect the drain with an absorbent bandage. Change the bandage and cleanse discharge from the neck as needed to prevent excoriation of the skin. Maintain the drain for 1 to 5 days, removing it when there is minimal discharge. Allow the stab incision to heal by second intention. **Redundant skin resumes its normal appearance within several weeks.** *Drain sublingual mucoceles (ranula) by excising an*

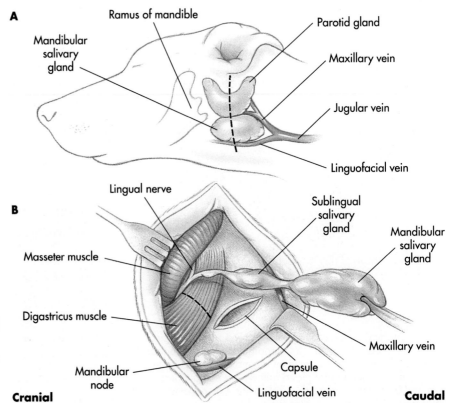

FIG. 16-34
A, To excise the mandibular and sublingual salivary glands, make an incision ventral to the external ear canal and over the mandibular salivary gland at the junction of the linguofacial and maxillary veins. **B,** Dissect the mandibular salivary gland after incising the capsule. Apply caudal traction on the mandibular gland and dissect the duct and sublingual gland until the lingual nerve is identified.

elliptical full-thickness section of the mucocele wall. Suture the granulation tissue lining to the sublingual mucosa (marsupialization) to encourage drainage for several days (Fig. 16-35). Drain pharyngeal mucoceles by aspiration or marsupialization. Excise redundant pharyngeal tissue to prevent airway obstruction after evacuation of the mucocele. Marsupialized ranulas contract and heal quickly by second intention. After bilateral mandibular and sublingual salivary gland excision, dogs still have sufficient saliva to adequately moisten their food.

Zygomatic Gland Excision

Zygomatic gland excision is required for zygomatic mucoceles, nonresponsive infections or inflammatory conditions, and neoplasia. *Position the patient in lateral or ventral recumbency. Protect the animal's eye from irritants with ophthalmic ointment. Incise skin and subcutaneous tissues over the dorsal rim of the zygomatic arch. Incise the palpebral fascia, retractor anguli oculi muscle, and orbital ligament and elevate them dorsally with the skin and globe. Further expose the gland by partially removing the zygomatic arch via ronguers or osteotomy. Retract the globe dorsally to expose the periorbital fat and underlying zygomatic gland. Remove the gland by blunt dissection (the gland is friable). Avoid the ventrally located anastomotic branch between the deep facial and external ophthalmic veins. Drain the mucocele if present. If possible, replace the zygomatic arch by securing the bone with suture placed through predrilled holes. Lavage the area and appose the palpebral fascia to the zygomatic periosteum with sutures. Close subcutaneous tissues and skin.*

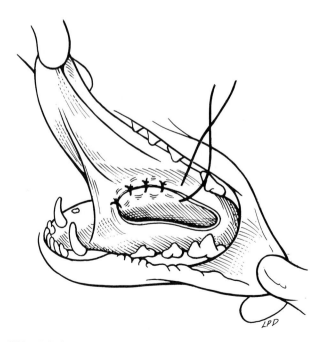

FIG. 16-35

Marsupialization of a ranula. After excising an elliptical piece of mucosa and granulation tissue from the mucocele wall, suture mucosa to the lining of the mucocele.

Parotid Gland Excision

Parotid gland excision is occasionally performed for neoplasia, fistula, chronic infection, or mucocele. The triangular shaped gland is located at the base of the auricular cartilage. *Position the patient in lateral recumbency. Incise skin from 1 to 2 cm ventral to the external acoustic meatus to a point midway between the ramus of the mandible and the bifurcation of the jugular vein. Incise the platysma muscle to expose the parotidoauricularis muscle, vertical ear canal, and parotid salivary gland. Sever and retract the parotidoauricularis muscle from its vertical ear canal attachment. Ligate and divide the caudal auricular vein. Begin dissection of the parotid gland at its dorsocaudal angle. Separate the parotid from the mandibular gland ventrally. Continue dissection between the gland and the vertical ear canal. Avoid traumatizing the facial nerve at the base of the horizontal ear canal. Ligate and divide the superficial temporal vein (a branch of the maxillary vein) coursing through the gland. Cauterize or ligate small vessels on the gland's medial surface. Ligate and transect the parotid duct as it leaves the gland. Lavage the area. Reappose the parotidoauricularis muscle. Complete closure by apposing subcutaneous tissues and skin.*

POSTOPERATIVE CARE AND ASSESSMENT

Change bandages daily if a Penrose drain has been placed. Depending on the amount of drainage, remove the drain 24 to 72 hours after surgery. Allow the drain site to heal by second intention. Soft food should be fed for 3 to 5 days following ranula marsupialization or excision of pharyngeal mucoceles.

COMPLICATIONS

Postoperative complications after salivary gland resection are uncommon but may include seroma formation, infection, and mucocele recurrence. Seromas can form in the dead space created by removal of the glands. They are resorbed and do not need to be aspirated or drained. Infection is rare if aseptic technique is used. Mucoceles recur if the side of mucocele origin was misdiagnosed or if inadequate gland was excised. Regional lymph nodes are sometimes mistaken for salivary glands. Dissection may be difficult if the mucocele was previously infected or injected. Attention to anatomic detail during surgery should minimize recurrence and complications associated with salivary gland excision.

PROGNOSIS

Rarely a mucocele will resolve without surgery. The prognosis is excellent if the disease is accurately diagnosed and excision is complete.

Suggested Reading

Bellenger CR, Simpson DJ: Canine sialocoeles—60 clinical cases, *J Small Animal Practice* 33:376, 1992.

Brown NO: Salivary gland diseases, *Problems in Veterinary Medicine: Gastrointestinal Surgical Complications* 1:281, 1989.

Carberry CA et al: Salivary gland tumors in dogs and cats: a literature and case review, *J Am Anim Hosp Assoc* 24:561, 1988.

Smith MM: Surgery of the canine salivary system, *Compend Contin Educ Pract Vet* 7:457, 1985.

Spangler WL, Culbertson MR: Salivary gland disease in dogs and cats: 245 cases (1985–1988), *J Am Vet Med Assoc* 198:465, 1991.

Weber WJ, Hobson HP: Pharyngeal mucocoeles in dogs, *Vet Surg* 15:5, 1986.

Surgery of the Esophagus

GENERAL PRINCIPLES AND TECHNIQUES

DEFINITIONS

Esophagotomy is an incision into the esophageal lumen, while **esophagectomy** is partial resection of the esophagus. **Regurgitation** is the passive expulsion of undigested food or fluid from the esophagus. **Vomiting** is a centrally-mediated reflex causing expulsion of food and/or fluid from the stomach and/or duodenum.

PREOPERATIVE CONCERNS

The esophagus carries food, water, and saliva from the pharynx to the stomach. Although less common than intestinal obstruction, esophageal obstruction may occur in dogs and cats secondary to foreign bodies, strictures, or masses. Esophageal surgery may be indicated if function is interrupted by obstruction or perforation (Table 16-14).

Diagnosis of esophageal disorders is based on history, clinical signs, and endoscopic or radiographic studies. The predominate clinical signs of esophageal pathology are regurgitation and dysphagia (Table 16-15). The patient's appetite may be normal, ravenous, or depressed. Regurgitation, ptyalism, and/or repeated swallowing attempts are frequent presenting signs. Undigested food may be regurgitated with either partial or complete obstructions. Partial esophageal obstruction causes progressive emaciation. Coughing, pulmonary crackles, mucopurulent nasal discharge, and/or fever suggest aspiration pneumonia secondary to regurgitation.

Aspiration pneumonia should be treated aggressively before esophageal surgery (see below). Esophageal perforations may cause septic mediastinitis evidenced by fever, pleural effusion, respiratory distress, and eventual death. Masses and foreign bodies may sometimes be palpated in the cervical esophagus. Distention of the cervical esophagus sometimes occurs with motility disorders. Compressing the thorax while the nostrils are occluded occasionally demonstrates cervical esophageal distention in animals with megaesophagus. Abnormalities of prehension and swallowing, regurgitation, or vomiting may be noted by observing the animal while it is eating. Vomiting is usually preceded by salivation, retching, and abdominal contractions and may contain bile or digested blood. The diagnosis of foreign bodies or masses is suggested by the history, clinical signs, and physical examination and confirmed by radiology, endoscopy, biopsy, and/or surgery.

Diagnosis of esophageal disorders may require a variety of techniques. Plain radiographs of the esophagus extending from the caudal portion of the oral cavity to the stomach should be assessed for radiopaque foreign bodies, esophageal size and location, periesophageal fluid or gas densities, and the presence or absence of aspiration pneumonia. The esophagus is not radiographically visible in most normal dogs and cats; however, small amounts of swallowed air may be seen in the cranial cervical and cranial thoracic esophagus when dogs are restrained in lateral recumbency. Mediastinitis, pneumomediastinum, and/or pleural effusion suggest esophageal perforation. Contrast fluoroscopic examination of the esophagus is indicated if plain radiographs are nondiagnostic. Fluoroscopic examination allows evaluation of swallowing, motility, and gastroesophageal sphincter function. Barium paste usually provides improved detail, but liquid is safer if aspirated. Food mixed with barium reveals some partial obstructions that are missed with barium paste.

Aqueous iodine or Iohexol, rather than barium, should be used if esophageal perforation is suspected. Esophagoscopy is useful in diagnosing esophageal obstruction, tumors, or inflammation. During esophagoscopy, mucosal lesions may be identified and biopsied, while foreign bodies can be removed or advanced into the stomach. Excessive force should never be used because the esophageal wall could be perforated. Esophagotomy or partial esophagectomy may be performed as a diagnostic and therapeutic procedure if a definitive diagnosis cannot be made by other means (p. 236).

TABLE 16-14
Surgical Diseases of the Esophagus
• Foreign bodies
• Tumors
• Perforation
• Hiatal hernia
• Fistulae
• Gastroesophageal intussusception
• Diverticula
• Cricopharyngeal achalasia
• Strictures

TABLE 16-15
Clinical Signs of Esophageal Disease
• Regurgitation
• Coughing
• Dysphagia
• Dyspnea
• Ptyalism
• Fever
• Altered appetite
• Weight loss

Treatment for aspiration pneumonia, esophagitis, and nutritional debilitation should be initiated before surgery (Table 16-16). For mild esophagitis, food and water should be withheld for 24 to 48 hours to reduce esophageal irritation. Water should be offered first; if there is no regurgitation, a low-fat gruel (which speeds gastric emptying and reduces reflux) should be fed for 3 to 4 days. Soft food should be fed for an additional 5 to 7 days, and then the animal should be gradually returned to its normal diet. For severe esophagitis, oral intake of food and water may need to be withheld for 7 days or longer. Hydration should be maintained with intravenous fluids; nutritional support may require feeding via a gastrostomy tube (see p. 74). Oral feeding with a low-fat gruel should be initiated as described for mild esophagitis and continued for 10 to 14 days. Feeding the animal with it standing on its hindlegs and with food elevated to mouth level may decrease regurgitation. Treatment with histamine-2 (H_2) antagonists such as cimetidine, ranitidine, or famotidine (Table 16-17) is useful to reduce gastric acidity and decrease esophageal mucosal damage if reflux occurs. However, omeprazole is needed in many patients with severe

esophagitis. Sucralfate slurries may be administered to protect denuded mucosa and reduce esophageal inflammation. Cisapride is used to increase the strength of gastric contractions, improve gastric emptying, and increase gastroesophageal sphincter pressure. Antibiotics should be provided that are effective against oral contaminants (e.g., ampicillin, amoxicillin, clindamycin, cephalosporins; Table 16-18). Concurrent corticosteroid therapy (i.e., prednisone at 0.5 mg/kg PO, BID) may decrease the risk of stenosis in animals with severe esophagitis; however, the benefit of this therapy is unproven.

NOTE • Lidocaine toxicity may be enhanced in patients who are given cimetidine concurrently.

Treatment of aspiration pneumonia should be initiated before esophageal surgery. If aspiration is observed while the animal is anesthetized, the airway should be suctioned to remove irritants. Fluid therapy is indicated if the animal is severely dyspneic or in shock. Nasal oxygen supplementation should be provided if the animal is severely dyspneic; positive pressure ventilation may be needed in unresponsive patients. Bronchodilators (i.e., aminophylline, oxtriphylline, terbutaline sulfate) may decrease bronchospasms and ventilatory muscle fatigue in these patients (see Table 16-18). Corticosteroids

TABLE 16-16

Preoperative Management of Patients with Esophageal Disorders

- Withhold food: mature animals—12 to 18 hours; pediatric animals—4 to 8 hours
- Correct fluid, electrolyte, and acid-base imbalances
- Give prophylactic antibiotics (i.e., ampicillin, cephalosporins)
- Support nutrition
- Treat esophagitis and aspiration pneumonia

TABLE 16-17

Treatment of Esophagitis

Cimetidine (Tagamet)
10 mg/kg PO, IV, SC, TID to QID

Ranitidine (Zantac)
2 mg/kg PO, IV, IM, BID

Famotidine (Pepcid)
0.5 mg/kg PO, SID to BID

Omeprazole (Prilosec)
0.7-1.5 mg/kg PO, SID

Sucralfate* (Carafate)
0.5-1.0 g PO, TID to QID

Cisapride (Propulsid)
Dogs—0.25-0.5 mg/kg PO, BID to TID
Cats—2.5-5.0 mg/cat PO, BID to TID

*Carafate impairs absorption and/or reduces bioavailability of cimetidine; give at different intervals.

TABLE 16-18

Treatment of Aspiration Pneumonia

Aminophylline
Dogs—11 mg/kg PO, IM, IV, TID
Cats—5 mg/kg PO, BID

Oxtriphylline Elixir (Choledyl SA)
Dogs—14-15 mg/kg PO, TID
Cats—6-8 mg/kg PO, BID to TID

Terbutaline (Brethine, Bricanyl)
Dogs—1.25-5.0 mg/dog SC, PO, BID to TID
Cats—1.25 mg/cat SC, PO, BID

Ampicillin
22 mg/kg IV, IM, SC, PO, TID to QID

Cefazolin (Ancef, Kefzol)
20 mg/kg IV, IM, TID

Clindamycin (Antirobe, Cleocin)
11 mg/kg PO, IV, BID

Enrofloxacin (Baytril)
5-10 mg/kg PO, IV, BID

Amikacin (Amiglyde-V)
10 mg/kg IV, IM, SC, TID or 30 mg/kg SID

Trimethoprim-Sulfadiazine (Tribrissen)
Dogs—15 mg/kg IM, PO, BID
Cats—15 mg/kg PO, BID

such as prednisone (0.25 mg/kg IV, BID) may be beneficial if the animal is in shock or severely dyspneic; however, they should be used with caution because they may interfere with host defense mechanisms. Expectorants (e.g., guaifenesin) are occasionally used in animals with productive coughs. Systemic antibiotic therapy is indicated in animals with pulmonary infection or sepsis. Broad-spectrum antibiotics (or combinations of antibiotics) effective against gram-negative and anaerobic bacteria should be used (e.g., clindamycin or ampicillin or cefazolin plus either enrofloxacin, amikacin, or trimethoprim-sulfadiazine; see Table 16-18). Antibiotic therapy should be based on results of culture and sensitivity, if possible.

☞ **N O T E** • Warning! Concurrent administration of aminophylline and ketamine lowers the seizure threshold.

ANESTHETIC CONSIDERATIONS

Fluid, electrolyte, and acid-base imbalances should be corrected before anesthetic induction. If feasible, mature animals should be fasted 12 to 18 hours before esophageal surgery; however, young puppies and kittens may be fasted for shorter periods (4 to 8 hours) to prevent hypoglycemia. Selected anesthetic protocols for stable patients undergoing cervical esophageal surgery are listed in Table 16-19. Procedures on the thoracic esophagus require modification of general anesthetic protocols to accommodate compromised function of the respiratory and cardiovascular systems. General recommendations for anesthesia in patients undergoing thoracic surgery are provided on p. 649. A mechanical ventilator is recommended. Nitrous oxide should not be used after the thorax is open because shunts develop. During lateral thoracotomy, large pulmonary shunts develop as the "up lung" receives most of the ventilation and the "down lung" receives more perfusion. Shunts can be minimized by compressing the up lung and increasing inflation pressures to 20 to 30 cm H_2O. The tidal volume (15 ml/kg) must be adequate to expand the lungs during thoracotomy. Inspiratory time should be kept between 1.0 and 1.5 seconds because prolonged duration may collapse alveolar capillaries and impede venous return. Respiratory rate should be between 6 to 10 breaths per minute. See p. 649 for recommendations for analgesics for patients undergoing thoracotomy. After anesthetic induction, suction of secretions and ingesta from the obstructed esophagus may help prevent aspiration and minimize contamination of the surgical site.

ANTIBIOTICS

Perioperative antibiotics may be given to prevent infection of periesophageal tissues. Prophylactic intravenous antibiotics should be given at the time of anesthetic induction and repeated 2 to 3 hours later. A third dose may be given 8 hours after the second dose. Broad-spectrum antibiotics effective against anaerobes (i.e., ampicillin, cephalosporins) are recommended. Animals with preoperative perforation or severe esophageal trauma should be treated with therapeutic antibiotics (see Table 16-18). Specimens collected from the surgical site or perforation should be submitted for bacterial culture and susceptibility. Duration of therapeutic antibiotics varies depending on the source of infection and contaminating organisms, but they should generally be continued for a minimum of 2 weeks.

SURGICAL ANATOMY

The cervical and proximal thoracic portions of the esophagus lie to the left of midline; however, the esophagus lies slightly to the right of midline from the tracheal bifurcation to the stomach. Layers of the esophageal wall include mucosa, submucosa, muscularis, and adventitia. The esophagus has no serosa; therefore early fibrin sealing of esophagotomy sites may be slower than other areas of the gastrointestinal tract. The submucosa is the holding layer of the esophagus and must be incorporated with all sutures. The normal canine esophagus has linear mucosal striations throughout its length. The distal portion of the feline esophagus usually has circular mucosal folds that form a herringbone pattern with positive contrast.

The vascular supply of the cervical esophagus is from branches of the thyroid and subclavian arteries. Bronchoesophageal arteries and segmental branches from the aorta supply the thoracic esophagus. The abdominal esophagus is supplied by branches from the left gastric and left phrenic arteries. Intramural branches ramify and anastomose within the submucosal layer. Collateral blood flow from the cervical and abdominal portions of the esophagus can provide the thoracic esophagus with adequate blood flow, provided the intramural esophageal vascular system is intact.

SURGICAL TECHNIQUES

Abnormalities of the cervical esophagus are approached using a ventral midline cervical incision. Thoracic esophageal abnormalities at the heart base are approached using a right

---

TABLE 16-19

Selected Anesthetic Protocols for Use in Animals with Cervical Esophageal Disorders

Premedication

Give atropine (0.02-0.04 mg/kg SC or IM) or glycopyrrolate (0.005-0.011 mg/kg SC or IM) plus oxymorphone* (0.05-0.1 mg/kg SC or IM) or butorphanol (0.2-0.4 mg/kg SC or IM), or buprenorphine (5-15 µg/kg IM).

Induction

Thiopental (10-12 mg/kg IV) or propofol (4-6 mg/kg IV). Alternately, use a combination of diazepam and ketamine (diazepam 0.27 mg/kg plus 5.5 mg/kg ketamine IV) titrated to effect.

Maintenance

Give isoflurane or halothane.

*Use 0.05 mg/kg in cats.

lateral thoracotomy, and those cranial or caudal to the heart, a left cranial or caudal thoracotomy. The abdominal esophagus is approached through a ventral midline celiotomy. Hair should be clipped from the entire ventral cervical area for surgery of the cervical esophagus and from the entire hemithorax for approaches to the thoracic esophagus. The skin should be aseptically prepared for surgery.

Approach to the Cervical Esophagus

Position the patient in dorsal recumbency (Fig. 16-36, A). Incise skin on the midline, beginning at the larynx and extending caudally to the manubrium. Incise and retract the platysma muscle and subcutaneous tissues. Separate the paired sternohyoid muscles along the midline to expose the underlying trachea (Fig. 16-36, B). Retract the thyroidea ima vein with the sternohyoid muscle or ligate it. If access is needed to the caudal cervical esophagus, separate and retract the sternocephalicus muscles. Retract the trachea to the right to expose the adjacent anatomic structures including the esophagus, the thyroid gland, cranial and caudal thyroid vessels, the recurrent laryngeal nerve, and the carotid sheath (vagosympathetic trunk, carotid artery, and internal jugular vein) (Fig. 16-36, C). Pass a stomach tube or esophageal stethoscope to facilitate identification of the esophagus and lesion. After completing the definitive procedure, lavage the surgical site with warmed sterile saline and return the trachea to its normal position. Close the incision by apposing the sternohyoid muscles using absorbable suture material (3-0 or 4-0) in a simple continuous suture pattern. Appose subcutaneous tissues with a simple continuous pattern (3-0 or 4-0) of absorbable suture material. Use nonabsorbable sutures (3-0 or 4-0 monofilament) and an appositional suture pattern to appose skin.

Approach to the Cranial Thoracic Esophagus via a Lateral Intercostal Thoracotomy

Position the patient in right lateral recumbency over a rolled towel placed perpendicular to the long axis of the

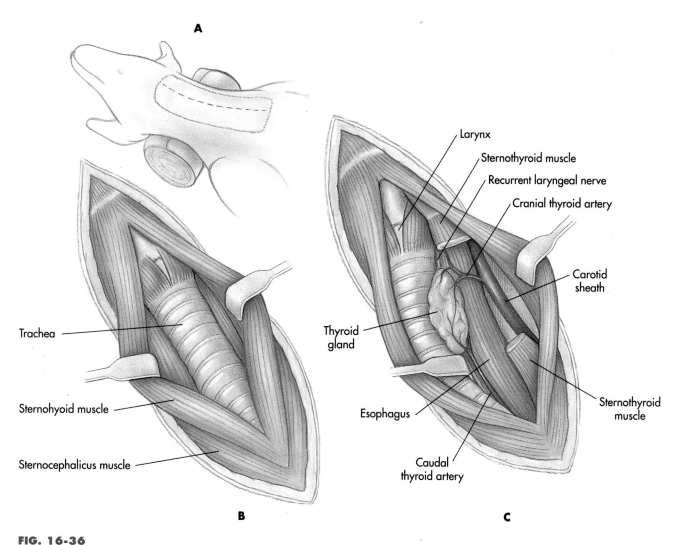

A

Larynx
Sternothyroid muscle
Recurrent laryngeal nerve
Cranial thyroid artery
Carotid sheath
Thyroid gland
Esophagus
Sternothyroid muscle
Caudal thyroid artery

Trachea
Sternohyoid muscle
Sternocephalicus muscle

B   **C**

FIG. 16-36
To approach the cervical esophagus, **A,** position the patient in dorsal recumbency with the neck resting on a rolled towel. **B,** Incise skin from the larynx to the manubrium and separate the sternohyoid muscles to expose the trachea. **C,** Retract the trachea to the right to expose the esophagus, thyroid, carotid sheath, and recurrent laryngeal nerve.

body (Fig. 16-37, A). Choose the appropriate intercostal space incision based on the radiographic location of the abnormality (Figs. 16-37, B–D). Most abnormalities cranial to the heart base can be accessed through a left third or fourth intercostal space incision (technique for thoracotomy is described on p. 651). *Identify the esophagus in the mediastinum dorsal to the brachiocephalic trunk (Fig. 16-37, E). Identification may be aided by passage of a stomach tube or by palpating the abnormality. Dissect the mediastinal pleura overlapping the esophagus to just above and below the proposed surgical site. Preserve the branch of the internal thoracic vein and the costocervical vein that cross the cranial esophagus.*

Approach to the Esophagus at the Heart Base via a Right Lateral Thoracotomy

The approach is the same as that for the cranial esophagus except the incision is made through the right fourth or fifth intercostal space (Fig. 16-38, A and B). *Identify the esophagus located just dorsal to the trachea in the mediastinum (Fig. 16-38, C). Dissect and retract the azygous vein from the esophagus to allow adequate exposure. Ligate the azygous vein if necessary to adequately expose the esophagus.* Closure is the same as for cranial thoracotomy.

Approach to the Caudal Esophagus via a Caudal Lateral Thoracotomy

Position the patient in lateral recumbency as described above for cranial lateral thoracotomy. Perform a caudal lateral thoracotomy (Fig. 16-39, A). Although the caudal esophagus can be approached through either a left or right eighth or ninth intercostal space incision, the left ninth space is preferred. *Expose the caudal esophagus by transecting the pulmonary ligament and packing the caudal lung lobes cranially. Identify the esophagus just ventral to the aorta (Fig. 16-39, B). Identify the dorsal and ventral vagal nerve branches on the lateral aspect of the esophagus and protect them.*

Esophagotomy

Pack off the esophagus from the remainder of the field with moistened laparotomy pads. Suction material from the cranial esophagus before making the esophagotomy incision to minimize contamination of the surgical site. If ingesta and secretions have not been completely suctioned, occlude the lumen cranial and caudal to the proposed esophagotomy site with fingers or noncrushing forceps. Place stay sutures adjacent to the proposed incision site to stabilize, aid manipulation, and avoid trauma to the esophageal edges. Make a stab incision into the lumen of the esophagus and extend the incision longitudinally as necessary to remove the foreign body or observe the lumen. Make the incision over the foreign body if the esophageal wall appears normal. If the wall appears compromised, make the incision caudal to the lesion or foreign body. Remove foreign bodies with forceps taking care to

avoid further esophageal trauma (tearing or perforation). Examine the esophageal lumen. Obtain culture specimens from necrotic and perforated areas. Debride and close perforations surrounded by healthy tissue that involve less than one fourth the circumference of the esophagus. Identify large necrotic areas or extensive perforations and perform a resection and anastomosis (see below).

Esophagotomy incisions may be closed with either a one- or two-layer closure. A two-layer simple interrupted closure results in greater immediate wound strength, better tissue apposition, and improved healing after esophagotomy but takes longer to perform than single-layer techniques. *Place each suture approximately 2 mm from the edge and 2 mm apart. Incorporate the mucosa and submucosa in the first layer of a two-layer simple interrupted closure. Place sutures so that the knots are within the esophageal lumen (Fig. 16-40, A). Incorporate adventitia, muscularis, and submucosa in the second layer of sutures with the knots tied extraluminally (Fig. 16-40, B and C). When a one-layer closure is used, pass each suture through all layers of the esophageal wall and tie the knots on the extraluminal surface. Check closure integrity by occluding the lumen, injecting saline, applying pressure, and observing for leakage between sutures.*

Partial Esophagectomy

Esophagectomy is performed to remove devitalized or diseased esophageal segments. Periesophageal tissues must be dissected from around the abnormal area to allow resection of diseased tissue and mobilization of normal esophagus; however, extensive dissection should be avoided to preserve vasculature. Excessive tension along the anastomosis may cause dehiscence. Although 20% to 50% of the esophagus has been resected and primarily anastomosed without tension relieving techniques, resection of more than 3 to 5 cm risks anastomotic dehiscence. Partial myotomy is recommended to relieve anastomotic tension when resecting large segments of esophagus (Fig. 16-41). Circumferential myotomy is a partial-thickness myotomy through the longitudinal muscle layers 2 to 3 cm cranial and caudal to the anastomosis. The inner circular muscle layers are not incised to avoid damaging the submucosal blood supply. Injection of saline into the muscularis may aid identification of the different muscle layers. The myotomy gap heals by second intention without stricture or dilation. Mobilizing the stomach cranially through an enlarged esophageal hiatus can also help reduce tension across the anastomosis. Other tension relieving techniques include interruption of the phrenic nerve and placement of "pexy" sutures between the esophagus and prevertebral fascia. Esophageal replacement may be necessary if segments of more than 3 to 5 cm are resected. Many replacement techniques have been described including microvascular anastomosis of the colon or small intestine to the esophagus, gastric tubes, skin tubes, and various prostheses. Replacement of the esophagus requires specialized training, techniques, and equipment to be successful.

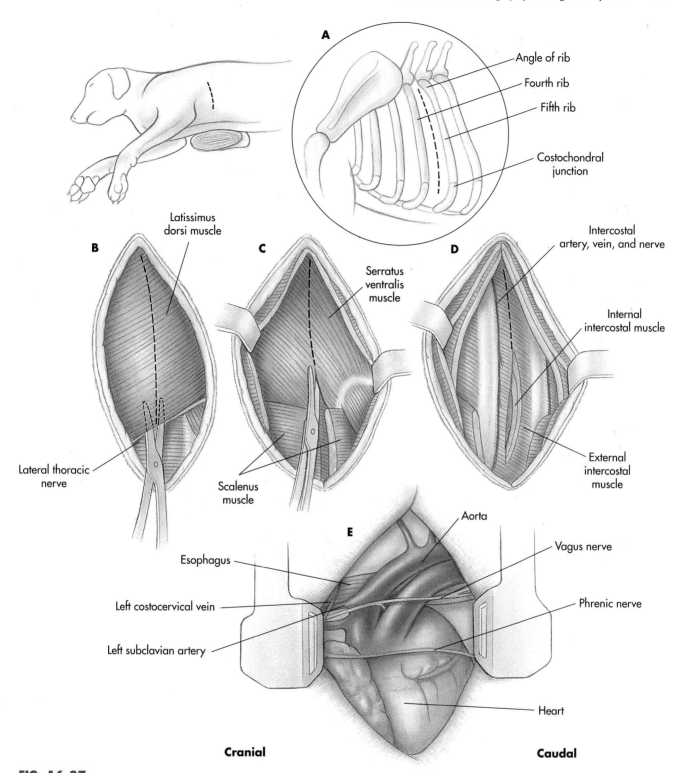

FIG. 16-37
To approach the cranial thoracic esophagus, **A,** position the patient in right lateral recumbency over a rolled towel placed perpendicular to the long axis of the body. **B,** Select the appropriate incision site based on the radiographic location of the lesion. Identify and transect the latissimus dorsi muscle. **C,** Identify and transect or retract the serratus ventralis and scalenus muscles. **D,** Expose and incise the intercostal muscles. **E,** Position rib retractors and identify the thoracic viscera.

FIG. 16-38
To approach the esophagus at the heart base, **A,** make an incision through the right fourth or fifth intercostal space. Identify and transect or retract the latissimus dorsi, serratus ventralis, scalenus, and external abdominal oblique muscles. **B,** Incise the intercostal muscles and **C,** expose the thoracic viscera.

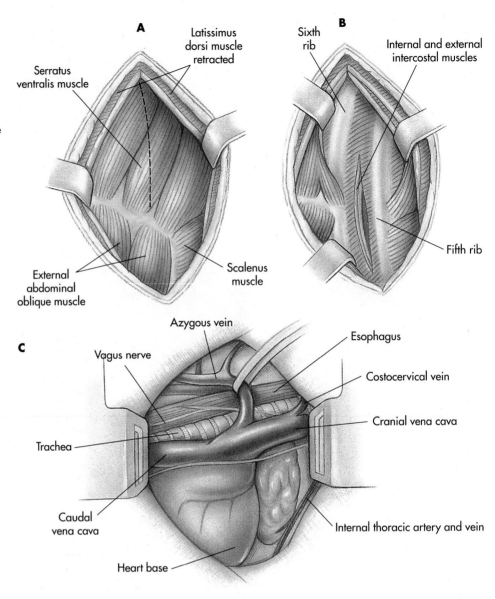

For esophagectomy occlude and stabilize the esophagus with fingers (scissor action of middle and index fingers) or noncrushing forceps. Resect the diseased portion of the esophagus (Fig. 16-42). Suction debris from the lumen of the remaining esophagus. Place three equally spaced stay sutures at each end of the remaining esophagus to facilitate gentle handling of the esophagus and help maintain apposition and alignment of the transected ends (see Fig. 16-42). Bring the esophageal ends into apposition with the stay sutures and suture it using a one- or two-layer closure as described for esophagotomy. Place sutures in the contralateral (far) wall first and then in the more accessible ipsilateral (near) wall. When using a two-layer closure, appose the esophagus in the following four steps (Fig. 16-43): (A) appose adventitia and muscularis of the contralateral wall around approximately one half of the esophageal circumference; (B) appose mucosa and submucosa of the contralateral wall; (C) appose mucosa and submucosa of the ipsilateral wall; and lastly (D) appose ad-

ventitia and muscularis of the ipsilateral wall. Check closure integrity by occluding the lumen, injecting saline, applying pressure, and observing for leakage between sutures.

Support or Patching Techniques

Augmentation of esophagotomy or esophagectomy sites with omentum or muscle can aid in healing by supporting, sealing, and revascularizing the surgical site. Muscle pedicles from the sternohyoid, sternothyroid, intercostal, diaphragm, or epaxial muscles can be mobilized and sutured over the primary repair or esophageal defect (Fig. 16-44, *A*). Alternatively, omentum can be mobilized from the abdomen, brought through a rent in the diaphragm, and sutured over the esophageal site (Fig. 16-44, *B*). Pedicles from the gastric wall and pericardium have also been used.

HEALING OF THE ESOPHAGUS

The esophagus is subject to constant movement from swallowing and respiration. This continuous motion may interfere

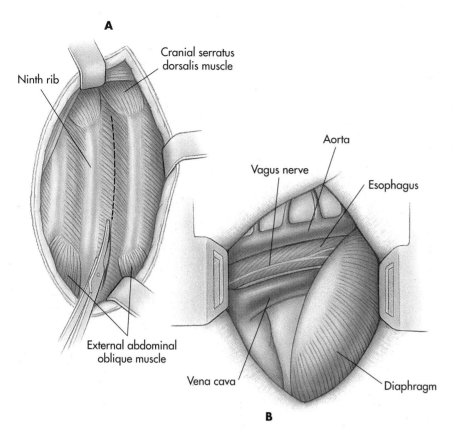

FIG. 16-39
To approach the caudal thoracic esophagus, position the animal in right lateral recumbency and make an eighth or ninth intercostal space incision. **A,** Identify and transect or retract the latissimus dorsi, cranial serratus dorsalis, external abdominal oblique, and intercostal muscles. **B,** Identify the diaphragm and other thoracic viscera.

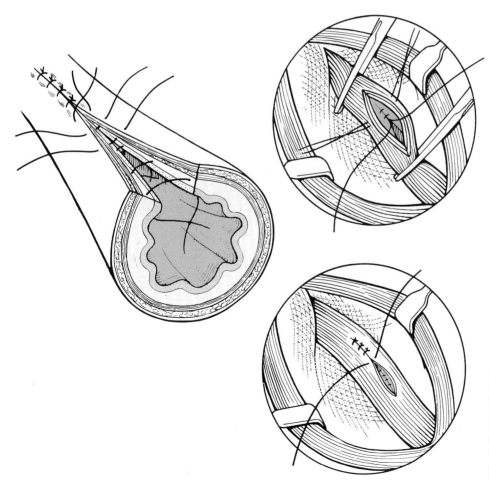

FIG. 16-40
A, For esophagotomy close mucosa and submucosa with simple interrupted sutures so the knots are intraluminal. **B** and **C,** Appose adventitia and muscularis with a second layer of simple interrupted sutures oriented with extraluminal knots.

FIG. 16-41
Tension relieving esophageal myotomy is performed 2 to 3 cm cranial and caudal to the anastomosis.

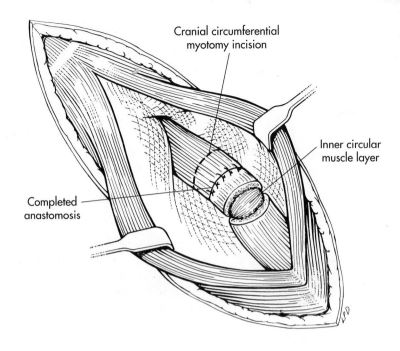

Cranial circumferential myotomy incision

Inner circular muscle layer

Completed anastomosis

Stay sutures

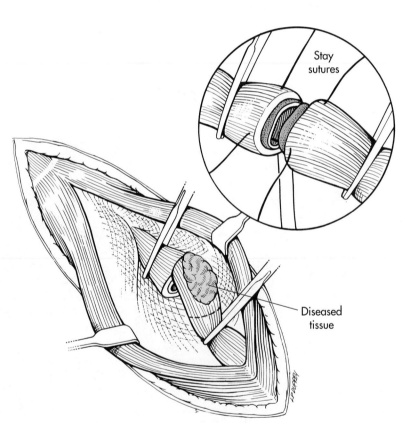

Diseased tissue

FIG. 16-42
For partial esophagectomy occlude the esophageal lumen with noncrushing forceps and mobilize and resect the diseased esophagus. Place stay sutures to manipulate the esophageal ends (*inset*). Anastomose the ends as illustrated in Fig. 16-43.

with healing and must be overcome with good surgical technique. Although large segments of the esophagus have been resected successfully, the esophagus does not tolerate longitudinal stretching well and may dehisce if tension is exces-

sive. Complications, particularly dehiscence, stricture, and fistulization, are common after esophageal surgery. The high complication rate has been blamed on the lack of serosal covering, lack of omentum, segmental blood supply, con-

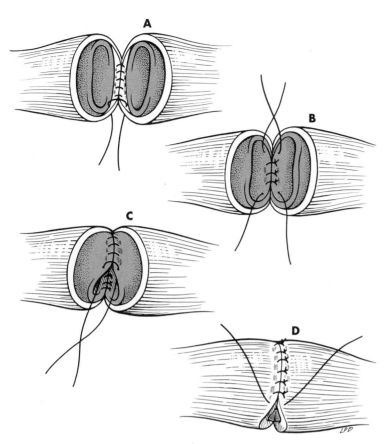

FIG. 16-43
During partial esophagectomy appose the ends with two layers of sutures in a four-step procedure. **A,** First, appose adventitia and muscularis on the far side with simple interrupted sutures and extraluminal knots. **B,** Then, appose submucosa and mucosa on the far side with simple interrupted sutures using intraluminal knots. **C,** Third, appose the near-side submucosa and mucosa, and **D,** lastly, appose the near-side muscularis and adventitia.

stant motion, and distention with passage of food boluses. Careful surgical technique and patient management can minimize most of the potential complicating factors.

SUTURE MATERIALS/ SPECIAL INSTRUMENTS

In addition to a general pack, special forceps (i.e., noncrushing Doyen forceps), delicate hemostats (i.e., Adson), Metzenbaum scissors, retractors (cervical approach—Gelpi retractors; thoracic approach—Finochietto retractors; malleable retractors), and tubes (chest tube, gastrostomy tube, stomach tube) may be necessary. A suction unit and laparotomy pads should also be available. Surgical stapling equipment (e.g., linear stapler, circular end-to-end stapler, ligate-and-divide vascular stapler, skin stapler) is beneficial but optional. Monofilament absorbable (polydioxanone, polyglyconate with a swaged-on taper point needle) and nonabsorbable (polypropylene, nylon with a reverse cutting needle) sutures (3-0 or 4-0) are recommended in the esophagus.

POSTOPERATIVE CARE AND ASSESSMENT

After esophageal surgery, analgesics should be provided as described for thoracotomy patients on p. 649. Air and fluid

must be evacuated via a thoracostomy tube or needle thoracentesis after thoracic procedures. Unless periesophageal or thoracic infection is anticipated, thoracostomy tubes can generally be removed within 8 to 12 hours after esophageal surgery. Nasal oxygen may benefit animals after thoracotomy (see Table 25-11 on p. 618).

Oral intake should be withheld for 24 to 48 hours. Intravenous fluids should be continued until oral intake resumes. Water may be offered 24 hours postoperatively if the esophagus is in good condition and regurgitation or vomiting does not occur. Blenderized food (gruel) may be offered during the next 24 hours if no vomiting or regurgitation occurs after water consumption. Blenderized food should be continued for 5 to 7 days and then the animal should be gradually returned to its normal diet over the next week. If oral intake is not anticipated or possible within 48 to 72 hours after surgery, feeding should be performed via a gastrostomy tube (see p. 74).

Esophagitis and aspiration pneumonia should be treated as described in the discussion on preoperative considerations (p. 232). Patients undergoing esophageal surgery should be closely monitored for fever and/or neutrophilia, which may indicate infection secondary to leakage. Dysphagia and regurgitation occurring 3 to 6 weeks after surgery may indicate esophageal stricture formation. It is extremely

FIG. 16-44

To patch the esophagus **A,** mobilize muscle adjacent to the esophagus and suture it over an esophageal incision to create an esophageal patch or **B,** mobilize omentum from the greater curvature of the stomach, pass it through an incision in the diaphragm, and suture it over the esophageal closure to create an omental patch.

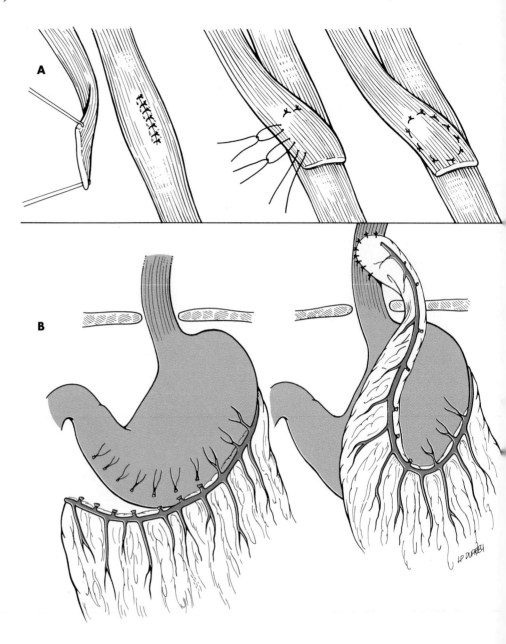

important that clients be informed of potential complications before and after surgery (Table 16-20).

COMPLICATIONS

Infection, regurgitation, pneumonia, esophagitis, dehiscence, fistula, stricture, and recurrence of disease are potential complications of esophageal surgery. Common errors in treating esophageal disorders include failure to immediately identify an esophageal foreign body, failure to recognize an esophageal perforation, failure to control esophagitis, selection of an inappropriate surgical approach, and failure to patch or support the esophagus appropriately.

SPECIAL AGE CONSIDERATIONS

Care must be used in anesthetizing young animals for esophageal surgery. Surgery is often performed in animals with persistent right aortic arches (see p. 258) or hiatal

TABLE 16-20

Client Education/Communication

- Regurgitating or vomiting may cause aspiration pneumonia, which can be fatal if not controlled.
- Surgery may not resolve all clinical signs of esophageal disease.
- Preventing oral intake, tube feeding, or elevated feeding may be necessary.
- Esophageal healing is poor compared to other parts of the gastrointestinal tract; therefore leakage, infection, dehiscence, and stricture are more common.
- Foreign bodies may perforate the esophagus or great vessels during extraction, with fatal results.
- Dogs should not be fed bones.

hernias (see p. 250) at 8 to 16 weeks of age. Perioperative hypothermia and hypoglycemia are common problems in these pediatric patients and may be life threatening.

Suggested Reading

Flanders JA: Problems and complications associated with esophageal surgery. In Matthiesen DT, editor: *Problems in veterinary medicine: gastrointestinal surgical problems,* Philadelphia, 1989, JB Lippincott.

Oakes MG et al: Esophagotomy closure in the dog: a comparison of a double-layer appositional and two single-layer appositional techniques, *Vet Surg* 22:451, 1993.

Stickle RL, Love NE: Radiographic diagnosis of esophageal disorders in dogs and cats, *Seminars in Veterinary Medicine and Surgery (Small Animal)* 4:179, 1989.

Waldron DR: Cervical and thoracic esophageal resection and anastomosis. In Bojrab MJ, editor: *Current techniques in small animal surgery,* ed 2, Philadelphia, 1983, Lea & Febiger.

SPECIFIC DISEASES

ESOPHAGEAL FOREIGN BODIES

DEFINITIONS

Foreign bodies are inanimate objects that may cause obstruction or partial obstruction of the esophageal lumen.

SYNONYMS

Foreign masses, foreign objects

GENERAL CONSIDERATIONS AND CLINICALLY RELEVANT PATHOPHYSIOLOGY

The most common foreign bodies are bones; although sharp metal objects (e.g., needles, fish hooks), balls, string, and an assortment of other objects have lodged in canine and feline esophagi. Foreign bodies lodge there because they are too large to pass or because they have sharp edges that become embedded in the esophageal mucosa. They are most commonly found at the thoracic inlet, heart base, or epiphrenic (diaphragm) area because extraesophageal structures limit esophageal dilation at these sites. The persistence of a foreign body (acting as a bolus) within the esophagus stimulates peristaltic activity. If the foreign body remains at one location for several days repeated peristaltic waves over the foreign body can produce pressure necrosis of the mucosa, submucosa, and external layers of the esophageal wall at contact points. Esophagitis results and interferes with esophageal motility and lower esophageal sphincter pressure. Food not passing the obstruction accumulates and may be regurgitated or cause proximal esophageal distention. Distention disrupts normal neuromuscular function and decreases peristalsis. Esophageal perforation is possible in any animal with an esophageal foreign body, and aspiration pneumonia (see p. 232) is a potential sequela in animals with regurgitation.

Sharp objects may abrade or lacerate the esophageal mucosa causing irritation and inflammation of the underlying tissues (esophagitis). Sharp objects may also perforate the esophageal wall and allow bacteria, ingesta, and secretions to contaminate the periesophageal tissues. Occasionally, sharp objects will perforate the esophageal wall and one of the great vessels at the heart base causing severe hemorrhage. Foreign bodies may penetrate the esophageal wall and establish a fistula with the trachea, bronchi, or pulmonary parenchyma.

DIAGNOSIS
Clinical Presentation

Signalment. Indiscriminate eaters (dogs) are more commonly affected than more particular eaters (cats). Although any breed of dog or cat may have an esophageal foreign body, small breed dogs are more frequently affected. Cats (having a tendency to play and hunt) more commonly present with string or needle foreign bodies than bones. Foreign bodies may occur in any age animal, but are most common during the first 3 years of life.

History. Animals may be presented within minutes of foreign body ingestion or weeks later. An acute onset of dysphagia and/or regurgitation are the initial clinical signs. Other signs may include gagging, excessive salivation, retching, inappetence, restlessness, depression, dehydration, and respiratory distress. Clinical signs are somewhat variable depending on duration, location, and type of obstruction. Patients with acute obstructions generally exhibit excess salivation and gag or regurgitate soon after eating. Weight loss and emaciation are sometimes seen in patients with long-term esophageal obstruction. Patients with complete obstructions regurgitate both solids and liquids while those with partial obstructions may retain liquids. Esophageal pain may cause anorexia. Foreign bodies impinging on the upper airways may cause acute respiratory distress. Sharp foreign bodies or those that have caused necrosis of the esophageal wall allow leakage of saliva and ingesta into the surrounding tissues causing inflammation and infection. These patients are likely to be anorexic, febrile, and/or dyspneic (due to pleural effusion). Hypovolemic shock can occur if a foreign body penetrates a major vessel adjacent to the esophagus. A history of being fed bones, getting into garbage, or roaming is consistent with foreign body ingestion.

Physical Examination Findings

Most patients are normal to slightly depressed and dehydrated on physical examination. If the foreign body is lodged in the cervical esophagus it may sometimes be palpated. Poor body condition may be present if the patient has been anorexic or regurgitating for several weeks. Abnormal lung sounds may be auscultated in patients with aspiration pneumonia.

Radiography/Ultrasonography/Endoscopy

Most foreign bodies (99%) are identified on good quality plain radiographs (Fig. 16-45). Foreign bodies are usually

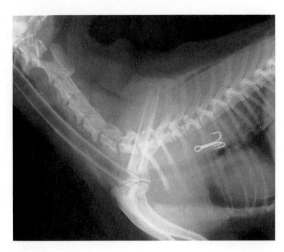

FIG. 16-45
Lateral thoracic radiograph showing an esophageal foreign body at the heart base in a dog.

found at or cranial to the thoracic inlet, heart base (approximately 10%), and diaphragm (approximately 85%). In addition to the foreign body there may be an adjacent soft tissue density (53%) and a dilated, air-filled cranial esophagus (21%) (Houlton et al, 1985). Pneumonia and tracheal distortion may also be present. Patients should be closely examined for signs of subcutaneous emphysema, pneumomediastinum, pleural effusion, or pneumothorax that suggest esophageal perforation. Esophograms are sometimes necessary to identify foreign bodies and perforations. Water-soluble, organic, iodine contrast materials or iohexol are recommended if esophageal perforation is suspected. However, if a bronchoesophageal fistula is suspected, an iodinated contrast agent should not be used because its hypertonicity may cause pulmonary edema. The presence of a foreign body may mask identification of a perforation during an esophogram. Foreign bodies can also be diagnosed endoscopically.

Laboratory Findings

With acute obstructions laboratory findings are normal. Perforation usually causes a neutrophilic leukocytosis. Hypoglycemia may be seen in young patients unable to eat and/or in septic shock.

DIFFERENTIAL DIAGNOSIS

Vascular ring anomalies, extraluminal masses, esophageal neoplasia, strictures, esophagitis, gastroesophageal intussusception, esophageal diverticula, hiatal hernias, megaesophagus, and cricopharyngeal dysfunction are other potential causes of regurgitation that must be differentiated from esophageal foreign bodies.

SURGICAL TREATMENT

Most esophageal foreign bodies (80% to 90%) can be successfully removed by nonsurgical means. During endoscopic procedures the neck is extended and the esophagus is insuf-

flated carefully to avoid rupturing weakened areas or causing tension pneumothorax. Forcing an object that is firmly embedded in the esophageal wall is contraindicated because doing so may cause perforation or enlargement of a preexisting perforation. Embedded fishhooks are an exception to this policy; however, care must be used to avoid lacerating vessels during their removal. After removal via endoscopy or gastrotomy, the esophagus must be reevaluated for evidence of perforation. This is done by careful endoscopic evaluation and/or radiography. Perforations should be surgically managed with debridement and closure (see p. 236).

Preoperative Management

Therapy to correct dehydration and electrolyte and acid-base imbalances should be initiated before surgery. Prophylactic antibiotics should be given (see p. 234).

Anesthesia

Anesthetic management of patients undergoing esophageal surgery is provided on p. 234. Deep general anesthesia or muscle relaxants that reduce esophageal tone facilitate endoscopic manipulations. Nitrous oxide should not be used in these patients. Animals with pneumonia should be given oxygen before anesthetic induction, and frequent ventilation and high inspired oxygen concentrations should be used during surgery.

Surgical Anatomy

Surgical anatomy of the esophagus is described on p. 234.

SURGICAL TECHNIQUE

Foreign bodies may be removed by extracting them endoscopically with grasping instruments or a balloon catheter as described below, advancing them into the stomach where they are allowed to dissolve, or they can be removed via gastrotomy (see p. 263 and p. 277), or by performing an esophagotomy or partial esophagectomy (see p. 236).

An alternative to grasping the foreign body is to pass a balloon catheter distal to the object (Fig. 16-46). The esophageal lumen is then dilated beyond its normal size by inflating the balloon, and the object is disengaged from the esophageal wall by endoscopic manipulations if necessary and removed as the catheter is pulled out through the mouth. This procedure is advisable only for foreign bodies with a relatively smooth contour. After nonsurgical foreign body removal, radiographs may be performed to look for evidence of perforation (e.g., pneumomediastinum, pneumothorax).

Distal esophageal foreign bodies are occasionally removed via a gastrotomy. An incision is made midway between the greater and lesser curvature. A forceps is directed into the distal esophagus, the object is grasped, and it is then pulled into the stomach and removed. Esophagotomy or partial esophagectomy is performed when foreign bodies are not successfully removed by other means, the risk of esophageal perforation or laceration is high, or evidence of mediastinitis, pleuritis, or esophageal necrosis exists. All esophageal disruptions are debrided if necessary and closed

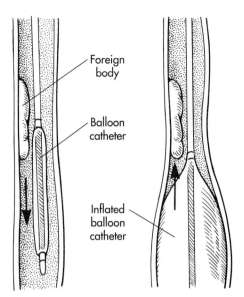

FIG. 16-46
Smooth esophageal foreign bodies can be removed via balloon retraction. Pass the catheter distal to the foreign body, then inflate the balloon and withdraw the catheter and foreign body.

in one or two layers as for esophagotomy. Abnormal communications between the alimentary and respiratory tracts (i.e., bronchoesophageal or tracheoesophageal fistula) must be closed. Partial or complete pulmonary lobectomy (see p. 655) is required with some bronchoesophageal fistulae.

POSTOPERATIVE CARE AND ASSESSMENT

All patients should be observed carefully for 2 to 3 days for signs of esophageal leakage and infection. Esophagitis and aspiration pneumonia should be treated as described on p. 232. Antibiotics should be continued for several days if the esophageal mucosa is severely eroded or lacerated. Intravenous fluids should be continued until feeding resumes. To avoid delays in healing, all oral intake (food, water, medications) should be withheld for a minimum of 24 hours after foreign body removal. If no regurgitation has been observed, water and then a bland gruel should be gradually introduced. Animals with minimal esophageal trauma may be offered water within 24 to 48 hours, followed by small meals of gruel. After 3 to 7 days of gruel feeding, soft, moist food should then be offered for 5 to 7 days, followed by a gradual return to a normal diet. Animals with moderate to severe esophageal trauma should avoid oral intake for 3 to 7 days. In debilitated patients or those requiring no oral intake for longer than 3 days, gastrostomy feeding tubes should be placed (see p. 74). Severe esophagitis should be treated with H_2 antagonists or proton pump inhibitors to reduce gastric acidity, sucralfate to protect denuded mucosa, and cisapride to empty the stomach (see p. 233). Antibiotics effective against oral anaerobes (ampicillin, amoxicillin, clindamycin; see p. 234) are indicated and corticosteroids may help prevent cicatrix forma-

tion. Analgesics should be provided to control pain (see Table 16-4).

Complications of foreign body removal include esophagitis, ischemic necrosis, dehiscence, leakage, infection, fistulae, esophageal diverticula, and stricture formation. Esophageal perforation may lead to mediastinitis, pleuritis, and pyothorax. Prolonged duration of clinical signs and increased numbers of immature neutrophils may suggest esophageal perforation; however, perforation is best diagnosed radiographically.

PROGNOSIS

Foreign body removal is essential. The prognosis is good if perforation has not occurred; however, it is guarded if perforation has resulted in mediastinitis and/or pyothorax. Foreign bodies that are removed often cause ischemic necrosis or perforation of the esophagus. Leakage of saliva and ingesta into the mediastinum or pleural cavity usually causes severe inflammation, infection, and death.

Reference

Houlton JEF et al: Thoracic esophageal foreign bodies in the dog: a review of ninety cases, *J Small Anim Pract* 26:521, 1985.

Suggested Reading

Parker NR, Walter PA, Gay J: Diagnosis and surgical management of esophageal perforation, *J Am Anim Hosp Assoc* 25:587, 1989.
Ryan WW, Greene RW: The conservative management of esophageal foreign bodies and their complications: a review of 66 cases in dogs and cats, *J Am Anim Hosp Assoc* 11:243, 1975.
Spielman BL, Shaker EH, Garvey MS: Esophageal foreign body in dogs: a retrospective study of 23 cases, *J Am Anim Hosp Assoc* 28:570, 1992.

ESOPHAGEAL STRICTURES

DEFINITIONS

Esophageal strictures are bands of intraluminal or intramural fibrous tissue that may cause obstruction or partial obstruction of the esophagus.

SYNONYMS

Esophageal stenosis, esophageal cicatrix

GENERAL CONSIDERATIONS AND CLINICALLY RELEVANT PATHOPHYSIOLOGY

Esophageal strictures may occur as a result of esophageal foreign bodies, surgery, esophagitis, or caustic agents. Stricture occurs more commonly after circumferential esophageal trauma. To produce a stricture, esophageal damage must involve the muscular layers and affect most of the circumference in a focal area. The mucosal defect is then replaced by epithelial migration. The gap in the muscle is filled by fibrous connective tissue, and the width of the scar is decreased by wound contraction and collagen remodeling. This leads to narrowing of the esophageal lumen and may cause obstruction. The degree of obstruction varies depending on the severity of the original lesion. Peristaltic waves carrying food boluses are disrupted by the obstruction. In cases of partial obstruction, part of each bolus passes the obstruction and moves down the esophagus. The other portion of the bolus accumulates proximal to the obstruction, and the proximal esophagus gradually distends. The distention disrupts normal neuromuscular function and decreases peristalsis. Accumulated food and secretions are frequently regurgitated.

Gastroesophageal reflux may occur during general anesthesia when protective mechanisms are decreased and the gastroesophageal sphincter loses tone. Gastric acid causes severe damage to the esophagus if not neutralized by saliva or removed by peristalsis within a few minutes. Signs of regurgitation may become evident 1 to 5 weeks after surgery because of stricture formation.

DIAGNOSIS
Clinical Presentation
Signalment. Any age, breed, or sex of dog or cat may be affected.

History. Regurgitation is the most common presenting sign, and stricture should be suspected in animals experiencing frequent regurgitation with a history of previous esophageal trauma or surgery. Some animals retain fluids but regurgitate solids. Pain may be experienced when solid food becomes lodged in the stricture by forceful esophageal peristaltic waves.

Physical Examination Findings
Although animals with esophageal strictures may be thin and depressed, physical examination is usually normal. Occasionally, the cervical esophagus is dilated.

Radiography/Ultrasonography/Endoscopy
Esophageal strictures can be difficult to identify. Positive contrast esophagrams facilitate diagnosis (Fig. 16-47). Partial strictures are more readily identified if barium is mixed with food. Dilation of the esophagus is identified proximal to an abrupt narrowing or stricture. Fluoroscopy can be used to assess esophageal motility during swallowing. It may be difficult to determine the entire extent of a stricture radiographically. Esophagoscopy allows visualization (plus biopsy usually) of the lesion. The mucosa is sometimes inflamed with erosions and ulcers, and sometimes the stricture is a ring of white fibrous tissue that narrows the esophageal lumen and fails to distend with insufflation. It may be impossible to advance the scope beyond the stricture in severe cases, and gastric overdistension can be a significant complication of esophagoscopy if the scope cannot be passed into the stomach to suction excess air. Biopsy and histologic examination rule out stricture secondary to neoplasia.

Laboratory Findings
Specific laboratory abnormalities are not present in animals with esophageal strictures.

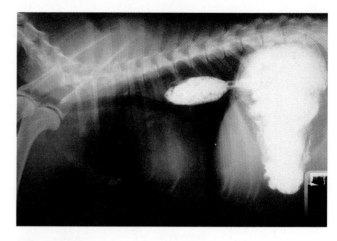

FIG. 16-47
Radiographic appearance of an esophageal stricture after administration of barium.

DIFFERENTIAL DIAGNOSIS
Vascular ring anomalies, extraluminal masses, esophageal neoplasia, foreign bodies, esophagitis, gastroesophageal intussusception, esophageal diverticulum, hiatal hernias, megaesophagus, and cricopharyngeal dysfunction are other potential causes of regurgitation that must be differentiated from esophageal stricture.

SURGICAL TREATMENT
Strictures are treated by correcting the cause and then reducing the narrowing with balloon catheter dilation or bouginage. Balloon catheter dilation is the preferred method for dilation of esophageal strictures because there is less chance of perforation and fewer dilations are required. Partial esophagectomy is usually not necessary and may not be possible, depending on the length of the stricture. Resistant cervical strictures may be corrected by the creation of a traction diverticulum.

Preoperative Management
Animals should be fasted before esophageal dilation. Treatment for esophagitis and aspiration pneumonia should be initiated before stricture treatment (see p. 232).

Anesthesia
General anesthesia is required for esophageal dilation or bouginage. Recommendations for anesthesia in patients with esophageal disorders are on p. 234.

Surgical Anatomy
Surgical anatomy of the esophagus is discussed on p. 234.

Positioning
Balloon dilation and bouginage are generally performed with the patient in lateral recumbency.

SURGICAL TECHNIQUE
Bouginage involves the dilation of a stricture using blunt dilators that are graduated in size. A thoroughly lubricated,

small, tapered probe (dilator) is initially pushed through the stricture into the distal esophagus. It is followed by a graduated series of successively larger probes until the desired lumen size is achieved or excess resistance is encountered. Bouginage exerts a longitudinal shearing force at the stricture site that is more likely than balloon dilation to result in perforation.

Balloon dilation of strictures may be done with the aid of an endoscope. *First, endoscopically place a guide wire through the stricture site. Use a wire that is stiff at one end and floppy at the other. Insert the floppy end of the wire through the scope's biopsy channel and through the stricture. Then withdraw the endoscope from the patient while continually feeding the wire into the patient, thus removing the endoscope from around the wire while the latter is kept in the stricture. Next place the balloon in the stricture by running the balloon catheter over the wire while observing it endoscopically. Once the balloon is positioned so that the middle of it is near the center of the stricture, inflate the balloon with fluid or air (depending on the type of balloon) and deflate it after a minute or so.* The balloon must stay in the stricture during this process. If the balloon is not correctly positioned, it will migrate out of the stricture as it is inflated and the stricture will not be dilated. Progressively larger balloons may be used until the desired degree of dilation is achieved.

POSTOPERATIVE CARE AND ASSESSMENT

Patients should be monitored closely for signs of perforation. Antibiotics may be used to help prevent infection. Corticosteroids (prednisolone, 0.5 mg/kg PO, BID) may be administered for a minimum of 2 weeks after the last dilation to help prevent stricture reformation, but the efficacy of this treatment is unknown. Repeat dilation is often necessary within 4 to 7 days. Preexisting esophagitis and aspiration pneumonia should be treated as described on p. 232. Nasal oxygen may benefit these animals postoperatively, and analgesics should be provided if necessary. Gastrostomy tube placement (see p. 74) may be beneficial in these patients so that oral feeding can be avoided for 7 to 10 days. If there is a substantial mucosal tear as a result of the procedure, antibiotics, antacids, and/or carafate may be administered (see Tables 16-17 and 16-18).

☞ **N O T E** • Clinical signs may be improved after therapy even though the stricture may not be resolved.

PROGNOSIS

Most patients with esophageal strictures can be helped by dilation, but strictures may reform. Thin stricture bands may require only one dilation. Patients with severe or long strictures often require multiple dilations. Care should be used because the stricture may perforate with excessive dilation. Resection of long strictures may result in dehiscence as a result of excessive anastomotic tension.

Suggested Reading

Burk RL, Zawie DA, Garvey MS: Balloon catheter dilation of intramural esophageal strictures in the dog and cat: a description of the procedure and a report of six cases, *Sem Vet Med Surgery* 2:241, 1987.

Golden DL, Henderson RA, Brewer WG: Use of an argon laser for transendoscopic radial incision of an esophageal web in a cat, *J Am Anim Hosp Assoc* 30:29, 1994.

Johnson KA, Maddison JE, Allan GS: Correction of cervical esophageal stricture in a dog by creation of a traction diverticulum, *J Am Vet Med Assoc* 201:1045, 1992.

Sooy TE et al: Balloon catheter dilatation of alimentary tract strictures in the dog and cat, *Radiology* 28:131, 1987.

ESOPHAGEAL DIVERTICULA

DEFINITIONS

Esophageal diverticula are saclike dilatations that produce pouches in the wall of the esophagus. A **pulsion diverticulum** is a herniation of the mucosa through the muscular layers of the esophagus. They are produced by exaggerated intraluminal pressure in association with abnormal regional peristalsis, or when obstruction interferes with normal peristalsis. **Traction diverticula** are distortions, angulations, or funnel-shaped bulges of the full-thickness wall of the esophagus, caused by adhesions resulting from an external lesion.

GENERAL CONSIDERATIONS AND CLINICALLY RELEVANT PATHOPHYSIOLOGY

Esophageal diverticula are rare. They may be acquired or congenital and are found most commonly in the distal cervical esophagus cranial to the thoracic inlet or in the distal thoracic esophagus just cranial to the diaphragm (epiphrenic). Congenital diverticula are believed to develop as a result of a congenital weakness of the esophageal wall, abnormal separation of tracheal and esophageal embryonic buds, or eccentric vacuole formation in the esophagus. Acquired forms are classified as pulsion or traction diverticula based on their cause. Pulsion diverticula are most common in the epiphrenic area but can form cranial to any diseased esophageal segment. Many conditions may initiate diverticulum formation, including esophagitis, esophageal stenosis, foreign bodies, vascular ring anomalies, neuromuscular dysfunction, and hiatal hernias. The esophageal mucosa herniates secondary to increased intraluminal pressure, food accumulation, and esophageal inflammation. The wall of a pulsion diverticulum consists of only esophageal epithelium and connective tissue.

Traction diverticula occur following an inflammatory process involving the trachea, bronchi, lymph nodes, or other extraesophageal structures. Inflammation causes fibrous tissue to form between the esophagus and the diseased structure. As the fibrous tissue matures it contracts and pulls an area of the esophagus outward to form a pouch. Most traction diverticula occur in the cranial and midthoracic esophagus. The wall of a traction diverticulum consists of adventitia, muscle, submucosa, and mucosa.

DIAGNOSIS
Clinical Presentation

Signalment. Any age, breed, or sex of dog or cat may be affected.

History. Small diverticula can be asymptomatic. Large, multilobulated diverticula are usually associated with clinical signs. Diverticula may result in esophageal impaction, chronic esophagitis, and diverticulum wall rupture with resultant mediastinitis or esophagotracheal/bronchial fistula formation. Clinical signs may include distress or gasping after eating, postprandial regurgitation, intermittent anorexia, fever, weight loss, thoracic or abdominal pain, and respiratory distress.

Physical Examination Findings

Physical examination is normal if the diverticulum is asymptomatic. Abnormal lung sounds may be auscultated if aspiration pneumonia has occurred.

Radiography/Ultrasonography/Endoscopy

Radiographs should be taken with the neck in an extended position to diminish "normal" esophageal redundancy in young and brachycephalic breeds. Diverticula appear as air-filled or food-filled masses in the area of the esophagus (Fig. 16-48). Dogs with generalized megaesophagus who tend to have greater out-pouching of the esophageal wall cranial to the heart base should not be misdiagnosed as having diverticula. An esophagram usually demonstrates a deviation or out-pouching of the esophageal lumen that fills partially or completely with contrast material. Esophagoscopy is helpful in confirming the radiographic diagnosis and identifying associated esophagitis, strictures, or other abnormalities. The esophageal wall may be very thin and esophagoscopy must be performed with care.

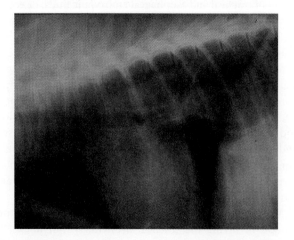

FIG. 16-48
Radiographic appearance of a caudal esophageal diverticulum. Note the air-distended esophageal pouch.

Laboratory Findings

Specific laboratory abnormalities are not found with esophageal diverticula. Laboratory findings consistent with pyothorax (see p. 699) may be found if the diverticulum has ruptured. Neutrophilia may be present if aspiration pneumonia has occurred.

DIFFERENTIAL DIAGNOSIS

Esophageal hiatal hernia, gastroesophageal intussusception, stricture, neoplasia, extraluminal masses, vascular ring anomaly, esophageal foreign body, esophagitis, and megaesophagus are other potential causes of regurgitation.

SURGICAL TREATMENT

Persistent underlying causes must be identified and treated. Asymptomatic, small diverticula may be treated by feeding a soft, bland diet with the animal in an upright position to avoid food accumulation in the pouch. Large diverticula should be surgically excised.

Preoperative Management

Esophagitis and aspiration pneumonia should be treated preoperatively as described on p. 232. Prophylactic antibiotics are indicated if esophageal resection is considered likely.

Anesthesia

Anesthetic recommendations for animals undergoing cervical esophageal surgery are discussed on p. 234. Anesthetic recommendations for thoracotomy are on p. 649.

Surgical Anatomy

Surgical anatomy of the esophagus is described on p. 234.

Positioning

Patients are positioned in dorsal or lateral recumbency, depending on the site of the diverticulum. Radiographs are important to help determine the best surgical approach. Diverticula in the cervical esophagus are approached via a ventral cervical midline incision with the animal in dorsal recumbency. Thoracic diverticula are usually approached via a lateral thoracotomy. Occasionally, a median sternotomy or thoracic wall flap may be necessary to approach diverticula at the thoracic inlet or cranial mediastinum.

SURGICAL TECHNIQUE

Following identification of the diverticulum, isolate it from surrounding structures with blunt and sharp dissection and then pack it off with laparotomy pads. Partial lung lobectomy may be necessary if adhesions are not easily separated. Position a TA or GIA stapling device along the base of the diverticulum and fire. Transect and remove the diverticulum without contaminating the surgical site. If stapling equipment is not available, suction the esophageal lumen and place noncrushing forceps across the proposed transection site. Transect the diverticulum and appose the edges as for esophagotomy with a one- or two-layer simple appositional pattern (see p. 236). Lavage the surgical site and, if possible, mobilize and place omentum over the incision. Thoracostomy tubes may be placed in animals having thoracotomies to evacuate residual air and fluid.

POSTOPERATIVE CARE AND ASSESSMENT

Postoperatively, these patients should be monitored for esophagitis and aspiration pneumonia and treated appropriately (see p. 232). Postoperative esophagoscopy and esophograms may be indicated if problems are detected. Regurgitation secondary to persistent esophagitis is a potential problem. Infection as a result of contamination of the surrounding tissues at surgery, dehiscence, or leakage at the surgical site are other potential problems. Postoperative analgesics should be provided to control pain (see p. 649 for recommendations after thoracotomy).

PROGNOSIS

Asymptomatic patients often continue to do well without surgery; feeding them in an upright position to avoid food accumulation in the diverticula may be helpful. It may be difficult to control clinical signs in symptomatic patients with medical therapy alone. If surgery is not possible, such patients should be treated for esophagitis and fed soft food in an upright position. The prognosis with surgical correction is good if thoracic contamination is avoided and good esophageal apposition is achieved.

Suggested Reading

Faulkner RT et al: Epiphrenic esophageal diverticulectomy in a dog: a case report and review, *J Am Anim Hosp Assoc* 17:77, 1981.

Lewis DT et al: What's your diagnosis? *J Am Vet Med Assoc* 196:1523, 1990.

ESOPHAGEAL NEOPLASIA

DEFINITIONS

Esophageal neoplasia is any abnormal, noninflammatory proliferation of cells in the esophagus.

GENERAL CONSIDERATIONS AND CLINICALLY RELEVANT PATHOPHYSIOLOGY

Neoplasia of the esophagus is rare. The most common types of tumors include sarcomas, squamous cell carcinomas, and leiomyomas. These tumors are usually advanced by the time clinical signs are recognized. Primary esophageal carcinomas are of unknown etiology. Primary esophageal sarcomas (osteosarcoma, fibrosarcoma) are often located in the vicinity of parasitic granulomas caused by *Spirocerca lupi*. The life cycle of *S. lupi* involves a coprophagous beetle that is eaten by the dog, or a transport host that is subsequently eaten by the dog. Regional tumors from the thyroid, thymus, heart base, or lung may invade the esophagus secondarily.

Esophageal tumors initially cause partial obstruction of the esophagus, which may interfere with motility and lead to dilation of the proximal esophagus. As the tumor enlarges, signs of complete esophageal obstruction become apparent. Most esophageal tumors are locally invasive and metastasize to draining lymph nodes.

DIAGNOSIS
Clinical Presentation

Signalment. In cats, squamous cell carcinomas are usually seen in females in the middle third of the esophagus just caudal to the thoracic inlet. Most esophageal tumors occur in dogs and cats over 6 to 8 years of age.

History. Chronic progressive signs of obstructive esophageal disease in middle-aged to older animals suggest esophageal neoplasia. Animals with primary tumors may be asymptomatic until the mass becomes large enough to cause signs of esophageal obstruction. These animals may present for regurgitation, drooling, dysphagia, anorexia, weight loss, and/or fetid breath. In animals with secondary tumors, clinical signs may include regurgitation, dyspnea, palpable masses, and/or systemic and local tumor effects.

Physical Examination Findings

Physical examination is usually normal. Some animals are thin and a dilated cervical esophagus may be identified. Hypertrophic osteopathy and spondylosis deformans may be noted, especially with *S. lupi*–induced sarcomas. Pneumonia secondary to aspiration may be present.

Radiography/Ultrasonography/Esophagoscopy

Aerophagia, displacement of the esophagus, and megaesophagus are signs of esophageal neoplasia. Survey thoracic radiographs may be normal or reveal a soft tissue density in the region of the esophagus (Fig. 16-49). The esophagus may retain

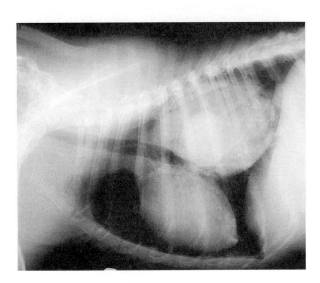

FIG. 16-49
Lateral thoracic radiograph of an 8-year-old dog with a large esophageal carcinoma.

air cranial to the tumor. The lungs should be evaluated for metastatic lesions. Contrast esophagrams may demonstrate an intraluminal mass (mucosal irregularities, filling defects, or stricture) with primary tumors, or an impinging extraluminal mass with secondary tumors. Fluoroscopic studies may reveal abnormal motility. Dogs with *S. lupi* commonly have spondylosis deformans plus or minus hypertrophic osteopathy. Esophagoscopy allows direct visualization of intraluminal masses and biopsy for definitive diagnosis (Fig. 16-50). An adult *S. lupi* is occasionally seen protruding into the lumen from the mass. Extraluminal masses cannot be visualized unless they have eroded into the lumen. It is difficult to inflate the lumen if it is being impinged on or invaded by extraluminal masses. Severe spondylosis of the cervical vertebrae is common with *Spirocerca* lesions.

Laboratory Findings

Laboratory values may indicate chronic disease or paraneoplastic syndromes. *S. lupi* eggs may be detected on a fecal sedimentation test but are usually difficult to find.

DIFFERENTIAL DIAGNOSIS

Esophageal stricture, extraluminal masses, vascular ring anomaly, esophageal foreign body, esophagitis, gastroesophageal intussusception, esophageal diverticulum, hiatal hernia, and megaesophagus are other potential causes of regurgitation.

SURGICAL TREATMENT

It is important to make an early diagnosis before metastasis or extensive esophageal involvement has occurred. Partial esophagectomy with end-to-end anastomosis is indicated when approximation can be accomplished without excess tension.

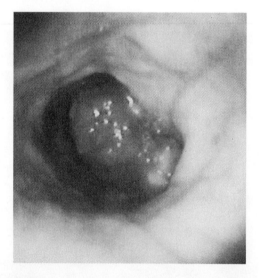

FIG. 16-50
Appearance of the mass in Fig. 16-49 on esophagoscopy. Esophagoscopy allows biopsy of intraluminal masses.

Preoperative Management

Medical treatment (anthelmentics; fenbendazole, 50 mg/kg PO; ivermectin, 50–200 µg/kg PO; disophenol, 10 mg/kg SC; or diethylcarbamazine, 20–500 mg/kg PO) can be attempted for *S. lupi,* but if a sarcoma is already present, treatment is not recommended.

Anesthesia

Anesthetic recommendations for animals undergoing cervical esophageal surgery are provided on p. 234. Selected anesthetic protocols for animals undergoing thoracic surgery are provided on p. 650.

Surgical Anatomy

Surgical anatomy of the esophagus is described on p. 234.

SURGICAL TECHNIQUE

Esophagectomy is described on p. 236.

POSTOPERATIVE CARE AND ASSESSMENT

Esophagitis and aspiration pneumonia should be monitored for and treated as needed postoperatively (see p. 232). Nasal oxygen may benefit these animals and analgesics should be provided to control pain. See p. 241 for recommendations for postoperative care of animals undergoing esophageal surgery. Dehiscence resulting from excessive tension at the anastomosis and tumor recurrence are potential complications of esophageal surgery.

PROGNOSIS

Most esophageal tumors are advanced at the time of diagnosis and do not respond well to radiation therapy or chemotherapy. Radiation therapy may be palliative, but radiation-induced esophagitis or damage to the heart, lungs, and great vessels are potential sequelae that are poorly tolerated. With surgery the prognosis is guarded for cure or palliation because resection is difficult as a result of the advanced nature of most tumors at the time of detection.

Suggested Reading

Fox SM, Burns J, Hawkins J: Spirocercosis in dogs, *Compend Cont Educ Pract Vet* 10:807, 1988.

Johnson RC: Canine spirocercosis and associated esophageal sarcoma, *Compend Cont Educ Pract Vet* 14:577, 1992.

Ridgway RL, Suter PF: Clinical and radiographic signs in primary and metastatic esophageal neoplasms of the dog, *J Am Vet Med Assoc* 174:700, 1979.

HIATAL HERNIAS

DEFINITIONS

Hiatal hernias are protrusions of the abdominal esophagus, gastroesophageal junction, and sometimes a portion of the gastric fundus through the esophageal hiatus into the caudal mediastinum cranial to the diaphragm.

GENERAL CONSIDERATIONS AND CLINICALLY RELEVANT PATHOPHYSIOLOGY

Hiatal hernias are usually caused by congenital abnormalities of the hiatus that allow cranial movement of the abdominal esophagus and stomach. The phrenicoesophageal ligament is lax or stretched and allows the gastroesophageal junction to be displaced through the hiatus into the caudal mediastinum. Malpositioning or lack of support of the gastroesophageal sphincter reduces gastroesophageal sphincter pressure and leads to gastroesophageal reflux. Gastroesophageal reflux and subsequent esophagitis and megaesophagus are responsible for most of the clinical signs. Hiatal hernia is occasionally secondary to trauma and has occurred concurrently with respiratory distress. Trauma may damage diaphragmatic nerves and muscles, resulting in hiatal laxity and subsequent herniation. In patients with upper respiratory obstruction, reduced intrathoracic pressure during inspiration has been theorized to contribute to esophageal reflux and visceral herniation. Hiatal hernia has been reported with tetanus.

With hiatal hernias, the stomach commonly slides in and out of the thorax. If the hernia is large enough, other abdominal viscera may also be cranially displaced into the thorax. Various types of hiatal abnormalities have been described (Fig. 16-51). In patients with sliding or axial hiatal hernias, the gastroesophageal junction is located within the thoracic cavity. In patients with paraesophageal or rolling hiatal hernias, the gastroesophageal junction is usually located in a normal position and the gastric fundus or other abdominal viscerae are displaced through the hiatus and located within the thorax. Some hiatal hernias are a combination of sliding and paraesophageal hernias with the gastroesophageal junction and gastric fundus both displaced.

DIAGNOSIS
Clinical Presentation

Signalment. Hiatal hernias may occur in a variety of dog and cat breeds; however, males and Chinese shar-pei dogs appear to be predisposed to this condition. Most symptomatic animals have signs relating to congenital hiatal hernia before reaching 1 year of age, although diagnosis may occur later. Patients with acquired hernias may develop signs at any age.

History. Regurgitation is the primary clinical sign in symptomatic individuals, but many patients are asymptomatic. Other signs may include vomiting, hypersalivation, dysphagia, respiratory distress, hematemesis, anorexia, and weight loss.

Physical Examination Findings

Affected patients may be thin upon physical examination.

Radiography/Ultrasonography

Hiatal hernias usually appear as a mass near the esophageal hiatus in the caudodorsal thoracic region on survey radiographs (Fig. 16-52). However, with sliding hernias, several radiographs may be necessary to identify the herniation because herniation may be intermittent. The presence of gas in the herniated portion aids in identification of the mass as herniated stomach. Varying degrees of megaesophagus and pneumonia may be noted. A positive contrast esophagram should show the gastroesophageal junction, rugal folds, or both cranial to the hiatus. Occasionally, strictures may be identified. Fluoroscopy may demonstrate hypomotility, delayed clearing of the distal esophagus, or gastroesophageal reflux. Compressing the abdomen while observing fluoroscopy may help identify hernias. Esophagoscopy can confirm mild to severe esophagitis (inflammation, mucosal erosion), gastric reflux, or strictures. Gastric mucosa that has entered the thoracic cavity can sometimes be identified. Some hiatal hernias are intermittent (sliding) and require multiple radiographs and/or flouroscopy to diagnose. Do not confuse hiatal hernias with peritoneopericardial (see p. 685) or traumatic (see p. 682) diaphragmatic hernias, despite their sometimes having a similar radiographic appearance.

Laboratory Findings

Hematology and serum chemistry results are nonspecific in affected animals.

DIFFERENTIAL DIAGNOSIS

Esophageal stricture, neoplasia, extraluminal masses, vascular ring anomaly, esophageal foreign body or perforation, esophagitis, esophageal intussusception, esophageal diverticulum, and megaesophagus are other potential causes of regurgitation.

SURGICAL TREATMENT

Affected patients may benefit from medical treatment for gastroesophageal reflux or esophagitis (see p. 232); however, surgery is generally recommended in symptomatic animals with congenital disease. A number of surgical techniques have been described for correction of this condition. Diaphragmatic hiatal reduction and plication, esophagopexy, and left-sided fundic gastropexy are described here. Gastropexy is probably the most important step in the repair. If esophagitis is severe and oral intake is to be prohibited for several days, a tube gastropexy (see p. 270) allows early alimentation without further esophageal irritation. Sphincter enhancing procedures such as a Nissen fundoplication (antireflux procedure) are performed by some surgeons instead of the aforementioned techniques. However, fundoplication or other antireflux procedures are only indicated in patients with evidence of gastroesophageal reflux. In dogs and cats, primary incompetence of the caudal esophageal sphincter has not been documented in association with hiatal hernia, and therefore antireflux procedures are not routinely recommended.

FIG. 16-51
Diagram of **A,** a normal gastroe-sophageal junction and **B–E,** hiatal abnormalities: **B,** sliding or axial hiatal hernia, **C,** parae-sophageal or rolling hiatal her-nia, **D,** combination of sliding and paraesophageal hernia, and **E,** gastroesophageal intussuscep-tion.

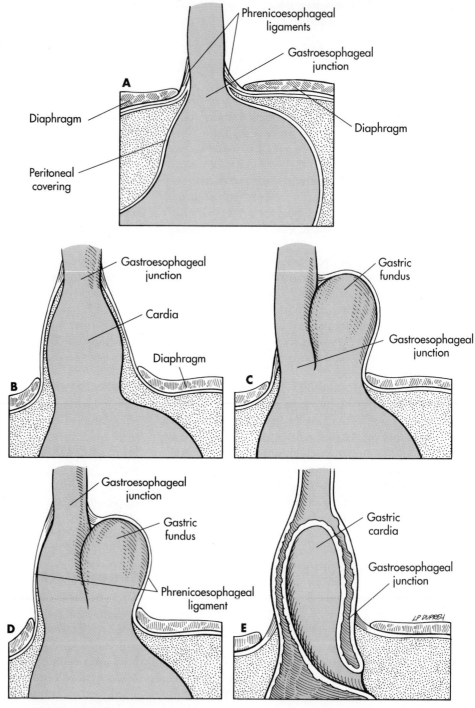

Preoperative Management

Reflux esophagitis and aspiration pneumonia should be treated before anesthetic induction (see p. 232). Feeding fre-quent, small meals of high-protein/low-fat foods may be ben-eficial. If megaesophagus is present, feeding affected animals in a standing, upright position may decrease regurgitation.

Anesthesia

Positive pressure ventilation may be necessary if pneumo-thorax is created during hiatal manipulations. Nitrous oxide should not be used in these patients. Negative intrathoracic pressure is reestablished by thoracentesis or tube thoracos-tomy after hiatal manipulations are complete. See p. 234 for anesthetic recommendations for patients undergoing esophageal surgery and p. 649 for those undergoing thoracic surgery.

Surgical Anatomy

The esophageal hiatus is one of three openings in the di-aphragm. The esophageal hiatus is more centrally located than the caval foramen (located ventrally) or aortic hiatus (located dorsally). The esophagus passes through the esophageal hiatus along with the vagal nerve trunks and esophageal vessels. The esophageal hiatus is surrounded by the phrenicoesophageal ligament, the thickened collagen fibers of which are weakened, stretched, or in some way defective in hiatal hernias. The terminal 1 to 2 cm of the esophagus lies within the abdominal cavity caudal to the diaphragm. The esophagogastric junction and gastroesophageal sphincter are in the abdomen and regulate movement of ingesta between the esophagus and stomach.

Positioning

Patients are positioned in dorsal recumbency, and the caudal thorax and ventral abdomen are prepared for aseptic surgery.

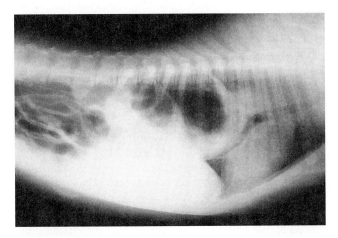

FIG. 16-52
Lateral radiograph of a 12-week-old shar-pei with a hiatal hernia. Note the air-filled mass (stomach) in the caudal thorax.

SURGICAL TECHNIQUE

Make a cranial ventral midline incision extending caudal to the umbilicus to expose the diaphragm and stomach. Retract the left lobes of the liver medially to expose the esophageal hiatus. Pass a stomach tube (28-32 French) to help identify and manipulate the esophagus. Grasp the stomach and reduce the hernia with gentle traction. Examine the hiatus. Dissect the phrenicoesophageal membrane, freeing the esophagus from the diaphragm ventrally. Preserve the vagal trunks and esophageal vessels during dissection. Place an umbilical tape sling around the abdominal esophagus to displace it caudally and facilitate manipulations. Perform a diaphragmatic hiatal plication/ reduction, esophagopexy, and left-sided fundic gastropexy. Accomplish diaphragmatic hiatal plication/reduction by excoriating or debriding the margins of the hiatus and then place three to five sutures (2-0 polydioxanone or polypropylene) to appose the edges and narrow the hiatus (Fig. 16-53, A). Plication should occur around a large stomach tube (28-32 French) (Fig. 16-53, B). The hiatus is reduced to 1 or 2 cm, a size that allows passage of one finger. Esophagopexy is accomplished by placing sutures (3-0 or 2-0 polydioxanone or polypropylene) from the remaining margin of the hiatus through the adventitia and muscular layers of the abdominal esophagus. Either a left-sided tube gastropexy or incisional gastropexy completes the repair (see pp. 270–271). The fundus is fixed with slight to moderate caudal traction to prevent cranial movement of the gastroesophageal junction into the thorax. Evacuate air from the chest via thoracentesis or tube thoracostomy and lavage and close the abdomen.

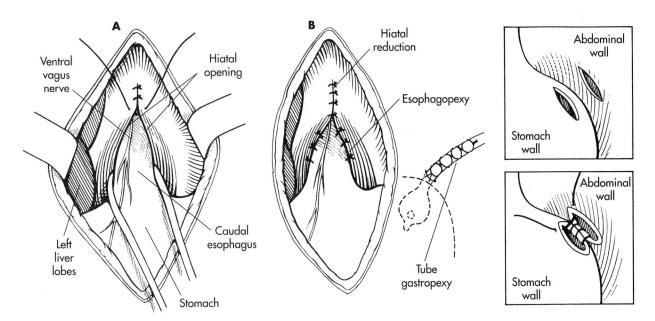

FIG. 16-53
A, Reduce hiatal hernias and decrease the size of the esophageal hiatus with plicating sutures. **B,** Suture the esophagus to the diaphragm (esophagopexy) and perform a tube or incisional gastropexy (*inset*) at the fundus.

POSTOPERATIVE CARE AND ASSESSMENT

Patients should be postoperatively monitored for dyspnea resulting from pneumothorax and air should be evacuated from the thorax as necessary. Nasal oxygen may benefit dyspneic animals. Analgesics should be provided as necessary to control pain (see Table 16-4). Affected animals may continue to regurgitate after surgery because of persistent esophagitis. Treatment of esophagitis and aspiration pneumonia should be continued postoperatively (see p. 232). Feeding from an elevated platform may be beneficial in animals with concurrent megaesophagus. Postoperative radiographic studies may be beneficial in patients with persistent clinical signs to identify persistent herniation, obstruction, or ulceration.

COMPLICATIONS

Dysphagia is common for several days; however, if it continues beyond that time, the hiatus may have been over-reduced, requiring reoperation. Infection may occur if the esophageal or gastric lumen is penetrated with sutures or tubes. Potential problems after antireflux procedures include gastric dilatation, necrotic gastritis, and acute death.

PROGNOSIS

Objective data comparing medical and surgical treatment in animals with hiatal hernias is not available. The prognosis without surgery is good in asymptomatic patients; however, symptomatic patients who are not surgically repaired may develop severe esophagitis and stricture. The prognosis is good with the described surgical repair; however, aspiration pneumonia must be controlled for a favorable outcome. Patients with gastroesophageal sphincter incompetence may benefit from additional antireflux procedures.

Suggested Reading

Bright RM et al: Hiatal hernia in the dog and cat: a retrospective study of 16 cases, *J Small Anim Pract* 31:244, 1990.

Ellison GW et al: Esophageal hiatal hernia in small animals: literature review and modified surgical technique, *J Am Anim Hosp Assoc* 23:391, 1987.

Prymak C, Saunders HM, Washabau RJ: Hiatal hernia by restoration and stabilization of normal anatomy: an evaluation in four dogs and one cat, *Vet Surg* 18:386, 1989.

Williams JM: Hiatal hernia in a shar-pei, *J Small Anim Pract* 31:251, 1990.

GASTROESOPHAGEAL INTUSSUSCEPTION

DEFINITIONS

Gastroesophageal intussusception is the invagination of the gastric cardia into the distal esophagus with or without the spleen, duodenum, pancreas, and omentum.

SYNONYMS

Esophageal intussusception, gastroesophageal invagination, esophageal invagination

GENERAL CONSIDERATIONS AND CLINICALLY RELEVANT PATHOPHYSIOLOGY

Gastroesophageal intussusception can be confused with esophageal hiatal hernia (see Fig. 16-51, *E* on p. 252). However, the gastroesophageal junction does not move cranially into the thorax as with sliding hiatal hernia, and the cardia is within the esophageal lumen rather than external to the esophagus as with paraesophageal hiatal hernia. Gastroesophageal intussusception usually occurs in immature animals with megaesophagus. The etiology of gastroesophageal intussusception is unknown. Idiopathic megaesophagus or incompetency of the gastroesophageal sphincter mechanism and subsequent regurgitation may predispose to this disorder. Vomiting and retching cause the esophagus to dilate. Experimental work in puppies has shown that vomiting can cause invagination of the gastric cardia into the esophagus. A large or lax esophageal hiatus may be necessary to allow the gastric cardia to move cranially into the esophagus. Entrapment or strangulation of the invaginated stomach occurs, causing esophageal obstruction, continued regurgitation, and rapid fluid loss. Discomfort is caused by stretching of gastric mesenteric attachments and esophagitis. Severe respiratory distress is caused by the greatly enlarged esophagus compressing the pulmonary parenchyma and/or aspiration pneumonia. Cardiovascular collapse occurs secondary to obstruction of venous return and eventually arterial blood supply. Resulting congestion, inflammation, and necrosis contribute to the animal's deterioration.

DIAGNOSIS
Clinical Presentation

Signalment. Although several breeds have been reported with gastroesophageal intussusception, German shepherds and other large breed dogs seem to be at increased risk. More cases have been reported in males than in females. Gastroesophageal intussusception has not been reported in cats. It is most common in young dogs, usually less than 3 months of age.

History. In most cases the onset of clinical signs is acute, with rapid deterioration and death with 1 to 3 days if the condition is not treated immediately. Signs may mimic those of aspiration pneumonia, making diagnosis difficult. Affected animals often have a history of esophageal disease (50%). An acute onset of clinical signs (i.e., regurgitation, vomiting, dyspnea, hematemesis, abdominal discomfort, rapid deterioration, death) is common.

Physical Examination Findings

Animals may be thin and evidence pain on abdominal palpation. Signs of shock (i.e., poor capillary refill, pale mucous membranes, labored breathing, tachycardia, and thready pulse) may be noted.

Radiography/Ultrasonography/Esophagoscopy

Radiographs show a dilated distal esophagus with a luminal soft tissue mass. Rugal folds may be associated with the soft tissue mass. The trachea may be deviated ventrally and signs of aspiration pneumonia may be apparent. The normal gastric gas bubble usually seen in the cranial abdomen may be absent or diminished in size. The intussusception can be outlined by either positive or negative contrast studies. Esophagoscopy reveals a dilated esophagus with gastric rugal folds within the distal esophageal lumen. Esophagitis may be apparent. It may not be possible to advance the endoscope into the distal esophagus or stomach.

Laboratory Findings

Laboratory findings are nonspecific and related to dehydration and shock.

DIFFERENTIAL DIAGNOSIS

Esophageal hiatal hernia, stricture, neoplasia, extraluminal masses, esophageal foreign body, or esophageal diverticulum are differential diagnoses.

SURGICAL TREATMENT

Surgical intervention should be performed as soon as possible after the gastroesophageal intussusception is diagnosed. Stabilization of the patient and treatment for shock should be performed before anesthetic induction; however, surgical treatment should not be delayed.

Preoperative Management

Shock treatment (i.e., fluid therapy, broad spectrum antibiotics, plus or minus steroids) should be initiated before anesthetic induction. Electrolyte and acid-base abnormalities should be identified and corrected before anesthetic induction, if possible. An ECG should be performed before anesthetic induction.

Anesthesia

Anesthetic recommendations for animals undergoing esophageal surgery are provided on p. 234.

Surgical Anatomy

See the discussion on surgical anatomy of the esophageal hiatus on p. 234.

Positioning

The animal is positioned in dorsal recumbency with the caudal thorax and ventral abdomen prepared for aseptic surgery.

SURGICAL TECHNIQUE

Make a ventral midline abdominal incision from the xiphoid process to several centimeters caudal to the um-
bilicus. Explore the abdomen and locate the duodenum and stomach. Apply gentle traction on the duodenum and stomach to reduce the intussusception. If necessary, digitally dilate or enlarge the esophageal hiatus to allow complete reduction of the intussusception. Examine the distal esophagus, stomach, and any other involved viscera for evidence of vascular thrombosis, avulsion, ischemia, or necrosis. Resect devitalized tissue. Reduce the size of the esophageal hiatus to 1 to 2 cm if it is too large or lax (see p. 253). Perform an incisional gastropexy (see p. 271) at the gastric fundus to prevent recurrence. Lavage and close the abdomen.

POSTOPERATIVE CARE AND ASSESSMENT

After surgery, fluids should be continued and acid-base and electrolyte imbalances corrected. Nasal oxygen may benefit animals that are dyspneic. Postoperative analgesics should be provided to control pain (see Table 16-4). Oral intake should be withheld initially to encourage resolution of esophagitis and gastritis (see p. 232). After 24 to 48 hours water can be offered. If vomiting or regurgitation does not occur, small amounts of a low-fat gruel can be offered several times a day. If megaesophagus is present, the animal should be fed in an upright position. However, esophageal weakness may not resolve. Gastrostomy tube feeding may be helpful. Continued deterioration and death may occur if the condition is not recognized and treated promptly. Devitalization of a portion of the esophagus or stomach may occur as a result of preoperative vascular compromise. Dysphagia is common for several days after surgery; however, persistent dysphagia may occur if the hiatus is overly narrowed by surgery. Such patients require reoperation.

PROGNOSIS

Antemortem diagnosis is rare (mortality approaches 95%); thus few cases of gastroesophageal intussusception have been diagnosed and treated successfully. Recurrence is not expected if an incisional gastropexy is performed and esophagitis is controlled.

Suggested Reading

Leib MS, Blass CE: Gastroesophageal intussusception in the dog: a review of the literature and a case report, *J Am Anim Hosp Assoc* 20:783, 1984.

CRICOPHARYNGEAL ACHALASIA

DEFINITIONS

Cricopharyngeal achalasia is one type of pharyngeal dysphagia. In it there is interruption of passage of a bolus from the oropharynx through the cranial esophageal sphincter into the cervical esophagus because of a failure of the sphincter to open correctly.

SYNONYMS

Congenital cricopharyngeal achalasia, cricopharyngeal dysphagia, cricopharyngeal dysfunction, cricopharyngeal asynchrony

GENERAL CONSIDERATIONS AND CLINICALLY RELEVANT PATHOPHYSIOLOGY

Cricopharyngeal achalasia is a rare cause of dysphagia; however, it is important that it be differentiated from other forms of oropharyngeal dysphagia because it is treatable. There are multiple swallowing disorders, and treatment for these conditions varies. The cause of cricopharyngeal achalasia is unknown but appears to be a congenital derangement in the coordination of the swallowing reflex. The cause is probably neurologic because the disorder can be reproduced by transecting the pharyngeal branch of the 10th cranial nerve. Cricopharyngeal achalasia is characterized by inadequate relaxation of the cricopharyngeal muscle in coordination with pharyngeal muscle contractions during swallowing. The small amount of food that succeeds in passing from the oropharynx into the proximal esophagus passes normally into the stomach. Repeated attempts to swallow are made until retained pharyngeal contents are swallowed, regurgitated, or aspirated. Food remaining in the pharynx may be aspirated into the trachea during inspiration, eliciting a cough and causing pneumonia.

In normal swallowing, food is grasped by the teeth and formed into a bolus by rapid tongue movements. The bolus is pushed up and back by the base of the tongue into the oropharynx. The pharyngeal muscles contract and force the bolus through the relaxed upper esophageal sphincter (cricopharyngeal muscles) into the cervical portion of the esophagus. The cricopharyngeal muscle contracts after the bolus passes. Cricopharyngeal muscle tone is linked to deglutition and the respiratory cycle. During swallowing the airways are protected by the soft palate closing the nasopharynx and the epiglottis flipping back to close the glottis.

DIAGNOSIS

Clinical Presentation

Signalment. The condition is rare. It seems to be more common in springer and cocker spaniels, but has been seen in a variety of breeds. Signs of dysphagia begin at weaning, although animals very rarely may not be diagnosed until they are older.

History. Most dogs appear normal until they begin eating solid food. At that time repeated unsuccessful attempts to swallow, with gagging, retching, and expulsion of saliva-covered food is noted. Regurgitation occurs immediately after swallowing. Most patients have a voracious appetite, but some become anorexic and lose weight.

Physical Examination Findings

Affected animals may appear normal or stunted at the time of examination. Some patients are emaciated. The animal should be observed eating and drinking to confirm dysphagia and to characterize it as oral or pharyngeal. Patients with oral dysphagia have difficulty with prehension and bolus formation. Those with pharyngeal dysphagia have difficulty transporting the bolus into the esophagus. Patients with cricopharyngeal dysphagia usually have more difficulty with food, whereas those with other types of pharyngeal dysphagias may have more difficulty (i.e., may aspirate more readily) when swallowing liquids.

Radiography/Ultrasonography

Survey thoracic radiographs should be evaluated for aspiration pneumonia and esophageal size. Definitive diagnosis requires fluoroscopic or cinefluoroscopic evaluation during a barium swallow. An experienced radiologist may need to differentiate cricopharyngeal achalasia from pharyngeal dysphagia. Patients with cricopharyngeal achalasia have adequate pharyngeal strength to push the food bolus into the esophagus, but the cricopharyngeal sphincter stays shut or opens at the wrong time during the swallowing reflex. Patients with pharyngeal dysphagia do not have adequate oropharyngeal strength to properly push the food bolus into the esophagus. Positive contrast within the trachea or outlining airways indicates aspiration. Esophageal motility should be evaluated during fluoroscopic studies to identify concurrent problems because many animals with pharyngeal dysphagia have concurrent esophageal dysfunction.

Laboratory Findings

Laboratory findings are normal unless the patient is severely debilitated or has aspiration pneumonia.

DIFFERENTIAL DIAGNOSIS

Pharyngeal dysphagia caused by inadequate pharyngeal contraction is difficult to differentiate from cricopharyngeal achalasia. Sometimes there is more than one abnormality contributing to dysphagia. Dental disease, oral masses, foreign bodies, stomatitis, cleft palate, and skeletal abnormalities should also be considered. Esophageal hypomotility and megaesophagus can also be associated with pharyngeal dysphagias. Other considerations include functional abnormalities resulting from rabies, central nervous system (CNS) disease, peripheral neuropathies, neuromuscular disease, myopathies, and myositis.

SURGICAL TREATMENT

Cricopharyngeal myectomy is curative for cricopharyngeal achalasia. Some surgeons also resect a portion of the thyropharyngeus muscle. Cricopharyngeal myectomy for patients with other pharyngeal dysphagias can be disastrous because it allows food retained in the proximal esophagus to more easily reenter the pharynx and be aspirated.

Preoperative Management

Supportive care is important; patients should be well hydrated and nourished before surgery. Preoperative nutritional support should be provided with a gastrostomy tube if necessary (see p. 74). Aspiration pneumonia should be treated with fluids, appropriate antibiotics, and expectorants. Perioperative antibiotics are recommended for debilitated patients.

Anesthesia

Recommendations for esophageal surgery are provided on p. 234. Hypothermia and hypoglycemia are serious problems in young patients and should be prevented during anesthesia and surgery.

Surgical Anatomy

The cranial esophagus is located dorsal to the larynx and slightly to the left of midline. The cricopharyngeal muscle lies on the larynx and pharynx immediately caudal to the thyropharyngeal muscle (Fig. 16-54). It arises from the lateral surface of the cricoid cartilage and passes dorsally to insert on the median dorsal raphe. The cricopharyngeal muscle can be identified as a bundle of transverse muscle fibers converging on the dorsal midline and blending into the longitudinal muscle fibers of the cranial esophagus. The thyropharyngeal muscle can be difficult to differentiate from the cricopharyngeal muscles because their muscle fibers are both oriented transversely. The thyropharyngeal muscle lies cranial to the cricopharyngeal muscle and is separated from it

by a thin septum of connective tissue. The separation is found dorsal to the attachment of the sternothyroideus muscle. The cricopharyngeal muscle controls most of the upper esophageal sphincter function. It is innervated by branches of the glossopharyngeal and vagus nerves. Blood supply to the cricopharyngeal muscles is primarily from branches of the cranial thyroid arteries.

Positioning

The animal is positioned in dorsal recumbency with the legs positioned lateral to the thorax. The ventral neck (from the angle of the mandible to the manubrium) should be prepared for aseptic surgery.

SURGICAL TECHNIQUE

Make a ventral midline cervical incision beginning cranial to the larynx and extending caudally to the mid-cervical area. Separate and retract the sternohyoid muscles laterally to expose the trachea. Rotate the larynx and trachea laterally via traction on the sternothyroid muscle to expose the cricopharyngeal musculature (Fig. 16-55, A). Place a suture through the lamina of the thyroid cartilage to maintain laryngeal rotation and exposure of the cricopharyngeal muscle and dorsal esophagus. Pass a gastric tube into

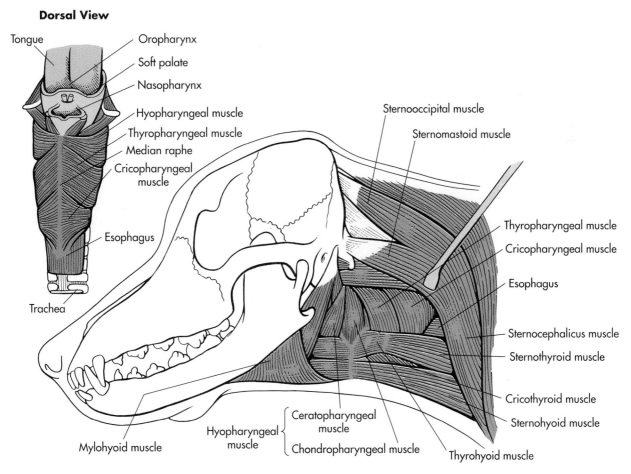

Dorsal View

Tongue
Oropharynx
Soft palate
Nasopharynx
Hyopharyngeal muscle
Thyropharyngeal muscle
Median raphe
Cricopharyngeal muscle
Esophagus
Trachea

Sternooccipital muscle
Sternomastoid muscle
Thyropharyngeal muscle
Cricopharyngeal muscle
Esophagus
Sternocephalicus muscle
Sternothyroid muscle
Cricothyroid muscle
Sternohyoid muscle

Mylohyoid muscle
Hyopharyngeal muscle
Ceratopharyngeal muscle
Chondropharyngeal muscle
Thyrohyoid muscle

FIG. 16-54
Surgical anatomy of the cranial esophagus and neck.

FIG. 16-55
During cricopharyngeal myectomy expose the cranial esophagus through a ventral midline cervical incision. **A,** Place a stay suture through the thyroid lamina and rotate the cricopharyngeal muscle into view. **B,** Resect the lateral portion of each cricopharyngeal muscle.

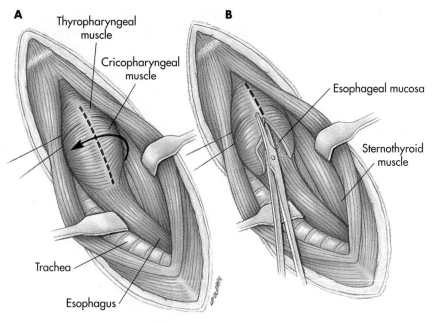

the esophagus to aid identification of the esophageal wall. Identify the cricopharyngeal muscles. Incise the cricopharyngeal muscle on its midline (Fig. 16-55, B). Elevate the muscle fibers from the underlying esophageal submucosa with care to avoid perforating the esophageal wall. Resect the lateral portion of each cricopharyngeus muscle. Inspect the esophageal wall for damage and lavage the area. Allow the larynx and trachea to return to their normal position. Appose the sternohyoid muscles with a continuous suture pattern. Close subcutaneous tissues and skin routinely.

POSTOPERATIVE CARE AND ASSESSMENT

A gruel or canned food should be fed for the first 1 to 2 days postoperatively, then the food should gradually be returned to normal food consistency over the next 3 to 4 days. If necessary, intravenous fluids should be continued to maintain hydration. Antibiotics should be continued if aspiration pneumonia is present. Inadequate or unilateral myectomy may not relieve signs of cricopharyngeal achalasia.

COMPLICATIONS

Recurrence of dysphagia because of fibrosis and constriction at the myectomy site can be prevented by adequate removal of muscle. Cricopharyngeal myectomy will worsen the patient's dysphagia and pneumonia if other concurrent pharyngeal dysphagias are present. Aspiration pneumonia may continue to be a problem if esophageal hypomotility exists.

PROGNOSIS

The prognosis is good if the only abnormality present is cricopharyngeal achalasia and guarded if other dysphagias are present. Persistent regurgitation may result in aspiration pneumonia. The prognosis without surgery is guarded because it is difficult to effectively nourish the patient and control pneumonia.

Suggested Reading

Allen SW: Surgical management of pharyngeal disorders in the dog and cat, *Problems in Veterinary Medicine: Head & Neck* 3:290, 1991.
Goring RL, Kagan KG: Cricopharyngeal achalasia in the dog: Radiographic evaluation and surgical management, *Compend Contin Educ Pract Vet* 4:438, 1982.

VASCULAR RING ANOMALIES

DEFINITIONS

Vascular ring anomalies are congenital malformations of the great vessels and their branches that cause constriction of the esophagus and signs of esophageal obstruction.

SYNONYMS

PRAA and **persistent fourth right aortic arch** are synonyms for persistent right aortic arch.

GENERAL CONSIDERATIONS AND CLINICALLY RELEVANT PATHOPHYSIOLOGY

The most common type of vascular ring anomaly is a persistent fourth right aortic arch, right dorsal aortic root, and rudimentary left ligamentum arteriosum (left sixth arch). The left pulmonary artery and the descending aorta are connected by the ligamentum arteriosum. The esophagus is encircled by the ligamentum arteriosum (or patent ductus arteriosus) on the left, the base of the heart and pulmonary artery ventrally, and the aortic arch on the right. The esophagus is constricted by this vascular "ring" and begins to dilate cranially as food accumulates. Food not passing beyond the constriction is intermittently regurgitated. Chronic regurgitation predisposes to aspiration pneumonia. Approximately

95% of those diagnosed with vascular ring anomalies will have a persistent right aortic arch (PRAA) (VanGundy, 1989). Persistent left vena cava occurs in conjunction with PRAA in about 40% of the cases (VanGundy, 1989).

Abnormal location of the great vessels mechanically interferes with function of the esophagus and sometimes the trachea and other adjacent structures. The severity of clinical signs and degree of esophageal stricture depend upon the vascular structures involved. Other types of vascular ring anomalies include: (1) persistent right aortic arch with persistent left subclavian artery, (2) persistent right aortic arch with persistent left ligamentum arteriosum and left subclavian artery, (3) double aortic arch, (4) normal left aortic arch with persistent right ligamentum arteriosum, (5) normal left aortic arch with persistent right subclavian artery, and (6) normal left aortic arch with persistent right ligamentum arteriosum and right subclavian artery.

Six pairs of aortic arches surround the esophagus and trachea during early fetal life. Normal maturation and selective regression of these arches form the adult vasculature. All vascular ring anomalies have resulted from abnormal development of arches three, four, and six. The mechanism of inheritance is thought to involve single or multiple recessive genes. In the embryo the first and second aortic arches disappear and the fifth arches are incomplete and inconsistent. The third arch joins the dorsal aortic arch and continues anteriorly as the right and left internal carotid arteries. The third arch also forms the brachiocephalic trunk. The dorsal aortas disappear between the third and fourth arches. Normally the left fourth aortic arch and the dorsal aortic root persist to form the permanent aortic arch. The left sixth arch becomes the ductus arteriosus and the right fourth arch contributes to the right subclavian artery.

DIAGNOSIS
Clinical Presentation

Signalment. Vascular ring anomalies occur in both dogs and cats, but are more common in dogs. German shepherds, Irish setters, and Boston terriers are the most commonly affected dog breeds. Siamese and Persian cats have been diagnosed more often than other cat breeds. Males and females are equally affected. The condition may affect multiple animals in a litter. Vascular ring anomalies are present at birth. Clinical signs are usually evident at the time of weaning, most being diagnosed between 2 and 6 months of age. The condition may not be recognized until later in life if obstruction is partial and signs are mild. Early diagnosis and treatment of PRAA may improve the prognosis.

History. The classic history is acute onset of regurgitation when solid or semisolid food is first fed. Regurgitation of undigested food occurs soon after eating early in the disease; later it may occur at variable times (minutes to hours). Affected animals may grow slower than litter mates and appear malnourished. They often have a voracious appetite, some immediately eating the regurgitated food. Coughing with respiratory distress may be a result of aspiration pneumonia and/or tracheal stenosis secondary to a double aortic arch.

Physical Examination Findings

Affected animals are often thin and small. An enlarged esophagus may sometimes be palpated at the thoracic inlet and neck. The thoracic inlet and caudal neck area may bulge when the chest is compressed. Murmurs are rare; an occasional patient may have a continuous murmur associated with concurrent patent ductus arteriosus (see p. 582). Pneumonia may be suggested by auscultating coarse crackles or finding fever.

Radiography/Ultrasonography/Endoscopy

Thoracic radiographs may reveal a dilated esophagus cranial to the heart containing air, water, or food. The trachea may be displaced ventrally and the esophagus may overlap it. Signs of pneumonia may be identified. Positive contrast radiography using a barium suspension or barium with food will demonstrate esophageal constriction at the base of the heart with varying degrees of esophageal dilatation extending cranially (Fig. 16-56). The caudal esophagus is usually a normal size, although sometimes it is dilated. Fluoroscopy is beneficial in evaluating esophageal motility. The dilated esophagus does not usually demonstrate normal peristaltic contractions. Although not routinely performed, angiography is beneficial in preoperatively identifying the type of vascular ring anomaly and other cardiac anomalies. Echocardiography may also be beneficial. Endoscopic examination of the esophagus helps rule out other causes of esophageal stricture or obstruction and may reveal esophageal ulceration. Tracheoscopy is not routinely performed, but may document tracheal lumen narrowing secondary to external compression.

Laboratory Findings

Laboratory findings are expected to be normal (for the animal's age) unless debilitation is severe or pneumonia is ongoing. In the latter patients neutrophilia may be present.

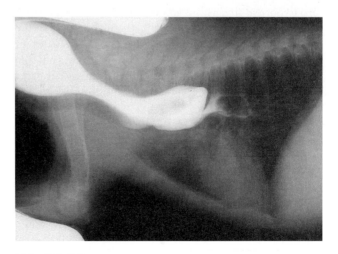

FIG. 16-56
Contrast esophagram of a dog with a persistent right aortic arch. Note the esophageal narrowing at the heart base. The cranial esophagus is dilated.

DIFFERENTIAL DIAGNOSIS

The primary differential diagnoses are generalized mega-esophagus and obstruction caused by a foreign body, stricture, mass, or hiatal hernia.

MEDICAL MANAGEMENT

Management of patients with vascular ring anomalies is both medical and surgical. Surgery should be performed as soon after onset of clinical signs as possible to reduce damage to the esophageal muscles and nerves. Clients should be informed that medical treatment without surgery is palliative at best and is not recommended. Medical management includes treating aspiration pneumonia (see p. 232) and improving the animal's nutritional status. An affected animal should be fed a gruel while standing on its hindlegs with the food dish elevated on a platform. The animal should be maintained in an upright position (standing on hindlegs) for 10 to 20 minutes after eating to allow gravity to assist emptying the dilated esophagus. Placement of a gastrostomy feeding tube may be beneficial for severely debilitated patients, particularly if aspiration is present and surgery is being considered.

SURGICAL TREATMENT

Surgical treatment of PRAA is described below. Other types of vascular ring anomalies can be managed in a similar fashion. A persistent left vena cava often covers the left ventral area of the vascular ring. A persistent right ligamentum arteriosum and some aberrant right subclavians should be approached from the right side. Angiograms are helpful in patients with double aortic arches to determine which arch is dominant and if adequate circulation can be maintained after transection of the other arch. It may not be possible to relieve constrictions caused by a double aortic arch. If the animal is severely debilitated, place a gastric feeding tube for several days before surgery.

Some surgeons attempt to decrease esophageal lumen size if the esophagus is severely dilated and not expected to return to normal size. This is accomplished by placing a series of nonpenetrating "plication" or "gathering" sutures in the accessible lateral esophageal wall. Alternatively a portion of the esophagus may be resected. These techniques are not recommended routinely because they increase the risk of complications.

Preoperative Management

Hydration, electrolyte, and acid-base abnormalities should be corrected before surgery if possible. If pneumonia is present or the animal is severely debilitated, nutrition should be provided via a gastrostomy feeding tube (see p. 74) for several days to a week. Antibiotics are indicated for animals with pneumonia and those that are debilitated (see p. 234).

Anesthesia

Anesthetic recommendations for animals undergoing thoracotomies are on p. 649. Pediatric patients must be kept warm and well hydrated during surgery and should be carefully monitored for hypoglycemia. Animals with pneumonia should be preoxygenated. Nitrous oxide should not be used in these patients.

Surgical Anatomy

Anatomy of the esophagus is provided on p. 234 and anatomy of the heart on p. 577. See also the discussion under General Considerations and Clinically Relevant Pathophysiology on p. 258.

Positioning

Most patients with vascular ring anomalies should be positioned in right lateral recumbency for a left lateral thoracotomy (see p. 651); however, those with persistent right ligamentum arteriosum are positioned in left lateral recumbency. Positioning of animals with double aortic arches varies depending on the dominant arch.

SURGICAL TECHNIQUE

Surgical transection of the constricting structure(s) is recommended before esophageal dilatation becomes severe. Transection is feasible with most vascular ring anomalies with the exception of some double aortic arches. *Perform a lateral thoracotomy at the left fourth (fifth) intercostal space for patients with PRAA. Pack the cranial lung caudally to expose the mediastinum dorsal to the heart. Identify the aorta, pulmonary artery, ligamentum arteriosum, vagus, and phrenic nerves (see Fig. 24-3 on p. 579 and Fig. 16-37 on p. 237). Identify the anomalous structure(s). If a persistent left cranial cava is present, dissect and retract the vena cava to improve visualization. If a prominent hemiazygous vein is also present, dissect, ligate, and divide it. If a constricting subclavian artery is identified, isolate, ligate, and transect it. Incise the mediastinum, dissect, and elevate the ligamentum arteriosum. Double ligate the ligamentum arteriosum and then transect it. Pass a ballooned catheter or large orogastric tube through the constricted esophagus to aid identification of constricting fibrous bands and to dilate the site. Dissect and transect these fibrous bands from the esophageal wall. Lavage the area, reposition the lung lobes, place a thoracostomy tube if necessary, and close the thorax routinely.*

POSTOPERATIVE CARE AND ASSESSMENT

Postoperative analgesics should be provided as described on p. 650. The patient should be closely monitored for dyspnea and the chest tapped if necessary. Nasal oxygen may benefit dyspneic patients. If a thoracostomy tube has been placed, the thorax should be aspirated at regular intervals (initially every 15 to 30 minutes) and the volume of air and fluid collected at each interval noted. Thoracostomy tubes can generally be removed the day of surgery or by the next morning in these patients. Antibiotics should be continued in debilitated patients if thoracic contamination occurred or if pneumonia exists.

Pediatric patients should be closely monitored for hypoglycemia in the postoperative period. Oral intake can be resumed within 12 to 24 hours of surgery. Initially a canned food gruel should be fed with the animal in an upright posture. This stance should be maintained for 10 to 20 minutes after eating to help prevent distention of the dilated esophagus and help reestablish esophageal muscle tone and esophageal size. Owners may gradually reduce the amount of water in the food 2 to 4 weeks after surgery if minimal regurgitation has occurred with gruel feeding. Hopefully, addition of water can ultimately be eliminated without increased regurgitation. Animals who can eat solid food without regurgitation should be allowed to eat with the bowl on the floor while standing normally. This feeding practice is continued unless regurgitation frequency increases. Some animals can eventually be fed any type food from a normal stance, while others must continue eating gruel from an elevated stand.

The esophagus should be reevaluated with an esophogram 1 to 2 months after surgery to assess persistent dilatation and motility. Sometimes the esophagus returns to a normal size and function. Other times the esophagus remains severely dilated with poor motility. If esophageal constriction occurs, balloon dilation (see p. 247) may be beneficial. Owners should be advised against breeding affected animals because it is believed to be a genetic disorder.

COMPLICATIONS

Surgical complications are common because of the initial malnourished and debilitated condition of affected animals and concurrent aspiration pneumonia. Approximately 80% of patients are expected to survive the initial postoperative period. Persistent regurgitation is the most common postoperative problem. Preoperative client education must emphasize the high incidence of continued regurgitation and the need for prolonged dietary management. Aspiration pneumonia and death may occur if regurgitation persists. Esophageal resection or imbrication increases the risk of contamination and infection secondary to esophageal leakage or dehiscence.

PROGNOSIS

Most patients surviving surgery improve (70% to 80%) (Van Gundy, 1989; Shires, 1981). They may not have completely normal esophageal function, but they generally regurgitate less and their body condition improves. If surgery is performed soon after signs appear, normal esophageal tone and function might return. The longer the delay before surgical correction, the more cautious the prognosis; some show little or no improvement. The prognosis is poor if there is esophageal dilatation caudal to the constriction because this area is often hypomotile and frequently does not regain normal size. Without surgery, regurgitation usually continues and worsens as the esophagus continues to dilate. Aspiration pneumonia will be a continuous threat. Animals may have difficulty maintaining adequate body condition.

References

Shires PK, Liu W: Persistent right aortic arch in dogs: a long term follow-up after surgical correction, *J Am Anim Hosp Assoc* 17:773, 1981.

VanGundy T: Vascular ring anomalies, *Compend Contin Educ Pract Vet* 11:36, 1989.

Suggested Reading

Fingeroth JM, Fossum TW: Late-onset regurgitation associated with persistent right aortic arch in two dogs, *J Am Vet Med Assoc* 191:981, 1987.

Helphrey ML: Vascular ring anomalies in the dog, *Vet Clin North Am* 9:207, 1979.

Surgery of the Stomach

GENERAL PRINCIPLES AND TECHNIQUES

DEFINITIONS

Gastrotomy is an incision through the stomach wall into the lumen. Partial **gastrectomy** is a resection of a portion of the stomach and **gastrostomy** is creation of an artificial opening into the gastric lumen. **Gastropexy** permanently adheres the stomach to the body wall. Removal of the pylorus (**pylorectomy**) and attachment of the stomach to the duodenum (**gastroduodenostomy**) is a **Billroth I** procedure. Attachment of the jejunum to the stomach (**gastrojejunostomy**) following a partial gastrectomy (including pylorectomy) is a **Billroth II** procedure. In a **pyloromyotomy,** an incision is made through the serosa and muscularis layers of the pylorus only. For a **pyloroplasty,** a full-thickness incision and tissue reorientation are performed to increase the diameter of the gastric outflow tract.

PREOPERATIVE CONCERNS

Gastric surgery is commonly performed for removal of foreign bodies (see p. 275) and to correct gastric dilatation-volvulus (see p. 277). Gastric ulceration or erosion (see p. 286), neoplasia (see p. 289), and benign gastric outflow obstruction (see p. 283) are less-frequent indications. Gastric disease may cause vomiting (intermittent or profuse and continuous) or just anorexia. Dehydration and hypokalemia are common in vomiting animals and should be corrected before anesthetic induction. Alkalosis may occur as a result of gastric fluid loss; however, metabolic acidosis may also be seen. Hematemesis may indicate gastric erosion or ulceration or coagulation abnormalities. Peritonitis resulting from perforation of the stomach due to necrosis or ulceration is often lethal if not treated promptly and aggressively (see p. 193). Aspiration pneumonia or esophagitis may also occur in vomiting animals. Treatment of severe aspiration pneumonia (see p. 232) should be done before anesthetic induction for gastric surgery, if possible.

Mild esophagitis can generally be treated by withholding food for 24 to 48 hours (see p. 233) and need not delay gastric surgery. However, severe esophagitis may necessitate withholding oral food for 7 to 10 days. A gastrostomy tube (see p. 74) placed during surgery may be considered if continued vomiting is not expected. If continued vomiting is likely, an enteral feeding tube should be placed (see p. 79). Treatment with H_2 antagonists (i.e., cimetidine, ranitidine, famotidine; Table 16-21) or omeprazole may be necessary. Orally administered sucralfate slurries protect denuded mucosa and reduce esophageal inflammation, and should be given 1 hour after other medications (see p. 288). Cisapride increases the strength of gastric contractions, improves gastric emptying, and increases gastroesophageal sphincter pressure. Antibiotics effective against oral contaminants (e.g., ampicillin, amoxicillin, clindamycin, cephalosporins) should be considered (Table 16-22).

When possible, food should be withheld for 8 to 12 hours before surgery to ensure that the stomach is empty. However, fasting for only 4 to 6 hours may help prevent hypoglycemia in pediatric patients (see the discussion on anesthetic and surgical management of pediatric patients below). Surgery for gastric obstruction, distension, malpositioning, or ulceration should be performed as soon as possible, once the animal is stabilized.

ANESTHETIC CONSIDERATIONS

Numerous anesthetic protocols have been used in animals with gastric disorders (Tables 16-23 and 16-24). Because vomiting, reflux, and aspiration are common, anticholinergics (i.e., atropine or glycopyrrolate) should be considered to decrease gastric secretion and reduce damage to the esophageal mucosa or respiratory tract. Nitrous oxide should be avoided whenever gastric or intestinal distention is present (e.g., gastric dilatation-volvulus, intestinal volvulus/torsion), because it rapidly diffuses into gas-filled areas, causing additional organ distention. Dogs may be premedicated with an anticholingeric and oxymorphone, butorphanol, or buprenorphine and induced with a thiobarbiturate, propofol, or a combination of diazepam and ketamine (given slowly intravenously). A combination of oxymorphone and diazepam intravenously may be sufficient for induction of severely depressed dogs. If additional drugs are needed for intubation, etomidate or a reduced dosage of a thiobarbiturate or propofol may be administered intravenously. Rapid induction and immediate intubation are essential if vomiting is a concern; however, mask induction is acceptable if vomiting is not a concern. Isoflurane is the inhalation agent of choice in arrhythmic patients.

Animals less than 6 months old should be anesthetized with care. Hepatic glycogen stores are rapidly depleted during fasting in puppies and kittens; therefore fasting longer than 4 to 6 hours is not generally recommended. If you are unable to monitor blood glucose, intravenous fluids contain-

---

TABLE 16-22

Antibiotic Therapy for Esophagitis

Ampicillin
22 mg/kg IV, IM, SC, PO, TID to QID

Amoxicillin (Amoxi-tabs, Amoxi-drops, Amoxi-inject)
22 mg/kg PO, IM or SC, BID or TID

Cefazolin (Ancef, Kefzol)
20 mg/kg IV, IM, TID

Clindamycin (Antirobe, Cleocin)
11 mg/kg PO or IV, BID

Enrofloxacin (Baytril)
5-10 mg/kg PO, IV, BID

TABLE 16-21

Treatment of Esophagitis

Cimetidine (Tagamet)
10 mg/kg PO, IV, SC, TID to QID

Ranitidine (Zantac)
2 mg/kg PO, IV, IM, SC, BID

Famotidine (Pepcid)
0.5 mg/kg PO, SID to BID

Omeprazole (Prilosec)
0.7-1.5 mg/kg PO, SID to BID

Sucralfate* (Carafate)
0.5-1.0 g PO, TID to QID

Cisapride (Propulsid)
Dogs—0.25-0.5 mg/kg PO, BID to TID
Cats—2.5-5.0 mg/cat PO, BID to TID

*Carafate impairs absorption and reduces bioavailability of H_2 antagonists; give at different times.

TABLE 16-23

Selected Anesthetic Protocols for Use in Stable Animals with Gastric Disorders

Premedication
Give atropine (0.02-0.04 mg/kg SC, IM) or glycopyrrolate (0.005-0.011 mg/kg SC, IM) plus oxymorphone (0.05-0.1 mg/kg SC, IM) or butorphanol (0.2-0.4 mg/kg SC, IM), or buprenorphine (5-15 µg/kg IM)

Induction
Thiopental (10-12 mg/kg IV) or propofol (4-6 mg/kg IV) or a combination of diazepam and ketamine (diazepam 0.27 mg/kg plus 5.5 mg/kg ketamine IV, titrated to effect)

Maintenance
Isoflurane or halothane

ing balanced electrolytes in a 2.5% dextrose solution should be given for surgeries longer than an hour or if anesthetic recovery is delayed. Hypothermia commonly develops in puppies and kittens during surgery because they have a higher surface area to body weight ratio, which results in greater heat loss by radiation and evaporation. Hypothermia may cause bradycardia, low cardiac output, and hypotension, which may prolong drug elimination and anesthetic recovery. Drugs that normally redistribute to muscle or fat will have prolonged effects in puppies and kittens after repeated administration. Reduced hepatorenal function may also prolong drug effects. Phenothiazine tranquilizers should be used with care in animals less than 3 months of age because the drugs may cause prolonged central nervous system depression. If used, phenothiazines should be given at one fourth to one half of the adult dose. Opioids can be used in young animals; however, they should be given at half the adult dose, and large or multiple doses should not be given.

ANTIBIOTICS

Perioperative antibiotics may be used if the gastric lumen will be entered; however, animals with normal immune function undergoing simple gastrotomy (i.e., proper aseptic technique and no spillage of gastric contents) rarely require them. If antibiotics (e.g., cefazolin; Table 16-25) are used, they should be given intravenously before anesthetic induction and continued for up to 12 hours postoperatively. Bacteria (besides *Helicobacter* sp.) are scarce in the stomach compared with other parts of the gastrointestinal tract because of the low gastric pH.

SURGICAL ANATOMY

The stomach can be divided into the cardia, fundus, body, pyloric antrum, pyloric canal, and pyloric ostium. The esophagus enters the stomach at the cardiac ostium. The fundus is dorsal to the cardiac ostium and, although it is relatively small in carnivores, is easy to identify on radiographs because it is typically gas-filled. The body of the stomach (or middle one third) lies against the left lobes of the liver. The pyloric antrum is funnel-shaped and opens into the pyloric canal. The pyloric ostium is the end of the pyloric canal that empties into the duodenum.

☞ **N O T E** · The gastric mucosa accounts for one half of its weight. It can be easily separated from the submucosa and serosa during gastropexy or pyloromyotomy.

The gastric (lesser curvature) and gastroepiploic (greater curvature) arteries supply the stomach and are derived from the celiac artery. The short gastric arteries arise from the splenic artery and supply the greater curvature. The portion of the lesser omentum that passes from the stomach to the liver is the hepatogastric ligament. The stomach of the beagle holds more than 500 ml of fluid when distended (a mature cat's stomach may hold 300 to 350 ml). When the stomach is highly distended it can be palpated beyond the costal arch.

☞ **N O T E** · The short gastric vessels are often avulsed in animals with gastric dilatation-volvulus (see the discussion of gastric dilatation-volvulus on p. 281).

SURGICAL TECHNIQUES

Gastric surgery is frequently performed in small animals. Generally, performing a gastrotomy is safer than performing an esophagotomy or enterotomy. Peritonitis infrequently occurs after gastrotomy if proper techniques are used. Stricture or obstruction is also rare.

Gastrotomy

The most common indication for gastrotomy in dogs and cats is removal of a foreign body (see p. 275). If endoscopy is available, removal of the foreign body with the appropriate retrieval device is preferred, when possible. Likewise, endoscopic gastric mucosal biopsy and exploration for ulceration,

---

TABLE 16-24

Selected Anesthetic Protocols for Use in Patients That Are Hypovolemic, Dehydrated, or Shocky*

Dogs
Induction

Oxymorphone (0.1 mg/kg IV) plus diazepam (0.2 mg/kg IV) Give in incremental dosages. Intubate if possible. If necessary give etomidate (0.5-1.5 mg/kg IV). Alternatively, give thiopental or propofol at extremely reduced dosages.

Maintenance

Isoflurane

Cats
Premedication

Butorphanol (0.2-0.4 mg/kg SC, IM) or buprenorphine (5-15 µg/kg IM) or oxymorphone (0.05 mg/kg SC, IM)

Induction

Diazepam (0.2 mg/kg IV) followed by etomidate (0.5-1.5 mg/kg IV). Alternatively, give thiopental or propofol at reduced dosages. If there are no contraindications to ketamine, reduced dosages of diazepam and ketamine may also be used.

Maintenance

Isoflurane

*Anticholinergics may be administered if indicated.

TABLE 16-25

Perioperative Antibiotic Therapy

Cefazolin (Ancef or Kefzol)
20 mg/kg IV at induction; repeat once or twice at 4-6 hr intervals

neoplasia, or hypertrophy are preferred over gastrotomy unless there is a scirrhous or submucosal lesion.

Make a ventral midline abdominal incision from the xiphoid to the pubis. Use Balfour retractors to retract the abdominal wall and provide adequate exposure to the gastrointestinal tract. Inspect the entire abdominal contents before incising the stomach. To decrease contamination, isolate the stomach from remaining abdominal contents with moistened laparotomy sponges. Place stay sutures to assist in manipulation of the stomach and help prevent spillage of gastric contents. Make the gastric incision in a hypovascular area of the ventral aspect of the stomach, between the greater and lesser curvatures (Fig. 16-57). Be sure that the

incision is not near the pylorus, lest closure of the incision causes excessive tissue to be infolded into the gastric lumen, producing outflow obstruction. Make a stab incision into the gastric lumen with a scalpel (Fig. 16-58, A), and enlarge the incision with Metzenbaum scissors (Fig. 16-58, B). Use suction to aspirate gastric contents and decrease spillage. Close the stomach with 2-0 or 3-0 suture material in a two-layer inverting seromuscular pattern, using an absorbable suture material such as polydioxanone or polyglyconate suture (Fig. 16-58, C). Include serosa, muscularis, and submucosa in the first layer, using a Cushing or simple continuous pattern, then follow it with a Lembert or Cushing pattern that incorporates the serosal and muscularis layers (Fig. 16-58, D). Alternatively, close the mucosa with a simple continuous suture pattern as a separate layer, to decrease postoperative bleeding. Substitute sterile instruments and gloves for ones contaminated by gastric contents, before closing the abdominal incision. Whenever you remove a gastric foreign body, be sure to check the entire intestinal tract for additional material that could cause an intestinal obstruction.

Partial Gastrectomy and Invagination of Gastric Tissue

Partial gastrectomy is indicated when necrosis, ulceration, or neoplasia involves the greater curvature, or middle portion, of the stomach. Necrosis of the greater curvature is primarily associated with gastric dilatation-volvulus (GDV) and may be treated by resection or invagination. Invagination does not require opening of the gastric lumen; however, obstruction from excessive intraluminal tissue is possible (but rare). The extent of necrosis is assessed by observing serosal color, gastric wall texture, vascular patency, and bleeding on incision; however, it is difficult to determine tissue viability in many cases with these techniques (see p. 295 for a discussion of methods to determine tissue viability). Necrotic tissue

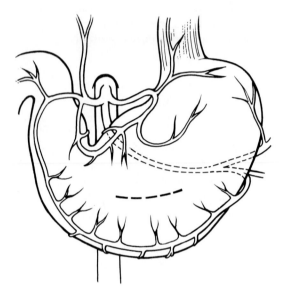

FIG. 16-57
Desired location of gastrotomy incisions.

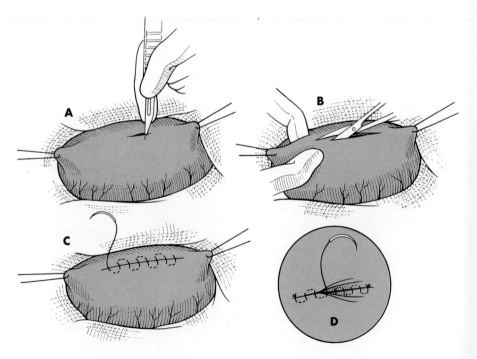

FIG. 16-58
For gastrotomy **A,** make a stab incision into the gastric lumen with a scalpel and **B,** enlarge the incision with Metzenbaum scissors. **C** and **D,** Close the stomach with a two-layer inverting seromuscular pattern.

may range in color from gray-green to black and often feels thin. A full-thickness incision can be made into the suspected necrotic tissue to assess arterial bleeding. Intravenous fluorescein dye has not proved to be an accurate method of determining gastric viability in dogs with GDV. Generally, if you question the viability of the gastric tissue, remove it or invaginate it. Failure to remove or invaginate necrotic tissue may cause perforation, peritonitis, and death. Melena is commonly observed for a few days after gastric invagination.

☞ **N O T E ·** Mucosal color cannot predict gastric tissue viability. It is commonly dark in dogs with GDV, even if the seromuscular layer is viable.

To remove the greater curvature of the stomach, ligate branches of the left gastroepiploic vessels and/or short gastric vessels along the section of the stomach to be removed (Fig. 16-59). Excise the necrotic tissue, leaving a margin of normal, actively bleeding tissue to suture. Close the stomach with a two-layer inverting suture pattern, using an absorbable suture (e.g., polydioxanone or polyglyconate suture; 2-0 or 3-0). Incorporate submucosa, muscularis, and serosal layers in a Cushing or simple continuous pattern in the first layer. Then use a Cushing or Lembert pattern to invert the serosa and muscularis over the first layer. Alternatively, you may use a thoracoabdominal (TA) stapling device to close the incision. To invaginate necrotic tissue, use a simple continuous suture pattern followed by an inverting suture pattern. Place sutures in healthy gastric tissue on both sides of the tissue that is to be invaginated, bringing the healthy tissue over the top of the necrotic tissue. Be sure that sutures are placed in healthy tissues to prevent dehiscence.

Removal of neoplasia (see p. 289) or ulceration (see p. 286) of the greater or lesser curvature is similar to that de-scribed for necrotic tissue. Most neoplasms in the gastric body have metastasized by the time they are diagnosed. If the abnormal tissue involves the dorsal or ventral aspect of the stomach, an elliptical incision encompassing the lesion and some adjacent normal tissue is used. Closure is as for a simple gastrotomy. Occasionally, the extent of the lesion requires resection of both the dorsal and ventral wall of the stomach. *In such cases, ligate branches of the right and left gastric artery and vein (lesser curvature) and left gastroepiploic artery and vein (greater curvature), and remove omental attachments. Following removal of the suspect tissues, perform a two-layer end-to-end anastomosis of the stomach. If the luminal circumferences are of disparate size, the larger circumference can be partially closed using a two-layer suture pattern (see Fig. 16-61, B). Close the mucosa and submucosa of the dorsal surface of the stomach with a simple continuous pattern, using an absorbable suture material (2-0 or 3-0), then close the ventral aspect. Suture the serosa and muscularis layers with an inverting suture pattern (e.g., Cushing or Lembert).*

Temporary Gastrostomy

Temporary gastrostomy is used to decompress the stomach and is occasionally indicated in dogs with GDV until more definitive surgery can be performed (see p. 280 for indications). It is recommended only if surgery must be delayed and alternative techniques fail to keep the stomach decompressed (see p. 280). **Gastric necrosis may continue in rotated stomachs, even after decompression.** Temporary gastrostomy can usually be performed with local anesthesia (i.e., 2% lidocaine), using a reverse-7 local block (Fig. 16-60, *A*) or direct infiltration over the proposed incision. Tranquilization or sedation may be necessary if the dog is fractious. *Make a 6- to 10-cm full-thickness incision in the right paracostal body wall, and identify the stomach (Fig. 16-60, B). Before incising into the gastric lumen, suture the*

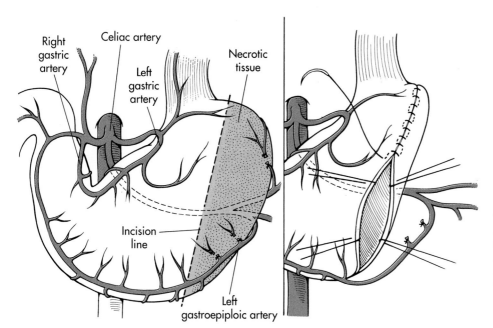

FIG. 16-59
To remove the greater curvature of the stomach, ligate branches of the left gastroepiploic vessels and/or short gastric vessels and excise the necrotic tissue. Close the stomach with a two-layer inverting suture pattern.

Right gastric artery
Celiac artery
Left gastric artery
Necrotic tissue
Incision line
Left gastroepiploic artery

FIG. 16-60
Temporary gastrostomy can usually be performed using **A,** a reverse-7 local block or direct infiltration over the proposed incision. **B,** Make a full-thickness incision in the right paracostal body wall and identify the stomach. **C,** Suture the stomach to skin using a simple continuous suture pattern, **D,** then make an incision in the stomach.

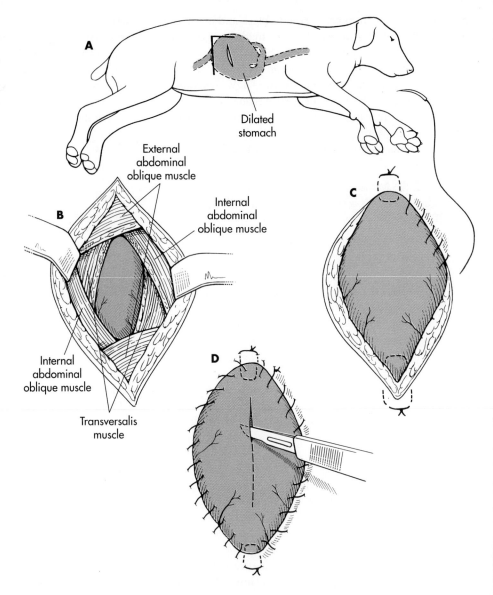

Dilated stomach

External abdominal oblique muscle

Internal abdominal oblique muscle

Internal abdominal oblique muscle

Transversalis muscle

stomach to skin using a simple continuous suture pattern (Fig. 16-60, C). Then make an incision in the stomach (Fig. 16-60, D). Be sure that the stomach is securely sutured to the skin to prevent leakage of gastric contents subcutaneously. Place Vaseline on the skin to prevent scalding from gastric contents.

Pylorectomy with Gastroduodenostomy (Billroth I)

Removal of the pylorus and gastroduodenostomy are indicated for neoplasia (see p. 289), outflow obstruction due to pyloric muscular hypertrophy (see p. 283), or ulceration of the gastric outflow tract (see p. 286). If neoplasia is present, at least 1- to 2-cm margins of normal tissue should be removed with the abnormal tissue. The margins of the resected tissue should be evaluated histologically for evidence of neoplasia. If damage to the common bile duct occurs, a cholecystoduodenostomy or cholecystojejunostomy may need to be performed (see p. 392). If the pancreatic ducts are inadvertently ligated, supplementation with pancreatic enzymes may be necessary postoperatively.

☞ **N O T E** · Be careful to avoid incising the common bile duct where it traverses the lesser omentum.

Identify the common bile duct and pancreatic ducts, then place stay sutures in the proximal duodenum and pyloric antrum. If increased caudoventral retraction of the pylorus is desired, identify and transect a portion of the hepatogastric ligament. Ligate branches of the right gastric and right gastroepiploic artery and vein to the affected tissues, and remove the omental and mesenteric attachments (Fig. 16-61, A). Use noncrushing forceps (Doyen) or fingers to occlude the stomach and duodenum proximal and distal to the area to be resected. Excise the area of pylorus to be removed, using Metzenbaum scissors or a scalpel blade, and inspect the remaining edges to ensure that all abnormal tissue has been excised. If there is marked disparity in the size of the gastric and duodenal lumens, incise the duodenum at an angle, or partially close the antrum (Fig. 16-61, B). Perform a one- or two-layer end-to-end anastomosis of the pyloric antrum to the duodenum, using 2-0 or

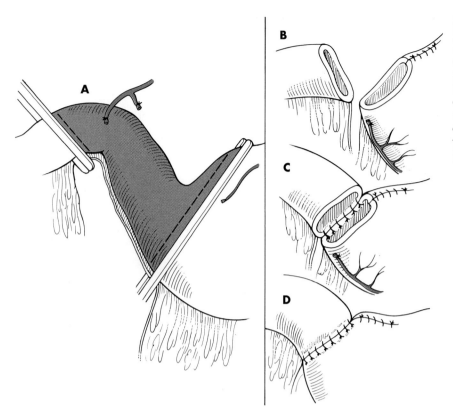

FIG. 16-61
For a Billroth I procedure, **A,** ligate vasculature, remove omental and mesenteric attachments, and excise the area of the pylorus to be removed. **B,** If there is marked disparity in the size of the gastric and duodenal lumens, incise the duodenum at an angle or partially close the antrum. **C,** Close the far (dorsal) aspect of the incision first, **D,** followed by the near (ventral) aspect.

3-0 absorbable suture material in a simple continuous, crushing, or simple interrupted pattern. In one study no difference was noted in the prevalence of postoperative leakage and incisional dehiscence between a one-layer and two-layer closure (Walter, Matthiesen, Stone, 1985). *Close the far (dorsal) aspect of the incision first (Fig. 16-61, C), followed by the near (ventral) aspect (Fig. 16-61, D). Avoid inverting excessive tissue, which might decrease the diameter of the gastric outflow tract.*

Partial Gastrectomy with Gastrojejunostomy (Billroth II)

If the extent of the lesion precludes performing an end-to-end anastomosis of the pyloric antrum to the duodenum, consider a Billroth II. If only mucosal hypertrophy is present, a Y-U pyloroplasty (see below) is easier to perform and is effective. Before undertaking this procedure, be sure that gross evidence of metastasis is not present (see p. 289 for information regarding gastric neoplasia). In most instances, a cholecystojejunostomy or cholecystoduodenostomy is required in addition to the gastrojejunostomy (see p. 392). Exocrine insufficiency may occur if the pancreatic ducts are damaged. Exocrine plus endocrine (i.e., diabetes mellitus) pancreatic insufficiency may occur as a result of pancreatic resection or severe damage to the pancreatic blood supply.

The procedure is similar to a Billroth I except that the distal stomach and proximal duodenum are closed after pylorectomy, and the jejunum is attached with a side-to-side anastomosis to the diaphragmatic surface of the stomach. *Resect the pylorus, antrum, and proximal duodenum as described above, ligating appropriate branches of the right*
and left gastric and gastroepiploic vessels (Fig. 16-62, A). Close the duodenal and pyloric antral stumps with a two-layer suture pattern. For the first layer, incorporate the mucosa and submucosa in a simple interrupted or simple continuous suture pattern of 2-0 or 3-0 absorbable suture material (Fig. 16-62, B). Then place an inverting suture pattern (e.g., Lembert) in the seromuscular layer. Identify an avascular area between the gastric incision and greater curvature. Bring a loop of proximal jejunum to the selected site, and attach it to the stomach with stay sutures. Suture the seromuscular layers of the stomach and intestine together, using a simple continuous suture pattern (Fig. 16-62, C). Make full-thickness, longitudinal incisions into the stomach and intestinal lumens, near the suture line (Fig. 16-62, D). Suture mucosa and submucosa of the stomach to the intestine with a continuous suture pattern (Fig. 16-62, E) of absorbable suture material (3-0 or 4-0). Next place a continuous suture pattern in the serosa and muscularis. Use of stapling devices has also been described for stump closure and creation of the gastrojejunostomy.

Pyloromyotomy and Pyloroplasty

Pyloromyotomy and pyloroplasty increase the diameter of the pylorus and are used to correct gastric outflow obstruction (i.e., chronic antral mucosal hypertrophy or pyloric stenosis). However, they should not be performed routinely in dogs without evidence of pyloric dysfunction (e.g., most dogs with GDV), because they can slow gastric emptying. Gastric draining procedures that increase the diameter of the pyloric lumen seem to favor early passage of viscous, nonhomogenous, and hyperosmolar gastric contents into the duodenum. This

FIG. 16-62
For a Billroth II procedure, **A,** resect the pylorus, antrum, and proximal duodenum. **B,** Close the duodenal and pyloric antral stumps with a two-layer suture pattern. **C,** Bring a loop of proximal jejunum to the stomach and suture the seromuscular layers of the stomach and intestine together. **D,** Make full-thickness, longitudinal incisions into the stomach and intestinal lumens. **E,** Suture mucosa and submucosa of the stomach to intestine with a continuous suture pattern.

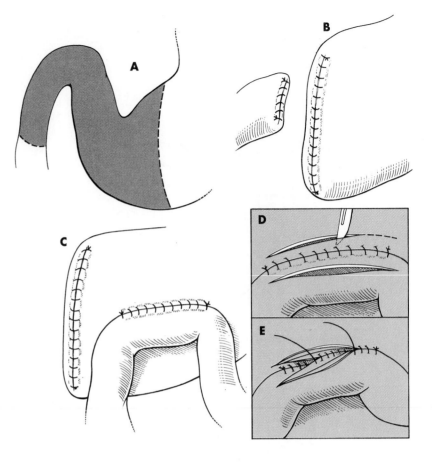

early passage may overstimulate the enterogastric reflex, prematurely inhibiting antral motor activity and delaying gastric emptying. Additionally, gastroduodenal reflux may occur if pyloric function is altered with surgery. Metoclopramide or cisapride (Table 16-26) may be beneficial in these cases.

Fredet-Ramstedt pyloromyotomy. Fredet-Ramstedt pyloromyotomy is the simplest and easiest of these procedures. It does not allow inspection or biopsy of the pyloric mucosa and probably provides only temporary benefit because healing may lessen the lumen size. *Hold the pylorus between the index finger and thumb in the nondominant hand. Select a hypovascular area of the ventral pylorus, and make a longitudinal incision through the serosa and muscularis, but not through the mucosa (Fig. 16-63). Make sure that the muscularis layer is completely incised, to allow the mucosa to bulge into the incision site. If the mucosa is inadvertently penetrated, suture it with interrupted sutures of 2-0 or 3-0 absorbable suture material.*

Heineke-Mikulicz pyloroplasty. Heineke-Mikulicz pyloroplasty allows limited exposure of the pyloric mucosa for biopsy and is easy to perform. *Make a full-thickness, longitudinal incision in the ventral surface of the pylorus (Fig. 16-64). Place traction sutures at the center of the incision, and orient the incision transversely. Suture the transverse incision with a one-layer suture pattern (simple interrupted or crushing) of 2-0 or 3-0 absorbable suture material. Place*

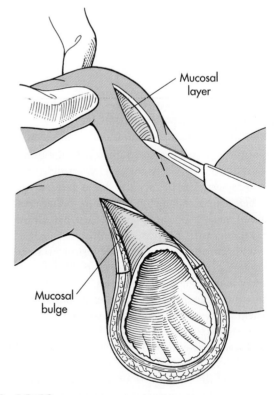

Mucosal layer

Mucosal bulge

FIG. 16-63
Fredet-Ramstedt pyloromyotomy.

TABLE 16-26
Prokinetic Drugs
Metoclopramide (Reglan)
0.25-0.5 mg/kg PO, IV or SC, SID to QID
Cisapride (Propulsid)
Dogs
0.25-0.5 mg/kg PO, BID to TID
Cats
2.5-5 mg/cat PO, BID to TID

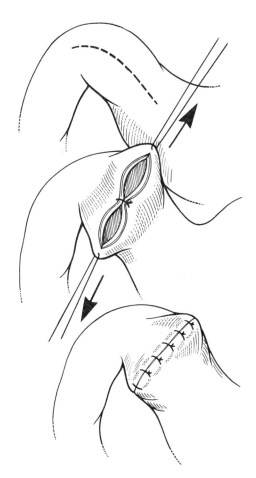

FIG. 16-64
Heineke-Mikulicz pyloroplasty.

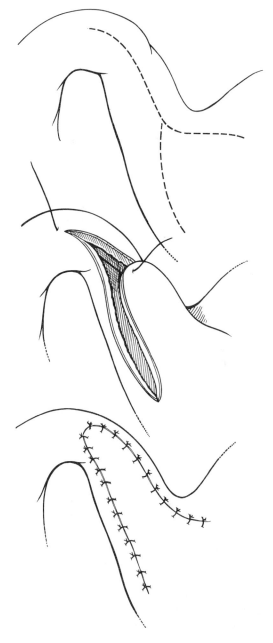

FIG. 16-65
Y-U pyloroplasty.

the sutures carefully, so that the incision edges are properly aligned and tissue inversion avoided.

Y-U pyloroplasty. The Y-U pyloroplasty allows greater accessibility for resection of the pyloric mucosa in dogs with mucosal hypertrophy, while simultaneously increasing the luminal diameter of the outflow tract. *Make a longitudinal incision (limb) in the serosa overlying the ventral pylorus, and extend it into the stomach by making two incisions (arms) that run parallel to the lesser and greater curvature of the stomach (creating a Y-shaped incision) (Fig. 16-65, A).*

Be sure that the angle of the Y is not overly narrow or necrosis may result. The limbs and arms of the Y-shaped incision should be approximately the same length. Make a full-thickness incision. Inspect the mucosa, and if necessary, resect it. If mucosa is resected, appose the remaining mucosal edges with a continuous suture pattern of absorbable suture material, before closing the Y incision. Suture the base of the antral flap to the distal end of the duodenal incision with a simple interrupted suture (absorbable 2-0 or 3-0 suture material), creating a U-shaped closure (Fig. 16-65, B). Close the remainder of the incision (the limbs) with simple interrupted sutures (Fig. 16-65, C). Be sure that tissue approximation is adequate to prevent leakage and that minimal tissue has been infolded into the pyloric lumen.

☞ **N O T E** · To decrease necrosis of the pointed tip of the gastric tissue flap, you may wish to excise the point of the "Y" before suturing it.

Gastropexy

Gastropexy techniques are designed to permanently adhere the stomach to the body wall. The most common indications are GDV (pyloric antrum to right body wall) and hiatal herniation (fundus to left body wall). Numerous gastropexy techniques have been described. Although the strength and extent of adhesions created by these various techniques differ, all of them (when properly performed) prevent movement of the stomach. To create a permanent adhesion, the gastric muscle must be in contact with the muscle of the body wall; **intact gastric serosa will not form permanent adhesions to an intact peritoneal surface.**

A technique for gastropexy has recently been described in which the stomach is incorporated into the abdominal incision during closure (Meyer-Lindenberg et al, 1993). Although this technique is easy, quick, and decreases recurrence of GDV, it results in the stomach being permanently adhered to the ventral body wall. The main advantage of this procedure is that it can be performed quickly. However, the subsequent abdominal exploration via a midline abdominal incision could perforate the stomach. Therefore, although this technique is preferable to not performing any type of "pexy," it is not generally recommended. Surgeons should become familiar with one of the techniques described below.

☞ **N O T E** · Always perform a permanent gastropexy in dogs with GDV!

Tube gastropexy. Tube gastropexy (gastrostomy) is quick and relatively simple (Fig. 16-66). Additionally, it allows postoperative gastric decompression and placement of medications directly into the stomach in inappetent animals. The tube should be left in place 7 to 10 days to form a permanent adhesion. Although this may increase the postoperative hospitalization period compared with other techniques, the tube can be capped, secured against the trunk, and the patient sent home on oral feeding. The risk of leakage is minimal if proper technique is used; however, improper placement may result in peritonitis.

☞ **N O T E** · Cut the tip off the end of the Foley catheter if food or viscous fluids are to be injected through it.

Make a stab incision into the right abdominal wall, caudal to the last rib and 4 to 10 cm lateral to the midline. Place a Foley catheter (18 to 30 French) through the stab incision (Fig. 16-67, A). Select a site in a hypovascular region of the seromuscular layer of the ventral surface of the pyloric antrum where the balloon of the catheter will not obstruct gastric outflow. Place a purse-string suture of 2-0 ab-

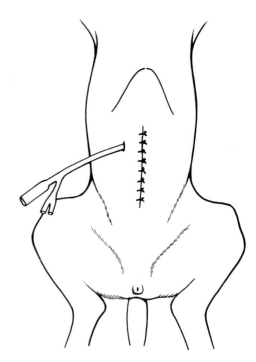

FIG. 16-66
Tube gastropexy.

sorbable suture (e.g., polydioxanone or polyglyconate suture) at this site. Make a stab incision through the purse-string suture and insert the Foley catheter tip into the gastric lumen. (NOTE: The Foley catheter can be placed through the omentum before entry into the stomach so that the omentum is secured between the stomach and body wall, or the omentum can be wrapped around the site after the stomach has been secured to the body wall.) Inflate the bulb of the Foley catheter with saline (not air), and secure the purse-string suture around the tube. Pre-place three to four absorbable sutures between the pyloric antrum and the body wall, where the tube exits (Fig. 16-67, B). Avoid penetrating the catheter or balloon when placing the sutures. Draw the stomach to the body wall by placing traction on the catheter, and tie the preplaced sutures (Fig. 16-67, C). Secure the tube to skin with a Roman sandal suture pattern (see p. 679), but avoid penetrating it with a suture. Place a bandage around the dog's abdomen and over the tube to prevent its premature removal (and use an Elizabethan collar if necessary). Leave the tube in place 7 to 10 days, then deflate the balloon and remove it. Leave the skin incision open to facilitate drainage. Place a light bandage over the open wound if desired.

Circumcostal gastropexy. Circumcostal gastropexy forms a stronger adhesion than most other techniques, but it is technically more challenging (Table 16-27). Because the lumen of the stomach is not entered, the risk for gastric leakage and abdominal contamination is decreased compared with tube gastropexy. Potential complications associated with circumcostal gastropexy include pneumothorax and rib fracture. *Make either a one- or two-layer hinged flap (ap-*

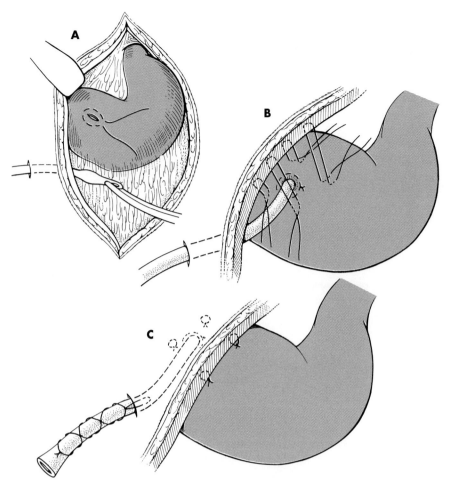

FIG. 16-67
For tube gastropexy **A,** insert a Foley catheter tip into the gastric lumen through a purse-string suture. **B,** Preplace three to four absorbable sutures between the pyloric antrum and the body wall where the tube exits. **C,** Draw the stomach to the body wall and tie the preplaced sutures. Secure the tube to skin with a Roman sandal suture pattern.

TABLE 16-27

Advantages and Disadvantages of Circumcostal Gastropexy

Advantages
- Strong
- Gastric lumen not opened

Disadvantages
- More difficult to perform
- Risk of pneumothorax
- Rib fractures may occur
- Does not provide direct access to gastric lumen if postoperative decompression is necessary

proximately 5 to 6 cm long in large dogs) by incising through the seromuscular layer of the pyloric antrum (Fig. 16-68, A). Do not incise the gastric mucosa or enter the lumen (if this occurs, suture the mucosa with 3-0 absorbable suture material). Elevate the flap by dissecting under the muscularis. If a one-hinged flap is made, place the hinge towards the lesser curvature. Make a 5- to 6-cm incision over the eleventh or twelfth rib at the level of the costochondral junction (Fig. 16-68, B). Be sure that the incision does not penetrate the diaphragmatic attachments to the

body wall, causing pneumothorax. Form a tunnel under the rib using a Carmalt clamp or hemostat (Fig. 16-68, C). Place stay sutures on the flap (if using a two-flap technique, place the sutures on the flap nearest the lesser curvature). Pass the gastric antral flap craniodorsal under the rib (Fig. 16-68, D) and suture it with 2-0 absorbable suture material to the original gastric margin (one-flap technique; Fig. 16-69, A) or the other flap (two-flap technique; Fig. 16-69, B).

Muscular flap (incisional) gastropexy. Muscular flap (incisional) gastropexy is easier than circumcostal gastropexy and avoids potential complications associated with tube gastropexy (Table 16-28). *Make two hinged flaps in the seromuscular layer of the gastric antrum (similar to that for a circumcostal gastropexy). Then make similar flaps in the right ventrolateral abdominal wall by incising the peritoneum and internal fascia of the rectus abdominis or transverse abdominis muscles (Fig. 16-70, A). Elevate flaps by dissecting ventral to the muscle layer (Fig. 16-70, B). Invert the flaps, and suture the edge of the abdominal flaps to the gastric flaps, using a simple continuous suture pattern of 2-0 absorbable or nonabsorbable suture (Fig. 16-70, C). Ensure that the muscularis layer of the stomach is in contact with the abdominal wall muscle (Fig. 16-70, D). Suture the cranial margin first, followed*

FIG. 16-68
For circumcostal gastropexy **A,** make either a one- or two-layer hinged seromuscular flap in the pyloric antrum. **B,** Make an incision over the eleventh or twelfth rib at the level of the costochondral junction. **C,** Form a tunnel under the rib using a Carmalt clamp or hemostat. **D,** Pass the gastric antral flap craniodorsal under the rib and suture it to the original gastric margin or the other flap (see Fig. 16-69).

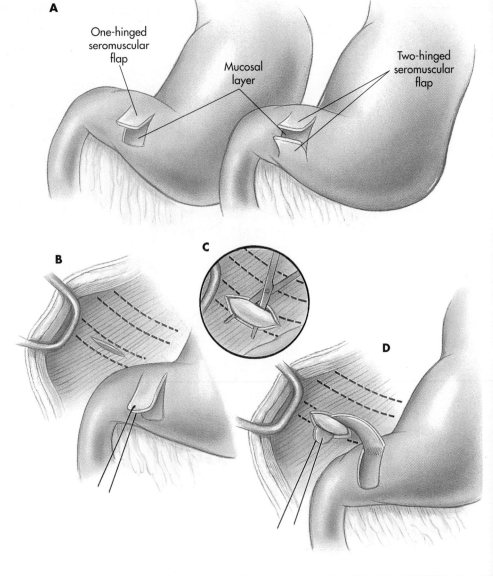

by the caudal margin. Be sure to place sufficient sutures so that a loop of bowel cannot become incarcerated between the flaps.

Belt-loop gastropexy. A belt-loop gastropexy is similar to a muscle flap gastropexy except that a single flap is elevated and passed beneath a tunnel created in the abdominal wall. It is technically simple and seems to result in adequate adhesions. *Elevate a seromuscular flap in the gastric antrum. Make two transverse incisions in the ventrolateral abdominal wall by incising the peritoneum and abdominal musculature (Fig. 16-71, A). The incisions should be 2.5 to 4 cm apart and 3 to 5 cm long. Create a tunnel under the abdominal musculature with forceps. Place stay sutures in the edge of the antral flap, and use them to pass the flap from cranial to caudal under the muscular flap (Fig. 16-71, B). Suture the flap to its original gastric margin, using a simple continuous suture pattern of 2-0 absorbable or non-absorbable suture material (Fig. 16-71, C).* You may wish to place additional sutures between the body wall and the stomach to decrease tension on the gastropexy.

GASTRIC WOUND HEALING

The extraordinarily rich blood supply, reduced bacterial numbers (as a result of gastric acidity), rapidly regenerating epithelium, and defense mechanisms provided by the omentum allow gastric incisions to heal quickly. Because the stomach has a thicker wall than the bowel, hemorrhage control is often more difficult because bleeders may be more difficult to locate. Gentle pressure applied to the bleeding tissues is usually effective; crushing clamps, forceps, and electrocautery should be avoided.

SUTURE MATERIALS/ SPECIAL INSTRUMENTS

Monofilament absorbable suture material (i.e., polydioxanone [PDS] or polyglyconate [Maxon]), is preferred for gastrointestinal surgery. These sutures are strong, have minimal

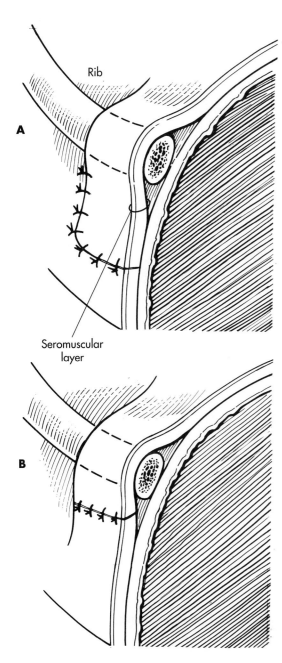

FIG. 16-69
A, With a one-flap technique suture the circumcostal flap to the original gastric margin. **B,** With a two-flap technique pass the seromuscular flap under the rib and suture it to the second flap.

tissue drag, and maintain tensile strength for longer than 45 days. Chromic gut suture is rapidly removed by digestion and phagocytosis and should be avoided. Nonabsorbable suture material that penetrates the lumen may cause gastric ulcers to form along the suture line if a continuous suture pattern is used. Therefore nonabsorbable suture material should be avoided in the stomach. Small-diameter swaged-on taper-point needles are generally preferred for gastrointestinal surgery. However, cutting needles are sometimes used because they more readily penetrate submucosa and require less stabilization of tissue (which might result in less crushing).

TABLE 16-28
Advantages and Disadvantages of Muscular Flap and Belt-Loop Gastropexy
Advantages
• Easy and quick to perform
• Gastric lumen not opened
Disadvantages
• Less strong than circumcostal gastropexy
• Does not provide direct access to gastric lumen if postoperative decompression is necessary

☞ **N O T E** • Do not use chromic gut suture for gastric surgery. It should also not be used for abdominal closure in very young animals or those that are hypoproteinemic.

Noncrushing forceps (e.g., Doyen forceps or some vascular clamps) are useful for occluding the gastric and duodenal stumps during gastroduodenostomy or gastrojejunostomy procedures (see p. 266). Pediatric Doyens are the appropriate size to occlude the duodenal lumen. If noncrushing forceps are not available, the straight portion of an Allis tissue forceps can be wrapped with a moistened sponge. Crushing forceps, such as Carmalt or Allen forceps, are useful to occlude the portion of the gastrointestinal tract that will be removed, but should not be placed on tissues that are not to be excised.

POSTOPERATIVE CARE AND ASSESSMENT

Electrolytes (especially potassium) should be monitored postoperatively. Analgesics should be provided as needed. Intravenous fluids are continued until the patient is drinking adequate amounts to maintain hydration. If prolonged vomiting or anorexia is anticipated, enteral hyperalimentation via a gastrostomy or enterostomy (if the animal is vomiting) tube (see Chapter 11) should be provided. With planning, feeding tubes can be placed during the initial surgery so as to avoid a second procedure. Food can be offered 12 hours postoperatively if there is no vomiting. ECGs should be monitored if arrhythmias were present before surgery or are anticipated postoperatively.

COMPLICATIONS

Complications associated with gastric surgery may include vomiting, anorexia, peritonitis secondary to intraoperative or postoperative leakage, ulceration at anastomotic sites, gastric outlet obstruction, and pancreatitis.

SPECIAL AGE CONSIDERATIONS

Young animals should not have food withheld for longer than 4 to 6 hours before surgery and should be fed as soon as they are fully recovered from the anesthesia. If they cannot

FIG. 16-70
For muscular flap gastropexy **A,** make hinged flaps in the seromuscular layer of the gastric antrum and in the right ventrolateral abdominal wall. **B,** Elevate the flaps by dissecting ventral to the muscle layer. **C,** Invert the flaps and suture the edge of the abdominal flaps to the gastric flaps using a simple continuous suture pattern. **D,** Ensure that the muscularis layer of the stomach is in contact with the abdominal wall muscle.

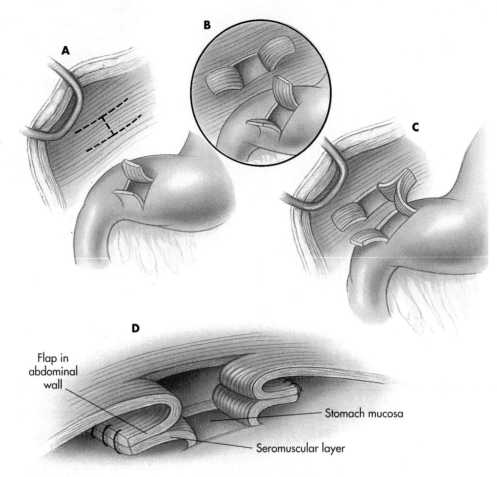

Flap in abdominal wall

Stomach mucosa

Seromuscular layer

FIG. 16-71
For a belt-loop gastropexy **A,** elevate a seromuscular flap in the gastric antrum. **B,** Make two transverse incisions in the ventrolateral abdominal wall and create a tunnel under the abdominal musculature with forceps. Pass the flap from cranial to caudal under the muscular flap. **C,** Suture the flap to its original gastric margin.

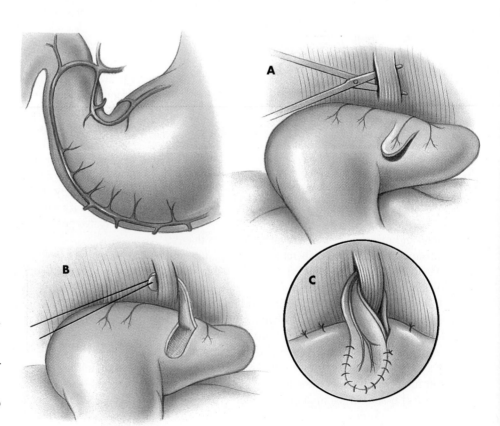

be fed, blood glucose concentrations should be maintained by adding glucose to the intravenous fluids (see the discussion of anesthesia on p. 262). Polydioxanone suture has been reported to cause calcinosis circumscripta in young dogs. Because the skin of puppies and kittens is delicate and elastic, skin sutures should be placed loosely. Geriatric animals may have delayed wound healing and may be immunosuppressed due to concurrent disease (e.g., diabetes mellitus, Cushing's disease). Strong absorbable or nonabsorbable suture material should be used in these patients and prophylactic antibiotic therapy initiated at anesthetic induction.

References

Meyer-Lindenberg A et al: Treatment of gastric dilatation-volvulus and a rapid method for prevention of relapse in dogs: 134 cases (1988–1991), *J Am Vet Med Assoc* 203: 1303, 1993.

Walter MC, Matthiesen DT, Stone EA: Pylorectomy and gastroduodenostomy in the dog: technique and clinical results in 28 cases, *J Am Vet Med Assoc* 187:909, 1985.

Suggested Reading

Ahmadu-Suka F et al: Billroth II gastrojejunostomy in dogs: stapling technique and postoperative complications, *Vet Surg* 17:211, 1988.

Beaumont PR: Anastomotic jejunal ulcer secondary to gastrojejunostomy in a dog, *J Amer Anim Hosp Assoc* 17:233, 1981.

Bright RM, Richardson DC, Stanton ME: Y-U antral flap advancement pyloroplasty in dogs, *Compend Contin Educ Pract Vet* 10:139, 1988.

Ellison GW: Wound healing in the gastrointestinal tract, *Semin Vet Med Surg (Small Anim)* 4:287, 1989.

Fossum TW, Rohn DA, Willard MD: Presumptive, iatrogenic gastric outflow obstruction associated with prior gastric surgery, *J Am Anim Hosp Assoc* 31:391, 1995.

Hosgood G: Surgical and anesthetic management of puppies and kittens, *Compend Cont Educ Pract Vet* 14:345, 1992.

Odonkor P, Mowat C, Himal HS: Prevention of sepsis-induced gastric lesions in dogs by cimetidine via inhibition of gastric secretion and by prostaglandin via cytoprotection, *Gastroenterology* 80:375, 1981.

Papageorges M, Bonneau NH, Breton L: Gastric drainage procedures: effects in normal dogs. III: Postmortem evaluation, *Vet Surg* 26:341, 1987.

Papageorges M, Breton L, Bonneau NH: Gastric drainage procedures: effects in normal dogs. II: Clinical observations and gastric emptying, *Vet Surg* 16:332, 1987.

Pearson H et al: Pyloric and oesophageal dysfunction in the cat, *Small Anim Pract* 15:487, 1974.

SPECIFIC DISEASES

GASTRIC FOREIGN BODIES

DEFINITIONS

A **gastric foreign body** is anything ingested by an animal that cannot be digested (i.e., rocks, plastic), or is slowly digested (bones). **Linear foreign bodies** are usually pieces of string, yarn, thread, cloth, or dental floss.

GENERAL CONSIDERATIONS AND CLINICALLY RELEVANT PATHOPHYSIOLOGY

Gastric foreign bodies usually cause vomiting due to outflow obstruction, gastric distention, and/or mucosal irritation (Table 16-29). Occasionally, however, gastric foreign bodies (i.e., pins, pieces of wire, surgical sponges) are asymptomatic, incidental findings on abdominal radiographs. Dogs are indiscriminate eaters and often ingest rocks, plastic toys, cooking bags, and other objects. Cats more commonly ingest linear material (e.g., sewing thread attached to a needle, yarn). In cats, linear foreign bodies are frequently anchored under the tongue or at the pylorus and often cause intestinal plication (Fig. 16-72). Noxious stimuli or distention of the duodenum or pyloric antrum stimulates vomiting, whereas similar stimulation of the gastric body often does not. Therefore vomiting is often intermittent, occurring when the object is forced into the pyloric antrum.

TABLE   16-29

Important Considerations for Gastric Foreign Bodies

- Initial clinical signs may not alert the owner to seriousness of disease.
- Linear foreign objects must be resolved as soon as possible to avoid intestinal perforation/peritonitis.
- Not all animals with gastric foreign objects vomit.
- Finding a foreign object in the stomach does not mean that it is always the cause of vomiting.
- Linear foreign bodies are more common in cats; always check under the tongue (this often requires sedation).
- Many foreign objects can be removed endoscopically.
- Complete exploration of the entire intestinal tract is mandatory.
- Always repeat the radiographs immediately before surgery to make sure that the object has not moved.

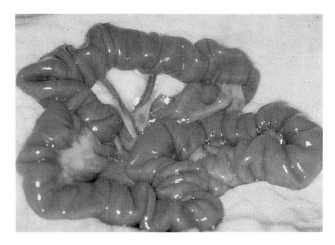

FIG. 16-72
Plication in the intestines of a cat caused by a string foreign body. (Courtesy Dr. J. Hauptman, Michigan State University.)

Foreign bodies may occur in the stomach and small intestine concurrently; therefore **complete exploration of the entire intestinal tract should be performed whenever surgery is done to remove a gastric foreign body.** If endoscopic removal is selected, be sure to examine the small intestine as far as possible. Small, blunt foreign bodies may pass through the digestive system without causing harm; however, most should be removed when they are diagnosed because of the risk of obstruction and perforation. **Repeat radiographs are indicated immediately before surgery.** Even if only a few hours have elapsed since the initial radiographs, the object may exit the stomach and be located in either the small intestine or colon. Foreign objects in the colon are usually eliminated without difficulty.

DIAGNOSIS
Clinical Presentation

Signalment. Young animals more commonly ingest foreign bodies than do older animals, and gastric or intestinal foreign bodies should be suspected in any puppy or kitten presenting for acute or persistent vomiting.

History. Most animals with gastric foreign bodies present for vomiting, anorexia, and/or depression. The vomiting may be intermittent and some animals may continue to eat and remain active. Vomiting is often absent if the foreign body is in the gastric fundus and does not obstruct the pylorus. Occasionally, abdominal pain is noted.

Physical Examination Findings

Physical examination is often unremarkable. The patient may be dehydrated; however, many animals with gastric foreign bodies continue to drink water. The object usually cannot be palpated because of the stomach's proximal location in the abdomen. Plicated intestines may be felt if there is a linear foreign object, and pain may be evident if gastric perforation has caused peritonitis. Thorough examination of the mouth, including ventral to the tongue, is mandatory in all animals with suspected linear foreign objects. General anesthesia is often necessary to properly evaluate the base of the tongue.

☞ **NOTE** · Don't forget to check under the tongue in cats with possible linear foreign objects.

Radiography/Endoscopy

Radiopaque foreign bodies can be diagnosed with plain films; however, many foreign bodies are radiolucent. Contrast studies may be necessary to delineate radiolucent foreign bodies. Barium should not be placed in the stomach if gastrointestinal perforation is suspected (i.e., pneumoperitoneum, abdominal effusion); a water-soluble contrast agent should be used in such cases. Double contrast studies, using both air and a positive contrast agent (i.e., barium sulfate), may be useful when the foreign object absorbs or is coated by the contrast material; however, if a radiolucent foreign body is suspected, endoscopy is preferred. Radiographic findings in cats with linear foreign bodies include plication and shortening of the small bowel, increased luminal gas bubbles, and peritonitis secondary to bowel perforation (see p. 192).

☞ **NOTE** · Do not do an upper GI if you will perform endoscopy within 24 hours. Do not use barium if perforation is likely!

Laboratory Findings

Laboratory findings depend on the severity and duration of the obstruction; they cannot be predicted. Laboratory parameters may be normal or may show only changes caused by dehydration (↑PCV, ↑TP, ↑BUN, ↑creatinine). If vomiting causes loss of gastric secretions, a hypochloremic, hypokalemic, metabolic alkalosis with paradoxical aciduria may occur. Sometimes a metabolic acidosis occurs because of dehydration and subsequent lactic acidosis.

DIFFERENTIAL DIAGNOSIS

Gastric neoplasms sometimes cause filling defects in the gastric lumen that could be confused with a foreign object. However, such lesions should remain in the same location when the animal is positioned for different radiographic views. Radiographs and endoscopy distinguish animals with gastric foreign objects from those with other causes of pyloric obstruction (e.g., chronic antral mucosal hypertropy or pyloric stenosis; see p. 283) or gastric ulceration (see p. 286).

MEDICAL MANAGEMENT

If the object is small and has rounded edges, vomition can be induced using apomorphine in the dog or xylazine in the cat (Table 16-30). However, this should only be attempted when the clinician is certain it will be expelled without causing harm. Factors that must be considered include whether the esophagus is apt to be lacerated, the likelihood of the object lodging in the esophagus, and whether aspiration of the object or gastric contents might occur. Esophageal surgery carries more risk than gastric surgery because the esophagus does not heal as readily as the stomach (see p. 238). Indiscriminate antibiotic use may mask clinical signs of peritonitis or pyothorax and delay treatment (see p. 192).

TABLE 16-30
Induction of Vomition

Dogs
Apomorphine
0.02-0.04 mg/kg IV or SC, respectively

Cats
Xylazine (Rompun)
0.4-0.5 mg/kg IV or SC, respectively

SURGICAL TREATMENT
Preoperative Management

If possible, metabolic and acid-base abnormalities should be identified and corrected, and food withheld for 12 hours. Radiographs should be taken immediately before surgery to verify the position of the object in the digestive tract. Perioperative antibiotics may be given at induction and continued for up to 12 hours postoperatively (see p. 263).

Anesthesia

See p. 262 for suggested anesthetic protocols for use in dogs with gastric disorders.

Surgical Anatomy

See p. 263 for surgical anatomy of the stomach.

Positioning

The animal is placed in dorsal recumbency and the abdomen prepared for a ventral midline incision. The prepped area should extend from midthorax to the pubis to allow the entire digestive system to be explored for foreign objects.

SURGICAL TECHNIQUE

Most gastric foreign bodies are easily removed via a gastrotomy incision (see p. 263 for technique). *Inspect the entire digestive system for material that could cause obstruction or perforation. If a linear foreign body is found in the pylorus and extends into the intestinal tract, do not try to pull it into the stomach unless it moves easily. Instead, make several incisions into the stomach and intestines to avoid causing further damage to the intestinal tract. Inspect the stomach for perforation or necrosis, and remove or patch abnormal tissue (see p. 301 for description of serosal patch), depending on the location. Close the gastric incision as described on p. 264.*

SUTURE MATERIALS/ SPECIAL INSTRUMENTS

Absorbable suture material (2-0 or 3-0) should be used to close the gastrotomy incision (see p. 264). Instruments helpful in performing gastric surgery are listed on p. 272.

POSTOPERATIVE CARE AND ASSESSMENT

The patient's fluid status should be monitored and hydration maintained with intravenous fluids postoperatively until the animal is drinking. Electrolyte abnormalities should be corrected. Hypokalemia is likely if the animal has been anorexic or had sustained vomiting. A bland diet should be fed for 12 to 24 hours after surgery if the patient is not vomiting. If vomiting continues, centrally acting antiemetics such as chlorpromazine, metoclopramide, or ondansetron (Table 16-31) may be administered, and oral food and water should be withheld. Refer to p. 288 for treatment of ulcers that may occur secondary to foreign bodies.

PROGNOSIS

The prognosis is good if the stomach has not perforated and the foreign body is removed. If perforation has occurred, the prognosis is guarded (see the discussion on peritonitis on p. 193).

Suggested Reading

Basher AWP, Fowler JD: Conservative versus surgical management of gastrointestinal linear foreign bodies in the cat, *Vet Surg* 16:135, 1987.

Felts JF, Fox PR, Burk RL: Thread and sewing needles as gastrointestinal foreign bodies in the cat: a review of 64 cases, *J Am Vet Med Assoc* 184:56, 1984.

GASTRIC DILATATION-VOLVULUS

DEFINITIONS

Enlargement of the stomach associated with rotation on its mesenteric axis is referred to as **gastric dilatation-volvulus (GDV)**. The term **simple dilatation** refers to a stomach that is engorged with air or froth, but not malpositioned. **Dilatation** refers to a condition in which an organ or structure is stretched beyond its normal dimensions; **dilation** is the act of stretching a cavity or orifice.

SYNONYMS

Gastric torsion, bloat, GDV

GENERAL CONSIDERATIONS AND CLINICALLY RELEVANT PATHOPHYSIOLOGY

Classically, the GDV syndrome is an acute condition with a mortality rate of 30% to 45% in treated animals. The gastric enlargement is thought to be associated with a functional or mechanical gastric outflow obstruction. The initiating cause of the outflow obstruction is unknown; however, once the stomach dilates, normal physiologic means of removing air (i.e., eructation, vomiting, and pyloric emptying) are hindered because the esophageal and pyloric portals are obstructed.

TABLE 16-31

Treatment of Vomiting

Chlorpromazine (Thorazine)
0.2-0.4 mg/kg IM, SC, or PO, TID to QID

Metoclopramide (Reglan)
0.25-0.5 mg/kg PO, IV, or SC, SID to QID or 1-2 mg/kg/day via continuous IV infusion

Ondansetron (Zofran)
0.1-0.3 mg/kg IV or SC, SID to BID

The stomach becomes enlarged as gas and/or fluid accumulate within the lumen. The gas probably comes from aerophagia, although bacterial fermentation of carbohydrates, diffusion from the bloodstream, and metabolic reactions may contribute. Normal gastric secretion and transudation of fluids into the gastric lumen as a result of venous congestion contribute to fluid accumulation. The cause of GDV is unknown, but exercise after ingestion of large meals of highly processed foods or water has been suggested to contribute. Epidemiologic studies have not supported a causal relationship between feeding soy-based or cereal-based dry dog food and GDV. Other contributing causes include an anatomic predisposition, ileus, trauma, primary gastric motility disorders, vomiting, and stress. Recommendations for clients of animals at high risk are provided in Table 16-32.

Generally, the stomach rotates in a clockwise direction when viewed from the surgeon's perspective (with the dog on its back and the clinician standing at the dog's side, facing cranially; Fig. 16-73). The rotation may be 90 to 360 degrees, but is usually 220 to 270 degrees. The duodenum and pylorus move ventrally and to the left of midline and become displaced between the esophagus and stomach. The spleen is usually displaced to the right ventral side of the abdomen.

Caudal vena cava and portal vein compression by the distended stomach decreases venous return and cardiac output, causing myocardial ischemia. Decreases in central venous pressure, stroke volume, mean arterial pressures, and cardiac output occur. Obstructive shock and inadequate tissue perfusion affect multiple organs, including the kidney, heart, pancreas, stomach, and small intestine. Cardiac arrhythmias occur in many dogs with GDV, particularly those with gastric necrosis. Arrhythmias may contribute to mortality and require appropriate monitoring and treatment (see discussion under Postoperative Care on p. 281). Myocardial depressant factor has also been recognized in affected dogs. Reperfusion injury has been implicated as causing much of the tissue damage that ultimately results in death after correction of GDV. Lazaroids, which inhibit lipid peroxidation, appear to decrease reperfusion injury and may eventually increase survival.

Partial or chronic gastric dilatation-volvulus may occur in dogs and is usually a progressive but non–life-threatening syndrome that may be associated with vomiting, anorexia, and/or weight loss. These dogs may have chronic, intermittent signs and appear normal between episodes. Gastric malpositioning may be intermittent or chronic but without dilatation. Plain or contrast radiographs are diagnostic, but repeat radiographs may be necessary if the stomach is intermittently malpositioned.

DIAGNOSIS
Clinical Presentation

Signalment. GDV primarily occurs in large, deep-chested breeds (i.e., Great Dane, weimaraner, Saint Bernard, German shepherd, Irish and Gordon setters, Doberman pinscher), but has been reported in cats and small breed dogs. Shar-peis may have an increased incidence compared with other medium-sized breeds. In a recent study, basset hounds had a high risk of GDV, despite their relatively small size (Glickman et al, 1994). Large breed size, degree of purity of breed, and increase of weight are significant risk factors for development of this disease. GDV may occur in any age dog, but is most common in middle-aged to older animals. Chest depth/width ratio appears to be highly correlated with the risk of bloat.

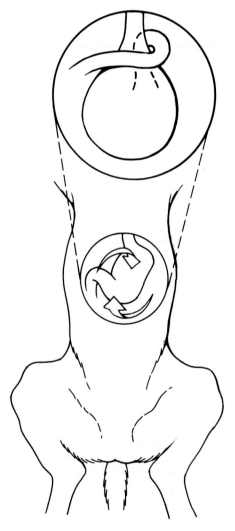

FIG. 16-73
Direction of gastric rotation in most dogs with GDV.

TABLE 16-32

Recommendations for Clients

- Feed several small meals a day, rather than one large meal.
- Avoid stress during feeding (if necessary, separate dogs in multiple-dog households during feeding).
- Restrict exercise before and after meals.
- For high-risk dogs, consider prophylactic gastropexy.
- Seek veterinary care as soon as signs of bloat are noted.

☞ **N O T E** · Although GDV usually occurs in large, deep-chested dogs, it should not be ruled out in cats or smaller dogs.

History. A dog with GDV may present with a history of a progressively distending and tympanic abdomen, or the owner may simply find the animal recumbent and depressed, with a distended abdomen. The dog may appear to be in pain and may have an arched back. Nonproductive retching, hypersalivation, and restlessness are common.

☞ **N O T E** · The diagnosis is often correctly made by owners who describe their animals as being "bloated."

Physical Examination Findings
Abdominal palpation often reveals various degrees of abdominal tympany or enlargement; however, it may be difficult to feel gastric distension in heavily muscled large-breed or very obese dogs. Splenomegaly is occasionally palpated. Clinical signs associated with shock, including weak peripheral pulses, tachycardia, prolonged capillary refill time, pale mucous membranes, or dyspnea, may be present.

Radiography
Radiographic evaluation is necessary to differentiate simple dilatation from dilatation plus volvulus. **Affected animals should be decompressed before radiographs are taken.** Right lateral and dorsoventral radiographic views are preferred. In normal dogs, the pylorus is located ventral to the fundus on the lateral view, and on the right side of the abdomen on the dorsoventral view. On a right lateral view of a dog with GDV, the pylorus lies cranial to the body of the stomach and is separated from the rest of the stomach by soft tissue (reverse C sign) (Fig. 16-74). On the dorsoventral view, the pylorus appears as a gas-filled structure to the left of

midline (Fig. 16-75). Free abdominal air suggests gastric rupture and warrants immediate surgery.

☞ **N O T E** · Caution! Positioning these animals for a ventrodorsal view may lead to aspiration.

Laboratory Findings
The CBC is seldom helpful unless DIC causes thrombocytopenia. Although normal or increased potassium concentrations may occur, hypokalemia is more common. Vascular stasis may cause increased lactic acid production, resulting in a metabolic acidosis. However, metabolic alkalosis caused by sequestration of hydrogen ions in the gastric lumen can offset the metabolic acidosis, causing the pH to be normal (i.e., a mixed acid-base disorder). Respiratory acidosis may be caused by hypoventilation secondary to gastric impingement on the diaphragm and decreased ventilatory compliance. Hence, routine use of sodium bicarbonate is inappropriate.

DIFFERENTIAL DIAGNOSIS
Simple gastric dilatation occurs commonly in young puppies from overeating and seldom requires specific treatment. The stomach, though greatly enlarged with ingesta and gas, is not malpositioned. Small intestine volvulus is a differential because it results in a tympanic and enlarged abdomen (see p. 316); however, dilatation of the intestinal tract is apparent on radiographs. Primary splenic torsion (see p. 454) often causes acute abdominal pain; however, gastric distention is

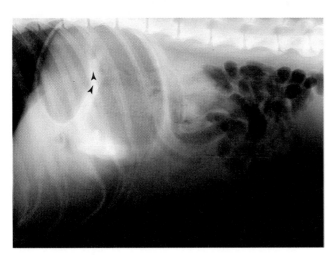

FIG. 16-74
Right lateral abdominal radiograph of a dog with GDV showing a distended, gas-filled stomach. Note the reverse C sign (*arrows*) caused by the shelf of soft tissue.

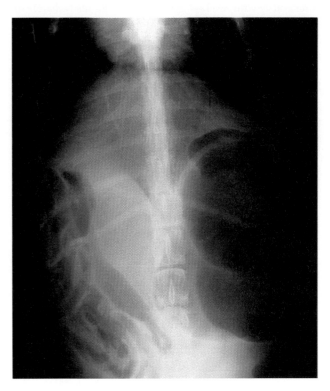

FIG. 16-75
Dorsoventral radiograph of a dog with GDV. The pylorus appears as a gas-filled structure to the left of midline.

usually mild, if present. Diaphragmatic herniation may produce clinical signs similar to GDV, particularly if the stomach is herniated and outflow is obstructed (see p. 682).

☞ **N O T E** · You cannot differentiate GDV from gastric dilatation without volvulus based on passing a stomach tube. Stomach tubes can often be passed in dogs with twisted stomachs.

MEDICAL MANAGEMENT

Patient stabilization is the initial objective (Table 16-33). A large-bore intravenous catheter(s) should be placed in either a jugular or both cephalic veins. Either isotonic fluids (90 ml/kg/hr), hypertonic 7% saline (4–5 ml/kg over 5 to 15 min), or hetastarch (5–10 ml/kg over 10 to 15 min) is administered. If hypertonic saline or hetastarch is given, adjustment of the rate of subsequent crystalloid administration is necessary. Blood should be drawn for blood gas analyses, a CBC, and a biochemical panel. Broad-spectrum antibiotics (e.g., cefazolin, ampicillin plus enrofloxacin) and possibly flunixin meglumine (for septic shock) should be administered. If the animal is dyspneic, oxygen therapy may be given by nasal insufflation or mask.

☞ **N O T E** · Use banamine with caution in dogs and cats, as it can cause severe gastrointestinal ulceration!

Gastric decompression should be performed while shock therapy is initiated. The stomach may be decompressed percutaneously with several large-bore intravenous catheters or a small trocar, or (preferably) a stomach tube may be passed. The stomach tube should be measured from the point of the nose to the xiphoid process and a piece of tape applied to the tube to mark the correct length. A roll of tape can be placed between the incisors and the tube passed through the center hole. Attempts should be made to pass the tube to the measured point. Placing the animal in different positions (i.e., sitting, reclining on a tilt-table) may help if it is difficult to advance the tube into the stomach. **Do not perforate the esophagus with overly rigorous attempts to pass the tube.** If these attempts fail, percutaneous decompression of the stomach should be attempted. This may relieve pressure on the cardia and allow the tube to enter the stomach. Once the air has been removed, the stomach should be flushed with warm water. If blood is seen in the fluid from the stomach,

prompt surgical intervention is warranted because this may indicate gastric necrosis. If the stomach tube can still not be passed, and immediate surgical correction is not possible, temporary decompression may be achieved by performing a temporary gastrostomy (see p. 265 for description of technique). **Placement of a Foley catheter into the stomach percutaneously should not be done unless the stomach is simultaneously tacked to the body wall (see p. 270) because of the high risk of peritonitis if the stomach pulls away from the tube.** Disadvantages of a temporary gastrostomy are that the stomach must be closed when the permanent gastropexy is performed, and there is a high risk of peritoneal contamination. However, a temporary gastrostomy will maintain gastric decompression if the animal is being referred, or surgery is delayed. If immediate surgery is not possible in an animal in which a stomach tube was passed but that dilates rapidly after decompression, the stomach tube can be exteriorized through a pharyngostomy approach. This will prevent the animal from chewing on the tube, until definitive surgery can be performed. **After the patient has been decompressed and is stable, radiographs may be taken.**

SURGICAL TREATMENT

Surgery should be performed as soon as the animal has been stabilized, even if the stomach has been decompressed. Rotation of a nondistended stomach interferes with gastric blood flow and may potentiate gastric necrosis.

Preoperative Management

The animal should be given intravenous fluids, antibiotics, and possibly flunixin meglumine before surgery (see discussion of Medical Management). Significant electrolyte and acid-base abnormalities should be corrected. A greatly enlarged stomach may hinder respiration and make it difficult for the animal to ventilate during anesthetic induction. An ECG should be monitored to detect cardiac arrhythmias, which, if significant, should be treated with lidocaine before surgery.

Anesthesia

Numerous anesthetic protocols have been described for dogs with GDV. If the animal has been decompressed and stabilized and cardiac arrhythmias are not present, the animal may be given oxymorphone and diazepam intravenously and induced with etomidate, thiobarbiturates, or propofol (Table 16-34). If the animal is depressed, oxymorphone and diazepam alone may be used for induction, or if necessary for intubation, etomidate may be given. Etomidate is a good choice for induction if the animal has not been well stabilized because it maintains cardiac output and is not arrhythmogenic. Alternatively, a combination of lidocaine and thiobarbiturate may be used if arrhythmias are present. For the latter, 9 mg/kg of each is drawn up and half is given initially, intravenously. Additional drug is given to effect to allow the dog to be intubated. Generally, no more than 6 mg/kg of lidocaine is given intravenously to prevent toxicity. If bradycardia occurs, anticholinergics (e.g., atropine or glycopyrro-

---

TABLE 16-33

Medical Management of GDV

- Fluids
- Antibiotics such as cefazolin (20 mg/kg IV) or a combination of enrofloxacin (Baytril)—5-10 mg/kg IV plus ampicillin at 22 mg/kg IV
- ± flunixin meglumine (Banamine) 1 mg/kg IV once or twice in dogs

(see p. 262)

TABLE 16-34
Selected Anesthetic Protocols for Dogs with GDV
Induction
Give oxymorphone (0.1 mg/kg IV) plus diazepam (0.2 mg/kg IV). Give in incremental dosages as necessary to intubate. If intubation is not possible, give etomidate (0.5-1.5 mg/kg IV) or thiopental or propofol (at reduced dosages) or (after diazepam and oxymorphone) use a combination of lidocaine and thiobarbiturates (see text)
Maintenance
Isoflurane

late) may be given. Nitrous oxide should not be used in dogs with GDV (see p. 262). Isoflurane is the inhalation agent of choice because it is less arrhythmogenic than halothane.

Surgical Anatomy

Normally, when viewed from the surgeon's perspective (i.e., with the animal in dorsal recumbency), the pylorus is located on the dog's right side, and the greater omentum arises from the greater curvature of the stomach and covers the intestines. The gastric (lesser curvature) and gastroepiploic (greater curvature) arteries supply the stomach and are derived from the celiac artery. The short gastric arteries arise from the splenic artery and supply the greater curvature. Rupture of the short gastrics in dogs with GDV is common and may contribute to blood loss and gastric infarction or necrosis. Eighty percent of the arterial flow is to the mucosa and the remainder is to the muscularis and serosa; therefore observation of mucosal color is not a reliable indicator of gastric wall viability. The mucosa often appears darkened due to vascular compromise, even when full-thickness necrosis is not present.

Positioning

The dog is placed in dorsal recumbency and the abdomen prepared for a midline abdominal incision. The prepped area should extend from midthorax to the pubis. If a tube gastropexy is being performed, the prepped area should be extended cranially and dorsally to allow the tube to be exteriorized behind the caudal right rib.

SURGICAL TECHNIQUE

The goals of surgical treatment are three-fold: (1) to inspect the stomach and spleen so as to identify and remove damaged or necrotic tissues, (2) to decompress the stomach and correct any malpositioning, and (3) to adhere the stomach to the body wall to prevent subsequent malpositioning. Upon entering the abdominal cavity of a dog with GDV, the first structure noted is the greater omentum, which usually covers the dilated stomach.

Decompress the stomach before repositioning, by using a large-bore needle (i.e., 14 or 16 gauge) attached to suc-

tion. If the needle becomes occluded with ingesta, have an assistant pass an orogastric stomach tube and perform gastric lavage. Intraoperative manipulation of the cardia will usually allow the tube to be passed into the stomach without difficulty. If adequate decompression is still not achieved, or an assistant is not available, a small gastrotomy incision can be performed to remove the gastric contents, although this should be avoided if possible. For a clockwise rotation, once the stomach has been decompressed, rotate it counterclockwise by grasping the pylorus (usually found below the esophagus) with the right hand and the greater curvature with the left. Push the greater curvature, or fundus, of the stomach towards the table while simultaneously elevating the pylorus (towards the incision). Check to make sure that the spleen is normally positioned in the left abdominal quadrant. If there is splenic necrosis or significant infarction, perform a partial or complete splenectomy (see p. 451). Remove or invaginate (see p. 264) necrotic gastric tissues. Avoid entering the gastric lumen, if possible. If you are uncertain whether gastric tissue will remain viable, invaginate the abnormal tissue (see p. 264). Verify that the gastrosplenic ligament is not torsed, and before closure, palpate the intraabdominal esophagus to ensure that the stomach is derotated.

☞ **NOTE** · Always perform a "permanent" gastropexy; do not suture intact gastric serosa to intact peritoneum (see p. 270).

To prevent recurrence of GDV, the stomach must be permanently adhered to the body wall. **Gastropexy should always be performed in conjunction with abdominal exploration and derotation of the stomach.** Techniques for permanent gastropexy are on pp. 270 to 272. Temporary gastrostomy is described on p. 265. Gastropexy is usually curative for dogs with partial or chronic GDV.

SUTURE MATERIALS/ SPECIAL INSTRUMENTS

Absorbable (polydioxanone or polyglyconate) or nonabsorbable (polypropylene) suture material may be used for the gastropexy (0 or 2-0). A Foley catheter is needed for a tube gastropexy. Balfour retractors, hand-held retractors (i.e., Army-Navy retractors or malleable retractors), and extra towel clamps (for placement on the rib when doing a circumcostal gastropexy) are helpful.

POSTOPERATIVE CARE AND ASSESSMENT

Electrolyte, fluid, and acid-basis status should be monitored closely postoperatively. Many dogs with GDV are hypokalemic postoperatively and require potassium supplementation (Table 16-35). Small amounts of water and soft, low-fat food should be offered 12 to 24 hours after surgery, and these patients should be observed for vomiting. Gastritis secondary to mucosal ischemia is common and may be associated with

TABLE 16-35

Intravenous Potassium Supplementation Guidelines

Serum Potassium* (mEq/L)	mEq KCL/L of fluid	Maximal infusion rate† (ml/kg/hr)
<2.0	80	6
2.1-2.5	60	8
2.6-3.0	40	12
3.0-3.5	28	16

*If serum potassium is not available, add potassium to a total concentration of 20 mEq/L.
†Do not exceed 0.5 mEq/kg/hr.

TABLE 16-36

H$_2$-Receptor Blockers

Cimetidine (Tagamet)

5-10 mg/kg PO, IV, SC, TID to QID

Ranitidine (Zantac)

2 mg/kg PO, IV, IM, SC, BID

Famotidine (Pepcid)

0.5 mg/kg PO, SID to BID

TABLE 16-37

Antiarrhythmic Therapy

Lidocaine (Xylocaine)

IV bolus (2 mg/kg increments up to total dose of 8 mg/kg) then IV drip at 50 µg/kg/min (500 mg in 500 ml of fluid, administered at maintenance rate [66 ml/kg/day])

Procainamide (Pronestyl)

10-15 mg/kg slow IV bolus or 25-60 µg/kg/min as a continuous IV infusion or 15 mg/kg IM, PO, BID to QID

Sotolol (Betapace)

1.0-2.0 mg/kg PO, BID

gastric hemorrhage or vomiting. If vomiting is severe or continuous, a centrally-acting antiemetic may be given (see p. 277). Secondary gastric ulcers may occur and require treatment (see p. 288). H$_2$ receptor blockers (e.g., cimetidine, ranitidine, or famotidine; Table 16-36) decrease gastric acidity and may be beneficial. Intravenous fluid therapy should be continued until oral fluid intake is adequate to maintain hydration. Patients should be monitored for hypoproteinemia and anemia in the early postoperative period.

Ventricular arrhythmias are common in dogs with GDV and usually begin 12 to 36 hours postoperatively. Their cause is unknown, but myocardial depressant factor, decreased cardiac output, and myocardial ischemia may contribute. Treatment of cardiac arrhythmias includes maintenance of normal hydration and correction of electrolyte imbalances [some antiarrhythmic drugs (i.e., lidocaine) are ineffective when the animal is hypokalemic; see Table 16-35]. If the arrhythmias: (1) interfere with cardiac output (as noted by poor peripheral pulses), (2) are multiform, (3) have subsequent premature beats inscribed on the wave of the previous complex (R on T), or (4) have a sustained ventricular rate greater than 160 beats per minute, they should be treated; usually with intravenous drugs. A test bolus of lidocaine, given intravenously (2 mg/kg bolus, up to 8 mg/kg total dose), can be used to determine responsiveness to this drug. If the arrhythmias decrease or stop, lidocaine should be given by a continuous intravenous infusion of 50 to 75 µg/kg/min (Table 16-37). Low doses should be used initially and only increased if necessary. Signs of lidocaine

toxicity include muscle tremors, vomiting, and seizures; lidocaine therapy should be discontinued if these signs occur. Other potentially effective antiarrhythmic drugs include procainamide and sotolol. Procainamide may be given as an intravenous bolus, by continuous infusion, intramuscularly, or orally (see Table 16-37). Sotolol may be effective in animals that have not responded to lidocaine and procainamide.

☞ **NOTE** · Lidocaine toxicity may be enhanced in patients who are given cimetidine concurrently.

COMPLICATIONS

Sepsis and peritonitis may be caused by gastric necrosis or perforation if devitalized tissue is not adequately removed. Diagnostic peritoneal lavage (see p. 198) may help diagnose peritonitis. Peritonitis mandates immediate surgical intervention. DIC may occur in dogs with GDV or peritonitis. Assessment of clotting parameters, plus appropriate treatment with fluids and heparin (see p. 195), may be necessary.

PROGNOSIS

With timely surgery, the prognosis is fair; however, mortality rates as high as 45% and greater have been reported (Matthiesen, 1985). A recent study reported a mortality rate of 15% among dogs with GDV; the mortality rate was 0.9% if gastric dilation without volvulus was present (or if GDV could not be verified at surgery) (Brockman, Washabau, Drobatz, 1995). The prognosis is poor if gastric necrosis or perforation occurs or if surgery is delayed. Recurrence rates for GDV differ, depending on techniques used, but most have reported rates of less than 10%. Tube gastropexy has the highest reported recurrence rate, varying from 5% to 29% (Fox et al, 1984; Johnson, Barrus, Greene, 1984).

Some dogs with GDV respond to tube decompression and medical stabilization alone. Occasionally, the stomach becomes normally positioned after the air is removed; or, it was only partially rotated (less than 180 degrees) or merely dilated. However, these dogs still have a high likelihood of recurrence. Therefore gastropexy should be recommended, even when conservative management successfully alleviates the gastric malpositioning. The reported recurrence rates of dogs operated on for GDV in which the stomach has been repositioned but gastropexy not performed approaches 80% (Meyer-Lindenberg et al, 1993; Whitney, 1989).

☞ **N O T E** • Always perform a permanent gastropexy because GDV will likely recur otherwise.

References

Brockman DJ, Washabau RJ, Drobatz KJ: Canine gastric dilatation/volvulus syndrome in a veterinary critical care unit: 295 cases (1986–1992), *J Am Vet Med Assoc* 207:460, 1995.

Fox SM et al: Circumcostal gastropexy versus tube gastrostomy: histological comparison of gastropexy adhesions, *J Am Anim Hosp Assoc* 24:273, 1988.

Glickman LT et al: Analysis of risk factors for gastric dilatation and dilatation-volvulus in dogs, *J Am Vet Med Assoc* 204:1465, 1994.

Johnson RG, Barrus J, Greene RW: Gastric dilatation-volvulus: recurrence rate following tube gastrostomy, *J Am Anim Hosp Assoc* 20:33, 1984.

Matthiesen DT: Partial gastrectomy as treatment of gastric volvulus: results in 30 dogs, *Vet Surg* 14:185, 1985.

Meyer-Lindenberg A et al: Treatment of gastric dilatation-volvulus and a rapid method for prevention of relapse in dogs: 134 cases (1988–1991), *J Am Vet Med Assoc* 203: 1303, 1993.

Whitney WO: Complications associated with the medical and surgical management of gastric dilatation-volvulus in the dog, *Probl Vet Med* 1:268, 1989.

Suggested Reading

Badylak SF, Lantz GC, Jeffries M: Prevention of reperfusion injury in surgically induced gastric dilatation-volvulus in dogs, *Am J Vet Res* 51:294, 1990.

Ellison GW: Gastric dilatation volvulus: surgical prevention, *Vet Clin North Am Small Anim Pract* 23:513, 1993.

Flanders JA, Harvey HJ: Results of tube gastrostomy as treatment for gastric volvulus in the dog, *J Am Vet Med Assoc* 185:74, 1984.

Frendin J, Funkquist B, Stavenborn M: Gastric displacement in dogs without clinical signs of acute dilatation, *J Small Anim Pract* 29:775, 1988.

Greenfield CL, Walshaw R, Thomas MW: Significance of the Heineke-Mikulicz pyloroplasty in the treatment of gastric dilatation-volvulus; a prospective clinical study, *Vet Surg* 18:22, 1989.

Hosgood G: Gastric dilatation-volvulus in dogs, *J Am Vet Med Assoc* 204:1742, 1994.

Lantz GC et al: Treatment of reperfusion injury in dogs with experimentally induced gastric dilatation-volvulus, *Am J Vet Res* 53:1594, 1992.

Leib MS, Blass CE: Gastric dilatation-volvulus in dogs: an update, *Compend Contin Educ Pract Vet* 6:961, 1984.

Leib MS et al: Circumcostal gastropexy for preventing recurrence of gastric dilatation-volvulus in the dogs: an evaluation of 30 cases, *J Am Vet Med Assoc* 187:245, 1985.

Leib MS, Monroe WE, Martin RA: Suspected chronic gastric volvulus in a dog with normal gastric emptying of liquids, *J Am Vet Med Assoc* 191:699, 1987.

Lindgren WG et al: Long-term follow-up and clinical results of incisional gastropexy for repair of gastric dilation-volvulus syndrome, *Vet Surg* 24:430, 1995 (abstract).

MacCoy DM et al: Partial invagination of the canine stomach for treatment of infarction of the gastric wall, *Vet Surg* 15:237, 1986.

Millis DL, Hauptman JG, Fulton RB: Abnormal hemostatic profiles and gastric necrosis in canine gastric dilatation-volvulus, *Vet Surg* 22:93, 1993.

Morgan RV: Acute gastric dilatation-volvulus syndrome, *Compend Contin Educ Pract Vet* 4:677, 1982.

Schulman AJ et al: Muscular flap gastropexy: a new surgical technique to prevent recurrences of gastric dilatation-volvulus syndrome, *J Am Anim Hosp Assoc* 22:339, 1986.

Woolfson JM, Kostolich M: Circumcostal gastropexy: clinical use of the technique in 34 dogs with gastric dilatation-volvulus, *J Am Anim Hosp Assoc* 22:825, 1986.

BENIGN GASTRIC OUTFLOW OBSTRUCTION

DEFINITIONS

Pyloric stenosis refers to benign muscular hypertrophy of the pylorus. **Chronic antral mucosal hypertrophy** refers to benign hypertrophy of the pyloric mucosa causing outflow obstruction (Fig. 16-76). **Chronic hypertrophic pyloric gastropathy (CHPG)** is a term that denotes pyloric hypertrophy, without specifying whether the mucosa or muscularis is involved. CHPG has been used specifically to refer to acquired mucosal hypertrophy by some authors and to either muscular (type I) or mucosal (types II and III) hypertrophy by others.

SYNONYMS

For pyloric stenosis—**benign antral muscular hypertrophy, congenital hypertrophic stenosis, congenital pyloric muscle hypertrophy;** for chronic antral mucosal hypertrophy—

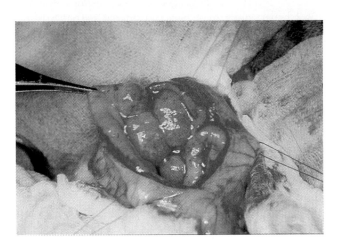

FIG. 16-76
Intraoperative photograph showing mucosal hypertrophy in a dog with chronic hypertrophic pyloric gastropathy. (From Willard MD: *Essentials of small animal medicine,* St. Louis, 1994, Mosby.)

pyloric or **gastric mucosal hypertrophy, chronic hypertrophic gastritis, multiple polyps of the gastric mucosa, acquired hypertrophy**

GENERAL CONSIDERATIONS AND CLINICALLY RELEVANT PATHOPHYSIOLOGY

Gastric outlet obstruction may be caused by pyloric abnormalities, disorders of gastric motility, or extrinsic lesions compressing the outflow tract (e.g., pancreatic, duodenal, or hepatic neoplasia; Table 16-38). Hypertrophy of the pyloric mucosa or muscle may be isolated, or may occur in conjunction with other abnormalities. A syndrome of polycystic kidneys, hepatic disease, polyneuropathy, and hypertrophic gastropathy has been described in the Drentse patrijshond breed.

The cause of pyloric stenosis is unknown, but excessive gastrin production has been implicated. Gastrin, the major regulator of gastric acid secretion, is trophic for gastric smooth muscle and mucosa, and congenital pyloric stenosis has been produced in puppies by administering gastrin to pregnant bitches. Neurogenic dysfunction may also play a role. Acute stress, inflammatory disease, or trauma might stimulate the sympathetic nervous system, reducing gastric motility and causing retention. Prolonged gastric distention may then lead to increased gastrin secretion and subsequent hypertrophy.

DIAGNOSIS
Clinical Presentation

Signalment. In dogs, pyloric stenosis is most commonly seen in brachycephalic (i.e., boxer, bulldogs, and Boston terrier) breeds. Siamese cats have also been reported with this condition. Affected cats may have both vomiting (due to gastric outlet obstruction) and regurgitation (due to secondary esophagitis and esophageal dysfunction). Chronic antral mucosal hypertrophy occurs most commonly in small-breed dogs (less than 10 kg), particularly Lhasa apso, shih tzu, and Maltese breeds. Some dogs reported with chronic antral mucosal hypertrophy have been considered particularly excitable or vicious. Males may be more commonly affected than females. Pyloric stenosis is more common in young animals; however, animals of any age may be affected. Chronic

---

TABLE 16-38

Important Considerations for Gastric Outlet Obstruction

- Not all older patients with proliferative masses causing outlet obstruction have malignancies
- Not all obstructed patients have hypokalemic, hypochloremic, metabolic alkalosis
- Benign gastric outflow obstruction usually has a good prognosis with appropriate therapy
- Gastroduodenoscopy is usually more appropriate than contrast radiographs; with endoscopy you can biopsy and *often* determine if malignancy is present

---

antral mucosal hypertrophy is more common in middle-aged to older dogs and may mimic neoplasia.

History. The clinical signs are caused by obstruction to gastric outflow. Vomiting is the most common sign; however, vomiting may be intermittent and/or delayed hours after feeding. Cats commonly have regurgitation and vomiting. Liquids often pass through the pylorus; therefore severe dehydration is uncommon and vomiting may occur for months to years before diagnosis. Animals with congenital pyloric stenosis often begin vomiting when they start eating solid food. The frequency of vomiting varies from several times daily to once or twice a week.

Physical Examination Findings

Physical examination findings are generally nonspecific. They may include weight loss, anorexia, depression, and/or dehydration. Abdominal pain is seldom present. Aspiration pneumonia and/or reflux esophagitis may occur secondary to chronic vomiting.

Radiography/Ultrasonography/Endoscopy

Survey abdominal radiographs may reveal gastric distention. If gastric outlet obstruction is suspected, endoscopy is usually recommended because it is diagnostic and allows biopsy. Radiography and ultrasonography are useful in eliminating extrinsic causes of pyloric obstruction. Contrast radiographs may show delayed emptying, pyloric wall thickening, and/or a filling defect in the pylorus. However, normal elimination of liquid barium does not rule out gastric outflow obstruction. Furthermore, it can be difficult to accurately interpret studies when barium is mixed with food. Ultrasonography usually reveals pyloric wall thickening and often detects neoplastic metastases. Ultrasonography also detects extrinsic lesions (e.g., abscess or neoplasia) that may cause gastric outflow obstruction.

☞ **N O T E** · Neoplastic pyloric disease and benign disease causing hypertrophy are often difficult to distinguish visually; biopsy is imperative!

Laboratory Findings

Hematologic and biochemical changes in animals with benign gastric outlet obstruction are usually nonspecific. If vomiting has caused loss of gastric secretions, a hypochloremic, hypokalemic, metabolic alkalosis may be present. Prerenal azotemia and/or hypoproteinemia may occur, particularly in young dogs with chronic and frequent vomiting.

DIFFERENTIAL DIAGNOSIS

Any condition that causes vomiting is a differential. Gastrointestinal foreign bodies, pythiosis, neoplasia, and ulceration may cause gastric outlet obstruction. Other causes of vomiting that should be eliminated before surgery, if possible, include uremia, hypoadrenocorticism, hypercalcemia, diabetic ketoacidosis, hepatic insufficiency, peritonitis, pancreatitis, feline hyperthyroidism, early right-sided heart failure in cats, gastritis, and inflammatory bowel disease.

MEDICAL MANAGEMENT

Dehydration and electrolyte and acid-base abnormalities should be corrected before surgery or endoscopy (see p. 261). H₂ receptor blockers (i.e., cimetidine, ranitidine, famotidine) or omeprazole may be used to treat esophagitis caused by frequent exposure of the esophagus to gastric acid (Table 16-39). Antibiotics may be indicated for esophagitis (see p. 233), ulceration (see p. 288), or aspiration (see p. 233).

SURGICAL TREATMENT

Surgery is recommended for benign pyloric obstruction. The goal is to remove the obstruction and reestablish normal gastric emptying. **A full-thickness biopsy should be submitted to ensure that the thickening is benign (Fig. 16-77).**

Preoperative Management

Food should be withheld for 24 hours before surgery. Presurgical endoscopy can define the extent of the lesion and confirm its benign or malignant nature by histologic or cytologic examination. Intravenous prophylactic antibiotics (e.g., cefazolin; Table 16-40) may be given at anesthetic induction if antibiotic therapy has not already been initiated, but is not essential.

Anesthesia

See p. 262 for suggested anesthetics to use in animals with gastric disorders.

Surgical Anatomy

See p. 263 for surgical anatomy of the stomach.

Positioning

The animal is placed in dorsal recumbency and the abdomen prepared for a ventral midline incision. The prepped area should extend from midthorax to near the pubis.

SURGICAL TECHNIQUE

Surgical procedures to correct outlet obstruction due to mucosal and/or muscular hypertrophy include pyloroplasty or Billroth I procedures. Pyloromyotomy (see p. 267) is often ineffective and is not recommended. If muscular hypertrophy without significant mucosal hypertrophy is present, a Heineke-Mikulicz pyloroplasty (see p. 268) is easy to perform. However, mucosal exposure is limited and it does not allow adequate resection of hypertrophied mucosa. When mucosal hypertrophy is present, a Y-U pyloroplasty (see p. 269) or Billroth I (see p. 266) procedure is preferred. A Y-U pyloroplasty allows hypertrophied mucosa to be removed and the outflow tract widened (Fig. 16-77). Alternatively, a Billroth I is more difficult and carries additional risk of dehiscence or leakage, but has been successfully performed in numerous dogs with benign outflow obstruction. A Billroth I, rather than a pyloroplasty, should be considered when the mucosa or muscular layers are so thickened that they are inflexible.

For mucosal hypertrophy, perform a Y-U pyloroplasty as described on p. 269. Be sure to perform a full-thickness biopsy and to resect the hypertrophied mucosa. Approximate incised edges of the mucosa with a continuous suture pattern of absorbable suture material (3-0), before closing the pyloroplasty.

SUTURE MATERIALS/ SPECIAL INSTRUMENTS

If the animal is severely hypoproteinemic or debilitated, wound healing may be delayed. Strong absorbable suture (2-0 or 3-0) should be used and chromic gut suture avoided.

TABLE 16-39
Histamine₂ Receptor Blockers and Protein Pump Inhibitors

Cimetidine (Tagamet)
5-10 mg/kg PO, IV, SC, TID to QID

Ranitidine (Zantac)
2 mg/kg PO, IV, IM, SC, BID

Famotidine (Pepcid)
0.5 mg/kg PO, SID to BID

Omeprazole (Prilosec)
0.7-1.5 mg/kg PO, SID to BID

TABLE 16-40
Perioperative Antibiotic Therapy

Cefazolin (Ancef or Kefzol)
20 mg/kg IV at induction; repeat once or twice at 4-6 hr intervals

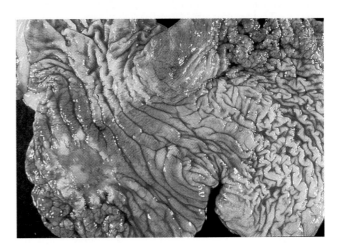

FIG. 16-77
Gastric ulceration associated with a gastric carcinoma.

POSTOPERATIVE CARE AND ASSESSMENT

Small amounts of water should be given the day following surgery and the patient observed for vomiting. If vomiting does not occur, small amounts of moist food can be given 24 hours postoperatively. Fluid therapy should be continued until the animal is eating and drinking normally. Electrolyte abnormalities should be monitored postoperatively and corrected, as necessary.

PROGNOSIS

The prognosis with surgical correction of these conditions is good. In one study of 39 dogs available for long-term evaluation, 85% had good or excellent outcomes (Matthiesen, Walter, 1986). A poor outcome is generally the result of technical failures (i.e., dehiscence or leakage) or choosing an inappropriate surgical technique for the lesion.

Reference

Matthiesen DT, Walter MC: Surgical treatment of chronic hypertrophic pyloric gastropathy in 45 dogs, *J Am Anim Hosp Assoc* 22:241, 1986.

Suggested Reading

Bellenger CR et al: Chronic hypertrophic pyloric gastropathy in 14 dogs, *Aust Vet J* 67:317, 1990.

Breitschwerdt EB et al: Hypergastrinemia in canine gastrointestinal disease, *J Am Anim Hosp Assoc* 22:585, 1986.

Dennis R et al: A case of hyperplastic gastropathy in a cat, *J Small Anim Pract* 28:491, 1987.

Happé RP, van der Gaag I, Wolvekamp WTC: Pyloric stenosis caused by hypertrophic gastritis in three dogs, *J Small Anim Pract* 22:7, 1981.

Huxtable CR et al: Chronic hypertrophic gastritis in a dog: successful treatment by partial gastrectomy, *J Small Anim Pract* 23:639, 1982.

Leib MS et al: Endoscopic diagnosis of chronic hypertrophic pyloric gastropathy in dogs, *J Vet Int Med* 7:335, 1993.

Pearson R: Pyloric stenosis in the dog, *Vet Rec* 393:1979.

Slappendel RJ et al: Familial stomatocytosis-hypertrophic gastritis (FSHG), a newly recognized disease in the dog, *The Veterinary Quarterly* 13:30, 1991.

Walter MC et al: Chronic hypertrophic pyloric gastropathy as a cause of pyloric obstruction in the dog, *J Am Vet Med Assoc* 186:157, 1985.

GASTRIC ULCERATION/EROSION

DEFINITIONS

An **ulcer** is a mucosal defect extending through the muscularis mucosae into the submucosa or deeper layers of the stomach, whereas an **erosion** does not penetrate the muscularis mucosae. **Gastrinomas** are gastrin-secreting tumors of the alimentary tract. **Zollinger-Ellison syndrome** is a condition in which gastroduodenal ulceration occurs as a result of hypersecretion of gastrin from a gastrinoma of the pancreas.

SYNONYMS

The terms **gastrinoma** and **Zollinger-Ellison syndrome** are often used interchangeably; however, gastrinomas can be located anywhere in the alimentary tract, while Zollinger-Ellison syndrome refers specifically to a gastrin-secreting tumor in the pancreas.

GENERAL CONSIDERATIONS AND CLINICALLY RELEVANT PATHOPHYSIOLOGY

Gastric ulceration in small animals is often iatrogenic (i.e., caused by nonsteroidal antiinflammatory drugs [NSAIDs]) or occurs secondary to an underlying disease process (e.g., mast cell disease, shock, tumor, hepatic failure) (Table 16-41). The most common sites for gastric ulcers are in the non-acid producing parts (i.e., fundus and pyloric antrum).

NSAIDs (e.g., aspirin, phenylbutazone, naproxen, flunixin meglumine, piroxicam, and ibuprofen) are common causes of gastrointestinal ulceration in dogs. The mechanism of ulcer formation secondary to these drugs is probably multifactorial, but prostaglandin synthesis inhibition seems important. Prostaglandins exert a protective effect on the mucosal barrier by stimulating mucus and bicarbonate production. Prostaglandin agonists (e.g., misoprostol) help prevent NSAID-induced lesions. Corticosteroids (particularly dexamethasone) may be ulcerogenic in dogs, especially when used at very high dosages. Prednisone, administered at appropriate dosages (2.2 mg/kg/day or less), infrequently causes gastric erosion or ulceration. Chronic steroid administration may decrease gastric mucus production, diminish the ability of mucosal cells to replicate, and increase exfolia-

---

TABLE 16-41

Important Considerations for Gastroduodenal Ulcers/Erosions

- Initial clinical signs (e.g., anorexia, depression) may not alert owner to seriousness of disease.
- Not all animals with ulcers vomit, and those that vomit may not vomit blood.
- NSAIDs are a very common cause, yet without careful questioning the history may not reveal their use.
- Look for underlying causes; do not just treat symptomatically.
- Anytime a patient with severe hepatic disease suddenly worsens, consider gastroduodenal ulceration even if there is no vomiting.
- Perforation may occur unexpectedly and cause potentially fatal peritonitis (see p. 192).
- Any patient with a spontaneous pneumoabdomen or septic peritonitis should be presumed to have a perforated ulcer and treated accordingly, regardless of lack of historical findings suggestive of ulceration.
- Surgical resection should be considered for ulcers that are resistant to medical therapy and those that are causing the patient to hemorrhage vigorously.
- Intraoperative endoscopy may be helpful in locating partial-thickness ulcers.

tion of mucosal cells into the gastric lumen. **The concurrent use of steroids and NSAIDs should be avoided.**

Gastric ulceration may be caused by neoplasia (see Fig. 16-77), either as a direct effect or by paraneoplastic mechanisms. Gastric adenocarcinoma and lymphoma are probably the most common infiltrative diseases causing ulceration. Paraneoplastic ulceration may be caused by mast cell tumors (common) or gastrinomas (rare). Gastroduodenal ulceration is a common complication of mast cell disease because histamine is a potent stimulator of gastric acid secretion. The cytoplasmic granules of mast cell tumors contain vasoactive amines (e.g., histamine and serotonin) and heparin. Histamine also causes vasodilation of gastric vessels and alters endothelial permeability, which promotes intravascular thrombosis and gastric necrosis.

Gastrin is normally secreted by the antral G cells in response to vagal stimulation and gastric distention, and is a potent stimulator of gastric acid secretion. Zollinger-Ellison syndrome is a condition in which there is hypersecretion of gastrin associated with neoplasia of the non-β pancreatic islet cells. Severe duodenal ulceration is seen with this disease, and removal of the pancreatic mass may be necessary to alleviate clinical signs (see p. 425). Because of the aggressive biological behavior of this malignant neoplasm, the prognosis for long-term cure is poor; however, aggressive medical management with omeprazole (0.7–1.5 mg/kg PO, SID) may be helpful. Thrombosis associated with disseminated intravascular coagulation (DIC) may decrease gastric blood flow and enhance ulcer formation. Both acute and chronic liver disease may be associated with gastrointestinal bleeding and ulcer formation. Chronic hepatic disease causes gastric mucosal injury through a variety of mechanisms, which are poorly understood.

Circulatory shock and the resultant poor gastric perfusion may cause "stress ulcers." Ulcers may also form secondary to septic shock and commonly occur in dogs with intervertebral disc disease (IVDD). Corticosteroid administration to dogs with severe neurologic disease probably contributes to the high prevalence of gastrointestinal ulcers in these patients. Other contributing factors in dogs with IVDD include alterations in mucosal blood flow, sympathetic and parasympathetic stimulation of the bowel, and the stress of major surgery and prolonged hospitalization. Colonic perforation of dogs with neurologic disease is associated with high mortality. Other conditions associated with gastrointestinal ulceration in small animals include inflammatory bowel disease, gastric or duodenal neoplasia, reflux of bile acid into the stomach, major surgery, uremia, pythiosis, recurrent pancreatitis, and possibly psychologic stress.

☞ **N O T E** • Use steroids with caution in patients with neurologic disease!

The stomach has an enormous ability to increase local blood flow, which helps remove caustic substances from the gastric lumen. Additionally, the rapid cell turnover rate of the gastric mucosa helps heal minor erosions in 1 to 2 days, providing the cause is removed. Other normal defenses that help prevent the formation of ulcers include those properties that interfere with absorption of hydrogen ions (i.e., phospholipid membranes, tight junctional complexes), neutralization of acid by bicarbonate (secreted by the oxyntic, pyloric, and duodenal mucosa), and a thick, alkaline mucus coating that traps and neutralizes hydrogen ions. For mucosal damage to occur, the gastric pH usually (but not always) must be lower than 3 to 5. Deep ulcers do not heal rapidly and heal by the formation of scar tissue rather than reepithelialization.

DIAGNOSIS
Clinical Presentation

Signalment. Gastric ulceration or erosion occurs more commonly in dogs than cats. Most noniatrogenic gastric ulcers in dogs occur in middle-aged or older dogs. There is no breed predisposition.

History. Although vomiting is a common clinical sign of gastrointestinal ulceration, some dogs present for anorexia and/or anemia, without vomiting. Vomitus may or may not contain digested blood, fresh blood, or blood clots. Digested blood looks like coffee grounds. Owners may or may not report that the stools of dogs with ulcers are black (melena) and that the dog has a poor appetite.

Physical Examination Findings

Abdominal pain may be present on abdominal palpation; however, many dogs with nonperforating gastric ulcers are not obviously in pain. Other signs of ulcer disease include anemia, edema (due to hypoproteinemia), melena, nausea, and weight loss.

Radiography/Ultrasonography/Endoscopy

Radiography and ultrasonography are seldom helpful in delineating gastric erosions. Positive contrast radiographs or ultrasonography may show abnormalities in the mucosal lining when deep ulcers are present. If gastroduodenal ulceration is suspected, the most sensitive and specific test is gastroduodenoscopy.

Laboratory Findings

A hemogram, serum biochemical profile, and urinalysis should be performed in animals in which gastric ulceration is suspected, to assess the severity of blood and protein loss and to identify underlying causes of ulceration (e.g., hepatic or renal failure). Animals with gastric ulcers may be anemic and/or hypoproteinemic. Clotting profiles should be performed when a coagulopathy is suspected. Electrolyte and acid-base abnormalities may occur if vomiting has been severe (e.g., hypochloremic, hypokalemic, metabolic alkalosis, or a metabolic acidosis). Gastrinomas (see p. 425) are uncommon, but if no other underlying cause is identified, serum gastrin levels can be measured (Table 16-42).

DIFFERENTIAL DIAGNOSIS

Gastric neoplasia, gastritis, and coagulopathies may mimic gastric ulceration/erosion. Gastric neoplasia and ulceration without neoplasia are best differentiated by endoscopy. Exploratory

TABLE 16-42

Basal Serum Gastrin Levels in Normal Dogs and Cats*

Dogs

<190 pg/ml†

Cats

<135 pg/ml

*These values may vary between laboratories.
†To convert from pg/ml to ng/L multiply pg/ml X 1.0.

TABLE 16-43

Medical Therapy of Animals with Gastric Ulceration

Sucralfate (Carafate)

0.5-1.0 g PO, TID to QID

Cimetidine (Tagamet)

5-10 mg/kg PO, IV, SC, TID to QID

Ranitidine (Zantac)

2 mg/kg PO, IV, IM, SC, BID

Famotidine (Pepcid)

0.5 mg/kg PO, SID to BID

Omeprazole (Prilosec)

0.7-1.5 mg/kg PO, SID to BID

Misoprostol (Cytotec)

1-5 µg/kg PO, TID to QID

gastrotomy is the next best test and is required if full-thickness biopsies are necessary. Full-thickness biopsies are usually required to diagnose scirrhous or submucosal lesions. Coagulopathies from ingestion of toxins, DIC, or inherent clotting abnormalities occasionally cause gastric bleeding. Coagulation profiles should be performed if a coagulopathy is suspected.

MEDICAL MANAGEMENT

Therapy depends on whether an underlying cause can be found, the severity of the bleeding, depth of the ulcer, likelihood of perforation, and the animal's status. Symptomatic therapy (i.e., fluids, antibiotics, blood, antiemetics) should be considered and underlying diseases identified and treated (i.e., discontinue ulcerogenic drugs, remove mast cell tumors or gastrinomas, treat renal or hepatic disease). Initially, medical treatment is recommended to control bleeding, if perforation seems unlikely. Agents used for treating ulcers include those that lessen gastric acidity and those that protect the gastric mucosa from damage (Table 16-43). Sucralfate forms a protective coating over the ulcer/erosion. However, its major drug actions that contribute to ulcer healing are related to stimulation of mucosal defense and reparative mechanisms and antipeptic effects, which are induced by both prostaglandin-dependent and prostaglandin-independent pathways. If bleeding is severe, a loading dose of 3 to 8 g of sucralfate may be given. Sucralfate should be given 1 hour after administration of other oral medications because it may interfere with their absorption. Drugs that interact with sucralfate include fluoroquinolones, tetracycline, theophylline, aminophylline, and digoxin. Cimetidine, ranitidine, and famotidine are H_2 receptor blockers that decrease acid secretion. Omeprazole and other proton-pump inhibitors are the most potent inhibitors of gastric acid secretion. Misoprostol is a prostaglandin analog that helps prevent ulceration in dogs receiving NSAIDs; it is unknown whether it helps cure gastric ulcers. Antacids (e.g., magnesium hydroxide) stimulate endogenous prostaglandin release, neutralize acids, and bind bile salts. Because they are most effective if administered frequently (i.e., up to 6 times per day) they are less useful in dogs and cats than in human beings. **Gastric foreign bodies should be removed promptly to allow the ulcer or erosion to heal.**

SURGICAL TREATMENT

If medical therapy is not successful in alleviating clinical signs within 5 to 7 days, bleeding is profuse and life-threatening, or perforation is believed imminent, surgery is indicated.

☞ **NOTE** · If possible, perform endoscopy before surgery to help identify the site and extent of the lesion(s).

Preoperative Management

If possible, the animal should be stabilized before surgery. Whole blood should be given if the animal is severely anemic (i.e., PCV less than 20%). If the animal is in DIC, heparin therapy may be considered. Electrolyte and acid-base abnormalities should be corrected and fluid therapy initiated.

Anesthesia

See p. 262 for anesthetic recommendations for animals undergoing gastric surgery.

Surgical Anatomy

Refer to p. 263 for surgical anatomy of the stomach.

Positioning

The dog is placed in dorsal recumbency and the abdomen prepared for a ventral midline incision. The prepped area should extend from midthorax to the pubis.

SURGICAL TECHNIQUE

If possible, remove the ulcer with a full-thickness gastric resection, and submit tissue for histopathologic examination. Assess the regional lymph nodes and liver for evidence of metastatic neoplasia or pythiosis, and biopsy them if they appear abnormal. Check both limbs of the pancreas for masses. Occasionally, the location of the ulcer near the pylorus makes full-thickness resection difficult. *If the ulcer is located at the pylorus and perforation is present or imminent, perform a serosal patch (see p. 301) over the site to help prevent leakage and promote ulcer healing.* A serosal patch is simpler to perform than a pylorectomy and gastroduodenostomy (Billroth I; see p. 266). Occasionally, a localized abscess will be noted where an ulcer has perforated, but the omentum or other abdominal structures have walled the site off. *If this is the case, carefully drain the abscess, and resect or patch the ulcer.* Preoperative or intraoperative endoscopy is helpful in locating ulcers; some are difficult to discern from the serosal surface. *If there is extensive disease secondary to something that may not resolve quickly (e.g., inflammatory bowel disease, hepatic failure, etc.) place an enterostomy feeding tube (see p. 79).*

SUTURE MATERIALS/ SPECIAL INSTRUMENTS

If the animal is severely hypoproteinemic or anemic, wound healing may be delayed. Polydioxanone, polyglyconate, polyglycolic acid, or polyglactin 910 suture (2-0 or 3-0) is preferred to close the gastrotomy incision (see p. 272). Gut suture should be avoided for gastric surgery.

POSTOPERATIVE CARE AND ASSESSMENT

Small amounts of water should be given the day following surgery and the patient observed for vomiting. If vomiting does not occur, small amounts of food can be given 24 hours postoperatively. The diet should be low fat and contain moderate amounts of protein and carbohydrates, to aid gastric emptying. If inflammatory bowel disease is possible, an elimination (e.g., hypoallergenic) diet should be considered. Moist diets are usually preferable to dry diets. Fluid therapy should be continued until the animal can maintain hydration with oral fluids.

PROGNOSIS

The prognosis depends on identification and treatment of underlying diseases and whether peritonitis is present. The prognosis is good if the ulcer is the result of treatable disease, and perforation has not occurred. If peritonitis is present, the prognosis is guarded (see the discussion of peritonitis on p. 193).

Suggested Reading

Barbar DL: Radiographic aspects of gastric ulcers in dogs, *Vet Rad* 23:109, 1982.

Jergens AE et al: Idiopathic inflammatory bowel disease associated with gastroduodenal ulceration-erosion: a report of nine cases in the dog and cat, *J Am Anim Hosp Assoc* 28:21, 1992.

Moreland KJ: Ulcer disease of the upper gastrointestinal tract in small animals: pathophysiology, diagnosis, and management, *Compend Contin Educ Pract Vet* 10:1265, 1988.

TABLE 16-44

Important Considerations for Gastric Neoplasia

- Most gastric tumors are malignant
- Anorexia, not vomiting, is the most common sign
- Many patients are anemic
- Most patients do not vomit until the neoplasm is well-advanced or is causing gastric outflow obstruction
- Neoplasia is a potential cause of ulceration in the dog and cat but many neoplasms do not cause ulceration
- Not all obstructed patients have hypokalemic, hypochloremic, metabolic alkalosis
- Gastroduodenoscopy is usually more appropriate than contrast radiographs; with endoscopy, you can biopsy and often (not always) diagnose malignancy

Stanton ME, Bright RM: Gastroduodenal ulceration in dogs, *J Vet Int Med* 3:238, 1989.

Willard MD, Toal RL, Cawley A: Gastric complications associated with correction of chronic diaphragmatic hernia in two dogs, *J Am Vet Med Assoc* 184:1151, 1984.

GASTRIC NEOPLASIA AND INFILTRATIVE DISEASE

DEFINITIONS

Adenocarcinomas arise from glandular tissue or are composed of tumor cells that form glandular structures. The term **lymphoma** denotes a malignant neoplasm arising from the lymphoid system. **Leiomyosarcomas** and **leiomyomas** are malignant and benign tumors, respectively, arising from smooth muscle. **Pythiosis** is a fungal infection, caused by *Pythiosis insidiosum*, that may cause a severe inflammatory and infiltrative lesion in the stomach. **Phycomycosis** is a more general term for mycoses caused by fungi of the group Phycomycetes.

SYNONYMS

Lymphoma and **lymphosarcoma** are used synonymously to denote a malignant neoplasm of the lymphoid system. **Pythiosis** and **phycomycosis** are technically different, but the terms are often used interchangeably.

GENERAL CONSIDERATIONS AND CLINICALLY RELEVANT PATHOPHYSIOLOGY

Benign gastric tumors are more commonly found in dogs than in cats; however, most gastric neoplasms are malignant (Table 16-44). Adenocarcinoma is the most common canine stomach tumor, accounting for 60% to 70% of reported cases (Withrow, 1989). Adenocarcinomas tend to metastasize to regional lymph nodes, liver, and/or lungs, and they may appear diffusely infiltrative or nodular. They usually occur in the pyloric antrum or lesser curvature. Other reported malignant gastric tumors in dogs include leiomyosarcoma, lymphosarcoma, and fibrosarcoma.

Lymphoma is the most common gastric tumor in cats; adenocarcinomas are rare. Most affected cats are FeLV negative. Lymphoma may be solitary or diffuse in the stomach and may or may not simultaneously affect the intestine.

Leiomyomas are the most common benign canine gastric tumor. They tend to be slow-growing, submucosal, and expansile. Clinical signs may not be apparent until the tumors are large. Leiomyomas usually occur at the cardia, and complete surgical excision may be possible because they are often pedunculated. Adenomatous polyps are occasionally found in dogs. They may be multiple and rarely cause clinical signs, but vomiting and/or anorexia may be seen if the polyps occur at the pylorus and cause obstruction. Other benign tumors rarely found in dogs include adenomas, lipomas, and fibromas.

Pythiosis is a fungal infection caused by *P. insidiosum* that affects any part of the alimentary tract (as well as skin). It is primarily found in the southeastern United States, particularly near the Gulf Coast. The fungus causes intensive submucosal infiltration of fibrous connective tissue and a profound inflammatory reaction in the mucosa (often with eosinophils) and deeper layers of the gastric wall (Fig. 16-78). The organism is often difficult to find histologically, and large tissue samples that include substantial submucosa should be submitted.

DIAGNOSIS
Clinical Presentation

Signalment. Belgian shepherd dogs (adenocarcinomas) and beagles (leiomyoma) may have an increased incidence of gastric neoplasia. Males appear to be more commonly affected than females. Adenocarcinoma is most common in dogs 8 to 9 years of age. Lymphoma affects primarily middle-aged and older dogs (average age is 6 years) and cats. Pythiosis may affect dogs of any age.

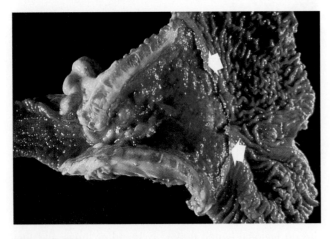

FIG. 16-78
Pythiosis affecting the pylorus and antrum of a dog's stomach. Note the sharp line of demarcation between normal and abnormal tissue (*arrows*).

History. Animals with gastric neoplasia or other infiltrative disease usually present with a history of anorexia. Chronic vomiting, hematemesis, melena, lethargy, weight loss, and/or edema may also occur. Many animals are asymptomatic until the tumor becomes large enough to cause gastric outlet obstruction. Clinical signs with pythiosis are generally the result of gastric outflow obstruction and gastric stasis.

Physical Examination Findings

Physical examination findings in animals with gastric neoplasia or pythiosis are often nonspecific (e.g., weight loss, anemia, and/or edema). Weight loss may be the result of anorexia, chronic vomiting, or cancer cachexia. Occasionally, a large mass may be palpated in the stomach; however, detailed palpation of the stomach is usually difficult. Abdominal pain may be present if there is ulceration or pancreatitis.

Radiography/Ultrasonography/Endoscopy

Noncontrast radiographs are generally nondiagnostic. Contrast radiographs may reveal filling defects, delayed gastric emptying, ulceration, loss of normal rugal folds, mucosal thickening, or loss of gastric wall compliance. If a gastric neoplasm is suspected, endoscopy allows mucosal biopsy of the stomach and duodenum. Tumors may be difficult to diagnose with endoscopy if they are scirrhous or completely submucosal. Pythiosis is particularly difficult to diagnose by flexible endoscopic biopsy because the organisms are found in the submucosa. Thoracic radiographs should be taken to rule out pulmonary metastasis. Ultrasonography may detect metastasis to the liver or regional lymph nodes and help define the gastric lesion.

Laboratory Findings

Clinical pathology changes in animals with gastric neoplasia are usually nonspecific. A microcytic, hypochromic or a normocytic, normochromic anemia may occur. The anemia may be the result of blood loss or chronic disease. If obstruction of biliary drainage is present, icterus ensues. If vomiting causes loss of gastric secretions, a hypochloremic, hypokalemic, metabolic alkalosis with or without paradoxical aciduria may occur.

> ☞ **N O T E** · If the animal is icteric, the lesion is probably near the pylorus. Be prepared to perform a cholecystoenterostomy (see p. 392).

DIFFERENTIAL DIAGNOSIS

Anorexia may be caused by many systemic diseases (e.g., uremia, hypoadrenocorticism, hepatic insufficiency, hypercalcemia, inflammatory disease). Gastric outlet obstruction due to nonneoplastic disease (i.e., chronic pyloric mucosal hypertrophy) may cause similar clinical signs (see p. 284). Cytologic and/or histologic examination of tissues is necessary to definitely differentiate these conditions. Gastric foreign bodies can be differentiated from neoplasia with radiography or endoscopy. Pythiosis and neoplasia may be differentiated by cytologic examination of tissue scrapings of the submucosa obtained by full-thickness biopsy (see Fig. 16-100 on p. 315).

☞ **N O T E** · Histologic diagnosis of pythiosis can be difficult. Submit at least two full-thickness biopsies.

MEDICAL MANAGEMENT

Medical management depends on the severity of clinical signs. If possible, electrolyte, acid-base, hydration, and coagulation abnormalities should be corrected before surgery.

SURGICAL TREATMENT
Preoperative Management

Food should be withheld for 12 hours before surgery. Perioperative antibiotics may be given at anesthetic induction and continued for up to 12 hours postoperatively.

Anesthesia

See p. 262 for suggested anesthetics to use in dogs with gastric disorders.

Surgical Anatomy

See p. 263 for surgical anatomy of the stomach.

Positioning

The animal is placed in dorsal recumbency and the abdomen prepared for a ventral midline incision. The prepped area should extend from midthorax to the pubis.

SURGICAL TECHNIQUE

With the exception of lymphoma, surgery is the only viable treatment for gastric neoplasia (Fig. 16-79). *Palpate the regional lymph nodes for evidence of metastasis. Inspect the liver and other abdominal structures for metastasis or thickening, and biopsy suspicious lesions.* If the lesion appears

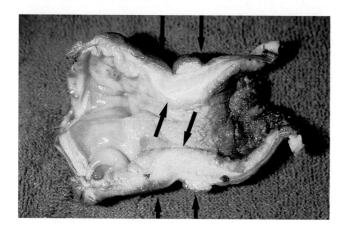

FIG. 16-79
A resected pylorus from a dog that had gastric outflow obstruction caused by a submucosal adenocarcinoma (*arrows*) that did not disrupt the mucosa.

localized to the stomach, gastric resection might be curative. If wide excision and bypass procedures such as gastrojejunostomy and cholecystojejunostomy are necessary (see p. 392), surgery is of dubious value because of the likelihood of tumor recurrence. Solitary gastric lymphoma is rarely cured by surgery alone, and chemotherapy is only palliative for diffuse lymphoma.

Wide surgical excision is currently the only potentially curative therapy available for pythiosis; however, obtaining wide surgical margins is difficult because of the extensive nature of the disease at diagnosis. Gastric drainage procedures, such as Billroth II procedures, may be warranted in some cases. Itraconazole therapy is being investigated and may help some patients.

Wide surgical margins (including some normal tissue) should be obtained for both gastric malignancies and pythiosis. Cytologic examination of tissues submitted during the surgical procedure or frozen sections are helpful to determine the adequacy of the tissue margins. Surgical techniques for gastric resection are described on pp. 264 to 267.

SUTURE MATERIALS/ SPECIAL INSTRUMENTS

Absorbable suture materials, such as polydioxanone or polyglyconate (2-0 or 3-0), should be used. Chromic gut suture should be avoided.

POSTOPERATIVE CARE AND ASSESSMENT

The electrolyte and fluid status of the patient should be monitored postoperatively, and deficiencies corrected. The animal can be fed a low-fat, bland diet beginning 24 hours after surgery if vomiting does not occur. If vomiting continues, centrally-acting antiemetics such as chlorpromazine, metoclopramide, or ondansetron (see Table 16-31) may be beneficial. An enterostomy feeding tube should be considered to help provide nutrition in the postoperative period.

PROGNOSIS

The prognosis is guarded for most gastric neoplasms because of their malignant characteristics and size at the time of diagnosis. For animals with benign lesions, surgery may be curative. Pythiosis may be difficult to treat surgically because of its rapid growth rate and extensive nature, but surgical cures have been achieved.

Reference

Withrow SJ: Tumors of the gastrointestinal system. In Withrow SJ, MacEwen EG: *Clinical veterinary oncology*, Philadelphia, 1989, J.B. Lippincott.

Suggested Reading

Comer KM: Anemia as a feature of primary gastrointestinal neoplasia, *Compend Cont Educ Pract Vet* 12:13, 1990.
Culbertson R, Branam PE, Rosenblatt LS: Esophageal/gastric leiomyoma in the laboratory beagle, *J Am Vet Med Assoc* 183:1168, 1983.

Fonda D, Gualtieri M, Scanziani E: Gastric carcinoma in the dog: a clinicopathological study of 11 cases, *J Small Anim Pract* 30:353, 1989.

Scanziani E et al: Gastric carcinoma in the Belgian shepherd dog, *J Small Anim Pract* 32:465, 1991.

Surgery of the Small Intestine

GENERAL PRINCIPLES AND TECHNIQUES

DEFINITIONS

Enterotomy is an incision into the intestine, and **enterectomy** is removal of a segment of intestine. **Intestinal resection and anastomosis** is an enterectomy with reestablishment of continuity between the divided ends. **Enteroenteropexy** or intestinal plication is surgical fixation of one intestinal segment to another, while **enteropexy** is fixation of an intestinal segment to the body wall or another loop of intestine.

PREOPERATIVE CONCERNS

Surgery of the small intestines is most often indicated for gastrointestinal obstruction (i.e., foreign bodies, masses). Other indications include trauma (i.e., perforation, is-chemia), malpositioning, infection, and diagnostic or supportive procedures (i.e., biopsy, culture, cytology, feeding tubes).

Diagnosis of small intestinal disease is based on history, clinical signs, physical examination, radiographs, ultrasound, laboratory data, endoscopy, and/or biopsy. Diet, medications, stressful events, and response to prior therapy should be ascertained from owners. Clinical signs of small intestinal disease are variable and nonspecific; vomiting, diarrhea, anorexia, depression, and/or weight loss are common (Table 16-45). Pain and shock may occur following trauma, vascular occlusion, or complete intestinal obstruction. Severe vomiting, shock, or an acute abdomen suggests intestinal malposition, ischemia, perforation, or upper intestinal obstruction. Chronic disease, however, is more typical of lower intestinal tract disease and/or partial obstruction. Visual examination provides information about the animal's mental state, temperament, nutritional state, and comfort. Abdominal palpation may identify pain, thickened small intestine, abdominal masses, or malpositioned organs.

Hematologic and biochemical profiles should be performed on animals with suspected small intestinal abnormalities to help identify concurrent systemic disease (e.g., renal disease, hepatic disease, hyperadrenocorticism, hypercalcemia, diabetes mellitus, and pancreatitis) and to direct preoperative therapy (Table 16-46). Dehydration, acid-base abnormalities, and electrolyte imbalances are common sequelae to vomiting, diarrhea, and fluid sequestration. These

TABLE   16-45

Clinical Signs of Chronic Intestinal Disease

Clinical Sign	Small Intestine	Large Intestine
Weight loss	Consistent	Infrequent
Appetite	Variable	Usually normal; variable
Vomiting	Occasional	Rare
Belching	Occasional	Rare
Flatulence and borborygmus	Occasional	Rare
Distended abdomen	Variable	Rare
Defecation quantity	Normal to large	Small to normal
Defecation frequency	Normal to slightly increased	Normal to very frequent
Blood in feces	If present, usually dark, black (melena)	If present, usually fresh, red (hematochezia)
Mucus in feces	Absent	Present or absent
Steatorrhea	Occasional	Absent
Fecalith	Absent	Sometimes
Urgency or tenesmus	Absent	Sometimes present
Dyschezia	Absent	Present with rectal disease
Rectal exam	Normal	May be normal or abnormal (blood, mucus, pain, mass)
Abdominal pain	Variable	Variable
Poor hair coat	Variable	Uncommon
Depression	Variable	Uncommon

abnormalities should be corrected before anesthetic induction, if possible. Profuse vomiting typically results in dehydration and may cause hypochloremia, hypokalemia, and/or hyponatremia. Vomitus originating from the duodenum results in greater sodium, potassium, and water losses than does gastric vomitus. Alkalosis generally occurs when there is a loss of gastric fluid; however, metabolic acidosis may occur as a result of fluid depletion from vomiting, insensible water losses, lack of intake, and/or catabolism of body stores. Crossmatched whole blood should be administered for acute hemorrhage when the packed cell volume (PCV) drops below 20%. Chronically ill, anemic patients should be given whole blood if hypovolemic and packed red blood cells (RBCs) if normovolemic. Clotting factor deficiencies should be corrected with whole fresh blood or fresh or fresh-frozen plasma. Platelet-rich plasma or platelet transfusions should be used if the animal is severely thrombocytopenic. Administration of plasma (5 to 20 ml/kg) or whole blood transfusions several hours before surgery should be considered if serum albumin concentrations are less than 1.5 g/dl. There is some evidence that blood transfusions may impair intestinal healing and increase susceptibility to intraabdominal sepsis (Tadros, Wobbes, Hendriks, 1992).

Plain radiographs may demonstrate abnormal gas-fluid patterns, masses, foreign bodies, abdominal fluid, or displaced viscera (Fig. 16-80). Right-lateral recumbent and ventrodorsal projections are preferred. Contrast studies are useful for demonstrating foreign bodies, obstructions, abnormal displacements, abnormal bowel wall thickness, irregular mucosal patterns, and distortion of the bowel wall. The positive contrast agent usually used for gastrointestinal radiology is micropulverized barium sulfate suspension; however, iodinated contrast or iohexol should be used when intestinal perforation is suspected but septic peritonitis cannot be demonstrated with abdominocentesis or diagnostic peritoneal lavage (see p. 198).

☞ **N O T E ·** Do not use barium for gastrointestinal (GI) series if intestinal perforation is suspected. Instead document peritonitis by abdominocentesis, diagnostic peritoneal lavage, or exploratory surgery.

TABLE 16-46

Preoperative Management of Patients Undergoing Intestinal Surgery

- Obtain minimum data base: complete blood cell count (CBC), chemistry profile, urinalysis, coagulation profile (if possible) ± electrocardiogram.
- Localize the lesion with abdominal palpation, radiographs, ultrasonography, and/or endoscopy.
- Correct hydration, electrolyte, and acid-base abnormalities.
- Transfuse if PCV is less than 20%.
- Withhold food from mature animals for 12 to 18 hours and from pediatric patients 4 to 8 hours before induction.
- Administer prophylactic antibiotics if indicated.

Ultrasonography can define intestinal and other abdominal masses and provide information about intestinal wall thickness (normal small intestine wall ranges from 2.0 to 3.0 mm), appearance and symmetry of the various wall layers, number of peristaltic contractions, pattern of intestinal contents (gas-hyperechoic, mucus-echogenic without acoustic shadowing, fluid-anechoic), lesion location, and extent of disease. Mucosal and muscular layers are hypoechoic; serosa is hyperechoic. Gastrointestinal endoscopy allows visualization and biopsy of the duodenum (and sometimes the upper jejunum and ileum) for detection of inflammation, ulcers, masses, and changes in wall thickness or texture.

ANESTHETIC CONSIDERATIONS

Mature animals should be fasted 12 to 18 hours before surgery, but pediatric patients should be fasted for only 4 to 8 hours. Special anesthetic considerations are needed when dealing with patients having bowel obstruction, ischemia, or perforation. Complications may arise because of uncorrected electrolyte, acid-base, and fluid imbalances. Enlarged viscera may compress the vena cava, causing circulatory and vascular compromise. Respiration may be compromised by viscera displacing the diaphragm cranially. Nitrous oxide increases the volume of air trapped in body viscera and therefore should be avoided in patients with intestinal obstruction. Visceral manipulation may induce bradycardia; however, atropine or glycopyrrolate can treat this. Water evaporates from exposed abdominal viscera at an increased rate; therefore fluid administration must be increased to replace this loss. Body heat is lost from exposed viscera and may lead to hypothermia, which reduces the need for anesthesia. Care should be taken during surgery to try to maintain body temperature at greater than 95°F. Selected anesthetic protocols for stable animals undergoing small intestinal surgery are provided in Table 16-47. Sick or debilitated animals should be anesthetized with care. Selected anesthetic protocols for use in animals with peritonitis are provided on p. 197.

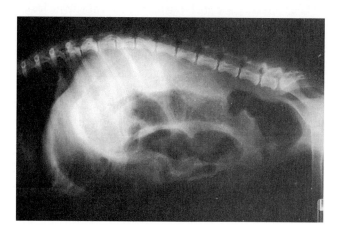

FIG. 16-80
Lateral radiograph of a depressed, anorexic, constipated, 2-year-old boxer with a "doughy" abdomen. Note massive intestinal distension with gas and ingesta. A corn cob was removed from the distal jejunum.

TABLE 16-47
Selected Anesthetic Protocols for Use in Stable Animals with Intestinal Disorders

Premedication

Give atropine (0.02-0.04 mg/kg SC or IM) or glycopyrrolate (0.005-0.011 mg/kg SC or IM) plus oxymorphone* (0.05-0.1 mg/kg SC or IM) or butorphanol (0.2-0.4 mg/kg SC or IM) or buprenorphine (5-15 μg/kg IM)

Induction

Thiopental (10-12 mg/kg IV) or propofol (4-6 mg/kg IV) or a combination of diazepam and ketamine (diazepam 0.27 mg/kg plus 5.5 mg/kg ketamine IV; titrated to effect)

Maintenance

Isoflurane or halothane
*Use 0.05 mg/kg in cats.

TABLE 16-48
Prophylactic Antibiotics in Animals Undergoing Intestinal Surgery

Cefazolin (Ancef, Kefzol)

20 mg/kg IV

Cefmetazole (Zefazone)

15 mg/kg IV

Cefoxitin (Mefoxin)

15-30 mg/kg IV

ANTIBIOTICS

A large flora of normal bacteria populate the gastrointestinal tract. Bacterial numbers are less in the duodenum and jejunum than in the ileum, colon, and rectum. The greatest number of bacteria (aerobic and anaerobic) are found in the colon. Few pathologic bacteria reside proximal to the ileocecal valve unless peristalsis is interrupted by ileus or obstruction and the normal flora is overgrown. An abnormal proliferation of resident bacteria occurs in the involved bowel because stagnant luminal contents and devitalized wall are excellent growth media. Six hours of abnormal conditions may allow numbers to increase from a range of 10^2 to 10^4/ml to a range of 10^8 to 10^{11}/ml of ingesta. The major gastrointestinal toxin-producing bacteria are *Escherichia coli* and *Clostridium* spp. Holding animals off food decreases bacterial numbers in the small intestine and stomach. Antibiotic therapy alters the normal intestinal flora and promotes resistant strains of bacteria. Nonetheless, antibiotics are indicated in animals with severe mucosal damage or acute gastrointestinal disease associated with bloody diarrhea, fever, leukocytosis, leukopenia, and/or shock.

Surgical techniques that involve entering the intestinal lumen are classified as clean-contaminated or contaminated procedures depending on the amount of spillage (see p. 59). Risk of infection in contaminated wounds increases with patient stress, organism pathogenicity, tissue susceptibility, and time. Common pathogens responsible for peritonitis following intestinal surgery are *E. coli*, *Enterococcus* spp., and coagulase-positive *Staphylococcus aureus*. Although less frequently isolated, anaerobes are also common and may cause peritonitis (see p. 193). Prophylactic antibiotics are indicated in animals with intestinal obstruction because there is an increased risk of contamination associated with bacterial overgrowth. They are also indicated when devascularized and traumatized tissue are present and when surgical times are expected to be greater than 2 to 3 hours. First generation cephalosporins (e.g., cefazolin; Table 16-48) should be administered before surgery on the upper and middle small intestine, while second generation cephalosporins (e.g., cefmetazole or cefoxitin; see Table 16-48) should be considered for procedures involving the distal small intestine and large intestine. Antibiotics should be redosed 2 hours after the initial dose.

SURGICAL ANATOMY

The intestines in dogs are approximately five times the body (crown-to-rump) length, with 80% being small intestine. Duodenum, jejunum, and ileum make up the small intestine. The duodenum is the most fixed portion, beginning at the pylorus to the right of midline and extending approximately 25 cm. It courses dorsocranially for a short distance, turns caudally at the cranial duodenal flexure, and continues on the right as the descending duodenum. The duodenum turns cranially at the caudal duodenal flexure where the duodenocolic ligament attaches. The ascending duodenum lies to the left of the mesenteric root. The common bile duct and pancreatic duct open in the first few centimeters of the duodenum at the major duodenal papilla in dogs. The accessory pancreatic duct enters caudal to this at the minor duodenal papilla.

The jejunum forms the majority of small intestinal coils lying in the ventrocaudal abdomen. It is the longest and most mobile segment of the small intestine. It begins to the left of the mesenteric root where the ascending duodenum turns to the right at the duodenojejunal flexure.

The ileum has an antimesenteric vessel and is approximately 15 cm long. It passes from the left to the right side in a transverse plane through the midlumbar region caudal to the root of the mesentery and joins the ascending colon on the right of the midline at the ileocolic orifice. The root of the mesentery attaches the jejunum and ileum to the dorsal body wall. Branches of the celiac and cranial mesenteric arteries supply the small intestine. Mesenteric lymph nodes lie along vessels in the mesentery.

Layers of the intestinal wall include mucosa, submucosa, muscularis, and serosa. Mucosa is an important barrier that separates the luminal environment from that of the abdominal cavity. Mucosal health and intestinal blood supply are important for normal intestinal secretion and absorption. Submucosa is the intestinal layer that provides mechanical strength; thus it must be engaged when suturing intestine to

TABLE 16-49

Principles of Intestinal Surgery

- Early diagnosis and good surgical technique avoid most complications.
- Perform surgery as soon as the diagnosis is made in patients with perforation, strangulation, or complete obstruction.
- Optimal healing requires a good blood supply, accurate mucosal apposition, and minimal surgical trauma.
- Systemic factors may delay healing and increase the risk of dehiscence, hypovolemia, shock, hypoproteinemia, debilitation, infections, etc.
- Use approximating suture patterns: simple interrupted, Gambee, crushing, or simple continuous.
- Engage submucosa in all sutures.
- Select a monofilament, synthetic absorbable suture such as polydioxanone or polyglyconate.
- Cover surgical sites with omentum or a serosal patch.
- Replace contaminated instruments and gloves before abdominal closure.

provide a secure closure. The submucosal layer provides blood vessels, lymphatics, and nerves. The muscularis is needed for normal motility. Serosa is important in forming a quick seal at a site of injury or incision.

SURGICAL TECHNIQUES

Surgical correction of mechanical obstructions is preferably performed within 12 hours of diagnosis, allowing time for partial to complete correction of fluid, acid-base, and electrolyte abnormalities. The benefits of stabilizing the patient must be weighed against the risk of ischemic necrosis caused by vascular disruption, which increases with time (Table 16-49). Consequences of perforation, loss of mucosal integrity, and systemic exposure to intestinal bacteria are life threatening. Surgery for penetrating abdominal wounds, intestinal perforation, volvulus, or peritonitis should be performed as soon as the diagnosis is made.

Ischemic necrosis of the bowel wall may occur with obstruction (complete or partial) or strangulation. Routine criteria to assess bowel viability include observation of intestinal color (pink to red rather than blue to black), wall texture, peristalsis, pulsation of arteries, and bleeding when incised. These factors are subjective; thus assessment of viability is often difficult. Bathing the involved segment in warm saline for a few minutes may improve color and peristalsis. However, normal appearance does not guarantee that the bowel will heal after surgery. Therefore bowel of questionable viability should be resected. A number of techniques have been proposed to increase the accuracy of standard clinical criteria for viability assessment, and their most common error is to indicate that viable bowel should be resected. Viability assessment techniques include using electromyography, radioactive microspheres, microtemperature probes, and pH measurements. These techniques are technically cumbersome, expensive, and not generally suited for clinical use. Doppler ultrasonic flow probes to detect pulsatile mural blood flow

have been used with an accuracy of 80% (Wheaton et al, 1983). Pulse oximetry measures oxygen saturation via pulse probes and may be superior to Doppler ultrasound in determining intestinal viability. Pulse oximetry of the intestinal wall as compared with peripheral oxygen saturation has shown that normal intestine remains within 1 cm of a normal pulse oximetry reading. Pulse oximetry is a reliable, reproducible means of assessing arterial perfusion of ischemic intestine, exceeding the overall accuracy of either standard clinical criteria or Doppler ultrasound when compared with fluorescein dye. Pulse oximetry is not as sensitive as fluorescein dye in detecting viability in segments with combined arterial and venous occlusion (Wheaton et al, 1983; Denobile, Guzzetta, Patterson, 1990). Intravenous injection of various agents (primarily fluorescein dye) is practical, but of limited accuracy (95% accurate in detecting nonviable bowel, less than 58% accurate in detecting viable bowel) (Wheaton et al, 1983). Fluorescein dye is injected intravenously (15 to 25 mg/kg), allowed to equilibrate for 2 to 3 minutes, and then the intestine is viewed with a Wood's lamp in a darkened operating room. Viable intestine has fluorescing areas of a smooth, uniform green-gold color or a finely mottled pattern with no areas of nonfluorescence greater than 3 mm. Fluorescein can be used only once in a 24-hour period. Dyes such as fluorescein assess only perfusion and not mucosal integrity, which is essential to maintain the mucosal barrier. Although this technique is a test of vascularity and not specifically viability, it can be a valuable adjunct in predicting viability.

Biopsy Techniques

Intestinal biopsy is indicated to diagnose intestinal diseases that have not been defined by other tests. The small intestine may be biopsied during endoscopy, ultrasonography, or laparotomy. All biopsy techniques require general anesthesia or sedation. The least invasive method of obtaining an intestinal biopsy is by endoscopy. Endoscopic biopsies are limited to infiltrative disease involving the mucosa and submucosa and to lesions located within the length of the endoscope. Fine-needle aspiration biopsy or automated microcore biopsy may be performed during ultrasonographic examination of intestinal lesions; however, it may be difficult to perform these procedures if mild or moderate infiltration is present. These procedures are applicable to the entire intestine and are generally safe and rapid. Sedation or general anesthesia is required during the procedure. Lesions smaller than 2 cm are aspirated with a 22-gauge, 3.5-inch spinal needle or a 20-gauge Westcott Style Biopsy needle. If aspirated samples are nondiagnostic, and the lesion is larger than 2 cm, an automated microcore biopsy is performed (Bard Bioptycut Biopsy needle). Potential complications include peritonitis, hematoma, tumor seeding, and adjacent organ trauma.

Localize the lesion with the transducer and aseptically prepare the skin over this site. Tense the skin and puncture with the needle. Using ultrasound guidance, direct the needle into the lesion but not through the mucosa. For aspiration biopsies remove the stylet and apply suction with a 6-cc syringe three to six times. After releasing suction, remove the needle and syringe. Collect two to four samples and evaluate the cytologic preparations. For a microcore biopsy select a site as far from the intestinal lumen as possible. Using the Tru-cut biopsy instrument with ultrasound guidance collect one or two biopsies. Transfer the samples to biopsy traps and place in 10% formalin. After sampling, observe the biopsy site with ultrasound for fluid collection suggestive of leakage or hemorrhage. Abdominal radiography may be used to look for pneumoperitoneum. Monitor mucous-membrane color, capillary refill time, pulse, and respiratory rate during recovery.

Enterotomy

Laparotomy and enterotomy should be performed if endoscopic or ultrasound biopsy is not possible or is nondiagnostic. Enterotomy allows collection of full-thickness biopsies from all areas of the intestine and other abdominal structures. Longitudinal or transverse enterotomy incisions can be made to collect biopsies. Multiple biopsies should be performed and samples should be reasonably large (4 to 5 mm) and contain adequate amounts of mucosa. The entire abdomen should be thoroughly explored before biopsies are performed. Biopsies or samples should be collected from lymph nodes, liver, kidney, or other tissues before gastric or intestinal procedures to prevent cross-contamination. Other indications for enterotomy include removal of foreign bodies and luminal examination.

Exteriorize and isolate the diseased or desired intestine from the abdomen by packing with towels or laparotomy sponges. Gently milk chyme (intestinal contents) from the lumen of the identified intestinal segment. To minimize spillage of chyme, occlude the lumen at both ends of the isolated segment by having an assistant use a scissorlike grip with the index and middle fingers, 4 to 6 cm on each side of the proposed enterotomy site (Fig. 16-81, A). If an assistant is not available, noncrushing intestinal forceps (Doyen) or a Penrose drain tourniquet can also be used to occlude the intestinal lumen. *Make a full-thickness stab incision into the intestinal lumen on the antimesenteric border with a No. 11 scalpel blade. Obtain full-thickness biopsies 2 to 3 mm wide by either making a second longitudinal incision parallel to the first with the scalpel blade or by removing an ellipse of intestinal wall at one margin of the first incision with Metzenbaum scissors (Figs. 16-81, B and C).* Transverse enterotomy incisions can also be made to obtain biopsies. *Place the biopsy serosal side down on a heavy piece of sterile paper to help prevent curling of the speci-*

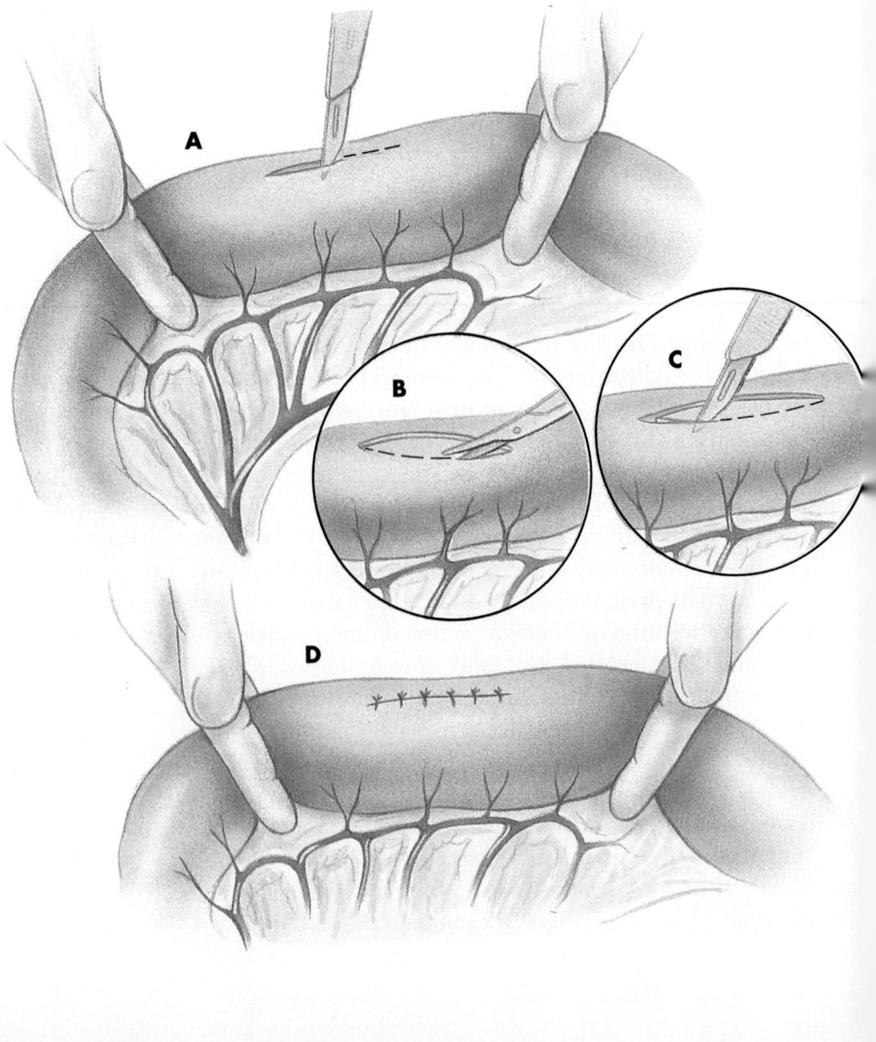

FIG. 16-81
For intestinal biopsy **A,** make a stab incision into the lumen with a No. 11 blade. **B,** Remove a 2- to 3-mm ellipse of tissue with Metzenbaum scissors or **C,** by making a second incision approximately parallel to the first with a scalpel. **D,** Close the incision with simple interrupted sutures.

men. Close the incision as described below with simple interrupted sutures (Fig. 16-81, D). Simple continuous or crushing sutures may also be used to close the enterotomy. *If a foreign body is present, make the incision in healthy-appearing tissue distal to the foreign body (Fig. 16-82). Lengthen the incision along the intestine's long axis with Metzenbaum scissors or scalpel as necessary to allow foreign body removal without tearing the intestine.*

After biopsy or foreign body removal prepare the incision for closure by trimming everted mucosa so that its edge is even with the serosal edge (if necessary). Suction the isolated lumen. Close the incision with gentle appositional force in a longitudinal or transverse direction using simple interrupted sutures (Fig. 16-83). Place sutures through all layers of the intestinal wall, 2 mm from the edge and 2 to 3 mm apart, with extraluminal knots. Angle the needle so the serosa is engaged slightly further from the edge than the mucosa (Fig. 16-84) to help reposition everting mucosa within the lumen. Tie each suture carefully without cutting through layers of the intestinal wall so as to gently appose all intestinal layers without crushing the tissue. Use a monofilament absorbable suture material (4-0 or 3-0 polydioxanone or polyglyconate) with a swaged-on taper or tapercut point needle. Consider a monofilament nonabsorbable suture (4-0 or 3-0 polypropylene or nylon) if the patient has an albumin level less than or equal to 2.0 g/dl. While maintaining luminal occlusion near the enterotomy site, moderately distend the lumen with sterile saline, apply gentle digital pressure, and observe for leakage between sutures or through needle holes. Place additional sutures if leakage occurs between sutures. Lavage the isolated intestine and the entire abdomen if contamination has occurred. Place omentum over the suture line before abdominal closure. Use a serosal patch (see p. 301) rather than omentum if intestinal integrity is questionable or if leakage occurs from needle holes. Replace contaminated instruments and gloves before abdominal closure.

Intestinal Resection and Anastomosis

Intestinal resection and anastomosis are recommended for removing ischemic, necrotic, neoplastic, or fungal-infected segments of intestine. Irreducible intussusceptions are also managed by resection and anastomosis. End-to-end anastomoses are recommended.

Sutured anastomoses. *Make an abdominal incision long enough to allow exploration of the abdomen. Thoroughly explore the abdomen and collect any nonintestinal specimens, then exteriorize and isolate the diseased intestine from the abdomen by packing with towels or laparotomy sponges. Assess intestinal viability and determine the amount of intestine needing resection. Double ligate and transect the arcadial mesenteric vessels from the cranial mesenteric artery that supplies this segment of intestine (Fig. 16-85). Double ligate the terminal arcade vessels and vasa recta vessels within the mesenteric fat at the points of proposed*

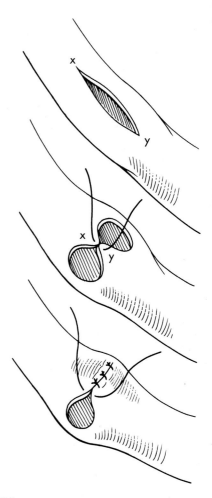

FIG. 16-83
Enterotomy incisions may be closed transversely if the intestinal lumen is small. Join the extremes (x and y) of the longitudinal incision with a simple interrupted suture to transpose the incision to a transverse orientation. Place remaining sutures 2 to 3 mm apart.

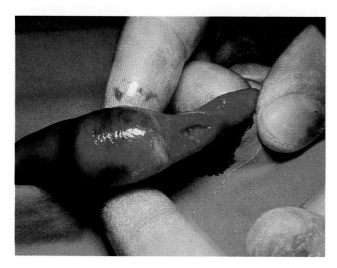

FIG. 16-82
Intestinal segment with a foreign body that was removed via an enterotomy. Note the dilated proximal intestine with some ischemic areas.

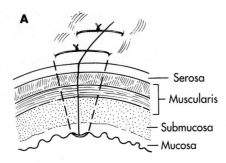

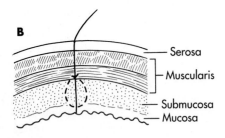

FIG. 16-84
A, For an approximating suture closure of the intestine place simple interrupted sutures 2 mm from the edge and 2 to 3 mm apart. Engage slightly more serosa than mucosa to force everted mucosa back into the lumen. **B,** Place crushing sutures similarly but pull them tight to cut through all layers except the submucosa when tying.

intestinal transection. Gently milk chyme (intestinal contents) from the lumen of the identified intestinal segment. Occlude the lumen at both ends of the segment to minimize spillage of chyme (see above). Place forceps across each end of the diseased bowel segment (these forceps may be either crushing or noncrushing because this segment of the intestine will be excised). Transect the intestine with either a scalpel blade or Metzenbaum scissors along the outside of the forceps. Make the incision either perpendicular or oblique to the long axis. Use a perpendicular incision (75 to 90 degree angle) at each end if the luminal diameters are the same. When luminal sizes of the intestinal ends are expected to be unequal, use a perpendicular incision across the intestine with the larger luminal diameter and an oblique incision (45- to 60-degree angle) across the intestine with the smaller luminal diameter to help correct size disparity (Figs. 16-86 and 16-87). **Make the oblique incision such that the antimesenteric border is shorter than the mesenteric border.** *Suction the intestinal ends and remove any debris clinging to the cut edges with a moistened gauze sponge. Trim everting mucosa with Metzenbaum scissors just before beginning the end-to-end anastomosis.*

Use 3-0 or 4-0 monofilament, absorbable suture (polydioxanone or polyglyconate) with a swaged-on taper or tapercut point needle. In peritonitis cases monofilament nonabsorbable suture (3-0 or 4-0 polypropylene or nylon) is sometimes used. Place simple interrupted sutures through all layers of the intestinal wall. Angle the needle so the serosa is engaged slightly further from the edge than the mucosa (see Fig. 16-84). This helps reposition everting mucosa

within the lumen. Tie each suture carefully so as to gently appose the edges of the intestine with the knots extraluminally. Tying sutures roughly or with too much tension causes the suture to cut through the serosa, muscularis, and mucosa and creates a crushing suture (see Fig. 16-84). Some surgeons prefer this suture, and others use a simple continuous pattern. Pulling continuous sutures too tight will have a purse-string effect, and significant stenosis may occur. A continuous pattern around the intestine may limit dilation at the anastomotic site and cause a partial obstruction. *Appose intestinal ends by first placing a simple interrupted suture at the mesenteric border (see Fig. 16-85, B) and then placing a second suture at the antimesenteric border approximately 180 degrees from the first (this divides the suture line into equal halves and allows determination of whether the ends are of approximately equal diameter).* The mesenteric suture is the most difficult suture to place in the anastomosis because of mesenteric fat. It is also the most common site of leakage. *If the ends are of equal diameter, space additional sutures between the first two sutures approximately 2 mm from the edge and 2 to 3 mm apart (see Fig. 16-85, C). If minor disparity still exists between lumen sizes, space the sutures around the larger lumen slightly further apart than the sutures in the intestine with the smaller lumen (see Fig. 16-87). To correct luminal disparity that cannot be accommodated by the angle of the incisions or by suture spacing, resect a small wedge (1 to 2 cm long and 1 to 3 mm wide) from the antimesenteric border of the intestine with the smaller lumen (Fig. 16-88).* This enlarges the perimeter of the stoma, giving it an oval shape. *Do not suture together the edges of the intestine with the larger lumen in an attempt to reduce luminal size to that of the smaller intestine.* Narrowing the larger lumen is not recommended because there is greater tendency for stricture at the anastomotic site when the dilated intestine contracts to a normal size. *After suture placement inspect the anastomosis and check for leakage. While maintaining luminal occlusion adjacent to the anastomotic site, moderately distend the lumen with sterile saline, apply gentle digital pressure, and observe for leakage between sutures or through needle holes.* This is a subjective test because all anastomoses can be made to leak if enough pressure is applied. *Place additional sutures if leakage occurs between sutures. Close the mesenteric defect with a simple continuous or interrupted suture pattern (4-0 polydioxanone or polyglyconate) being careful not to penetrate or traumatize arcadial vessels near the defect. Lavage the isolated intestine and the entire abdomen if abdominal contamination has occurred. Wrap the anastomotic site with omentum before abdominal closure or use a serosal patch (see p. 301) if intestinal integrity is questionable and leakage is likely.*

Stapled anastomoses. Resection may also be accomplished with staples. Three stapled anastomosis techniques are available: (1) triangulating end-to-end, (2) inverting end-to-end, and (3) side-to-side or functional end-to-end anastomoses. The small size of the intestine (less than 20 mm) often precludes the use of triangulating and inverting

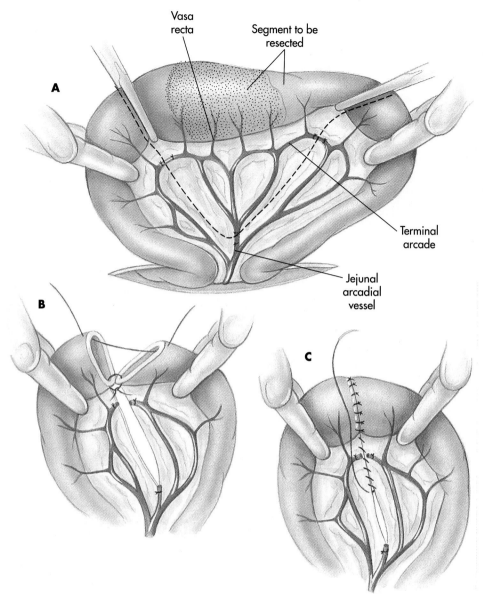

Vasa recta

Segment to be resected

A

Terminal arcade

Jejunal arcadial vessel

B

C

FIG. 16-85
During small intestinal resection and anastomosis place forceps transversely across the dilated proximal intestine and obliquely across the distal intestine. **A,** Transect the intestine and mesentery where the *dotted lines* indicate. **B,** Place the first suture at the mesenteric border and the second at the antimesenteric border. **C,** Place additional simple interrupted sutures to complete the anastomosis. Appose mesentery with a simple continuous pattern.

staple techniques. A functional end-to-end anastomosis creates a larger stoma than the original intestinal lumen and is the preferred technique because the other two stapling techniques decrease lumen size. Stapled anastomoses result in a higher tensile strength than sutured anastomoses after 7 days. They heal by primary intention with minimal inflammation. Thick, inflamed, and edematous tissues may prevent proper firing of the stapler by preventing complete penetration and formation of the staples into a B-shaped configuration. Dilation causes thinning of the visceral walls and may result in tissues too thin for the staples to be effective.

☞ **N O T E** · Staples are expensive; weigh the cost vs. the value of your time and the condition of the patient.

A triangulating end-to-end anastomosis is performed with a transverse stapling instrument (thoracoabdominal

[TA]). *Remove the diseased intestine, then place three stay sutures to divide the stoma into three equal segments and appose the divided intestinal ends. Apply the TA stapler across each segment, partially overlapping the previous staple line. Trim protruding tissue before the instrument is removed.* Each application of the stapler applies a double staggered row of staples. This technique everts the edges. *Inspect the anastomosis for potential leakage and lavage. Appose the mesentery with a continuous suture pattern.*

An end-to-end anastomosis is performed using a circular, inverting, end-to-end anastomosis stapler (EEA, Premium CEEA, or ILP staplers [see Product Appendix]). These instruments are composed of a staple cartridge with a circular blade attached to a dome-shaped anvil and rod (Fig. 16-89). They are available in several sizes that create anastomotic stomas approximately 10 mm smaller than their cartridge size (EEA—31 mm, 28 mm, 25 mm, 21 mm; ILP—33 mm, 29 mm, 25 mm, 21 mm). The intestinal lumen size should be

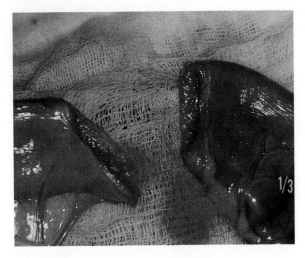

FIG. 16-86
To perform an end-to-end anastomosis when the intestinal segments are of disparate size, transect the dilated intestine at a right angle and the smaller segment at an oblique angle (45 to 60 degrees).

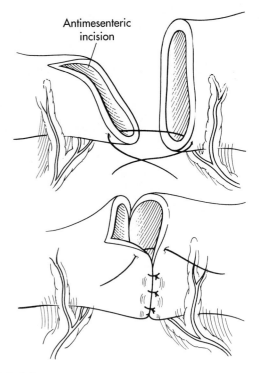

FIG. 16-88
If incision angling and suture spacing do not totally accommodate the luminal size differences, remove a wedge from the antimesenteric border of the distal intestine.

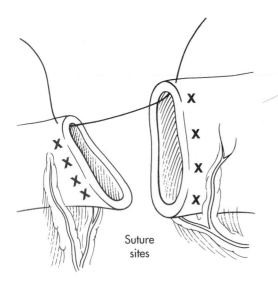

FIG. 16-87
In addition to angling the incisions (see Fig. 16-86), further correct for size disparity by spacing sutures around the larger lumen slightly further apart than around the smaller lumen.

0.6 mm larger in diameter than the stapler. Activation applies a circular double row of staples and simultaneously resects a doughnut of intestinal wall at the anastomotic site. End-to-end staplers are used less frequently in the small intestine than in other areas of the gastrointestinal tract because of the small lumen size of the small intestine. End-to-end staplers are used commonly during Billroth I, esophageal, and large bowel anastomosis procedures. Do not use the stapler if the tissue is too thick (will not compress to 2.0 mm) or too thin (compresses to less than 2.0 mm) and only if there is sufficient tissue to allow proper inversion of tissue edges. *Ligate and divide vessels to the diseased intestine as usual. Dissect the mesentery away from each intestinal segment*

(31-mm cartridge—1.5-cm, 28-mm—1.0-cm, 25- or 21-mm—0.5 cm) because these tissues or ligatures may interfere with instrument closure. Place the purse-string instrument around the proximal intestine at the point of desired transection. Place the purse-string suture and transect the intestine using the purse-string instrument as the cutting guide. Place a purse-string suture and make the distal transection using the same technique. Insert a lubricated ovoid sizer through an enterotomy to determine the appropriate staple cartridge size and to dilate the intestine. Insert the stapler cartridge into the intestinal lumen through an enterotomy 3 to 4 cm from the transection site. Insert the anvil into the other intestinal end. Facilitate placement by placing three to four stay sutures at the edge of the intestine. Using the stay sutures, first pull the mesenteric border of the intestine over the anvil and then over the antimesenteric border. If it appears that the lumen of the intestine will not easily accommodate the anvil or the sizer of the desired diameter, insert a well-lubricated 26-30 French Foley catheter with a 30-ml balloon. Slowly inflate the balloon with sterile water to adequately dilate the intestine. After this dilation procedure, insert the stapler components.

Tie both purse-string sutures securely around the shaft of the stapler (see Fig. 16-89, p. 301). Twist the wing nut to compress the intestinal segments between the cartridge and anvil until the unit is aligned. Examine the anastomotic site for evidence of intestinal slippage. Release the safety and activate the instrument by squeezing the handles. Partially separate the anvil and cartridge by loosening the

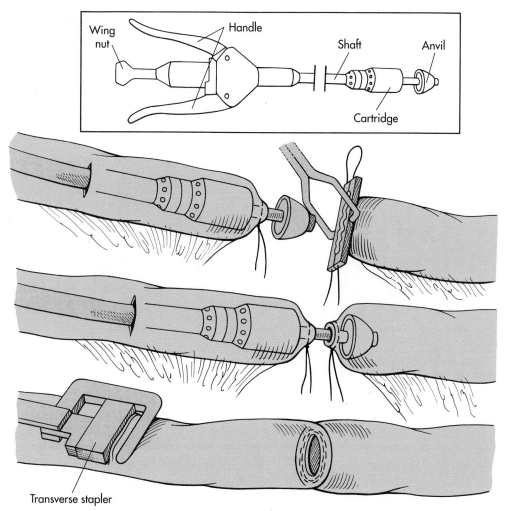

FIG. 16-89
For an inverting end-to-end anastomosis use an end-to-end anastomosis stapler and a transverse stapler. Insert the stapler cartridge into the intestinal lumen through an enterotomy 3 to 4 cm from the transection site. Insert the anvil into the other intestinal end. Tie purse-string sutures securely around the shaft of the stapler. After completing the anastomosis, close the enterotomy with sutures or a transverse stapler.

wing nut and remove the stapling instrument. Facilitate instrument removal by placing a traction suture around the staple line and lift the edge of the staple line over the anvil while gently rotating the instrument.

Inspect the severed, inverted intestinal segment; all tissue layers should be present if leakage is to be prevented. Inspect the anastomotic site for hemorrhage and integrity. Close the enterotomy with sutures or a transverse stapler. Close the mesenteric defect with a continuous pattern. Lavage the surgical site and place an omental or serosal patch (see below) before closing the abdomen.

A side-to-side anastomosis or a functional end-to-end anastomosis is created using a linear cutting stapler (gastrointestinal anastomosis [GIA] stapler) and a transverse anastomotic stapler (thoracoabdominal [TA] or RU 60). This is the preferred technique for small intestinal anastomosis because the resulting stoma is larger than the original, and luminal size disparity is easily accommodated.

Resect diseased intestine and use the linear cutting stapler to join the bowel segments at their antimesenteric borders, creating an antiperistaltic side-to-side anastomosis. Fully insert (50 mm) the linear cutting stapler into the stomas of

each intestinal loop and activate it (Fig. 16-90). Activation results in the placement of two double staggered staple lines that join the intestinal loops as the knife simultaneously incises between them. *Separate the stapled suture line and apply the transverse stapling instrument to close the anastomosis.* The transverse stapler places a double staggered row of staples but has no cutting action. *Transect protruding intestinal wall flush with the stapler. Remove the stapler and place an anchoring suture at the base of the staple line where tension is greatest to discourage staple pullout. Close the mesenteric defect with a continuous pattern before lavaging, patching, and closing the abdomen.*

Serosal Patching

Serosal patching is placement of an antimesenteric border of the small intestine over a suture line or organ defect and securing it with sutures (Fig. 16-91). Serosal patching serves to provide support, a fibrin seal, resistance to leakage, and blood supply to the damaged area, and may prevent intussusception. Patches are commonly used after intestinal surgery when closure integrity is questioned or when dehiscence is repaired. Patches that span visceral defects are covered with mucosal epithelium within 8 weeks. Most commonly, jejunum adjacent to the defect or area of questionable viability

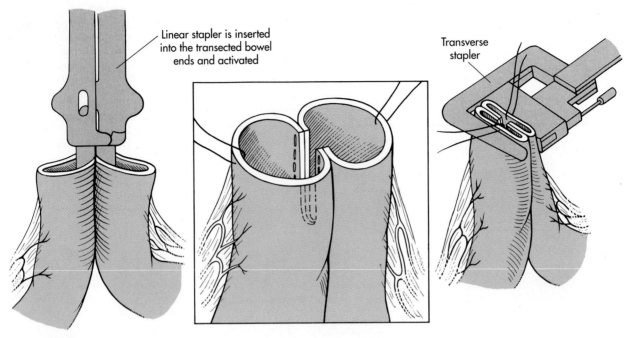

Linear stapler is inserted into the transected bowel ends and activated

Transverse stapler

FIG. 16-90
For a functional end-to-end anastomosis use a linear cutting stapler and a transverse stapler. Fully insert (50 mm) the linear cutting stapler into the stomas of each intestinal loop and activate it. Separate the stapled suture line and apply the transverse stapling instrument to close the anastomosis.

is used for the serosal patch, although other sources could include stomach, other intestinal segments, or urinary bladder.

Use one or more loops of intestine to form the patch. Use gentle loops to avoid stretching, twisting, or kinking the intestine and mesenteric vessels. If using more than one loop of intestine, suture these loops together before securing the patch to the damaged area (see Fig. 16-91). All sutures used to create or secure the patch engage the submucosa, muscularis, and serosa; they should not penetrate the intestinal lumen. Place interrupted or continuous sutures in healthy tissue to secure the patch and isolate the damaged area.

Bowel Plication

Enteroenteropexy or bowel plication is performed to prevent recurrence of intussusception. Serosa-to-serosa adhesions are formed by suturing adjacent loops of intestine together. The small intestine from the duodenocolic ligament to the ileocolic junction should be sutured to decrease the potential for intestinal strangulation. *Place small intestinal loops side by side to form a series of gentle loops from the distal duodenum to the distal ileum. Secure the loops by placing sutures that engage the submucosa, muscularis, and serosa 6 to 10 cm apart (Fig. 16-92). Use 3-0 or 4-0 monofilament absorbable or nonabsorbable sutures with a swaged-on taper point needle. Avoid positioning the intestinal loops at acute angles lest intestinal obstruction occurs.* Entering the lumen with "pexy" sutures may increase the risk of leakage and abdominal contamination.

HEALING OF THE SMALL INTESTINE

Optimal intestinal healing is dependent on a good blood supply, accurate mucosal apposition, and minimal surgical trauma. Approximating suture patterns facilitate rapid healing. Everting and inverting suture patterns retard intestinal healing and may result in greater stricture formation. Healing is facilitated by adjacent serosal surfaces and omentum, which help to seal wounds and contribute to the blood supply. Healing of the intestine is generally rapid but can be delayed by local and systemic factors. Systemic factors such as hypovolemia, shock, hypoproteinemia, debilitation, and concurrent infections may delay healing and increase the risk of incisional breakdown. Tension on the repair caused by accumulated ingesta, fluid, gas, or poor mobilization of the bowel increases the potential for intestinal suture breakdown.

The three overlapping phases of healing are lag, proliferative, and maturation. The lag phase occurs during days 0 to 4 and is associated with inflammation and edema of the healing intestine. A fibrin seal forms during the first few hours. Although the fibrin clot contributes to wound strength, most of the wound strength is attributed to sutures during this phase. Healing is functionally weakest at the end of the lag phase because of fibrinolysis and collagen deposition; thus dehiscence most commonly occurs between 3 and 5 days after intestinal surgery. Everted intestinal anastomoses have reduced tensile and bursting strength during the lag phase of healing and therefore have an increased tendency for leakage. The proliferative phase of healing occurs between days 3 and 14. Fi-

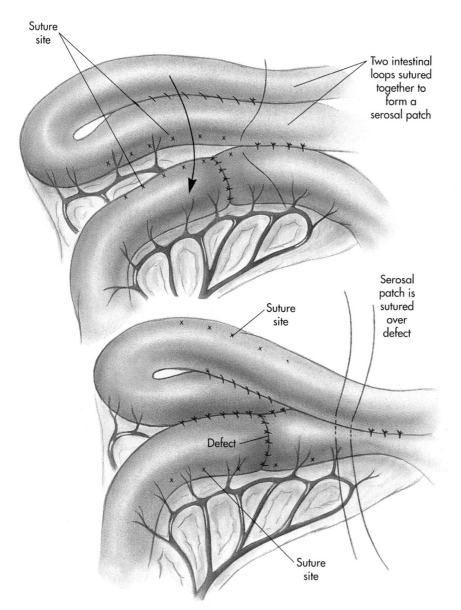

Suture
site

Two intestinal
loops sutured
together to
form a
serosal patch

FIG. 16-91
Create a serosal patch by suturing adjacent intestinal loops together with simple continuous or interrupted sutures. Suture the patch over the defect or suture line.

Serosal
patch is
sutured
over
defect

Suture
site

Defect

Suture
site

brous repair occurs, accompanied by a rapid gain in wound strength. The strength of the repair site approximates that of normal intestine 10 to 17 days after surgery. The maturation phase of healing occurs between 10 to 180 days. Collagen is reorganized and remodeled during this healing phase.

SUTURE MATERIALS/ SPECIAL INSTRUMENTS

Instruments recommended to facilitate intestinal surgery include self-retaining abdominal retractors, malleable retractors, Doyen noncrushing forceps, Babcock forceps, Metzenbaum scissors, No. 11 scalpel blade, Penrose drains, and suction. Although most absorbable sutures can be used, 3-0 or 4-0 monofilament polydioxanone or polyglyconate is preferred. Long-lasting monofilament absorbable (polydioxanone or polyglyconate) or nonabsorbable (nylon or polypropylene) sutures should be selected for patients with low albumin levels. Patching techniques should also be consid-

ered in these patients to reinforce and facilitate healing of the surgical site. Alternatively, surgical stapling equipment (transverse stapling instrument, end-to-end anastomosis stapler, linear stapler, ligate and divide instrument, and skin stapler) can be used for some procedures. Other instruments useful for diagnosis of digestive disorders are Westcott Style Biopsy needles and Bard Biopty-Cut needles (see Product Appendix).

☞ **N O T E** · Do not use catgut or multifilament suture for closing intestinal incisions.

POSTOPERATIVE CARE AND ASSESSMENT

Postoperative care must be individualized to each specific patient and its concurrent problems. The animal should be monitored closely for vomiting during recovery. Analgesics

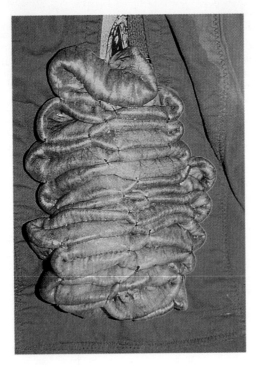

FIG. 16-92
Intraoperative photograph showing the appearance of intestinal loops after intestinal plication.

TABLE 16-50

**Antibiotic Therapy for
Treatment of Postoperative Peritonitis**

Cefazolin (Ancef, Kefzol)
20 mg/kg IV

Cefmetazole (Zefazone)
15 mg/kg IV

Cefoxitin (Mefoxin)
15-30 mg/kg IV

Enrofloxacin (Baytril)
5-10 mg/kg PO or IV, BID

Ampicillin
22 mg/kg IV, IM, SC, or PO, TID to QID

TABLE 16-51

**Common Errors in Treating Animals
with Small Intestinal Disorders**

- Failure to diagnose and treat the condition before ischemia and necrosis occur
- Failure to prevent abdominal contamination
- Failure to prevent intestinal leakage
- Failure to maintain hydration and nutritional homeostasis

(i.e., oxymorphone, butorphanol, or buprenorphine; see Table 16-4) should be provided as needed (see p. 209). Hydration should be maintained with intravenous fluids, and electrolyte and acid-base abnormalities should be monitored and corrected. Small amounts of water may be offered 8 to 12 hours after surgery. If no vomiting occurs, small amounts of food may be offered 12 to 24 hours after surgery. Animals should be fed a bland, low-fat food (e.g., i/d or boiled rice, potatoes and pasta combined with boiled skinless chicken, yogurt, or low-fat cottage cheese) three to four times daily. The normal diet should be reintroduced gradually, beginning 48 to 72 hours after surgery. Debilitated patients may require enteral or parenteral nutrition. Antibiotics should be discontinued within 2 to 6 hours of surgery unless peritonitis is present. Early ambulation and feeding should be encouraged to minimize ileus.

After intestinal surgery, clinical signs (e.g., depression, high fever, excessive abdominal tenderness, vomiting, and/or ileus) and response to abdominal palpation should be monitored for evidence of leakage and subsequent peritonitis or abscess formation. If peritonitis is suspected, an abdominocentesis, chemistry profile, and complete blood cell count (CBC) should be performed. Abdominal fluid should be submitted for culture and sensitivity, and antibiotics (e.g., cefazolin, cefmetazole, cefoxitin, or enrofloxacin and ampicillin; Table 16-50) and fluid therapy should be initiated. Continuation of antibiotics should be based on results of culture and susceptibility testing. The abdomen should be explored if toxic neutrophils with engulfed bacteria or intestinal debris are present. Aggressive treatment of general-

ized peritonitis by open peritoneal drainage may be necessary (see p. 198). The small intestinal dehiscence rate approaches 16%, with 74% of those patients dying (Allen, Smeak, Schertel, 1992).

COMPLICATIONS

Shock, leakage, ileus, dehiscence, perforation, peritonitis, stenosis, short bowel syndrome, recurrence, and death are potential complications of intestinal surgery (Table 16-51). Hypoalbuminemic dogs have the same complication rate following intestinal surgery as dogs with normal plasma albumin levels. Clinically significant strictures are rare unless inverting or everting suture patterns are used or excessive tension exists at the resection site. Short-bowel syndrome may occur if large segments of intestine (more than 70% to 80%) must be resected. Weight loss, diarrhea, and malnutrition are the predominate clinical signs. Treatment is based on the severity of clinical signs and must be planned individually and modified as needed. The goal of treatment is to provide nutritional support until intestinal adaptation occurs (1 to 2 months) and diarrhea is controlled. Acute signs should be treated by correcting hydration and electrolyte imbalances, providing adequate nutrition (an enteral elemental diet or total parenteral nutrition may be necessary), and controlling diarrhea. A highly digestible diet (e.g., i/d or k/d) should be fed several times daily when oral feeding begins. Daily vitamin-mineral supplements should be given. Opiate

TABLE 16-52

Treatment of Short-Bowel Syndrome

Loperamide (Imodium)
Dogs
0.1-0.2 mg/kg PO, BID to TID

Cats
0.08-0.16 mg/kg PO, BID

Cimetidine (Tagamet)
5-10 mg/kg PO, IV, SC, TID to QID

Ranitidine (Zantac)
2 mg/kg PO, IV, IM, or SC, BID

Famotidine (Pepcid)
0.5 mg/kg PO, SID to BID

antidiarrheals (e.g., loperamide; Table 16-52) and H_2 antagonists (cimetidine, ranitidine, or famotidine) may be useful in decreasing gastric hypersecretion, which causes diarrhea and damages duodenal mucosa. Intestinal bacterial overgrowth should be controlled with antibiotics (e.g., tetracycline). Surgical attempts to control short-bowel syndrome should be used only when medical and dietary therapy fail. The prognosis depends on the extent and site of resection, degree of intestinal adaptation, preoperative condition, and postoperative care. Preservation of the ileocolic valve helps prevent bacterial overgrowth and prolongs intestinal transit time. The remaining intestine should be allowed 1 to 2 months to adapt.

SPECIAL AGE CONSIDERATIONS

Young animals more frequently have gastrointestinal parasite infestations or garbage- or foreign body-induced gastroenteritis and intussusceptions. Young animals can quickly become hypothermic and hypoglycemic during surgery and require special care. Healing may be delayed in old animals because of concurrent problems.

References

Allen DA, Smeak DD, Schertel ER: Prevalence of small intestinal dehiscence and associated clinical factors: a retrospective study of 121 dogs, *J Am Anim Hosp Assoc* 28:70, 1992.

DeNobile J, Guzzetta P, Patterson K: Pulse oximetry as a means of assessing bowel viability, *J Surg Res* 48:21, 1990.

Tadros T, Wobbes T, Hendriks T: Blood transfusion impairs the healing of experimental intestinal anastomoses, *Ann Surg* 215:276, 1992.

Wheaton LG et al: A comparison of three techniques for intraoperative prediction of small intestinal injury, *J Am Anim Hosp Assoc* 19:897, 1983.

Suggested Reading

Bellah JR, Bell G: Serum amylase and lipase activities after exploratory laparotomy in dogs, *Am J Vet Res* 50:1638, 1989.

Crowe DT: The serosal patch: clinical use in 12 animals, *Vet Surg* 13:29, 1984.

Ferrara JJ et al: Surface oximetry: a new method to evaluate intestinal perfusion, *Amer Surg* 54:10, 1988.

Harvey HJ: Complications of small intestinal biopsy in hypoalbuminemic dogs, *Vet Surg* 19:289, 1990.

Penninck DG et al: The technique of percutaneous ultrasound-guided fine-needle aspiration biopsy and automated microcore biopsy in small animal gastrointestinal disease, *Vet Radiol Ultrasound* 34:433, 1993.

Penninck DG et al: Ultrasonography of the normal canine gastrointestinal tract, *Vet Radiol* 30:272, 1989.

Penninck DG et al: Ultrasonographic evaluation of gastrointestinal diseases in small animals, *Vet Radiol* 31:134, 1990.

Ritchey ML, Lally KP, Ostericher R: Comparison of different techniques of stapled bowel anastomosis in a canine model, *Arch Surg* 128:1365, 1993.

Thompson JS, Bragg LE, West WW: Serum enzyme levels during intestinal ischemia, *Ann Surg* 211:369, 1990.

Ullman SL, Pavletic MM, Clark GN: Open intestinal anastomosis with surgical stapling equipment in 24 dogs and cats, *Vet Surg* 20:385, 1991.

United States Surgical Corporation: *Stapling techniques: general surgery with Auto Suture instruments,* ed 3, Norwalk, Conn, 1988, United States Surgical Corporation.

Yanoff SR et al: Short-bowel syndrome in four dogs, *Vet Surg* 21:217, 1992.

SPECIFIC DISEASES

INTESTINAL FOREIGN BODIES

DEFINITIONS

Intestinal foreign bodies are ingested objects that may cause complete or partial intraluminal obstruction.

SYNONYMS

Foreign object

GENERAL CONSIDERATIONS AND CLINICALLY RELEVANT PATHOPHYSIOLOGY

The oropharyngeal opening is larger than any other orifice in the gastrointestinal tract. Foreign bodies that traverse the esophagus and stomach may become lodged in the smaller diameter intestine. Bones, balls, toys, rocks, corncobs, cloth, metal objects (e.g., fishhooks, needles), peach pits, acorns, pecans, and linear objects (i.e., string or thread) are common intestinal foreign bodies. Some foreign bodies continue to move slowly through the intestine, while others become lodged in an intestinal segment where they cause complete or partial obstruction.

Partial or incomplete obstructions allow limited passage of fluid or gas, whereas complete obstructions do not allow fluid or gas to advance past the obstruction (Fig. 16-93). The clinical course and signs are more severe in animals with complete intraluminal obstructions, particularly

FIG. 16-93
Pathophysiologic events occurring with mechanical obstruction of the intestinal lumen.

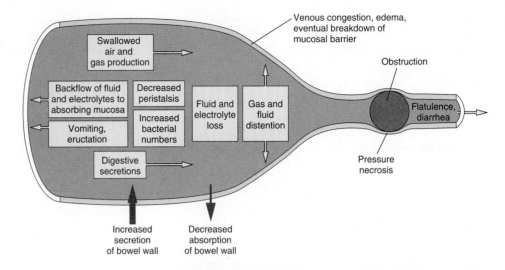

Venous congestion, edema, eventual breakdown of mucosal barrier

Obstruction

Swallowed air and gas production

Backflow of fluid and electrolytes to absorbing mucosa

Decreased peristalsis

Vomiting, eructation

Increased bacterial numbers

Fluid and electrolyte loss

Gas and fluid distention

Flatulence, diarrhea

Digestive secretions

Pressure necrosis

Increased secretion of bowel wall

Decreased absorption of bowel wall

"higher" obstructions, than in those with partial obstructions. With complete intraluminal obstruction, the intestine oral to the lesion distends with gas and fluid. Fluid accumulation is caused by both retention of fluid in the intestinal lumen and secretion of fluid by intestinal glands. During obstruction, secretion increases and absorption decreases (secretions are normally reabsorbed in the lower jejunum and ileum). Gas accumulating in the intestine proximal to the obstruction consists of swallowed air, and gas formed in the lumen by fermentation. Intraluminal pressure proximal to the obstruction gradually increases because of the accumulation of fluid and gas. Lymphatic and capillary stasis occurs when intraluminal pressures reach 30 mm Hg (normal is 2 to 4 mm Hg with peristaltic pressures of 15 to 25 mm Hg); venous drainage is prevented when pressures reach 50 mm Hg. The arterial supply is not affected, and hydrostatic pressure increases at the capillary bed producing a net shift of fluid into the interstitium and causing intestinal wall edema. Eventually fluid shifts not only into the lumen, but from the serosa into the peritoneal cavity. Circulation in the mucosa and submucosa is impaired, oxygen consumption decreases, arteriovenous shunting occurs, and the mucosa becomes ischemic. Full-thickness wall necrosis may occur at the obstruction site. Small intestinal stasis leads to luminal bacterial overgrowth. If the normal mucosal barrier is impaired by distension and ischemia, there is potential for increased permeability with bacterial migration and absorption of toxins into the systemic circulation and/or peritoneal cavity.

More proximal and complete obstructions cause more acute and severe signs, with increased likelihood of dehydration, electrolyte imbalance, and shock. Proximal or high obstructions (i.e., duodenum or proximal jejunum) cause persistent vomiting, loss of gastric secretions, electrolyte imbalances, and dehydration. The major cause of mortality from upper small intestinal obstruction is severe, rapid hypovolemia. Untreated dogs with high, complete obstructions usually die within 3 to 4 days. Distal or low obstructions (i.e., distal jejunum, ileum, or ileocecal junction) cause varying degrees of metabolic acidosis. Clinical signs of dis-

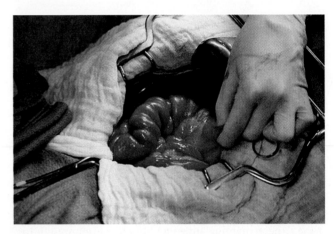

FIG. 16-94
Intraoperative appearance of bunched intestines secondary to a towel "string" foreign body.

tal and incomplete obstructions may be insidious, with vague, intermittent anorexia, lethargy, and occasional vomiting spanning several days or weeks. These animals usually lose weight, but may live for more than 3 weeks if water is available.

Linear foreign bodies cause similar signs. A number of objects can assume a linear configuration, including string, thread, nylon stockings, cloth, and sacks. Part of the object lodges (usually at the base of the tongue or pylorus), while the remainder advances into the intestine. As peristaltic waves attempt to advance the object, the intestine gathers around it causing partial or complete obstruction (Fig. 16-94). Continued peristalsis may cause the object to become taut, cut into the mucosa, and then lacerate the mesenteric border of the intestine. Multiple perforations may occur. Such perforation causing peritonitis is associated with high mortality.

☞ **N O T E** • Linear foreign bodies usually perforate the mesenteric border of the small intestine.

DIAGNOSIS
Clinical Presentation

Signalment. There is no breed or sex predisposition; however, cats more commonly ingest linear foreign bodies than dogs. Most cats with linear foreign bodies are less than 4 years old. Other types of foreign bodies are more commonly found in dogs. Playful young animals seem more prone to foreign body ingestion.

History. Presentation and clinical signs depend on the location, completeness, and duration of the obstruction, and the vascular integrity of the involved segment. Acute onset of vomiting, anorexia, and depression are the most common presenting complaints. Diarrhea and abdominal pain are sometimes noted. Occasionally, the animal has been observed swallowing the object.

Physical Examination Findings

Physical examination may reveal abdominal distention, diarrhea, abdominal pain, abnormal posture, and/or shock. Animals with high obstructions may be severely dehydrated; those with low obstructions may be thin as a result of severe weight loss. Abdominal palpation may identify an abnormal intestinal mass with gas- and fluid-filled loops of intestine proximal to the mass. Linear foreign bodies may sometimes be visualized around the base of the tongue. Abdominal pain is common if linear foreign bodies have caused bunching of intestines.

Radiography/Ultrasonography/Endoscopy

Radiography will often diagnose complete or near complete obstructions and may identify the cause. Obstructed intestinal loops become distended with air, fluid, and/or ingesta (Figs. 16-95 and 16-96). "Stacking" of distended intestines and sharp bends or turns in the dilated intestine suggest anatomic ileus. Linear foreign bodies cause the intestines to appear bunched or pleated together with small gas bubbles in the lumen and without gas-distended intestinal loops (Fig. 16-97). Contrast studies may be necessary to differentiate anatomic from physiologic ileus. Contrast may delineate the foreign body, reveal luminal filling defects, or demonstrate delayed transit time or displacement of intestinal loops. Ultrasonography may identify foreign objects with a hyperechoic margin plus or minus fluid accumulation. It also allows motility to be assessed. Many intestinal foreign bodies are not identified endoscopically because the scope can seldom be advanced beyond the descending duodenum. However, linear foreign bodies lodged at the pylorus that prevent scope passage into the duodenum may be recognized.

☞ **N O T E** · Radiographs of animals with gastrointestinal foreign bodies should be repeated immediately before surgery to ensure that the foreign body is still located in the stomach or small intestine. Most foreign bodies that enter the large intestine will be eliminated in the feces.

Laboratory Findings

Fluid, electrolyte, and acid-base abnormalities are often identified on complete blood counts and biochemistry profiles. Leukocytosis with a left shift or degenerative leukopenia accompanied by septic abdominal effusion indicates intestinal ischemia or perforation with peritonitis.

DIFFERENTIAL DIAGNOSIS

The differential diagnosis includes all other causes of intestinal obstruction: intussusception, intestinal volvulus/torsion, intestinal incarceration, adhesions, strictures, abscesses, granuloma, hematoma, neoplasia, or congenital malformations. Other causes might include physiologic ileus secondary to inflammation (e.g., parvovirus or peritonitis).

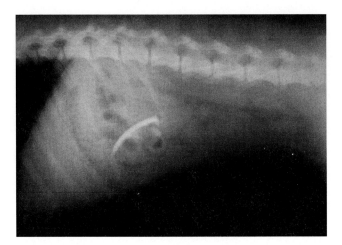

FIG. 16-95
Lateral abdominal radiograph of a 3-year-old, female Labrador retriever. Note the radiopaque foreign body in the proximal small intestine. The multiple, well-circumscribed, soft tissue masses visible throughout the caudal abdomen are fetuses within the uterus. One-fourth of a tennis ball was removed from the proximal duodenum.

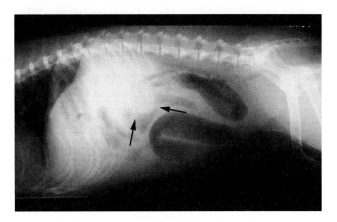

FIG. 16-96
Lateral abdominal radiograph of a dog with segmental ileus. Note the gas and fluid accumulation and the midabdominal, 2.5-cm circular, radiopaque foreign body (*arrows*). A hazelnut was removed from the jejunum.

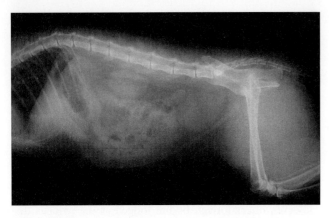

FIG. 16-97
Lateral abdominal radiograph of a 6-month-old cat that had been vomiting for 2 days. Note bunching of the small intestine and numerous circular intestinal opacifications containing small air bubbles. A string foreign body was surgically removed.

MEDICAL MANAGEMENT

Some foreign bodies pass through the intestine without requiring therapy. Foreign body advancement may be monitored radiographically unless vomiting is severe, debilitation occurs, or there is evidence of peritonitis (i.e., abdominal pain, fever, neutrophilia; see also p. 193). Radiographs should always be repeated before surgery (even if they were taken the previous evening) because the foreign body may have moved into the colon or passed in the feces.

SURGICAL TREATMENT

In cases of partial obstruction, failure to radiographically demonstrate foreign body movement within the intestine over an 8-hour period, or failure to pass the object within approximately 36 hours indicates the need for surgery. Surgery should not be delayed to observe for passage of the object through the intestinal tract if abdominal pain, fever, vomiting, or lethargy is apparent. Most foreign bodies can be removed by enterotomy rather than resection and anastomosis unless intestinal necrosis or perforation is present. If a linear object has been present a long time, it may become embedded in the mucosa, necessitating intestinal resection. Multiple enterotomies (two to four) are often necessary to remove linear foreign bodies. Iatrogenic laceration of the mesenteric border may occur if excessive tension causes the object to saw through the wall before or during extraction.

☞ **N O T E ·** Foreign body removal is one of the most common indications for gastric and intestinal surgery.

Preoperative Management

Fluid, electrolyte, and acid-base deficits should be corrected before surgery if possible. Prophylactic antibiotics should be administered according to the recommendations on p. 294.

Anesthesia

Anesthetic recommendations for animals undergoing intestinal surgery are provided on p. 293. Nitrous oxide should be avoided in animals with obstructions to prevent further gas accumulation in the intestinal tract.

Surgical Anatomy

Surgical anatomy of the small intestine is described on p. 294.

Positioning

The patient should be positioned in dorsal recumbency for a ventral midline celiotomy. The surgically prepared area should extend from mid-thorax to perineum.

SURGICAL TECHNIQUE

Make an incision through the linea alba that is sufficient to allow complete exploration of the abdomen. Explore the entire abdomen and gastrointestinal tract to avoid overlooking concurrent abnormalities or multiple foreign bodies. Once the foreign body has been located, isolate this loop of intestine from the remainder of the abdominal cavity with laparotomy pads or sterile towels. Complete obstructions may cause the bowel to be severely distended and appear cyanotic; however, reserve determination of intestinal viability until the bowel has been decompressed and the foreign body has been removed by enterotomy. Bathe the intestine in warm saline for a few minutes to help improve its color and peristalsis. Normally the appearance of the intestine improves rapidly after decompression. If the intestinal segment is determined to be viable, close the enterotomy with simple interrupted sutures as described on p. 297. Resect nonviable or questionable intestine and reestablish bowel continuity by end-to-end anastomosis (see p. 297). After foreign body removal carefully examine the intestine for evidence of perforation that might necessitate resection of the involved segment(s).

A single-enterotomy catheter technique has been described to remove linear foreign bodies (Anderson and Lippincott, 1992). *Make an incision into the stomach or intestine at the site at which the object is fixed. Suture the linear object to a soft catheter, then completely advance the catheter into the distal intestine. Close the enterotomy site and milk the catheter and foreign body through the intestinal tract and out through the anus.* This technique limits the number of enterotomies and may thereby reduce the risk of leakage and dehiscence.

SUTURE MATERIALS/ SPECIAL INSTRUMENTS

Instruments for enterotomy or intestinal resection and anastomosis are discussed on p. 303. Polydioxanone or polyglyconate (3-0 or 4-0) are preferred sutures for these procedures; however, nonabsorbable (nylon or polypropylene) sutures are sometimes used in hypoalbuminemic animals.

POSTOPERATIVE CARE AND ASSESSMENT

Postoperative treatment includes further correction of fluid, electrolyte, and acid-base deficits. Analgesics should be given as needed to control pain (see Table 16-4). Antibiotics should be continued if peritonitis was diagnosed or if gross abdominal contamination occurred. If no vomiting has occurred, water can be offered 8 to 12 hours, and food, 12 to 24 hours after surgery. These animals should be monitored for signs of leakage and peritonitis (see p. 193).

COMPLICATIONS

Early diagnosis of intestinal foreign bodies and good surgical technique are necessary to avoid complications (e.g., intestinal necrosis, perforation, leakage, dehiscence, peritonitis, endotoxic shock, and stenosis). The risk of peritonitis and death is much higher if free gas is present on preoperative radiographs. Resecting large segments of intestine may result in a patient with short-bowel syndrome (see p. 304) and a guarded prognosis.

PROGNOSIS

The prognosis is good if peritonitis and extensive resections are avoided. The prognosis without surgery is guarded because animals may die from hypovolemic or endotoxic shock, septicemia, peritonitis, or starvation.

Reference

Anderson S, Lippincott CL: Single enterotomy removal of gastrointestinal linear foreign bodies, *J Am Anim Hosp Assoc* 28:487, 1992.

Suggested Reading

Basher AWP, Fowler JD: Conservative versus surgical management of gastrointestinal linear foreign bodies in the cat, *Vet Surg* 16:138, 1987.

Evans KL, Smeak DD, Biller DS: Gastrointestinal linear foreign bodies in 32 dogs: a retrospective evaluation and feline comparison, *J Am Anim Hosp Assoc,* 30:445, 1994.

Felts JF, Fox PR, Burk RL: Thread and sewing needles as gastrointestinal foreign bodies in the cat: a review of 64 cases, *J Am Vet Med Assoc* 184:56, 1984.

Muir P, Rosin E: Failure of the single enterotomy technique to remove a linear intestinal foreign object in a cat, *Vet Rec* 136:75, 1995.

INTESTINAL NEOPLASIA

DEFINITIONS

Intestinal neoplasia includes those tumors that arise from one of the layers of the intestinal wall, its glands, or associated cells or lymphatics.

GENERAL CONSIDERATIONS AND CLINICALLY RELEVANT PATHOPHYSIOLOGY

Intestinal tumors occur most commonly in the canine rectum and colon and the feline small intestine. Most intestinal tumors are malignant. Intestinal tumors may cause intramural or intraluminal mechanical obstruction. They most commonly invade the muscular layer of the intestinal wall, where they compromise the lumen diameter and reduce distensibility. The proximal bowel distends with fluid and gas, and its function is compromised as with foreign body obstructions. At the time of diagnosis the disease is usually advanced, and most malignant tumors have metastasized. Malignant tumors spread by local invasion (e.g., serosa, mesentery, omentum, local lymph nodes) and distant metastasis (i.e., lung, liver, spleen). The most common small intestinal malignancies are adenocarcinoma (Fig. 16-98) and lymphosarcoma. Other small intestinal neoplasms include leiomyoma, leiomyosarcoma, fibrosarcoma, mast cell tumor, hemangiosarcoma, anaplastic sarcoma, carcinoids, plasmacytoma, neurolemmoma, adenomas, and adenomatous polyp.

Adenocarcinomas are locally invasive and slow growing. They most commonly arise in the duodenum and colon in dogs and distal jejunum and ileum in cats. There are three morphologic forms: (1) infiltrative adenocarcinomas cause a thickened stenotic area that obstructs the intestinal lumen; (2) ulcerative adenocarcinomas have a deep indurated mucosal ulcer with raised edges; and (3) proliferative adenocarcinomas are lobulated, expanding intraluminal masses. Mucosal ulceration may cause melena and iron-deficiency anemia. These tumors spread to adjacent serosal surfaces, mesentery, omentum, and regional lymph nodes by local invasion and may metastasize distally (i.e., lung, liver).

Lymphosarcoma (lymphoma) is a neoplastic proliferation of lymphocytes. In cats it may be caused by feline leukemia virus (FeLV) or feline immunodeficiency virus (FIV). In dogs the etiology is unknown. Affected animals may have multicentric disease. There are two intestinal types of lymphoma: diffuse and nodular. Diffuse infiltration of the lamina propria and submucosa with neoplastic lymphocytes

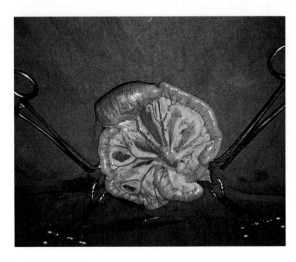

FIG. 16-98
Intraoperative photograph of an adenocarcinoma that was partially obstructing the jejunum of a 15-year-old cat.

causes malabsorption and occasional deep ulceration. Nodular lymphoma is an expanding intestinal mass causing obstruction that occurs most often in the ileocecocolic area. Involvement of regional lymph nodes and other organs is common.

☞ **N O T E ·** Assess FeLV/FIV status in cats with intestinal neoplasia.

Adenomatous polyps are found in the feline duodenum and canine rectum. Recurrence after complete resection is not expected. Intestinal leiomyosarcomas are malignant smooth-muscle tumors of older dogs and most commonly occur in the cecum and jejunum. Neoplastic spread is by local invasion, and metastasis is slow to occur. Survival of approximately 12 months is expected after resection of a localized lesion.

DIAGNOSIS
Clinical Presentation

Signalment. Adenocarcinoma is more common in dogs than in cats. In dogs adenocarcinoma is the most common intestinal tumor, and leiomyosarcoma is the most common sarcoma. Boxers, collies, and German shepherds may be predisposed to intestinal tumors. In cats lymphosarcoma is most common, followed by adenocarcinoma and mast cell tumor. Siamese cats may be predisposed to small intestinal adenocarcinomas. Intestinal tumors generally occur in older animals. Carcinomas are seen at a mean age of 9 years in dogs and 10 years in cats. Leiomyosarcomas occur at a mean age of 11 years in dogs. Lymphosarcoma occurs in dogs and cats at a mean age of 10.6 years. The mean age for cats with intestinal mast cell tumors is 13 years.

History. Patients initially have vague clinical signs of depression, anorexia, and lethargy, which may progress to diarrhea and/or vomiting. Weight loss is progressive. Other clinical signs may include dehydration, melena, hematemesis, anemia, fever, icterus, and/or abdominal effusion. Signs of intestinal obstruction, abscessation, and malabsorption may also occur. Lymphatic obstruction may cause steatorrhea from lymphangiectasia. Signs involving other organs may develop secondary to metastasis.

Physical Examination Findings

The animal may be in poor body condition. Abdominal palpation may reveal a firm abdominal mass, thickened intestinal loops, or mesenteric lymphadenopathy.

Radiography/Ultrasonography/Endoscopy

Radiographs should be taken of the thorax and abdomen if neoplasia is suspected. Masses, abnormal gas/fluid patterns, visceral displacement, and abdominal fluid may be seen on plain films. Contrast radiographs are helpful for delineating regions of mucosal irregularity, luminal narrowing, intramural infiltration, thickening, or nodularity. Abdominal ul-

trasonography often delineates the mass and may facilitate percutaneous biopsy. Intestinal tumors produce a broad spectrum of ultrasonic patterns. Ultrasonographic findings may include intestinal wall thickening and loss of discrete wall layers, but the intestine may also appear normal. Ileus, fluid accumulation, and lymphadenopathy may be recognized. Mucosal irregularity, inflammation, ulceration, and a narrowed lumen may be identified during endoscopy. Mucosal biopsies can be diagnostic if the tumor involves the mucosa.

Laboratory Findings

Hematologic and biochemical profiles are often normal. Laboratory evaluation may reveal blood-loss anemia, neutrophilic leukocytosis with left shift, hypoalbuminemia, or elevated serum hepatic enzyme concentrations. A definitive diagnosis of intestinal neoplasia can only be made on histologic examination of tissue.

DIFFERENTIAL DIAGNOSIS

The differential diagnosis includes all other causes of intestinal obstruction (i.e., foreign bodies, intussusception, intestinal volvulus/torsion, adhesions, strictures, abscesses, granuloma, hematoma, or congenital malformation). Other causes might include physiologic ileus secondary to inflammation (parvovirus or peritonitis).

MEDICAL MANAGEMENT

Lymphosarcoma may respond to chemotherapy. (Refer to a medicine text for additional information and chemotherapeutic protocols.) The response of other tumor types to chemotherapy is unknown or poor. Radiation therapy is used primarily for tumors in the distal half of the rectum and anal canal.

SURGICAL TREATMENT

Surgical resection is the treatment of choice for intestinal tumors; however, many tumors are too advanced to allow complete resection by the time they are diagnosed. If metastasis has occurred surgical resection may be palliative.

Preoperative Management

Fluid, electrolyte, and acid-base deficits should be corrected before surgery if possible. Transfusions should be considered if the packed cell volume (PCV) is less than 20%. Prophylactic antibiotics should be given according to recommendations on p. 294. Debilitated animals or those that are likely to remain anorexic or have continued vomiting should have enteral feeding tubes placed at the time of surgery (see p. 79).

Anesthesia

General anesthetic recommendations for animals undergoing intestinal surgery are provided on p. 293. Many tumor patients are debilitated; therefore balanced anesthesia using injectable agents (i.e., opioids) and isoflurane is recommended. Nitrous oxide should be avoided if there is ileus.

Surgical Anatomy

Surgical anatomy of the small intestine is provided on p. 294.

Positioning

Patients should be positioned in dorsal recumbency for a ventral midline celiotomy. The entire abdomen and caudal thorax should be clipped and prepped for aseptic surgery.

SURGICAL TECHNIQUE

Make an incision through the linea alba from the xiphoid process to the pubis to allow complete abdominal exploration. Explore the entire abdomen and gastrointestinal tract to avoid overlooking concurrent abnormalities. Biopsy mesenteric lymph nodes and other organs as needed before incising intestine. Resect the mass with 4- to 8-cm margins of grossly normal tissue and perform an end-to-end anastomosis (see p. 297). Pay special attention to surgical technique because these patients are frequently debilitated. Submit tissues for histopathologic evaluation and tumor staging.

SUTURE MATERIALS/ SPECIAL INSTRUMENTS

Instruments for enterotomy or intestinal resection and anastomosis are discussed on p. 303. Polydioxanone or polyglyconate (3-0 or 4-0) are preferred sutures for these procedures; however, nonabsorbable (nylon or polypropylene) sutures may be used in hypoalbuminemic animals.

POSTOPERATIVE CARE AND ASSESSMENT

Postoperative care should be individualized according to patient status and concurrent diseases. Fluid support should be maintained until the animal is drinking enough to maintain hydration. Electrolyte and acid-base deficits should be corrected. Analgesics should be provided as necessary (see Table 16-4). If peritonitis, abdominal contamination, and/or severe debilitation occur, therapeutic antibiotics should be given. Nutritional support should be provided via enterostomy tube if vomiting or anorexia persists (see p. 79). Adjuvant chemotherapy has been recommended for some malignant intestinal tumors, but efficacy is unproven (see previous page under Medical Management), except for lymphoma.

COMPLICATIONS

Leakage, dehiscence, and peritonitis are potential complications and may occur more frequently in debilitated patients. Stenosis after surgical resection or tumor recurrence may cause recurrent signs of obstruction. Short bowel syndrome (see p. 304) is a potential complication if large portions of the bowel are resected.

PROGNOSIS

The prognosis is excellent when benign tumors or polyps are completely excised. The prognosis is good for patients with localized intestinal adenocarcinoma if complete resection is possible. Cats with intestinal adenocarcinoma may live more than 2 years after surgery. The prognosis for solitary nodular lymphoma is better than for diffuse lymphoma (which carries a poor prognosis). A guarded to poor prognosis should be given if nonresectable tumors are present because other modes of therapy are ineffective, of questionable value, or not advised because of severe side effects. An exception is lymphosarcoma, which may respond well to chemotherapy.

Suggested Reading

Feeney DA, Klausner JS, Johnston GR: Chronic bowel obstruction caused by primary intestinal neoplasia: a report of five cases, *J Am Anim Hosp Assoc* 18:67, 1982.

Groaten AM et al: Ultrasonographic appearance of feline alimentary lymphoma, *Vet Radiol Ultrason* 35:468, 1994.

Kosovsky JE, Matthiesen DT, Patnaik AK: Small intestinal adenocarcinoma in cats: 32 cases (1978–1985), *J Am Vet Med Assoc* 192:233, 1988.

MacDonald JM, Mullen HS, Moroff SD: Adenomatous polyps of the duodenum in cats: 18 cases (1985–1990), *J Am Vet Med Assoc* 202:647, 1993.

Straw RC: Tumors of the intestinal tract. In Withrow SJ, MacEwen EG, editors: *Clinical veterinary oncology*, Philadelphia, 1989, JB Lippincott.

INTUSSUSCEPTION

DEFINITIONS

Intussusception is the telescoping or invagination of one intestinal segment (**intussusceptum**) into the lumen of an adjacent segment (**intussuscipiens**) (Fig. 16-99, *A*).

SYNONYMS

Intestinal telescoping, intestinal invagination

GENERAL CONSIDERATIONS AND CLINICALLY RELEVANT PATHOPHYSIOLOGY

Gastrointestinal tract intussusceptions may occur anywhere; however, ileocolic and jejuno-jejunal intussusceptions are most common. Intussusceptions are frequently associated with enteritis (i.e., parasitism, viral or bacterial infections, dietary indiscretion or change, foreign bodies, and/or masses) or systemic illness; however, the cause of most intussusceptions is unknown. They have also been reported after environmental change and surgery. Intussusceptions after surgery may be associated with ileus, adhesions, or anastomosis malfunction. Intestinal irritation resulting in hypermotility may cause one intestinal loop to invaginate into another. The direction of the intussusception can be from proximal to distal or vice versa. The intussusceptum is more commonly a proximal intestinal segment and the intussuscipiens a more distal segment (i.e., the intussusception occurs in the direction of normal peristalsis). Intussusceptions can occur at multiple sites and are sometimes double (two invaginations at same site). Reverse peristalsis may increase the length of intestine involved in the

FIG. 16-99
A, Configuration of an intussusception: neck, intussusceptum, apex, intussuscipiens. **B,** To reduce an intussusception place traction on the neck as you milk the apex out of the intussuscipiens.

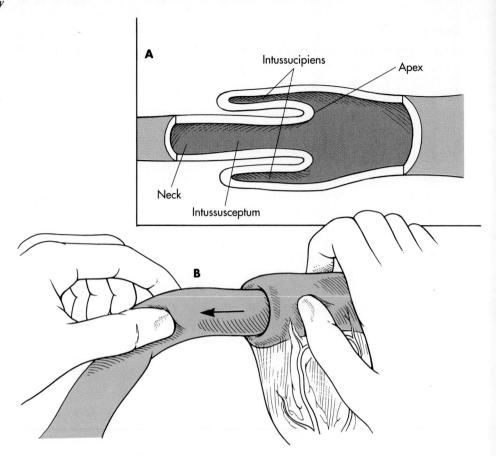

intussusception. The amount of available mesentery limits the extent of intestinal involvement and the degree of vascular compromise.

Initially, invagination produces partial intestinal obstruction, which may progress to complete obstruction. Vessels attached to the intussusceptum collapse because of increased intraluminal pressure or kinking and those vessels may avulse. The wall becomes edematous, ischemic, and turgid. Blood extravasates into the lumen and the serosa fissures. Fibrin seals the layers of the intestine together and may help localize peritonitis as wall necrosis occurs. Eventually, intestinal devitalization occurs with subsequent abdominal cavity contamination. Intussusceptions may occur as agonal events (i.e., are incidental findings and not the cause of death). Agonal intussusceptions are easily reduced and are associated with minimal inflammation; intestinal walls are not edematous and fibrin does not seal the layers of intestine together.

DIAGNOSIS
Clinical Presentation

Signalment. Intussusceptions occur more commonly in dogs. German shepherd dogs and Siamese cats may be more commonly affected than other breeds. Intussusceptions appear to be more common in immature animals (younger than 1 year). Parasitism or enteritis should be suspected as a cause for intussusception in young dogs and intestinal thickening or masses should be suspected in adults.

History. Most animals have been ill, changed environments, or had recent surgery before signs of intussusception begin. The severity and type of clinical signs depend on the location, completeness, vascular integrity, and duration of intestinal obstruction. Scant bloody diarrhea, vomiting, abdominal pain, and a palpable mass may occur with intussusceptions. Acute intussusceptions must be considered in puppies with parvoviral enteritis that suddenly become worse. Chronic cases can have less marked clinical signs. Patients with chronic intussusception often have intractable, intermittent diarrhea, and hypoalbuminemia. Other clinical signs include depression and emaciation. Chronic intussusception is one reason why a puppy with an apparently acute episode of enteritis has persisting diarrhea.

Physical Examination Findings

A presumptive diagnosis of intussusception can be made when an elongated, thickened intestinal loop (sausage-shaped mass) is palpated. Jejuno-jejunal intussusceptions are easier to palpate than ileocolic intussusceptions because they are usually more caudal and ventral in the abdomen. Some intussusceptions slide in and out of the colon and can be missed during palpation. Others may protrude from the rectum and can be mistaken for a rectal prolapse (see Fig. 16-128 on p. 361). To distinguish rectal prolapse from protruding intussusception, the area around the protruding tissue should be palpated. If a fornix exists, rectal prolapse rather than an intussusception is present.

Radiography/Ultrasonography/Endoscopy

Radiographic signs of intestinal obstruction may occur. Intussusceptions causing partial obstruction may be missed on plain radiographs if there is little gas accumulation. Jejunal intussusceptions more often result in obstructive patterns than ileocolic intussusception. A tubular soft tissue mass may be identified. The apex of the intussusception may be outlined if sufficient gas accumulates in the distal intestinal segment. A barium enema or upper gastrointestinal tract study can localize the obstruction. A ribbon of contrast material may be seen in the intussusceptum aboral to a dilated intestinal segment. Occasionally, contrast material accumulates in the lumen between the intussusceptum and intussuscipiens.

Ultrasonography is useful in detecting intussusceptions. The ultrasonographic appearance of an intussusception in the transverse plane is that of a multilayered, targetlike lesion (concentric hyperechoic and hypoechoic rings) with associated proximal fluid accumulation and decreased intestinal motility. Longitudinal scans demonstrate a layered appearance with alternating parallel hyperechoic and hypoechoic lines. Colonoscopy may identify invaginated intestine protruding into the colon in patients with ileocolic or cecocolic intussusception.

Laboratory Findings

Abnormal laboratory findings may include dehydration, stress leukograms, anemia, and electrolyte and acid-base abnormalities. Chronic intussusception may cause hypoalbuminemia because of protein loss from congested mucosa. Fecal examination sometimes reveals parasite infestation.

DIFFERENTIAL DIAGNOSIS

The differential diagnosis includes all other causes of intestinal obstruction (i.e., foreign bodies, intestinal volvulus/torsion, intestinal incarceration, adhesions, strictures, abscesses, granuloma, hematoma, tumors, or congenital malformation). Other causes might include physiologic ileus secondary to inflammation (i.e., parvovirus or peritonitis).

MEDICAL MANAGEMENT

Occasionally, percutaneous manual reduction of the intussusception is successful and the intussusception does not recur. Rarely, intussusceptions self-correct by forming adhesions and sloughing the intussusceptum. However, most intussusceptions require surgical reduction and ancillary procedures to prevent recurrence. Medical therapy should be aimed at correcting fluid and electrolyte imbalances and determining the underlying cause of the intussusception (i.e., enteritis, parasitism).

SURGICAL TREATMENT

Because recurrence is common, intussusceptions should be treated surgically even if they can be manually reduced. Biopsying the intestine at the time of surgical correction may help identify the cause of the intussusception. The tip of the intussusceptum should be evaluated for masses.

Preoperative Management

Hydration, electrolyte, and acid-base deficits should be corrected before surgery if possible. Pediatric patients should not be fasted for more than 4 to 8 hours in order to reduce the likelihood of hypoglycemia. Prophylactic antibiotics should be given according to the recommendations on p. 294.

Anesthesia

General anesthetic recommendations for animals undergoing intestinal surgery are provided on p. 293. Nitrous oxide should be avoided if ileus is present. Care must be used to prevent hypothermia, especially in pediatric patients. Blood glucose concentrations should be monitored during and after surgery in young patients.

Surgical Anatomy

Surgical anatomy of the small intestine is provided on p. 294.

Positioning

Animals should be positioned in dorsal recumbency for a ventral midline celiotomy. The entire abdomen and caudal thorax should be clipped and prepared for aseptic surgery.

SURGICAL TECHNIQUE

*Explore the abdomen, collect specimens, and isolate the involved intestine with laparotomy pads. Reduce intussusceptions manually if possible by gently applying traction on the neck of the intussusceptum while milking its apex (leading edge) out of the intussuscipiens (Fig. 16-99, B). Avoid excessive traction because this may tear the compromised intestine. Manual reduction is successful only if fibrin has not formed firm serosal adhesions. Evaluate the reduced intestine for viability and perforation. Carefully palpate the leading edge of the intussusceptum to detect mass lesions. Perform a resection and anastomosis if manual reduction is impossible, tissue is devitalized, or mesenteric vessels have been avulsed from a portion of the involved intestine. Submit biopsies of the involved intestine to identify the cause of the intussusception. **Perform an enteroenteropexy** (see p. 302) **to prevent recurrence.***

SUTURE MATERIALS/ SPECIAL INSTRUMENTS

Instruments for enterotomy or intestinal resection and anastomosis are discussed on p. 303. Polydioxanone or polyglyconate (3-0 or 4-0) are preferred sutures for these procedures; however, nonabsorbable (nylon or polypropylene) sutures may be used in hypoalbuminemic animals. Chromic gut suture should be avoided in young animals and in those that are debilitated because the suture may be rapidly catabolized and weakened.

POSTOPERATIVE CARE AND ASSESSMENT

Postoperative management should be individualized according to patient's status and concurrent diseases. Hydration, electrolyte, and acid-base abnormalities should continue to be corrected postoperatively until the animal resumes adequate oral intake. Analgesics should be provided according to the recommendations in Chapter 12. Therapeutic antibiotics are appropriate if peritonitis, abdominal contamination, or severe debilitation is present. Nutritional support via an enterostomy tube (see p. 79) may be necessary if the patient is debilitated, vomiting, or remains anorexic.

PROGNOSIS

The patient's prognosis depends on the cause, location, completeness, and duration of the intussusception. Animals with intestinal intussusceptions may die within 3 to 4 days or live for several weeks. Those who die acutely usually have high obstructions or enterotoxemia; death is due to hypovolemia, and electrolyte and acid-base imbalances. Animals with an intussusception may live for several weeks if obstruction is partial or distal, vasculature is functional, and adequate fluid intake is maintained. Rarely, an animal will self-cure if the neck of the intussusception seals, a firm adhesion forms to the intussuscipiens, and the intussusceptum sloughs, reestablishing luminal patency. The prognosis with surgery is good if recurrence is prevented and extensive resections are avoided. Recurrence is expected in 20% to 30% of affected animals without enteropexy (Oakes et al, 1994). Leakage, dehiscence, peritonitis, and death are potential complications that occur more frequently in debilitated patients. Stenosis and short-bowel syndrome may occur if large segments of the bowel are removed (see p. 304).

Reference

Oakes MG et al: Enteroplication for the prevention of recurrent intussusceptions in dogs, *J Am Vet Med Assoc* 205:72, 1994.

Suggested Reading

Bellinger CR, Beck JA: Intussusception in 12 cats, *J Small Anim Pract* 35:295, 1994.

Lewis DD, Ellison GW: Intussusception in dogs and cats, *Compend Contin Educ Pract Vet* 9:523, 1987.

Watson DE, Mahaffey MB, Neuwirth LA: Ultrasonographic detection of duodenojejunal intussusception in a dog, *J Am Anim Hosp Assoc* 27:367, 1991.

INFECTIOUS AND INFLAMMATORY CONDITIONS

DEFINITIONS

Enteritis is inflammation of the intestine. Organisms or syndromes causing chronic enteritis may produce obstruction, diarrhea, and/or vomiting.

GENERAL CONSIDERATIONS AND CLINICALLY RELEVANT PATHOPHYSIOLOGY

Lymphocytic-plasmacytic enteritis, eosinophilic gastroenterocolitis, granulomatous enteritis, intestinal lymphangiectasia, intestinal bacteria overgrowth, and fungal infections such as *Histoplasma capsulatum*, *Pythium* spp., and other saprophytes are potential causes of infectious and inflammatory conditions of the intestines. Biopsy of the intestine may be required to diagnose and differentiate them from noninflammatory diseases (i.e., hyperthyroidism, giardiasis, lymphosarcoma, adenocarcinoma, exocrine pancreatic insufficiency, functional intestinal disorders, and feline infectious peritonitis with gastrointestinal involvement). One of the more common inflammatory lesions of the intestine requiring surgery for diagnosis and treatment is pythiosis (phycomycosis). *Pythium* spp. are ubiquitous, being found in water, soil, vegetable matter, and feces. *Pythium* is an aquatic organism to which animals in contact with swamp water are commonly exposed. High water temperatures may enhance *Pythium* growth and asexual reproduction (motile, biflagellated zoospores), predisposing to infection during the summer and fall months. *Pythium* lesions are slow growing and commonly involve the stomach, small and large intestine, rectum, mesentery, skin, and mesenteric lymph nodes. *Pythium* may invade traumatized (devitalized, necrotic, or ulcerated) tissue, but the motile spores may also penetrate intact mucosa. Fungal hyphae invade the intestinal wall causing infarction, necrosis, and a granulomatous tissue reaction. The intestinal wall thickens and signs of partial intestinal obstruction or malabsorption occur. Invasion by extension occurs along blood vessels, nerves, lymphatics, and fascial planes to other areas and organs. Invasion into blood vessels causes thrombosis and visceral infarction.

DIAGNOSIS
Clinical Presentation

Signalment. Pythiosis most commonly occurs in large-breed male dogs living in the southern Gulf states. The disease is rare in cats, but may cause ulcerative gastroenteritis. Young dogs (1 to 3 years) are most frequently affected.

History. Diarrhea and weight loss are the most common complaints. Clinical signs include diarrhea, vomiting, anorexia, depression, and/or progressive weight loss. Intestinal ulceration and necrosis may cause bloody diarrhea.

Physical Examination Findings

Affected animals are frequently thin. An abdominal mass or marked regional intestinal thickening may be detected on abdominal palpation or rectal examination.

Radiography/Ultrasonography/Endoscopy

An abdominal mass, thickened intestine, and/or signs of partial obstruction may be visualized on plain radiographs; however, severe weight reduction and loss of abdominal fat may cause poor abdominal contrast. Contrast radiography may delineate thickened, stenotic areas. Intestinal thickening and abnormal wall layering are common on ultrasonography. Ultrasonography or fluoroscopy may show a lack of motility in the involved segment. A narrowed, nondistensible gastric or intestinal lumen, with or without ulceration, may be visualized on endoscopy. Rigid endoscopic biopsies are more likely to be diagnostic than flexible endoscopic mucosal biopsies because the latter typically samples mucosa but not the fibrous submucosa, where hyphae are found.

Laboratory Findings

A complete blood count may reveal mild to moderate nonregenerative anemia and mild neutrophilia, with or without a left shift. Definitive diagnosis depends on identification of broad-branching, nonseptate or sparsely septate hyphae in tissues (Fig. 16-100). Hyphae are most easily found within necrotic granulomas of the submucosa and muscularis. Biopsies of enlarged mesenteric lymph nodes generally reveal granulomatous inflammation. Culture of the intestinal lesion should be performed to more specifically identify the fungal organism.

DIFFERENTIAL DIAGNOSIS

Pythiosis must be differentiated from other causes of partial intestinal obstruction, especially intussusception. Other differentials include neoplasia, other fungal lesions, and regional enteritis. Pythiosis may cause lesions similar to perianal fistulae.

MEDICAL MANAGEMENT

Antifungal agents have not proven efficacious; therefore, radical surgical excision is required for potential cure. However, the extensive nature of many of the lesions limits complete resection.

SURGICAL TREATMENT
Preoperative Management

Fluid, electrolyte, and acid-base abnormalities should be corrected before surgery. Prophylactic antibiotics should be given based on recommendations provided on p. 294.

Anesthesia

General anesthetic recommendations are provided on p. 293. The majority of affected animals are debilitated;

therefore, balanced anesthesia using injectable agents (i.e., opioids) and isoflurane is recommended. Nitrous oxide should be avoided if ileus is present.

Surgical Anatomy

Surgical anatomy of the small intestine is discussed on p. 294.

Positioning

The animal should be positioned in dorsal recumbency for exploratory celiotomy. The ventral abdomen and caudal thorax should be clipped and prepped for aseptic surgery.

SURGICAL TECHNIQUE

Expose the abdomen from the xiphoid process to the pubis. Explore the abdomen; the intestinal lesion may be extensive or multicentric, and mesenteric lymph nodes are generally enlarged. Intestinal lesions are firm, granulomatous masses with mural thickening (Fig. 16-101). Biopsy lymph nodes and any other abnormal tissues. Resect the entire intestinal lesion with 4 to 8 cm of grossly normal intestine surrounding it because fungal hyphae have been found to extend several centimeters into normal appearing tissue. Reappose intestinal ends with an end-to-end anastomosis (see p. 297).

SUTURE MATERIALS/ SPECIAL INSTRUMENTS

Instruments for enterotomy or intestinal resection and anastomosis are discussed on p. 303. Polydioxanone or polyglyconate (3-0 or 4-0) are preferred sutures for these procedures. Nonabsorbable (i.e., nylon or polypropylene) sutures should generally be avoided in infected sites. Chromic gut suture should be avoided in infection, young animals, and those that are debilitated.

POSTOPERATIVE CARE AND ASSESSMENT

Fluid, electrolyte, and acid-base abnormalities should be monitored and corrected after surgery. Analgesics should be

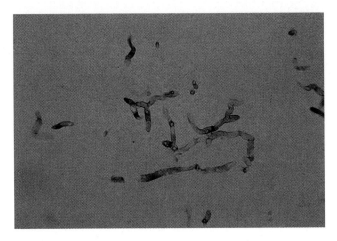

FIG. 16-100
Photomicrograph of *Pythium* hyphae that are broad-branching, nonseptate, or sparsely septate.

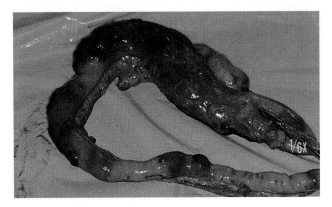

FIG. 16-101
Multiple small, firm masses causing partial intestinal obstruction associated with pythiosis in a dog.

provided as needed (see Table 16-4). Therapeutic antibiotics should be given if the animal has evidence of peritonitis, if abdominal contamination occurs during surgery, or if severe debilitation is present. Nutritional support via an enteral feeding tube or parenteral hyperalimentation may be necessary postoperatively if the patient is debilitated or unlikely to eat (see Chapter 11). Adjuvant antifungal therapy (e.g., itraconazole) has been recommended, but its efficacy is uncertain. Vaccines made from fungal cultures have been used as adjuvant therapy in horses. Leakage, dehiscence, peritonitis, stenosis, and short-bowel syndrome are potential complications of surgery. Signs of pythiosis may recur if tissue margins are not free of fungal hyphae.

PROGNOSIS

The prognosis with complete resection is fair to good. Some dogs will have recurrence and others will be clinically normal without adjuvant therapy. The prognosis is guarded if the disease is advanced and mesenteric vessels have thrombosed or adjacent structures have been invaded. The prognosis for nonresectable lesions is poor to guarded because current antifungal drugs are of questionable efficacy.

Suggested Reading

Ader PL: Phycomycosis in fifteen dogs and two cats, *J Am Vet Med Assoc* 174:1216, 1979.

Dennis JS, Kruger JM, Mullaney TP: Lymphocytic/plasmacytic gastroenteritis in cats: 14 cases (1985–1990), *J Am Vet Med Assoc* 200:1712, 1992.

Jergens AE et al: Idiopathic inflammatory bowel disease in dogs and cats: 84 cases (1987–1990), *J Am Vet Med Assoc* 201:1603, 1992.

Miller RI: Gastrointestinal phycomycosis in 63 dogs, *J Am Vet Med Assoc* 186:473, 1985.

Pavletic MM, Miller RI, Turnwald GH: Intestinal infarction associated with canine phycomycosis, *J Am Anim Hosp Assoc* 19:913, 1983.

INTESTINAL VOLVULUS/TORSION

DEFINITIONS

Intestinal **volvulus** is defined as twisting of the intestine, which causes obstruction. Intestinal **torsion** is twisting of the intestines about the root of the mesentery. The terms *torsion* and *volvulus* are often used interchangeably.

SYNONYMS

Mesenteric torsion, mesenteric volvulus

GENERAL CONSIDERATIONS AND CLINICALLY RELEVANT PATHOPHYSIOLOGY

Intestinal volvulus/torsion is uncommon in small animals because they have short mesenteric attachments. When it does occur the jejunum is most commonly involved. Intestinal volvulus causes both mechanical and strangulation obstruction—a medical and surgical emergency (Fig. 16-102). Areas of the intestines not fixed in location by attachments to parietal peritoneum or adjacent viscera are suspended by mesentery, which provides greater freedom of movement. Movement and physiologic twisting or turning of suspended intestine occurs during physical activity and normal peristalsis. Twisting occurs around the mesenteric axis or root. If mesenteric attachments fail to prevent excessive rotation, vascular compromise, tissue ischemia, and luminal obstruction occur. Rotation may exceed 360 degrees in either a clockwise or counterclockwise direction. Predisposing factors in man include absence of mesenteric fat, narrow mesenteric root, excessive mesenteric length, and increased bowel length. Twisting compromises the cranial mesenteric artery and all its branches resulting in impediment of blood flow to the distal duodenum, jejunum, ileum, cecum, ascending colon, transverse colon, and proximal descending colon. After mesenteric twisting the rapid cascade of vascular obstruction, intestinal anoxia, circulatory shock, endotoxemia, and cardiovascular failure results in death if the condition is not corrected immediately. Mesenteric twisting decreases venous return and arterial perfusion. The arteries and veins may thrombose. Edema and congestion of the intestinal wall lead to anoxia. Blood is lost both into the intestinal lumen and abdominal cavity. Motility is disrupted and normal bacterial flora proliferate rapidly (especially aerobic coliforms and anaerobic species), both proximal to and within the strangulated intestine. Small intestinal bacterial concentrations that normally range from 10^2 to 10^4 per milliliter liquid secretion may increase to 10^8 to 10^{11} per milliliter within 6 hours of strangulation. Endotoxins primarily from *Escherichia coli* and exotoxins from *Clostridia* spp. are produced. These toxins and bacteria escape into the abdomen through the damaged mucosal barrier and are absorbed into the systemic circulation. Death from strangulation obstruction is usually the result of a combination of hypovolemic shock, sepsis, and products of tissue necrosis. Reperfusion injury caused by oxygen-derived free radicals following derotation and tissue reoxygenation may be severe and contribute to mortality.

DIAGNOSIS
Clinical Presentation

Signalment. Male, medium-to-large, sporting or working breeds have most commonly been diagnosed with intestinal volvulus/torsion. German shepherds (with pancreatic insufficiency) and English pointers appear predisposed to intestinal volvulus/torsion. Young adult dogs (2 to 3 years) are most commonly affected.

History. Vigorous activity, dietary indiscretion, or trauma often precedes volvulus. Other factors that might be associated with intestinal volvulus include recent gastrointestinal surgery, enteritis, parasitism, foreign bodies, obstructive masses, exocrine pancreatic insufficiency, and concurrent gastric dilatation-volvulus. Some animals have been ill for several days and then suddenly deteriorate. Others progress from appearing normal to near death in less than 6 hours. Clinical signs range from peracute to acute and are commonly associated with partial obstruction and ischemia. Signs include acute pain, shock (tachycardia, pale to injected

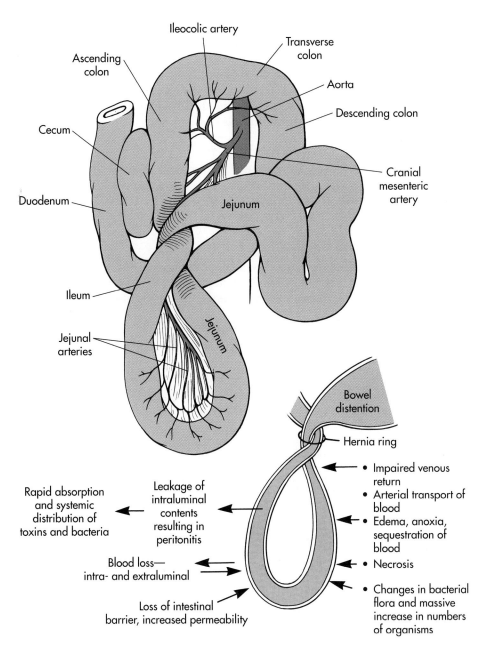

Ileocolic artery

Transverse colon

Ascending colon

Aorta

Descending colon

Cecum

Cranial mesenteric artery

Duodenum

Jejunum

Ileum

Jejunum

Jejunal arteries

Bowel distention

Hernia ring

- Impaired venous return
- Arterial transport of blood
- Edema, anoxia, sequestration of blood
- Necrosis
- Changes in bacterial flora and massive increase in numbers of organisms

Rapid absorption and systemic distribution of toxins and bacteria

Leakage of intraluminal contents resulting in peritonitis

Blood loss— intra- and extraluminal

Loss of intestinal barrier, increased permeability

mucous membranes, prolonged capillary refill, weak pulses), and mild abdominal enlargement. There is an acute onset of nausea, retching, vomiting, hematochezia, depression, weakness, and/or recumbency.

Physical Examination Findings

Affected animals usually present in shock with an acute abdomen. Pain and dilated loops of intestine may be detected by abdominal palpation. Occasionally, abdominal fluid is found, the amount varying with duration of clinical signs.

Radiography/Ultrasonography

Plain radiographs are often diagnostic with the entire intestinal tract uniformly distended with gas. Intestinal fluid, free abdominal fluid, and generalized loss of serosal detail are expected. Definitive diagnosis of intestinal volvulus/torsion is made at surgery or necropsy.

Laboratory Findings

Common laboratory findings are normal packed cell volume (PCV), leukocytosis, hypoproteinemia, hypoalbuminemia, and hypokalemia. Serosanguineous fluid may be collected on abdominocentesis. A modified transudate (increased red blood cells and protein) with an absence of platelets indicates an acute vascular insult.

DIFFERENTIAL DIAGNOSIS

Any systemic or mechanical cause of acute abdomen should be included in the differential diagnosis. Surgical differentials include gastric dilatation-volvulus, cecocolic volvulus, splenic torsion and rupture, physiologic ileus, mechanical obstruction, abdominal trauma, and peritonitis. Systemic illnesses may include hemorrhagic gastroenteritis, viral enteritis, and pancreatitis.

MEDICAL MANAGEMENT

Shock therapy (fluids, antibiotics, plus or minus corticosteroids; see below) is essential but not curative. Immediate diagnosis and surgery are necessary if the patient is to survive.

SURGICAL TREATMENT
Preoperative Management

Initial treatment consists of aggressive shock therapy and correction of electrolyte and acid-base abnormalities. Shock doses of fluids (i.e., 90 ml/kg/hr) should be administered rapidly; however, if possible, central venous pressure should be monitored to avoid volume overload. Alternatively, hypertonic saline or hetastarch may be given (see p. 280). Broad-spectrum antibiotic therapy and possibly a nonsteroidal antiinflammatory drug should be administered. Blood transfusions may be warranted if massive blood loss has taken place. Drugs that block formation of or scavenge oxygen free radicals (e.g., superoxide dismutase, allopurinol, dimethylsulfoxide, corticosteroids, gold compounds) may prove to be beneficial in the future.

Anesthesia

These patients are extreme anesthetic risks. A balanced anesthetic protocol (e.g., opioids plus isoflurane) should be used. Selected anesthetic protocols for use in dogs with intestinal volvulus/torsion are provided in Table 16-53. They should be preoxygenated before surgery. Placing two venous catheters (i.e., two cephalic or a cephalic and jugular catheter) before surgery is recommended to allow fluids, blood, pressors, or other agents to be given simultaneously if needed. Hypotension should be corrected before and prevented during and after surgery. If the total protein is less than 4.0 g/dl or albumin is less than 1.5 g/dl, perioperative colloid administration may be indicated. Colloids may be given preoperatively, intraoperatively, and/or postoperatively for a total dose of 20 ml/kg/day (Table 16-54). If colloids are given during surgery, acute intraoperative hypotension should be treated with crystalloids. Dobutamine (2 to 10 µg/kg/min, IV) or dopamine (2 to 10 µg/kg/min, IV) may be given during surgery for inotropic support. Dobutamine is less arrythmogenic and chronotropic than dopamine and is preferred if the patient is hypotensive and anuric. If they are anuric and normotensive, low dose dopamine (0.5 to 1.5 µg/kg/min, IV) plus furosemide (0.2 mg/kg, IV) may be preferable. These patients should be monitored for arrhythmias or tachycardia. An ECG, pulse oximeter, and direct and indirect blood pressure measurements should be monitored throughout surgery. **Nitrous oxide is contraindicated.**

Surgical Anatomy

Surgical anatomy of the small intestine is provided on p. 294. The cranial mesenteric artery branches to form the caudal pancreaticoduodenal, jejunal, ileocolic, right colic, and middle colic arteries.

Positioning

The patient should be positioned in dorsal recumbency for a ventral midline celiotomy. The caudal thorax and entire abdomen should be prepped for aseptic surgery.

SURGICAL TECHNIQUE

Quickly explore the abdomen to confirm the diagnosis and determine the direction of twisting. The intestine will appear dilated, edematous, and discolored with the serosal surfaces ranging from red to black in color. Decompress the intestine if necessary to allow derotation and reposition the intestines. Allow the intestine to reperfuse and stabilize while the abdomen is more thoroughly explored. Evaluate intestinal viability and resect devitalized tissue. Thoroughly lavage the abdomen with warm physiologic saline or balanced electrolyte solution. Perform open peritoneal drainage (see p. 198) if intestinal necrosis and peritonitis are identified.

SUTURE MATERIALS/ SPECIAL INSTRUMENTS

Suction is useful for decompressing the intestine before derotating and repositioning.

POSTOPERATIVE CARE AND ASSESSMENT

Fluid, electrolyte, and acid-base abnormalities should continue to be corrected after surgery. These patients may benefit from nasal oxygen postoperatively, and they should be monitored for signs of continued abdominal discomfort. Analgesics should be used if necessary (see Table 16-4). Continuation of perioperative antibiotics is reasonable, particularly if full-thickness necrosis of the intestine was present. Nutritional support should be provided via parenteral hyperalimentation if the animal is likely to be anorexic or continue to vomit.

TABLE 16-53

Selected Anesthetic Protocols for Use in Dogs with Intestinal Volvulus/Torsion

Induction

Oxymorphone (0.1 mg/kg IV) plus diazepam (0.2 mg/kg IV). Give in incremental dosages. Intubate if possible. If necessary, give etomidate (0.5-1.5 mg/kg IV). Alternately give thiopental or propofol at reduced doses.

Maintenance

Isoflurane

TABLE 16-54

Colloid Administration (Hetastarch, Dextrans)

Total daily dose—20 ml/kg/day
Surgical dose—7-10 ml/kg

PROGNOSIS

Mortality approaches 100%. Vomiting, diarrhea, shock, intestinal necrosis, dehiscence, and peritonitis are common. Patients that survive may develop short bowel syndrome following massive intestinal resection (see p. 304). Most animals who have survived have been incidentally diagnosed during celiotomy for another problem, had rotation limited to 180 degrees, and were operated on within a few hours of occurrence.

Suggested Reading

Carberry CA, Flanders JA: Cecal-colic volvulus in two dogs, *Vet Surg* 22:225, 1993.

Harvey HJ, Rendano VT: Small bowel volvulus in dogs: clinical observations, *Vet Surg* 13:91, 1984.

Nemzek JA, Walshaw R, Hauptman JG: Mesenteric volvulus in the dog: a retrospective study, *J Am Anim Hosp Assoc* 29:357, 1993.

Shealy PM, Henderson RA: Canine intestinal volvulus: a report of nine new cases, *Vet Surg* 21:15, 1992.

Westermarck E, Rimaila-Pärnänen E: Mesenteric torsion in dogs with exocrine pancreatic insufficiency: 21 cases (1978–1987), *J Am Vet Med Assoc* 195:1404, 1989.

Surgery of the Large Intestine

GENERAL PRINCIPLES AND TECHNIQUES

DEFINITIONS

Colopexy is surgical fixation of the colon. **Colectomy** is partial or complete resection of the colon, and **typhlectomy** is resection of the cecum. **Tenesmus** is straining to defecate, while **dyschezia** is pain or discomfort on defecation. **Hematochezia** is the passage of stools that contain red blood, and **melena** is passage of tarry stools (i.e., digested blood).

PREOPERATIVE CONCERNS

Surgery of the large intestine is indicated for lesions causing obstruction, perforations, colonic inertia, or chronic inflammation. The most common causes of obstruction are tumors, intussusceptions, and granulomatous masses. Foreign bodies that have reached the colon are generally expelled with the feces unless the distal colon or rectum is obstructed.

Differentiation of large bowel disease from small intestinal disorders is usually based on history and physical examination (see Table 16-45 on p. 292); however, in some cases (i.e., fungal, infectious, neoplastic), radiographs, ultrasonography, endoscopy, and/or biopsy may be necessary. Differentiation of the various causes of large intestinal disorders is made based on history, physical examination, fecal exam, endoscopy and biopsy, therapeutic trials, and culture. With the exception of patients with histoplasmosis, pythiosis, megacolon, and tumor, most patients with disease localized to the large bowel do not have significant weight loss. Affected patients may pass small quantities of feces, or they may be constipated. Tenesmus, dyschezia, fresh fecal blood, and/or fecal mucus may be observed. Other clinical signs may include diarrhea, vomiting, anorexia, abdominal enlargement, abdominal pain, fecaliths, abnormal fecal shape, rectal prolapse, depression, and/or poor hair coat (see Table 16-45 on p. 292).

Physical examination findings vary depending on the disease and its location in the large bowel (see Table 16-46). The colon is palpable in the dorsocaudal abdomen. Feces can often be differentiated from masses (e.g., tumor) by applying gentle pressure. Normal feces deform; however, animals with constipation/obstipation have hard and dry feces. Sublumbar lymph node enlargement can sometimes be detected by palpation of the caudal abdomen or occasionally on rectal examination. Enlargement is suggestive of metastatic neoplasia. The shape and symmetry of the pelvis and any masses in the pelvic canal should be noted on rectal exam. Intraluminal masses, thickening of the wall, and strictures can often be detected. The anus and anal sacs should be checked for thickening, enlargement, and pain. Feces should be examined for parasites.

Laboratory data may reveal hydration, electrolyte, acid-base, or serum biochemical abnormalities (see Table 16-46). Anemia and hypoalbuminemia are rare in these patients. Although nonspecific, elevation of serum alkaline phosphatase, creatinine phosphokinase, lactic dehydrogenase, and serum glutamic oxaloacetic transaminase may be seen in animals with intestinal ischemia.

Plain colonic radiographs rarely contribute significantly and are most useful in animals with megacolon. Withholding food (24 hours) and evacuating the colon improve visualization. Luminal masses may be identified if the colon contains gas. Properly performed barium enemas may identify dilations, constrictions, wall thickening, filling defects, infiltrative disease, extraluminal compression, intraluminal masses, intussusceptions, or cecal inversion. A coiled spring appearance when the colon is filled with air or barium is indicative of a possible cecal inversion/intussusception. Ultrasonography gives information about large bowel wall thickness, wall layers, wall symmetry, peristalsis, and echogenicity of intestinal contents. Biopsies may be obtained with ultrasound guidance. Computed tomography and magnetic resonance imaging are beneficial in some cases, but these diagnostic techniques are often unavailable. Colonoscopy is safe and more sensitive than radiography. It allows for direct visualization of the lumen, for culture sampling and cytology, and for mucosal biopsy.

If the patient is not rapidly deteriorating, hydration, acid-base, and electrolyte deficits should be corrected before anesthetic induction. Crossmatched whole blood should be administered when the PCV drops below 20% to 22% as a result of acute hemorrhage. Chronically ill, anemic patients should be given whole blood if hypovolemic and packed RBCs if normovolemic. Clotting factor deficiencies should be corrected with fresh whole blood (Table 16-55) or fresh or fresh-frozen plasma; platelet-rich plasma or platelet transfu-

TABLE 16-55
Blood Transfusions

ml of Donor Blood Needed

$$\text{Recipient blood volume}^{\dagger} \times \frac{\text{Desired PCV} - \text{actual patient PCV}}{\text{PCV of anticoagulated donor blood}}$$

†Total blood volume is estimated at 90 ml/kg for dogs and 70 ml/kg for cats. A rough estimate is that 2.2 ml of blood/kg of body weight will increase the recipient's PCV by 1%.

TABLE 16-56
Bowel Preparation for Large Intestinal and Rectal Surgery

Polyethylene Glycol Electrolyte Solution (Colyte or GoLytely)

25-40 ml/kg; PO via stomach tube approximately 24 hours and 18-20 hours before colonoscopy or surgery.

Bisacodyl (Dulcolax)
Dogs

5-20 mg PO, SID to BID

Cats

2.5-5 mg PO, SID to BID

sions should be used if the animal is thrombocytopenic. Plasma (5 to 20 ml/kg) or whole blood (20 ml/kg) administration should be considered if albumin levels are less than 1.5 g/dl. There is some evidence that blood transfusions may impair intestinal healing and increase susceptibility to intraabdominal sepsis (Tadros, Wobbes, Hendriks, 1992).

The colon contains more bacteria (i.e., more than 10^{10}/gm of feces) than the rest of the gastrointestinal tract. Mechanical emptying and cleansing are indicated to reduce bacterial numbers unless the colon is perforated or obstructed. Feeding an elemental diet that requires no digestion (composed of glucose, amino acids, etc.) will reduce colonic bacterial numbers to 10^{3}/gm of feces. If possible, an elemental diet or a low residue diet of hamburger and white rice should be fed for 2 to 3 days before surgery. Holding animals off feed also reduces bacterial numbers in the colon. Food should be withheld 24 hours before surgery, but free access to water should be allowed. Laxatives, cathartics, and warm water enemas should be given 24 hours before surgery. Colon electrolyte solutions (i.e., Colyte or GoLytely; Table 16-56) more effectively cleanse the colon than enemas; the only contraindication to their use is obstruction. Bisacodyl, a stimulant laxative, may be administered to facilitate colonic evacuation. Although colonic electrolyte solutions work well alone, enemas facilitate complete cleansing. A warm water enema should be given the day before surgery and one 10% povidone-iodine enema given 3 hours before surgery. Enemas given any closer to surgery than 3 hours are contraindicated because they liquefy intestinal contents and may add to dissemination of contaminated material during surgery. Be careful; enemas can cause further deterioration of debilitated, anorexic patients and rarely cause colonic perforation. They may be ineffective in cats with megacolon.

ANESTHETIC CONSIDERATIONS

Anesthetic complications may arise because of uncorrected hydration, electrolyte, or acid-base abnormalities. Large masses or visceral displacement may impair circulation and respiration. Nitrous oxide increases the volume of air trapped in hollow viscera and therefore should be avoided in patients with intestinal obstruction. Atropine or glycopyrrolate may prevent bradycardia induced by visceral manipulation. Water evaporates from exposed abdominal viscera at an increased rate; therefore fluid administration must be increased to replace this loss. Body heat is lost because of va-

sodilation and visceral exposure causing hypothermia, which reduces the need for anesthesia. Patients should be kept dry to minimize the effects of hypothermia. Selected protocols for stable animals undergoing large intestinal surgery are provided in Table 16-47 on p. 294.

ANTIBIOTICS

There is a high risk of infection after colorectal surgery. Although controversial, the use of antibiotics in colorectal surgery reduces morbidity and mortality associated with infection. Systemic perioperative antibiotics effective against gram-negative aerobes and anaerobes should be given (Table 16-57). Recommended drugs include second generation cephalosporins (i.e., cefmetazole, cefoxitin, cefotetan) given at the time of induction. Third generation cephalosporins effective against gram-positive and gram-negative aerobes and some anaerobes are available, albeit expensive. Gentamicin plus cefazolin can be given intravenously at induction. Aminoglycosides (i.e., neomycin, kanamycin) and metronidazole can be given orally in combination beginning 24 hours before surgery. Metronidazole is absorbed from the gastrointestinal tract and is effective against anaerobes. Aminoglycosides are only effective against aerobic bacteria. Gastrointestinal absorption of aminoglycosides is minimal in normal patients, but can be substantial if the bowel is eroded or inflamed. The use of such nonabsorbable antibiotics has been linked with the emergence of resistant infections. A combination of neomycin and erythromycin can be given beginning 24 hours before surgery to rapidly reduce aerobes and anaerobes. Metronidazole combined with first generation cephalosporins (cephazolin), aminoglycosides, or trimethoprim-sulfa is also useful.

SURGICAL ANATOMY

The cecum, ascending colon, transverse colon, descending colon, and rectum are segments of the large bowel. The ascending colon and cecum are located at the termination of the ileum. In dogs the cecum is an S-shaped, blind pouch located to the right of the mesenteric root; in cats it is a short, straight, blind pouch. The cecum is ventral to the right

TABLE 16-57

Prophylactic Antibiotic Use in Animals Undergoing Perineal, Rectal, or Colonic Surgery

Cefmetazole (Zefazone)
15 mg/kg IV; repeat every 1.5 to 2 hr for 2 to 3 doses

Cefoxitin (Mefoxin)
15-30 mg/kg IV; repeat every 1.5 to 2 hr for 2 to 3 doses

Cefotetan (Cefotan)
30 mg/kg IV; repeat every 8 hr for 24 hr

Gentamicin (Gentocin)
6 mg/kg IV, SID

Cefazolin (Ancef, Kefzol)
20 mg/kg IV; QID for 24 hr

Neomycin (Biosol)
20 mg/kg PO, TID

Kanamycin (Kantrim)
11 mg/kg PO, TID

Metronidazole (Flagyl)
10 mg/kg IV or PO, TID

Erythromycin
10-20 mg/kg PO, BID to TID

Trimethoprim-Sulfadiazine (Tribrissen)
Dogs
15 mg/kg IM or PO, BID

Cats
15 mg/kg PO, BID

TABLE 16-58

Approximate Lengths of Colonic Segments

Ascending Colon
Dogs
3-9 cm

Cats
1-2 cm

Transverse Colon
Dogs
6-8 cm

Cats
2-4 cm

Descending Colon
10-16 cm long; varies with animal size

kidney, dorsal to the small intestine, and medial to the descending duodenum. A short antimesenteric vessel helps identify the ascending colon lying to the right of the mesenteric root (Table 16-58). The ascending colon communicates with the ileum via the ileocolic orifice and with the cecum via the cecocolic orifice (approximately 1 cm caudal to the ileocolic orifice). The short ascending colon turns from right to left at the right colic flexure (hepatic flexure) and becomes the transverse colon, traveling cranial to the mesenteric root. The colon turns caudally at the left colic flexure (splenic flexure) and becomes the descending colon. The descending colon is the longest segment of colon (see Table 16-58). It begins on the left where it is dorsal to the small intestine and continues caudally to the pelvic inlet. The large bowel continues through the pelvic canal to the anus as the rectum. The colorectal junction is difficult to identify. Landmarks include the pubic brim, pelvic inlet, seventh lumbar vertebra, and the seromuscular point of penetration of the cranial rectal artery. The mesocolon is the short mesenteric attachment of the colon to the body wall. The layers of the large intestinal wall are the same as the layers of the small intestinal wall (mucosa, submucosa, muscularis, and serosa).

The blood supply to the large bowel is from the ileocolic artery, a branch of the cranial mesenteric artery, and the caudal mesenteric artery. These major branches run parallel to the intestine giving off short vasa recta vessels, which penetrate the intestinal wall. Branches of the ileocolic and left colic artery anastomose. The ileocolic artery supplies the ileum, cecum, and ascending and transverse colon. It gives rise to the middle colic and right colic arteries. The right colic artery supplies the cecum, ascending colon, and part of the transverse colon. The middle colic artery supplies part of the transverse colon and half of the descending colon; it anastomoses with the left colic artery, which supplies the distal half of the descending colon. The left colic and cranial rectal arteries originate from the caudal mesenteric artery. The cranial rectal artery primarily supplies the cranial rectum, but also sends several vasae rectae to a short segment of the terminal colon. The internal iliac artery supplies branches to the rectum via prostatic or vaginal artery branches. Venous drainage essentially mirrors arterial supply. The caudal mesenteric vein is short and enters the portal vein. The vagus and pelvic nerves supply the colon with parasympathetic innervation. Sympathetic innervation is supplied from the paravertebral sympathetic trunk via the sympathetic ganglia.

SURGICAL TECHNIQUES

Surgical principles for large intestinal surgery are similar to those for small intestinal surgery (Table 16-59). Assessment of bowel viability can be difficult, but it is important that necrotic or avascular areas of the colon be removed at surgery and that unnecessary resection be avoided. Because of the short mesocolon, avulsion of colonic blood supply is less common than avulsion of the mesenteric blood supply. Techniques for assessing bowel viability are provided on p. 295.

Resection and anastomosis may be performed using sutures or staples. Four stapled anastomosis techniques are available: (1) the triangulating end-to-end anastomosis, (2)

TABLE 16-59

Principles of Large Intestinal Surgery

- Reduce colonic bacterial numbers by eliminating oral intake, preparing the colon, and giving antibiotics.
- Early diagnosis and good surgical technique avoid most complications.
- Perform surgery as soon as the diagnosis is made in patients with perforation, strangulation, or complete obstructions.
- Optimal healing requires a good blood supply, accurate mucosal apposition, and minimal surgical trauma.
- Systemic factors may delay healing and increase the risk of dehiscence: hypovolemia, shock, hypoproteinemia, debilitation, infections, etc.
- Use approximating suture patterns: simple interrupted, Gambee, crushing, or simple continuous.
- Engage submucosa in all sutures.
- Select a monofilament, synthetic absorbable suture: polydioxanone, polyglyconate.
- Cover surgical sites with omentum or a serosal patch.
- Replace contaminated instruments and gloves before abdominal closure.

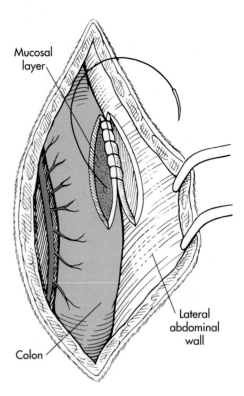

FIG. 16-103
To "pexy" the colon to the abdominal wall make a 3- to 5-cm seromuscular incision along the antimesenteric border of the colon. Make a similar incision 2 to 3 cm lateral to the linea alba through peritoneum and underlying muscle of the left abdominal wall. Appose the edges of the seromuscular incision to the edges of the abdominal wall incision with two simple continuous suture lines.

inverting end-to-end anastomosis, (3) side-to-side or functional end-to-end anastomosis, and (4) end-to-side anastomosis. Inverting end-to-end anastomoses (see p. 298) are most commonly performed during colonic anastomosis. Although more expensive, stapled anastomoses show less tissue reaction, more mature fibrous connective tissue, greater tensile strength, fewer mucoceles and necrotic areas, and less luminal stenosis than suture techniques. The staples in the cartridge are bent against the anvil into a B shape when fired, providing a degree of hemostasis without collapsing the microcirculation. Thick, inflamed, and edematous tissues may prevent proper firing of the stapler by preventing complete penetration and formation of the staples into a B-shaped configuration. Dilatation causes thinning of the visceral walls and may result in tissues too thin for the staples to be effective. In these cases a suture anastomosis should be performed. Circular, inverting, end-to-end staplers are often used to anastomose the colon. It is easier to use end-to-end staplers in the colon than in other areas of the gastrointestinal tract because the instrument can be introduced through the anus rather than a separate enterotomy or gastrotomy incision. The colon of most adult animals can accommodate the size of available staplers. Transanal introduction of the stapler may not be possible in all cats and small dogs because of their small anus and narrow pelvic canal.

Biopsy Techniques

Intestinal biopsy is indicated to establish a diagnosis for intestinal diseases that have not been diagnosed by other means. Large intestine may be biopsied during endoscopy, ultrasonography, or laparotomy. The least invasive method of obtaining an intestinal biopsy is by colonoscopy. Samples can also be collected for culture and exfoliative cytology during colonoscopy. Flexible endoscopic biopsies are limited to

infiltrative disease involving the mucosa and submucosa, and to lesions located within the length of the endoscope; rigid proctoscopes allow biopsy of the muscular layer.

Colopexy

Colopexy is done to create permanent adhesions between the serosal surfaces of the colon and abdominal wall so as to prevent caudal movement of the colon and rectum (Fig. 16-103). The most common indication for colopexy is to prevent recurring rectal prolapse. Incisional and nonincisional techniques have been described and both are equally effective. A potential complication is infection as a result of suture penetration into the colonic lumen.

Expose and explore the abdomen. Locate and isolate the descending colon from the remainder of the abdomen. Pull the descending colon cranially to reduce the prolapse. Verify prolapse reduction by having a nonsterile assistant inspect the anus visually and perform a rectal examination. Make a 3- to 5-cm longitudinal incision along the antimesenteric border of the distal descending colon through only the serosal and muscularis layers. Create a similar incision on the left abdominal wall several centimeters lateral (2.5 cm or more) to the linea alba through the peritoneum and underlying muscle. Appose each edge of the colonic and abdominal wall incisions with two simple continuous or simple interrupted rows of sutures using 2-0 or 3-0 monofilament absorbable (e.g., polydioxanone or polyglyconate) or nonabsorbable (nylon, polypropylene) suture material (see Fig. 16-107). Engage the submucosa as each suture is placed. Lavage the surgical site and surround it with omentum before abdominal closure. Alternatively, scarify an 8- to 10-cm antimesenteric segment of the descending colon by scraping the serosa with a scalpel blade or rubbing it with a gauze sponge. On the left abdominal wall opposite the prepared colon, scarify the peritoneum in the same manner. Preplace, then tie, six to eight horizontal mattress sutures between the two scarified surfaces. Roll the colon toward the midline and place a second row of six to eight sutures. Use 2-0 to 3-0 monofilament absorbable or nonabsorbable sutures that engage the submucosa, but do not penetrate the colonic mucosa. Tie the sutures apposing the scarified surfaces.

Colon Resection and Anastomosis

Colectomy or colonic resection and anastomosis are primarily performed to excise colonic masses or to treat megacolon. Other surgical indications include trauma, perforation, intussusception, and cecal inversion. The procedure is much the same as for small intestinal resection and anastomosis (see p. 297) with the exception of vascular ligation. During subtotal colectomy, 90% to 95% of the colon is resected; the primary adverse effect is frequent and soft stools.

☞ **N O T E** · Up to 70% of the colon can be resected in animals without adverse side effects.

Explore the entire abdomen through a ventral midline celiotomy. Collect nonintestinal specimens before entering the bowel lumen. Carefully isolate the diseased bowel with laparotomy pads or sterile towels. Assess intestinal viability and determine resection sites. Double ligate all the vasa recta vessels to the diseased segment (Fig. 16-104), but do not ligate the major colic vessels running parallel to the mesenteric border of the bowel unless performing a colectomy. Gently milk fecal material from the lumen of the isolated bowel. Occlude the lumen at both ends to minimize fecal contamination by having an assistant use a scissorlike grip with the index and middle fingers positioned 4 to 6 cm from the diseased tissue on the colonic wall. Noncrushing intestinal forceps (Doyen) or a Penrose drain tourniquet can also be used to occlude the intestinal lumen. Place another pair of forceps (either crushing [Carmalt] or noncrushing [Doyen]) across each end of the diseased bowel segment. Transect through healthy colon using a scalpel blade or Metzenbaum scissors along the outside of the crushing forceps (see Fig. 16-85 on p. 299). Make the incision perpendicular to the long axis if the lumen sizes are about equal. Use an oblique (45- to 60-degree angle) incision across the smaller intestinal segment when lumen sizes are expected to be unequal. Angle the incision so the antime-senteric border is shorter than the mesenteric border. Suction the intestinal ends and remove any debris clinging to the cut edges with a moistened gauze sponge. Trim everting mucosa with Metzenbaum scissors just before beginning the anastomosis.

Sutured anastomoses. *Reappose intestinal ends with a one- or two-layer suture closure or with staples. Use 3-0 or 4-0 monofilament absorbable (polydioxanone, polyglyconate) or nonabsorbable (nylon, polypropylene) suture with a taper or tapercut, swaged-on needle. Place simple interrupted sutures through all layers of the wall and position knots extraluminally when a one-layer closure is used. Angle the needle so slightly more serosa than mucosa is engaged with each bite to help prevent mucosa from protruding between sutures (see Fig. 16-84 on p. 298). Begin by placing one suture at the mesenteric border and one at the antimesenteric border. If the intestinal ends are of equal diameter, space additional sutures between the first two sutures approximately 2 mm from the edge and 2 to 3 mm apart. Gently appose the tissue edges when tying knots to prevent tissue strangulation and disruption of blood supply. If minor disparity still exists between lumen sizes, space sutures around the larger lumen slightly further apart than the sutures in the intestinal segment with the smaller lumen.* Luminal disparity that cannot be accommodated by the angle of the incisions or suture spacing is usually correctable by resecting a small wedge (1 to 2 cm long, 1 to 3 mm wide) from the antimesenteric border of the intestine with the smaller lumen (see Fig. 16-88 on p. 300). This enlarges the stomal perimeter and gives it an oval shape. *After completing the anastomosis, check for leakage by moderately distending the lumen with saline and applying gentle digital pressure. Look for leakage between sutures or through suture holes. Place additional sutures if leakage occurs between sutures. Close the mesenteric defect. Lavage the isolated intestine thoroughly without allowing the fluid to seep into the abdominal cavity. Remove the laparotomy pads and change gloves and instruments. Lavage the abdomen with sterile, warm saline, then use suction to remove the fluid. Wrap the anastomotic site with omentum or create a serosal patch (see p. 301).* A two-layer anastomosis is occasionally recommended if there is tension at the anastomotic site. A two-layer anastomosis is performed in the same manner as a one-layer closure except that the serosa and muscularis are apposed in a separate layer. All sutures engage the submucosa. The first layer of simple interrupted sutures is placed to appose mucosa and submucosa, with the knots tied within the lumen. The second layer of interrupted sutures apposes muscularis and serosa, with knots positioned extraluminally.

Stapled anastomoses. Anastomosis of the distal colon to the ileum or jejunum using inverting end-to-end, functional end-to-end, or end-to-side stapling techniques may be used. The inverting end-to-end and functional end-to-end techniques are performed the same as for small intestinal anastomoses (see p. 298). *For an end-to-side technique first insert the end-to-end stapling instrument (without anvil) through the open transected end of the colon. Advance the*

FIG. 16-104

To perform a partial colectomy (*dashed lines*) double ligate the vasa recta vessels (preserve the major colonic vessels). Perform a subtotal colectomy with preservation of the ileocolic junction by double ligating the paired arteries and veins (*open red circles*). Perform a subtotal colectomy and ileocolic anastomosis by double ligating the paired arteries and veins (*shaded dark circles*). Transection sites are identified by the corresponding symbol. In dogs do not ligate the cranial rectal artery; ligate the left colic and vasa recti from the cranial rectal artery.

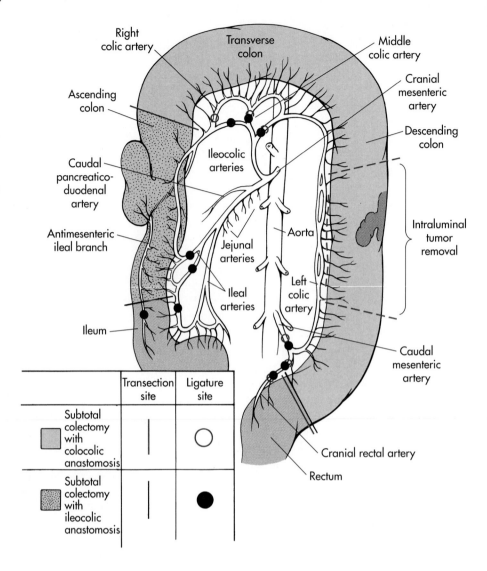

	Transection site	Ligature site
Subtotal colectomy with colocolic anastomosis	|	○
Subtotal colectomy with ileocolic anastomosis	|	●

center rod through an antimesenteric stab wound surrounded by a purse-string suture. Tie the suture and place the anvil on the center rod. Introduce the anvil into the lumen of the ileum. Tie the ileal purse-string suture, close the instrument, and fire the staples. Gently rotate and remove the instrument. Inspect the anastomotic site for hemostasis and integrity. Close the transected colon with a transverse stapler. Lavage the surgical sites and place an omental or serosal patch (see p. 301).

Typhlectomy

Typhlectomy or cecal resection is performed when the cecum becomes impacted, inverted, perforated, neoplastic, or is severely inflamed. *Begin typhlectomy for a noninverted cecum by ligating cecal branches of the ileocecal artery within the ileocecal mesenteric attachment (ileocecal fold) (Fig. 16-105, A). Dissect the ileocecal fold freeing the cecum from the ileum and colon (Fig. 16-105, B). Place a clamp across the base of the cecum (Fig. 16-105, C). Milk intestinal contents from the ascending colon and ileum adjacent to the cecocolic orifice and occlude the lumen. Tran-*

sect the cecum where it joins the ascending colon. Close the defect with simple interrupted sutures. Alternatively, place a transverse or linear cutting stapling instrument across the base of the cecum. Activate the stapler. Transect the cecum before removing the transverse stapling instrument. Lavage, then cover the surgical site with an omental or serosal patch (see p. 301). The cecum may be difficult to locate if it is inverted, but its location may be identified by a small indentation where it can be palpated within the colonic lumen (Fig. 16-106). *Manually reduce the cecum, if possible, before resection. Perform an antimesenteric colotomy and exteriorize the cecum if it cannot be manually reduced (Fig. 16-107). Resect the cecum and close the cecocolic orifice with sutures or staples as described above (Fig. 16-108).*

HEALING OF THE LARGE INTESTINE

Colonic healing is similar to that in the small intestine (see p. 302), but delayed. Wound tensile strength lags behind return of strength in the small intestine, and dehiscence is more likely. Optimal healing is dependent on a good blood supply, accurate mucosal apposition, minimal surgical

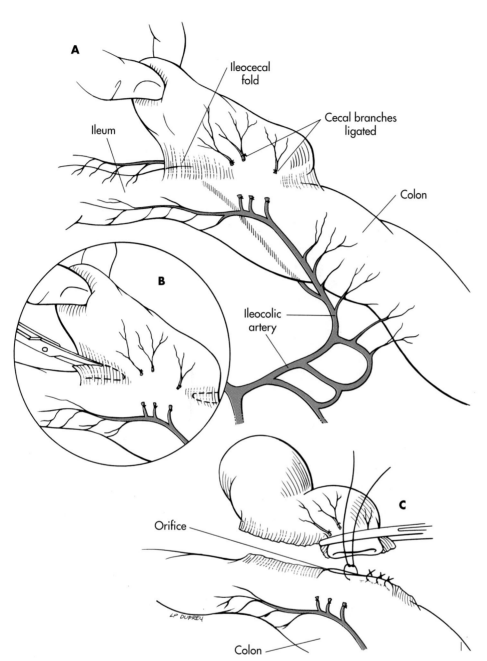

FIG. 16-105
To perform typhlectomy **A,** double ligate the cecal branches of the ileocolic vessels. **B,** Dissect the ileocecal fold of mesentery. **C,** Place a clamp across the base of the cecum near the cecocolic orifice and transect. Close the colonic defect with simple interrupted sutures.

Labels in figure: Ileocecal fold; Ileum; Cecal branches ligated; Colon; Ileocolic artery; Orifice; Colon; LP DUPREY

trauma, and a tension-free closure. Delayed healing may occur for a number of reasons. Collateral circulation to the large intestine is poor compared with the small intestine. There are large numbers of anaerobic and aerobic intraluminal bacteria composing up to 10% of the dry fecal weight. Normal colon bacterial counts range from 10^{10} to 10^{11} bacteria per gram of feces. More anaerobes (Table 16-60) than aerobes populate the colon. High intraluminal pressure develops during passage of a solid fecal bolus. This mechanical stress on the suture line may lead to dehiscence. Risk of dehiscence during the first 3 to 4 days is high because collagen lysis exceeds synthesis. Using antibiotics and avoiding sutures that strangulate tissue may improve healing.

Stapled anastomoses have a higher bursting pressure during the early lag phase of healing and a higher tensile strength after 7 days than hand-sutured anastomoses. Min-

imal inflammation and a double row of staples increase wound strength. The β-shaped staples provide hemostasis without collapsing the microcirculation, and their alignment assures equal tension around the circumference of the anastomosis. However, unhealthy tissues should not be stapled.

SUTURE MATERIALS/ SPECIAL INSTRUMENTS

Instruments and suture materials are the same as those required for small intestinal surgery (see p. 303).

POSTOPERATIVE CARE AND ASSESSMENT

Postoperative care should be individualized for each patient. Animals should be closely monitored for vomiting or

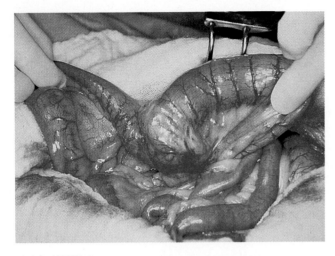

FIG. 16-106
Note the appearance of a cecum that is inverted into the colonic lumen.

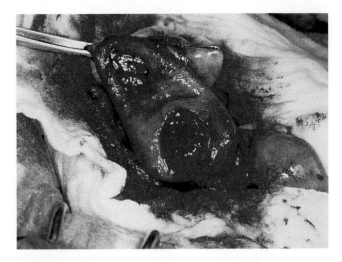

FIG. 16-108
The inverted cecum is excised and the colonic defect is closed with simple interrupted sutures.

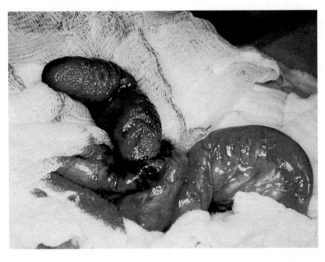

FIG. 16-107
During typhlectomy an incision is made on either side of the cecal dimple and the inverted cecum is exteriorized.

TABLE 16-60
Colonic Bacteria

Anaerobes
- *Bacteroides* spp.
- *Bifidobacteria* spp.
- *Lactobacilli* spp.
- *Clostridium* spp.
- *Fusobacteria* spp.
- Anaerobic *Streptococci* spp.

Aerobes
Gram-Negative
- *Escherichia coli*
- *Klebsiella* spp.
- *Proteus* spp.

Gram-Positive
- *Staphylococcus* spp.
- *Corynebacterium* spp.

regurgitation during recovery to prevent aspiration pneumonia. Analgesics (i.e., oxymorphone, butorphanol, buprenorphine; Table 16-4) should be given as needed. Hydration, electrolyte, and acid-base abnormalities should be monitored and corrected. Intravenous fluid therapy should be continued until the animal is eating and drinking normally. Antibiotics may be discontinued 2 to 4 hours after surgery, unless peritonitis is present. Small amounts of water may be offered 8 to 12 hours after surgery. If vomiting does not occur, small amounts of food can be given beginning 12 to 24 hours after surgery. A bland, low-fat diet (i/d or boiled rice, potatoes and pasta combined with boiled skinless chicken, yogurt, or low-fat cottage cheese) may be fed three to four times daily. The animal's normal diet can be gradually reintroduced beginning 48 to 72 hours after surgery. Debilitated patients may require enteral or parenteral nutrition (see Chapter 11). Stool softeners and/or laxatives should be administered when oral intake begins (Table 16-61). They may be given orally as a supplement (e.g., dioctyl sulfosuccinate/docusate sodium, bisacodyl, lactulose, magnesium salts) or added to food (e.g., psyllium, pumpkin, bran cereal, coarse wheat bran). Appetite can be stimulated in some cats by an intravenous injection of diazepam (0.5 mg) or oral cyproheptadine (Periactin—2 mg/cat PO, BID).

Abdominal palpation and measurement of body temperature should be performed postoperatively to monitor for peritonitis or abscess formation. Depression, high fever, excessive abdominal tenderness, vomiting, and ileus may indicate peritonitis. If peritonitis is suspected, an abdominocentesis or diagnostic peritoneal lavage should be performed (see p. 198). A threefold or greater increase in serum lipase activity may occur after routine exploratory laparotomy in dogs without pancreatitis (Bellah, Bell, 1989). Early ambulation and oral intake should be encouraged to reduce postop-

TABLE 16-61
Stool Softeners and Laxatives

Dioctyl Sodium Sulfosuccinate or Docusate Sodium (Colace)
Dogs
50 to 200 mg PO, BID to TID
Cats
50 mg PO, SID to BID

Bisacodyl (Dulcolax)
Dogs
5-20 mg PO, SID to BID
Cats
2.5-5 mg PO, SID to BID

Lactulose (Chronulac)
Dogs
1 ml/4.5 kg PO, TID to effect
Cats
5 ml/cat PO, TID

Psyllium (Metamucil)
Dogs
2-10 g PO, SID to BID or 1 tsp per 10 kg, twice daily in food
Cats
1-4 g PO, SID to BID or 1 tsp per 10 kg, twice daily in food

Magnesium Hydroxide (Milk of Magnesia) (cathartic dose)
Dogs
15-50 ml per dog PO, SID
Cats
2-6 ml PO, SID

Canned Pumpkin
1-4 tablespoons PO, SID

Coarse Wheat Bran
Dogs
1-2 tablespoons PO, SID

erative ileus. Color, consistency, and presence or absence of blood in the stool should be noted after surgery. Tenesmus and hematochezia may be observed. Subtotal colectomy generally increases the frequency of defecation 30% to 50%. Stools frequently remain loose for days to weeks and then become more semiformed.

COMPLICATIONS

Hemorrhage and fecal contamination of the abdomen are the most common complications of large intestinal surgery. Other potential complications include shock, leakage, dehiscence, perforation, peritonitis, stenosis, incontinence, or death. Fecal contamination can be avoided by preoperative colon preparation or by manually displacing the contents of

the colon away from the resection sites, properly using atraumatic intestinal forceps, and performing copious lavage before closure. The frequency of leakage at the anastomotic site is similar for staple and suture anastomosis techniques. Leakage may be minimized by placing a serosal patch around the anastomosis (see p. 301). Long-term corticosteroid use in man is associated with a high incidence of abscesses after colonic anastomosis and may predispose to dehiscence. Hemorrhage can be avoided with proper ligature placement and careful inspection of the anastomosis. Clinically significant strictures are rare unless inverting or everting suture patterns are used, or excessive tension exists at the resection site. Strictures may be managed by incision with an electrosurgical tip or laser ablation. Dilation by balloon or bougienage may also be effective (see p. 247). If these techniques do not alleviate signs of obstruction, surgical resection may be required. Incontinence is rarely associated with colectomy.

SPECIAL AGE CONSIDERATIONS

Young animals more frequently have prolapsed rectum or intussusception as a result of parasite infestation or garbage or foreign body ingestion. They are prone to hypoglycemia and hypothermia during surgery. Neoplasia is more common in older animals.

References

Bellah JR, Bell G: Serum amylase and lipase activities after exploratory laparotomy in dogs, *Am J Vet Res* 50:1638, 1989.
Tadros T, Wobbes T, Hendriks T: Blood transfusion impairs the healing of experimental intestinal anastomoses, *Ann Surg* 215:276, 1992.

Suggested Reading

Ellison GW: Wound healing in the gastrointestinal tract, *Semin Vet Med Surg (Small Animal)* 4:287, 1989.
Goldsmid SE et al: Colorectal blood supply in dogs, *Am J Vet Res* 54:1948, 1993.
Harvey HJ: Complications of small intestinal biopsy in hypoalbuminemic dogs, *Vet Surg* 19:289, 1990.
Kudish M, Pavletic MM: Subtotal colectomy with surgical stapling instruments via a trans-cecal approach for treatment of acquired megacolon in cats, *Vet Surg* 22:457, 1993.
Popovitch CA, Holt D, Bright R: Colopexy as a treatment for rectal prolapse in dogs and cats: a retrospective study of 14 cases, *Vet Surg* 23:115, 1994.
Thompson JS, Gragg LE, West WW: Serum enzyme levels during intestinal ischemia, *Ann Surg* 211:369, 1990.

SPECIFIC DISEASES

NEOPLASIA

DEFINITIONS

Tumors occurring in the colon or rectum are termed **colorectal neoplasia. Polyps** are grossly visible protrusions from the mucosal surface of either neoplastic or nonneoplastic cells.

GENERAL CONSIDERATIONS AND CLINICALLY RELEVANT PATHOPHYSIOLOGY

Intestinal tumors occur most commonly in the rectum or colon of dogs and the small intestine of cats. Adenomatous polyps and adenocarcinomas are the most common colorectal neoplasms. Other reported tumors include lymphosarcoma, leiomyoma, leiomyosarcoma, plasmacytoma, mast cell tumors, and carcinoids. Intestinal wall tumors usually invade the muscular layer of the intestines, causing obstruction via luminal compromise and/or interference with peristalsis. The proximal bowel may become distended by feces, fluid, and/or gas, compromising its function. Clinical signs of tenesmus, dyschezia, and hematochezia can be attributed to the presence of a friable luminal mass that bleeds when abraded by the passage of feces. In some animals tenesmus and dyschezia are caused by partial luminal obstruction by a full-thickness annular mass. Physical examination, endoscopy, ultrasound, computed tomography, and magnetic resonance imaging are the principal ways to assess abdominal and pelvic structures for neoplasia.

The cause of colorectal polyps is unknown. Most polyps occur in the dog's rectum near the anorectal junction, although they may occasionally be found in the colon. Most appear dark red or pink, soft, friable, and hemorrhagic. They are usually sessile or slightly pedunculated and may be single or multiple. Single masses may be so large as to suggest a broad base mass when they actually have a small stalk. Most polyps are hyperplastic or adenomatous, and epithelial changes do not cross the lamina muscularis; however, some have atypia and are considered carcinoma in situ. Intraepithelial carcinomatous change or malignant transformation may occur.

Adenocarcinomas of the colon and rectum are rare in dogs and cats; in man most are believed to rise from preexisting adenomatous polyps. Most adenocarcinomas of the large intestine are located in the canine and feline rectum (more than 50% are mid-rectum). They may be annular (intramural) or intraluminal. Intraluminal masses may be multiple, pedunculated, nodular, and/or ulcerated. Annular masses typically infiltrate all layers of the intestinal wall causing circumferential narrowing. These tumors are firm, grayish white in color, and often ulcerated. Tumors of the large intestine usually grow slowly and spread to adjacent serosal surfaces, mesentery, omentum, and regional lymph nodes by local invasion. Distant metastases may occur to lymph nodes, lungs, liver, spleen, pancreas, adrenals, and peritoneal surfaces.

Leiomyomas are benign neoplasms of smooth muscle occurring sporadically in the large intestine. They are well encapsulated, circumscribed, and light in color with a smooth glistening cut surface. Clinical signs (i.e., tenesmus) may not be seen until the mass reaches an appreciable size. Mucosa is usually not involved; therefore melena is uncommon. Removal is usually accomplished by blunt dissection from the colorectal wall via an anal, perineal, or abdominal approach. Recurrence is uncommon and long-term survival is expected.

Leiomyosarcomas are invasive, malignant smooth muscle tumors that are usually slow to metastasize. Most reported cecal tumors are leiomyosarcomas. Cecal leiomyosarcomas occur most commonly in old, larger breed dogs of either sex. Some patients present acutely with cecal rupture and peritonitis and others because of lethargy and anorexia. Prognosis for long-term survival is poor. Survival without metastasis approximates 12 months after resection, with most patients eventually being euthanized because of tumor recurrence or metastasis (Gibbons, Murtaugh, 1989).

DIAGNOSIS
Clinical Presentation

Signalment. Colorectal tumors are more frequent in dogs than cats. The incidence of polyps is equal in males and females with an increased prevalence suggested in poodles, Airedale terriers, German shepherds, and collies. Colonic carcinomas are two to three times more common in males than females. Mixed breed dogs, poodles, German shepherds, collies, West Highland white terriers, Airedales, and Lhasa apsos appear to be most commonly affected. Leiomyomas and leiomyosarcomas occur more frequently in medium to large breeds, with no particular breed or sex predilection. Most large intestinal tumors occur in middle-aged to old dogs; however, dogs as young as 2 years of age have been affected. Mean ages reported for colorectal tumors are 6.9 years for polyps, 10.9 years for leiomyomas, 11.4 years for leiomyosarcomas, and 8.5 years for carcinomas (Gibbons, Murtaugh, 1989).

History. Most dogs present because owners have noticed blood and mucus in feces. Common clinical signs include straining to defecate, passage of blood and mucus with feces, painful defecation, and passage of ribbonlike feces. Constipation, vomiting, anorexia, weight loss, depression, septic peritonitis, and/or malabsorption occur occasionally. Some animals are asymptomatic and masses are found during routine physical examination. Tenesmus is often present and can cause prolapse of the mass or rectum. Sometimes the only sign is prolapse of a mass during defecation. Signs involving other organ systems may develop secondary to metastasis and paraneoplastic syndromes.

Physical Examination Findings

Animals with colorectal neoplasia may be thin. Colorectal masses are often identified during abdominal or rectal palpation. More than 60% of anal and rectal canal masses are diagnosed during rectal palpation (Gibbons, Murtaugh, 1989). Masses may bleed and fragment during palpation, and they may be pedunculated, sessile, nodular, firm, soft, or friable. Prolapse of the mass is often possible to allow visual inspection. During rectal examination it should be determined whether the mass is fixed or moveable and whether the sublumbar lymph nodes are enlarged.

Radiography/Ultrasonography/Endoscopy

Thoracic and abdominal radiographs should be taken to evaluate the extent of disease. It is difficult to evaluate the rectum and anus on plain radiographs; however, a mass may be identified protruding into the lumen if surrounded by intraluminal gas. Sublumbar lymph node size should be evaluated because enlargement is often indicative of metastasis. A barium enema may help delineate the mass, but proctoscopy is generally more valuable. In man, intrarectal ultrasonography appears to be the most accurate imaging technique for staging rectal cancers. Intrarectal ultrasonography helps predict the degree of tumor invasion allowing for better treatment planning. Proctoscopy/colonoscopy should be performed to identify diffuse or multiple lesions and to localize lesions to the distal colon and rectum. Size, location, distribution, and multiplicity of lesions should be determined. Examination may reveal a pedunculated or sessile mass, irregular luminal narrowing, and/or ulceration. All lesions should be biopsied, and submucosa should be included in biopsies with obvious, deep infiltrating disease. Presurgical biopsies are useful prognostic tools; therefore unnecessary surgery can be avoided in patients with poor prognoses. Endoscopic snare polypectomy is frequently performed in man with sessile masses smaller than 15 mm and pedunculated masses smaller than 35 mm, and can occasionally be performed in dogs.

Laboratory Findings

Results of complete blood cell counts and biochemical profiles are nonspecific for colorectal tumors. Anemia and hypoproteinemia are rarely present if chronic bleeding has occurred from an ulcerated mass.

DIFFERENTIAL DIAGNOSIS

Differential diagnosis includes all other causes of large bowel obstruction or irritation including intussusception, constipation, obstipation, colitis, perforation, benign stricture, congenital stricture, granuloma, hematoma, or congenital malformation.

MEDICAL MANAGEMENT

Lymphosarcoma may respond to chemotherapy. The response of other tumors to chemotherapy is unknown. Radiation therapy is restricted to masses smaller than 3 cm that are confined to the rectal wall and located in the distal half of the rectum and anal canal.

SURGICAL TREATMENT

Surgical resection is the treatment of choice for intestinal tumors. Unfortunately many tumors are too far advanced for successful resection when diagnosed. Incontinence may occur after resection.

Preoperative Management

Hydration, electrolyte, and acid-base abnormalities should be corrected before surgery. Transfusion should be performed if the patient's packed cell volume (PCV) is lower than 20% (see p. 320). If the animal has no obstruction, bacterial numbers may be reduced by evacuating the colon with oral cathartics, enemas, and fasting (see p. 320). Antibiotics effective against aerobic and anaerobic intestinal bacteria flora should be given (see p. 320).

Anesthesia

General anesthetic recommendations for animals undergoing large intestinal surgery are provided on p. 320. Patients with tumors may be debilitated; therefore balanced anesthesia using injectable agents and isoflurane is recommended. Epidural anesthesia may be advantageous (see Chapter 12).

Surgical Anatomy

Surgical anatomy of the large intestine is on p. 320.

Positioning

Tumors of the cecum and colon are approached via a ventral celiotomy with the patient in dorsal recumbency. Rectal tumors may be approached using either a ventral midline celiotomy with pelvic osteotomy, anal eversion, or perineal dissection. Tumors of the cranial to middle rectum are approached with the patient in dorsal recumbency using a ventral celiotomy and pelvic osteotomy. Tumors of the caudal rectum and anal canal are approached with the patient in ventral recumbency using the DePage position and anal eversion, or a dorsal (see p. 340) or lateral (see p. 341) perineal approach. For the DePage position, the perineum is elevated by tilting the table, padding the hindquarters, and securing the tail over the back.

SURGICAL TECHNIQUE

Surgical resection is the most common treatment for large intestinal neoplasia. Margins of 4 to 8 cm are recommended during partial colectomy (see p. 323) for malignant tumors. Noninvasive anal or rectal masses are often everted through the anus and excised with limited normal tissue margins. In human beings local excision is performed when rectal tumors are limited to the submucosa or muscularis, mobile, 3 cm or smaller, and well or moderately differentiated. Full-thickness resection of the involved colon or rectum is required for large, sessile masses. Tumors invading the serosa or perirectal tissue that are fixed, 3 cm or larger, poorly differentiated, or atypical should be excised via an abdominal incision, rectal pull-through (see p. 339), or perineal resection (see p. 338) with lymph node excision. Abdominal resection may require a pelvic osteotomy to remove a pubic bone flap (see p. 338) (Graham, Garnsey, Jessup, 1990). *Dilate and retract the anus to allow visualization of the mass. Place stay sutures in the rectal mucosa near the mass to facilitate eversion through the anus (see Fig. 16-112 on p. 341). Use an electrosurgical electrode, laser, or scalpel blade to incise mucosa and submucosa surrounding the mass. Remove the mass and appose mucosa and submucosa with simple interrupted 4-0 absorbable (i.e., polydioxanone, polyglyconate, or polyglactin 910) sutures.*

SUTURE MATERIALS/ SPECIAL INSTRUMENTS

Absorbable (i.e., polydioxanone, polyglyconate, polyglactin 910) sutures are preferred when removing masses from the rectum. Absorbable or nonabsorbable sutures may be used for colectomy (see p. 303), but the former is preferred.

POSTOPERATIVE CARE AND ASSESSMENT

Care and management after surgery should be individualized. Hydration and electrolyte balance are maintained with fluid therapy. Analgesics should be provided as necessary. Therapeutic antibiotics are appropriate when contamination, peritonitis, or severe debilitation is present. Nutritional support (see Chapter 11) may be necessary if the patient is debilitated and refuses to eat. Adjuvant chemotherapy has been recommended for malignant tumors, but efficacy is unknown.

COMPLICATIONS

Leakage, dehiscence, and peritonitis are potential complications. Tenesmus, dyschezia, and hematochezia are expected after colorectal surgery. Incontinence may be seen in animals after rectal pull-through procedures. Stricture or tumor recurrence may cause signs of intestinal obstruction.

PROGNOSIS

A guarded prognosis should be given to animals with nonresectable tumors because other modes of therapy are ineffective, of questionable value, or nonapplicable because of severe side effects. Some lymphosarcoma cases respond well to chemotherapy. Tumor control of 46% (median, 6 months) and survival of 67% (median, 7 months) at 1 year were reported from a small group of dogs (n=6) with distal rectal and anal canal carcinomas receiving a single dose of orthovoltage radiation from 15 to 25 Gy (Turrel, Theon, 1986). In another study, dogs with adenocarcinoma not having treatment survived a mean of 15 months (Church, Mehlhaff, Patnaik, 1987).

The prognosis for patients with benign masses is generally good to excellent if excision is complete; however, recurrence and malignant transformation are possible when polyp excision is incomplete. Contrary to those in man, most canine colorectal polyps do not have carcinoma in situ. The prognosis for patients with malignant tumors is fair to guarded depending on the tumor type, location, stage, and resectability. Leiomyoma excision is expected to be curative with a median survival of 26 months (mean, 31.6 months) (McPherron et al, 1992). Leiomyosarcoma patients live approximately 12 months before signs of recurrence or metastasis. Complete surgical excision of colorectal adenocarcinomas is curative; however, the prognosis is poor because most cannot be completely excised due to local infiltration, spread to lymph nodes, and pelvic canal location. Dogs with colorectal adenocarcinomas are usually euthanized because of failure to control dyschezia and hematochezia. In one study, dogs with single, pedunculated, polypoid masses survived a mean of 32 months, those with nodular lesions survived a mean of 12 months, and those with annular masses causing strictures survived a mean of 1.6 months (Church, Mehlhaff, Patnaik, 1987). Adjuvant chemotherapy and/or radiation therapy is suggested for patients with adenocarcinoma and leiomyosarcoma, but efficacy is unproven.

References

Church EM, Mehlhaff CJ, Patnaik AK: Colorectal adenocarcinoma in dogs: 78 cases (1973–84), *J Am Vet Med Assoc* 191:727, 1987.

Gibbons GC, Murtaugh RJ: Cecal smooth muscle cell neoplasia in the dog: report of 11 cases and literature review, *J Am Anim Hosp Assoc* 25:191, 1989.

Graham RA, Garnsey L, Jessup JM: Local excision of rectal carcinoma, *Am J Surg* 160:306, 1990.

McPherron MA et al: Colorectal leiomyomas in seven dogs, *J Am Anim Hosp Assoc* 28:43, 1992.

Turrel JM, Theon AP: Single-high dose irradiation for selected canine rectal tumors, *Vet Radiology* 27:141, 1986.

Suggested Reading

Sentovich SM et al: Transrectal ultrasound of rectal tumors, *Am J Surg* 166:638, 1993.

Shirouzu K et al: Treatment of rectal carcinoid tumors, *Am J Surg* 160:262, 1990.

COLITIS

DEFINITIONS

Colitis is inflammation of the colon caused by a variety of organisms, diets, and syndromes. **Inflammatory bowel disease** is an idiopathic inflammation of the bowel.

SYNONYMS

Although the terms **colitis, acute colitis, chronic colitis, ulcerative colitis,** and **inflammatory bowel disease** are often used interchangeably, they are different.

GENERAL CONSIDERATIONS AND CLINICALLY RELEVANT PATHOPHYSIOLOGY

Underlying causes for acute infectious and inflammatory conditions of the large intestine are often not diagnosed because they are self-limiting. However, with chronic diseases, determination of the cause is often necessary in order to resolve them. A variety of factors including bacteria, viruses, fungi, parasites, diet, and immunologic agents may cause colitis. Mucosa may be infiltrated by various inflammatory cells (lymphocytes, plasma cells, eosinophils, neutrophils, or macrophages). Lymphocytic-plasmacytic colitis is the most common cause of inflammatory bowel disease (IBD) of the feline colon; IBD is less common in dogs.

Colonic inflammation disrupts normal secretory and absorptive functions of the colon so there is increased net secretion and decreased absorption of sodium, chloride, and water. Colonic motility patterns change so that segmental contractions, which provide resistance to flow of feces, are reduced, while peristaltic contractions are normal or reduced. The colon is usually hypomotile, and diarrhea results from decreased resistance to flow, accelerated transit, increased secretion of water and electrolytes, and accentuated reflux urge to defecate as a result of mucosal irritation. Mucosal ulceration and smooth muscle spasms may be present. Microbial populations are altered.

DIAGNOSIS
Clinical Presentation

Signalment. Boxers have been identified as having a high incidence of histiocytic colitis, although this is currently an infrequent diagnosis. Young and middle-aged dogs are most likely to be affected by infiltrative fungal disease.

History. Patients usually present with a history of constant or intermittent large intestinal diarrhea. They sometimes void small amounts frequently, have a sense of urgency to defecate, and/or have accidents in the house. Hematochezia, fecal mucus, and tenesmus are common but not consistent. Other less common signs include vomiting, depression, weight loss (rare except for fungal infections and neoplasia), dyschezia, and constipation. The animal's diet should be investigated and alterations made to eliminate food as the cause.

Physical Examination Findings

Physical examination findings are often normal. Rectal examination may be normal or abnormal (e.g., painful, roughened mucosa).

Radiography/Ultrasonography/Endoscopy

Plain radiographs, contrast studies, and ultrasonography sometimes show intestinal wall thickening, but are seldom performed in these patients. Colonoscopy with mucosal biopsy provides a definitive diagnosis for fungal infections, neoplasia, and IBD.

Laboratory Findings

Fecal examination may be positive for parasites (e.g., whipworms, *Giardia*). Complete blood counts (CBCs) and serum biochemical profiles are usually normal. Hemograms may reflect chronic inflammation, stress, or anemia. Hypoalbuminemia may be seen in patients with histoplasmosis or pythiosis.

DIFFERENTIAL DIAGNOSIS

Food allergy, lymphocytic-plasmacytic colitis, eosinophilic colitis, ulcerative colitis, intestinal neoplasia (especially lymphoma), granulomatous colitis, coccidia, giardiasis, whipworms, histoplasmosis, protethecosis, pythiosis, bacterial colitis (neutrophilic enterocolitis), clostridial colitis, feline immunodeficiency virus, feline leukemia virus (FeLV), irritable bowel syndrome (i.e., fiber responsive disease), and ileocolic or cecocolic intussusception are potential diagnoses.

MEDICAL MANAGEMENT

Inflammatory diseases of the large intestine are generally managed with medical therapy directed at the causative agent. Therapy for acute colitis is initially symptomatic.

Food should be withheld for 24 to 48 hours and then a bland, easily digested, low-fat, and nonallergenic diet should be introduced (e.g., i/d, d/d, or homemade rice/potato and lean meat, cottage cheese, or eggs). Anthelmintics are appropriate if parasites are present. Motility modifiers are sometimes used on a short-term basis. For patients with chronic disease, medical therapy may include anthelmintics, dietary modification (i.e., feline supplemental diets and/or elimination diets), corticosteroids, metronidazole, antimetabolites (azathioprine, chlorambucil; Table 16-62), nonsteroidal antiinflammatories (sulfasalazine, mesalamine, osalazine), and antimicrobials. Colonic resection is rarely needed or considered in dogs with colonic inflammatory disease. However, partial or complete colectomy may be required in very severe cases (mucosal sloughing) where medical therapy has not or is not expected to stop severe protein losses.

SURGICAL TREATMENT
Preoperative Management

Preoperative care should be provided as discussed on p. 319. Fluids and transfusions should be given before surgery if indicated (see p. 320). Prophylactic antibiotics should be given before surgery. If surgery is indicated, antibiotics effective against colonic aerobes and anaerobes should be given (see p. 320).

TABLE 16-62
Medical Management of Colitis

Metronidazole
10-15 mg/kg PO, BID

Prednisolone
1-2 mg/kg SID

Azathioprine (Imuran)
Dogs
2.2 mg/kg PO SID initially, then 2.2 mg/kg, EOD

Cats
0.3 mg/kg every second day; however, must be given with extreme care.

Chlorambucil (Leukeran)
Cats < 3 kg
1 mg twice a week for 6 to 8 weeks; if effective, taper dose

Cats > 3 kg
2 mg twice a week for 6 to 8 weeks; if effective, taper dose

Sulfasalazine (Azulfidine)
25 mg/kg PO, BID

Mesalamine (Asacol, Mesasal)
10-20 mg/kg PO, BID to TID

Osalazine (Dipentum)
10-20 mg/kg PO, BID to TID

Anesthesia

General anesthetic recommendations for large intestinal surgery are provided on p. 320.

Surgical Anatomy

Surgical anatomy of the large intestine is described on p. 320.

Positioning

Patients should be positioned in dorsal recumbency for a ventral midline celiotomy. The entire ventral abdomen should be clipped and prepped for aseptic surgery.

SURGICAL TECHNIQUE

Surgical biopsy may be required to establish appropriate medical therapy; however, colonic biopsy during exploratory laparotomy is seldom indicated. Biopsies should instead be obtained by endoscopy. Techniques for large intestinal biopsy are the same as for the small intestine (see p. 295). Colectomy is described on p. 323.

SUTURE MATERIALS/SPECIAL INSTRUMENTS

Refer to p. 303 for instruments for large intestinal surgery. Polydioxanone or polyglyconate (3-0 or 4-0) are preferred sutures for colectomy or colonic biopsy; however, nonabsorbable (e.g., nylon or polypropylene) sutures may be used in hypoalbuminemic animals. Chromic gut suture should be avoided in young animals and in those that are debilitated because the suture may rapidly catabolize and weaken.

POSTOPERATIVE CARE AND ASSESSMENT

Severely affected patients may benefit from enteral or parenteral nutritional support after surgery. Analgesics, antibiotics, and fluids should be given as necessary. After surgery, animals should be monitored for evidence of peritonitis (see p. 193).

COMPLICATIONS

Colonic perforation is a rare complication of colonoscopic or ultrasonographic biopsy and may occur because of leakage from colotomy biopsy or colectomy sites. Strictures may occur after partial colectomy.

PROGNOSIS

Signs of acute colitis are frequently alleviated by a 24- to 36-hour fast (see discussion of Medical Management on p. 331). The prognosis for chronic colitis depends on the underlying cause; it is poor for prototothecosis, nonresectable pythiosis, and nonresectable malignancy. Lifetime treatment may be needed for some patients with chronic colitis. Prognosis for recovery after surgical biopsy of the large intestines is good if appropriate surgical principles are followed. The patient may need lifetime medical treatment for the underlying cause of colitis.

Suggested Reading

Willard MD: Inflammatory bowel disease: perspectives on therapy, *J Am Anim Hosp Assoc* 28:27, 1992.

MEGACOLON

DEFINITIONS

Megacolon is a descriptive term for persistent increased large intestinal diameter and hypomotility associated with severe constipation. A diagnosis of **idiopathic megacolon** is made if mechanical, neurologic, or endocrine causes cannot be identified. **Constipation** is difficult or infrequent defecation with passage of unduly hard and dry fecal material, and **obstipation** is extreme constipation (no feces may be passed).

GENERAL CONSIDERATIONS AND CLINICALLY RELEVANT PATHOPHYSIOLOGY

Megacolon is most frequently diagnosed in cats. It is not a specific disease but a clinical sign associated with failure to normally void feces. It may be congenital or acquired and occurs secondary to colonic inertia and outlet obstruction. Causes of colonic inertia may be prolonged distension, neurologic trauma, congenital dysfunction, endocrine disease, behavioral abnormalities, or it may be idiopathic. Outlet obstruction can be caused by pelvic fracture malunion, large intestinal strictures or neoplasia, anal atresia or stricture, compressive extraluminal masses, foreign bodies, or improper diet. Idiopathic megacolon in cats associated with colonic inertia is thought to be the result of an abnormality of either the intrinsic or extrinsic innervation to the lower large intestine.

Feces that are retained in the colon for prolonged periods dehydrate and solidify because of continued water absorption. Fecal concretions are produced that are difficult and painful to eliminate. The fecal mass may become so large and hard that passage through the pelvic canal is impossible. Prolonged severe colonic distension eventually causes irreversible changes in colonic smooth muscles and nerves, causing inertia. Absorption of bacterial toxins from the retained feces may cause depression, anorexia, and weakness. Vomiting occurs secondary to prolonged obstruction, absorbed toxins, and/or vagal stimulation. Liquid may pass around fecal concretions and cause diarrhea. Blood and mucus from mucosal irritation may be seen in the feces.

DIAGNOSIS
Clinical Presentation

Signalment. Idiopathic megacolon is primarily seen in cats but rarely occurs in dogs. There is no sex predisposition; however, Manx cats were overrepresented in one study (de Haan, Ellison, Bellah, 1992). Megacolon secondary to neurologic, obstructive, or medical disease may occur in any animal. Middle-aged and older cats are most commonly diagnosed with idiopathic megacolon (range, 1 to 16 years; mean age, approximately 5 to 7.5 years).

History. Affected animals present for evaluation of constipation or obstipation. They may be depressed, anorexic, have tenesmus, weakness, lethargy, poor hair coat, vomiting, weight loss, and occasionally watery, mucoid, or bloody diarrhea. Clinical signs are often severe and chronic because many clients pay little attention to their pet's elimination habits.

Physical Examination Findings

A lean body condition and poor hair coat may be evident on physical examination. Some animals are depressed and dehydrated. Abdominal palpation reveals a distended colon. Rectal examination reveals hard feces at the pelvic inlet.

Radiography/Ultrasonography

Abdominal radiographs demonstrate a distended colon impacted with fecal material. Radiographs should be performed to rule out obstructive diseases (i.e., pelvic fracture malunions, sacrocaudal spinal trauma or deformities, and intramural or mural colonic or rectoanal obstructive lesions; Fig. 16-109).

Laboratory Findings

Nonspecific changes in the CBC and biochemistry profile may be evident. Histologic examination of colons removed from most cats with idiopathic megacolon usually reveals normal colonic wall ganglion cells.

DIFFERENTIAL DIAGNOSIS

Idiopathic megacolon must be differentiated from congenital, obstructive, neurologic, and systemic causes of megacolon. Causes of constipation include drugs (e.g., opiates, anticholinergics, barium), severe dehydration, environmental changes, perianal pain (e.g., from perineal hernia), inappropriate diet, perineal hernia, colorectal masses or strictures, hypercalcemia, hypokalemia, hypothyroidism, and spinal cord or nerve damage.

MEDICAL MANAGEMENT

Constipation is difficult to treat once megacolon develops; however, medical management should be attempted before colectomy. Initial management includes correction of hydration, electrolyte, and acid-base abnormalities in severely affected animals. The colon should be evacuated with stool softeners, enemas, and/or digital evacuation. General anesthesia is typically required for digital evacuation. Mucosal damage may occur with evacuation; therefore, antibiotics may be indicated to protect against systemic absorption of bacteria and toxins. To control constipation, long-term high-fiber diets, stool softeners, bulk laxatives, and enemas are needed. Osmotic laxatives (e.g., lactulose or ice cream, or milk in some cats; Table 16-63) and prokinetic drugs (i.e., cisapride) may help prevent recurrence once the colon is evacuated by enemas. If recurrent obstipation necessitates frequent fecal extraction, surgery may be indicated. Some owners find medical therapy intolerable and opt for euthanasia if surgery is not available.

SURGICAL TREATMENT

Surgery for megacolon entails removing all of the colon except a short distal segment needed to reestablish intestinal continuity. Megacolon secondary to pelvic fracture malunion should be treated with subtotal colectomy, pelvic reconstruction, or both. Pelvic reconstruction involves partial pelvectomy and bone repositioning to widen the pelvic canal. Pelvic reconstruction is recommended before irreversible myoneural damage has occurred secondary to chronic colonic distention. Reconstruction should be performed as soon as pelvic narrowing and constipation/obstipation are diagnosed. Signs of obstruction are generally eliminated if the pelvic canal is widened within 6 months of the injury; however, reconstruction alone may not alleviate clinical signs if megacolon is severe. A subtotal colectomy in addition to a pelvectomy may be necessary to alleviate signs

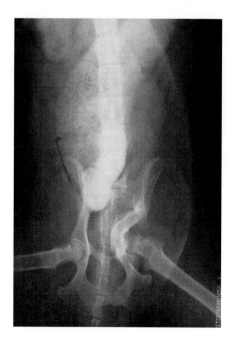

FIG. 16-109
Radiograph of a dog with megacolon secondary to malunion of pelvic fractures and narrowing of the pelvic canal.

TABLE 16-63
Drugs Used for Constipation in Dogs and Cats
Lactulose (Chronulac)
Dogs
1 ml/4.5 kg PO, TID to effect
Cats
5 ml/cat PO, TID
Cisapride (Propulsid)
Dogs
0.25-0.5 mg/kg PO, BID to TID
Cats
2.5-5 mg/cat PO, BID to TID

in these patients. Care should be taken during pelvectomy to protect adjacent soft tissue structures (i.e., urethra, rectum, blood vessels, and nerves). After colectomy the small intestine adapts by increasing stool capacity and water absorption.

Preoperative Management

Preoperative intestinal preparation using multiple enemas to evacuate the large colon is ineffective and unnecessary. Prophylactic antibiotics effective against aerobic and anaerobic colonic bacteria should be given (see p. 320).

Anesthesia

General anesthetic recommendations for large intestinal surgery are given on p. 320.

Surgical Anatomy

Surgical anatomy of the large intestine is provided on p. 320.

Positioning

The animal should be positioned in dorsal recumbency with the entire ventral abdomen clipped and prepared for aseptic surgery. The prepped area should extend caudal to the pubic brim.

SURGICAL TECHNIQUE
Subtotal Colectomy

Explore the abdomen and biopsy abnormal tissues. Isolate the distal small intestine, cecum, and colon from the remainder of the abdomen with several moistened laparotomy pads. Identify resection sites at the distal jejunum or proximal ileum and distal 1 to 2 cm of colon. Choose sites that will allow apposition without tension. Ligate and transect branches of the ileal artery and vein, ileocolic artery and vein, caudal mesenteric artery and vein, and cranial rectal artery and vein (see Fig. 16-104). An alternative procedure is to preserve the ileocolic sphincter; however, it is more difficult to achieve a tension-free apposition if the ileocolic sphincter is preserved. Ileocolic anastomosis is technically easier and allows removal of more colon. *If the ileocolic valve is preserved, ligate the right colic, middle colic, and caudal mesenteric vessels. If the ileum is partially or completely removed, also ligate the ileocolic and terminal ileal arcadial vessels.*

☞ **N O T E** · Do not ligate the cranial rectal artery in dogs. Instead ligate the left colic artery and vasa recta from the cranial rectal artery.

Milk feces into the dilated colon, which will be resected. Place intestinal forceps proximal and distal to the planned resection site. Resect the dilated colon at its junction with the small intestine or just distal to the cecum. Perform an end-to-end anastomosis with either a circular stapler or sutures. Correct for luminal size disparity when performing a suture anastomosis by altering the angle of transection (oblique angles on small lumens and perpendicular angles

on large lumens) using unequal suture spacing (further apart on the large lumen) and/or resecting an antimesenteric wedge from the intestine (see p. 300).

If a staple technique is used, place purse-string sutures at each colonic end before resection. Insert the stapler into the colon transanally or through an antimesenteric incision in the cecum or colon. Transanal introduction of the stapler may not be possible in all cats because of their small anus and narrow pelvic canal. *Lavage the anastomotic site and close the mesenteric defect. Remove laparotomy pads, lavage the abdomen, and place omentum over the surgical site.*

SUTURE MATERIALS/ SPECIAL INSTRUMENTS

Instruments for large intestinal surgery are discussed on p. 303. Polydioxanone or polyglyconate (3-0 or 4-0) are preferred sutures for colectomy; however, nonabsorbable (e.g., nylon or polypropylene) sutures may be used in debilitated or hypoalbuminemic animals.

POSTOPERATIVE CARE AND ASSESSMENT

Hydration should be maintained with intravenous or subcutaneous fluids for 1 to 3 days after surgery, and analgesics should be given as necessary. Prophylactic antibiotics should be continued if gross abdominal contamination occurred or if the patient is extremely debilitated. Patients should be monitored frequently for signs of anastomotic leakage. Food may be offered within 24 hours of surgery, although anorexia may persist for 5 or more days. Diazepam or cyproheptadine (Table 16-64) may be used to stimulate eating in some cats. It may be necessary to keep animals on a low-volume, high-caloric diet for 10 to 14 days. Liquid, tarry feces and tenesmus should be expected immediately after surgery. The character of the feces changes gradually from diarrhea to soft, formed stool in 80% of cats by 6 weeks after surgery. Semiformed stools and, rarely, diarrhea persist in some cats. The frequency of defecation is usually increased (30% to 50%) compared with normal cats; however, most cats are continent. The litter pan should be kept clean to encourage defecation.

COMPLICATIONS

Leakage, dehiscence, peritonitis, ischemic necrosis, stricture, and abscess formation are potential complications of subtotal colectomy. Sometimes diarrhea persists and other times constipation recurs. Persistent diarrhea may be the result of

TABLE 16-64

Appetite Stimulants in Cats

Diazepam (Valium)
0.5 mg/cat IV

Cyproheptadine (Periactin)
2.0 mg/cat PO, BID

small intestinal bacterial overgrowth or hypersecretion, or it may be bile-salt and fatty-acid mediated. Treatment for persistent diarrhea includes antidiarrheal agents, a low-fat diet, oral antibiotics, and bile salt binding agents. Constipation after subtotal colectomy is easily controlled by dietary management, stool softeners, and occasionally manual extraction.

PROGNOSIS

Long-term results of subtotal colectomy for idiopathic megacolon in cats are usually good to excellent. The prognosis is fair to guarded without surgery. Medical management of chronic constipation is possible; however, the frequency of enemas and the need for manual evacuation often become intolerable, prompting euthanasia. Dogs may not do as well with subtotal colectomy as cats.

Reference

de Haan JJ, Ellison GW, Bellah JR: Surgical correction of idiopathic megacolon in cats, *Feline Pract* 20:6, 1992.

Suggested Reading

Bertoy RW et al: Total colectomy with ileorectal anastomosis in the cat, *Vet Surg* 18:204, 1989.

Gregory CR et al: Enteric function in cats after subtotal colectomy for treatment of megacolon, *Vet Surg* 19:216, 1990.

Kudish M, Pavletic MM: Subtotal colectomy with surgical stapling instruments via a trans-cecal approach for treatment of acquired megacolon in cats, *Vet Surg* 22:457, 1993.

Matthiesen DT, Scavelli TD, Whitney WO: Subtotal colectomy for the treatment of obstipation secondary to pelvic fracture malunion in cats, *Vet Surg* 20:113, 1991.

Rosin E et al: Subtotal colectomy for treatment of chronic constipation associated with idiopathic megacolon in cats: 38 cases (1979–1985), *J Am Vet Med Assoc* 193:850, 1988.

Schrader SC: Pelvic osteotomy as a treatment for obstipation in cats with acquired stenosis of the pelvic canal: six cases (1978–1989), *J Am Vet Med Assoc* 200:208, 1992.

Surgery of the Perineum, Rectum, and Anus

GENERAL PRINCIPLES AND TECHNIQUES

DEFINITIONS

Rectal resection is removal of a portion of the terminal large intestine. **Rectal pull-through** is resection of the terminal colon and/or mid-rectum using an anal approach, with or without an abdominal approach. **Anal sacculectomy** is removal of the anal sac(s).

PREOPERATIVE CONCERNS

Rectal surgery is usually performed to resect masses or non-functional bowel and to repair rectal prolapse, perforations,

or fistulae (Table 16-65). Perineal surgery is most often performed to treat perineal hernias, perianal fistulae, anal sac disease, tumors, rectovaginal or rectourethral fistulae, and other traumatic or congenital anomalies (e.g., atresia ani, anovaginal cleft). Scooting, anal licking, constipation, tenesmus, and dyschezia are typical presenting complaints associated with perineal and rectal disease (Table 16-66). Fresh blood may be seen in the feces or perianal region. Perianal tumors and perineal fistulae often cause perianal thickening and ulceration, whereas perineal swelling is usually associated with perineal hernias. Pelvic sacroiliac fractures/separations occasionally cause rectal perforation (less than 1%). Fresh blood and omentum may be found during rectal examination in animals with rectal laceration or perforation.

Diagnosis of rectal, perianal, or perineal disease is primarily based on history, clinical signs, physical examination, imaging (i.e., radiology, ultrasound, computed tomography [CT scan], magnetic resonance imaging [MRI]), endoscopy, and histopathology. Suspected impaired anorectal innervation necessitates myelographic, manometric, and electrodiagnostic evaluations. Many conditions can be diagnosed on physical examination and a thorough rectal examination is crucial (Table 16-67). Anesthesia may be required for adequate rectal examination of animals with pain. Visual inspection of the perineum may reveal unilateral or bilateral swelling, perianal masses, ulceration, fistulae, fecal soiling, or prolapsed mucosa.

Results of complete blood counts (CBC) and serum biochemistry tests are nonspecific. Neoplastic masses may be associated with hypercalcemia, anemia, and other paraneoplastic syndromes. Azotemia plus or minus hyperkalemia may occur with bladder entrapment secondary to perineal hernia. Hypercalcemia is common with some anal sac tumors (see p. 344) and may be reduced preoperatively with fluids and diuretics (see p. 346).

Rectal and perineal radiographs may confirm physical examination findings. If possible, the colon and rectum should be evacuated with enemas, laxatives, and/or cathartics before radiographic studies. The rectum should be evaluated for size, location, and masses. Enlarged sublumbar lymph nodes suggest metastasis. The prostate may be enlarged and malpositioned. The urinary bladder may be identified within a perineal hernia. A perforated rectum may allow gas in the perineal, intrapelvic or caudal retroperitoneal soft tissues, or peritoneal cavity. Gastrointestinal barium studies (enema or oral), urethrograms, and cystograms sometimes help evaluate

---

TABLE 16-65

Potential Indications for Rectal, Anal, and Perineal Surgery

• Diagnostic biopsy	• Perianal fistulae
• Anal sac disease	• Rectal ischemia
• Colonic obstruction	• Rectal prolapse
• Perineal hernia	• Neoplasia
• Rectal perforation	• Fecal incontinence

TABLE 16-66

Clinical Signs of Rectal, Anal, and Perineal Disease

	Anal Tumor	Anal Sacculitis	Perineal Hernia	Perianal Fistula	Rectal Prolapse	Fecal Incontinence
Anal Biting/Scooting	+	+	−	+	±	−
Anal Licking	+	+	−	+	±	−
Tenesmus	+	+	+	+	+	±
Thickening/Swelling	+	+	+	+	±	±
Constipation/Obstipation	±	±	+	±	±	±
Diarrhea	−	±	−	±	±	±
Hemorrhage/Hematochezia	+	+	−	±	±	±
Mass	+	±	+	−	+	−
Pain/Dyschezia	+	+	+	+	+	−
Ulceration/Fistula	±	±	−	+	±	±
Pelvic diaphragm weakness	−	−	+	−	±	±
Decreased Anal Tone	−	−	−	±	±	±
Fecal Incontinence	−	−	±	±	±	+
Stricture	±	−	−	±	±	±
Abnormal Discharge	−	+	−	+	−	−
Febrile	−	±	−	±	−	−
Inflammation	±	+	±	+	±	±
Rectal Prolapse	−	−	±	−	+	−
Other	± hypercalcemia	dermatitis, odor, tail chasing	shock, uremia, stranguria, vomiting	odor, ↓ weight, ↓ appetite, lethargy, poor hair coat		self-trauma, hyper- or paraesthesia

TABLE 16-67

Abnormalities That May Be Noted During Rectal Examination

- Masses
- Strictures
- Perianal thickening
- Anal sac enlargement
- Pain
- Reduced sphincter tone
- Pelvic diaphragm weakness
- Rectal deviation or sacculation
- Sublumbar lymph node enlargement
- Prostatomegaly
- Pelvic canal distortion
- Thickening or irregularity of rectal mucosa

patients with perineal hernias. In human beings, ultrasonography using a rectal probe is more accurate than a CT scan or MRI evaluation of rectal wall thickness and tumor depth (Sentovich et al, 1992). Ultrasound guided biopsies and aspi-

rates can be collected from rectal masses. Proctoscopy helps define rectal disease, but should be combined with colonoscopy because tumors and inflammatory disease may also affect the colon (see p. 327). Samples should be collected for culture, cytology, and biopsy. Normal tissue should be biopsied in addition to thickened folds, masses, strictures, or ulcers. Perforation is an uncommon complication of proctoscopy.

Preoperative patient preparation is similar to that used before colon surgery (see p. 320). Warm compresses should be applied to inflamed or infected areas 2 to 3 times daily, and stool softeners should be used if surgery is delayed (see Table 16-61). The location of fistulae and tumors should be mapped before surgery. Unless the colon is perforated or obstructed, mechanical emptying and cleansing help reduce bacterial numbers. Rectal perforation should be corrected as soon as it is diagnosed. Minimally, all patients should have their terminal rectum digitally evacuated while under anesthesia, just before surgery. For some surgeries (e.g., extensive rectal resection), more complete patient preparation is necessary. If possible an elemental diet or a low residue diet (e.g., hamburger and white rice) should be fed for 2 to 3 days before surgery. Food should be withheld 24 hours before surgery in adult patients (4 to 8 hours in pediatric patients), but free access to water should be allowed. Bisacodyl, a stimulant laxative, facilitates colonic evacuation (see Table 16-56). Laxatives, cathartics, and warm water enemas should be given 24 hours before surgery (see Table 16-61). Colyte or GoLytely should be administered orally by stomach tube 24 hours and 18 to 20 hours before surgery. Although these colonic lavage solutions work well, enemas facilitate complete cleansing. A warm water enema should be given the day before surgery and a 10% povidone-iodine enema given 3 hours before surgery. Patients with perianal disease may be in too much pain to allow preoperative enemas. Furthermore, enemas may cause perforation or trauma, further deteriorating debilitated, anorexic patients. Enemas given any closer to surgery than 3 hours are contraindicated because they liquefy intestinal contents and may promote dissemination of contaminated material during surgery. After large bowel evacuation using laxatives, cathartics, and/or enemas, feces may remain in a deviated or dilated rectal area and should be removed manually.

After anesthetic induction, a urinary catheter should be placed to aid intraoperative identification of the urethra, the rectum should be manually cleaned (if necessary), and the anal sacs expressed. The entire perineum (from dorsal to the tail head and including the ventral tail) should be clipped and aseptically prepared for surgery. If a celiotomy is planned, the ventral abdomen should also be clipped and prepared for aseptic surgery.

ANESTHETIC CONSIDERATIONS

Anesthetic complications may arise from uncorrected hydration, electrolyte, or acid-base abnormalities. Nitrous oxide increases the volume of air trapped in body viscera and should be avoided in patients with intestinal obstruction. Atropine or glycopyrrolate (Table 16-68) may prevent bradycardia induced by visceral manipulation. Water evaporates from exposed abdominal viscera at an increased rate; therefore fluid administration should be increased to replace this loss. Hypothermia occurs because of vasodilation and visceral exposure, reducing the need for anesthetics. These patients should be kept dry and warm. Opioid premedicants (e.g., butorphanol, oxymorphone, or buprenorphine) may also provide pre- and postoperative analgesia. Ketamine gives poor visceral analgesia and should not be used alone for surgical procedures. It is also contraindicated in cats with renal dysfunction.

If there are no contraindications (e.g., sepsis, bleeding diatheses, hypovolemia [for epidurals using local anesthetics]), epidurals (see Chapter 12) may be used in dogs to supplement general anesthesia. It is rare that epidural anesthesia alone is sufficient for surgery. If general anesthesia is not used, heavy sedation (i.e., oxymorphone) is needed. Epidural doses should be decreased if a spinal has been inadvertently performed, if the patient is pregnant or obese, or if there are space-occupying vertebral canal lesions. Opioids may be pre-

TABLE 16-68
Selected Anesthetic Protocols for Use in Animals Undergoing Perineal, Rectal, or Anal Surgery
Dogs
Premedication
Atropine (0.02-0.04 mg/kg IV, IM, SC) or glycopyrrolate (0.005-0.011 mg/kg IV, IM, SC) plus butorphanol (0.2-0.4 mg/kg SC or IM) or buprenorphine (5-15 µg/kg IM) or oxymorphone (0.05-0.1 mg/kg SC or IM)
Induction
Thiopental (10-12 mg/kg) or propofol (4-6 mg/kg) administered IV to effect
Maintenance
Isoflurane or halothane
Cats
Premedication
Atropine (0.02-0.04 mg/kg IV, IM, SC) or glycopyrrolate (0.005-0.011 mg/kg IV, IM, SC) plus ketamine (5mg/kg IM) plus butorphanol (0.2-0.4 mg/kg SC, IM)
Induction
Diazepam (0.27 mg/kg) plus ketamine (5.5 mg/kg) combined and administered IV to effect *or* thiopental (10-12 mg/kg) or propofol (4-6 mg/kg) administered IV to effect or mask or chamber induction
Maintenance
Isoflurane or halothane

ferred over local anesthetic drugs in epidurals because opioids cause sensory loss without motor block and do not promote hypotension. Because local anesthetics in epidurals may cause hypotension, dehydration should be corrected before performing the procedure.

ANTIBIOTICS

There is a high risk of infection after colorectal surgery. Although controversial, the use of antibiotics in colorectal surgery reduces morbidity and mortality associated with infection. Systemic perioperative antibiotics effective against gram-negative aerobes and anaerobes should be given (see Table 16-57). Recommended drugs include second generation cephalosporins (i.e., cefmetazole, cefoxitin, cefotetan) given at the time of induction. Third generation cephalosporins effective against gram-positive and gram-negative aerobes and some anaerobes are available, albeit expensive. Gentamicin plus cefazolin can be given intravenously at induction. Aminoglycosides (i.e., neomycin, kanamycin) and metronidazole can be given orally in combination beginning 24 hours before surgery.

Metronidazole is absorbed from the gastrointestinal tract and is effective against anaerobes. Aminoglycosides are only effective against aerobic bacteria. Gastrointestinal absorption of aminoglycosides is minimal in normal patients, but can be substantial if the bowel is eroded or inflamed. The use of such nonabsorbable antibiotics has been linked with the emergence of resistant infections. A combination of neomycin and erythromycin can be given beginning 24 hours before surgery to rapidly reduce aerobes and anaerobes. Metronidazole combined with first generation cephalosporins (cefazolin), aminoglycosides, or trimethoprim-sulfa is also useful (see Table 16-57).

SURGICAL ANATOMY

The rectum is the segment of large intestine coursing through the pelvic canal and ending at the anus. The colorectal junction is difficult to identify. Landmarks used to estimate the location of the colorectal junction include the pubic brim, pelvic inlet, seventh lumbar vertebra, and seromuscular penetration point of the cranial rectal artery. The cranial rectum is attached to the sacrum by the mesorectum. The mesorectum does not cover the entire rectum; the terminal rectum is retroperitoneal. At the level of the second caudal vertebra the mesorectum reflects onto the sides of the pelvis as parietal peritoneum, forming a pararectal fossa on each side. The peritoneal reflection is cranial to the rectococcygeus muscles and contains the autonomic nerve fibers of the pelvic plexus that innervate the rectum. The pelvic plexus is paired, composed of parasympathetic pelvic and sympathetic hypogastric nerves, and lies dorsal to the prostate in males (see p. 487). The caudal part of the rectum is supported by the levator ani muscles medially and coccygeus muscles laterally. The external anal sphincter muscle demarcates the caudal limit of the rectum.

The anal canal is a continuation of the rectum to the anus and is only 1 to 2 centimeters long. It is divided into three zones: (1) columnar, (2) intermediate, and (3) cutaneous. The innermost zone (columnar) has a series of longitudinal mucosal and submucosal ridges called anal columns or pillars. The pockets between these columns are the anal sinuses, which extend caudally and end in blind pouches under the anocutaneous line. The length of the columnar zone varies from 3 to 25 mm. The intermediate zone is usually less than 1 to 2 mm wide but forms a distinct, raised, circumferential ridge called the *anocutaneous line.* Anal glands are found in the columnar and intermediate zones. The cutaneous zone is outermost and has very fine hairs but appears as hairless skin. Sebaceous, circumanal, and apocrine sweat glands are only found in the cutaneous zone. The anus is the external opening of the anal canal.

The cranial rectal artery is a branch of the caudal mesenteric artery and is the major blood supply to the rectum. Blood supply from the middle rectal artery (from the internal pudendal branch of the internal iliac artery) and caudal rectal artery (from the middle caudal branch of the median sacral artery or from the internal pudendal branch of the internal iliac artery) are variable and relatively insignificant. To ensure adequate anastomotic blood supply, it is recommended that the cranial rectal artery in dogs be preserved unless the intrapelvic rectum is resected (Goldsmid et al, 1993). Lymphatics from the anal canal and rectum drain cranially into the medial iliac lymph node.

The internal and external sphincter muscles surround the terminal rectum and anal canal to control defecation. The anal sacs lie between these two muscles on each side of the anus (see p. 350). The internal anal sphincter is a caudal thickening of the circular smooth muscle lining the anal canal. It is an involuntary, smooth muscle that works with other muscles of defecation to prevent indiscriminate defecation. It is innervated by the parasympathetic branches of the pelvic nerve (S_{1-3}), which are inhibitory. Motor fibers from the hypogastric nerves are sympathetic to the internal anal sphincter. The external anal sphincter is a large, circumferential band of skeletal (striated) muscle chiefly responsible for fecal continence. It is wider dorsally than ventrally where its fibers decussate and spread to insert on the urethra and bulbospongiosus muscle. The only voluntary nerve supply to the external anal sphincter comes from the caudal rectal branches of the pudendal nerves. The blood supply to the external anal sphincter is from the perineal arteries. See p. 354 for surgical anatomy of the pelvic diaphragm.

SURGICAL TECHNIQUES

For optimal healing, a monofilament, synthetic absorbable suture (e.g., polydioxanone, polyglyconate) and approximating suture patterns (i.e., simple interrupted, Gambee, crushing, or simple continuous) should be used for rectoanal surgery. A monofilament, nonabsorbable suture (e.g., polypropylene or nylon) or absorbable suture material (e.g., polydioxanone or polyglyconate) may be used for herniorrhaphy. Fecal incontinence usually occurs if more than 4 cm or the final 1.5 cm of the terminal rectum are resected, if the perineal nerves are damaged, or if more than half the external anal sphincter is damaged.

☞ **N O T E** • Be sure to engage the submucosa in all sutures.

Rectal Resection

The primary indication for rectal resection is to excise a neoplastic, necrotic, traumatized (e.g., prolapse, fistula, or diverticulum), or strictured segment of rectum. Other indications include congenital anomalies and perforations or lacerations. The rectum may be exposed using a ventral, dorsal, rectal pull-through, lateral, or anal approach. The diseased rectum is resected and the remaining rectum reapposed to the rectum, colon, or ileum using techniques described for colectomy on p. 323.

Ventral approach. Lesions at the colorectal junction are resected using this approach. A ventral approach to the rectum must be accompanied by a pubic symphysiotomy or pubic osteotomy (Fig. 16-110; also see p. 488) to gain access to the pelvic canal. Pubic symphysiotomy provides more limited exposure than pubic osteotomy. *For pubic symphysiotomy, incise the entire length of the adductor aponeurosis. Divide the pubis and ischium on the midline with an osteotome and mallet or an oscillating saw. Separate the*

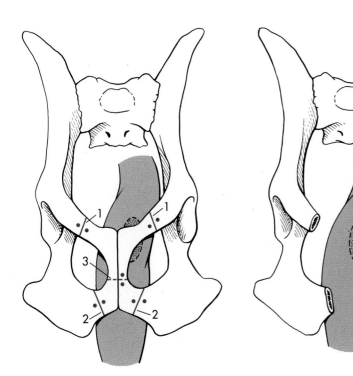

FIG. 16-110
For a ventral rectal approach extend the ventral celiotomy incision over the symphysis of the pelvis. Incise and elevate the aponeurosis of the adductor and gracilis muscles. Predrill holes on each side of proposed osteotomy sites. Perform a pubic osteotomy at sites 1 and 2 to expose the entire intrapelvic rectum. Perform an osteotomy at sites 1 and 3 if exposure of the caudal intrapelvic rectum is unnecessary.

pubis and ischium with a self-retaining retractor (e.g., pediatric Finochietto).

Anal approach. An anal approach is suitable for excision of small, noninvasive, pedunculated polyps and broad-based rectal masses that can be exteriorized through the anus. Lesions involving the caudal rectum or anal canal can be exteriorized using this approach. Perforations of the terminal rectum may be apposed through this approach, although a lateral approach (see below) allows lavage and drainage of contaminated adjacent tissues. The mucocutaneous junction and skin must be resected if they are diseased but fecal incontinence is a common sequela. *With the patient in ventral recumbency, dilate the anus with three or four stay sutures placed through the mucocutaneous junction (Figs.16-111, A and B). Evert the rectal wall by placing stay sutures (e.g., 3-0 nylon or other monofilament suture) in the rectal mucosa cranial or caudal to the mass/lesion and applying caudal traction. Place additional stay sutures to further retract the mass/lesion if necessary (Fig. 16-111, C). Use electrosurgery, laser, or scalpel incisions to remove masses. Make a partial or full-thickness incision, depending on malignancy and need for wide borders. Appose cut edges with simple interrupted sutures (e.g., 3-0 or 4-0 polydioxanone or polyglyconate; Fig. 16-111, D). Remove the stay sutures and allow the surgical site to retract within the pelvic canal.*

Rectal pull-through approach. The primary indication for performing a rectal pull-through is to resect a distal colonic or mid-rectal lesion not approachable through the abdomen and too large or cranial for an anal approach. *Position the animal in ventral recumbency with the hindquarters elevated. Evert the rectum with stay sutures placed cranial to the mucocutaneous junction (1.5 cm or more if possible; Fig. 16-112, A). Using the stay sutures, apply caudal traction to the cranial rectum. Begin a full-thickness 360-degree incision through the rectum, leaving a 1.5-cm cuff of nondiseased rectal wall attached to the anus if possible. Place three or four stay sutures in the rectal cuff. Mobilize the rectum by bluntly dissecting along the external wall (Fig. 16-112, B). Continue dissection as far cranially as the cranial rectal artery if necessary.* If dissection occurs cranial to the second caudal vertebrae, the peritoneal cavity will be entered. *Ligate or coagulate rectal vessels as they are encountered. Split the rectum longitudinally until normal tissue is identified if the lesion is diffuse (Fig. 16-112, C). Transect the diseased rectum in stages with 1 to 2 cm of normal tissue at each end. Transect one fourth to one third of the circumference and then appose the cranial end of the rectum to the caudal rectal cuff with simple interrupted sutures (e.g., 3-0 or 4-0 polydioxanone or polyglyconate; Fig. 16-112, D). Continue transecting and apposing until all diseased tissue has been excised.* Some surgeons prefer a two-layer closure: first appose the seromuscular layer and then the mucosa/submucosal layer.

A Swenson's pull-through is performed when disease extends into the colon. *For this procedure position the patient in dorsal recumbency so both a ventral abdominal and anal approach may be used. Transect the colon proximal to the mass. Oversew the ends of the colon and rectum.* Linear cutting or transverse stapling instruments may be used to reappose the colon and rectum. *Ligate vessels supplying the distal colon and rectum (see p. 324). Place stay sutures through the end of the remaining colon or ileum and rectum. Grasp the sutures with transanally placed forceps and evert the rectum through the anus. Advance colon or ileum through the pelvic canal with stay sutures. Resect*

FIG. 16-111
For an anal approach to the rectum **A,** position the patient in a perineal position. **B,** Place stay sutures around the anus to dilate it and expose the lesion. **C,** Place additional stay sutures near the lesion and apply caudal traction to exteriorize it. **D,** Resect the mass and suture the defect.

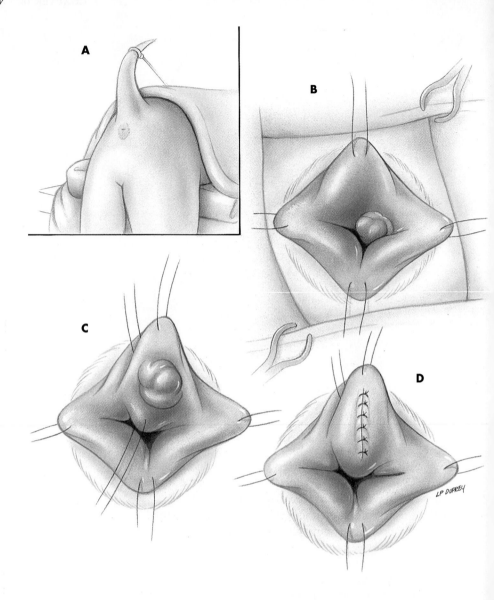

the lesion and anastomose the end of the colon or ileum to the terminal rectum as described above. Gently replace the intestine into the pelvic canal.

Dorsal approach. A dorsal approach is used if the lesion involves the caudal or middle rectum and not the anal canal. *Position the patient in ventral recumbency with the pelvis elevated and the tail fixed over the back. Pad the cranial aspect of the hindlimbs to prevent pressure on the femoral nerves. Make a curvilinear incision from one ischiatic tuberosity to the other curving dorsal to the anus (Fig. 16-113, A). Incise subcutaneous fat and perineal fascia. Locate the rectum, external anal sphincter, levator ani, and coccygeus muscles laterally and the rectococcygeus muscles dorsally. Transect the paired rectococcygeus muscles near their origin on the rectal wall or insertion on the caudal vertebrae (Fig. 16-113, B). Elevate the external anal sphincter and caudal edge of the levator ani to the level of the caudal rectal nerve. Partially transect the levator ani muscles for more cranial rectal resections if necessary. Position a self-retaining retractor (i.e., Gelpi or Weitlaner) to* improve visualization if necessary. Gently retract the rectum caudally and mobilize the rectum cranially to normal bowel. Repair the lacerated rectum or resect the diseased bowel. Ligate or cauterize vessels to the diseased bowel. Place stay sutures in the cranial bowel before transection. Appose the bowel ends with interrupted appositional sutures (e.g., 3-0 or 4-0 polydioxanone or polyglyconate, Fig. 16-113, C) or an end-to-end stapling device (see p. 298). Reappose transected levator ani muscle with appositional cruciate or mattress sutures.* Some surgeons reattach the rectococcygeus muscles and external anal sphincter to the rectus muscle. *Thoroughly lavage the area and place drains if significant contamination has occurred.* Placement of a drain against the anastomotic site may cause dehiscence. *Separately appose the subcutaneous tissue and skin with continuous or interrupted sutures of 3-0 or 4-0 polydioxanone and 3-0 or 4-0 nylon or polypropylene, respectively.*

☞ **N O T E ·** If contamination is severe, consider delayed primary closure.

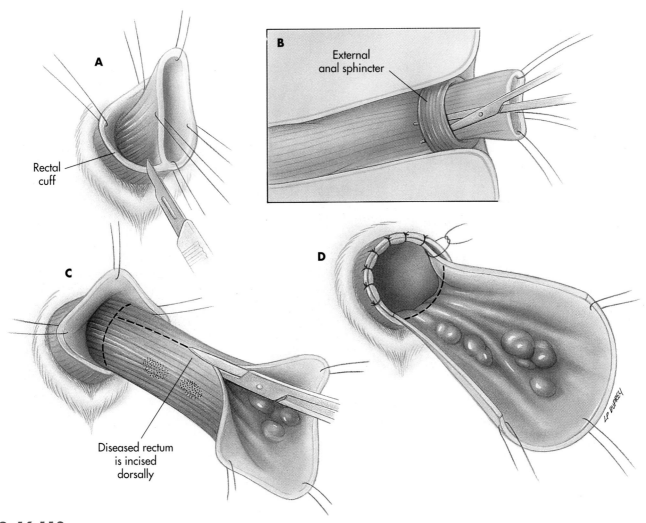

FIG. 16-112
To perform a rectal pull-through **A,** evert the rectal wall through the anus with stay sutures.
B, Make a full-thickness incision through the rectal wall, preserving a 1.5-cm cuff of distal
rectum. Mobilize the rectum by dissecting directly against the rectal wall to separate it from
the external anal sphincter and surrounding tissue. **C,** Pull the mobilized rectum caudally
and incise longitudinally to normal tissue. **D,** Appose the cut edge of the normal cranial
rectum to the preserved rectal cuff with simple interrupted sutures.

Lateral approach. The lateral approach limits exposure to one side of the rectum and may be suitable for laceration repair or diverticulum resection. *Make a curvilinear*
incision 2 to 3 cm lateral to the anus, beginning dorsal
to the tail head and extending ventral to the anus
(Fig. 16-114, A). Incise subcutaneous tissues to expose the
pelvic diaphragm. Separate the fascia between the exter-
nal anal sphincter and the levator ani muscle. Preserve the
caudal rectal nerve to the external anal sphincter
(Fig. 16-114, B). Repair the laceration with a one- or two-
layer closure using simple interrupted sutures (e.g., 3-0 or
4-0 polydioxanone or polyglyconate). Thoroughly lavage
the area and place a Penrose or closed suction drain if soft
tissues were contaminated with feces. Resect diverticula
with a linear stapling device. Reappose the external anal
sphincter and levator ani muscles with interrupted apposi-

tional sutures. Place additional sutures between the exter-
nal anal sphincter and internal obturator muscle if this fas-
cial plane is disrupted. Close subcutaneous tissues and skin
routinely.

Anal Sacculectomy

Anal sacculectomy is performed to remove chronically infected or impacted anal sacs, anal sac fistulae, or neoplasia.
Meticulous dissection is required to prevent fecal incontinence by preserving the anal sphincter muscles and nerves. A
closed or open technique may be used. The closed technique
is preferred because the external anal sphincter muscle is not
transected and the lumen of the anal sac remains closed, preventing contact between secretions and adjacent tissues. See
p. 350 for a description of open and closed anal sacculectomy techniques.

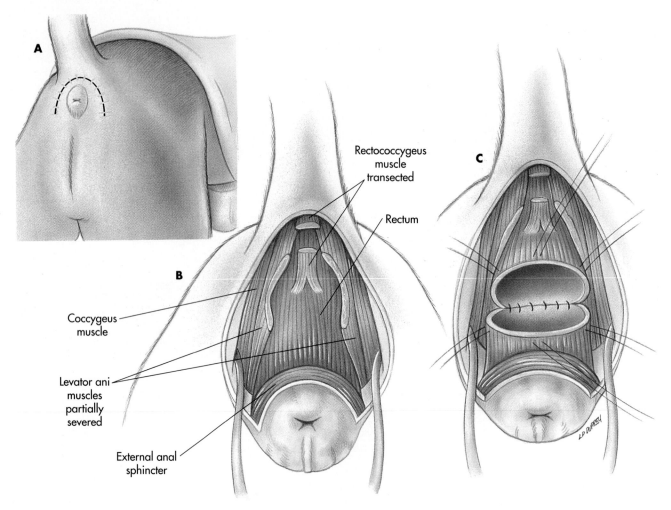

FIG. 16-113
For a dorsal rectal approach **A,** make a curvilinear incision from one ischial tuberosity to the other, curving dorsally to the anus. **B,** Identify the rectococcygeus, levator ani, and coccygeus muscles. **C,** Transect the rectococcygeus muscle and partially incise the levator ani. Resect the diseased rectum and appose the ends with a suture triangulation technique or end-to-end stapling instrument.

☞ **N O T E** · It is wise to perform histologic evaluation to rule out anal sac tumors.

HEALING OF THE RECTUM

Rectal healing is affected by the same factors that affect colonic healing (see p. 324). Optimal healing requires a good blood supply, accurate mucosal apposition, and minimal surgical trauma. Systemic factors that may delay healing and increase the risk of dehiscence include hypovolemia, shock, hypoproteinemia, debilitation, and/or infection.

SUTURE MATERIALS/SPECIAL INSTRUMENTS

In addition to a general pack, abdominal (i.e., Balfour), perineal (e.g., Gelpi), and pelvic (e.g., Finochietto) retractors are recommended to aid in exposing the surgical field. Doyen, Babcock, and Carmalt forceps may be needed to occlude or retract the intestine. Metzenbaum and iris scissors are indi-cated for dissection. Penrose or closed suction drains are used in contaminated areas. Other special instruments or equipment that may be necessary for rectal or perianal surgery include a probe or groove director, fulguration unit, laser unit, silicone elastomer, and surgical stapling equipment.

POSTOPERATIVE CARE AND ASSESSMENT

Postoperative care is individualized for the patient. They should be observed closely during recovery for vomiting. Analgesics (see Table 16-4) should be given as necessary. Hydration should be maintained with intravenous fluids until the animal is eating and drinking normally and electrolyte and acid-base abnormalities have been corrected. Ileus may be minimized by encouraging early ambulation and eating. An Elizabethan collar, bucket, or side-bars should be used to protect the surgical site. Purse-string sutures should be removed immediately or within 2 to 3 days postoperatively. Prophylactic antibiotics can generally be discontinued 2 to 4

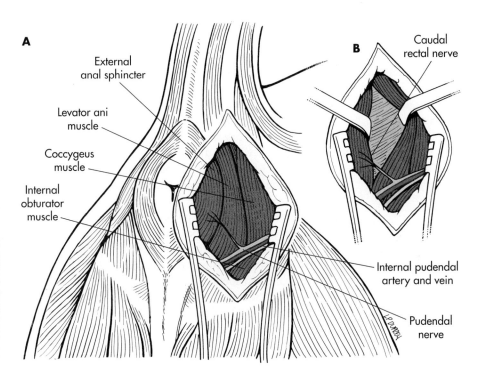

FIG. 16-114
For a lateral rectal approach **A,** make an incision 1 to 2 cm lateral to the anus. **B,** Identify the internal pudendal artery and vein and pudendal nerve crossing the internal obturator muscle. Note the caudal rectal nerve to the external anal sphincter. Separate fascia between the external anal sphincter and levator ani muscles to expose the lateral aspect of the rectum.

A

External anal sphincter

Levator ani muscle

Coccygeus muscle

Internal obturator muscle

B

Caudal rectal nerve

Internal pudendal artery and vein

Pudendal nerve

---

hours postoperatively; however, they should be continued if contamination has occurred (see above under antibiotics).

A stool softener should be given when oral intake begins (see Table 16-61) and continued for 2 weeks, or as needed. If vomiting does not occur, water should be offered 8 to 12 hours postoperatively. After rectal surgery a bland low-fat food (i/d or boiled rice, potatoes and pasta combined with boiled skinless chicken, yogurt, or low fat cottage cheese) should be fed three to four times daily. The patient's normal diet should be gradually reintroduced, beginning 48 to 72 hours after surgery. Patients having perineal surgery may resume their normal diet with the first feeding. Debilitated patients may require enteral or parenteral nutrition.

☞ **NOTE** · Warn owners that rectal, perianal, or perineal disease can cause fecal incontinence.

Warm compresses should be applied two to three times daily for 15 to 20 minutes to minimize postoperative swelling after perianal or perineal surgery. Incisional site redness and pain may indicate early infection. Anal sphincter function, continence, perineal swelling, and drainage should be assessed daily. Color, consistency, and presence or absence of fecal blood should be noted. Increased frequency of defecation may occur after major colorectal resections. Perianal and perineal area surgeries are predisposed to infection because of high bacterial numbers in these areas. Depression, high fever, abdominal tenderness, vomiting, ileus, or perineal inflammation may indicate infection or peritonitis. If peritonitis is suspected, abdominocentesis or diagnostic peritoneal lavage (see p. 198), chemistry profile, and CBC should be performed and antibiotic and fluid therapy initiated. The abdomen should be explored if toxic neutrophils with en-

TABLE 16-69	
Potential Complications of Perianal and Rectal Surgery	
• Infection	• Recurrence
• Dehiscence	• Metastasis
• Tenesmus	• Nerve damage (pudendal,
• Rectal prolapse	sciatic, femoral)
• Dyschezia	• Urethral obstruction
• Hematochezia	• Stranguria
• Temporary or permanent	• Dysuria
incontinence	• Urinary incontinence
• Anal stricture	• Bladder atony
• Flatulence	• Death
• Hemorrhage	

gulfed bacteria or intestinal debris are present. Aggressive treatment of generalized peritonitis by open peritoneal drainage (see p. 198) may be necessary.

COMPLICATIONS

Potential complications after rectoanal, perianal, and perineal surgery are numerous (Table 16-69). Postoperative tenesmus, hematochezia, and fecal incontinence are common. Postoperative tenesmus and hematochezia should resolve in most animals after suture removal or absorption. Incontinence with extensive rectal resection results from loss of rectal afferent nerves or from disruption of the pelvic plexus at the peritoneal reflection. Removal of the distal 1.5 cm of rectum may cause fecal incontinence even if the external anal sphincter is preserved. Fecal incontinence is uncommon when 4 cm or less of the rectum is resected, preserving the terminal rectal cuff. Longer rectal resections (6 cm or longer) disrupt the peritoneal reflection and frequently result in incontinence. Other potential complications include rectal prolapse, perirectal abscesses, dehiscence, and stenosis.

Significant strictures occur more commonly after rectal than colonic resection, probably because of excessive tension at the resection site. They can usually be managed by incision with an electrosurgical tip or laser or by balloon dilation. If these techniques do not alleviate obstruction, surgical resection may be required. Anal stricture is a complication of anal sac disease, perianal fistula, neoplasia, and surgical or nonsurgical trauma. Anal strictures may be treated by anoplasty, balloon dilation, incision with electrosurgery, laser, or scalpel, or resection.

SPECIAL AGE CONSIDERATIONS

Young animals may have congenital abnormalities such as atresia ani or imperforate ani. Neoplasia is more common in older animals.

References

Goldsmid SE et al: Colorectal blood supply in dogs, *Am J Vet Res* 54:1948, 1993.

Sentovich SM et al: Transrectal ultrasound of rectal tumors, *Am J of Surgery* 166:638, 1992.

Suggested Reading

Anderson GI et al: Rectal resection in the dog: a new surgical approach and the evaluation of its effects on fecal continence, *Vet Surg* 16:119, 1987.

Anson LW, Betts CW, Stone EA: A retrospective evaluation of the rectal pull-through technique, *Vet Surg* 17:141, 1988.

Deen KI et al: Anal sphincter defects: correlation between endoanal ultrasound and surgery, *Ann Surg* 218:201, 1993.

McKeown DB et al: Dorsal approach to the caudal pelvic canal and rectum: effect on normal dogs, *Vet Surg* 13:181, 1984.

SPECIFIC DISEASES

ANAL NEOPLASIA

DEFINITION

Perianal glands are modified sebaceous glands.

SYNONYMS

For perianal gland adenomas—**circumanal tumors** and **hepatoid tumors;** for anal sac tumors—**apocrine gland tumors**

GENERAL CONSIDERATIONS AND CLINICALLY RELEVANT PATHOPHYSIOLOGY

The most common perianal tumors are adenomas and carcinomas of the perianal and apocrine glands. Apocrine gland tumors usually involve the anal sacs. Perianal glands are located primarily around the anus and base of the tail; however, they are also found in the thigh, prepuce, and dorsal and ventral midline from the base of the skull to the umbilicus. Perianal tumors may occur at any of these locations. The most common malignant tumors are perianal gland adenocarcinomas and apocrine gland adenocarcinomas. Other common tumors are listed in Table 16-70.

Perianal adenomas are the most common canine perianal tumors (80%). They are the third most frequent tumor in male dogs. They occur 12 times more often in intact males than in intact females and are more common in ovariohysterectomized females than in intact females. They are hormone dependent and usually decrease in size after castration. They may be single or multiple and are usually small, raised, firm, and well circumscribed; however, some are large and ulcerated. Many dogs with perianal adenomas also have testicular interstitial cell tumors (see p. 562).

Perianal gland adenocarcinomas cannot be grossly differentiated from adenomas. They are usually solitary, ulcerated, locally invasive, and can be confused with perianal fistulae or ruptured anal sacs. These tumors are not hormone responsive. Both primary and metastatic sites grow more slowly than many other malignancies. They usually metastasize to the intrapelvic and sublumbar lymph nodes. Other metastatic sites include the liver, lungs, kidney, spleen, bone, and abdominal lymph nodes.

Anal sac apocrine gland adenocarcinomas (anal sac adenocarcinoma, apocrine gland adenocarcinoma) arise in the anal sac. Most patients have unilateral tumors, but bilateral involvement occurs. These tumors can release parathyroid hormone-like activity, causing hypercalcemia, polyuria, and polydipsia. Initially, anal sac adenocarcinomas grow slowly and are confined to the anal sac; however, invasion into surrounding tissues, rectum, and pelvic canal occurs with continued growth. Most show evidence of stromal and lymphatic invasion. Metastasis to the iliac, sacral, and sublumbar lymph nodes may occur. Distant metastasis may develop in any organ although the lung, liver, and spleen are the most common sites.

☞ **N O T E ·** Suspect perianal gland adenomas in male dogs. Suspect anal sac adenocarcinomas in intact female dogs, particularly if the dog is hypercalcemic.

TABLE 16-70

Common Tumors of the Perianal Region

- Perianal gland adenoma
- Perianal gland adenocarcinoma
- Apocrine gland adenocarcinoma
- Lipoma
- Leiomyoma
- Squamous cell carcinoma
- Melanoma
- Lymphoma
- Mast cell tumor
- Miscellaneous skin tumors

Anal squamous cell carcinomas arise from the anocutaneous line. They are typically malignant and metastasize quickly. Extensive fistula or mucosal-cutaneous ulcer-like lesions occur and are often covered with mucus. Anal function is impaired, and pain, tenesmus, and hemorrhage are typical. The prognosis is grave because of their malignant nature. Treatment is often discouraged.

DIAGNOSIS
Clinical Presentation

Signalment. Perianal tumors are common in middle-aged and older male dogs, but rare in females. The mean age for anal sac apocrine gland adenocarcinoma is 10.8 years (Ross et al, 1991). Adenomas are more prevalent in cocker spaniels, beagles, bulldogs, and Samoyeds. Cats do not have perianal/circumanal glands. Apocrine gland adenocarcinomas usually occur in dogs; especially old, ovariohysterectomized females.

History. Tumors in the perianal region cause irritation with subsequent licking, scooting, and tenesmus. Continued tumor growth or excoriation of the thin perianal skin causes mild hemorrhage, which may be noted in the feces or where the animal sits. Constipation, obstipation, and dyschezia may occur with large, invasive tumors. Some tumors are asymptomatic and found incidentally on physical examination. Benign tumors are usually slow growing and non-painful. Malignant tumors are usually fast growing, firm, invasive, and are commonly ulcerated. Perianal tumors in castrated males should be considered malignant until proven otherwise. Paraneoplastic hypercalcemia is common with anal sac adenocarcinomas (Table 16-71). Fecal incontinence may occur with aggressive tumors. Other signs potentially associated with metastatic lesions include chronic cough, limb edema, and urethral and rectal obstruction.

Physical Examination Findings

Multiple perianal masses are often identified around the circumference of the anus in the hairless area. They may be of variable size, covered with epithelium or ulcerated, friable, and broad-based (Fig. 16-115). Most adenomas are well circumscribed, whereas carcinomas are invasive. Careful palpation of the perianal tissues during rectal examination often identifies masses that are difficult to visually differentiate from normal perianal tissue. Anal sac tumors are not always obvious when the anal sacs are palpated.

TABLE 16-71
Signs of Hypercalcemia
• Anorexia
• Weight loss
• Vomiting
• Polyuria
• Polydipsia
• Muscle weakness
• Constipation

☞ N O T E · Check the sublumbar and other regional lymph nodes for enlargement and asymmetry.

Radiography/Ultrasonography

Radiographs of the abdomen and thorax help stage the disease. Enlarged sublumbar lymph nodes suggest metastasis. Abdominal ultrasonography allows lymph node evaluation.

Laboratory Findings

Cytology helps, but histology is necessary to differentiate perianal adenomas from carcinomas. However, it can be difficult to distinguish benign and malignant tumors, even with histopathology. Anal sac tumors often cause hypercalcemia and renal dysfunction. Some hypercalcemic patients are also hypophosphatemic.

DIFFERENTIAL DIAGNOSIS

Differential diagnoses of anal and perianal irritation include anal sacculitis, dermatitis, endoparasites, perianal fistula, or tumors. Differential diagnoses for perianal swelling include perineal hernia, perianal neoplasia, perianal gland

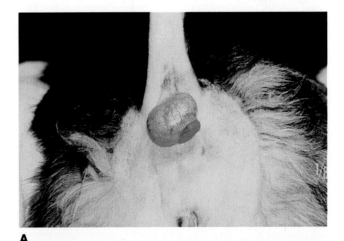
A

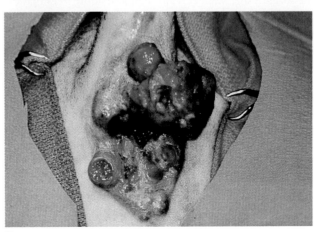
B

FIG. 16-115
Perianal tumors. **A,** A single tumor with intact epithelium. **B,** Multiple ulcerated perianal tumors.

hyperplasia, anal sacculitis, anal sac neoplasia, atresia ani, rectal pythiosis, and vaginal tumors. Differential diagnoses for dyschezia include rectal foreign body, perineal hernia, perianal fistula, anal stricture, rectal stricture, anal sac abscess, rectal or anal neoplasia, anal trauma, anal dermatitis, anorectal prolapse, inflammatory bowel disease, histoplasmosis, and pythiosis.

MEDICAL TREATMENT

Some perianal tumors respond to chemotherapy or radiation therapy, but reports documenting effectiveness are lacking. Perianal gland adenomas may shrink after a short course of diethylstilbestrol (Table 16-72). Radiation therapy or chemotherapy is recommended for nonresectable malignancies. Vincristine, doxorubicin, and cyclophosphamide (VAC) or melphalan have also been recommended. Radiation or chemotherapy may convert a marginally operable tumor to an operable tumor.

SURGICAL TREATMENT

Surgical excision is the treatment of choice for perianal tumors. Generally, perianal masses not involving the anal sacs are perianal adenomas. Therefore castration and resection of small masses, or biopsy of multiple or large masses is recommended. Patients should be reevaluated 4 to 6 weeks after castration/biopsy. Adenomas will be smaller at this time and can generally be resected with less trauma to the external anal sphincter. Some adenomas regress completely after castration. If malignancy is identified histologically, wide resection should be promptly performed.

Preoperative Management

Fluid, electrolyte, and acid-base abnormalities should be corrected before surgery. Perioperative antibiotics are indicated in old or debilitated patients. They should be given intravenously at induction and discontinued within 12 to 24 hours of surgery. Enemas should not be administered on the day of surgery because they may increase contamination of the surgical site. Manual removal of remaining feces may be done after induction but before preparing the animal for aseptic surgery. Mildly to moderately hypercalcemic animals should first be rehydrated with physiologic saline solution. If they are urinating, furosemide and prednisone (Table 16-73) may be given. Severely affected animals may also be treated with alkalinizing agents (e.g., sodium bicarbonate) and bone resorption inhibitors (i.e., etidronate disodium or salmon calcitonin). The effectiveness and dose of etidronate disodium are unproven in dogs; it should be used with caution. Peritoneal dialysis may be performed in oliguric patients.

Anesthesia

Patients with perianal tumors may be old, debilitated, and have other serious medical problems, requiring special care during anesthesia. Anesthetic recommendations for animals undergoing perianal surgery are on p. 337. An antihistamine (e.g., diphenhydramine [Benadryl]; 0.5 mg/kg, intravenously) should be administered to patients with mast cell tumors before surgery to decrease the effects of tumor histamine release. It may be given intravenously immediately before surgery, but should be given extremely slowly to avoid hypotension. Alternately, it may be administered intramuscularly 30 minutes before anesthetic induction.

Surgical Anatomy

Anatomy of the rectum and perianal region is on p. 338. Cats do not have perianal/circumanal glands.

Positioning

Position the patient in ventral (preferred) or dorsal recumbency to allow access to the tumors and scrotal region. Fix the tail over the back, elevate the pelvis, and pad the hindlegs when using a perineal position.

SURGICAL TECHNIQUE

Removal of one half of the anal sphincter is possible with some return of fecal continence within a few weeks. Resection of metastatic sites (e.g., lymph nodes) from patients with anal sac adenocarcinomas may help control hypercalcemia. *Begin by performing a prescrotal or caudal castration on intact male dogs with perianal adenomas (see p. 527). Incise perianal skin surrounding perianal adenomas with minimal margins of normal tissue. Dissect the tumor from subcutaneous tissues and the external anal sphincter with minimal trauma. Thoroughly lavage the area. Close dead space with monofilament absorbable sutures (e.g., 3-0 to 4-0 polydioxanone or polyglyconate), and skin with interrupted appositional sutures (e.g.,*

TABLE 16-72

Diethylstilbestrol Administration

0.5-1.0 mg daily for 2 to 3 weeks

TABLE 16-73

Treatment of Hypercalcemia

Furosemide (Lasix)
2-4 mg/kg IV, PO, SC; BID to TID

Prednisone
1-2 mg/kg IV, PO, SC; BID

Sodium Bicarbonate
0.5-2 mEq/kg given in IV fluids (check blood gas)

Etidronate Disodium (Didronel)
Dogs—5 mg/kg/day, PO
Cats—10 mg/kg/day, PO

Salmon Calcitonin
4 U/kg IV; then 4-8 U/kg, SC; SID to BID

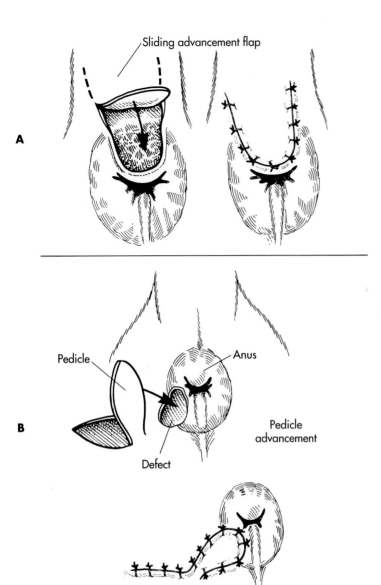

FIG. 16-116
Resect perianal masses with involved muscle. Close large defects in the sphincter with **A,** a sliding advancement flap or **B,** a local pedicle flap to help prevent anal stenosis.

monofilament, 3-0 to 4-0 nylon or polypropylene). Submit the excised masses and testicles for histologic evaluation.

Resect malignant tumors with a minimum of 1 cm of normal tissue on all borders (Fig. 16-116). This includes partial resection of the external anal sphincter, anal canal, and anal sacs in some cases. Appose the epithelial edges to avoid anal stricture.

POSTOPERATIVE CARE AND ASSESSMENT

Give systemic analgesics (see Table 16-4 on p. 209) as necessary for pain. Hypercalcemia should be treated until serum calcium is normal. Most animals are normocalcemic within 24 hours of primary tumor resection. The perianal area should be kept clean, and an Elizabethan collar or similar restraint device should be used to keep the patient from licking at surgical sites. Animals not vomiting may receive water and food within 8 to 12 hours. A stool softener may be added to the food for 2 to 3 weeks (see Table 16-61 on p. 327). Chemotherapy may slow recurrence and metastatic tumor growth

but its efficacy is unknown. The rectum and perianal area should be palpated for evidence of stricture or tumor recurrence when sutures are removed at 7 to 10 days. Patients with malignancies should be reevaluated for recurrence or metastasis at 2, 4, and 6 months, and then yearly. Rectal palpation, serum calcium values, and abdominal radiography or ultrasonography are indicated during reevaluation. Recurrence of malignant tumors is often detected by 3 months after surgery. Potential complications of perianal surgery are listed in Table 16-74.

PROGNOSIS

Prolonged estrogen therapy is not recommended because of its myelotoxic and temporary effects. Radiation therapy is an option, but surgery is less expensive, faster, and safer. The prognosis after surgery is good for benign perianal tumors but guarded to poor for malignant tumors, although some malignant tumors may be slow growing and late to metastasize. Palliation for nonresectable malignant tumors may involve partial resection, cryosurgery, chemotherapy, or radiation therapy. The prognosis for perianal gland adenomas is good to excellent after castration. Adenomas occasionally recur (less than 10%) and should be rebiopsied. Early, complete excision of perianal gland adenocarcinomas can be curative, but most carcinomas are invasive or metastasize to lymph nodes. Recurrence is common but may take many months; therefore the prognosis is poor.

Anal sac adenocarcinomas in female dogs warrant a poor prognosis because they frequently spread locally and to lymph nodes by the time of diagnosis. Recurrent hypercalcemia suggests recurrence or metastasis. Of 11 dogs with metastasis at the time of surgery, a mean survival of 9.9 months (median, 6 months; range, 1.5 to 39 months) was reported (Ross et al, 1991). Ten dogs in the same study that did not have detectable metastasis before surgery had a mean survival of 15.8 months (median, 15.5 months; range, 3 to 35 months). The prognosis for anal squamous cell carcinoma is grave with or without surgery.

Reference

Ross JT et al: Adenocarcinoma of the apocrine glands of the anal sac in dogs: a review of 32 cases, *J Am Anim Hosp Assoc* 27:349, 1991.

Suggested Reading

Hause WR et al: Pseudohyperparathyroidism associated with adenocarcinomas of anal sac origin in four dogs, *J Am Anim Hosp Assoc* 17:373, 1981.

Isitor GN: Comparative ultrastructural study of normal, adenomatous, carcinomatous, and hyperplastic cells of canine hepatoid circumanal glands, *Am J Vet Res* 44:463, 1983.

Liska WD, Withrow SJ: Cryosurgical treatment of perianal gland adenomas in the dog, *J Am Anim Hosp Assoc* 14:457, 1978.

Sentovich SM et al: Transrectal ultrasound of rectal tumors, *Am J Surgery* 166:638, 1992.

Wilson GP, Hayes HM: Castration for treatment of perianal gland neoplasms in the dog, *J Am Vet Med Assoc* 174:1301, 1979.

ANAL SAC INFECTION/IMPACTION

DEFINITIONS

Anal sac impaction is an abnormal accumulation of anal sac secretions secondary to inflammation, infection, or duct obstruction.

SYNONYMS

Anal sacculitis, abscess. Anal sacs are sometimes erroneously referred to as anal glands.

GENERAL CONSIDERATIONS AND CLINICALLY RELEVANT PATHOPHYSIOLOGY

Anal sac diseases include impaction, infection, abscessation, and neoplasia. The anal sacs are modified adnexal skin structure. They are paired, lying between the fibers of the anal sphincter, and are lined by squamous epithelium with modified apocrine and sebaceous glands. They serve as reservoirs for their malodorous, pastelike secretions. Excretions are expelled through the ducts during normal defecation and extreme excitement. Forceful contractions of the sphincter are necessary for anal sac emptying.

Anal sacculitis is common, affecting approximately 10% of dogs, and is usually caused by infection or duct obstruction. Ductal obstruction leads to bacterial overgrowth, infection, and inflammation. Inflammation enhances secretions, which serve as an ideal medium for bacterial growth. Secretions continue to accumulate despite ductal obstruction, and the sacs become impacted and eventually rupture. Distention causes pain. Chronic fistulation may result if infection or duct obstruction persists. Anal sacculitis also occurs without duct obstruction. In these cases hypersecretion occurs and the sac is easy to express. Secretions are more liquid than normal with yellowish-white granules. Factors that may cause chronic hypersecretion include infectious, endocrine, allergic, behavioral, and idiopathic mechanisms. Malfunction of the anal sphincter mechanism secondary to chronic diarrhea, anal laxity, constipation, and obesity may contribute to retention of anal sac secretions and development of anal sacculitis.

DIAGNOSIS
Clinical Presentation

Signalment. Anal sacculitis may occur in any age, breed, or sex of animal; however, it is most common in small and toy breed dogs and rare in cats. Anal sacculitis may be associated with seborrheic dermatitis or other dermatoses in some animals.

History. Many animals have a history of recent (1 to 3 weeks) diarrhea or soft stools or estrus. They usually evidence anal irritation (e.g., scooting, licking, and biting at the tailhead or anus). Other complaints include tail chasing, malodorous perianal discharge, pain or tenderness, and behavioral change. Tenesmus, dyschezia, constipation, and hematochezia occasionally occur. Generalized dermatitis or dermatitis at a secondary site are sometimes recognized.

Physical Examination Findings

The anal sac region may appear swollen and inflamed. Abscesses or impaction may cause the anal sac to rupture and create a draining lesion at the 4 o'clock or 7 o'clock position. The animal may be febrile with abscesses or severe sacculitis. Palpation of the perianal tissue during rectal examination may identify an enlarged, firm, and sometimes painful anal sac. Digital expression of the anal sac may expel normal (serous, slightly viscid and granular, pale-yellow liquid) or abnormal secretions (whitish-gray, brown, yellow or green, bloody, purulent, gritty, turbid, opaque). It may be impossible to express material from diseased sacs. Animals with untreated anal sac abscesses may be debilitated, have other perianal or rectal abscesses, or develop anal stricture. Perineal fistulae occasionally occur.

☞ **N O T E** · Routine palpation and expression of the anal sacs during physical examinations may allow early detection of anal sac disease.

Impaction is diagnosed when the sac is distended, mildly painful, and not readily expressed. Anal sacculitis is diagnosed when moderate or severe pain is elicited on palpation, and secretions are liquid, yellowish, blood-tinged, or purulent. Diagnosis of anal sac abscessation is made when there is marked distention of the sac with a purulent exudate, cellulitis of surrounding tissues, erythema of overlying skin, pain, and fever. An anal sac rupture is diagnosed by finding a draining tract associated with the anal sac.

Radiography/Ultrasonography

Plain radiographs are recommended if neoplasia is suspected (see p. 345). A fistulogram may help determine whether a draining tract is associated with the anal sac region or some other perineal location.

Laboratory Findings

Hematology and serum biochemistry changes are nonspecific. Leukocytosis with a left shift may be noted with anal sac abscesses. Cytology from diseased anal sac secretions reveals cellular debris, large numbers of leukocytes, and numerous bacteria. Culture and sensitivity testing of the anal sac is recommended. The normal bacterial flora of the anal sacs include small numbers of micrococci, *Escherichia coli, Streptococcus faecalis,* and *Staphylococcus* spp. Bacteria typically cultured from diseased anal sacs include: *S. faecalis, Clostridium perfringens, E. coli, Proteus* spp., *Staphylococcus* spp., micrococci, and diphtheroids.

DIFFERENTIAL DIAGNOSIS

The primary differentials for anal sacculitis are flea allergy (from licking and biting), perianal tumor (caused by swelling and ulceration), perianal fistulae, or tail fold pyoderma (the result of abscessation and draining tracts). Differential diagnoses for anal or perianal irritation include anal sacculitis, dermatitis, endoparasites, perianal fistulae, or tumors. Differential diagnoses for perianal swelling include perianal hernia, perianal neoplasia, perianal gland hyperplasia, anal sacculitis, anal sac neoplasia, atresia ani, rectal pythiosis, and vaginal tumors. Differential diagnoses for dyschezia include rectal foreign body, perineal hernia, perianal fistulae, anal stricture, rectal stricture, anal sac abscess, rectal neoplasia, anal neoplasia, anal trauma, anal dermatitis, rectal pythiosis, and anorectal prolapse.

MEDICAL TREATMENT

Treatment depends on the stage of infection. Most anal sac problems can be medically managed by manual expression, lavage, antibiotics, and dietary change. Treatment of concomitant dermatoses facilitates treatment of anal sacculitis. Mild sacculitis or impaction is treated by expressing, lavaging (with saline), and infusing the glands with an antibiotic-corticosteroid preparation. Dry secretions may be softened by lavaging with saline or infusing a ceruminolytic agent. If the anal sacs are infected, 0.5% chlorhexidine or 10% povidone-iodine may be added to saline flushes. Adding fiber (e.g., w/d, pumpkin, bran, or psyllium) to the diet makes the feces firm and bulky, which may stretch the anus during defecation causing the anal sacs to be compressed and emptied. In more severe cases, weekly evaluation, expression, and lavage with a dilute antiseptic solution or saline may be required. Oral antibiotics in chronic cases are chosen based on sensitivity results. Anal sac abscesses should be lanced, drained, and flushed. Hot compresses, applied two to three times daily for 15 to 20 minutes each are beneficial for abscesses. Appropriate oral antibiotics should be administered to patients with anal sac abscesses. Chemical cauterization is not recommended because severe perineal sloughing may result (Fig. 16-117).

SURGICAL TREATMENT

Failure of medical therapy and suspicion of neoplasia are indications for anal sacculectomy. If a draining tract persists after anal sac rupture, surgery should be delayed until inflammation is controlled. Both anal sacs should be removed, even if only one is obviously involved, to avoid a second surgery. Either an open or closed technique may be used; however, there is more risk of fecal incontinence and local infection with the open technique.

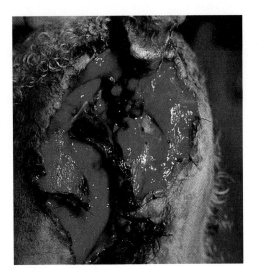

FIG. 16-117
Note the extensive perineal sloughing that occurred after chemical cauterization to treat anal sacculitis. This dog was euthanized because of deep vascular erosion and hemorrhage. Chemical cauterization is not recommended for treatment of anal sacculitis.

☞ **NOTE** • Warn owners of the risk of incontinence.

Preoperative Management

Anal sacculitis, abscessation, or fistulation should be treated for several days as described above to reduce inflammation before surgery. Inflammation and fibrosis present at the time of surgery increase the risk of damage to the anal sphincter. Temporary or permanent fecal incontinence may result secondary to sphincter damage.

Anesthesia

Anesthetic recommendations for animals undergoing perianal surgery are on p. 337.

Surgical Anatomy

One anal sac lies on each side of the anus between the internal and external anal sphincters. The anal sac is a cutaneous diverticulum lined by microscopic glands. Secretions of these sebaceous and aprocrine glands accumulate in the anal sac and are normally expelled through the ducts during defecation or contraction of the anal sphincter. The ducts of the anal sacs open in the cutaneous zone at approximately the 4 o'clock to 5 o'clock and 7 o'clock to 8 o'clock positions. The duct opening in cats is more lateral to the anocutaneous line than in dogs. They are visible lateral to the anus in the normal contracted state.

Positioning

Position the patient in ventral recumbency with the tail fixed dorsally over the back. Elevate the pelvis and pad the hindlegs when using a perineal position.

SURGICAL TECHNIQUE

Palpate the anal sacs to determine their location and extent by placing the index or middle finger in the rectum and the thumb over the sac. Manually evacuate feces from the rectum if present. Prepare the perineal area for surgery.

Closed technique. *Insert a small probe or hemostat into the orifice of the anal sac duct (Fig. 16-118, A). Advance the instrument until the lateral extent of the sac is identified.* Alternately, wax or synthetic resin may be infused to distend the sac before resection. *Make a curvilinear incision over the anal sac. Dissecting directly against the anal sac, separate the internal and external anal sphincter muscle fibers from the sac's exterior with small Metzenbaum or iris scissors. Avoid excising or traumatizing the muscles or the caudal rectal artery medial to the duct. Continue dissecting to free the sac and duct to its mucocutaneous junction at the anal canal (Fig. 16-118, B). Perforation of the sac may occur during dissection, and tissues may be contaminated with secretions. Place a ligature around the duct at the mucocutaneous junction (e.g., 4-0 polydioxanone or*

Closed technique

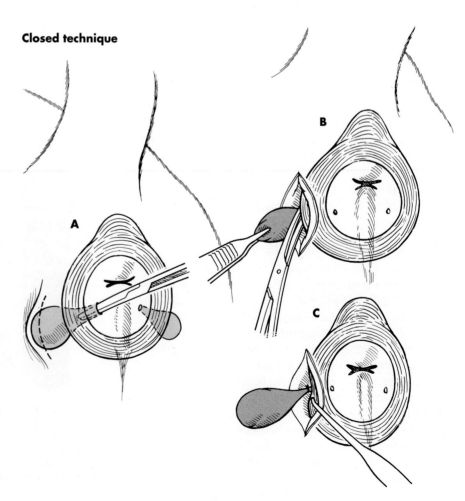

FIG. 16-118
Anal sacculectomy may be performed closed or open. For the closed technique locate the anal sacs at the 4 o'clock to 5 o'clock and 7 o'clock to 8 o'clock positions between the internal and external anal sphincter muscles. **A,** Insert a hemostat into the anal sac. **B,** Make an incision at the lateral aspect of the anal sac and carefully dissect the sac from the sphincter muscle fibers. **C,** Ligate the duct near the orifice.

polyglyconate) (Fig. 16-118, C). Excise the anal sac and duct, then inspect for completeness of removal. Control hemorrhage with ligatures, electrocoagulation, or pressure. Lavage the tissues thoroughly. Appose subcutaneous tissues with interrupted sutures of 4-0 polydioxanone or polyglyconate and skin with 3-0 or 4-0 nylon or polypropylene.

Open technique. *Place a scissors blade or groove director into the duct of the anal sac (Fig. 16-119, A). Apply medial traction on the duct while incising through skin, subcutaneous tissue, external anal sphincter, duct, and sac. Continue the incision to the lateral extent of the anal sac (Fig. 16-119, B). Elevate the cut edge of the sac and use small Metzenbaum or iris scissors to dissect the sac free of its attachments to muscle and surrounding tissue.* The lining of the anal sac is grayish and glistening and is easily distinguished from surrounding tissue. *Complete the procedure as for closed sacculectomy (Fig. 16-119, C).*

POSTOPERATIVE CARE AND ASSESSMENT

Systemic analgesics (see Table 16-4 on p. 209) should be given as necessary. The perianal area should be kept clean, and an Elizabethan collar or similar restraint device should be used to keep the patient from licking the sites. Food and water may be offered within 8 to 12 hours if no vomiting has been noted. A stool softener may be added to the food for 2 to 3 weeks (see Table 16-61 on p. 327). The surgical site should be monitored for signs of infection or drainage, and the rectum and perianal area should be palpated for evidence of stricture when sutures are removed at 7 to 10 days. Fecal continence may be impaired during the healing process, but usually returns to normal within several weeks.

COMPLICATIONS

A draining tract after surgery suggests a piece of anal sac was left at the surgical site. This occurs more commonly with inexperienced surgeons or inflamed and fibrotic tissues. Surgical excision is necessary or drainage will continue. Other complications include infection, dehiscence, tenesmus, rectal prolapse, dyschezia, hematochezia, permanent incontinence, and anal stricture. Fecal incontinence after anal sacculectomy may be temporary or permanent.

PROGNOSIS

The prognosis for nonneoplastic anal sac disease is good if it is not associated with perianal fistulae. Most cases of anal sacculitis can be treated medically if they are recognized early, treated appropriately, and not associated with neoplasia or perianal fistulae.

Open technique

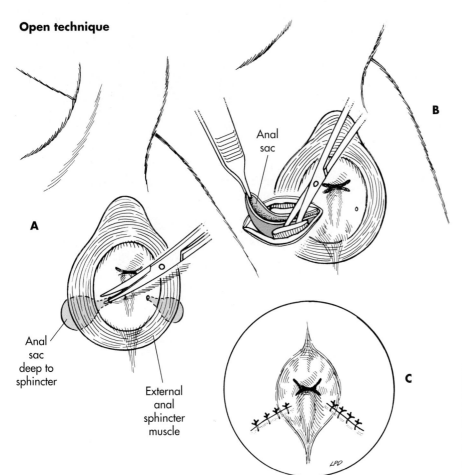

Anal sac

B

A

Anal sac deep to sphincter

External anal sphincter muscle

C

FIG. 16-119
For the open technique **A,** insert the blade of the scissors into the sac and incise through skin, subcutaneous tissues, external anal sphincter, and anal sac. **B,** Elevate the cut edge of the sac and dissect it from the anal sphincter. **C,** Appose the sphincter, subcutaneous tissues, and skin.

Suggested Reading

Anderson RK: Anal sac disease and its related dermatoses, *Compend Contin Educ Pract Vet* 6:829, 1984.

Hause WR et al: Pseudohyperparathyroidism associated with adenocarcinomas of anal sac origin in four dogs, *J Am Anim Hosp Assoc* 17:373, 1981.

Ross JT et al: Adenocarcinoma of the apocrine glands of the anal sac in dogs: a review of 32 cases, *J Am Anim Hosp Assoc* 27:349, 1991.

PERINEAL HERNIA

DEFINITIONS

Perineal hernias occur when the perineal muscles separate allowing rectum, pelvic, and/or abdominal contents to displace perineal skin.

SYNONYMS

Caudal hernia, sciatic hernia, dorsal hernia, ventral hernia

GENERAL CONSIDERATIONS AND CLINICALLY RELEVANT PATHOPHYSIOLOGY

Perineal hernia occurs when pelvic diaphragm muscles fail to support the rectal wall, allowing persistent rectal distension and impaired defecation. The cause of pelvic diaphragm weakening is poorly understood but believed to be associated with male hormones, straining, and congenital or acquired muscle weakness or atrophy. The pelvic diaphragm is stronger in female dogs than males. Atrophy of the pelvic diaphragm muscles, possibly of neurologic origin, has been identified in some animals with hernias. Any condition that causes straining may stress the pelvic diaphragm (see Table 16-75).

Herniation may be unilateral or bilateral (Fig. 16-120). Most occur between the levator ani, external anal sphincter, and internal obturator muscles (caudal hernia); however, some are between the sacrotuberous ligament and coccygeus muscle (sciatic hernia), levator ani and coccygeus muscles (dorsal hernia), or ischiourethralis, bulbocavernosus, and ischiocavernosus muscles (ventral hernia). Hernial contents are surrounded by a thin layer of perineal fascia (hernial sac), subcutaneous tissue, and skin. The hernial sac may contain pelvic or retroperitoneal fat, serous fluid, a deviated or dilated rectum, a rectal diverticulum, prostate, urinary bladder, or small intestine (Fig. 16-121). Cats usually only have rectum within the hernial sac. Organs displaced into the hernia may become obstructed and strangulated. Visceral obstruction or strangulation is associated with rapid deterioration unless the obstruction or entrapment is corrected.

DIAGNOSIS
Clinical Presentation

Signalment. Perineal hernias are common in dogs and rare in cats. They occur almost exclusively in intact, male dogs (93%) (Hayes, Wilson, Tarone, 1978). Perineal hernias in female dogs are often related to trauma. Feline perineal hernias usually occur in neutered males; however, female cats are more prone to perineal hernias than female dogs. Dogs with short tails may be predisposed to herniation. Breeds most commonly affected are Boston terriers, boxers, Welsh

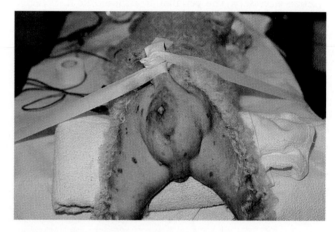

FIG. 16-120
Bilateral perineal hernias in a dog.

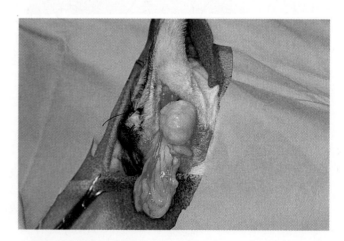

FIG. 16-121
Perineal hernia in a dog. Note the urinary bladder and pelvic fat occupying this hernial sac.

TABLE 16-75
Conditions That Cause Straining and May Predispose to Perineal Herniation

- Prostatitis
- Cystitis
- Urinary tract obstruction
- Colorectal obstruction
- Rectal deviation/dilation
- Perianal inflammation
- Anal sacculitis
- Diarrhea
- Constipation

corgis, Pekingese, collies, poodles, and mongrels. Most perineal hernias occur in dogs older than 5 years. The median age (range) in two studies of 76 and 100 dogs, respectively, was 9 years (5 to 13 years) and 10 years (3 to 16 years) (Orsher, 1986; Hosgood et al, 1995). Risk of occurrence increases with age until 14 years in intact males (Hayes et al, 1978). The median age at diagnosis in 40 cats was 10 years (range, 3 to 18.5 years) (Welches et al, 1991).

History. Affected animals usually present because of difficulty defecating. Some owners notice a swelling lateral to the anus. Occasionally animals present as emergencies because of postrenal uremia associated with bladder entrapment or shock associated with intestinal strangulation. Clinical signs may include perineal swelling, constipation, obstipation, dyschezia, tenesmus, rectal prolapse, stranguria, anuria, vomiting, flatulence, and fecal incontinence.

Physical Examination Findings

Diagnosis is based on finding a perineal swelling lateral to the anus and a weakened pelvic diaphragm (see Fig. 16-120). Some reports indicate a right-sided predominance. The swelling may appear to surround the anus and cause it to bulge. A rectal deviation often contains impacted feces. Cats typically have bilateral hernias, which seldom cause obvious perineal swelling. Rectal palpation of the pelvic diaphragm reveals a weakness or separation of the muscles. The prostate is sometimes found in the hernia. Severe straining can produce rectal prolapse. Some animals are systemically ill and shocky because of visceral strangulation. If ballottement suggests liquid is present and the animal is dysuric, perineal centesis should be performed to determine if urine is present.

☞ **N O T E** • A soft swelling in the perineal region may indicate that the bladder is entrapped in the hernia. Prompt therapy may be necessary to relieve urinary obstruction in these animals.

Radiography/Ultrasonography

Plain radiographs are seldom needed; however, they may reveal the position of the urinary bladder and prostate and asymmetry or enlargement. Radiographically documenting retroflexion of the urinary bladder often requires a urethrogram and/or cystogram. Administration of oral or rectal barium demonstrates the position of the colon and rectum. In one study where oral barium was given to assess rectal abnormalities, all dogs had rectal deviation (30/30) and some also had rectal dilatation (12/30) (Hosgood et al, 1995). Rectal diverticula were not documented radiographically or at surgery. Ultrasonographic identification of the urinary bladder and prostate is also possible.

Laboratory Findings

Patients with bladder retroflexion often have azotemia, hyperkalemia, hyperphosphatemia, and neutrophilic leukocytosis.

DIFFERENTIAL DIAGNOSIS

Differential diagnoses for perianal swelling include perineal hernia, perianal neoplasia, perianal gland hyperplasia, anal sacculitis, anal sac neoplasia, atresia ani, and vaginal tumors. Differential diagnoses for dyschezia include rectal foreign body, perineal hernia, perianal fistula, anal stricture, rectal stricture, anal sac abscess, rectal neoplasia, anal neoplasia, anal trauma, anal dermatitis, rectal pythiosis, and anorectal prolapse.

MEDICAL TREATMENT

The goal of treatment is to relieve and prevent constipation and dysuria, and to prevent organ strangulation. Causative factors (i.e., urinary tract obstruction or infection, megacolon, prostatitis) should be corrected. Normal defecation can sometimes be maintained using laxatives, stool softeners, dietary changes, periodic enemas, and/or manual rectal evacuation. The urinary bladder can be decompressed by centesis or catheterization. However, long-term use of these treatments is contraindicated because life-threatening visceral entrapment and strangulation may occur.

SURGICAL TREATMENT

Herniorrhaphy should always be recommended. Retroflexion of the urinary bladder and visceral entrapment are emergencies requiring immediate surgery. Castration, although controversial, is recommended during herniorrhaphy because it has been reported to reduce recurrence. Noncastrated dogs have a recurrence rate 2.7 times greater than castrated dogs (Hayes, Wilson, Tarone, 1978).

The two most commonly used techniques are the traditional or anatomic reapposition and the internal obturator roll-up or transposition technique. It is more difficult to close the ventral aspect of the hernia using the former technique. Temporary deformity of the anus occurs and is especially pronounced after bilateral herniorrhaphy. Postoperative tenesmus and rectal prolapse may be more frequent in these cases. The internal obturator transposition technique is more difficult, especially if internal obturator muscle atrophy is severe. However, it causes less tension on sutures, less deformity of the anus, and creates a ventral patch/sling for the defect. Other herniorrhaphy techniques have included using the superficial gluteal or semitendinous muscles, placement of synthetic mesh, or a combination of techniques. Bilateral herniorrhaphy is possible, but postoperative discomfort and tenesmus may be greater than after unilateral procedures. If accessible, the prostate should be biopsied. Either a caudal or prescrotal castration may be performed (see p. 527). Rectal imbrication or sacculectomy is rarely indicated and significantly increases the risk of postoperative infection. Fixation of the ductus deferens may help prevent recurrence when the bladder or prostate has been displaced into perineal hernias (Bilbrey, Smeak, DeHoff, 1990).

☞ **N O T E** • Some surgeons prefer waiting 4 to 6 weeks before performing the second herniorrhaphy in dogs with bilateral disease.

Preoperative Management

Stool softeners (see Table 16-61 on p. 327) should be given 2 to 3 days before surgery. The large intestine should be evacuated with laxatives, cathartics, enemas, and manual extraction (see p. 320). Prophylactic antibiotics effective against gram-negative and anaerobic organisms (see Table 16-57 on p. 321) should be given intravenously after anesthetic induction. If the urinary bladder is retroflexed into the hernia, a urinary catheter should be placed or cystocentesis performed via the perineum to relieve distress and prevent further physiologic deterioration.

Anesthesia

Anesthetic recommendations for animals undergoing perineal surgery are on p. 337. Many affected animals are geriatric and have concurrent abnormalities that may influence drug selection. See p. 346 for management of hypercalcemic animals.

Surgical Anatomy

The pelvic diaphragm is composed of the paired medial coccygeal and levator ani muscles. The paired levator ani muscle originates from the floor of the pelvis and medial shaft of the ilium, fans out around the sides of the rectum, and then narrows and inserts ventrally on the seventh caudal vertebra. The paired coccygeus muscle is a thick muscle lying lateral to the thin levator ani. The coccygeus originates from the ischiatic spine on the pelvic floor and inserts ventrally on caudal vertebrae two through five.

The paired rectococcygeus muscle arises from the external longitudinal musculature of the rectum caudal to the levator and coccygeus muscles and inserts on the ventral surface of the fifth to sixth caudal vertebrae. The rectococcygeus muscle shortens the rectum when the tail is raised during defecation. The peritoneal reflection is cranial to the rectococcygeus muscles. The sacrotuberous ligament in the dog is a fibrous band running from the transverse process of the last sacral and first caudal vertebrae to the lateral angle of the ischiatic tuberosity rostral to the pelvic diaphragm. Cats do not have a sacrotuberous ligament. The sciatic nerve lies just cranial and lateral to the sacrotuberous ligament. The internal obturator muscle is a fan-shaped muscle covering the dorsal surface of the ischium. It originates from the dorsal surface of the ischium and pelvic symphysis. Its tendon of insertion passes over the lesser ischiatic notch, ventral to the sacrotuberous ligament. The internal pudendal artery and vein and the pudendal nerve run caudomedially through the pelvic canal on the dorsal surface of the internal obturator muscle, lateral to the coccygeus and levator ani muscles. The pudendal nerve is dorsal to the vessels and divides into the caudal rectal and perineal nerves. The obturator nerve passes through the ventral aspect of the levator ani in a caudolateral direction.

> ☞ **N O T E** • Perineal vessels and nerves may be displaced from their normal anatomic location by the hernial contents. Careful observation and dissection is required to preserve these structures.

Positioning

Clip and aseptically prepare the perineum for surgery. The prepared area should extend 10 to 15 cm cranial to the tail base, laterally beyond the ischial tuberosity, and ventrally to include the scrotum. The animal should be positioned in ventral recumbency with the tail fixed over the back, the pelvis elevated, and the hindlegs padded. Alternatively, a well-padded perineal stand may be used.

SURGICAL TECHNIQUE
Approach

Make a curvilinear incision beginning cranial to the coccygeus muscles, curving over the hernial bulge 1 to 2 cm lateral to the anus, and extending 2 to 3 cm ventral to the pelvic floor (Fig. 16-122). Incise subcutaneous tissue and hernial sac. Identify and reduce hernial contents by dissecting subcutaneous and fibrous attachments. Biopsy any abnormal structures within the hernia (e.g., prostate, masses). Maintain hernial reduction by packing the defect with a moistened, tagged sponge. Identify the muscles involved in the hernia, internal pudendal artery and vein, pudendal nerve, caudal rectal vessels and nerve, and sacrotuberous ligament. Repair the hernia with one of the described techniques. After herniorrhaphy perform a caudal castration through a median perineal incision (see p. 527).

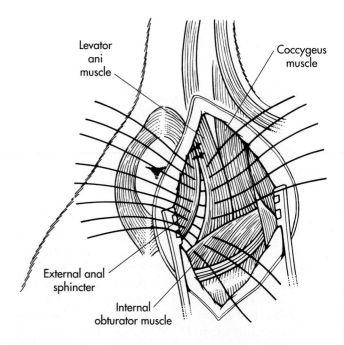

Levator ani muscle

Coccygeus muscle

External anal sphincter

Internal obturator muscle

FIG. 16-122
For perineal hernia repair using the traditional technique make a curvilinear incision 1 to 2 cm lateral to the anus from dorsal to the tailhead to ventral to the anus. Appose the external anal sphincter to the combined levator ani and coccygeus muscles (plus or minus the sacrotuberous ligament) laterally and the external anal sphincter and internal obturator muscles ventrally.

☞ **NOTE** · Do not mistake the prostate for a mass and attempt to excise it!

Traditional or Anatomic Herniorrhaphy

Preplace simple interrupted 0 or 2-0 monofilament sutures using a large, curved needle (see Fig. 16-122). Begin suture placement between the external anal sphincter and levator ani, coccygeus, or both muscles. Space sutures less than 1 cm apart. As placement progresses ventrally and laterally, incorporate the sacrotuberous ligament for a secure repair if necessary. **Place sutures through rather than around the sacrotuberous ligament to avoid sciatic nerve entrapment.** *Direct ventral sutures between the external anal sphincter and the internal obturator muscle. Be cognizant of the pudendal vessels and nerves at all times to prevent traumatizing these structures. Tie sutures beginning dorsally and progressing ventrally. Remove the sponge used to maintain reduction before tying the last few sutures. Evaluate the repair; place additional sutures if weaknesses or defects persist. Lavage the area. Close subcutaneous tissues with an interrupted or continuous appositional pattern (e.g., 3-0 or 4-0 polydioxanone or polyglyconate), and skin with an appositional interrupted pattern (e.g., 3-0 or 4-0 nylon).*

Internal Obturator Transposition Herniorrhaphy

Incise fascia and periosteum along the caudal border of the ischium and origin of the internal obturator muscle. Using a periosteal elevator, elevate the periosteum and internal obturator muscle from the ischium (Fig. 16-123, A). Transpose dorsomedially or roll up the muscle into the defect to allow apposition between the coccygeus, levator ani, and external anal sphincter. Transect the internal obturator tendon of insertion if necessary to get adequate coverage of the defect. The internal obturator tendon is often difficult to visualize, making transection difficult. Use care to avoid transection of the caudal gluteal vessels and perineal nerve. *Preplace simple interrupted sutures as with the traditional technique. Begin by apposing the combined levator ani and coccygeus muscles with the external anal sphincter muscle dorsally. Then place sutures between the internal obturator and external anal sphincter medially and the levator ani and coccygeus muscles laterally (Fig. 16-123, B).*

Ductus Deferopexy

After castration and herniorrhaphy in dogs with bladder or prostate retroflexion, the ductus deferens can be secured to the abdominal wall to prevent recurrent caudal organ displacement.

Approach the abdomen through a caudal ventral midline incision. Retroflex the urinary bladder caudally through the incision to expose the ductus deferens. Separate the ligated ductus deferens from the testicular artery and vein and gently pull it through the inguinal ring. Dissect each ductus deferens from its peritoneal attachments to the level of the prostate. Pull the urinary bladder and prostate forward by applying moderate traction on the ductus deferens. At an adjacent site on the ventrolateral abdominal wall make two incisions (1.5 to 2 cm apart) through the peritoneum and transversus abdominis muscle. Tunnel between these incisions and draw the ductus deferens through the tunnel. Suture the ductus deferens to itself and the abdominal wall with three or four 3-0 monofilament sutures. Repeat the procedure on the opposite side to fix the bladder and prostate in a more cranial position.

☞ **NOTE** · Although prolonging surgery time, this procedure is worthwhile in dogs with bladder retroflexion.

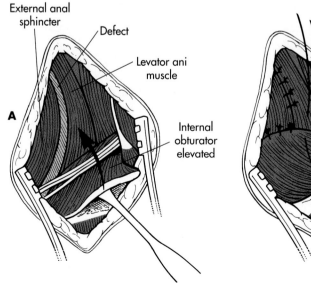

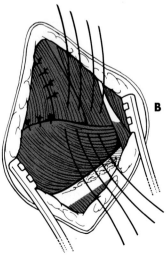

FIG. 16-123
A, Elevate the internal obturator muscle from the ischium when using the internal obturator transposition technique. **B,** Appose the external anal sphincter muscle and combined levator ani and coccygeus muscles dorsally. Transpose the internal obturator muscle dorsomedially to fill the ventral defect and suture it to the external anal sphincter muscle medially and the coccygeus muscle and sacrotuberous ligament laterally.

POSTOPERATIVE CARE AND ASSESSMENT

Analgesics (see Table 16-4 on p. 209) should be given as necessary to minimize straining and rectal prolapse. If rectal prolapse occurs a purse-string suture should be placed. Fluid therapy should be continued in uremic patients. Warm compresses applied to the surgical site two to three times daily diminish swelling and perianal irritation. Antibiotics may be discontinued within 12 hours unless ischemic, necrotic, or contaminated tissues were present before surgery or the patient is debilitated. After herniorrhaphy these patients should be monitored for signs of wound infection (i.e., redness, pain, swelling, discharge). Stool softeners (see Table 16-61 on p. 327) should be continued for 1 to 2 months.

COMPLICATIONS

Most postoperative complications are prevented by meticulous surgical technique. Hernia recurrence or contralateral herniation is believed to be reduced by castration during herniorrhaphy. Recurrence is related to the expertise of the surgeon; inexperienced surgeons have higher recurrence rates. Infection and dehiscence can usually be prevented by appropriate antibiotic prophylaxis and surgical technique. Marked pain, non–weight-bearing lameness, and knuckling after surgery suggest sciatic nerve entrapment. If this is suspected the offending suture should be removed immediately via a caudolateral approach to the hip. Other potential complications are listed in Table 16-76.

PROGNOSIS

Defecation in affected patients is facilitated by medical and dietary management. The danger of prolonged medical therapy is that the bladder, intestine, or prostate will become trapped in the hernia with life-threatening consequences. The prognosis is fair to good when surgery is performed by an experienced surgeon. Patients with bladder retroflexion have the poorest prognosis. Preexisting neurologic abnormalities (i.e., anal sphincter incompetence or compromised urinary bladder innervation) will not be corrected by the herniorrhaphy.

References

Bilbrey SA, Smeak DD, DeHoff W: Fixation of the deferent ducts for retrodisplacement of the urinary bladder and prostate in canine perineal hernia, *Vet Surg* 19:24, 1990.

TABLE 16-76

Potential Complications of Herniorrhaphy

• Hemorrhage	• Fecal incontinence
• Depression	• Urethral damage
• Anorexia	• Dysuria
• Tenesmus	• Stranguria
• Dyschezia	• Bladder atony
• Flatulence	• Bladder necrosis
• Hematochezia	• Urinary incontinence
• Rectal prolapse	

Hayes HM, Wilson GP, Tarone RE: The epidemiologic features of perineal hernia in 771 dogs, *J Am Anim Hosp Assoc* 14:703, 1978.

Hosgood G et al: Perineal herniorrhaphy: perioperative data for 100 dogs, *J Am Anim Hosp Assoc* 31:331, 1995.

Orsher RJ: Clinical and surgical parameters in dogs with perineal hernia: analysis of internal obturator transposition, *Vet Surg* 15:253, 1986.

Welches CD et al: Perineal hernia in the cat: a retrospective study in 40 cases, *J Am Anim Hosp Assoc* 28:431, 1991.

Suggested Reading

Matthiesen DT: Diagnosis and management of complications occurring after perineal herniorrhaphy in dogs, *Compend Contin Educ Pract Vet* 11:797, 1989.

PERIANAL FISTULAE

DEFINITION

Perianal fistulae are suppurative, progressive, deep, ulcerating tracts in the perianal tissues.

SYNONYMS

Perianal sinuses, perineal fistulae, perianal fissures, furunculosis, pararectal fistulae, anusitis, fistulae-in-ano, anorectal abscesses

GENERAL CONSIDERATIONS AND CLINICALLY RELEVANT PATHOPHYSIOLOGY

The etiology of perianal fistulae is unknown. The combination of infection and abscessation of glands around the anus, the moist, contaminated anal environment, and a broad-based, low-set tail conformation are believed to contribute to perianal fistula formation. German shepherd dogs have a greater density of apocrine glands in the cutaneous zone of the anal canal, which may predispose them to perianal fistulae. Bacterial infection may occur after development of cutaneous lesions. Immunologic and endocrine studies have found no abnormalities in affected dogs.

Fistulae first appear as small draining holes in perianal skin that is inflamed and hyperpigmented. As the disease progresses these punctate holes enlarge and coalesce forming large areas of ulceration and granulation. Tracts may extend into the deep perirectal tissues and anal sacs. Hidradenitis, chronic necrotizing pyogranulomatous inflammation of the skin and hair follicles, cellulitis, dilated and inflamed lymphatics, necrosis, and fibrosis occur. Partial rectal stricture may occur.

DIAGNOSIS
Clinical Presentation

Signalment. Perianal fistulae occur most commonly in German shepherd dogs, but Irish setters also are predisposed. Various other breeds have been diagnosed with this condition. The disease appears to be more common in males than females (approximately 2:1), with a predominance in intact animals. Perianal fistulae are extremely rare in cats. Perianal fistulae may occur at any age; however, the mean age of 44 dogs with perianal fistulae was 5.2 years (range, 0.5 to 13 years) (Killingsworth et al, 1988a).

History. Dogs with perianal fistulae usually present because of anal discomfort, constipation, diarrhea, odor, licking, scooting, tenesmus, dyschezia, ulceration, and/or purulent perianal discharge. Many owners have noticed perianal ulcers or tracts. Pain may cause dogs to become vicious when the tail or perineum is examined or manipulated. Weight loss, decreased appetite, and lethargy may occur.

Physical Examination Findings

Dogs with perianal fistulae often appear normal; however, some are thin with a poor hair coat. The perianal area should be examined for fistulae. The perineum is often painful, and affected dogs may snap, bite, or cry when the tail is lifted, necessitating sedation or general anesthesia for thorough perineal examination. Tracts may be single but are typically multiple (Fig. 16-124). Fistulae can be difficult to identify if there are only a few punctate lesions and minimal ulceration. The condition becomes more evident as tracts coalesce and swelling and inflammation develop. The entire circumference of the anus may be ulcerated in severe cases. Previously unidentified tracts often become obvious when the dog is anesthetized and clipped. A rectal exam should determine the depth of involvement, degree of fibrosis, and relationship of anal sacs to fistulae. Anal stenosis and rectocutaneous fistulae may be identified during rectal examination.

☞ **N O T E ·** Examination of the perineal area establishes the tentative diagnosis; however, histologic examination is necessary to rule out squamous cell carcinoma, pythiosis, and other erosive conditions.

Radiography

Radiographs are not necessary unless there is a strong suspicion of neoplastic involvement.

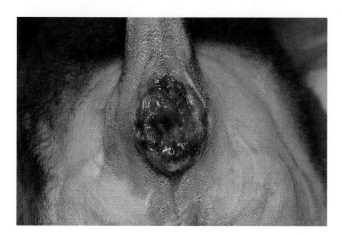

FIG. 16-124
Appearance of coalescing ulcers that characterize perianal fistulae of moderate severity.

Laboratory Findings

Minimum database results are nonspecific. Commonly isolated bacteria from deep, intraoperative perianal fistulae samples are *Escherichia coli, Staphylococcus aureus,* β-hemolytic streptococci, and *Proteus mirabilis* (Killingsworth et al, 1988a). Bacterial contamination is believed to occur after ulceration. Acute and chronic inflammation with fibrosis and granulation tissue are expected. Some tracts have an epithelial lining; others involve the anal crypts and rectal mucosa.

DIFFERENTIAL DIAGNOSIS

In its early stages anal squamous cell carcinoma may resemble perianal fistulae. Other important differential diagnoses include perianal tumors, anal sac fistulae, pythiosis, and fistulae associated with tail fold pyoderma.

MEDICAL TREATMENT

Management of perianal fistulae requires diligence, is frustrating for veterinarians and clients, and is uncomfortable for patients. Medical therapy alone often allows the condition to progress. Regular perianal cleansing and antibiotic therapy reduce inflammation but seldom allow healing of fistulae. Stool softeners may reduce dyschezia.

SURGICAL TREATMENT

Surgery is recommended. The goals of surgery are to eliminate necrotic or unhealthy tissue and stimulate second intention healing without causing fecal incontinence or anal stenosis. Numerous surgical procedures have been used for treating perianal fistulae, including superficial or radical excision, cryotherapy, fulguration, chemical cautery, and tail amputation. Staged procedures may be necessary during the initial months of treatment and may need to be repeated intermittently for life. Dogs with mild to moderate disease usually respond better to treatment than those with severe disease.

Radical resection is the excision of all diseased skin, subcutaneous tissue, muscle, and fascia. The rectum is apposed to remaining skin with widely spaced interrupted sutures. The remainder of the defect is allowed to heal by second intention. Fecal incontinence is a common postoperative problem. Superficial resection (i.e., excision of all skin involved in the inflammatory process) is recommended with severe or nonresponsive perianal fistulae. Debridement and fulguration of fistulae have less potential for causing fecal incontinence than extensive resection but tend to be ineffective in severe cases. Concurrent tail amputation is recommended by some surgeons. Anal sacculectomy (see p. 350) is needed when fistulae involve the anal sacs. Debridement and chemical cauterization (resection of epithelium overlying coalescing fistulous tracts, followed by the application of an irritant chemical to the underlying granulation tissue) may be performed using a strong iodine solution (Table 16-77). This technique is less effective than debridement and fulguration/ablation but may be selected for patients with mild disease or when healing begins to lag or small fistulae are identified after debridement and fulguration/ablation. Use of chemical cauterization at this time may eliminate the need for general anesthesia and reoperation.

Cryotherapy of perianal fistulae involves the application of a cryogen to destroy diseased tissue. Tissue that has been frozen will necrose and then slough off during the subsequent 1 to 2 weeks. The wounds heal by second intention. Appropriately controlling the freeze by using thermocouples is helpful. However, cryosurgery is not recommended because it is very difficult to control the freeze; muscles and nerves are often inadvertently destroyed. Up to one half of the patients have severe anal stenosis after cryosurgery. Other complications include flatulence, tenesmus, incontinence, diarrhea, and constipation.

Preoperative Management

The expected results of treatment and their important postoperative role should be thoroughly explained to the owner. A firm commitment of their ability and willingness to provide long-term postoperative care must be obtained from the owner. The location of the fistula(e) should be mapped on a chart of the perianal region. Administration of stool softeners should be initiated several days before surgery (see Table 16-61 on p. 327). The colon should be evacuated and food withheld the day before surgery. Hot compresses should be applied to the perineum to help remove exudate and debris. Analgesics may be necessary if the patient objects to perianal manipulations. Prophylactic antibiotics effective against gram-negative and anaerobic bacteria should be given during anesthetic induction.

> ☞ **N O T E** · Before any surgical procedure the dog's owner must commit to rigorous postoperative care, otherwise the benefits of surgery may be negated. Owners not willing to make financial and care commitments or those who become frustrated during treatment usually request euthanasia of their pet.

Anesthesia

Anesthetic recommendations for animals undergoing perianal surgery are on p. 337.

Surgical Anatomy

Anatomy of the perianal region is on p. 338.

TABLE 16-77

Chemical Cauterizing Agents

Silver nitrate
4.5%-5.0% phenol
7% iodine

Positioning

The patient should be positioned in ventral recumbency with the hindlegs over the end of the table. The pelvis should be elevated with padding and the tail secured over the back. The end of the table should be padded to avoid pressure on the femoral nerves. Alternatively a padded perineal stand may be used.

SURGICAL TECHNIQUE
Debridement and Fulguration/Ablation

Probe and explore the direction of each fistula (Fig. 16-125). Connect all communicating fistulae by excising the overlying epithelium (Fig. 16-126) to expose the underlying infected granulation bed. Superficially "char" (surface dehydration) this bed with a fulguration current or laser. Leave all areas open to heal by second intention. Expect to repeat this technique once or twice during the first months of therapy to resolve the fistulae.

Tail Amputation

Tail amputation performed in conjunction with debridement and fulguration/ablation may improve perineal ventilation and drying. The benefits of tail amputation are controversial. Many owners refuse amputation initially but agree to have it after they discover healing has not been ideal after the initial treatment(s). *Make an elliptical incision around the base of the tail (Fig. 16-127, A). Incise the subcutaneous tissues to expose the muscles. Separate the attachments of*

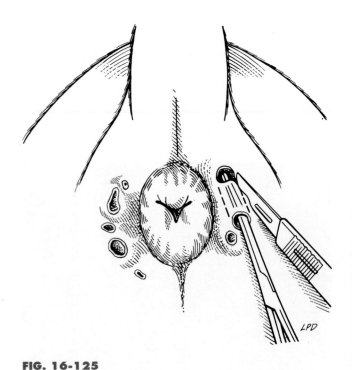

FIG. 16-125
During debridement and fulguration of perineal fistulae, probe each tract and excise overlying epithelium between communicating tracts to expose the underlying granulation tissue.

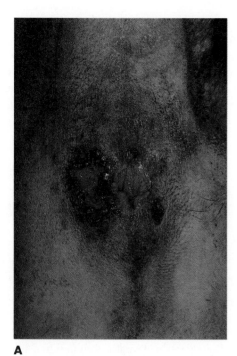

FIG. 16-126
Appearance of perianal fistulae in a dog
A, before surgery, **B,** after debridement,
and **C,** after fulguration.

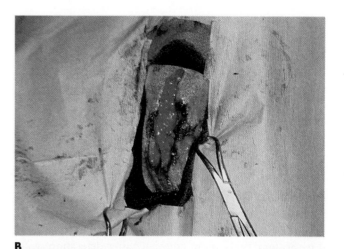

B

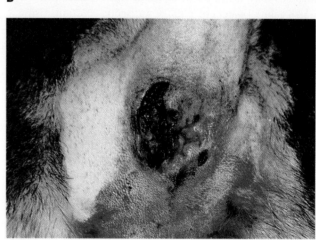

C

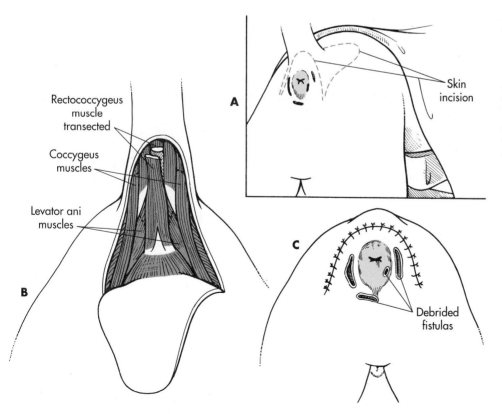

Rectococcygeus
muscle
transected

Coccygeus
muscles

Levator ani
muscles

Skin
incision

Debrided
fistulas

A

B

C

FIG. 16-127
Treatment of perianal fistulae
may be facilitated by tail amputation. **A,** Make an elliptical
incision around the base of the
tail. **B,** Expose, identify, and
transect the coccygeal musculature. **C,** Disarticulate the tail
at the second or third caudal
vertebra and close dead space
and skin.

the levator ani, rectococcygeus, and coccygeus muscles to the caudal vertebrae (Fig. 16-127, B). Transect the tail by disarticulation at the second or third caudal vertebra. Ligate the medial and lateral caudal arteries and veins. Appose the levator ani muscles and lavage the site. Appose subcutaneous tissues with a simple interrupted or continuous pattern. Excise redundant skin if necessary and appose skin edges with approximating, nonabsorbable sutures (Fig. 16-127, C).

POSTOPERATIVE CARE AND ASSESSMENT

Systemic (see Table 16-4 on p. 209) or epidural analgesics should be used as needed. The perineum should be cleaned three to four times daily, especially after defecation, with warm saline (water) or a dilute antiseptic solution. Using a hose and warm tap water is a convenient and acceptable method of cleaning. An Elizabethan collar, bucket, or side bars should be used to prevent self-mutilation, and stool softeners should be given to facilitate fecal passage during the first 3 to 4 weeks (see Table 16-61 on p. 327). The stool softener should make the stool soft but not sticky or pasty. A low-bulk diet should be fed. Giving antibiotics effective against gram-negative and anaerobic bacteria is helpful, albeit not essential. The size of the debrided areas should be mapped immediately after surgery and at each reevaluation to allow accurate monitoring. Patient reevaluation should be performed every 2 to 4 weeks, and nonhealing or new fistulae should be treated as needed. After fistula resolution, owners should keep the perineum clipped and clean. They should check for new fistulae on a monthly basis.

> ☞ **NOTE** · It is essential that the perineum be kept clean!

COMPLICATIONS

Fecal incontinence, anal stenosis, and recurrence sometimes precipitate euthanasia. These are common complications with some surgical techniques. Flatulence, tenesmus, constipation, and diarrhea may also occur. Complications are more common and severe after radical resection (Table 16-78) vs. superficial resection or fulguration/ablation.

PROGNOSIS

Medical therapy alone is rarely effective. Mild perianal fistulae may be controlled if owners are diligent about daily perianal care. The area must be kept clean and dry to prevent dis-

---

TABLE 16-78

Potential Complications of Wide Resection of Fistulae

• Fecal incontinence	• Dyschezia
• Flatulence	• Constipation
• Diarrhea	• Anal stenosis
• Tenesmus	• Recurrence

---

ease progression. The prognosis after surgery is fair to poor, depending on the severity of the disease at the time of surgery and postoperative owner compliance. Early diagnosis and surgery allow less radical procedures with fewer postoperative complications. Recurrence is common, and multiple surgeries may be needed. Many animals are euthanized because of pain, nonresponse to treatment, recurrence, and/or client frustration.

Reference

Killingsworth CR et al: Bacterial population and histologic changes in dogs with perianal fistula, *Am J Vet Res* 49:1736, 1988a.

Suggested Reading

Budsberg SC, Spurgeon TL, Liggitt HD: Anatomic predisposition to perianal fistulae formation in the German shepherd dog, *Am J Vet Res* 46:1468, 1985.

Elkins AD, Hobson HP: Management of perianal fistulae: a retrospective study of 23 cases, *Vet Surg* 11:110, 1982.

Goring RL, Bright RM, Stancil ML: Perianal fistulas in the dog: retrospective evaluation of surgical treatment by deroofing and fulguration, *Vet Surg* 15:392, 1986.

Killingsworth CR et al: Thyroid and immunologic status in dogs with perianal fistula, *Am J Vet Res* 49:1742, 1988b.

Matushek KJ, Rosin E: Perianal fistulas in dogs, *Compend Contin Educ Pract Vet* 13:621, 1991.

van Ee RT, Palminteri A: Tail amputation for treatment of perianal fistula in dogs, *J Am Anim Hosp Assoc* 23:95, 1987.

Vasseur PB: Perianal fistulae in dogs: a retrospective of surgical techniques, *J Am Anim Hosp Assoc* 17:177, 1981.

Vasseur PB: Results of surgical excision of perianal fistulas in dogs, *J Am Vet Med Assoc* 185:60, 1984.

RECTAL PROLAPSE

DEFINITIONS

Rectal prolapse is a protrusion of rectal mucosa from the anus.

SYNONYMS

Everted rectum, everted anus, anal prolapse

GENERAL CONSIDERATIONS AND CLINICALLY RELEVANT PATHOPHYSIOLOGY

Rectal prolapse is principally associated with endoparasitism or enteritis in young animals, and tumors or perineal hernias in middle-aged to older animals. However, any condition causing tenesmus may result in rectal prolapse (Table 16-79). Weakness of perirectal and perianal connective tissues or muscles, uncoordinated peristaltic contractions, and inflammation or edema of rectal mucous membranes predispose patients to rectal prolapse.

Rectal prolapse may be complete or incomplete. Incomplete prolapse involves only mucosa. A part of the entire anorectal circumference may be affected. Complete pro-

TABLE 16-79

Conditions Associated with Rectal Prolapse

- Endoparasitism
- Enteritis
- Intestinal foreign bodies
- Dystocia
- Urolithiasis
- Constipation
- Congenital defects
- Sphincter laxity
- Prostatic disease

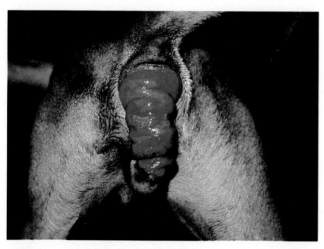

FIG. 16-128
Appearance of a rectal prolapse. Note the large amount of everted rectum that must be differentiated from an intussusception.

lapse involves all layers of the rectal wall and the entire circumference. The amount of eversion increases with continued straining, varying from a few millimeters to many centimeters. Everted tissue becomes edematous, preventing spontaneous retraction into the pelvic canal. Continued exposure causes excoriation, bleeding, desiccation, and necrosis.

DIAGNOSIS
Clinical Presentation

Signalment. Rectal prolapse occurs in dogs and cats, with no documented breed predispositions. However, it may occur more often in Manx cats because of their anal laxity. It may occur at any age but is more common in young animals.

History. Straining or recent perineal surgery are common. Constipation, diarrhea, prostatitis, urinary tract infections, dyspnea, and dystocia may produce tenesmus. Perineal or perianal irritation from trauma or surgery may also cause straining and rectal prolapse.

Physical Examination Findings

The physical status of the patient is unpredictable because of the numerous potential causes of rectal prolapse. Protrusion

of anorectal mucosa is obvious on physical examination. The degree of prolapse may vary from a few millimeters to several centimeters (Fig. 16-128). Rectal prolapse must be differentiated from ileocolic intussusception (see below).

Radiography

Radiography may help identify the cause of the prolapse.

Laboratory Findings

Laboratory tests are nonspecific for rectal prolapse but may identify the cause and define the patient's physiologic status. Parasites and viral enteritis are common in young animals.

DIFFERENTIAL DIAGNOSIS

The primary differential diagnosis for rectal prolapse is intussusception. Insertion of a probe (i.e., thermometer or smooth tube) alongside the prolapsed mass is possible with an intussusception but not with a rectal prolapse.

MEDICAL TREATMENT

Treatment and prognosis depend on the cause, degree of prolapse, chronicity, and whether it is a recurrent prolapse. Acute rectal prolapse is easily treated, but chronic disease may require resection. Manual reduction and placement of a purse-string suture around the anus are recommended for acute prolapses with minimal tissue damage and edema (Fig. 16-129, *A*). Warm saline lavages, massage, and lubrication (e.g., with a water soluble gel) should be applied to the everted tissue before digital reduction. A purse-string suture tight enough to maintain prolapse reduction without interfering with passage of soft stool should be placed. Most rectal prolapse patients respond well to manual reduction when the cause is treated and resolved.

SURGICAL TREATMENT

Nonreducible or severely traumatized prolapses necessitate amputation. Colopexy should be performed when rectal prolapse repeatedly recurs after manual reduction or amputation (see p. 322).

☞ **NOTE** • You must attempt to identify the underlying cause and treat it.

Preoperative Management

Surgery should be prompt to prevent further trauma to the everted tissues. Extensive colorectal preparation is unnecessary. Prophylactic antibiotics effective against gram-negative and anaerobic bacteria (see Table 16-57 on p. 321) should be given at the time of anesthetic induction. The exposed tissue should be lavaged with warm sterile saline and lubricated with a water soluble gel.

Anesthesia

Anesthetic recommendations for animals undergoing rectal and perineal surgery are on p. 337.

Surgical Anatomy

Surgical anatomy of the rectum and perineum are on p. 338.

Positioning

After the perianal area has been clipped and aseptically prepared for surgery, the everted tissue should again be lavaged and lubricated. The patient should be positioned in ventral recumbency with the hindlegs over the end of the table. The pelvis should be elevated with padding, and the tail secured over the back. The end of the table should be padded to avoid pressure on the femoral nerves. Alternatively a perineal stand may be used.

SURGICAL TECHNIQUE

Place a sterile test tube or syringe case into the rectal lumen to serve as a guide (Fig. 16-129, B). Place three horizontal mattress stay sutures (at the 12 o'clock, 5 o'clock, and 8 o'clock positions) through all layers of the prolapse just cra-

nial to the proposed transection site. These sutures should enter the rectal lumen with the needle being deflected by the probe before being passed through the rectal tissues again. Transect the traumatized tissue in stages caudal to the stay sutures. Anatomically appose the transected edges with simple interrupted sutures (e.g., 3-0 or 4-0 polydioxanone or polyglyconate) after each stage of the resection. Space sutures approximately 2 mm apart and 2 mm from the cut edge. Inspect the anastomosis for gaps between sutures. Remove the stay sutures and gently replace the anastomotic site within the pelvic or anal canal. Place a purse-string suture around the anus if postoperative tenesmus is anticipated.

POSTOPERATIVE CARE AND ASSESSMENT

The cause of the prolapse must be treated to prevent recurrence. Epidural opioids may eliminate postoperative tenesmus for several hours (see p. 337). Systemic analgesics should

FIG. 16-129
A, Digitally reduce small prolapses with healthy mucosa and place a purse-string suture around the rectum. Resect irreducible or traumatized prolapses. **B,** Place a probe in the rectal lumen and three to four stay sutures in the rectal wall. Make a full-thickness incision through the prolapsed tissue. Appose the edges with simple interrupted sutures.

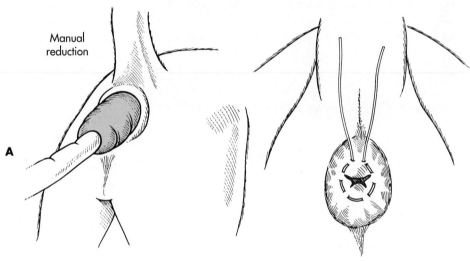

Manual reduction

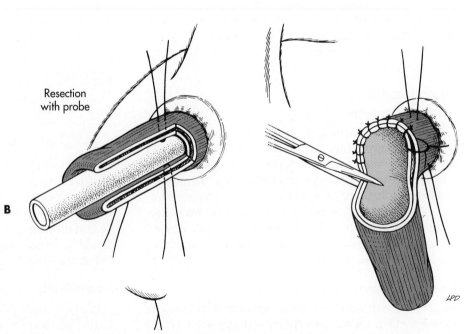

Resection with probe

be given if necessary (see Table 16-4 on p. 209). A low-fiber diet should be fed while the purse-string suture is in place. The purse-string suture can generally be removed 3 to 5 days after manual reduction and 1 to 2 days after resection. Stool softeners should be given for 2 to 3 weeks after resection (see Table 16-61 on p. 327). Amputees must be monitored for leakage from the surgical site.

COMPLICATIONS

Potential complications of manual reduction of rectal prolapses are tenesmus, dyschezia, hematochezia, and recurrence. Additional complications of resection include hemorrhage, leakage, anal stenosis, infection, dehiscence, and fecal incontinence.

PROGNOSIS

Incomplete prolapses occurring during defecation may reduce spontaneously. The prognosis for chronic rectal prolapse without manual reduction or surgery is poor. Chronically exposed rectal mucosa is traumatized by licking, sitting, and environmental exposure, ultimately becoming necrotic with secondary sepsis. The prognosis for most animals treated surgically is good, provided the primary cause of tenesmus or irritation is appropriately treated.

Suggested Reading

Popovitch CA, Holt D, Bright R: Colopexy as a treatment for rectal prolapse in dogs and cats: a retrospective study of 14 cases, *Vet Surg* 23:115, 1994.

FECAL INCONTINENCE

DEFINITIONS

Fecal incontinence is the inability to voluntarily control defecation. **Reservoir incontinence** results from a failure of the large bowel to adapt to and contain the colorectal contents. **Sphincter incontinence** is a failure of the sphincter mechanism to resist propulsive forces in the rectum so that feces are involuntarily passed.

GENERAL CONSIDERATIONS AND CLINICALLY RELEVANT PATHOPHYSIOLOGY

Fecal incontinence is uncommon in dogs and cats. Fecal continence depends on maintenance of colonic reservoir function and anal sphincter control. Muscles involved in fecal continence include the internal anal sphincter, external anal sphincter, rectococcygeus, levator ani, and coccygeus muscles. As fecal material is propelled distally into the terminal rectum, the rectum distends and the internal anal sphincter dilates while the external anal sphincter and caudal portion of the levator ani muscles contract. Subsequently, propulsive contractions decrease, and normal resting tone is restored in 2 to 3 minutes. Thus the rectum distends and adapts with each new bolus to increase its storage capacity, and a resting

anorectal high-pressure zone is created by the internal anal sphincter, external anal sphincter, and caudal portion of the levator ani muscles. The internal anal sphincter contributes 50% to 80% of the resting tone in the high-pressure zone. The external anal sphincter is tonically active but contributes minimally to the resting tone; its short contractions resist peristaltic waves. The role of the levator ani is uncertain. Animals posture and increase abdominal pressure by closing the glottis, fixing the diaphragm, and contracting the abdominal wall when defecation is appropriate. This causes the external anal sphincter to relax and the rectococcygeus, levator ani, and coccygeus muscles to contract.

Reservoir incontinence (Table 16-80) is usually characterized by frequent, conscious defecation. Loss of reservoir continence causes production of abnormally soft, unformed, or liquefied feces. Loss of reservoir continence may be caused by diffuse colonic disease resulting in decreased distensibility, or it may be secondary to reduced colonic length after resection (e.g., two thirds or more). The small intestine increases water absorption and capacity after subtotal colectomy; therefore many animals regain reservoir continence.

Sphincter incontinence (see Table 16-80) may be neurogenic or nonneurogenic. Partial fecal incontinence may occur if only one muscle group malfunctions. Loss of sensory receptors and the afferent limb of the continence mechanism can be secondary to rectal resection. An adequate cuff of rectal muscularis must be preserved to maintain sphincter continence. Loss of efferent neural control occurs when caudal rectal nerves are damaged. Sacral spinal cord lesions of S_{1-3} cord segments (L_5 vertebral level in dogs and L_6 in cats) damage the cell bodies of the pudendal nerve. Peripheral pudendal nerve damage can occur anywhere from the cauda equina distally. Unilateral pudendal nerve damage causes fecal incontinence for only 3 to 4 weeks because of

TABLE 16-80

Causes of Fecal Incontinence

Reservoir Incontinence
- Diffuse colonic disease resulting in decreased distensibility
- Reduced colonic length after resection (e.g., two thirds or more)

Sphincter Incontinence
- Rectal resection (within 4 cm of terminal rectum)
- Inadequate cuff of rectal muscularis (less than approximately 1.5 cm)
- Damage to the caudal rectal nerves
- Sacral spinal cord lesions of S_{1-3} cord segments (L_5 vertebral level in dogs and L_6 in cats)
- Peripheral pudendal nerve damage
- Physical disruption of the external anal sphincter after:
  —anorectal trauma
  —rectal prolapse
  —severe perianal disease (e.g., inflammation, tumors)
  —surgical resection
- Resection of more than half the external anal sphincter

cross innervation and muscle fiber decussation. Bilateral pudendal nerve damage causes permanent incontinence. Nonneurogenic sphincter incontinence occurs secondary to physical disruption of the external anal sphincter after anorectal trauma, rectal prolapse, severe perianal disease (inflammation, tumors), or surgical resection. The incidence of incontinence increases as external anal sphincter resection approaches 180 degrees. Resection of more than half of the external anal sphincter usually results in fecal incontinence.

DIAGNOSIS
Clinical Presentation

Signalment. Any breed or sex of dog or cat may have fecal incontinence. Manx cats may be predisposed because of anal laxity secondary to abnormal innervation. Dogs with perineal fistulae (see p. 356) may develop fecal incontinence. Fecal incontinence may occur in any age animal, although 50% of affected animals are 11 years or older (Guilford, 1990).

History. History is important in differentiating reservoir from sphincter incontinence and determining potential causes. Animals present because of inappropriate defecation. Some affected animals posture and void normally despite having inappropriate defecation. A fecal bolus may be voided when barking, coughing, or rising from a recumbent position, without posturing or recognition of the event. It is important to find out if the onset of incontinence is associated with recent colorectal or perineal surgery, trauma, perianal disease, or neurologic disease. Signs of incontinence vary from occasional incontinence to perineal soiling and fecal dribbling. Reservoir incontinence may be associated with frequent defecation, tenesmus, hematochezia, and mucoid stools.

☞ **N O T E** · Owners may not be aware of their pet's incontinence, particularly if the animal resides primarily outdoors.

Physical Examination Findings

Patients with fecal incontinence often appear normal. Rectal and perineal examination may reveal colorectal or perianal disease. Anal sphincter tone may be diminished and the anus dilated, and/or rectal mucosa prolapsed. The abdomen should be palpated to determine colonic size and bladder tone, and a thorough neurologic examination should be performed. Self-inflicted skin trauma suggests paresthesia. Hyperesthesia may be detected in the lumbosacral area. Hindlimb paresthesia, urinary incontinence, and hyperesthesia suggest cauda equina syndrome.

Radiography/Ultrasonography/Endoscopy

Plain radiographs should be evaluated for colorectal or pelvic canal masses, vertebral abnormalities (e.g., lumbosacral stenosis or fracture), or pelvic fractures. Myelography, epidurography, computed tomography (CT scan), or mag-

netic resonance imaging (MRI) help diagnose spinal cord or cauda equina lesions. Endoanal ultrasonography helps evaluate anal sphincter morphology and localize weak areas (Deen et al, 1993). An external anal sphincter muscle defect is identified as either a hypoechogenic or hyperechogenic wedge-shaped area. An internal sphincter defect is identified as a loss of continuity of the normal hypoechoic ring. Colonoscopy and proctoscopy are indicated if reservoir incontinence is suspected.

Laboratory Findings

Hemogram, serum biochemistry profile, urinalysis, and fecal exam are recommended. Hematology and serum biochemistry values may suggest the etiology. Electromyography and manometry help assess the anorectal sphincter complex in some cases. These exams help differentiate reservoir incontinence from sphincter incontinence and neurogenic incontinence from nonneurogenic incontinence. Electromyography can reveal denervation or myopathy. Manometry gives anal and colorectal pressure profiles and evaluates the degree of anorectal tone impairment and internal and external anal sphincter function. Presence of an intact reflex arch may be determined more simply by inflating a Foley catheter in the rectum and observing the response.

DIFFERENTIAL DIAGNOSIS

Differential diagnoses and potential causes of fecal incontinence include anal disease (e.g., anal sacculitis, dermatitis, endoparasites, perianal fistulae, or tumors), colorectal disease (e.g., colitis, neoplasia), poor diet, trauma or denervation to the muscles of continence, damage to somatic peripheral nerves (i.e., pudendal, or S_{2-3} C_1 spinal nerves), damage to autonomic peripheral nerves (i.e., pelvic plexus, pelvic nerves), cauda equina syndrome, central nervous system injury (e.g., sacral spinal segments, spinothalamic tracts, frontal cortex), and behavioral abnormalities.

MEDICAL TREATMENT

The causative disease or condition should be treated if possible. Owner acceptance may require that the pet be kept outdoors. Many patients are euthanized because owners are unable or unwilling to tolerate incontinence. Goals of medical management are to reduce fecal water content, decrease fecal bulk, slow transit time, and increase anal sphincter tone. Symptomatic medical management includes dietary change, pharmacologic therapy, and induced defecation. A low residue diet (i.e., cottage cheese and rice) reduces fecal volume by up to 85% and lessens defecation frequency. Opioids (Table 16-81) promote segmental contractions, slowing bowel transit time and increasing water absorption. Enemas and rectal stimulation can promote colonic evacuation at appropriate times and help prevent inappropriate defecation.

SURGICAL TREATMENT

Sphincter-enhancing procedures for treating fecal incontinence in animals have been inadequately investigated; described surgical techniques must be considered investigational.

TABLE 16-81
Opioids That Slow Bowel Transit Time
Diphenoxylate Hydrochloride (Lomotil)
Dogs—0.1-0.2 mg/kg PO, BID to TID
Cats—0.05-0.1 mg/kg PO, BID
Loperamide Hydrochloride (Imodium)
Dogs—0.1-0.2 mg/kg PO, BID to TID
Cats—0.08-0.16 mg/kg PO, BID

Anal sphincter function has been enhanced by using either a fascial sling (Leeds, Renegar, 1981) or silicone elastomer (Silastic sheeting #501-3) (Dean et al, 1988).

Preoperative Management

The colon should be evacuated with laxatives, oral cathartics, and enemas, and remaining fecal material should be manually evacuated after anesthetic induction. Antibiotics effective against gram-negative and anaerobic bacteria (see Table 16-57 on p. 321) should be given after anesthetic induction.

FIG. 16-130
Fecal continence may be improved by enhancing the function of the anal sphincter with an implant. **A,** Make 3- to 4-cm incisions on each side of the anus. Connect the incisions with a tunnel dorsal and ventral to the anus. **B,** Direct the implant through the tunnels. **C,** Secure the implant to the coccygeus muscle, pull it snug around a probe, and secure it to itself. (Modified from Dean PW et al: *Vet Surg* 17:304, 1988.)

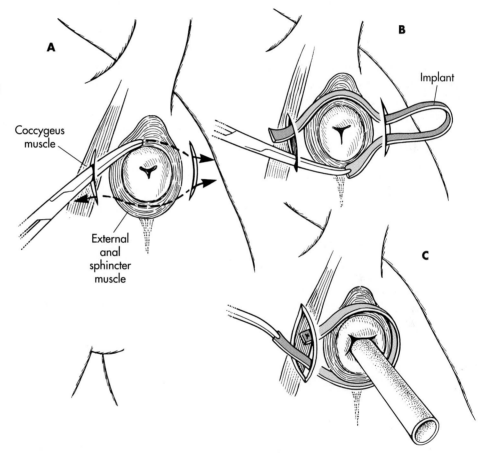

Anesthesia

General anesthesia is recommended. Anesthetic recommendations for animals undergoing rectal and perineal surgery are on p. 337.

Surgical Anatomy

Surgical anatomy of the rectum and perineum is on p. 338.

Positioning

Clip and aseptically prepare the perineum or ventral abdomen. The patient should be positioned in ventral recumbency with the hindlegs over the end of the table. The pelvis should be elevated with padding, and the tail should be secured over the back. The end of the table should be padded to avoid pressure on the femoral nerves. Alternatively, a perineal stand may be used.

SURGICAL TECHNIQUE
Fascial Sling

Harvest two strips of tensor fasciae latae (6 cm × 0.5 cm) from the lateral thigh, suture them together, and transfer to the anus. Close the fascial defect and appose subcutaneous tissues and skin. Make a 4-cm incision on each side of the anus just lateral to the tail base. Connect the two incisions by undermining the tissue ventral to the anus with a curved hemostat. Direct the fascial strip around the ventral anus using curved hemostats. Suture the fascia to the coccygeus muscle at the base of the tail on one side, pull it snug, and suture it to the tail base on the opposite side (e.g., 2-0 or 3-0 monofilament nylon or polypropylene). Alternatively, secure one end to the coccygeus muscle and direct the other end of the fascial strip over the base of the tail, pull it snug, and suture it to itself at the tail base. Lavage the area and reappose subcutaneous tissues and skin.

Implantation of a Silicone Elastomer

Make two incisions lateral to the anus as described above (Fig. 16-130, A). Make a tunnel ventral and dorsal to the anus with curved hemostats. Insert the implant through the tunnels (Fig. 16-130, B). Overlap the implant ends and pull it snug around the anus. To prevent overtightening place a 1-cm probe in the rectum while the implant is tightened (Fig. 16-130, C). Suture the overlapping ends of the implant together with nonabsorbable monofilament suture (e.g., 2-0 or 3-0 nylon or polypropylene). Lavage the area and reappose subcutaneous tissues and skin.

POSTOPERATIVE CARE AND ASSESSMENT

Analgesics should be given as needed, and antibiotics should be continued for several days to minimize the risk of implant infection. Stool softeners should be administered (see Table 16-61 on p. 327), and a low-residue diet fed. The animal should be monitored for infection and effectiveness of the procedure. Tenesmus is expected for several days.

COMPLICATIONS

The major complications associated with these procedures are failure or recurrence of incontinence. Slings often loosen slightly after implantation. Correction of incontinence may only be partial, and some signs may persist. Infection, dehiscence, and sloughing of the implant are risks. Persistent tenesmus and potential obstruction may occur if the sling is too snug.

PROGNOSIS

Prognosis depends on the type and extent of the incontinence. Complete neurogenic incontinence is incurable. Improved sphincter function is anticipated after surgery, although signs may worsen with implant loosening. Muscle trauma or irritation often causes partial or temporary incontinence, which improves as the muscles heal.

References

Dean PW et al: Silicone elastomer for fecal incontinence in dogs, *Vet Surg* 17:304–310, 1988.

Deen KI et al: Anal sphincter defects: correlation between endoanal ultrasound and surgery, *Ann Surg* 218:201, 1993.

Guilford WG: Fecal incontinence in dogs and cats, *Compend Cont Educ Pract Vet* 12:313, 1990.

Leeds EB, Renegar WR: A modified fascial sling for the treatment of fecal incontinence—surgical technique, *J Am Anim Hosp Assoc* 17:663, 1981.

CHAPTER 17

Surgery of the Liver

GENERAL PRINCIPLES AND TECHNIQUES

DEFINITIONS

Hepatectomy refers to removal of either the entire liver (**total hepatectomy**) or a portion (**partial hepatectomy**).

PREOPERATIVE CONCERNS

The liver is the largest gland in the body. It is the primary site of the metabolism (detoxification) of many substances and plays a central role in the metabolism of protein, fat, and carbohydrates. Unfortunately, clinical signs of hepatic disease may not be apparent until the disease is advanced and dysfunction is irreversible. Hepatic failure may affect many other organ systems, including the CNS, kidney, intestines, and heart.

☞ **N O T E** · Animals with severe or chronic hepatic disease may bleed excessively. Evaluate clotting before surgery and give blood transfusions if necessary.

The liver produces most of the plasma proteins, including albumin, alpha and beta globulins, fibrinogen, and prothrombin. Hypoalbuminemia is common in patients with advanced hepatic disease that may also be dehydrated due to vomiting. Fluid therapy may further dilute albumin; plasma or colloid infusions should be considered in these patients, in addition to electrolyte solutions. Albumin levels less than 2.0 g/dl may delay wound healing. Severe electrolyte abnormalities are uncommon with hepatic disease, but assessment of potassium levels is warranted. Coagulopathies may occur because of decreased synthesis of clotting factors. Evaluation of clotting parameters preoperatively is warranted, and transfusions with fresh whole blood may decrease intraoperative hemorrhage in selected patients. Some patients with hepatic disease are anemic due to nutritional deficiencies, coagulation abnormalities, or gastrointestinal hemorrhage. Animals with hematocrits less than 20% should be given preoperative blood transfusions (Table 17-1). Many patients with liver disease are anorexic and may require nutritional supplementation before surgery (see Chapter 11). Hypoglycemia occurs with severe hepatic insufficiency; monitoring of blood glucose levels and supplementing fluids with glucose may be needed. Patients with massive ascites may have ventilatory disturbances due to diaphragmatic displacement and restriction of lung expansion. Removal of some abdominal fluid in such patients before anesthetic induction may help prevent hypoventilation. Patients with hepatic encephalopathy should be treated with dietary therapy, appropriate antibiotics, enemas, fluids, and other medications (see p. 377) to decrease or eliminate clinical signs before surgery.

☞ **N O T E** · Monitor serum albumin, glucose, and electrolytes closely in patients with severe hepatic disease.

ANESTHETIC CONSIDERATIONS

Animals with hepatic dysfunction may have impaired ability to metabolize and inactivate some drugs due to a decreased hepatic metabolic rate, decreased hepatic blood flow, decreased volume of distribution (i.e., of drugs that are highly protein-bound), and a decreased extraction efficiency. Prolonged duration of action or altered function of drugs commonly used to anesthetize veterinary patients may result. Acetylpromazine lowers the seizure threshold and should

---

TABLE 17-1

Blood Transfusions

ml of Donor Blood Needed

$$\text{recipient blood volume}^* \times \frac{\text{desired PCV} - \text{actual patient PCV}}{\text{PCV of anticoagulated donor blood}}$$

*Total blood volume is estimated at 90 ml/kg for dogs and 70 ml/kg for cats.

Note: A rough estimate is that 2.2 ml of blood/kg of body weight will increase the recipient's PCV by 1%.

TABLE 17-2

Selected Anesthetic Agents for
Animals with Hepatic Disease*

Premedication

Give atropine (0.02-0.04 mg/kg SC or IM) or glycopyrrolate
(0.005-0.011 mg/kg SC or IM) plus oxymorphone[†] (0.05-
0.1 mg/kg SC or IM) or butorphanol (0.2-0.4 mg/kg SC
or IM) or buprenorphine (5-15 μg/kg IM)

Induction

Diazepam (0.2 mg/kg IV) plus etomidate (0.5-1.5 mg/kg
IV). Alternatively, if not vomiting, mask induction can be
used or give thiopental or propofol at reduced doses.

Maintenance

Isoflurane

*See p. 378 for recommendations for patients with portosystemic
shunts.
[†]Use 0.05 mg/kg in cats.

TABLE 17-3

Antibiotics in Animals with
Hepatocellular Compromise

Ampicillin

22 mg/kg IV, IM, or SC, TID to QID

Metronidazole (Flagyl)

10 mg/kg PO, TID

Cefazolin (Ancef, Kefzol)

20 mg/kg IV or IM, TID to QID

Clindamycin (Antirobe)

11 mg/kg PO, BID

not be used in patients with hepatic encephalopathy. It also
lowers systemic vascular resistance and blood pressure and
may alter the metabolism of some drugs (i.e., procaine, suc-
cinylcholine); it should be avoided in patients with severe hepatic dysfunction. Diazepam is useful as a premedicant in
patients with hepatic dysfunction because it causes mild,
dose-related CNS depression, does not depress the cardiopulmonary system, raises the seizure threshold, and can
be antagonized with flumazenil (Table 17-2). Diazepam is
best used in conjunction with an opioid because it may disinhibit some behaviors when used alone. It should be used
with caution in hypoalbuminemic patients. Most opioids
have little or no adverse effect on the liver; however, intravenous morphine should be avoided in dogs with hepatic
dysfunction because it may cause hepatic congestion due to
histamine release and hepatic vein spasm. Although some
opioid analgesics may have prolonged action when hepatic
function is reduced, their effects can be antagonized. Barbiturates (e.g., thiopental) should be used cautiously or
avoided in patients with significant hepatic disease because
these drugs may have a prolonged duration of action. Ketamine is metabolized in the liver of dogs (it is excreted largely
unchanged in the urine of cats) and its central stimulant action may precipitate seizures in encephalopathic patients.
Thus ketamine should be administered at reduced dosages to
dogs with mild hepatic dysfunction and avoided in patients
with severe dysfunction. See recommendations on p. 378 for
anesthetic management of animals with portosystemic
shunts.

Inhalation anesthetics are the preferred method of maintaining anesthesia in patients undergoing hepatic surgery.
Heart rate and rhythm, respiratory rate, and urine output
should be monitored. Hyperventilation may cause a significant decrease in portal blood flow. Halothane and isoflurane
cause decreases in portal blood flow, but hepatic arterial
blood flow tends to increase during isoflurane anesthesia,

preserving hepatic oxygenation. Isoflurane, unlike
halothane, has not been associated with postoperative hepatic dysfunction. Isoflurane is the inhalation agent of choice
for patients with severe hepatic disease. Monitoring of blood
gases, blood pressures, blood glucose concentrations, hematocrit, and total protein is advantageous in these patients.

ANTIBIOTICS

Anaerobic bacteria normally reside in the liver but may proliferate if there is hepatic ischemia or hypoxia. Thus prophylactic antibiotics are warranted in most patients undergoing
hepatic surgery. The pharmacokinetics of antibiotics may be
altered in these patients by depressed hepatic metabolism, alterations in hepatic arterial or portal blood flow, hypoalbuminemia, or reductions in biliary excretion. Antibiotics are
specifically indicated in the treatment of hepatic encephalopathy (see p. 377), bacterial hepatitis, and hepatic abscesses. Broad-spectrum antibiotics that are effective against
anaerobes (i.e., penicillin derivatives, metronidazole, clindamycin) are appropriate and relatively safe in patients with
hepatocellular compromise (Table 17-3). Metronidazole,
when administered at doses greater than 60 mg/kg of body
weight, has caused neurologic signs (e.g., ataxia, nystagmus,
head tilt, and seizures) in some dogs. Potentially hepatotoxic
antibiotics (e.g., chloramphenicol, chlortetracycline, or erythromycin) should be avoided, if possible.

SURGICAL ANATOMY

The diaphragmatic surface (parietal surface) of the liver is
convex and lies mainly in touch with the diaphragm. The visceral surface faces caudoventrally and to the left and contacts
the stomach, duodenum, pancreas, and right kidney. There
are six hepatic lobes (Fig. 17-1). The borders of the liver are
normally sharp, but they appear more rounded in young animals and in those with infiltrated, congested, or scarred liv-
ers. The liver has two afferent blood supplies: a low-pressure
portal system and a high-pressure arterial system. The portal
vein drains the stomach, intestines, pancreas, and spleen and
supplies four fifths of the blood that enters the liver. The remainder of the afferent blood supply is from the proper he-

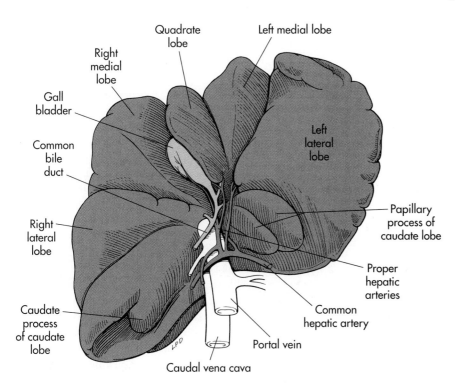

FIG. 17-1
Anatomy of the liver.

Quadrate lobe

Left medial lobe

Right medial lobe

Gall bladder

Common bile duct

Left lateral lobe

Right lateral lobe

Papillary process of caudate lobe

Proper hepatic arteries

Common hepatic artery

Caudate process of caudate lobe

Portal vein

Caudal vena cava

patic arteries. The proper hepatic arteries are branches of the common hepatic artery and may number between two and five. The efferent drainage of the liver is through the hepatic veins. In the fetal pup, the ductus venosus shunts blood from the umbilical vein to the hepatic venous system. The ductus venosus becomes fibrotic after birth and is known as the ligamentum venosum. Bile, formed in the liver, is discharged into bile canaliculi lying between the hepatocytes. These canaliculi unite to form interlobular ducts that ultimately merge to form lobar or bile ducts (see p. 390). The portal vein, bile ducts, hepatic artery, lymphatics, and nerves are contained in the lace-like and nonsupporting portion of the lesser omentum known as the hepatoduodenal ligament.

☞ **N O T E** · The cranial location of the liver makes biopsy somewhat difficult in large, deep-chested breeds. Extend the incision as far cranially as possible for maximal exposure.

SURGICAL TECHNIQUES

Surgery of the liver is complicated by the fact that hepatic tissue is friable. Because of the sparsity of fibrous protein in the liver, sharp dissection is difficult and results in retraction of blood vessels and bile ducts within the friable stroma. Ligation of structures (i.e., blood vessels and bile ducts) after they have been cut is extremely difficult. Packing the liver firmly enough to obtain hemostasis may cause compressed cells to become ischemic and necrotic. Maintaining hepatic blood supply is important because the liver normally harbors pathogenic anaerobes. Thus surgery of the liver requires different techniques than are used in surgery on most other abdominal organs.

☞ **N O T E** · Obtain a liver biopsy during abdominal exploration in all animals with possible hepatic dysfunction or a liver that appears grossly abnormal.

Hepatic biopsies are commonly indicated in patients with known or suspected hepatic disease. The biopsies may be obtained percutaneously, with laparoscopy, or at surgery. Partial hepatectomies are less commonly performed but may be indicated for focal neoplasms or trauma. The standard approach for hepatic surgery is a cranial ventral midline abdominal incision. The caudal aspect of the sternum can be split if additional exposure is needed.

Percutaneous Liver Biopsy

Percutaneous core biopsies or fine-needle aspirations are most successful in patients with diffuse hepatic disease; however, ultrasound guidance will allow some focal lesions to be biopsied. Animals with clinical bleeding, severe thrombocytopenia (i.e., less than 20,000 platelets/μl), cavitary lesions, or highly vascular lesions (determined with ultrasound) should not have percutaneous core biopsies performed due to the risk of uncontrollable hemorrhage or abdominal infection. Caution is also recommended with fine-needle aspiration in these patients. Tissue core biopsies may be obtained with a Tru-cut biopsy (Fig. 17-2) or an automated biopsy device (e.g., Bard Biopty Instrument). Fine-needle aspirates may be obtained with a hand-held syringe or an aspiration gun with syringe attached to a 20- to 25- gauge, 1- to 3-inch needle. For histopathology, the needle should be removed from the syringe or gun and placed in formalin. Once the sample has been fixed, it should be removed from the needle for processing. Fine-needle aspiration is most likely to be diagnostic

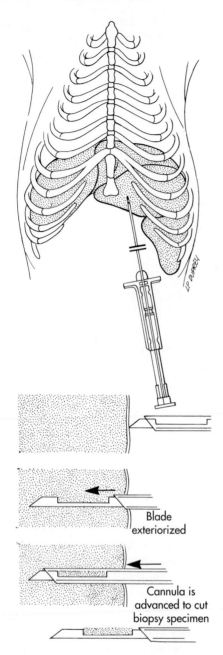

FIG. 17-2
Tissue core biopsy.

Blade exteriorized

Cannula is advanced to cut biopsy specimen

the biopsy needle through the skin incision in a craniodorsal direction, angling it slightly toward the left of midline. Advance the needle until resistance is met or ultrasound guidance shows the needle to be positioned at the surface of the liver. Advance the biopsy needle into the hepatic tissue and obtain the biopsy (Fig. 17-2).

Surgical Liver Biopsy

Biopsies of the liver should be routinely obtained during exploratory laparotomy in animals with known or suspected liver disease. Surgical biopsy allows the entire liver to be thoroughly inspected and palpated, and focal lesions to be biopsied for histopathology, culture, or copper analysis. Furthermore, hemorrhage from the biopsy site can be readily identified and controlled with proper technique. If generalized hepatic disease is present, the biopsy can be taken from the most accessible site (marginal biopsy samples). With focal disease, the entire liver should be carefully palpated for the presence of intraparenchymal nodules or cavities and representative samples obtained. The information gained from histologic examination of the liver may prove beneficial in determining prognosis, diagnosis, and long-term management of patients with hepatic dysfunction.

A biopsy of the hepatic margin may be obtained by the "guillotine" method. *Place a loop of suture around the protuding margin of a liver lobe. Pull the ligature tight and allow it to crush through the hepatic parenchyma before tying it (Fig. 17-3, A). As the suture tears through the soft hepatic tissue, vessels and biliary ducts are ligated. Hold the liver gently between the fingers and, using a sharp blade, cut the hepatic tissue approximately 5 mm distal to the ligature (allowing the stump of crushed tissue to remain with the ligature). To avoid crushing the biopsy sample and causing artifacts, do not handle it with tissue forceps. Place a portion of the sample in formalin for histologic examination; reserve the remainder for culture and cytologic examination. Check the biopsy site for hemorrhage. If hemorrhage continues, place a pledget of absorbable gelatin foam over the site. Alternatively, if a focal (nonmarginal) area of the liver is to be biopsied, use a punch biopsy or Tru-cut biopsy (see Fig. 17-2) or place several overlapping guillotine sutures around the margin of the lesion and excise it (Fig. 17-3, B). Use caution with a punch biopsy to avoid penetrating more than half the thickness of the liver with each biopsy. Apply pressure to the site until bleeding stops. If hemorrhage continues, place a pledget of absorbable gelatin foam over the site.*

Partial Lobectomy

Partial lobectomy may be indicated in some conditions in which disease involves only a portion of a liver lobe (e.g., peripheral hepatic arteriovenous fistulae, focal neoplasia, hepatic abscesses, or trauma). Partial lobectomy may be challenging because of the difficulty in obtaining hemostasis and should be done with extreme caution in animals with bleeding disorders. Stapling instruments have been used for both

in patients with diffuse hepatic neoplasia (e.g., lymphosarcoma), fungal disease, and idiopathic hepatic lipidosis. However, inability to diagnose these conditions on a fine-needle aspirate does not preclude disease. If core biopsies are performed, two or three (2-cm long) samples should be obtained. Percutaneous biopsies may be obtained under tranquilization or heavy sedation using a transthoracic or transabdominal approach. The latter is described here.

With the animal in dorsal recumbency, clip the hair from the area surrounding the xiphoid process and prepare it for aseptic surgery. Make a small incision in the skin on the left side between the costal arch and xiphoid process. Insert

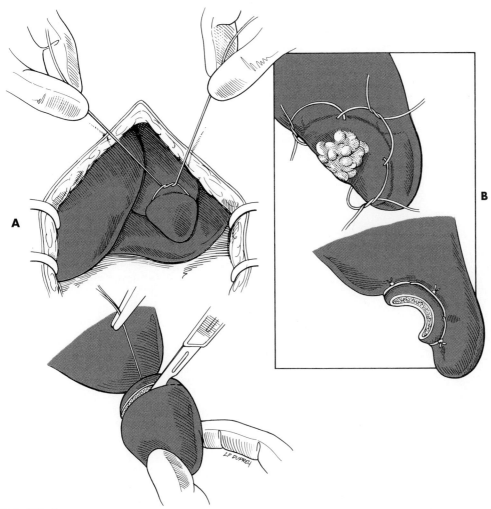

FIG. 17-3

A biopsy of the hepatic margin may be obtained by the "guillotine" method. **A,** Place a loop of suture around the protruding margin of a liver lobe. Pull the ligature tight and allow it to crush through the hepatic parenchyma before tieing it. Using a sharp blade, cut the hepatic tissue approximately 5 mm distal to the ligature. **B,** Alternatively, place several overlapping guillotine sutures around the margin of the lesion and excise it.

partial and complete lobectomies, but discretion should be used in their application because hemorrhage may occur if the staples do not adequately compress hepatic tissue.

Determine the line of separation between normal hepatic parenchyma and that to be removed and sharply incise the liver capsule along the selected site (Fig. 17-4, A). Bluntly fracture the liver with fingers (Fig. 17-4, B) or the blunt end of a Bard Parker scalpel handle and expose parenchymal vessels. Ligate large vessels (hemoclips may be used) and electrocoagulate small bleeders that are encountered during the dissection (Fig. 17-4, C). Alternately, place a stapling device (Autosuture TA 90, 55, or 30) across the base of the lobe and deploy the staples. Excise the hepatic parenchyma distal to the ligatures or staples. Before closing the abdomen ensure that the raw surface of the liver is dry and free of hemorrhage. In small dogs and cats you may place several overlapping guillotine sutures (as de-

scribed above) along the entire line of demarcation (Fig. 17-5). Be sure the entire width of the hepatic parenchyma is included in the sutures. After tightening the sutures securely, use a sharp blade to cut the hepatic tissue distal to the ligature, allowing a stump of crushed tissue to remain with the ligature.

Complete Lobectomy

Complete lobectomy may be indicated in some focal lesions involving one or two hepatic lobes (e.g., traumatic lacerations of the liver or hepatic arteriovenous fistulae). The left lobes (i.e., left lateral and left medial lobes) of the liver maintain their separation near the hilus more than do the other lobes; therefore these lobes can often be removed in small dogs and cats by placing a single encircling ligature around the base of the lobe. For the right lateral and caudate lobes, careful dissection around the hepatic caudal vena cava is usually necessary.

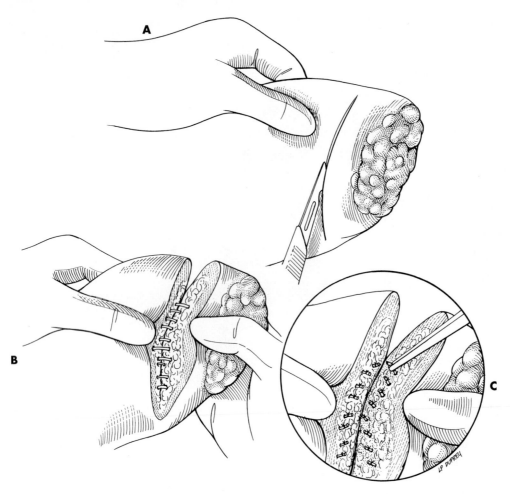

FIG. 17-4
A, For partial lobectomy, determine the line of separation between normal hepatic parenchyma and that to be removed and sharply incise the liver capsule along the selected site. **B,** Bluntly fracture the liver and expose parenchymal vessels. **C,** Ligate large vessels and electrocoagulate small bleeders.

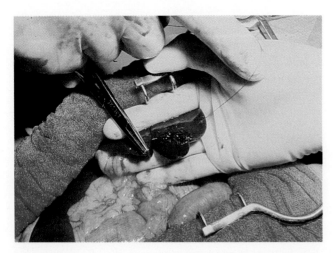

FIG. 17-5
In small dogs and cats, partial hepatectomy may be performed by placing several overlapping guillotine sutures proximal to the tissue to be excised.

☞ **N O T E ·** Complete lobectomy can be challenging, particularly in large dogs. Monitor these patients carefully for postoperative hemorrhage.

For the left lobes in small dogs and cats crush the parenchyma near the hilus with fingers or forceps. Place an encircling ligature around the crushed area and tie. For the left lobes in larger dogs and right and caudate lobes carefully dissect, if necessary, the lobe from the caudal vena cava. Isolate the blood vessels and biliary ducts near the hilus and ligate them. Double ligate or oversew the ends of large vessels. Resect the parenchymal tissue, leaving a stump of tissue distal to the ligatures to prevent retraction of the hepatic tissue from the ligatures and subsequent hemorrhage. Before performing the dissection, umbilical tape can be passed around the portal vein, celiac artery, cranial mesenteric arteries, and the caudal vena cava in front of and behind the liver. The umbilical tape is passed through rubber tubing, which can be used to occlude the hepatic blood supply if uncontrollable hemorrhage occurs.

HEALING OF THE LIVER

The liver is uniquely different in its healing properties from other visceral organs. It has a relative absence of connective tissue stroma, is highly susceptible to small changes in blood flow, and has an enormous regenerative capacity. With regeneration, adequate liver function is possible in patients even after 80% of the organ has been removed or destroyed. Lacerations of the liver should be closed only when bleeding is profuse. If lacerations are sutured, they should be closed in a manner that does not create an internal pocket of bile or blood or cause ischemia of the surrounding cells. Ligation of the proper hepatic artery can be performed as an emergency measure to control hemorrhage from extensive liver lacerations. Complex fractures or severe contusions should be treated by hepatic lobectomy if ligation of the hepatic artery does not result in hemostasis.

SUTURE MATERIALS/SPECIAL INSTRUMENTS

Guillotine biopsies are often performed with large (0 or 2-0) chromic gut suture or polyglactin 910. Suture with good knot security (e.g., silk suture) may facilitate partial hepatectomy. Polydioxanone or polyglyconate suture may also be used for vessel ligation in complete and partial lobectomies.

POSTOPERATIVE CARE AND ASSESSMENT

Recovery from anesthesia should be closely monitored in animals with severe hepatic dysfunction. Because of the increased half-life of some drugs in patients with hepatic dysfunction, recoveries may be prolonged. Intravenous fluids should be provided until the patient is able to maintain hydration. Blood glucose levels should be monitored; transient hypoglycemia is common after removal of large portions of the liver. Albumin levels should be maintained (i.e., > 2.0 g/dl) by the administration of plasma or whole blood, and clotting factors should be assessed if hemorrhage or petechiation occurs. Antibiotics given during surgery should be continued for 2 to 3 days if partial hepatectomy has been performed. Nutritional supplementation may be necessary in some patients during the early postoperative period, particularly if the animal is anorexic or has severe vomiting or diarrhea (see Chapter 11).

Analgesics (e.g., oxymorphone, butorphanol, buprenorphine) should be provided to patients who exhibit pain after surgery (Table 17-4).

COMPLICATIONS

Nondiagnostic biopsies may occur if the tissue sample is crushed, fragmented, or is of insufficient quantity, or if the specimen contains predominantly blood or necrotic portions of mass lesions. Bile peritonitis may occur if the gallbladder or bile ducts are inadvertently penetrated. A recent study found the complication rate in 246 animals undergoing ultrasound-guided biopsy of abdominal structures to be 1.2% (Leveille et al, 1993).

TABLE 17-4
Postoperative Analgesics
Oxymorphone (Numorphan) 0.05-0.1 mg/kg IV, IM every 4 hours (as needed)
Butorphanol (Torbutrol, Torbugesic) 0.2-0.4 mg/kg IV, IM, or SC every 2 to 4 hours (as needed)
Buprenorphine (Buprenex) 5-15 μg/kg IV, IM every 6 hours (as needed)

The most common and serious complication of hepatic surgery is hemorrhage. This may result from ligatures slipping off of friable hepatic tissue. Care should be exercised to ensure that a stump of tissue remains distal to the ligature when encircling sutures are used for biopsy or partial hepatectomy. Following hepatic trauma, anaerobic bacteria may proliferate in hypoxic portions of the liver and cause sepsis. Therefore broad-spectrum antibiotics should be used in patients with severe hepatic trauma and in those undergoing hepatic surgery. Complications following major hepatic resections may include portal hypertension, ascites, fever, coagulopathies, and/or persistent bile drainage.

SPECIAL AGE CONSIDERATIONS

Portosystemic shunt ligation (see p. 378) is often performed in young animals. These young animals are particularly prone to hypoglycemia, and serum glucose concentrations should be carefully monitored. Hypothermia, a particular problem in young patients, decreases the minimum alveolar concentration (MAC) of inhalants used for anesthetic maintenance.

Reference

Leveille R et al: Complications after ultrasound-guided biopsy of abdominal structures in dogs and cats: 246 cases (1984-1991), *J Am Vet Med Assoc* 203:413, 1993.

Suggested Reading

Bjorling DE, Prasse KW, Holmes RA: Partial hepatectomy in dogs, *Compend Contin Educ Pract Vet* 7:257, 1985.

Bunch SE, Polak DM, Hornbuckle WE: A modified laparoscopic approach for liver biopsy in dogs, *J Am Vet Med Assoc* 187:1032, 1985.

Davenport D: Antimicrobial therapy for gastrointestinal, pancreatic, and hepatic disorders, *Probl Vet Med* 2:374, 1990.

Fry PD, Rest JR: Partial hepatectomy in two dogs, *J Small Anim Pract* 34:192, 1993.

Hitt ME, Hanna P, Singh A: Percutaneous transabdominal hepatic needle biopsies in dogs, *Am J Vet Res* 53:785, 1992.

Kosovsky JE et al: Results of partial hepatectomy in 18 dogs with hepatocellular carcinoma, *J Am Anim Hosp Assoc* 25:203, 1989.

Lewis DD et al: Hepatic lobectomy in the dog: a comparison of stapling and ligation techniques, *Vet Surg* 19:221, 1990.

Pavletic MM: Surgical stapling devices in small animal surgery, *Compend Contin Educ Pract Vet* 12:1724, 1990.

PORTOSYSTEMIC VASCULAR ANOMALIES

DEFINITIONS

Portosystemic vascular anomalies (PSVA) or **portosystemic shunts (PSS)** are anomalous vessels that allow normal portal blood draining the stomach, intestines, pancreas, and spleen to pass directly into the systemic circulation without first passing through the liver. **Extrahepatic shunts** are those in which the vascular anomaly is located outside the hepatic parenchyma; **intrahepatic shunts** are those within the liver.

SYNONYMS

The term **portocaval shunt** is frequently used; however, this term technically refers to a specific type of vascular anomaly (i.e., portal vein to caudal cava).

GENERAL CONSIDERATIONS AND CLINICALLY RELEVANT PATHOPHYSIOLOGY

When portal blood bypasses the liver, "toxins" that are normally deactivated in the liver enter the systemic circulation. Additionally, important hepatotrophic substances from the pancreas and intestines do not reach the liver, resulting in hepatic atrophy or failure of the liver to obtain normal size. Hepatic insufficiency or hepatic encephalopathy frequently occurs. Hepatic encephalopathy is a clinical syndrome of altered central nervous system function resulting from hepatic insufficiency. A variety of substances (i.e., ammonia, methionine/mercaptans, short-chain fatty acids, alterations in the ratio between circulating levels of branched-chain and aromatic amino acids, and γ-aminobutyric acid) have been incriminated in the resulting elaboration of false neurotransmitters.

Portosystemic shunts (PSS) may be broadly categorized as intrahepatic or extrahepatic. Extrahepatic shunts may be congenital or acquired. Congenital extrahepatic shunts are usually single anomalous vessels that allow abnormal blood flow to occur from the portal vein to the systemic circulation. Extrahepatic PSS account for nearly 63% of single shunts in dogs; they also occur in cats. Many different PSS have been described in dogs and cats, including (1) portal vein to caudal vena cava, (2) portal vein to azygous, (3) left gastric vein to caudal vena cava, (4) splenic vein to caudal vena cava, (5) left gastric, cranial mesenteric, caudal mesenteric, or gastroduodenal vein to the caudal vena cava, and (6) combinations of the above (Fig. 17-6). Intrahepatic shunts are usually congenital, singular shunts that occur due to a failure of the ductus venosus to close following birth, or they may arise when other portal to hepatic vein or caudal vena cava anastomoses exist. Congenital intrahepatic PSS constitute about 35% of single shunts in dogs.

Acquired extrahepatic shunts are typically multiple and represent about 20% of all canine PSS. They are thought to

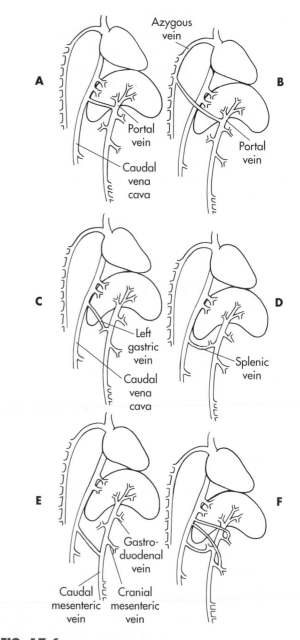

FIG. 17-6
Portosystemic shunts described in dogs and cats. **A,** Portal vein to caudal vena cava. **B,** Portal vein to azygous. **C,** Left gastric vein to caudal vena cava. **D,** Splenic vein to caudal vena cava. **E,** Left gastric, cranial mesenteric, caudal mesenteric, or gastroduodenal veins to the caudal vena cava. **F,** Combinations of the above.

arise in part due to increased resistance to portal blood flow and subsequent portal hypertension. This hypertension causes normal, nonfunctional microvascular connections that are present at birth between portal and systemic veins to become functional. Multiple shunts are most commonly associated with chronic, severe hepatic disease (i.e., cirrhosis), but have been reported secondary to hepatoportal fibrosis in young dogs. Veno-occlusive hepatic disease has also been reported as a cause of multiple PSS in young cocker spaniels. Multiple shunts most commonly occur in the left renal area

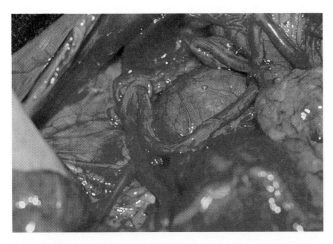

FIG. 17-7
Multiple shunts near the left kidney in a dog with hepatic disease and portal hypertension.

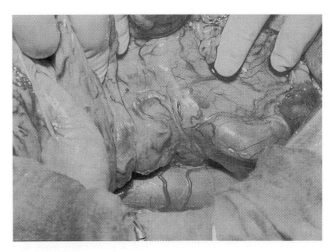

FIG. 17-9
Multiple collateral shunting vessels in the dog in Fig. 17-8.

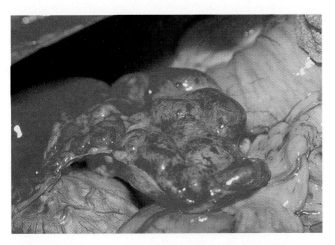

FIG. 17-8
Hepatic arteriovenous fistula in a 1-year-old Labrador. Note the dilated vessels in the hepatic parenchyma. The fistula was found during surgery for a gastric foreign body.

and root of the mesentery (Fig. 17-7), and connections to the caudal vena cava or azygous veins are usually observed.

Arteriovenous (A-V) fistulae account for about 2% of single shunts and may be congenital or acquired. Acquired A-V fistulae occur secondary to trauma, tumors, surgical procedures, or degenerative processes that cause arteries to rupture into adjacent veins. They form between branches of the hepatic artery and portal vein. As congenital lesions, they are believed to develop as a result of failure of the common embryologic capillary plexus to differentiate into an artery or a vein. Affected animals usually develop portal hypertension and multiple collateral shunting vessels and frequently have ascites (Figs. 17-8 and 17-9).

DIAGNOSIS
Clinical Presentation

Signalment. Purebred dogs are at increased risk to have aberrations of the portal circulation. Domestic shorthair cats

are most commonly affected, although these aberrations also occur in purebred cats. Single PSS are usually congenital and are most commonly diagnosed in animals less than 1 year of age. Extrahepatic shunts have been most frequently diagnosed in miniature and toy-breed dogs (e.g., miniature schnauzers, Yorkshire terriers, poodles, Lhaso apsos, and Pekingese). Intrahepatic PSS are more commonly diagnosed in large-breed dogs (e.g., German shepherds, golden retrievers, Doberman pinschers, Labrador retrievers, Irish setters, Samoyeds, and Irish wolfhounds). Congenital extrahepatic and intrahepatic shunts have been reported in cats. There is no convincing sex predisposition for these anomalies in either species.

☞ **N O T E** · Suspect extrahepatic shunts in small-breed dogs and intrahepatic shunts in larger dogs. Although congenital PSS are usually diagnosed in young dogs, occasionally they are found in dogs developing clinical signs when they reach middle age. Some affected dogs have had numerous cystotomies to remove urate calculi.

Multiple shunts are commonly diagnosed in animals between 1 and 7 years of age; however, multiple acquired PSS secondary to hepatoportal fibrosis have been reported in dogs as young as 4 months of age. Breeds most commonly affected include the German shepherd, Doberman pinscher, and cocker spaniel. Multiple acquired shunts have been described in cats.

Most dogs with hepatic A-V fistulae have been young (i.e., younger than 1.5 years) at the time of diagnosis. A 1.5-year-old male domestic shorthair cat has also been described with what was assumed to be a congenital hepatic A-V fistula (Legendre et al, 1976).

History. The presenting history for animals with PSS is highly variable. Affected animals are usually evaluated because of failure to grow, small body stature, or weight loss. Other common abnormalities include intermittent anorexia, depression, vomiting, polydipsia or polyuria, ptyalism (especially in cats), pica, amaurosis, and behavioral changes. Some animals present for evaluation of urinary dysfunction (i.e., hematuria, dysuria, pollakiuria, stranguria, urethral obstruction) associated with urate urolithiasis (see below). Occasionally, the first abnormality noted is prolonged response to anesthetic agents or tranquilizers that require hepatic metabolism for clearance. Signs of hepatic encephalopathy (i.e., ataxia, weakness, stupor, head pressing, circling, amaurosis, pacing, seizures, or coma) are often intermittent and usually worsen after the animal has been fed a high-protein diet. However, failure to find such a temporal relationship should not deter one from making a diagnosis. Signs vary tremendously and sometimes the patient simply appears overly quiet. Hepatic encephalopathy may also worsen after gastrointestinal hemorrhage (e.g., parasites or ulceration).

☞ **N O T E** · Consider PSS in any young dog that has a prolonged recovery from anesthesia, but appears otherwise healthy.

The most common presenting sign in dogs with hepatic A-V fistula is sudden onset of depression, ascites, and vomiting. Often the animal presents with an acute onset of gastrointestinal or neurologic signs, despite the chronic nature of this condition. The ascites is typically a pure transudate despite a serum albumin greater than 1.8 g/dl. Many animals have concurrent gastrointestinal foreign bodies; presumably gastric irritation causes pica in these animals.

☞ **N O T E** · Gastric foreign bodies are not uncommon in dogs with hepatic A-V fistulae and are occasionally the reason the dog presents for veterinary care.

Physical Examination Findings

Most animals with PSS have microhepatica and the kidneys may feel prominent or "plump." A golden or copper color to the iris has been observed in many cats with PSS. Neurologic abnormalities may be noted (see above). Ptyalism is a common finding in cats, but rare in dogs. Animals with hepatic A-V fistulae may have a palpably enlarged liver (rare) or ascites. An audible bruit can sometimes be auscultated in the cranial abdomen of affected animals.

Radiography, Ultrasonography, Nuclear Imaging

The definitive diagnosis of PSS is made via surgical identification of the shunt, intraoperative positive contrast portography, ultrasound, or nuclear hepatic scintigraphy. Various positive contrast techniques have been described including splenoportography, cranial mesenteric arterial portography, celiac arteriography, transsplenic portal catheterization, and jejunal vein portography. Jejunal vein portography is the simplest and most effective portographic technique (see below). The most consistent finding on plain abdominal radiographs is microhepatica.

Both intrahepatic and extrahepatic shunts have been identified with ultrasound. Occasionally a dilated intrahepatic vessel, or the communication of an intrahepatic shunt with the caudal vena cava, will be noted. With extrahepatic shunts, overlying bowel may obscure the shunt, but a small liver with few detectable hepatic or portal veins may be noted. The bladder and renal pelves should be assessed for calculi because urate stones are usually radiolucent and difficult to see on plain abdominal radiographs. Ultrasound is also useful to identify the anechoic, tortuous vessels seen with hepatic A-V fistulae.

Nuclear scintigraphy is a rapid, noninvasive method of documenting abnormal hepatic blood flow. Sodium pertechnetate Tc 99m (^{99m}Tc) and N-isopropyl-p iodoamphetamine (IMP) have been used for analysis of PSS. After colonic administration of ^{99m}Tc, the time when activity in the region of the liver is first noted is compared with the time when activity appears in the region of the heart. Animals with liver-to-heart time intervals greater than 2 seconds have been considered clinically normal (Koblik, Hornof, 1995). False positive results have not been reported; however, false negative results may occur if a small shunt involves only a peripheral portion of the portal system or if the animal has microvascular hepatic dysplasia. IMP is rapidly absorbed across the colonic mucosa and allows calculation of the percentage of portal blood flow bypassing the liver. In normal dogs, IMP should be completely extracted by the liver and lung activity should not be visible on static images. With PSS, liver activity is variable and less prominent than in normal dogs.

☞ **N O T E** · Nuclear scintigraphy is a useful noninvasive tool for diagnosing shunts, but is not accurate in animals with hepatic microvascular dysplasia.

Laboratory Findings

Hematologic, serum biochemical, and urine analysis of animals with PSS may disclose various abnormalities. Hematologic abnormalities may include microcytosis with normochromic erythrocytes, mild nonregenerative anemia, target cell formation, or poikilocytosis. Biochemical tests often reveal reduction in serum albumin and blood urea nitrogen (BUN) concentrations. Low plasma albumin is a common finding in dogs; however, some dogs (and most cats) with PSS have normal albumin levels. Low BUN results from reduced conversion of ammonia to urea in the hepatic urea cycle. Other abnormalities occasionally include mild increases in serum alanine aminotransferase, aspartate aminotransferase, and alkaline phosphatase. Serum bilirubin concentration is usually normal. Hypocholesterolemia and fasting hypoglycemia may occur in some animals. Functional measurements of coagulation (i.e., prothrombin time, activated partial thromboplastin time, and activated coagulation time) are usually normal. Routine urinalysis may disclose dilute urine or ammonium biurate crystals. Hyperuricemia and hyperammonemia lead to increased urinary excretion of urate and ammonia, promoting urinary precipitation of ammonium biurate crystals. Hematuria, pyuria, and proteinuria may occur if urate calculi form. The hematologic and biochemical profiles of canine hepatic A-V fistulae can be similar to those of dogs with single or multiple PSS.

The most reliable tests for diagnosing PSS in dogs and cats are liver function tests and nuclear scintigraphy (see above). Measurement of fasting and postprandial serum bile acids and the ammonia tolerance test (ATT) are sensitive indicators of hepatic insufficiency. Of these, serum bile acids (Table 17-5) are most commonly measured because of the relative ease of performing this test compared to the ATT. A normal liver rapidly clears bile acids by first-pass extraction so that little or no increase is noted in postprandial samples, when compared to fasting samples. In animals with PSS, the abnormal blood flow results in abnormal hepatic clearance of bile acids and elevated postprandial concentrations. It is imperative that fasting and postprandial samples are obtained because fasting samples often have normal bile acid concentrations. Abnormalities in serum bile acids are also noted with other diseases, but young dogs with elevated (e.g., greater than or equal to 100 μmol/L) postprandial serum bile acids in conjunction with microhepatica often have PSS. Ammonia is labile in blood and therefore blood samples have to be refrigerated immediately and transported on ice, and the plasma and blood cells separated promptly in a refrigerated centrifuge. This has limited the usefulness of the ATT in many practices.

DIFFERENTIAL DIAGNOSIS

PSS must be differentiated from other diseases causing hepatic insufficiency (e.g., cirrhosis) or neurologic abnormalities (e.g., hydrocephalus, epilepsy) in dogs and cats.

MEDICAL MANAGEMENT

Surgery is the treatment of choice for animals with PSS because continued deterioration of hepatic function will occur as long as the majority of blood is shunted away from the liver. Life expectancy of animals that are managed medically is generally reported to be 2 months to 2 years. Restoring hepatotrophic factors to the liver will result in hepatic regeneration; however, surgical therapy of this condition is not without risk. Medical management should be initiated prior to surgical intervention in animals with signs of hepatic en-

cephalopathy. The goals of medical therapy are to identify and correct precipitating factors, to decrease absorption of toxins produced by intestinal bacteria, and to decrease the interaction between enteric bacteria and nitrogenous substances. Precipitating factors for hepatic encephalopathy include high-protein meals, bacterial infections, gastrointestinal bleeding, blood transfusions, inappropriate drug therapy, and electrolyte/acid-base abnormalities.

☞ **N O T E** • Surgery is associated with a relatively high mortality; but is more apt to allow a normal life span than long-term medical management.

General supportive care should include fluid therapy (0.9% NaCl or 0.45% NaCl and 2.5% dextrose), normalization of acid-base disturbances, and supplementation of potassium as needed to maintain normal serum potassium concentrations. A highly digestible diet in which the primary source of calories is carbohydrates should be fed. For long-term dietary management, feed the highest-protein diet the animal will tolerate. Moderately protein-restricted diets (i.e., k/d or in some animals u/d; Hill's Pet Products) that contain high levels of branched-chain amino acids and arginine are often used. Antibiotics (Table 17-6) are used to reduce the enteric flora responsible for the production of many of the toxins (i.e., ammonia) that are thought to cause hepatic encephalopathy. Oral neomycin is frequently used for this purpose, but it should be avoided in animals that are azotemic. Metronidazole or ampicillin, given either orally or parenterally, will also reduce intestinal ammonia concentrations. Lactulose is a synthetic disaccharide that acts to acidify colonic contents and trap ammonium ions in the lumen (see Table 17-6). It is also an osmotic cathartic that reduces intestinal transit time and decreases production and absorption of ammonia. Lactulose may be given orally or as a retention en-

TABLE 17-5
Measurement of Serum Bile Acids

1. Fast the animal for 12 hours.
2. Collect a serum sample.
3. Feed 1-2 tbsp. p/d* (dogs) or c/d* (cats).
4. Collect a serum sample 2 hours after feeding.

*Hill's Pet Products, Topeka, Kan.; if the animal is extremely sensitive to protein, feed a protein-restricted diet mixed with a small amount of corn oil.

TABLE 17-6
Drugs Used in the Management of Animals with PSS

Neomycin (Biosol)
10-20 mg/kg PO, BID to TID

Metronidazole (Flagyl)
10 mg/kg PO or IV, TID

Ampicillin
22 mg/kg PO, IV, IM, or SC, TID to QID

Lactulose (Cephalac, Chronulac)
2.5 to 25 ml PO, TID so that the animal has two or three soft stools a day

Dogs
0.5 ml/kg PO, TID

Cats
2.5-5 ml/cat PO, TID

ema. Side effects of lactulose administration may include diarrhea, vomiting, anorexia, and increased gastrointestinal loss of potassium and water. Treatment of animals presenting in hepatic coma must be prompt and aggressive; cleansing enemas (warm water) and retention enemas with neomycin and/or lactulose should be given. Acid-base and electrolyte abnormalities and hypoglycemia must be identified and corrected. The reader is referred to a medical text for additional recommendations on the management of coma secondary to hepatic insufficiency.

SURGICAL TREATMENT

The goal of surgery is to identify and ligate or attenuate the abnormal vessel. In many cases it is not possible to totally occlude shunts without producing life-threatening portal hypertension; these shunts should only be attenuated. When total ligation is not possible, a second surgery several months after the first operation to totally occlude the shunt may be necessary; however, in some animals the shunts will thrombose. If the shunt(s) is identified during abdominal exploration, positive contrast portography examination is not always necessary. Direct intraoperative shunt identification without portography has the advantages of decreased operative time, decreased client cost, and avoidance of large amounts of hypertonic contrast material. However, if a shunt is not identified visually, intraoperative portography is necessary.

☞ **NOTE** • Portography localizes the lesion, but is not necessary in all animals with PSS. If done, it is often best to perform portography at a separate surgery to avoid prolonged surgical times.

Preoperative Management

Encephalopathic patients should be stabilized prior to surgery. Perioperative antibiotics (e.g., cephalosporins) are recommended in patients with PSS. Fluid and electrolyte imbalances should be corrected before surgery. Refer to Medical Management (above) for other recommendations.

Anesthesia

Extreme care must be exercised when anesthetizing an animal that has PSS. Because of their reduced liver function and abnormal hepatic blood flow, drug absorption, metabolism, and clearance are markedly reduced. In addition, drugs that are highly protein bound are affected by the low albumin concentrations that may accompany PSS (i.e., increased levels of circulating unbound drug). Therefore drugs that are metabolized by the liver (e.g., barbiturates and phenothiazine tranquilizers) and those that are highly protein bound (e.g., diazepam) should be avoided. Benzodiazepines may also negatively affect neurologic function in hepatoencephalopathic patients. A reversible opioid may be administered with an anticholinergic, followed by mask or chamber induction with isoflurane and oxygen and endotracheal in-

tubation (Table 17-7). Blood glucose levels should be monitored because patients with PSS may have reduced hepatic glycogen stores. Care should be taken to prevent hypothermia. Inotropic support (i.e., dobutamine [2-10 μg/kg/min; IV] or dopamine [2-10 μg/kg/min; IV]) may be necessary in some patients. These patients should be monitored for arrhythmias or tachycardia.

Surgical Anatomy

The canine portal vein varies from 3 to 8 cm long, depending on the animal's size. On a radiographic contrast study of the normal portal system, the portal system usually originates at the level of the first lumbar vertebra (Fig. 17-10). It is formed by confluence of the cranial and caudal mesenteric veins and splenic vein. The splenic vein enters the portal vein at the level of the thoracolumbar junction. The phrenicoabdominal veins terminate in the caudal vena cava about 1 cm cranial to the renal veins. Any vein entering the caudal vena cava cranial to the phrenicoabdominal veins (before the hepatic veins) may be considered an anomalous structure.

☞ **NOTE** • Examine the caudal vena cava carefully. The only vessels that should enter the caudal vena cava between the renal veins and hepatic veins are the small phrenicoabdominal veins.

Positioning

A standard ventral midline celiotomy is performed from the xiphoid cartilage caudally, and the portal system examined.

TABLE 17-7

Selected Anesthetic Protocols for Animals with PSS

Dogs
Premedication

Give atropine (0.02-0.04 mg/kg SC or IM) or glycopyrrolate (0.005-0.011 mg/kg SC or IM) plus oxymorphone (0.05-0.1 mg/kg SC or IM)

Induction

Mask induce with isoflurane

Maintenance

Isoflurane

Cats
Premedication

Give atropine (0.02-0.04 mg/kg SC or IM) or glycopyrrolate (0.005-0.011 mg/kg SC or IM) plus butorphanol (0.2-0.4 mg/kg SC or IM) or buprenorphine (5-15 μg/kg IM) or oxymorphone (0.05 mg/kg SC or IM)

Induction

Chamber induce with isoflurane

Maintenance

Isoflurane

For intrahepatic shunts and A-V fistulae, the incision may need to extend cranially through the xiphoid process and caudal sternebrae.

SURGICAL TECHNIQUE

Single extrahepatic and intrahepatic shunts are treated by ligating or attenuating the anomalous vessel. Animals with multiple hepatic shunts may benefit from caudal vena cava banding. Arteriovenous fistulae are treated by removing the affected liver lobe. Measurement of portal pressures should be done in conjunction with occlusion of intrahepatic or extrahepatic shunts or vena cava banding. Normal portal pressure in dogs is 8 to 13 cm H_2O, which is 7 to 8 cm H_2O higher than systemic venous pressure (Table 17-8). However, in animals with single PSS, resting portal pressures are often closer to systemic venous pressures. Excessive portal venous pressures can result in splanchnic congestion, portal hypertension, and death.

Ligation of Single Extrahepatic Shunts

Perform a midline abdominal incision. Identify the portal vein by retracting the duodenum to the left and ventrally. Locate the caudal vena cava, renal veins, phrenicoabdominal veins, and portal vein (ventral to the caudal vena cava at the most dorsal aspect of the mesoduodenum). Note any

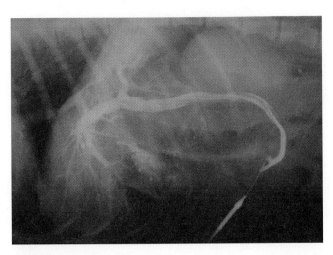

FIG. 17-10
Mesenteric portogram in a dog with a normal portal system. The portal system originates at the level of the first lumbar vertebra. Note the hepatic vasculature.

TABLE 17-8
Normal Pressures in Dogs
Portal Pressures
8-13 cm H_2O
6-10 mm Hg
Systemic Venous Pressures
0-6 cm H_2O
0-4 mm Hg

veins entering the caudal vena cava proximal to the phrenicoabdominal veins. If the shunt has not been identified, open the omental bursa and retract the stomach cranially, the duodenum to the right and ventrally, and the left lobe of the pancreas caudally. Identify shunts that communicate with the caudal vena cava through the epiploic foramen by observing abnormal tributaries of the portal vein, left gastric vein, or splenic vein. Once the anomalous vessel is identified, isolate it and pass 2-0 silk suture around the vessel (Fig. 17-11). If jejunal portography was not performed (see below), exteriorize a segment of jejunum and insert a 20- to 22-gauge over-the-needle catheter (Angiocath, Abbocath) into a jejunal vein. Do not damage the corresponding jejunal artery. Obtain baseline portal pressures. Temporarily occlude the shunt and observe portal pressures during this manipulation. Occlusion of the shunt should result in a rapid increase in portal pressure, which aids in confirmation of the anomalous vessel. Check portal pressures carefully before and during shunt ligation. If you are unsure whether complete ligation should be attempted, err on the conservative side and only attenuate the shunt. If you are uncertain whether the vessel you have occluded is the shunt, perform jejunal portography.

Once you have positively identified the shunt, slowly tighten the ligature while monitoring portal pressures. If possible, completely occlude the shunting vessel but do not allow postligation portal pressures to exceed 10 cm H_2O (8 mm Hg) above baseline pressures or 20 to 23 cm H_2O (15 to 18 mm Hg). You may be able to only attenuate the vessel. Observe the viscera for evidence of splanchnic congestion for 5 to 10 minutes. If excessive splanchnic congestion is noted, loosen the suture. Remove the jejunal vein catheter and ligate the vein. Examine the kidneys and bladder for the presence of calculi. If cystic calculi are present and the patient is stable, remove the calculi during the

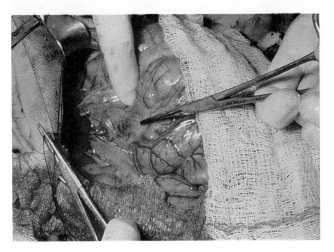

FIG. 17-11
To identify the portal vein, retract the duodenum to the left and ventrally. Note any vessels entering the caudal vena cava proximal to the phrenicoabdominal veins (*hemostat*).

shunt ligation surgery. If operative time has been lengthy or renal calculi are present, it may be best to schedule a second surgery. Obtain a liver biopsy (see p. 370) before closing the abdomen.

Jejunal Portography

Positive contrast radiographs can determine if the shunt is extrahepatic or intrahepatic. If the caudal extent of the PSS is cranial to T_{13}, the shunt is probably intrahepatic. If the caudal extent of the shunt is caudal to T_{13}, it is probably extrahepatic. *Exteriorize a loop of jejunum. Identify a jejunal vein near the mesenteric border of the intestine and place two sutures around the vessel. Insert a 20- to 22-gauge over-the-needle catheter into the vessel (Fig. 17-12) and use the preplaced sutures to secure it to the vessel. Attach a heparinized extension set and three-way stop-cock to the catheter. Close the abdominal incision temporarily. Inject a water-soluble contrast agent (e.g., Renovist) (2 ml/kg body weight) as a bolus into the catheter and make an exposure when the last milliliter is being injected. Making a lateral and ventrodorsal projection will help more fully define the location of the shunt (Fig. 17-13). The catheter can also be used for pressure measurement.*

With multiple hepatic shunts, radiographic confirmation of the shunts is rarely necessary. The technique of intraoperative mesenteric portography in these patients is the same as for single PSS, except that exposures should be delayed approximately 3 or 4 seconds after the start of injection of the contrast material, to enable adequate filling of the shunting vessels.

Ligation of Intrahepatic Shunts

Both intravascular and extravascular methods have been described for ligation of intrahepatic shunts. Ligation of intrahepatic shunts can be extremely challenging because the vessel is often difficult to locate. Occasionally, the shunt can be identified as a palpable depression or soft spot in a liver lobe,

or it may be seen entering into the caudal vena cava if it is not completely encircled by hepatic parenchymal tissue. Intraoperative ultrasound has been used to help identify the shunt in hepatic tissue, but this technique is not always successful. Isolation and obstruction of the specific branch of the portal vein supplying the intrahepatic PSS shunt have been described. An intravascular technique involving temporary hepatic vascular occlusion (see below, under A-V fistula) in conjunction with caudal caval venotomy has also been described for intrahepatic shunt occlusion (Breznock et al, 1983). With this technique, the shunting vessel is identified entering the lumen of the caudal cava cranial to the liver. The vessel is completely occluded or attenuated by suturing the ostium. Isolation of shunts involving the left medial or lateral liver lobes that are not completely surrounded by hepatic tissue is described here.

☞ **N O T E** • Warn owners that ligation of intrahepatic shunts is difficult because the shunts are hard to locate during surgery.

Extend the abdominal incision proximally into the caudal sternebrae. Incise the left triangular ligament and free the left lateral liver lobe so that it can be retracted to the right. Use a combination of sharp and blunt dissection to isolate the anomalous vessel at its junction with the hepatic vein. Place a single silk ligature around the vessel and attenuate flow while measuring portal pressures.

Caudal Vena Cava Banding for Multiple Shunts

Surgical management of multiple PSS involves suture attenuation (or banding) of the abdominal vena cava, just caudal to the hepatic hilus. The intent of this procedure is to raise the systemic venous pressure within the abdomen to, or slightly above, that of the portal venous system. The beneficial result of such an elevation in systemic intraabdominal

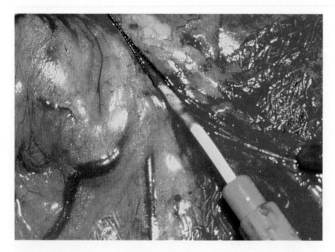

FIG. 17-12
To catheterize a jejunal vein, place two sutures around the selected vessel. Insert a 20- to 22-gauge over-the-needle catheter into the vein and use the preplaced sutures to secure it to the vessel.

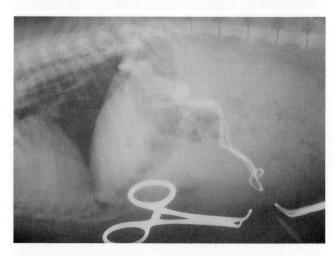

FIG. 17-13
Portogram in a dog with a portoazygous shunt.

venous pressure is improved hepatic portal blood flow. Potential negative results of vena caval banding include accentuation of ascitic fluid formation and subcutaneous edema in the rear quarters. Such problems are usually short term. Because of the need to simultaneously monitor both the portal venous and the abdominal caudal vena caval pressures, two venous catheters are needed. The mesenteric catheter previously described is used to monitor portal venous pressure. A second catheter placed either through a purse-string suture in the abdominal vena cava, caudal to the banding ligature, or percutaneously into the lateral or medial saphenous vein and extending into the caudal vena cava, is used to monitor systemic venous pressure.

Multiple extrahepatic PSS are usually evident at exploratory laparotomy. Findings that may be noted include enlarged mesenteric veins, a larger-than-normal portal vein, and anomalous connections between the portal venous system and the systemic venous circulation. The most common location for multiple PSS is in the area of the left kidney; however, anomalous venous connections between the mesenteric circulation and the caudal vena cava or its tributaries may be noted throughout the abdomen (Fig. 17-14). Portoazygous connections have also been observed in clinical cases. Care should be taken when incising the abdominal wall in patients with suspected multiple PSS because large, dilated vessels may be present in the falciform ligament and/or the greater omentum. Trauma to these vessels upon abdominal entry may produce significant hemorrhage. Dissection of the falciform ligament usually requires ligation or cauterization of multiple vessels. Because many patients with multiple extrahepatic PSS have ascites, suction should be available upon abdominal entry to evacuate ascitic fluid.

☞ **N O T E** • Finding multiple shunts indicates hepatic disease; biopsy the liver in these animals.

Explore the abdominal cavity and observe the mesenteric circulation. Examine the portal system as described above for single PSS. Examine the left renal area by temporarily exteriorizing the spleen and using the descending colon and associated mesocolon to retract the remaining intestines to the right. Evaluate the left paravertebral area and note vascular connections between the portal system and the azygous vein. Use right-angled forceps to isolate the abdominal vena cava as close to the liver as possible. Place silk suture (0 or No. 1) around the vena cava and constrict it. Monitor vena cava and portal venous pressures using a two-channel pressure transducer or two water manometers (NOTE: Fine modulations in ligature tension are more difficult with the latter technique because the water manometers respond more slowly to changing pressures). Partially attenuate the caudal vena cava until systemic venous pressures caudal to the ligation equal or just exceed (by 1 to 2 mm Hg) portal venous pressures. Pressures should be closely monitored at the time of knot-tieing as the vena caval pressure will often drop rapidly for a time after suture attenuation. Following banding, closely observe the mesen-

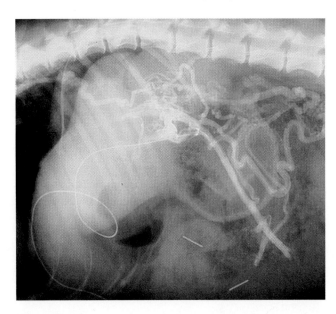

FIG. 17-14
Portogram in a dog with multiple extrahepatic shunts. (Courtesy L. Howe, Texas A&M University.)

teric circulation for up to 20 minutes for signs of excessive congestion. Within a few minutes of occlusion, vena caval pressures will transiently drop to less than those recorded at the time of banding. Do not attempt to individually or collectively ligate the anomalous vessels. Remove the venous catheters and obtain a liver biopsy (see p. 370).

Partial Hepatectomy for Removal of Hepatic A-V Fistula

Treatment of hepatic A-V fistulae involves removal of the affected lobes and abnormal vascular structures. This has been done with or without temporary hepatic vascular occlusion. If temporary vascular occlusion is used, the vascular clamps and occlusive ligatures should be released within 15 minutes. In some animals, caudal vena cava banding has also been performed to increase hepatic blood flow.

Extend the abdominal incision cranially through the caudal sternebrae and incise the diaphragm down to and partially around the hiatus of the caudal vena cava. Place moistened umbilical tapes around the thoracic portion of the caudal vena cava, abdominal portion of the caudal vena cava (between the liver and renal veins), and the portal vein (just proximal to the first hepatic branch). Pass the umbilical tapes through a piece of rubber tubing (Rumel tourniquet). Identify, isolate, and ligate the phrenicoabdominal veins and isolate the celiac and cranial mesenteric arteries. Place a purse-string suture in the portal vein or a splenic tributary and pass a 3.5 or 5 French catheter into the vessel to monitor portal pressures. Monitor blood pressure carefully during surgery; manipulation and ligation of the fistula may cause sudden, severe fluctuations. Isolate the affected lobes by dissection of the triangular, coronary, and hepatorenal ligaments and ligaments of the lesser omentum. Identify the hepatic arterial branch supplying the affected lobe and temporarily occlude it to see if pressure within the fistula diminishes. Double ligate the arterial supply of the fistula with nonabsorbable suture (e.g., 2-0 silk). Isolate the portal branch and biliary ducts to the affected lobe and double ligate them. Temporarily occlude the vasculature by tightening the preplaced umbilical tape ligatures and by placing vascular clamps on the celiac and cranial mesenteric arteries. Sharply dissect the liver parenchyma to resect the affected lobe. Ligate any vascular structures not already occluded and control hemorrhage by packing the area for several minutes. Sometimes the affected portion of the liver can be removed by partial hepatectomy without performing vascular occlusion as described here.

SUTURE MATERIALS/SPECIAL INSTRUMENTS

Blunt-tipped, right-angled, or Mixter forceps are useful for dissecting around venous structures. Shunt ligation is usually performed with silk suture because of the relative knot security this suture affords. Delayed wound healing may be a potential problem if the patient is hypoproteinemic. To prevent dehiscence, a long-lasting absorbable suture material such as polydioxanone or a nonabsorbable suture material should be used to close the linea alba.

Right-angled forceps (such as Mixter forceps, gallbladder or gallduct forceps, or thoracic forceps) are widely available from many instrument manufacturers or suppliers, including Weck, Miltex, V. Mueller, Scanlan, and Codman.

POSTOPERATIVE CARE AND ASSESSMENT

Numerous complications may be associated with the surgical procedure and immediate postoperative period in PSS patients. Intensive care management and close observation of the postoperative single PSS patient are extremely important. Portal hypertension can develop several hours postoperatively and may not be evident immediately after shunt ligation or attenuation. Hypertension and splanchnic congestion may be evidenced as a painful abdomen, hemorrhagic diarrhea, endotoxic shock, and death. Because many of the shunt patients experience painful abdomens during the early postoperative period, recognition of life-threatening portal hypertension may be difficult. However, should signs of endotoxic shock or hemorrhagic diarrhea or other signs of a deteriorating condition occur, emergency surgery to remove or loosen the ligature around the shunting vessel is advisable. Portal vein thrombosis may occur in single PSS cases in which the shunt has been partially ligated; it is a potentially life-threatening complication. If a shunt is only partially ligated, some authors recommend a single anticoagulant dose of heparin at the time of shunt attenuation. Ascites may occur following single shunt ligation. The ascites is self-limiting and usually resolves in 1 to 3 weeks. Diuretics may be used if drainage from the surgical incision site is

present or if the animal experiences discomfort secondary to the abdominal distention. Status epilepticus after PSS ligation has been reported. These seizures generally are first noted 2 to 3 days after shunt ligation; their etiology is unknown. Long-term anticonvulsant therapy may be needed to control the seizures and some permanent neurologic abnormalities may be noted (e.g., blindness). Medical management of hepatic encephalopathy should be continued postoperatively until the hepatic parenchyma regenerates (this may take several months). If there is no improvement in clinical signs within 2 to 3 months, nuclear scintigraphy or jejunal portography should be repeated.

☞ **NOTE** · Warn owners that some animals recover well from anesthesia and then suddenly die. Most animals who survive 24 hours have a good prognosis.

Postoperative management of the patient with multiple PSS is often less demanding than for a patient with single PSS. A commonly observed postoperative problem following vena caval banding is the accelerated production of ascitic fluid. Ascites can be modulated by the intermittent use of diuretics. Abdominocentesis should be performed only if absolutely necessary. Dietary management (low-salt diet) may also be helpful. The formation of ascites often decreases as hepatic function improves in association with improved hepatic portal circulation. This, in turn, provides a more favorable plasma oncotic pressure due to enhanced albumin production. Less common problems following vena caval banding are subcutaneous edema and peripheral venous congestion, particularly in the rear quarters or ventral abdomen. Both problems are usually transient.

PROGNOSIS

Surgical mortality associated with the treatment of single PSS is high, a fact that is a reflection of the many variables and unknown factors that exist in relation to portal physiology and dynamics. A mortality rate of 14% to 21% has been reported for single, extrahepatic shunts (Johnson, Armstrong, Hauptman, 1987; Scavelli et al, 1986; VanGundy, Boothe, Wolf, 1990). In animals in which complete occlusion of the shunting vessel is performed, an excellent quality of life and normal life span are customary. In some patients that tolerate only partial occlusion of the shunt, clinical signs may continue postoperatively and require dietary and medical management. In such animals with continued signs, reoperation and total shunt occlusion are recommended. In a recent study of 20 dogs that underwent partial ligation of a single PSS, long-term outcome was completely satisfactory in 10 (Komtebedde et al, 1995). However, 10 dogs developed complications (i.e., central nervous system, gastrointestinal, or urinary tract abnormalities) at 4 to 79 months after surgery. Hemorrhage, hypotension, and acute hepatic congestion have been reported as common complications during surgical correction of intrahepatic PSS in dogs. A 25% mortality rate associated with surgery has been reported in these dogs (Breznock et al, 1983); however, this may be optimistic, even for most large referral institutions.

☞ **N O T E** · Ligation of intrahepatic shunts is more difficult than ligation of extrahepatic shunts. Intraoperative death may occur with the former but is unusual with the latter. Most dogs with extrahepatic shunts that die do so in the early postoperative period.

The prognosis following venal caval banding in patients with multiple PSS depends, in part, on the reversibility of the primary inciting cause and the degree of portal hypertension present at surgery. The long-term effects of vena caval banding in clinical patients are largely undetermined. Breznock reported that approximately 60% of his patients with multiple PSS improved following vena caval banding. If shunts are secondary to primary hepatocellular disease, caudal vena cava banding is of questionable benefit. Patients that have severe portal hypertension such that banding does not sufficiently elevate vena caval pressures to approximate that of the portal system do not benefit from vena caval banding. The long-term prognosis is good for dogs with hepatic A-V fistulae that survive surgery.

References

Breznock EM et al: Surgical manipulation of intrahepatic portocaval shunts in dogs, *J Am Vet Med Assoc* 182:798, 1983.

Johnson CA, Armstrong PJ, Hauptman JG: Congenital portosystemic shunts in dogs: 46 cases (1979-1986), *J Am Vet Med Assoc* 191:1478, 1987.

Koblik PD, Hornof WJ: Transcolonic sodium pertechnetate Tc 99m scintigraphy for diagnosis of macrovascular portsystemic shunts in dogs, cats, and potbellied pigs: 176 cases (1988-1992), *J Am Vet Med Assoc* 207:729, 1995.

Komtebedde J et al: Intrahepatic portosystemic venous anomaly in the dog: perioperative management and complications, *Vet Surg* 20:2379, 1995.

Legendre AM et al: Ascites associated with intrahepatic arteriovenous fistula in a cat, *J Am Vet Med Assoc* 168:589, 1976.

Scavelli TD et al: Portosystemic shunts in cats: seven cases (1976-1984), *J Am Vet Med Assoc* 189:317, 1986.

VanGundy TE, Boothe HW, Wolf A: Results of surgical management of feline portosystemic shunts, *J Am Anim Hosp Assoc* 26:55, 1990.

Suggested Reading

Bailey MQ et al: Ultrasonographic findings associated with congenital hepatic arteriovenous fistula in three dogs, *J Am Vet Med Assoc* 192:1009, 1988.

Berger B et al: Congenital portosystemic shunts, *J Am Vet Med Assoc* 188:517, 1986.

Birchard SJ: Surgical management of portosystemic shunts in dogs and cats, *Compend Contin Educ Pract Vet* 6:795, 1984.

Birchard SJ, Biller DS, Johnson SE: Differentiation of intrahepatic versus extrahepatic portosystemic shunts in dogs using positive-contrast portography, *J Am Anim Hosp Assoc* 25:13, 1989.

Blaxter AC et al: Congenital portosystemic shunts in the cat: a report of nine cases, *J Small Anim Pract* 29:631, 1988.

Breznock EM: Surgical manipulation of portosystemic shunts in dogs, *J Am Vet Med Assoc* 174:819, 1979.

Butler LM, Fossum TW, Boothe HW: Surgical management of extrahepatic portosystemic shunts in the dog and cat, *Semin Vet Med Surg (Small Anim)* 5:127, 1990.

Center SA: Liver function tests in the diagnosis of portosystemic vascular anomalies, *Semin Vet Med Surg (Small Anim)* 5:94, 1990.

Center SA, Magne ML: Historical, physical examination, and clinicopathologic features of portosystemic vascular anomalies in the dog and cat, *Semin Vet Med Surg (Small Anim)* 5:83, 1990.

Easley JC, Carpenter JL: Hepatic arteriovenous fistula in two Saint Bernard pups, *J Am Vet Med Assoc* 166:167, 1975.

Flanders JA et al: Adjustment of total serum calcium concentration for binding to albumin and protein in cats: 291 cases (1986-1987), *J Am Vet Med Assoc* 194:1609, 1989.

Grauer GF, Pitts RP: Primary polydipsia in three dogs with portosystemic shunts, *J Am Anim Hosp Assoc* 23:197, 1987.

Griffiths GL, Lumsden JH, Valli VEO: Hematologic and biochemical changes in dogs with portosystemic shunts, *J Am Anim Hosp Assoc* 17:705, 1981.

Hardie EM, Kornegay JN, Cullen JM: Status epilepticus after ligation of portosystemic shunts, *Vet Surg* 19:412, 1990.

Hardy RM: Pathophysiology of hepatic encephalopathy, *Semin Vet Med Surg (Small Anim)* 5:100, 1990.

Hottinger HA, Walshaw R, Hauptman JG: Long-term results of complete and partial ligation of congenital portosystemic shunts in dogs, *Vet Surg* 24:331, 1995.

Koblik PD, Hornof WJ, Breznock EM: Use of quantitative hepatic scintigraphy to evaluate spontaneous portosystemic shunts in 12 dogs, *Vet Radiol* 24:232, 1983.

Koblik PD et al: Use of transcolonic 123 I-iodoamphetamine to diagnose spontaneous portosystemic shunts in 18 dogs, *Vet Radiol* 30:67, 1989.

Komtebedde J et al: Long-term clinical outcome after partial ligation of single extrahepatic vascular anomalies in 20 dogs, *Vet Surg* 24:2379, 1995.

Martin RA, Freeman LE: Identification and surgical management of portosystemic shunts in the dog and cat, *Sem Vet Med Surg (Small Anim)* 2:302, 1987.

Matsushek KJ, Bjorling D, Mathews K: Generalized motor seizures after portosystemic shunt ligation in dogs: five cases (1981-1988), *J Am Vet Med Assoc* 196:2014, 1990.

Moore PF, Whiting PG: Hepatic lesions associated with intrahepatic arterioportal fistulae, *Vet Pathol* 23:57, 1986.

Rand JS, Best SJ, Mathews KA: Portosystemic vascular shunts in a family of American Cocker Spaniels, *J Am Anim Hosp Assoc* 24:265, 1988.

Rogers WA et al: Intrahepatic arteriovenous fistulae in a dog resulting in portal hypertension, portacaval shunts, and reversal of portal blood flow, *J Am Anim Hosp Assoc* 13:470, 1977.

Roy RG et al: Portal vein thrombosis as a complication of portosystemic shunt ligation in two dogs, *J Am Anim Hosp Assoc* 28:53, 1992.

Schmidt S, Suter PF: Indirect and direct determination of the portal vein pressure in normal and abnormal dogs and normal cats, *Vet Rad* 21:246, 1980.

Schulz KS, Martin RA, Henderson RA: Transsplenic portal catheterization: surgical technique and use in two dogs with portosystemic shunts, *Vet Surg* 22:363, 1993.

Swalec KM, Smeak DD: Partial versus complete attenuation of single portosystemic shunts, *Vet Surg* 19:406, 1990.

Taboada J: Medical management of animals with portosystemic shunts, *Semin Vet Med Surg (Small Anim)* 5:107, 1990.

van den Ingh TSGAM, Rothuizen J: Hepatoportal fibrosis in three young dogs, *Vet Rec* 110:575, 1982.

CAVITARY HEPATIC LESIONS

DEFINITIONS

Cavitary hepatic lesions are usually cysts or abscesses; however, large neoplastic lesions (i.e., hemangiomas, adenomas) occasionally cavitate. **Hepatic abscesses** are localized collections of pus in the hepatic parenchyma. **Hepatic cysts** are closed, fluid-filled sacs lined by secretory epithelium.

GENERAL CONSIDERATIONS AND CLINICALLY RELEVANT PATHOPHYSIOLOGY

Hepatic abscesses are rare in dogs and cats and are usually associated with extrahepatic infection (i.e., ascending biliary tract infections, hematogenous infection via the portal vein or hepatic artery, or direct extension from areas adjacent to the liver), hepatic trauma (i.e., surgical biopsy, penetrating wounds, or blunt trauma), or neoplasia. Despite the normal presence of bacteria in the liver of dogs, hepatic abscesses seldom occur. This may be related to a well-developed local defense system provided by the liver's rich blood supply and the phagocytic ability of reticuloendothelial cells.

Hepatic abscesses are most frequently recognized as a complication of omphalophlebitis in puppies and are usually diagnosed at necropsy. Diabetes mellitus has been associated with hepatic abscesses. Most hepatic abscesses are caused by pyogenic bacteria. Small abscesses may not be associated with clinical signs and may resorb without therapy.

Hepatic cysts are usually incidental findings, although rarely they will obtain such size that they interfere with normal function of adjacent organs. A single hepatic cyst may be noted, or several cysts may be present in the same or different lobes. Concurrent polycystic renal disease has been reported in cats. If hepatic cysts are present in an animal with clinical evidence of hepatic dysfunction, liver biopsy is often warranted to determine the cause.

DIAGNOSIS
Clinical Presentation

Signalment. There is no reported sex or breed predisposition for hepatic abscesses or cysts.

History. Clinical signs of hepatic abscessation vary and may include anorexia, lethargy, weight loss, and intermittent abdominal pain. Most animals with hepatic cysts are asymptomatic; however, some cysts cause abdominal distention. Secondary infections of hepatic cysts may cause clinical signs similar to those of hepatic abscesses.

Physical Examination Findings

Physical examination findings commonly noted in animals with hepatic abscessation include persistent fever, hepatomegaly, and abdominal enlargement. Palpation of a firm abdominal mass and marked abdominal distention may be noted in some animals with hepatic cysts.

Radiography/Ultrasonography

Small hepatic cysts are often incidental findings on abdominal radiographs or ultrasonography. Large hepatic cysts are usually well-defined radiopaque structures located in the cranial abdomen (Fig. 17-15). Abdominal radiographs may demonstrate hepatomegaly in animals with hepatic abscesses, but a well-defined hepatic mass is seldom evident. Occasionally, gas within the hepatic parenchyma will be noted, which strongly suggests abscessation due to gas-forming bacteria. Ultrasonography is the most useful diagnostic test for defining hepatic abscesses and cysts in dogs and cats. Hepatic abscesses appear as hypoechoic or anechoic structures that may contain mixed echo densities, depending on cellularity. Scintigraphy and computed tomography are also highly sensitive, but less commonly used. Ultrasound-guided fine-needle aspirations of hepatic abscesses can be performed before surgery; however, there is a risk that the abscess will rupture or drain into the abdomen and cause diffuse peritonitis. Fluid removed from cysts during fine-needle aspiration is usually transudative in nature.

☞ **NOTE •** In cats with hepatic cysts evaluate the kidneys for concurrent cystic disease.

Laboratory Findings

Laboratory abnormalities are seldom present with hepatic cysts. They are variable in animals with hepatic abscesses, but may include an inflammatory leukogram and nonregenerative anemia. Serum biochemical abnormalities may include hypoalbuminemia, hypokalemia, hyperglycemia, and elevated hepatic enzymes; however, elevation of alanine transaminase activity is not a consistent finding.

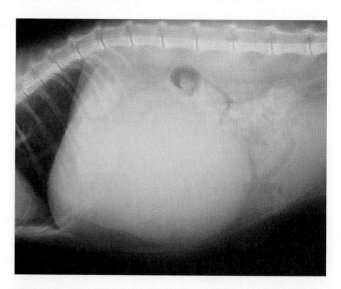

FIG. 17-15
Lateral abdominal radiograph of a 2-year-old cat with a large hepatic cyst. The cat was asymptomatic.

DIFFERENTIAL DIAGNOSIS

Hepatic cysts, abscesses, neoplasms, and parasitic lesions must be differentiated. Hepatic abscesses are often difficult to diagnose because they produce nonspecific signs that may be masked by associated disease processes. Large neoplastic hepatic lesions may necrose and become secondarily infected. Infection of hepatic cysts is also possible. Therefore histologic evaluation of surgically resected tissue is important.

MEDICAL MANAGEMENT

Medical management of hepatic abscesses entails fluid therapy, correcting electrolyte and acid-base abnormalities, and initiating appropriate antibiotics. Resection of hepatic abscesses is indicated as soon as the animal has been stabilized. Preoperative antibiotic therapy may be based on culture and sensitivity results if fine-needle aspiration has been performed, or antibiotics with bactericidal activity against anaerobes and gram-negative bacteria (e.g., amoxicillin plus clavulanic acid, cefoxitin, cefazolin plus metronidazole; Table 17-9) may be given empirically. Parenteral antibiotics are indicated in the perioperative period. Combination therapy may be necessary, particularly if multiple organisms are isolated. Percutaneous drainage of hepatic cysts and sclerosis of the cyst lining have not been reported in dogs or cats.

SURGICAL TREATMENT

Whether hepatic cysts should be removed when diagnosed in asymptomatic animals is not clear. Although these cysts could enlarge or become infected and cause clinical signs, little information is available regarding the long-term follow-up of nonsurgically resected large hepatic cysts in dogs or cats. Hepatic cysts associated with clinical signs and hepatic abscesses should be promptly resected.

Preoperative Management

Symptomatic animals should be stabilized before surgery. Antibiotics may be initiated before surgery, or in some animals they may be administered after intraoperative cultures have been taken.

Anesthesia

Refer to p. 367 for the anesthetic management of animals with hepatic disease.

Surgical Anatomy

Refer to p. 368 for surgical anatomy of the liver.

Positioning

The animal is positioned in dorsal recumbency for a midline abdominal incision. The prepped area should extend from mid-thorax to the pubis.

SURGICAL TECHNIQUE

Hepatic abscesses and cysts are generally treated by partial hepatectomy (see p. 370). Although there is less concern regarding spillage of cystic contents into the abdomen, it is wise to try to remove the cyst without entering the lumen. Culturing hepatic cysts may be optional if the fluid does not appear infected cytologically; however, some cysts can develop secondary bacterial infections.

Pack the area surrounding the liver with moistened laparotomy sponges to decrease intraoperative contamination if the lumen of the abscess or cyst is entered. If possible, resect the affected portion of the liver without entering the lesion. Culture the lesion and submit it for histologic examination. Palpate the remainder of the liver parenchyma for other nodules and explore the abdominal cavity for associated infections or disease.

SUTURE MATERIALS/SPECIAL INSTRUMENTS

See p. 373 for recommendations for suture choices during partial hepatectomy.

POSTOPERATIVE CARE AND ASSESSMENT

Fluid therapy for animals with hepatic abscesses should be continued until the animal is drinking normally. Antibiotic therapy should be continued for 7 to 10 days. The animal should be monitored for peritonitis (i.e., leukocytosis, fever, abdominal fluid, abdominal pain) if abdominal contamination occurred. Minimal postoperative care is needed for most animals with hepatic cysts.

PROGNOSIS

The prognosis for animals with hepatic abscesses depends on the rapidity with which the abscess is diagnosed, whether concurrent peritonitis is present, and the overall health of the animal. With prompt surgical intervention, the prognosis is good. The prognosis for animals with hepatic cysts (with or without surgery) is good unless there is concurrent hepatic or renal disease.

TABLE 17-9

Antibiotics in Animals with Hepatic Abscesses

Amoxicillin plus clavulanate
(Clavamox)

Dogs
12.5-25 mg/kg PO, BID

Cats
62.5 mg PO, BID

Cefoxitin (Mefoxin)
30 mg/kg IV, TID to QID

Cefazolin (Ancef, Kefzol)
20 mg/kg IV or IM, TID to QID

Metronidazole (Flagyl)
10 mg/kg IV or PO, TID

Suggested Reading

Black AP: A solitary congenital hepatic cyst in a cat, *Aust Vet Pract* 13:166, 1983.

Grooters AM, Sherding RG, Johnson SE: Hepatic abscesses in dogs, *Comp Cont Educ Pract Vet* 17:833, 1995.

Grooters AM et al: Hepatic abscesses associated with diabetes mellitus in two dogs, *J Vet Intern Med* 8:203, 1994.

Hargis AM, Thomassen RW: Hepatic abscesses in beagle puppies, *Lab Anim Sci* 30:689, 1980.

Lord PF et al: Emphysematous hepatic abscess associated with trauma, necrotic hepatic nodular hyperplasia and adenoma in a dog: a case history report, *Vet Radiol* 23:46, 1982.

Stebbins KE: Polycystic disease of the kidney and liver in an adult Persian cat, *J Comp Path* 100:327, 1989.

Valentine BA, Porter WP: Multiple hepatic abscesses and peritonitis caused by eugonic fermenter-4 bacilli in a pup, *J Am Vet Med Assoc* 183:1324, 1983.

van den Ingh TSGAM, Rothuizen J: Congenital cystic disease of the liver in seven dogs, *J Comp Path* 95:405, 1985.

HEPATOBILIARY NEOPLASIA

DEFINITIONS

Hepatocellular tumors arise from hepatocytes; **cholangiocellular neoplasms** arise from intahepatic or extrahepatic bile duct epithelium.

SYNONYMS

The term **hepatoma** has been used to refer to both hepatocellular carcinomas and hepatocellular adenomas. Cholangiocellular carcinomas are also known as **bile duct carcinomas.**

GENERAL CONSIDERATIONS AND CLINICALLY RELEVANT PATHOPHYSIOLOGY

Primary hepatic neoplasms are uncommon in dogs and cats (Table 17-10). They may be of epithelial or mesenchymal (see Table 17-10) origin. Hepatocellular carcinomas and cholangiocellular carcinomas are the most commonly diagnosed primary hepatic malignancies in dogs. Hepatocellular carcinomas may involve a single liver lobe or may be nodular or diffuse and involve multiple lobes. In cats, cholangiocellular adenomas are the most common primary tumor. Hepatic carcinoids are rare tumors that arise from neuroectodermal cells in the liver. Benign hepatic masses (i.e., adenomas or cysts) are often incidental findings at necropsy. They may be more common than malignant tumors in both species but often go undiagnosed because they seldom cause clinical signs. Cholangiocellular carcinomas arise primarily from intrahepatic bile duct epithelium; neoplasms of the extrahepatic bile duct and gallbladder are rare.

Most malignant primary hepatic tumors are highly metastatic. They may metastasize by direct extension to other parts of the liver or to adjacent organs or via lymphatics or blood to distant sites. The most common sites for epithelial tumors to metastasize are the regional lymph nodes and lungs. Mesenchymal tumors most often metastasize to the spleen.

Metastatic neoplasia is more common in the liver than are primary tumors. The liver is a common site for metastasis because it acts as a filter between the abdominal organs and the systemic circulation. Lymphosarcoma is the most common secondary hepatic tumor. Other tumors that commonly metastasize to the liver include pancreatic adenocarcinomas, hemangiosarcomas, insulinomas, and tumors of the alimentary and urinary tracts.

DIAGNOSIS
Clinical Presentation

Signalment. Primary hepatic neoplasia is usually a disease of aged dogs and cats. There is no known breed predisposition. Hepatocellular carcinomas may be more common in male dogs, while cholangiocellular carcinomas may be more common in cats and female dogs. Dogs with metastatic liver cancer may be slightly younger than those presenting with primary hepatic malignancy (7.8 years vs. 10 years).

History. Many animals with primary hepatic neoplasia present for signs associated with hepatic failure. The animal may be lethargic, weak, anorexic, losing weight, or vomiting, and/or have polyuria/polydipsia. The clinical signs associated with metastatic hepatic neoplasia are highly variable.

Physical Examination Findings

The most significant finding on physical examination of most primary hepatic tumors is an enlarged liver; however, hepatic carcinoids may not cause significant hepatomegaly. Additional findings may include jaundice and ascites. Hepatocellular adenomas may rupture and cause hemoperitoneum. Marked hepatomegaly is less common with metastatic neoplasia; however, lymphosarcoma often causes diffuse hepatic enlargement.

Radiography/Ultrasonography

Survey radiographs help localize the mass to the liver (Fig. 17-16) and may reveal extrahepatic metastasis; however,

---

TABLE 17-10

Primary Hepatic Neoplasia in Dogs and Cats

Epithelial
- Hepatocellular carcinoma
- Hepatocellular adenoma
- Cholangiocellular carcinoma
- Cholangiocellular adenoma
- Hepatic carcinoids

Mesenchymal
- Hemangiosarcoma
- Fibrosarcoma
- Extraskeletal osteosarcoma
- Leiomyosarcoma

radiographs may be useless if ascites is present. Thoracic radiographs should be taken whenever hepatic neoplasia is suspected, because pulmonary metastasis is common. Ultrasonography localizes and defines the extent of disease. It is particularly useful in animals with ascites. Ultrasound-guided biopsies may allow presurgical diagnosis (see p. 369).

Laboratory Findings

Neutrophilia and biochemical abnormalities compatible with hepatic disease ($\uparrow$ serum alanine transaminase, $\uparrow$ aspartate transaminase, $\uparrow$ serum alkaline phosphate) are common but inconsistent findings in animals with hepatic neoplasia. They are nonspecific, but their recognition may prompt further evaluation of the hepatobiliary system. Mild to moderate anemia is less commonly associated with hepatic neoplasia. Serum bilirubin concentrations may be increased, particularly if extrahepatic biliary obstruction occurs. Occasionally, hypoglycemia causes clinical signs. Albumin levels are usually normal in patients with primary hepatic neoplasia. Biochemical abnormalities seldom correlate with the extent of hepatic involvement with either primary or metastatic tumors.

☞ **N O T E** · Laboratory abnormalities often do not occur until the neoplasm is large, making surgical resection difficult.

DIFFERENTIAL DIAGNOSIS

Primary hepatobiliary tumors must be differentiated from nodular hyperplasia, abscesses, hematomas, or cysts. Histologic and/or cytologic evaluation of fine-needle aspirates or biopsy specimens is necessary to definitely distinguish between these lesions (see p. 369). Percutaneous biopsies should not be performed in animals with clinical bleeding

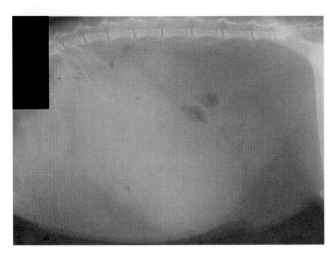

FIG. 17-16
Lateral abdominal radiograph of a dog with a large, malignant hepatic tumor. Note the similarities between the radiographic appearance of this tumor and the benign hepatic cyst in Fig. 17-15. Benign and malignant hepatic masses cannot be differentiated radiographically.

disorders, or if the lesions appear cavitary or highly vascular. Cytologic evaluation of abdominal fluid is seldom helpful in differentiating between these lesions.

MEDICAL MANAGEMENT

Surgical excision of primary malignant hepatic tumors is the treatment of choice. Unfortunately, these tumors are often not diagnosed until they are large and metastasis has occurred. Because they are usually diagnosed in older animals, concurrent cardiac, renal, or other metabolic problems are common. Medical therapy should aim at correcting fluid and electrolyte imbalances and providing nutrition to improve chances of surviving surgery.

SURGICAL TREATMENT

If the tumor is localized to a single lobe or confined to the gallbladder, surgical resection may be curative. Partial hepatectomy and cholecystectomy are described on pp. 370 and 391. Surgical biopsies should be performed on all animals with hepatomegaly or nodularity because differentiation of lesions requires histopathology. Finding multiple hepatic masses does not indicate metastatic disease because primary hepatic tumors may spread to other portions of the liver. If neoplasia is suspected, the draining lymph nodes and surrounding organs should be carefully assessed for metastasis. Hepatocellular tumors are most commonly found in the left medial and left lateral liver lobes.

Preoperative Management

The animal should be stabilized before surgery, if possible. Fluid therapy should be initiated and electrolyte imbalances corrected. Blood transfusions (see Table 17-1) should be given to animals that are severely anemic (i.e., PCV less than 20%), especially if bleeding tendencies are present (i.e., petechiation, ecchymosis, or hemorrhage). If the animal has clinical evidence of coagulopathy or is severely thrombocytopenic (i.e., less than 20,000 platelets/μl), consider plasma or whole blood transfusions and ensure hemostasis at surgery. Patients with prolonged one-stage prothrombin time (OSPT or PT) and partial thromboplastin time (PTT) should be monitored for bleeding before, during, and after surgery. If the patient has massive ascites, slow removal of some fluid before anesthetic induction may help prevent hypoventilation associated with positioning the patient while it is being prepared for surgery.

Anesthesia

Ventilation of patients with ascites will require support (i.e., intermittent positive-pressure ventilation; IPPV). Compression of the caudal vena cava in patients with large hepatic masses or massive ascites may cause decreased venous return and reduced cardiac output. Refer to p. 367 for additional comments regarding the anesthetic management of patients with hepatic disease.

Surgical Anatomy

Refer to p. 368 for surgical anatomy of the liver.

Positioning

Exploration of the liver is generally performed through a cranial ventral midline abdominal incision (see p. 180). The incision may be extended paracostally to allow enhanced visualization and manipulation of large tumors. The prepped area should extend from mid-thorax to the pubis.

SURGICAL TECHNIQUE

See pp. 370-371 for a description of surgical techniques for partial hepatectomy or cholecystectomy, respectively.

SUTURE MATERIALS/SPECIAL INSTRUMENTS

Absorbable suture material is used for hepatic biopsy (see p. 373). Ligation of the cystic duct for cholecystectomy is generally done with nonabsorbable suture material (see p. 391).

POSTOPERATIVE CARE AND ASSESSMENT

Postoperative nutritional support of patients with hepatic neoplasia is often necessary (see p. 373). Nonresectable primary hepatic tumors seldom respond to chemotherapy or radiation therapy. Chemotherapy may palliate hepatic lymphosarcoma. For other considerations in animals undergoing partial hepatectomy refer to p. 373.

PROGNOSIS

The prognosis for dogs and cats with primary hepatobiliary malignancies is often poor; however, in a study of 18 dogs with hepatocellular carcinomas, 8 dogs had a mean survival of 308 days, and 10 additional dogs were alive 377 days after surgery (range, 195 days to more than 1025 days) (Kosovsky et al, 1989). In a recent report of cats with malignant nonlymphomatous hepatobiliary disease that underwent surgery, the median length of the survival was 0.1 months (range, less than 1 day to 4 months) (Lawrence, Erb, Harvey,

1994). The high rate of metastasis and degree of invasion make surgical resection unlikely to be curative in most patients. Benign tumors may be surgically resected, and long-term survival of patients with benign hepatic tumors has been reported. Survival times in four cats with hepatobiliary cystadenomas ranged from 12 to 44 months after surgery (Trout et al, 1995).

☞ **NOTE** · Cures are uncommon, but dogs with hepatocellular carcinoma may live for a year or longer following surgery.

References

Kosovsky JE et al: Results of partial hepatectomy in 18 dogs with hepatocellular carcinoma, *J Am Anim Hosp Assoc* 25:203, 1989.

Lawrence HJ, Erb HN, Harvey HJ: Nonlymphomatous hepatobiliary masses in cats: 41 cases, *Vet Surg* 23:365, 1994.

Trout NJ et al: Surgical treatment of hepatobiliary cystadenomas in cats: five cases (1988-1993), *J Am Vet Med Assoc* 206:505, 1995.

Suggested Reading

Fry PD, Rest JR: Partial hepatectomy in two dogs, *J Small Anim Pract* 34:192, 1993.

Haines DM et al: Multifocal telangiectatic osteosarcoma and malignant mixed hepatic tumor in a dog, *J Am Anim Hosp Assoc* 23:509, 1987.

Leveille R et al: Complications after ultrasound-guided biopsy of abdominal structures in dogs and cats: 246 cases (1984-1991), *J Am Vet Med Assoc* 203:413, 1993.

Magne ML: Primary epithelial hepatic tumors in the dog, *Compend Contin Educ Pract Vet* 6:506, 1984.

McCaw DL, da Silva Curiel JMA, Shaw DP: Hepatic myelolipomas in a cat, *J Am Vet Med Assoc* 197: 243, 1990.

Post G, Patnaik AK: Nonhematopoietic hepatic neoplasms in cats: 21 cases (1983-1988), *J Am Vet Med Assoc* 201:1080, 1992.

CHAPTER 18

Surgery of the Extrahepatic Biliary System

GENERAL PRINCIPLES AND TECHNIQUES

DEFINITIONS

Cholecystotomy is the creation of an opening into the gallbladder for drainage; **cholecystectomy** is removal of the gallbladder. **Choledochotomy** is incision of the common bile duct for exploration or removal of a calculus. **Choledochoduodenostomy** is a rarely indicated procedure in dogs and cats that involves surgical anastomosis of the common bile duct to the duodenum. **Cholecystoduodenostomy** and **cholecystojejunostomy** are surgical anastomoses of the gallbladder to the duodenum or jejunum, respectively. Calculi may form in the gallbladder (**cholelithiasis**) or the common bile duct (**choledocholithiasis**).

PREOPERATIVE CONCERNS

Biliary disease may be due to obstruction of the extrahepatic biliary system, neoplasia, infection, or trauma. Lesions that cause obstruction of the extrahepatic biliary system may be extraluminal or intraluminal. Extraluminal obstruction may be caused by pancreatic neoplasia, duodenal or pyloric neoplasia, hepatic or biliary neoplasia, pancreatitis, or pancreatic abscessation. Intraluminal obstruction is less common but may occur in association with cholelithiasis, choledocholithiasis, or inspissated bile. Pancreatic disease is the most common cause of extrahepatic biliary obstruction in dogs. Scar formation may occur in or around the duct, or the duct may be compressed by fibrotic or inflamed pancreatic tissue. Pancreatic abscesses and cysts may also cause biliary obstruction.

Animals with obstructive biliary disease should have electrolyte and fluid abnormalities corrected preoperatively. Prolonged biliary obstruction may cause vitamin K malabsorption, resulting in deficiencies of factors VII, IX, and X. Animals with clinical evidence of bleeding should be administered vitamin K_1 for 24 to 48 hours before surgery (Table

TABLE 18-1

Dosage for Vitamin K_1 (AquaMephyton, Mephyton)

0.1-0.2 mg/kg SC,* SID

*Do not give IV or IM.

18-1), or given fresh whole blood. Partial or complete biliary obstruction may allow ascending aerobic and anaerobic infection and subsequent bacteremia. Therefore perioperative antibiotic therapy is indicated (see Chapter 10).

Extrahepatic biliary injury may occur due to blunt or penetrating trauma. Common bile duct, gallbladder, cystic duct, or hepatic duct lacerations may cause bile peritonitis, or (if the infection is "walled-off") a localized inflammatory process with adherence to surrounding organs. Necrotizing cholecystitis occurs when bacteria damage the gallbladder wall, often resulting in peritoneal spillage of bile (Fig. 18-1). This frequently produces a severe, generalized septic peritonitis. Sometimes bile becomes inspissated before the gallbladder ruptures and spillage of the relatively thick, gelatinous mass into the cranial abdomen causes a localized peritonitis. Adhesions or fistulous tracts around the gallbladder occasionally occur. See p. 398 for a discussion of the preoperative management of animals with bile peritonitis.

ANESTHETIC CONSIDERATIONS

The anesthetic requirements and concerns for patients with biliary disease are similar to those with hepatic disease. Please refer to p. 367. An additional concern in patients with obstructive biliary disease relates to the effect of mu-agonists (e.g., oxymorphone, morphine) on smooth muscle tone. In human beings with biliary obstruction, these drugs increase sphincter tone and enhance pain. Mixed agonist antagonists (e.g., butorphanol; Table 18-2) may be preferable as premedicants and analgesics in these patients.

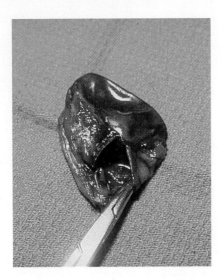

FIG. 18-1
Ruptured gallbladder in a dog with necrotizing cholecystitis.

ANTIBIOTICS

Prophylactic antibiotics are recommended in patients undergoing biliary surgery because of the detrimental effects of bacterial infection on healing. Antibiotic therapy for biliary infections should be based on results of culture and sensitivity testing of liver parenchyma and/or bile. The most common organisms isolated from biliary infections are *E. coli*, *Klebsiella* spp., *Enterobacter* spp., *Proteus* spp., and *Pseudomonas* spp. Antibiotics that are excreted in active form in the bile and are commonly used to treat biliary disease include amoxicillin, cefazolin, and enrofloxacin (Table 18-3). Chloramphenicol is dependent on hepatic metabolism and should be avoided in patients with severe hepatic dysfunction.

SURGICAL ANATOMY

The hepatic and cystic ducts, bile duct (also known as common bile duct), plus the gallbladder, constitute the extrahepatic biliary system (Fig. 18-2). Bile drains from the hepatic ducts into the bile duct and is stored and concentrated in the gallbladder. The gallbladder lies between the quadrate lobe of the liver medially and the right medial lobe laterally. It is a pear-shaped organ that, in medium-sized dogs, holds approximately 15 ml of bile. The rounded end is the fundus. Between the neck of the gallbladder (i.e., the tapering end leading into the cystic duct) and the fundus is the body, or middle portion, of the gallbladder.

The cystic duct extends from the neck of the gallbladder to the junction with the first tributary from the liver. From this point to the opening of the biliary system into the duodenum, the duct is termed the *bile duct*. The bile duct runs through the lesser omentum for approximately 5 cm and enters the mesenteric wall of the duodenum. The canine bile duct terminates in the duodenum near the opening of the minor pancreatic duct. This combined opening of the minor pancreatic duct and bile duct is the major duodenal papilla. The feline bile duct usually joins the major pancreatic duct before entering the duodenum.

TABLE 18-2
Dose of Butorphanol (Torbutrol, Torbugesic) in Animals with Biliary Disease
0.2-0.4 mg/kg IV, IM, or SC as a preanesthetic
0.2-0.4 mg/kg IV, IM, or SC every 2 to 4 hours as needed for analgesia

TABLE 18-3
Antibiotics Commonly Used in the Treatment of Biliary Disease
Amoxicillin (Amoxi-Tabs, AmoxiDrops, Amoxi-inject)
20 mg/kg PO, IM or SC, BID to TID
Cefazolin (Ancef, Kefzol)
20 mg/kg IV or IM, TID to QID
Enrofloxacin (Baytril)
5-10 mg/kg PO, IM, or IV, BID

SURGICAL TECHNIQUES

Exploratory laparotomy should be performed in animals in whom leakage of bile into the abdomen is suspected, in animals with obstruction of bile flow that is not clearly due to pancreatitis, and in animals with suspected neoplasia (biliary tract, intestinal, or pancreatic), parasitic disease, or biliary calculi. During exploration, patency of the common bile duct needs to be ensured by manually expressing the gallbladder, or by retrograde (i.e., from the duodenum; see below) or occasionally normograde (i.e., from the gallbladder) catheterization of the duct.

Treatment of animals with biliary obstruction secondary to benign pancreatic disease initially consists of medical management of the pancreatitis. If clinical or laboratory improvement is not seen within 7 to 10 days of initiating appropriate therapy, or if clinical deterioration occurs despite appropriate medical therapy, cholecystoduodenostomy or cholecystojejunostomy may be considered. In extremely ill patients with biliary obstruction who cannot undergo surgical exploration, temporary decompression of the gallbladder using ultrasound-guided aspiration, or a Foley or self-retaining accordion catheter, may be warranted.

☞ **NOTE** • Biliary obstruction due to pancreatitis usually resolves with appropriate medical management.

Cholecystotomy

Cholecystotomy is rarely performed but may be indicated to remove some choleliths (see p. 395) or when the gallbladder contents are inspissated and cannot be aspirated into a syringe. *Pack the area surrounding the gallbladder with ster-*

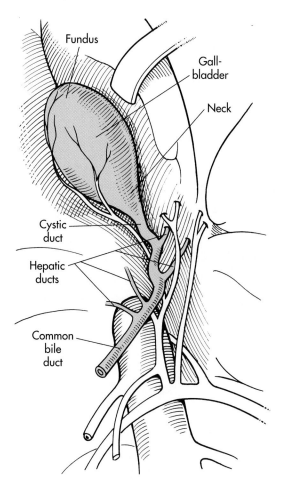

FIG. 18-2
Anatomy of the extrahepatic biliary system.

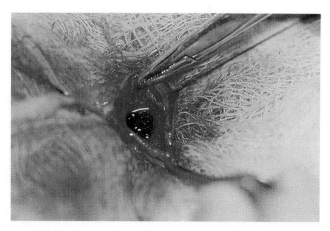

FIG. 18-3
Before cholecystotomy, place stay sutures in the gallbladder to facilitate manipulation and decrease spillage. Then make an incision in the fundus of the gallbladder.

ile, moistened laparotomy sponges. Place stay sutures in the gallbladder to facilitate manipulation and decrease spillage. Make an incision in the fundus of the gallbladder (Fig. 18-3). Remove the gallbladder contents and submit for culture. Lavage the gallbladder with warmed, sterile saline. Catheterize the common bile duct via the cystic duct with a 3.5 or 5 French soft catheter and flush it to ensure patency. Close the incision with a one- or two-layer inverting suture pattern using absorbable suture material (3-0 to 5-0).

Cholecystectomy

Diseases such as cholecystitis and cholelithiasis are best treated by cholecystectomy (see p. 395). Cholecystectomy may also be indicated for primary neoplasia or traumatic rupture of the gallbladder. Always determine the patency of the common bile duct before performing this technique. *Expose the gallbladder and incise the visceral peritoneum along the junction of the gallbladder and liver with Metzenbaum scissors (Fig. 18-4, A). Apply gentle traction to the gallbladder and, using blunt dissection, free it from the liver. Free the cystic duct to its junction with the common bile duct. Be sure to identify the common bile duct and avoid damaging it during the procedure. If necessary, identify the common bile duct by placing a 3.5 or 5 French soft*

catheter into the duct via the duodenal papilla. Make a small enterotomy in the proximal duodenum, locate the duodenal papilla, and place a small red rubber tube into the common bile duct (Fig. 18-4, B). Flush the duct to ensure its patency. Clamp and double ligate the cystic duct and cystic artery (Fig. 18-4, C) with nonabsorbable suture material (2-0 to 4-0). Sever the duct distal to the ligatures and remove the gallbladder. Submit a portion of the wall, plus bile, for culture if infection is suspected. Submit the remainder of the gallbladder for histologic analysis if indicated (for cholecystitis or neoplasia). Close the duodenal incision with simple interrupted sutures of absorbable suture material.

Choledochotomy

Direct incision of the bile duct should be performed only in animals in which the duct is markedly dilated, such as may occur with chronic obstruction, and where the obstruction can be removed (i.e., choledocholithiasis, biliary sludge). An attempt should first be made to remove the obstruction by flushing the common bile duct, using a catheter placed via an enterotomy or cholecystotomy. Extraluminal obstruction or stricture of the duct is best treated with biliary diversion techniques (see below).

Pack the area surrounding the common bile duct with sterile, moistened laparotomy sponges. Place traction sutures into the distended duct. Make a small incision into the duct and remove the obstruction (Fig. 18-5). Flush the duct with copious amounts of warmed, sterile saline and pass a 3.5 to 5 French soft catheter into the gallbladder and duodenum to ensure patency. Close the incision with a simple continuous or simple interrupted suture pattern of absorbable suture material (4-0 or 5-0). If leakage is a concern, pass a catheter into the duct via an incision in the proximal duodenum (see above). Small leaks may be treated by stenting the incision with a 3.5 to 5 French soft catheter (see discussion on repairing common bile duct injuries).

FIG. 18-4
For cholecystectomy, **A,** expose the gallbladder and incise the visceral peritoneum along the junction of the gallbladder and liver with Metzenbaum scissors. **B,** Identify the common bile duct and avoid damaging it during the procedure. If necessary, cannulate the duct via the duodenal papilla. **C,** Clamp and double ligate the cystic duct and cystic artery.

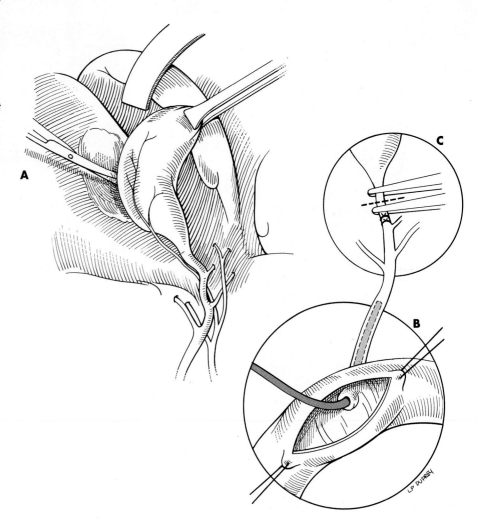

Bile Flow Diversion

Bile flow diversion is indicated when common bile duct obstruction is present or the duct is severely traumatized and the gallbladder is not directly involved in the disease process. Cholecystojejunostomy or cholecystoduodenostomy is preferred over choledochoduodenostomy in dogs and cats because the latter procedure is often difficult to perform successfully, due to the small size of the common bile duct in these species. If cholecystojejunostomy is performed, the proximal jejunum should be used to decrease the incidence of postoperative maldigestion of lipids. Additionally, duodenal ulceration may occur more commonly as a sequela to cholecystojejunostomy than to cholecystoduodenostomy. In dogs, it has been recommended that the stoma between the bowel and the gallbladder be at least 2.5 cm long to minimize the potential for obstruction of bile flow or retention of bowel contents in the gallbladder. Making the stoma too small is more apt to result in ascending or chronic cholecystitis than is making the stoma too large.

Mobilize the gallbladder from the liver as described for cholecystectomy. Place stay sutures approximately 3 cm apart in the gallbladder. Bring the gallbladder into apposition with the antimesenteric surface of the descending duodenum so that there is little or no tension on the gallbladder or intestine. Pack the area surrounding the gallbladder and duodenum with sterile, moistened laparotomy sponges. Place a continuous suture of absorbable suture material between the serosa of the gallbladder and the serosa of the duodenum, near the mesentery (referred to as original suture line; Fig. 18-6, A). Make the suture line 3 to 4 cm in length. Leave the ends of the suture long and use them to manipulate the intestine and gallbladder. Drain the gallbladder and make a 2.5- to 3-cm incision into it, parallel to the preplaced suture line (Fig. 18-6, B). Have an assistant occlude the duodenum proximal and distal to the proposed incision site. Make a similar parallel incision in the antimesenteric surface of the duodenum (Fig. 18-6, C). Place a continuous suture line of absorbable suture material (2-0 to 4-0) from the mucosa of the gallbladder to the mucosa of the duodenum, beginning with the edges closest to the original suture line (Fig. 18-6, D). Then use the same suture material to suture the mucosal edges of the stoma farthest from the original suture line (Fig. 18-6, E). Complete the stoma by suturing the serosal edges of the gallbladder and intestine over the near side of the stoma (i.e., the side farthest from the original suture line; Fig. 18-6, F).

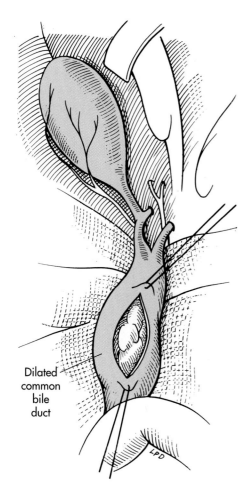

FIG. 18-5
Choledochotomy.

Repair of Common Bile Duct Injuries

The surgical technique used to repair lacerations of the common bile duct depends on the location and severity of the lesion. Severely damaged ducts, particularly if there has been bile leakage or adhesion formation, are difficult to repair primarily. Incisional dehiscence, leakage, and stricture formation are common. If the injury is distal to the entrance of the hepatic ducts, the common bile duct should be ligated proximal and distal to the injury and biliary diversion performed (i.e., cholecystoduodenostomy or cholecystojejunostomy; see above). If the duct has been cleanly severed and the luminal diameter is greater than 4 to 5 mm, primary suturing and anastomosis are possible. Similarly, proximal lacerations or perforations may be treated with primary suturing. The mucosa of the bile duct should be accurately reapposed. Small sutures should be used and tension on the suture line avoided. The use of stenting catheters in the common bile duct is controversial, but temporary bile diversion may allow bile duct injuries to heal that would otherwise dehisce, leak, or stricture. The tube acts to decompress the biliary tree and minimizes bile leakage from the site during healing. Disadvantages of tubes placed in the bile duct include an increased potential for stricture due to the presence of a foreign body

at the injured site, obstruction of the tube, and ascending infection. If the bile duct is stented, a soft tube that is smaller than the diameter of the duct should be used to minimize irritation to the duct wall. The use of rubber tubes or catheters that enter the duodenum and T-tubes that exit the duct and are exteriorized through the abdominal wall has been described in the veterinary literature. The use of a straight catheter (i.e., Sovereign feeding tube, Dover red rubber Robinson catheter) has been described here.

Identify the common bile duct. This may be facilitated by passing a catheter into the duct from the duodenum (see above discussion of cholecystectomy). Be careful to not interfere with the blood supply to the duct during manipulation. Carefully debride the transected ends of the duct, but be sure to leave adequate duct length to avoid having tension on the suture line when the ends are reapposed. Reappose the ends of the duct with absorbable suture material using simple interrupted sutures (4-0 to 6-0). Place a 3.5 to 5 French soft catheter in the duct from the duodenum to stent the suture line (Fig. 18-7). Suture the distal end of the catheter to the duodenal lumen with a small chromic gut suture (3-0 or 4-0). As the suture dissolves, peristalsis will cause the catheter to enter the intestinal lumen, where it will pass in the feces.

HEALING OF THE BILIARY TRACT

Studies have shown that if just a small strip of the common bile duct wall remains intact, the duct will regenerate. However, longitudinal tension on the suture line of a repaired biliary duct causes severe stenosis. In addition to promoting stricture of the duct, there is some suggestion that intraluminal tubes may interfere with normal biliary drainage, thus promoting cholangitis. Because of uncertainties regarding healing of the duct in the presence of infection, leakage, or tension, drainage procedures such as cholecystojejunostomies are commonly performed in lieu of direct repair of the common bile duct (see above).

SUTURE MATERIALS/SPECIAL INSTRUMENTS

Absorbable suture material should be used in the biliary tree because nonabsorbable suture may act as a nidus for stone formation. Biliary duct surgery is aided by the use of small instruments such as those that are used for ophthalmic surgery. The gallbladder should be emptied with a syringe and needle or a needle attached to suction before surgical manipulations to decrease spillage of bile during biliary diversion surgery.

POSTOPERATIVE CARE AND ASSESSMENT

Fluid therapy should be continued until the animal is able to maintain hydration with oral fluids. Electrolytes and acid-base status should be assessed and corrected during the postoperative period. Many patients with bile peritonitis (see p. 397) are debilitated before surgery, and nutritional supplementation

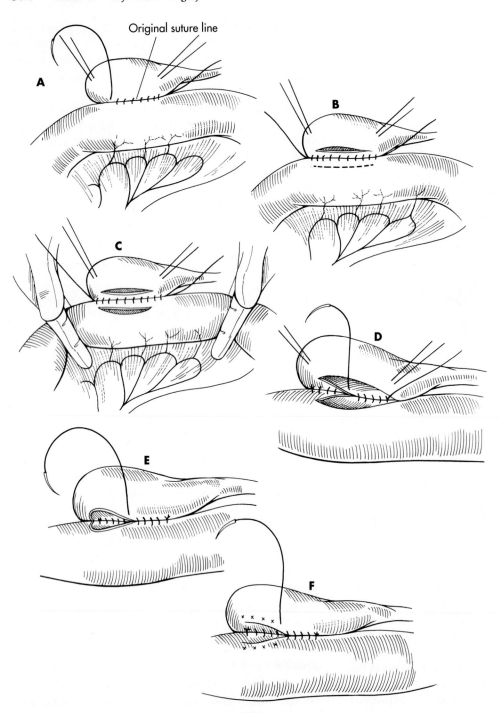

FIG. 18-6

For cholecystoduodenostomy (or cholecystojejunostomy), bring the gallbladder into apposition with the antimesenteric surface of the descending duodenum. **A,** Place a 3- to 4-cm continuous suture line between the serosa of the gallbladder and the serosa of the duodenum (original suture line). **B,** Drain the gallbladder and make a 2.5- to 3-cm incision into it, parallel with the preplaced suture line. **C,** Have an assistant occlude the duodenum proximal and distal to the proposed incision site and make a parallel incision in the antimesenteric surface of the duodenum. **D,** Place a continuous suture line from the mucosa of the gallbladder to the mucosa of the duodenum, beginning with the edges closest to the original suture line. **E,** Then suture the mucosal edges of the stoma farthest from the original suture line. **F,** Complete the stoma by suturing the serosal edges of the gallbladder and intestine over the near side of the stoma.

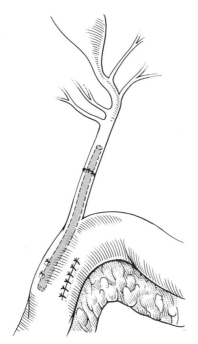

FIG. 18-7
Lacerations in the common bile duct may be sutured over a stent placed via a duodenotomy.

may be beneficial (see Chapter 11). Antibiotic therapy should be continued for 7 to 10 days if cholecystitis was present or bile leakage occurred before or during surgery. Open abdominal drainage may be considered in patients with generalized bile peritonitis. Refer to p. 399 for analgesic recommendations in patients with bile peritonitis.

COMPLICATIONS

Surgery of the extrahepatic biliary tree requires technical competence, manual dexterity, and sound surgical judgment to prevent serious complications. Potential complications after cholecystectomy (particularly if perforation was present) include generalized peritonitis, shock, sepsis, hypoglycemia, hypoproteinemia, and hypokalemia. Stricture, bile leakage, and dehiscence may occur after surgery of the common bile duct. Ascending cholangiohepatitis may occur in some animals after biliary diversion, particularly if the stoma of the enteric-biliary anastomosis is too small and intestinal contents remain in the gallbladder lumen for prolonged periods. Intermittent antibiotic therapy may be necessary in such animals.

SPECIAL AGE CONSIDERATIONS

Trauma should be suspected in young animals presenting with bile peritonitis. Obstruction secondary to pancreatitis or neoplasia is more common in middle-aged or older animals.

Suggested Reading

Bjorling DE: Surgical management of hepatic and biliary diseases in cats, *Compend Contin Educ Pract Vet* 13:1419, 1991.

Blass CE: Surgery of the extrahepatic biliary tract, *Compend Contin Educ Pract Vet* 5:801, 1983.

Blass CE, Seim HB: Surgical techniques for the liver and biliary tract, *Vet Clin North Am Small Anim Pract* 15:257, 1985.

Fossum TW, Willard MD: Diseases of the gallbladder and the extrahepatic biliary system. In Ettinger SJ: *Textbook of veterinary internal medicine,* ed 4, Philadelphia, 1995, WB Saunders.

Herzog U et al: Surgical treatment for cholelithiasis, *Surg Gynecol Obstet* 175:238, 1992.

Hunt CA, Gofton N: Primary repair of a transected bile duct, *J Am Anim Hosp Assoc* 20:57, 1984.

Johnson SE: Liver and biliary tract, In Anderson NV: *Veterinary gastroenterology,* ed 2, Philadelphia, 1992, Lea & Febiger.

Kirpensteijn J et al: Cholelithiasis in dogs: 29 cases (1980-1990), *J Am Vet Med Assoc* 202:1137, 1993.

Lawrence D et al: Temporary bile diversion in cats with experimental extrahepatic bile duct obstruction, *Vet Surg* 21:446, 1992.

Martin RA, MacCoy DM, Harvey HJ: Surgical management of extrahepatic biliary tract disease: a report of eleven cases, *J Am Anim Hosp Assoc* 22:301, 1986.

Matthiesen DT: Complications associated with surgery of the extrahepatic biliary system, *Probl Vet Med* 1:295, 1989.

Neer TM: A review of disorders of the gallbladder and extrahepatic biliary tract in the dog and cat, *J Vet Intern Med* 6:186, 1992.

SPECIFIC DISEASES

CHOLELITHIASIS

DEFINITIONS

Calculi in the gallbladder are **choleliths** and those found in the common bile duct are **choledocholiths.**

SYNONYMS

Gallstones

GENERAL CONSIDERATIONS AND CLINICALLY RELEVANT PATHOPHYSIOLOGY

Choleliths are often fortuitous findings at necropsy or during imaging with radiographs or ultrasound. They are frequently clinically silent; however, they may cause cholecystitis, vomiting, anorexia, icterus, fever, or abdominal pain. Whereas human beings usually develop dietary-induced cholesterol gallstones, cholesterol, bilirubin, and mixed stones have been reported in dogs and cats. The rarity of canine cholelithiasis may be due to (1) decreased concentrations of cholesterol in canine bile, (2) absorption of ionized calcium from the gallbladder, limiting the amount of free ionized calcium in bile, and (3) failure to recognize them. Calcium salts are the major components of pigment gallstones; thus availability of ionized calcium may be important in gallstone formation in dogs. Pigment gallstones can be experimentally produced in dogs after 6 weeks of a methionine-deficient diet or with a high-cholesterol diet that is deficient in taurine.

☞ **NOTE** · Most choleliths are asymptomatic; treatment is indicated only when the calculi cause clinical signs.

DIAGNOSIS
Clinical Presentation

Signalment. Aged female small-breed dogs appear to be at increased risk for development of choleliths.

History. Most animals with choleliths are asymptomatic; however, they may be presented because of fever, vomiting, icterus, or abdominal pain if cholecystitis or biliary obstruction occurs. Clinical signs may be mild and intermittent in some animals.

Physical Examination Findings

Icterus may be noted if the calculus causes biliary obstruction or ascending cholangitis. Abdominal pain and vomiting may also occur. Choleliths have rarely been associated with perforation of the gallbladder or common bile duct (see p. 397).

Radiography/Ultrasonography

Gallstones are seldom radiodense (Fig. 18-8), but they are readily identified by ultrasound. A mass or acoustic shadowing originating from the gallbladder may be noted (Fig. 18-9). The latter may be indicative of a stone that is too small to see with ultrasound. If obstruction is present, dilation of the common bile duct or hepatic ducts may also be detected. Contrast radiographs of the biliary tree are rarely useful in icteric patients. Endoscopic retrograde pancreatography is difficult and rarely performed in dogs. Direct injection of contrast into dilated bile ducts via transabdominal placement of a "slim" needle has been accomplished in people, but is seldom done in dogs.

Laboratory Findings

Abnormalities are uncommon; however, symptomatic animals may show abnormalities compatible with extrahepatic biliary obstruction. Increased serum alkaline phosphatase (SAP), usually with hyperbilirubinemia, is typical in partial or complete obstructions and when ascending cholangitis occurs. Cats tend to have lesser elevations of SAP than do dogs. Hypercholesterolemia may be found secondary to biliary tract obstruction, especially in cats. Urinalysis is helpful early in the disease course because bilirubinuria usually occurs before hyperbilirubinemia.

DIFFERENTIAL DIAGNOSIS

Evidence of concurrent cholecystitis should be sought in symptomatic animals with choleliths. Sludge and true concretions may be difficult to differentiate in some animals before surgery.

MEDICAL MANAGEMENT

Medical dissolution of gallstones in dogs and cats has not been reported and is probably not feasible due to the expected content of most gallstones. Medical management of animals with biliary obstruction is discussed on p. 389. Concurrent cholecystitis should be treated with appropriate antibiotics.

SURGICAL TREATMENT

Because choleliths may be associated with cholecystitis and cause vomiting, anorexia, icterus, fever, or abdominal pain, they should be removed if they are found in a patient with biliary tract disease.

Preoperative Management

Refer to p. 389 for the preoperative management of patients with biliary obstruction.

Anesthesia

Refer to pp. 367 and 389 for discussions of the anesthetic management of patients with hepatic or obstructive biliary disease, respectively.

Surgical Anatomy

Surgical anatomy of the biliary tract is described on p. 390.

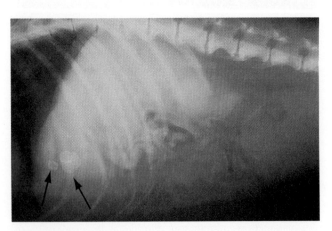

FIG. 18-8
Lateral abdominal radiograph in a dog with radiodense choleliths (*arrows*). (From Ettinger, Feldman: *Textbook of veterinary internal medicine*, ed 4, Philadelphia, 1995, WB Saunders.)

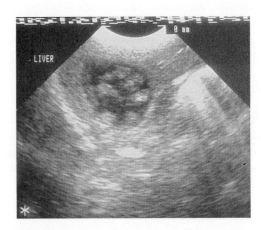

FIG. 18-9
Abdominal ultrasound showing multiple choleliths and sludge in the gallbladder of an asymptomatic dog.

Positioning

Choleliths are generally removed via a cranial midline abdominal incision.

SURGICAL TECHNIQUE

Cholecystectomy (see p. 391) is the surgical treatment of choice in dogs with clinical signs secondary to cholelithiasis. If stones are also present in the common bile duct, the duct can be catheterized via the duodenum and the stones flushed into the gallbladder (see p. 391). Alternatively, if the bile duct is enlarged, the duct can be incised (choledochotomy) and the stones removed directly; however, care is needed when suturing the common bile duct, to avoid stricture formation (see p. 391). Clinical studies have found a greatly increased mortality in human patients with cholelithiasis when choledochotomy is performed vs. cholecystectomy. Bile should be cultured.

SUTURE MATERIALS/SPECIAL INSTRUMENTS

The gallbladder and common bile duct should be sutured with absorbable suture material to decrease the likelihood of suture serving as a nidus for calculi formation.

POSTOPERATIVE CARE AND ASSESSMENT

Refer to p. 393 for the postoperative management of patients with obstructive biliary disorders.

PROGNOSIS

The prognosis is excellent with proper surgical technique.

Suggested Reading

Fossum TW, Willard MD: Diseases of the gallbladder and the extrahepatic biliary system. In Ettinger SJ: *Textbook of veterinary internal medicine*, ed 4, Philadelphia, 1995, WB Saunders.

Heidner GL, Campbell KL: Cholelithiasis in a cat, *J Am Vet Med Assoc* 186:176, 1985.

Johnson SE: Liver and biliary tract. In Anderson NV: *Veterinary gastroenterology*, ed 2, Philadelphia, 1992, Lea & Febiger.

Jorgenson LS et al: Recurrent cholelithiasis in a cat, *Compend Contin Educ Pract Vet* 9:265, 1987.

Kipnis RM: Cholelithiasis, gallbladder perforation, and bile peritonitis in a dog, *Canine Practice* 13:15, 1986.

Kirpensteijn J et al: Cholelithiasis in dogs: 29 cases (1980-1990), *J Am Vet Med Assoc* 202:1137, 1993.

Rege RV: Absorption of biliary calcium from the canine gallbladder: protection against the formation of calcium-containing gallstones, *J Lab Clin Med* 110:381, 1987.

BILE PERITONITIS

DEFINITIONS

Bile peritonitis is an inflammation of the peritoneum caused by bile leakage into the abdomen.

SYNONYMS

Bilious ascites

GENERAL CONSIDERATIONS AND CLINICALLY RELEVANT PATHOPHYSIOLOGY

Acute abdomen (i.e., shock and/or pain due to severe abdominal disease) may be caused by leakage of bile into the abdominal cavity, particularly if there is concurrent septic peritonitis. Leakage of bile into the abdominal cavity may occur with traumatic rupture of any portion of the extrahepatic biliary tree or may be secondary to necrotizing cholecystitis or chronic obstruction (rare).

Untreated bile peritonitis is often lethal; hence early diagnosis is imperative. If rupture is associated with biliary tract infection, clinical signs of bile peritonitis usually develop quickly. However, in dogs with sterile bile peritonitis (i.e., rupture due to trauma), clinical signs other than ascites and icterus may not be noted for weeks. Bile in the abdominal cavity causes chemical peritonitis, which may not be associated with overt clinical signs initially; however, changes in intestinal mucosal permeability may lead to secondary bacterial infection of the effusion. If diagnosis of a ruptured biliary tract is delayed, repair of the biliary tract will be complicated by necrotic tissues and adhesions. Diagnostic peritoneal lavage (see p. 198) may assist in the early diagnosis of bile peritonitis (before onset of clinical signs) in animals sustaining abdominal trauma.

☞ **N O T E** · Repair ruptured bile ducts or gallbladders as soon as possible because the surgery becomes more difficult when adhesions and necrotic tissue are present.

Rupture of the extrahepatic biliary ducts or gallbladder may be due to blunt abdominal trauma, cholecystitis, or obstruction secondary to calculi, neoplasia, or parasites. Trauma usually causes rupture of the common bile duct rather than the gallbladder. Ductal rupture probably occurs when a force is applied adjacent to the gallbladder sufficient to cause rapid emptying, combined with a shearing force on the duct. In human beings, biliary duct rupture has been reported in persons previously having undergone cholecystectomy, suggesting that shearing of the duct alone is sometimes sufficient. The most common site of ductal rupture appears to be the common bile duct just distal to the entrance of the last hepatic duct; however, rupture may occur in the distal common bile duct, cystic duct (rare), or hepatic ducts. Gallbladder rupture is principally due to necrotizing cholecystitis or cholelithiasis. Many dogs with necrotizing cholecystitis have obstruction of the common bile duct; however, rupture can be due to necrosis and perforation of only the gallbladder wall.

DIAGNOSIS
Clinical Presentation

Signalment. Traumatic rupture of the common bile duct or gallbladder may occur in animals of any age.

Necrotizing cholecystitis is more common in middle-aged or older animals.

History. The animal may have sustained trauma several weeks prior to presentation. Clinical signs may be slowly progressive or acute if the bile becomes infected (see below).

Physical Examination Findings

Clinical signs of bile peritonitis depend on the presence of bacteria and on whether the peritonitis is diffuse or localized. Animals with infected bile peritonitis generally present in shock with acute abdominal pain, fever, vomiting, and anorexia. Animals that develop localized peritonitis secondary to inspissated bile tend not to be as sick as those with diffuse peritonitis. Sometimes pain can be localized to the anterior abdomen. Some animals are diagnosed before a diseased gallbladder ruptures, in which case signs are similar to those with localized peritonitis.

> ☞ **NOTE** · Perform diagnostic peritoneal lavage to help identify bile peritonitis in dogs sustaining trauma, before the onset of clinical signs.

Radiography/Ultrasonography

Radiographs of animals with bile peritonitis can show a generalized loss of abdominal detail if the peritonitis is diffuse, or a soft-tissue density in the cranial abdomen if the infection is localized. Plain radiographs may reveal radiodense gallstones or air in the gallbladder wall or lumen. Ultrasonography may also delineate the location of mass-lesions and evaluate the gallbladder and biliary ducts. Exploratory laparotomy is indicated in any patient with bile peritonitis and negates the need for extensive diagnostic workups.

> ☞ **NOTE** · Ultrasonography provides more information regarding biliary tract structure than plain radiographs and is particularly useful if abdominal effusion is present.

Laboratory Findings

Bilious effusions should have bilirubin concentrations greater than those found in serum. Neutrophilia is often noted if the peritonitis is generalized; however, with localized infections, the white blood cell count may be normal. Other findings are inconsistent and depend on the severity of the peritonitis. The most common bacterial isolate from animals with bilious effusion in one study was *E. coli* (Ludwig et al, 1995).

DIFFERENTIAL DIAGNOSIS

A bilious effusion is obvious because the fluid looks like bile; it is usually easy to distinguish from an effusion that is due to another cause and that has been stained by bilirubin. However, if there is any doubt as to whether the fluid is bilious or bile-stained, simultaneous bilirubin concentrations in the serum and effusion should be compared (see above).

> ☞ **NOTE** · Compare fluid bilirubin levels to those in serum.

MEDICAL MANAGEMENT

Animals with bile peritonitis may be anemic, hypoproteinemic, dehydrated, or have electrolyte imbalances. The irritating effects of bile on the peritoneum cause inflammation and fluid transudation into the abdominal cavity, and the animal may present in hypovolemic and/or septic shock. Aggressive fluid therapy may be needed and electrolyte imbalances should be corrected. Broad-spectrum antibiotics should be administered before, during, and after surgery. Whole-blood transfusions (see Table 17-1 on p. 367) may be indicated (i.e., hematocrit less than 20%). Vitamin K$_1$ administration (or fresh whole blood) should also be considered in these patients, because disruption of bile flow occasionally causes vitamin K malabsorption and coagulation disturbances (see Table 18-1 on p. 389).

SURGICAL TREATMENT

Surgical treatment options for common bile duct rupture include ductal repair or biliary diversion (see pp. 392–393). Repair is possible if the rupture is diagnosed early but becomes difficult once adhesions develop. Cholecystoduodenostomy or cholecystojejunostomy is usually easier and safer. Rupture of a hepatic duct can be treated by ligation of the leaking duct. Gallbladder rupture secondary to infective processes should be treated by cholecystectomy (see p. 391).

Treatment of necrotizing cholecystitis includes early surgical exploration, once the animal has been stabilized. Treatment consists of cholecystectomy, antibiotics, and appropriate therapy for peritonitis. Generally, attempts to salvage the gallbladder by closing the defect are inappropriate because the wall is usually necrotic. Be sure that the common bile duct is not ligated when the gallbladder is removed. In one study of 23 dogs with necrotizing cholecystitis, the mortality rate was 39%; delayed diagnosis probably contributed to the high mortality (Church, Matthiesen, 1988).

> ☞ **NOTE** · Animals with necrotizing cholecystitis have infected bile; therefore clinical signs often begin soon after gallbladder rupture occurs. Unless diagnosis and surgical intervention are prompt, mortality is high.

Preoperative Management

Surgery should be performed as soon as the animal has been stabilized. Electrolyte and fluid abnormalities should be corrected before surgery. See also medical management of patients with bile peritonitis, above.

Anesthesia

Hypovolemic, septic, or shocky dogs may be induced with oxymorphone plus diazepam (Table 18-4), given to effect. If intubation is not possible, etomidate may be given or mask induction with isoflurane used if the patient is not vomiting.

TABLE 18-4
Selected Anesthetic Protocol for Dogs with Biliary Disease
Induction
Oxymorphone (0.1 mg/kg IV) plus diazepam (0.2 mg/kg IV). Give in incremental dosages. Intubate if possible. If necessary, give etomidate (0.5-1.5 mg/kg IV) to effect.
Maintenance
Isoflurane

TABLE 18-5
Postoperative Analgesics
Oxymorphone (Numorphan)
0.05-0.1 mg/kg IV, IM every 4 hours (as needed)
Butorphanol (Torbutrol, Torbugesic)
0.2-0.4 mg/kg IV, IM, or SC every 2 to 4 hours (as needed)

For stable patients, please refer to the anesthetic management of patients with hepatobiliary disease on p. 367.

Surgical Anatomy

See p. 390 for surgical anatomy of the extrahepatic biliary system.

Positioning

Exposure of the gallbladder is generally via a cranial midline abdominal incision (see p. 180). The caudal thorax and entire abdomen should be prepared for aseptic surgery.

SURGICAL TECHNIQUE

Cholecystectomy is discussed on p. 391. Laceration or transection of the bile ducts may be treated by primary repair (see p. 393) or biliary diversion (p. 392). A damaged hepatic duct may be ligated because alternative routes for biliary drainage from a single liver lobe will develop. The abdominal fluid and/or site of rupture/perforation should be cultured during surgery. Once the site of leakage has been identified and corrected, the abdomen should be flushed with copious amounts of warmed, sterile fluids. Open abdominal drainage (see p. 198) may be considered if generalized peritonitis is present.

SUTURE MATERIALS/SPECIAL INSTRUMENTS

A Poole suction tip is useful to remove abdominal fluid and help identify the site of leakage. It is also used to remove fluid instilled in the abdomen during lavage.

POSTOPERATIVE CARE AND ASSESSMENT

Fluid therapy should be continued until the animal is able to maintain hydration on its own. Electrolytes and acid-base status should be monitored. Many patients with bile peritonitis are extremely debilitated before surgery. Animals with bile peritonitis are in extreme pain. Postoperative analgesia

may be provided with oxymorphone (Table 18-5). Butorphanol is also effective, but analgesia is of shorter duration than when oxymorphone is given. Nutritional supplementation via a needle-catheter jejunostomy or parenterally is beneficial in these patients (see Chapter 11). Antibiotic therapy based on culture of bile should be continued for at least 7 to 14 days postoperatively.

PROGNOSIS

The prognosis for patients with diffuse, septic bile peritonitis is guarded. Without aggressive surgical management, most of these patients will die. The prognosis is better if the condition is diagnosed and treated early and is better in animals with nonseptic biliary effusions. In a recent study of 24 dogs and 2 cats with bile peritonitis, overall survival was 46% (Ludwig et al, 1995).

References

Church EM, Matthiesen DT: Surgical treatment of 23 dogs with necrotizing cholecystitis, *J Am Anim Hosp Assoc* 24:305, 1988.

Ludwig LL et al: Surgical treatment of bile peritonitis in 24 dogs and 2 cats: a retrospective study (1987-1994), *Vet Surg* 24:430, 1995 (abstract).

Suggested Reading

Fossum TW, Willard MD: Diseases of the gallbladder and the extrahepatic biliary system. In Ettinger SJ: *Textbook of veterinary internal medicine,* ed 4, Philadelphia, 1995, WB Saunders.

Hunt CA, Gofton N: Primary repair of a transected bile duct, *J Am Anim Hosp Assoc* 20:57, 1984.

Kipnis RM: Cholelithiasis, gallbladder perforation, and bile peritonitis in a dog, *Canine Practice* 13:15, 1986.

Lawrence D et al: Temporary bile diversion in cats with experimental extrahepatic bile duct obstruction, *Vet Surg* 21:446, 1992.

Watkins PE, Pearson H, Denny HR: Traumatic rupture of the bile duct in the dog: a report of seven cases, *J Small Anim Pract* 24:731, 1983.

CHAPTER 19

Surgery of the Endocrine System

Surgery of the Adrenal and Pituitary Glands

GENERAL PRINCIPLES AND TECHNIQUES

DEFINITIONS

Adrenalectomy is the removal of one or both adrenal glands. **Hypophysectomy** is removal of the pituitary gland (hypophysis). **Hyperadrenocorticism** is a multisystemic disorder that results from excessive glucocorticoids. **Cushing's disease** refers to hyperadrenocorticism caused by a pituitary adenoma. **Addison's disease** is due to deficiency of glucocorticoids and/or mineralocorticoids.

PREOPERATIVE CONCERNS

Adrenocortical insufficiency may be naturally occurring (primary or secondary to other diseases) or iatrogenic, following administration of glucocorticoids, progestins, or adrenocorticolytic drugs (e.g., o,p'-DDD). The history should include dosages of corticosteroids or other drugs given, type of corticosteroids, duration of administration, and time since last dose. It is easier to inhibit glucocorticoid than mineralocorticoid secretion (see the discussion of anatomy on p. 402). When glucocorticoid secretion is severely suppressed, the patient may experience collapse and weakness without evidence of electrolyte abnormalities. If secretion of mineralocorticoids is suppressed, electrolyte abnormalities (i.e., hyponatremia, hyperkalemia) and azotemia may occur. Reduced ability to retain sodium results in volume depletion, decreased cardiac output, and reduced vascular tone, which may manifest as acute vascular collapse. Gastrointestinal disturbances and prolonged vomiting may also contribute to electrolyte abnormalities and volume depletion. Electrolyte concentrations should be corrected before surgery. Some dogs with hypoadrenocorticism are hypoalbuminemic. A protective steroid release normally occurs during surgery, which prevents circulatory collapse. However, animals with hypoadrenocorticism may be unable to respond to such stress and often require glucocorticoid supplementation before and during surgery. When minor elective surgery is performed in animals with adrenocortical insufficiency, glucocorticoid therapy may be given intravenously before induction of anesthesia (Table 19-1). The same dose can be given intravenously or intramuscularly after recovery from anesthesia, and then the animal returned to its oral maintenance glucocorticoid therapy the day following surgery. For major surgery, a similar protocol is used, except that glucocorticoid therapy is continued at approximately five times the maintenance dose for 2 to 3 days (Table 19-2). Normal maintenance doses are then reinstituted. Once the animal is eating, medications can be given orally, rather than by injection.

Iatrogenic hyperadrenocorticism is the most common form. Spontaneous hyperadrenocorticism is usually caused by excessive pituitary secretion of ACTH, resulting in

---

> **TABLE** 19-1
>
> **Protocol for Glucocorticoid Administration in Animals with Adrenocortical Insufficiency Undergoing Minor Elective Procedures***
>
> 1. 1 hr before surgery give *one* of the following IV:
>
> **Prednisolone Sodium Succinate**
>
> 1.0-2.0 mg/kg, or
>
> **Dexamethasone**
>
> 0.1-0.2 mg/kg, or
>
> **Soluble hydrocortisone**
>
> 4-5 mg/kg
>
> 2. Repeat dose at recovery IV or IM
> 3. Resume maintenance glucocorticoid therapy on first postoperative day, if needed
>
> *Modified from Short CE: *Principles and practice of veterinary anesthesia,* Los Angeles, 1987, Williams & Wilkins.

TABLE 19-2

Protocol for Glucocorticoid Administration in Animals with Adrenocortical Insufficiency Undergoing Major Elective Procedures*

1. Administer preoperative steroids as described in Table 19-1
2. Repeat dose at recovery IV or IM
3. Days 1 and 2 postoperatively—administer one of the following IV or IM:

Prednisolone

0.5 mg/kg BID, or

Dexamethasone

0.1 mg/kg SID, or

Prednisone

0.5 mg/kg BID, or

Cortisone Acetate

2.5 mg/kg BID

4. Resume maintenance glucocorticoid therapy on third postoperative day, unless complications arise

*Modified from Short CE: *Principles and practice of veterinary anesthesia,* Los Angeles, 1987, Williams & Wilkins.

bilateral adrenocortical hyperplasia (80% to 90% of noniatrogenic cases). Functional adrenocortical tumors are less common (10% to 20% of noniatrogenic cases). Patients with hyperadrenocorticism are catabolic and have protein depletion and connective tissue abnormalities. Muscle wasting, weakness, and thin, fragile skin are common. Electrolyte and/or acid-base abnormalities, hyperglycemia, and hypertension may be present. Intraabdominal fat deposition, combined with muscular weakness, sometimes causes ventilatory abnormalities. Concurrent abnormalities (e.g., congestive heart failure, diabetes mellitus) increase the anesthetic risk in these patients. Cardiovascular abnormalities may occur secondary to hypertension; a thorough preoperative cardiac examination is warranted. Electrolyte and acid-base abnormalities should be corrected before surgery. Animals with hyperadrenocorticism are at increased risk for postoperative pulmonary thromboembolism. If hypercoagulopathies are suspected preoperatively, preventative measures (e.g., low-dose heparin therapy) may be indicated. Most animals with hyperadrenocorticism have urinary tract infection, even when the urinalysis shows no evidence of it. Urine should routinely be cultured in these patients.

ANESTHETIC CONSIDERATIONS

A variety of anesthetic protocols may be used in adrenocortical-insufficient or hyperadrenal animals. Maintenance of electrolyte and glucose levels is important. Glucocorticoid supplementation is often necessary in animals with adrenocortical insufficiency undergoing surgery (see above). Glucocorticoid therapy should be instituted preoperatively in

patients with hyperadrenocorticism that are undergoing adrenalectomy. Because of the close association of the adrenals and caudal vena cava, retraction of the caudal cava is often necessary for adrenalectomy. Vascular pressures should be closely monitored during surgery, and retraction should be done carefully to prevent obstructing venous return. Animals with pheochromocytomas require special anesthetic considerations to avoid complications associated with excessive catecholamine secretion (see p. 409).

ANTIBIOTICS

Animals with hyperadrenocorticism are at increased risk to develop postoperative infections as a result of high levels of circulating glucocorticoids and immunosuppression. Therefore perioperative prophylactic antibiotics are recommended in such animals undergoing surgery.

SURGICAL ANATOMY

The adrenal glands are located near the craniomedial pole of the kidneys (Fig. 19-1). The left adrenal is slightly larger than the right. The left gland lies beneath the lateral process of the second lumbar vertebra, while the right adrenal is more cranial, lying beneath the lateral process of the last thoracic vertebra. Because of the proximity of the right adrenal to the caudal vena cava, surgical removal of neoplastic glands can be difficult. The phrenicoabdominal vessels cross the ventral surface of the adrenal. The adrenal glands are composed of two functionally and structurally different regions. The outer cortex produces mineralocorticoids (e.g., aldosterone), glucocorticoids, and small amounts of androgenic hormones. Mineralocorticoids regulate sodium and potassium concentrations. Aldosterone causes transport of sodium and potassium through the renal tubular walls and also causes hydrogen ion transport.

The adrenal medulla is functionally related to the sympathetic nervous system and secretes epinephrine and norepinephrine in response to sympathetic stimulation. Epinephrine and norepinephrine have almost the same effects as direct sympathetic stimulation (e.g., vascular constriction, resulting in increased arterial pressures; inhibition of the gastrointestinal tract; pupillary dilation; increased rates of cellular metabolism throughout the body), except that their effects last significantly longer because they are slowly removed from circulation.

SURGICAL TECHNIQUES

Adrenalectomy is usually performed for adrenal tumors. Bilateral adrenalectomy for treatment of Cushing's disease is controversial and not commonly performed. Two approaches may be used. A ventral midline approach allows the entire abdomen to be explored for metastasis and bilateral adrenalectomy to be performed with a single surgical incision, if necessary. However, exposure and dissection of the adrenal may be difficult with this approach, particularly in large dogs. A paracostal incision provides improved access to the adrenal gland but does not allow evaluation of the liver or other organs for metastasis. It may be considered in

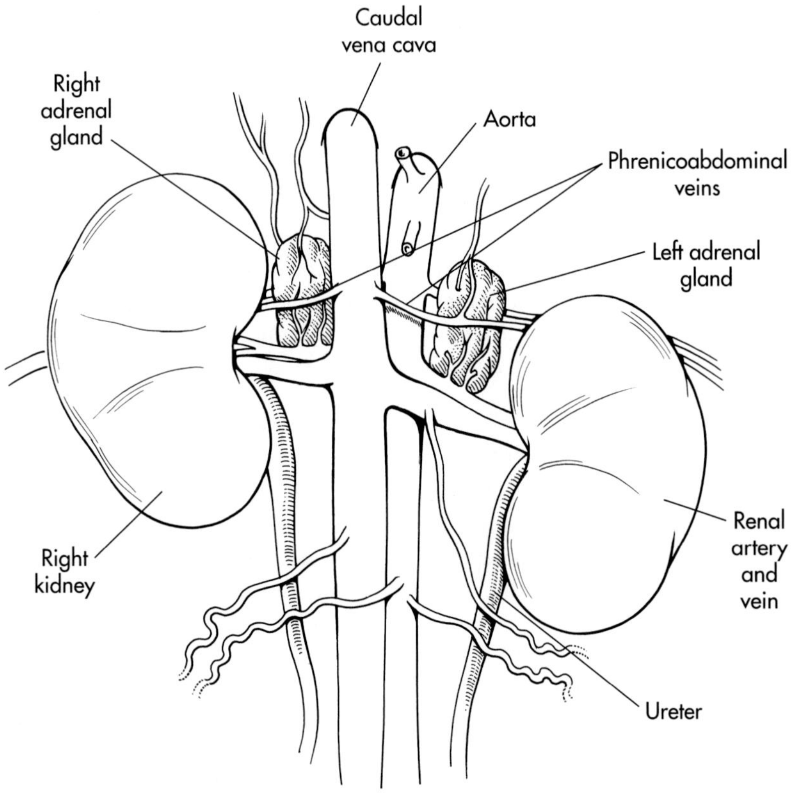

FIG. 19-1
Location of the adrenal glands.

Location of the adrenal glands.

Labels: Right adrenal gland; Caudal vena cava; Aorta; Phrenicoabdominal veins; Left adrenal gland; Renal artery and vein; Ureter; Right kidney

animals with unilateral lesions, without evidence of metastasis on ultrasound, computed tomography, or magnetic resonance imaging. Adrenalectomy is not advised if extensive tumor metastasis is present, or if invasion of the caudal cava and surrounding organs makes complete removal of neoplastic tissue unlikely. Concurrent diabetes mellitus might be a contraindication to bilateral adrenalectomy because lack of endogenous catecholamines may make it difficult to regulate the diabetes.

Adrenalectomy Via a Midline Abdominal Approach

Prepare the entire ventral abdomen and caudal thorax for aseptic surgery. Perform a ventral midline abdominal incision that extends from the xiphoid cartilage to near the pubis. Identify the enlarged adrenal, and carefully inspect the entire abdomen (including the other adrenal) for abnormalities or evidence of metastasis. Palpate the liver for evidence of nodularity and biopsy if indicated. Palpate the caudal vena cava near the adrenals for evidence of tumor invasion or thrombosis. If additional exposure is needed for adrenalectomy, extend the incision paracostally on the side of the affected gland by incising the fascia of the rectus abdominis muscle and fibers of the external abdominal oblique, internal abdominal oblique, and transversus abdominis muscles, respectively. Use self-retaining retractors to improve visualization of the abdominal cavity. Retract liver, spleen, and stomach cranially, kidney caudally, and vena cava medially, to expose the entire gland. Identify the blood supply and ureter to the ipsilateral kidney, and avoid these structures during

dissection. Ligate the phrenicoabdominal vein, and divide it between sutures. Carefully dissect the adrenal gland from surrounding tissues, using a combination of sharp and blunt dissection (Fig. 19-2). Numerous vessels may be encountered. Obtain hemostasis with electrocautery if the vessels are small or with hemoclips if they are large. If possible, do not invade the adrenal capsule. Removing the adrenal in one piece will decrease the chance of leaving small pieces of neoplastic tissue within the abdominal cavity. *If tumor thrombosis is present in the caudal cava, but extensive metastasis is not apparent, perform temporary occlusion of the cava using Rumel tourniquets (see p. 578). Make a longitudinal incision in the vein and remove the thrombus. Close the cava with a continuous suture pattern of 5-0 or 6-0 vascular suture, and close the abdomen routinely (see discussion of suture material on p. 404). If a paracostal incision was made, begin the closure by approximating the abdominal wall at the junction of the combined ventral and paracostal incisions. After closing the linea alba, suture each muscle layer of the paracostal incision with a continuous pattern of synthetic absorbable sutures. Close skin and subcutaneous tissue routinely.*

Adrenalectomy Via a Paralumbar Approach

Place the animal in lateral recumbency, with a rolled towel or sandbag between the abdomen and operating table. Prepare the caudal hemithorax and lateral abdomen for aseptic surgery. Make an incision just caudal to the thirteenth rib, which extends from the lateral vertebral processes to within 3 to 4 cm of the ventral midline (approximately 10 to 14 cm long, depending on the animal's size [Fig. 19-3]]). Incise the abdominal muscles individually and identify the adrenal gland cranial to the kidney. Retract the kidney ventrally, and ligate any vascular structures that cross its surface. Dissect the gland free from surrounding tissues (Fig. 19-4). Suture each muscle layer of the paracostal incision with a continuous pattern of synthetic absorbable sutures. Close skin and subcutaneous tissues routinely.

HEALING OF THE ADRENAL AND PITUITARY GLANDS

Because adrenal or pituitary biopsies are rarely performed, there is little information regarding healing of these glands following surgery.

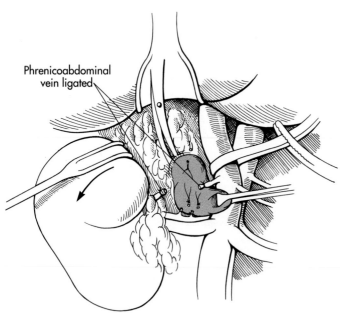

Phrenicoabdominal vein ligated

FIG. 19-2
To resect the right adrenal gland, retract the vena cava medially. Ligate the phrenicoabdominal vein, and divide it between sutures. Carefully dissect the adrenal gland from surrounding tissues.

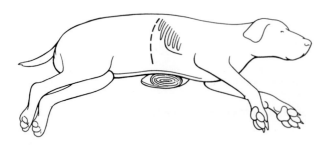

FIG. 19-3
Adrenalectomy may be performed via a paralumbar approach. Place the animal in lateral recumbency, with a rolled towel or sandbag between the abdomen and operating table. Make an incision just caudal to the thirteenth rib, which extends from the lateral vertebral processes to within 3 to 4 cm of the ventral midline.

SUTURE MATERIALS/SPECIAL INSTRUMENTS

Hyperadrenocorticism may cause delayed wound healing; therefore abdominal closure should be performed with strong, slowly absorbed or nonabsorbable suture material (e.g., polydioxanone, polyglyconate, polypropylene, or nylon). Self-retaining retractors such as Balfour abdominal retractors are recommended, to improve abdominal visualization. Malleable retractors, covered with moistened sponges, are used to retract viscera from the adrenal glands. Electrocautery and hemoclips make hemostasis easier, compared with suture ligation of vessels.

POSTOPERATIVE CARE AND ASSESSMENT

After adrenalectomy, hydration status and electrolyte balance should be monitored carefully and corrected as necessary. Permanent adrenal insufficiency occurs in animals after bilateral adrenalectomy, and these animals require life-long glucocorticoid (prednisone or prednisolone) and/or mineralocorticoid (desoxycorticosterone or fludrocortisone) replacement (Table 19-3). These animals should be closely monitored for hypoadrenocortical collapse. They are most likely to have an addisonian crisis after they have been released to the owner's care. Owners must be advised to watch for malaise, inappetence, or other clinical signs suggesting decompensation. Temporary adrenal insufficiency occurs after unilateral removal of functional adrenal tumors, because of suppression of the opposite adrenal's function by the tumor. Glucocorticoids should be supplemented postoperatively (see Table 19-3), but may be discontinued when the remaining adrenal begins to function normally, as determined by results of an ACTH-stimulation test.

Pulmonary thromboembolism is a potentially life-threatening complication of adrenal surgery (particularly in dogs with adrenal neoplasia). Sudden, severe, postoperative respiratory distress may indicate pulmonary thromboembolism. Lung perfusion scans may help identify lung regions that are

TABLE 19-3
Postoperative Drug Therapy After Adrenalectomy in Dogs
Fludrocortisone acetate (Florinef)
0.02 mg/kg PO, SID to BID
Prednisone or Prednisolone
0.5 mg/kg BID for 7-14 days, then 0.2 mg/kg SID or
Cortisone
2.5 mg/kg BID for 7-14 days, then 0.5 mg/kg BID
Heparin
75 units/kg SC, TID
Streptokinase
Loading dose—5000 IU/kg IV over 30 min; then 2000 IU/kg/hr IV over 24 hrs (constant rate infusion)

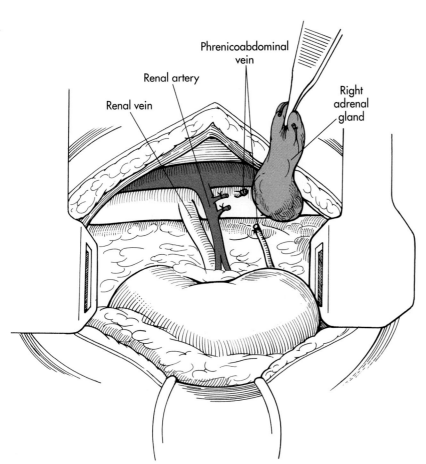

FIG. 19-4
To expose the adrenal gland via a paralumbar approach, retract the kidney ventrally, and ligate any vascular structures that cross its surface.

Phrenicoabdominal vein

Renal artery

Renal vein

Right adrenal gland

underperfused. Treatment with strict cage rest, oxygen, anticoagulants (e.g., heparin), and thrombolytic agents (e.g. streptokinase) may be beneficial (see Table 19-3). These animals should be assessed frequently for signs of hemorrhage, and the hematocrit should be checked every 2 hours. If the PCV drops or hemorrhage is noted, the streptokinase infusion should be discontinued.

COMPLICATIONS

The main complications of adrenalectomy are hemorrhage, fluid and electrolyte imbalances, pancreatitis, wound infections, delayed wound healing, and thromboembolism. Postoperative hemorrhage is usually associated with incomplete occlusion of small vessels surrounding an enlarged, highly vascular tumor. Judicious use of electrocautery and hemoclips helps avoid this complication. Delayed wound healing is often encountered in animals with hyperadrenocorticism, as a result of the negative effect of steroids on wound healing. Care should thus be used in performing abdominal closure in these animals (see above). Strong monofilament absorbable (i.e., polydioxanone, polyglyconate) or nonabsorbable (i.e., polypropylene) suture should be used.

SPECIAL AGE CONSIDERATIONS

Animals with adrenal neoplasia are usually old and often have concurrent abnormalities (e.g., hypertension, cardiovascular abnormalities); therefore extreme care should be used during anesthesia. These animals also require extensive postoperative monitoring. If the animal is debilitated, anorexic, or vomiting,

placement of an enteral feeding tube during surgery (see p. 79) or providing parenteral nutrition is advised.

Suggested Reading

Emms SG et al: Adrenalectomy in the management of canine hyperadrenocorticism, *J Am Anim Hosp Assoc* 23:557, 1987.

Kaplan AJ, Peterson ME: Effects of desoxycorticosterone pivilate administration on blood pressure in dogs with primary hypoadrenocorticism, *J Am Vet Med Assoc* 206:327, 1995.

Langais-Burgess L, Lumsden JH: Concurrent hypoadrenocorticism and hypoalbuminemia in dogs: a retrospective surgery, *J Am Anim Hosp Assoc* 31:307, 1995.

Rakich PM, Lorenz MD: Clinical signs and laboratory abnormalities in 23 dogs with spontaneous hypoadrenocorticism, *J Am Anim Hosp Assoc* 20:647, 1984.

van Sluijs FJ, Sjollema BE: Adrenalectomy in 36 dogs and 2 cats with hyperadrenocorticism, *Tijdschr Diergeneeskd* 117:29s, 1992.

SPECIFIC DISEASES

ADRENAL NEOPLASIA

DEFINITIONS

Adrenal carcinomas are autonomously functioning malignant tumors of the adrenal cortex; **adrenal adenomas** are benign adrenocortical tumors. **Pheochromocytomas** are catecholamine-secreting tumors of the chromaffin tissue that usually arise in adrenal medullary tissue.

SYNONYMS

For pheochromocytoma—**paraganglioma**

GENERAL CONSIDERATIONS AND CLINICALLY RELEVANT PATHOPHYSIOLOGY

The most common tumors of the canine adrenal glands are adrenal adenomas, carcinomas, and pheochromocytomas. Noniatrogenic hyperadrenocorticism (not due to excessive administration of glucocorticoids) may be caused by excessive pituitary secretion of ACTH (pituitary-dependent hyperadrenocorticism) or primary adrenocortical tumors, which secrete excessive cortisol. Pituitary-dependent hyperadrenocorticism is more common than adrenal neoplasia, accounting for approximately 80% of cases (see p. 401). Most adrenal tumors are not functional, and clinical signs are caused by local invasion of the tumor into surrounding tissue and/or distant metastases. Functional tumors secrete excessive amounts of cortisol, which inhibits pituitary ACTH secretion, causing atrophy of the contralateral adrenal. Adrenocortical adenomas and carcinomas appear to occur with equal frequency. They are usually unilateral; however, bilateral adrenocortical neoplasia rarely occurs. Dogs with bilateral adrenal neoplasia do not have historical or physical examination findings or laboratory abnormalities differentiating them from dogs with unilateral disease. Ultrasonographic evaluation of the adrenals often identifies adrenomegaly and localizes the tumor to one side of the body (see below). Colonic perforation is a rare sequel of excessive glucocorticoid secretion. Corticosteroids may inhibit collagen synthesis and increase collagen breakdown. Additionally, they may cause breakdown of the mucosal barrier and inhibit normal immune responses.

☞ **N O T E** • Most hyperadrenocortical animals have pituitary, rather than adrenal, tumors.

Pheochromocytomas are tumors of the adrenal medulla that secrete excessive amounts of catecholamines (primarily norepinephrine, but also epinephrine and dopamine) and other vasoactive peptides (i.e., vasoactive intestinal polypeptide, somatostatin, enkephalin, corticotropin). Excessive catecholamine and vasoactive peptide levels may manifest as cardiovascular, respiratory, or central nervous system disease. Although these tumors have classically been reported as benign, recent reports suggest that regional invasion and distant metastases (liver, regional lymph nodes, lungs, spleen, ovary, diaphragm, vertebrae) occur in 50% of affected dogs. Invasion of the caudal vena cava, phrenicoabdominal artery or vein, renal artery or vein, or hepatic vein may cause signs of ascites, edema, or venous distention. Pheochromocytomas are usually unilateral, although bilateral tumors occur. These masses are usually reddish tan, multilobulated, firm or friable, and may be completely or partially encapsulated. Occasionally, pheochromocytomas may be associated with neoplastic transformation of multiple endocrine tissues of neuroectoderm origin (e.g., pituitary, adrenocortical, or thyroid adenomas, or pancreatic islet cell tumors). Extraadrenal pheochromocytomas have been reported in dogs and cats. Other tumors that arise from the adrenal medulla are neuroblastomas and ganglioneuromas; however, they are rare.

DIAGNOSIS
Clinical Presentation

Signalment. Adrenocortical tumors usually occur in older, large-breed dogs and appear to be diagnosed more commonly in females. A definitive breed predisposition has not been identified. Pheochromocytomas usually occur in older dogs but have been reported in dogs as young as 1 year of age. Both sexes appear to be equally affected. Boxers may be predisposed to this tumor. Adrenal tumors are rarely diagnosed in cats.

History. Functional adrenocortical tumors commonly cause hyperadrenocorticism (i.e., polyuria, polydipsia, polyphagia, abdominal enlargement, endocrine alopecia, muscle wasting, weakness, lethargy, panting, and/or hyperpigmentation). Signs of nonfunctional adrenocortical tumors include anorexia, abdominal enlargement, abdominal pain, diarrhea, vomiting, and lethargy. Vomiting has been associated with intestinal perforation in a dog with adrenocortical adenoma. High circulating levels of glucocorticoids may make diagnosis of intestinal perforation difficult because signs of peritonitis (i.e., abdominal discomfort, restlessness, panting, weakness, and/or dyspnea) are obscured. Occasionally dogs are asymptomatic, and the adrenal mass is a fortuitous finding at surgery or necropsy.

Physical Examination Findings

Clinical findings in animals with adrenocortical tumors depend on whether the tumors are functional. Clinical findings supportive of a diagnosis of hyperadrenocorticism are usually present in those with functional tumors (see above), whereas ascites, abdominal pain, edema, diarrhea, and vomiting are common with nonfunctional tumors.

Clinical findings in animals with pheochromocytomas may include tachycardia/cardiac arrhythmias, acute collapse, polypnea, panting, cough, lethargy, anorexia, dyspnea, weakness, abdominal distention, congestive heart failure, ataxia, incoordination, polyuria-polydipsia, and alopecia. Hypertension (paroxysmal or sustained) is frequently present. In one study, six of eight dogs with invasive tumors died within hours of initial examination of apparent sudden cardiovascular collapse that was believed to be related to hypertension and/or cardiac arrhythmias (Bouayad et al, 1987).

Radiography/Ultrasonography

Adrenal tumors are difficult to detect radiographically unless they are associated with significant adrenal enlargement (greater than or equal to 20 mm) or calcification. For best results, food should be withheld for 24 hours before radiography to allow the gastrointestinal tract to empty. In

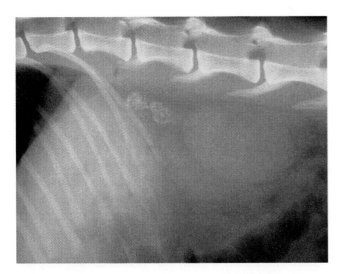

FIG. 19-5
Lateral abdominal radiograph of a cat with a mineralized, neoplastic adrenal gland. (Courtesy L. Homco, Texas A&M University.)

some animals, mineralization of tissue cranial to the kidney may be seen on plain radiographs and may or may not be associated with obvious adrenal enlargement (Fig. 19-5). This finding is suggestive of adrenocortical neoplasia (adenoma or carcinoma). The incidence of nonneoplastic mineralization of adrenal glands is low; however, bilateral adrenal calcification may occur with pituitary-dependent hyperadrenocorticism. Hepatomegaly, calcinosis cutis, or osteoporosis may also be noted radiographically in some animals with adrenocortical neoplasia, but can also be seen with pituitary-dependent disease. Enhanced abdominal contrast secondary to increased fat distribution in the abdomen may be found. Pheochromocytomas may be detected radiographically if sufficiently enlarged; however, ultrasonography is more sensitive.

> **☞ NOTE ·** Mineralization of an adrenal gland suggests neoplasia.

Ultrasonography is useful to assess adrenal gland size, echogenicity, and shape. The normal canine adrenal gland (in mature dogs) is 2 to 3 cm long, 1 cm wide, and 0.5 cm thick. Some authors have reported abdominal ultrasonography to be an inconsistent diagnostic aid in dogs with adrenal neoplasia. However, others reported ultrasonography correctly identifying the involved gland in 76% of dogs with adrenal carcinomas and 62% of dogs with adrenal adenomas (Reusch, Feldman, 1991). Pheochromocytomas have been reported to have mixed echo patterns and cannot be definitively differentiated from adrenocortical tumors. Bilateral adrenal enlargement is suggestive of pituitary-dependent hyperadrenocorticism because functional adrenocortical tumors typically cause atrophy of the contralateral gland. Adrenal metastasis may be diagnosed with ultrasound.

> **☞ NOTE ·** Ultrasound is more useful than radiographs in identifying adrenal abnormalities.

X-ray computed tomography (CT) and magnetic resonance imaging enable accurate localization of adrenal neoplasia; however, they do not allow adrenal adenomas, carcinomas, and pheochromocytomas to be differentiated. Adrenal carcinomas may appear as well-demarcated, homogeneous masses, or they may be poorly demarcated, with irregular texture and contrast enhancement. Masses that are poorly demarcated, have irregular shape, and are nonhomogeneous with mineralization are usually carcinomas. Determination of caudal vena cava invasion is not usually possible with CT. Caudal vena caval angiography should be performed preoperatively if caudal caval thrombosis is suspected. Excretory urography may help identify tumor invasion necessitating nephrectomy (i.e., ureteral obstruction or renal invasion).

> **☞ NOTE ·** CT and MRI do not differentiate adrenal adenomas, carcinomas, or pheochromocytomas.

Laboratory Findings

Laboratory abnormalities are inconsistent and nonspecific in animals with pheochromocytomas. There are no consistent changes in animals with hyperadrenocorticism; however, common laboratory abnormalities include increased serum alkaline phosphatase, neutrophilic leukocytosis, lymphopenia, eosinopenia, mild polycythemia, increased alanine aminotransferase, and hypercholesterolemia. Urinary tract abnormalities may include hyposthenuria (urine specific gravity less than 1.007) or isosthenuria (1.008 to 1.012). Urinary tract infections are common in hyperadrenal dogs, even when bacteria and inflammatory cells are absent on urinalysis.

Spontaneous hyperadrenocorticism is diagnosed based on the results of an ACTH-stimulation test (Table 19-4), low-dose dexamethasone suppression (LDDS) test, or both. ACTH-stimulation and LDDS tests are the best initial diagnostic tests for hyperadrenocorticism, but should be performed after exogenous steroids have been eliminated. Approximately 85% of dogs with pituitary-dependent hyperadrenocorticism and adrenocortical tumors have increased post-ACTH plasma cortisol concentrations. Pre-ACTH and post-ACTH cortisol concentrations tend to be elevated or in the high-normal range in animals with adrenocortical neoplasia (Table 19-5). False positive tests may occur in dogs that are chronically stressed or ill. If plasma cortisol concentrations are normal, but clinical signs are suggestive of hyperadrenocorticism, an LDDS test should be performed. Once a definitive diagnosis of hyperadrenocorticism has been made, differentiation of adrenal-dependent and pituitary-dependent causes can be made by LDDS, high-dose dexamethasone suppression test, ultrasonography, or measurement of endogenous ACTH. Readers are referred to a medical text for further information.

DIFFERENTIAL DIAGNOSIS

Pheochromocytomas and adrenocortical tumors must be differentiated because the operative management of these cases is different. Generally, clinical signs and laboratory analysis allow preoperative differentiation (see above). At surgery, pheochromocytomas may be identified grossly by application of Zenker's solution (potassium dichromate or iodate), which results in oxidation of catecholamines, forming a dark brown pigment within 10 to 20 minutes after application to the surface of a freshly sectioned tumor. Although adrenal carcinomas are apt to be large and invasive, differentiation of adenomas and carcinomas is impossible without histopathology. Apparent metastatic lesions in the liver or draining lymph nodes may suggest malignancy, but care should be used to differentiate benign hepatic nodules from neoplastic disease.

☞ **NOTE** • Definitive diagnosis of adrenal tumors requires histopathology.

MEDICAL MANAGEMENT

Adrenergic blockage (i.e., phenoxybenzamine, phentolamine, prazosin) is used in patients with pheochromocytomas to control blood pressure. These drugs are also used intraoperatively (see discussion of anesthetic management on p. 409). If tachycardia or cardiac arrhythmias are present, β-adrenergic blockage may also be used; however, unopposed β-blockage may result in severe hypertension.

Mitotane (o,p'-DDD) can be used to control clinical signs in animals with adrenocortical tumors; however, tumors are more resistant to the adrenocorticolytic effects of mitotane than are normal or hyperplastic adrenal cortices. Larger doses (Table 19-6) are required to obtain and maintain control in these dogs than in those with pituitary-dependent hy-

peradrenocorticism, and greater side effects (i.e., gastric irritation, vomiting) can be expected. Ketoconazole is an alternative to mitotane because it is less toxic, causes reversible inhibition of adrenal steroid production, and has little effect on mineralocorticoid production. Ketoconazole (Table 19-7) may be used in animals with malignant adrenocortical tumors who are not surgical candidates because of metastasis. Ketoconazole may be used preoperatively to reduce the risk of anesthesia and surgery in animals with uncontrolled hyperadrenocorticism, and as a diagnostic trial in dogs in whom equivocal test results make the diagnosis of hyperadrenocorticism difficult. It should be given for a minimum of 4 to 8 weeks, if used for the latter purpose. It must be given for the duration of the animal's life if it is used to control clinical signs. Adverse reactions (i.e., anorexia, depression, vomiting, diarrhea, icterus) may necessitate stopping the drug or reducing the dosage. If an overdose is suspected of causing acute illness or collapse, administer glucocorticoids. Rechecks (including ACTH-stimulation) are recommended every 3 to 6 months.

SURGICAL TREATMENT

The overall health of the animal, presence of unresectable metastases, and apparent invasiveness of the tumor (i.e., evidence of caudal cava thrombosis on CT or ultrasound) should be considered when determining the appropriateness of surgery for adrenal tumors. Prolonged survival has been reported in dogs with invasive, malignant tumors that required caudal caval venotomy; however, some owners elect euthanasia if complete resection is not possible or guaranteed. Long-term survival (i.e., greater than 1 year) may be possible, even in dogs with widespread metastatic lesions. If

---

TABLE 19-4

ACTH-Stimulation Test in Dogs

1. Obtain serum for pre-ACTH.
2. Administer 0.25 mg synthetic ACTH (Cortosyn)/dog IV.
3. Obtain serum 1 hr post-ACTH administration.

TABLE 19-5

Patterns of ACTH-Stimulation Tests (Post-ACTH Cortisol)*

>24 µg/dl—strongly suggestive of hyperadrenocorticism
19-24 µg/dl—suggestive of hyperadrenocorticism
8-18 µg/dl—normal
<8 µg/dl—suggestive of iatrogenic Cushing's

*There may be substantial variation between laboratories.
To convert µg/dl to nmol/L, multiply µg/dl × 27.59.

TABLE 19-6

Mitotane (Lysodren) Treatment for Adrenal Tumors

- Administer 50-75 mg/kg/day for 14 days.
- If needed, increase dose by another 50 mg/kg for another 14 days.
- Repeat this increment every 14 days until the disease is controlled or the animal does not tolerate this drug.

TABLE 19-7

Ketoconazole Treatment for Adrenal Tumors

1. Administer 5 mg/kg with food BID for 7 days.
2. Increase dose to 10 mg/kg BID for 7-14 days.
3. Perform ACTH-stimulation test 2 to 4 hrs after giving ketoconazole dose.
4. If there is a lack of adrenocortical response to ACTH and clinical improvement without causing illness, continue same dosage.
5. If there is a response to ACTH or no clinical improvement, increase the dosage to 15 mg/kg BID.

the tumor appears invasive, a midline abdominal approach is preferred, to allow evaluation of the caudal cava and other abdominal structures. Thrombus removal may require that the midline incision be extended into the caudal thorax via a caudal median sternotomy approach (see p. 654). Small tumors, or those that do not appear invasive, may be removed from a paralumbar approach (see p. 403).

☞ N O T E • Preoperative MRI helps determine whether caudal vena caval invasion is present.

Preoperative Management

Renal function should be determined before surgery, in case ipsilateral nephrectomy is necessary. Electrolyte or acid-base abnormalities, hyperglycemia, and hypertension should be corrected before surgery, if possible. Fluid therapy should be initiated before anesthetic induction. Animals with hyperadrenocorticism are at increased risk to develop pulmonary thromboembolism postoperatively. If hypercoagulopathies are suspected, preventative low-dose heparin therapy may be indicated (Table 19-8). Perioperative antibiotics should be administered and continued postoperatively in hyperadrenal animals. Particular emphasis should be placed on preoperative examination of the cardiovascular system for evidence of arrhythmias or congestive heart failure in animals with pheochromocytomas.

Anesthesia

Anesthetic complications are common during adrenalectomy for pheochromocytomas, and wide fluctuations in heart rate and blood pressure are frequent. Cardiac rhythm, arterial blood pressure, and pulse oximetry should be closely monitored. Treatment for several days before surgery with an α-adrenergic blocker (i.e., phenoxybenzamine; Table 19-9) is recommended. The dose of phenoxybenzamine is increased until blood pressure is within the normal range. Heart rate can be controlled with a β-blocker (i.e., propranolol, esmolol); however, it should not be initiated until adequate α-blockade is established (i.e., normal blood pressure). Intraoperative β-blockage with esmolol (see Table 19-9) is preferred because of its short half-life. Cardiac arrhythmias may be treated with lidocaine (Table 19-10). Hypertension may result from tumor manipulation and can be minimized by isolating the tumor's blood supply before manipulating the tumor. Hypertension may be treated with phentolamine given as an IV bolus (see Table 19-9). Sodium nitroprusside may also be infused for maintenance of blood pressure. Hypotension frequently occurs after tumor removal, and high doses of crystalloids may be necessary to maintain perfusion. If hypotension persists, dobutamine should be given. These tumors tend to be highly vascular, and significant intraoperative hemorrhage may require blood transfusions (particularly if caudal caval venotomy is performed to remove a thrombus).

Atropine, xylazine, and ketamine should be avoided in patients with suspected pheochromocytomas. Atropine potentiates the chronotropic effects of epinephrine and lowers

TABLE 19-8

Heparin Therapy for DIC

Heparin

50-100 U/kg SC, BID

Heparin-Activated Plasma

(Incubate 5-10 U heparin/kg body weight with 1 U fresh plasma for 30 min) give 10 ml/kg IV

TABLE 19-9

Drugs Used During Perioperative Management of Animals with Pheochromocytomas

Phenoxybenzamine (Dibenzyline)

0.2-0.4 mg/kg PO, BID

Esmolol (Brevibloc)

0.05-0.1 mg/kg slow IV boluses every 5 min to total cumulative dose of 0.5 mg/kg or 50-200 μg/kg/min constant rate infusion

Phentolamine (Regitine)

0.02-0.1 mg/kg IV

Sodium Nitroprusside (Nipride)

0.5-5 μg/kg/min IV

TABLE 19-10

Lidocaine Administration

Give IV (2 mg/kg bolus, up to 8 mg/kg total dose) to determine responsiveness to this drug. If the arrhythmias decrease or stop, lidocaine should be given by a continuous intravenous infusion of 50-75 μg/kg/min (for 50 μg/kg/min, place 500 mg lidocaine in 500 ml of fluids and administer at maintenance rate [66 ml/kg/day])

its arrhythmogenic threshold. Xylazine (an α$_2$ agonist) may cause transient hypertension followed by hypotension, may increase the sensitivity of the myocardium to catecholamines, and may potentiate cardiac arrhythmias. Ketamine increases circulating catecholamine levels, heart rate, and blood pressure, and should be avoided. Isoflurane is the inhalation agent of choice because it does not sensitize the myocardium to epinephrine-induced arrhythmias.

Surgical Anatomy

See p. 402 for the discussion of the surgical anatomy of the adrenal gland.

Positioning

The animal is positioned in either dorsal recumbency or lateral recumbency with the affected side up, depending on the operative approach chosen. With large or invasive tumors, a generous area should be clipped and prepped for surgery, to allow a caudal thoracotomy to be performed if necessary.

SURGICAL TECHNIQUE

Perform an adrenalectomy as described on pp. 403 and 404 via either a midline abdominal or a paralumbar approach. Concurrent nephrectomy may be necessary in some patients with invasive tumors. Surgical resection of adrenal tumors should be aggressive, to ensure complete tumor removal. En bloc resection should be performed, if possible, to avoid leaving small fragments of neoplastic tissue. The vascular supply to pheochromocytomas should be isolated before tumor manipulation, to decrease catecholamine release or to help prevent shedding of tumor cells. Exploration of the entire abdomen should be performed, with special attention paid to the bladder, pelvic canal, kidney, aorta, and near the junction of the caudal mesenteric artery, where extraadrenal neoplasia is reported to occur.

SUTURE MATERIALS/SPECIAL INSTRUMENTS

Delayed wound healing may occur in any debilitated animal (see comments on p. 405). Self-retaining retractors (e.g., Balfour abdominal retractors) and malleable retractors are useful to improve visualization of the adrenal glands. With vascular tumors, electrocautery and hemoclips allow hemostasis to be obtained more easily than does suture ligation of vessels.

POSTOPERATIVE CARE AND ASSESSMENT

Animals with hyperadrenocorticism often develop hypoadrenocorticism postoperatively as a result of atrophy of the contralateral gland. These animals require glucocorticoid therapy postoperatively (see discussion of postoperative care on p. 404). If hyperadrenocorticism continues postoperatively, therapy with mitotane should be considered. Fluid therapy should be continued until the animal is able to maintain hydration. Blood pressure and heart rate and rhythm should be carefully monitored postoperatively. Blood transfusions may be required intraoperatively or postoperatively in some patients. Dogs should be reevaluated periodically for tumor recurrence.

PROGNOSIS

Prolonged survivals (1 to 2 years) have been reported in dogs with invasive, metastatic pheochromocytomas after aggressive surgical resection (Gilson, Withrow, Orton, 1994). Prognosis for dogs with adrenocortical carcinomas depends on the tumor's size and invasiveness, but generally the prognosis is poor. In one study of 14 dogs with adrenocortical carcinomas, only 3 were alive at 6 months (Scavelli, Peterson, Matthiesen, 1987). In a more recent study of 36 dogs with adrenocortical tumors (presumably both adenomas and carcinomas), 10 of 18 dogs that were discharged from the hospital died from unrelated causes between 6 and 49 months (mean, 22 months) and the remaining 8 dogs

were alive at 3 to 48 months after surgery (mean, 16 months) (Van Sluijs and Sjollema, 1992).

☞ **N O T E ·** Warn owners that animals with pheochromocytomas may die suddenly as a result of arrhythmias and hypertension.

References

Bouayad H et al: Pheochromocytoma in dogs: 13 cases (1980–1985), *J Am Vet Med Assoc* 191:1610, 1987.

Gilson SD, Withrow SJ, Orton EC: Surgical treatment of pheochromocytoma: technique, complications, and results in 6 dogs, *Vet Surg* 23:195, 1994.

Reusch CE, Feldman EC: Canine hyperadrenocorticism due to adrenocortical neoplasia, *J Vet Int Med* 5:3, 1991.

Scavelli TD, Peterson ME, Matthiesen DT: Results of surgical treatment for hyperadrenocorticism caused by adrenocortical neoplasia in the dog: 25 cases (1980–1984). *J Am Vet Med Assoc* 189:1360, 1986.

Van Sluijs FJ, Sjollema BE: Adrenalectomy in 36 dogs and 2 cats with hyperadrenocorticism, *Tijdschrift voor Diergeneeskunde* 117:29S, 1992.

Suggested Reading

Ford SL, Feldman EC, Nelson RW: Hyperadrenocorticism caused by bilateral adrenocortical neoplasia in dogs: four cases (1983–1988), *J Am Vet Med Assoc* 202:789, 1993.

Kipperman BS et al: Pituitary tumor size, neurologic signs, and relation to endocrine test results in dogs with pituitary-dependent hyperadrenocorticism: 43 cases (1980–1990), *J Am Vet Med Assoc* 201:762, 1992.

Moore MP, Robinette JD: Cecal perforation and adrenocortical adenoma in a dog, *J Am Vet Med Assoc* 191:87, 1987.

Patnaik AK et al: Extra-adrenal pheochromocytoma (paraganglioma) in a cat, *J Am Vet Med Assoc* 197:104, 1990.

Penninck DG, Feldman EC, Nylant TG: Radiographic features of canine hyperadrenocorticism caused by autonomously functioning adrenocortical tumors: 23 cases (1978–1986), *J Am Vet Med Assoc* 192:1604, 1988.

Poffenbarger EM, Feeney DA, Hayden DW: Gray-scale ultrasonography in the diagnosis of adrenal neoplasia in dogs: six cases (1981–1986), *J Am Vet Med Assoc* 192:228, 1988.

Voorhout et al: Nephrotomography and ultrasonography for the localization of hyperfunctioning adrenocortical tumors in dogs, *Am J Vet Res* 51:1280, 1990.

Voorhout G, Stolp R, Rijnberg A, et al: Assessment of survey radiography and comparison with x-ray computed tomography for detection of hyperfunctioning adrenocortical tumors in dogs, *J Am Vet Med Assoc* 196:1799, 1990.

PITUITARY NEOPLASIA

DEFINITIONS

Pituitary tumors arise from the hypophysis in the sella turcica.

SYNONYMS

For pituitary—**hypophysis**

GENERAL CONSIDERATIONS AND CLINICALLY RELEVANT PATHOPHYSIOLOGY

Pituitary tumors are the most common cause of canine hyperadrenocorticism. They may be functional (60%) or nonfunctional (40%). Clinical signs are usually due to hypersecretion of ACTH from tumors in the pars distalis (adenohypophysis) or pars intermedia. Large pituitary tumors often grow dorsally into the brain because the diaphragm of the sella is incomplete. Thus nonfunctional tumors may cause clinical signs by impinging on adjacent brain tissue (i.e., optic chiasm, hypothalamus, thalamus, infundibular recess, and third ventricle). Tumor size and development of neurologic signs do not always correlate. Adenomas and carcinomas may arise from pituitary tissue; however, carcinomas represent less than 3% of all pituitary neoplasms. Adenomas are usually classified as *microadenomas* (less than 1 cm in diameter) or *macroadenomas* (greater than 1 cm in diameter). Microadenomas are most common, accounting for nearly 70% of all pituitary tumors.

DIAGNOSIS
Clinical Presentation

Signalment. Poodles, dachshunds, and boxers may be predisposed to pituitary-dependent hyperadrenocorticism. Middle-aged and older dogs are most commonly affected; however, young dogs may occasionally develop pituitary tumors.

History. Most dogs present for evaluation of typical signs of hyperadrenocorticism (i.e., polyuria, polydipsia, polyphagia, abdominal enlargement, endocrine alopecia, muscle wasting, weakness, lethargy, panting, and/or hyperpigmentation). Concurrent neurologic signs may also be noted (seizures, visual deficits, ataxia, incoordination, facial hemiplegia, head tilt, somnolence, compulsive walking, depression). The diversity of neurologic signs in dogs with pituitary tumors is probably a result of impingement on various parts of the brain responsible for differing functions. Mental depression and stupor were reported as the most common abnormalities in two studies describing 19 dogs with large pituitary tumors. In animals with nonfunctional macroadenomas or carcinomas, neurologic signs may be the only presenting abnormality.

☞ **N O T E ·** Large, nonfunctional pituitary tumors may cause neurologic abnormalities. Functional tumors usually cause hyperadrenocorticism but may also cause neurologic signs.

Physical Examination Findings

Typical signs of hyperadrenocorticism (see above) are expected in animals with functional pituitary tumors. Neurologic abnormalities (e.g., papillary edema, ataxia, incoordination) occasionally occur.

Radiography/Imaging

Diagnosis of pituitary neoplasia is best made with computed tomography (CT) or magnetic resonance imaging. Pituitary adenomas and carcinomas cannot be differentiated with CT; however, differentiation of animals with microadenomas, which might benefit from hypophysectomy, and those with macroadenomas (in which surgical therapy is seldom indicated) is possible. Bilateral adrenal enlargement, diagnosed by ultrasonography, is usually indicative of pituitary-dependent hyperadrenocorticism.

Laboratory Findings

Laboratory abnormalities are generally consistent with hyperadrenocorticism. Small, nonfunctional pituitary tumors seldom cause laboratory abnormalities. Large tumors may cause increased intracranial pressure, measured on a CSF tap. See p. 407 for differentiation of pituitary-dependent hyperadrenocorticism from adrenocortical neoplasia.

DIFFERENTIAL DIAGNOSIS

Animals with Cushing's syndrome must be differentiated from those with iatrogenic hyperadrenocorticism or adrenocortical neoplasms (see p. 407). Once a diagnosis of pituitary dysfunction has been made, pituitary neoplasms must be differentiated from other lesions that may arise in the pituitary (i.e., cysts, abscesses, craniopharyngiomas); however, such lesions are extremely rare.

MEDICAL MANAGEMENT

Clinical signs of hyperadrenocorticism may be treated with mitotane or ketoconazole (see p. 408). External-beam radiation therapy appears to be an effective treatment for large pituitary tumors, when combined with concurrent adrenal-suppressive treatment (mitotane or ketoconazole). Long-term survival (mean, 740 plus or minus 372 days) was reported in one study with radiation therapy (Dow et al, 1990).

SURGICAL TREATMENT

Hypophysectomy can be performed in animals with pituitary microadenomas and functional adenohypophyseal hyperplasia (rare); however, it is seldom performed by veterinary surgeons. Advocates of this procedure suggest that the majority of dogs with pituitary-dependent hyperadrenocorticism tumors are surgical candidates for hypophysectomy and that this technique is preferable to long-term medical management. However, if concurrent neurologic signs are present, or tumor has extended intracranially or transsphenoidally, hypophysectomy is not indicated. Hypophysectomy should not be considered in animals intended for breeding purposes because it renders them infertile. There are no clinical or experimental data suggesting that hypophysectomy is safe and effective in cats. Because there are no reliable anatomic landmarks for hypophysectomy, radiographic markers, combined with a cranial sinus venogram, are necessary to identify the pituitary location in some animals. Placement of the endotracheal tube via a tracheotomy and use of an operating microscope are recommended by some authors.

☞ **N O T E** • Hypophysectomy should be performed only by surgeons familiar with the regional anatomy and technique.

Preoperative Management

If surgery is considered for a pituitary neoplasm, extensive preoperative workup is indicated to confirm and localize the lesion and help define landmarks for surgery. Catheterization of the angularis oculi vein preoperatively has been recommended to help identify landmarks. Radiographic markers are placed on the sphenoid bone in conjunction with venous sinus angiography (Niebauer, 1993). Animals with hyperadrenocorticism are at increased risk to develop postoperative infections because of the high levels of circulating glucocorticoids. Perioperative prophylactic antibiotics are recommended. See p. 401 for additional comments on the preoperative management of animals with hyperadrenocorticism.

Anesthesia

Most animals with pituitary tumors do not require special anesthetic consideration; however, patients that have large masses increasing intracranial pressures need special precautions. Fluid therapy should be restricted to the volume required to maintain adequate circulation. Isoflurane interferes with autoregulation of cerebral blood flow less than does halothane, and is the inhalant of choice. Although most injectable anesthetics decrease cerebral metabolic oxygen requirements, cerebral blood flow, and intracranial pressure, ketamine does not. Its use should be avoided in patients with intracranial masses and other conditions in which increased intracranial pressures may occur as a result of surgery. Patients with increased intracranial pressures should be hyperventilated during surgery.

Surgical Anatomy

The pituitary is a small appendage of the diencephalon (Fig. 19-6). It occupies a shallow, oval recess in the basisphenoid bone called the *sella turcica*. Pituitary size varies greatly among breeds of dogs and within the same breed, but it is usually approximately 1 cm in length. The pituitary is composed of the adenohypophysis and neurohypophysis. The former is further subdivided into the pars proximalis, pars intermedia, and pars distalis. The arterial supply of the pituitary arises from the internal carotid arteries and caudal communicating arteries.

Positioning

Position the animal in dorsal recumbency, with the neck flexed and the hard palate at 30 degrees to the horizontal surface of the table (Fig. 19-7). Open the mouth maximally and secure the jaw with tape. The lower jaw should be approximately 80 degrees to the table surface. Retract the tongue against the lower jaw with tongue forceps. Flush the oral cavity and wipe it with a sterile surgical sponge impregnated with 0.05% dilute chlorhexidine solution.

SURGICAL TECHNIQUE

Transsphenoidal, intracranial, and peripharyngeal approaches have been described for hypophysectomy. Only the transsphenoidal approach is described here. Bleeding can be excessive with this technique. Have bone wax handy to fill the burr hole.

Make a midline incision along the rostral two thirds of the soft palate, and retract the palate with Gelpi retractors. Use electrocautery to control hemorrhage. Make a midline incision in the nasopharyngeal mucoperiosteum, and subperiosteally elevate the mucoperiosteum to expose the caudal aspect of the presphenoid and rostral aspect of the basisphenoid bones. Identify a small vascular foramen on the midline of the rostral portion of the basisphenoid bone, 2 to 6 mm caudal to the suture line between the presphenoid and basisphenoid bones (Fig. 19-8, A). Use a 2- to 4-mm diameter egg-shaped drill to burr a hole centered on the vascular foramen. With the drill positioned 45 degrees to the horizontal plane, remove the

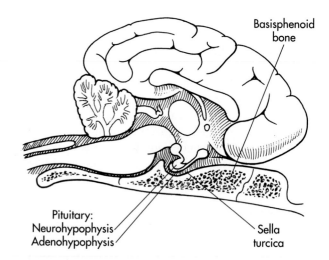

FIG. 19-6
Location of the pituitary gland.

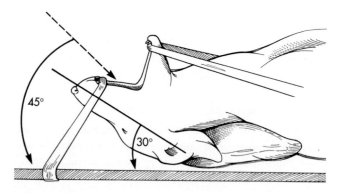

FIG. 19-7
For transsphenoidal hypophysectomy, position the animal in dorsal recumbency, with the neck flexed and the hard palate at 30 degrees to the horizontal surface of the table.

outer cortex of bone (Fig.19-8, B). Control bleeding with continuous suction, and occlude larger bleeders with bone wax. Partially remove the inner cortex with the drill; use a curette to excise the remaining portion of the cortex and expose the dura mater. Make a cruciate incision in the dura mater, but avoid the cavernous venous sinuses that lie lateral to the hypophysis. Break or loosen the dural attachments with a fine, blunt instrument. Apply traction to the hypophysis, using a 2- to 4-mm diameter suction tip. To prevent small tissue fragments from being lost in the suction, place a tissue filter as an interphase between the suction tip and tubing. Excise any visible remnant of the pituitary stalk. Fill the burr hole with bone wax or a muscle graft harvested from the soft palate incision. Appose the nasopharyngeal mucoperiosteum over the hole (do not suture). Close the soft palate incision with a two-layer simple interrupted pattern.

SUTURE MATERIALS/SPECIAL INSTRUMENTS

Delayed wound healing may occur in animals with hyperadrenocorticism; therefore incisions should be closed with strong, slowly absorbed or nonabsorbable suture material (e.g., polydioxanone, polyglyconate, polypropylene, or nylon). A drill with a 2- to 4-mm egg-shaped burr is required for hypophysectomy. Bone wax, a suction device, a tissue filter (approximately 150 μm), and a fine, blunt instrument (e.g., Steven's tenotomy hook) are also recommended.

POSTOPERATIVE CARE AND ASSESSMENT

After hypophysectomy, fluid therapy should be continued until the animal is able to maintain its hydration. Beginning immediately after surgery, desmopressin acetate (DDAVP) should be given for up to 2 weeks (Table 19-11). Corticosteroid therapy should be instituted before surgery and continued postoperatively. Thyroid hormone supplementation should be initiated after surgery and will need to be given for life. If bone wax was used to control hemorrhage, antibiotic therapy should be continued for 7 to 10 days. Nasal discharge and impaired swallowing may be observed for the first few days postoperatively. Persistence of these signs may indicate palate dehiscence.

COMPLICATIONS

Life-threatening complications of hypophysectomy include severe hemorrhage and nervous system abnormalities related to surgical damage of the hypothalamus or adjacent brain. Dehiscence of the palate incision may occur and re-

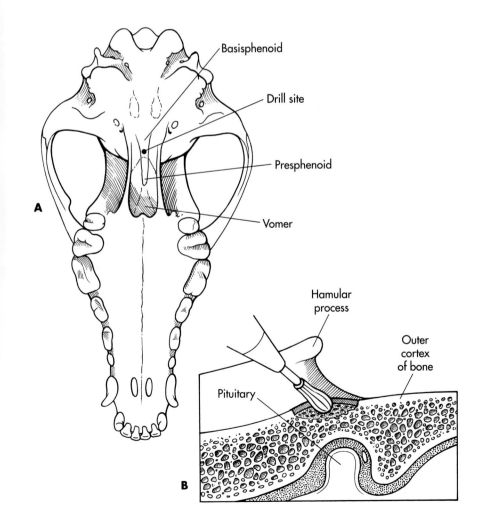

FIG. 19-8
A, For transsphenoidal hypophysectomy, identify a small vascular foramen on the midline of the rostral portion of the basisphenoid bone. **B,** With a drill positioned 45 degrees to the horizontal plane, remove the outer cortex of bone.

TABLE 19-11

Postoperative Drug Therapy Following Hypophysectomy

Desmopressin Acetate

2 µg/dog (2-4 drops of 100 µg/ml) intranasally or in conjunctiva SID to BID

Prednisone or Prednisolone

0.2 mg/kg SID

Thyroid Hormone (Soloxine, Thyrotabs, Synthroid)

22 µg/kg PO, BID

quire reoperation. Keratoconjunctivitis sicca due to development of iatrogenic damage of the pterygopalatine nerves has been reported uncommonly.

PROGNOSIS

Long-term survival is possible following hypophysectomy, radiation therapy plus chemotherapy, or chemotherapy alone in dogs with pituitary-dependent hyperadrenocorticism due to microadenomas. Long-term survival has also been reported in dogs with large, functional tumors, following radiation therapy.

References

Dow SW et al: Response of dogs with functional pituitary macroadenomas and macrocarcinomas to radiation, *J Small Anim Pract* 31:287, 1990.

Niebauer GW: Hypophysectomy. In Slatter D, ed: *Textbook of small animal surgery,* vol 2, Philadelphia, 1993, WB Saunders.

Suggested Reading

Lantz GC et al: Transsphenoidal hypophysectomy in the clinically normal dog, *Am J Vet Res* 49:1134, 1988.

Nelson RW, Ihle SL, Feldman EC: Pituitary macroadenomas and macroadenocarcinomas in dogs treated with mitotane for pituitary-dependent hyperadrenocorticism: 13 cases (1981–1986), *J Am Vet Med Assoc* 194:1612, 1989.

Surgery of the Pancreas

GENERAL PRINCIPLES AND TECHNIQUES

DEFINITIONS

Pancreatectomy is surgical removal of all or part of the pancreas. **Insulinoma** is a functional tumor of pancreatic β-islet cells; excessive insulin production commonly causes hypoglycemia in affected animals (see p. 421). **Zollinger-Ellison syndrome** is a condition caused by non–β-islet cell tumors, in which excess gastrin is secreted (see p. 425).

PREOPERATIVE CONCERNS

Animals with pancreatic inflammation often present with vomiting and may also have weight loss and debilitation; however, cats with pancreatitis do not show vomiting as reliably as do dogs. Vomiting animals require fluid therapy and correction of electrolyte and acid-base abnormalities before surgery. Diabetic animals (which may be prone to pancreatitis) are often anesthetized for elective and nonelective procedures. These animals should be carefully evaluated for overall metabolic status before surgery. Preoperative laboratory analysis includes CBC, serum biochemical panel (including fasting blood glucose, BUN, and creatinine), and urinalysis. Severe hyperglycemia (greater than 300 mg/dl) or ketoacidosis should be corrected before surgery with insulin administration, intravenous fluids, and electrolytes. Animals with pancreatic tumors may present with a wide variety of metabolic disorders.

ANESTHETIC CONSIDERATIONS

Many protocols have been described for anesthetic management of diabetic animals. Blood glucose concentrations ideally should be maintained between 100 and 300 mg/dl during surgery. Hypoglycemia may occur if animals are given their regular insulin dose and food is withheld before surgery; however, the stress of surgery usually results in hyperglycemia. Animals should be fed their normal diet the day before surgery, and their regular dose of insulin should be administered. Food should be withheld 12 hours before surgery or a small meal given after the morning insulin. Surgery should be performed in the morning. Blood glucose concentrations should be measured the morning of surgery. One to 2 hours before surgery, if the blood glucose concentration is between 150 and 300 mg/dl, the animal should be administered one half of its usual morning dose of insulin, subcutaneously. Blood glucose should be checked at induction and hourly thereafter. If the blood glucose level is low, administer 0.45% saline and 2.5% dextrose (5 ml/kg for the first hour and then 2.5 ml/kg thereafter). If blood glucose is normal, administer lactated Ringer's solution (at the same rate). Fluids should be changed to 5% dextrose and an additional small dose of regular insulin given if the blood glucose concentration is greater than 300 mg/dl.

☞ **N O T E ·** It is important to maintain excellent perfusion during surgery to help prevent postoperative pancreatitis.

Selected anesthetic protocols for animals with pancreatic disease that are stable are provided in Table 19-12. These animals may be premedicated with an anticholinergic and opioid, induced with thiobarbiturates or propofol, and maintained on either halothane or isoflurane inhalants. If the animal is shocky, dehydrated, or hypovolemic, anesthesia must be induced and maintained with greater care. Suggested anesthetic protocols are provided in Table 19-13. Alternatively, animals that are not vomiting may be induced with a mask or placed in a chamber, or they may be given thiopental or propofol at reduced dosages. If there are no contraindications to ketamine, reduced dosages of diazepam and ketamine may also be used in cats.

ANTIBIOTICS

The role of antibiotics in the treatment of noninfected pancreatic conditions (e.g., pancreatitis) is a matter of debate; however, they are often used to help prevent secondary infections in necrotic pancreatic and peripancreatic tissues. Prophylactic antibiotic therapy is indicated in animals undergoing pancreatic biopsy or partial pancreatectomy, to prevent pancreatic abscessation. Because pancreatic infections may be polymicrobial, broad-spectrum antimicrobial therapy (e.g., cefazolin; Table 19-14) is recommended. Antibiotic therapy should be based on results of culture and sensitivity of infected tissues in animals with pancreatic abscessation.

SURGICAL ANATOMY

The pancreas of dogs and cats is composed of a right and left limb and a small central body (Fig. 19-9). The right limb of the pancreas lies within the mesoduodenum and is closely associated with the duodenum, particularly at its cranial aspect. The dorsal aspect of the right pancreatic lobe is visualized by retracting the duodenum ventrally and toward the midline; the ventral aspect of the right pancreatic lobe is examined by retracting the duodenum laterally. The pancreatic body (angle) lies in the bend formed by the pylorus and duodenum. The left pancreatic lobe is viewed within the deep leaf of the greater omentum by retracting the stomach cranially and the transverse colon caudally.

☞ **N O T E** · Visualize the left lobe of the pancreas by looking in the deep leaf of the greater omentum, while retracting the stomach cranially.

The main blood supply to the left pancreatic lobe is via branches of the splenic artery; however, branches from the common hepatic and gastroduodenal arteries also supply portions of it. The main vessels of the right lobe of the pancreas are the pancreatic branches of the cranial and caudal pancreaticoduodenal arteries that anastomose in the gland. The cranial pancreaticoduodenal artery is a terminal branch of the hepatic artery; the caudal pancreaticoduodenal arises from the cranial mesenteric vessel. These vessels also provide branches that supply the duodenum. Because they are closely associated with the proximal portion of the right lobe of the pancreas, care must be used to avoid damaging these vessels during pancreatic surgery, or devitalization of the duodenum may occur.

☞ **N O T E** · The proximity and shared blood supply of the pancreas and duodenum make duodenal resection difficult, if pancreatic function is to be maintained.

The pancreas has both endocrine (insulin) and exocrine (digestive secretions) functions. Digestive secretions enter the duodenum via one of two ducts. These ducts may

---

TABLE 19-12

Selected Anesthetic Protocols for Use in Stable Dogs and Cats with Pancreatic Disease

Premedication

Give atropine (0.02-0.04 mg/kg SC or IM) or glycopyrrolate (0.005-0.011 mg/kg SC or IM) plus oxymorphone* (0.05-0.1 mg/kg SC or IM) or butorphanol (0.2-0.4 mg/kg SC or IM) or buprenorphine (5-15 μg/kg IM)

Induction

Thiopental (10-12 mg/kg IV) or propofol (4-6 mg/kg IV)

Maintenance

Isoflurane or halothane

*Use 0.05 mg/kg in cats.

TABLE 19-13

Selected Anesthetic Protocols for Use in Hypovolemic, Dehydrated, or Shocky Animals with Pancreatic Disease

Dogs
Induction

Oxymorphone (0.1 mg/kg IV) plus diazepam (0.2 mg/kg IV). Give in incremental dosages. Intubate if possible. If necessary, give etomidate (0.5-1.5 mg/kg IV). (See text also.)

Maintenance

Isoflurane

Cats
Premedication

Butorphanol (0.2-0.4 mg/kg SC or IM) or buprenorphine (5-15 μg/kg IM) or oxymorphone (0.05 mg/kg SC or IM)

Induction

Diazepam (0.2 mg/kg IV) followed by etomidate (0.5-1.5 mg/kg IV). (See text also.)

Maintenance

Isoflurane

TABLE 19-14

Prophylactic Antibiotic Therapy

Cefazolin (Ancel, Kefzol)

20 mg/kg IV at induction; repeat in 2-3 hr

---

communicate within the gland, or may cross each other. When the two ducts do not communicate, the pancreatic duct drains the right lobe and the accessory pancreatic duct drains the left lobe. The accessory pancreatic duct is the largest excretory pancreatic duct in dogs. It opens into the duodenum at the minor duodenal papilla. The smaller pancreatic duct is occasionally absent. The latter usually enters the duodenum on the major duodenal papilla, adjacent to the common bile duct. The pancreatic duct is the principal, and oftentimes only, duct in cats.

FIG. 19-9
Vascular supply to the pancreas.

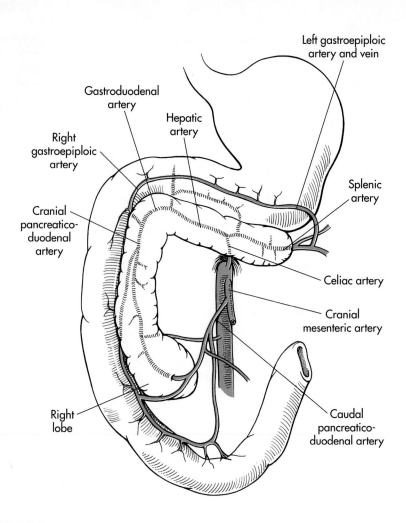

Left gastroepiploic
artery and vein

Gastroduodenal
artery

Hepatic
artery

Right
gastroepiploic
artery

Splenic
artery

Cranial
pancreatico-
duodenal
artery

Celiac artery

Cranial
mesenteric artery

Right
lobe

Caudal
pancreatico-
duodenal artery

☞ **N O T E** • Extrahepatic biliary obstruction may occur secondary to pancreatic swelling or masses because of impingement of the common bile duct as it enters the major duodenal papilla.

SURGICAL TECHNIQUES

After performing a ventral midline abdominal incision that extends from the xiphoid cartilage to caudal to the umbilicus, examine the pancreas using a combination of gentle palpation and visual examination. It must be handled gently to avoid causing pancreatitis. The free portion of the greater omentum is retracted cranially and covered with moist sponges. The omental leaf overlying the pancreas can be bluntly separated to allow direct visualization of the left pancreas. When neoplasia is suspected, lymph nodes that lie along the splenic vessels and portal vein and those at the hilus of the liver and head of the pancreas should be examined for evidence of metastasis.

☞ **N O T E** • Handle the pancreas gently to avoid causing pancreatitis!

Pancreatic biopsy and partial pancreatectomy are more frequently performed in dogs than in cats. However, because of the difficulty in diagnosing feline pancreatitis, biopsy may be more commonly indicated than presently used. Laparoscopic biopsy is possible in cats and seems to be well tolerated in this species. Pancreatic biopsy is occasionally performed in dogs to differentiate benign pancreatic conditions (e.g., pancreatitis, pancreatic fibrosis) from neoplastic disease. Although ultrasound-guided biopsies of large pancreatic lesions may be possible, exploratory laparotomy and direct visualization of pancreatic tissue are usually indicated. Partial pancreatectomy is indicated in animals with insulin-secreting or gastrin-secreting tumors or for pancreatic adenocarcinoma (see p. 427). Total pancreatectomy is infrequently performed in veterinary patients. Removal of the pancreas without duodenectomy requires that pancreatic tissue be bluntly dissected from the pancreaticoduodenal vessels without damaging branches supplying the duodenum. In animals with pancreatic disease this is difficult because of adhesions, fibrosis, and edema. Therefore total pancreatectomy is usually performed in conjunction with resection and anastomosis of the proximal duodenum, common bile duct ligation, and cholecystojejunostomy. These procedures are associated with high morbidity and mortality. Pancreatic drainage is indicated in some conditions (e.g., large abscesses or cysts) in which pancreatectomy is not feasible. A Penrose drain or double-lumen sump drain is sutured to the surrounding tissues with chromic gut suture and exteriorized lateral to the abdominal incision (see also p. 421).

☞ **N O T E** · Total pancreatectomy is difficult because it usually necessitates cholecystoenterostomy and removal of the duodenum.

Pancreatic Biopsy

If diffuse pancreatic disease is present, a biopsy is best obtained by removing a small portion of the caudal aspect of the right pancreatic limb (see the discussion of partial pancreatectomy below). Focal lesions near the extremity of the pancreas may be removed similarly. *For focal lesions within the pancreatic parenchyma, use a Tru-Cut or Vim-Silverman needle (see p. 463), or shave off a portion of the lesion with a scalpel to obtain a small sample of pancreatic tissue. Use care to avoid damaging adjacent blood vessels or pancreatic ducts.*

Partial Pancreatectomy

Focal lesions near the extremity of the pancreas can be removed by the suture fracture technique. *Incise the mesoduodenum or omentum on each side of the pancreas to be removed. Pass nonabsorbable suture material from one side of the pancreas to the other, through the incisions, so*

that the suture is just proximal to the lesion being excised. Tighten the suture and allow it to crush through the parenchyma, which ligates vessels and ducts (Fig. 19-10). Excise the specimen, distal to the ligature. Close any holes in the mesoduodenum with absorbable suture material.

Blunt separation of pancreatic lobules and ligation of ducts can be performed for lesions anywhere within the pancreas. With small lesions it may be possible to identify and preserve the pancreatic ducts. *Identify the lesion to be removed, and gently incise the mesoduodenum or omentum overlying it (Fig. 19-11, A). For lesions involving the pancreatic body or proximal aspect of the right lobe, bluntly dissect pancreatic tissue from the pancreaticoduodenal vessels, using gauze sponges. Ligate or cauterize small pancreatic vessels, but avoid damaging the pancreaticoduodenal vessels. Separate the affected lobules from adjoining tissue by blunt dissection, using sterile Q-tips or Halsted mosquito hemostats (Fig. 19-11, B). Identify blood vessels and ducts supplying the portion of pancreas to be removed and ligate them (Fig. 19-11, C). Excise the affected pancreatic tissue, and close any holes in the mesoduodenum.*

☞ **N O T E** · Ligate the pancreatic ducts with nonabsorbable suture.

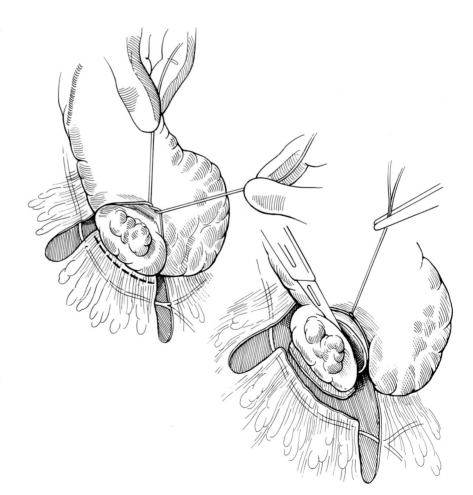

FIG. 19-10
Focal lesions near the extremity of the pancreas can be removed by the suture fracture technique. Incise the mesoduodenum or omentum *(dotted line)*, and pass nonabsorbable suture material from one side of the pancreas to the other, through the incisions. Tighten the suture, and allow it to crush through the parenchyma.

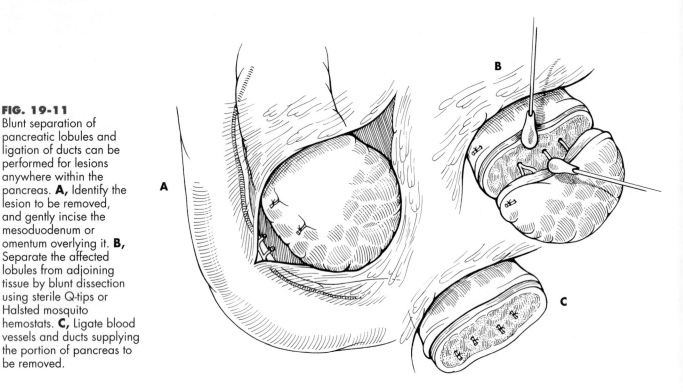

FIG. 19-11
Blunt separation of pancreatic lobules and ligation of ducts can be performed for lesions anywhere within the pancreas. **A,** Identify the lesion to be removed, and gently incise the mesoduodenum or omentum overlying it. **B,** Separate the affected lobules from adjoining tissue by blunt dissection using sterile Q-tips or Halsted mosquito hemostats. **C,** Ligate blood vessels and ducts supplying the portion of pancreas to be removed.

HEALING OF THE PANCREAS

The fibrous stroma of the pancreas allows healing to occur by protein synthesis, epithelialization, and fibrin polymerization. Pancreatic duct obstruction is seldom caused by wound contraction; rather, parenchymal edema or obstruction at the duodenal papilla is usually responsible. The main concern associated with pancreatic healing following surgery is related to the effect of healing on the flow and drainage of pancreatic secretions. As much as 80% of the pancreas can be removed without causing deleterious decreases in exocrine or endocrine function, if the duct to the remaining portion is left intact.

SUTURE MATERIAL/SPECIAL INSTRUMENTS

Duct ligation is performed with nonabsorbable suture material (i.e., polypropylene, nylon) in animals with inflammatory, aseptic, or neoplastic conditions. In septic conditions of the pancreas, monofilament absorbable suture material (e.g., polydioxanone, polyglyconate) may be used; braided suture material should be avoided. Chromic gut suture should be avoided because it may be rapidly digested by pancreatic enzymes.

POSTOPERATIVE CARE AND ASSESSMENT

Oral feedings should be delayed for 2 to 5 days after extensive pancreatic surgery and hydration and electrolytes maintained with intravenous fluid therapy. Feeding should be initiated first with water to observe whether vomiting occurs. If the animal does not vomit, small amounts of low-fat (less than 2% fat on a dry-matter basis), bland food (e.g., rice and defatted chicken) may be given. Animals with diffuse pancreatic dis-

TABLE 19-15
Octreotide Administration for Prevention of Pancreatitis
1-2 µg/kg SC before surgery

TABLE 19-16
Treatment of Exocrine Pancreatic Insufficiency
Pancrelipase (Festal II)
1 tablet before or with meals (do not crush or break tablet) **OR**
Viokase
1-2 tsp with food

ease or those that develop pancreatitis postoperatively may require total parenteral nutrition postoperatively. With septic conditions, broad-spectrum antibiotic therapy is generally continued for 10 to 14 days postoperatively.

COMPLICATIONS

The most common complication of pancreatic surgery is pancreatitis. This can be minimized with gentle tissue handling. Octreotide (Table 19-15) may be useful in preventing postoperative pancreatitis. Exocrine pancreatic insufficiency (EPI) may occur if pancreatic drainage is completely obstructed. EPI is treated with pancreatic supplements of commercial pancreatic extract (e.g., Pancrelipase; Table 19-16); feeding low-fat, highly digestible meals; and antibiotics for associated small intestine bacterial overgrowth. Endocrine pancreatic insufficiency (diabetes) may result when greater than 80% to 90% of pancreatic tissue is removed. Supplementation with insulin may be necessary.

SPECIAL AGE CONSIDERATIONS

Pancreatic disease is usually found in middle-aged or older animals. Special care needs to be taken to meet the nutritional and metabolic needs of geriatric patients, particularly when disease may have caused inappetence or chronic vomiting. Parenteral hyperalimentation may be necessary before and after surgery in these patients.

Suggested Reading

Allen SW, Cornelius LM, Mahaffey EA: A comparison of two methods of partial pancreatectomy in the dog, *Vet Surg* 18:274, 1989.

Hall JA, Macy DW, Husted PW: Acute canine pancreatitis, *Compend Contin Educ Pract Vet* 10:403, 1988.

Jacobs RM, Murtaugh RJ, DeHoff WD: Review of the clinicopathological findings of acute pancreatitis in the dog: use of an experimental model, *J Am Anim Hosp Assoc* 21:795, 1985.

Macky ED: Pancreatic disease of cats, *Compend Contin Educ Pract Vet* 15:589, 1993.

Schaer M: Acute pancreatitis in dogs, *Compend Contin Educ Pract Vet* 13:1769, 1991.

Simpson KW: Current concepts of the pathogenesis and pathophysiology of acute pancreatitis in the dog and cat, *Compend Contin Educ Pract Vet* 15:247, 1993.

Simpson KW et al: Circulating concentrations of trypsin-like immunoreactivity and activities of lipase and amylase after pancreatic duct ligation in dogs, *Am J Vet Res* 50:629, 1989.

SPECIFIC DISEASES

PANCREATIC ABSCESSES AND PSEUDOCYSTS

DEFINITIONS

Pancreatic abscesses are a collection of purulent material and necrotic tissue within, and extending from, the pancreatic parenchyma. **Pancreatic pseudocysts** are collections of pancreatic fluid enclosed within a wall of granulation tissue.

SYNONYMS

Pancreatic cyst

GENERAL CONSIDERATIONS AND CLINICALLY RELEVANT PATHOPHYSIOLOGY

Pancreatic abscesses (Fig. 19-12) are a pancreatic or peripancreatic collection of purulent, necrotic, and hemorrhagic tissues that usually occur as a consequence of acute pancreatitis. Pancreatic abscesses may also occur in human beings as a consequence of chronic ductal obstruction. Bacteria probably gain entrance to the pancreas from enteric reflux or hematogenously.

Pancreatic pseudocysts (Fig. 19-13) are only rarely diagnosed in small animals. They may be associated with recurrent bouts of pancreatitis or trauma. The fluid contained within the cysts is a combination of blood and pancreatic fluids and enzymes. They are not true cysts because the fluid is thought to leak from damaged pancreatic ducts and vessels, rather than being secreted by the lining of the cyst. Pancreatic pseudocysts may be incidental findings or may be associated with nonspecific abdominal signs (e.g., pain, vomiting).

☞ **N O T E** · Large pancreatic masses in symptomatic or asymptomatic animals may be pseudocysts. Don't recommend euthanasia based solely on the radiographic finding of a large abdominal mass.

DIAGNOSIS
Clinical Presentation

Signalment. Pancreatic abscesses generally arise following acute bouts of pancreatitis; therefore the signalment of animals presenting with pancreatic abscesses closely parallels

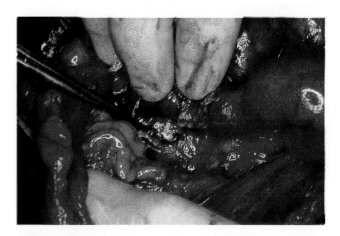

FIG. 19-12
Pancreatic abscess in a dog.

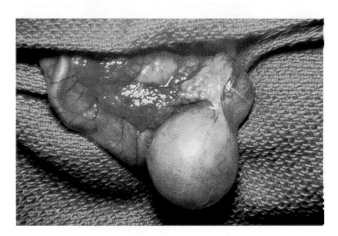

FIG. 19-13
Pancreatic pseudocyst. (Courtesy HP Hobson, Texas A&M University.)

that of animals diagnosed with acute pancreatitis (see p. 414). Most animals are middle-aged to older, and dogs are more commonly affected than cats.

History. Most animals with pancreatic abscesses have a previous history of acute onset of anorexia, depression, diarrhea, or vomiting, and most have previously been treated for gastroenteritis that was probably pancreatitis. Other clinical findings may include ataxia, anorexia, or pyrexia. Animals with pancreatic cysts may be asymptomatic or show vague signs of abdominal discomfort.

☞ **NOTE** · Animals with pancreatic abscesses often vomit far less than animals with "classic" pancreatitis.

Physical Examination Findings

Typical findings with pancreatic abscesses may include pain during abdominal palpation, depression, icterus, pyrexia, palpable cranial abdominal mass, or abdominal distention. However, the animal may have none of these findings. Some animals may be weak and reluctant to stand. Pyrexia is inconsistent.

Radiography/Ultrasonography

The most consistent finding with pancreatic abscesses on survey abdominal radiographs is an ill-defined increase in soft tissue density in the right cranial abdominal quadrant (Fig. 19-14). If peritonitis is present, a generalized increase in soft tissue density and loss of visceral contrast throughout the abdomen may be observed. Abdominal ultrasonography is more sensitive and usually reveals a mass in the area of the pancreas. Gallbladder and bile duct distention may also be noted. Gastric outflow obstruction is occasionally observed on contrast studies of the upper gastrointestinal tract. Ultrasound examination is the best tool to identify pancreatic pseudocysts; however, differentiation of pseudocysts from other fluid-filled masses is not possible without fluid evaluation. Percutaneous fine-needle aspiration of masses can be considered; however,

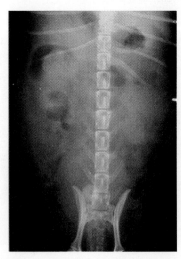

FIG. 19-14
Abdominal radiograph of the dog in Fig. 19-12 with a pancreatic abscess. Note the ill-defined increase in soft-tissue density in the right cranial abdominal quadrant.

the risk of abdominal contamination usually outweighs any advantages of a preoperative diagnosis.

☞ **NOTE** · Fine-needle aspiration of cavitary pancreatic masses is risky.

Laboratory Findings

Hematologic and serum biochemical findings with pancreatic abscesses are inconsistent but may include leukocytosis, neutrophilia with or without a left shift, lymphopenia, or monocytosis. Serum biochemical abnormalities may include hyperbilirubinemia and high serum alkaline phosphatase due to extrahepatic cholestasis, high alanine aminotransferase, hypocholesterolemia, hyponatremia, hypochloremia, and hypokalemia. Serum lipase and serum amylase activity is variable. Bilirubinuria is often present. Blood work in animals withpseudocysts may be consistent with pancreatitis or may be normal.

☞ **NOTE** · Lack of neutrophilia does not exclude pancreatic abscessation.

DIFFERENTIAL DIAGNOSIS

Pancreatic abscesses must be differentiated from other causes of vomiting and cranial abdominal pain (e.g., pancreatitis, gastric foreign bodies, intestinal foreign bodies, gastritis, cholecystitis, pancreatic neoplasia, gastrointestinal neoplasia). Ultrasound evaluation of the pancreas is the most useful test to differentiate these abnormalities preoperatively; however, exploratory surgery may be required to make a definitive diagnosis in some animals. Pancreatic pseudocysts must be differentiated from pancreatic abscesses or neoplasia, based on gross appearance, culture results, and histopathologic examination.

MEDICAL MANAGEMENT

Pancreatic abscesses are surgical diseases. The mortality rate in human beings with pancreatic abscesses is nearly 100% when medical therapy alone is used. With surgical treatment, mortality has been reduced to 14% to 67% (Stricker, Hunt, 1986). Similar studies have not been reported in dogs or cats. Small pancreatic pseudocysts may resolve spontaneously without therapy.

SURGICAL TREATMENT

Generalized peritonitis is present in some dogs with pancreatic abscesses. On opening the abdomen, a mass is observed originating from the pancreas in the cranial portion of the abdomen. The mass may be firm and fibrotic or friable. Multiple adhesions to omentum and adjacent loops of small or large intestine are frequently present. Adhesions may be present with pseudocysts, if the cyst has ruptured and reformed; however, fewer adhesions are expected than with pancreatic abscesses. Pseudocysts may be drained at surgery or by fine-needle aspiration. The former is associated with a lower rate of recurrence.

Preoperative Management

With pancreatic abscesses, medical management should be initiated before surgery. Fluid therapy should be initiated, based on results of serum biochemical analyses. Supplemental potassium chloride may be necessary if the animal is hypokalemic. A broad-spectrum antibiotic should be administered intravenously before surgery and continued for at least 10 to 14 days postoperatively.

Anesthesia

Refer to the discussion of the anesthetic management of animals with pancreatic disease on p. 414.

Surgical Anatomy

Refer to the discussion of the surgical anatomy of the pancreas on p. 415.

Positioning

The animal is positioned in dorsal recumbency, and the caudal thorax and entire abdomen are prepared for aseptic surgery.

SURGICAL TECHNIQUE
Pancreatic Abscesses

Perform a midline abdominal laparotomy that extends from the xiphoid cartilage caudally to distal to the umbilicus. Gently explore the abdomen. Locate the pancreatic mass and obtain cultures of infected tissues. Gently break down adhesions to the intestine and omentum. Try to preserve the pancreatic ducts, common bile ducts, and adjacent vascular structures during dissection. Debride necrotic or purulent areas of the pancreas using a combination of sharp and blunt dissection. Resect as much of the infected and necrotic pancreas as possible. If the mass is not resectable, debride it and place a Penrose drain(s) into the mass, and exteriorize it lateral to the abdominal incision. Determine common bile duct patency by gently expressing the gallbladder. If the common bile duct is not patent, catheterize the duct and try to obtain flow, or perform a cholecystoenterostomy (see p. 392). **Make sure you do not ligate the common bile duct.** *If generalized peritonitis is present, lavage the abdomen thoroughly with warmed, sterile saline or lactated Ringer's solution. The abdomen may be closed or left open for drainage (see p. 198).*

Pancreatic Pseudocysts

Explore the abdominal cavity as described above. Locate the pancreatic mass and obtain cultures of the cystic fluid. Gently break down adhesions, if present. Resect as much of the fibrous wall surrounding the pseudocyst as possible. If the mass is not resectable, aspirate the fluid. A Penrose can be placed; however, this will increase the risk of iatrogenic infection. Close the abdomen routinely.

SUTURE MATERIALS/SPECIAL INSTRUMENTS

Absorbable suture material should be used for the partial pancreatectomy in animals with pancreatic abscesses. Aerobic and anaerobic culture swabs should be available. Copious amounts of warmed fluids should be available for abdominal flushing; suction allows complete removal of instilled fluid and facilitates dilution of infected fluids in the abdominal cavity.

POSTOPERATIVE CARE AND ASSESSMENT

Antibiotic therapy should be continued, based on results of culture and sensitivity of abdominal fluid or infected pancreatic tissues. Fluid therapy should be continued until the animal is eating and drinking normally. If prolonged recovery is anticipated, or the animal is severely malnourished before surgery, needle-catheter jejunostomy or parenteral feeding should be initiated postoperatively. Potassium supplementation may be necessary until the animal is eating normally. Animals should be closely observed postoperatively for signs of continued infection (continued pyrexia, worsening or lack of improvement in CBC). **Repeat surgeries may be necessary in such animals.** Hypoproteinemia and hypoalbuminemia may be severe (particularly if open abdominal drainage is performed) and warrant plasma transfusions. Prolonged fever or sudden deterioration may indicate sepsis. Blood cultures are warranted if bacteremia is suspected. Pancreatitis is a potential complication of any surgery involving the pancreas (see p. 418).

☞ **N O T E** • Warn owners that repeat surgery may be necessary with pancreatic abscesses.

PROGNOSIS

The prognosis in animals with pancreatic abscesses is guarded. In one study of six dogs, three animals recovered and were discharged (Salisbury et al, 1988). Early recognition and aggressive therapy may improve the survival of animals with pancreatic abscesses. The prognosis for pancreatic pseudocysts is good. Many will resolve spontaneously.

References

Salisbury SK et al: Pancreatic abscess in dogs: six cases (1978–1986), *J Am Vet Med Assoc* 193:1104, 1988.
Stricker PD, Hunt DR: Surgical aspects of pancreatic abscess, *Br J Surg* 73:644, 1986.

Suggested Reading

Bellenger CR et al: Pancreatic pseudocyst in a dog, *Aust Vet Pract* 13:67, 1983.
Rutgers C, Herring DS, Orton EC: Pancreatic pseudocyst associated with acute pancreatitis in a dog: ultrasonographic diagnosis, *J Am Anim Hosp Assoc* 121:411, 1985.

INSULINOMAS

DEFINITIONS

Insulinomas are functional tumors of the β-cells of the islands of Langerhans that secrete insulin despite the presence of hypoglycemia.

SYNONYMS

Pancreatic β-cell tumors, **adenomas,** or **adenocarcinomas** of the pancreatic islets

GENERAL CONSIDERATIONS AND CLINICALLY RELEVANT PATHOPHYSIOLOGY

Insulinomas are pancreatic islet cell tumors that secrete excessive amounts of insulin, causing hypoglycemia. They are more commonly recognized in dogs than in cats. Unlike human beings, in whom up to 90% of insulinomas are benign, malignant tumors predominate in dogs. They are slow growing tumors that compress adjacent pancreatic parenchyma. They are usually sharply delineated and encapsulated, and, although most are malignant, surgical excision is often palliative, prolonging survival.

☞ **N O T E** • More than 90% of canine insulinomas are malignant.

DIAGNOSIS
Clinical Presentation

Signalment. These tumors generally occur in middle-aged to older dogs, with no sex predisposition. Medium- to large-breed dogs (e.g., Irish setters, German shepherds, Labrador retrievers, standard poodles, and boxers) appear to be more commonly affected.

History. Clinical signs are attributable to hypoglycemia and include muscle tremors, muscle weakness, ataxia, mental dullness, disorientation, collapse, and/or convulsions. Dogs may be easily agitated and may have intermittent periods of excitability and restlessness. These clinical signs suggest hypoglycemia of any cause, not just insulinoma. Owners may notice clinical signs for months before presenting the animals for evaluation. Clinical signs are often intermittent initially, but occur more commonly as the disease progresses. Owners often report that clinical signs diminish or resolve with feeding. Many animals are treated for seizures with anticonvulsant agents before the diagnosis is made.

☞ **N O T E** • Warn owners that chronic hypoglycemia may cause permanent neurologic abnormalities.

Physical Examination Findings

Physical examination findings may reveal a normal or ataxic animal, muscle weakness, mental dullness, or disorientation. Affected dogs do not usually have physical examination abnormalities between hypoglycemic episodes, a fact that may help differentiate insulinoma from other causes of hypoglycemia. Withholding food before and during the evaluation may precipitate seizures in affected animals. Neuronal demyelination and axonal degeneration may occur from chronic hypoglycemia. Although the cause is not known for certain, direct toxic effects of hypoglycemia on peripheral nerves or a paraneoplastic neuropathy has been postulated.

Signs of peripheral polyneuropathy (i.e., ataxia, weakness) may continue despite appropriate therapy.

Radiography/Ultrasonography

Thoracic and abdominal radiographs do not contribute to the diagnosis; however, the location of the tumor within the pancreas can sometimes be determined with ultrasound. Ultrasonography may also indicate metastasis to the liver and regional lymph nodes in some affected animals. Thoracic radiographs are indicated to look for metastasis, although pulmonary metastasis is rare.

Laboratory Findings

Tentative diagnosis of insulinoma is based on demonstration of Whipple's triad (Table 19-17). Fasting or nonfasting blood glucose concentrations are often less than 70 mg/dl. If blood glucose concentrations are initially within the normal range, most affected dogs can be made hypoglycemic by fasting for 12 to 24 hours. Blood glucose measurements should be determined every 2 to 3 hours in these animals, until hypoglycemia is detected.

Once hypoglycemia has been confirmed, serum insulin levels should be measured. If food has been withheld from the animal to induce hypoglycemia, serum insulin concentrations should be measured on the first hypoglycemic sample (i.e., less than 60 mg/dl). Normal fasting serum immunoreactive insulin concentrations range from 5 to 26 μU/ml, whereas insulin levels in affected animals often exceed 70 μU/ml. If insulin levels fall within the normal range, an amended insulin/glucose ratio can be determined; however, false positive results are possible (Table 19-18). Definitive diagnosis of insulinoma may require exploratory surgery.

DIFFERENTIAL DIAGNOSIS

Insulinomas should be considered a differential in any dog with persistent and progressive seizures. Once hypoglycemia has been verified, these tumors must be differentiated from other causes of hypoglycemia, including extrapancreatic neoplasms, hunting dog or puppy hypoglycemia, sepsis, hepatic failure, hypoadrenocorticism, and hypopituitarism. Laboratory error should be considered in animals that do not have clinical signs of hypoglycemia.

MEDICAL MANAGEMENT

Dogs with insulinomas should be fed frequent small meals. Three to six meals per day of a diet that is high in protein and complex carbohydrates, but low in refined sugar, reduces clinical signs. Exercise restriction may also help alleviate clinical signs. Glucocorticoid therapy (Table 19-19) may also help prevent hypoglycemia due to islet cell tumors by increasing hepatic glucose production and decreasing cellular glucose uptake. The lowest possible dose that controls hypoglycemia should be used, to avoid iatrogenic hyperadrenocorticism (e.g., polyphagia, polydipsia, bilateral symmetric alopecia, thin epidermis). If clinical signs of hyperadrenocorticism occur, glucocorticoid therapy may be decreased and alternate drugs used; however, hyperadreno-corticism may be preferable to hypoglycemia. Diazoxide (see Table 19-19) is an oral hyperglycemic agent that acts to inhibit pancreatic insulin secretion and glucose uptake by tissues. It is effective in raising blood glucose concentrations in some dogs with insulinomas; however, side effects (e.g., anorexia, vomiting, aplastic anemia, cataracts, bone marrow suppression, thrombocytopenia, anorexia, diarrhea, tachycardia, and fluid retention) may occur. Diazoxide should be used with caution in animals with hepatic dysfunction. If hypoglycemia is severe and unresponsive, intravenous 5% or 10% dextrose may be necessary to maintain blood glucose concentrations in the normal range until surgery can be performed. Streptozotocin has been used in human beings with insulinomas; however, this drug is nephrotoxic in dogs. Alloxan and a somatostatin analog (octreotide) have been used in a few dogs with insulinomas; however, there are too few data to recommend their use at this time. Despite previous reports of a beneficial effect of octreotide in a few dogs with insulinomas, a recent study reported no clinical improvement in two of three dogs and minimal benefit in the third dog when treated with this drug (Simpson et al, 1995).

NOTE • Streptozotocin is nephrotoxic in dogs.

TABLE 19-17

Whipple's Triad

- Clinical signs associated with hypoglycemia (usually neurologic abnormalities)
- Fasting blood glucose concentrations ≤ 40 mg/dl
- Relief of neurologic signs with feeding or glucose administration

---

TABLE 19-18

Amended Insulin Glucose Ratio (μU/mg)

$$\frac{\text{Serum insulin } (\mu U/ml \times 100)}{\text{Plasma glucose } (mg/dl) - 30^*}$$

*If the blood glucose is less than or equal to 30 mg/dl use 1 for the denominator.

TABLE 19-19

Oral Hyperglycemic Agents

Prednisone or Prednisolone

0.25 to 2 mg/kg BID

Diazoxide (Proglycem)

Start with 10 mg/kg divided BID with meals. May gradually increase to 60 mg/kg divided BID. Concurrent administration of hydrochlorothiazide may enhance effects of diazoxide.

SURGICAL TREATMENT
Preoperative Management

Fluid therapy with 5% glucose should be initiated 12 to 24 hours before surgery. Food is withheld 12 hours before surgery. Blood glucose concentrations should be measured immediately before surgery and additional glucose given if the concentration is less than 75 to 100 mg/dl.

Anesthesia

The goal of surgery is to maintain blood glucose concentrations greater than 75 to 100 mg/dl. Thiobarbiturates or etomidate may be used for anesthetic induction because they decrease cerebral glucose metabolism. After intubation, anesthesia should be maintained with isoflurane or halothane. Isoflurane decreases cerebral metabolic rate more than does halothane. Blood glucose concentrations should be monitored regularly during surgery (i.e., every 20 to 40 minutes) to avoid intraoperative hypoglycemia.

Surgical Anatomy

Refer to the discussion of the surgical anatomy of the pancreas on p. 415.

Positioning

The animal is positioned in dorsal recumbency and the caudoventral thorax and entire abdomen are prepared for aseptic surgery.

SURGICAL TECHNIQUE

Explore the cranial abdominal cavity thoroughly for evidence of neoplasia. Carefully and gently palpate the entire pancreas for evidence of tumor nodules. Most dogs have solitary nodules (Fig. 19-15). Tumors are located with equal frequency in the left and right lobes of the pancreas and in the body. Metastasis is noted in approximately 50% of cases at the time of surgery. Metastasis usually occurs to the regional lymph nodes and liver; however, duodenal, mesenteric, and omental metastasis may also occur. *Perform a partial pancreatectomy (see p. 417), removing tumor nodules*

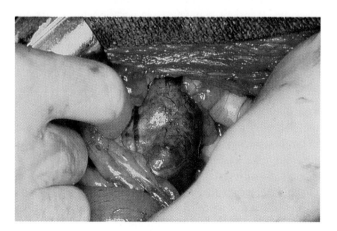

FIG. 19-15
Functional islet-cell adenocarcinoma in a dog.

with as wide a margin of normal tissue as possible. Submit excised lesions for histopathologic examination. Excise metastatic nodules, if possible.

If the tumor cannot be identified, intravenous methylene blue may be administered (Table 19-20). Methylene blue may stain neoplastic islet cells, helping to differentiate them from surrounding normal tissue. Maximal staining occurs within 30 minutes. A common side effect of methylene blue administration is hemolytic anemia due to Heinz body formation.

☞ **NOTE** • Fatal canine Heinz body anemia has been reported as resulting from the use of methylene blue.

SUTURE MATERIALS/SPECIAL INSTRUMENTS

Balfour abdominal retractors are useful for abdominal exploration. Sterile Q-tips or fine hemostats are useful for separating pancreatic tissues during partial pancreatectomy. Duct ligation is performed using 3-0 or 4-0 nonabsorbable suture material (see p. 418). Methylene blue administration may be used to help identify primary and metastatic nodules (see above).

POSTOPERATIVE CARE AND ASSESSMENT

Blood glucose concentrations should be measured frequently during the first 24 hours postoperatively. Pancreatitis may result from surgical manipulation of the pancreas. Small amounts of water may be administered the day following surgery, and if vomiting does not occur, feeding of small frequent meals may be initiated. Once the blood glucose concentration stabilizes at 75 to 100 mg/dl or greater, the glucose infusion can be discontinued (Table 19-21). If persistent hypoglycemia continues, medical therapy (glucocorticoids, diazoxide; see Table 19-19) should be initiated. Prolonged hypoglycemia may cause cerebral laminar necrosis. Neurologic signs (i.e., ataxia, bizarre behavior, coma, seizures) may persist in such animals despite normoglycemia. Transient hyperglycemia occasionally occurs and may persist for years after surgery. Insulin therapy may be indicated if blood glucose concentrations greater than 180 mg/dl persist for more than 3 to 5 days.

COMPLICATIONS

Complications of surgery in animals with insulinomas include persistent hypoglycemia, pancreatitis, diabetes mellitus, epilepsy, and diffuse polyneuropathy. The most common causes of postoperative hypoglycemia are unrecognized or unresectable metastases or multiple or incompletely resected primary tumors. Persistent hyperglycemia occurs in up to one third of dogs undergoing surgical removal of insulinomas and is thought to be due to suppression of normal β-cells by tumor insulin, resulting in loss of insulin production.

TABLE 19-20

Methylene Blue Administration

Dilute 3 mg/kg of 1% methylene blue in 250 ml of 0.9% sterile saline and give IV over 30-40 min.

TABLE 19-21

Postoperative Recommendations for Maintaining Glucose Concentrations

- Initially monitor blood glucose every 2-3 hrs.
- Continue providing glucose-containing fluids until the blood glucose is > 75 mg/dl.
- If hypoglycemia persists, administer steroids or diazoxide.

PROGNOSIS

The long-term survival of animals with insulinomas depends on the clinical stage of the tumor at the time of surgery. Nearly 50% of all dogs that do not have evidence of metastasis at the time of surgery will be normoglycemic for at least 1 year after partial pancreatectomy. Survival rates are similar for dogs with and without evidence of lymph node metastasis; however, hepatic metastasis leads to decreased survival times. Long-term disease-free periods can be obtained in some dogs with multiple surgeries to remove hepatic nodules as clinical signs occur. Young dogs may have a poorer prognosis than older dogs.

☞ **NOTE** • If metastasis is inapparent at surgery, survival of longer than 1 year may occur (even though cures are unlikely).

Reference

Simpson KW et al: Evaluation of the long-acting somatostatin analogue octreotide in the management of insulinoma in three dogs, *J Sm Anim Pract* 36:161, 1995.

Suggested Reading

Caywood DD et al: Pancreatic insulin-secreting neoplasms: clinical, diagnostic, and prognostic features in 73 dogs, *J Am Anim Hosp Assoc* 24:577, 1988.

Dunn JK et al: Insulin-secreting tumors of the canine pancreas: clinical and pathological features of 11 cases, *J Small Anim Pract* 34:325, 1993.

Fingeroth JM, Smeak DD: Intravenous methylene blue infusion for intraoperative identification of pancreatic islet-cell tumors in dogs. II: Clinical trials and results in four dogs, *J Am Anim Hosp Assoc* 24:175, 1988.

Fingeroth JM, Smeak DD, Jacobs RM: Intravenous methylene blue infusion for intraoperative identification of parathyroid gland and pancreatic islet-cell tumors in dogs. I: Experimental determination of dose-related staining efficacy and toxicity, *J Am Anim Hosp Assoc* 24:165, 1988.

Leifer CE, Peterson ME, Matus RE: Insulin-secreting tumor: diagnosis and medical and surgical management in 55 dogs, *J Am Vet Med Assoc* 188:60, 1986.

Leifer CE et al: Hypoglycemia associated with nonislet cell tumor in 13 dogs, *J Am Vet Med Assoc* 186:53, 1985.

McMillan FD, Barr B, Feldman EC: Functional pancreatic islet cell tumor in a cat, *J Am Anim Hosp Assoc* 21:741, 1985.

Mehlhaff CJ et al: Insulin-producing islet cell neoplasms: surgical considerations and general management in 3 dogs, *J Am Anim Hosp Assoc* 21:607, 1985.

Parker AJ, O'Brien D, Musselman EE: Diazoxide treatment of metastatic insulinoma in a dog, *J Am Anim Hosp Assoc* 18:315, 1982.

Wilson, JW, Caywood DD: Functional tumors of the pancreatic beta cells, *Compend Contin Educ Pract Vet* 3:458, 1981.

GASTRINOMAS

DEFINITIONS

Gastrinomas are tumors that secrete excessive gastrin. **Zollinger-Ellison syndrome** is a term used to describe a syndrome of gastric acid hypersecretion, gastrointestinal ulceration, and non–β-cell pancreatic tumors.

SYNONYMS

Non–β-cell tumors, gastrin-secreting tumors. The terms *gastrinoma* and *Zollinger-Ellison syndrome* are often used interchangeably; however, gastrinomas can arise in other parts of the alimentary tract. Zollinger-Ellison syndrome refers specifically to gastrinomas arising in the pancreas.

GENERAL CONSIDERATIONS AND CLINICALLY RELEVANT PATHOPHYSIOLOGY

Gastrinomas are rare tumors in dogs and cats. They are derived from ectopic amine precursor uptake decarboxylase (APUD) cells in the pancreas and produce an excess of the hormone gastrin. Gastrin is normally secreted by cells of the antral and duodenal mucosa, in response to antral distention and stimulation by amino acids. The excess gastrin causes hyperacidity, which can cause multiple ulcerations in the duodenal mucosa. Pancreatic gastrin-secreting tumors are usually locally invasive into adjacent parenchyma and frequently metastasize to regional lymph nodes and/or liver.

DIAGNOSIS
Clinical Presentation

Signalment. Dogs and cats may be affected. Too few cases have been reported to determine breed or sex predisposition.

History. Most animals present with clinical signs of anorexia, vomiting (which is occasionally blood-tinged), regurgitation, intermittent diarrhea, weight loss, and/or dehydration. Clinical signs may be present for several days or months before diagnosis. Animals may have been treated for gastric ulcers for months without response.

Physical Examination Findings

Clinical findings are nonspecific and may include dehydration, diarrhea, melena, hematemesis (coffee-ground appearance), steatorrhea, and/or weight loss. Abdominal pain is not a consistent finding. Perforation of a gastric ulcer may lead to signs of generalized peritonitis (see p. 193).

Radiography/Ultrasonography/Endoscopy

Radiographs and ultrasonography are nondiagnostic for gastrinomas because pancreatic masses are generally too small to be visualized. Endoscopy is the most useful technique for diagnosing esophagitis, gastric mucosal hypertrophy, and/or duodenal ulceration in dogs with suggestive clinical signs. Ulcers are most commonly located in the proximal duodenum.

Laboratory Findings

Nonspecific laboratory abnormalities noted in animals with gastrinomas include anemia, hypoproteinemia, and/or leukocytosis. Electrolyte and acid-base abnormalities may occur if vomiting has been severe (e.g., hypochloremic, hypokalemic, metabolic alkalosis or metabolic acidosis). Preoperative diagnosis of gastrinoma is based on demonstration of hypergastrinemia. Blood samples for serum gastrin analysis should be obtained after a 12-hour fast. Baseline serum gastrin levels are provided in Table 19-22. Serum gastrin levels of animals with Zollinger-Ellison syndrome may exceed 1000 pg/ml.

DIFFERENTIAL DIAGNOSIS

Gastrinomas must be differentiated from other causes of peptic ulceration, including nonsteroidal antiinflammatory drugs (NSAIDs), corticosteroids, gastric neoplasia, infiltrative disease, mast cell tumors, disseminated intravascular coagulation, hepatic disease, circulatory shock, and septic shock (see also p. 286). Other causes of hypergastrinemia include renal failure, gastric outflow obstruction, and current H_2-blocker therapy.

MEDICAL MANAGEMENT

Because of the aggressive biologic behavior of this malignant neoplasm, the prognosis for long-term cure is poor; however, aggressive medical management with omeprazole (Table 19-23) may be helpful. Proton-pump inhibitors (e.g., omeprazole) are the most potent inhibitors of gastric-acid secretion known. Other agents that may be used to help treat

TABLE 19-22
Basal Serum Gastrin Levels in Normal Dogs and Cats (pg/ml)*

Dogs
< 190

Cats
< 135

*To convert from pg/ml to ng/L, multiply pg/ml × 1.0.
NOTE: These values may vary between laboratories.

TABLE 19-23

Medical Therapy for Animals with Gastrinoma

Omeprazole (Prilosec)
0.7-1.5 mg/kg PO, SID to BID (preferred)

Sucralfate (Carafate)
0.5-1.0 g PO, TID to QID

Famotidine (Pepsid)
0.5 mg/kg PO, SID to BID

ulcers in dogs with gastrinomas include those that lessen gastric acidity and those that protect the gastric mucosa from damage (see Table 19-23). However, the effectiveness of these drugs in animals with gastrinomas is limited, and beneficial effects may be short-lived.

Sucralfate forms a protective coating over the ulcer or erosion. If bleeding is severe, a loading dose of 3 to 8 g of sucralfate may be given. Cimetidine, ranitidine, and famotidine are H$_2$ receptor blockers that decrease acid secretion; however, they tend to be much less effective than omeprazole (see Table 19-23).

SURGICAL TREATMENT

Exploratory laparotomy is often required to confirm the diagnosis. Surgical resection of the pancreatic mass may provide a cure if metastasis is not present. If metastasis is present, surgical debulking of the mass and removal of operable metastatic lesions may improve efficacy of medical therapy and prolong survival. The gastrointestinal tract should be closely inspected during surgery for evidence of ulcerations that may perforate. Any such lesions should be removed or have a serosal patch performed over them (see p. 301). Total gastrectomy has been recommended in animals that are unresponsive to medical therapy preoperatively; however, because of long-term complications (i.e., malnutrition, dysphagia, or bile reflux), this procedure is seldom performed.

Preoperative Management

If possible, the animal should be stabilized before surgery. Whole blood should be given if the animal is severely anemic (i.e., PCV less than 20%). Anemic animals should be oxygenated before induction. Electrolyte and acid-base abnormalities should be corrected and fluid therapy initiated before surgery.

Anesthesia

See p. 414 for anesthetic recommendations for animals undergoing pancreatic surgery.

Surgical Anatomy

Please refer to p. 415 for discussion of the surgical anatomy of the pancreas and p. 263 for discussion of the surgical anatomy of the stomach.

Positioning

The animal is placed in dorsal recumbency and the abdomen prepared for a ventral midline incision. The caudal thorax and entire ventral abdomen should be prepped for aseptic surgery.

SURGICAL TECHNIQUE

Perform a thorough abdominal exploration. Inspect the draining lymph nodes, liver, duodenum, and mesentery for evidence of metastasis. Inspect the entire pancreas for a mass lesion. Perform a partial pancreatectomy (see p. 417) and resect metastatic lesions that are accessible. Submit excised tissues for histopathologic examination.

SUTURE MATERIALS/SPECIAL INSTRUMENTS

If the animal is severely hypoproteinemic or anemic, wound healing may be delayed. In such cases, polydioxanone or polyglyconate suture (2-0 or 3-0) is preferred, to close gastrotomy and abdominal incisions (see p. 182). These sutures may also be used to perform a serosal patch.

POSTOPERATIVE CARE AND ASSESSMENT

Anemic animals will benefit from nasal oxygen postoperatively. Small amounts of water should be given the day following surgery and the patient observed for vomiting. If vomiting does not occur, small amounts of food can be given 24 hours postoperatively. The diet should be low-fat and contain moderate amounts of protein and carbohydrates to aid gastric emptying. Fluid therapy should be continued until the animal is eating and drinking. Medical therapy for ulcers should be continued until clinical signs resolve. Long-term medical therapy may be necessary to control gastric hypersecretion as a result of hypergastrinemia, and to decrease the incidence and severity of ulcers.

PROGNOSIS

Because of the metastatic nature of this tumor, the long-term prognosis is generally guarded.

Suggested Reading

Feldman EC, Nelson RW: Gastrointestinal endocrinology. In Feldman EC, Nelson RW, eds: *Canine and feline endocrinology and reproduction,* ed 2, Philadelphia, 1996, WB Saunders.

Gabbert NH, et al: Serum immunoreactive gastrin concentration in the dog: basal and postprandial values measured by radioimmunoassay, *Am J Vet Res* 45:2351, 1984.

Happe RP, et al: Zollinger-Ellison syndrome in three dogs, *Vet Path* 17:177, 1980.

Jin G, Braasch JW, Rossi RL: Surgical management of gastrinoma, *Surg Clin North Am* 65:285, 1985.

Jones, BR: Peptic ulceration in a dog associated with an islet cell carcinoma of the pancreas and an elevated plasma gastrin level, *J Sm Animal Pract* 17:593, 1976.

Middleton DJ, Watson ADJ, Culvenor JE: Duodenal ulceration associated with gastrin-secreting pancreatic tumor in a cat, *J Am Vet Med Assoc* 183:461, 1983.

Williams DA: Exocrine pancreatic disease. In Ettinger SJ: *Textbook of veterinary internal medicine*, ed 3, Philadelphia, 1989, WB Saunders.

EXOCRINE PANCREATIC NEOPLASIA

DEFINITIONS

Exocrine pancreatic carcinomas are malignant tumors that arise from either acinar or ductular epithelial cells.

SYNONYMS

Pancreatic adenocarcinoma

GENERAL CONSIDERATIONS AND CLINICALLY RELEVANT PATHOPHYSIOLOGY

Exocrine pancreatic tumors are slightly more common than tumors of the pancreatic islet cells in dogs and cats. Pancreatic tumors are more common in human beings than in dogs and are associated with an extremely high mortality rate (approximately 90% within 1 year of diagnosis). Most pancreatic tumors are malignant (adenocarcinoma); they are aggressive tumors that invade locally and metastasize readily. The most common sites for metastasis are liver, lungs, peritoneum, and regional lymph nodes. Metastatic pancreatic carcinoma was diagnosed in one dog that presented for evaluation of diabetes insipidus. Benign pancreatic tumors (i.e., adenomas) are extremely rare.

DIAGNOSIS
Clinical Presentation

Signalment. Pancreatic adenocarcinomas may be slightly more common in cats than in dogs. They occur more commonly in older animals, and Airedale terriers and boxers have been reported to have higher risk for this tumor. A sex predisposition has not been proved in dogs; however, pancreatic carcinoma seems to be more common in males.

☞ **N O T E** · You cannot differentiate pancreatic adenocarcinoma from benign pancreatic disease on the basis of clinical signs.

History. Animals with pancreatic adenocarcinoma may present with vomiting, abdominal pain, anorexia, weight loss, lethargy, abdominal distention, and/or diarrhea. The history may be acute or chronic. Adenomas are usually incidental findings at surgery or at necropsy and are not associated with clinical signs.

Physical Examination Findings

Physical examination findings for exocrine pancreatic carcinoma may include abdominal pain on palpation and/or ascites (secondary to compression of the portal vein or other vessels or due to widespread abdominal metastasis). A palpable abdominal mass is present in some animals. In some animals the first clinical sign noted is icterus due to common bile duct obstruction.

Radiography/Ultrasonography

An ill-defined increase in soft tissue density in the right cranial abdominal quadrant may be noted on survey abdominal radiographs. If ascites is present, a loss of visceral contrast throughout the abdomen may be observed. Abdominal ultrasonography often reveals a mass in the area of the pancreas. Distention of the gallbladder and bile ducts may be noted if there is extrahepatic biliary tract obstruction. Gastric outflow obstruction may be observed on contrast studies of the upper gastrointestinal tract.

Laboratory Findings

Laboratory abnormalities have not been well defined in animals with exocrine pancreatic neoplasia. Abnormalities consistent with extrahepatic cholestasis (i.e., elevated alkaline phosphatase and hyperbilirubinemia) are often present. Mild leukocytosis, dehydration, and hemoconcentration may be present in some animals.

DIFFERENTIAL DIAGNOSIS

Exocrine pancreatic carcinoma must be differentiated from benign and metastatic pancreatic disease. Nodular pancreatic hyperplasia, a condition seen in older animals, is characterized by multiple small, white lesions that protrude minimally from the pancreatic surface. Adenomas are usually small masses that may contain cysts. These conditions are not associated with clinical signs. Pancreatic carcinomas are usually well advanced at the time of diagnosis, and it may be difficult to determine the site of origin of the neoplastic masses grossly.

MEDICAL MANAGEMENT

Although numerous modalities have been used in human beings in an attempt to improve the survival of patients with pancreatic adenocarcinoma, only those patients who have resectable lesions at the time of laparotomy have a fair prognosis. Chemotherapeutic agents have not prolonged the life of people or animals with this tumor.

SURGICAL TREATMENT

Surgical resection is the treatment of choice; however, most animals are presented with advanced disease and surgical resection is not possible.

Preoperative Management

The animal should be stabilized before surgery with intravenous fluids and correction of acid-base and electrolyte abnormalities.

Anesthesia

Refer to the discussion of anesthetic management of animals with pancreatic disease on p. 414

Surgical Anatomy

Surgical anatomy of the pancreas is described on p. 415.

Positioning

The animal is prepared for a ventral midline exploratory. The entire abdomen and caudal thorax should be prepared for aseptic surgery.

SURGICAL TECHNIQUE

Make an abdominal incision that extends from the xiphoid cartilage as far caudally as necessary to allow complete exploration of the abdominal cavity. After identifying the pancreatic mass, explore abdominal organs, peritoneum, and regional nodes for evidence of metastasis (Fig. 19-16). Euthanasia should be considered in animals with widespread metastasis. *Perform a partial pancreatectomy, if possible. Confirm the patency of the common bile duct before abdominal closure.*

SUTURE MATERIALS/SPECIAL INSTRUMENTS

A standard soft-tissue pack or general surgery pack is generally all that is required. Refer to p. 417 for requirements for partial pancreatectomy.

POSTOPERATIVE CARE AND ASSESSMENT

Animals presenting with pancreatic carcinomas are often debilitated and require special attention to ensure that their nutritional needs are met postoperatively. Enteral or parenteral hyperalimentation should be considered. See also p. 418 for postoperative care of patients with pancreatic disease.

PROGNOSIS

The prognosis is extremely poor for animals with pancreatic carcinomas. Most have widespread disease at the time of diagnosis, and many are euthanized at surgery. Survival of less than 3 months should be expected for most of the remaining animals.

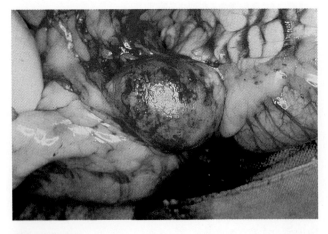

FIG. 19-16
Pancreatic carcinoma in a dog.

Suggested Reading

Anderson NV, Johnson KH: Pancreatic carcinoma in the dog, *J Am Vet Med Assoc* 150:286, 1967.

Bright JM: Pancreatic adenocarcinoma in a dog with maldigestion syndrome, *J Am Vet Med Assoc* 187:420, 1985.

Davenport DJ, Chew DJ, Johnson GC: Diabetes insipidus associated with metastatic pancreatic carcinoma in a dog, *J Am Vet Med Assoc* 189:204, 1986.

O'Brien TD et al: Pancreatic endocrine tumor in a cat: clinical, pathological, and immunohistochemical evaluation, *J Am Anim Hosp Assoc* 26:453, 1990.

Popp JA: Tumors of the liver, gall bladder, and pancreas. In Moulton JE: *Tumors in domestic animals*, ed 3, Berkeley, California, 1990, University of California Press.

Surgery of the Thyroid and Parathyroid Glands

GENERAL PRINCIPLES AND TECHNIQUES

DEFINITIONS

Thyroidectomy is removal of a thyroid gland. **Hypothyroidism** is deficient secretion of thyroxine. **Goitrous hypothyroidism** is caused by an abnormal iodine uptake or by defects in iodine uptake, organification, or thyroglobulin formation. **Nongoitrous hypothyroidism** is spontaneous hypothyroidism that may be immune-mediated (i.e., lymphocytic thyroiditis) or a result of idiopathic atrophy. **Hyperthyroidism** is excessive secretion of thyroxine. **Primary hyperparathyroidism** is excessive secretion of parathyroid hormone (PTH) by one or more abnormal parathyroid glands.

PREOPERATIVE CONCERNS

Hypothyroidism is common in dogs. It is usually due to thyroid dysfunction (primary hypothyroidism), although pituitary and hypothalamic causes are occasionally diagnosed. Secretion of thyroid hormones, triiodothyronine (T_3) and thyroxine (T_4), from the thyroid is controlled by a feedback mechanism between the hypothalamus, pituitary, and thyroid glands. Thyrotropin (thyroid-stimulating hormone; TSH) is produced in the pars distalis of the pituitary gland. It stimulates the synthesis and release of thyroglobulin (precursor of T_3 and T_4), T_3, and T_4. Release of thyrotropin is controlled by a neuropeptide produced in the hypothalamus, thyrotropin-releasing hormone (TRH). TRH secretion is inhibited by high circulating levels of glucocorticoids (e.g., hyperadrenocorticism) or thyroid hormone. Primary hypothyroidism is usually caused by idiopathic follicular atrophy or lymphocytic thyroiditis. Dogs with lymphocytic thyroiditis have circulating thyroglobulin antibodies that form antigen-antibody complexes within the gland, causing functional glandular tissue to be replaced by fibrous tissue. Hypothyroidism in cats is usually caused by surgical removal of the thyroid glands or damage to their blood supply during thyroidectomy (see p. 431); however, congenital hypothyroidism in a family of Abyssinian cats has been reported (Jones et al, 1992). The disease was inherited as an autosomal recessive trait and appeared to be the result of a defect of iodide organification. Congenital hypothyroidism has also been reported in dogs.

Hypothyroidism may be manifested as lethargy, exercise intolerance, weight gain, constipation, nonpruritic symmetric alopecia, peripheral neuropathies (i.e., laryngeal paralysis, vestibular deficits, megaesophagus), reproductive problems, cardiovascular changes (i.e., bradycardia, weak apex beat), and/or coagulopathies. Hypothyroidism may also result in decreased activity of factor VIII or VIII-related antigen, which may predispose to spontaneous bleeding or serious hemorrhage during surgery in animals with von Willebrand disease. The mean von Willebrand factor/antigen concentration in hypothyroid dogs has been found to be significantly decreased compared with that in euthyroid dogs. Thus it appears that reduced concentrations of plasma von Willebrand factor/antigen can be found in dogs, in association with congenital von Willebrand disease or with von Willebrand disease acquired through hypothyroidism. Animals with untreated hypothyroidism undergoing emergency procedures should be given oral 1-triiodothyronine (Table 19-24) 3 to 4 times a day or a single intravenous dose of 1-thyroxine. Elective procedures should be postponed until replacement therapy has been maintained for a minimum of 2 weeks. If excessive bleeding is noted despite thyroid supplementation, whole blood or plasma should be given (Table 19-25).

> ☞ **N O T E** • See p. 433 for preoperative concerns in animals with hyperthyroidism.

> ☞ **N O T E** • Hypothyroid animals may bleed excessively during surgery. Monitor hemostasis carefully!

Animals with hyperparathyroidism often present for abnormalities associated with hypercalcemia. Parathyroid hormone (PTH) is synthesized by chief cells of the parathyroid glands. PTH stimulates renal reabsorption of calcium, mobilizes calcium from bone, and promotes intestinal calcium reabsorption. PTH also controls hydroxylation of 25-hydroxyvitamin D_3 to 1,25 dihydroxyvitamin D_3 in the proximal renal tubules. 1,25-Dihydroxyvitamin D_3 regulates PTH secretion through a negative feedback mechanism. PTH is synthesized and secreted in response to decreases in circulating calcium levels. Functional parathyroid neoplasms (primary hyperparathyroidism; see p. 436) cause hypercalcemia through excessive secretion of PTH, which results in increased renal calcium reabsorption and increased renal phosphorus excretion, increased calcium and phosphorus release from bone, and increased intestinal absorption of calcium and phosphorus. Description of preoperative management of animals with functional parathyroid tumors is provided on p. 437. Primary hypoparathyroidism is a rare cause of hypocalcemia in dogs and cats. It has been reported to affect primarily middle-aged female dogs, secondary to lymphocytic parathyroiditis. Most affected animals have a history of neurologic (particularly seizures) or neuromuscular disease.

ANESTHETIC CONSIDERATIONS

Hypothyroidism may cause prolonged anesthetic recovery. Dosages of premedications and anesthetics may need to be decreased in moderately or severely affected animals. Blood pressure, cardiac function, and hematocrit should be closely monitored during anesthesia and in the early postoperative period. Blood should be available in the event that excessive bleeding occurs intraoperatively. Hypothermia may be of greater concern in these patients because of their inability to regulate body temperature normally; care should be taken to maintain body temperature intraoperatively and to rewarm these patients after surgery. See pp. 434 and 440 for anesthetic recommendations for animals undergoing thyroidectomy.

> ☞ **N O T E** • Hypothyroid animals may require reduced dosages of anesthetics.

ANTIBIOTICS

Guidelines for appropriate perioperative antibiotic use should be followed in hypothyroid patients (see Chapter 10). Prophylactic antibiotic therapy should be considered in animals that are debilitated, obese, and/or have concurrent hyperadrenocorticism.

TABLE 19-24

Treatment of Canine Hypothyroidism

Maintenance

Levothyroxine (Soloxine) 22 μg/kg PO, BID

Before surgery (if not on maintenance therapy)

1. Oral—liothyronine (T_3; Cytobin or Cytomel) 4 to 6 μg/kg PO, TID or QID **OR**
2. IV—L-thyroxine; 20-40 μg/kg (1 dose)

TABLE 19-25

Blood Transfusions

ml of Donor Blood Needed:

$$\text{recipient blood volume*} \times \frac{\text{desired PCV} - \text{actual patient PCV}}{\text{PCV of anticoagulated donor blood}}$$

*Total blood volume is estimated at 90 ml/kg for dogs and 70 ml/kg for cats.
NOTE: A rough estimate is that 2.2 ml of blood/kg of body weight will increase the recipient's PCV by 1%.

SURGICAL ANATOMY

The thyroid glands (or lobes) are dark red, elongated structures attached to the outer surface of the proximal portion of the trachea (Fig. 19-17). They are usually positioned laterally and slightly ventral to the fifth to eighth cartilage rings. The left lobe is usually located one to three tracheal rings caudal to the right lobe. In adult dogs they are approximately 5 cm in length and 1.5 cm wide; in cats they are 2.0 cm long and 0.3 cm wide. Occasionally the right and left lobes are connected by a ventral isthmus. Unlike most glandular organs, they can often be palpated when enlarged. Thyroid secretions (i.e., thyroxine, triiodothyronine, and calcitonin) exert a major effect on metabolism. Thyroid hormone is synthesized by follicular cells, stored intercellularly, and released into the circulation. In adults, it causes an increase in overall metabolic rate; in juveniles it stimulates growth. Calcitonin (formed by parafollicular C cells) lowers blood calcium by stimulating calcium uptake. Functional accessory thyroid tissue is common along the trachea, thoracic inlet, mediastinum, and thoracic portion of the descending aorta. Thyroid follicular cells arise from a midline outpouching known as the *thyroid diverticulum* on the ventral pharyngeal floor. The diverticulum's pharyngeal connections usually separate completely; however, a persistent connection that has functional glandular epithelium and cysts along its course may remain (thyroglossal duct).

The cranial and caudal thyroid arteries are the thyroid's principal blood supply. The cranial thyroid artery arises from the common carotid artery; the caudal thyroid artery typically arises from the brachiocephalic artery. The cranial and caudal thyroid arteries anastomose on the dorsal surface of the gland, where they send numerous vessels that supply the gland. The cranial thyroid artery in dogs usually sends a branch that supplies the external parathyroid gland before entering the thyroid parenchyma. In cats the branch that supplies the external parathyroid gland may arise from the cranial thyroid artery after it has perforated the capsule. Caudal thyroid arteries may not be present in cats. Innervation to the thyroid is via the thyroid nerve, which is formed from the cranial ganglion and cranial laryngeal nerve.

The parathyroid glands are small ellipsoid disks, usually occurring as four structurally independent glands in close association with the thyroid glands. The external parathyroid glands (so named because they lie outside the thyroid capsule) are normally found on the cranial dorsolateral surface of the respective thyroid. The internal parathyroid glands are embedded within the thyroid parenchyma, usually at the caudomedial pole.

SURGICAL TECHNIQUES

Thyroidectomy may be performed via an intracapsular or extracapsular approach. The extracapsular approach is used in dogs with malignant thyroid tumors (e.g., carcinomas; see p. 440), and no attempt is made to spare the ipsilateral parathyroid glands. Intracapsular and modified extracapsular approaches have been described for thyroidectomy in cats (see p. 434). These techniques spare the external parathyroid glands in an attempt to avoid complications associated with hypoparathyroidism. Modification of the original intracap-

FIG. 19-17
The thyroid glands are located lateral and slightly ventral to the fifth to eighth cartilage rings.

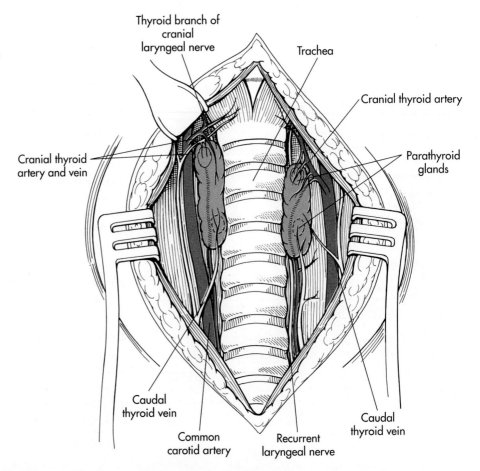

Thyroid branch of cranial laryngeal nerve

Trachea

Cranial thyroid artery

Parathyroid glands

Cranial thyroid artery and vein

Caudal thyroid vein

Caudal thyroid vein

Common carotid artery

Recurrent laryngeal nerve

sular approach (developed to decrease the incidence of post-thyroidectomy hyperthyroidism) involves excising the majority of the thyroid capsule once the thyroid tissue has been removed. Recurrence of hyperthyroidism in cats following thyroidectomy is thought to be the result of hypertrophy of small nests of functional thyroid tissue attached to the capsule and not removed.

HEALING OF THE THYROID AND PARATHYROID GLANDS

Abnormal thyroid tissue (i.e., adenomatous tissue) appears to regenerate and hypertrophy following incomplete feline thyroidectomy. Parathyroid tissue may be able to revascularize and regain function, even if it has been totally separated from its blood supply. Hence, many surgeons recommend implanting an inadvertently excised parathyroid gland into surrounding muscle, rather than discarding it. Ectopic parathyroid tissue may also hypertrophy following parathyroid gland removal, resulting in normal parathyroid function.

SUTURE MATERIALS/SPECIAL INSTRUMENTS

Delayed wound healing may occur in animals with hypothyroidism, and care should be used in closing surgical wounds in these patients. See p. 435 and p. 438 for a discussion of the instruments for thyroidectomy and parathyroidectomy, respectively.

POSTOPERATIVE CARE AND ASSESSMENT

Postoperative care and assessment of animals undergoing thyroidectomy for hyperthyroidism or neoplasia are given on p. 435 and p. 438, respectively.

Reference

Jones BR et al: Preliminary studies on congenital hypothyroidism in a family of Abyssinian cats, *Vet Rec* 131:145, 1992.

Suggested Reading

Avgeris S, Lothrop CD, McDonald TP: Plasma von Willebrand factor concentration and thyroid function in dogs, *J Am Vet Med Assoc* 196:921, 1990.

Jaggy A et al: Neurological manifestations of hypothyroidism: a retrospective study of 29 dogs, *J Vet Int Med* 8:328, 1994.

Matthiesen DT, Mullen HS: Problems and complications associated with endocrine surgery in the dog and cat, *Probl Vet Med* 2:627, 1990.

Medleau L et al: Congenital hypothyroidism in a dog, *J Am Anim Hosp Assoc* 21:341, 1985.

SPECIFIC DISEASES

FELINE HYPERTHYROIDISM

DEFINITIONS

Hyperthyroidism is a multisystemic disease that results from excessive production and secretion of thyroxine (T_4).

SYNONYMS

Goiter is an enlargement of the thyroid gland. **Graves' disease** describes an autoimmune disorder of human beings in which circulating autoantibodies stimulate thyroid tissue. It is the most common cause of human hyperthyroidism.

GENERAL CONSIDERATIONS AND CLINICALLY RELEVANT PATHOPHYSIOLOGY

Hyperthyroidism may occur in dogs or cats; however, it is much more common in cats, in whom it is generally associated with adenomatous hyperplasia of one or both thyroid glands. Approximately 80% of affected cats have bilateral thyroid gland involvement, although the enlargement is usually asymmetric. In approximately 5% of cats the thyroid mass is ectopic (i.e., at the thoracic inlet or in the cranial mediastinum). Feline hyperthyroidism secondary to malignant thyroid carcinomas is rare. The cause of feline hyperthyroidism is unknown. Suggested causes have included circulating thyroid-stimulating immunoglobulins, serum thyroid growth-stimulating immunoglobulins, dietary goitrogens, and viral causes. Excessive circulating thyroxine causes multisystemic organ dysfunction. Thyrotoxicosis increases the metabolic rate and sensitivity to catecholamines and causes significant cardiovascular and metabolic abnormalities. Up to 80% of affected cats may have thyrotoxic heart disease, and approximately 20% of these may have congestive heart failure.

Multifactorial mechanisms may cause neuromuscular and central nervous system dysfunction in some hyperthyroid cats. Neurologic signs associated with feline hyperthyroidism are listed in Table 19-26. T_4 and T_3 bind to receptor sites in the sarcoplasm that increase skeletal muscle heat production and mitochondrial oxygen consumption. The hyperthyroid state may reduce muscle contraction by uncoupling oxidative phosphorylation. Thyroid hormones may decrease the threshold for cerebral tissue activation, alter activity of some brain enzymes, and interact with catecholamines to alter the mental state of some affected animals. Abnormalities of the central nervous system may include hyperexcitability, irritability, aggression, seizures, confusion, and stupor.

TABLE 19-26

Neurologic Abnormalities in Hypokalemic, Hyperthyroid Cats

- Generalized weakness
- Neck ventroflexion
- Fatigue
- Muscle tremors
- Ataxia
- Incoordination
- Inability to jump
- Muscle atrophy
- Breathlessness
- Collapse

DIAGNOSIS
Clinical Presentation

Signalment. Hyperthyroidism generally affects cats older than 8 years of age (mean age, 13 years). There is no sex predisposition.

History. Most affected cats are presented because of weight loss despite a normal or voracious appetite, restlessness, and/or hyperactivity. Occasionally, a small mass is noted in the ventral cervical region. Vomiting, diarrhea, polyuria, polydipsia, aggression, and/or a rough hair coat may also occur. There is sometimes an increased frequency of defecation. Body temperature may be slightly elevated. Approximately 10% of hyperthyroid cats are depressed, lethargic, inappetent, and/or weak (i.e., "apathetic" hyperthyroidism).

Physical Examination Findings

A palpable cervical mass is present in most affected cats. The weight of the enlarged gland often causes it to gravitate ventrally, because the thyroid is loosely attached to tracheal fascia. Occasionally, the gland may descend into the thoracic inlet, where it can no longer be palpated. Additional physical examination findings may include emaciation, a thin and/or roughened hair coat, and cardiac abnormalities (e.g., tachycardia, gallop rhythms, murmurs, left anterior fascicular block, and/or atrial and ventricular tachyarrhythmias). Electrocardiographic abnormalities may include tachycardia, prolonged QRS duration, increased R-wave amplitudes in lead II, and ventricular preexcitation.

Radiography/Ultrasonography/Thyroid Imaging

An enlarged heart, consistent with hypertrophic cardiomyopathy, is often found on thoracic radiographs and echocardiography. If the cat is in congestive heart failure, pleural effusion and/or pulmonary edema may occur. Ectopic thyroid tissue is rarely visible radiographically. Thyroid imaging can confirm the diagnosis by detecting functional ectopic thyroid tissue. With this procedure a radionuclide (technetium 99m) is administered intravenously. The drug accumulates in functional thyroid tissue; scanning with a scintillation camera provides an image of functional thyroid tissue (Figs. 19-18 and 19-19). Percent thyroid uptake of technetium 99m is correlated with total serum thyroxine concentrations.

☞ **N O T E** · For animals undergoing thyroidectomy, take thoracic radiographs and/or perform echocardiography.

Laboratory Findings

Most affected cats have high serum T_4 (and T_3) concentrations; however, the diagnosis of hyperthyroidism cannot be excluded on the basis of normal thyroxine concentrations. Other abnormalities may include mild elevations in red blood cell numbers, increased PCV, neutrophilic leukocytosis, eosinopenia, lymphopenia, and elevated alanine aminotransferase and alkaline phosphatase. If baseline

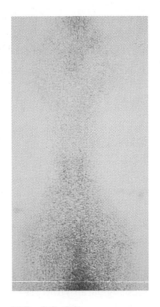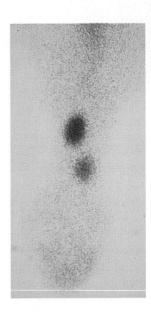

FIG. 19-18
Thyroid imaging may be used to identify functional thyroid tissue. Compare the normal scan in this cat with that of the hyperthyroid cat in Fig. 19-19.

FIG. 19-19
Thyroid scan in a cat with bilateral thyroid adenomas.

TABLE **19-27**

T_3 Suppression Test

Day 1
Obtain morning baseline serum T_4 and T_3 concentrations

Days 1 and 2
Give sodium liothyronine,* 25μg/cat PO, TID for 2 days

Morning of Day 3
Administer sodium liothyronine, wait 2-4 hrs, then measure serum T_4 and T_3

Modified from Bunch SE: *Essentials of small animal medicine,* St. Louis, 1992, Mosby.
*Cytobin.

---

serum thyroid hormone concentrations are normal in a cat with appropriate clinical signs and a palpable ventral cervical mass, serum T_4 concentration should be repeated in 3 to 4 weeks. Alternatively, a T_3 suppression test (Table 19-27) or a thyrotropin-releasing hormone (TRH) stimulation test may be performed. In normal cats the serum T_4 concentration should decrease by greater than 50% after administration of sodium liothyronine (i.e., less than 1.5 μg/dl), whereas in hyperthyroid cats there should be a minimal decrease in serum T_4 concentrations. T_3 concentrations should increase in both hyperthyroid and euthyroid cats, if the medication was given appropriately. For the TRH test, serum T_3 and T_4 concentrations are measured before and 4 hours after IV administration of 0.1 mg/kg TRH. Hyperthyroid cats usually have a relative increase of T_4 of less than 50%; normal cats have a relative increase of greater than 50%. Alternatively, response to oral antithyroid drugs or results of a sodium pertechnetate scan may be used to help confirm the diagnosis.

DIFFERENTIAL DIAGNOSIS

Cats presenting with weight loss or vomiting as a result of hyperthyroidism must be differentiated from those with intestinal lymphoma or inflammatory bowel disease. Those with neurologic signs must be differentiated from cats with primary CNS abnormalities. Cardiac dysfunction secondary to hyperthyroidism should be differentiated from that resulting from other acquired or congenital causes.

MEDICAL MANAGEMENT

Treatment of feline hyperthyroidism may include long-term administration of antithyroid drugs (see Preoperative Management below), iodine-131 (^{131}I), or surgical removal of the affected glands (Table 19-28). The choice of treatment regimen for the individual cat depends on the age and condition of the cat (i.e., presence of cardiovascular or renal disease) and the treatment modalities available to the practitioner.

The long-term administration of antithyroid drugs (e.g., methimazole) can cause remission; however, clinical signs return once the drug is discontinued. The drug inhibits synthesis of thyroid hormones. Although administration of methimazole may be associated with side effects (Table 19-29), the drug is generally well tolerated, and many side effects resolve with continued therapy. Rarely, drug-induced hepatopathy, thrombocytopenia, and agranulocytosis occur with chronic therapy. If thyroid carcinoma is suspected, medical therapy with antithyroid drugs may palliate clinical signs while allowing tumor growth. Propylthiouracil (PTU) is an effective oral antithyroid drug in cats; however, because its use has been associated with development of autoimmune hemolytic anemia and immune-mediated thrombocytopenia, it is not recommended.

Iodine-131 is a safe and effective method of treating hyperthyroidism; however, it requires facilities to safely handle the isotope. The cat must be confined for several weeks, during which it is a human health hazard. It is therefore important to eliminate other diseases before treating with ^{131}I, so that minimal contact with the cat is required during treatment. Radioactive iodine is trapped in the thyroid gland and causes local tissue destruction. The efficacy of radioactive iodine therapy is reduced by recent administration of antithyroid drugs because these drugs reduce incorporation of the radioactive iodine into the thyroid gland. If carcinoma is present, larger doses of ^{131}I may be necessary.

SURGICAL TREATMENT

Surgical treatment of hyperthyroidism involves thyroidectomy. The major complication of thyroidectomy is hypoparathyroidism secondary to removal or damage of the parathyroid glands. The procedure must be performed carefully to avoid this complication.

Preoperative Management

Metabolic and cardiovascular abnormalities associated with hyperthyroidism make anesthesia risky. Therefore cats should be made euthyroid preoperatively by administering methimazole (Tapazole; Table 19-30). Generally, administration for 1 to 3 weeks before surgery is sufficient; however, the T_4 concentration should be repeated to ensure that it is within the normal range before surgery is performed (see comment on side effects above). If preoperative therapy with methimazole is not tolerated, propranolol may be given for 1 to 2 weeks before surgery (see Table 19-30) to decrease the heart rate. Propranolol should be discontinued 24 to 48 hours before surgery because of its β-blocking effects, which may interfere with treatment of hypotension.

Because cardiac abnormalities are common, an electrocardiogram, chest x-ray, and echocardiogram should be performed before surgery. Many hyperthyroid cats have concurrent renal disease, hypokalemia and/or azotemia. These cats should be given fluids before, during, and after surgery, and care should be used to ensure that further deterioration of renal function does not occur during surgery (see the discussion of anesthetic management of animals with renal disease on p. 462) or after surgery, when cardiac output drops

TABLE 19-28
Treatment Options
• Long-term administration of antithyroid drugs   • Iodine-131   • Surgical removal of the affected glands

TABLE 19-29
Potential Side Effects of Methimazole Therapy (See Text)
• Anorexia   • Vomiting   • Pruritus   • Lethargy   • Development of serum antinuclear antibodies   • Hepatopathy   • Thrombocytopenia ± bleeding   • Agranulocytosis   • Leukopenia   • Coombs positive

TABLE 19-30
Preoperative Drug Therapy for Cats with Hyperthyroidism
Methimazole (Tapazole)
5 mg/cat PO, BID or TID* followed by 2.5-5.0 mg/cat PO, BID or TID
Propranolol† (Inderal)
2.5-5 mg/cat (0.4-1.2 mg/kg) PO, BID or TID
*If long-term administration is considered, this dose should be adjusted to maintain the T_4 concentration within the normal range.   †Propranolol should be used with care in hyperthyroid cats. Administration of propranolol to hypokalemic cats may cause sudden death.

because the cat becomes euthyroid. Fluid therapy should be adjusted if the cat is in congestive heart failure.

Anesthesia

Inhalants that sensitize the heart to arrhythmias should be avoided (e.g., halothane). Cats with cardiomyopathy may be premedicated with butorphanol (0.2 mg/kg intramuscularly or subcutaneously) and induced with diazepam (0.2 mg/kg intravenously) followed by etomidate (1 to 3 mg/kg intravenously). Maintenance on isoflurane in oxygen should be used. If the cat does not have cardiomyopathy, a variety of anesthetic protocols can be used (e.g., premedicate similarly and chamber induce with isoflurane in oxygen). If arrhythmias occur during surgery that are not due to hypoxemia or the anesthetic, esmolol may be given as an intravenous bolus (Table 19-31).

Surgical Anatomy

Refer to p. 430 for a description of the surgical anatomy of the thyroid glands.

Positioning

Clip and prepare the entire ventral neck and cranioventral thorax for aseptic surgery. Place the animal in dorsal recumbency, with the neck slightly hyperextended and forelimbs pulled caudally.

SURGICAL TECHNIQUE
Intracapsular Thyroidectomy

Make a skin incision from the larynx to a point cranial to the manubrium. Bluntly separate the sternohyoid and sternothyroid muscles. Use a self-retaining retractor (i.e., Gelpi) to maintain exposure. Identify the enlarged thyroid gland and external parathyroid gland (Fig. 19-20). Make an incision on the caudoventral surface of the gland in an avascular area (Fig. 19-21), and extend it cranially with small scissors (i.e., iris scissors). Carefully remove the thyroid tissue from the capsule, using a combination of blunt and sharp dissection. Perform the dissection carefully to avoid damaging the parathyroid gland or its blood supply. Use bipolar cautery to achieve hemostasis but avoid damaging the gland's blood supply. After the thyroid parenchyma has been removed, excise the majority of the thyroid capsule; however, do not excise capsule that is intimately associated with the external parathyroid gland. Close subcutaneous tissues with a simple continuous suture pattern. Close skin with either a simple continuous or a simple interrupted suture pattern.

☞ **N O T E** · Sterile Q-tips are useful to help separate the gland from the capsule.

Modified Extracapsular Approach for Thyroidectomy

Position the animal as described above. Locate the thyroid gland as described above, and ligate or cauterize the caudal thyroid vein. Cauterize the thyroid capsule approximately

TABLE 19-31

Esmolol (Brevibloc) Therapy in Dogs and Cats

Give a loading dose of 75-100 μg/kg over 3 min IV, then give by constant infusion 25-150 μg/kg/min

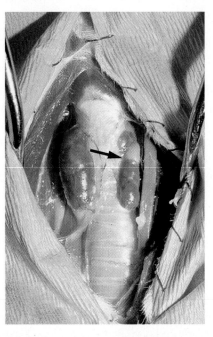

FIG. 19-20
Unilateral thyroid enlargement in a cat. Note the parathyroid gland at the cranial pole of the left thyroid gland (*arrow*).

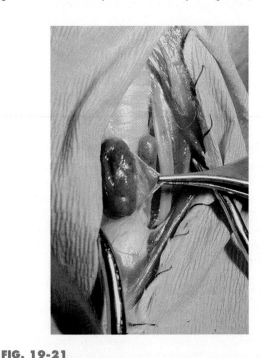

FIG. 19-21
For intracapsular thyroidectomy, make an incision on the caudoventral surface of the gland in an avascular area, and extend it cranially with small scissors (i.e., iris scissors). Carefully remove the thyroid tissue from the capsule, using a combination of blunt and sharp dissection.

2 mm from the external parathyroid gland, using fine-tipped bipolar cautery forceps (Fig. 19-22, A). With small, fine scissors cut the gland at the cauterized area, and remove the gland by sharp and blunt dissection from the parathyroid gland (Fig. 19-22, B). Carefully dissect all thyroid gland from the surrounding tissues and parathyroid gland (Fig. 19-22, C). Do not damage the cranial thyroid artery or its branches to the external parathyroid gland. Close as described above.

☞ **N O T E** • Take special care to avoid damaging the cranial thyroid artery, or hypocalcemia may occur.

SUTURE MATERIALS/SPECIAL INSTRUMENTS

Small, fine instruments, such as iris scissors and Bishop-Harmon thumb forceps, facilitate removal of the thyroid glands. Bipolar cautery forceps are advantageous for providing hemostasis because they allow finer control of coagulation than do unipolar forceps. Sterile Q-tips are useful for dissecting the thyroid glands from the parathyroid glands.

POSTOPERATIVE CARE AND ASSESSMENT

Complications may include hypocalcemia, hypothyroidism, recurrence of hyperthyroidism, Horner's syndrome, and/or laryngeal paralysis. Hypocalcemia due to hypoparathyroidism may be permanent or temporary. Persistent hypocalcemia may occur if all four parathyroid glands are removed or their blood supply is irreversibly damaged. Temporary hypocalcemia is usually caused by disruption of the parathyroid blood supply. Hypocalcemia should not occur

after unilateral thyroidectomy. Recurrent hyperthyroidism may result from hypertrophy of adenomatous tissue not removed during thyroidectomy, or from adenomatous changes in ectopic thyroid tissue. Hyperthyroidism has been reported within 2 to 3 years in 5% to 11% of cats having bilateral thyroidectomy. If possible, a thyroid scan should be performed to localize hyperfunctioning tissue in these animals, before repeat surgery.

☞ **N O T E** • Hypocalcemia is extremely rare after unilateral thyroidectomy for feline hyperthyroidism.

Hypocalcemia (serum calcium level less than 9 mg/dl in adult dogs and less than 8.5 mg/dl in adult cats) is the most important, acute, life-threatening complication of thyroidectomy. Most animals do not develop clinical signs until the serum calcium level is less than 7.5 mg/dl. Animals should be closely observed for signs of hypocalcemia (i.e., panting, nervousness, facial rubbing, muscle twitching, ataxia, seizures) for 2 to 4 days. In cats, early signs may include lethargy, anorexia, panting, and facial rubbing. Clinical signs are usually noted within 24 to 96 hours, although delayed signs have been reported up to 5 to 6 days later. Acute signs of hypocalcemia may be treated with intravenous 10% calcium gluconate. Calcium should be given slowly intravenously (Table 19-32) and cardiac rate and rhythm monitored during administration. It should be discontinued if bradycardia develops. Calcium gluconate can also be added to the fluids, or the intravenous dose can be diluted in an equal volume of saline and given subcutaneously every 6 to 8 hours (Table 19-32), until the animal is eating and able to be given oral medications. Subcutaneous or intravenous calcium should be discontinued when the

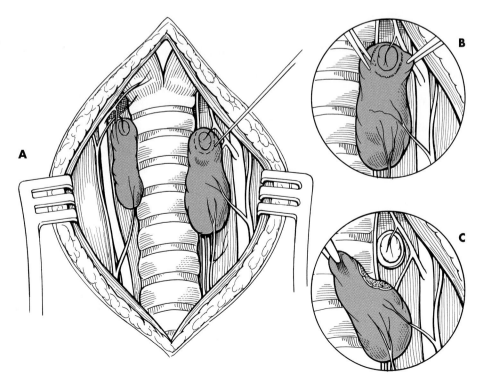

FIG. 19-22
A, To perform a modified extracapsular thyroidectomy, cauterize the thyroid capsule approximately 2 mm from the external parathyroid gland, using fine-tipped bipolar cautery forceps. **B,** With small, fine scissors cut the gland at the cauterized area and remove from the parathyroid gland. **C,** Carefully dissect all thyroid gland from the surrounding tissues and parathyroid gland.

serum calcium level is greater than 8 mg/dl. Maintenance therapy consists of oral calcium and vitamin D administration (Table 19-32). The form of vitamin D most commonly used is dihydrotachysterol. It does not accumulate in fat and has a more rapid onset of action than vitamin D_3. Serum calcium levels should be monitored weekly and the dosage of calcium changed accordingly. Vitamin D supplementation can often be discontinued once the parathyroid gland revascularizes. Some animals will need to be maintained on vitamin D for months before the dose can be reduced; others require lifelong therapy.

Suggested Reading

Birchard SJ, Peterson ME, Jacobson A: Surgical treatment of feline hyperthyroidism: results of 85 cases, *Vet Surg* 14:47, 1985.

Broussard JD, Petersen ME, Fox PR: Changes in clinical and laboratory findings in cats with hyperthyroidism from 1983 to 1993, *J Am Vet Med Assoc* 206:302, 1995.

Ferguson DC, Hoeing M: Hyperthyroidism in the cat, *Feline Pract* 18:10, 1990.

Flanders JA, Harvey HJ, Erb HN: Feline thyroidectomy: a comparison of postoperative hypocalcemia associated with three different surgical techniques, *Vet Surg* 16:362, 1987.

Jacobs G et al: Congestive heart failure associated with hyperthyroidism in cats, *J Am Vet Med Assoc* 188:52, 1986.

Joseph RJ, Petersen ME: Review and comparison of neuromuscular and central nervous system manifestations of hyperthyroidism in cats and humans, *Prog Vet Neurol* 3:114, 1992.

Kintzer PP, Peterson MK: Thyroid scintigraphy in small animals, *Semin Vet Med Surg (Small Anim)* 6:131, 1991.

Meric SM: Diagnosis and management of feline hyperthyroidism, *Compend Contin Educ Pract Vet* 11:1053, 1989.

Meric SM: The three therapeutic options for feline hyperthyroidism, *Vet Med* 84:969, 1989.

Mooney CT et al: Qualitative and quantitative thyroid imaging in feline hyperthyroidism using technetium-99m as pertechnetate, *Vet Radiol Ultras* 33:313, 1992.

Peterson ME, Brousard JD, Gamble DA: Use of the thyrotropin releasing hormone stimulation test to diagnose mild hyperthyroidism in cats, *J Vet Int Med* 8:279, 1994.

Peterson ME, Graves TK, Gamble DA: Triiodothyronine (T_3) suppression test: an aid in the diagnosis of mild hyperthyroidism in cats, *J Vet Int Med* 4:233, 1990.

Peterson ME et al: Electrocardiographic findings in 45 cats with hyperthyroidism, *J Am Vet Med Assoc* 180:934, 1982.

Swalec KM, Birchard SJ: Recurrence of hyperthyroidism after thyroidectomy in cats, *J Am Anim Hosp Assoc* 26:433, 1990.

Welches CD et al: Occurrence of problems after three techniques of bilateral thyroidectomy in cats, *Vet Surg* 18:392, 1989.

HYPERPARATHYROIDISM

DEFINITIONS

Primary hyperparathyroidism is a disorder resulting from excessive secretion of parathyroid hormone (PTH) by the parathyroid gland(s).

TABLE 19-32
Treatment of Hypocalcemia Following Thyroidectomy

Management of Acute Signs

Give 0.5-1.5 ml/kg (5-15 mg Ca/kg) of 10% calcium gluconate slowly IV (over 10-20 min) and monitor the heart, then add 10 ml of 10% calcium gluconate into 250 ml of lactated Ringer's solution and drip at maintenance rate or give IV dose diluted in equal volume of saline SC (in multiple sites). Monitor serum calcium frequently (2-3 times a day, if necessary).

Maintenance Therapy

Give calcium lactate 0.2-0.5 g/cat/day in divided doses PO and give vitamin D (dihydrotachysterol) PO 0.02-0.03 mg/kg/day for 5-7 days, then 0.01 mg/kg/day for 5-7 days, then 0.005 mg/kg/day for 1-4 mo.

GENERAL CONSIDERATIONS AND CLINICALLY RELEVANT PATHOPHYSIOLOGY

Primary hyperparathyroidism is uncommon in dogs and cats. It is usually caused by parathyroid adenomas, although parathyroid carcinomas and parathyroid hyperplasia have also been reported. Parathyroid adenomas are typically small, well-encapsulated tumors that appear brown or red and are located near the thyroid glands; however, ectopic adenomas may be located near the thoracic inlet or in the cranial mediastinum. Clinical signs are caused by PTH increasing calcium absorption and phosphorus excretion in the kidney, and enhancing bone resorption. The net result is to increase serum calcium levels and decrease serum phosphorus levels. Clinical abnormalities caused by hypercalcemia may include dystrophic calcification, impaired renal tubular concentrating ability, nephrolithiasis, and calcium oxalate urolithiasis.

DIAGNOSIS
Clinical Presentation

Signalment. Parathyroid tumors usually occur in older dogs. There is no sex predisposition. Keeshonden (and possibly German shepherds and Norwegian elkhounds) may be predisposed. Primary gland hyperplasia has been reported in young dogs.

History. Dogs may be asymptomatic or may present for nonspecific signs (e.g., polyuria, polydipsia, vomiting, weakness, constipation, lethargy, and/or inappetence). Clinical signs may be insidious in onset. The most common clinical signs in cats with primary hyperparathyroidism are anorexia, lethargy, vomiting, weakness, and weight loss; polyuria and polydipsia are less common in cats than dogs. Occasionally bone and joint pain and pathologic fractures may occur secondary to skeletal demineralization. Cystic calculi may occur secondary to hypercalcemia.

☞ **N O T E** · Consider primary hyperparathyroidism in animals with hypercalcemia, dystrophic calcification, calcium oxalate urolithiasis, and/or nephrolithiasis.

Physical Examination Findings

Physical examination findings are usually nonspecific. The enlarged parathyroid gland can seldom be palpated in dogs; however, a cervical mass may be palpated in some cats.

Radiography/Ultrasonography

Cervical radiographs seldom identify the neoplasm; however, ultrasonographic evaluation of the cervical region occasionally reveals a parathyroid mass. Marked demineralization of the skeleton, nephrolithiasis, and/or nephrocalcinosis may be noted radiographically.

Laboratory Findings

Serum biochemical abnormalities in dogs with primary hyperparathyroidism include hypercalcemia and hypophosphatemia. Hypercalcemia is the most consistent finding in affected cats. Measurement of PTH in animals with normal renal function helps confirm hyperparathyroidism. High-normal or increased serum concentrations of PTH in hypercalcemic animals with normal renal function are suggestive of hyperparathyroidism. Other causes of hypercalcemia (see below) are usually associated with low or low-normal levels of PTH. Renal dysfunction (which may occur secondary to hypercalcemia or be a primary disorder) may also elevate serum concentrations of PTH. If renal function is abnormal, serum PTH concentrations should be evaluated in conjunction with serum ionized calcium concentration. Serum ionized calcium levels are increased in hyperparathyroidism but low to low-normal in renal failure (Table 19-33). Definitive diagnosis of primary hyperparathyroidism requires surgical exploration of the parathyroid glands.

DIFFERENTIAL DIAGNOSIS

Thoracic and abdominal radiographs, abdominal ultrasonography, routine blood work, and lymph node aspirations should be performed in animals with hypercalcemia to identify possible neoplastic causes (e.g., lymphosarcoma, apocrine gland adenocarcinoma) before pursuing hyperparathyroidism. Other causes of hypercalcemia include granulomatous disease, renal failure, hypoadrenocorticism, and hypervitaminosis D. Thyroglossal cysts (formed when the embryonic thyroglossal duct fills with fluid) may be confused with parathyroid masses on palpation.

☞ **N O T E** • Paraneoplastic syndrome is a more common cause of hypercalcemia than primary hyperparathyroidism.

MEDICAL MANAGEMENT

Hypercalcemia may be treated by diuresis (see the discussion of Preoperative Management below). Surgical removal of the neoplastic parathyroid tissue is the definitive treatment for primary hyperparathyroidism. Initially glucocorticoid therapy is usually effective in lowering serum calcium

TABLE 19-33

Serum Parathyroid (PTH) and Calcium (Ca²⁺) Levels with Primary Hyperparathyroidism (HPTH) and Renal Disease

	PTH	Ca²*
HPTH	↑	↑
Renal failure	↑	↓

*Serum ionized calcium

concentrations in animals with lymphosarcoma; it may also occasionally lower calcium concentrations in animals with other disorders.

SURGICAL TREATMENT

Parathyroidectomy is the treatment of choice for hyperparathyroidism caused by parathyroid neoplasia and primary hyperplasia. If the parathyroid glands are uniformly enlarged, secondary hyperparathyroidism should be suspected and other diagnostic tests performed to identify the cause (i.e., renal or nutritional secondary hyperparathyroidism); however, enlargement of all four glands may occur with primary hyperplasia. If one or several glands are slightly enlarged, parathyroid adenomas or primary hyperplasia should be suspected. Most dogs with primary hyperparathyroidism have a single parathyroid adenoma. If the parathyroid glands appear normal, ectopic parathyroid tissue may be located near the base of the heart.

☞ **N O T E** • If you cannot find any other cause of hypercalcemia and the parathyroid glands appear normal, look for ectopic parathyroid tissue.

Preoperative Management

Before anesthetic induction, diuresis should be instituted with physiologic saline solution to help lower serum calcium levels (Table 19-34). Fluids should be used with caution in animals with severe renal dysfunction. Once the animal has been appropriately hydrated, furosemide administration may promote further calciuresis. Electrolytes should be monitored to prevent iatrogenic hypokalemia.

Anesthesia

Theoretically, marked hypercalcemia may cause bradycardia, peripheral vasoconstriction, and hypertension. Hypotension may occur during anesthesia associated with relaxation of peripheral vascular tone. Hypercalcemia also may predispose to cardiac arrhythmias. Anesthetic agents that potentiate arrhythmias (i.e., thiobarbiturates, halothane) should be avoided.

Surgical Anatomy

A discussion of the anatomy of the parathyroid glands is provided on p. 430.

Positioning

Clip and prepare the entire ventral neck and cranioventral thorax for aseptic surgery. Place the animal in dorsal recumbency, with the neck slightly hyperextended and forelimbs pulled caudally.

SURGICAL TECHNIQUE

All four parathyroid glands should be carefully inspected. If the external parathyroid gland is involved, the gland can be removed without removing the thyroid gland; however, removal of the internal parathyroid gland requires that thyroidectomy be performed (see p. 434). The external parathyroid gland should be spared when the internal parathyroid gland is neoplastic. Visualization of the abnormal parathyroid gland may be facilitated with infusion of intravenous methylene blue in saline solution (see Table 19-20). Abnormal parathyroid tissue may stain dark blue with this procedure. A common side effect of methylene blue administration is hemolytic anemia because of Heinz body formation. Severe and occasionally fatal Heinz body anemia has been reported after the use of methylene blue. If carcinoma is suspected, based on apparent invasiveness of the tumor, complete thyroidectomy and removal of draining lymph nodes are indicated.

SUTURE MATERIALS/SPECIAL INSTRUMENTS

Small, fine instruments, such as iris scissors and Bishop-Harmon thumb forceps, facilitate removal of the parathyroid glands. Bipolar cautery forceps are advantageous for providing hemostasis because they allow finer control of coagulation than do unipolar forceps. Sterile Q-tips are useful for dissecting the parathyroid glands from the thyroid glands.

POSTOPERATIVE CARE AND ASSESSMENT

Hypocalcemia is the most frequent postoperative complication in dogs; it may be less common in cats. Hypocalcemia may occur after removal of a single parathyroid adenoma because negative feedback from high circulating levels of PTH suppresses function in the other normal glands. PTH has a functional half-life of 20 minutes; thus PTH levels fall rapidly once neoplastic tissue has been removed. Hypocalcemia may be most pronounced in animals with higher preoperative serum calcium levels and those with marked skeletal demineralization. Treatment of hypocalcemia is

---

TABLE 19-34

Diuresis of Hypercalcemic Dogs

0.9% Physiologic Saline Solution
90 ml/kg/day

Furosemide (Lasix)
2-4 mg/kg IV, BID or TID

---

given in Table 19-32. Treatment of hypocalcemia should not be necessary for prolonged periods in these patients. Renal function should be monitored postoperatively in patients with hypercalcemia. The prognosis for long-term survival following parathyroidectomy for hyperparathyroidism secondary to adenomas or hyperplasia is excellent, if there is not severe renal damage.

Suggested Reading

Berger B, Feldman EC: Primary hyperparathyroidism in dogs: 21 cases (1976–1986), *J Am Vet Med Assoc* 191:350, 1987.

Bland KI et al: Intraoperative localization of parathyroid glands using methylthionine chloride and tetramethylthionine chloride in secondary hyperparathyroidism, *Surg Gynecol Obstet* 160:42, 1985.

DeVries SE et al: Primary parathyroid gland hyperplasia in dogs: six cases (1982–1991), *J Am Vet Med Assoc* 202:1132, 1993.

Fingeroth JM, Smeak DD, Jacobs RM: Intravenous methylene blue infusion for intraoperative identification of parathyroid gland and pancreatic islet-cell tumors in dogs. I: Experimental determination of dose-related staining efficacy and toxicity, *J Am Anim Hosp Assoc* 24:165, 1988.

Kallet AJ et al: Primary hyperparathyroidism in cats: seven cases (1984–1989), *J Am Vet Med Assoc* 199:1767, 1991.

Klausner JS, O'Leary TP, Osborne CA: Calcium urolithiasis in two dogs with parathyroid adenomas, *J Am Vet Med Assoc* 191:1423, 1987.

Marquez GA, Klausner JS, Osborne CA: Calcium oxalate urolithiasis in cat with a functional parathyroid adenocarcinoma, *J Am Vet Med Assoc* 206:817, 1995.

Mueller DL, Noxon JO: Primary hyperparathyroidism in a dog, *Comp Anim Prac* 19:36, 1989.

THYROID CARCINOMAS IN DOGS

DEFINITIONS

Thyroid neoplasms may be **carcinomas** (malignant) or **adenomas** (benign). Carcinomas may arise from follicular cells and be classified as follicular, compact, papillary, or mixed, or they may arise from parafollicular or C-cells (medullary thyroid carcinomas).

GENERAL CONSIDERATIONS AND CLINICALLY RELEVANT PATHOPHYSIOLOGY

Thyroid neoplasms make up 1% to 4% of all tumors in dogs. Canine thyroid carcinomas are more common than adenomas (63% to 87% of canine thyroid tumors are carcinomas), whereas, functional adenomas prevail in cats (see the discussion of feline hyperthyroidism on p. 431). Adenocarcinomas are generally rapidly growing, highly invasive tumors that frequently metastasize to the draining lymph nodes and lungs. Reportedly, large tumors (i.e., those greater than 100 cm^3) are always associated with pulmonary metastasis. Although histologic classification of thyroid tumors based on the predominant microscopic pattern has been done (e.g., compact cellular or solid, follicular, mixed solid follicular, or anaplastic), the histologic pattern has been thought to correlate poorly with prognosis. However, a recent study suggests that medullary thyroid carcinomas are more apt to be well circumscribed and resectable, and possess gross and histologic characteristics of a less malignant nature than other thyroid carcinomas (Carver et al, 1995). Ectopic thyroid tumors have been reported at the heart base, caudal mediastinum, and tongue.

☞ **N O T E** · Surgical excision of canine thyroid tumors is usually difficult because of their invasiveness.

Tumors arising in cystic remnants of the thyroglossal duct are rarely reported in dogs. They are usually well-circumscribed, fluctuant, moveable enlargements in the ventral midline cervical region. Histologically, they are usually well-differentiated papillary carcinomas.

DIAGNOSIS
Clinical Presentation

Signalment. Thyroid neoplasia is most common in medium- to large-breed dogs; boxers, beagles, and golden retrievers may be predisposed. Most affected dogs are middle-aged or older (mean age, 9 years). A sex predisposition is not apparent.

History. Affected animals often present for evaluation of a palpable cervical enlargement, dysphagia, dyspnea, coughing, voice change, and/or exercise intolerance. Respiratory abnormalities may be the result of tracheal compression or pulmonary metastasis. Hyperthyroidism (i.e., polydipsia, polyuria, weakness, restlessness, and a propensity to seek cool places) is rarely associated with canine thyroid carcinomas.

Physical Examination Findings

A ventral cervical mass is often palpable. Carcinomas usually appear firm and poorly encapsulated; adenomas are typically small and freely moveable. Abnormal lung sounds may occur secondary to pulmonary metastasis. Bilateral ptosis and prolapse of the nictitating membrane can be associated with paralysis of the extraocular and intraocular muscles secondary to thyroid adenocarcinoma invasion of the cavernous sinuses in dogs.

Radiography/Ultrasonography/Thyroid Imaging

Cervical radiographs or ultrasonography usually reveals diffuse cervical edema and soft-tissue swelling caudal to the mandible and surrounding the trachea. The mass may be partially mineralized. Thoracic radiographs should be taken to identify pulmonary metastasis. Thyroid imaging (see p. 432) may reveal abnormal thyroid gland uptake (heterogenous uptake with "hot" and "cold" regions, compared with normal thyroids or salivary gland uptake) and focal accumulations of the radiopharmaceutical in the lungs, indicative of pulmonary metastasis.

Laboratory Findings

Cytologic evaluation of a fine-needle aspirate of the cervical mass may reveal bizarre, pleomorphic cells, consistent with neoplasia. Nondiagnostic samples may be obtained if the sample is contaminated with blood or is hypocellular. Additionally, neoplastic follicular epithelial cells are fragile and are often broken during sample preparation. Hyperthyroidism and hypothyroidism are occasionally associated with thyroid carcinomas; therefore measuring T_4 and T_3 concentrations is warranted. Hematologic and serum biochemical results are often normal. Hypocalcemia has been reported in a dog with a thyroid medullary carcinoma.

DIFFERENTIAL DIAGNOSIS

Cervical swelling because of thyroid neoplasia must be differentiated from abscesses, lymphadenopathy, or sialoadenopathy. This can usually be done by cytologic evaluation of fine-needle aspirates.

MEDICAL MANAGEMENT

Dogs with thyroid carcinomas, particularly if the dogs are hyperthyroid, may be palliated with radioactive iodine (^{131}I); however, much larger doses of ^{131}I appear to be necessary in dogs than in cats with thyroid adenomas. These large doses necessitate lengthy hospital stays and make this treatment prohibitively expensive for many owners. Chemotherapy with doxorubicin may benefit animals for whom complete excision is not possible. External-beam (cobalt) irradiation appears beneficial in reducing tumor volume in animals, after debulking procedures; however, large doses are required.

SURGICAL TREATMENT

Surgical excision of thyroid adenomas is the treatment of choice. Surgical removal of thyroid carcinomas is often difficult because of their invasive nature and pronounced vascularity (Fig. 19-23) but should be considered if metastasis is not evident, and the lesion is localized. Marginal excision (i.e., just outside the tumor pseudocapsule) in tumors that are freely moveable results in fewer complications than more extensive resection and does not appear to affect the local recurrence rate. Adjunctive radiation therapy or chemotherapy may be warranted if complete surgical excision is not possible. Chemotherapy may be indicated if debulking is being done in animals with metastasis.

☞ **N O T E** · Have blood for transfusion available during surgery because hemorrhage is often excessive.

Preoperative Management

Electrolyte and acid-base abnormalities should be corrected before surgery. Fluid therapy should be initiated before surgery in geriatric patients with reduced renal function and in those that are dehydrated.

Anesthesia

In human beings, life-threatening thyroid storms are reported intraoperatively and postoperatively after surgery of thyroid tumors. Clinical signs of tachycardia or arrhythmias may occur because of catecholamine release; treatment should be anticipated. It may be wise to avoid drugs that are arrhythmogenic (e.g., barbiturates and halothane) in these patients.

Surgical Anatomy

Surgical anatomy of the thyroid glands is discussed on p. 430. Important structures that may adhere to or surround the tumor include carotid artery, internal jugular vein, recurrent laryngeal nerve, and esophagus. These structures should be identified and preserved, if possible, during the dissection.

Positioning

The animal is placed in dorsal recumbency, with the neck slightly hyperextended. The front limbs should be tied back away from the neck. The entire neck, cranial thorax, and caudal intermandibular space should be clipped and prepared for aseptic surgery.

SURGICAL TECHNIQUE

Make a ventral midline incision over the thyroid glands. Identify the neoplastic mass and adjacent structures. If necessary, ligate the carotid artery and jugular vein. Remove the mass (thyroid and parathyroid glands) by a combination of sharp and blunt dissection. Identify and remove abnormal cervical lymph nodes. Use electrocautery and ligation to provide hemostasis. Inspect the contralateral thyroid, and biopsy or remove if indicated. Close the incision routinely. Submit tissue for histologic evaluation (Fig. 19-24).

SUTURE MATERIALS/SPECIAL INSTRUMENTS

These tumors are frequently very vascular, and electrocautery is useful for obtaining hemostasis.

POSTOPERATIVE CARE AND ASSESSMENT

A light pressure wrap may be used postoperatively to help decrease hemorrhage and swelling; however, it should be placed with care and monitored, to avoid causing airway obstruction. The hematocrit should be monitored postoperatively and transfusions given as needed. If unilateral thyroparathyroidectomy is performed, the animal should be observed for hypocalcemia or hypothyroidism, but supplementation is usually not necessary. If bilateral thyroparathyroidectomy is performed, vitamin D, calcium, and thyroid supplementation should be initiated postoperatively (see p. 435).

PROGNOSIS

The prognosis is guarded for thyroid carcinomas and depends on tumor size, resectability, and presence of metastasis. The mean survival in one study of 17 dogs with thyroid tumors treated with surgical excision was 7 months (Harari, Patterson, Rosenthal, 1986). In another study of freely moveable carcinomas the mean survival was 20 months (Klein et al, 1995). Prognosis for thyroid adenomas is excellent.

References

Carver JR, Kapatkin A, Patnaik AK: A comparison of medullary thyroid carcinoma and adenocarcinoma in dogs: a retrospective study of 38 cases, *Vet Surg* 24:315, 1995.

Harari J, Patterson JS, Rosenthal RC: Clinical and pathologic features of thyroid tumors in 26 dogs, *J Am Vet Med Assoc* 188:1160, 1986.

Klein MK et al: Treatment of thyroid carcinoma in dogs by surgical resection alone: 20 cases (1981–1989), *J Am Vet Med Assoc* 206:1007, 1995.

Suggested Reading

Haley PJ et al: Thyroid neoplasms in a colony of beagle dogs, *Vet Pathol* 26:438, 1989.

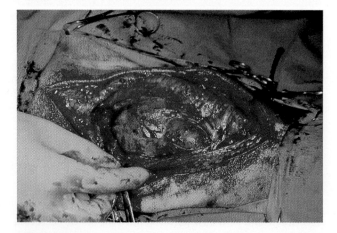

FIG. 19-23
Thyroid carcinoma in a dog. Note the invasiveness of the tumor.

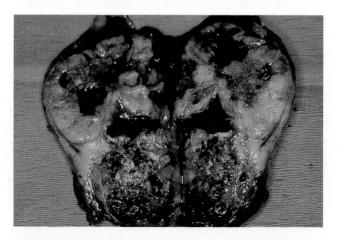

FIG. 19-24
Appearance of a well-encapsulated thyroid carcinoma in a dog. Note the areas of necrosis within the gland.

Harari J: Canine thyroid tumors, *Calif Vet* 7:9, 1984.

Jeglum KA, Whereat A: Chemotherapy of canine thyroid carcinoma, *Compend Contin Educ Pract Vet* 5:96, 1983.

Sullivan M et al: Thyroid tumors in the dog, *J Small Anim Pract* 28:505, 1987.

Susaneck SJ: Thyroid tumors in the dog, *Compend Contin Educ Pract Vet* 5:35, 1983.

Walsh KM, Diters RW: Carcinoma of ectopic thyroid in a dog, *J Am Anim Hosp Assoc* 20:665, 1984.

CHAPTER 20

Surgery of the Hemolymphatic System

Surgery of the Lymphatic System

GENERAL PRINCIPLES AND TECHNIQUES

DEFINITIONS

Tissue for histopathologic examination of lymph nodes may be obtained by removing the entire node (**lymphadenectomy**) or by excising a portion of it. **Lymphangiomas** and **lymphangiosarcomas** are benign and malignant tumors of peripheral lymphatics, respectively.

PREOPERATIVE CONCERNS

Lymphadenopathy is one of the more common lymphatic abnormalities of dogs and cats. Lymphadenopathy may be the result of focal infection, inflammation, neoplasia (metastic or primary), or systemic disease. When examining an animal with lymphadenopathy, it is important to determine whether the enlargement is generalized or localized (regional). With localized lymphadenopathy, areas drained by the node should be examined for evidence of infection, inflammation, or neoplasia. Cytological evaluation of lymph node aspirates may help determine the underlying disease process. Fine-needle aspirates should be done before lymph node biopsy because occasionally neoplastic cells or fungal elements will be noted. However, nondiagnostic aspirates may be obtained in animals with well-differentiated tumors and in those with focal infection or neoplasia. The reader is referred to a medicine text for an in-depth discussion of lymph node cytology.

The mandibular, superficial cervical, superficial inguinal, and popliteal lymph nodes are palpable in most animals (Fig. 20-1). The tonsils may be visualized within the oral cavity and facial lymph nodes may be found in some normal animals. The axillary, accessory axillary, cervical, femoral, and retropharyngeal lymph nodes are usually only palpable when

enlarged in dogs; however, the axillary node may be readily located in cats, even when its size is only moderately increased. Unless the animal is extremely thin or cachectic, sublumbar and mesenteric lymph nodes must be enlarged to be detected on rectal or abdominal palpation. The texture of the enlarged node and sensitivity to pressure or manipulation should be noted. Acute enlargement (i.e., suppurative lymphadenitis) can be associated with pain, but lymphoid neoplasia usually causes painless enlargement. Metastic neoplasia and fungal infections sometimes cause nodes to become fixed to surrounding tissues. Clinical signs may result from lymphadenopathy (e.g., coughing because of tracheal compression by enlarged hilar lymph nodes or constipation as a result of sublumbar lymphadenopathy). Survey radiographs may detect internal lymphadenopathy. Thoracic films should be examined for evidence of mediastinal, hilar, or sternal lymphadenopathy; abdominal radiographs may reveal ventral deviation of the colon as a result of sublumbar lymphadenopathy.

Lymphangiomas are rare, benign neoplasms originating from lymphatic capillaries. They are believed to be developmental anomalies associated with failure of primitive

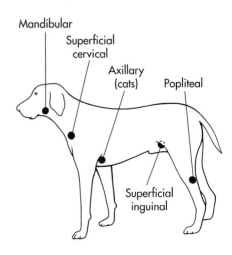

FIG. 20-1
Location of palpable lymph nodes.

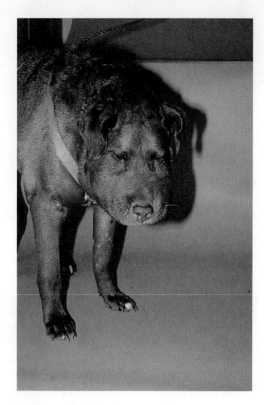

FIG. 20-2
Massive head and neck swelling in a dog with diffuse lymphangiosarcoma.

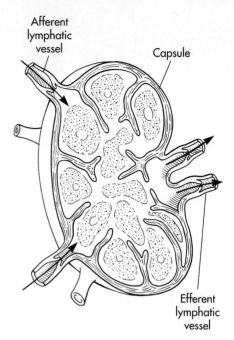

FIG. 20-3
Structure of a lymph node showing afferent and efferent drainage.

lymphatic sacs to establish venous communication. These endothelial sprouts continue to grow, infiltrate surrounding tissues, produce pressure and subsequent necrosis, and form cystic structures. They typically present as large, fluctuant swellings that are noticed incidentally or because of interference with normal structures as a result of expansive growth. They have been identified arising from subcutaneous tissue, nasopharynx, and the retroperitoneal space of dogs. Affected dogs are usually middle-aged or older. Treatment for lymphangioma is complete surgical excision or marsupialization. Lymphangiosarcomas (Fig. 20-2) are malignant tumors that arise from lymphatic capillaries. They are locally aggressive and metastasis has been reported to regional lymph nodes, lungs, spleen, kidneys, and bone marrow. Even without metastasis, the local invasiveness of this tumor often calls for euthanasia. Surgical management may be considered; however, cures are unlikely. Histologically, lymphangiomas and lymphangiosarcomas are composed of vascular spaces lined by endothelial cells and focal lymphoid aggregates divided by connective tissue stroma. Unlike hemangiomas, the cystic spaces are not filled with blood.

ANESTHETIC CONSIDERATIONS

Excision of superficial nodes (e.g., popliteal) can be performed under local anesthesia and sedation if the patient's condition dictates; however, short-duration general anesthesia usually facilitates extirpation.

ANTIBIOTICS

Perioperative antibiotics are seldom indicated in animals undergoing lymph node biopsy or removal.

SURGICAL ANATOMY

Lymph nodes are bean-shaped structures with a convex surface and a small flat or concave hilus (Fig. 20-3). They are usually found encased in fat at flexor angles or joints, in the mediastinum and mesentery, and in the angle formed by the origin of larger blood vessels.

SURGICAL TECHNIQUES

Lymph node biopsy is easy, relatively inexpensive, and provides valuable information. There are no absolute contraindications to lymph node biopsy. Significant hemostatic disorders should be corrected preoperatively, if possible, and care taken to properly ligate blood vessels.

The selection of a lymph node to be biopsied is based on clinical findings. With generalized lymphadenopathy the popliteal, inguinal, and prescapular lymph nodes are preferred sites; at least two nodes should be biopsied. The mandibular lymph node and nodes draining the gastrointestinal tract should not be chosen for biopsy in these patients because their morphologic appearance is often distorted by reactive hyperplasia caused by constant antigenic exposure.

Incisional Biopsy

Incisional (wedge) biopsy of lymph nodes is indicated when lymphadenectomy may be difficult because of a node's size or location (i.e., nodes that are located close to major vessels or nerves). *Use a No. 15 scalpel blade to remove a wedge-shaped section of the parenchyma (Fig. 20-4, A), and*

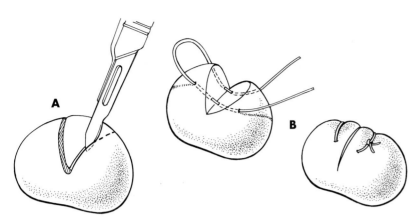

FIG. 20-4
A, Incisional (wedge) biopsy of lymph nodes is occasionally performed. Use a No. 15 scalpel blade to remove a wedge-shaped section of the parenchyma. **B,** Place a horizontal mattress suture of absorbable suture material to close the incision.

place the sample in a buffered formalin solution. In order to provide hemostasis, place a horizontal mattress suture of absorbable suture material (i.e., 3-0 chromic catgut) to close the incision (Fig. 20-4, B).

Lymphadenectomy

Prepare the skin overlying the lymph node for aseptic surgery. Immobilize the lymph node firmly in one hand, and make an incision in the overlying skin. Bluntly dissect the node from surrounding tissue. Generally, a vessel near the hilus of the node requires ligation to prevent postoperative hemorrhage. Handle the node gently to prevent damage and distortion of the lymph node tissue. Section the node to provide samples for aerobic and anaerobic cultures, fungal cultures, histopathology, and cytology. Make impression smears by lightly blotting the cut edge of the node with absorbent paper and touching the sample lightly to a glass slide before placing it in formalin. Close dead space and suture skin routinely.

HEALING OF THE LYMPHATIC SYSTEM

Healing of lymphatics is usually rapid. Lymphedema rarely occurs following lymphadenectomy because collateral pathways form. If lymphedema occurs, it is usually transient and seldom requires specific therapy. Frequently, prolonged obstruction of lymphatics may cause a lymphaticovenous anastomosis to open or form, providing an alternate pathway for lymph flow.

SUTURE MATERIALS/SPECIAL INSTRUMENTS

Special instruments are not required for lymph node biopsy or removal. Absorbable suture should be used in the lymph node parenchyma.

POSTOPERATIVE CARE AND ASSESSMENT

After lymphadenectomy, the patient should be observed for swelling at the surgical site. Swelling is usually associated with hematoma formation as a result of inadequate hemostasis or with seroma formation, if dead space was not obliterated.

COMPLICATIONS

Manipulation of a tumor during biopsy procedures may transiently increase the number of neoplastic cells present in the lymphatic and vascular systems; however, subsequent metastasis has seldom been substantiated. A hematoma may develop if vessels are not ligated adequately.

SPECIAL AGE CONSIDERATIONS

The age and physical condition of animals with lymphadenopathy must be considered. Increased lymph node size may be expected in young animals as a part of an appropriate immunologic response. As the animal ages, lymph node size usually decreases, making nodes difficult to palpate. Loss of fat that normally surrounds the nodes in cachectic patients may make the nodes prominent.

Suggested Reading

Mooney SC et al: Generalized lymphadenopathy resembling lymphoma in cats: six cases (1972-1976), *J Amer Vet Med Assoc* 190:897, 1987.

Moore FM et al: Distinctive peripheral lymph node hyperplasia of young cats, *Vet Pathol* 23:386, 1986.

Perman V et al: Lymph node biopsy, *Vet Clin N Amer* 4:281, 1974.

Rudd RG et al: Lymphangiosarcoma in dogs, *J Am Anim Hosp Assoc* 25:695, 1989.

Stobie D, Carpenter JL: Lymphangiosarcoma of the mediastinum, mesentery, and omentum in a cat with chylothorax, *J Am Anim Hosp Assoc* 29:78, 1993.

SPECIFIC DISEASES

LYMPHEDEMA

DEFINITIONS

Lymphedema is an accumulation of fluid in the interstitial space. **Primary lymphedema** is caused by an abnormality or disease of lymph vessels or lymph nodes; **secondary lymphedema** occurs as a result of lymphatic obstruction of the nodes or vessels by neoplasia, filariasis, lymphoproliferative disorders, or surgery.

GENERAL CONSIDERATIONS AND CLINICALLY RELEVANT PATHOPHYSIOLOGY

Lymphedema results from a disturbance of the equilibrium between the amount of fluid in the interstitial space that needs to be cleared (capillary filtrate) and the capacity of the lymphatic and venous systems to remove this fluid. Possible etiologies include: (1) overload of the lymphatic system, (2) inadequate collection by the lymphatic terminal buds, (3) abnormal lymphatic contractility, (4) insufficient lymphatics, (5) lymph node obstruction, and (6) central vessel (i.e., thoracic duct) defects. Regardless of cause, when capillary filtration exceeds the combined resorptive capabilities of the venous and lymphatic systems, edema results. This edema is relatively protein-rich (2 to 5 g/dl). Because of the resultant high osmotic pressure, additional fluid is pulled into the interstitial space, worsening the edema. If the lymphatic system cannot adequately drain this interstitial fluid, collagen deposition and fibrosis may result. Hence, although the early stages are reversible, chronic edema is associated with thickening and fibrosis of tissues, making treatment difficult. The domestic species most commonly reported to have lymphedema is the dog.

Lymphedema may occur as a result of a primary defect in the lymphatic system or may be secondary to other diseases or surgical procedures. Distinguishing between primary and secondary lymphedema is often difficult. Lymph node obstruction, although more commonly associated with secondary lymphedema, has been associated with primary lymphedema. Many of the dogs reported with primary lymphedema have had small or absent lymph nodes. Perhaps the initial defect in some dogs with lymphedema is fibrosis of the lymph nodes, leading to secondary obstructive changes in the lymphatic vessels. As the vessels dilate, they lose contractility, and the lymphatic valves become permanently nonfunctional. Secondary lymphedema may be caused by conditions that increase the rate of interstitial fluid formation as a result of altered capillary permeability (e.g., trauma, heat, irradiation, or infection). Venous congestion (i.e., because of heart failure) may also cause lymphedema by decreasing fluid resorption. Examples of secondary lymphedema include that resulting from neoplasia or infiltration of lymph nodes by filaria (such as *Wuchereria bancrofti, Brugia timori*) and that which is secondary to lymphoproliferative disorders.

☞ **NOTE** · Lymphedema may be caused by primary lymphatic abnormalities or may be secondary to other diseases or surgery. It is often difficult to distinguish between primary and secondary lymphedema. Age of onset of clinical signs does not help distinguish in many cases because middle-aged animals may have acute signs of lymphedema secondary to congenital lymphatic abnormalities.

Clinical Presentation

Signalment. Primary lymphedema is usually noted at birth or shortly thereafter; however, older animals may develop lymphedema associated with congenital abnormalities. The lymphatic system may function normally until a precipitating cause (e.g., infection or trauma) overwhelms the marginal lymphatic system. Congenital, hereditary lymphedema has been reported in bulldogs and poodles. A sex predisposition is not evident.

☞ **NOTE** · Congenital lymphatic abnormalities may not cause lymphedema until the animal is several years old. Clinical signs of primary lymphedema may be precipitated by infection, trauma, or surgery.

History. The age of onset, progression of disease, extent of involvement (unilateral versus bilateral, pelvic limb versus forelimb), and history of previous surgery, trauma, or exposure to infectious agents should be ascertained. Lymphedema typically presents as a spontaneous, painless swelling of the extremities, with pitting edema. The onset may be insidious. The rear limbs are more commonly affected, and unilateral swelling may be present. Lymphedema usually begins in the distal extremity and progresses proximally. In severely affected animals, all four limbs and the trunk may be edematous. Although the patient may be less active than normal because of the weight of the limb or may carry the limb when ambulating, lameness and pain are uncommon without massive enlargement or cellulitis.

Physical Examination Findings

The diagnosis of lymphedema is usually made on the basis of clinical signs (Fig. 20-5). The limb is generally not excessively warm or cool. Although frequently bilateral, the degree of swelling is often greater in one limb. Occasionally, the swelling may be precipitated by minor trauma and/or superficial skin infections. As the edema becomes chronic, fibrosis occurs, and the edema will tend to progressively pit less, until pitting is absent. With chronic edema, massage and rest will not appreciably decrease the size of the limb.

Lymphography/Lymphoscintigraphy

The classic diagnostic tool has been direct lymphography (see below for a description of the technique). Oil-based contrast media are contraindicated in patients with primary lymphedema, because the high volume of contrast medium necessary to visualize the lymphatics and the propensity for extravasation may further damage existing lymphatics. Lymphoscintigraphy is an alternative approach for imaging peripheral lymphatics that involves the intradermal injection of high-molecular weight, radiolabeled colloids.

Laboratory Findings

Specific laboratory abnormalities are not found.

DIFFERENTIAL DIAGNOSIS

The key differential diagnosis is abnormality of the venous system, such as venous stasis or arteriovenous fistula. Clinical signs are usually adequate to differentiate lymphedema from edema caused by venous obstruction. Typical changes in the latter include varices, stasis hyperpigmentation, and cutaneous ulceration. Arteriovenous fistulae are vascular ab-

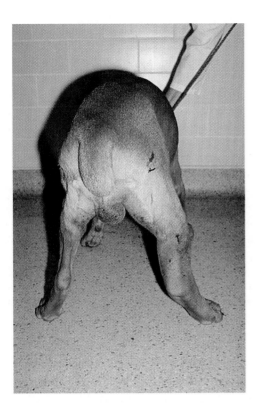

FIG. 20-5
A 2-year-old boxer with lymphedema. Note the massive swelling of the right rear limb.

TABLE 20-1
Benzopyrones for the Treatment of Lymphedema
Rutin*
50 mg/kg PO, TID
*This is one drug in the family of benzopyrones; other drugs may be as or more effective. The dose is an extrapolation of that used in people; side effects appear rare, but controlled studies have not been performed.

by removing fluid from the tissues; proteins that are not reabsorbed become increasingly concentrated, causing further tissue damage.

☞ **NOTE** • Medical therapy is often ineffective in substantially reducing swelling caused by lymphedema; however, medical management has received little attention in veterinary medicine. Amputation is a reasonable alternative for unilateral lymphedema, particularly when it interferes with limb function and initial medical management is ineffective.

The benzopyrones comprise a group of drugs that can be used to successfully treat experimental lymphedema in dogs and spontaneous lymphedema in human beings. All drugs in this group appear to reduce high-protein edema. Their main action appears to be stimulation of macrophages, which promotes proteolysis. Protein fragments can then be reabsorbed into the blood. These drugs are active orally and topically, are inexpensive, and are relatively free of side effects. Included in this category of drugs are coumarin (5,6 benzo-[alpha]-pyrone), O-(B-hydroxy-ethyl)-rutosides, diosmin, and rutin. Recommended dosages for human beings are 440 mg/day of coumarin and 3 g/day for rutosides, diosmin, and rutin (Table 20-1). Although these drugs (e.g., rutin) are being investigated in spontaneous lymphedema in dogs, their efficacy is currently uncertain.

normalities in which there are direct communications between an adjacent artery and vein. They may be acquired (following trauma, neoplasia, infection, or iatrogenic ligation of an artery and vein together) or congenital. Clinical signs with arteriovenous fistulae vary, depending on location; however, palpation of strong pulsatile vessels, often with a fremitus or "thrill," and auscultation of a machinery murmur, or bruit, are classic findings. Angiography is necessary to confirm the diagnosis and determine the size, extent, and location of the fistula. Physical examination should eliminate systemic causes of bilateral edema, including heart failure, renal failure, cirrhosis, and hypoproteinemia. Other differential diagnoses include trauma, neoplasia, and foreign bodies.

MEDICAL MANAGEMENT

In the early stages of lymphedema, before the development of fibrosis, nonsurgical therapy may decrease the swelling and make the patient more comfortable. Nonsurgical therapy consists of heavy bandages or splints that exert pressure on the limb, meticulous care of the skin to avoid infection, weight control, and appropriate use of antibiotics to treat and prevent cellulitis and lymphangitis. Drugs that have been used to treat human patients with lymphedema include steroids, diuretics, anticoagulants, and fibrinolysin inhibitors. For the most part, the proposed benefits of these pharmaceuticals have not been substantiated. Long-term treatment of lymphedema with diuretics, which initially decrease the size of the limb, is contraindicated. Diuretics act

SURGICAL TREATMENT

With the exception of amputation, no current surgical treatment offers a cure for lymphedema. Numerous therapies have been described in human patients, including lymphangioplasty, bridging procedures, lymphaticovenous shunts, omental transposition, superficial to deep anastomosis, and excision (with or without skin grafting). These techniques have not been adequately evaluated in dogs with spontaneous lymphedema. Lymphangiography rarely provides information that helps manage animals with spontaneous lymphedema, but occasionally defines the underlying lymphatic abnormality (i.e., hypoplasia, aplasia, or hyperplasia of lymphatics). It is a tool that must be correlated with other historical and physical findings. Biopsies of affected tissues should be submitted because lymphangiosarcoma, a highly malignant neoplasm, has been reported to occur in human beings with long-standing lymphedema. The technique for lymphangiography is described below.

> ☞ **N O T E** • Biopsies should be performed in lymphedematous animals to rule out neoplasia. Neoplastic transformation of chronically edematous tissue may occur.

Preoperative Management

Perioperative antibiotics are indicated in patients undergoing lymphangiography because there is a high risk of subsequent lymphangitis. Before other preoperative procedures, inject 1 ml of 3% Evans Blue dye between the second and third or third and fourth digits, to aid in the visualization and cannulation of lymphatics.

Anesthesia

General anesthesia is required for direct lymphangiography.

Surgical Anatomy

The lymphatic system of the extremities can be divided into two parts, the superficial lymphatics and the deep, or muscular, lymphatics. The superficial system appears to be the one most commonly involved in lymphedema. This is the system of lymphatics observed during pedal lymphangiography (Fig. 20-6). These lymphatics empty into a valved group of vessels that are found at the junction of the dermis and subcutaneous tissue. Lymph then drains into afferent lymphatics located in the subcutaneous fat. The superficial lymphatics of the pelvic limb consist of a larger medial group and a smaller lateral group. Lymphatics follow the branches of the medial saphenous vein and drain into the superficial inguinal lymph nodes. Efferent lymphatics from the lymph nodes drain into the larger lymphatic ducts. The deeper lymphatics drain the fascial planes surrounding skeletal muscles (lymphatics are not found within skeletal muscle bundles), joints, and synovium. Deep lymphatic collector vessels accompany the main blood vessels of the extremities. Controversy exists as to whether the two lymphatic systems (superficial and deep) communicate; however, communications usually appear to be a result of lymphatic pathology or a response to abnormal lymph flow. The lumbar lymph trunks receive vessels from the pelvic limbs, abdominal lymph nodes, and the intestines before uniting to form the cisterna chyli.

Positioning

Position the animal on the radiology table in lateral recumbency, with the affected limb down and the opposite limb retracted from the x-ray field. Prepare and drape the dorsomedial aspect of the metatarsus for aseptic surgery.

Technique for Direct Lymphangiography

Make a 5-cm skin incision over the middorsomedial metatarsal region. Use sharp and blunt dissection until a blue-stained superficial metatarsal lymphatic vessel is identified (Fig. 20-7). Meticulously dissect the lymphatic

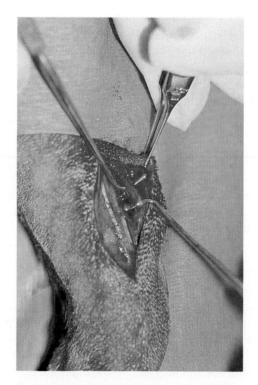

FIG. 20-7
Pedal lymphangiography. Evans' Blue dye is injected interdigitally before pedal lymphangiography. Then a 5-cm longitudinal incision is made on the dorsomedial aspect of the metatarsus. A combination of sharp and blunt dissection is used to identify the blue-stained superficial metatarsal lymphatic vessel. The lymphatic must be meticulously cleared of all subcutaneous tissues, using small blunt probes.

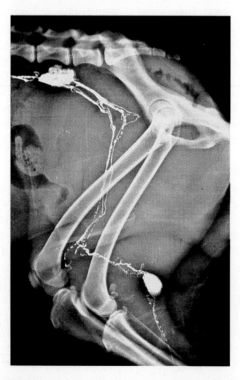

FIG. 20-6
Pedal lymphangiogram in a dog. The superficial lymphatic system is filled with contrast.

free from surrounding tissue with fine, blunt dissection probes, and cannulate the lymphatic, using a lymph duct cannulator or a 27- or 30-gauge over-the-needle catheter. Inject a small amount of sterile saline into the catheter or cannulator to verify patency. Then manually infuse an aqueous-based radiographic contrast agent into the lymphatic vessel. Take radiographs immediately following the injection (Fig. 20-8); additional radiographs may be made, depending on the rate of lymphatic transport of the contrast agent, which varies from patient to patient. Upon completion of the lymphangiogram, withdraw the cannulator, ligate the lymphatic vessel, and close the incision in a routine fashion.

SUTURE MATERIALS/SPECIAL INSTRUMENTS

A commercial lymphatic duct cannulator, such as a Tegtmeyer lymph duct cannulator, may facilitate cannulation of the lymphatic vessel.

POSTOPERATIVE CARE AND ASSESSMENT

If the lymphatics appear abnormal in character or quantity, or if an obvious obstruction is not noted on the lymphangiogram, then medical therapy or amputation should be considered. The patient should be observed for swelling or worsening of the edema, following the procedure.

PROGNOSIS

Primary lymphedema seldom resolves spontaneously. Neoplastic alteration of chronic lymphedematous tissue has been reported in human beings and may be a concern in animals.

Suggested Reading

Fossum TW, Miller MW: Lymphedema. I. Etiopathogenesis, *J Vet Int Med* 6:283, 1992.

Fossum TW et al: Lymphedema. II. Clinical signs, diagnosis, and treatment, *J Vet Int Med* 6:312, 1992.

Leighton RL, Suter PF: Primary lymphedema of the hindlimb in the dog, *J Amer Vet Med Assoc* 175:369, 1975.

Prier JE, Schaffer B, Skelley JF: Direct lymphangiography in the dog, *J Amer Vet Med Assoc* 140:943, 1962.

Takahashi JL, Farrow CS, Presnell KR: Primary lymphedema in a dog: a case report, *J Amer Anim Hosp Assoc* 20:849, 1984.

Surgery of the Spleen

GENERAL PRINCIPLES AND TECHNIQUES

DEFINITIONS

Splenomegaly is enlargement of the spleen as a result of any cause. **Splenectomy** is surgical removal of the spleen. **Splenosis** is the congenital or traumatic presence of multiple nodules of normal splenic tissue in the abdomen. **Siderotic plaques** are brown or rust-colored deposits of iron and calcium that may be found on the splenic surface (Fig. 20-9).

PREOPERATIVE CONCERNS

Animals presenting with surgical diseases of the spleen often have either diffuse or focal splenomegaly. Diffuse (symmetric) splenomegaly may be attributed to congestion (e.g., splenic torsion, right-sided heart failure, gastric dilatation-volvulus, or drugs) or infiltration as a result of infection (e.g., fungal, bacteria, or viral), immune-mediated disease (e.g., immune-mediated thrombocytopenia), or neoplasia (e.g., lymphosarcoma or feline mastocytosis). Focal (asymmetric) splenomegaly may be caused by benign (e.g., nodular regeneration, hematoma [see p. 456], or trauma) or

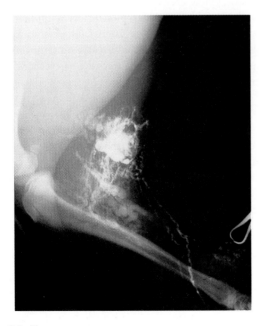

FIG. 20-8
Lymphangiogram of a dog with lymphedema. Note the dilated, tortuous lymphatics. Compare this to the lymphangiogram of a normal dog in Fig. 20-6.

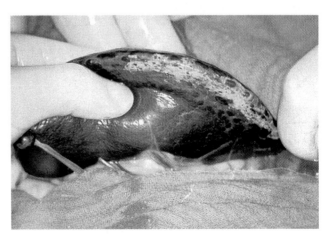

FIG. 20-9
Siderotic plaques on the splenic surface.

neoplastic processes (e.g., hemangiosarcoma [see p. 456]). Infiltrative splenomegaly resulting from neoplasia is one of the most common causes of spontaneous (noniatrogenic) splenomegaly in dogs and cats.

Anemia may be present because of acute hemorrhage associated with splenic trauma or hematoma rupture, or associated with the underlying disease (i.e., chronic infection, immune-mediated disease, or disseminated intravascular coagulation). Coagulation profiles should be performed in animals with evidence of bleeding not thought to be the result of trauma. Normally hydrated animals with a PCV less than 20% or hemoglobin less than 5 to 7 g/dl may benefit from preoperative blood transfusions (Table 20-2). If disseminated intravascular hemolysis is suspected, heparin therapy may be indicated (Table 20-3). Intravenous fluids should be administered to dehydrated animals before surgery.

ANESTHETIC CONSIDERATIONS

Anemic patients should be given oxygen before induction and during recovery. Anticholinergic drugs may be used to prevent bradycardia. Barbiturates that cause splenic congestion should be avoided. Acepromazine should also be avoided in these patients because of potential red blood cell sequestration, hypotension, and impact on platelet function. There may be a hypotensive episode as a result of volume depletion after splenectomy, and arterial blood pressure should be monitored carefully during surgery.

ANTIBIOTICS

Antibiotic use in most animals with splenic disease is dictated by the nature of the underlying disease. The merit of perioperative prophylactic antibiotics for splenectomy in dogs is largely unknown and depends on the animal's age,

concurrent disease, and length of surgery. Perioperative antibiotics in healthy animals are usually unnecessary, but may be given at induction and discontinued within 24 hours. Longer-term antibiotic therapy may be warranted in animals that are immunosuppressed or severely debilitated. A case of multiple abscessation, septicemia, and death associated with splenectomy performed in conjunction with dental cleaning and extraction has been reported.

SURGICAL ANATOMY

The spleen is situated in the left cranial abdominal quadrant. It usually lies parallel to the greater curvature of the stomach; however, its exact location is dependent on its size and on the position of other abdominal organs. When the stomach is contracted, the spleen usually lies within the rib cage, but with massive gastric enlargement it may be in the caudal abdomen. The splenic capsule is composed of elastic and smooth muscle fibers. The parenchyma consists of a white pulp (i.e., lymphoid tissue) and red pulp (i.e., venous sinuses and cellular tissue filling the intravascular spaces). Large numbers of α-adrenergic receptors are responsible for splenic contraction. When the spleen is contracted, it feels firm in consistency. The spleen is normally red in color, but siderotic plaques or fibrin deposits may alter its appearance.

The arterial supply of the spleen is usually the splenic artery, a branch of the celiac artery. The splenic artery is generally over 2 mm in diameter and gives off three to five long primary branches as it courses in the greater omentum toward the ventral third of the spleen. The first branch is usually to the pancreas and is the main supply of the left limb of that organ. The two remaining branches run toward the proximal half of the spleen, where they send 20 to 30 splenic branches that enter the parenchyma. The branches then continue in the gastrosplenic ligament to the great curvature of the stomach, where they form the short gastric arteries (supplies fundus) and left gastroepiploic artery (supplies greater curvature of the stomach) (Fig. 20-10). Other branches supply the splenocolic ligament and greater omentum. Venous drainage is via the splenic vein into the gastrosplenic vein, which empties into the portal vein.

SURGICAL TECHNIQUES

The spleen is approached via a ventral midline abdominal incision that extends from the xiphoid to a point caudal to the umbilicus. The incision may need to be lengthened for large lesions or to allow complete abdominal exploration. Complete abdominal exploration should be performed in any animal with suspected neoplasia.

Splenic Biopsy

Splenic biopsies are indicated to ascertain the cause of clinically significant splenomegaly or suspected metastatic lesions to the spleen. They may be obtained percutaneously, by fine-needle aspiration, or at surgery. Ultrasound-guided biopsies improve the likelihood of obtaining diagnostic samples percutaneously. Percutaneous biopsies are often diagnostic for diffuse lesions (e.g., mastocytosis or lymphosar-

---

TABLE 20-2

Blood Transfusions

ml of Donor Blood Needed

$$\text{Recipient blood volume*} \times \frac{\text{Desired PCV} - \text{Actual patient PCV}}{\text{PCV of anticoagulated donor blood}}$$

*Total blood volume is estimated at 90 ml/kg for dogs and 70 ml/kg for cats.
Note: A rough estimate is that 2.2 ml of blood/kg of body weight will increase the recipient's PCV by 1%.

TABLE 20-3

Heparin Therapy for DIC

Heparin
50-100 U/kg SC, BID or TID

Heparin-Activated Plasma
(Incubate 5-10 U heparin/kg body weight with 1 U fresh plasma for 30 minutes); give 10 ml/kg IV

coma); however, focal or nodular lesions may be missed. Differentiation of hemangiosarcoma and hematoma with cytologic analysis of samples obtained by fine-needle aspiration is rarely possible (see p. 457). When cavitary lesions are identified with ultrasound, fine-needle aspiration should be performed with care, or not at all. Rupture of cavitary lesions may occur during aspiration and be fatal, especially in animals with coagulopathies.

Biopsy samples should be placed in 10 volumes of formalin to 1 part tissue for routine hematoxylin and eosin staining. Special preservatives may be required if additional staining techniques are desired (e.g., for identification of viral inclusions, Bouin's fixative is preferred). Samples that are larger than 5 cm should be scored (cut into) before placement in formalin, to allow the sample to fix properly. Large splenic masses should be scored at multiple sites, but left intact to allow identification of the entire lesion and its relationships by the pathologist. If this is not possible, multiple representative samples should be submitted from diverse sites, including the margin of the abnormal and normal-appearing tissues. If the lesion is cavitary (i.e., splenic mass, cyst, or abscess), it should be ruptured before placing in formalin.

Splenic aspiration. *Place the animal in right lateral or dorsal recumbency, using manual restraint or mild sedation. Avoid using phenothiazine tranquilizers or barbiturates because the resultant splenic congestion may cause a nondiagnostic sample as a result of blood dilution. Surgically prep a small area on the left side of the abdomen, and isolate the spleen. Using a plastic syringe attached to a small needle (23 or 25 gauge, 1 to 1.5 in), penetrate the abdominal wall and advance the needle into the spleen. Apply suction on the syringe several times. Before removing the needle from the abdomen, relieve suction on the syringe to prevent aspirating the contents of the needle into the syringe. Remove the needle from the abdomen, and place the specimen on a slide for evaluation.*

Surgical biopsy. During celiotomy, focal lesions may be biopsied by fine-needle aspiration or with a Tru-cut (see p. 370), Jamshidi, modified Franklin-Silverman, or punch biopsy. *To remove focal lesions near the center of the spleen, make a rectangular or oval incision through the capsule and into the parenchyma, to sufficient depth to remove the lesion. Close the defect by placing simple interrupted or mattress sutures of absorbable material (3-0 or 4-0) in the splenic capsule.* Partial splenectomy may be performed if more diffuse lesions are present (see below).

Repair of Lacerations

Splenorrhaphy is indicated to provide hemostasis in superficial traumatic lesions of the splenic capsule. *Explore the lesion and ligate any large traumatized vessels. Place simple interrupted or mattress sutures of absorbable material (3-0 or 4-0) in the splenic capsule. Apply gentle pressure to the area for several minutes. If bleeding continues, ligate the splenic branches supplying the lesion as close to the hilus of the spleen as possible. Small areas of ischemia will revascularize as a result of collateralization.*

Partial Splenectomy

Partial splenectomy is indicated in animals with traumatic or focal lesions of the spleen, to preserve splenic function. *Define the area of the spleen to be removed, and double ligate and incise hilar vessels supplying the area (Fig. 20-11, A). Note the extent of ischemia that develops, and use this as a guideline for the resection. Squeeze the splenic tissue at this line between a thumb and forefinger, and milk the splenic pulp toward the ischemic area. Place forceps on the flattened portion, and divide the spleen between the forceps (Fig. 20-11, B). Close the cut surface of the spleen adjacent to the forceps with a continuous suture pattern of absorbable suture material (3-0 or 4-0 [Fig. 20-11, C]). Alternatively, place two rows of mattress sutures in a continuous overlapping fashion at the line of demarcation. If hemorrhage continues, oversew the end of the spleen with a continuous suture of absorbable suture material.* Automated stapling devices (e.g., TA staplers) may also

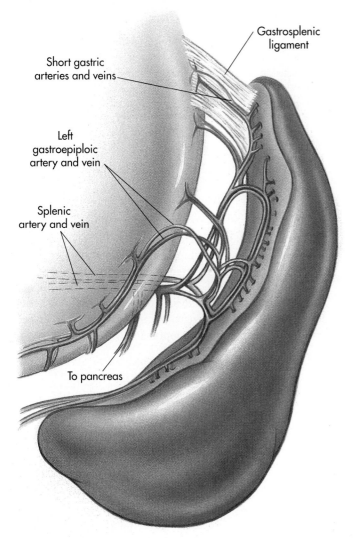

FIG. 20-10
Splenic vasculature. Note the short gastric arteries, which are often avulsed in dogs with gastric dilatation-volvulus.

Labels on figure:
Gastrosplenic ligament
Short gastric arteries and veins
Left gastroepiploic artery and vein
Splenic artery and vein
To pancreas

FIG. 20-11
Partial splenectomy preserves splenic function in animals with traumatic or focal lesions. **A,** Define the area of the spleen to be removed and double ligate and incise hilar vessels supplying the area. **B,** Transect the spleen between forceps, and **C,** close the cut surface with a continuous suture pattern.

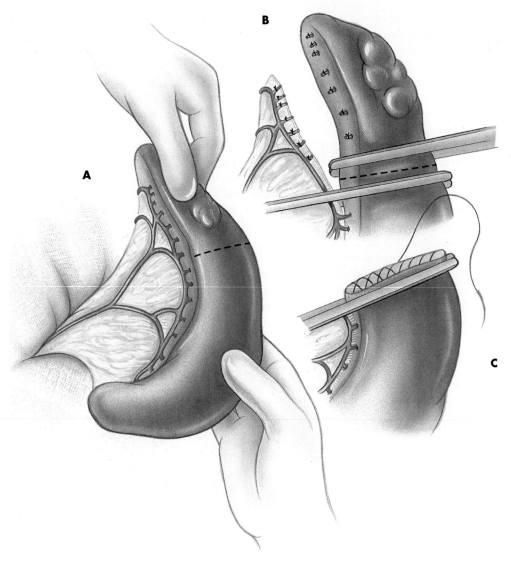

be used for partial splenectomy; however, there is some risk that if the staples are not secured in sufficient tissue, they will loosen and allow hemorrhage to occur from the splenic stump. Either 3.5- or 4.8-sized stainless steel staples are recommended. When properly performed, surgical stapling for partial splenectomy significantly decreases surgical time and decreases omental adhesion to the spleen.

Total Splenectomy

Total splenectomy is most commonly performed in animals with splenic neoplasia, torsion (stomach or spleen), or severe trauma. Splenectomy has previously been advocated for immune-mediated hematologic disorders refractory to medical therapy (e.g., thrombocytopenia or hemolytic anemia); however, proper use of immunosuppressive drugs and corticosteroids has decreased the need for splenectomy. However, splenectomy may be used if drug therapy is unsuccessful or unacceptable. Although life-threatening sepsis has been associated with total splenectomy in humans, this has not been recognized in dogs. However, partial splenectomy is preferred over total splenectomy, when possible. The major dis-

advantages of total splenectomy are loss of its reservoir, immune-defense, and hematopoiesis and filtration functions. Elective splenectomy is often performed in dogs used as blood donors, to reduce the risk of transferring *Ehrlichia* sp., *Hemobartonella* sp., or *Babesia* sp. to noninfected animals during transfusions. Splenectomy is contraindicated in patients with bone marrow hypoplasia in which the spleen is a main site of hematopoiesis.

After exploring the abdomen, exteriorize the spleen, and place moistened abdominal sponges or laparotomy pads around the incision under the spleen. Double ligate and transect all vessels at the splenic hilus with absorbable (preferred) or nonabsorbable suture material (Fig. 20-12). Preserve the short gastric branches supplying the gastric fundus, if possible. Alternatively, open the omental bursa, and isolate the splenic artery. Identify the branch(es) supplying the left limb of the pancreas. Double ligate and transect the splenic artery distal to this vessel(s). Interference with blood flow through the pancreatic branch of the splenic artery may result in ischemic pancreatitis and peritonitis.

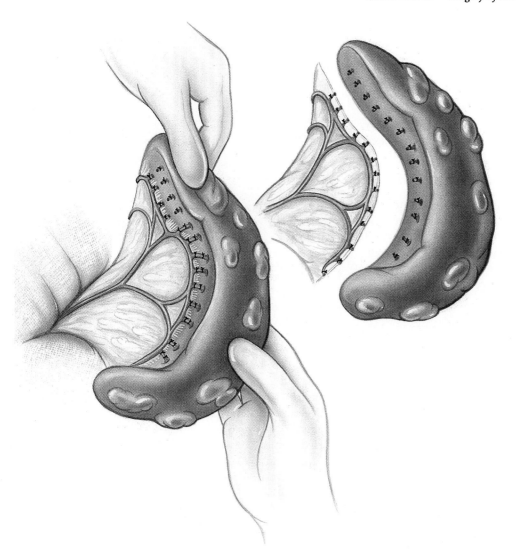

FIG. 20-12
For total splenectomy, double ligate and transect all vessels at the splenic hilus. Preserve the short gastric branches supplying the gastric fundus, if possible.

☞ **NOTE** • Spare the short gastric arteries when performing splenectomy, if possible.

SUTURE MATERIALS/SPECIAL INSTRUMENTS

Other than a general soft-tissue pack, special instruments are not required; however, a large number of clamps should be available for splenectomy. Absorbable suture material is generally used for splenic surgery. If generalized peritonitis is present, monofilament synthetic absorbable suture material should be used for vessel ligation (e.g., polydioxanone or polyglyconate).

POSTOPERATIVE CARE AND ASSESSMENT

Following splenic biopsy or splenectomy, the animal should be closely observed for 24 hours for evidence of hemorrhage. The hematocrit should be evaluated every few hours until the animal is stable. Nasal oxygen should be administered to anemic patients and analgesics given, if necessary (see Table 21-5 on p. 469). Hemorrhage may be indicative of technical failures or disseminated intravascular coagulation (which may occur following removal of large neoplastic lesions or torsed spleens). Fluid therapy should be continued until the animal is able to maintain its own hydration, and electrolytes and acid-base abnormalities should be corrected. Mild postoperative leukocytosis may occur following splenectomy in dogs because the spleen influences bone-marrow leukocyte production; however, large or prolonged elevations may indicate infection (i.e., splenic abscess or peritonitis). Increased numbers of Howell-Jolly bodies, nucleated erythrocytes, target cells, or platelets may also be found postsplenectomy.

COMPLICATIONS

The major complication of splenic surgery is hemorrhage. This is more of a problem with splenic biopsies or partial splenectomy than with total splenectomy, providing proper technique is used for vessel ligation. In one study of 31 dogs undergoing total splenectomy, 19 showed postoperative complications, although none were thought to be directly related to the splenectomy or asplenism (Hosgood, 1987). Reported complications of splenectomy in dogs include abscessation, traumatic pancreatitis, and gastric fistulation (as a result of impairment of gastric blood flow). The risk of developing septic complications following splenectomy appears to be significant only in those animals that are immunosuppressed before surgery (e.g., immunosuppressive therapy for immune-mediated hemolytic anemia).

SPECIAL AGE CONSIDERATIONS

Splenic surgery is most commonly performed in middle-aged or older animals. Special care must be taken to meet the metabolic and nutritional needs of these animals. Physical examinations and laboratory analyses should be thorough, to determine if concurrent disease exists that may influence the surgery or postoperative care.

Reference

Hosgood G: Splenectomy in the dog: a retrospective study of 31 cases, *J Am Anim Hosp Assoc* 23:275, 1987.

Suggested Reading

Couto CG: A diagnostic approach to splenomegaly in cats and dogs, *Vet Med* 85:220, 1990.
Feldman BF, Handagama P, Lubberink AAME: Splenectomy as adjunctive therapy for immune-mediated thrombocytopenia and hemolytic anemia in the dog, *J Am Vet Med Assoc* 187:617, 1985.
Hosgood G et al: Splenectomy in the dog by ligation of the splenic and short gastric arteries, *Vet Surg* 18:110, 1989.
Waldron DR, Robertson J: Partial splenectomy in the dog: a comparison of stapling and ligation techniques, *J Am Anim Hosp Assoc* 31:343, 1995.

SPECIFIC DISEASES

SPLENIC TORSION

DEFINITIONS

Splenic torsion occurs when the spleen twists on its vascular pedicle.

GENERAL CONSIDERATIONS AND CLINICALLY RELEVANT PATHOPHYSIOLOGY

Splenic torsion most commonly occurs in association with gastric dilatation-volvulus. Isolated splenic torsion is rare, but is reported in dogs (Fig. 20-13). Typically, the thin-walled splenic vein is occluded, although the splenic artery remains partially patent, resulting in congestive splenomegaly. Vascular thrombosis (particularly of the splenic vein) may occur. In some dogs, clinical signs are acute, although in others the torsion is presumably intermittent, and abnormalities are first noted weeks before diagnosis.

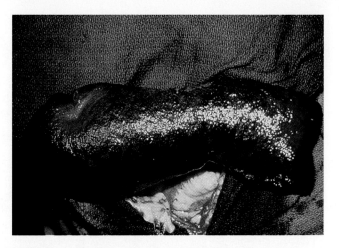

FIG. 20-13
Torsed spleen in a dog with acute cardiovascular collapse and shock. Note the dark, congested appearance of the spleen.

The cause of isolated splenic torsion is uncertain. It may be related to congenital abnormalities or traumatic disruption of the gastrosplenic or splenocolic ligaments. It also has been hypothesized that splenic torsion may occur after partial gastric torsion (i.e., an intermittently malpositioned stomach), in which it is thought that the spleen remains torsed despite repositioning of the stomach.

Splenic infarction may be associated with other diseases (e.g., liver disease, renal disease, hyperadrenocorticism, neoplasia, or thrombosis associated with cardiovascular disease). Splenic infarction in these dogs appears to be a sign of altered blood flow and coagulation, rather than of the primary disease. In such cases, splenectomy should be reserved for those animals that have life-threatening complications, such as hemoabdomen or sepsis.

☞ **N O T E** · Splenic torsion can be acute and life-threatening, requiring prompt diagnosis and treatment.

DIAGNOSIS
Clinical Presentation

Signalment. Splenic torsion usually occurs in large-breed dogs (e.g., Great Danes), with no age or sex predilection.

History. Most animals present because of some combination of vomiting, weakness or depression, icterus, hematuria or hemoglobinuria, abdominal pain, and/or diarrhea. Clinical signs may be acute or chronic. Some owners have reported chronic intermittent signs for up to 3 weeks before evaluation. Acute torsion may cause signs of cardiovascular collapse and shock.

Physical Examination Findings

The most prominent physical examination finding is splenic enlargement or a midabdominal mass. Abdominal pain, fever, dehydration, pale mucous membranes, and/or icterus are sometimes found. Dogs with cardiovascular collapse and shock present with tachycardia, pale mucous membranes, prolonged capillary refill times, and/or weak peripheral pulses.

Radiography/Ultrasonography

The most common radiographic findings are decreased visceral detail associated with peritoneal effusion and small intestine displacement. The splenic outline is often difficult to discern; however, if the dorsal extremity or body of the spleen is not observed in its normal position, splenic torsion is suggested. Occasionally, gas bubbles within the spleen may be identified, presumably formed by gas-producing bacteria (e.g., *Clostridium* sp.). Ultrasonography may reveal a markedly enlarged spleen that is diffusely hypoechoic, with linear echoes separating large, anechoic areas. This pattern may be unique to splenic torsion. Enlargement of hilar splenic vessels may also be suggestive of this condition.

☞ **NOTE** · Ultrasonography is the most useful noninvasive diagnostic tool for evaluating the spleen.

Laboratory Findings

Laboratory analysis may reveal anemia, leukocytosis, hemoglobinuria, elevated serum alkaline phosphatase activity, and/or elevated alanine transaminase activity.

DIFFERENTIAL DIAGNOSIS

Differentials include other causes of splenomegaly (i.e., neoplasia, trauma, hematoma, abscess, or immune-mediated disease), peritoneal effusion (i.e., peritonitis or ascites), other midabdominal masses (e.g., gastrointestinal, pancreatic, renal, or lymph node enlargement), and gastric dilatation-volvulus.

MEDICAL MANAGEMENT

Splenic torsion is a surgical disease; medical management is usually limited to stabilizing the animal for surgery (see discussion below under Preoperative Management). If the animal is shocky, intravenous fluids and antibiotic therapy should be initiated.

SURGICAL TREATMENT

The timing of surgical therapy is influenced by the animal's status at presentation. Animals presenting with signs of shock should be operated on as quickly as possible after they have been stabilized. Surgery may be reasonably delayed for short periods in animals with chronic disease; however, prompt surgical intervention is recommended. Gastric dilatation-volvulus may occur in dogs following splenic torsion and stretching of the gastric ligaments. Thus prophylactic gastropexy (see p. 270) may be warranted at the time of splenectomy.

Preoperative Management

Fluid deficits and electrolyte and acid-base abnormalities should be corrected before surgery, if possible. Whole blood administration is warranted in animals with hematocrits less than 20% (see Table 20-2). Perioperative antibiotic therapy is recommended, because vascular occlusion and necrosis may allow proliferation of bacteria within the spleen. Electrocardiograms are warranted to determine if cardiac arrhythmias are present that may require therapy before anesthetic induction or during surgery. The enlarged and congested spleen may rupture with handling, causing abdominal hemorrhage; therefore blood transfusion products should be available.

Anesthesia

See gastric dilatation-volvulus on p. 277 for anesthetic recommendations. Avoid barbiturates or other drugs that cause splenic congestion.

Surgical Anatomy

Refer to p. 450 for surgical anatomy of the spleen.

Positioning

The animal is positioned in dorsal recumbency, and the entire ventral abdomen is prepared for aseptic surgery. The ventral incision should extend from the xiphoid and should be long enough to allow the enlarged spleen to be manipulated and exteriorized.

SURGICAL TECHNIQUE

The treatment of splenic torsion is somewhat controversial. Some authors recommend that in animals with acute torsion, the splenic pedicle be untwisted and the spleen repositioned. If vascular patency is present, restoration of blood flow will cause the spleen to decrease to near-normal size within a few minutes. Splenectomy (see p. 452) may be safer, because there is no good way to secure the spleen in its normal position, and torsion may recur. Splenectomy is the only viable option in animals in whom the vascular pedicle cannot be untwisted because of fibrosis, splenic rupture, or vascular thrombosis.

SUTURE MATERIALS/SPECIAL INSTRUMENTS

Refer to p. 453 for suture materials for splenectomy.

POSTOPERATIVE CARE AND ASSESSMENT

Most animals recover quickly following repositioning or removal of the torsed spleen. Intravenous fluid therapy should be continued until the animal is able to maintain its own hydration. Vomiting may occur postoperatively, associated with pancreatic ischemia and pancreatitis. The blood supply to the left limb of the pancreas arises from the splenic artery, and the vascular obstruction may extend to this pancreatic branch.

PROGNOSIS

The prognosis is generally good following surgical management of splenic torsion. Delayed diagnosis may result in splenic necrosis, sepsis, peritonitis, and/or disseminated intravascular coagulation.

Suggested Reading

Hardie EM et al: Splenic infarction in 16 dogs: a retrospective study, *J Vet Int Med* 9:141, 1995.

Konde LJ et al: Sonographic and radiographic changes associated with splenic torsion in the dog, *Vet Radiol* 30:41, 1989.

Maxie MG et al: Splenic torsion in three Great Danes, *Can Vet J* 11:249, 1970.

Mills DL et al: Gastric dilatation-volvulus after splenic torsion in two dogs, *J Am Vet Med Assoc* 207:314, 1995.

O'Neill JA: Managing an unusual case of splenic torsion, *Vet Med* 80:35, 1985.

Stickle GRL: Radiographic signs of isolated splenic torsion in dogs: eight cases (1980-1987), *J Am Vet Med Assoc* 194:103, 1989.

Wright RP, Callahan KE: Surgically treating a case of splenic torsion, *Vet Med* 82:532, 1987.

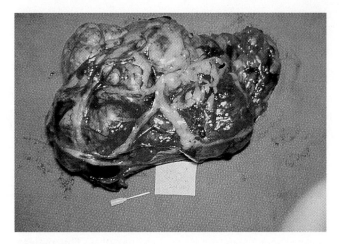

FIG. 20-14
Splenic leiomyosarcoma in a 6-year-old mixed-breed dog.

SPLENIC NEOPLASIA

DEFINITIONS

Hemangiosarcomas are malignant neoplasms that arise from blood vessels; **hemangiomas** are benign tumors of dilated blood vessels. A **hematoma** is a swelling, or mass of blood (usually clotted), confined to an organ, tissue, or space, and caused by seepage as a result of coagulopathy.

SYNONYMS

For hemangiosarcoma—**angiosarcoma, hemangioendothelioma**

GENERAL CONSIDERATIONS AND CLINICALLY RELEVANT PATHOPHYSIOLOGY

The spleen is composed of a variety of tissues, and splenic neoplasia may arise from blood vessels, lymphoid tissues, smooth muscle, or the connective tissue that makes up the fibrous stroma. The most common tumor in dogs is hemangiosarcoma. Other malignant (e.g., lymphosarcoma, mast cell tumor, leiomyosarcoma, fibrosarcoma, liposarcoma, osteosarcoma, chondrosarcoma, myxosarcoma, rhabdomyosarcoma, and fibrous histiocytoma) and benign (e.g., hemangiomas and myelolipidomas) neoplasms may also occur (Fig. 20-14). The most frequently recognized nonneoplastic lesions of the spleen are nodular hyperplasia and hematomas (Fig. 20-15). It has been hypothesized that splenic hematoma and nodular hyperplasia are related diseases. Nodular hyperplasia may cause bleeding by disrupting splenic blood flow.

Canine splenic hemangiosarcoma is more common than all other types of malignant splenic tumors combined. Hemangiosarcomas are observed in 0.3% to 2% of all canine necropsies. In one study of 1372 splenic samples submitted over a 4-year period, hyperplastic nodules were diagnosed most commonly (Spangler, Culbertson, 1992). Because hemangiosarcomas arise from blood vessels, they may form in several different sites of the body. Between

24% and 45% of dogs presenting with splenic hemangiosarcoma have concurrent right atrial hemangiosarcoma (Waters et al, 1988). Splenic hemangiosarcomas are aggressive tumors that frequently metastasize to liver, omentum, and mesentery. As many as 50% or more of affected dogs have gross evidence of metastatic disease on initial presentation. Lung metastases may be more common in dogs with right atrial tumors than in those without (Waters et al, 1988).

Splenic hematomas are variably sized, encapsulated, blood and fibrin-filled masses that are often grossly indistinguishable from hemangiosarcomas. Histologically, the cavities are surrounded by congestion, fibrosis, and areas of necrosis. They may result from trauma, occur spontaneously, or may be secondary to other diseases (e.g., nodular hyperplasia). Hemangiomas and hemangiosarcomas may be difficult to distinguish histologically, but because the prognosis for these lesions is very different (see below), it is important that they be accurately differentiated. Splenic masses with evidence of malignant neoplastic endothelial cell proliferation can be easily identified as hemangiosarcoma. However, multiple sections of a malignant mass may be studied without seeing obvious malignancy. More importantly, proliferation of plump endothelial cells that resemble neoplastic endothelium, but do not have evidence of mitotic activity, may be misdiagnosed as hemangiosarcoma.

Mastocytoma, lymphosarcoma, myeloproliferative disease, and hemangiosarcoma are the most common neoplasms of the feline spleen. Splenic involvement is a consistent finding in cats with noncutaneous systemic mastocytosis. It is not associated with FeLV and is primarily a disease of older cats. Mast cell infiltrates may also be recognized in other organs (i.e., liver, lymph nodes, and bone marrow), and circulating mastocytosis may be present in 50% of affected cats. Splenomegaly is one of the most common gross findings in mast cell disease, which is usually diagnosed by finding neoplastic cells in the circulation or on bone marrow examination. Splenic hemangiosarcoma is less commonly recognized in cats than in dogs. Extraabdominal

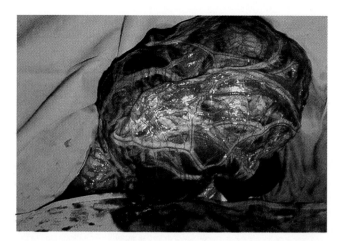

FIG. 20-15
Splenic hematoma in a 10-year-old Labrador retriever. Note the similar appearance of this benign mass to the malignant tumor in Fig. 20-14.

metastasis, particularly to the myocardium, appears to be common.

DIAGNOSIS
Clinical Presentation

Signalment. Splenic tumors (including hematomas) usually occur in medium-to-large sized dogs. German shepherd dogs are at increased risk for hemangiosarcoma and hemangioma. Some authors have reported that spayed female dogs have increased risk, although others have reported this tumor to occur more commonly in male dogs. No obvious breed or sex predilection has been observed in dogs with nonangiogenic and nonlymphomatous splenic sarcomas.

History. Dogs with hemangiosarcoma may present for abdominal enlargement, anorexia, lethargy, depression, and/or vomiting or may have acute signs of weakness, depression, anorexia, and hypovolemic shock caused by splenic rupture and hemorrhage. Clinical signs with splenic hematoma are similar, except that rupture leading to collapse and anorexia are less common because large masses frequently become apparent before rupture occurs. The most common clinical signs of disease with other types of sarcomas are decreased appetite, abdominal distention (as a result of peritoneal effusion and/or tumor mass), polydipsia, vomiting, and/or lethargy. In contrast to dogs with hemangiosarcoma, splenic rupture and hemorrhage are uncommon in dogs with nonangiogenic and nonlymphomatous splenic tumors.

Physical Examination Findings

Physical examination findings include lethargy, weakness, abdominal distention, and possibly splenomegaly or a splenic mass. If abdominal effusion is present, it is not always possible to palpate the enlarged spleen. If rupture occurs, the animal may present with signs of hypovolemic shock (tachycardia, pale mucous membranes, and weak peripheral pulses).

Radiography/Ultrasonography

Abdominal masses are usually detected radiographically in dogs with hemangiosarcoma and nonangiogenic and nonlymphomatous sarcomas; however, peritoneal fluid may make locating the lesion in the spleen difficult. Ultrasonography is more definitive in locating lesions in the spleen and detecting abdominal metastases. Differentiation of hematoma from neoplastic lesions is difficult with ultrasound. Finding internal septation and encapsulation or apparent metastasis helps differentiate hematoma from hemangiosarcoma. Thoracic radiographs should be taken to detect pulmonary or thoracic neoplasia.

☞ **NOTE** • Before surgery, echo the heart to look for right atrial hemangiosarcoma.

Laboratory Findings

Neutrophilic leukocytosis may be present in some dogs. Mild or moderate anemia associated with chronic disease and/or hemoperitoneum is also common. Other hematologic abnormalities resulting from hemangiosarcomas may include numerous nucleated blood cells (inappropriate numbers for the degree of anemia), Howell-Jolly bodies, poikilocytosis, acanthocytosis, schistocytosis, and/or thrombocytopenia. Hemostatic disorders, particularly thrombocytopenia caused by disseminated intravascular coagulation, are frequent in dogs with splenic tumors. Abdominal effusion is generally serosanguineous or hemorrhagic. Cytologic analysis of abdominal fluid rarely reveals tumor cells.

DIFFERENTIAL DIAGNOSIS

Splenic hematoma and hemangioma must be differentiated from hemangiosarcoma and other neoplastic diseases of the spleen (see comments above). When cavitary lesions are identified with ultrasound, fine-needle aspiration should be performed cautiously, or not at all. Diagnosis of hemangiosarcoma is difficult with fine-needle aspirates because the cells exfoliate poorly. Additionally, cytologic differentiation of hematoma and hemangiosarcoma with samples obtained by fine-needle aspiration is often impossible because large numbers of neoplastic cells are often necessary to make an accurate diagnosis. Further, rupture of cavitary lesions may occur during aspiration and be fatal. Exploratory surgery is usually indicated to differentiate them; however, it is difficult to differentiate these lesions by direct visualization. Although the presence of hepatic nodules may indicate metastasis and malignancy in dogs with splenic masses, the hepatic nodules may also represent extramedullary hematopoiesis or nodular hyperplasia in animals with benign or malignant tumors. Other causes of hemoperitoneum include hepatocellular carcinoma and rodenticide poisoning.

☞ **NOTE** • Diagnosis of splenic hemangiosarcoma may require that multiple histologic sections be reviewed.

MEDICAL MANAGEMENT

Surgical resection is the mainstay of therapy in dogs with splenic hemangiosarcoma, and there are few reports of postoperative chemotherapy or immunotherapy significantly prolonging survival. Readers are referred to an oncology text for discussion of protocols and treatment regimens used in dogs with hemangiosarcoma.

SURGICAL TREATMENT

Splenectomy is the treatment of choice for animals with splenic hematoma and hemangioma. It is also the treatment of choice for animals with hemangiosarcoma, in whom evidence of extensive metastasis or other organ failure does not preclude the short-term benefits of removing the enlarged and/or ruptured spleen. The median survival time of dogs with splenic hemangiosarcoma is between 10 and 23 weeks after splenectomy, depending on the stage of the disease (Johnson et al, 1989; Hammer, Couto, 1992). With nonangiogenic and nonlymphomatous sarcomas, the median survival times after splenectomy were 2.5 months for all dogs that survived the early postoperative period, and 9 months for the subset of dogs that did not have evidence of metastasis at surgery (Weinstein, Carpenter, Schunk, 1989). Splenectomy may not be warranted in dogs with concurrent right atrial tumors. Thus careful preoperative examination of patients is warranted. Dogs with splenic lymphoma and clinical signs associated with massive splenomegaly, splenic rupture, and hemoperitoneum may also benefit from splenectomy.

Preoperative Management

Anemic animals may require blood transfusions before surgery and should be preoxygenated. An ECG should be performed to determine if ventricular arrhythmias requiring preoperative or intraoperative therapy are present. Ventricular arrhythmias were documented in 22 of 78 dogs with splenic masses in one study, and anemia and hemoabdomen were found to be strongly associated with arrhythmia development (Keyes, 1992). Hydration, electrolyte, and acid-base abnormalities should be corrected before anesthesia. Perioperative antibiotics may be indicated in some animals undergoing splenectomy (see p. 450).

Anesthesia

See gastric dilatation-volvulus on p. 277 for recommendations for anesthesia. Avoid barbiturates or other drugs that cause splenic congestion.

Surgical Anatomy

Refer to p. 450 for surgical anatomy of the spleen.

Positioning

The animal is placed in dorsal recumbency for a ventral midline celiotomy (see p. 455).

SURGICAL TECHNIQUE

Splenectomy is described on p. 452. Total splenectomy, rather than partial splenectomy, is warranted in animals with malignant tumors or large benign masses.

☞ **NOTE** · It is difficult to differentiate hemangiosarcoma and hematoma. You must submit multiple samples for histopathology.

SUTURE MATERIALS/SPECIAL INSTRUMENTS

Surgical instruments for diseases of the spleen are described on p. 450. Poor healing may occur in patients with neoplasia (particularly in debilitated animals); thus care should be used in closing abdominal incisions, and strong, monofilament absorbable or nonabsorbable suture should be used.

POSTOPERATIVE CARE AND ASSESSMENT

Animals with splenic hemangiosarcoma should be closely observed for disseminated intravascular coagulation following splenectomy. Fluid therapy should be continued until the animal is able to maintain its own hydration. The hematocrit should be monitored and blood transfusions provided if the PCV is less than 20%. Septic complications following splenectomy appear to be rare, and antibiotic therapy can be discontinued within 24 hours in most animals.

☞ **NOTE** · Be prepared to treat cardiac arrhythmias, particularly if hemoabdomen and/or anemia are present.

PROGNOSIS

The prognosis for animals with hemangiosarcoma depends on whether clinical signs are apparent at the time of surgery. In one study, 76.4% of dogs that had hemoperitoneum at surgery had a median survival time of 17 days; whereas the median survival time was 121 days if splenectomy was performed before development of hemoperitoneum (Prymak et al, 1988). Most dogs with splenic hemangioma lived 1 year or more after surgery; however, the median survival for affected dogs was less than that of the control population in the aforementioned study.

References

Hammer AS, Couto CG: Diagnosing and treating canine hemangiosarcoma, *Vet Med* 87:188, 1992.

Johnson KA et al: Predictors of neoplasia and survival after splenectomy, *J Vet Intern Med* 3:160, 1989.

Keyes ML: Ventricular arrhythmias in dogs with splenic masses. *J Vet Intern Med* 6:140, 1992 (abstract).

Prymak C et al: Epidemiologic, clinical, pathologic, and prognostic characteristics of splenic hematoma in dogs: 217 cases (1985) *J Am Vet Med Assoc* 193:706, 1988.

Spangler WL, Culbertson MR: Prevalence, type, and importance of splenic diseases in dogs: 1,480 cases (1985-1989), *J Am Vet Med Assoc* 200:829, 1992.

Waters DJ et al: Metastatic pattern in dogs with splenic haemangiosarcoma: clinical implications, *J Small Anim Pract* 29:805: 1988.

Weinstein MJ, Carpenter JL, Schunk CJM: Nonangiogenic and nonlymphomatous sarcomas of the canine spleen: 57 cases (1975-1987), *J Am Vet Med Assoc* 195:784: 1989.

Suggested Reading

Brooks MB et al: Use of splenectomy in the management of lymphoma in dogs: 16 cases (1976-1985), *J Am Vet Med Assoc* 191:1008, 1987.

Read HM, Middleton DJ: Non-endothelial primary splenic sarcomas in two dogs, *Vet Rec* 122:440, 1988.

Spangler WL, Culbertson MR: Prevalence and type of splenic disease in cats: 455 cases (1985-1991), *J Am Vet Med Assoc* 201:773, 1992.

Srebernik N, Appleby EC: Breed prevalence and sites of haemangioma in dogs, *Vet Rec* 129:408, 1991.

Wrigley RH et al: Ultrasonographic features of splenic lymphosarcoma in dogs: 12 cases (1980-1986), *J Am Vet Med Assoc* 193:1565, 1988.

Wrigley RH et al: Clinical features and diagnosis of splenic hematomas in dogs: 10 cases (1980-1987), *J Am Anim Hosp Assoc* 26:371, 1990.

Wrigley RH et al: Ultrasonographic features of splenic hemangiosarcoma in dogs: 18 cases (1980-1986), *J Am Vet Med Assoc* 192:1113, 1988.

Zimmer MA, Stair EL: Splenic myelolipomas in two dogs, *Vet Pathol* 20:637, 1983.

CHAPTER 21

Surgery of the Kidney and Ureter

GENERAL PRINCIPLES AND TECHNIQUES

DEFINITIONS

Nephrectomy is excision of the kidney; **nephrotomy** is a surgical incision into the kidney. **Nephrostomy** is the creation of a permanent fistula leading into the pelvis of the kidney; temporary nephrostomy tubes (**nephropyelostomy**) are occasionally used to divert urine when obstructive uropathy occurs, or when the proximal ureter has been avulsed from the kidney. **Pyelolithotomy** is an incision into the renal pelvis and proximal ureter; a **ureterotomy** is an incision into the ureter; both are generally used to remove calculi. **Neoureterostomy** is a surgical procedure performed to correct intramural ectopic ureters; **ureteroneocystostomy** involves implantation of a resected ureter into the bladder.

PREOPERATIVE CONCERNS

Renal disease or ureteral trauma or obstruction may cause signs of acute or chronic renal failure. The minimum database for urinary dysfunction includes BUN, creatinine, urinalysis, hematocrit, total protein, albumin, electrolytes (especially potassium), total CO_2, and an ECG, if electrolytes are not readily available. These animals may have significant metabolic derangements, besides azotemia. Acute renal disease usually causes moderate or severe dehydration. Although most oliguric animals have acute renal failure, many animals with nonobstructive acute renal failure are not oliguric. Preoperative intravenous fluid therapy is needed to restore circulating blood volume and urine production; however, fluids must be administered judiciously to avoid overloading these patients. Diuretics may also be helpful to enhance urine production in animals that are adequately hydrated. Urine production of hydrated animals on maintenance fluids that do not have abnormal extrarenal losses should be at least 50 ml/kg/day or greater than 2 ml/kg/hr.

☞ **N O T E** · Abnormalities in serum potassium levels may lead to cardiac arrhythmias, so correct these abnormalities before surgery.

Various electrolyte and acid-base abnormalities may occur, depending on the severity and duration of the renal or ureteral disease. Hyperkalemia is often present in acute obstructive renal disorders and some acute renal parenchymal disorders. Hypokalemia may occur with acute or chronic renal disease and diuretic therapy. Both conditions predispose to cardiac arrhythmias and should be corrected before surgery. Clinically important hypocalcemia is occasionally associated with chronic renal disease. Metabolic acidosis may also be present in animals with acute or chronic renal disease.

Animals with chronic renal failure may be anemic because of decreased levels of erythropoietin. Erythropoietin is produced by the kidneys and acts to stimulate red cell production in the bone marrow. Elevated plasma levels of parathyroid hormone may have a negative effect on erythropoietin concentrations. Gastric ulceration, bleeding, or increased red cell fragility may occur in uremic patients. Coagulation profiles may be warranted in animals with chronic renal disorders. Normally hydrated animals with a PCV of less than 20% or hemoglobin of less than 5 g/dl may benefit from preoperative blood transfusions (Table 21-1).

TABLE 21-1

Blood Transfusions

ml of Donor Blood Needed

$$\text{Recipient blood volume}^* \times \frac{\text{Desired PCV} - \text{Actual patient PCV}}{\text{PCV of anticoagulated donor blood}}$$

*Total blood volume is estimated at 90 ml/kg for dogs and 70 ml/kg for cats.
Note: A rough estimate is that 2.2 ml of blood/kg of body weight will increase the recipient's PCV by 1%.

ANESTHETIC CONSIDERATIONS

Anemic patients should be given oxygen before induction and during recovery. Anticholinergic drugs are used to prevent bradycardia. Systemic arterial blood pressure and urine output should be monitored during surgery. Because of intrinsic properties of the kidney, renal blood flow tends to remain constant, despite variations in systemic arterial pressure between 75 and 160 mm Hg, a phenomenon termed *autoregulation*. However, hypotension during surgery may cause renal vasoconstriction, decreased blood flow, and subsequent renal damage. Hypotensive drugs (e.g., acetylpromazine) should be avoided in animals with renal impairment. If the animal is oliguric but normotensive, low-dose dopamine (1 to 2 µg/kg/min intravenously), with or without furosemide (0.2 mg/kg intravenously), can be used. Alternatively, mannitol (¼ to ½ g/kg intravenously) may be used in cats. If both oliguria and hypotension coexist, dopamine (2 to 10 µg/kg/min intravenously) or dobutamine (2 to 10 µg/kg/min intravenously) may be administered. Thiobarbiturates should be avoided if arrhythmias are present. Isoflurane is the inhalation agent of choice in arrhythmic patients.

General anesthetic principles that should be considered in animals with renal disease include the following. They may be premedicated with an anticholinergic (i.e., atropine or glycopyrrolate; Table 21-2) and oxymorphone, butorphanol, or buprenorphine (Tables 21-2 and 21-3). If the animal has minimal renal compromise, a thiobarbiturate, propofol, or a mask can be used for induction. Ketamine should be avoided in cats with renal compromise. If the dog is severely depressed, oxymorphone plus diazepam (Table 21-3) may allow intubation. If additional drugs are needed, etomidate (Table 21-3) or a reduced dose of thiobarbiturate or propofol may be administered intravenously, or mask induction may be used if the animal is not vomiting. Urine output should be monitored during and after surgery.

ANTIBIOTICS

Perioperative antibiotic therapy should be considered in animals with renal disease or obstruction, even if there is no evidence of infection. Animals with renal calculi or ectopic ureters may have concurrent infections and should be placed on appropriate antibiotics, based on urine culture and susceptibility. Alternatively, antibiotics can be withheld until appropriate intraoperative cultures have been taken. If possible, potentially nephrotoxic antibiotics (i.e., aminoglycosides, tetracycline [except doxycycline], and sulfonamides) should be avoided. Penicillin drugs (i.e., penicillin G, ampicillin, amoxicillin, and combinations of clavulanic acid and amoxicillin; Table 21-4) are highly concentrated in urine. They are bactericidal and generally effective against gram-positive organisms. Cephalosporins (e.g., cefazolin, 20 mg/kg intravenously at induction) have an enhanced gram-negative spectrum, are excreted in the urine, and are often used for perioperative antibiotic therapy. Fluoroquinolones (e.g., enrofloxacin; Table 21-4) have a broad activity against aerobic gram-negative bacteria. Drug doses or dosing frequency should be altered as required by the degree of renal compromise.

SURGICAL ANATOMY

The kidneys lie in the retroperitoneal space lateral to the aorta and caudal vena cava. They have a fibrous capsule and are held in position by subperitoneal connective tissue. The cranial pole of the right kidney lies at the level of the thirteenth rib. In an average-sized dog, the cranial pole of the left kidney lies about 5 cm caudal to the upper third of the last rib. The renal pelvis is the funnel-shaped structure that receives urine and directs it into the ureter. There are generally five to six diverticula that curve outward from the renal pelvis. The renal artery normally bifurcates into dorsal and ventral branches; however, variations are common. The ureter begins at the renal pelvis and enters the dorsal surface

---

TABLE 21-2

Selected Anesthetic Protocols for Use in Stable Dogs and Cats with Renal Disease

Premedication

Give atropine (0.02-0.04 mg/kg SC or IM) or glycopyrrolate (0.005-0.011 mg/kg SC or IM) plus oxymorphone* (0.05-0.1 mg/kg SC or IM); or butorphanol (0.2-0.4 mg/kg SC or IM); or buprenorphine (5-15 µg/kg IM)

Induction

Thiopental (10-12 mg/kg IV) or propofol (4-6 mg/kg IV) (see text also)

Maintenance

Isoflurane or halothane
*Use 0.05 mg/kg in cats.

TABLE 21-3

Selected Anesthetic Protocols for Use in Decompensated Patients in Renal Failure or in Hypovolemic, Dehydrated, or Shocky Animals

Dogs
Induction

Oxymorphone (0.1 mg/kg IV) plus diazepam (0.2 mg/kg IV) Give in incremental dosages. Intubate if possible. If necessary, give etomidate (0.5-1.5 mg/kg IV).

Maintenance
Isoflurane

Cats
Premedication

Butorphanol (0.2-0.4 mg/kg SC or IM) or buprenorphine (5-15 µg/kg IM) or oxymorphone (0.05 mg/kg SC or IM)

Induction

Diazepam (0.2 mg/kg IV) followed by etomidate (0.5-1.5 mg/kg IV) (see text also)

Maintenance
Isoflurane

of the bladder obliquely, by means of two slit-like orifices. The blood supply to the ureter is from the cranial ureteral artery (from the renal artery) and the caudal ureteral artery (from the prostatic or vaginal artery).

☞ **N O T E** · The anatomy of the renal vasculature is highly variable, so use care when ligating these vessels during nephrectomy.

SURGICAL TECHNIQUES

For the kidney, a ventral midline abdominal incision is performed from the xiphoid to caudal to the umbilicus. If the distal ureter must be transected (i.e., for nephrectomy) or a cystotomy is necessary, the incision should extend to the pubis. Balfour retractors are used to retract the abdominal wall and expose the kidney. The entire abdominal contents should be inspected before exploring the urinary tract. The right kidney is exposed by elevating the duodenum and displacing the other loops of intestine toward the animal's left side. Similarly, the left kidney is exposed by elevating the mesocolon so that the small intestine is retracted to the animal's right side. The kidney can be isolated from the remaining abdominal contents with moistened laparotomy sponges.

Renal Biopsy

Renal biopsy may be indicated to diagnose the cause of renal insufficiency (especially acute renal failure), hematuria (rare), or proteinuria. It may be performed at surgery, or percutaneously, with the aid of ultrasound, laparoscopy, a keyhole ab-

dominal incision, or blindly. Of the percutaneous techniques, ultrasound-guided biopsy is preferable. Percutaneous biopsy should be avoided in patients with bleeding disorders, large intrarenal cysts, perirenal abscesses, or obstructive uropathy. Giving fluids before, during, and shortly after biopsy to initiate and maintain a mild diuresis may decrease the formation of blood clots within the renal pelvis, that could cause hydronephrosis. Surgical biopsies may be performed using a biopsy instrument (e.g., Vim Tru-Cut or Franklin modified Vim-Silverman biopsy needles; Fig. 21-1) or a wedge resection. The latter allows a larger sample to be obtained.

Needle biopsy. *Perform a needle biopsy with a Tru-Cut instrument by placing the tip of the instrument on the kidney capsule, with the obturator specimen rod fully retracted within the outer cannula. Push the specimen rod into the lesion by advancing the plastic handle. Then advance the outer sheath of the needle into the tissue to sever the biopsy sample. Withdraw the needle, with the outer sheath over the specimen rod. Apply digital pressure to the site to control hemmorhage.* **Be sure that the sample is primarily cortical tissue.**

Wedge biopsy. *For a wedge biopsy, make an incision into the renal parenchyma with a No. 15 scalpel blade. Make another incision at an angle to the first incision to remove a wedged-shaped piece of parenchyma (Fig. 21-2).* **Be sure to include cortex in the sample.** *Close the incision with a mattress suture of 3-0 absorbable suture material.*

Nephrectomy

Nephrectomy is indicated for renal neoplasia, severe trauma resulting in uncontrollable hemorrhage or urine leakage, pyelonephritis that is resistant to medical therapy, hydronephrosis, and ureteral abnormalities (i.e., avulsion, stricture, rupture, or calculi) that defy surgical repair. Before nephrectomy, renal function in the opposite kidney should be assessed by determining its glomerular filtration rate (GFR), if possible. **Excretory urograms are not innocuous and can produce anuric/oliguric renal failure in animals**

TABLE 21-4

Selected Antibiotics of Use in Animals with Renal Disease

Ampicillin
22 mg/kg IV, IM, SC, or PO, TID

Amoxicillin Plus Clavulanate (Clavamox)
Dogs
12.5-25 mg/kg PO, BID
Cats
62.5 mg PO, BID

Cefazolin (Ancef, Kefzol)
20 mg/kg IV or IM, TID to QID

Trimethoprim-Sulfadiazine (Tribrissen)
Dogs
15 mg/kg IM or PO, BID
Cats
15 mg/kg PO, BID

Enrofloxacin (Baytril)
5-10 mg/kg PO or IV, BID

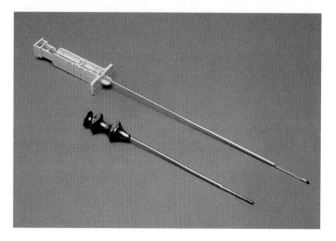

FIG. 21-1
Vim Tru-Cut *(top)* and Franklin modified Vim-Silverman biopsy needles *(bottom).*

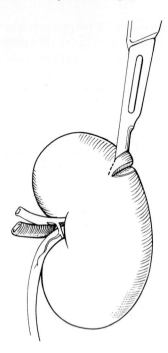

FIG. 21-2
Wedge biopsies provide larger samples than do needle
biopsies.

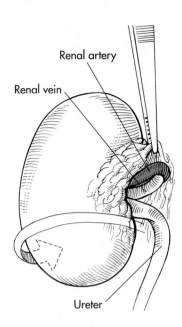

FIG. 21-3
During nephrectomy, elevate the kidney and retract it medially to locate the renal artery and vein on the dorsal surface
of the renal hilus.

with previously mild or moderate renal disease. If excretory
urograms are done, avoid large doses of contrast material
and maintain good renal perfusion. Bilateral renal dysfunction may warrant a guarded prognosis. If renal neoplasia is
suspected, radiography (thoracic and abdominal) and ultrasonography should be performed to help rule out metastasis
(including to the opposite kidney). To avoid unintentional
transection, the opposite ureter should always be identified;
this is particularly critical when removing large neoplasms.

*Grasp the peritoneum over the kidney and incise it. Free
the kidney from its sublumbar attachments, using a combination of blunt and sharp dissection. Elevate the kidney
and retract it medially to locate the renal artery and vein on
the dorsal surface of the renal hilus (Fig. 21-3). Identify any
branches of the renal artery. Double ligate the renal artery
with absorbable (e.g., polydioxanone or polyglyconate) or
nonabsorbable (e.g., cardiovascular silk) suture close to
the abdominal aorta, to ensure that all branches have been
ligated. Identify the renal vein and ligate it similarly. The
left ovarian and testicular veins drain into the renal vein
and should not be ligated in intact dogs. Avoid ligating the
renal artery and vein together to prevent an arteriovenous
fistula from forming. Ligate the ureter near the bladder with
absorbable suture material. Remove the kidney and ureter,
and after procuring appropriate culture specimens, submit
them for histologic examination.*

Partial Nephrectomy

Partial nephrectomy is occasionally warranted for focal renal
lesions, particularly if optimal preservation of renal function
is necessary because of bilateral renal dysfunction. However,

in most cases total nephrectomy is easier and has less risk of
postoperative hemorrhage. If partial nephrectomy is performed, electrocoagulation of bleeding vessels should be
avoided because this results in excessive parenchymal damage. Avoid partial nephrectomy in animals with clinically significant coagulopathies, as excessive blood loss may occur
following this procedure.

*If possible, strip the renal capsule from the area of the kid-
ney to be excised. Use absorbable suture (No. 0 or 1) with
two long, straight needles attached. Thread the needles
into the kidney at the proposed resection site (Figs. 21-4, A
and B). Tie the thread into three separate ligatures, but
avoid damaging the renal vessels or ureter (Fig. 21-4, C).
Excise the renal tissue distal to these ligatures. Ligate any
bleeders and suture the exposed diverticula with absorbable suture material (2-0 or 3-0). Approximate the capsule over the end of the kidney (Fig. 21-4, D), and anchor
it to the sublumbar tissues to prevent rotation of the kidney.
Alternatively, clamp the renal vessels with vascular forceps,
and excise the kidney parenchyma. Ligate parenchymal
vessels, and close the renal pelvis and diverticula. Suture
the capsule as described above, and remove the clamps
from the renal vessels.*

Nephrotomy

Nephrotomy is usually performed to remove calculi (see p.
475) that are lodged within the renal pelvis, but it may also
be performed to explore the renal pelvis for neoplasia or
hematuria. Nephrotomy should be avoided in patients with
severe hydronephrosis because ample parenchyma may not
be available to prevent postoperative urine leakage. Additionally, nephrotomy may temporarily decrease renal func-

CHAPTER 21 *Surgery of the Kidney and Ureter* **465**

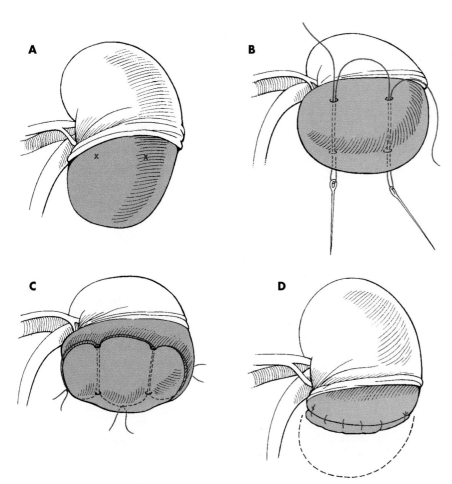

FIG. 21-4
For partial nephrectomy, use large, absorbable suture with two long, straight needles attached. **A** and **B,** Thread the needles into the kidney at the proposed resection site. **C,** Tie the thread into three separate ligatures, but avoid damaging the renal vessels or ureter. Excise the renal tissue distal to these ligatures. **D,** Approximate capsule over the end of the kidney, and anchor it to the sublumbar tissues, to prevent rotation of the kidney.

tion by 25% to 50%. Although bilateral nephrotomies can be performed, this could precipitate acute renal failure if renal function is sufficiently compromised preoperatively. Staged procedures are indicated in such patients.

Closure of nephrotomy incisions may be accomplished without sutures or with transparenchymal horizontal mattress sutures. The latter may cause increased vascular strangulation, pressure necrosis, infarction, and postoperative hemorrhage. Cyanoacrylate adhesive provides rapid hemostasis; however, if the adhesive enters the renal diverticula, calculus formation may occur.

Locate the renal vessels, and temporarily occlude them with vascular forceps, a tourniquet, or an assistant's fingers. Mobilize the kidney to expose the convex lateral surface. Make a sharp incision along the midline of the convex border of the kidney sufficient to allow removal of the calculi and inspection of the entire renal pelvis (Fig. 21-5). Extend the incision from the capsule to the pelvic diverticula (Fig. 21-5). Alternatively, make a sharp incision through the capsule, and bluntly separate the renal parenchyma with forceps. Culture the renal pelvis. Remove the calculi and flush the kidney with warm saline or lactated Ringer's solution. Assess the ureter for patency by placing a 3½ French soft rubber catheter down the ureter and flushing it with warm fluids. Close the nephrotomy by apposing the

cut tissues and applying digital pressure (for approximately 5 min), while restoring blood flow through the renal vessels (sutureless technique). Alternatively, appose the capsule with a continuous pattern of absorbable suture material (Fig. 21-5). If adequate hemostasis is not achieved or urine leakage is a concern, place absorbable sutures through the cortex in a horizontal mattress fashion (see comments above; Fig. 21-5). Then suture the capsule with a continuous pattern of absorbable suture material. Replace the kidney in its original location. Sutures may be placed in the peritoneum where the kidney was elevated to help stabilize it.

Pyelolithotomy

Pyelolithotomy may be performed to remove renal calculi if the proximal ureter and renal pelvis are sufficiently dilated. This procedure avoids renal parenchymal trauma associated with nephrotomy. Pyelolithotomy is extremely difficult if the ureter is not dilated.

Dissect the kidney from its sublumbar attachments, and expose the dorsal surface. Identify the ureter and renal vessels (Fig. 21-6, A). Make an incision over the dilated pelvis and proximal ureter, and remove the calculi (Fig. 21-6, B). Flush the renal pelvis and diverticula with warm saline to remove small debris. Next flush the ureter to ensure its

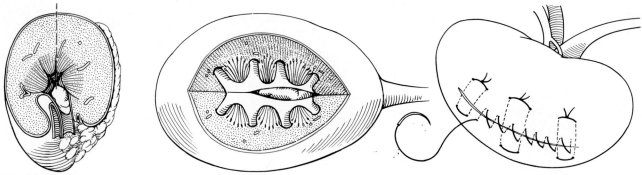

FIG. 21-5
Nephrotomy is usually performed to remove calculi lodged within the renal pelvis. Make a sharp incision along the midline of the convex border of the kidney. Close the nephrotomy by apposing the cut tissues and suturing the capsule with a continuous pattern of absorbable suture material (see text for sutureless technique). If adequate hemostasis is not achieved or urine leakage is a concern, place absorbable sutures through the cortex in a horizontal mattress fashion. Then suture the capsule with a continuous pattern of absorbable suture material.

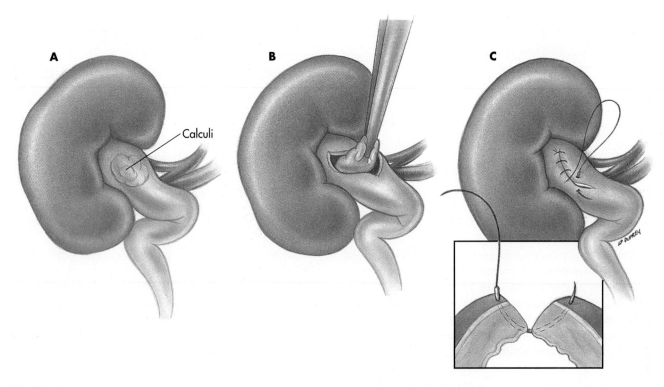

FIG. 21-6
Pyelolithotomy may be performed when the proximal ureter is dilated. **A,** Expose the dorsal surface of the kidney, and identify the ureter and renal vessels. **B,** Make an incision over the dilated pelvis and proximal ureter, and remove the calculi. **C,** Close the incision with a continuous suture pattern.

patency. Close the incision with a continuous suture of 4-0 or 5-0 absorbable suture material (Fig. 21-6, C).

Ureterotomy

Ureterotomy is occasionally performed to remove obstructive calculi. Because there is a risk of postoperative leakage and stricture formation, ureterotomy should be performed with care. If obstruction is not present, dietary dissolution of stru-

vite calculi may be attempted. However, removal of calculi is indicated if obstruction occurs or seems likely (e.g., hydroureter or hydronephrosis). Depending on the size of the animal, removal of the stones with a ureteroscope may be possible. Some stones located in the distal ureter may be flushed or pulled into the bladder through a cystotomy, making a ureterotomy unnecessary. Although ureteral mucosa will regenerate over a stent if the mucosa has not been completely disrupted, the use of stenting catheters is controversial because they may promote stricture formation and infection. If stents are used, they should be smaller than the diameter of the ureter. In some animals, ureteral stents may be placed so that they exit the urethral orifice and are sutured to the exterior. Transverse or longitudinal incisions may be made in the ureter; however, there may be less tension on transverse ureterotomies, and thus they may heal more readily.

Make a transverse or longitudinal incision in the dilated ureter proximal to the calculi and remove them (Fig. 21-7, A). Place a small, soft rubber catheter into the ureter proximal and distal to the incision, and flush the ureter with warm fluid. Be certain that all calculi have been removed and that the ureter is patent. Close the incision with simple interrupted sutures of 5-0 to 7-0 absorbable suture material (Fig. 21-7, B). Alternatively, if the ureter is not dilated and stricture formation seems likely, make a longitudinal incision over the calculi, and close the incision in a transverse fashion (Fig. 21-7, C). If the ureter has been damaged, perform a resection and anastomosis or proximal urinary diversion (see below).

Ureteral Anastomosis

Ureteral anastomosis is technically difficult in small patients (i.e., small dogs and cats) and has a high rate of postoperative obstruction. If the ureter is transected or damaged near the bladder, ureteroneocystostomy may be performed (see below). If the ureter is avulsed from the renal pelvis, urinary drainage can be performed by placing a catheter through the renal parenchyma into the ureter (Fig. 21-8). The end of the catheter is exteriorized through the body wall. If function is adequate in the opposite kidney, nephrectomy may be considered, to minimize possible complications of leakage, stricture, or infection. Minimal dissection should be done around the ureter to avoid compromising its blood supply. To avoid damaging the ureter, stay sutures should be placed for manipulation, and traumatic forceps should be avoided. The amount of tension that can be placed on the ureter without causing stricture formation is unknown; therefore tension across the anastomotic site should be avoided. Various synthetic materials have been used to replace the ureter, but most are unacceptable because they promote fibrosis, calculus formation, or infection. A bladder-flap ureteroplasty has been described for ureteral trauma near the bladder (Fig. 21-9). With this technique, a flap is elevated from the ventral surface of the bladder, and the ureter reimplanted into the flap. The flap is then closed as a tube. As with ureterotomy, stenting catheters should be used with caution because they may promote stricture formation.

For ureteral anastomosis, suture the ureter directly, or spatulate it by making a longitudinal incision on opposite sides of each end of the ureter (Fig. 21-10, A). Pre-place absorbable sutures (5-0 or 6-0) at the apex of the spatulated incisions and align the ureteral ends (Fig. 21-10, B). Appose the ureteral ends with simple interrupted sutures, using the preplaced sutures. Close the remainder of the ureter with simple interrupted sutures (Fig. 21-10, C). Ensure that the ends of the ureter are not twisted and

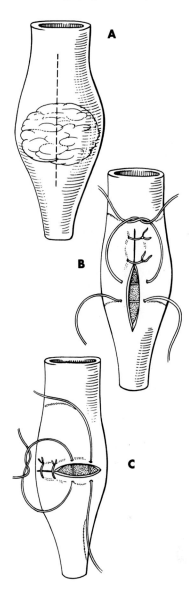

FIG. 21-7
Ureterotomy is occasionally performed to remove obstructive calculi. **A,** Make a transverse or longitudinal incision in the dilated ureter proximal to the calculi and remove them. **B,** Close the incision with simple interrupted sutures. **C,** Alternatively, make a longitudinal incision over the calculi, and close the incision in a transverse fashion.

that sufficient sutures have been placed to prevent leakage (Fig. 21-10, D).

Neoureterostomy

Neoureterostomy (see p. 473) is performed for intramural ectopic ureters. Although some ectopic ureters completely bypass the bladder, most travel under the bladder mucosa before exiting and opening into the urethra or vagina.

Ureteroneocystostomy

Ureteroneocystostomy is performed for extraluminal ectopic ureters and to repair ureters that are damaged near the bladder. The ureter is resected or debrided and reimplanted into the bladder lumen (see p. 473).

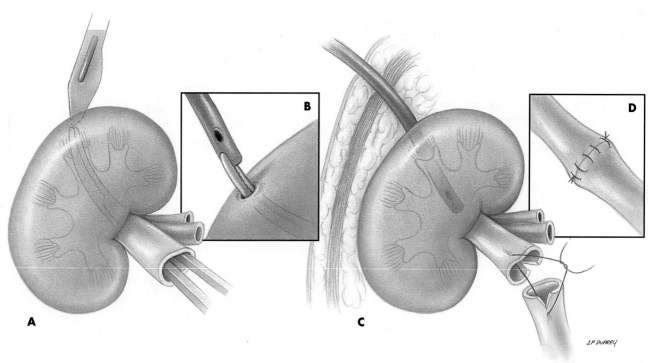

FIG. 21-8
Urinary drainage can be performed by placing a catheter through the renal parenchyma into the renal pelvis. **A,** Place a hemostat into the renal pelvis via the ureter, and incise over its tip with a scalpel blade. **B,** Grasp a catheter with the hemostat, and **C,** pull it into the renal pelvis. **D,** Anastomose the torn ureteral ends.

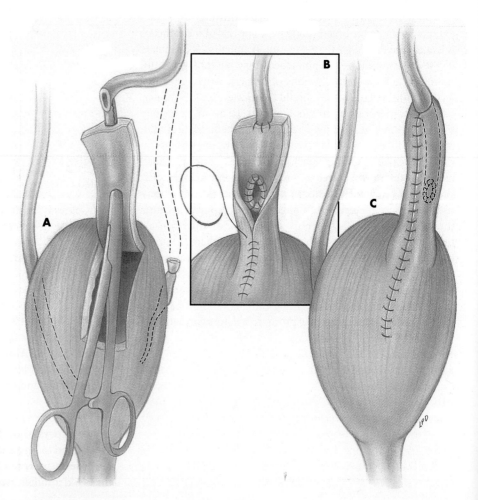

FIG. 21-9
A bladder-flap ureteroplasty may be performed when ureteral trauma occurs near the bladder. **A,** Elevate a flap from the ventral surface of the bladder, and **B,** reimplant the ureter into the flap. **C,** Close the flap as a tube.

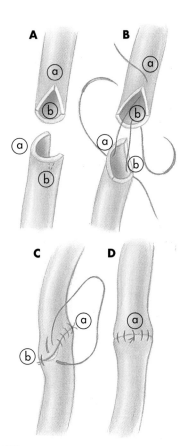

FIG. 21-10
For ureteral anastomosis, suture the ureter directly, or **A,** spatulate it by making a longitudinal incision on opposite sides of each end of the ureter. **B,** Pre-place absorbable sutures at the apex of the spatulated incisions, and align the ureteral ends. Appose the ureteral ends with simple interrupted sutures using the preplaced sutures. **C** and **D,** Close the remainder of the ureter with simple interrupted sutures.

HEALING OF THE KIDNEY AND URETER

Mild contusions or fractures of the kidney parenchyma heal primarily by fibrous connective tissue synthesis. Although scar production occurs and may obliterate some functional nephrons, wound contraction is usually minimal. However, renal pelvis and collecting ducts experience wound contraction and scar tissue formation, resulting in strictures. Uroepithelium has enormous proliferative potential and may seal a damaged area within 48 hours. If at least 50% of the ureteral circumference remains, the ureter will heal by epithelization, fibrous connective tissue synthesis, and longitudinal vs. circumferential wound contraction. Peristalsis is absent in the distal segment of a transected ureter for at least 10 days after repair. This may promote hydroureter in the proximal segment and subsequent hydronephrosis. Immobilizing the ureter to surrounding structures will also inhibit peristalsis and diminish urine flow.

☞ **NOTE** • The uroepithelium has enormous regenerative capacity, but improper technique may produce strictures.

TABLE 21-5		
Postoperative Analgesics		
Oxymorphone (Numorphan)		
0.05-0.1 mg/kg IV, IM, every 4 hours (as needed)		
Butorphanol (Torbutrol, Torbugesic)		
0.2-0.4 mg/kg IV, IM, or SC, every 2 to 4 hours (as needed)		
Buprenorphine (Buprenex)		
5-15 µg/kg, IV, IM, every 6 hours (as needed)		

SUTURE MATERIALS/SPECIAL INSTRUMENTS

Absorbable suture material such as polyglactin 910 (Vicryl), polyglycolic acid (Dexon), polydioxanone (PDS), or polyglyconate (Maxon) should be used. Nonabsorbable suture materials may promote calculus formation and infection. Although PDS and Maxon maintain tensile strength and are more slowly absorbed than is desirable for most urinary surgery, they have less tissue drag than Dexon or Vicryl. The use of pediatric or ophthalmic instruments will facilitate surgery of the ureter. These instruments tend to be smaller and more delicate and may cause less tissue trauma than larger instruments.

POSTOPERATIVE CARE AND ASSESSMENT

The hematocrit should be monitored postoperatively, and abdominocentesis performed if hemorrhage or leakage is suspected. Significant hemorrhage may require blood transfusions (see Table 21-1) or repeat surgery. Anemic animals should have nasal oxygen during the anesthetic recovery period. Central venous pressure and urine output may be monitored to evaluate hydration postoperatively. Indwelling urinary catheters allow urine output measurement. Animals (particularly young animals) should be closely monitored for urethral obstruction following repair of ectopic ureters. Ureteral obstruction as a result of surgical swelling or stomal stenosis may occur; however, unless the surgery was performed bilaterally, this will typically go undetected unless abdominal radiographs or ultrasonography documents significant hydroureter or hydronephrosis. Urinary leakage may be diagnosed by abdominocentesis and measurement of fluid creatinine levels (not BUN). With uroperitoneum, creatinine levels in the abdominal fluid will be greater than serum creatinine levels (see p. 496). Electrolyte and acid-base abnormalities should be monitored and corrected postoperatively. Postoperative analgesics should be given as necessary (Table 21-5).

COMPLICATIONS

The major complications of surgery of the kidney are renal failure, hemorrhage, and urinary leakage. Urinary leakage or obstruction as a result of stenosis or stricture is common after ureteral surgery. Complications of renal biopsy may include microscopic hematuria, gross hematuria, hemorrhage, and hydronephrosis secondary to the formation of blood clots in the renal pelvis.

SPECIAL AGE CONSIDERATIONS

Older animals often have some degree of renal compromise and require careful monitoring during any surgical procedure. Hypotension should be avoided during surgery and the postoperative period to avoid further renal damage. If cardiac disease is also present, fluids should be used judiciously to prevent overhydration while maintaining renal blood flow.

Suggested Reading

Bellah JR: Wound healing in the urinary tract, *Semin Vet Med Surg (Small Anim)* 4:294, 1989.

Dupre GP, Dee LG, Dee JF: Ureterotomies for treatment of ureterolithiasis in two dogs, *J Am Anim Hosp Assoc* 26:500, 1990.

Jeraj K, Osborne CA, Stevens JB: Evaluation of renal biopsy in 197 dogs and cats, *J Am Vet Med Assoc* 181:367, 1982.

Kochin EG et al: Evaluation of a method of ureteroneocystostomy in cats, *J Am Vet Med Assoc* 202:257, 1993.

Waldron DR et al: Ureteroneocystostomy: a comparison of the submucosal tunnel and transverse pull through techniques, *J Am Anim Hosp Assoc* 23:285, 1987.

SPECIFIC DISEASES

ECTOPIC URETER

DEFINITIONS

Ectopic ureter is a congenital anomaly in which one or both ureters empty outside the bladder. **Extraluminal** ectopic ureters are those that completely bypass the bladder; **intraluminal** ectopic ureters course submucosally in the bladder to open in the urethra or vagina.

SYNONYMS

Ureteral ectopia

GENERAL CONSIDERATIONS AND CLINICALLY RELEVANT PATHOPHYSIOLOGY

The ureter normally enters the dorsolateral, caudal surface of the bladder and empties into the trigone after a short intramural course (Fig. 21-11). Abnormalities in embryogenesis of the urinary system may cause ureteral ectopia. Associated abnormalities (i.e., urethral sphincter incompetence, bladder hypoplasia, vestibulovaginal abnormalities, or ureteroceles; Fig. 21-12) may occur concurrently with ectopic ureters. Surgical correction of ureteral ectopia is recommended; however, the presence of other abnormalities increases the likelihood of postoperative incontinence.

Approximately 70% to 80% of affected dogs have unilateral intramural (Fig. 21-13, *A*) or extramural (Fig. 21-13, *B*) ectopia. Of these, intramural lesions are more common. Other abnormalities noted in some dogs include double

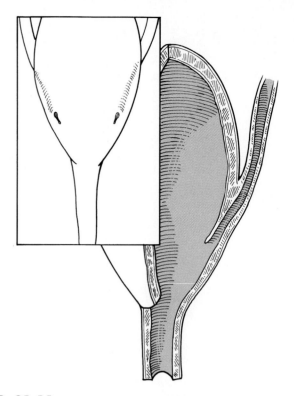

FIG. 21-11
The ureters normally enter the dorsolateral, caudal surface of the bladder and empty into the trigone after a short intramural course.

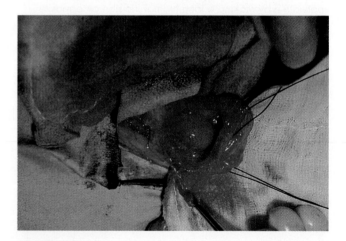

FIG. 21-12
A ureterocele in the bladder of a dog. The contralateral ureter was ectopic.

ureteral openings (i.e., where the ureter opens in the bladder plus more distally; Fig. 21-13; *C*) or ureteral troughs (Fig. 21-13, *D*). Although ureteral ectopia is less common in cats, bilateral ectopia may occur more frequently in cats than in dogs. Diagnosis of ureteral ectopia is important because it can be corrected surgically.

Pyelonephritis and cystitis are common in dogs with ureteral ectopia. Small kidneys may be the result of end-stage pyelonephritis, congenital dysplasia, or congenital cystic dis-

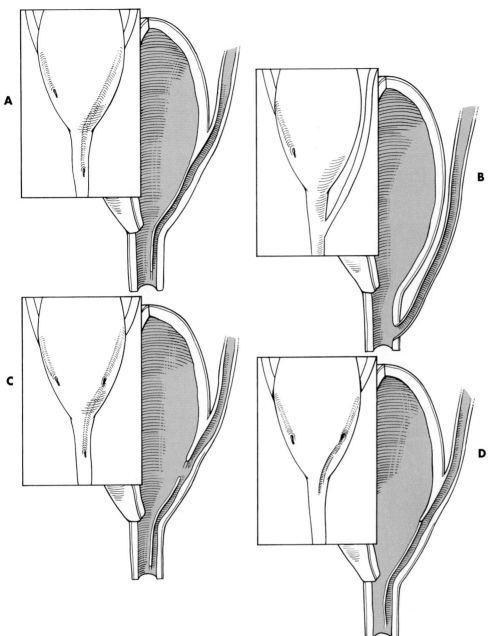

ease. Hydronephrosis may be caused by chronic pyelonephritis or ureteral obstruction (e.g., stenosis or absence of a functional opening). Hydroureter is the most frequent urogenital abnormality in dogs with ureteral ectopia and may be caused by chronic infection, obstructed urine outflow, or a primary lack of ureteral peristalsis. Hypoplastic bladders or intrapelvic bladders may be congenital or secondary to lack of normal filling of the bladder. With unilateral ectopia, hydroureter and hydronephrosis may occur in the contralateral ureter as a result of chronic ascending urinary tract infections.

DIAGNOSIS
Clinical Presentation

Signalment. Ectopic ureters are usually seen in female dogs (female:male ratio of 20:1). However, affected males may be less commonly diagnosed because the opening of the ectopic ureter is closer to the bladder than to the tip of the penis, and distal urethral pressures may prevent urine dribbling. Siberian huskies have an increased incidence of ureteral ectopia. Golden retrievers, Labrador retrievers, miniature poodles, and some terrier breeds may also have a higher-than-expected incidence. Ureteral ectopia should be suspected in any young animal that presents with a history of incontinence since birth; however, this condition should also be included as a differential in older animals with life-long urinary incontinence.

☞ **N O T E** · Ectopic ureters should not be excluded as a possible diagnosis even if urinary incontinence is intermittent or the animal seems to urinate normal volumes.

History. Urinary incontinence is usually constant, but may be intermittent. Many affected animals are able to urinate normally, particularly if the condition is unilateral, the ureters open near the trigone and retrograde filling of the bladder occurs, or the bladder is of sufficient size to act as a reservoir. Even animals with bilateral ectopia may have normal voiding associated with intermittent urine dribbling.

Physical Examination Findings

Physical examination findings include wetness of perivulvar hair, odor, and irritation or urine-scalding of surrounding skin. Some dogs may have a persistent hymen that is detected digitally or with vaginoscopy. Other findings are unremarkable unless pyelonephritis is present.

Radiography/Ultrasonography

The size and shape of the kidneys, bladder, and prostate should be assessed with survey abdominal radiographs. Excretory urography is the most commonly used method for confirming ectopic ureters (Fig. 21-14) and defining associated urogenital abnormalities (i.e., hydronephrosis, hydroureter, hypoplastic bladder, and ureteroceles; see Fig. 21-12). Radiographs should be made both early and late after contrast administration because extramural ectopia is best identified before the bladder completely fills with contrast. However, contrast radiography does not accurately identify all ectopic ureters and often fails to differentiate between intramural and extramural lesions. The colon should

be emptied to enhance visualization of the ureters and their site of termination. Retrograde cystography, pneumocystography (with animal in dorsoventral position to allow gas contrast to rise adjacent to ureters), and vaginoscopy may help correctly define ectopic ureter morphology. Cystoscopy may be the most reliable method for diagnosing ectopic ureters in females. Ultrasonography is also useful for defining ureteral and renal abnormalities.

☞ **N O T E ·** Excretory urography is not 100% sensitive and does not accurately differentiate all intramural and extramural lesions.

Laboratory Findings

A CBC, serum chemistry profile, and urinalysis (with microbial culture) should be performed. Concomitant urinary tract infection is common. Renal failure may be present because of chronic pyelonephritis, obstructive uropathy, or concurrent congenital abnormalities (see p. 461).

DIFFERENTIAL DIAGNOSIS

Ureteral ectopia should be considered likely in any young animal presenting for incontinence. Behavioral incontinence is also common in young animals because of exaggerated submissiveness. Other causes of incontinence include urge incontinence (associated with inflammation or infection), neurogenic disorders (i.e., lower- and upper-motor neuron disorders or reflex dyssynergia), anatomic outflow obstruction (i.e., paradoxical incontinence), and urethral sphincter incontinence (i.e., hormone-responsive incontinence). Behavioral, urge, neurogenic, and hormone-responsive incontinence should be eliminated before considering tests for ectopia in older animals.

MEDICAL MANAGEMENT

Incontinence may persist after surgical correction if there is concomitant urethral sphincter incompetence. Urethral pressure profilometry can detect sphincter incompetence before surgery. α-Adrenergic agonists (i.e., phenylpropanolamine or ephedrine; Table 21-6), or perhaps diethylstilbestrol, may be used to increase urethral sphincter tone.

SURGICAL TREATMENT

Surgical correction is the treatment of choice for ectopic ureters, even if marginal improvement occurs with medical management. Surgery should be performed as soon as possi-

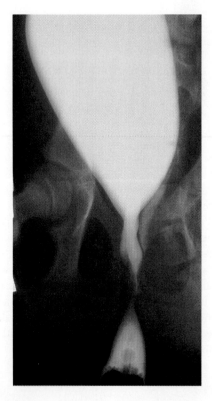

FIG. 21-14
Excretory urogram in a dog with an ectopic ureter. Note the dilated ureter filled with contrast agent adjacent to the proximal urethra. (Courtesy L. Homco, Texas A&M University.)

TABLE 21-6
Phenylpropanolamine (Propagest) Dosages
Dogs
1.5-2.0 mg/kg PO, BID
Cats
1.5 mg/kg PO, TID

ble to prevent secondary abnormalities (i.e., hydroureter, hydronephrosis) resulting from ascending urinary tract infections or outflow obstruction. Neoureterostomy is performed for intramural ectopic ureters. Although some ectopic ureters completely bypass the bladder, most travel under the bladder mucosa before exiting and opening into the urethra or vagina. If the ureter is extraluminal, the ureter must be resected and reimplanted into the bladder lumen.

Preoperative Management

Hydration, acid-base, and electrolytes abnormalities should be corrected before surgery (see p. 461). Patients should be placed on appropriate antibiotics, as indicated by urine culture and susceptibility testing. If antibiotic therapy has not been initiated before surgery, antibiotics (e.g., cefazolin) should be administered after intraoperative cultures have been taken. Renal function should be determined before surgery if there is hydronephrosis or renal fibrosis. Nonfunctional kidneys should be removed (see below).

☞ **N O T E** • Be sure to determine before surgery whether the kidney is functional.

Anesthesia

If renal impairment is not present, many different anesthetic regimens can be used safely. If renal impairment is present, see p. 462 for suggested anesthetic protocols.

Surgical Anatomy

Surgical anatomy of the kidney and ureter are described on p. 462.

Positioning

The animal is placed in dorsal recumbency and the abdomen prepared for a ventral midline incision. The prepped area should extend from above the xiphoid to below the pubis.

SURGICAL TECHNIQUE

The entire urinary system should be explored before the ureter is repaired. Nonfunctional kidneys and their ureter should be removed; otherwise, the ureter and kidney should be preserved. If nephrectomy is considered, bilateral ectopia should first be ruled out. With nephrectomy, the end of the ectopic ureter should be ligated as close to its termination as possible.

Neoureterostomy

Handle the bladder tissues with extreme care, and use stay sutures whenever possible. Once the bladder has been emptied of urine, use sterile Q-tips to absorb urine (rather than a sponge) to avoid abrading the mucosal surface. The use of pediatric instruments may help decrease tissue trauma. Swelling or hyperemia will make the ureters difficult to locate beneath the mucosa.

Make an incision into the ventral bladder, near the urethra (Fig. 21-15, A). Place stay sutures to facilitate retraction of the bladder wall edges. Inspect the trigone for ureteral openings. Identify a submucosal swelling or ridge within the bladder wall; this may be facilitated by digitally occluding the urethra to cause ureteral dilatation. Use a No. 15 scalpel blade to make a 3- to 5-mm longitudinal incision through the bladder mucosa into the ureteral lumen. Use simple interrupted sutures to suture the ureteral mucosa to the bladder with 5-0 to 7-0 absorbable suture material (Fig. 21-15, B). Place a 3½ or 5 French catheter into the distal ureter (Fig. 21-15, C). Just distal to the new stoma, pass one or two nonabsorbable sutures (3-0 or 4-0) from the serosal surface circumferentially around the tube, staying beneath the mucosa (Fig. 21-15, D). Be sure that the suture does not penetrate the bladder lumen. Use this suture to ligate the distal ureter after removing the catheter. Close the proximal urethra with simple interrupted or simple continuous sutures (single or double layer), **but ensure that the urethral diameter is not compromised.** *Close the bladder in such a manner as to ensure a water-tight seal (i.e., simple continuous or inverting suture pattern, depending on the bladder wall thickness; see p. 484).*

Ureteroneocystostomy

If the ureter is extraluminal, it must be resected and reimplanted into the bladder lumen. In dogs, the ureter may be implanted into the bladder using a simple transverse pull-through or an intramural tunnel (3:1 tunnel length to ureteral orifice diameter) technique. The latter technique may cause less fibrosis and quicker return of normal ureteral function. The diameter of the feline ureter is approximately 0.4 mm at the level of the bladder, and standard ureteroneocystostomy techniques often cause ureteral obstruction. Microsurgical techniques may be necessary to prevent ureteral obstruction in cats.

Perform a ventral cystotomy as described above for neoureterostomy. Ligate the ureter and transect it, preserving as much length as possible (Fig. 21-16). Place a stay suture on the proximal end of the transected ureter. Incise the bladder mucosa, and create a short oblique submucosal tunnel in the bladder wall. Use the stay suture to draw the ureter into the bladder lumen to avoid damaging the ureter. Make a 1- to 2-mm longitudinal incision in the ureter end (i.e., spatulate it) and suture it to the bladder mucosa with absorbable suture (e.g., polyglycolic acid or polyglactin 910).

SUTURE MATERIALS/SPECIAL INSTRUMENTS

Absorbable suture material such as polyglactin 910 (Vicryl), polyglycolic acid (Dexon), polydioxanone (PDS), or polyglyconate (Maxon) should be used in the bladder because nonabsorbable suture materials may promote calculus formation or infection. Small suture (i.e., 4-0 or 5-0) is preferred to suture the ureter to the bladder mucosa. The distal ureter should be ligated with nonabsorbable suture because

FIG. 21-15
Neoureterostomy is performed for intramural ectopic ureters. **A,** Perform a cystotomy, and make a 3- to 5-mm longitudinal incision through the bladder mucosa into the ureteral lumen. **B,** Use simple interrupted sutures to suture the ureteral mucosa to the bladder. **C,** Place a 3½ or 5 French catheter into the distal ureter. **D,** Just distal to the new stoma, pass one or two nonabsorbable sutures from the serosal surface circumferentially around the tube, staying beneath the mucosa.

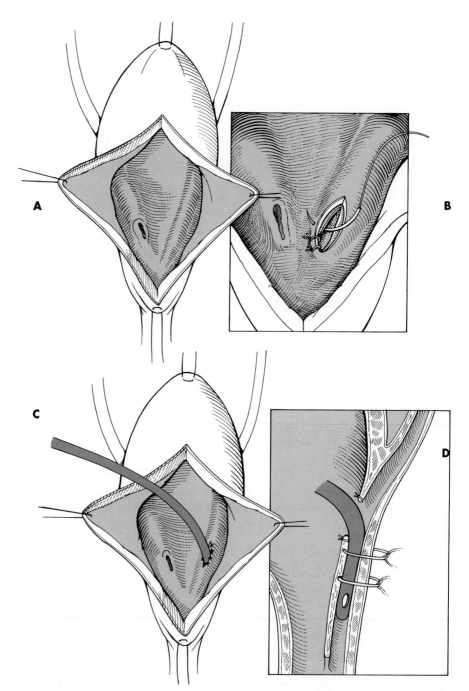

incontinence may recur as a result of recanalization of the distal ureter, following the use of absorbable suture material.

POSTOPERATIVE CARE AND ASSESSMENT

The animal should be observed closely after surgery for signs of urinary obstruction or leakage. If urethral obstruction occurs because of postoperative swelling, an indwelling urinary catheter should be placed for 3 to 4 days, until normal voiding occurs. If bilateral ectopia is corrected during the same surgery (or significant renal impairment exists in the contralateral kidney with unilateral surgery), the animal should be monitored for signs of renal failure as a result of ureteral swelling and subsequent obstruction. If incontinence continues for longer than 2 to 3 months postoperatively, an excretory urogram or cystoscopy should be performed to evaluate the ureters. Occasionally the distal end (i.e., ligated end) will be patent, or bilateral ectopia was missed initially.

☞ **NOTE** • Ureteral stoma swelling is probably common after this surgery and may cause some obstruction to ureteral flow, but it usually goes undetected and resolves without therapy.

PROGNOSIS

Up to 30% to 55% of patients will continue to show some degree of incontinence following surgery. In one study, functional abnormalities of the urinary bladder or urethra were detected in 8 of 9 dogs with congenital ectopic ureters, using cystometrographic studies and urethral pressure profiles (Lane, Lappin, Seim, 1995). Obtaining urethral pressure

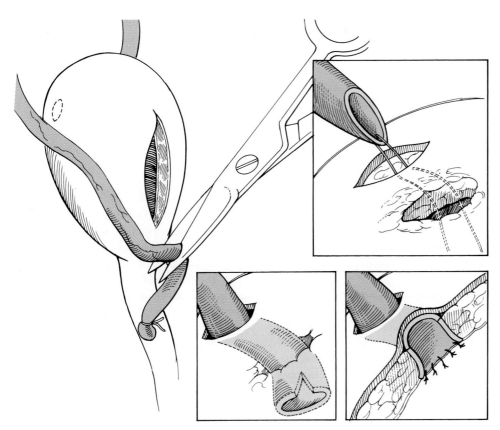

FIG. 21-16
Ureteroneocystostomy is performed when the ureter is extraluminal. Ligate the ureter and transect it. Place a stay suture on the proximal end of the transected ureter. Incise the bladder mucosa, and create a short oblique submucosal tunnel in the bladder wall. Spatulate the ureter end, and suture it to the bladder mucosa with absorbable suture.

measurements before surgery and after phenylpropanolamine therapy (see above) is instituted may help predict the likelihood of continence after surgery. Siberian huskies are particularly prone to postoperative incontinence because of a high incidence of urethral sphincter incompetence. These dogs may respond to α-adrenergic agonists. If bladder hypoplasia is present, incontinence may continue until the bladder enlarges and properly functions as a reservoir. Dogs with ureteral troughs may have a poorer prognosis than dogs with nondistended intramural ectopic ureters.

Reference

Lane IF, Lappin MR, Seim HB: Evaluation of results of preoperative urodynamic measurements in nine dogs with ectopic ureters, *J Am Vet Med Assoc* 206:1348, 1995.

Suggested Reading

Dean PW, Bojrab MJ, Constantinescu GM: Canine ectopic ureter, *Compend Contin Educ Pract Vet* 10:146, 1988.

Lane IF, Lappin MR, Seim HB: Predictive value of urodynamic measurements in the management of ectopic ureters in the dog, *J Vet Intern Med* 6:119, 1992.

Mason LK et al: Surgery of ectopic ureters: pre- and postoperative radiographic morphology, *J Am Anim Hosp Assoc* 26:73, 1990.

McLaughlin R, Miller CW: Urinary incontinence after surgical repair of ureteral ectopia in dogs, *Vet Surg* 20:100, 1991.

Stone, EA, Mason LK: Surgery of ectopic ureters: types, method of correction, and postoperative results, *J Am Anim Hosp Assoc* 26:81, 1990.

Waldron DR: Ectopic ureter surgery and its problems, *Probl Vet Med* 1:85, 1989.

RENAL AND URETERAL CALCULI

DEFINITIONS

Urolithiasis refers to having urinary calculi or **uroliths** (kidney, ureter, bladder, or urethra). The condition of having renal or ureteral calculi (i.e., **nephroliths** or **ureteroliths**) is **nephrolithiasis** or **ureterolithiasis,** respectively. **Nephrolithotomy** is performed to remove renal calculi from the renal pelvis by incising through kidney parenchyma; **pyelolithotomy** is an incision into the renal pelvis and proximal ureter. **Ureterolithotomy** is removal of calculi from the ureter by incision. A **staghorn** calculus is one that occurs in the renal pelvis and extends into the diverticula.

SYNONYMS

For nephrolithotomy—**lithonephrotomy**

GENERAL CONSIDERATIONS AND CLINICALLY RELEVANT PATHOPHYSIOLOGY

Only 5% to 10% of canine uroliths are in the kidney and ureter; calculi are found even less commonly at these sites in cats. Uroliths are named according to their mineral content. Struvite (magnesium ammonium phosphate) uroliths are most common, but other types include calcium oxalate, urate, silicate, cystine, and mixed stones. Some disease processes (i.e., portosystemic shunts or hepatic cirrhosis) are associated with a high rate of urolithiasis (see p. 376). Certain breeds (i.e., dalmatians and dachshunds) also have a high incidence of urolithiasis because of metabolic abnormalities (see p. 499).

Whether all renal or ureteral stones should be removed is controversial. If they are associated with infection, they should be removed; however, removal of noninfected stones from the renal pelvis may produce more renal damage than the stone caused. Other facts that must be considered include the effectiveness of medical therapy in dissolving the stone, renal function in the affected and contralateral kidney, the overall health of the animal, and the presence of obstructive uropathy (i.e., hydronephrosis, hydroureter, or renal failure). Ureteral calculi frequently cause obstruction and often require prompt surgical removal.

Although nonsurgical removal of renal calculi is common in human beings (i.e., lithotripsy), these techniques are less available to pets and may be less effective. Any stone that is surgically removed should be submitted for analysis (Fig. 21-17). Knowledge of the stone's mineral composition will direct appropriate treatment to prevent recurrence. Because of the relationship between infection and calculi, microbial cultures of urine (and possible calculi) are mandatory for patients with uroliths. Factors contributing to the formation of uroliths include a favorable urine pH, infection, high concentration of crystalloids in the urine, and decreased concentration of urine crystallization inhibitors (see p. 499 for a more detailed discussion of stone formation and treatment). In general, it is difficult to eliminate urinary tract infections if calculi are present.

DIAGNOSIS
Clinical Presentation

Signalment. Some breeds have a higher incidence of urolithiasis because of metabolic abnormalities or underlying disease processes (see p. 499). Siamese cats may have an increased incidence of nephrolithiasis. Middle-aged to older animals have a higher rate of urolithiasis than young animals. However, some calculi occur in young animals (i.e., urate calculi associated with portosystemic shunts, struvite calculi in schnauzers).

History. The history varies, depending on whether or not the stone has caused obstruction or there is concurrent infection. Clinical signs may be intermittent, particularly if the animal has been treated with antibiotics. A previous history of urolithiasis is common if stone analysis was not performed or appropriate therapy not instituted following previous surgery.

Physical Examination Findings

Renal calculi may be asymptomatic or associated with hematuria, flank pain, or renomegaly. Hematuria is often the clinical sign noted in cats with nephrolithiasis; these cats may be erroneously diagnosed as having feline urologic syndrome (FUS). Animals with pyelonephritis may be polyuric or polydipsic, lethargic, depressed, febrile, or anorexic. If there is substantial destruction of renal tissue, the animal may be uremic (i.e., anorexic, depressed, dehydrated, and vomiting). Dysuria or stranguria may occur if there is concurrent cystitis. Signs associated with ureteral calculi are usually caused by concurrent pyelonephritis or obstructive uropathy (i.e., uremia).

Radiography/Ultrasonography

Renal calculi may be incidental findings on abdominal radiographs or with ultrasonography. Most renal and ureteral calculi are radiopaque and thus appear as increased densities in the renal pelvis or ureter (Fig. 21-18). Whenever renal calculi are diagnosed, the ureters, bladder, and urethra should also be examined carefully for the presence of calculi. Associ-

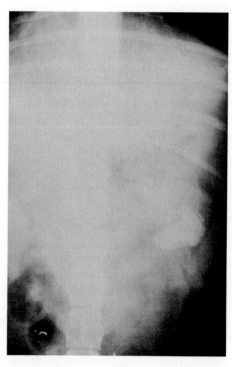

FIG. 21-18
Radiopaque renal calculus in a dog.

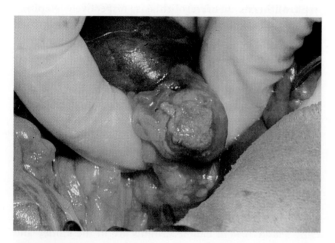

FIG. 21-17
Intraoperative photograph of a renal calculus in a dog.

ated abnormalities (i.e., hydronephrosis or hydroureter) may be assessed by ultrasonography (preferred) or excretory urography (see p. 463).

Laboratory Findings

A CBC, serum chemistry profile, urinalysis, and urine culture should be performed. Concomitant urinary tract infection is common. Renal failure may be present as a result of chronic pyelonephritis or obstructive uropathy (see p. 461). Findings associated with hepatic disease (low BUN or hypoproteinemia) may be present in some animals with urate calculi (see p. 367).

DIFFERENTIAL DIAGNOSIS

Uroliths should be considered in any animal presenting for chronic urinary tract infection, hematuria, stranguria, pollakiuria, or acute obstructive uropathy.

MEDICAL MANAGEMENT

Potential underlying causes of renal or ureteral calculi should be identified and treated (i.e., infection, portosystemic shunts, or metabolic abnormalities). Some stones can be managed with dietary therapy or pharmacologic agents (see the discussion on bladder calculi, p. 500). If dietary therapy is used to dissolve renal calculi, there is a risk that the stones will become small enough to enter the ureter and cause obstruction. Therefore these animals should be monitored carefully for evidence of ureteral obstruction during such therapy. Dry, extracorporeal shock-wave lithotripsy has been reported for treatment of calcium oxalate ureterolithiasis and nephrolithiasis in a dog (Bailey, Burk, 1995).

SURGICAL TREATMENT

Surgical removal of renal and ureteral calculi should be considered when they are infected or cause obstruction. Surgery should be performed as soon as possible once the animal has been stabilized, to prevent irreversible renal damage.

Preoperative Management

If possible, hydration, acid-base, and electrolyte abnormalities should be corrected before surgery. Patients should be placed on appropriate antibiotics, as indicated by urine culture and susceptibility testing. If antibiotic therapy has not been initiated before surgery, antibiotics (e.g., cefazolin) should be administered after intraoperative cultures have been taken. Renal function should be determined before surgery. Nephrectomy, rather than stone removal, is indicated in nonfunctional kidneys; otherwise the kidney and ureter should be preserved.

☞ **N O T E** · Make sure you determine before surgery whether the kidney is functional!

Anesthesia

If renal impairment is not present, many anesthetic regimens can be used safely. If renal impairment is present, see p. 462 for suggested anesthetic protocols.

Surgical Anatomy

Surgical anatomy of the kidney and ureter are discussed on p. 462.

Positioning

The animal is placed in dorsal recumbency and the abdomen prepared for a ventral midline incision. The prepped area should extend from above the xiphoid to caudal to the pubis. If nephrectomy is performed, the incision will need to extend caudally, to allow the ureter to be ligated near the bladder.

SURGICAL TECHNIQUE

The entire urinary system should be explored before the calculi are removed (including the contralateral kidney and ureter). Occasionally, multiple ureteral or renal plus ureteral calculi are found. Additionally, stones may be found in the bladder or urethra. Renal calculi can be removed via a nephrotomy (see p. 464) or pyelolithotomy (see p. 465). If the renal pelvis and proximal ureter are sufficiently dilated, a pyelolithotomy is preferred because it avoids renal parenchymal incision and subsequent nephron damage. However, if the stone is large and involves the diverticula plus pelvis, nephrotomy is usually necessary. Occasionally, soft stones can be crushed and removed through the renal pelvis, but care is necessary to prevent ureteral damage that may cause subsequent stricture formation.

☞ **N O T E** · ALWAYS submit the stones for analysis.

Bilateral nephrotomy can be performed; however, there is risk that renal failure will occur postoperatively. If possible, staged procedures should be considered. Cultures of the renal pelvis or ureter should be submitted. The stones should be submitted for analysis and possibly microbial culture. Rarely, fungal elements will be seen on cytologic analysis of material (grit, exudate) found in the renal pelvis.

SUTURE MATERIALS/SPECIAL INSTRUMENTS

Absorbable suture material such as polyglactin 910 (Vicryl), polyglycolic acid (Dexon), polydioxanone (PDS), or polyglyconate (Maxon) should be used in the kidney and ureter.

POSTOPERATIVE CARE AND ASSESSMENT

The animal should be observed closely after surgery for signs of urinary obstruction or leakage. Renal failure may occur if bilateral nephrotomy was performed, or if significant renal impairment was present in the contralateral kidney preoperatively. See p. 469 for postoperative care of patients with renal disease.

COMPLICATIONS

The major complications of renal surgery are renal failure, hemorrhage, and urinary leakage. Urinary leakage or obstruction caused by stenosis or stricture are common with ureteral surgery.

SPECIAL AGE CONSIDERATIONS

Older animals often have some degree of renal compromise and require careful monitoring during any surgical procedure. Hypotension should be avoided during surgery and the postoperative period to avoid further renal damage. If cardiac disease is also present, fluids should be used judiciously to prevent overhydration while maintaining renal blood flow.

PROGNOSIS

If the underlying disease, infection, or metabolic abnormality is not treated, most uroliths will recur. A recurrence rate of 25% has been reported in dogs (Brown et al, 1977). The subsequent episodes may occur within a few months.

References

Bailey G, Burk RL: Dry extracorporeal shock wave lithotripsy for treatment of ureterolithiasis and nephrolithiasis in a dog, *J Am Vet Med Assoc* 207:592, 1995.

Brown NO, et al: Canine urolithiasis: retrospective analysis of 438 cases, *J Am Vet Med Assoc* 170:44, 1977.

Suggested Reading

Carter WO, Hawkins EC, Morrison WB: Feline nephrolithiasis: eight cases (1984 through 1989), *J Am Anim Hosp Assoc* 29:247, 1993

Clark TP, Panciera R: Calcium phosphate urolithiasis and renal dysplasia in a young dog, *J Am Vet Med Assoc* 200:1509, 1992.

Dupre GP, Dee LG, Dee JF: Ureterotomies for treatment of ureterolithiasis in two dogs, *J Am Anim Hosp Assoc* 26:500, 1990.

Gregory CR et al: Oxalate nephrosis and sclerosis after renal transplantation in a cat, *Vet Surg* 22:21, 1993.

RENAL AND URETERAL NEOPLASIA

DEFINITION

Nephroblastomas are rapidly developing malignant mixed tumors that arise from embryonal elements of the kidney.

SYNONYMS

For nephroblastoma—**embryonal adenomyosarcoma, nephroma, Wilms' tumor**

GENERAL CONSIDERATIONS AND CLINICALLY RELEVANT PATHOPHYSIOLOGY

Primary renal tumors are uncommon in dogs and cats, accounting for 0.6% to 1.7% of reported neoplasms (Klein et al, 1988). They are usually malignant in both species. In dogs, carcinomas are most common (Table 21-7). Benign renal tumors occasionally occur. Lymphoma is the most common renal neoplasm in cats and may be primary or metastatic, associated with the alimentary form of this disease. Renal carcinomas are common in cats.

Bilateral renal involvement occurs in nearly 30% of dogs with primary renal neoplasia. Metastasis to liver, adrenal

TABLE 21-7

Types of Canine Renal Tumors

Malignant
- Carcinomas
- Hemangiosarcomas
- Fibrosarcomas
- Transitional cell carcinomas
- Nephroblastomas
- Squamous cell carcinomas
- Undifferentiated carcinomas

Benign
- Adenomas
- Hemangiomas
- Teratomas

glands, lung, lymph nodes, bone, and brain is common with renal tumors. With renal carcinoma, pulmonary metastasis is detected radiographically in nearly half of affected dogs. Pulmonary metastasis occurs with some nephroblastomas; but is infrequent for transitional cell tumors. Renal metastasis of other primary abdominal tumors is also common. Renal neoplasia may cause local signs, or systemic manifestations of renal failure. Tumors arising from the renal pelvis are more apt to cause hematuria or hydronephrosis than signs of renal failure. Unilateral renal damage may not be associated with systemic clinical signs, even if the kidney becomes nonfunctional. Large renal neoplasms may compress or invade the caudal vena cava, causing vascular obstruction. Collateral circulation usually develops in such cases, preventing clinical signs (i.e., rear limb edema or ascites).

☞ **N O T E** · Primary renal neoplasia may occur bilaterally.

DIAGNOSIS
Clinical Presentation

Signalment. Renal carcinomas occur more commonly in males than females and may be hormonally induced. In German shepherd dogs, renal cystadenocarcinomas have been associated with generalized nodular dermatofibrosis. This syndrome occurs most commonly in middle-aged dogs of either sex and appears to be inherited in an autosomal-dominant fashion. Renal neoplasia most commonly occurs in middle-aged to older animals. Nephroblastomas and undifferentiated renal sarcomas occur most commonly in young dogs and cats; however, they may also occur in older animals. Teratomas may occur in the kidneys of young dogs.

History. The history of animals with primary renal tumors is often vague and nonspecific. Although the owner may relate intermittent or chronic signs associated with the urinary tract or systemic signs of renal failure, the most common signs are anorexia, depression, and weight loss. Occasionally, the only abnormality noted is abdominal enlargement associated with a renal mass. Renal failure is primarily seen with bilateral involvement (e.g., lymphoma in cats). Dyspnea related to pulmonary metastasis is occasionally noted. With some benign neoplasms (i.e., hemangioma), intermittent or constant hematuria is common.

Physical Examination Findings

An abdominal mass is often palpated in dogs and cats with renal neoplasia. The kidney may feel enlarged, firm, or nodular. Other findings are often nonspecific, and may include weight loss, anorexia, depression, anemia, dyspnea, and pyrexia. Lameness has been associated with bony metastasis and hypertrophic osteopathy.

Radiography/Ultrasonography

Renal enlargement may be identified on survey abdominal radiographs; however, ultrasonography is more sensitive and specific. Excretory urography may allow localization of renal neoplasia and assessment of parenchymal involvement. If vascular involvement is suspected, selective angiography can be used to detect intravascular or extravascular (compressive) lesions. Thoracic radiographs should be taken to detect pulmonary metastasis.

Laboratory Findings

Laboratory findings are often nonspecific; however, anemia and azotemia are common. A CBC (including platelet count), serum chemistry profile, and urinalysis should be performed. Rarely, polycythemia may be found. Gross hematuria may occur with mesenchymal (i.e., anaplastic sarcomas fibromas, hemangiosarcomas, and lymphosarcoma) and transitional cell tumors; however, microscopic hematuria is more common. Proteinuria may also be noted.

DIFFERENTIAL DIAGNOSIS

Renal neoplasia must be differentiated from other causes of renomegaly (i.e., hydronephrosis, polycystic disease, or abscess) or abdominal enlargement (e.g., neoplasia of the adrenal glands, spleen, liver, or lymph nodes). Abdominal ultrasonography is the most useful diagnostic tool. Ultrasound-guided biopsy can be performed if the kidney does not appear fluid-filled; however, the biopsy may cause peritonitis, uncontrollable hemorrhage, or may seed the abdomen with tumor cells.

MEDICAL MANAGEMENT

Preoperative medical management of animals with renal neoplasia is necessary if renal failure is present or anemia is severe (i.e., a PCV of less than 20%). Medical management of animals with renal failure is discussed on p. 461.

SURGICAL TREATMENT

Nephrectomy is indicated for malignant renal tumors if they are unilateral and there is no evidence of metastasis (Fig. 21-19). Dogs with renal carcinoma have lived for up to 4 years after removal of the affected kidney (Klein et al, 1988). However, typically metastasis is present at the time of diagnosis because of the late onset of clinical signs. Adjuvant

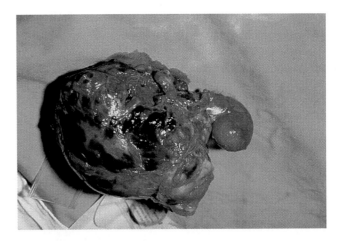

FIG. 21-19
Renal hemangioendothelioma in a 6-year-old dog.

chemotherapy or radiation therapy may prolong the lives of dogs and cats with malignant renal neoplasia, but little data are available on which to base recommendations at this time. Cats with renal lymphoma may respond to chemotherapy for variable time periods.

Preoperative Management

If possible, hydration, acid-base, and electrolyte abnormalities should be corrected before surgery. Perioperative antibiotic therapy is indicated in some patients (i.e., large neoplasms that may be secondarily infected or immunosuppressed or chronically debilitated patients). Animals with preexisting infection (i.e., urinary tract infections) should be treated with antibiotics before surgery. If the patient is anemic, preoxygenation is beneficial. Preoperative blood transfusions should be considered in moderately to severely anemic patients, and blood should be available for intraoperative and postoperative transfusions, if needed.

Anesthesia

If renal impairment is not present, many anesthetic regimens can be used safely. If renal impairment is present, see p. 462 for suggested anesthetic protocols.

Surgical Anatomy

Surgical anatomy of the kidney and ureter is discussed on p. 462.

Positioning

The animal is placed in dorsal recumbency and the abdomen prepared for a ventral midline incision. The prepped area should extend from above the xiphoid to below the pubis.

SURGICAL TECHNIQUE

The entire abdomen should be explored for metastasis before performing a nephrectomy (see p. 463). The other kidney should be palpated and biopsies performed if bilateral involvement is suspected. Intraoperative cytology or examination of frozen sections is helpful to determine if the tumor is malignant. The adjacent ureter should be located to ensure that it is not inadvertently ligated. Occasionally, the tumor will invade surrounding tissues (e.g., sublumbar musculature or caudal vena cava) making removal of the entire kidney difficult. The entire ureter should be removed with the kidney. Careful handling of the neoplastic kidney and ligation of the renal vein may help prevent seeding of neoplastic cells via the vasculature or directly into adjacent tissues.

SUTURE MATERIALS/SPECIAL INSTRUMENTS

Absorbable suture material such as polyglactin 910 (Vicryl), polyglycolic acid (Dexon), polydioxanone (PDS), or polyglyconate (Maxon), or nonabsorbable cardiovascular silk can be used to ligate the renal vessels and ureter.

POSTOPERATIVE CARE AND ASSESSMENT

See p. 469 for postoperative care of patients with renal disease.

COMPLICATIONS

The major complications of nephrectomy are hemorrhage and urinary leakage if the vessels or ureter are not adequately ligated. If the animal had preexisting renal dysfunction, renal failure may occur postoperatively. With large renal tumors, ligation of the opposite ureter is possible if care is not taken to determine its location intraoperatively.

SPECIAL AGE CONSIDERATIONS

Older animals may have some degree of renal dysfunction in the contralateral kidney and require careful monitoring during the surgical procedure. Additionally, many animals have bilateral renal neoplasia. Renal neoplasia should not be excluded as a potential diagnosis in young animals with renomegaly.

PROGNOSIS

Because of the aggressive, malignant nature of most renal tumors and the fact that they are seldom diagnosed early, the prognosis is typically poor. However, if nephrectomy is performed early before metastasis, long-term survival is possible. Long-term survival (i.e., longer than 20 months) with nephroblastoma has been reported (Klein MK et al, 1988). With benign neoplasia, nephrectomy is usually curative.

Reference

Klein MK et al: Canine primary renal neoplasms: a retrospective review of 54 cases, *J Am Anim Hosp Assoc* 24:443, 1988.

Suggested Reading

Atlee BA et al: Nodular dermatofibrosis in German shepherd dogs as a marker for renal cystadenocarcinoma, *J Am Anim Hosp Assoc* 27:481, 1991.

Clark WR, Wilson RB: Renal adenoma in a cat, *J Am Vet Med Assoc* 193:1557, 1988.

Cosenza SF, Seely JC: Generalized nodular dermatofibrosis and renal cystadenocarcinomas in a German shepherd dog, *J Am Vet Med Assoc* 189:1587, 1986.

Gilbert PA, Griffin CE, Walder EJ: Nodular dermatofibrosis and renal cystadenoma in a German shepherd dog, *J Am Anim Hosp Assoc* 26:253, 1990.

Goldsmid SE et al: Renal transitional cell carcinoma in a dog, *J Am Anim Hosp Assoc* 28:241, 1992.

Gregory CR et al: Feline leukemia virus-associated lymphosarcoma following renal transplantation in a cat, *Transplantation* 52:1097, 1991.

Madewell BR et al: Leukemoid blood response and bone infarcts in a dog with renal tubular adenocarcinoma, *J Am Vet Med Assoc* 197:1623, 1990.

Rudd RG, Whitehair JG, Leipold HW: Spindle cell sarcoma in the kidney of a dog, *J Am Vet Med Assoc* 198:1023, 1991.

Widmer WR, Carlton WW: Persistent hematuria in a dog with renal hemangioma, *J Am Vet Med Assoc* 197:237, 1990.

CHAPTER 22

Surgery of the Urinary Bladder and Urethra

GENERAL PRINCIPLES AND TECHNIQUES

DEFINITIONS

Cystotomy is surgical incision into the urinary bladder whereas **urethrotomy** is an incision into the urethra. **Cystectomy** is removal of a portion of the urinary bladder. **Cystolithiasis** and **cystolithectomy** refer to the development of urinary bladder calculi and their removal, respectively. The **trigone** of the bladder is a smooth triangular portion of the mucous membrane at the base of the bladder (i.e., near the urethra) where the ureters empty. **Cystostomy** is the creation of an opening into the bladder; prepubic catheterization (temporary cystostomy) is usually performed to provide cutaneous urinary diversion in animals with urethral obstruction or trauma. **Uroabdomen** is the condition of having urinary leakage into the abdominal cavity; the urine may be from the kidneys, ureters, bladder, or urethra. **Urethrostomy** is the creation of a permanent fistula into the urethra and is generally performed for irreparable or recurrent urethral stricture, or to prevent repeated obstruction (i.e., with feline urologic syndrome or sterile cystitis).

PREOPERATIVE CONCERNS

Cystolithiasis, neoplasia, and rupture are the most common abnormalities of the urinary bladder in small animals. Urinary obstruction may occur if calculi become lodged in the urethra or a tumor obstructs the proximal urethra or trigone. Male cats with sterile cystitis may develop penile urethral obstruction (see p. 512). Obstruction to urinary flow may result in a distended urinary bladder, postrenal uremia, and hyperkalemia. Bladder rupture is common after motor vehicular trauma; urine leakage may also occur from necrotic bladders (i.e., following damage to its blood supply) or as a complication of bladder surgery (Fig. 22-1). Urinary leakage into the abdominal cavity results in uremia, dehydration, hypovolemia, hyperkalemia, and death if undiagnosed or untreated. **Urinary obstruction and uroperitoneum are medical emergencies, not surgical emergencies.** Hyperkalemia associated with these conditions makes the animal prone to cardiac arrhythmias; therefore fluid and electrolyte abnormalities should be corrected prior to induction of anesthesia (see p. 496).

Hyperkalemia, besides causing a predisposition to cardiac arrhythmias, causes bradycardia, absent or flattened P waves, prolongation of the P-R interval, widened QRS complexes, and/or "tented" or spiked T waves. Potassium concentrations greater than 7.0 mEq/L may be associated with irregular idioventricular rhythms, and when potassium concentrations exceed 9.0 mEq/L, atrial standstill is common. Mild or moderate hyperkalemia may be treated with IV fluids (i.e., 0.9% saline for dilution; Table 22-1). If the animal has concurrent hyponatremia, 5% dextrose solutions (i.e., D5W) and half-strength saline should be

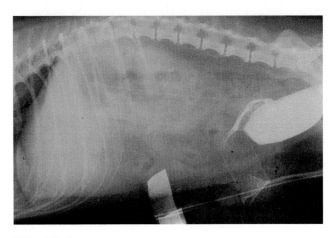

FIG. 22-1
Positive contrast cystourethrogram in a dog 3 days after a cystotomy was performed. Note contrast leaking from the incision at the dorsal aspect of the bladder.

TABLE 22-1

Treatment of Hyperkalemia in Cats

1. Dilute by giving 0.9% saline IV
2. If necessary give sodium bicarbonate (see Table 22-2) or insulin (0.5 units/kg regular insulin IV) plus dextrose (2 g per unit of insulin)
3. If hyperkalemia is life-threatening may give 10% calcium gluconate (0.5-1.0 ml/kg) for transient cardiac protection. Give slowly (over 5-10 min) while monitoring the patient's ECG.

TABLE 22-2

Sodium Bicarbonate Therapy

1-2 mEq/kg IV; repeat only if indicated based on assessment of acid-base balance and potassium concentration

or

0.3 × base deficit (mEq)* × b.w. (kg) (give half IV and remainder over 4-6 hr if necessary)

*Desired bicarbonate–patient's bicarbonate

TABLE 22-3

Selected Anesthetic Protocols for Use in Stable Dogs and Cats with Urinary Abnormalities

Premedication

Oxymorphone* (0.05-0.1 mg/kg SC or IM) or butorphanol (0.2-0.4 mg/kg SC or IM) or buprenorphine (5-15 μg/kg IM)

Induction

Thiopental (10-12 mg/kg IV) or propofol (4-6 mg/kg IV) (see text also)

Maintenance

Isoflurane or halothane

*Use 0.05 mg/kg in cats.

avoided. Although seldom required, severe hyperkalemia may be treated with sodium bicarbonate (Table 22-2). Bicarbonate therapy drives potassium into cells in exchange for hydrogen ions. Alternatively, some clinicians prefer insulin and dextrose administration (see Table 22-1). Insulin facilitates cellular uptake of potassium, while dextrose prevents hypoglycemia following insulin administration. If the hyperkalemia appears immediately life-threatening, 10% calcium gluconate given slowly intravenously may protect the heart until other therapy lowers the plasma potassium concentration.

In animals with uroperitoneum, hyperkalemia and azotemia are best treated with fluids (dilution) and prevention of reabsorption of electrolytes and waste products by providing abdominal drainage. Penrose drains are ineffective for long-term abdominal drainage (i.e., more than 12 to 24 hours) because they are quickly isolated from the abdominal cavity by omentum and fibrin (see p. 196); however, they can be used for short-term management in patients with uroabdomen. The goal of abdominal drainage in these patients is to normalize serum electrolytes and decrease azotemia, making the animal a better candidate for anesthesia. Abdominal drainage for 6 to 12 hours is often adequate for this purpose. Alternately, peritoneal drainage may be accomplished by placement of a peritoneal dialysis catheter. Peritoneal dialysis may be especially useful when treating patients with concurrent renal dysfunction.

Urethral trauma (e.g., gunshot or bite wounds, rupture due to vehicular trauma) or neoplasia may result in urinary obstruction. If the prostatic or penile urethra is torn, subcutaneous urine leakage may occur. Initial signs of subcutaneous urine leakage are bruising and/or swelling of the tissues. The skin and subcutaneous tissues can necrose if left untreated. Management of patients with urethral rupture

prior to surgery may necessitate placement of an indwelling urinary catheter and/or cutaneous urinary diversion (tube cystostomy).

ANESTHETIC CONSIDERATIONS

Electrolyte (i.e., hyperkalemia) and acid-base abnormalities in patients with urinary obstruction or leakage should be corrected prior to anesthetic induction (see above and pp. 461 and 512). Fluids are given intravenously to restore normal hydration and combat postobstruction diuresis. Relief of obstruction without appropriate parenteral fluids commonly results in hypovolemic shock and possibly death. An ECG should be monitored before, during, and after surgery for cardiac arrhythmias. If the animal is hyperkalemic, 0.9% saline should be used for fluid therapy. If the serum potassium is normal, a balanced electrolyte solution should be administered.

Anticholinergics are not routinely recommended for trauma patients because they may increase heart rate and oxygen consumption, and cause a predisposition to cardiac arrhythmias. If analgesia is needed, butorphanol, oxymorphone, or buprenorphine may be given in small, incremental doses (Table 22-3). Acetylpromazine should only be used if volume replacement has been adequate and shock or severe blood loss are unlikely. Thiobarbiturates are arrhythmogenic and should therefore be used cautiously in animals with preexisting arrhythmias. Combinations of opioids and benzodiazepines (diazepam) do not cause severe vasodilation or myocardial depression and are useful for inducing anesthesia despite hypovolemia or dehydration (Table 22-4). Etomidate may be used for induction since it maintains cardiovascular stability and is not arrhythmogenic. Alternatively, if the patient is not vomiting, mask or chamber induction can be used, or thiopental or propofol may be administered at reduced dosages. Cats may be premedicated using low dosages of butorphanol, buprenorphine, or oxymorphone and induced with etomidate. Because cats excrete in their urine the active form of ketamine it should be used very cautiously (if at all) in this species if urinary obstruction or renal dysfunc-

TABLE 22-4
Selected Anesthetic Protocols for Use in Decompensated Patients in Renal Failure or Hypovolemic, Dehydrated, or Shocky Animals with Urinary Abnormalities
Dogs
Induction
Oxymorphone (0.1 mg/kg IV) plus diazepam (0.2 mg/kg IV). Give in incremental dosages. Intubate if possible. If necessary, give etomidate (0.5-1.5 mg/kg IV). (See text also.)
Maintenance
Isoflurane
Cats
Premedication
Butorphanol (0.2-0.4 mg/kg SC or IM) or buprenorphine (5-15 µg/kg IM) or oxymorphone (0.05 mg/kg SC or IM)
Induction
Diazepam (0.2 mg/kg IV) followed by etomidate (0.5-1.5 mg/kg IV). (See text also.)
Maintenance
Isoflurane

tion is present. Isoflurane is the least cardiodepressant inhalation anesthetic.

ANTIBIOTICS

Perioperative antibiotic therapy should be considered in animals with urinary obstruction or leakage because infection prolongs healing and may promote stricture formation. Animals with cystic or urethral calculi often have concurrent infections and should be placed on appropriate antibiotics based on urine culture and susceptibility. Alternately, antibiotics can be withheld until appropriate intraoperative cultures have been taken. Potentially nephrotoxic antibiotics (i.e., aminoglycosides, tetracycline) should be avoided in patients with obstructions (see p. 462).

SURGICAL ANATOMY

The bladder location varies depending on the amount of urine it currently contains; when empty it lies entirely, or almost entirely, within the pelvic cavity. In a 12-kg dog it holds up to 120 ml of urine without becoming overly distended. The bladder is divided into a neck, which connects it to the urethra, and a body. The bladder receives its blood supply from the cranial and caudal vesical arteries, which are branches of the umbilical and urogenital arteries, respectively. Sympathetic innervation is from the hypogastric nerves, while parasympathetic innervation is via the pelvic nerve. The pudendal nerve supplies somatic innervation to the external bladder sphincter and striated musculature of the urethra. The urethra in male dogs is divided into a prostatic and a penile portion (see below).

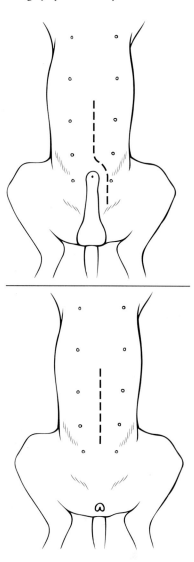

FIG. 22-2
To expose the bladder, make an incision from the umbilicus to the pubis.

SURGICAL TECHNIQUES

For the bladder, an incision is made from the umbilicus caudal to the pubis (Fig. 22-2). The proximal urethra (i.e., prostatic urethra) can be reached by this approach; however, pelvic osteotomy or symphysiotomy is required for adequate exposure of the membranous urethra (i.e., from the caudal edge of the prostate to the ischial arch; Figs. 22-3 and 22-4). The penile urethra begins at the ischial arch and extends to the external urethral penile orifice. The penile urethra may be approached in the perineal (perineal urethrotomy) or scrotal (scrotal urethrotomy) regions, or between the scrotum and the external urethral orifice (prescrotal urethrotomy). The skin overlying the site is prepared for aseptic surgery in the standard fashion before using either approach.

Cystotomy

Cystotomy may be performed for removal of cystic and urethral calculi (see p. 499), identification and biopsy of mass lesions (see p. 505), repair of ectopic ureters (see

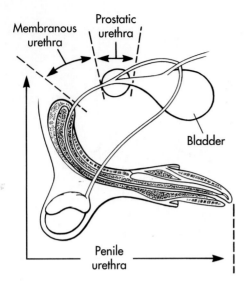

FIG. 22-3
The urethra of male dogs is composed of prostatic, membranous, and penile portions.

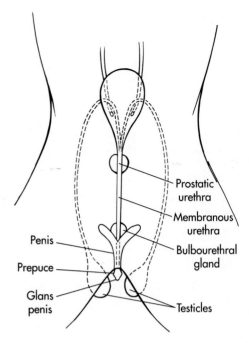

FIG. 22-4
Anatomy of the bladder, urethra, and reproductive system in male cats.

p. 470), or diagnosis of urinary tract infection resistant to treatment. The incision is generally made on the dorsal or ventral surface of the bladder, away from the urethra; however, ventral exposure is performed if identification and/or catheterization of the ureteral openings is necessary. The goal of cystotomy closure is to obtain a water-tight seal that will not promote calculi formation. This can be accomplished using a single- or double-layer appositional pattern or by inverting suture patterns using absorbable suture material. If the bladder wall is thick, a single-layer appositional closure is sufficient and, ideally, the suture should not penetrate the bladder lumen. In normal bladders, however, a double-layer inverting suture pattern is frequently used and luminal penetration is common. Suturing the bladder mucosa as a separate layer (in a simple continuous suture pattern) seems to decrease postoperative bleeding in dogs with bleeding tendencies (see the discussion on suture materials below).

Isolate the bladder from the rest of the abdominal cavity by placing moistened laparotomy pads beneath it. Place stay sutures on the bladder apex to facilitate manipulation (Fig. 22-5, A). Make the incision in the dorsal or ventral aspect of the bladder, away from the ureters and urethra and between major blood vessels. Remove urine by suction (perform intraoperative cystocentesis prior to cystotomy if suction is not available). Excise a small section of the bladder wall adjacent to the incision and submit it for culture. Check the bladder apex for a diverticulum and remove it if necessary. Examine the mucosa for defects and pass a catheter down the urethra to check for patency. Close the bladder in two or three layers with absorbable suture material. For a two-layer closure, suture the seromuscular layers with two continuous inverting suture lines (i.e., Cushing, followed by Lembert; Fig. 22-5, B). If a three-layer closure

is used, suture the mucosa as a separate layer with a simple continuous suture pattern.

☞ **NOTE** · If removing cystic calculi, be sure to catheterize the urethra and flush until you are certain that the urethra is free of calculi. Leaving stones in the urethra is a common error.

Cystostomy (Prepubic Catheterization)

Temporary cystostomy or prepubic catheterization is performed to provide cutaneous urinary diversion in animals with urinary obstruction, or traumatized or surgically repaired urethras. It may also be advisable for animals with bladder atony secondary to neurologic disease or to prevent overdistention of the bladder after surgery. Cystostomy may be performed by placing a Foley catheter (6 to 12 French) via a small abdominal incision, or percutaneously by placing a Stamey Malecot catheter (10 to 14 French) into the bladder (Fig. 22-6). Premature removal of the Stamey Malecot catheter was reported in experimental dogs (Dhein et al, 1989); therefore surgically placed Foley catheters may be preferred for long-term catheterization in ambulatory patients. The catheters can generally be placed under local anesthesia (augmented by chemical restraint or mask inhalation anesthesia, if necessary). They can also be placed during exploratory laparotomy. Removal of the Stamey catheter can be performed by gentle traction within 3 or 4 days after placement without risk of urinary leakage; however, it is recommended that a Foley catheter be left in 5 to 7 days.

To place a Foley catheter, make a small midline incision caudal to the umbilicus in females or adjacent to the pre-

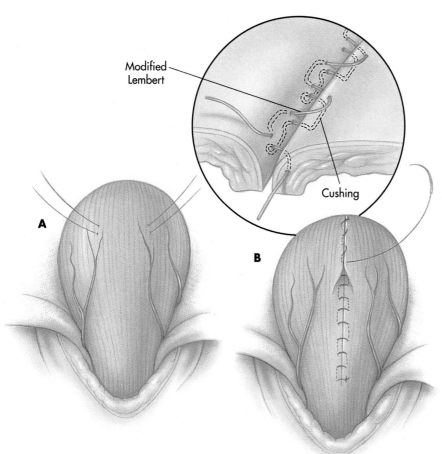

Modified Lembert

Cushing

A

B

FIG. 22-5
Cystotomy is indicated to remove calculi, repair trauma, resect or biopsy neoplasms, or correct congenital abnormalities. **A,** Isolate the bladder and place stay sutures in it to facilitate manipulation. Make the incision in the dorsal or ventral aspect of the bladder. **B,** For a two-layer closure, suture the seromuscular layer with two continuous inverting suture lines.

puce in males. Locate the bladder and place stay sutures and a purse-string suture into it (Fig. 22-7, A). Place the tip of the Foley catheter into the abdominal cavity through a separate stab incision in the abdominal wall (Fig. 22-7, B). Make a small stab incision into the bladder (within the purse-string suture) and place the Foley catheter into the bladder lumen. Inflate the balloon with saline and secure the catheter within the lumen by tieing the purse-string suture around it with a Roman sandal suture (see p. 679 and Fig. 22-7, C). Tack the bladder to the body wall with several absorbable sutures (Fig. 22-7, D). Close the initial incision and tack the catheter to the skin by placing sutures through a piece of tape attached to the catheter.

For a Stamey catheter (see Fig. 22-6), place the dog in right– or left–lateral recumbency and prep the ventrolateral aspect of the caudal abdominal wall. Do not evacuate the bladder prior to catheter placement. Make a small skin incision over the bladder and with the stylet securely fixed within the catheter (with the Malecot wings twisted flat), direct it through the stab incision. Thrust the catheter into the bladder lumen making sure that the entire flanged portion of the catheter is within the bladder lumen (once urine is obtained, advance the catheter 1 cm further). Release the Luer-lock to open the Malecot wings and remove the obturator. Secure the catheter to the skin.

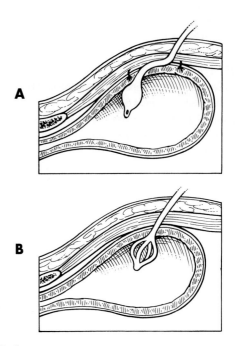

A

B

FIG. 22-6
Temporary cystostomy or prepubic catheterization may be performed by placing a **A,** Foley catheter or **B,** Stamey Malecot catheter into the bladder.

FIG. 22-7
A, To place a Foley catheter, make a small incision and locate the bladder. Place stay sutures and a purse-string suture in the bladder. Place the tip of the Foley catheter into the abdominal cavity through a separate stab incision in the abdominal wall. **B,** Make a small stab incision into the bladder and place the Foley catheter into the bladder lumen. **C,** Inflate the balloon with saline and secure the catheter within the lumen by tieing the purse-string suture around it with a Roman sandal suture. **D,** Tack the bladder to the body wall with several absorbable sutures.

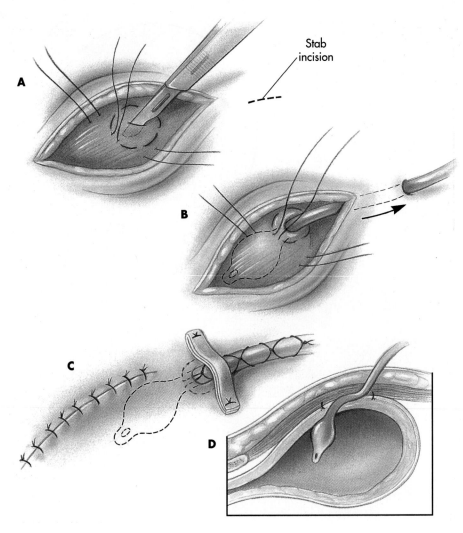

Stab incision

Intrapelvic Urethral Anastomosis

The intrapelvic urethra may be torn secondarily to pelvic fracture or other trauma, or it may be damaged during surgery. Primary suture repair of a completely transected urethra is indicated whenever possible. Dependent on size, small lacerations or partial ruptures may heal if urine is diverted through a urethral catheter or tube cystostomy for 7 to 21 days. *Perform a caudal ventral midline abdominal incision and, if necessary, a pubic symphysiotomy or bilateral pubic and ischial osteotomy (see below). Locate the transected ends of the urethra and debride them. Minimize dissection around the urethra and bladder to avoid damaging the vascular or nerve supply to these structures (Fig. 22-8). Suture the ends with six to eight absorbable interrupted sutures over a transurethral catheter (preferably a Foley catheter or other soft catheter). Leave the catheter in place for 7 to 10 days. If the urethral tissues do not hold suture due to prolonged urine extravasation and subsequent tissue devitalization, delayed repair is indicated. Place a transurethral catheter to divert urine flow for 5 to 7 days. If a catheter cannot be placed from the penile orifice into the bladder, pass a catheter from the bladder into the traumatized tissue, tie it to a catheter placed from the penile urethral orifice,* and use it to pull the penile catheter into the bladder. If the urethra does not heal completely in 7 to 10 days or stricture occurs, resect the urethral ends and suture them over a catheter as described for primary repair. Tube cystostomy can also be used to provide urinary diversion while the urethra is healing, but take care to ensure that the bladder is not allowed to distend or urethral flow of urine will occur.

Adequate urethral exposure can be obtained in some dogs by splitting the symphysis on the midline. In other dogs the cranial aspect of the pubis can be removed. Bilateral pubic and ischial osteotomy allows exposure of the entire urogenital tract in female dogs. *Make a ventral midline incision from the umbilicus to the vulva. Perform a celiotomy from the umbilicus to the pubis, then sharply separate the adductor muscles on the midline of the pubis and ischium. Subperiostally elevate the adductor muscles until the obturator nerves and half of the obturator foramen are exposed (Fig. 22-9, A). Transect the prepubic tendon along the left pubis to the proposed pubic osteotomy site. Predrill holes in the pubis and ischium on both sides of the four proposed osteotomy sites and craniocaudally along the left pubis (Fig. 22-9, B). Osteotomize the pubis and elevate the internal obturator mus-*

Male

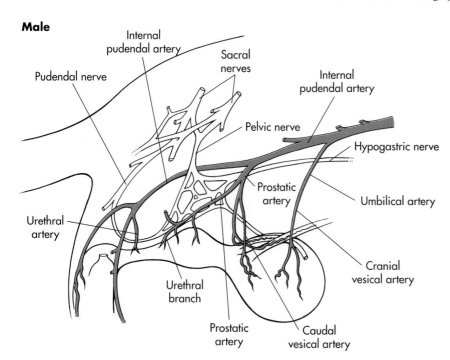

FIG. 22-8
Vascular and nerve supply to the bladder and urethra.

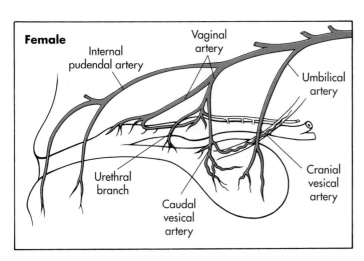

cle from the left pubis and ischium allowing reflection of the entire central bony plate to the right (Fig. 22-9, C). To close the osteotomy sites, preplace orthopedic wire through the previously drilled holes on the right side. Then, before replacing the bone plate, place sutures through the lines of holes in the left pubis and ischium, through the left internal obturator muscle, and back through the adjacent holes in the pubis or ischium. Place orthopedic wire through the left osteotomy sites, then secure the preplaced wires and sutures (Fig. 22-9, D). Reappose the adductor muscles and prepubic tendon before closing the linea alba.

Urethrotomy

Urethrotomy is performed in male dogs to remove urethral calculi that cannot be retrohydropropulsed into the bladder (see p. 501) and to facilitate placement of catheters into the bladder. Occasionally urethrotomy is performed to biopsy obstructive lesions (i.e., strictures, scar tissue, neoplasms).

Prescrotal or perineal urethrotomy may be performed. To avoid possible postoperative urethral stricture cystotomy, rather than urethrotomy, should be performed preferentially if calculi can be dislodged into the bladder by urohydropropulsion.

Prescrotal urethrotomy. Prescrotal urethrotomy (Fig. 22-10) is used to remove calculi from the distal penile urethra, or to place Foley catheters into the urinary bladder if the catheter is of sufficient length and the obstruction is distal to the proposed urethrotomy incision. Occasionally, urethrotomy can be performed under local anesthesia with narcotic sedation in severely depressed or uremic patients. Prescrotal urethrotomies can be left to heal by second intention; however, hemorrhage should be expected from the surgical site for 3 to 5 days (particularly during urination). Primary closure is preferred to decrease postoperative bleeding if the mucosa is healthy and adequate apposition of the urethral mucosa can be achieved.

FIG. 22-9
A, For bilateral pubic and ischial osteotomy elevate the adductor muscles until the obturator nerves and half of the obturator foramen are exposed. **B,** Predrill holes in the pubis and ischium on both sides of the four proposed osteotomy sites and craniocaudally along the left pubis. **C,** Osteotomize the pubis and elevate the internal obturator muscle from the left pubis and ischium allowing reflecting of the entire central bony plate. **D,** Close the osteotomy with orthopedic wire.

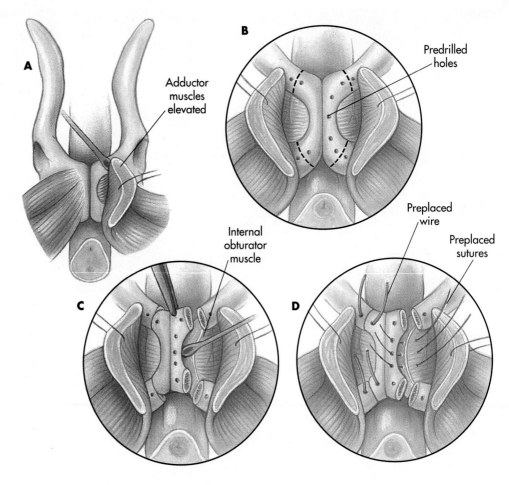

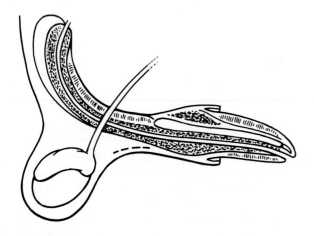

FIG. 22-10
Prescrotal urethrotomy.

With the dog in dorsal recumbency, place a sterile catheter into the penile urethra to the scrotum or to the obstruction. Make a ventral midline incision through the skin and subcutaneous tissues, between the caudal aspect of the os penis and scrotum. Identify, mobilize, and retract the retractor penis muscle laterally to expose the urethra (Fig. 22-11). Using a No. 15 scalpel blade, make an incision into the urethral lumen over the catheter (Fig. 22-12). Iris scissors can be used to extend the incision, if necessary. Remove calculi with forceps and gently flush the urethra with warm saline. The incision may be left to heal by second intention or the urethra may be closed with simple interrupted absorbable sutures (4-0 or 5-0). Place the first layer in the urethral mucosa and corpus spongiosum, then appose subcutaneous tissues and skin with simple interrupted sutures or a continuous subcuticular suture pattern. Some surgeons prefer a continuous suture pattern in the urethra to promote hemostasis. *Remove the urinary catheter following surgery, regardless of whether the urethra is sutured or not.*

Perineal urethrotomy. Perineal urethrotomy (Fig. 22-13) is occasionally used to remove calculi lodged at the ischial arch and to place catheters into the bladder of large, male dogs. Perineal urethrotomy is less commonly indicated than urethrotomy at other sites. They should be closed to prevent potential subcutaneous urine leakage.

Place a purse-string suture in the anus. Place a sterile catheter into the urethra to the level of the bladder or the site of the obstruction. With the dog in sternal recumbency and the rear limbs hanging over the edge of the table, make a

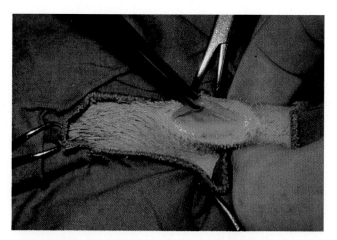

FIG. 22-11
For prescrotal urethrotomy, make a ventral midline incision through the skin and subcutaneous tissues, between the caudal aspect of the os penis and scrotum. Identify, mobilize, and retract the retractor penis muscle laterally to expose the urethra.

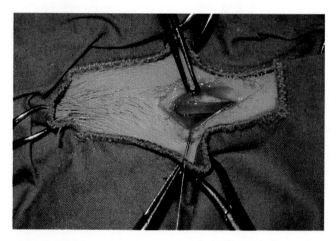

FIG. 22-12
Use a No. 15 scalpel blade to make an incision into the urethral lumen over the catheter (see Fig. 22-11).

midline incision over the urethra, midway between the scrotum and anus. Identify the retractor penis muscle, elevate, and retract it (Fig. 22-14, A). Separate the paired bulbospongiosus muscles at their raphe to expose the corpus spongiosum, then incise the corpus spongiosum to enter the urethral lumen (Fig. 22-14, B and C). Close the incision as described above for prescrotal urethrotomy (Fig. 22-14, D).

Urethrostomy

Urethrostomy is indicated for: (1) recurrent, obstructive calculi that cannot be managed medically; (2) calculi that cannot be removed by retrohydropropulsion or urethrotomy; (3) urethral stricture; (4) urethral or penile neoplasia or severe trauma; and (5) preputial neoplasia requiring penile amputation. Depending on the site of the lesion it can be prescrotal, scrotal, perineal, or prepubic in dogs. Scrotal ure-

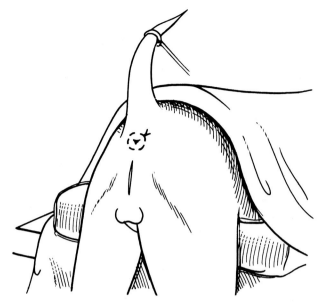

FIG. 22-13
Perineal urethrotomy.

throstomy is preferred if castration is an option and the lesion is distal to the scrotum. Perineal urethrostomy is routinely performed in cats; however, prepubic and subpubic urethrostomy have also been described.

Prescrotal urethrostomy. Prescrotal urethrostomy is performed similarly to prescrotal urethrotomy except that the urethral mucosa is sutured to the skin. *Make a 3- to 4-cm incision in the urethral mucosa as described above. The length of the urethral incision should be 6 to 8 times its luminal diameter. Periurethral sutures can be placed to the subcutaneous tissues using a simple continuous suture pattern of absorbable suture material. Place simple interrupted absorbable sutures (3-0 to 5-0) from the urethral mucosa to the skin beginning at the caudal aspect of the incision. Suture the remainder of the urethral mucosa to the skin with simple interrupted sutures (Fig. 22-15). Suture skin at either end of the incision with simple interrupted sutures.*

Scrotal urethrostomy. Scrotal urethrostomy (Fig. 22-16) is preferred over perineal or prepubic urethrostomy because the urethra is wider, more superficial, and surrounded by less cavernous tissues here than at other sites. Therefore, postoperative hemorrhage is often less than with the other techniques and stricture is less likely.

If the dog is intact, castrate him and excise the scrotum; otherwise, perform a scrotal ablation (Fig. 22-17, A). Place a sterile catheter into the urethra to the level of the ischial arch or beyond. Make a midline incision over the urethra through the subcutaneous tissues. Identify the retractor penis muscle, mobilize, and retract it laterally to expose the urethra. Using a No. 15 scalpel blade, make a 3- to 4-cm incision into the urethral lumen over the catheter

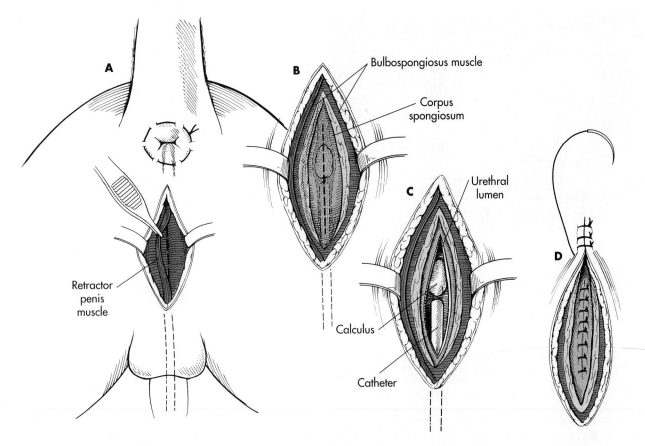

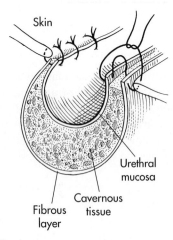

FIG. 22-14
For perineal urethrotomy **A,** make a midline incision over the urethra, midway between the scrotum and anus. Identify the retractor penis muscle, elevate, and retract it. **B,** Separate the paired bulbospongiosus muscles at their raphe to expose the corpus spongiosum, **C,** then incise the corpus spongiosum to enter the urethral lumen. **D,** Close the urethra with simple interrupted absorbable sutures. Place the first layer in the urethral mucosa and corpus spongiosum, then appose subcutaneous tissues and skin with simple interrupted sutures or a continuous subcuticular suture pattern.

FIG. 22-15
For urethrostomy, place simple interrupted absorbable sutures from the urethral mucosa to skin. To improve hemostasis, avoid incorporating cavernous tissue in the sutures.

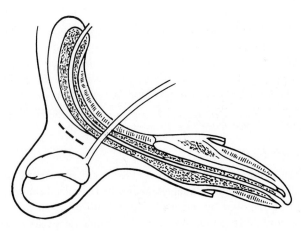

FIG. 22-16
Scrotal urethrostomy.

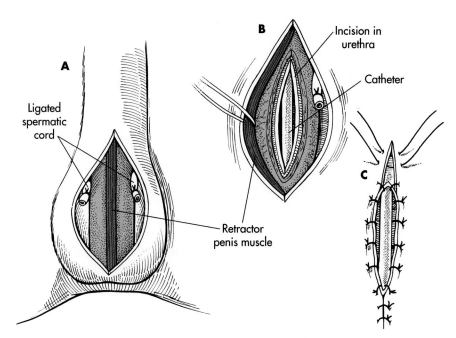

FIG. 22-17
Scrotal urethrostomy is preferred over other sites because there is less hemorrhage. Perform a scrotal ablation. **A,** Make a midline incision over the urethra through the subcutaneous tissues. Identify the retractor penis muscle, mobilize, and retract it laterally to expose the urethra. **B,** Using a No. 15 scalpel blade, make a 3- to 4-cm incision into the urethral lumen over the catheter. **C,** Suture urethral mucosa to skin with simple interrupted sutures.

(Fig. 22-17, B). Suture the urethra as described above for prescrotal urethrostomy (Fig. 22-17, C).

Canine perineal urethrostomy. Because it often causes unacceptable urine scalding, perineal urethrostomy is only used in dogs that have urinary problems that a scrotal or prescrotal urethrostomy will not solve. Additionally, the surrounding cavernous tissue is large at this location, and hemorrhage can be profuse. Furthermore, the urethra is less superficial here and mobilizing it can result in excessive suture-line tension causing dehiscence.

Make a 4- to 6-cm incision in skin and overlying tissues and incise the perineal urethra as described above for perineal urethrotomy. The urethral incision should be 1.5 to 2.0 cm in length. Suture the urethral mucosa to the skin as described above for prescrotal urethrostomy (Fig. 22-18).

Prepubic urethrostomy. Prepubic (antepubic) urethrostomy is a salvage procedure performed when damage to the membranous or penile urethra is irreparable (this is rare), or removal of these tissues is necessary (i.e., neoplasia). Unless nerve damage occurs (this is most likely if prostatic resection is performed), most animals are continent following this procedure.

Make a ventral midline incision from the umbilicus to the pubis. Free the intrapelvic urethra from the pelvic floor using blunt dissection. Be sure to preserve the urethral artery and its branches. Sever the distal aspect of the intrapelvic urethra. It may be necessary to carefully dissect the prostate from the urethra to ensure that there is ample urethra to exteriorize in some male dogs. Preserve the blood supply to the neck of the bladder. In male dogs, exteriorize the urethra through a small stab incision 2 to 3 cm lateral to the

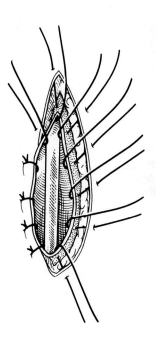

FIG. 22-18
For urethrostomy, place simple interrupted absorbable sutures from the urethral mucosa to skin beginning at the caudal aspect of the incision. Suture the remainder of the urethral mucosa to skin with simple interrupted sutures. Suture skin at either end of the incision with simple interrupted sutures.

prepuce or within the prepuce. In females, exteriorize the urethra through the ventral midline incision or 2 to 3 lateral to the linea alba (Fig. 22-19, A). Spatulate the distal end of the urethra to increase the luminal diameter (Fig. 22-19, B), then suture the urethral mucosa to skin with interrupted sutures of absorbable (e.g., polyglyconate or polydioxanone suture) or nonabsorbable (e.g., nylon or polypropylene) suture. Be sure that there is little tension on the urethrostomy site and that the urethra is not bent

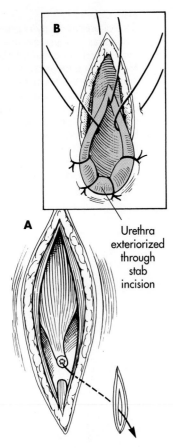

FIG. 22-19
Prepubic urethrostomy may be performed when distal urethral lesions are present. **A,** Sever the distal aspect of the intrapelvic urethra and exteriorize it through a small stab incision 2 to 3 cm lateral to the linea alba. **B,** Spatulate the distal end of the urethra to increase the luminal diameter and suture the urethral mucosa to skin with interrupted sutures.

sharply. A Foley catheter can be placed into the bladder through the urethrostomy to divert urine during initial healing (i.e., 24 to 48 hours).

Subpubic urethrostomy. Subpubic urethrostomy is similar to prepubic urethrostomy except that the urethra is exteriorized caudal to the brim of the pubis. In cats, this procedure may be less likely to cause postoperative stricture, recurrent UTI, or chronic urine-scald dermatitis. It is indicated when repeated stricture occurs after perineal urethrostomy.

Perform this procedure similarly to the one described above, but retract the skin caudally past the brim of the pubis. Expose the medial boundary of the obturator foramen by elevating the adductor muscle and cranial portion of the gracilis muscle from the periosteum of the pubis. Partially incise the prepubic tendon and reflect it laterally to expose the pubic rami (Fig. 22-20). Osteotomize the pubic rami 1.5 cm lateral to the pubic symphysis. Make a transverse incision through the body of the pubic bone and across the pubic symphysis. Rotate the pubic flap ventrally to visualize

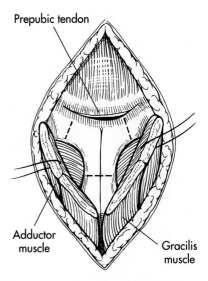

FIG. 22-20
For pubic osteotomy, partially incise the prepubic tendon and reflect it laterally to expose the pubic rami. Osteotomize the pubic rami 1.5 cm lateral to the pubic symphysis. Make a transverse incision through the body of the pubic bone and across the pubic symphysis.

the intrapelvic urethra. Transect the urethra cranial to the lesion (i.e., stricture) and replace the pubic flap (Fig. 22-21, A). Reappose the muscular aponeuroses of the gracilis and adductor muscles with interrupted or horizontal mattress sutures. Make a 1-cm stab incision 3 cm distal to the caudal extent of the abdominal incision. Tunnel through the subcutaneous tissues and exteriorize the urethra (Fig. 22-21, B). Spatulate the urethral end and suture it to the skin with 4-0 suture material. Close the abdominal incision but leave the caudal 1 cm of the linea alba open to avoid crimping the urethra as it passes over the pubic flap. Resect the tissues at the perineal urethrostomy site and either close them or leave them open to heal by second intention.

Feline perineal urethrostomy. Perineal urethrostomy (see p. 513) is indicated to prevent recurrence of obstruction in male cats or to treat obstruction that cannot be eliminated by catheterization. It is also useful when treating strictures that occur following urethral obstruction and catheterization.

Urinary Diversion

Permanent urinary diversion may be indicated when neoplasia involves the bladder trigone. After cystectomy, the ureters may be anastomosed to an isolated bowel conduit or reservoir or into the intact colon, jejunum, or ileum (Fig. 22-22). Complications associated with ureteral anastomosis to the bowel include reabsorption of electrolytes and nitrogenous waste products, upper UTI, and neurologic dysfunction. Azotemia, hyperammonemia, hyperchloremia, and metabolic acidosis are common after these procedures. **Because it is a salvage procedure commonly associated with life-threatening complications, clients should be carefully**

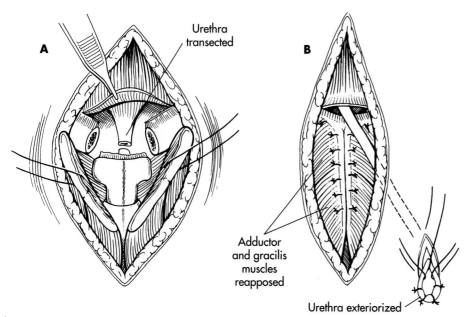

FIG. 22-21
For subpubic urethrostomy, perform a pubic osteotomy (see Fig. 22-20) and rotate the pubic flap ventrally to visualize the intrapelvic urethra. **A,** Transect the urethra cranial to the lesion and replace the pubic flap. **B,** Exteriorize the urethra through a stab incision, spatulate the urethral end, and suture it to skin.

counseled when considering this treatment option. Ureterocolonic anastomosis is the most commonly performed technique for permanent urinary diversion. The patient should be fasted for 48 hours and saline enemas given 12 to 24 hours before surgery. Prophylactic antibiotics are given and should be continued for at least 8 weeks after surgery.

Excise the bladder and proximal urethra (1 to 2 cm distal to the suspected area of neoplasia) and ligate and transect the ureters. Dissect the ureters from their retroperitoneal attachments. Determine the length of the ureters and choose a site for each to be implanted into the colon. Stagger the sites for anastomosis of the right and left ureters so that they are at different sites in the colon. Express feces from the proposed site of ureteral anastomoses and place atraumatic forceps on the colon. Make a three-sided seromuscular colonic flap for each ureter (Fig. 22-23, A), then create a 4-mm circular defect in the colonic mucosa with tenotomy scissors (Fig. 22-23, B). Transect the end of the ureter, spatulate it, and tunnel the ureters through the seromuscular flap into the colonic lumen. Suture the ureter to the colonic mucosa with simple interrupted sutures (5-0 or 6-0 absorbable suture material; Fig. 22-23, C). Close the flap over the ureter, but be sure to avoid compromising the ureteral lumen (Fig. 22-23, D).

HEALING OF THE BLADDER AND URETHRA

Compared with other organs, the urinary bladder heals quickly, regaining 100% of normal tissue strength in 14 to 21 days. Complete reepithelization of the bladder occurs in 30 days. Substantial portions of the bladder can be safely resected. As long as the undamaged trigone persists, the bladder will expand (due to epithelial regeneration, scar tissue formation and remodeling, hypertrophy, and proliferation

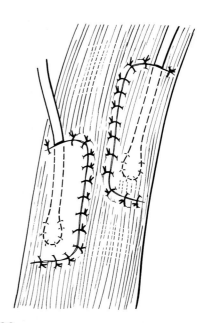

FIG. 22-22
Permanent urinary diversion may be performed by anastomosing the ureters into the intact colon, jejunum, or ileum.

of smooth muscle) until it again functions as an effective reservoir.

If urethral continuity is not completely disrupted, the urethra can heal by regeneration of urethral mucosa in as little as 7 days. Urine extravasation (particularly if infected) delays wound healing and promotes periurethral fibrosis and stricture formation. Urinary diversion via a urethral catheter or tube cystostomy is therefore indicated for small urethral lacerations. When complete transection of the urethra occurs, fibrous tissue proliferation occurs in the gaps between the severed ends. Contraction of the fibrous tissue often leads to stricture and urinary obstruction. Primary anastomosis over an indwelling catheter (or proximal urinary

FIG. 22-23
For colonic urinary diversion, **A,** make
a three-sided seromuscular flap for
each ureter, **B,** then create a 4-mm
circular defect in the colonic mucosa
with tenotomy scissors. Transect the end
of the ureter, spatulate it, and tunnel the
ureters through the seromuscular flap
into the colonic lumen. **C,** Suture the
ureter to colonic mucosa with simple
interrupted sutures. **D,** Close the flap
over the ureter but be sure to avoid
compromising the ureteral lumen.

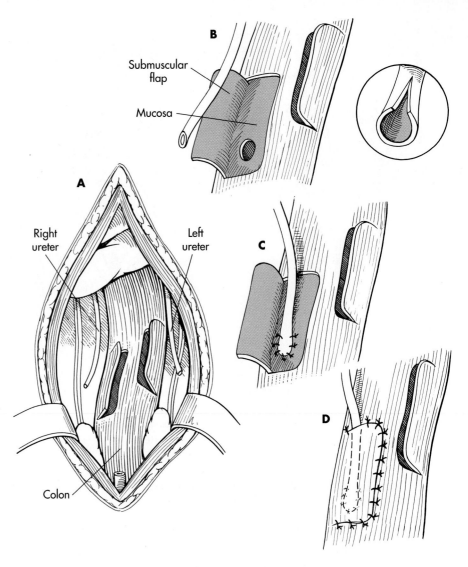

diversion) should be performed to decrease the likelihood of
stricture formation. The catheter should be left in place for 3
to 5 days.

SUTURE MATERIALS/SPECIAL INSTRUMENTS

Absorbable suture material (e.g., polydioxanone [PDS],
polyglyconate [Maxon], polyglycolic acid [Dexon] or
polyglactin-910 [Vicryl]) is preferred for bladder and urethral surgery. Most sutures appear to lose tensile strength
faster in alkaline urine (such as that seen with *Proteus* infections) than in infected, acidic urine or sterile urine. Polyglycolic acid and polyglactin-910 cause less inflammation than
chromic gut suture; however, in some infections (i.e., *Proteus
mirabilis*) they may lose tensile strength very quickly (i.e., less
than 24 hours). Experimentally, in an *in vitro* setting, PDS
maintains greater than 90% and 87% of its original tensile
strength at 28 days in sterile urine and *Escherichia coli* inoculated urine, respectively, but loses all strength by 7 days in
Proteus mirabilis inoculated urine (Schiller, Stone, Gupta,
1993). Nonabsorbable sutures should be avoided due to their
potential to promote calculi formation.

POSTOPERATIVE CARE AND ASSESSMENT

Urination should be closely monitored in patients after urethral surgery to detect obstruction due to tissue swelling, fibrosis, or necrosis. Following removal of the urinary obstruction, intravenous fluid therapy should be maintained
until postobstructive diuresis ceases. Electrolytes should be
monitored (particularly potassium) as hypokalemia may occur secondary to diuresis or medical therapy of hyperkalemia. Patients should be monitored for pain postoperatively and analgesics provided as necessary (Table 22-5).
Elizabethan collars should be used in patients with indwelling urinary catheters, urethrotomies, or urethrostomies
to prevent early catheter removal or self-mutilation. With
urethrotomy the patient should be observed for postoperative hemorrhage. Digital pressure on the surgical site may be
necessary to stop bleeding immediately after surgery or after
urination (for 3 to 5 days). Bladder atony may occur in as little as 12 hours if the animal is sedated or given narcotic analgesics postoperatively, or does not void due to pain. The
bladder should be kept decompressed by manually expressing it until the patient is urinating normally.

TABLE 22-5

Postoperative Analgesics

Oxymorphone (Numorphan)

0.05-0.1 mg/kg IV, IM, every 4 hours (as needed)

Butorphanol (Torbutrol, Torbugesic)

0.2-0.4 mg/kg IV, IM, or SC, every 2 to 4 hours (as needed)

Buprenorphine (Buprenex)

5-15 µg/kg IV, IM, every 6 hours (as needed)

In cats with urethrostomies, paper instead of gravel litter should be used until the wound is healed and urinary cultures should be performed routinely to check for UTI. An indwelling catheter may promote stricture formation and UTI in cats following surgery; therefore their use is not recommended. Animals with ureterocolonic anastomoses should be checked regularly for pyelonephritis. Inappetence may result in increased absorption of urine due to lack of fecal bulk; therefore, animals should be encouraged to eat as soon as possible after surgery. Excretory urography (e.g., presence of hydroureter and/or hydronephrosis) may help determine the long-term need for antibiotics in these patients.

COMPLICATIONS

The most common complications of urethral wound repair are stricture formation and urinary leakage. Indwelling catheters may allow ascending bacterial infection or cause fibrosis and stricture. Oversized stents (those that distend the urethra) should be avoided. Complications of prepubic catheterization (temporary cystostomy) may include bowel perforation from improper percutaneous placement, urinary tract infection, transient hematuria, uroabdomen, premature catheter removal, and breakage or incomplete removal of the catheter. Stricture formation in cats following perineal urethrostomy is generally due to making the stoma too small (i.e., making the stoma in the proximal penile urethra instead of the distal pelvic urethra), or postoperative subcutaneous urine leakage and subsequent granulation tissue formation (see p. 513). Urinary and fecal incontinence may occur if the nerves are damaged during dissection around the pelvic urethra. Perineal urethrostomy is associated with a high prevalence of UTI postoperatively. Rectal prolapse has also been reported following perineal urethrostomy in cats. Pyelonephritis, renal failure due to end-stage kidney disease, neurologic dysfunction, hyperchloremic metabolic acidosis, and diarrhea with subsequent perineal irritation are possible complications of ureterocolonic urinary diversion (see p. 492).

SPECIAL AGE CONSIDERATIONS

Older animals may have preexisting cardiac or renal dysfunction and should be monitored closely. Young animals may have very small urethras, making surgical repair of complete transections difficult.

References

Dhein CR et al: Prepubic (suprapubic) catheterization of the dog, *J Am Anim Hosp Assoc* 25:261, 1989.

Schiller TD, Stone EA, Gupta BS: *In vitro* loss of tensile strength and elasticity of five absorbable suture materials in sterile and infected canine urine, *Vet Surg* 22:208, 1993.

Suggested Reading

Allen SW, Crowell WA: Ventral approach to the pelvic canal in the female dog, *Vet Surg* 20:118, 1991.

Anson LW: Urethral trauma and principles of urethral surgery, *Compend Contin Educ Pract Vet* 9:981, 1987.

Bellah JR: Problems of the urethra, *Probl Vet Med* 1:17, 1989.

Bellah JR: Wound healing in the urinary tract, *Semin Vet Med Surg (Small Anim)* 4:294, 1989.

Bilbrey SA, Birchard SJ, Smeak DD: Scrotal urethrostomy: a retrospective review of 38 dogs (1973 through 1988), *J Am Anim Hosp Assoc* 27:560, 1991.

Bjorling DE, Howard PE: Urinary salvage procedures, *Probl Vet Med* 1:93, 1989.

Bjorling DE, Petersen SW: Surgical techniques for urinary tract diversion and salvage in small animals, *Compend Contin Educ Pract Vet* 12:1699, 1990.

Bradley RL: Prepubic urethrostomy, *Probl Vet Med* 1:120, 1989.

Cooley AJ et al: The effects of indwelling transurethral catheterization and tube cystostomy on urethral anastomoses in dogs, *Vet Surg* 24:423, 1995 (abstract).

Crowe DT: Ventral versus dorsal cystotomy: an experimental investigation, *J Am Anim Hosp Assoc* 22:382, 1986.

Dean PW et al: Canine urethrotomy and urethrostomy, *Compend Contin Educ Pract Vet* 12:1541, 1990.

Ellison GW, Lewis DD, Boren FC: Subpubic urethrostomy to salvage a failed perineal urethrostomy in a cat, *Compend Contin Educ Pract Vet* 11:946, 1989.

Gregory CR: The effects of perineal urethrostomy on urethral function in male cats, *Compend Contin Educ Pract Vet* 9:895, 1987.

Griffin DW, Gregory CR: Prevalence of bacterial urinary tract infection after perineal urethrostomy in cats, *J Am Vet Med Assoc* 200:681, 1992.

Hosgood G, Hedlund CS: Perineal urethrostomy in cats, *Compend Contin Educ Pract Vet* 14:1195, 1992.

Kusba JK, Lipowitz AJ: Repair of strictures following perineal urethrostomy in the cat, *J Am Anim Hosp Assoc* 18:308, 1982.

Layton CE et al: Intrapelvic urethral anastomosis: a comparison of three techniques, *Vet Surg* 16:175, 1987.

Radasch RM et al: Cystotomy closure: a comparison of the strength of appositional and inverting suture patterns, *Vet Surg* 19:283, 1990.

Scavelli TD: Complications associated with perineal urethrostomy in the cat, *Probl Vet Med* 1:111, 1989.

Smith JD, Stone EA, Gilson SD: Placement of a permanent cystostomy catheter to relieve urine outflow obstruction in dogs with transitional cell carcinoma, *J Am Vet Med Assoc* 206:496, 1995.

Stone EA et al: Ureterocolonic anastomosis in clinically normal dogs, *Am J Vet Res* 49:1147, 1988.

Stone EA et al: Ureterocolonic anastomosis in ten dogs with transitional cell carcinoma, *Vet Surg* 17:147, 1988.

Waldron DR et al: The canine urethra: a comparison of first and second intention healing, *Vet Surg* 14:213, 1985.

Weber WJ et al: Comparison of the healing of prescrotal urethrotomy incisions in the dog: sutured versus nonsutured, *Am J Vet Res* 46:1309, 1985.

Yoshioka MM, Carb A: Antepubic urethrostomy in the dog, *J Am Anim Hosp Assoc* 18:290, 1982.

SPECIFIC DISEASES

UROABDOMEN

DEFINITIONS

Uroabdomen is an accumulation of urine in the peritoneal cavity. Urine may leak from the kidney, ureter, bladder, and/or proximal urethra.

SYNONYMS

Uroperitoneum

GENERAL CONSIDERATIONS AND CLINICALLY RELEVANT PATHOPHYSIOLOGY

Bladder rupture is the most common cause of uroabdomen in dogs and cats. It may occur spontaneously (associated with tumor, severe cystitis, or urethral obstruction), be due to blunt or penetrating abdominal trauma, or be iatrogenic following cystocentesis or bladder catheterization. Urinary tract leakage may also be a complication of surgery. Any animal presenting after vehicular trauma should be assessed for possible urinary tract trauma. The impact of the collision may cause the bladder, urethra, or ureter to rupture or necrose. The sharp ends of pelvic fractures may sever or lacerate the urethra. Diagnosis is usually delayed because clinical signs are rarely present at initial examination (see below).

Immediate surgery is contraindicated in animals with uroabdomen that are hyperkalemic or uremic. They should first be treated medically to normalize electrolytes and decrease circulating nitrogenous waste products. Intravenous fluids should be given and abdominal drainage performed (see p. 482). Penrose drains can be placed in the ventral abdomen under local anesthesia (sedate if necessary) to allow drainage for 6 to 12 hours. This will stabilize most animals with previously normal renal function. If there is concurrent renal dysfunction, a peritoneal dialysis catheter may be placed instead of Penrose drains, and the abdominal cavity flushed with dialysis solution.

When urine leaks into the abdominal cavity, some nitrogenous waste products and electrolytes are reabsorbed across the peritoneal membrane and reenter the circulation. Whether molecules are reabsorbed depends on their size. Urea is a small molecule that rapidly equilibrates across the peritoneal surface; however, some larger molecules (e.g., creatinine) cannot pass back into the bloodstream and therefore remain concentrated in the abdominal fluid. **To diagnose uroabdomen, creatinine levels in the abdominal fluid should be measured and compared to serum levels.** If the fluid is urine, the creatinine concentration in the fluid will be substantially greater than that found in serum. Because urea rapidly equilibrates across the peritoneum, BUN may be approximately the same in both abdominal fluid and serum, regardless of the cause of the abdominal effusion.

☞ **NOTE** • Creatinine does not equilibrate across the peritoneal surface; BUN does! Compare creatinine levels (not BUN) in the fluid and serum.

DIAGNOSIS
Clinical Presentation

Signalment. It has been suggested that urinary bladder rupture occurs more frequently in male dogs than female dogs because their long, narrow urethras cannot dilate rapidly; however, ruptured bladders are common in females that have sustained vehicular trauma. Urethral rupture in female dogs following trauma is uncommon. Male dogs and cats with obstruction due to calculi or sterile cystitis (FUS) have a high risk of bladder rupture if the obstruction is not alleviated promptly (see pp. 499 and 512).

History. Clinical signs of urinary tract trauma are often vague and may be masked by other signs of trauma. In one study of dogs with pelvic trauma in addition to urinary tract trauma, the urinary trauma went clinically undetected in one third of dogs. The animal may present for azotemia (i.e., vomiting, anorexia, depression, lethargy), or hematuria, dysuria, abdominal pain, and/or abdominal swelling or herniation may be noted. Abdominal and perineal bruising are common with vehicular trauma, particularly if there are pelvic fractures. Bruising in this region, however, may also indicate subcutaneous urine leakage. Further evaluation of the urinary tract is therefore warranted in such patients. In female dogs, there may be a history of previous catheterization using a rigid catheter. Rupture of the urethra is most frequently associated with pelvic fractures in male dogs. Often urinary tract rupture is overlooked in the initial workup of traumatized patients and the diagnosis is not made until the animal shows signs of azotemia. **It is important to remember that animals with ruptured bladders or unilateral ureteral trauma may urinate normal volumes, without evidence of hematuria.** If the rupture is located dorsally or is small, leakage may only occur when the bladder becomes distended. Similarly the ability to retrieve fluid while performing bladder catheterization does not preclude the diagnosis of a ruptured bladder.

☞ **NOTE** • Don't rule out bladder rupture in animals that appear to urinate normal volumes.

Physical Examination Findings

Abdominal palpation should be performed to determine the size and shape of the bladder. The animal should be closely examined for abdominal swelling or fluid accumulation. Urine quantity and character (i.e., hematuria, dysuria) and bruising on the ventral abdomen or perineum should be monitored.

Radiography/Ultrasonography

Survey radiographs may show reduced size or absence of the urinary bladder, lack of contrast and increased size of the retroperitoneal space, and/or lack of normal intraabdominal contrast. If a ruptured bladder is suspected a positive contrast cystourethrogram should be performed. A balloon-tipped catheter is placed in the distal urethra (just past the os penis in male dogs) and the balloon is inflated. While palpating the bladder for distention, approximately 2.2 ml/kg of diluted (1 part contrast medium to 2 parts sterile saline) aqueous organic iodide contrast medium is injected into the catheter. A radiograph is taken while the last few milliliters of contrast is being injected. Fluoroscopy, if available, can be used to determine when the bladder is distended. Taking a radiograph while the contrast agent is being injected may show a "jet" lesion of contrast agent from the bladder (Fig. 22-24). Free contrast agent in the abdominal cavity will coat and highlight abdominal organs. If a lesion is not identified in the bladder or urethra and the animal is well-hydrated, an excretory urogram can be performed (see p. 463). Contrast leakage into the retroperitoneal space (for proximal lesions) or abdomen (for distal lesions) occurs with ureteral rupture or laceration (Fig. 22-25). If periureteral fibrosis has occurred, obstruction rather than leakage may be noted. Leakage of contrast from the renal capsule may be noted with renal parenchymal trauma. Parenchymal trauma of the right kidney should be suspected in dogs with uroabdomen and fractures of the thirteenth right rib.

Laboratory Findings

A CBC and serum biochemical profile with electrolytes should be performed. Hyperkalemia and azotemia may be noted. Analysis of abdominal fluid should be performed if urinary tract rupture is suspected. With uroabdomen, creatinine levels of the abdominal fluid will be greater than those in the blood (see above). Renal failure may be present if obstruction preceded the rupture (see p. 461). Bladder rupture secondary to urinary tract infection may result in septic peritonitis (see p. 193).

DIFFERENTIAL DIAGNOSIS

Other causes of abdominal effusion or azotemia should be considered differentials. Peritonitis may cause vomiting, dehydration, and prerenal azotemia. Vomiting may be due to pancreatic, peritoneal, renal, splenic, hepatobiliary, or gastrointestinal abnormalities. In animals with abdominal effusion subsequent to trauma, uroabdomen, bile peritonitis, and septic peritonitis should be considered.

MEDICAL MANAGEMENT

If the animal is not hyperkalemic or azotemic (i.e., the diagnosis is made within 12 to 18 hours after rupture), it should be rehydrated with 0.9% saline and immediate surgical repair should be considered. Occasionally, concurrent trauma (e.g., traumatic myocarditis, pulmonary contusions) will delay surgery. In such patients, abdominal drainage and/or urinary diversion (i.e., urethral catheter and/or tube cystostomy; see p. 484) may be necessary until the animal is stable. With delayed diagnosis, correction of electrolytes, hydration, and acid-base balance should be performed prior to surgery (see above and p. 481). Antibiotics may be administered based on culture results if infection is present, or prophylactically if abdominal drains are placed.

☞ **N O T E** · Animals with acid-base and electrolyte abnormalities are poor anesthetic candidates. Correct these abnormalities prior to surgery!

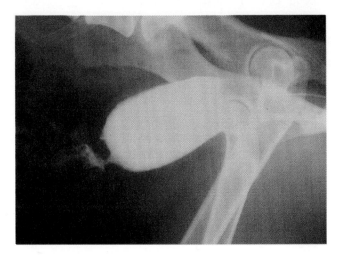

FIG. 22-24
Positive contrast cystourethrogram in a dog with a ruptured bladder. The radiograph was taken while the contrast agent was being injected and shows a "jet" lesion of contrast agent from the bladder. (Courtesy L. Homco, Texas A&M University.)

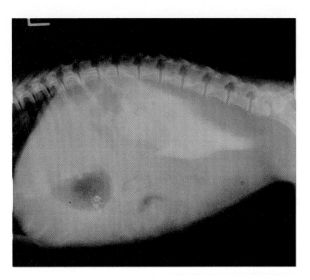

FIG. 22-25
Excretory urogram in a dog with a ruptured ureter. Note accumulation of contrast in the retroperitoneal space. The contralateral ureter was avulsed from its blood supply.

SURGICAL TREATMENT

Urethral trauma may be repaired by primary anastomosis (immediate or delayed) or the urethra may be allowed to heal over a urinary catheter if it is not completely transected. Ureteral rupture may be repaired by anastomosis or reimplantation into the bladder, depending on location of the damage (see p. 467). Bladder rupture generally occurs near the apex. Although small ruptures may heal if the bladder is kept decompressed, surgical exploration and repair are indicated in most patients. The entire abdomen should be explored to determine the reason for rupture and/or identify concurrent trauma. If bladder rupture is secondary to severe cystitis, tumor, or obstruction, the bladder may be extremely friable or large areas may be necrotic making excision and primary closure of the rent difficult. In such cases, prolonged urinary diversion (see p. 484) may be beneficial. If cystitis or tumor is present, a biopsy of the bladder mucosa should be submitted for culture and histologic examination. In animals with rupture due to obstruction from calculi, the urethra should be carefully checked for calculi and its patency verified prior to repairing the bladder defect.

Preoperative Management

An ECG should be evaluated for arrhythmias. If possible, hydration, acid-base, and electrolyte abnormalities should be corrected prior to surgery (see above and p. 481). If antibiotic therapy has not been initiated prior to surgery, perioperative antibiotics (e.g., cefazolin) may be administered at induction.

Anesthesia

If renal impairment is not present, many different anesthetic regimens can be used safely. If renal impairment is present, see p. 462 for suggested anesthetic protocols. If the animal is vomiting, avoid mask or chamber induction.

Surgical Anatomy

Refer to p. 483 for surgical anatomy of the bladder and urethra.

Positioning

The animal is placed in dorsal recumbency and the abdomen prepared for a ventral midline incision. For bladder rupture, the entire ventral abdomen should be prepped to allow complete exploration of the abdomen.

SURGICAL TECHNIQUE

Cystotomy is described on p. 483. *Excise devitalized or necrotic bladder tissue and suture the rent with a one- or two-layer continuous suture pattern. If the bladder is markedly thickened, perform a single-layer anastomosing pattern; otherwise, use a two-layer inverting pattern. If tissues are friable and a water-tight seal is not achieved, perform a serosal patch over the incision line (see p. 301).*

SUTURE MATERIALS/SPECIAL INSTRUMENTS

Absorbable suture material (e.g., polydioxanone [PDS], polyglyconate [Maxon], polyglycolic acid [Dexon] or polyglactin-910 [Vicryl]), is preferred for bladder and urethral surgery (see p. 494).

POSTOPERATIVE CARE AND ASSESSMENT

Intravenous fluids should be given until the animal is able to drink adequate fluids to maintain hydration. The patient should be observed closely after surgery for signs of urinary obstruction or peritonitis. If bladder atony is present, the bladder should be kept decompressed by intermittent urinary catheterization or by manual expression. Urinary tract infection is common with indwelling or repeated catheterization. An α-blocker (e.g., phenoxybenzamine; Table 22-6) and/or a somatic muscle relaxant (e.g., diazepam) can be used to decrease urethral sphincter tone. Bethanechol is a cholinergic that increases detrusor contractility and may aid voiding. Manual expression of the bladder should be done with care following surgery (particularly in patients with friable bladders secondary to infection or obstruction) to avoid disrupting the suture line.

COMPLICATIONS

The major complication of bladder surgery is urinary leakage, especially if a water-tight seal is not achieved or devitalized tissues are sutured and subsequently dehisce. Occasionally, peritonitis may occur from infected urine or secondary to surgically induced contamination.

PROGNOSIS

The prognosis is excellent for animals with traumatic bladder rupture. Occasionally rupture secondary to obstruction may have a guarded prognosis if the majority of the bladder is necrotic.

TABLE 22-6

Drugs Used to Improve Urination

Phenoxybenzamine (Dibenzyline)
Dogs
0.25 mg/kg PO, BID-TID

Cats
0.5 mg/kg PO, BID (may cause hypotension)

Diazepam (Valium)
Dogs
0.2 mg/kg PO, TID

Cats
2-5 mg/cat PO, BID-TID (duration of action is 1 to 2 hours when given orally)

Bethanechol (Urecholine)
Dogs
5-15 mg/dog PO, BID-TID

Cats
1.25-5 mg/cat PO, BID-TID

Suggested Reading

Pechman RD Jr: Urinary trauma in dogs and cats: a review, *J Am Anim Hosp Assoc* 18:33, 1982.

Selcer BA: Urinary tract trauma associated with pelvic trauma, *J Am Anim Hosp Assoc* 19:785, 1982.

BLADDER AND URETHRAL CALCULI

DEFINITIONS

When urine becomes supersaturated with dissolved salts, the salts may precipitate to form **crystals (crystalluria).** If the crystals are not excreted, they may aggregate into solid concretions known as **calculi. Urolithiasis** is a term that refers to having urinary calculi or **uroliths** (kidney, ureter, bladder, or urethra). **Cystolithiasis** and **cystolithectomy** refer to the development of urinary bladder calculi, and their removal, respectively. **Cystotomy** is a surgical incision into the urinary bladder, while **urethrotomy** is an incision into the urethra.

SYNONYMS

Stones

GENERAL CONSIDERATIONS AND CLINICALLY RELEVANT PATHOPHYSIOLOGY

The large majority of canine uroliths are found in the bladder or urethra. Struvite (i.e., magnesium ammonium phosphate) calculi are the most common canine uroliths, followed by calcium oxalate, urate, silicate, cystine, and mixed types. Urinary tract infections are an important predisposing cause for the formation of struvite calculi in dogs. Urease-producing bacteria split urea to ammonia and carbon dioxide. Hydrolysis of ammonia forms ammonium ions and hydroxyl ions, which alkalinize the urine and decrease struvite solubility. Bacterial cystitis also increases organic debris, which can serve as a nidus for crystallization. Feline struvite formation usually occurs despite lack of UTI.

Calcium oxalate calculi occur most commonly in dogs with transient, postprandial hypercalcemia and hypercalciuria. Many affected dogs have low-to-normal parathyroid hormone concentrations. Although rare, they may also occur in dogs with defective tubular resorption of calcium, primary hyperparathyroidism, lymphoma, vitamin D intoxication, decreased urine concentrations of citrate, or increased dietary oxalate. Concurrent UTI is rare. Acidic urine favors calcium oxalate crystal formation.

☞ **N O T E** · Struvite calculi are frequently associated with infection; UTI is less common with calcium oxalate stones.

Urate calculi are usually composed of ammonium acid urate derived from metabolic degradation of endogenous purine ribonucleotides and dietary nucleic acids. Dalmations have defective hepatic transport of uric acid resulting in decreased production of allantoin and increased urinary excretion of uric acid. Dalmations also have decreased proximal tubular resorption and distal tubular secretion of uric acid making urate urolithiasis common in this breed. Dogs with hepatic insufficiency (i.e., portosystemic shunts, hepatic cirrhosis) may form ammonium acid urate stones due to increased renal excretion of ammonium urates. Secondary UTI may occur as a result of mucosal irritation. Silicate uroliths are often jack-shaped and are probably related to increased dietary intake of silicates, silicic acid, or magnesium silicate (Fig. 22-26). Cystine uroliths occur due to an inherited disorder of renal tubular transport. Cystine stones usually occur in acid urine.

Although dissolution of some stones is possible, surgical removal is often necessary initially to allow a diagnosis of stone type. Appropriate medical management may help decrease the recurrence of canine uroliths (Table 22-7). Supersaturation of urine with salts appears to be the primary factor favoring calculi formation. Other factors (i.e., presence of a nidus on which the stone can form, decreased concentrations of urine crystallization inhibitors) also appear to contribute to stone formation.

☞ **N O T E** · It is necessary to remove and analyze stones to determine type; subsequent medical management is important to prevent recurrence.

DIAGNOSIS
Clinical Presentation

Signalment. Struvite calculi are more common in female dogs than males because females more commonly have UTI; however, urethral obstruction from stones is more common in males (Table 22-8). Uroliths may occur in dogs of any age, but they are most frequently observed in middle-aged dogs. Calculi in dogs less than 1 year of age are often struvite due to UTI. Calcium oxalate uroliths are more common in male dogs, particularly miniature

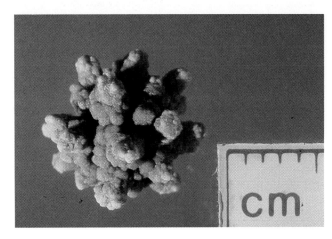

FIG. 22-26
Silicate urolith from a 12-year-old cat with chronic hematuria.

TABLE 22-7

Treatment and Prevention of Canine Urolithiasis

Urolith Type	Treatment Options	Prevention
Struvite	Surgical removal or dissolution Hill's s/d diet Control infection Urease inhibitor? Keep urine pH <6.5, BUN <10 mg/dl, and urine specific gravity <1.020	Hill's c/d diet Monitor urine pH and urine sediment, treat any infections quickly and appropriately
Calcium oxalate	Surgical removal	Hill's u/d diet? Potassium citrate?
Urate	Surgical removal or dissolution Hill's u/d diet Allopurinol Control infection	Hill's u/d diet Allopurinol if necessary Correct congenital portosystemic shunts
Silicate	Surgical removal	Hill's u/d diet Prevent consumption of dirt
Cystine	Surgical removal or dissolution Hill's u/d diet D-penicillamine N-(2-Mercaptopropionyl)-glycine (MPG)	Hill's u/d diet Thiol-containing drugs if necessary

Modified from Nelson R, Couto G: *Essentials of small animal internal medicine*, St. Louis, 1995, Mosby.

TABLE 22-8

Breed, Sex, and Age Predispositions for Urinary Calculi

Struvite
- Miniature schnauzers, Bischon Frises, cocker spaniels
- Females more than males, middle-aged dogs
- UTI

Calcium Oxalate
- Miniature schnauzers, Lhasa apsos, Yorkshire terriers
- Males, middle-aged to older dogs

Calcium Phosphate
- Yorkshire terriers

Urate
- Dalmatians, English bulldogs
- Dogs with portosystemic shunts

Silicate
- German shepherds, golden retrievers, Labradors
- Males, middle-aged dogs

Cystine
- Dachshunds, English bulldogs (maybe basset hounds and rottweilers)
- Males, middle-aged dogs

schnauzers, miniature poodles, Yorkshire terriers, Lhasa apsos, and shih tzus. Middle-aged to older dogs are most commonly affected. Sixty percent of urate uroliths occur in dalmatians—most of the remainder are seen in breeds that commonly have portosystemic shunts (i.e., Yorkshire terri-ers, Pekingese, Lhasa apsos). Middle-aged, male German shepherds seem to be at increased risk for silicate urolithia-sis. Cystine uroliths most frequently occur in middle-aged, male dachshunds. Other breeds that appear to be at in-creased risk for cystine urolithiasis include basset hounds, English bulldogs, Yorkshire terriers, Irish terriers, and Chi-huahuas.

History. Clinical signs of UTI (i.e., hematuria, pollaki-uria, stranguria) are common in dogs with bladder or ure-thral calculi. Small stones may lodge in the urethra of male dogs and cause partial or complete urinary obstruction. Bladder distention, abdominal pain, stranguria, para-doxical incontinence, and/or signs of postrenal azotemia (i.e., anorexia, vomiting, depression) may develop. Occa-sionally bladder rupture will occur and result in uroab-domen (see p. 496).

Physical Examination Findings

The bladder wall is often thickened and the stones them-selves are occasionally palpable. Signs consistent with UTI may be noted. Abdominal pain, anorexia, vomiting, and/or depression may be noted if urinary tract obstruction occurs.

Radiography/Ultrasonography

Survey abdominal radiographs and/or ultrasonography are indicated in any animal with urolithiasis. In addition to defining the number and location of bladder and urethral calculi, the procedures may indicate the presence of calculi in the kidney and/or ureter. Calcium-containing uroliths (i.e., calcium phosphate and calcium oxalate) are the most radio-dense, while cystine and urate uroliths are the least radiopaque. Struvite calculi are normally radiodense and are usually observed with plain radiography (Fig. 22-27). Retrograde cystourethrography may help identify radiolucent stones in the bladder or urethra. Ultrasonography may be used to identify calculi and evaluate the kidneys and ureters for concurrent abnormalities.

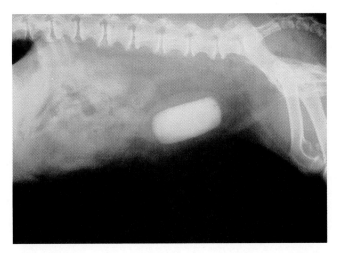

FIG. 22-27
A large radiodense struvite calculus in the bladder of a dog with chronic cystitis.

Laboratory Findings

A CBC, serum chemistry profile (including electrolytes), urinalysis, and urine culture should be performed. Concomitant urinary tract infection is common (i.e., pyuria, hematuria, proteinuria, and/or bacteriuria). Renal failure may be present due to chronic pyelonephritis or obstructive uropathy (see p. 461). Findings associated with hepatic insufficiency (low BUN, hypoalbuminemia) may be present in some animals with urate calculi.

☞ **N O T E** • Always identify and treat concurrent urinary tract infections!

DIFFERENTIAL DIAGNOSIS

Uroliths should be considered in any animal presenting for chronic urinary tract infection, hematuria, stranguria, pollakiuria, or obstructive uropathy. Other differentials include neoplasia and granulomatous inflammation.

MEDICAL MANAGEMENT

Urethral obstruction should be relieved and/or bladder decompression performed if necessary. Using a finger inserted in the rectum and massaging a urethral urolith toward the vagina may dislodge uroliths in female dogs. Urohydropropulsion may be used to propel urethral stones back into the bladder in both male and female dogs (Fig. 22-28, *A*). A

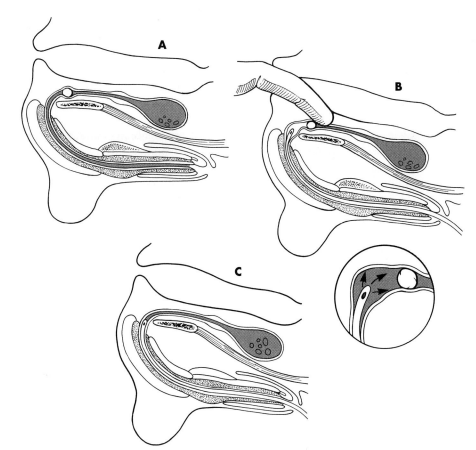

FIG. 22-28
A, Urohydropropulsion may be used to propel urethral stones back into the bladder. **B,** Place a catheter in the urethra distal to the stone and inject sterile saline while the urethra is occluded by a finger in the rectum (or vagina in females). **C,** Once the urethra is dilated remove the finger, allowing the stone to be flushed into the bladder.

catheter is placed in the urethra distal to the stone and sterile saline or a combination of sterile saline and a 1:1 mixture of aqueous lubricant (e.g. Lubafax surgical lubricant) is injected while the urethra is occluded by a finger in the rectum (or vagina in females) (Fig. 22-28, *B*). Once the urethra is dilated, the finger should be removed, allowing the stone to be flushed into the bladder (Fig. 22-28, *C*). Stones lodged within the urethra causing obstruction that cannot be hydropropulsed into the bladder can be removed via urethrotomy (see p. 487).

☞ **N O T E ·** Always try to flush urethral calculi into the bladder so that cystotomy (rather than urethrotomy) can be performed.

SURGICAL TREATMENT

When the urolith has not been typed, surgery should be considered if there are concurrent or predisposing anatomic abnormalities (e.g., urachal diverticula), if medical dissolution is not possible, or if a bladder mucosal culture is required. Although medical dissolution of struvite, urate, and cystine calculi is possible, surgical removal of calcium oxalate, calcium phosphate, and silicate stones is necessary. Disadvantages of medical dissolution may include cost, necessity of frequent rechecks, and poor owner compliance for maintaining a suitable dietary regimen. **Cystotomy should be performed preferentially over urethrotomy if the stones can be flushed into the bladder either preoperatively or intraoperatively.** Calculi should be submitted for stone analysis (and possibly culture) to guide postoperative management and help prevent recurrence, particularly if stone type was not determined based on identification of urine crystals.

Preoperative Management

Postrenal azotemia and hyperkalemia should be treated prior to surgery (see p. 481). Fluid therapy should be initiated to promote diuresis. An ECG should be evaluated for arrythmias. UTI should be eradicated prior to surgery, and perioperative antibiotics should be considered if the animal is not already receiving antibiotics. Prophylactic antibiotics, however, may be withheld until after bladder mucosa has been excised for culture in animals with negative urine cultures.

☞ **N O T E ·** If possible, eradicate concurrent UTI prior to surgery. Otherwise submit bladder mucosa and stones for culture.

Anesthesia

If renal impairment is not present, many different anesthetic regimens can be used safely. If renal impairment is present, see p. 462 for suggested anesthetic protocols. Avoid mask or chamber induction if the patient is vomiting.

Surgical Anatomy

Refer to p. 483 for surgical anatomy of the bladder and urethra.

Positioning

The animal is placed in dorsal recumbency and the abdomen prepared for a ventral midline incision. The prepped area should extend from below the pubis proximally to the thorax.

SURGICAL TECHNIQUE

Bladder calculi are removed via cystotomy (see p. 483). *Perform a cystotomy and incise a small piece of bladder at the incision and submit it for culture and possibly histologic examination. Remove the bladder stones and carefully check the urethra for additional calculi. In male dogs, place a catheter into the urethra from the penile orifice and occlude the vesicourethral opening with a finger from within the bladder lumen. Have an assistant gently occlude the penile urethra around the catheter with fingers to minimize fluid leakage. Flush the catheter with sterile saline to maximally dilate the urethra (i.e., when additional saline cannot be flushed into the catheter). While fluid is still being flushed into the catheter, remove the finger at the vesicourethral opening. Repeat this procedure until it is certain that no stones remain in the urethral lumen. Check the bladder for urachal diverticula and excise if necessary. Submit the stones for mineral analysis and possibly for microbial culture.*

SUTURE MATERIALS/SPECIAL INSTRUMENTS

Absorbable suture material (e.g., polydioxanone [PDS], polyglyconate [Maxon], polyglycolic acid [Dexon] or polyglactin-910 [Vicryl]) is preferred for bladder and urethral surgery (see p. 494).

POSTOPERATIVE CARE AND ASSESSMENT

The animal should be closely monitored for urinary obstruction or leakage following surgery. Urine sediment and pH should be monitored regularly and UTI treated promptly. Preventive treatment specific to the stone type should be implemented to help prevent recurrence of urolithiasis (Table 22-9). D-penicillamine may inhibit wound healing and should not be initiated earlier than 2 weeks after surgery. Readers are referred to other sources for specific recommendations regarding medical treatment and prevention of urolithiasis.

TABLE 22-9

Drugs Used in the Treatment of Urinary Calculi

Allopurinol (Zyloprim)
7-10 mg/kg PO, SID-TID*

D-Penicillamine (Cuprimine)
10-15 mg/kg PO, BID

N-(2-Mercaptopropionyl)-glycine (MPG)
15 mg/kg PO, BID

*If possible, adjust dosage based on measurement of uric acid excretion

COMPLICATIONS

Complications associated with cystotomy are uncommon; however, urine leakage is possible. The main complication of urethrotomy is hemorrhage, which may persist up to 7 days postoperatively. Urethral stricture is uncommon.

PROGNOSIS

The recurrence rate for calculi formation is estimated at 12% to 25% (DiBartola, Chew, 1981). Recurrence is more common in dogs with cystine and urate stones than in those with oxalate or phosphate stones. Appropriate medical management (i.e., prevention of UTI) is necessary to decrease the recurrence of struvite calculi.

Reference

DiBartola SP, Chew DJ: Canine urolithiasis, *Compend Contin Educ Pract Vet* 3:226, 1981.

Suggested Reading

Bartges JW, Osborne CA, Polzin DJ: Recurrent sterile struvite urocystolithiasis in three related English cocker spaniels, *J Am Anim Hosp Assoc* 28:459, 1992.

Case LC, Ling GV, Franti CE, et al: Cystine-containing urinary calculi in dogs: 102 cases (1981-1989), *J Am Vet Med Assoc* 201:129, 1992.

Grauer GF: Canine urolithiasis. In Nelson RW, Couto CG, editors: *Essentials of small animal medicine*, St. Louis, 1993, Mosby.

Ling GV et al: Epizootiologic evaluation and quantitative analysis of urinary calculi from 150 cats, *J Am Vet Med Assoc* 196:1459, 1990.

Ling GV et al: Xanthine-containing urinary calculi in dogs given allopurinol, *J Am Vet Med Assoc* 198:1935, 1991.

Lulich JP, Osborne CA: Catheter-assisted retrieval of urocystoliths from dogs and cats, *J Am Vet Med Assoc* 201:111, 1992.

Sorenson JL, Ling GV: Metabolic and genetic aspects of urate urolithiasis in dalmations, *J Am Vet Med Assoc* 203:857, 1993.

URETHRAL PROLAPSE

DEFINITIONS

Urethral prolapse is a protrusion of the urethra mucosa beyond the end of the penis.

GENERAL CONSIDERATIONS AND CLINICALLY RELEVANT PATHOPHYSIOLOGY

Urethral prolapse is uncommon. It may occur after excessive sexual excitement or masturbation, or may be associated with genitourinary infections.

DIAGNOSIS
Clinical Presentation

Signalment. Dogs most commonly affected are young English bulldogs, but it has also been reported in a Boston terrier and a Yorkshire terrier.

History. The owner may notice a reddened protrusion at the tip of the penis and/or intermittent penile bleeding which may worsen when the dog becomes excited. Prolapse may be intermittent, occurring only when the dog has an erection. Some affected dogs lick at the preputial orifice and may traumatize the exposed urethral mucosa.

☞ **N O T E** • Penile bleeding may be intermittent (e.g., during erection).

Physical Examination Findings

When the penis is extruded from the preputial orifice a small, reddened mass may be visible protruding from the tip of the penis (Fig. 22-29). Penile erection may cause the protrusion to enlarge. Necrosis of the prolapsed urethra may occur secondary to drying or self-inflicted trauma. The prepuce should be checked for evidence of balanoposthitis or neoplasia.

Laboratory Findings

Anemia may occur in dogs with intermittent or chronic bleeding. Urinalysis should be performed to exclude urinary tract infection. Exclusion of a coagulopathy in dogs with intermittent prolapse may be indicated.

DIFFERENTIAL DIAGNOSIS

Urethral prolapse may be differentiated from other causes of preputial bleeding by extruding the penis and examining the urethral orifice. Urethritis, fractures of the os penis, urethral calculi, and urethral stricture may be associated with hematuria and/or preputial bleeding. Other possible causes of penile bleeding include preputial, penile, or urethral neoplasia and prostatic lesions.

MEDICAL MANAGEMENT

Concurrent infection of the genitourinary tract should be treated. If the urethral mucosa is not necrotic, the prolapse can occasionally be reduced by gently manipulating it with a

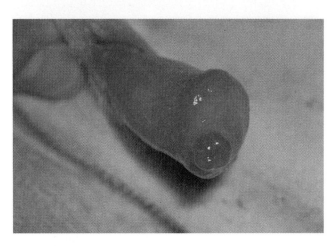

FIG. 22-29
Urethral prolapse in a dog. Note the small, reddened mass (urethra) protruding from the tip of the penis. (Courtesy H.P. Hobson, Texas A&M University.)

sterile cotton swab or by placing a lubricated catheter into the urethral orifice. A purse-string suture of 5-0 or 6-0 suture material can be placed in the penis around the orifice and tightened to prevent the prolapse from recurring without obstructing urination. The suture should be removed after 5 days and the patient monitored for recurrence. Spontaneous recovery has not been reported.

SURGICAL TREATMENT

Surgical resection of the prolapsed urethra is the treatment of choice. Bilateral orchiectomy should be performed, particularly in dogs that have prolapse associated with erection or sexual excitement.

Preoperative Management

The animal should be kept from traumatizing the urethra prior to surgery.

Anesthesia

Many different anesthetic regimens can be used safely if the animal is otherwise healthy.

Surgical Anatomy

Surgical anatomy of the urethra is discussed on p. 483.

Positioning

The animal is placed in dorsal or lateral recumbency and the penis extruded and gently cleaned with dilute chlorhexidine solution.

SURGICAL TECHNIQUE

Place stay sutures in the urethral mucosa and apply gentle traction to straighten the prolapsed material. Place one or two straight needles through the penile tissues (Fig. 22-30) or use stay sutures in the urethral mucosa distal to the proposed site of transection to prevent the urethra from re- *tracting within the penis. Transect the urethra along its circumference and suture it to the penis with 4-0 to 6-0 simple interrupted sutures of monofilament absorbable or nonabsorbable suture (Fig. 22-31). Alternately, make an incision on the ventral surface of the penis through both penile and urethral mucosa, extending halfway around the circumference of the urethra. Suture the urethral mucosa to the penile mucosa, then incise the dorsal surface of the urethral mucosa and suture it to the penis. This prevents retraction and the need for stay sutures.* Concurrent excision of the distal end of the penis may be necessary in some dogs.

SUTURE MATERIALS/SPECIAL INSTRUMENTS

Monofilament, nonreactive suture material such as polydioxanone, polyglyconate, or polypropylene can be used.

POSTOPERATIVE CARE AND ASSESSMENT

An Elizabethan collar or side-bar should be used postoperatively to prevent the dog from licking. Tranquilizers may be helpful to prevent postoperative hemorrhage but should only be used in patients in which pain has been appropriately managed. Nonabsorbable sutures should be removed in 7 to 10 days.

COMPLICATIONS

Hemorrhage from the surgical site may occur for 7 to 14 days. The dog should be prevented from becoming excited during the early postoperative period.

PROGNOSIS

Without surgery, the prolapse will not spontaneously resolve. Recurrence is uncommon following surgical resection, however.

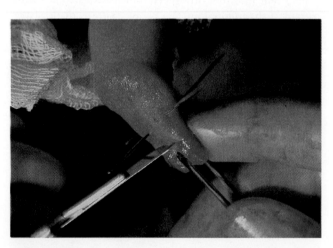

FIG. 22-30
To resect a urethral prolapse, place stay sutures in the urethral mucosa and apply gentle traction to straighten the prolapsed tissue. Place one or two straight needles through the penile tissues to prevent the urethra from retracting within the penis and circumferentially transect the urethra. (Courtesy H.P. Hobson, Texas A&M University.)

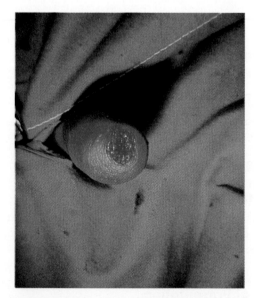

FIG. 22-31
After resecting the prolapsed urethra, suture the urethral mucosa to the penis with simple interrupted sutures. (Courtesy H.P. Hobson, Texas A&M University.)

Suggested Reading

Hobson HP, Heller RH: Surgical correction of prolapse in the male urethra, *Vet Med/Small Anim Clin* 66:1177, 1971.

McDonald RK: Urethral prolapse in a Yorkshire terrier, *Compend Small Anim Pract Vet* 11:682, 1989.

Sinibaldi KR, Greene RW: Surgical correction of prolapse of the male urethra in three English bulldogs, *J Am Anim Hosp Assoc* 9:450, 1973.

BLADDER AND URETHRAL NEOPLASIA

DEFINITIONS

Transitional cell carcinomas are malignant tumors arising from a transitional type of stratified epithelium that usually affect the urinary bladder. **Rhabdomyosarcomas** are highly malignant tumors of striated muscle that may develop from pluripotent stem cells of the primitive urogenital ridge—remnants of the müllerian or wolffian ducts.

GENERAL CONSIDERATIONS AND CLINICALLY RELEVANT PATHOPHYSIOLOGY

Bladder neoplasia occurs more frequently than neoplasia of the remainder of the urinary system in dogs. In cats, renal lymphosarcoma is more common than bladder neoplasia. It has been hypothesized that the prevailing variation of bladder tumors between dogs and cats is due to differences in metabolism of tryptophan and its carcinogenic intermediary metabolites. Although dogs excrete aromatic amine metabolites of tryptophan in appreciable quantities into their urine, feline urine is almost devoid of them. Prolonged contact of the bladder mucosa with such carcinogenic substances may be important in the development of tumors. Cyclophosphamide may also cause bladder neoplasia in dogs. Most bladder tumors are malignant; metastasis to the sublumbar lymph nodes and lungs is common. Local extension to the ureters and/or urethra is also common.

Transitional cell carcinoma is the most common tumor type in canine and feline bladders; other malignant bladder tumors include squamous cell carcinoma, adenocarcinoma, fibrosarcoma, leiomyosarcoma, neurofibrosarcoma, rhabdomyosarcoma, and hemangiosarcoma. Fibromas, leiomyomas, hemangiomas, rhabdomyoma, myxomas, and neurofibromas are benign bladder tumors. Inflammatory polyps may also be found in the bladder. Metastasis of other tumors to the bladder is uncommon although extension of prostatic or urethral tumors may occur. Dogs with bladder tumors commonly have other concurrent, primary tumors elsewhere in the body. Fibromas are benign tumors of mesenchymal origin that may occur in the bladder. They may be incidental findings or cause clinical signs similar to urinary tract infection. Frequently they are pedunculated, single, or multiple—surgical excision is often curative. Single or multiple bladder papillomas may occur in older dogs and cause hematuria when ulcerated.

Transitional cell carcinomas are the most common canine urethral neoplasm; urethral tumors are exceedingly rare in cats. Other urethral tumors include squamous cell carcinoma and adenocarcinoma. These tumors may be primary urethral masses or they may be extensions of prostatic or bladder neoplasia. Malignant urethral tumors are frequently locally invasive and may metastasize to the sublumbar lymph nodes and lungs. Granulomatous inflammation of the urethra in female dogs may cause clinical signs similar to urethral neoplasia (i.e., stranguria, hematuria, pollakiuria, vaginal discharge, and/or urinary obstruction). Neoplasia and granulomatous inflammation may be differentiated by cytologic evaluation of urethral aspirates or surgical biopsies. The cause of granulomatous urethritis is unknown. Affected dogs respond favorably to immunosuppressive therapy (i.e., prednisone or prednisone plus cyclophosphamide) plus antibiotics.

☞ **N O T E** • Granulomatous inflammation may cause clinical signs similar to urethral tumors. These lesions must be differentiated.

DIAGNOSIS
Clinical Presentation

Signalment. Bladder tumors are more common in dogs than cats. Older, neutered dogs weighing more than 10 kg are most commonly affected; however, botryoid rhabdomyosarcoma often occurs in young large-breed dogs. In one study of feline bladder tumors, males were affected three times more commonly than females (Schwarz, Greene, Patnaik, 1985). Bladder tumors usually occur in older cats. Urethral tumors are more common in older female dogs.

History. Most dogs with bladder or urethral tumors are examined because of hematuria, pollakiuria, stranguria, and/or dysuria. Other signs include incontinence, polyuria/polydipsia, lameness, and dyspnea. Lameness may be due to bone metastasis or hypertrophic osteopathy. The most common clinical sign in cats is intermittent or persistent hematuria. If the tumor causes urethral or bladder obstruction, signs of uremia (i.e., vomiting, anorexia, depression) may occur.

Physical Examination Findings

The most common physical exam findings include a urethral or caudal abdominal mass, prostatomegaly, bladder distention, abdominal pain, weakness, lymphadenopathy, cough or dyspnea, and/or lameness. Urethral masses in females may be palpated rectally or by digital examination of the vagina. Physical examination findings are normal in nearly one third of dogs with bladder neoplasia.

Radiography/Ultrasonography

Survey abdominal radiographs are rarely diagnostic, but may exclude prostatic disease or urolithiasis. The sublumbar lymph nodes, pelvis, and vertebrae should be examined for metastasis. Diffuse thickening or calcification of the bladder wall is occasionally noted. Positive-contrast urography and ultrasonography are the most useful tools for diagnosing

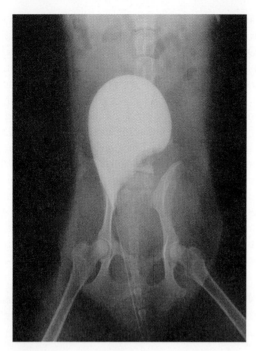

FIG. 22-32
Cystourethrogram in a dog with a large transitional cell carcinoma. Note the filling defect near the bladder trigone.

urethral or bladder neoplasia (Fig. 22-32.) Excretory urography may show hydroureter and/or hydronephrosis, and irregular filling defects in the bladder. Double-contrast cystography is most effective for delineating masses in the bladder wall and lumen. Retrograde urethrography (see p. 497) should be performed in dogs with suspected urethral neoplasia to determine the length of the urethra affected and to check for evidence of trigonal involvement. Thoracic radiographs should be performed to identify pulmonary metastasis. Ultrasonography is useful to evaluate the abdomen for metastasis. Although fine-needle aspirates of the mass may provide a presurgical diagnosis, it may cause seeding of the tumor along the needle tract. Cystoscopy is useful for identifying lesions and obtaining biopsies in female dogs.

Laboratory Findings

A CBC, serum biochemical profile, and urinalysis should be performed in animals with bladder tumors. Hematuria, pyuria, proteinuria, and/or bacteriuria are common. Although malignant cells may be found in the urine sediment of some dogs with bladder or urethral tumors, they are not detected in most cats with bladder neoplasia. Care should be taken to avoid confusing neoplastic cells from those that are merely dysplastic; atypical transitional cells are common in animals with cystitis. Also, prolonged exposure to urine may make interpretation of abnormal cells difficult. Emptying the bladder and performing cytologic evaluation of a saline wash may be helpful in some animals. Hematologic and biochemical parameters are usually normal; however, elevations in serum creatinine and BUN may occur with partial obstruction of the lower urinary tract. Anemia is common in cats with bladder

tumors. Hypereosinophilia has been reported in a cat with transitional cell carcinoma of the bladder (Sellon et al, 1992).

DIFFERENTIAL DIAGNOSIS

Other causes of hematuria and/or bacteriuria (e.g., urolithiasis, prostatic disease, polypoid cystitis) should be excluded. Many cats with lower urinary tract neoplasia are treated presumptively for sterile cystitis with antibiotics, urinary acidifiers, and/or dietary changes for months prior to making the diagnosis. Nonneoplastic (granulomatous) infiltrative urethral disease should be differentiated from neoplasia by cytologic and/or histopathologic evaluation of biopsy specimens.

MEDICAL MANAGEMENT

If partial or complete urinary obstruction is present, the animal should be stabilized prior to surgery with fluids and cutaneous urinary diversion (urethral catheter or tube cystostomy). Electrolyte and acid-base abnormalities should be corrected and concurrent UTI treated with appropriate antibiotics. An ECG should be evaluated for arrhythmias. Treatment of malignant bladder tumors with excision and/or adjuvant chemotherapy has also been reported. Piroxicam (Table 22-10) has been used to treat nonresectable transitional cell carcinoma of the urinary bladder in dogs. In one study, partial or complete remission of tumor was noted in 6 of 34 dogs; many other dogs subjectively had an improved quality of life, despite lack of tumor remission (Knapp et al, 1994). The exact mechanism of piroxicam antitumor activity is unknown; however, decreased inflammation and PGE_2-mediated immunosuppression may be involved. The most common side effect of piroxicam administration is gastrointestinal irritation (i.e., anorexia, melena, and/or vomiting). Concurrent use of misoprostol may be beneficial in these cases (see Table 22-10).

SURGICAL TREATMENT

Surgical therapy is difficult because the most common site for urinary bladder neoplasia is the trigone. Although the ureters can be transected and implanted into the apex of the bladder following partial cystectomy, incontinence typically occurs if the trigone is removed. Similarly, implantation of the ureters at a distant site (i.e., the colon) following complete cystectomy typically causes pyelonephritis and/or incontinence (see p. 492). Tumor spread beyond the primary site is also common. Transplantation of transitional cell carcinoma to the subcutaneous tissues of the surgical incision has been reported in dogs; therefore, the same instruments should not be used on other tissues that are used to resect or biopsy bladder tumors. Surgical excision of neoplastic lesions may be curative if the tumor is benign (Fig. 22-33).

Resection of focal lesions of the urethra is possible with a transpubic surgical approach and urethral resection and anastomosis (see p. 488). Prepubic urethrostomy (see p. 491) with resection of neoplastic tissues may be performed if the distal urethra is involved. Urethral tumors that involve the entire length of the urethra or the bladder trigone are generally inoperable.

TABLE 22-10
Medical Treatment of Canine Cystic Transitional Cell Carcinoma
Piroxicam (Feldene)
0.3 mg/kg PO, EOD to SID*
Misoprostol (Cytotec)
1-5 µg/kg PO, TID
*Start with EOD administration and observe response; SID administration may be associated with gastrointestinal ulceration.

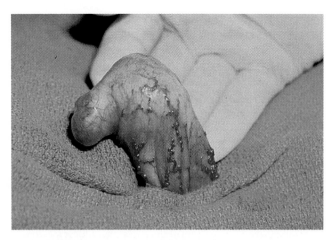

FIG. 22-33
Leiomyoma of the bladder. Surgical excision of benign tumors or those located at the bladder apex may be curative.

Preoperative Management

See discussion on medical management on p. 506.

Anesthesia

If renal impairment is not present, many different anesthetic regimens can be used safely. If renal impairment is present, see p. 462 for suggested anesthetic protocols.

Surgical Anatomy

Refer to p. 483 for the surgical anatomy of the bladder and urethra.

Positioning

The animal is placed in dorsal recumbency and the abdomen prepared for a ventral midline incision. For bladder neoplasia, the incision should extend from above the umbilicus to the brim of the pelvis. With urethral neoplasia, the incision should be extended caudally to allow a pubic osteotomy to be performed.

SURGICAL TECHNIQUE

Examine the sublumbar lymph nodes, ureters, and other abdominal organs for evidence of tumor extension or metastasis. For bladder neoplasia, locate the entrance of the ureters into the trigone and excise the tumor, removing at least 1 cm of normal tissue. Be sure to avoid damaging the ureters. If a large portion of the bladder has been removed, place a urinary catheter and suture the bladder with a continuous appositional suture pattern. Otherwise, a two-layer inverting pattern can be used (see p. 483). If the bladder trigone is involved, consider ureterocolonic urinary diversion (see p. 492), chemotherapy, or euthanasia.

For urethral neoplasia, check the trigone, ureters, sublumbar lymph nodes, and other abdominal tissues for evidence of neoplasia. Perform a pelvic osteotomy and carefully examine the entire urethra. If the tumor does not involve the entire urethra or trigone, perform a urethral resection and anastomosis (see p. 486). If only the distal urethra is involved and neoplastic tissues can be resected, consider a prepubic urethrostomy (see p. 491). Rarely a benign, pedunculated urethral tumor may be removed through a urethrotomy incision (see p. 487).

SUTURE MATERIALS/SPECIAL INSTRUMENTS

Absorbable suture material (e.g., polydioxanone [PDS], polyglyconate [Maxon], polyglycolic acid [Dexon] or polyglactin-910 [Vicryl]), is preferred for bladder and urethral surgery (see p. 494).

POSTOPERATIVE CARE AND ASSESSMENT

The animal should be observed for urinary leakage or obstruction following surgery. With ureterocolonic anastomosis, intravenous fluids should be continued for 24 to 72 hours to ensure diuresis and the animal should be encouraged to eat the day following surgery (see p. 492). The kidneys should be monitored for function and infection postoperatively. If neurologic dysfunction occurs, blood ammonia levels should be measured and the animal treated appropriately (see p. 492). The addition of 0.5 to 2.0 g of sodium bicarbonate to the food twice daily may result in improvement of clinical signs associated with hyperchloremia and metabolic acidosis following this procedure. Placement of Vaseline on the perineum may help prevent urine scalding.

COMPLICATIONS

The most common complications of bladder and urethral surgery are urinary leakage or obstruction (see p. 495). Pyelonephritis, renal failure, neurologic dysfunction, electrolyte abnormalities, metabolic acidosis, and diarrhea with subsequent perineal irritation are possible complications of ureterocolonic urinary diversion (see p. 495).

PROGNOSIS

Because of the malignant nature of most lower urinary tract tumors, the prognosis is guarded. Many tumors have already metastasized at diagnosis. With aggressive surgery, urethral tumors may have a better prognosis than bladder tumors. Chemotherapy may allow dogs with bladder tumors to survive for significantly longer periods than if they undergo surgery. Dogs with transitional cell carcinoma of the bladder treated with doxorubicin and cyclophosphamide had a median survival time of 259 days compared to 86 days with surgery alone (Helfand et al, 1994). The results of ureterocolonic anastomosis in a large number of dogs have not been reported, but with improved techniques and the prevention of the deleterious effects of pyelonephritis on renal function, long-term survival might be possible. Newer treatment methods such as photodynamic therapy may improve the prognosis of animals with bladder tumors in the future.

References

Helfand SC et al: Comparison of three treatments for transitional cell carcinoma of the bladder in the dog, *J Am Anim Hosp Assoc* 30:270, 1994.

Knapp DW et al: Piroxicam therapy in 34 dogs with transitional cell carcinoma of the urinary bladder, *J Vet Intern Med* 8:273, 1994.

Schwarz PD, Greene RW, Patnaik AK: Urinary bladder tumors in the cat: a review of 27 cases, *J Am Anim Hosp Assoc* 21:237, 1985.

Sellon RK et al: Hypereosinophilia associated with transitional cell carcinoma in a cat, *J Am Vet Med Assoc* 201:591, 1992.

Suggested Reading

Anderson WI et al: Presumptive subcutaneous surgical transplantation of a urinary bladder transitional cell carcinoma in a dog, *Cornell Vet* 79:263, 1989.

Bjorling DE, Howard PE: Urinary salvage procedures, *Probl Vet Med* 1:93, 1989.

Bojrab MJ, Perry L, Tamas SP: Transitional cell carcinomas of the canine bladder: diagnosis and management, *J Am Vet Med Assoc* 8:495, 1986.

Crow SE: Urinary tract neoplasms in dogs and cats, *Compend Contin Educ Pract Vet* 7:607, 1985.

Davies JV, Read HM: Urethral tumours in dogs, *J Small Anim Pract* 21:131, 1990.

Esplin DG: Urinary bladder fibromas in dogs: 51 cases (1981-1985), *J Am Vet Med Assoc* 190:440, 1987.

Krawiec DR: Canine bladder tumors: the incidence, diagnosis, therapy, and prognosis, *Vet Med* 1:47, 1991.

Moroff SD et al: Infiltrative urethral disease in female dogs: 41 cases (1980–1987), *J Am Vet Med Assoc* 199:247, 1991.

Norris AM et al: Canine bladder and urethral tumors: a retrospective study of 115 cases (1980–1985), *J Vet Intern Med* 6:145, 1992.

Van Vechten M, Goldschmidt MH, Wortman JA: Embryonal rhabdomyosarcoma of the urinary bladder in dogs, *Compend Contin Educ Pract Vet* 12:783, 1990.

URINARY INCONTINENCE

DEFINITIONS

Urinary incontinence is due to failure of voluntary control of the vesical and urethral sphincters with constant or frequent involuntary passage of urine. Incontinence may be caused by neurogenic abnormalities, or anatomic outflow obstruction (**paradoxical** or **overflow incontinence**), may be hormone responsive (**urethral sphincter mechanism incontinence**), or may be due to inflammation (**urge incontinence**), congenital abnormalities (e.g., ectopic ureters), or behavioral problems.

GENERAL CONSIDERATIONS AND CLINICALLY RELEVANT PATHOPHYSIOLOGY

No true bladder sphincter exists in the bitch, so continence is maintained by multiple, interacting factors. Poor urethral tone, marked urethral hypoplasia, "pelvic" bladders, ovariohysterectomy, obesity, and congenital abnormalities have all been implicated as potential causes of urinary sphincter mechanism incontinence in female dogs. Congenital urethral sphincter mechanism incontinence has also been described in cats. Some animals respond to estrogen supplementation or drugs that act on the autonomic nervous system. Sympathomimetic drugs, particularly α-adrenergic stimulants (e.g., ephedrine, phenylpropanolamine, and imipramine) have been used to increase urethral sphincter tone. Surgical alternatives to improve urethral resistance include urethral slings, artificial sphincters, urethral lengthening procedures, periurethral injections of polytetrafluoroethylene, colposuspension, and cystourethropexy. Because these techniques are not uniformly successful, or because success has not been well documented in a large number of animals with urinary incontinence, surgical treatment (other than for congenital abnormalities such as ectopic ureters; see p. 470) should be reserved for animals that do not respond to medical management (see below), or when the owners refuse to consider long-term drug therapy.

☞ **N O T E** · Ectopic ureters (see p. 470) should be considered a differential in any young animal with urinary incontinence.

Estrogens probably exert their beneficial effect by improving smooth muscle contractility and sensitivity to α-adrenergic innervation. Bladder neck position may affect continence; increases in intraabdominal pressure are transmitted to both the bladder and proximal urethra in bitches with an intraabdominal bladder neck. Dogs, however, with more caudal (pelvic) bladders have this pressure transmitted to the bladder, but not the urethra. Experimentally, a rise in intraabdominal pressure leads to shortening of the functional urethral length, which might increase the adverse effect of bladder neck position in these dogs, thereby worsening incontinence.

DIAGNOSIS
Clinical Presentation

Signalment. Medium-sized and large-breed dogs seem to be at increased risk, particularly Doberman pinschers, Old English sheepdogs, and springer spaniels. Among small-breed dogs, miniature poodles may be at increased risk. Incontinence may be first noted at any age, depending on the cause.

History. Animals may have a life-long history of urinary incontinence or it may occur after ovariohysterectomy. The incontinence may be continuous, intermittent, or occur only during excitement or when asleep.

Physical Examination Findings

Physical examination findings are usually unremarkable. In some animals the bladder may be caudally displaced in the abdominal cavity. Signs of concurrent urinary tract infection (i.e., hematuria, dysuria, stranguria) may be noticed. In cats with urethral hypoplasia, vaginal aplasia is common with the uterine horns emptying in the caudal part of the dorsal wall of the bladder.

Radiography

Excretory urography should be performed to identify the termination of the ureters into the bladder. The vesicourethral junction may appear blunted and abnormally dilated, or the urethra may seem abnormally short. In cats with vaginal aplasia, radiographic evidence of a communication between the lumen of the uterus and the bladder may be noted.

Laboratory Findings

Other than findings consistent with urinary tract infection in some animals, laboratory findings are unremarkable. Urine cultures should be performed in all animals with incontinence, even if the urinalysis is not suggestive of a UTI.

DIFFERENTIAL DIAGNOSIS

The various causes of urinary incontinence must be differentiated. Urge incontinence secondary to cystic or urethral infection/inflammation should be excluded (e.g., response with appropriate antibiotics). Ectopic ureters should be detected and corrected surgically (see p. 470). Paradoxical incontinence (e.g., partial obstruction due to urethral calculi, neoplasia, or strictures) and neurogenic incontinence should be differentiated from urethral sphincter mechanism incompetence based on radiographic findings, neurologic examination, and/or catheterization. Urethral sphincter profilometry and cystometry can determine urethral sphincter tone and bladder emptying pressures.

MEDICAL MANAGEMENT

Dogs with suspected urethral sphincter mechanism incompetence should be treated with estrogens and/or sympathomimetic drugs initially. Diethylstilbestrol (DES) and/or α-adrenergic agonists (i.e., phenylpropanolamine or ephedrine; Table 22-11) may be used to increase urethral sphincter tone. If the animal responds to DES, the frequency of administration should be decreased to the lowest effective dose. High doses of DES may cause estrus-like signs, bone marrow toxicity, and/or alopecia; therefore, dosages greater than 1 mg daily should be used with caution. Use of α-adrenergic agonists with DES may allow lower dosages to

TABLE 22-11
Drugs Used in the Treatment of Urinary Incontinence
Phenylpropanolamine (Propagest, Dexatrim)
Dogs
1.5-2.0 mg/kg PO, BID to TID
Cats
1.5 mg/kg PO, TID
Ephedrine
Dogs
4 mg/kg or 12.5-50 mg/dog PO, BID to TID
Cats
2-4 mg/kg PO, BID to TID
Diethylstilbestrol (DES)
Dog
0.1-1.0 mg daily PO for 3-5 days, then same dose once weekly
Testosterone Cypionate (Depotestosterone)
Dog
2.2 mg/kg IM, every 30 days

be used. Phenylpropanolamine is used more frequently than ephedrine because it has fewer side effects (i.e., hyperexcitability, panting, and/or anorexia) and greater efficacy over time. Some male dogs with testosterone-responsive urinary incontinence may be managed by parenteral testosterone. Repositol forms (i.e., testosterone cypionate; see Table 22-11) are most commonly used. If prostatic enlargement or perianal adenomas are present (or occur during therapy), phenylpropanolamine or ephedrine should be used rather than testosterone.

SURGICAL TREATMENT

There is presently no single surgical procedure that will cure incontinence in all female dogs with urethral sphincter mechanism incontinence. Colposuspension has been performed on a large number of patients, with 53% of 150 dogs in one study becoming continent after surgery (Holt, 1990). Cystourethropexy resulted in continence in 9 of 10 bitches immediately following surgery; however, incontinence recurred in 7 of these dogs within 5 months of the surgery (Massat et al, 1993). The addition of phenylpropanolamine to these 7 dogs further controlled incontinence in 6 of them, despite their being unresponsive to it before surgery. Urinary incontinence was treated by urethral submucosal Teflon injection in 22 dogs (Arnold et al, 1989). Continence was achieved in all dogs for at least 2 months; however, incontinence recurred in 64% (14 dogs). A second Teflon injection was effective in controlling the incontinence in 11 of 12 dogs. In animals with marked urethral hypoplasia, reconstruction of the bladder neck may be effective in eliminating or decreasing incontinence (see below).

☞ **N O T E ·** Rule out other causes of incontinence and determine efficacy of medical management before attempting surgical correction.

Preoperative Management

Concurrent urinary tract infections should be treated before surgery.

Anesthesia

If renal impairment is not present, many different anesthetic regimens can be used safely. If renal impairment is present, see p. 462 for suggested anesthetic protocols.

Surgical Anatomy

See p. 483.

Positioning

The animal is placed in dorsal recumbency and the abdomen prepared for a ventral midline incision. The prepped area should be sufficient to allow the incision to extend from the pubis proximally to the umbilicus.

SURGICAL TECHNIQUE

Although numerous techniques have been described to correct urethral sphincter mechanism incontinence, only bladder flap reconstruction for treatment of hypoplastic urethras and colposuspension will be described here.

Bladder Flap Reconstruction of a Hypoplastic Urethra

Perform a ventral cystotomy that extends into the proximal aspect of the hypoplastic urethra. Identify the ureteral openings. Make two stab incisions into the bladder wall caudal and lateral to the ureteral stoma, with the distance between the stab incisions representing the desired circumference of the new urethral tube, in addition to an allowance for suturing (Fig. 22-34). A 4 French (cats) or 8 French (dogs) catheter should pass easily into the newly created urethral tube. Use scissors to extend the incision towards the urethra, creating two full-thickness flaps. Reflect the flaps cranially (Fig. 22-35, A). Suture the defect from the urethral end cranially to form the urethral tube (Fig. 22-35, B) with a two-layer simple continuous suture pattern or a simple continuous suture pattern and a Cushing's pattern. Use absorbable suture material (2-0 to 4-0). If the urethral lumen is compromised by placing two layers of sutures, suture the urethral tube with a single-layer appositional pattern using care to ensure sufficient apposition of sutures such that urine leakage will not occur. Suture the flaps together. Perform ovariohysterectomy in intact cats in which the uterine horns empty into the bladder.

Colposuspension

Place a Foley catheter into the bladder and empty it of urine. Make a caudal midline abdominal skin incision extending onto the pubis. Undermine subcutaneous fascia

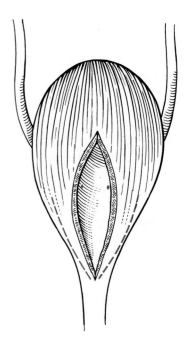

FIG. 22-34
For bladder flap reconstruction of a hypoplastic urethra, make two stab incisions into the bladder wall caudal and lateral to the ureteral stoma. Then, make two full-thickness flaps (see Fig. 22-35).

and fat and expose the prepubic tendon bilaterally. Extend the abdominal incision through the linea alba and expose the bladder. Place traction on the bladder and identify the bladder neck by inflating the bulb of the Foley catheter. Bluntly dissect the tissues between the urethra and the pelvic floor. Have an assistant displace the vagina cranially by placing a finger in the vulva. Separate the fat and fascia around the ventral bladder neck and proximal urethra and expose the vaginal wall dorsolateral to the urethra. While maintaining cranial traction on the vagina (Fig. 22-36, A), place two sutures (0 or 1 monofilament nonabsorbable suture) on each side from the vagina to the prepubic tendon (Fig. 22-36, B). Place sutures full-thickness through the vaginal wall taking care to ensure that the urethra is not compressed or displaced by the sutures.

SUTURE MATERIALS/SPECIAL INSTRUMENTS

Absorbable suture material (e.g., polydioxanone [PDS], polyglyconate [Maxon], polyglycolic acid [Dexon] or polyglactin-910 [Vicryl]) is preferred for bladder and urethral surgery (see p. 494).

POSTOPERATIVE CARE AND ASSESSMENT

The animal should be closely monitored for urinary obstruction or leakage following surgery. If urinary obstruction occurs, an indwelling urinary catheter should be placed and maintained for 3 to 5 days. Animals should be monitored for urinary tract infections periodically after surgery.

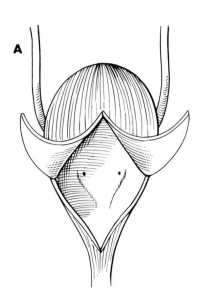

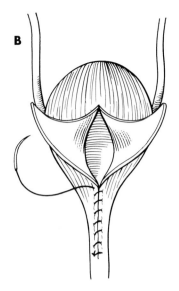

FIG. 22-35
Use scissors to extend the incisions illustrated in Fig. 22-34 towards the urethra, creating two full-thickness flaps. **A,** Reflect the flaps cranially and **B,** suture the defect from the urethral end cranially to form a urethral tube.

COMPLICATIONS

If the urethral lumen is of insufficient width or swelling is excessive, urinary obstruction may occur. Other complications include return of incontinence and urinary leakage.

PROGNOSIS

Urinary continence or decreased frequency and volume of urine dribbling appear to occur in most animals with urethral hypoplasia following bladder flap reconstruction.

References

Arnold S et al: Treatment of urinary incontinence in dogs by endoscopic injection of Teflon, *J Am Vet Med Assoc* 195:1369, 1989.

Holt PE: Long-term evaluation of colposuspension in the treatment of urinary incontinence due to incompetence of the urethral sphincter mechanism, *Vet Rec* 127:537, 1990.

Massat BJ et al: Cystourethropexy to correct refractory urinary incontinence due to urethral sphincter mechanism incompetence: preliminary results in ten bitches, *Vet Surg* 22:260, 1993.

Suggested Reading

Dean PW, Novotny MJ, O'Brien DP: Prosthetic sphincter for urinary incontinence: results in three cases, *J Am Anim Hosp Assoc* 23:447, 1989.

Gregory SP, Holt PE: The immediate effect of colposuspension on resting and stressed urethral pressure profiles in anesthetized incontinent bitches, *Vet Surg* 23:330, 1994.

Holt PE: Urinary incontinence in the bitch due to sphincter mechanism incompetence: prevalence in referred dogs and retrospective analysis of sixty cases, *J Small Anim Pract* 26:181, 1985.

Holt PE: Urinary incontinence in the bitch due to sphincter mechanism incompetence: surgical treatment, *J Small Anim Pract* 26:237, 1985.

Holt PE: Surgical management of congenital urethral sphincter mechanism incompetence in eight female cats and a bitch, *Vet Surg* 22:98, 1993.

Holt PE, Gibbs C: Congenital urinary incontinence in cats: a review of 19 cases, *Vet Rec* 130:437, 1992.

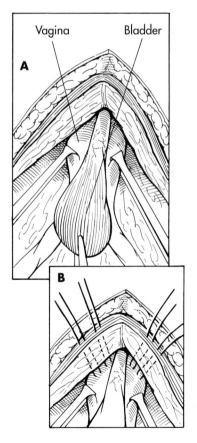

FIG. 22-36
Colposuspension is occasionally performed for urinary incontinence. Separate the fat and fascia around the ventral bladder neck and proximal urethra and expose the vaginal wall dorsolateral to the urethra. **A,** While maintaining cranial traction on the vagina, **B,** place two sutures on each side from the vagina to the prepubic tendon.

FELINE UROLOGIC SYNDROME (STERILE CYSTITIS)

DEFINITIONS

Feline urologic syndrome (FUS) is a term used to describe an idiopathic inflammatory process of the feline lower urinary tract that sometimes results in partial or complete urethral obstruction. The current accepted terminology is **sterile cystitis.**

SYNONYMS

Feline obstructive uropathy, blocked

GENERAL CONSIDERATIONS AND CLINICALLY RELEVANT PATHOPHYSIOLOGY

Cats with sterile cystitis may account for as many as 10% of all feline admissions to veterinary hospitals. They may or may not have struvite crystals or calculi, and struvite crystalluria may be found in some cats without evidence of associated signs of sterile cystitis. Urinary tract infection is uncommon in obstructed cats. Dietary factors (i.e., high dietary magnesium or ash content, feeding dry food), obesity, urine alkalinity, UTI, decreased urine volume and decreased frequency of urination, viruses (e.g., feline calicivirus, bovine herpesvirus 4, feline synctia-forming virus), and vesicourachal diverticula have all been implicated as causes of sterile cystitis in cats; however, the etiology is not defined and is probably multifactorial.

☞ **N O T E** • Struvite crystals are not always associated with signs of sterile cystitis and some cats with sterile cystitis do not have struvite crystals or calculi.

DIAGNOSIS
Clinical Presentation

Signalment. Overweight cats may be predisposed to sterile cystitis. Males and females are equally affected; however, male cats are more likely to obstruct due to the small diameter of their urethras. Middle-aged cats are more commonly affected and indoor cats may be at increased risk.

History. Unobstructed cats usually present for evaluation of pollakiuria, stranguria, hematuria, and/or inappropriate urination. Cats with obstruction may appear uncomfortable or anxious, restless, may attempt to urinate frequently, lick their genitalia, and may have abdominal pain. If obstruction has been present for greater than 36 to 48 hours, anorexia, dehydration, vomiting, collapse, stupor, hypothermia, and/or bradycardia may be noted (see p. 481).

Physical Examination Findings

If the cat is obstructed, the bladder will feel distended and firm (unless it has ruptured) and cannot be expressed. Abdominal palpation may elicit signs of pain. Care should be taken when palpating the bladder of obstructed cats to prevent iatrogenic rupture.

Laboratory Findings

Laboratory findings may be normal or may show evidence of uremia, metabolic acidosis, and/or hyperkalemia.

DIFFERENTIAL DIAGNOSIS

Other causes of urethral obstruction (e.g., neoplasia, trauma) should be excluded based on clinical signs, physical examination findings, and history.

MEDICAL MANAGEMENT

For obstructed cats, fluid therapy should begin before laboratory data is returned. Fluids should be given intravenously to restore normal hydration and treat hyperkalemia (see p. 481). 0.9% saline should be used in case the cat is hyperkalemic. If serum potassium is later found to be normal, a balanced electrolyte solution should be administered. Obstruction should be promptly relieved by urethral catheterization or gentle penile massage, if possible. If the cat is severely depressed, minimal restraint may be necessary. In other cats, general anesthesia may be required (see below). Sterile isotonic fluid should be used to flush plugs or calculi into the bladder. Nonmetal, smooth, well-lubricated catheters are preferred to minimize urethral trauma. If the catheter cannot be advanced, cystocentesis may be helpful. If a normal stream is not present following catheterization or detrusor atony is present, an indwelling, soft urinary catheter may be sewn in place; however, this often promotes UTI. The cat should be stabilized prior to performing a perineal urethrostomy.

SURGICAL TREATMENT

Perineal urethrostomy is indicated to prevent recurrence of obstruction in male cats or to treat obstruction that cannot be eliminated by catheterization. It is also useful to treat strictures that occur following urethral obstruction and catheterization. With appropriate nonsurgical treatment of obstructed cats, this procedure is less commonly indicated than previously. There is a high incidence of postoperative bacterial urinary tract infection after urethrostomy due to anatomic alterations of the urethral meatus, compromised intrinsic defense mechanisms, and the underlying uropathy. Many cats have a permanent loss of striated urethral sphincter function after this procedure, although incontinence is rare.

Preoperative Management

Electrolyte (i.e., hyperkalemia) and acid-base abnormalities should be corrected prior to anesthetic induction (see p. 482). Fluids should be given intravenously to restore normal hydration and combat postobstruction diuresis. Cats that were initially severely uremic will often have a marked post obstruction diuresis during which time they require large volumes of intravenous fluids to prevent severe hypovolemia. Serum potassium concentrations must be monitored to avoid hypokalemia.

Anesthesia

An ECG should be monitored before, during, and after surgery for cardiac arrhythmias. If the cat has been adequately stabilized (i.e., hydration and potassium are normal), diazepam followed by ultra–short-acting thiobarbiturates (thiamylal sodium, thiopental sodium), or propofol, or mask induction may be used (after premedicating with an opioid; Table 22-12). Thiobarbiturates are arrhythmogenic and should therefore be used cautiously in animals with pre-existing arrhythmias. Isoflurane is the least cardiodepressant inhalation anesthetic and should be used for maintenance. Shocky, dehydrated, or hypovolemic patients should be induced with diazepam followed by etomidate, after premedicating with an opioid. Because ketamine is excreted in the urine in its active form it should be used very cautiously (if at all) and at low dosages in cats with urinary obstruction. Mask induction should not be used if the cat is vomiting.

Surgical Anatomy

For a description of the surgical anatomy of the urethra, refer to p. 484.

Positioning

The cat is placed in sternal recumbency with the perineal region elevated slightly. Ventilation may need to be assisted when the cat is positioned in this manner.

SURGICAL TECHNIQUE
Perineal Urethrostomy

Place a purse-string suture in the anus and catheterize the penis if possible. Make an elliptical incision around the scrotum and prepuce and excise them. Place an Allis tissue forceps on the end of the prepuce or around the catheter to help manipulate the penis. Reflect the penis dorsolaterally and sharply dissect the surrounding loose tissue on either side (Fig. 22-37, A). Extend the dissection ventrally and laterally toward the penile attachments at the ischial arch. Elevate the penis dorsally and sharply sever the ventral penile ligament. Then, transect the ischiocavernosus muscles and ischiourethralis muscles at their insertion on the ischium to avoid damaging branches of the pudendal nerves

*and to minimize hemorrhage (Fig. 22-37, B). Reflect the penis ventrally to expose the dorsal surface. Expose the bulbourethral glands proximal and dorsal to the bulbospongiosus muscle and cranial to the severed ischiocavernosus and ischiourethralis muscles. Avoid excessive dorsal dissection to prevent damaging the nerves and vessels supplying the urethral muscle. Elevate and remove the retractor penis muscle over the urethra (Fig. 22-37, C) and longitudinally incise the penile urethra using a No. 11 blade or sharp tenotomy scissors. **Continue the urethra incision proximal to the pelvic urethra approximately 1 cm beyond the level of the bulbourethral glands** (Fig. 22-37, D). Pass a closed Halsted mosquito hemostat up the urethra to ensure that the urethral width is adequate. The hemostat should be able to be passed to the level of the box-locks without resistance. Suture the urethral mucosa to the skin using 4-0 absorbable (polydioxanone or polyglyconate) or nonabsorbable (nylon or polypropylene) suture on a taper-cut, swaged-on needle. Be sure to suture the urethral mucosa to skin (it is sometimes difficult to identify mucosa). Place the most proximal sutures at a 45-degree angle to the skin first, then place the remainder. Suture the proximal two thirds of the penile urethra to the skin and amputate the distal end by placing a horizontal mattress suture through the skin and penile tissues and severing the penis distal to this ligature. Close the remaining skin with simple interrupted sutures (Fig. 22-38).*

SUTURE MATERIALS/SPECIAL INSTRUMENTS

A urinary catheter is placed in the urethra to help locate it during the operation. Monofilament absorbable (polydioxanone or polyglyconate) or nonabsorbable (polypropylene or nylon) suture is preferred. The sutures should be removed 10 to 14 days after the surgery. Tenotomy scissors and small, atraumatic forceps are useful.

POSTOPERATIVE CARE AND ASSESSMENT

Paper, instead of gravel litter, should be used until the wound is healed. Urinary cultures should be performed periodically to check for UTI. Indwelling catheters should not be routinely used following surgery as they may promote stricture formation and/or UTI.

☞ **N O T E** • Evaluate these cats periodically for UTI.

COMPLICATIONS

The most serious complication of perineal urethrostomy is stricture formation. Stricture formation in cats following perineal urethrostomy is generally due to making the stoma too small (i.e., making the stoma in the proximal penile urethra instead of the distal pelvic urethra), or to postoperative subcutaneous urine leakage and subsequent granulation tissue formation (see p. 495). Urinary and fecal incontinence

---

TABLE 22-12

Selected Anesthetic Protocols for Use in Shocky, Dehydrated, or Hypovolemic Cats with Sterile Cystitis

Premedication

Butorphanol (0.2-0.4 mg/kg SC or IM) or buprenorphine (5-15 µg/kg IM) or oxymorphone (0.05 mg/kg SC or IM)

Induction

Diazepam (0.2 mg/kg IV) followed by etomidate (0.5-1.5 mg/kg IV)

Maintenance

Isoflurane

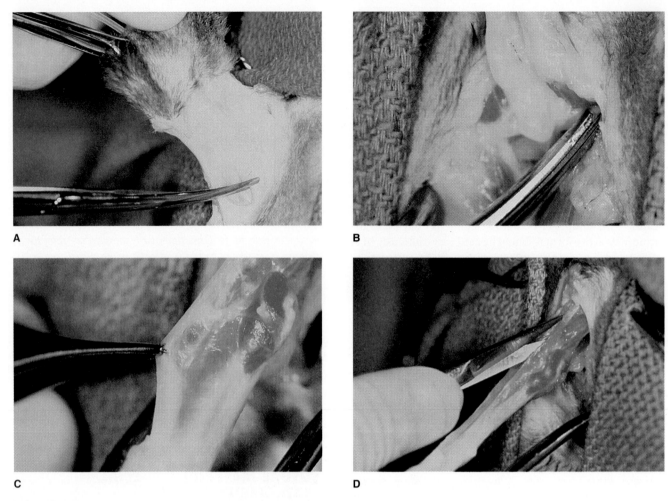

A

B

C

D

FIG. 22-37
Perineal urethrostomy may be performed in male cats with urinary obstruction. **A,** Reflect the penis dorsolaterally and sharply dissect surrounding loose tissue on either side. **B,** Transect the ischiocavernosus muscles and ischiourethralis muscles at their insertion on the ischium to avoid damaging branches of the pudendal nerves and to minimize hemorrhage. **C,** Elevate and remove the retractor penis muscle over the urethra, before making a longitudinal incision in the penile urethra. **D,** To ensure that the urethral width is adequate, extend the urethral incision approximately 1 cm beyond the level of the bulbourethral glands. (From Hosgood G, Hedlund CS: Perineal urethrostomy in cats, *Compend Contin Educ Pract Vet* 14:1195, 1992.)

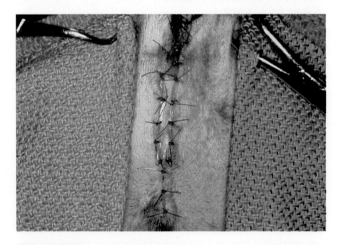

FIG. 22-38
Appearance of a completed perineal urethrostomy in a cat. (From Hosgood G, Hedlund CS: Perineal urethrostomy in cats, *Compend Contin Educ Pract Vet* 14:1195, 1992.)

may occur if the nerves are damaged during dissection around the pelvic urethra (see Surgical Technique). Perineal urethrostomy is associated with a high prevalence of UTI postoperatively due to anatomic alterations of the urethral meatus, compromised intrinsic defense mechanisms, and the underlying uropathy. Indwelling catheters may allow ascending bacterial infection and/or cause fibrosis and stricture. Although incontinence is rare, many cats have a permanent loss of striated urethral sphincter function after this procedure. Rectal prolapse has been reported following perineal urethrostomy in cats.

☞ **NOTE** • Stricture formation following perineal urethrostomy is usually due to making the stoma too small.

PROGNOSIS

The mortality rate of obstructed cats may exceed 35%. This high rate is often due to the financial constraints of owners reluctant to finance multiple or prolonged hospitalizations. Recurrence of obstruction is uncommon if perineal urethrostomy is performed properly; however, the cat should be monitored periodically for UTI for the remainder of its life.

Suggested Reading

Gregory CR: The effects of perineal urethrostomy on urethral function in male cats, *Compend Contin Educ Pract Vet* 9:895, 1987.

Griffin DW, Gregory CR: Prevalence of bacterial urinary tract infection after perineal urethrostomy in cats, *J Am Vet Med Assoc* 200:681, 1992.

Hosgood G, Hedlund CS: Perineal urethrostomy in cats, *Compend Contin Educ Pract Vet* 14:1195, 1992.

Kusba JK, Lipowitz AJ: Repair of strictures following perineal urethrostomy in the cat, *J Am Anim Hosp Assoc* 18:308, 1982.

Scavelli TD: Complications associated with perineal urethrostomy in the cat, *Probl Vet Med* 1:111, 1989.

CHAPTER 23

Surgery of the Reproductive and Genital Systems

GENERAL PRINCIPLES AND TECHNIQUES

DEFINITIONS

Neutering, or **castration,** refers to either **ovariohysterectomy** (surgical removal of the ovaries and uterus) or **orchiectomy** (surgical removal of the testicles). **Mastectomy** is excision of one or more mammary glands or mammary tissue. **Episiotomy** is incision of the vulvar orifice to expose the vulva and vagina, while **episioplasty** is reconstruction of the vulva. **Prostatectomy** is removal of all or a portion of the prostate gland. **Hysterotomy** is a surgical incision into the uterus (e.g., cesarean section).

PREOPERATIVE CONCERNS

Reproductive surgery encompasses a variety of techniques designed to alter the ability of the animal to reproduce, aid parturition, and/or treat or prevent disease of the reproductive organs (Table 23-1). The primary indication for reproductive tract surgery is to limit reproduction, but it may also be done to relieve dystocia, prevent or treat tumors influenced by reproductive hormones (e.g., mammary tumors, testicular tumors, perianal adenomas), help control certain diseases of the reproductive tract (e.g., pyometra, metritis, prostatitis, prostatic abscessation), and help stabilize systemic disease (e.g., diabetes, epilepsy). Neutering is performed in some animals to prevent or alter behavioral abnormalities and to reconstruct traumatized, diseased, or malformed tissue.

History and clinical signs of animals needing reproductive surgery depend on the gender and the disease. Most animals presenting for elective reproductive surgery (i.e., castration, ovariohysterectomy [OHE]) are healthy. Asymptomatic animals with neoplasia may have a mass found incidentally on physical examination. Those with genital tract infections may be severely ill and have fever, toxemia, incontinence, or obstruction. Prostatic disease is common in male

dogs; clinical signs may be nonspecific (i.e., fever, malaise, vomiting, dehydration, caudal abdominal pain, and/or gait abnormalities). Hematuria caused by reflux of blood from the prostatic urethra into the bladder and/or concurrent urinary tract infection may occur. Urethral discharge (preputial/urethral drip) is caused by passive release of blood, pus, or prostatic fluid into the prostatic urethra. Stranguria occurs when the prostate compresses or obstructs the urethra. Urinary incontinence may be caused by prostatic impingement on the pelvic nerves. Prostatic enlargement compressing the rectum results in tenesmus or smaller stool diameter. Constipation may occur secondary to obstruction or pain during defecation.

Diagnosis of reproductive tract disease is based on history, clinical signs, physical examination, diagnostic imaging (e.g., radiographs, ultrasound, computed tomography, magnetic resonance imaging, bone scan), endoscopy, cytology,

---

TABLE 23-1

Surgical Procedures of the Reproductive Tract

- Ovariohysterectomy
- Castration
- Cesarean section
- Cryptorchid castration
- Mastectomy
- Scrotal ablation
- Episiotomy
- Vasectomy
- Episioplasty
- Prostatic drainage
  - Drains
  - Omentalization
  - Marsupialization
- Prostatectomy
- Penile amputation
- Preputial reconstruction
- Biopsy

microbiology, hormonal assay, hematology, serum biochemistry profile, urinalysis, and/or other laboratory results. In females, physical examination should include inspection and palpation of the abdomen, vulva, and mammary glands. Abdominal palpation may reveal an enlarged uterus, mass, visceral displacement, and/or pain. Abnormal vulvar skin folds, conformation, discharge, or enlargement may be noted. During estrus and proestrus, the vulva is swollen to two or three times normal size, appears turgid, and has a hemorrhagic to straw-colored discharge. The swelling and turgidity diminish during estrus and diestrus. A vaginal examination is recommended when vaginal discharge or enlargement is detected. The vestibule and vagina should be visualized and digitally palpated. An otoscope or vaginal speculum allows visual inspection of the vestibule and caudal vagina; however, an endoscope is needed for evaluation of the cranial vagina and cervix. The vagina must be insufflated with air to distend mucosal folds and allow thorough evaluation. Vaginography may help evaluate vaginal anomalies, masses, or injuries if vaginoscopy fails to define the problem. Positive-contrast vaginography using a Foley catheter and a water-soluble contrast agent is easily performed. Mammary glands should be inspected for symmetry, texture, size, mobility, and discharge. If masses are identified, cytology of aspirates or discharges may help differentiate inflammation from neoplasia. Vaginal, uterine, or mammary gland cultures are recommended if infection is suspected. Cystometrograms and urethral pressure profiles may help assess urinary incontinence. Histologic evaluation is necessary to confirm the diagnosis and allow a more accurate prognosis with most conditions.

Vaginal cytology should be consistent with the bitch's estrus cycle. The normal vaginal flora includes numerous aerobic and anaerobic bacteria (Table 23-2). Persistent vaginal discharge indicates a need for brucellosis testing. Assessment of hormone levels is occasionally helpful. In female dogs, estradiol levels are ≤ 10 pg/ml during late anestrus, ≥ 10 pg/ml at onset of proestrus, and 50-100 pg/ml at late proestrus. Progesterone levels are 0.5-1.0 ng/ml during anestrus and proestrus, 2-5 ng/ml at ovulation, peak at 15-90 ng/ml after the luteinizing hormone (LH) peaks, and remain elevated during gestation. For mean serum concentrations of luteinizing hormone and follicle-stimulating hormone (FHS) see Table 23-3.

Thoracic and abdominal radiographs are needed if reproductive tract tumors are suspected. The normal nongravid uterus is rarely identified by plain radiographs or ultrasonography. Radiographically, an enlarged gravid uterus can be detected within 31 to 38 days and fetal skeletal mineralization by 45 days after the luteinizing hormone peak (within a mean of 0.5 days of onset of estrus). If the cervix is open or the animal is in estrus, positive contrast may be injected to outline the endometrium. The mucosa will appear smooth during estrus and scalloped with endometritis. Ovarian masses and follicular changes can be detected in the periovulatory period using ultrasonography while it is difficult to identify the normal, nongravid uterus. Using a fluid-distended urinary bladder as an acoustic window may reveal fluid-distended horns and a thickened uterine wall. Pregnancy and fetal viability can be detected ultrasonographically as early as 20 to 28 days into gestation. Ultrasonography can also detect uterine cysts, masses or fluid, premature placental separation, and a thickened uterine wall.

Thorough abdominal and rectal palpation is needed to evaluate prostatic size, symmetry, texture and mobility, and sublumbar lymph node size. Prostatic palpation sometimes elicits pain in animals with prostatitis. Abdominal radiographs define prostatic size, shape, and location. Radiographically, the normal prostate is near the cranial brim of the pubis and should not displace the colon or bladder. Its contour should be smooth and symmetric. Abnormal prostates may be asymmetric, irregular, and/or displace adjacent viscera. Sublumbar lymph nodes, lumbar vertebrae, and the bony pelvis should be evaluated for evidence of metastases. A positive-contrast cystourethrogram helps evaluate prostatic position in relation to the bladder, urethral size, mucosal contour, and prostatic reflux. Ultrasonography defines parenchymal homogeneity, contour, disease distribution, and urethral diameter. Cytology and biopsy specimens can be collected with ultrasound guidance. Cytologic evaluation of prostatic fluid is one of the most informative tests. Prostatic fluid is best obtained by ejaculation, but prostatic washes or fine-needle aspiration is often acceptable. Prostatic massage or ejaculation fluid in normal dogs has few transitional cells, rare neutrophils, and a varying number of erythrocytes. Fine-needle aspiration cytology is more likely to demonstrate neoplastic cells, increased neutrophils, bacteria, and other debris. Urine and prostatic fluid should be cul-

---

TABLE 23-2

Normal Vaginal Flora

- α and β-hemolytic *Streptococcus*
- *Staphylococcus* spp.
- *Proteus* spp.
- *Escherichia coli*
- *Bacillus* spp.
- *Bacteroides* spp.
- *Pasteurella* spp.
- Anaerobic enterococci
- *Mycoplasma*

TABLE 23-3

Serum Hormone Concentrations in Female Dogs (ng/ml)

	Intact	Neutered
LH	1.2 (±0.9)	28.7 (±25.8)
FSH	98 (+49)	1219 (+763)

From Olson PN, Mulinix JA, Nett TM: Concentrations of luteinizing hormone and follicle-stimulating hormone in the serum of sexually intact and neutered dogs, *Am J Vet Res* 53:762, 1992.

tured to detect bacterial infections. A bone scan and thoracic radiographs help stage the disease if neoplasia is suspected. It occasionally helps to evaluate urinary incontinence with a cystometrogram and urethral pressure profile. The scrotum should be examined for size, symmetry, thickening, masses, sensitivity, and scrotal adhesions. Testicles should be palpated for size, consistency, contour, symmetry, and sensitivity. Ultrasonography helps evaluate scrotal swelling and detects testicular abnormalities including cryptorchidism, testicular torsion, and neoplasia. The normal testicular architecture is coarse and homogeneous with the mediastinum testis represented as a central hyperechoic band. The epididymis is anechoic to hypoechoic, relative to the testicular parenchyma. The prepuce and penis are observed for signs of trauma, wounds, masses, irritation, and congenital abnormalities. The penis should be completely extruded from the prepuce for thorough examination. Occasionally, radiographs help evaluate os penis fractures and urethral extension of disease. Cytologic evaluation should be performed on all accessible masses. A biopsy is necessary to definitively diagnose prostatic, testicular, penile, preputial, or scrotal masses.

Measurement of serum hormone concentrations may aid in determining whether a male dog has been neutered or has a hormone-producing tumor; however, episodic release of gonadotropins makes interpretation of hormone assays difficult, and reference values vary between laboratories. Expected serum concentrations of LH and FSH in intact and castrated male dogs are provided in Table 23-4. In intact male dogs, serum testosterone concentrations range between 0.5 and 9.0 ng/ml, while serum estrogen concentrations are generally less than 15 pg/ml.

ANESTHETIC CONSIDERATIONS

General anesthesia is recommended for elective surgeries involving the reproductive tract. Careful preoperative screening of animals undergoing elective surgery is important; anesthetic complications in apparently healthy animals may arise due to uncorrected hydration or electrolyte or acid-base abnormalities. Numerous anesthetic protocols may be used for elective surgery in healthy animals; suggested anesthetic protocols are provided in Table 23-5. Atropine or glycopyrrolate may prevent bradycardia induced by visceral manipulation. Opioid premedicants (e.g., butorphanol, oxymorphone, or buprenorphine) may also provide pre- and postoperative analgesia. Ketamine gives poor visceral analgesia and should not be used alone for surgical procedures. During abdominal surgery, water evaporates from exposed viscera at an increased rate; therefore, fluid administration must be increased to replace this loss. Body heat loss due to vasodilation and visceral exposure causes hypothermia, which reduces the need for anesthesia. Be careful to maintain body temperature during surgery and rewarm the patient postoperatively.

Neutering has traditionally been recommended at 5 to 7 months of age. Early neutering (i.e., 6 to 16 weeks) gives good results if precautions are taken to prevent hypoglycemia, hypothermia, and hemorrhage. Animals less than 6 months of age should be premedicated with an anticholinergic. If tranquilization is needed in dogs in addition to analgesia, oxymorphone should be used but acepromazine avoided. Butorphanol may be used as a premedicant in young cats, but provides little sedation. Mask or chamber inductions are useful in very young animals. Depending on the patient's tractability, reduced dosages of thiopental or propofol, or a combination of diazepam and ketamine may be used for intravenous induction. Isoflurane is preferred for maintenance of anesthesia.

If there are no contraindications (e.g., sepsis, bleeding diatheses, hypovolemia [for epidurals using local anesthetics]), epidurals may be used in dogs to supplement general

---

TABLE 23-4

Serum Hormone Concentrations in Male Dogs (ng/ml)

	Intact	Neutered
LH	6.0 (±5.2)	17.1 (±9.9)
FSH	89 (+28)	858 (+674)

From Olson PN, Mulinix JA, Nett TM: Concentrations of luteinizing hormone and follicle-stimulating hormone in the serum of sexually intact and neutered dogs, *Am J Vet Res* 53:762, 1992.

TABLE 23-5

Selected Anesthetic Protocols for Elective Surgery in Healthy Animals Older Than 6 Months of Age

Dogs
Premedication

Atropine (0.02-0.04 mg/kg SC or IM) or glycopyrrolate (0.005-0.011 mg/kg SC, IM) plus acepromazine (0.05 mg/kg SC or IM; not to exceed 1 mg) and butorphanol* (0.2-0.4 mg/kg SC, IM)

Induction

Thiopental (10-12 mg/kg) administered IV to effect

Maintenance
Isoflurane or halothane

Cats
Premedication

Atropine (0.02-0.04 mg/kg SC or IM) or glycopyrrolate (0.005-0.011 mg/kg SC, IM) plus ketamine (5 mg/kg IM) and butorphanol (0.2-0.4 mg/kg SC, IM)

Induction

Diazepam (0.27 mg/kg) plus ketamine (5.5 mg/kg) combined and administered IV to effect or thiopental (10-12 mg/kg) administered IV to effect or mask or chamber induction

Maintenance

Isoflurane or halothane

*Other opioids may be substituted for butorphanol (see text).

TABLE 23-6

Epidural Anesthesia in Dogs

Drug	Dose	Onset of Action	Duration of Action
Lidocaine 2%*	1 ml/3.4 kg (T_5) 1 ml/4.5 kg (T_{13}-L_1)[†]	10 min	1 to 1.5 hr
Bupivacaine 0.25% or 0.5%* (preservative free)	1 ml/4.5 kg	20 to 30 min	4.5 to 6 hr
Fentanyl	0.001 mg/kg	4 to 10 min	6 hr
Oxymorphone	0.1 mg/kg	15 min?	10 hr
Morphine (preservative free)	0.1 mg/kg[‡]	23 min	20 hr
Buprenorphine	0.005 mg/kg	30 min?	12 to 18 hr

*Avoid head-down position after epidural.
[†]A block to T_1 leads to intercostal nerve paralysis; a block to C_7-C_5 leads to phrenic nerve paralysis.
[‡]The dose for epidural morphine in cats is 0.03 mg/kg.

anesthesia (Table 23-6). It is rare that epidural anesthesia alone is sufficient for surgery. If general anesthesia is not used, heavy sedation (i.e., oxymorphone, diazepam) is needed. Epidural doses should be decreased if a spinal has been inadvertently performed, the patient is pregnant or obese, or there are space-occupying vertebral canal lesions. Opioids can be better than local anesthetic drugs in epidurals because opioids cause sensory loss without motor block, and they do not promote hypotension. Because local anesthetics in epidurals may cause hypotension, dehydration should be corrected prior to performing the procedure.

Patients requiring cesarean section are often greater anesthetic risks because of hypovolemia, hypoglycemia, hypocalcemia, and/or toxemia. A distended uterus may decrease tidal volume. Drugs that depress the mother also depress the fetus. The rate of placental transfer is directly related to lipid solubility and concentration of nonionized drug. Anesthetic time should be kept to a minimum and return to consciousness should be rapid. Ideally, inhalation agents should be used only after the neonates are removed and at minimal concentrations. Nitrous oxide crosses the placental barrier, but lower levels are found in the fetus than the mother. Nitrous oxide may also promote hypoxemia. Epidural anesthesia is safe for the fetus, but must be used with other drugs and may induce maternal hypovolemia (see above). Before making the skin incision, a lidocaine line block may be used in dogs. Suggested anesthetic protocols for cesarean section are provided in Table 23-7. See below under techniques for cesarean section for neonate care.

ANTIBIOTICS

Perioperative antibiotics are not needed for elective OHE or castration. Antibiotic choice should be based on culture and susceptibility or on expected pathogens in patients with pyometra, metritis, or bacterial prostatitis. Until culture results are available, antibiotics used to treat pyometra should be efficacious against *E. coli* (e.g., cefazolin, cefoxitin, amoxicillin plus clavulanate, trimethoprim-sulfadiazine; Table 23-8) because

this is the most common pathogen. Aminoglycosides are nephrotoxic and should be avoided due to the prevalence of renal dysfunction with pyometra. Choice of prophylactic antibiotics for surgery involving tumors or trauma depends on the patient's condition and surgeon's preference (see Chapter 10).

Antibiotic selection for prostatic diseases should be based on culture results and expected blood:prostate barrier penetration. Antibiotics should be lipid-soluble (usually nonionized), non–protein bound, and have a high pKa (degree of drug ionization; high pKa = more basic). Those with a high degree of lipid solubility are best at crossing the blood:prostate barrier. Antibiotics with a high pKa concentrate in the prostate are less ionized at physiologic conditions. Prostatic infections produce acidic prostatic fluid, which helps trap antibiotics in the fluid. Basic antibiotics that concentrate in the prostate include erythromycin, clindamycin, carbenicillin, and trimethoprim (see Table 23-8). Enrofloxacin also achieves high prostatic fluid concentrations and is effective against some resistant gram-negative urogenital pathogens. Tetracyclines (e.g., doxycycline) are also useful.

SURGICAL ANATOMY
Female Reproductive Tract

The female reproductive tract includes the ovaries, oviduct, uterus, vagina, vulva, and mammary glands. The ovaries are located within a thin-walled peritoneal sac, the ovarian bursa, just caudal to the pole of each kidney. The uterine tube or oviduct courses through the wall of the ovarian bursa. The right ovary lies further cranially than the left. The right ovary lies dorsal to the descending duodenum, and the left ovary dorsal to the descending colon and lateral to the spleen. Medial retraction of the mesoduodenum or mesocolon exposes the ovary on each side. Each ovary is attached by the proper ligament to the uterine horn and via the suspensory ligament to the transversalis fascia medial to the last one or two ribs. The ovarian pedicle (mesovarium) includes the suspensory ligament with its artery and vein, ovarian artery and vein, and variable amounts of fat and connective

TABLE 23-7
Selected Anesthetic Protocols for Cesarean Section

General Principles

1. Place an IV catheter
2. Immediately begin volume replacement with IV crystalloids (10-20 ml/kg)
3. Preoxygenate before induction

Dogs
Premedication

Glycopyrrolate (0.005-0.011 mg/kg SC, IM)

Induction

Oxymorphone (0.1 mg/kg IV) plus diazepam (0.2 mg/kg IV); intubate if possible. If necessary, give etomidate (0.5-1.5 mg/kg IV). Alternatively, small doses of thiopental or propofol may be used.

Maintenance

Isoflurane

Cats
Premedication

Glycopyrrolate (0.005-0.011 mg/kg SC, IM) and butorphanol (0.2-0.4 mg/kg SC, IM)

Induction

Diazepam (0.2 mg/kg IV) followed by etomidate (0.5-1.5 mg/kg IV). Alternately, a combination of diazepam (0.27 mg/kg) plus ketamine (5.5 mg/kg) may be administered IV to effect or reduced dosages of thiopental or propofol may be used.

Maintenance

Isoflurane

TABLE 23-8
Antibiotics for Treatment of Reproductive Disorders

Cefazolin (Ancef, Kefzol)
20 mg/kg IV, IM, TID

Cefoxitin (Mefoxin)
15-30 mg/kg IV, TID to QID

Amoxicillin plus Clavulanate (Clavamox)
Dogs
12.5-25 mg/kg PO, BID
Cats
62.5 mg/cat PO, BID

Ampicillin
22 mg/kg IV, IM, or SC, TID to QID

Trimethoprim-Sulfadiazine (Tribrissen)
Dogs
15 mg/kg IM or PO, BID
Cats
15 mg/kg PO, BID

Erythromycin
10-20 mg/kg PO, BID to TID

Clindamycin (Antirobe)
11 mg/kg PO, BID

Doxycycline (Vibramycin)
5 mg/kg PO, BID

Enrofloxacin (Baytril)
5-10 mg/kg PO or IV, BID

Carbenicillin (Geocillin)
(For urinary tract infections) 10 mg/kg PO, TID

tissue. Canine ovarian pedicles contain more fat than in cats, making it more difficult to visualize the vasculature. The ovarian vessels take a tortuous path within the pedicle. Ovarian arteries originate from the aorta. The left ovarian vein drains into the left renal vein; the right vein drains into the caudal vena cava. The suspensory ligament is a tough, whitish band of tissue that diverges as it travels from the ovary to attach on the last two ribs. The broad ligament (mesometrium) is the peritoneal fold that suspends the uterus. The round ligament travels in the free edge of the broad ligament from the ovary through the inguinal canal with the vaginal process. The uterus has a short body and long narrow horns. The blood supply to the uterus is from the uterine arteries and veins. The cervix is the constricted caudal part of the uterus and is thicker than the uterine body and vagina. It is oriented in a nearly vertical position with the uterine opening dorsal. The vagina is long and connects with the vaginal vestibule at the urethral entrance. The clitoris is broad, flat, vascular, infiltrated with fat, and lies on the floor of the vestibule near the vulva. The clitoral fossa is a depression on the floor of the vestibule that is sometimes mistaken for the urethral orifice. The vulva is the external opening of the genital tract. The vulvar lips are thick and form a pointed commissure. The constrictor vulvae and constrictor vestibule muscles encircle the vulva and vestibule. See p. 541 for anatomy of the mammary glands.

NOTE • Fatty broad ligaments are more vascular and may require ligation after transection.

Male Reproductive Tract

The major components of the male genital tract are the testicles, penis, and prostate. The prostate gland completely surrounds the neck of the bladder and beginning of the urethra. In dogs less than 4 years of age, the prostate is usually located in the pelvic cavity at the brim of the pubis. The prostate begins to enlarge at puberty, becoming intraabdominal in location. It varies greatly in size at maturity. The prostate is encapsulated by fibromuscular tissue and is bilobate with a prominent middorsal sulcus. The dorsal sulcus continues into the prostatic parenchyma as the median septum. The ventrolateral surfaces of the prostate are covered by a fat pad. The parenchyma is lobulated with tubuloalveolar glands that empty through small ducts (12 to 20) into the prostatic urethra. The ductus deferens enters the craniodorsal surface of the prostate and courses caudoventrally to enter the urethra at the colliculus seminalis. The blood and nerve supply (pelvic and hypogastric nerves) are located in the lateral pedicles (peritoneal reflection) entering the prostate at the 10 o'clock and 2 o'clock positions when viewed in a transverse plane. The prostatic arteries originate from the urogenital artery (branch of internal iliac artery) and supply branches to the ductus deferens, urethra, urinary bladder, ureters, and rectum. The hypogastric (sympathetic) and pelvic (parasympathetic) nerves follow the vasculature and are essential for micturition and continence (Fig. 23-1). The pudendal nerve sends branches along the ventral surface of the urethra extending to the bladder neck. The pudendal nerve innervates the skeletal muscle of the external urethral sphincter. The iliac lymph nodes drain the prostate. In cats, bulbourethral glands are found caudal to the prostate at the ischial arch.

The penis has a root, body, and glans. The root of the penis is formed by the right and left crura, which originate from the ischiatic tuberosity. Each crus is composed of corpus cavernosum penis surrounded by tunica albuginea. The two corpora extend side by side, separated by a median septum, along the length of the penile body to the os penis in the glans penis. The distal end of the penis or glans penis is covered by the prepuce, a mucosal lined fold of integument. The distal end of the dog's penis is directed cranially and located ventral to the abdominal wall. The distal end of the cat's penis is directed caudal and ventral in the perineum. The glans of the feline penis is covered with caudally directed cornified spines that are more prominent in intact males. The feline os penis is very small, whereas in dogs it is a long, grooved, rough bone. The urethra travels through the ventral groove in the os penis and penis. The corpus spongiosum surrounds the urethra. The ischiocavernosus muscle arises from the ischiatic tuberosity and inserts on the crus. The retractor penis muscles originate from the ventral surface of the sacrum or the first two caudal vertebrae and extend distally on the ventral surface of the penis to insert at the level of the glans. The retractor and external anal sphincter muscles share muscle fibers. The bulbospongiosus muscle bulges between the ischiocavernosus muscles ventral to the external anal sphincter.

☞ **N O T E** • Scotties generally have larger prostates than other similarly sized breeds.

☞ **N O T E** • Surgery of the penis is often associated with significant hemorrhage because of the vascular nature of the cavernosus tissue.

The scrotum is located between the inguinal region and anus. In dogs, scrotal skin is thin and sparsely haired. The feline scrotum is more dorsal and densely haired than the canine scrotum. The scrotum is a membranous pouch with a midline septum that houses the testes, epididymis, and distal spermatic cords. The testis, epididymis, ductus deferens, and associated vessels and nerves are covered by visceral and parietal vaginal tunic and spermatic fascia. The testes are relatively small and ovoid. The epididymis is large, convoluted, and attached to the lateral side of the testis. The head of the epididymis communicates with the testis, and the caudal extremity or tail is continuous with the ductus deferens. The tail is attached to the testis by the proper ligament of the testis. The ligament of the tail of the epididymis attaches the epididymis to the vaginal tunic and the spermatic fascia. The ductus deferens loops around the ureter as it travels from the inguinal ring, enters the dorsal prostate, and terminates in the prostatic urethra. The ureter is dorsal to the ductus deferens. The spermatic cord begins at the inguinal ring where the testicular artery, testicular veins (pampiniform plexus), lymphatics, testicular autonomic nerve plexus, ductus deferens and its artery and vein, smooth muscle, and visceral layer of the vaginal tunic come together. The cremaster muscle travels along the external surface of the parietal tunic. The cremaster is a thin, flat extension of the internal abdominal oblique muscle.

☞ **N O T E** • The epididymis can often be palpated in dogs with epididymitis.

FIG. 23-1
Innervation to the prostate and bladder.

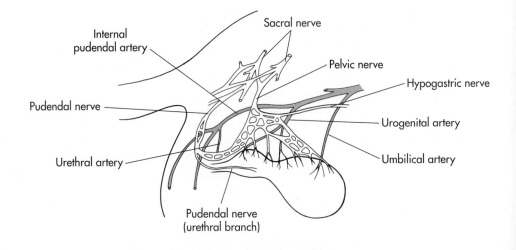

Internal pudendal artery

Sacral nerve

Pelvic nerve

Hypogastric nerve

Pudendal nerve

Urogenital artery

Umbilical artery

Urethral artery

Pudendal nerve (urethral branch)

SURGICAL TECHNIQUES

For elective surgeries, food should be withheld from adults for 12 to 18 hours and from pediatric patients for 4 to 8 hours prior to surgery. The ventral abdomen should be clipped and aseptically prepared for all procedures that may require a celiotomy. The urinary bladder should be expressed if the patient has not voided immediately prior to induction. In male dogs, the prescrotal area should be clipped and prepared for aseptic surgery; however, trauma to the scrotum (i.e., with clippers, antiseptic soaps, or solutions) should be avoided. Canine scrotal skin is sensitive and swells with minimal trauma or irritation. In cats, hair can be plucked or pulled from the scrotum. The prepuce or vestibule should be flushed with dilute antiseptic solutions before procedures involving these areas. For some procedures of the perineum, prostate, or penis, placement of a urethral catheter helps identify the urethra.

☞ **NOTE** • Many techniques are used for ovariohysterectomy and castration. However, the goals are the same: removal of the ovaries, plus uterine horns and body, or the testes with placement of secure ligatures.

Pediatric tissues are more fragile than adult tissues and must be handled gently. 3-0 to 5-0 ligatures should be used in young animals. Early neutering delays growth plate closure by an average of 9 weeks, resulting in increased bone length in male and female dogs (Salmeri et al, 1991). Infantile vulva and mammary glands or penis, prepuce, and os penis persist following early neutering. Early neutering does not affect weight gain, daily food consumption, or activity level.

Ovariohysterectomy

The most common reason to perform ovariohysterectomy (OHE) is to prevent estrus and unwanted offspring. Other reasons include prevention of mammary tumors or congenital anomalies, prevention and treatment of pyometra, metritis, neoplasia (i.e., ovarian, uterine, or vaginal), cysts, trauma, uterine torsion, uterine prolapse, subinvolution of placental sites, vaginal prolapse, vaginal hyperplasia, and control of some endocrine abnormalities (i.e., diabetes, epilepsy) and dermatoses (e.g., generalized *Demodex*). Many technical variations of OHE have been described—only one technique is described here.

☞ **NOTE** • In dogs, make the incision immediately caudal to the umbilicus to allow ligation of the ovarian pedicle. Make the incision more caudal in cats to allow ligation of the uterine body.

Clip and surgically prepare the ventral abdomen from the xiphoid to the pubis. Identify the umbilicus and visually divide the caudal abdomen into thirds. In dogs, make the incision just caudal to the umbilicus in the cranial third of the caudal abdomen. More caudal incisions make it difficult to exteriorize canine ovaries. In deep-chested dogs or those with an enlarged uterus, extend the incision cranially or caudally to allow exteriorization of the tract without exces-

sive traction. In cats, the body of the uterus is more caudal and difficult to exteriorize; therefore make the incision in the middle third of the caudal abdomen. Make a 4- to 8-cm incision through skin and subcutaneous tissues to expose the linea alba. Grasp the linea alba or ventral rectus sheath, tent it outward, and make a stab incision into the abdominal cavity. Extend the linea incision cranial and caudal to the stab with Mayo scissors. Elevate the left abdominal wall by grasping the linea or external rectus sheath with thumb forceps. Slide the ovariectomy hook (e.g., Covault, Snook), with the hook against the abdominal wall, 2 to 3 cm caudal to the kidney (Fig. 23-2, A). Turn the hook medially to ensnare the uterine horn, broad ligament, or round ligament and gently elevate it from the abdomen. Anatomically confirm the identification of the uterine horn by following it to either the uterine bifurcation or ovary. If the uterine horn cannot be located with the hook, retroflex the bladder through the incision and locate the uterine body and horns between the colon and bladder. With caudal and medial traction on the uterine horn, identify the suspensory ligament by palpation as the taut fibrous band at the proximal edge of the ovarian pedicle (Fig. 23-2, B). Stretch or break the suspensory ligament near the kidney, without tearing the ovarian vessels, to allow exteriorization of the ovary. Use the index finger to apply caudolateral traction on the suspensory ligament while maintaining caudomedial traction on the uterine horn (Fig. 23-2, C).

Make a hole in the broad ligament caudal to the ovarian pedicle. Place one or two Rochester Carmalt forceps across the ovarian pedicle proximal (deep) to the ovary and one across the proper ligament of the ovary (Fig. 23-2, D). The proximal (deep) clamp serves as a groove for the ligature, the middle clamp holds the pedicle for ligation, and the distal clamp prevents backflow of blood after transection. When using two clamps, the ovarian pedicle clamp serves both to hold the pedicle and make a groove for the ligature. Place a "figure 8" ligature proximal to (below) the ovarian pedicle clamps (Fig. 23-2, E). Choose an absorbable suture material for ligatures (i.e., 2-0 or 3-0 chromic catgut, polydioxanone, polyglyconate, or polyglactin 910). Begin by directing the blunt end of the needle through the middle of the pedicle, loop the suture around one side of the pedicle, then redirect the needle through the original hole from the same direction and loop the ligature around the other half of the pedicle. Securely tie the ligature. Remove one clamp or "flash" a single clamp while tightening the ligature to allow pedicle compression. Place a second circumferential ligature proximal to (below) the first to control hemorrhage, which may occur from puncturing a vessel as the needle is passed through the pedicle. Place a mosquito hemostat on the suspensory ligament near the ovary (Fig. 23-2, F). Transect the ovarian pedicle between the Carmalt and ovary. Open the ovarian bursa and examine the ovary to be certain that it has been removed in its entirety. Remove the Carmalt from the ovarian pedicle and observe for hemorrhage. Replace the Carmalt and religate the pedicle if hemorrhage is noted.

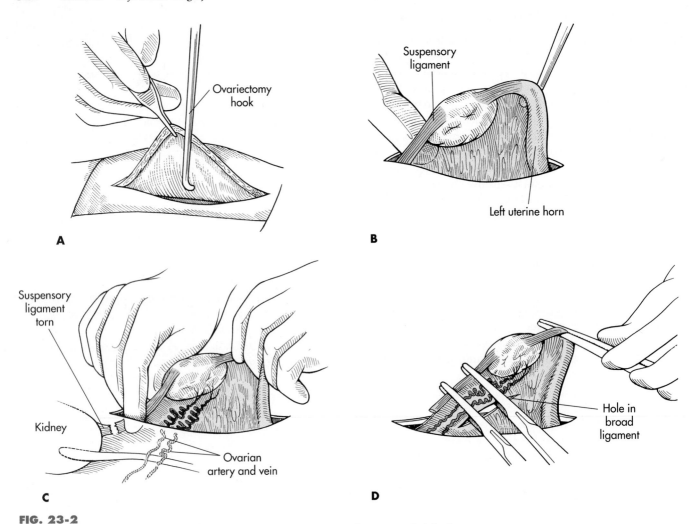

A

B

C

D

FIG. 23-2
A, For ovariohysterectomy, elevate the abdominal wall with thumb forceps and slide the ovariectomy hook against the abdominal wall, 2 to 3 cm caudal to the kidney. **B,** Exteriorize the uterine horn with the hook and identify the suspensory ligament at the cranial edge of the ovarian pedicle. **C,** Stretch or tear the suspensory ligament to allow exteriorization of the ovary using the index finger to apply caudolateral traction on the suspensory ligament while maintaining caudomedial traction on the uterine horn. **D,** Place two Carmalt forceps across the ovarian pedicle proximal to the ovary and one across the proper ligament (or place three forceps proximal to the ovary). Remove the most proximal clamp and place a figure-8 ligature at this site. *Continued*

Trace the uterine horn to the uterine body. Grasp the other uterine horn and follow it to the opposite ovary. Place clamps and ligatures as described above. Make a window in the broad ligament adjacent to the uterine body and uterine artery and vein. Place a Carmalt across the broad ligament on each side and transect (Fig. 23-2, G). Apply a ligature around the broad ligament if the patient is in estrus, pregnant, or the broad ligament is heavily infiltrated with vessels or fat. Apply cranial traction on the uterus and ligate the uterine body cranial to the cervix. Place a figure-8 suture through the body using the point of the needle and encircling the uterine vessels on each side. Place a circumferential ligature nearer the cervix (Fig. 23-2, H). Place a Carmalt across the uterine body cranial to the ligatures. Grasp the uterine wall with forceps or mosquito hemostats cranial to the ligatures. Transect the uterine body and observe for hemorrhage. Religate if hemorrhage is observed. Some surgeons place one to three Carmalts across the uterine body prior to ligation. In cats, clamps may cut rather than crush a friable or engorged uterus and cause transection prior to ligature placement. *Replace the uterine stump into the abdomen before releasing the hemostats or forceps. Close the abdominal wall in three layers (fascia/linea alba, subcutaneous tissue, and skin).*

Orchiectomy

Castration reduces overpopulation by inhibiting male fertility and decreases male aggressiveness, roaming, and undesirable urination behavior. It helps prevent androgen-related diseases including prostatic diseases, perianal adenomas, and perineal hernias. Other indications for castration include congenital abnormalities, testicular or epididymal abnor-

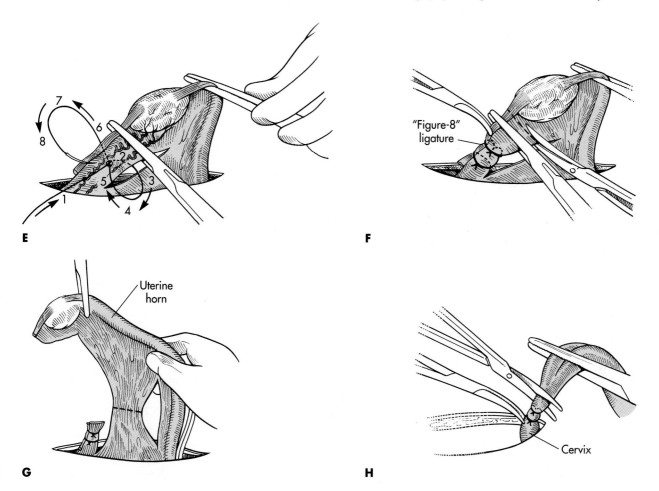

FIG. 23-2 (CONT'D)
E, Direct the blunt end of the needle through the middle of the pedicle (*1* to *2*), loop the suture around one side of the pedicle (*3* to *4*), then redirect the needle through the original hole from the same direction (*5* to *6*), and loop the ligature around the other half of the pedicle (*7* to *8*). Securely tie the ligature (*1* and *8*). **F,** Place a circumferential ligature proximal to the first ligature, then place a hemostat on the suspensory ligament near the ovary. Transect the ovarian pedicle distal to the clamp across the ovarian pedicle. **G,** Separate the broad ligament from the uterine horn. Clamp and ligate the broad ligament (*dashed line*) if it appears vascular. **H,** To ligate the uterus, place a figure-8 suture through the uterine body near the cervix. Place a second circumferential ligature closer to the cervix, place a Carmalt forceps distal to the ligatures, and transect between the Carmalt forceps and ligatures. Inspect the uterine stump for hemorrhage (use a mosquito hemostat attached to the uterine wall to prevent retraction of the uterus into the abdomen).

malities, scrotal neoplasia, trauma or abscesses, inguinal-scrotal herniorrhaphy, scrotal urethrostomy, epilepsy control, and control of endocrine abnormalities.

Canine castration. Either a prescrotal or perineal approach may be used for castration. A prescrotal approach is most common and more easily performed. The testicles are more difficult to exteriorize with a perineal approach, but it may be selected to avoid repositioning and aseptically preparing a second surgical site when the patient is in a perineal position for another surgical procedure (e.g., perineal hernia repair).

Open, prescrotal castration. *Position the patient in dorsal recumbency. Verify the presence of both testicles in the scrotum. Clip and aseptically prepare the caudal abdomen and medial thighs. Avoid irritating the scrotum with clippers or antiseptics. Drape the surgical area to exclude the scrotum from the field. Apply pressure on the scrotum to advance one testicle as far as possible into the prescrotal area. Incise skin and subcutaneous tissues along the median raphe over the displaced testicle (Fig. 23-3, A). Continue the incision through spermatic fascia to exteriorize the testicle. Incise the parietal vaginal tunic over the testicle (Fig. 23-3, B). Do not incise the tunica albuginea, which would expose the testicular parenchyma. Place a hemostat across the vaginal tunic where it attaches to the epididymis. Digitally separate the ligament of the tail of the epididymis from the tunic while applying traction with the hemostat on the tunic (Fig. 23-3, C). Further exteriorize the*

FIG. 23-3
A, To perform an open canine castration, advance one testicle into the prescrotal area by applying pressure over the scrotum. Make an incision over the testicle. **B,** Incise the spermatic fascia and parietal vagina tunic. **C,** Place a hemostat across the tunic where it attaches to the epididymis and digitally separate the ligament of the tail of the epididymis from the tunic. **D,** Ligate the ductus deferens and vascular cord individually and then encircle both with a proximal circumferential ligature. Apply a Carmalt forceps distal to the ligatures and transect between the clamp and ligatures.

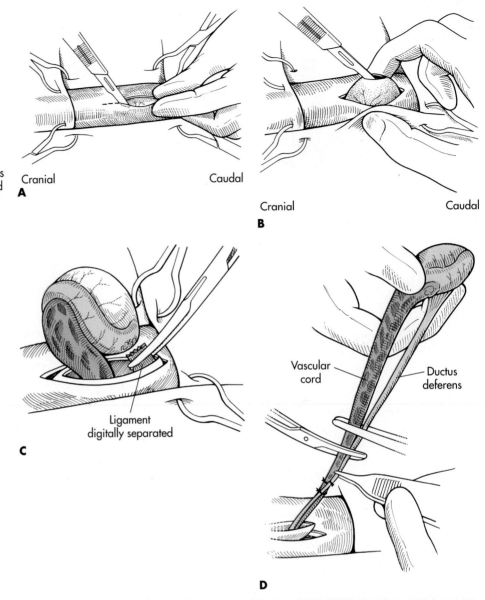

testicle by applying caudal and outward traction. Identify the structures of the spermatic cord. Individually ligate the vascular cord and ductus deferens, then place an encircling ligature around both. Many surgeons ligate the ductus deferens and pampiniform plexus together. Use 2-0 or 3-0 absorbable suture (e.g., chromic catgut, polyglactin 910, polydioxanone, or polyglyconate) for ligatures. Alternatively, use hemostatic staples. Place a hemostat across the cord near the testicle. Grasp the ductus deferens with thumb forceps above the ligature and transect both the ductus deferens and vascular cord between the hemostat and ligatures (Fig. 23-3, D). Inspect the cord for hemorrhage and replace the cord within the tunic. Encircle the cremaster muscle and tunic with a ligature. Advance the second testicle into the incision, incise the fascial covering, and remove the testicle as described. Appose the incised dense fascia on either side of the penis with interrupted or continuous sutures. Close subcutaneous tissues with a continuous pattern. Appose skin with an intradermal, subcuticular, or simple interrupted suture pattern.

☞ **N O T E** · The risk of ligature slippage and loosening may be greater with closed than with open techniques; however, removal of the tunics may reduce postoperative swelling.

Closed, prescrotal castration. "Closed" castration is performed similarly to the "open" technique described above except that the parietal vaginal tunics are not incised. Maximally exteriorize the spermatic cord by reflecting fat and fascia from the parietal tunic with a gauze sponge. Place traction on the testicle while the fibrous attachments between the spermatic cord tunic and scrotum are torn. Place mass ligatures (e.g., 2-0 or 3-0 absorbable) around the entire spermatic cord and tunics. Pass the needle through the cremaster muscle if a transfixation ligature is desired. Hemostatic staples may also be used.

Perineal castration. Perineal castration is performed using the same techniques as for an open, prescrotal castration. It is more difficult to displace the testicles into a caudal incision than into a prescrotal incision. An "open" technique must be used. *Make a midline skin and subcutaneous tissue incision dorsal to the scrotum in the perineum ventral to the anus. Advance one testicle to the incision and incise the spermatic fascia and tunic. Exteriorize the testicle and ligate the spermatic cord as described for an open, prescrotal castration.*

Scrotal Ablation

Scrotal ablation is necessary for neoplastic scrotal diseases and for castration performed in conjunction with scrotal urethrostomy in dogs and perineal urethrostomy in cats. Other indications include severe scrotal trauma, abscesses, or ischemia. Scrotal ablation may improve the postcastration appearance of dogs if they have a pendulous scrotum. Surgical time is somewhat longer when scrotal ablation is performed. *Elevate the scrotum and testicles from the body wall. Make an elliptical skin incision at the base of the scrotum, being careful not to excise too much skin. Control hemorrhage with electrocoagulation, ligation, or pressure. Incise the vaginal tunics and remove the testicles as described for open castration. Remove the scrotum after incising its median septum. Appose subcutaneous tissues with a simple continuous suture pattern (e.g., 3-0 absorbable suture). Appose skin edges with approximating interrupted sutures (e.g., 3-0 or 4-0 nonabsorbable suture).*

Feline Castration

Pluck hair from the scrotum rather than clipping (Fig. 23-4, A). In kittens less than 16 to 20 weeks of age, plucking scrotal hair may be difficult. Use clippers to gently remove scrotal hair. Position the cat in dorsal or lateral recumbency with the hind legs pulled cranially. Mobilize a testicle in the scrotum by applying pressure with the thumb and index finger at the base of the scrotum. Make a 1-cm incision over each testicle at the end of the scrotum from cranial to caudal (Fig. 23-4, B). Incise the parietal vaginal tunic over the testicle. Digitally separate the attachment of the ligament of the tail of the epididymis to the vaginal tunic (Fig. 23-4, C). Double ligate the spermatic cord with absorbable suture (e.g., 3-0 chromic catgut) or hemoclips or remove the ductus deferens from the testicle and tie it with the vessels (see below). Alternatively, use a figure-8 knot (see below). Transect the cord, inspect for bleeding, and replace it within the tunic. Excise the second testicle in a similar fashion. Resect any tags of tissue protruding from the scrotum. Allow the scrotal incision to heal by second intention.

To ligate the ductus deferens with the vessels, separate the ductus deferens from the testicle. Using the remainder of the spermatic cord (testicular vessels and testicle) as one strand and the ductus deferens as the other, tie two to three square knots (five to six throws) (Fig. 23-4, D). Sever the vessels with attached testicle and ductus deferens distal to the knot. Inspect for hemorrhage.

For an overhand or figure-8 knot, the spermatic cord is tied on itself with the aid of a curved mosquito hemostat. *Place the hemostat on top of the cord (Fig. 23-5, A). Wrap the distal (testicle) end of the cord over the hemostat once (Fig. 23-5, B). Direct the wrapped hemostat ventral to the cord while holding the testicle in the opposite hand (Fig. 23-5, C). Open the tips of the hemostat and grasp the distal end of the cord (Fig. 23-5, D). Transect the spermatic cord near the testicle and manipulate the severed end of the cord through the loops around the hemostat (Fig. 23-5, E). Snug the knot, resect excess cord, inspect for bleeding, and replace the cord within the tunic before releasing (Fig. 23-5, F).*

Cryptorchid Castration

Cryptorchidism is a congenital failure of the testicle(s) to descend into the scrotum. Testes normally are pulled into the scrotum soon after birth by fibrosis and contraction of the gubernaculum. There is little hope of further testicular descent after 2 months of age. One or both testicles may be in an abnormal position, although unilateral cryptorchidism is most common. Testicular agenesis (failure of testis development [one, monorchism; two, anorchism]) is rare. Cryptorchid testes are frequently small, soft, and proportionally misshapen. They may be in the inguinal area or abdominal cavity. Bilateral castration is recommended for cryptorchid animals because the condition is believed to be a sex-linked autosomal recessive trait in dogs. Retained canine testes are predisposed to neoplasia (seminomas and Sertoli cell tumors). If the testicle is in the inguinal region, it can often be palpated between the inguinal ring and scrotum once the animal is anesthetized; however, large inguinal fat pads may obscure testes in this area. *Advance unilateral, mobile inguinal testicles to the prescrotal incision and remove. Remove nonmobile testicles by making an incision over the inguinal ring. Dissect through subcutaneous fat and mobilize and remove the testicle.* Submit the testicles for histological examination to verify removal of testicular tissue and to rule out neoplasia.

Nonpalpable testes must be located via exploratory laparotomy. *Make a ventral midline incision from the umbilicus to the pubis or a paramedian incision adjacent to the prepuce. Find the testicle(s) by retroflexing the bladder, locating the ductus deferens dorsal to the neck of the bladder, and following the ductus deferens to the testicle. If the ductus deferens travels into the inguinal ring and the testicle cannot be manipulated into the abdomen, perform an inguinal incision. Avulse the ligament of the tail of the epididymis. Double ligate the testicular artery and vein and ductus deferens separately. Transect and remove the testicle. Inspect for hemorrhage and close the abdomen in three layers.*

FIG. 23-4

A, For feline castration, pluck hair from the scrotum and aseptically prepare the scrotum for surgery. **B,** Make cranial to caudal skin incisions over each testicle. **C,** Incise and separate the parietal tunic from the testicle, then transect the ductus deferens near the testicle. **D,** Tie two to three square knots with the ductus deferens and the spermatic vessels.

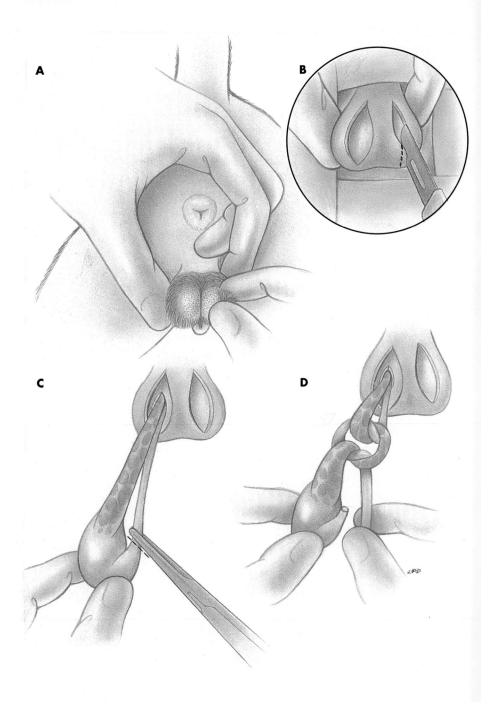

Vasectomy

Vasectomy inhibits male fertility while maintaining male behavioral patterns. Androgens continue to be produced because Leydig's cells are not significantly altered. The technique is rarely recommended because roaming, aggression, and urine marking persist while reduction of hormonally associated diseases does not occur. Spermatozoa persist in canine ejaculates for 3 weeks and feline ejaculates for 7 weeks after vasectomy (Pineda, Dooley, 1984). In dogs, the time to azoospermia is shortened by flushing the ductus deferens at the time of vasectomy (Frenette, Dooley, Pineda, 1986). Vasectomized males should be evaluated after the procedure to document azoospermic ejaculates before contact with intact bitches. This technique should be discouraged as a means of population control.

Make a 1- to 2-cm incision over the spermatic cord between the scrotum and inguinal ring (Fig. 23-6, A). Locate the spermatic cord, incise the vaginal tunic, and isolate the ductus deferens by blunt dissection (Fig. 23-6, B). Double ligate the ductus deferens and resect a 0.5-cm section of ductus between ligatures (Fig. 23-6, C). Repeat the procedure on the contralateral spermatic cord. Appose subcutaneous tissues and skin.

Cesarean Section

The goal of cesarean section (hysterotomy) is to remove all fetuses from the gravid uterus as quickly as possible. The primary indications for cesarean section are dystocia (i.e., oversized, malpositioned, or maldeveloped fetuses, small pelvic canal size, uterine inertia), or fetal putrefaction. Elective ce-

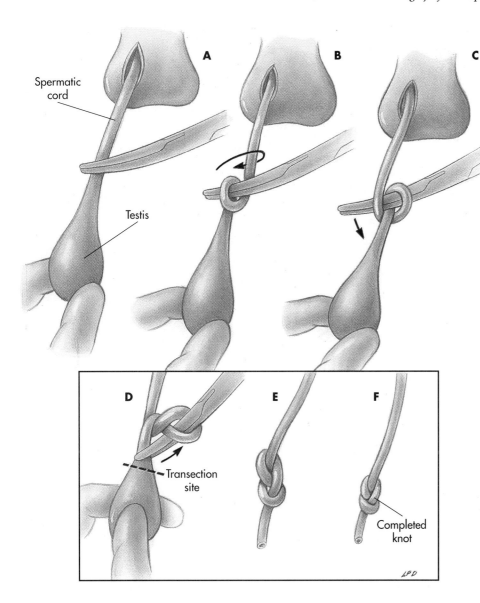

FIG. 23-5
An overhand technique may be used for feline castration. **A,** Place a curved hemostat on top of the cord and wrap the spermatic cord over it. Direct the hemostat's tip **B,** dorsally and then **C,** ventrally around the cord opposite the testicle. **D,** Next, grasp the cord near the testicle. **E,** Transect the testicle and pull the end of the cord through the wrap. **F,** Digitally snug the knot. Note: Tieing the knot closer to the scrotum than shown leaves less of a "tag."

sarians are often scheduled for brachycephalic breeds and other animals with a history of dystocia or those with pelvic fracture malunion. Cesarean section is more common in small dogs and brachycephalic breeds. Animals with dystocia often have fluid and electrolyte abnormalities that should be corrected prior to surgery. Although usually a postpartum problem, prepartum eclampsia causes hypocalcemia. Prophylactic antibiotics (e.g., cefazolin, 20 mg/kg IV) should be given if fetal death or uterine infection is suspected. Anesthetize these animals carefully (see p. 521); fetal depression and decreased viability are directly proportional to the degree of maternal depression.

Ovariohysterectomy can be safely performed in conjunction with a cesarean section if the patient receives adequate fluid therapy. The cesarean section may be performed as described and followed by OHE, or an en bloc resection can be performed (Robbins and Mullens, 1994). En bloc ovariohysterectomy is performed before hysterotomy (uterine incision) and removal of the neonates. Neonatal survival with en bloc resection is similar to that for other techniques for managing dystocia. Changes in blood pressure and hematocrit

are minimal following en bloc ovariohysterectomy, and mothering and lactation are normal following OHE. En bloc removal of the gravid uterus may be elective or necessary due to fetal death or questionable uterine integrity or health. Advantages of en bloc ovariohysterectomy of the gravid uterus include minimal anesthetic time, minimal potential for abdominal contamination, and population control with avoidance of a second surgery. The disadvantage of this technique is that a second team is required to resuscitate the neonates.

Cesarean without ovariohysterectomy. *Clip and perform a preliminary abdominal prep before anesthetic induction to minimize time from induction to delivery. Preoxygenate the bitch/queen if possible before induction. Anesthetize the patient using a general or regional protocol that is appropriate for the bitch/queen and minimizes neonatal depression (see discussion on anesthesia on p. 519). Position the patient in dorsal recumbency. Apply a final aseptic scrub to the ventral abdomen. Make a ventral midline incision from just cranial to the umbilicus to near the pubis. Elevate the external rectus sheath prior to making a stab incision through the linea alba to avoid inadvertent*

FIG. 23-6
A, For vasectomy, incise skin over the spermatic cord between the inguinal ring and scrotum. **B,** Incise the vaginal tunic and isolate the ductus deferens. **C,** Ligate the ductus deferens and remove a small segment.

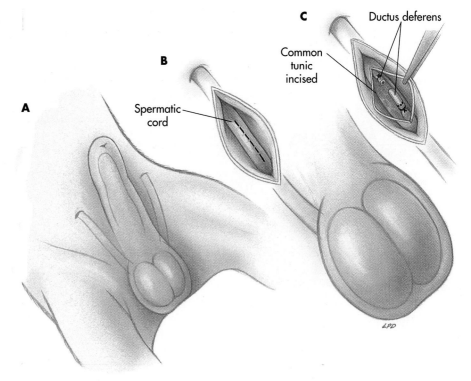

laceration of the uterus. *Exteriorize the gravid uterine horns by carefully lifting rather than pulling them out of the abdomen (Fig. 23-7) because uterine vessels are easily avulsed and the uterine wall readily tears. Isolate the uterus from the remainder of the abdomen with sterile towels or laparotomy pads. Tent and then incise the uterine body to avoid lacerating the neonate. Extend the incision with Metzenbaum scissors. The incision should be long enough to prevent tearing during extraction of the fetus. Empty each horn by gently squeezing (milking) cranial to each fetus to move it toward the incision, then grasping and gently pulling it from the uterus (Fig. 23-8). Rupture the amniotic sac and clamp the umbilical cord as each neonate is presented. Avoid contaminating the abdomen and surgical field with amniotic fluids. Aseptically pass each neonate to an assistant (see below for neonatal care). At term the placenta is often expelled with the neonate; however, if the placenta has not separated, gently pull it from the endometrium. Do not forcibly separate the placenta from the uterine wall or severe hemorrhage may occur. Palpate the pelvic canal and remove any fetus from this location.*

Uterine contraction usually begins when the fetuses are removed. *Administer oxytocin or ergonovine maleate (Table 23-9) if contraction has not occurred. Give oxytocin and compress the uterine walls if endometrial hemorrhage is severe. Lavage the external uterus to remove debris. Close the uterine incision with 3-0 or 4-0 absorbable sutures using an appositional pattern in a single-layer simple continuous pattern, a double-layer appositional closure (mucosa and submucosa followed by muscularis and serosa), or an appositional closure followed by a second layer inverting pattern (Cushing or Lembert). Lavage the surgical site and replace contaminated towels, sponges, instruments, and gloves. Inspect for uterine vessel avulsion*

and control hemorrhage. Lavage the abdomen if contamination or spillage of uterine contents has occurred. Cover the uterine incision with omentum. Appose the abdominal wall in three layers (rectus fascia, subcutaneous tissue, and skin). Use subcuticular or intradermal skin closure to eliminate suture ends that may irritate neonates. Lavage all antiseptics, blood, and debris from the ventral abdomen and mammae.

En bloc resection. *Perform en bloc ovariohysterectomy of the gravid uterus by first exteriorizing and isolating the ovarian pedicles and separating the broad ligament from the uterus to the point of the cervix. Manipulate fetuses in the vagina or cervix into the uterine body. Then, double or triple clamp the ovarian pedicles and uterus just cranial to the cervix. Quickly transect between clamps and remove the ovaries and uterus. Give the uterus to a team of assistants to open and resuscitate the neonates.* The time from clamping the uterus to removal of the neonates should be 30 to 60 seconds. *Double ligate ovarian and uterine pedicles. Inspect for hemorrhage and close the abdomen.*

Neonatal care. *Firmly cradle the neonate and gently swing downward to help clear fluid from the upper airways. Gently suction the nares and nasopharynx. Briskly rub and dry each neonate to stimulate the respiratory drive. If necessary, antagonize opioids (place a drop of naloxone under the tongue) and give doxapram (place a drop under the tongue) to stimulate respiration. Ligate, transect, and disinfect the umbilical cord. Inspect each neonate for congenital or developmental anomalies (i.e., cleft palate, limb deformity, hernia, imperforate anus). Place neonates in a warm environment (32° C, 90° F) until their mother is able to care for them. Allow nursing as soon as possible to ensure colostrum intake. Closely observe the mother and her behavior toward the neonates during the first few hours;*

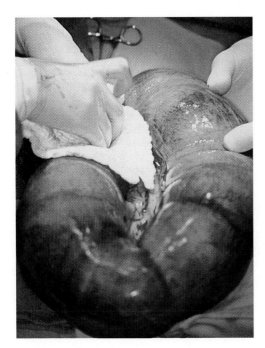

FIG. 23-7
Gravid horns should be carefully exteriorized from the abdomen to avoid tearing the uterine wall or vessels.

some mothers will reject or kill their neonates. Discharge the bitch/queen and neonates from the hospital as soon as possible to reduce stress and exposure to potential pathogens.

Mastectomy

Mastectomy or removal of the mammary gland(s) is usually performed to remove tumors. One gland (simple mastectomy), several glands (regional mastectomy), or an entire chain (complete unilateral mastectomy) may be excised and the defect closed. Simultaneous removal of both mammary chains (complete bilateral mastectomy) causes significant suture line tension and is not recommended. Staged procedures are advised to facilitate defect closure and reduce patient discomfort when bilateral mastectomy is needed. Ovariohysterectomy during the same anesthesia is performed before mastectomy to prevent seeding the abdomen with tumor cells. If the tumor crosses the midline, however, it may be excised first—clean instruments and gloves should be used for the OHE. The technique for mastectomy is described on p. 542.

Episiotomy

An episiotomy is an incision of the vulvar orifice to allow access to the vestibule and vagina. It is indicated to surgically explore the vagina, excise vaginal masses, repair lacerations, modify congenital defects or strictures, expose the urethral papilla, and facilitate manual fetal extraction. *With the animal in a perineal position, place a noncrushing clamp (i.e., Doyen) with one shaft in the vagina on each side of the perineal midline (Fig. 23-9, A). Make a midline skin incision through the dorsal commissure of the vulvar lips to just distal to the external anal sphincter muscle with a scalpel*

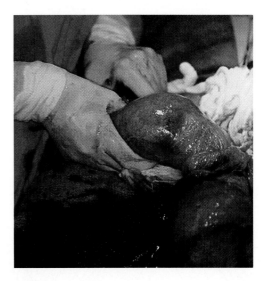

FIG. 23-8
Gently "milk" puppies toward the uterine incision by squeezing cranial to them.

TABLE 23-9
Drugs That Initiate Uterine Contraction
Oxytocin
Dogs
1-5 units IM or IV
Cats
0.5 units IM or IV (can be repeated but do not exceed 3 units total dose)
Ergonovine Maleate
0.02-0.1 mg/kg IM

blade. Continue the incision through the muscle and vaginal wall with Mayo scissors (see Fig. 23-9, A). Control hemorrhage with hemostats, electrocoagulation, and ligatures. Place two or three horizontal mattress stay sutures full-thickness through the skin and vaginal mucosa on each side of the incision to facilitate retraction and hemostasis. Then, remove the Doyen clamps and position a self-retaining retractor (e.g., Gelpi) to improve exposure, if necessary. Evaluate the vagina and vestibule and perform any needed procedures. Close the episiotomy incision in three layers. Preplace an interrupted suture to realign and reappose the dorsal vulvar commissure. First, reappose the vaginal mucosa with simple interrupted or continuous sutures (e.g., 3-0 or 4-0 polydioxanone or polyglyconate), tieing the knots in the lumen (Fig. 23-9, B). Then, reappose muscles and subcutaneous tissues in a continuous pattern (Fig. 23-9, C). Lastly, reappose skin with interrupted appositional sutures (e.g., 3-0 or 4-0 nylon or polypropylene). Place an Elizabethan collar, bucket, or sidebars after surgery to prevent self-trauma. To reduce inflammation and edema, apply cold compresses immediately after surgery and warm compresses the following day.

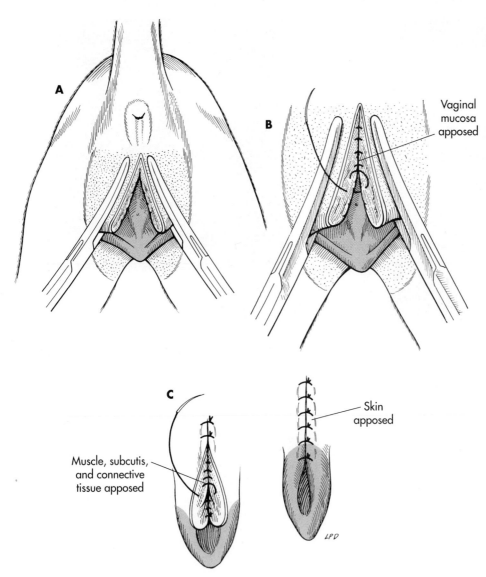

FIG. 23-9
A, For episiotomy, place non-crushing forceps on each side of the proposed incision site. **B,** Make a full-thickness incision from the dorsal vulvar commissure to near the external anal sphincter muscle. Explore the vagina and vestibule. Appose vaginal mucosa with a simple continuous suture pattern. **C,** Appose muscle, subcutis, and connective tissue with a second layer of sutures and skin with a third layer of appositional sutures.

Vaginal mucosa apposed

Skin apposed

Muscle, subcutis, and connective tissue apposed

Episioplasty

Episioplasty is a reconstructive procedure most commonly performed to excise excess skin folds around the vulva that cause perivulvar dermatitis. Skin fold pyoderma should be treated medically prior to surgical reconstruction. *With the patient in a perineal position, assess the amount of skin to be excised by elevating the skin fold and evaluating expected tension (Fig. 23-10, A). Beginning near the ventral vulvar commissure, make a crescent-shaped incision encircling the vulva at the proposed lateral and dorsal borders of the resection. Make a second crescent-shaped incision medial and parallel to the first to outline the ellipse of skin to be removed (Fig. 23-10, B). Excise the outlined segment of skin and excess subcutaneous tissue (Fig. 23-10, C). Place interrupted sutures at the 3 o'clock, 9 o'clock, and 12 o'clock positions to assess the effectiveness of the resection (Fig. 23-10, D). Resect more skin along the outer margin if the vulva is still recessed or skin folds persist. Bring the skin edges into approximation by first apposing the subcutaneous tissues using interrupted sutures with buried knots (e.g., 3-0 or 4-0 polydioxanone or polygly-conate). Place the first sutures at the 12, 3, and 9 o'clock positions to symmetrically align the edges. Appose skin edges with simple interrupted sutures (e.g., 3-0 or 4-0 nylon or polypropylene; Fig. 23-10, E). Place an Elizabethan collar or bucket over the head to prevent licking and chewing at the surgical site. Continue antibiotics if necessary to control the pyoderma.*

Testicular Biopsy

Testicular biopsy may be performed in valuable breeding animals to help determine the etiology of infertility or reduced fertility. Biopsies are obtained using a biopsy needle directed through the scrotal skin or by wedge resection. A wedge of tissue is collected by making a prescrotal incision and then incising the spermatic fascia and tunics. Large blood vessels should be avoided to minimize hemorrhage. *Make a 1-cm incision through the tunica albuginea of one testicle with a sterile, thin razor blade or No. 11 scalpel blade. Excise a wedge of testicular parenchyma with the razor blade. Appose the tunica albuginea with 4-0 to 6-0 absorbable suture (i.e., polydioxanone or polyglyconate). Appose skin*

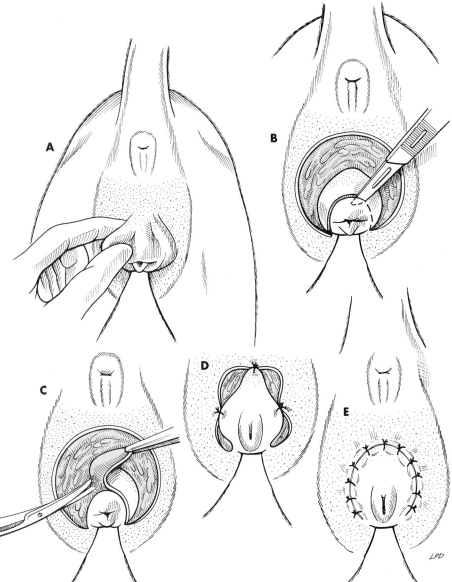

FIG. 23-10
A, Episioplasty is performed after assessing the amount of skin to be excised. **B,** Make two parallel crescent-shaped incisions encircling the vulva and, **C,** excise the outlined segment of skin and underlying subcutaneous tissues. **D,** Appose skin edges by placing the initial sutures at the 3 o'clock, 9 o'clock, and 12 o'clock positions. **E,** Appose remaining skin with simple interrupted sutures.

edges with intradermal (subcuticular) or simple interrupted sutures. Better preservation of architectural detail is obtained by placing the sample in Bouin's, Zenker's, or Stieve's fixative, rather than formalin.

Prostatic Biopsy

Prostatic biopsy is needed to definitively diagnose some prostatic diseases. Percutaneous techniques are preferred because they are less invasive, less expensive, and have reduced morbidity. However, operative techniques allow collection of larger samples from more specific sites. The prostatic urethra must not be damaged, and specimens should be submitted for both histologic and microbiologic evaluation. Percutaneous biopsies are performed using Tru-Cut, Biopty needle (see Product Appendix), or Franklin-Silverman biopsy needles. They may be guided by palpation (blind) or with the aid of ultrasonography. The latter is preferred because it facilitates guiding the needle to abnormal areas. Biopsy should not be performed if abscesses or cysts are suspected.

Ultrasound guided biopsy. *Position the patient in dorsal or lateral recumbency and ultrasonographically evaluate the prostate. Aseptically prepare the abdominal wall in the area the biopsy needle will be inserted. Nick the skin (3- to 5-mm incision) with a scalpel blade at the needle insertion site. Identify the desired biopsy site with ultrasound and visualize needle placement into the prostate. Collect two to three biopsies with a Biopty needle/instrument. Observe the prostate for hemorrhage or fluid leakage with ultrasound.*

Palpation guided biopsy. *Position the patient in a perineal position with the tail fixed over the back. Aseptically prepare the perineum around the anus. Mobilize and reposition the prostate in a more caudal position by having an assistant apply gentle pressure on the caudal abdomen. Make a nick incision (3 to 5 mm) slightly lateral to the midline, midway between the anus and ischial tuberosity. Confirm the location of the prostate by rectal examination. Insert the needle through the soft tissues ventral to the rectum. Guide the needle to the prostate digitally via rectal* *palpation. Penetrate the capsule at the caudal margin of the prostate with the needle in the closed position, then fully insert the inner cannula into the prostatic parenchyma. Quickly advance the outer cannula over the stationary inner cannula, or fire the trigger when using an automatic instrument, to cut the specimen. Remove the needle from the prostate in the closed position. Evaluate the specimen size and collect additional samples, if necessary.*

Open biopsy. *Collect prostatic biopsies during exploratory laparotomy with a biopsy needle or wedge excision. Via a caudal midline abdominal incision, retract the urinary bladder cranially using stay sutures. Isolate the prostate from the remainder of the abdomen with sterile laparotomy pads. Palpate the prostate and select a biopsy site. Dissect periprostatic fat from the desired site. Excise a wedge of prostatic tissue using a No. 11 scalpel blade. Appose edges of the defect by placing cruciate or simple continuous absorbable sutures (e.g., 3-0 or 4-0 polydioxanone or polyglyconate) in the prostatic capsule. Lavage the surgical site(s) and replace periprostatic fat. Close the abdomen in three layers.*

Prostatectomy

Total prostatectomy. Total prostatectomy is indicated for patients with tumors that have not metastasized; it is rarely performed for severe trauma or chronic prostatic disease that has been nonresponsive to other treatments. The procedure is infrequently performed because urinary incontinence commonly results. *Expose the prostate through a caudal ventral midline celiotomy and pubic osteotomy (see p. 488). Place a urethral catheter. Retract the urinary bladder cranially with stay sutures. Dissect the lateral pedicles and periprostatic fat directly from the capsule without damaging the dorsal plexus of vessels and nerves (Fig. 23-11, A). Control hemostasis by ligation and electrocoagulation. Ligate and divide the prostatic vessels and ductus deferens as close to the prostate as possible. Dissect the prostate from the urinary bladder and extrapelvic urethra. Transect the urethra on both ends as close to the prostate as possible (Fig. 23-11, B). Avoid the trigone and neck of the bladder. Remove the prostate. Advance the urethral catheter into the urinary bladder. Approximate the urethral ends with simple interrupted sutures using 4-0 to 6-0 synthetic absorbable suture (i.e., polydioxanone, polyglyconate) on a taper point swaged-on needle. Place the first two sutures at the 12 o'clock and 6 o'clock positions, leaving the ends long to aid rotation of the urethra during suturing (Fig. 23-11, C). Place the dorsal suture first. Space sutures approximately 2 mm apart and 1.5 to 2.0 mm from the edge. Place a cystostomy tube (see p. 484) or transurethral Foley catheter to divert urine for 5 to 7 days. Biopsy an iliac or sublumbar lymph node to evaluate for metastasis. Replace contaminated instruments and gloves. Lavage the surgical site and abdomen. Place omentum around the anastomosis. Wire the pubic segment into place. Perform a three-layer abdominal wall closure.* Place an Elizabethan collar, bucket, or sidebars after surgery to prevent displacement of the catheter and surgical site trauma.

Subtotal prostatectomy. Subtotal prostatectomy is indicated in stable patients for recurrent abscessation or cysts that have not responded to drainage procedures. A urinary catheter should be placed to aid urethral identification. The prostate is approached and exposed as for total prostatectomy (see above). Submit excised tissue for histologic evaluation.

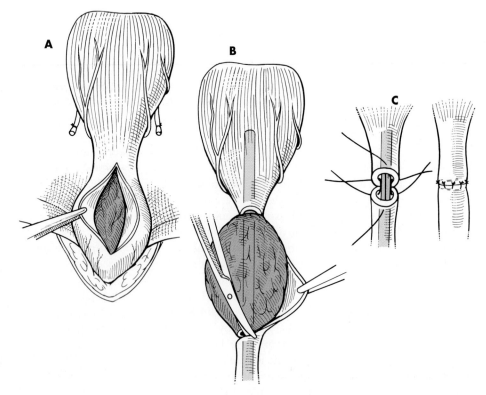

FIG. 23-11
A, To perform total prostatectomy, separate the fascia, vessels, and nerves from the prostate by dissecting directly against the capsule. **B,** Then dissect the cranial and caudal edges of the prostate from the urethra and transect the urethra as close to the prostate as possible. **C,** Stent the urethra with a catheter and appose the ends with approximating sutures.

Subtotal prostatectomy with capsulectomy. *Isolate and ligate or cauterize all vessels as they enter the prostatic capsule. Excise the prostate within 5 mm of the urethra using scissors, an electrosurgical unit, or laser (Fig. 23-12, A). Place a cystostomy tube if the urethral catheter is to be removed (see p. 484). Assess hemostasis and lavage the surgical site. Surround the prostatic urethra with omentum or prostatic fat. Close the abdomen routinely.*

Intracapsular subtotal prostatectomy. *Incise the ventral median septum with an electroscalpel. Continue the incision through the parenchyma into the ventral urethra. Using the electroscalpel, resect all parenchyma except a 2- to 3-mm shell attached to the capsule (Fig. 23-12, B). Resect all the urethra except a 3- to 5-mm dorsal strip. Lavage the prostatic shell and close the capsule over a urethral catheter positioned in the urinary bladder. Use an approximating pattern for the first layer and an inverting pattern for the second layer of closure (e.g., 3-0 or 4-0 polydioxanone or polyglyconate). Maintain the catheter for 10 days. Alternatively, use an ultrasonic surgical aspirator to remove parenchyma and preserve the urethra.*

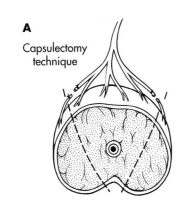

A
Capsulectomy technique

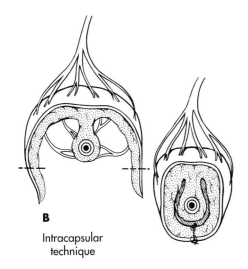

B
Intracapsular technique

FIG. 23-12
Subtotal prostatectomy may be performed using, **A,** capsulectomy or, **B,** intracapsular techniques.

HEALING OF THE REPRODUCTIVE AND GENITAL SYSTEMS

Reproductive organs heal like other visceral tissues. Incisions into testicular parenchyma may cause an immunologic response and subsequent sperm granuloma. Scarring of the uterus may inhibit placentation. To decrease uterine adhesions, omentum can be placed over incisions. Failure of postpartum uterine involution may be caused by excessive collagen breakdown due to uterine collagenase activity. Optimal healing requires a good blood supply, accurate mucosal apposition, and minimal surgical trauma. Systemic factors (i.e., hypovolemia, shock, hypoproteinemia, debilitation, infection) may delay healing and increase the risk of dehiscence.

SUTURE MATERIALS/SPECIAL INSTRUMENTS

Instruments needed for reproductive surgery include an ovariohysterectomy hook (i.e. Covault, Snook), retractors (i.e., Balfour [abdominal procedures], Gelpi or Weitlander [perineal procedures], Finochietto [pelvic procedures], vaginal speculum or otoscope [vaginal procedures]), scissors (i.e., Metzenbaum, Mayo), forceps (i.e., Doyen, Carmalt, curved mosquito), biopsy instruments (Bard Biopty-cut Biopsy Needle with a Bard Biopsy Instrument; see Product Appendix), and drains. Orthopedic instruments are needed if a pelvic osteotomy is performed. An electrosurgical unit and laser unit are sometimes beneficial.

Monofilament absorbable and nonabsorbable sutures are recommended for most reproductive tract procedures (i.e., 2-0 to 6-0 polydioxanone, polyglyconate, polypropylene, or nylon) (Table 23-10). Chromic catgut (2-0 to 0) or polyglactin-910 (Vicryl) is preferred by some for ligatures. Stapling equipment (transverse, ligate and divide, and skin staplers) are sometimes used.

POSTOPERATIVE CARE AND ASSESSMENT

Animals undergoing reproductive tract surgery should be monitored postoperatively for hemorrhage and infection. The incision site should be assessed twice daily for redness, swelling, or discharge. Activity should be limited to leash walks until sutures are removed (generally 10 to 14 days). Water is usually offered 8 to 12 hours after surgery, unless vomiting occurs. If the animal does not vomit, food can be given 12 to 24 hours postoperatively. Analgesics should be given as necessary to alleviate discomfort (see Table 23-25, p. 548). Nonelective procedures are often performed on sick animals having fluid, electrolyte, and acid-base abnormalities which need monitoring and continued treatment in the

---

TABLE 23-10

Suture Recommendations for Reproductive Suture

- Select a monofilament, synthetic, absorbable suture for visceral closure (i.e., polydioxanone, polyglyconate)
- Select an absorbable suture for ligatures (i.e., chromic catgut, polydioxanone, polyglyconate, polyglactin 910)

postoperative period. Therapeutic antibiotics should be continued in patients with preoperative infections. Surgical sites should be protected by using an Elizabethan collar, bucket, sidebars, or bandage to prevent self-trauma. Stool softeners may be administered after prostatic or perineal surgery to minimize discomfort during defecation (Table 23-11). After perineal surgery, warm compresses should be applied to the surgical site two to three times daily.

COMPLICATIONS

Most complications associated with reproductive surgery can be avoided by using good surgical technique (i.e., gentle tissue handling, good hemostasis, and aseptic technique) (Table 23-12). OHE is difficult in larger dogs and is associated with more complications. Hemorrhage primarily occurs from the ovarian pedicles, uterine vessels, or uterine wall when ligatures are improperly placed; it rarely occurs from vessels that accompany the suspensory ligament or those within the broad ligament. Excessive hemorrhage may occur when OHE is performed during estrus. Ureter ligation or trauma may result from ligation of a dropped or hemorrhaging ovarian pedicle if exposure of the caudal renal pole is inadequate. The ureter may also be ligated when the urinary bladder is distended and the trigone and ureterovesical junction are displaced cranially. Hydronephrosis, necessitating ureteronephrectomy, results unless the offending ligature is promptly removed. Signs of estrus may recur if some ovarian tissue remains in the abdominal cavity. If this occurs, abdominal exploration during estrus may help identify the ovarian tissue. Fistulous tracts and granulomas may form when nonabsorbable multifilament suture material is used for ligations. These fistulae are usually located in the flank, but may also occur along the medial thigh or inguinal region. They intermittently discharge blood-tinged fluid or pus. A reduction in discharge may occur after antibiotic therapy;

however, the discharge recurs when antibiotic therapy is discontinued. These fistulae will not resolve until the suture material is removed. Caution must be exercised during dissection as there may be adhesions to the vena cava and other vital structures.

Urinary incontinence is uncommon after OHE but may occur soon after surgery or in geriatric bitches. Causes of urinary incontinence include low estrogen levels, uterine stump adhesions, or granulomas to the urinary bladder and vaginoureteral fistula (see p. 508). Although some owners believe that OHE causes obesity, properly fed and exercised neutered animals should not gain excessive weight. Juvenile behavior and external genitalia may persist in animals that are neutered at a very young age (6 to 12 weeks). Other possible complications of OHE include self-trauma, incisional swelling, seroma, infection, delayed healing, dehiscence, trauma to intestines or spleen, cervical pyometra, endocrine alopecia, behavioral change, and eunuchoid syndrome.

Serious complications following properly performed castrations are rare but may include incisional problems (i.e., swelling, seroma formation, cellulitis, infection, self-trauma, dehiscence), hemorrhage, scrotal hematoma, scrotal bruising, abscess, granuloma, urinary incontinence, endocrine alopecia, behavior change, and eunuchoid syndrome. Trauma to the penis and urethra may occur during dissection, especially with scrotal ablation. Although unlikely, an unwanted pregnancy may occur if a recently castrated male copulates with a female in estrus because spermatozoa persist in the ductus deferens for as long as 21 days in dogs and 49 days in cats (Pineda, Dooley, 1984).

Complications of cesarean section, with or without OHE, include hemorrhage, hypovolemia, hypothermia, hypocalcemia, anorexia, anemia, agalactia, metritis, and vomiting. Severe hemorrhage may necessitate OHE. Calcium levels should be monitored if eclampsia is suspected. Eclampsia may occur anytime during the first postpartum month. An odorless, dark red-brown to serous uterine discharge or lochia is expected for 4 to 6 weeks postpartum. Incisional complications, such as swelling, infection, seroma, self-trauma, and dehiscence, may occur. Uterine scarring may prevent future placentation and adhesions may interfere with uterine motility. Complications are rare after mastectomy (see p. 542), episiotomy, episioplasty, testicular biopsy, and prostatic biopsy, but may occur (Table 23-13). Dehiscence after episioplasty may occur if skin resection results in excessive suture line tension. Perivulvar dermatitis will persist or recur if an inadequate amount of skin is excised.

Early postoperative complications of prostatectomy may include hemorrhage, urine leakage, infection, and urethral

TABLE 23-11
Stool Softeners

Dioctyl Sodium Sulfosuccinate or Docusate Sodium (Colace)
Dogs
50 to 200 mg PO, BID to TID

Cats
50 mg PO, SID to BID

Lactulose (Chronulac)
Dogs
1 ml/4.5 kg PO, TID to effect

Cats
5 ml/cat PO, TID

Psyllium (Metamucil)
Dogs
2-10 g PO, SID to BID or 1 tsp per 10 kg; twice daily in food

Cats
1-4 g PO, SID to BID or 1 tsp per 10 kg; twice daily in food

TABLE 23-12
Common Errors in Reproductive Surgery

- Failure to support septic or debilitated patients with fluids, antibiotics, and/or nutrition
- Failure to completely resect tumors
- Failure to obtain a histologic diagnosis
- Failure to prevent self-mutilation of the surgical site

catheter displacement; later complications may include dehiscence, urethral stricture, and urinary incontinence. Urinary incontinence is expected (more than 85%) in dogs after prostatectomy, unless the prostate is of normal size and dissection does not traumatize trigonal innervation or vascularity (Basinger et al, 1989). Incontinence due to diminished urethral sphincter tone may be treated with α-adrenergic agonists (i.e., phenylpropanolamine or ephedrine), which increase urethral sphincter tone or diethylstilbestrol (DES) (Table 23-14). Phenylpropanolamine is used more frequently than ephedrine because it has fewer side effects (i.e., hyperexcitability, panting, and/or anorexia) and greater efficacy over time (see also p. 509).

SPECIAL AGE CONSIDERATIONS

The greatest benefit from elective neutering is obtained when the animal is less than a year of age. Undesirable behaviors are usually not learned by this age and some tumors can be prevented. Pediatric tissues are more fragile than adult tissues and must be handled gently. Tumors, pyometra, and prostatic infections are more common in geriatric patients.

References

Basinger RR et al: Urodynamic alterations associated with clinical prostatic diseases and prostatic surgery in 23 dogs, *J Am Anim Hosp Assoc* 25:385, 1989.

Frenette MD, Dooley MS, Pineda MH: Effect of flushing the vas deferentia at the time of vasectomy on the rate of clearance of spermatozoa from ejaculates of dogs and cats, *Am J Vet Res* 47:463, 1986.

Pineda MH, Dooley MP: Surgical and chemical vasectomy in the cat, *Am J Vet Res* 45:291, 1984.

Robbins MA, Mullens HS: En bloc ovariohysterectomy as a treatment for dystocia in dogs and cats, *Vet Surg* 23:48, 1994.

Salmeri KR et al: Gonadectomy in immature dogs: effects on skeletal, physical and behavioral development, *J Am Vet Med Assoc* 198:1193, 1991.

Suggested Reading

Aronsohn MG, Faggella AM: Surgical techniques for neutering 6- to 14-week-old kittens, *J Am Vet Med Assoc* 202:53, 1993.

Berzon JL: Complications of elective ovariohysterectomy in the dog and cat at a teaching institution: clinical review of 853 cases, *Vet Surg* 8:89, 1979.

Freshman JL et al: Clinical evaluation of infertility in dogs, *Compend Contin Educ Pract Vet* 10:443, 1988.

Gaudet DA: Retrospective study of 128 cases of canine dystocia, *J Am Anim Hosp Assoc* 21:813, 1985.

Hardie EM: Selected surgeries of the male and female reproductive tracts, *Vet Clin North Am Small Anim Pract* 14:109, 1984.

Hardie EM et al: Subtotal canine prostatectomy with the neodymium:yttrium-aluminum-garnet laser, *Vet Surg* 19:348, 1990.

Johnston SD: Questions and answers on the effects of surgically neutering dogs and cats, *J Am Vet Med Assoc* 198:1206, 1991.

O'Farrell V, Peachey E: Behavioral effects of ovariohysterectomy on bitches, *J Small Anim Pract* 31:595, 1990.

Olson PN, Mulinix JA, Nett TM: Concentrations of luteinizing hormone and follicle-stimulating hormone in the serum of sexually intact and neutered dogs, *Am J Vet Res* 53:762, 1992.

Pugh CR, Konde LJ, Park RD: Testicular ultrasound in the normal dog, *Vet Radiol* 31:195, 1990.

Pugh CR, Konde LJ: Sonographic evaluation of canine testicular and scrotal abnormalities: a review of 26 case histories, *Vet Radiol* 32:243, 1991.

Rawlings CA et al: Subcapsular subtotal prostatectomy in normal dogs: use of an ultrasonic surgical aspirator, *Vet Surg* 23:182, 1994.

Richardson EA, Mulled H: Cryptorchidism in cats, *Compend Cont Educ Pract Vet* 15:1342, 1993.

Robertson JJ, Bojrab MJ: Subtotal intracapsular prostatectomy: results in normal dogs, *Vet Surg* 13:6, 1984.

Salmeri KR, Olson PN, Bloomberg MS: Elective gonadectomy in dogs: a review, *J Am Vet Med Assoc* 198:1183, 1991.

Yeager AE et al: Ultrasonographic appearance of the uterus, placenta, fetus, and fetal membranes throughout accurately timed pregnancy in beagles, *Am J Vet Res* 53:342, 1992.

TABLE 23-13

Potential Complications after Reproductive Surgery

Episiotomy
- Pain, swelling, inflammation, hemorrhage, infection, dehiscence, self-trauma

Episioplasty
- Inflammation, swelling, infection, dehiscence, recurrent perivulvar dermatitis

Testicular Biopsy
- Hemorrhage, infection, local hyperthermia, scarring, adhesions, immune-mediated orchitis, testicular atrophy, reduced sperm count (temporary)

Prostatic Biopsy
- Hemorrhage, hematuria, urine leakage, infection

TABLE 23-14

Treatment of Urinary Incontinence

Phenylpropanolamine (Propagest, Dexatrim)
Dogs
1.5-2.0 mg/kg PO, BID to TID

Cats
1.5 mg/kg PO, TID

Ephedrine
Dogs
4 mg/kg or 12.5-50 mg/dog PO, BID to TID

Cats
2-4 mg/kg PO, BID to TID

Diethylstilbestrol (DES)
Dogs
0.1 to 1.0 mg daily PO for 3-5 days, then same dose once weekly

Surgery of the Female Reproductive Tract

SPECIFIC DISEASES

UTERINE NEOPLASIA

DEFINITIONS

Leiomyoma and **leiomyosarcoma** are benign and malignant smooth muscle tumors, respectively, that may occur in the uterus. Uterine **adenocarcinomas** are malignant tumors of the uterine glands.

GENERAL CONSIDERATIONS AND CLINICALLY RELEVANT PATHOPHYSIOLOGY

Uterine neoplasia is rare in dogs and cats; most tumors are incidental findings at necropsy. Tumors that may occur in the uterus are listed in Table 23-15. They may develop in the remnant of the uterine body following ovariohysterectomy (OHE). Concurrent pathology may include cystic ovaries, cystic endometrial hyperplasia, and pyometra, suggesting a common hormonal influence.

Most uterine tumors are leiomyomas that arise from the myometrium. Leiomyomas are benign and generally noninvasive and slow growing. They may protrude into the uterine lumen on a stalk or cause the wall to bulge externally. German shepherd dogs have a syndrome characterized by multiple uterine leiomyomas, bilateral renal cystadenocarcinomas, and nodular dermatofibrosis. The most common malignant tumors of bitches and queens are leiomyosarcoma and endometrial adenocarcinoma, respectively. Leiomyosarcomas are grossly difficult to distinguish from leiomyomas. They are invasive tumors that are usually slow to metastasize. Adenocarcinomas cause the endometrium to become thickened and nodular. The tumor may be solid or cystic, sessile, or polypoid, and may obliterate the uterine lumen. Multicentric adenocarcinoma has been reported. Metastasis is usually present at the time of diagnosis and may occur to the cerebrum, eyes, ovaries, adrenal glands, thyroid glands, lungs, liver, kidneys, bladder, intestines, pancreas, pericardium, myocardium, diaphragm, and/or regional lymph nodes.

DIAGNOSIS
Clinical Presentation

Signalment. No breed predilections have been reported. Most affected animals are middle-aged or older.

History. Most uterine tumors are asymptomatic unless they are large and compress the gastrointestinal or urinary tracts. Animals may have a history of abnormal estrus cycles and/or a mucoid or hemorrhagic vaginal discharge as a result of tumor irritation and vascular erosion. Uterine tumors may obstruct the cervix and cause pyometra, thus presenting clini-

TABLE 23-15	
Uterine Tumors	
• Leiomyoma	• Fibroma
• Leiomyosarcoma	• Adenoma
• Adenocarcinoma	• Fibrosarcoma
• Lipoma	

cal signs may include a purulent vaginal discharge, pyrexia, anorexia, vomiting, polydipsia, and/or polyuria. Tumor growth may compress the colon, bladder, or urethra causing straining or obstruction. Other signs may include abdominal distention, dysuria, hematuria, dyspnea, and/or loss of consciousness.

Physical Examination Findings

Physical examination is often normal although large masses may be palpated. A hemorrhagic vaginal discharge may be noted. Some uterine masses are palpable during rectal examination. Enlarged, asymmetric sublumbar lymph nodes may be palpated if the tumor has metastasized. Digital vaginal examination is usually normal. Animals with pyometra may be depressed, febrile, painful on abdominal palpation, and have a purulent vaginal discharge (see p. 545).

Radiography/Ultrasonography/Endoscopy

Radiography and ultrasonography may show a mass in the uterine area. The echogenicity of uterine masses is variable. Ultrasound-guided biopsies may provide information regarding tumor type. Abdominal radiographs should be evaluated for evidence of lymph node enlargement or visceral metastasis, and thoracic radiographs should be evaluated for metastasis. Vaginoscopy may reveal abnormal discharge.

Laboratory Findings

Hematologic and serum biochemical profile results are nonspecific. The patient may be anemic if a chronic hemorrhagic discharge or paraneoplastic syndrome is present. Neoplastic cells are rarely identified on vaginal cytology. Definitive diagnosis requires histopathology.

DIFFERENTIAL DIAGNOSIS

Differential diagnoses for uterine masses include intestinal foreign bodies, tumor or fungal lesions, urinary tract masses, or lymph node enlargement secondary to neoplasia or inflammation. Differential diagnoses for vaginal discharge include estrus, parturition, abortion, normal lochia, vaginitis, metritis, pyometra, placental subinvolution, mucometra, uterine torsion, or trauma.

MEDICAL MANAGEMENT

Effectiveness of chemotherapy and radiation therapy on uterine masses is unknown.

SURGICAL TREATMENT

Ovariohysterectomy is the treatment of choice for uterine tumors.

Preoperative Management

Hydration, electrolyte, and acid-base abnormalities should be corrected before surgery. Patients with elevated blood urea nitrogen or creatinine concentrations should be diuresed before surgery. If pyometra is present, antibiotic therapy should be initiated (see Table 23-8 on p. 521). Mature patients should be fasted for 12 to 18 hours before anesthetic induction.

Anesthesia

A variety of anesthetic protocols can be used in animals with uterine tumors if they are not debilitated and do not have concurrent pyometra. Anesthetic recommendations for animals with pyometra are provided on p. 546.

Surgical Anatomy

Surgical anatomy of the reproductive tract is on p. 520.

Positioning

Patients are positioned in dorsal recumbency for a ventral midline celiotomy. The entire ventral abdomen and caudal thorax should be clipped and prepared for aseptic surgery.

SURGICAL TECHNIQUE

Perform a ventral midline celiotomy. Explore the abdomen for evidence of metastasis or other abnormalities. Biopsy or excise abnormal structures. Perform an OHE (see p. 523), removing the cervix if it is within 1 to 2 cm of the tumor. Culture the uterus if metritis or pyometra is suspected.

POSTOPERATIVE CARE AND ASSESSMENT

Fluid therapy should be continued if the patient was dehydrated or uremic and postoperative analgesics given as needed (see Table 23-25, p. 548). Antibiotics are not necessary unless a uterine infection was identified. Thoracic and abdominal radiographs should be evaluated periodically (e.g., 1 to 2 months, 6 months) if a malignant tumor was present. Complications of OHE are discussed on p. 536. The tumor may recur locally or metastasize.

PROGNOSIS

The prognosis for asymptomatic benign tumors without surgery is good unless the mass enlarges sufficiently to impinge on the gastrointestinal or urinary tracts. The prognosis following OHE is excellent for benign tumors and good for malignant tumors if there is no evidence of metastasis or local infiltration. The prognosis for uterine adenocarcinomas is guarded due to its propensity to metastasize prior to diagnosis. The effectiveness of other treatment modalities for uterine tumors is unknown.

Suggested Reading

Baldwin CJ, Roszel JF, Clark TP: Uterine adenocarcinoma in dogs, *Compend Contin Educ Pract Vet* 14:731, 1992.

Herron MA: Tumors of the canine genital system, *J Am Anim Hosp Assoc* 17:981, 1983.

Stein BS: Tumors of the feline genital tract, *J Am Anim Hosp Assoc* 17:1022, 1981.

MAMMARY NEOPLASIA

DEFINITIONS

Lumpectomy is removal of a mass or part of a mammae, **simple mastectomy** is excision of an entire gland, and **regional mastectomy** is excision of the involved gland and adjacent glands. **Unilateral mastectomy** is the removal of all mammary glands, subcutaneous tissues, and associated lymphatics on one side of the midline, while **bilateral mastectomy** is the simultaneous removal of both mammary chains.

GENERAL CONSIDERATIONS AND CLINICALLY RELEVANT PATHOPHYSIOLOGY

Mammary tumors are uncommon in male dogs but the most common tumor in female dogs. They are less common in cats, but still account for nearly one third of all tumors in this species. Approximately 35% to 50% of canine mammary tumors and 90% of feline mammary tumors are malignant (Ogilvie, Moore, 1995). Canine mammary tumor types are listed in Table 23-16. Malignant mammary tumors spread via lymphatics and blood vessels to the regional lymph nodes and lungs. Other less common metastatic sites include the adrenal glands, kidneys, heart, liver, bone, brain, and skin.

The cause of mammary gland neoplasia is unknown; however, many are hormone-dependent and most can be prevented if OHE is performed before 1 year of age. The risk of mammary tumors for dogs spayed before their first estrus is 0.05%. This risk increases to 8% after one estrus cycle and 26% after the second estrus (Ogilvie, Moore, 1995). Cats ovariectomized prior to one year of age have a 0.6% risk of developing mammary carcinomas compared with intact cats. Estrogen and/or progesterone receptors are found in 50% or more of canine mammary carcinomas and 70% of benign canine mammary tumors (Sartin et al, 1992). Dogs with tumors containing estrogen or progesterone receptors live longer than those without (Ogilvie, Moore, 1995). Progesterone receptors are found in some feline mammary tumors (Johnston et al, 1984). Progesterone administration may be associated with the development of malignant mammary tumors in cats and benign tumors in dogs. Dogs with benign mammary tumors have more than a threefold risk of developing malignant mammary tumors.

In dogs, benign tumors are usually classified as benign mixed tumors (fibroadenomas), adenomas, or benign mesenchymal tumors (Fig. 23-13). Most canine malignant mammary tumors are carcinomas (see Table 23-16); however, sarcomas (less than 5%) and carcinosarcomas (malignant mixed tumors) also occur. Sarcomas have a higher incidence of metastasis than carcinomas. Some "malignant" mammary tumors do not recur or spread after surgery. Papillary or tubular carcinomas have a better prognosis than solid or

TABLE 23-16
Canine Mammary Masses

• Benign mixed tumors
• Carcinomas
   Solid carcinomas
   Tubular adenocarcinomas
   Papillary adenocarcinomas
   Anaplastic carcinomas
• Hyperplasia
• Adenomas
• Malignant mixed tumors
• Sarcomas
• Myeloepitheliomas

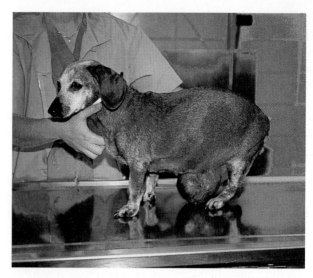

FIG. 23-13
A large mammary tumor in a 13-year-old female dachshund.

anaplastic carcinomas. Inflammatory carcinomas are poorly differentiated carcinomas with extensive mononuclear and polymorphonuclear cellular infiltrates. It may be difficult to differentiate mastitis from inflammatory carcinoma on physical examination or with cytology. These tumors grow rapidly, invading cutaneous lymphatics and causing marked edema and inflammation. They are poorly demarcated, firm, often ulcerated, and may involve both mammary chains. Some areas of involvement appear rash-like. Extensive lymphedema of the limbs may occur secondary to lymphatic occlusion or infiltration. Disseminated intravascular coagulation is common in dogs with inflammatory carcinoma and this tumor indicates a poor prognosis.

Most feline mammary tumors are adenocarcinomas; however, other types of carcinomas and sarcomas are common. Feline mammary tumors grow rapidly and metastasize to local lymph nodes and lungs early in the course of disease. Feline mammary tumors are not as well circumscribed as their canine counterparts; they are firm and often ulcerated. Feline mammary tumors must be differentiated from lobular hyperplasia and fibroepithelial hyperplasia. Hyperplasia is often associated with exogenous progesterone administration. A unilateral mastectomy is recommended to remove feline mammary tumors because local recurrence is common with less radical procedures. Cats with malignant mammary tumors generally survive less than 1 year.

DIAGNOSIS
Clinical Presentation

Signalment. Mammary tumors are common in female dogs and cats. The greatest frequency of mammary tumors is found in poodles, Boston terriers, fox terriers, Airedale terriers, dachshunds, Great Pyrenees, Samoyeds, keeshonden, and sporting breeds (pointers, retrievers, setters, spaniels). Almost all feline mammary tumors (99%) occur in intact females. Most mammary tumors occur in middle-aged or older animals; they are rare in young animals. The incidence of mammary tumors increases markedly after 6 years of age. Dogs develop mammary tumors at a median age of 10 to 11 years, while feline carcinomas occur most often between 8 to 12 years of age.

History. Many mammary tumors are discovered during routine physical examination. Animals may be presented because of a lump and/or abnormal discharge from the mammae. A delay of several months is common before the animal is evaluated by a veterinarian. Occasionally, an animal with advanced disease presents because of dyspnea or lameness secondary to pulmonary or bone metastasis, respectively.

Physical Examination Findings

Mammary masses may be of various sizes (2 to 3 mm to 8 cm). The most common site for canine mammary tumors is the caudal mammary glands. Multiple masses may be found in one or both mammary chains. Most masses are easily moveable but occasionally are fixed to the underlying muscle or fascia. Masses may be sessile or pedunculated, solid or cystic, and ulcerated or covered with skin and hair. Inflammatory carcinoma or mastitis should be suspected if the glands are diffusely swollen with poor demarcation between normal and abnormal tissue. Inflammatory carcinomas are often ulcerated. Axillary or inguinal lymph node enlargement may be palpable and sublumbar lymph node enlargement detected on rectal examination. Lameness or limb edema is suggestive of metastasis.

Radiography/Ultrasonography

Thoracic radiographs (both lateral views and a ventrodorsal view) should be evaluated for pulmonary metastasis. Thoracic metastasis occurs in 25% to 50% of dogs with malignant mammary tumors by the time of diagnosis (Ogilvie, Moore, 1995). Pleural fluid may occur in cats with metastatic pulmonary disease. Abdominal radiographs should be evaluated for iliac lymph node enlargement with caudal tumors. Abdominal ultrasonography may help detect abdominal metastasis.

Laboratory Findings

Minimum database (CBC, biochemistry profile, urinalysis) results are nonspecific for mammary neoplasia, but are important in identifying concurrent geriatric problems or paraneoplastic syndromes. Aspiration or exfoliative cytology helps distinguish inflammatory, benign, and malignant masses. Detection of neoplastic cells in lymph node aspirates helps stage the disease. If pleural fluid is present, it should be evaluated cytologically. Bone scans help confirm bone metastasis. Definitive diagnosis is dependent on histopathology of tissue. Each mass should be evaluated histologically as different tumor types may occur in the same individual.

DIFFERENTIAL DIAGNOSIS

Mammary hypertrophy, mastitis, granulomas, skin tumors, or foreign bodies (e.g., BB pellet or shot) are differential diagnoses. Mammary hypertrophy results from endogenous or exogenous progesterone stimulation and commonly occurs in young intact female cats 2 to 4 weeks after estrus (when progesterone concentrations are elevated). Hypertrophy can usually be ruled out based on history and cytologic findings. Mastitis occurs after estrus, parturition, or false pregnancy; the swelling is usually more localized than with inflammatory carcinoma.

MEDICAL MANAGEMENT

Reports on the efficacy of treatment modalities other than surgery are lacking. Chemotherapy may be beneficial in controlling some malignant tumors. Neither chemotherapy, radiation therapy, nor hormonal therapy is routinely recommended as an adjunct to surgery.

SURGICAL TREATMENT

Surgical excision is the treatment of choice for all mammary tumors except inflammatory carcinomas. Surgical excision allows histological diagnosis and can be curative, improve quality of life, or modify disease progression. Inflammatory carcinomas are extremely aggressive and surgery is of no value in controlling or palliating the disease. Selection of a surgical technique for removing the tumor and variable amounts of mammary tissue depends on tumor size, location and consistency, patient status, and surgeon preference. Survival is not influenced by technique unless incomplete resection is performed. However, local recurrence is decreased in cats when unilateral mastectomy is performed rather than a lumpectomy (Ogilvie, Moore, 1995). A combination of different techniques may be selected if an animal has several masses in glands of both chains. All tumors should be excised, as each mass may be a different tumor type. If complete excision is not possible with a single surgery, a second procedure should be delayed 3 to 4 weeks to allow healing and relaxation of stretched skin. Ovariohysterectomy may be performed at the time of tumor removal. Ovariohysterectomy should be done prior to mastectomy to prevent seeding the abdominal cavity with tumor cells. Although it will not prevent the further development of mammary tumors, it will prevent uterine disease (e.g., pyometra, metritis) and eliminate female hormonal influence on existing tumors.

Lumpectomy or partial mammectomy is excision of a mass and a surrounding margin of grossly normal mammary tissue (greater than or equal to 1 cm). It is used when the mass is small (less than 5 mm), encapsulated, noninvasive, and at the periphery of the gland. Milk and lymph leakage from incised mammary tissue into the wound may cause postoperative inflammation and discomfort. Simple mastectomy is excision of the entire gland containing the tumor. It is used when the tumor involves the central area of the gland or the majority of the gland. Removal of the entire gland may be easier than incising mammary tissue and avoids postoperative problems with milk and lymph leakage. Regional mastectomy involves excision of the involved and adjacent glands. This technique is selected when multiple tumors occur in adjacent glands in the chain or when the mass occurs between two glands. It is sometimes technically easier to remove the confluent caudal abdominal and inguinal glands than either gland alone. Unilateral mastectomy is performed when numerous tumors occur throughout the chain. A unilateral mastectomy may take less time and be less traumatic than multiple lumpectomies or mastectomies. Bilateral mastectomy can be performed when numerous masses occur in both chains; however, skin closure can be extremely difficult or impossible. Therefore it is not recommended. Instead, staged unilateral mastectomies are preferred.

> ☞ **N O T E** · Separate mammary masses on the same dog may be of different histologic types; therefore, excise all masses and submit for histologic examination. Be sure you can determine which mass came from which site when the biopsy report returns.

Preoperative Management

A complete workup is indicated in all patients to stage the disease and identify other problems that may alter the prognosis. Ulcerated, infected masses should be treated with warm compresses and antibiotics for several days prior to surgery to reduce inflammation and allow the gross tumor margins to be more accurately assessed. Preoperative antibiotics are necessary only in severely debilitated patients or those with evidence of infection. If renal disease (e.g., secondary to hypercalcemia of malignancy) is present, preoperative fluids should be administered. The entire ventral abdomen and caudal thorax should be clipped. Each mammary chain should be carefully palpated and the location of each mass mapped. Additional masses are frequently identified once the hair has been removed.

Anesthesia

A variety of anesthetic protocols can be used in animals with mammary masses. General anesthesia is usually less stressful to the patient than local anesthesia, even when small lumps are resected.

Surgical Anatomy

Dogs usually have five pairs and cats four pairs of mammary glands. Mammary glands are compound, tubuloalveolar, apocrine glands. The caudal superficial epigastric arteries and veins supply the caudal glands (Table 23-17). The caudal superficial epigastric artery arises from the external pudendal artery near the superficial inguinal lymph node. Branches

TABLE 23-17

Major Blood Vessels Supplying the Mammary Glands of Dogs and Cats

Mammary Glands 1 & 2
Ventral and lateral branches of the intercostal, internal thoracic, and lateral thoracic vessels

Mammary Glands 2 & 3
Cranial superficial epigastric vessels

Mammary Glands 4 & 5
Caudal superficial epigastric vessels

of the cranial and caudal superficial epigastric arteries anastomose. The cranial thoracic mammae are supplied by the fourth, fifth, and sixth ventral and lateral cutaneous vessels and nerves (from intercostals) and branches of the lateral thoracic vessels (from axillary artery). The caudal thoracic mammae are supplied by the sixth and seventh cutaneous nerves and vessels and branches of the cranial superficial epigastric vessels. The cranial superficial epigastric vessels supply the cranial abdominal mamma and skin over the rectus abdominis muscle. The axillary lymph node drains the three cranial glands and the inguinal lymph node drains the two caudal glands; however, there are lymphatic connections between glands and across the midline.

Positioning

Position the patient in dorsal recumbency with the thoracic limbs fixed cranially and the pelvic limbs fixed caudally in a relaxed position. The entire ventral abdomen, caudal thorax, and inguinal areas should be clipped and prepared for aseptic surgery.

SURGICAL TECHNIQUE

Make an elliptical incision around the involved mammary gland(s), a minimum of 1 cm from the tumor (Fig. 23-14, A). Continue the incision through subcutaneous tissues to the fascia of the external abdominal wall. Avoid incising mammary tissue; however, this is often impossible, as mammary tissue may be confluent between adjacent glands. The midline separation between mammary chains is distinct. *Control superficial hemorrhage with electrocoagulation, hemostats, and/or ligation. Perform an en bloc excision by elevating one edge of the incision and dissecting subcutaneous tissue from the pectoral and rectus fascia using a smooth gliding motion of the scissors (Fig. 23-14, B). Use traction on the elevated skin segment to facilitate dissection.* Abdominal and inguinal glands are loosely attached by fat and connective tissue and easily separated from rectus fascia. Thoracic glands adhere to the underlying pectoral muscles with little intervening fat or connective tissue. *Resect the inguinal fat pad and lymph node(s) with the inguinal mammary gland.* The axillary lymph node is not included with en bloc resection of the thoracic glands. *Excise fascia if the tumor has invaded subcutaneous tissues.* Some neoplastic lesions will invade the

abdominal musculature and excision must include a portion of the abdominal wall. *Continue gliding scissor dissection until major vessels (i.e., cranial superficial epigastrics and caudal superficial epigastrics) to the gland are encountered. Isolate and ligate these vessels (Fig. 23-14, C). Ligate the cranial superficial epigastric vessel where it penetrates the rectus abdominis between the caudal thoracic and cranial abdominal (third) mammary glands (see Table 23-17). Ligate the caudal superficial epigastric vessel adjacent to the inguinal fat pad near the inguinal ring (see Table 23-17). Ligate branches supplying the first and second thoracic mammary glands (see Table 23-17) as they are encountered penetrating the pectoral muscles. Lavage the wound and evaluate for abnormal tissue. Undermine the wound edges and advance skin toward the center of the defect with walking sutures (Fig. 23-14, D). If dead space is extensive, place a Penrose drain to help prevent fluid accumulation. Appose skin edges with a subcutaneous or subcuticular suture pattern (Fig. 23-14, E). Use 3-0 or 4-0 absorbable suture (polydioxanone or polyglyconate) on a swaged-on taper-point needle in either an interrupted or continuous pattern.* Skin apposition is most difficult in the thoracic region because the ribs make the area less compressible than the abdomen and the skin is less mobile. *Use appositional skin sutures (e.g., 3-0 or 4-0 nylon or polypropylene) or staples. Place a padded circumferential bandage to compress dead space, mobilize tissue, and support the wound.*

POSTOPERATIVE CARE AND ASSESSMENT

Analgesics (see Table 23-25, p. 549) and supportive care should be given as needed. An abdominal bandage should be used to support the wound, compress dead space, and absorb fluid. Bandages are changed daily for the first 2 to 3 days, or as needed to keep it dry. The wound should be inspected for inflammation, swelling, drainage, seroma, dehiscence, and necrosis. If a Penrose drain was used, it should be removed when drainage diminishes to a minimal amount (usually within 3 to 5 days). Bandages and sutures are generally removed 5 to 7 days and 7 to 10 days after surgery, respectively. Patients with malignant tumors should be reevaluated for local recurrence and metastasis every 3 to 4 months.

COMPLICATIONS

Complications include pain, inflammation, hemorrhage, seroma formation, infection, ischemic necrosis, self-trauma, dehiscence, hind limb edema, and tumor recurrence. In dogs, local recurrence occurs within 2 years and varies from 20% to 73%.

PROGNOSIS

Significant prognostic factors in dogs are provided in Table 23-18. Significant prognostic factors in cats are tumor size, extent of surgery, and histologic grading (Ogilvie, Moore, 1995). The prognosis for dogs with benign tumors is good with surgery. The prognosis for dogs with malignant tumors is variable and depends on several factors including tumor type and stage. Most dogs with malignant tumors, but without obvious metastasis at the time of surgery, die or are euthanized for tumor-related problems within 1 to 2 years. In dogs, tumors less than 3 cm have a better prognosis (35% recurrence at 2 years) than tumors greater than 3 cm in diameter (80% recurrence at 2 years). In cats, tumors less than 2 cm have less local recurrence than those greater than 2 to 3 cm. Cats with mammary carcinoma greater than 3 cm have a median survival of 6 months, while those with tumors less than 2 cm have a median survival of about 3 years (MacEwen et al, 1984). Queens with tumors less than or equal to 8 cm³ in volume have the longest disease-free interval and median survival times (4.5 years after surgery). The presence of multiple tumors does not affect the prognosis in dogs, but may decrease survival in cats.

Adenocarcinomas that are confined to the duct epithelium have a good prognosis after surgery. The prognosis worsens when neoplastic cells extend beyond the duct system and is poorest when neoplastic cells are found in blood or lymphatic vessels. Poorly differentiated adenocarcinomas have a 90% recurrence rate 2 years after surgery. The recurrence rate for moderately differentiated tumors is 68% and for well-differentiated tumors, 24% 2 years after surgery (Kurzman, Gilbertson, 1986). Treatment modalities other than surgery may slow tumor progression, but few data are available to allow predictions of their effectiveness. Mammary gland sarcoma and inflammatory carcinoma have a very poor prognosis.

TABLE 23-18
Significant Prognostic Factors for Mammary Tumors in Dogs
• Histologic type
• Degree of invasion
• Degree of nuclear differentiation
• Evidence of lymphoid cellular reactivity
• Tumor size
• Lymph node involvement
• Hormone receptor activity
• Presence of ulceration
• Fixation

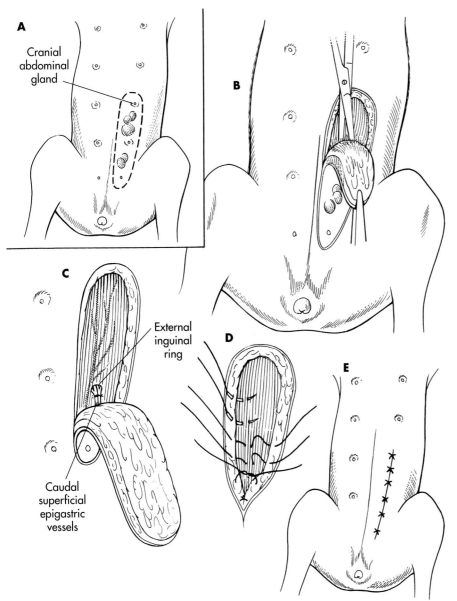

FIG. 23-14
A, For caudal mastectomy, make an elliptical incision around the glands to be excised. **B,** Incise subcutaneous tissue to expose the abdominal fascia. Elevate the cranial edge of the segment and separate subcutaneous tissue from the fascia by sliding sharp scissors along the abdominal fascia. **C,** Ligate and divide the caudal superficial epigastric vessels near the inguinal ring. **D,** Advance skin edges to the center of the defect with walking sutures and subcuticular sutures. **E,** Appose skin edges with appositional sutures.

References

Johnston SD et al: Progesterone receptors in feline mammary adenocarcinomas, *Am J Vet Res* 45:379, 1984.

Kurzman ID, Gilbertson SR: Prognostic factors in canine mammary tumors, *Semin Vet Med Surg (Small Animal)* 1:25, 1986.

MacEwen EG et al: Prognostic factors for feline mammary tumors, *J Am Vet Med Assoc* 185:201, 1984.

Ogilvie GK, Moore AS: Managing the veterinary cancer patient: a practice manual, Trenton, N.J., 1995, Veterinary Learning Systems.

Sartin EA et al: Estrogen and progesterone receptor status of mammary carcinomas and correlation with clinical outcome in dogs, *Am J Vet Res* 53:2196, 1992.

Suggested Reading

Allen SW, Prasse KW, Mahaffey EA: Cytologic differentiation of benign from malignant canine mammary tumors, *Vet Pathol* 23:649, 1986.

Allen SW, Mahaffey EA: Canine mammary neoplasia: prognostic indicators and response of surgical therapy, *J Am Anim Hosp Assoc* 25:540, 1989.

Susaneck SJ et al: Inflammatory mammary carcinoma in a dog, *J Am Anim Hosp Assoc* 19:971, 1983.

Weijer K, Hart AM: Prognostic factors in feline mammary carcinoma, *J National Cancer Institute* 70:709, 1983.

PYOMETRA

DEFINITIONS

Pyometra is an accumulation of purulent material within the uterus. Uterine distention with sterile fluid is referred to as **hydrometra** (watery secretions) or **mucometra** (mucoid secretions).

GENERAL CONSIDERATIONS AND CLINICALLY RELEVANT PATHOPHYSIOLOGY

Pyometra is a potentially life-threatening condition associated with cystic endometrial hyperplasia. Cystic endometrial hyperplasia and pyometra both develop during diestrus. In dogs, the diestrual period of a normal, nongravid bitch lasts approximately 70 days. The uterus is influenced by progesterone produced by ovarian corpora lutea. Progesterone stimulates the growth and secretory activity of the endometrial glands and reduces myometrial activity. Cystic endometrial hyperplasia is an abnormal uterine response developing during diestrus (luteal phase of cycle) when there is high or prolonged ovarian production of progesterone or exogenously administered progesterone. Excessive progesterone influence or an exaggerated progesterone response causes the uterine glandular tissue to become cystic, edematous, thickened, and infiltrated by lymphocytes and plasma cells. Fluid accumulates in endometrial glands and the uterine lumen with cystic endometrial hyperplasia. Uterine drainage is hindered by progesterone inhibition of myometrial contractility. This abnormal uterine environment allows bacterial colonization and pyometra.

Estrogen increases the number of uterine progesterone receptors, which may explain why there is an increased incidence of pyometra after estrogens are administered to prevent pregnancy. Uterine tumors sometimes obstruct the outflow of uterine secretions and may contribute to the development of pyometra. Feline pyometra is less frequent than canine pyometra because development of luteal tissue requires copulation or artificially induced ovulation; however, cats treated with progestins for skin disease have an increased incidence of pyometra.

Infection causes the morbidity and mortality associated with pyometra. Leukocyte response to bacteria is inhibited in a progesterone-primed uterus. *Escherichia coli* is the most common organism identified in canine and feline pyometra. *E. coli* has an affinity for the endometrium and myometrium. Bacterial invasion is thought to be opportunistic because the most commonly isolated organisms are also the normal flora of the vagina (Table 23-19). Other bacterial sources include the urinary tract and transient bacteremia. Vaginal discharge occurs if the cervix is patent or "open." A closed cervix prevents discharge of infected fluid and causes more serious disease. Animals may become dehydrated and toxic. Septicemia and endotoxemia can develop if pyometra is untreated. Compression or overdistention of the uterus may allow infected uterine contents to leak and cause peritonitis.

Concurrent abnormalities in animals with pyometra may include hypoglycemia, renal and hepatic dysfunction, anemia, and cardiac abnormalities (Table 23-20). Hypoglycemia is common in dogs with pyometra. Sepsis and septic shock deplete glycogen stores, increase peripheral glucose use, and decrease gluconeogenesis. Transient hyperglycemia occasionally occurs due to excessive catecholamine and glucagon release. Progesterone-induced growth hormone production may cause persistent hyperglycemia and glucosuria. Judicious insulin treatment may be required in patients with persistent hyperglycemia (i.e., greater than 300 mg/dl), after appropriate medical and surgical treatment.

Renal dysfunction associated with pyometra may be caused by prerenal azotemia, primary glomerular disease, reduced tubular concentrating ability, tubular interstitial disease, reduced glomerular filtration, and concurrent renal disease. Prerenal azotemia is due to poor perfusion, dehydration, and shock. Primary glomerular disease occurs secondary to immune-complex glomerulonephritis. Bacterial antigens also interfere with renal tubular concentrating ability. Once the bacterial antigen is removed, these changes resolve and normal renal function returns. Reduced tubular concentrating ability is related to inhibition of antidiuretic hormone at the level of the renal tubule by bacterial endotoxins, obligatory solute load from decreased glomerular filtration rate, and other unknown factors. Normal tubular concentrating ability usually returns in 2 to 8 weeks after OHE. Hepatocellular injury may be secondary to intrahepatic cholestasis and retention of bile pigments, toxicity from sepsis and endotoxemia, or poor perfusion.

Anemia may be caused by chronic inflammation suppressing erythropoiesis, loss of red cells into the uterine

TABLE 23-19

Organisms Most Commonly Cultured from Dogs with Pyometra

* *Escherichia coli*
* *Staphylococcus aureus**
* *Streptococcus* spp.*
* *Pseudomonas* spp.*
* *Proteus* spp.*
* *Pasteurella* spp.
* *Klebsiella* spp.
* *Haemophilus* spp.
* *Serratia* spp.
* *Moraxella* spp.

*Also found as normal vaginal flora.

TABLE 23-20

Potential Abnormalities in Animals with Pyometra

* Hypoglycemia
* Renal dysfunction
* Hepatic dysfunction
* Anemia
* Cardiac arrhythmias
* Coagulation abnormalities

lumen, hemodilution, or surgical blood loss. Nonregenerative anemia should spontaneously resolve a few weeks after OHE. Coagulation deficits are infrequent, but may occur secondary to concurrent metabolic imbalances. Cardiac arrhythmias result from toxic effects of pyometra, shock, acidosis, and electrolyte imbalance.

DIAGNOSIS
Clinical Presentation

Signalment. Pyometra affects intact dogs more commonly than cats. In dogs, there is no breed predisposition. Domestic shorthair and Siamese cats are affected more commonly than other breeds (Kenney et al, 1987). Pyometra generally occurs in older (7 to 8 years) intact bitches and queens; however, it may occur in younger animals who have been given exogenous estrogen or progestins.

History. Pyometra usually occurs several weeks (i.e., in cats 1 to 4, in dogs 4 to 8) after estrus, or following mismating injections or exogenous administration of estrogens or progestins. The animal may present because of a purulent, sometimes bloody, vaginal discharge. Others have obvious abdominal distention, fever, partial-to-complete anorexia, lethargy, polyuria, polydipsia, vomiting, diarrhea, and/or weight loss. Animals with closed pyometra more commonly have vomiting and diarrhea.

Physical Examination Findings

A purulent blood-tinged vaginal discharge may occur if the cervix is open. Uterine enlargement may be detected on abdominal palpation. Dehydration is frequent. Animals with endotoxemia or septicemia may be in shock, hypothermic, and moribund. Fever is infrequent.

Radiography/Ultrasonography

A fluid-filled uterus should be detected on abdominal radiographs (Fig. 23-15) and/or ultrasonography. The enlarged uterus is located in the caudal abdomen and may displace intestine cranially and dorsally. Occasionally, with open pyometra or uterine rupture, enough drainage occurs so that the uterus is not radiographically detected. Displacing the intestines with a wooden spoon or abdominal bandage may improve uterine visualization. Signs of uterine rupture and peritonitis (i.e., poor serosal contrast) should be noted. It is important to rule out pregnancy. Radiographically, fetal calcification can be identified after approximately 45 days of gestation. Ultrasonography can identify fetal structures (Table 23-21), assess fetal viability, identify uterine fluid, and determine uterine wall thickness. Pyometra, hydrometra, mucometra, or hematometra appear the same ultrasonographically. The uterus is identified as a well-defined linear or convoluted tubular structure with a hypoechoic to anechoic lumen and thin echogenic walls.

Laboratory Findings

Metabolic abnormalities may be identified from a complete blood count, biochemistry profile, and urinalysis. The most common hemogram findings are neutrophilia with a left shift, monocytosis, and evidence of white blood cell toxicity. White blood cell numbers usually exceed 30,000/µL with closed pyometras and may be as high as 100,000 to 200,000/µL. However, normal numbers of WBCs are often seen with open pyometras. Leukopenia may indicate overwhelming infection and septicemia or be secondary to uterine sequestration of neutrophils. Mild normocytic, normochromic, nonregenerative anemia may also occur. Clotting abnormalities and disseminated intravascular coagulation may occur in severely affected patients.

☞ **N O T E •** Do not rule out pyometra in animals with normal numbers of WBCs or leukopenia. Sequestration of neutrophils in the enlarged uterus may cause neutropenia despite severe infection.

Common biochemical abnormalities include hyperproteinemia, hyperglobulinemia, and azotemia. Electrolyte abnormalities may occur with severe vomiting or diarrhea. Less common abnormalities include increased alanine aminotransferase and alkaline phosphatase activities (secondary to toxemia-induced hepatocellular damage or dehydration). Hyperglycemia or hypoglycemia may be associated with concurrent diabetes or sepsis. Urinalysis may reveal isosthenuria, proteinuria, and bacteriuria. Cystocentesis should not be performed if pyometra is suspected to avoid uterine puncture and abdominal contamination. Vaginal cytology confirms a septic exudate with open pyometra and is abnormal even when the cervix is closed. Bacterial culture and susceptibility are essential for selection of appropriate antibiotics.

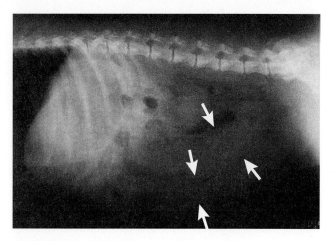

FIG. 23-15
Lateral abdominal radiograph of a dog with pyometra. Note the enlarged uterus *(arrows)* in the caudoventral abdomen displacing viscera cranially and dorsally.

DIFFERENTIAL DIAGNOSIS

Differential diagnoses include mucometra, hydrometra, pyovagina, pregnancy, metritis, uterine torsion, and peritonitis (Figs. 23-16 and 23-17).

MEDICAL MANAGEMENT

Medical evacuation of the uterus with prostaglandin therapy (PGF$_{2\alpha}$) is inappropriate for critically ill patients because evacuation is neither immediate nor complete.

Medical therapy with antibiotics for 2 to 3 weeks and PGF$_{2\alpha}$ (Table 23-22) should be considered only for metabolically stable, valuable, breeding animals. More than one series of prostaglandin injections may be necessary. Owners must be informed that PGF$_{2\alpha}$ therapy is not approved for use in dogs and cats and that serious complications (e.g., uterine rupture or leakage of intraluminal contents into the abdomen and sepsis) are possible. Short-term side effects (30 to 60 minutes) include panting, salivation, emesis, defecation, urination, mydriasis, nesting, tenesmus, lordosis, vocalization, and intensive grooming. High doses of prostaglandin may result in ataxia, collapse, hypovolemic shock, respiratory distress, or death. PGF$_{2\alpha}$ therapy may cause reduced fertility.

SURGICAL TREATMENT

Treatment (OHE) should not be delayed more than is absolutely necessary. Morbidity and mortality are associated with concurrent metabolic abnormalities and organ dysfunction (see above). Surgical drainage of the uterus without OHE is not recommended, but has been successful in a few cases (Ewing et al, 1970). The corpora lutea are removed and each horn lavaged and suctioned. Indwelling drains are placed through the cervix to allow daily lavage with dilute antiseptics.

Preoperative Management

Surgery should not be delayed more than a few hours while medical therapy is instituted, especially in patients with closed pyometra. Urine output, glucose, and arrhythmias should be monitored preoperatively. Hydration, electrolyte, and acid-base imbalances should be corrected prior to sur-

TABLE 23-21

Radiographic and Ultrasonographic Evaluation of Pregnancy

Radiographs
- Fetal calcification detected—45 days of gestation

Ultrasonography
- Fetal structures visualized 23 to 25 days after luteinizing hormone peak or 21 days after onset of diestrus
- Assess fetal viability at 24 to 30 days of gestation

gery, if possible (the prognosis is improved when azotemia is corrected before surgery). A broad-spectrum antibiotic effective against *E. coli* (e.g., cefazolin, cefoxitin, amoxicillin plus clavulanate, ampicillin, or trimethoprim-sulfonamides; Table 23-23) should be given while awaiting antibiotic susceptibility results. Aminoglycosides are nephrotoxic and not recommended due to the prevalence of renal dysfunction with pyometra. In addition to fluid volume replacement, endotoxic or septicemic patients may also be given corticosteroids (15 to 30 mg/kg prednisolone sodium succinate or 4 to 6 mg/kg dexamethasone intravenously) or flunixin meglumine (but not both). Fluid input and urine output should be monitored to help assess renal function. Low-dose dopamine (0.5 to 1.5 µg/kg/min intravenously) may be used to improve renal function (see below) or diuretics (e.g., furosemide, 2 to 4 mg/kg intravenously, intramuscularly, or subcutaneously or 20% mannitol, 0.5 to 1.0 g/kg intravenously) may be administered in volume-overloaded patients with reduced urine production. Administration of antiarrhythmics may occasionally be necessary.

Anesthesia

Anesthetic protocols vary greatly depending on patient status. Animals that are systemically ill need to be closely monitored during anesthesia. They may be induced with an opioid plus diazepam, given in incremental dosages as necessary to intubate (Table 23-24). If intubation is not possible, etomidate or reduced dosages of thiopental or propofol may be given. If etomidate is not available, arrhythmic dogs may be premedicated with oxymorphone and induced with thiopental and lidocaine. For the latter, 9 mg/kg of each is drawn up and half is given initially, intravenously. Additional drug is given to allow the dog to be intubated. Generally, no more than 6 mg/kg of lidocaine is given intravenously to prevent toxicity. Isoflurane is the inhalant of choice because it causes minimal cardiac depression, and induction and recovery are usually rapid. The anesthetic depth should be monitored closely in these patients. Anesthetic management of stable animals is described on p. 519.

Hypotension should be corrected prior to and prevented during and after surgery in animals with pyometra. Animals with total protein less than 4.0 g/dl or albumin less than 1.5 g/dl may benefit from perioperative colloid administration. Colloids may be given preoperatively, intraoperatively, and/or postoperatively for a total dose of 20 ml/kg/day. If

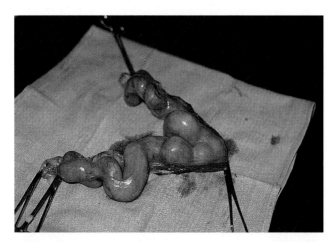

FIG. 23-16
An enlarged, friable uterus in an animal with pyometra. Compare this to the enlarged uterus in an animal with mucometra in Fig. 23-17. The two cannot be differentiated radiographically.

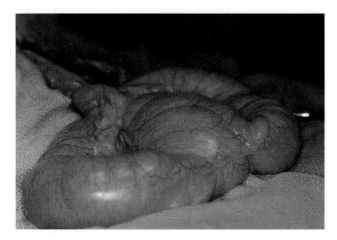

FIG. 23-17
Intraoperative appearance of the uterus in an animal with mucometra.

colloids are given during surgery (7 to 10 ml/kg), acute intraoperative hypotension should be treated with crystalloids. Dobutamine (2 to 10 µg/kg/min intravenously) or dopamine (2 to 10 µg/kg/min intravenously) may be given during surgery for inotropic support. Dobutamine is less arrhythmogenic and chronotropic than dopamine and is preferred if the patient is hypotensive and anuric. If they are anuric and normotensive, low-dose dopamine (0.5 to 1.5 µg/kg/min intravenously) plus furosemide (0.2 mg/kg intravenously) may be preferable. These patients should be monitored for arrhythmias or tachycardia.

Positioning

Position the patient in dorsal recumbency for a ventral midline celiotomy. The entire ventral abdomen should be clipped and prepared for aseptic surgery.

Surgical Anatomy

Surgical anatomy of the reproductive tract is on p. 520.

TABLE 23-22
PGF2$_\alpha$ Therapy of Pyometra*

0.1-0.25 mg/kg SC, SID or BID for 3–5 days.
*Dosages and efficacy of treatment are not definitively established.
NOTE: Breeding should be attempted during the next estrus.

SURGICAL TECHNIQUE

Expose the abdomen through a ventral midline incision beginning 2 to 3 cm caudal to the xiphoid and extending to the pubis. Explore the abdomen and locate the distended uterus. Observe for evidence of peritonitis (i.e., serosal inflammation, increased abdominal fluid, petechiation). Obtain abdominal fluid for culture, evacuate the urinary bladder by cystocentesis, and collect a urine specimen for culture and analysis if not previously submitted. Carefully exteriorize the uterus without applying pressure or excessive traction. A fluid-filled uterus is often friable; therefore, lift rather than pull the uterus out of the abdomen. Do not use a spay hook to locate and exteriorize the uterus because the uterus may tear. Do not correct uterine torsion because this will release bacteria and toxins. *Isolate the uterus from the abdomen with laparotomy pads or sterile towels. Place clamps and ligatures as previously described for OHE except that the cervix may be resected in addition to ovaries, uterine horns, and uterine body. Ligate the pedicles with absorbable monofilament suture material (i.e., 2-0 or 3-0 polydioxanone or polyglyconate) and transect at the junction of the cervix and vagina. Thoroughly lavage the vaginal stump. Culture the contents of the uterus without contaminating the surgical field. Remove laparotomy pads and replace contaminated instruments, gloves, and drapes. Lavage the abdomen and close the incision routinely. Submit the tract for pathologic evaluation.*

POSTOPERATIVE CARE AND ASSESSMENT

Give analgesics as necessary (Table 23-25). These patients should be monitored closely for 24 to 48 hours for sepsis and shock, dehydration, and electrolyte or acid-base imbalances. Severe hypoproteinemia or anemia may require plasma or blood transfusions, respectively. Fluid therapy should be continued postoperatively until the animal is eating and drinking normally. Antibiotic therapy based on culture and sensitivity results should be continued for 10 to 14 days. Low-dose dopamine or diuretics (Table 23-26) may be given postoperatively if urine production is reduced. Evidence of abdominal discomfort, elevated temperature, and pain suggests peritonitis.

COMPLICATIONS

Complications associated with elective OHE may also occur following OHE for pyometra (see p. 536). Death occurs in 5% to 8% of patients despite appropriate therapy and is common after uterine rupture. Septicemia, endotoxemia, peritonitis, and cervical or stump pyometra may occur.

TABLE 23-23

Selected Antibiotics of Use in Animals with Pyometra

Cefazolin (Ancef, Kefzol)
20 mg/kg IV or IM, TID

Cefoxitin (Mefoxin)
15-30 mg/kg IV, TID to QID

Amoxicillin plus Clavulanate (Clavamox)
Dogs
12.5-25 mg/kg PO, BID

Cats
62.5 mg/cat PO, BID

Ampicillin
22 mg/kg IV, IM, SC, or PO, TID to QID

Trimethoprim-Sulfadiazine (Tribrissen)
Dogs
15 mg/kg IM or PO, BID

Cats
15 mg/kg PO, BID

Enrofloxacin (Baytril)
5-10 mg/kg PO or IV, BID

TABLE 23-24

Selected Anesthetic Protocols for Debilitated or Shocky Animals with Pyometra

Dogs
Induction

Oxymorphone (0.1 mg/kg IV) plus diazepam (0.2 mg/kg IV). Give in incremental dosages. Intubate if possible. If necessary, give etomidate (0.5-1.5 mg/kg IV). Alternatively, if not vomiting, mask induction can be used or give thiopental or propofol at reduced doses.

Maintenance
Isoflurane

Cats
Premedication

Butorphanol (0.2-0.4 mg/kg SC or IM) or buprenorphine (5-15 µg/kg IM) or oxymorphone (0.05 mg/kg SC or IM)

Induction

Diazepam (0.2 mg/kg IV) followed by etomidate (0.5-1.5 mg/kg IV). Alternatively, if not vomiting, mask or chamber induction can be used or give thiopental or propofol at reduced dosages. If there are no contraindications to ketamine (i.e., renal dysfunction), reduced dosages of diazepam and ketamine may also be used.

Maintenance
Isoflurane

TABLE 23-25

Postoperative Analgesics

Oxymorphone (Numorphan)
0.05-0.1 mg/kg IV, IM, every 4 hours (as needed)

Butorphanol (Torbutrol, Torbugesic)
0.2-0.4 mg/kg IV, IM, or SC, every 2 to 4 hours (as needed)

Buprenorphine (Buprenex)
5-15 µg/kg IV, IM, every 6 hours (as needed)

TABLE 23-26

Diuretic Therapy

Dopamine (low-dose)
1-2 µg/kg/min IV

Furosemide (Lasix)
2-4 mg/kg IV, IM, or SC (SID to QID as needed)

Stump pyometra may be associated with residual ovarian tissue. In these cases, the remaining stump should be excised and residual ovarian tissue removed. Other complications may include anorexia, lethargy, anemia, pyrexia, vomiting, and icterus. Most complications resolve within 2 weeks of surgery.

PROGNOSIS

Death usually occurs without surgical or medical therapy; however, a few animals recover following corpus luteum regression and spontaneous uterine drainage. Pyometra recurrence at subsequent diestrus is common in these animals. Pyometra commonly persists or recurs after prostaglandin therapy in dogs (77% bitches at 27 months) (Meyers-Wallen, Goldschmidt, Flickinger, 1987). However, after prostaglandin therapy at least one normal litter is produced in 40% to 74% of bitches (Meyers-Wallen, Goldschmidt, Flickinger, 1987) and 81% of queens (Davidson, Feldman, Nelson, 1992). Prognosis following surgery is good if abdominal contamination is avoided, shock and sepsis are controlled, and renal damage reversed by fluid therapy and bacterial antigen elimination (84% recovery) (Hardy, Osborne, 1974). Death may occur when metabolic abnormalities are severe and unresponsive to appropriate therapy.

References

Davidson AP, Feldman EC, Nelson RW: Treatment of pyometra in cats, using prostaglandin F$_{2\alpha}$: 21 cases (1982-1990), *J Am Vet Med Assoc* 200:825, 1992.

Ewing GO et al: Therapy of canine pyometra, *J Am Anim Hosp Assoc* 6:218, 1970.

Hardy RM, Osborne CA: Canine pyometra: pathophysiology, diagnosis, and treatment of uterine and extra-uterine lesions, *J Am Anim Hosp Assoc* 10:245, 1974.

Kenney KJ et al: Pyometra in cats: 183 cases (1979–1984), *J Am Vet Med Assoc* 191:1130, 1987.

Meyers-Wallen VN, Goldschmidt MH, Flickinger GL: Prostaglandin F$_{2\alpha}$ treatment of canine pyometra, *J Am Vet Med Assoc* 189:1557, 1987.

Suggested Reading

Fayrer-Hosken RA et al: Early diagnosis of canine pyometra using ultrasonography, *Vet Radiol* 32:287, 1991.

Nelson RW, Feldman ED, Stabenfeldt GH: Treatment of canine pyometra and endometritis with prostaglandin F$_{2\alpha}$, *J Am Vet Med Assoc* 181:899, 1982.

Potter K, Hancock DH, Gallina AM: Clinical and pathologic features of endometrial hyperplasia, pyometra, and endometritis in cats: 79 cases (1980–1985), *J Am Vet Med Assoc* 198:1427, 1991.

Stone EA et al: Renal dysfunction in dogs with pyometra, *J Am Vet Med Assoc* 193:457, 1988.

Wheaton LG et al: Results and complications of surgical treatment of pyometra: a review of 80 cases, *J Am Anim Hosp Assoc* 25:563, 1989.

VAGINAL PROLAPSE/HYPERPLASIA

DEFINITION

Vaginal prolapse/hyperplasia occurs during estrus or proestrus as a result of edematous enlargement of vaginal tissue.

SYNONYMS

Vaginal hypertrophy, vaginal edema, estral eversion, estral hypertrophy

GENERAL CONSIDERATIONS AND CLINICALLY RELEVANT PATHOPHYSIOLOGY

Vaginal hyperplasia/hypertrophy is uncommon, but may occur during proestrus and estrus. The mucosa is not truly hyperplastic; it enlarges because of edema. Normal estrogenic stimulation causes vaginal mucosa to become hyperemic, edematous, and keratinized. These normal effects are accentuated with vaginal prolapse/hyperplasia causing edematous mucosa to evert during proestrus and estrus and occasionally at the end of diestrus or parturition. Prolapse may occur with hyperestrogenism or weakness of vaginal connective tissue. The amount of edema and eversion is extremely variable. Severe edema causes vaginal tissue to protrude from the vulva. Although the protruding mass may be large, the origin of the mass is usually small (approximately 1 cm) and located on the vaginal floor cranial to the urethral orifice. The width of the mass varies from stalk-like to involving the circumference of the vaginal floor. Prolapsing tissue promotes straining, which further increases the amount of prolapsed tissue. The edematous tissue mechanically obstructs and interferes with normal breeding. Tissue protruding from between the vulvar lips is often traumatized by abrasion, licking, or drying. Trauma results in ulceration and bleeding. The mass may compress surrounding structures and cause stranguria, hematuria, or tenesmus. Although edema resolves spontaneously when the follicular phase of the cycle and ovarian production of estrogen have elapsed, prolapse may recur with each succeeding estrus cycle.

☞ **N O T E ·** Vaginal prolapse/hyperplasia appears to be familial. Affected animals should not be bred.

DIAGNOSIS
Clinical Presentation

Signalment. Although rare, vaginal prolapse/hyperplasia is most common in large-breed dogs. It most commonly occurs in young bitches (2 years or younger) during one of their first three estrus cycles. Vaginal prolapse/hyperplasia is extremely rare in cats.

History. The most common historical findings are protrusion of a mass from the vulva, vulvar discharge, or bleeding. Bitches may present because they refuse to allow intromission during breeding. The history should indicate if the animal is in estrus or proestrus. Other signs of vaginal disease include frequent perineal licking, pollakiuria, dysuria, and perineal enlargement/swelling.

Physical Examination Findings

A mass may be seen protruding between the vulvar lips or the perineum may bulge. Acute prolapse and nonprotruding prolapses are characterized by a glistening, edematous, pale pink mucosal surface. Chronic prolapses appear leathery (i.e., dry and dull), corrugated, and sometimes ulcerated or fissured. The mass should be examined carefully to determine origin, size at the base, locations of the vaginal lumen and urethral opening, and extent of tissue damage. Vaginal palpation should identify a mass arising from the ventral vaginal floor, if it is not protruding. Vaginal areas other than just cranial to the urethral orifice should feel normal.

Radiography

Radiographs are unnecessary unless neoplasia is suspected.

Laboratory Findings

Vaginal cytology should confirm estrogen stimulation (i.e., RBCs in the absence of cornified vaginal epithelial cells). Aspiration cytology helps differentiate prolapse from neoplasia.

DIFFERENTIAL DIAGNOSIS

Uterine prolapse (see p. 551) and vaginal tumors are the most difficult to differentiate from vaginal prolapse/hyperplasia. The most common types of vulvar-vaginal tumors are fibroleiomyoma, lipoma, leiomyosarcoma, squamous cell carcinoma, and transmissible venereal tumor. Most vulvar-vaginal tumors occur in old (10 years or older), intact females. Benign vulvar-vaginal tumors are most common and respond to local excision and OHE. Fibroleiomyoma is the most common benign tumor. Fibroleiomyomas originate around the urethral papilla and are usually pedunculated, smooth, firm, and pale. The most common malignant tumors are transmissible venereal tumors. These tumors tend to be broad-based, irregular, friable, and bleed easily. Malignant vulvar-vaginal tumors are often locally invasive and metastasize early to local lymph nodes.

MEDICAL MANAGEMENT

If protrusion is not circumferential, vaginal prolapse will spontaneously resolve when estrogen influence diminishes. Animals with vaginal prolapse/hyperplasia should not be used for breeding because the disease has a familial predisposition. Artificial insemination may be considered when a valuable bitch will not allow intromission and the owners insist on breeding. Transmissible venereal tumors (TVTs) can be treated with vincristine (0.025 mg/kg up to 1 mg or 0.5 mg/m^2 intravenously, weekly for 3 to 6 weeks) or combination chemotherapy. TVTs also respond to local excision, radiation therapy, and immunotherapy. In addition, TVTs sometimes regress spontaneously.

SURGICAL TREATMENT

Ovariohysterectomy is recommended to prevent recurrence and injury to the everted mucosa. Large, protruding masses may require manual reduction via an episiotomy and vulvar sutures to prevent recurrence until the edematous tissue shrinks. Resection of the protruding tissue without OHE is not recommended because the procedure is associated with significant hemorrhage and does not prevent recurrence during subsequent estrus cycles. Resection of protruding tissue is recommended when the tissue is severely damaged or necrotic. Ovariohysterectomy and mass excision or biopsy are recommended for all vaginal tumors except TVT. Many vaginal tumors are under hormonal influence and regress after OHE.

Preoperative Management

Protruding mucosa should be lavaged with warm saline or water to remove debris and necrotic tissue. An antibiotic or antibiotic/steroid ointment can be applied to the exposed tissue and the mass replaced within the vagina or vestibule, if possible. An Elizabethan collar, bucket, or sidebars should be used to prevent self-trauma before surgery.

Anesthesia

Anesthetic recommendations for animals undergoing reproductive surgery are on p. 519.

Surgical Anatomy

Anatomy of the reproductive system is on p. 520. Vaginal lymphatic drainage is to the internal iliac lymph nodes.

Positioning

The patient is positioned in dorsal recumbency for OHE. The entire ventral abdomen and perineum should be clipped and prepared for aseptic surgery. Episiotomy requires that they be repositioned in a perineal position (i.e., ventral recumbency, pelvic limbs over the edge of a padded table, tail fixed dorsally over the back).

SURGICAL TECHNIQUE

Perform an OHE (see p. 523) and biopsy the mass to rule out neoplasia. Perform an episiotomy if necessary to allow biopsy. Replace the protruding mass into the vagina or vestibule. Lavage, lubricate, and reduce the prolapsed tissue by digital manipulation. Maintain reduction by placing two to three horizontal mattress sutures (e.g., 2-0 nylon or polypropylene) between the vulvar lips.

If resection of necrotic or severely traumatized tissue is necessary, position the patient in a perineal position and perform an episiotomy to expose the mass. Place and maintain a urethral catheter during the procedure. In stages, incise the base of the edematous tissue. Control hemorrhage with pressure, ligatures, and electrocoagulation. Appose adjacent mucosal edges with interrupted or continuous approximating sutures (e.g., 3-0 or 4-0 polydioxanone or polyglyconate). Edema should resolve within 5 to 7 days of OHE.

POSTOPERATIVE CARE AND ASSESSMENT

Patients should be supported postoperatively with fluids and analgesics (see Table 23-25) as needed. Cold compresses should be applied immediately after episiotomy and warm compresses the following day to reduce inflammation and swelling. Self-trauma may result in dehiscence due to perineal discomfort associated with episiotomy and/or vulvar sutures; an Elizabethan collar, bucket, or sidebars should be used postoperatively. The vagina should be palpated 5 to 7 days after mass reduction and/or OHE, and vulvar sutures removed if tissue eversion has regressed with minimal threat of reprotrusion. Hemorrhage may occur following amputation of the protruding edematous tissue but is self-limiting if good surgical technique was employed.

PROGNOSIS

The prognosis is excellent following OHE; without OHE recurrence during subsequent estrus and difficult conception are common. Edema will resolve when estrogen levels diminish at the end of estrus. Offspring may be predisposed to the condition.

Suggested Reading

Bilbrey SA et al: Vulvovaginectomy and perineal urethrostomy for neoplasms of the vulva and vagina, *Vet Surg* 18:450, 1989.

Hardie EM: Selected surgeries of the male and female reproductive tracts, *Vet Clin North Am Small Anim Pract* 14:109, 1984.

Kydd DM, Burnie AG: Vaginal neoplasia in the bitch: a review of forty clinical cases, *J Small Anim Pract* 27:255, 1986.

Manothaiudom K, Johnston SD: Clinical approach to vaginal/vestibular masses in the bitch, *Vet Clin North Am Small Anim Pract* 21:509, 1991.

Memon MA, Pavletic MM, Kumar SA: Chronic vaginal prolapse during pregnancy in a bitch, *J Am Vet Med Assoc* 202:295, 1993.

Schutte AP: Vaginal prolapse in the bitch, *J S Afr Vet Med Assoc* 38:197, 1967.

Thacher C, Bradley RL: Vulvar and vaginal tumors in the dog: a retrospective study, *J Am Vet Med Assoc* 183:690, 1983.

UTERINE PROLAPSE

DEFINITIONS

Uterine prolapse is an eversion and protrusion of a portion of the uterus through the cervix into the vagina during or near parturition.

SYNONYMS

Uterine eversion

GENERAL CONSIDERATIONS AND CLINICALLY RELEVANT PATHOPHYSIOLOGY

Uterine prolapse is rare. It is similar to estrus-associated vaginal prolapse/hyperplasia (see p. 549); however, uterine prolapse is associated with parturition and involves the entire vaginal circumference. The cervix must be dilated for uterine prolapse to occur. One or both uterine horns may prolapse and reside in the cranial vagina or be everted through the vulva. Uterine prolapse usually occurs with prolonged labor. The everted tissue is doughnut-shaped and discolored from venous congestion, trauma, and debris. Uterine prolapse may result in tearing of the broad ligament and uterine artery hemorrhage. Hemorrhage may lead to hypovolemic shock unless controlled quickly.

DIAGNOSIS
Clinical Presentation

Signalment. The condition is rare but may occur near or at parturition. There is no recognized age predisposition.

History. Uterine prolapse is associated with excessive straining during parturition. A mucosal mass is generally noticed protruding from the vulva. Vague signs of abdominal distress and tenesmus may be noted. Signs of hemorrhagic shock may occur if the ovarian or uterine vessels have ruptured. Other signs may include restlessness, abnormal posture, pain, perineal bulging, licking, and dysuria.

Physical Examination Findings

Uterine prolapse is diagnosed on physical examination by digital examination of the vagina. Perineal bulging may be recognized. Everted mucosa may protrude through the vulva or be digitally palpated in the vagina. A fornix will be identified by inserting a probe or finger along the protruding mass if it is a vaginal mass or prolapse, but not if it is a uterine prolapse. The animal may be stable or show signs of hemorrhagic shock (e.g., pale mucous membranes, tachycardia, weak pulse).

Radiography/Ultrasonography/Vaginoscopy

A gravid uterus or postpartum uterus may be identified on radiographs or ultrasonography. Vaginoscopy may be used to confirm the diagnosis.

Laboratory Findings

Specific laboratory abnormalities are not seen. Anemia may be present if the uterine artery has ruptured.

DIFFERENTIAL DIAGNOSIS

Differential diagnoses include vaginal prolapse/hyperplasia (see p. 549), vaginal tumor (see p. 549), and uterine torsion.

MEDICAL MANAGEMENT

Medical treatment is rarely successful. Shock should be treated with fluids (plus or minus corticosteroids). Acid-base and electrolyte imbalances should be corrected. The protruding mass should be lavaged with warm saline and gently massaged to reduce edema. Lavaging with hypertonic dextrose solution may reduce swelling. The mass should then be lubricated with a water-soluble gel and manually replaced.

SURGICAL TREATMENT

The goals of treatment are to replace the uterus (see above under medical management) and prevent infection. Treatment options include manual reduction, manual reduction with immediate OHE, reduction during celiotomy, and amputation of the mass. Ovariohysterectomy should be performed if tissue is devitalized, irreducible, or vessels in the broad ligament have ruptured. Laparotomy may be necessary to facilitate manual reduction by placing cranial traction on the broad ligament or uterus. Occasionally, uterine amputation is necessary to allow reduction. Everted uterine tissue may be amputated similarly to that described for vaginal prolapse/hyperplasia (see p. 549); however, the uterine arteries must be ligated. After uterine amputation, an OHE should be performed. Vaginapexy may be performed during cesarean section, celiotomy, or when the patient is stable.

☞ **N O T E** • The urethra should be catheterized during uterine amputation to prevent traumatizing it or the urethral papilla.

Preoperative Management

Shocky patients should have surgery performed as soon as they have been stabilized. Shock should be treated with fluids (plus or minus corticosteroids), and acid-base and electrolyte imbalances corrected. Prophylactic antibiotics should be given when the prolapse is contaminated or traumatized. Hair should be clipped from the abdomen and perineum and the areas prepared for aseptic surgery. Viability of the prolapsed tissue should be assessed and, if the tissue appears healthy, the mass lavaged and replaced. Use techniques described above, under Medical Management.

Anesthesia

Anesthetic recommendations for animals undergoing reproductive surgery are provided on p. 519. Animals that are in shock require special care during induction and anesthesia. Anesthetic protocols for debilitated and shocky patients are provided in Table 23-24, p. 548. Epidural anesthesia (see p. 520) may facilitate prolapse reduction and reduce postoperative straining. Local anesthetics should not be used in an epidural unless volume depletion has been corrected.

Positioning

Manual reduction may be accomplished with the patient in ventral, dorsal, or lateral recumbency. A perineal position is recommended for episiotomy and dorsal recumbency for celiotomy.

Surgical Anatomy

Surgical anatomy of the reproductive tract is provided on p. 520.

SURGICAL TECHNIQUE

Reduce acute prolapses manually. Lavage the protruding tissue with warm saline or water and diluted antiseptic. Hypertonic agents (e.g., sugar) may help reduce edema and facilitate reduction. *Gently compress the mass to reduce edema while attempting to reduce the prolapse. If necessary, perform an episiotomy to assist reduction. Insert a urethral catheter. Place horizontal mattress sutures between the vulvar lips to maintain reduction and prevent recurrence. If necessary, perform celiotomy to facilitate reduction by cranial uterine traction, ensure proper alignment of the uterine horns, and assess integrity of the vasculature.*

POSTOPERATIVE CARE AND ASSESSMENT

Shock, dehydration, and blood loss should be treated and analgesics given as necessary (see Table 23-25). Urination should be monitored because swelling and pain may cause urethral obstruction. If dysuria or anuria is anticipated, a urinary catheter should be placed. Antibiotics should be continued postoperatively if the uterus appeared moderately to severely traumatized and OHE was not performed. Complications may include hemorrhage, shock, dehydration, infection, necrosis, urethral obstruction, recurrence, and death.

PROGNOSIS

Complete uterine prolapse will not regress spontaneously. Survival following successful manual reduction of uterine prolapses is common, but infertility and dystocia may occur with subsequent breeding. The prognosis following OHE is excellent if shock and hemorrhage are treated appropriately.

Suggested Reading

Manothaiudom K, Johnston SD: Clinical approach to vaginal/vestibular masses in the bitch, *Vet Clin North Am Small Anim Pract* 21:509, 1991.

Surgery of the Male Reproductive Tract

SPECIFIC DISEASES

PROSTATIC HYPERPLASIA

DEFINITIONS

Prostatic hyperplasia is a benign enlargement of the prostate. Increased numbers of prostatic cells occur secondary to androgenic hormone stimulation.

SYNONYMS

Benign prostatic hyperplasia, prostatic "hypertrophy," BPH

GENERAL CONSIDERATIONS AND CLINICALLY RELEVANT PATHOPHYSIOLOGY

Benign prostatic hyperplasia is the most common canine prostatic disorder. Potential causes of hyperplasia include an abnormal ratio of androgens to estrogens, increased number of androgen receptors, and increased tissue sensitivity to androgens. The primary androgen promoting hyperplasia is dihydrotestosterone. Benign prostatic hyperplasia may be a normal aging change; however, marked enlargement may cause constipation, tenesmus, altered stool shape, and/or dysuria. Prostatic enlargement rarely causes urinary obstruction. Pressure on the pelvic diaphragm may contribute to the development of a perineal hernia.

Hyperplasia may be glandular or complex. Glandular hyperplasia affects dogs as young as 1 year of age and peaks at 5 to 6 years. There is a uniform proliferation of secretory structures with glandular hyperplasia, and gland consistency is normal. Complex hyperplasia is seen in dogs as young as 2 years of age, but predominately occurs between 8 and 9 years. Cystic dilated alveoli are present with heterogeneous epithelial cells varying from normal to nonfunctional cuboidal cells. Acini are filled with eosinophilic material, and plasma cells and lymphocytes are present in the hyperplastic stroma.

DIAGNOSIS
Clinical Presentation

Signalment. Sexually intact male dogs are affected. Doberman pinschers may be predisposed to prostatic disease (Krawiec, Heflin, 1992). Benign prostatic hyperplasia is found in most sexually intact male dogs over 6 years of age. Mean age at diagnosis is 8.9 years for most prostatic diseases (Krawiec, Heflin, 1992).

History. Dogs may present for tenesmus, hematuria, and/or urethral bleeding.

Physical Examination Findings

Most dogs are asymptomatic, but tenesmus, hematuria, or urethral bleeding may occur. Rectal palpation reveals symmetric, nonpainful prostatic enlargement.

Radiography/Ultrasonography

Radiographically, the prostate appears symmetrically enlarged. Ultrasonography shows diffuse, symmetric prostatic involvement, and small, multiple, diffuse cysts are common. The overall echogenicity of the gland is normal to increased.

Laboratory Findings

Cytology reveals hemorrhage and mild inflammation without sepsis. Prostatic epithelial cells, erythrocytes, and a few leukocytes are identified. Definitive diagnosis requires histopathology to confirm hyperplastic changes.

DIFFERENTIAL DIAGNOSIS

Differential diagnoses include prostatic squamous metaplasia, prostatic cysts (see p. 558), periprostatic cysts (see p. 558), prostatitis (see p. 554), prostatic neoplasia (see p. 560), and prostatic abscesses (see below). Prostatic aspiration or biopsy (see p. 533) may be necessary to differentiate benign and malignant prostatic enlargement. Ultrasonography may differentiate benign prostatic enlargement from that due to cysts or abscesses.

MEDICAL MANAGEMENT

Estrogen therapy has been used to reduce prostatic size, but is not recommended because it causes infertility, squamous metaplasia, abscessation, and aplastic anemia. Medroxyprogesterone acetate (Table 23-27) alleviated signs of hyperplasia within 4 to 6 weeks in 16 of 19 (84%) dogs treated (Bamberg-Thalén, Linde-Forsberg, 1993). Most, however, had recurrence at an average of 13.6 months. Potential progestin side effects include increased appetite, weight gain, mammary neoplasia and dysplasia, and diabetes mellitus. Ketaconazole may be safer but requires life-long therapy.

SURGICAL TREATMENT

Asymptomatic animals do not require therapy. Castration is the best treatment for dogs with clinical disease. Castration permanently involutes the prostate within 3 to 12 weeks.

Preoperative Management

Constipation, tenesmus, and urine retention should be treated symptomatically. Stool softeners may facilitate defecation (see p. 536).

Anesthesia

Anesthetic recommendations for animals undergoing elective reproductive surgery are provided on p. 519.

Surgical Anatomy

Surgical anatomy of the prostate is provided on p. 521.

TABLE 23-27
Medical Management of Benign Prostatic Enlargement

Medroxyprogesterone Acetate (DepoProvera)

3 mg/kg (minimum dose of 50 mg) SC; repeat dose in 4 to 6 weeks if signs persist

*From Bamberg-Thalén B, Linde-Forsberg C: Treatment of canine benign prostatic hyperplasia with medroxyprogesterone acetate, *J Am Anim Hosp Assoc* 29:221, 1993.

Positioning

The patient is positioned in dorsal recumbency for prescrotal castration (see p. 525) and a perineal position for perineal castration (see p. 527). See p. 525 for recommendations for clipping and surgically prepping for castration.

SURGICAL TECHNIQUE

Castration is described on p. 524.

POSTOPERATIVE CARE AND ASSESSMENT

Analgesics should be provided for pain (see Table 23-25, p. 548), if necessary. Symptomatic treatment for constipation, tenesmus, and urine retention may be necessary until involution is sufficient to diminish clinical signs. Prostatic involution can be evaluated ultrasonographically.

PROGNOSIS

The prognosis following castration is excellent. Although symptomatic therapy alone may initially be helpful, clinical signs recur or worsen without castration.

References

Bamberg-Thalén B, Linde-Forsberg C: Treatment of canine benign prostatic hyperplasia with medroxyprogesterone acetate, *J Am Anim Hosp Assoc* 29:221, 1993.

Krawiec DR, Heflin D: Study of prostatic disease in dogs: 177 cases (1981–1986), *J Am Vet Med Assoc* 200:1119, 1992.

Suggested Reading

Basinger RR, Rawlings CA, Barsanti JA, et al: Urodynamic alterations associated with clinical prostatic diseases and prostatic surgery in 23 dogs, *J Am Anim Hosp Assoc* 25:385, 1989.

PROSTATIC ABSCESSES

DEFINITIONS

Prostatic abscesses are localized accumulations of purulent material within the prostatic parenchyma. **Prostatitis** is an infection of the prostate gland, with or without abscess formation.

GENERAL CONSIDERATIONS AND CLINICALLY RELEVANT PATHOPHYSIOLOGY

Prostatitis is common in dogs but rare in cats. Infection occurs when bacteria colonize the prostatic parenchyma. The source of bacteria is usually the urethra, although a hematogenous infection is possible. Factors predisposing to infection include disruption of normal parenchymal architecture, urethral disease, urinary tract infections, altered urine flow, altered prostatic secretions, and reduced host immunity. Prostatic cystic hyperplasia, squamous metaplasia, and cysts increase the risk of infection. Androgenic hormones are necessary for prostatic secretions; estrogenic hormones decrease secretory activity and may cause prostatic squamous metaplasia leading to cyst formation with subsequent abscessation. Microabscesses form and coalesce, causing large abscesses if not treated promptly. Enlargement of the prostate compresses the colon (and rarely the urethra), causing obstruction. Abscess rupture may cause septicemia, peritonitis, and cardiovascular collapse. A high prostatic secretion concentration of zinc probably provides antibacterial activity and normal sperm function. The prostatic epithelium creates a blood/prostate barrier because of its lipid bilayer. Bacterial colonization of the prostate is reduced by normal defense mechanisms (Table 23-28).

DIAGNOSIS
Clinical Presentation

Signalment. Abscesses primarily occur in older, sexually intact males with prostatitis, squamous metaplasia, or cysts. Although prostatic abscesses may occur in dogs as young as 2 years of age, 81 of 92 affected dogs (88%) in one study were older than 8 years (mean, 10.8 years) (Mullen, Matthiesen, Scavelli, 1990).

History. The dog may have recurrent or nonresponsive urinary tract infections. Animals are usually presented because of an acute onset of depression/lethargy, straining to urinate or defecate, hematuria, vomiting, discomfort or pain, and polyuria/polydipsia (Table 23-29). Other clinical signs may include fever, anorexia, diarrhea, and dehydration.

Physical Examination Findings

Abscessed prostates are generally enlarged, painful, and asymmetric with fluctuant areas (Tables 23-30 and 23-31). Rectal palpation is often painful, and caudal abdominal pain, lumbar pain, and pelvic limb stiffness may also occur. Peritonitis may cause abdominal distention. The scrotum and testicles should be palpated for evidence of masses, enlargement, or increased sensitivity. Some animals have perineal hernias, subcutaneous edema, and/or feminization. Depression, fever, anorexia, vomiting, diarrhea, and dehydration are associated with severe infections. Additionally, signs of tachycardia, pale or injected mucous membranes, delayed capillary refill, and/or weak pulses suggest sepsis and shock.

Radiography/Ultrasonography

Radiographic changes include prostatomegaly, indistinct borders, and occasional mineralization (Table 23-32). Loss of abdominal detail suggests peritonitis (see p. 193). Contrast procedures may show reflux into the prostatic parenchyma and alteration in urethral diameter. Ultrasonographic evaluation identifies hyperechoic, intraparenchymal, fluid-filled spaces.

Laboratory Findings

Neutrophilic leukocytosis with a left shift, toxic neutrophils, and monocytosis may occur. Additional abnormalities may include elevated serum alkaline phosphatase and alanine transaminase activities, creatinine concentrations, hyperglobulinemia, hypoglycemia, and hypokalemia. Hematuria, pyuria, and bacteriuria are common on urinalysis. Prostatic wash or fine-needle aspiration cytology yields highly cellular smears with large numbers of neutrophils and smaller numbers of macrophages and epithelial cells. Squamous metaplasia, hyperplasia, or normal epithelial cells may be detected. The most commonly isolated bacteria are listed in Table 23-33. Occasionally, anaerobic organisms or *Mycoplasma* are isolated. Urine culture (in addition to prostatic fluid culture) should be performed because concurrent infections are

TABLE 23-28

Normal Prostatic Defense Mechanisms Against Infection

- Local production of IgA and IgG prostatic antibacterial factor
- Mechanical urethral flushing during urination
- Urethral high-pressure zone
- Urethral peristalsis
- Surface characteristics of the urethral mucosa

TABLE 23-29

Frequency of Clinical Signs in 92 Dogs with Prostatic Abscesses

Depression/lethargy	85%
Straining to urinate or defecate	65%
Hematuria	54%
Vomiting	35%
Discomfort or pain	26%
Polyuria/polydipsia	18%

From Mullen, Matthiesen, Scavelli: *J Am Anim Hosp Assoc* 26:369, 1990.

TABLE 23-30

Frequency of Physical Examination Findings on Rectal Palpation in 92 Dogs with Prostatic Abscesses

Prostatomegaly	93%
Pain	73%
Asymmetry with fluctuant areas	49%

*From Mullen, Matthiesen, Scavelli: *J Am Anim Hosp Assoc* 26:369, 1990.

common. Antimicrobial sensitivity should be determined for all pathogens. Histologic evaluation may show localized or diffuse inflammation; glandular lumens are typically filled with neutrophils, bacteria, and necrotic debris. Fibrosis, atrophy, and stromal accumulations of lymphocytes and plasma cells are found with chronic prostatitis.

DIFFERENTIAL DIAGNOSIS

Differential diagnoses include prostatitis, prostatic cyst, periprostatic cyst, prostatic neoplasm, prostatic hyperplasia, rectal mass, and intrapelvic masses.

MEDICAL MANAGEMENT

Prostatitis and small prostatic abscesses are treated with antibiotics, fluid therapy, and nutritional support. If the animal is in septic shock (systemic inflammatory response syndrome), fluid replacement therapy should be initiated as soon as possible (Table 23-34). Flunixin meglumine may also be administered. If hypokalemia (see Table 16-35, p. 282) and hyponatremia are present, intravenous supplementation is required. Hypoglycemia is common in septic shock, and glucose may need to be added to the fluids (i.e., 2.5% to 5% dextrose) or given as a slow IV bolus if rapid replacement is necessary (see Table 23-34). Severe metabolic acidosis requires bicarbonate therapy (see Table 22-2, p. 482). Corticosteroid administration in septic patients is controversial and its use with flunixin meglumine increases the risk of gastrointestinal ulceration. Urine output should be monitored (normal urine output is more than 1 to 2 ml/kg/hr).

Broad-spectrum antibiotic therapy should be initiated as soon as the diagnosis is made. Ampicillin plus enrofloxacin (Table 23-35) is an effective combination in most animals with septic shock. However, amikacin plus clindamycin or amikacin plus metronidazole may be necessary if anaerobic infection is suspected. A second-generation cephalosporin (e.g., cefoxitin sodium) may also be used if gram-negative aerobic plus anaerobic infection is suspected. If resistant bacterial infection is present in an animal with renal compromise, imipenem may be considered (see Table 23-35). Initial antibiotic therapy should be altered based on results of aerobic and anaerobic culture of prostatic or abdominal fluids obtained at surgery.

SURGICAL TREATMENT

Acute bacterial prostatitis and prostatic abscesses are potentially life-threatening. Shock therapy must be initiated promptly (see above). Large abscesses should be drained and castration performed when the patient is stable. Castration may reduce the duration of infection. Prostatic biopsy should be performed during drainage or resection. Subtotal prostatectomy (see p. 534) is indicated in stable patients for recurrent abscessation or cysts that have not responded to drainage procedures. Rarely, total prostatectomy (see p. 534) is performed for recurrent prostatic infections.

TABLE 23-31

Clinical Signs of Prostatic Disease

Signs	Diagnosis			
	Hyperplasia	**Infection Abscess**	**Cyst**	**Neoplasia**
Prostatomegaly	+	+	+	±
Symmetric prostatic enlargement	+	±	±	±
Pain on prostatic palpation	−	±	−	±
Fluctuant prostate	−	±	+	−
Lymph node enlargement	−	±	−	±
Ultrasound	normal to ↑ echogenicity	hypoechoic cavities	anechoic cavities	hyperechoic or heterogenous irregular urethra
Cytology	hemorrhage	inflammation, bacteria	hemorrhage	atypical cells ± inflammation & bacteria
Peripheral leukocytosis	−	+	−	±
Pyuria	rare	+	rare	±
Systemic signs	±	+	±	±

+ = present; − = absent; ± = variable

Preoperative Management

The animal should be stabilized before surgery (see above). Place a urinary catheter before surgery to facilitate intraoperative identification of the urethra.

Anesthesia

Anesthetic recommendations for animals in shock are provided in Table 23-24. Anesthetic recommendations for animals undergoing reproductive surgery are on p. 519.

TABLE 23-32

Radiographic Changes in 92 Dogs with Prostatic Abscesses

Prostatomegaly	85%
Indistinct prostatic borders	27%

From Mullen, Matthiesen, Scavell: *J Am Anim Hosp Assoc* 26:369, 1990.

TABLE 23-33

Most Commonly Isolated Bacterial Organisms in Animals with Prostatic Abscesses

- *Escherichia coli*
- *Pseudomonas* spp.
- *Staphylococcus* spp.
- *Streptococcus* spp.
- *Proteus* spp.

TABLE 23-34

Shock Treatment

Lactated Ringer's Solution or Physiologic Saline Solution
Dogs
Up to 90 ml/kg/hr (to effect)

Cats
Up to 60 ml/kg/hr (to effect)

OR

Hetastarch
5-10 ml/kg (up to 20 ml/kg/day)

OR

7% Hypertonic Saline
4-5 ml/kg (up to 10 ml/kg/day), then isotonic crystalloids at 10-20 ml/kg/hr (to effect)

OR

7% Saline and Dextran 70
3-5 ml/kg (up to 10 ml/kg/day), then isotonic crystalloids at 10-20 ml/kg/hr (to effect)

Flunixin Meglumine (Banamine)
1 mg/kg IV, once or twice if in septic shock

50% Dextrose
1-2 ml/kg IV

Surgical Anatomy

Surgical anatomy of the prostate is provided on p. 521.

Positioning

The ventral abdomen and medial thighs should be clipped and aseptically prepared for surgery and the prepuce flushed with a 0.1% povidone-iodine or a 1:40 dilution of 2% chlorhexidine solution. The patient is positioned in dorsal recumbency for a midline celiotomy.

SURGICAL TECHNIQUE

Large abscesses or cysts should be drained. The choice of drainage procedures depends on the size and location of the abscess/cyst. Marsupialization (see p. 559) is an option if the abscess/cyst can be mobilized to the ventral abdominal wall and the capsule is capable of holding sutures. It is more commonly used for cysts than for abscesses. Prostatic omentalization is a recently described technique that may decrease postoperative care for patients with prostatic abscesses (White, Williams, 1995). Perform castration before performing the abdominal exploration.

Multiple Drain Technique

Place a urethral catheter. Expose the prostate through a ventral midline celiotomy from umbilicus to the pubis. Extend the incision caudally and perform a pubic osteotomy if necessary to adequately expose the prostate (see p. 488). Place Balfour retractors to facilitate exposure. Explore the abdomen and isolate the bladder and prostate with laparotomy sponges. Place traction sutures through the bladder wall to retract the prostate cranially. Dissect the ventral fat pad from the prostatic capsule. Insert a large-gauge needle into the abscess/cyst, collect a sample for culture and susceptibility testing, and suction its contents. Avoiding vessels and nerves, incise the ventral aspect of

TABLE 23-35

Antibiotic Therapy in Animals with Septic Shock

Ampicillin
22 mg/kg IV, TID

Enrofloxacin (Baytril)
5-10 mg/kg IV, BID

Amikacin (Amiglyde-V)
30 mg/kg IV, SID

Clindamycin (Cleocin)
11 mg/kg IV, TID

Metronidazole (Flagyl)
10 mg/kg IV, TID

Cefoxitin (Mefoxin)
15-30 mg/kg IV, TID to QID

Imipenem (Primaxin)
3-10 mg/kg IV, TID to QID

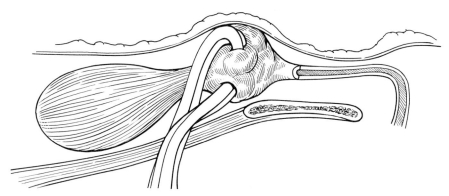

FIG. 23-18
Prostatic abscesses and cysts may be treated using multiple Penrose drains that exit the abdomen in the prepubic area.

the prostate over the abscess/cyst cavity. Digitally break down all trabecula and fibrous bands to connect adjacent abscesses/cysts, creating a common cavity. Suction and lavage the cavity to remove fluid accumulations. Debride necrotic tissue. Place two to four Penrose drains (½ inch) transversely across the ventrolateral aspect of both lobes of the prostate (Fig. 23-18). Periprostatic drains may also be placed. Alternatively, place a tube drain into the abscess/cyst cavity for continuous suction drainage. Exteriorize the end of the drain(s) 2 to 3 cm lateral to the abdominal incision and prepuce. Biopsy the prostatic parenchyma. Secure the drains to the skin with cruciate sutures (e.g., 3-0 nylon). Lavage the surgical site and entire abdomen if contamination has occurred. Surround the surgical site with omentum and periprostatic fat. Close the abdomen routinely. Remove drains in 1 to 3 weeks.

Omentalization

Expose, isolate, and culture the prostate as described above for drain insertion. Make stab incisions bilaterally in the lateral aspects of the prostate gland and remove the purulent material by suction. Explore and digitally break down any loculated abscesses within the parenchyma. Identify the prostatic urethra by palpation of the previously placed urethral catheter. Place a Penrose drain around the prostatic urethra within the parenchyma to elevate the gland and facilitate irrigation of the abscess cavities with warm saline. Enlarge the stab incisions by resection of the lateral capsular tissue. Submit excised tissue for histopathologic examination. Introduce omentum through one capsulotomy wound with forceps introduced through the contralateral wound. Pass the omentum around the prostatic urethra, exit it through the same incision, and anchor it to itself with absorbable mattress sutures. Close the abdomen routinely.

POSTOPERATIVE CARE AND ASSESSMENT

Analgesics should be given as necessary (see Table 23-25) and the patient monitored for sepsis, shock, and anemia. Fluid and nutritional support should be provided until the patient is stable and eating. Appropriate antibiotics should be given for 2 to 3 weeks. Ideally, urine or prostatic fluid culture should be performed 3 to 5 days after starting antibiotics and 2 to 3 days after antibiotics are discontinued. The abdomen should be bandaged to protect drains or suction apparatus, and an Elizabethan collar, bucket, or sidebars used to prevent self-trauma and drain removal. Water-insoluble ointments may be applied around drains to prevent skin scalding. Bandages should be changed daily or when "strike-through" is detected. Drains may be removed when the discharge becomes serosanguineous and diminished in volume (1 to 3 weeks). Recurring or persistent infection should be identified by culturing prostatic fluid and performing ultrasonography every 3 to 4 months for 1 year.

COMPLICATIONS

The most common short-term complications following drainage are provided in Table 23-36. Urine may be voided through the drains for a few days if urethral erosion is present. Scalding around drains and subcutaneous edema may occur. Drains may be prematurely removed by the patient. Subtotal prostatectomy may cause shock, urine leakage, and urinary incontinence. Death or urinary incontinence is more common following subtotal prostatectomy than drainage procedures.

Long-term complications following drainage and resection include recurrent prostatitis, abscesses, urinary tract infections, urinary incontinence, urethrocutaneous fistula formation, and periprostatic cyst formation. In one study, recurrence of prostatic disease was 18%, urinary tract infections was 33%, and urinary incontinence was 46% following implantation of drains (Mullen, Matthiesen, Scavelli, 1990).

PROGNOSIS

Antibiotics and supportive therapy may resolve small abscesses. Large, untreated abscesses will eventually cause septicemia, toxemia, and death. Immediate postoperative mortality may approach 25% (Mullen, Matthiesen, Scavelli, 1990). If a prostatic abscess has ruptured, mortality approaches 50% (Mullen, Matthiesen, Scavelli, 1990). Fair to excellent results are expected if the patient survives 2 weeks after surgery. Peritonitis may occur after abscess rupture or surgical contamination. The prognosis after omentalization appears good if sufficient omentum is placed within the prostate.

References

Mullen HS, Matthiesen DT, Scavelli TD: Results of surgery and postoperative complications in 92 dogs treated for prostatic abscessation by a multiple Penrose drain technique, *J Am Anim Hosp Assoc* 26:369, 1990.

TABLE 23-36
Short-Term Complications after Prostatic Drainage

- Hypoproteinemia
- Subcutaneous edema
- Hypoglycemia
- Anemia
- Sepsis
- Shock
- Hypokalemia
- Incisional infections
- Urine leakage
- Urinary incontinence

White RAS, Williams JM: Intracapsular prostatic omentalization: a new technique for management of prostatic abscesses in dogs, *Vet Surg* 24:390, 1995.

Suggested Reading

Basinger RR et al: Urodynamic alterations associated with clinical prostatic diseases and prostatic surgery in 23 dogs, *J Am Anim Hosp Assoc* 25:385, 1989.

Cowan LA et al: Effects of castration on chronic bacterial prostatitis in dogs, *J Am Vet Med Assoc* 199:346, 1991.

Cowan LA et al: Effects of bacterial infection and castration on prostatic tissue zinc concentration in dogs, *Am J Vet Res* 52:1262, 1991.

Klausner JS, Obsorne CA: Management of canine bacterial prostatitis, *J Am Vet Med Assoc* 182:292, 1983.

Krawiec DR, Heflin D: Study of prostatic disease in dogs: 177 cases (1981–1986), *J Am Vet Med Assoc* 200:1119, 1992.

Matthiesen DT, Manfra Marretta S: Complications associated with the surgical treatment of prostatic abscessation, *Problems in Vet Med: Urogenital Surgical Conditions* 1:63, 1989.

PROSTATIC CYSTS

DEFINITIONS

A **prostatic cyst** is a nonseptic, fluid-filled cavity within or attached to the prostate.

SYNONYMS

Retention cyst, true cyst, cystic hyperplasia, hematocyst, and **periprostatic cysts** are terms used for different types of prostatic cysts.

GENERAL CONSIDERATIONS AND CLINICALLY RELEVANT PATHOPHYSIOLOGY

Parenchymal prostatic cysts occur within or have a physical communication with the prostatic parenchyma (Fig. 23-19). They are common in dogs and may be associated with benign prostatic hyperplasia (see p. 552). Their etiology is unknown, but some are congenital. Sertoli cell tumors or exogenous estrogens may cause squamous metaplasia, which occludes ducts resulting in secretory stasis with progressive acinar dilation. Cysts coalesce as they enlarge and are surrounded by dense collagen that can ossify. Small cysts often become confluent, forming larger cavities. Parenchymal cysts are typically found throughout the gland. Histologically, parenchymal prostatic cysts are lined by compressed epithelium (transitional, cuboidal, or squamous) and filled with secretory material and cellular debris.

Periprostatic cysts are rare compared to other types of prostatic disease. Periprostatic cysts are adjacent and attached to the prostate, but seldom communicate with the parenchyma. They may originate from the uterus masculinus, an embryonic structure derived from the müllerian duct system and attached on the dorsal prostatic midline. These cysts are often large, extending into the perineal fossa or abdomen. They may displace and compromise adjacent viscera and its function. Periprostatic cysts are usually filled with pale yellow to orange fluid; hemorrhage will cause it to be brownish-red. Histologically, the wall of a periprostatic cyst resembles the wall of a parenchymal cyst (compressed epithelium and dense collagen). Some walls are calcified. Prostatic cysts may become infected and abscess.

DIAGNOSIS
Clinical Presentation

Signalment. Prostatic cysts are most common in older, intact male, large-breed dogs.

History. Dogs are often asymptomatic until the cysts become large enough to cause rectal, bladder, or urethral obstruction. A perineal bulge or abdominal distention may occur with large cysts. Presenting complaints include depression, inappetence, stranguria, tenesmus, and/or bloody penile discharge.

Physical Examination Findings

Clinical signs and examination findings due to prostatic cysts are similar to those due to prostatic hyperplasia (see p. 552). However, periprostatic cysts are asymmetric, fluctuant, and sometimes cause abdominal distention. The most common physical finding is a palpable abdominal mass. Sterile prostatic cysts are not painful. The scrotum and testicles should be palpated for evidence of concurrent masses, enlargement, or increased sensitivity, which suggest Sertoli cell tumor.

Radiography/Ultrasonography

Prostatic cysts and periprostatic cysts may be difficult to differentiate from the urinary bladder without a cystourethrogram. Prostate or cyst wall calcification may be detected on plain films. Ultrasonography helps detect and define cavitary changes. Periprostatic cysts are usually large anechoic structures with internal septa. Some communicate with large anechoic cavities within the prostatic parenchyma. Ultrasound guided aspirates can be obtained; however, be careful to prevent iatrogenic peritonitis if infection is likely.

Laboratory Findings

Specific laboratory abnormalities are rare. Aspiration of a sterile, yellow to serosanguineous fluid with minimal inflammation suggests a periprostatic cyst. Cytologic evaluation reveals prostatic epithelial cells and few leukocytes, but more erythrocytes and hemosiderophages than with prostatic hy-

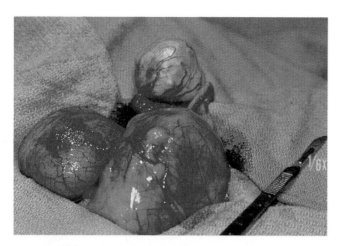

FIG. 23-19
Intraoperative appearance of a large prostatic cyst with squamous metaplasia. Note the enlarged, nodular cryptorchid testicle (*dorsal*) in which a Sertoli cell tumor was diagnosed histologically.

perplasia. The presence of numerous squamous epithelial cells suggests squamous metaplasia.

DIFFERENTIAL DIAGNOSIS

Differential diagnoses include prostatic abscess, squamous metaplasia, neoplasia, or hyperplasia.

MEDICAL MANAGEMENT

Medical therapy includes treatment of constipation and urine retention. Stool softeners (see p. 536) may be given and the bladder drained by centesis or catheterization as needed. Percutaneous drainage by centesis is palliative but may cause abscessation.

SURGICAL TREATMENT

Treatment for small parenchymal cysts is castration. Dogs with large cysts should be castrated and the cyst either drained, resected, or debulked. Incomplete resection may be necessary to avoid incontinence.

Preoperative Management

Animals with prostatic cysts are generally stable. Perioperative antibiotics are reasonable if marsupialization or a prolonged surgery are anticipated.

Anesthesia

Anesthetic recommendations for animals undergoing reproductive surgery are provided on p. 519.

Positioning

The ventral abdomen, ventral perineum, and medial thighs are clipped and prepared for aseptic surgery. The dog is positioned in dorsal recumbency for a midline celiotomy.

SURGICAL TECHNIQUE

Castration should be performed and large cysts resected or drained. Cystic fluid should be cultured and a prostatic biopsy obtained (see p. 533). Nonresectable cysts may be drained by marsupialization or multiple drains (see p. 556). Subtotal prostatectomy (see p. 534) may be appropriate for recurring cysts.

Marsupialization

Expose and isolate the prostate as described on p. 556 for drain insertion. Make a second incision (5 to 8 cm) through the abdominal wall lateral to the prepuce over the abscess/cyst cavity (Fig. 23-20, A). Excise 0.5 to 1 cm of abdominal muscle (Fig. 23-20, B). Suture capsule or cyst wall to the external rectus fascia (Fig. 23-20, C). Use continuous or interrupted 3-0 to 4-0 polydioxanone or polyglyconate sutures. Facilitate suturing by having an assistant elevate the prostate toward the abdominal wall. Incise the abscess/cyst wall and suction the contents. Place a second layer of simple continuous or interrupted sutures (e.g., 3-0 or 4-0 nylon, polypropylene) between the skin edge and capsule/cyst edge (Fig. 23-20, D and E). Biopsy the prostatic parenchyma. Digitally break down trabeculae and fibrous bands to create a confluent cavity. Lavage the cavity and surgical site, place omentum around the marsupialization, and close the abdomen in three layers. An alternative technique is to incise the ventrolateral aspect of the cyst/abscess wall and suction the cavity before suturing it to the rectus fascia. The capsule/cyst wall is then sutured 5 mm from the incised edge of the cavity to the rectus fascia. This variation has a higher risk of abdominal contamination.

POSTOPERATIVE CARE AND ASSESSMENT

Analgesics (see Table 23-25) and supportive care (e.g., fluids, electrolytes) should be given as necessary. Monitor closely for shock and infection. Medical therapy may manage urine retention, constipation, and discomfort. See p. 557 for postoperative care and potential complications following prostatic or cystic drain placement. Drains should be left in place for 1 to 3 weeks. Marsupialization may result in a permanent fistula or may close prematurely. Urine may be voided through the marsupialization for a few days if urethral erosion is present.

PROGNOSIS

The prognosis is good to fair after castration and surgical drainage. Some prostatic and periprostatic cysts recur and require repeated drainage; however, this is rare if the dog is castrated. Overzealous resection may cause detrusor atony, incontinence, or bladder ischemia.

Suggested Reading

Aultman SH, Betts CW: An unusual case of a prostatic cyst: utilization of a suprapubic catheter, *J Am Anim Hosp Assoc* 14:638, 1978.

Krawiec DR, Heflin D: Study of prostatic disease in dogs: 177 cases (1981–1986), *J Am Vet Med Assoc* 200:1119, 1992.

Stowater JL, Lamb CR: Ultrasonographic features of paraprostatic cysts in nine dogs, *Vet Radiol* 30:232, 1989.

FIG. 23-20
A, To marsupialize a prostatic cyst or abscess, make a longitudinal incision lateral to the prepuce over the enlarged mass. **B,** Excise an ellipse of abdominal muscle, **C,** then suture the prostatic capsule to the external rectus sheath. Make an incision through the prostatic capsule and, **D** and **E,** suture the edge of the capsule to skin.

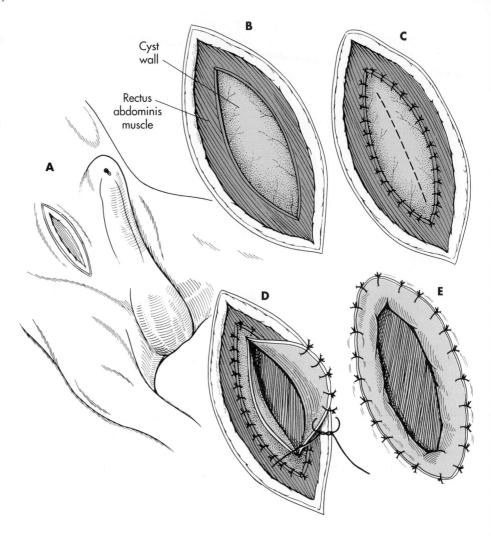

Cyst wall

Rectus abdominis muscle

PROSTATIC NEOPLASIA

DEFINITIONS
Prostatic tumors may originate from epithelial tissue (carcinomas), smooth muscle tissue (leiomyosarcoma), or vascular structures (hemangiosarcoma).

GENERAL CONSIDERATIONS AND CLINICALLY RELEVANT PATHOPHYSIOLOGY
While prostatic neoplasia is the most common prostatic disease in neutered, male dogs, it is still uncommon in dogs and rare in cats. Testicular hormones are not believed to cause prostatic tumors, but adrenal and pituitary hormones may be influential. Most prostatic tumors are adenocarcinomas (Table 23-37). Prostatic carcinomas are locally invasive and metastasize early to regional lymph nodes (iliac, pelvic, and sublumbar), lung, and bone. They frequently invade bone, bladder, colon, and surrounding tissues by direct extension. Other metastatic sites include liver, spleen, kidney, heart, and adrenal glands. Bone involvement may cause pain or pathologic fractures. Hypertrophic osteopathy has occasionally been associated with prostatic tumors. Prostatic enlargement causes compression and partial obstruction of the colon, rec-

tum, and sometimes urethra. Pitting edema of the pelvic limbs may occur secondary to lymphatic invasion of the tumor. Most tumors involve the trigone and urethra and have metastasized at the time of diagnosis. The behavior of feline prostatic tumors is unknown.

DIAGNOSIS
Clinical Presentation
Signalment. Prostatic neoplasia occurs in both intact and neutered males. Medium- to large-breed dogs are over-represented, but there is no obvious predisposition. The average age of occurrence is 8 to 10 years.

History. Signs may include weight loss, pelvic limb lameness or weakness, tenesmus, dyschezia, urine retention or incontinence, stranguria, dysuria, polyuria, polydipsia, hematuria, pelvic limb edema, and abdominal, pelvic, or lumbar pain. Prostatic neoplasia may cause marked emaciation and debility. Metastasis may produce other signs (e.g., dyspnea).

Physical Examination Findings
The animal may be debilitated and weak. Lymph node infiltration and lymphatic obstruction can cause pelvic limb edema. The prostate may be normal sized, but is often asymmetrically enlarged. Pain, firmness, fixation, and nodular ir-

regularity are characteristic of prostatic neoplasia. Sublumbar lymph node enlargement may be detected during rectal examination. Skeletal palpation sometimes elicits pain secondary to bone metastasis.

Radiography/Ultrasonography

Thoracic radiographs should be evaluated for metastasis. Abdominal and pelvic radiographs should be evaluated for prostatic size and mineralization, lymph node enlargement, colon displacement, and osteolytic or proliferative vertebral or pelvic lesions. Retrograde urethrocystography may determine urethral size and mucosal smoothness, prostatic symmetry, and urethroprostatic reflux. Most prostatic tumors involve the urethra and trigone. Ultrasonography defines the prostatic mass as cystic or solid. It also evaluates abdominal lymph nodes. Most prostatic adenocarcinomas are hyperechoic. Prostatic aspiration and biopsy are facilitated by ultrasound guidance. Nuclear bone scans can locate metastatic sites.

Laboratory Findings

Hematology, serum biochemistry profile, urinalysis, urine culture, and electrocardiography are used to assess the patient's condition. Results are nonspecific for prostatic neoplasia, although paraneoplastic syndromes and concurrent problems may be identified. Anemia, hematuria, and/or pyuria may be detected.

Fine-needle aspiration of prostatic neoplasia may yield a moderately cellular sample with abnormal epithelial cells. Neoplastic-appearing epithelial cells have large, prominent, multiple nuclei with multiple nucleoli and cytoplasmic vacuolation. Additional cytologic criteria of malignancy are provided in Table 23-38. Prostatic washes are less reliable in obtaining neoplastic cells. Biopsy is needed for definitive diagnosis.

DIFFERENTIAL DIAGNOSIS

Differential diagnoses include prostatic hyperplasia, abscesses, cysts, periprostatic cysts, prostatitis, rectal masses, or pelvic masses.

MEDICAL MANAGEMENT

Efficacy of chemotherapy and radiation therapy has not been reported for prostatic tumors. Ketoconazole and luteinizing hormone-releasing hormone agonists have been suggested. Ketoconazole inhibits testicular and adrenal testosterone synthesis. Luteinizing hormone-releasing hormone agonists ultimately decrease FSH, LH, and testosterone release.

SURGICAL TREATMENT

Treatment is rarely successful. Treatment protocols combining surgery, chemotherapy, and radiation therapy are being investigated, but their efficacy is presently unknown.

Preoperative Management

Clip and aseptically prepare the ventral abdomen, ventral perineum, and medial thighs.

TABLE 23-37
Prostatic Tumor Types

Carcinomas
- Adenocarcinoma
- Transitional cell carcinoma
- Squamous cell carcinoma
- Undifferentiated

Leiomyosarcomas

Hemangiosarcomas

TABLE 23-38
Additional Cytologic Criteria of Malignancy

- Variation in nuclear and nucleolar size
- Variable and increased nuclear cytoplasmic ratio
- Nuclear molding
- Abnormal mitotic figures
- Coarsely clumped chromatin

Anesthesia

Anesthetic recommendations for animals undergoing reproductive surgery are on p. 519.

Surgical Anatomy

Surgical anatomy of the male reproductive tract is on p. 521.

Positioning

The patient is positioned in dorsal recumbency for a midline celiotomy. The entire ventral abdomen and inguinal area should be clipped and prepared for aseptic surgery.

SURGICAL TECHNIQUE

Castration may temporarily slow tumor growth. Prostatectomy may be curative if the tumor is diagnosed early. Unfortunately, most tumors are advanced when diagnosed, making preservation of trigonal innervation impossible. Such dogs often are unacceptable pets after prostatectomy because of urinary incontinence.

POSTOPERATIVE CARE AND ASSESSMENT

Analgesics (see Table 23-25) and fluids should be given as necessary. The bladder should be decompressed and urine diverted for 4 to 5 days with a urinary catheter or cystostomy tube after prostatectomy (see p. 534). Patients should be monitored for urine leakage, incontinence, and/or infection. Reevaluation at frequent intervals for local recurrence and metastasis is recommended. Complications and treatment of animals following prostatectomy are on p. 536.

PROGNOSIS

The prognosis is poor because of metastasis, recurrence, and poor quality of life associated with urinary incontinence.

Hormonal therapy has not been useful in dogs. Most untreated dogs are euthanized within 1 to 3 months because of progressive clinical signs.

Suggested Reading

Basinger RR et al: Urodynamic alterations associated with clinical prostatic diseases and prostatic surgery in 23 dogs, *J Am Anim Hosp Assoc* 25:385, 1989.

Bell RW et al: Clinical and pathologic features of prostatic adenocarcinoma in sexually intact and castrated dogs: 31 cases (1970–1987), *J Am Vet Med Assoc* 199:1623, 1991.

Durham SK, Dietze AE: Prostatic adenocarcinoma with and without metastasis to bone, *J Am Vet Med Assoc* 188:1432, 1986.

Hubbard BS, Vulgamott JC, Liska WD: Prostatic adenocarcinoma in a cat, *J Am Vet Med Assoc* 197:1493, 1990.

Krawiec DR, Heflin D: Study of prostatic disease in dogs: 177 cases (1981–1986), *J Am Vet Med Assoc* 200:1119, 1992.

Turrel JM: Intraoperative radiotherapy of carcinoma of the prostate gland in ten dogs, *J Am Vet Med Assoc* 190:48, 1987.

TESTICULAR AND SCROTAL NEOPLASIA

DEFINITIONS

Sertoli cells are supporting elongated cells of seminiferous tubules that nourish spermatids. **Leydig cells** are interstitial tissue cells, believed to be responsible for internal secretion of testosterone.

GENERAL CONSIDERATIONS AND CLINICALLY RELEVANT PATHOPHYSIOLOGY

Scrotal tumors are most commonly mast cell tumors (MCT) or melanomas. Mast cells are normal immune system cells and are important in inflammatory responses to tissue trauma. Cytoplasmic granules in mast cells contain heparin, histamine, platelet-activating factor, and eosinophilic chemotactic factor. The number and type of granules in MCT depends on the degree of tumor differentiation. Well-differentiated MCT contain more heparin, while undifferentiated tumors have more histamine. The cause of MCT is unknown, although chronically inflamed areas have been reported to be at increased risk for tumor development. In dogs, 50% of MCT are malignant, especially those in the preputial, inguinal, and perineal areas. Regional lymph nodes, spleen, liver, and bone marrow are common metastatic sites. Mast cell tumors have no distinctive appearance. They may be raised, hairless, ulcerated, erythematous, well-defined, and/or diffuse skin thickenings. Manipulation of MCT may cause degranulation, erythema, and wheal formation. Gastroduodenal ulcers occur in up to 80% of dogs with MCT due to histamine release (Howard et al, 1969). Ulcers may cause anorexia, vomiting, diarrhea, and/or melena (see p. 286). Heparin and proteolytic enzyme release may prolong coagulation and delay wound healing after resection. Melanomas originate from melanocytes and melanoblasts, cells of neuroectodermal origin. Masses may be brown-to-black or occasionally nonpigmented. Melanomas are more common in dogs than cats. Tumors originating in the skin tend to be benign. Local recurrence and distant metastasis are common with malignant melanomas. Metastasis usually occurs first to the lymph nodes and then to the lungs.

The most common testicular neoplasms are Sertoli cell tumors, interstitial (Leydig) cell tumors, and seminomas; they occur with equal frequency. Other types of testicular tumors are rare (Table 23-39). Many old dogs have multiple tumors in one or both testicles. Tumors involving scrotal testes are usually benign, while those in cryptorchid testes may be malignant. Metastases are slow growing, but are occasionally detected in the lumbar, deep inguinal, and external iliac lymph nodes. Visceral metastasis is rare. Testicular tumors interfere with testicular function by invading or compressing seminiferous tubules or producing excessive estrogen or testosterone. Interstitial cell tumor production of excess testosterone may contribute to perianal adenomas, perineal hernia, and benign prostatic hyperplasia. Sertoli cell tumors producing excess estrogens may cause squamous metaplasia of the prostate, feminization, and/or myelotoxicity.

Sertoli cell tumors arise from sustentacular cells. Normal and neoplastic Sertoli cells produce estrogenic hormones. Sertoli cell tumors are usually solitary, but may be multiple and bilateral. Sertoli cell tumors are more common in cryptorchid than scrotal testes. Tumors are discrete with expansile growth, compressing and destroying surrounding testicular tissue. Large tumors may cause distention or destruction of the tunic and growth may extend along the spermatic cord. They are firm, multilobulated, and gray-white with areas of necrosis, hemorrhage, or cysts. Dogs with Sertoli cell tumors often have signs of hyperestrogenism (Table 23-40), especially those with large tumors. Signs regress with castration and tumor removal. Persistence or recurrence of clinical signs suggests estrogen-producing metastasis. Sertoli cell tumors have a higher rate of metastasis than other testicular tumors.

Interstitial (Leydig) cell tumors occur in scrotal testes as multiple or solitary forms and frequently coexist with Sertoli cell tumors. Most interstitial cell tumors are benign, soft, encapsulated, and rarely exceed 1 to 2 cm diameter. Interstitial cell tumors may cause the testicle to enlarge but are difficult to palpate. On cut surfaces they are discrete, round, tan to yellow-orange masses with foci of hemorrhage or cystic spaces. Dogs with interstitial cell tumors may be infertile. These tumors produce androgens or contribute to androgenic hormone imbalance. Perineal hernia, perianal adenomas and hyperplasia, and prostatic disease have been associated with interstitial cell tumors.

Seminomas arise from testicular germ cells and occur commonly in cryptorchid and scrotal testicles. They are usually solitary, but may be multiple, bilateral, and coexist with other tumor types. Seminomas can be large, replacing most testicular tissue. They are softer than Sertoli cell tumors with a glistening, pinkish gray-tan, multilobulated, unencapsulated cut surface. Signs of feminization rarely occur. They rarely metastasize.

TABLE 23-39

Scrotal and Testicular Tumors

Scrotal Tumors
- Mast cell tumors (MCT)
- Melanomas

Testicular Tumors
- Sertoli cell
- Interstitial cell
- Seminoma
- Embryonal carcinoma
- Lipoma
- Fibroma
- Hemangioma
- Chondroma
- Teratoma

TABLE 23-40

Signs of Hyperestrogenism

- Bilateral symmetrical alopecia
- Brittle hair
- Poor hair regrowth
- Thin skin
- Hyperpigmentation
- Nipple elongation
- Mammary enlargement
- Penile atrophy
- Preputial swelling and sagging
- Squatting micturition
- Reduced libido
- Male attraction
- Testicular atrophy
- Prostatic atrophy or cystic enlargement
- Myelotoxicosis

DIAGNOSIS
Clinical Presentation

Signalment. Scrotal and testicular tumors are more common in dogs than cats. They usually occur in dogs older than 10 years; however, tumors in cryptorchid animals may occur earlier. Cryptorchidism predisposes to development of Sertoli cell tumors and seminomas. Cryptorchid dogs are 13.6 times more likely to develop testicular tumors than normal dogs (Hayes, Pendergrass, 1976). A breed predisposition for developing testicular tumors has not been identified. Dogs predisposed to MCT include English bulldogs, English bull terriers, boxers, and Boston terriers.

History. Affected, asymptomatic animals may present for evaluation of a mass that has been seen or felt in the scrotal or inguinal areas or for endocrine abnormalities (e.g., changes in hair coat, infertility, lethargy, feminization [see Table 23-40], perianal tumors, or prostatic disease).

Physical Examination Findings

The scrotal skin should be examined for inflammation, nodules, masses, and ulceration. Scrotal skin should be of uniform thickness. Both testicles should be evaluated for symmetry, firmness, irregularity, scrotal adhesions, and sensitivity. Small or deep intraparenchymal testicular tumors are not detectable on palpation, but the testis may be firm and hard. If the animal is cryptorchid, the inguinal area should be checked for a retained testicle and the abdomen for a mass. Enlarged sublumbar lymph nodes and prostate may be detected by rectal examination. The abdomen should be palpated for splenomegaly, hepatomegaly, and lymph node enlargement, signs of metastasis (i.e., with MCT). Sertoli cell tumors and seminomas may cause feminization (see Table 23-40).

Radiography/Ultrasonography

Intraabdominal testicles may be seen radiographically as caudal abdominal masses if they are at least twice the diameter of the small intestine. Radiographs also help identify intraabdominal lymph node enlargement and organomegaly.

Ultrasound delineates scrotal and testicular neoplasia, abscess, ischemia, testicular torsion, and scrotal hernia. Testicular tumors have variable echogenicity.

Laboratory Findings

Complete laboratory analysis (i.e., CBC, panel, urinalysis) is indicated in animals with scrotal or testicular tumors. Non-regenerative anemia, leukopenia, and thrombocytopenia may be associated with hyperestrogenism and myelotoxicosis. Fine-needle aspiration cytology of scrotal and testicular lesions helps identify neoplastic cells, fungal elements, abnormal sperm, bacteria, and inflammation. Fine-needle aspiration of the testicle is rarely performed, but can help differentiate neoplasia from abscesses or granulomas. Cytology of the preputial mucosa may reveal cornification secondary to Sertoli cell tumor estrogen production. Fine-needle aspiration cytology is usually diagnostic for MCT. Animals with MCT should be checked for circulating mast cells, eosinophilia, and basophilia via CBC and buffy coat smear. Microcytic-hypochromic anemia suggests gastrointestinal hemorrhage. More than 10 mast cells per 1000 nucleated cells in the bone marrow is abnormal. Tumor histopathology is necessary to grade the tumor and determine prognosis. Cytology from melanomas usually reveals round to spindle-shaped cells, frequently containing brown-to-black granules.

Brucella canis infections may be diagnosed with an agar-gel immunodiffusion test. Semen evaluation to determine fertility is rarely performed when neoplasia is diagnosed. Serum testosterone levels are sometimes elevated with interstitial cell tumors (Table 23-41). Sertoli cell tumors and seminomas sometimes increase serum estradiol concentrations.

DIFFERENTIAL DIAGNOSIS

Other differentials for testicular masses include sperm granuloma, fibrosis, hematoma, spermatocele, varicocele, orchitis, and epididymitis. Other differential diagnoses for scrotal disease include dermatitis, self-trauma, chemical burn, and laceration. *Brucella canis* infection should be considered in animals presented for scrotal dermatitis, orchitis, reproductive failure, epididymitis, or testicular atrophy.

☞ **N O T E** · Test for *Brucella canis* infection in dogs with unexplained scrotal or testicular disease.

MEDICAL MANAGEMENT

Mast cell tumors may respond to chemotherapy or radiation therapy. The efficacy of chemotherapy or radiation therapy for other scrotal or testicular tumors is unknown.

SURGICAL TREATMENT

Tumor excision gives the best chance for a good prognosis. Removal of both testicles is recommended for testicular neoplasia. Castration is described on p. 524. If the owner insists on preserving breeding potential, unilateral castration of the neoplastic testicle may be performed. The testicles should be submitted for histologic examination. Scrotal ablation (see p. 527) and castration are recommended to treat scrotal tumors and testicular tumors with scrotal adhesions. Even discrete MCT extend deep into surrounding tissue; therefore, 3-cm margins on all sides are recommended.

Preoperative Management

Few patients with testicular tumors are debilitated except those with myelosuppression, testicular torsion, or concurrent diseases. Anemic and thrombocytopenic animals may need blood transfusions and antibiotics to prevent infections. An antihistamine (e.g., diphenhydramine [Benadryl], 0.5 mg/kg intravenously, slowly) should be administered to patients with MCT before surgery, to decrease the effects of tumor histamine release. It may be given intravenously immediately prior to surgery, but should be given extremely slowly to avoid hypotension. Alternately, it may be administered intramuscularly 30 minutes before anesthetic induction. An H_2 antagonist (i.e., ranitidine, cimetidine, or famotidine) or a proton pump inhibitor (i.e., omeprazole) will reduce gastric acid secretion and decrease the incidence and severity of gastrointestinal ulceration. Sucralfate may be given for existing ulcers (Table 23-42). Sucralfate should be given 1 hour after administration of other oral medications because it *may* interfere with their absorption.

Anesthesia

Anesthetic recommendations for animals undergoing reproductive surgery are on p. 519.

Positioning

Position the patient in dorsal recumbency for a prescrotal castration or an exploratory laparotomy. The entire ventral abdomen should be clipped and prepared for exploratory laparotomy; see p. 525 for recommendations for surgical preparation of animals undergoing castration.

SURGICAL TECHNIQUE

Castration and scrotal ablation are described on pp. 524 and 527, respectively.

POSTOPERATIVE CARE AND ASSESSMENT

Analgesics (see Table 23-25) and supportive care should be given as necessary. Patients with MCT should be continued on an H_2 antagonist, proton pump inhibitor, and/or protectant if gastrointestinal ulceration occurs (see Table 23-42). Adjunctive therapy for malignant tumors may prove beneficial. Patients with malignant tumors should be reevaluated every 3 to 4 months for recurrence or metastasis. Complications associated with paraneoplastic syndromes and metastasis may become evident or persist following castration.

PROGNOSIS

Surgery is curative for most testicular tumors. The prognosis for interstitial cell tumors, Sertoli cell tumors without metastasis or myelotoxicity, and seminomas without signs of hyperestrogenism is excellent. Myelotoxicity may be fatal despite appropriate therapy, but usually improves within 2 to 3 weeks of tumor removal. Chemotherapy should be instituted if Sertoli cell tumors or seminomas have metastasized. Low-grade MCT are less likely to recur or metastasize. Nonresectable or incompletely resected MCT may respond to radiation therapy or chemotherapy. Efficacy of nonsurgical treatment modalities for other tumors is unknown.

TABLE 23-41

Normal Serum Testosterone Levels in Males (ng/ml)

Dog (intact)	0.4-10
Dog (castrated)	<0.015
Cat (intact)	1.0-6.0
Cat (castrated)	<0.5

From Rosen DK, Carpenter JL: *J Am Vet Med Assoc* 202:1865, 1993.

TABLE 23-42

Medical Therapy of Gastroduodenal Ulcers

Sucralfate (Carafate)
0.5-1.0 g PO, TID to QID

Cimetidine (Tagamet)
5-10 mg/kg PO, IV or SC, TID to QID

Ranitidine (Zantac)
2 mg/kg PO, IV, IM, SC, BID

Famotidine (Pepcid)
0.5 mg/kg PO, SID to BID

Omeprazole (Prilosec)
0.7-1.5 mg/kg PO, SID to BID

References

Hayes HM, Pendergrass TW: Canine testicular tumors: epidemiologic features of 410 cases, *Int J Cancer* 18:482, 1976.

Howard EB et al: Mastocytoma and gastroduodenal ulceration, *Vet Pathol* 6:146, 1969.

Rosen DK, Carpenter JL: Functional ectopic interstitial cell tumor in a castrated male cat, *J Am Vet Med Assoc* 202:1865, 1993.

Suggested Reading

Johnston GR et al: Ultrasonographic features of testicular neoplasia in dogs: 16 cases (1980–1988), *J Am Vet Med Assoc* 198:1779, 1991.

HYPOSPADIAS

DEFINITION

Hypospadias is a developmental anomaly in males where the urethra opens ventral and caudal to the normal orifice.

GENERAL CONSIDERATIONS AND CLINICALLY RELEVANT PATHOPHYSIOLOGY

Hypospadias is rare and many affected animals have other congenital or developmental anomalies. It occurs as a result of failure of the genital folds and genital swellings to fuse normally during fetal development. This causes abnormal development of the penile urethra, penis, prepuce, and/or scrotum. Hypospadias is accompanied by hypoplasia of the corpus cavernosum urethra. The urethra opens anywhere along its length at one or more locations. Hypospadias is classified based on the location of the urethral opening as glandular, penile, scrotal, perineal, or anal. The prepuce is similarly affected and ventrally incomplete. In some cases the penis may be underdeveloped and abnormal (ventral or caudal deviation, blunt) and the scrotum may be divided. Urine may pool within the prepuce causing irritation and infection of the penis and preputial lining (balanoposthitis).

☞ **N O T E** • Do not use animals with hypospadias for breeding.

DIAGNOSIS
Clinical Presentation

Signalment. Breed predisposition has not been documented. The defect is present at birth.

History. Small defects and those occurring in the glans may not cause problems. Some patients with hypospadias of the glans and abnormal preputial development may present because of a chronically exposed penis. Larger and more caudal urethral openings cause urine pooling within the prepuce or dermatitis due to urine contact. A preputial discharge may occur. There may be a history of urinary incontinence or infection.

Physical Examination Findings

Skin irritation or preputial inflammation may be identified. The preputial opening may be incompletely formed and the scrotum divided. The penis should be completely extruded from the prepuce and examined. A fibrous band may be noted running from the glans to the urethral opening and deviating the penis. The urethral opening is identified on the ventral aspect of the penis along the normal urethral path.

Radiography

Radiographs are unnecessary, but occasionally identify other congenital anomalies.

Laboratory Findings

Urine culture may be positive. Other laboratory results are nonspecific.

DIFFERENTIAL DIAGNOSIS

Differential diagnoses include pseudohermaphrodite, true hermaphrodite, urethral fistula or trauma, persistent penile frenulum, and penile hypoplasia.

MEDICAL MANAGEMENT

Urine scalding should be treated by frequent bathing and application of water-impermeable ointments near the urethral opening. The penile mucosa should be kept moist with ointments. If urine pooling occurs the prepuce should be flushed daily with physiologic saline solution.

SURGICAL TREATMENT

Abnormal urethral openings near the penile tip may not require surgery. In other cases, reconstruction (with or without penile amputation) is advised. Preputial reconstruction is needed in patients with an incompletely formed preputial orifice and hypospadia at the glans. Constant penile exposure is prevented by closing the preputial orifice to its normal extent. Excision of the external genitalia is recommended for major developmental defects involving the urethra, prepuce, and penis. Penile amputation is also indicated for severe trauma and neoplasia. Neutering affected animals is recommended.

Preoperative Management

A preoperatively placed urethral catheter facilitates urethral identification.

Anesthesia

Surgery on pediatric patients should be delayed until they are approximately 8 weeks old. Recommendations for anesthetic management of neonates for reproductive surgery are on p. 519.

Surgical Anatomy

Surgical anatomy of the penis is provided on p. 522.

Positioning

Dorsal recumbency is recommended unless the urethra opens in the perineal or anal regions and a perineal position is preferred. The ventral abdomen, medial thighs, and ventral perineum should be clipped and prepared for aseptic surgery.

SURGICAL TECHNIQUE
Prepuce Reconstruction

Incise the mucocutaneous junction on the caudoventral aspect of the prepuce (Fig. 23-21). Separate mucosa from skin. Reappose the mucosa beginning at a more cranial location with simple interrupted sutures (e.g., 4-0 to 6-0 polydioxanone or polyglyconate). Appose skin with a second layer of simple interrupted sutures (e.g., 3-0 or 4-0 nylon or polypropylene). If this creates an orifice that is too small to allow penile extrusion, incise the dorsocranial aspect of the prepuce and suture the mucosa to the skin on each side with interrupted sutures (e.g., 4-0 nylon or polypropylene).

Urethral Reconstruction

Close small urethral defects by incising the margins of the defect and apposing the urethral edges over a urethral catheter. Use 4-0 to 6-0 monofilament absorbable suture (e.g., polydioxanone, polyglyconate) in a simple interrupted or continuous pattern. Close skin over the urethral repair with 3-0 or 4-0 nonabsorbable suture (e.g., nylon or polypropylene) using an appositional pattern.

Subtotal Penile Amputation

Make an elliptical incision around the prepuce, penis, and scrotum preserving adequate skin for closure (Fig. 23-22, A). Dissect the penis from the body wall from cranial to caudal (Fig. 23-22, B). Ligate or cauterize preputial vessels. Perform a castration as with scrotal ablation (see p. 527).

Locate and ligate the dorsal penile vessels just caudal to the desired amputation site. Perform a urethrostomy; scrotal urethrostomy (see p. 489) is preferred. Reflect or transect the retractor penis muscle. Make a midline urethral incision over the catheter. Place a circumferential catgut ligature around the penis just caudal to the proposed amputation site and just cranial to the urethrostomy site. Amputate the penis in a wedge fashion (Fig. 23-22, C). Appose the tunica albuginea to close the end of the penis with 3-0 or 4-0 absorbable suture (e.g., polydioxanone or polyglyconate). Appose urethral mucosa to skin at the urethrostomy site with simple interrupted 4-0 to 6-0 absorbable or nonabsorbable sutures (e.g., polydioxanone, polyglyconate, polypropylene, nylon) (Fig. 23-22, D). Close subcutaneous tissue and skin cranial and caudal to the urethrostomy in two layers (Fig. 23-22, E).

POSTOPERATIVE CARE AND ASSESSMENT

Analgesics should be given as necessary (see Table 23-25) and urination monitored by observing for a nonrestricted urine stream. Hemorrhage may occur from cavernous tissue for days, especially during excitement or urination. Hemorrhage may be minimized by keeping the animal quiet and calm during the early postoperative period. An Elizabethan collar, bucket, or sidebars should be used to prevent self-trauma. Hemorrhage, urine leakage, infection, seroma, and dehiscence are potential incisional complications. Urethral or preputial reconstruction may cause stricture formation. Urethral stricture may interfere with urine flow and produce obstruction. Preputial stricture may prevent extrusion of the penis.

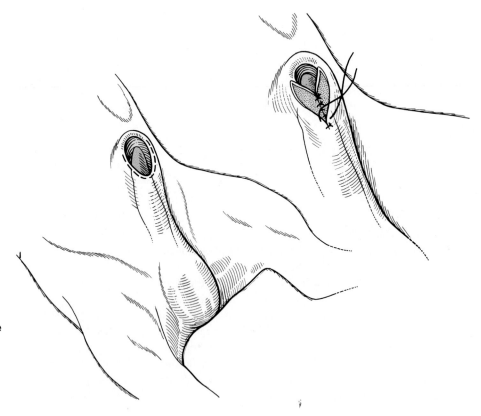

FIG. 23-21
Preputial reconstruction to narrow the orifice is accomplished by incising the mucocutaneous junction (*dashed line*) and reapposing mucosa and skin in separate layers beginning at a more cranial location.

PROGNOSIS

Hypospadias is not life-threatening; however, penile exposure and urine-induced dermatitis cause discomfort. Surgery usually salvages an animal as a pet, improves cosmesis, and reduces urine-induced dermatitis.

Suggested Reading

Ader PL, Hobson HP: Hypospadias: a review of the veterinary literature and a report of three cases in the dog, *J Am Anim Hosp Assoc* 12:721, 1978.

Howard PE, Bjorling DE: The intersexual animal, *Problems in Vet Med: Urogenital Surgical Conditions* 1:74, 1989.

Smith MM, Gourley IM: Preputial reconstruction in a dog, *J Am Vet Med Assoc* 196:1493, 1990.

PHIMOSIS

DEFINITION

Phimosis is the inability of the penis to protrude from the prepuce or sheath.

SYNONYMS

Preputial stenosis

GENERAL CONSIDERATIONS AND CLINICALLY RELEVANT PATHOPHYSIOLOGY

Phimosis is rare. It is usually the result of too small (or absent) a preputial opening. Phimosis may be developmental

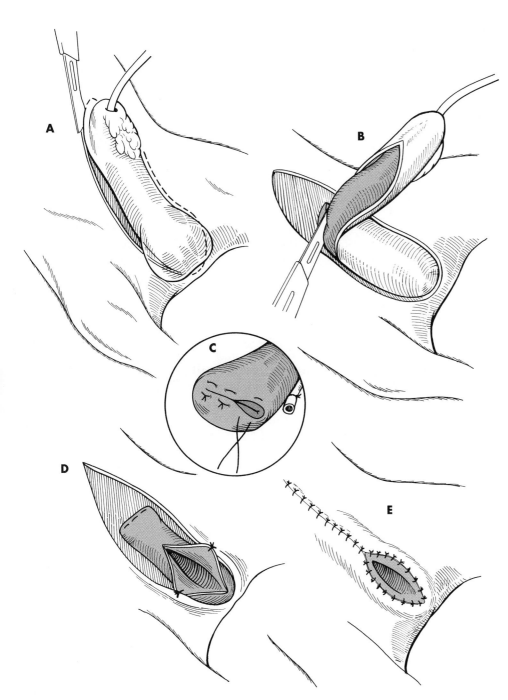

FIG. 23-22
Penile neoplasia, trauma, or congenital anomalies may be treated by subtotal penile amputation and scrotal urethrostomy. **A,** Make an elliptical incision around the base of the scrotum and prepuce and remove the testicles. **B,** Separate the penis from the external abdominal wall to just caudal to the os penis. **C,** Amputate the distal penis and appose the tunica albuginea over the cavernous tissue. **D** and **E,** Incise the urethra in the scrotal area and suture urethral mucosa to skin.

or due to trauma. It may also occur secondary to penile or preputial neoplasia or preputial cellulitis. Inability to extrude the penis causes preputial irritation and infection secondary to urine pooling within the prepuce. Balanoposthitis causes preputial discharge.

DIAGNOSIS
Clinical Presentation

Signalment. There is no known breed predisposition. Congenital phimosis is recognizable in neonates, but may go undetected for months. Acquired phimosis may occur at any age.

History. Affected animals may dribble urine or be unable to copulate. Animals without a preputial opening cannot void urine appropriately and have preputial swelling.

Physical Examination Findings

Affected animals have a small or nonexistent preputial opening. There may be evidence of previous preputial trauma, and a purulent or hemorrhagic preputial discharge is common. The prepuce may be distended with urine, inflamed, and infected. Manual extrusion or palpation of the penis may reveal a mass preventing advancement of the penis.

Radiography

Radiographs are unnecessary unless neoplasia is suspected.

Laboratory Findings

Results of laboratory tests are nonspecific. Preputial cytology may reveal inflammation and infection. Bacteria may be cultured from the prepuce.

DIFFERENTIAL DIAGNOSIS

Differential diagnoses include penile hypoplasia and hermaphroditism.

MEDICAL MANAGEMENT

Phimosis caused by an inflammatory or infectious disease may be relieved by warm compresses, antibiotic therapy, and urine diversion with a catheter. The prepuce should be lavaged daily with physiologic saline solution to reduce urine scalding.

SURGICAL TREATMENT

Phimosis caused by a developmental anomaly or stricture is managed by reconstruction of the preputial orifice. The goal of surgery is to enlarge the preputial orifice and allow unrestricted movement of the penis in and out of the prepuce.

☞ **N O T E** • Neuter animals with small preputial openings.

Preoperative Management

The prepuce should be lavaged with a dilute antiseptic solution before surgery and a urinary catheter placed to divert urine.

Anesthesia

Anesthetic recommendations for animals undergoing reproductive surgery are provided on p. 519.

Surgical Anatomy

Surgical anatomy of the male reproductive system is on p. 521.

Positioning

The patient is positioned in dorsal recumbency and the end of the prepuce clipped and prepared for aseptic surgery.

SURGICAL TECHNIQUE

Enlarge the preputial opening by making a full-thickness incision at the craniodorsal aspect of the prepuce. Determine the desired length and width of the preputial incision based on the severity of phimosis. *Remove a small wedge (3 to 5 mm) of prepuce with the base at the mucocutaneous junction (Fig. 23-23, A). Appose mucosa to the ipsilateral skin edge on each side with a simple interrupted suture pattern (e.g., 4-0 to 6-0 polydioxanone or polyglyconate) (Fig. 23-23, B and C). Extrude the penis completely to examine for other developmental defects, injuries, or masses. Amputate the tip of the prepuce if stenosis is too long to be relieved by incision and adequate preputial length can be maintained.* Amputation may cause a shortened prepuce, allowing chronic penile protrusion and exposure. *Identify the site of resection and amputate the preputial tip (Fig. 23-24, A). Circumferentially appose preputial mucosa to skin with a simple interrupted or continuous suture pattern (e.g., 4-0 to 6-0 polydioxanone or polyglyconate) (Fig. 23-24, B and C). Neuter affected animals.*

POSTOPERATIVE CARE AND ASSESSMENT

Analgesics and supportive care should be given as needed. Warm compresses and antibiotics may be used to treat balanoposthitis. An Elizabethan collar, bucket, or sidebars should be used to prevent self-trauma. Phimosis may persist if the incision is not long enough. Persistent protrusion of the glans may occur if the ventrocaudal prepuce is incised. Self-trauma may cause dehiscence and stricture formation.

PROGNOSIS

Without surgery, balanoposthitis may become severe and cause discomfort. A second surgical procedure may be necessary after the animal matures.

Suggested Reading

Ader PL, Hobson HP: Hypospadias: a review of the veterinary literature and a report of three cases in the dog, *J Am Anim Hosp Assoc* 14:721, 1978.

Proescholdt TA, DeYoung DW, Evans LE: Preputial reconstruction for phimosis and infantile penis, *J Am Anim Hosp Assoc* 725, 1977.

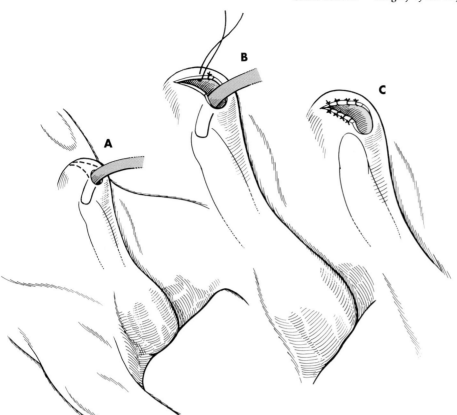

FIG. 23-23
A, For phimosis, enlarge the preputial orifice by resecting a full-thickness wedge from the craniodorsal aspect. **B** and **C,** Appose mucosa to the ipsilateral skin edge on each side.

PARAPHIMOSIS

DEFINITION

Paraphimosis is the inability to retract the penis into the sheath/prepuce. **Priapism** is persistent erection of the penis without sexual excitement.

GENERAL CONSIDERATIONS AND CLINICALLY RELEVANT PATHOPHYSIOLOGY

Paraphimosis may be associated with copulation, trauma, penile hematoma, neoplasia, or foreign bodies. The penis may be unable to retract within the prepuce because the edges of the prepuce roll inward or the preputial orifice is too small to accommodate the swollen or engorged penis. Initially the penis appears normal. However, when the penis cannot be retracted it is easily traumatized and circulation is impaired. Impaired circulation causes the penis to become edematous, which further compromises circulation. Vascular engorgement may progress to thrombosis of the corpus spongiosum and necrosis. A moderately compromised, chronically protruded penis will become dry, fissured, and cornified.

DIAGNOSIS
Clinical Presentation

Signalment. The condition occurs more often in dogs than cats. Sexual hyperactivity preceding paraphimosis may be noted in young dogs.

History. Paraphimosis can result from priapism, masturbation, or excessive sexual activity. Canine paraphimosis oc-

curs most commonly after an erection. It may occur in long-haired cats if the penis becomes entangled in hairs. It may also be associated with posterior paralysis or the inability of preputial muscles to pull the prepuce over the penis after an erection.

Physical Examination Findings

Paraphimosis is diagnosed by visual inspection. The exposed, swollen, edematous penis is painful. The traumatized penis may be fissured, lacerated, and/or bleeding. The animal may require sedation or anesthesia before penile examination. The severity of penile trauma and vascular compromise should be determined. The prepuce should be evaluated to determine whether it is too short or the orifice too small or too large. The retracted penis should normally be covered by at least 1 cm of prepuce cranial to its termination.

Radiography

Radiographs are unnecessary unless urethral trauma is suspected.

Laboratory Findings

Laboratory findings are nonspecific.

DIFFERENTIAL DIAGNOSIS

Paraphimosis must be differentiated from priapism, vascular thrombosis, chronic urethritis, stretching or weakness of the retractor penis muscles, and hypoplastic or surgically damaged preputial muscles. Mechanical, vascular, or neural causes should be suspected when the penis is easily reduced.

FIG. 23-24
A, To enlarge the preputial orifice, resect the tip of the prepuce and, **B** and **C,** suture preputial mucosa to skin.

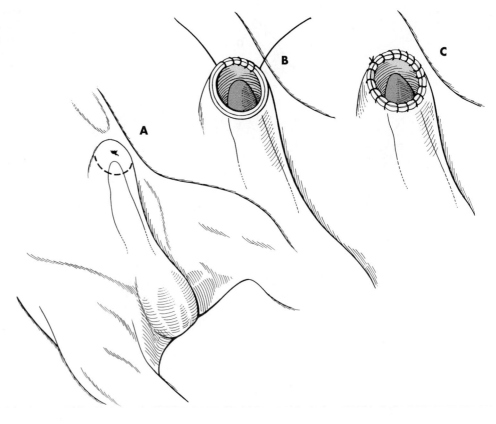

MEDICAL MANAGEMENT

Initially, the prepuce should be pulled back until it unfolds and the preputial mucocutaneous junction identified. This allows restoration of penile circulation and resolution of edema. The penis should be examined carefully for constricting foreign bodies and the protruded, edematous penis cleaned with warm physiologic saline solution or water. To reduce edema, gently massage the penis and apply a hypertonic or hygroscopic agent (sugar). Corticosteroids and diuretics may reduce edema after the constriction is relieved. When swelling has decreased, the prepuce should be flushed with a mild antiseptic soap or lubricant, and the preputial edges dilated or retracted thus allowing the penis to retract within the prepuce.

SURGICAL TREATMENT

Patients with acute paraphimosis are often managed conservatively. Others may require preputial reconstruction or penile amputation. A preputiotomy may be necessary to allow retraction of the penis into the prepuce if conservative measures fail. If the prepuce is of adequate length and the orifice too large, narrow it (see Fig. 23-21). Enlarge the preputial opening if the prepuce is of adequate length and the orifice too small (see Figs. 23-23 and 23-24). When the prepuce is too short it may be lengthened or the penis may be amputated. Preputial deficiencies of less than 1 to 2 cm may be corrected by cranial advancement of the prepuce. Partial amputation of the penis is indicated for severe trauma or abnormalities of the penis or prepuce, neoplasia, recurring urethral prolapse, and recurring paraphimosis. Partial penile

amputation is applicable when the site of transection is cranial to the caudal end of the os penis. Castration is recommended to prevent recurrence of paraphimosis due to sexual activity.

☞ **NOTE ·** Castration may prevent recurrent paraphimosis caused by sexual activity.

Preoperative Management

See the discussion on medical treatment above.

Anesthesia

Anesthetic recommendations for animals with reproductive disorders are on p. 519.

Surgical Anatomy

The prepuce covers the nonerect penis in dogs and cats. The dog's prepuce should normally extend approximately 1 cm beyond the end of the penis.

Positioning

Position the patient in dorsal recumbency. Clip the prepuce and surrounding skin and prepare them for aseptic surgery.

SURGICAL TECHNIQUE
Preputiotomy

Make a full-thickness dorsal or ventral linear incision in the prepuce. If the preputial orifice is of normal size, anatomically reappose mucosa (e.g., 4-0 to 6-0 polydioxanone or

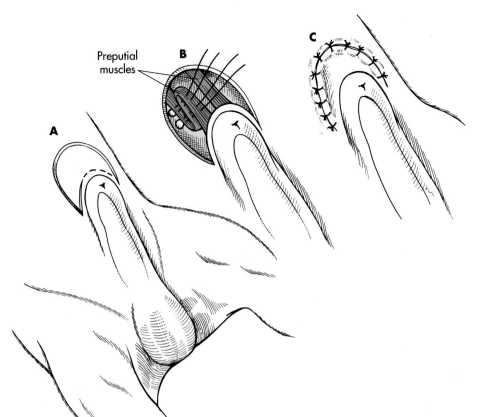

Preputial muscles

polyglyconate, approximating sutures) and skin (e.g., 3-0 or 4-0 nylon or polypropylene, approximating sutures) in separate layers.

Preputial Lengthening

Lengthen or translocate the prepuce cranially by resecting a crescent-shaped piece of skin from the body wall just cranial to the prepuce (Fig. 23-25, A). Preserve the preputial vessels. Identify the preputial muscles and shorten them by overlapping and suturing or segmental excision and reapposition (Fig. 23-25, B). Close subcutaneous tissues and skin in two layers to further advance the skin cranially (Fig. 23-25, C). Alternatively, the prepuce can be lengthened with a two-stage procedure in which oral mucosa is transplanted cranial to the prepuce and later rolled into a tube to cover the end of the penis (Smith, Gourley, 1990).

Partial Penile Amputation

Place a urethral catheter to facilitate orientation and prevent urethral trauma. Extrude the penis from the prepuce and maintain this position by snugly closing the preputial orifice around the penis with a towel clamp. Place a Penrose drain tourniquet caudal to the proposed amputation site. Make a lateral "V" incision through the tunica albuginea and cavernous tissue on each side of the urethra and os penis (Fig. 23-26, A). Transect the os penis with bone cutters as far caudally as possible being careful not to traumatize the urethra (Fig. 23-26, B). Transect the urethra 1 to 2 cm cranial to the penile transection and spatulate the dorsal aspect. Identify and ligate the dorsal artery of the penis after loosening the tourniquet. Fold the spatulated urethra over the transected

end of the penis (Fig. 23-26, C). Appose urethral mucosa to tunic albuginea; include some cavernous tissue with each bite (Fig. 23-26, D). Use 4-0 to 6-0 polydioxanone or polyglyconate with a swaged-on, taper-point needle in a simple interrupted or continuous pattern. Shorten the prepuce if the new penile tip cannot be extruded from the prepuce; the prepuce should extend approximately 1 cm cranial to the retracted penis. *Resect an ellipse of prepuce approximately the same length as the amount of penis that was amputated (Fig. 23-26, E). Make an elliptical, transverse, full-thickness incision in the midportion of the prepuce (beginning approximately 2 cm caudal to the cranial junction of the prepuce and body wall). Remove this ventral skin and mucosal segment, reflect the penis caudally, and resect a similar segment of dorsal preputial mucosa. Close the defect by first apposing the dorsal and then ventral preputial mucosa with 4-0 or 5-0 monofilament absorbable suture (e.g., polydioxanone or polyglyconate) in a simple interrupted or continuous pattern. Then appose skin with approximating 3-0 or 4-0 nonabsorbable sutures (e.g., nylon, polypropylene).*

POSTOPERATIVE CARE AND ASSESSMENT

Analgesics should be given as necessary and an Elizabethan collar, bucket, or sidebars used to prevent self-trauma. Dehiscence, stricture, infection, and recurrence are potential complications of treatment. Hemorrhage usually occurs during urination or excitement for several days after penile amputation. Ventral preputial incisions may lead to chronic exposure of the glans penis. Preputial advancements may relax postoperatively allowing the distal penis to be reexposed.

PROGNOSIS

The prognosis with manual reduction or reconstruction plus castration is good; however, recurrence is common if the animal is not castrated.

Reference

Smith MM, Gourley IM: Preputial reconstruction in a dog, *J Am Vet Med Assoc* 196:1493, 1990.

Suggested Reading

Ader PL, Hobson HP: Hypospadias: a review of the veterinary literature and a report of three cases in the dog, *J Am Anim Hosp Assoc* 14:721, 1978.
Hardie EM: Selected surgeries of the male and female reproductive tracts, *Vet Clin North Am Small Anim Pract* 14:109, 1984.

Pope ER, Swaim SF: Surgical reconstruction of a hypoplastic prepuce, *J Am Anim Hosp Assoc* 22:73, 1986.
Swalec KM, Smeak DD: Priapism after castration in a cat, *J Am Vet Med Assoc* 195:963, 1989.

PENILE AND PREPUTIAL TRAUMA AND NEOPLASIA

DEFINITIONS

A **penile hematoma** is a localized collection of blood that accumulates secondary to laceration or puncture of the cavernous tissues.

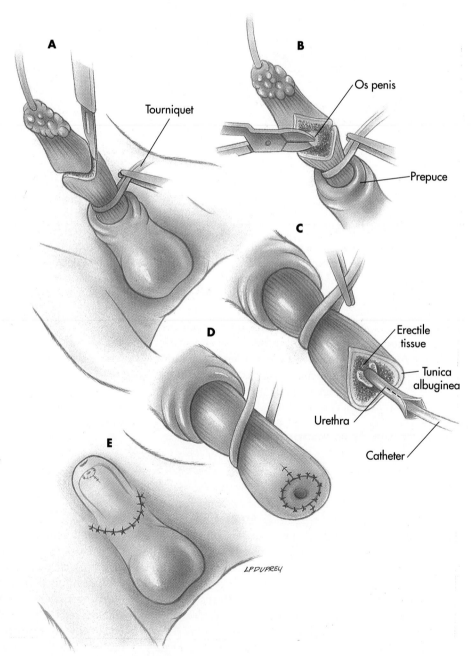

FIG. 23-26
A, During partial penile amputation, retract the prepuce, place a tourniquet around the penis, and make a lateral V incision through the tunica albuginea and cavernous tissue. **B,** Transect the os penis as far caudal as possible. **C,** Transect the urethra 1 to 2 cm cranial to the penile transection and spatulate the end. **D,** Appose urethral mucosa to the tunica albuginea. **E,** Shorten the prepuce to allow extrusion of the distal penis by removing a full-thickness segment from the midsection.

GENERAL CONSIDERATIONS AND CLINICALLY RELEVANT PATHOPHYSIOLOGY

The prepuce and penis may be traumatized by animal bites, vehicular or other accidents, and human attacks (Fig. 23-27). Trauma may cause penile hematomas or os penis fracture. The hematoma swelling may cause the penis to protrude. Lacerations or punctures may bleed for days.

Neoplasms commonly found on skin occur on the prepuce (Table 23-43). Neoplasms of the penis and mucosal lining of the prepuce include transmissible venereal tumors (TVT), squamous cell carcinoma, hemangiosarcoma, and papillomas. Transmissible venereal tumors are contagious tumors spread by sexual contact or licking. They are wart-like, friable, and bleed easily (Fig. 23-28).

DIAGNOSIS
Clinical Presentation

Signalment. Trauma and tumors are more common in intact males. Young animals are more commonly traumatized and old animals more commonly have tumors.

History. Signs of penile or preputial disease include a serosanguineous, hemorrhagic, or purulent preputial discharge, inability or unwillingness to copulate, and/or pain. Some animals present with phimosis (see p. 567) or paraphimosis (see p. 569). The urethra may be obstructed or lacerated, causing dysuria, anuria, or urine extravasation. Many dogs are asymptomatic.

Physical Examination Findings

An injury or abnormal mass may be detected on physical examination. The prepuce may appear swollen, inflamed, nodular, lacerated, ischemic, and/or necrotic. Abnormalities involving preputial skin are usually apparent; preputial mucosal lesions may be detected only by palpation. It may be impossible to exteriorize the penis for examination if there is a mass within the prepuce or on the penis. In other cases, paraphimosis is present because of injury causing inflammation, edema, and engorgement; or a mass prevents penile retraction. Penile deviation may occur secondary to traumatic fractures of the os penis. Rectal palpation may reveal enlarged lymph nodes.

Radiography/Ultrasonography

Radiographs of the abdomen and thorax are indicated to stage tumors. Plain radiographs may reveal os penis fractures. A urethrogram helps assess urethral involvement with penile trauma or tumors.

Laboratory Findings

Laboratory results are nonspecific for penile trauma or neoplasia. Cytology of preputial discharges may show toxic neutrophils, excess bacteria, fungi, or foreign material, but these findings must be interpreted cautiously because they can be found in normal animals. Cytology of preputial or penile masses may help identify the tumor type. Transmissible venereal tumors have large round cells with numerous mitotic figures.

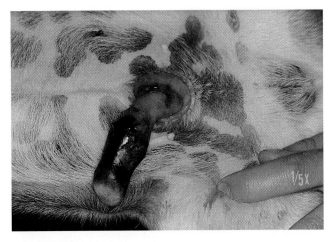

FIG. 23-27
Penile necrosis that occurred after trauma and necessitated partial penile amputation and preputial reconstruction.

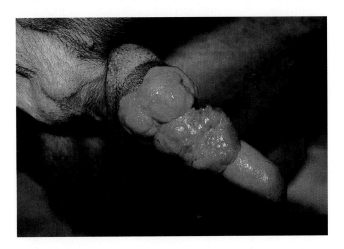

FIG. 23-28
Penile transmissible venereal tumors.

DIFFERENTIAL DIAGNOSIS

Hematomas, abscesses, granulomas, and fungal infections may cause similar lesions.

MEDICAL MANAGEMENT

Some injuries heal spontaneously. Penile hematomas should be allowed to resolve spontaneously, unless they cause persistent paraphimosis. Transmissible venereal tumors are treated with vincristine, 0.5 mg/m^2 intravenously, or 0.025 mg/kg up to 1 mg intravenously, weekly for 3 to 6 weeks.

SURGICAL TREATMENT

Transmissible venereal tumors respond well to chemotherapy or radiation therapy; however, other tumors are best resected. Partial or complete penile amputation is necessary for severely traumatized, necrotic, or neoplastic lesions (see pp. 567 and 571). Hematomas causing persistent paraphimosis can be surgically exposed and evacuated; however, they may recur. Os penis fractures with minimal displacement require

TABLE 23-43

Preputial Tumors

Benign
- Hemangiomas
- Papillomas
- Histiocytomas

Malignant
- Melanomas
- Mast cell tumors
- Hemangiosarcomas
- Squamous cell carcinomas

no surgery. Displaced fractures may be splinted with an indwelling polypropylene urethral catheter spanning the os penis and sutured to the tip of the urethra. More comminuted fractures may be stabilized with small plates, or the penis may be amputated.

Preoperative Management

The prepuce and penis should be lavaged with dilute antiseptic solutions. Antibiotics should be given if the penile or preputial tissue is severely damaged or necrotic.

Anesthesia

Anesthetic management of animals undergoing reproductive surgery is on p. 519.

Surgical Anatomy

Surgical anatomy of the male reproductive tract is on p. 521.

Positioning

Position the patient in dorsal recumbency. The ventral abdomen, ventral perineum, and medial thighs should be clipped and prepared for aseptic surgery.

SURGICAL TECHNIQUE
Preputial Lacerations

Debride, lavage, and appose preputial lacerations. Close full-thickness injuries in two layers, first apposing the preputial mucosa (e.g., 4-0 to 6-0 polydioxanone or polyglyconate) and then skin (e.g., 3-0 or 4-0 nylon or polypropylene) with approximating sutures. Hematomas that cause

persistent paraphimosis can be surgically exposed and evacuated. *Incise the tunic albuginea over the hematoma. Remove blood clots and fibrin. Lavage the cavity and snugly appose the tunic albuginea.* Take care to maintain an adequate preputial orifice and length when reconstructing preputial lacerations.

Penile Lacerations or Punctures

Suture the tunica albuginea to close penile lacerations or punctures and minimize hemorrhage during excitement or urination. Use 4-0 to 6-0 absorbable (e.g., polyglyconate or polydioxanone), simple interrupted sutures on a swaged-on, taper-point needle. Bleeding from small penile punctures or lacerations during penile engorgement is minimized by suturing the tunica albuginea.

POSTOPERATIVE CARE AND ASSESSMENT

Analgesics and antibiotics should be given as needed and the animal monitored for hemorrhage and/or urine leakage. An Elizabethan collar, bucket, or sidebars should be used to prevent self-trauma. Reevaluation for tumor recurrence or metastasis should be performed every 3 to 4 months for 1 year. Hemorrhage, seroma, infection, urine leakage, dehiscence, stricture, recurrence, and metastasis are potential complications. Urethral obstruction may occur due to callus formation following os penis fractures.

PROGNOSIS

Some injuries heal by second intention without complications; however, nonsutured preputial lacerations may fistulate. In other cases, persistent hemorrhage, urine extravasation, infection, and stricture may cause morbidity. The prognosis is good following appropriate surgical treatment for most injuries. The prognosis following tumor excision depends on the biologic behavior of the tumor and the tumor stage at presentation.

Suggested Reading

Bjorling DE: Traumatic injuries of the urogenital system, *Vet Clin North Am: Small Anim Pract* 14:61, 1984.

Herron MA: Tumors of the canine genital system, *J Am Anim Hosp Assoc* 19:981, 1983.

Richardson RC: Canine transmissible venereal tumor, *Compend Contin Educ Pract Vet* 3:951, 1981.

CHAPTER 24

Surgery of the Cardiovascular System

GENERAL PRINCIPLES AND TECHNIQUES

DEFINITIONS

Cardiac surgery includes procedures performed on the pericardium, cardiac ventricles, atria, venae cavae, aorta, and main pulmonary artery. **Closed cardiac procedures** (i.e., those that do not require opening major cardiac structures) are most commonly performed; however, some conditions require **open cardiac surgery** (i.e., a major cardiac structure must be opened to accomplish the repair). Open cardiac surgery necessitates that circulation be arrested during the procedure by inflow occlusion or cardiopulmonary bypass. **Venous inflow occlusion** provides brief circulatory arrest, allowing short procedures (less than 5 min) to be performed. Longer open cardiac procedures require establishing an extracorporeal circulation by **cardiopulmonary bypass** to maintain organ perfusion during surgery.

PREOPERATIVE CONCERNS

Animals requiring cardiac surgery often have prior cardiovascular compromise that should be corrected or controlled medically when possible, prior to anesthetic induction (Table 24-1). Congestive heart failure, particularly pulmonary edema, should be managed with diuretics (e.g., furosemide) and ACE inhibitors (e.g., enalapril, lisinopril) before surgery. Cardiac arrhythmias should be recognized and treated (see also postoperative care below). Ventricular tachycardia should be suppressed before surgery with class I antiarrhythmic drugs (i.e., lidocaine, procainamide). Lidocaine is effective for management of ventricular tachyarrhythmias during and immediately after surgery. Supraventricular tachycardia may require management with digoxin, beta-adrenergic blockers (e.g., esmolol, propranolol, atenolol), or calcium channel blocking drugs (e.g., diltiazem) prior to surgery. Atrial fibrillation should be controlled prior to surgery with digoxin to lower the ventricular response rate below 140 bpm. This may require the addition

TABLE 24-1

Selected Drugs Used in the Management of Animals with Cardiac Disease

Furosemide (Lasix)

2-4 mg/kg PO, IV, SC, SID to QID as needed

Enalapril (Vasotec, Enacard)

0.25-0.5 mg/kg PO, SID to BID

Lisinopril (Prinovil, Zestril)
Dogs

0.25-0.5 mg/kg PO, SID

Procainamide (Pronestyl)
Dogs

10-15 mg/kg slow IV bolus or 25-60 µg/kg/min as a continuous IV infusion or 15 mg/kg IM, PO, BID to QID

Lidocaine (Xylocaine)
Dogs

IV bolus (2mg/kg increments up to total dose of 8 mg/kg/hr) then IV drip at 50-75 µg/kg/min (500 mg in 500 ml of fluid administered at maintenance rate [66 ml/kg/day] equals 50 µg/kg/min)

Esmolol (Brevibloc)

100 µg/kg/min constant rate infusion or 0.05-0.1 mg/kg slow IV bolus every 5 min (up to 0.5 mg/kg total cumulative dose)

Propranolol (Inderal)

0.2-2.0 mg/kg PO, BID to TID

Atenolol (Tenormin)
Dogs

6.25-50 mg/dog PO, SID to BID

Cats

6.25-12.5 mg/cat PO, SID to BID

Diltiazem (Cardizem)

1.0-1.5 mg/kg PO, TID

of beta-adrenergic blockade or calcium channel blocking drugs if digoxin alone does not decrease the ventricular rate sufficiently. Animals with bradycardia should undergo an atropine response test before surgery. If bradycardia is not responsive to atropine, temporary transvenous pacing or constant intravenous infusion of isoproterenol (see management of bradycardia on p. 605) may be required.

Most animals should undergo evaluation by echocardiography prior to cardiac surgery as an incomplete or inaccurate diagnosis can have devastating consequences. With the advent of Doppler echocardiography, cardiac catheterization is no longer routinely necessary prior to cardiac surgery.

ANESTHETIC CONSIDERATIONS

Preanesthetic medication is appropriate for most animals undergoing cardiac surgery (Tables 24-2 and 24-3). Parenteral opioids (i.e., oxymorphone, butorphanol, buprenorphine, or fentanyl) induce sedation with minimal cardiovascular effects. All opioids have the potential to produce respiratory depression and/or bradycardia. Anticholinergics (i.e., atropine or glycopyrrolate) should be administered as needed to treat bradycardia when using an opioid. Benzodiazepines (i.e., diazepam, 0.2 mg/kg up to 5 mg; and midazolam, 0.2 mg/kg up to 5 mg) have minimal cardiopulmonary effects and can be combined with opioids to enhance sedation. There may be an unpredictable behavioral response (e.g., excitation, aggressiveness) to benzodiazepine administration in some animals.

Induction of anesthesia should be undertaken with caution in animals with cardiopulmonary compromise. Thiobarbiturates should be avoided in patients with significant cardiac disease because they cause dose-dependent cardiac depression and are arrhythmogenic. Propofol (Diprivan, Rapinovet) produces rapid induction but causes essentially the same cardiovascular compromise as thiobarbiturates. Ketamine combined with diazepam also is appropriate for induction of compromised patients but should be avoided in animals with mitral insufficiency because it increases the regurgitant fraction. Diazepam has minimal cardiopulmonary

effects and helps offset the negative effects of ketamine (i.e., muscle rigidity and potential for seizures). Time to intubation is longer than with other agents but is still considered relatively fast. Opioids can be used for induction of very sick and compromised dogs; however, opioids do not truly induce anesthesia, so intubation may be difficult in alert animals. Etomidate is not arrhythmogenic, maintains cardiac output, and offers rapid induction. Mask induction with isoflurane is discouraged in patients with cardiopulmonary disorders because of the high inspired concentrations and time necessary to achieve intubation.

Anesthesia can be maintained with an inhalation agent in most cardiac patients. For compromised patients, isoflurane is the inhalation agent of choice. The insoluble nature of isoflurane allows rapid induction, recovery, and change in the depth of anesthesia. It depresses contractility less than other inhalation agents and is less arrhythmogenic. Adjunct intravenous opioids can be administered to decrease the levels of isoflurane necessary to achieve adequate anesthesia. Opioids combined with low concentrations of isoflurane may not produce adequate muscle relaxation, which may make administration of a nondepolarizing muscle relaxant desirable. Atracurium (0.1-0.2 mg/kg IV) is a short-acting muscle relaxant that is not dependent on metabolism or excretion to terminate its action (it must be used with intermittent positive pressure ventilation).

TABLE 24-2

Selected Anesthetic Protocols for Use in Stable Animals with Cardiovascular Disease

Premedication

Give atropine (0.02-0.04 mg/kg SC or IM) or glycopyrrolate (0.005-0.011 mg/kg SC or IM) if indicated plus oxymorphone* (0.05-0.1 mg/kg SC or IM) or butorphanol (0.2-0.4 mg/kg SC or IM) or buprenorphine (5-15 μg/kg IM)

Induction

Thiopental (10-12 mg/kg IV) or propofol (4-6 mg/kg IV)

Maintenance

Isoflurane or halothane
*Use 0.05 mg/kg in cats.

TABLE 24-3

Selected Anesthetic Protocols for Use in Animals with Heart Failure, Hypovolemia, Dehydration, or Those in Shock

Dogs
Induction

Oxymorphone (0.1 mg/kg IV) plus diazepam (0.2 mg/kg IV). Give in incremental dosages. Intubate if possible. If necessary, give etomidate (0.5-1.5 mg/kg IV). Alternately, give thiopental or propofol at reduced dosages. If there are no contraindications to ketamine, reduced dosages of diazepam and ketamine may also be used.

Maintenance

Isoflurane

Cats
Premedication

Butorphanol (0.2-0.4 mg/kg SC or IM) or buprenorphine (5-15 μg/kg IM) or oxymorphone (0.05 mg/kg SC or IM)

Induction

Diazepam (0.2 mg/kg IV) followed by etomidate (0.5-1.5 mg/kg IV). Alternately, if not vomiting, mask or chamber induction can be used or give thiopental or propofol at reduced dosages. If there are no contraindications to ketamine, reduced dosages of diazepam and ketamine may also be used.

Maintenance

Isoflurane

Thoracic surgery always requires controlled ventilation. Controlled ventilation can be achieved by manually squeezing the reservoir bag or by a mechanical ventilator attached to the anesthetic machine. Ideally, mechanical ventilation should achieve a tidal volume of 10 to 15 ml/kg of body weight at an inspiratory pressure of 20 cm of water. Assuring adequate ventilation is accomplished by optimizing tidal volume, inspiratory pressure, and respiratory rate to achieve ventilation with the least risk of causing pulmonary injury or cardiovascular compromise. Ultimately, the goal of mechanical ventilation is to maintain normocapnia. Ventilation can be monitored by measurement of end tidal CO_2 by capnography, or arterial CO_2 by blood gas analysis.

Successful inflow occlusion requires meticulous anesthesia. Balanced anesthetic techniques that minimize inhalation anesthetic agents are indicated. Animals should be hyperventilated for 5 minutes before inflow occlusion. Ventilation is discontinued during inflow occlusion and resumed immediately upon release of inflow occlusion. Drugs and equipment for full cardiac resuscitation must be immediately available after inflow occlusion. Gentle cardiac massage may be necessary after inflow occlusion to reestablish cardiac function. Digital occlusion of the descending aorta during this period helps direct available cardiac output to the heart and brain. If ventricular fibrillation occurs, immediate internal defibrillation is necessary as soon as inflow occlusion is discontinued. Constant intravenous infusion of lidocaine (Table 24-4) should be initiated before inflow occlusion and continued as needed. Epinephrine, administered as a constant rate infusion, should be given as the animal is being weaned off inflow occlusion or a pump (see Table 24-4). If long-term inotropic support is necessary, dobutamine should be given (see Table 24-4).

ANTIBIOTICS

Perioperative antibiotics are indicated for cardiac procedures lasting more than 90 minutes. First-generation cephalosporins (e.g., cefazolin sodium, cephapirin sodium) can be administered intravenously at induction and repeated once or twice every 4 to 8 hours (Table 24-5). For cardiac procedures involving circulatory arrest or cardiopulmonary bypass, intravenous cefoxitin sodium should be administered before surgery and continued for 24 to 48 hours after surgery (see Table 24-5).

SURGICAL ANATOMY

The heart is the largest mediastinal organ. It generally extends from the third rib to the caudal border of the sixth rib; however, variations exist among breeds and between individuals. The heart base (i.e., craniodorsal aspect that receives the great vessels) faces dorsocranially, while the apex (i.e., formed by muscles of the left ventricle) points caudoventrally. Except for a portion of the right side of the heart (cardiac notch), most of its surface is covered by lung. The right ventricular wall accounts for approximately 22% of the total heart weight; the left ventricular wall accounts for nearly 40%.

The right atrium receives blood from the systemic circulation. The coronary sinus enters the left aspect of the atrium, ventral to the caudal vena cava. The caudal vena cava returns blood from the abdominal viscera, pelvic limbs, and a portion of the abdominal wall (Fig. 24-1). The cranial vena cava returns blood to the heart from the head, neck, thoracic limbs, ventral thoracic wall, and a portion of the abdominal wall. The azygous vein usually enters in the cranial vena cava; it carries blood from the lumbar regions and caudal thoracic wall. The brachycephalic trunk is the first large artery from the aortic arch. The common carotid arteries usually arise from it as separate vessels. The left subclavian artery arises from the aortic arch distal to the brachycephalic trunk (the right subclavian is a branch of the brachycephalic trunk). The vertebral arteries, costocervical trunk, internal thoracic arteries, and axillary arteries branch from the subclavian vessels.

The pericardium is a thick, two-layered sac composed of outer fibrous and inner serous layers. The pericardial cavity is located between two layers (visceral and parietal) of serous pericardium and normally contains a small amount of fluid. The fibrous pericardium blends with the adventitia of the large vessels, and its apex forms the sternopericardiac ligament. Phrenic nerves lie in a narrow plica of pleura adjacent to the pericardium at the heart base. Complete pericardiectomy requires that these nerves be elevated to avoid incising them. The vagus nerves lie dorsal to the phrenic nerve. They divide to form dorsal and ventral branches that lie on the esophagus in the caudal thorax. The left recurrent laryngeal nerve leaves the vagus and loops around the arch distal to the ligamentum arteriosum to run cranially along the ventrolateral tracheal surface.

TABLE 24-4
Drugs for Inflow Occlusion
Lidocaine
50-75 µg/kg/min IV infusion (see also Table 24-1)
Dobutamine
2-10 µg/kg/min IV
Epinephrine
0.1-0.4 µg/kg/min IV

TABLE 24-5
Prophylactic Antibiotics for Cardiac Surgery
Cefazolin (Ancef, Kefzol)
20 mg/kg IV at induction
Cephapirin (Cefadyl)
22 mg/kg IV at induction
Cefoxitin (Mefoxin)
30 mg/kg IV at induction

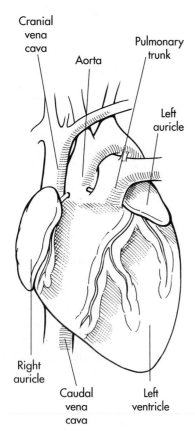

FIG. 24-1
Cardiac anatomy.

SURGICAL TECHNIQUES

Cardiac surgery is not fundamentally different from other types of general surgery and similar principles of good surgical technique (i.e., atraumatic tissue handling, good hemostasis, and secure knot tieing) apply. Consequences of poor surgical technique are often devastating. Cardiac surgery differs from other surgeries in that motion from ventilation and cardiac contractions adds to the technical difficulty of performing these procedures. Approaches that provide limited access to dorsal structures (e.g., median sternotomy; see p. 654) require that surgeons incise, suture, and/or ligate structures located deep within the thorax. Ligature placement using hand ties (see p. 52) are useful in such situations and the ability to place hand-tied knots (vs. instrument tieing) should be considered a fundamental skill for cardiac surgeons. Secure knot tieing is critically important to successful cardiac surgery. Hand tieing knots is fast and produces tighter and more secure knots than instrument tieing. The one-handed knot tie technique (see p. 53) is best suited to the fine sutures used in cardiac surgery. Tight knots are facilitated by throwing the first two or three throws in the same direction before finishing with square knots for security.

Closure of cardiovascular structures requires precise suturing techniques and good instrument handling skills to minimize hemorrhage. Using fine suture with swaged-on atraumatic needles (see discussion on suture materials on p. 45) and carefully following the needle contour when suturing (to minimize the size of needle tracts) are important. "Palming" of needle holders is a good skill for fast suturing, but should be avoided when suturing inside the thoracic cavity. Finer control is gained by grasping instruments with fingers placed in the instrument rings.

Inflow Occlusion

Inflow occlusion is a technique used for open heart surgery where all venous flow to the heart is temporarily interrupted. Because inflow occlusion results in complete circulatory arrest, it allows limited time to perform cardiac procedures. Ideally, circulatory arrest in a normothermic patient should be less than 2 minutes, but can be extended to 4 minutes if necessary. Circulatory arrest time can be extended up to 6 minutes with mild, whole-body hypothermia (30° to 34° C).

Depending on the cardiac procedure being done, perform a left or right thoracotomy (see p. 652), or median sternotomy (see p. 654). With a right thoracotomy or median sternotomy, occlude the cranial and caudal venae cavae and azygous vein with vascular clamps or Rumel tourniquets (Fig. 24-2). Make a Rumel tourniquet by passing umbilical tape around the vessel, then thread the umbilical tape through a piece of rubber tubing that is 1 to 3 inches long. When the umbilical tape has been adequately tightened to occlude the vessel, place a clamp above the rubber tubing to hold it securely in place. Take care to avoid injuring the right phrenic nerve during placement of the clamps or tourniquets. For left thoracotomies, pass separate tourniquets around the cranial and caudal venae cavae. Then, dissecting dorsal to the esophagus and aorta, occlude the azygous vein by placing a tourniquet around it (Fig. 24-3).

Cardiopulmonary Bypass

Cardiopulmonary bypass is a procedure whereby an extracorporeal system provides flow of oxygenated blood to the patient while blood is diverted away from the heart and lungs. This greatly extends the time available for open cardiac surgery. Several advances (i.e., development of membrane oxygenators, improved methods of myocardial protection, increased availability of monitoring technologies, and improved veterinary critical care) have made cardiopulmonary bypass increasingly feasible in dogs. Cardiopulmonary bypass can be used to treat dogs with congenital or acquired cardiac defects. Readers are referred to a cardiovascular surgery text for details of performing cardiopulmonary bypass.

HEALING OF CARDIOVASCULAR STRUCTURES

Vascular structures heal quickly, forming a fibrin seal within minutes. Epithelialization and early endothelial regeneration occur in veins used for grafts. Thrombosis commonly occurs in small veins that have been traumatically occluded for short periods of time; however, thrombosis of large veins occluded during inflow occlusion or cardiac bypass procedures has not been a clinically recognized problem. To avoid

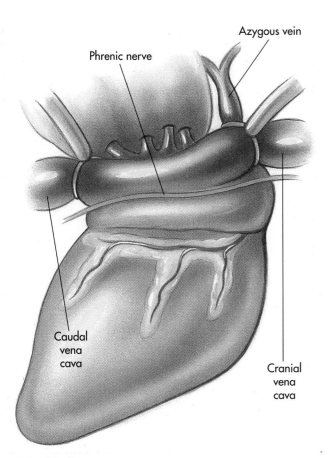

FIG. 24-2
To occlude cardiac inflow from the right side of the thorax, pass tapes around the caudal vena cava and the common drainage of the azygous veins and cranial vena cava. Fashion tourniquets for inflow occlusion by passing the tapes through rubber tubing. (Illustration modified from Orton EC: *Small animal thoracic surgery,* Philadelphia, 1995, Williams & Wilkins.)

thrombosis of vascular structures, they should be handled gently as trauma may lead to the deposition of platelets, fibrin, and red cells on the intimal surface. If the torn intima is lifted upward, a flap may develop that partially or completely occludes the distal lumen. This in turn can lead to accumulation of blood within the vessel wall, vascular sludging, and thrombosis.

SUTURE MATERIALS/SPECIAL INSTRUMENTS

Polypropylene is the standard suture used for cardiovascular procedures. The most common sizes used are 3-0, 4-0, and 5-0. These sutures should be available with swaged-on taper-point cardiovascular needles in a variety of sizes. Some procedures require that suture be double-armed (i.e., with needles at both ends). Teflon pledgets are useful for buttressing mattress sutures in ventricular myocardium or great vessels.

Successful cardiac surgery requires proper surgical instrumentation. Most of the basic instruments required for general surgery can be used for cardiac surgery; however, a few specialized instruments are desirable for thoracic surgery.

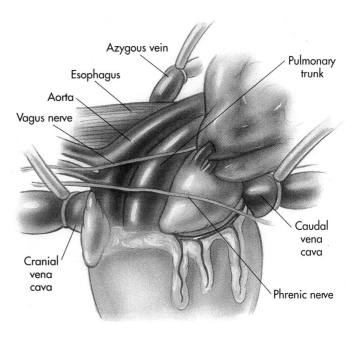

FIG. 24-3
During inflow occlusion from the left side of the thorax, pass tapes around the cranial and caudal vena cava and azygous vein. Fashion tourniquets as described in Fig. 24-2. (Illustration modified from Orton EC: *Small animal thoracic surgery,* Philadelphia, 1995, Williams & Wilkins.)

The standard thoracic retractor is a Finochietto retractor (Fig. 24-4, *A*). It is helpful to have at least two sizes to accommodate different-sized animals. Self-retaining orthopedic retractors can substitute as thoracic retractors in small dogs and cats. The standard tissue forceps for thoracic surgery is a DeBakey tissue forceps (Fig. 24-4, *B*). At least two DeBakey forceps should be available, and it is helpful if one has a carbide inlay for grasping suture needles. Metzenbaum scissors are the standard operating scissors for cardiac surgery. Curved Metzenbaum scissors are more versatile than the straight design. Potts scissors (45-degree angle) are desirable for some cardiac surgery (Fig. 24-4, *C*). Needle holders should be long and available in different sizes to accommodate a variety of suture needle sizes. Mayo-Heger, Crile-Wood, and Castroviejo needle holders represent a good selection of sizes for thoracic surgery in animals. Angled thoracic forceps are an important instrument for cardiac surgery and should be available in a variety of sizes (Fig. 24-4, *D*). Vascular clamps are noncrushing clamps used for temporary occlusion of cardiovascular and pulmonary structures. They come in a variety of sizes and shapes including straight, angled, curved, and tangential (Fig. 24-5). The most versatile shape for most cardiac surgery is a medium-width tangential clamp.

POSTOPERATIVE CARE AND ASSESSMENT

Patient monitoring and postoperative care are the cornerstones of successful cardiac surgery. The level of supportive care required for cardiac surgeries depends on the patient

FIG. 24-4
Instruments for cardiovascular surgery: **A,** Finochietto retractor; **B,** DeBakey tissue forceps; **C,** Potts scissors; and **D,** angled thoracic forceps.

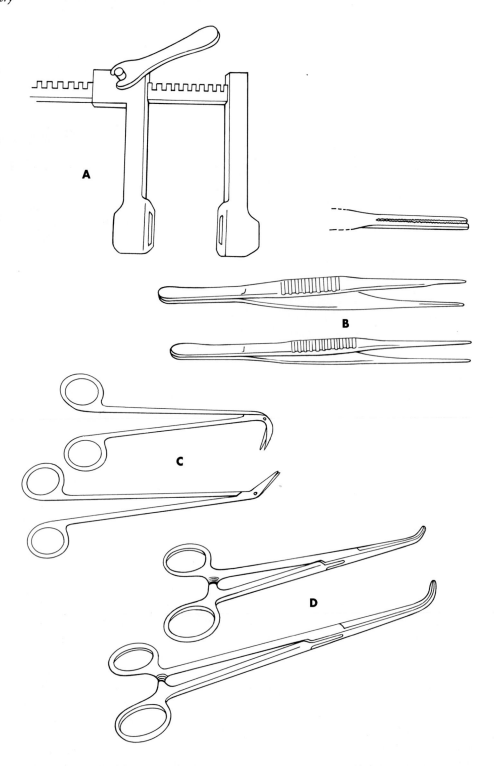

and surgical procedure performed. A working knowledge of cardiopulmonary function and good patient observation skills are as important to successful patient management as advanced monitoring devices.

Evaluation of ventilation is important after any thoracic surgery. Poor ventilatory efforts may first be noted in the period after surgery when the influence of anesthetic drugs is still present, but ventilatory support has been discontinued. Hypoventilation may also occur from uncontrolled pain. Total ventilation can be assessed directly by measuring the vol-

ume of expired gas with a respirometer. Tidal volume should be at least 10 ml per kg of body weight. Ultimately, the best measure of alveolar ventilation is arterial CO_2 tension ($PaCO_2$). Alveolar hypoventilation is present when $PaCO_2$ is increased above 40 mm of Hg. Treatment of hypoventilation should be directed at correcting its underlying cause if possible. Drugs that are known to depress ventilation (i.e., opioids and muscle relaxants) should be used with caution in the perioperative period, and the risk of ventilatory depression weighed against the risk of hypoventilation due to pain (see

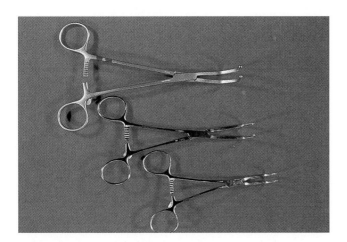

FIG. 24-5
Tangential vascular clamps.

p. 649 for analgesia after thoracotomy). Pleural air or fluid should be evacuated if present. Injury or dysfunction of the neuromuscular ventilatory apparatus should be corrected, if possible. If hypoventilation is severe and the cause is not immediately correctable, positive-pressure ventilation is indicated.

Under physiologic conditions, gas exchange between the alveolus and pulmonary capillary blood is efficient, and alveolar oxygen tension (P_AO_2) and arterial oxygen tension (PaO_2) are nearly equal. In patients with impaired gas exchange, hypoxemia occurs because P_AO_2 and PaO_2 are not equal. The most common causes of impaired pulmonary gas exchange in the postoperative setting are ventilation/perfusion (V_A/Q) mismatch and pulmonary shunt secondary to alveolar collapse. Impaired pulmonary gas exchange may or may not be responsive to supplemental oxygen therapy depending on its underlying cause. Therefore, response to supplemental oxygen therapy must be evaluated for each individual patient, preferably by blood gas analysis. The therapeutic goal of supplemental oxygen should be to keep PaO_2 above 80 mm of Hg. Positive end-expiratory pressure (PEEP) therapy is indicated for patients with severe gas exchange impairment that is not responsive to supplemental oxygen therapy alone.

Maintaining an adequate PaO_2 in a patient is important because it is the major determinant of hemoglobin oxygen saturation (SaO_2). SaO_2 can be measured by pulse oximetry. The therapeutic goal should be to maintain SaO_2 at or above 90%. Oxygen content of the blood is a function of SaO_2 and hemoglobin concentration. Thus, maintenance of an adequate oxygen content requires not only adequate pulmonary function (SaO_2 greater than 90%), but also an adequate hemoglobin concentration. Maintenance of the packed cell volume above 30% is an important therapeutic goal for animals undergoing cardiac surgery, especially if cardiopulmonary compromise is present.

Systemic blood pressure is directly proportional to cardiac output and systemic vascular resistance. Measurement of blood pressure provides a good assessment of cardiovascular function especially during and immediately after

TABLE 24-6

Postoperative Analgesics

Oxymorphone (Numorphan)
0.05-0.1 mg/kg IV, IM, every 4 hours (as needed)

Butorphanol (Torbutrol, Torbugesic)
0.2-0.4 mg/kg IV, IM, or SC, every 2 to 4 hours (as needed)

Buprenorphine (Buprenex)
5-15 µg/kg IV, IM, every 6 hours (as needed)

surgery. Indirect techniques for measuring blood pressure include the oscillometric method, the basis of monitors such as the Dinamap, or Doppler method. Doppler technique provides only systolic pressure, but is useful for evaluating blood pressure trends during and after surgery. Indirect methods of blood pressure assessment are less invasive, but are also less accurate than direct measurements. Direct measurement of blood pressure requires placement of an arterial catheter. Arterial catheters have the additional advantage of providing access for arterial blood gas analysis. An arterial catheter can be placed percutaneously into a dorsal pedal artery of the hind limb. Direct blood pressure measurement also requires a pressure transducer and monitor, or a manometer. The therapeutic goal is to maintain a mean blood pressure above 65 mm of Hg and systolic blood pressure above 90 mm of Hg. Blood pressure can be elevated by increasing either cardiac output or systemic vascular resistance. In most instances, the more appropriate therapeutic strategy to correct hypotension is to improve cardiac output. Maintenance of adequate vascular volume is the most important aspect of maintaining adequate cardiac output. Central venous pressure should be maintained between 5 and 10 cm of water. Indications for arterial pressor therapy are rare. Inotropic and pressor support can be obtained by constant intravenous infusion of epinephrine (see Table 24-4). Long-term inotropic support is maintained by dobutamine (see Table 24-4).

Monitoring the electrocardiogram for disturbances in cardiac rhythm is important for animals undergoing cardiac surgery. Sinus tachycardia is the most common rhythm disturbance in surgery patients. Therapy for sinus tachycardia should be directed at correction of its underlying cause and improvement of cardiac output. Ventricular dysrhythmias including premature ventricular complexes (PVCs) and nonsustained or sustained ventricular tachycardia are frequently encountered during and after cardiac surgery. Frequent PVCs, particularly when they occur with a short coupling interval (i.e., R on T phenomena), and rapid ventricular tachycardia should be suppressed in the perioperative period. Continuous intravenous infusion of lidocaine is effective in most instances. Ventricular fibrillation is a form of cardiac arrest that requires immediate electrical defibrillation. If cardiac surgery is performed frequently, equipment for defibrillation should be available. Recommendations for postoperative analgesics are provided in Table 24-6.

COMPLICATIONS

The major complication associated with cardiac surgery is hemorrhage. Severe hemorrhage may be encountered intraoperatively or postoperatively. Materials for blood transfusion should be available. Fresh whole blood should be collected as close as possible to the time that it is needed and should not be cooled as this may reduce platelet content. If possible, a compatible donor should be identified by crossmatching with the patient before surgery. Autotransfusion can be undertaken in animals that are bleeding after surgery by collecting blood from the pleural space directly into CPDA (citrate, phosphate, dextrose, adenine) collection bags and returning the blood to the patient with a standard blood administration filter. In most cases, autotransfusion of bleeding patients is preferred over returning the patient to surgery to control bleeding.

SPECIAL AGE CONSIDERATIONS

Most animals undergoing surgery for congenital cardiac defects are young. Special care must be taken during surgery and postoperatively in these animals. Young animals should not have food withheld for greater than 4 to 6 hours before surgery and should be fed as soon as they are fully recovered from anesthesia. If they cannot be fed, glucose concentrations should be supported by adding glucose to intravenous fluids, and serum glucose concentrations should be monitored intraoperatively. Hypothermia is common in young patients during thoracotomy and is protective during cardiac procedures. However, the temperature should be monitored closely and they should be actively rewarmed postoperatively.

☞ **N O T E** · Remember, hypothermia decreases the minimum alveolar concentration (MAC) of inhalants used for maintenance.

Suggested Reading

Gravlee GP, Davis RF, Utley JR: *Cardiopulmonary bypass: principles and practice,* Philadelphia, 1993, Williams & Wilkins.

Kaplin JA: *Cardiac anesthesia,* ed 3, Philadelphia, 1993, WB Saunders.

Orton EC: *Small animal thoracic surgery,* Philadelphia, 1995, Williams & Wilkins.

SPECIFIC DISEASES

PATENT DUCTUS ARTERIOSUS

DEFINITIONS

The **ductus arteriosus** is a fetal vessel that connects the main pulmonary artery and descending aorta. During development it shunts blood away from the collapsed fetal lungs. Normally it closes shortly after birth during the transition from fetal to extrauterine life. Continued patency of the ductus arteriosus for more than a few days after birth is termed **patent ductus arteriosus.**

SYNONYMS

Persistent ductus arteriosus, PDA

GENERAL CONSIDERATIONS AND CLINICALLY RELEVANT PATHOPHYSIOLOGY

PDA is the most common congenital heart defect of dogs; it also occurs in cats. PDA causes a left-to-right shunt that results in volume overload of the left ventricle and produces left ventricular dilation and hypertrophy. Progressive left ventricular dilation distends the mitral valve annulus causing secondary regurgitation and additional ventricular overload. This severe volume overload leads to left-sided congestive heart failure and pulmonary edema, usually within the first year of life. Atrial fibrillation may occur as a late sequela due to marked left atrial dilation.

Rarely, dogs with PDA develop suprasystemic pulmonary hypertension that reverses the direction of flow through the shunt causing severe hypoxemia and cyanosis (Eisenmenger's physiology). Right-to-left PDA can occur as a late sequela to untreated PDA. When right-to-left PDA is noted in very young animals it may be due to persistent pulmonary hypertension after birth. Reversal of PDA lessens the risk for developing progressive left-sided heart failure, but causes severe debilitating systemic hypoxemia, exercise intolerance, and progressive polycythemia.

DIAGNOSIS
Clinical Presentation

Signalment. PDA is seen more commonly in purebred, female dogs. Maltese, Pomeranians, Shetland sheepdogs, English springer spaniels, keeshonden, bichons frises, miniature and toy poodles, and Yorkshire terriers are at increased risk to develop PDA. A genetic basis has been established in poodles.

History. Most young animals with PDA are asymptomatic or have only mild exercise intolerance. The most common complaint in symptomatic animals with left-to-right shunts is cough or shortness of breath (or both) due to pulmonary edema. Animals with right-to-left or reverse PDA may be asymptomatic or have exercise intolerance and hind limb collapse on exercise.

Physical Examination Findings

The most prominent physical finding associated with PDA is a characteristic continuous (machinery) murmur heard best at the left heart base. The left apical cardiac impulse is prominent and displaced caudally and a palpable cardiac "thrill" often is present. Femoral pulses are strong or hyperkinetic (water hammer pulse) due to a wide pulse pressure caused by diastolic runoff of blood through the ductus. Tall R waves (greater than 2.5 mV) or wide P waves on a lead II electrocardiogram are supportive of the diagnosis, but not always present. Atrial fibrillation or ventricular ectopy may be present in advanced cases.

The physical examination findings in animals with right-to-left or reverse PDA differ from those with left-to-right shunts. "Differential" cyanosis is typically present (i.e., cyanosis is most apparent in the caudal mucous membranes), but cyanosis may also be noted in the cranial half of the body in some animals. Cyanosis occurs because there is admixture of nonoxygenated blood (from the pulmonary artery) with the oxygenated aortic blood. Femoral pulses are normal. A systolic cardiac murmur, rather than a machinery murmur, is often present. However, a murmur may not be auscultated if polycythemia is present (see below under Laboratory Findings) or if left and right sided pressures are nearly equal and shunting of blood through the ductus is minimal.

Radiography/Echocardiography

Thoracic radiographs typically show left atrial and ventricular enlargement, enlargement of pulmonary vessels, and a characteristic dilation of the descending aorta on the dorsoventral view. Echocardiography provides information that further confirms PDA and helps exclude concurrent cardiac defects, but is not invariably required to establish the diagnosis. Echocardiographic findings that support a diagnosis of PDA include left atrial enlargement, left ventricular dilation and hypertrophy, pulmonary artery dilation, increased aortic ejection velocity, and a characteristic reverse turbulent Doppler flow pattern in the pulmonary artery.

With right-to-left PDA, thoracic radiographs show evidence of biventricular enlargement and marked enlargement of the pulmonary artery segment. Pulmonary arteries may also appear tortuous. A right-to-left PDA can be documented by performing a saline bubble contrast echocardiogram. Observing bubbles in the descending aorta, but not in any left-sided cardiac chamber, is diagnostic.

Laboratory Findings

Laboratory abnormalities are uncommon in animals with left-to-right shunting PDA; however, animals with right-to-left shunts are commonly polycythemic. Polycythemia occurs in response to increased erythropoietin production due to chronic hypoxemia.

DIFFERENTIAL DIAGNOSIS

The characteristic physical examination findings (i.e., continuous murmur, bounding arterial pulses) make diagnosis of PDA straightforward in most affected animals. A combination of aortic stenosis/aortic insufficiency (see p. 588) or ventricular septal defect/aortic insufficiency (see p. 591) results in a to-and-fro murmur that may be difficult to differentiate from continuous PDA murmurs. In some animals where the diastolic component of the PDA murmur is difficult to detect, other differentials would include subaortic stenosis, pulmonic stenosis, atrial septal defect, and ventricular septal defect. Differentials for dogs with right-to-left PDA include tetralogy of Fallot, right-to-left shunting atrial or ventricular septal defects, or other complex forms of cyanotic heart disease (rare).

TABLE 24-7
Perioperative Diuretics
Furosemide (Lasix)
2-4 mg/kg IM or IV, QID

MEDICAL MANAGEMENT

Animals with pulmonary edema should be given furosemide (Table 24-7) for 24 to 48 hours before surgery. If atrial fibrillation is present, the ventricular response rate should be controlled using digoxin (with or without beta-adrenergic blockers or calcium channel blockers) before surgery. If hemodynamically significant arrhythmias are present they must be controlled. Complete resolution of clinical signs of congestive heart failure may be difficult with medical management alone.

SURGICAL TREATMENT

Surgical correction of PDA is accomplished by ligation of the ductus arteriosus. Ligation of PDA is considered curative and should be performed as soon as possible after diagnosis. Secondary mitral regurgitation usually regresses after surgery due to reduction in left ventricular dilation. Inadvertent ductal rupture during dissection is the most serious complication associated with PDA repair. The risk of this complication decreases as the surgeon's experience increases. Small ruptures, especially those on the back side of the ductus, often respond to gentle tamponade, but will enlarge and worsen if dissection is continued. Large ruptures must be controlled immediately with vascular clamps and then repaired with pledget-buttressed mattress sutures. Once bleeding is controlled, a decision must be made whether to continue surgery or to abandon surgery in favor of repair at a later time. Second surgeries are more difficult due to adhesions at the surgical site, so complete occlusion should be attempted during the initial procedure, if possible. Often, simple ductal ligation is not possible after a rupture has occurred. In such instances, surgical alternatives include ductal closure with pledget-buttressed mattress sutures or ductal division and closure between vascular clamps. The divided ductal ends are closed with a continuous mattress suture oversewn with a simple continuous pattern. Ductal closure without division is safer than surgical division, but recannulation of the ductus may occur. Because ductal division requires added technical expertise, it should be undertaken only by experienced surgeons.

Preoperative Management

Preoperative arrhythmias should be controlled prior to surgery. If the animal has signs of congestive heart failure treatment with positive inotropes (i.e., digoxin), vasodilators (i.e., hydralazine, enalapril), and diuretics (i.e., furosemide) should be initiated preoperatively. Excessive diuretics and/or vasodilators may cause hypotension and should be avoided.

Anesthesia

Bradycardia occasionally occurs during PDA ligation. An anticholinergic (i.e., atropine or glycopyrrolate) should be available and given if the heart rate drops below 60 bpm. Blood should be available for transfusion if excessive hemorrhage occurs during the surgical procedure. Techniques for anesthetic management of cardiovascular patients are discussed on p. 576.

Surgical Anatomy

The ductus arteriosus in dogs and cats is usually wide (approximately 1 cm), but relatively short (less than 1 cm). It is located between the aorta and main pulmonary arteries, caudal to the origin of the brachycephalic and left subclavian arteries. As a result, most mixing of oxygenated and nonoxygenated blood occurs in the descending aorta in dogs with reverse PDA. Thus normally oxygenated blood is supplied to the head and neck, while desaturated blood is presented to the caudal half of the body (see comments on Differential Diagosis on p. 583). The left vagus nerve always passes over the ductus arteriosus and must be identified and retracted during dissection. The left recurrent laryngeal nerve can often be identified as it loops around the ductus.

Positioning

The animal is positioned in right lateral recumbency and the left thorax prepared for aseptic surgery.

SURGICAL TECHNIQUES

Perform a left fourth space intercostal thoracotomy (see p. 652). Identify the left vagus nerve as it courses over the ductus arteriosus and isolate it using sharp dissection at the level of the ductus. Place a suture around the nerve and gently retract it (Fig. 24-6). Isolate the ductus arteriosus by bluntly dissecting around it without opening the pericardial sac. Pass a right-angle forceps behind the ductus, parallel to its transverse plane, to isolate the caudal aspect of the ductus. Then, dissect the cranial aspect of the ductus by angling the forceps caudally approximately 45 degrees (Fig. 24-7). Complete dissection of the ductus by passing forceps from medial to the ductus in a caudal to cranial direction. Grasp the suture with right-angle forceps. Slowly pull the suture beneath the ductus. If the suture does not slide easily around the ductus, do not force it. Regrasp the suture and repeat the process, being careful not to include surrounding soft tissues in the forceps. Pass a second suture using the same maneuver. Alternatively, the suture may be passed as a double loop and the suture cut so that you have two strands (Fig. 24-8). Slowly tighten the suture closest to the aorta first. Then tighten the remaining suture.

SUTURE MATERIALS/SPECIAL INSTRUMENTS

Heavy silk (No. 1 or 0) or cotton tape is a suitable material for ductal ligation. Right-angle forceps are best suited for blunt dissection of the PDA and passing ligatures. Angled or tangential vascular clamps are required for surgical division of PDA, or for repair of inadvertent ruptures. Polypropylene

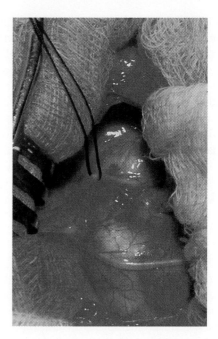

FIG. 24-6
During PDA ligation, elevate and retract the left vagus nerve to expose the ductus arteriosus. The left recurrent laryngeal nerve may be seen as it separates from the vagus nerve and courses caudally around the ductus arteriosus.

mattress sutures (4-0), buttressed with Teflon pledgets, are used for repair of ruptured PDA.

POSTOPERATIVE CARE AND ASSESSMENT

Postoperative pain should be treated with systemic opioids and local anesthetic techniques. Bupivacaine may be used intercostally or intrapleurally to supplement analgesia (see p. 650). Young animals should be fed as soon as they are fully recovered from surgery. Thoracostomy tubes are occasionally placed prior to thoracic closure (e.g., if intraoperative bleeding occurred). They can generally be removed within 12 to 24 hours after surgery.

PROGNOSIS

Dogs with untreated PDA usually develop progressive left-sided congestive heart failure and pulmonary edema. Seventy percent of dogs with untreated PDA die before 1 year of age. Dogs with PDA may also develop suprasystemic pulmonary hypertension that reverses the direction of the shunt causing severe hypoxemia, cyanosis, and exercise intolerance. Ligation of a completely reversed PDA is contraindicated.

Suggested Reading

Birchard SJ, Bonagura JD, Fingland RB: Results of ligation of patent ductus arteriosus in dogs: 201 cases (1969–1988), *J Am Vet Med Assoc* 196:2011, 1990.

Breznock EM et al: A surgical method for correction of patent ductus arteriosus in the dog, *J Am Vet Med Assoc* 158:753, 1971.

Jackson WF, Henderson RA: Ligature placement in closure of patent ductus arteriosus, *J Am Anim Hosp Assoc* 15:55, 1979.

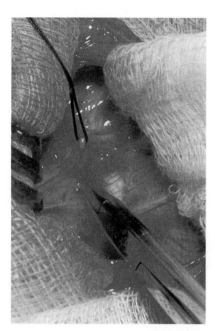

FIG. 24-7
Isolate the craniomedial aspect of the ductus arteriosus by bluntly dissecting with an angled forceps. The forceps should be directed at a 45-degree angle from the transverse plane.

Jones CL, Buchanan J: Patent ductus arteriosus: anatomy and surgery in a cat, *J Am Vet Med Assoc* 179:364, 1981.

O'Brien SE et al: Right-to-left patent ductus arteriosus with dysplastic left ventricle in a dog, *J Am Vet Med Assoc* 192:1435, 1988.

Oswald GP, Orton EC: Patent ductus arteriosus and pulmonary hypertension in related Pembroke Welsh Corgis, *J Am Vet Med Assoc* 202:761, 1993.

Partington BP et al: Transvenous coil embolization for treatment of patent ductus venosus in a dog, *J Am Vet Med Assoc* 202:281, 1993.

Russo EA: Iatrogenic metabolic alkalosis with respiratory alkalosis in a dog with patent ductus arteriosus, *J Am Vet Med Assoc* 183:889, 1983.

PULMONIC STENOSIS

DEFINITIONS

Pulmonic stenosis is a congenital narrowing of the pulmonic valve, pulmonary artery, or right ventricular outflow tract.

SYNONYMS

Pulmonic valve dysplasia, right outflow tract obstruction, PS

GENERAL CONSIDERATIONS AND CLINICALLY RELEVANT PATHOPHYSIOLOGY

Pulmonic stenosis (PS) is a common congenital heart defect in dogs and an uncommon defect in cats. In dogs, the condition is usually valvular, although supravalvular and subvalvular defects have been reported. Subvalvular stenosis can occur as a primary isolated defect, but more often occurs from infundibu-

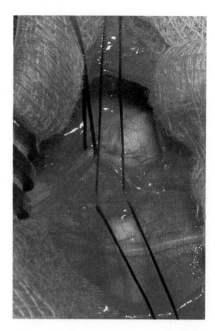

FIG. 24-8
Ligate the PDA by passing two ligatures around the ductus arteriosus. Tie the ligatures separately.

lar hypertrophy secondary to a primary valvular stenosis. Valvular stenosis may be simple, consisting of incomplete separation of valve leaflets, or due to valve dysplasia characterized by a hypoplastic valve annulus and thickened immobile valve leaflets. Greater than 80% of dogs with valvular PS have some degree of valve dysplasia (Fingland, Bonagura, Myer, 1986).

PS causes pressure overload and hypertrophy of the right ventricle. Right ventricular hypertrophy often compounds right ventricular outflow obstruction by narrowing the right ventricular outflow tract. Narrowing of the right ventricular outflow tract is greatest during systole, producing a dynamic obstruction that contributes to the fixed stenosis. Dynamic stenosis has important implications for surgical repair of PS. Dogs with mild to moderate obstructions may remain asymptomatic, whereas dogs with severe obstructions may show exercise intolerance, syncope, progressive right-sided congestive heart failure, or sudden death.

DIAGNOSIS
Clinical Presentation

Signalment. English bulldogs, beagles, miniature schnauzers, cocker spaniels, Samoyeds, mastiffs, and terrier breeds are at increased risk to develop PS. English bulldogs and boxers have a high concurrent incidence of aberrant left coronary artery (due to a single right coronary artery), which has important surgical implications.

History. Young animals with PS are often asymptomatic. Advanced cases may present with exercise intolerance, syncope, or abdominal distention from ascites.

Physical Examination Findings

The predominate physical finding is a systolic ejection murmur heard best at the left heart base. The electrocardiogram may show prominent S waves in leads I, II, III, and aVF indicative of a right axis shift and right ventricular hypertrophy.

Radiography/Echocardiography

Thoracic radiographs show varying degrees of right ventricular enlargement and main pulmonary artery segment enlargement. Diagnosis of PS can be confirmed by echocardiography. Cardiac catheterization is usually only necessary if abnormal coronary anatomy is suspected or an intervention procedure (e.g., percutaneous balloon valvuloplasty) is performed. Echocardiographic findings include right ventricular hypertrophy, poststenotic dilation of the main pulmonary artery, malformation of the pulmonic valve, and a high pulmonary flow velocity. A systolic pressure gradient across the stenosis can be measured directly by right heart catheterization or calculated from the Doppler derived peak systolic pulmonic flow velocity ($\Delta P = 4 V^2$).

Laboratory Findings

Specific laboratory abnormalities are not found in animals with PS.

DIFFERENTIAL DIAGNOSIS

Differential diagnoses include subvalvular aortic stenosis, ventricular septal defect, atrial septal defect, and tetralogy of Fallot.

MEDICAL MANAGEMENT

There is no specific medical therapy for PS other than symptomatic treatment for congestive heart failure, if it occurs. Percutaneous balloon valvuloplasty is a nonsurgical alternative for correction of moderate to severe PS, if facilities and expertise for cardiac catheterization are available. Simple valvular PS is more amenable to balloon valvuloplasty than severe pulmonic valve dysplasia or severe PS with dynamic obstruction.

SURGICAL TREATMENT

Therapy for PS is based on its degree of severity and on type of lesion present. Severity is judged by the presence of signs, extent of right ventricular hypertrophy, and magnitude of systolic pressure gradient. Systolic pressure gradients measured in unsedated or unanesthetized animals are considered mild when they are less than 50 mm Hg, moderate when they are between 50 and 75 mm Hg, and severe when they are greater than 75 mm Hg. Animals with PS that have no signs, mild hypertrophy, and a pressure gradient less than 50 mm of Hg generally do not require surgical intervention. If the pressure gradient is greater than 50 mm Hg and right ventricular hypertrophy is significant, surgical correction should be considered.

English bulldogs with PS present a therapeutic dilemma because of the possibility of concurrent aberrant left coronary artery. In dogs with this defect, the left coronary artery courses across the right ventricular outflow tract and is at risk for injury during valve dilation. Sudden death due to rupture of the coronary artery has occurred during balloon

valvuloplasty. Aberrant left coronary artery also precludes patch-graft valvuloplasty. A valved or nonvalved conduit placed between the right ventricle and pulmonary artery is a possible surgical option for this condition.

Preoperative Management

Right-sided congestive heart failure or cardiac arrhythmias should be managed medically prior to surgery. See preoperative management of animals with cardiovascular disease on p. 575.

Anesthesia

Refer to p. 576 for anesthetic management of cardiac patients.

Surgical Anatomy

The pulmonary valve is approached through a left fourth or fifth intercostal thoracotomy or median sternotomy. The valve consists of right, left, and intermediate semilunar cusps. The area in which sounds associated with lesions of the pulmonary valve may be heard best is located at the fourth intercostal space, slightly below a line drawn through the point of the shoulder. See also comments about concurrent aberrant left coronary arteries above.

Positioning

Animals are positioned in right lateral recumbency and the entire left hemithorax is prepared for aseptic surgery.

SURGICAL TECHNIQUES

Surgical options for correction of PS include valve dilation and patch-graft valvuloplasty. Animals with moderate pressure gradients, simple valvular lesions, and moderate infundibular hypertrophy are most likely to benefit from valve dilation techniques, whereas animals with severe pressure gradients, dysplastic valve lesions, or severe hypertrophy are less likely to respond. Patch-graft valvuloplasty is indicated for severe PS, particularly if marked infundibular hypertrophy and dynamic stenosis are suspected. Patch-graft valvuloplasty also can be used effectively to relieve concurrent or isolated supravalvular PS.

Valve Dilation

Perform a left fourth intercostal thoracotomy. Open the pericardium over the right outflow tract and suture it to the thoracotomy incision. Place a buttressed mattress suture in the right ventricular outflow tract and pass it through a tourniquet. Make a stab incision in the ventricle and pass a dilating instrument into the right ventricular outflow tract and across the pulmonic valve (Fig. 24-9). Dilate the pulmonic valve several times by opening and closing the dilating instrument. Remove the instrument and close the ventricular incision by tieing the mattress suture.

Open-Patch Graft Correction

Open-patch graft correction of PS is performed with inflow occlusion and mild hypothermia (32° to 34° C). Circulatory arrest time should be less than 5 minutes.

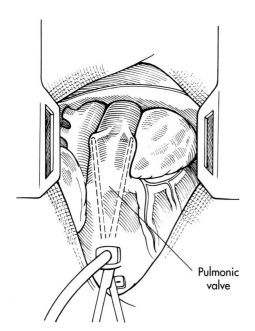

FIG. 24-9
Perform transventricular dilation of the pulmonic valve by placing a pledget-buttressed mattress suture in the right ventricular wall, ventral to the pulmonic valve. Pass the suture ends through tubing to form a tourniquet. Make a stab incision in the ventricle and pass a dilating instrument into the right ventricle and across the pulmonic valve. Dilate the pulmonic valve three to five times. (Illustration modified from Orton EC: *Small animal thoracic surgery*, Philadelphia, 1995, Williams & Wilkins.)

Perform a left fifth intercostal thoracotomy. Pass tape tourniquets around the vena cavae and azygous vein (see Inflow Occlusion on p. 578). Make a partial-thickness incision in the right ventricular outflow tract (Fig. 24-10, A). Suture an autogenous pericardial or synthetic patch to the ventriculotomy incision and the cranial aspect of the pulmonary artery (Fig. 24-10, B). Initiate venous inflow occlusion and make full-thickness incisions into the pulmonary artery and right ventricle (Fig. 24-10, C). Incise or excise dysplastic pulmonic valve leaflets, as necessary. Complete suturing of the pulmonary artery to the patch-graft and discontinue inflow occlusion (Fig. 24-10, D and E). Resuscitate the heart. It is important to remove air from the heart by discontinuing inflow occlusion just prior to tieing the last suture.

SUTURE MATERIALS/SPECIAL INSTRUMENTS

Polypropylene (3-0) suture buttressed with Teflon pledgets is suitable for transventricular valve dilation. Valve dilation can be accomplished with a Cooley or Tubbs valve dilating instrument or with an appropriate size hemostatic forceps. Synthetic materials such as polytetrafluoroethylene (PTFE) or autogenous pericardium can be used for the patch-graft procedure. Polypropylene (4-0) suture is appropriate for suturing the patch-graft.

POSTOPERATIVE CARE AND ASSESSMENT

Postoperative pain should be treated with systemic opioids and local anesthetic techniques (see p. 649) for postthoracotomy analgesia). Animals should be monitored for pulmonary edema after surgery. If pulmonary edema occurs, it should be treated with furosemide.

PROGNOSIS

Valve dilation is associated with minimal risk of complications and carries a low operative mortality, but is less likely to be effective for severe PS. Patch grafting is effective in relieving severe PS, but is unforgiving of technical errors during surgery. Operative mortality for this procedure is approximately 15% to 20% in the hands of an experienced surgeon. The most common problem encountered is inability to resuscitate the heart after inflow occlusion.

Prognosis for dogs with PS depends on its severity. Animals with systolic pressure gradients greater than 75 mm of Hg are likely to experience heart failure or sudden death early in life. The prognosis after surgery depends on the degree of gradient reduction achieved. Valve dilation procedures are effective in relieving moderate to severe stenosis, but may not sufficiently reduce the pressure gradient across severely dysplastic valves. Patch-graft valvuloplasty is highly effective at relieving the pressure gradient across the pulmonic valve regardless of severity, but carries a higher risk of operative mortality. Successful patch-graft valvuloplasty results in substantial pulmonic valve insufficiency, but this has minimal consequence as long as the tricuspid valve is competent and pulmonary hypertension is not present.

Reference

Fingland RB, Bonagura JD, Myer CW: Pulmonic stenosis in the dog: 29 cases (1975–1984), *J Am Vet Med Assoc* 189:218, 1986.

Suggested Reading

Breznock EM, Wood GL: A patch-graft technique for correction of pulmonic stenosis in dogs, *J Am Vet Med Assoc* 169:1090, 1976.
Brownlie SE et al: Percutaneous balloon valvuloplasty in four dogs with pulmonic stenosis, *J Small Anim Pract* 32:165, 1991.
Buchanan JW: Pulmonic stenosis caused by single coronary artery in dogs: four cases (1965–1984), *J Am Vet Med Assoc* 196:115, 1990.
Orton EC, Bruecker KA, McCracken TO: An open patch-graft technique for correction of pulmonic stenosis in the dog, *Vet Surg* 19:148, 1990.
Shores A, Weirich WE: A modified pericardial patch graft technique for correction of pulmonic stenosis in the dog, *J Am Anim Hosp Assoc* 21:809, 1985.
Sisson DD, MacCoy DM: Treatment of congenital pulmonic stenosis in two dogs by balloon valvuloplasty, *J Vet Intern Med* 2:92, 1988.
Whiting PG et al: Double-outlet right ventricle for relief of pulmonic stenosis: an experimental study, *Vet Surg* 13:64, 1984.

FIG. 24-10
To place a transvalvular patch for pulmonic stenosis, pass tapes for inflow occlusion as described in Fig. 24-3.
A, Partially incise the right ventricular outflow tract just ventral to the pulmonic valve. **B,** Suture a synthetic or pericardial patch to the ventriculotomy and cranial aspect of the pulmonary artery. **C,** Initiate inflow occlusion and incise the pulmonary artery, extending the incision across the pulmonary valve. **D,** Make the ventriculotomy incision full thickness. **E,** Finish suturing the patch-graft to the pulmonary artery. (Illustration modified from Orton EC: *Small animal thoracic surgery*, Philadelphia, 1995, Williams & Wilkins.)

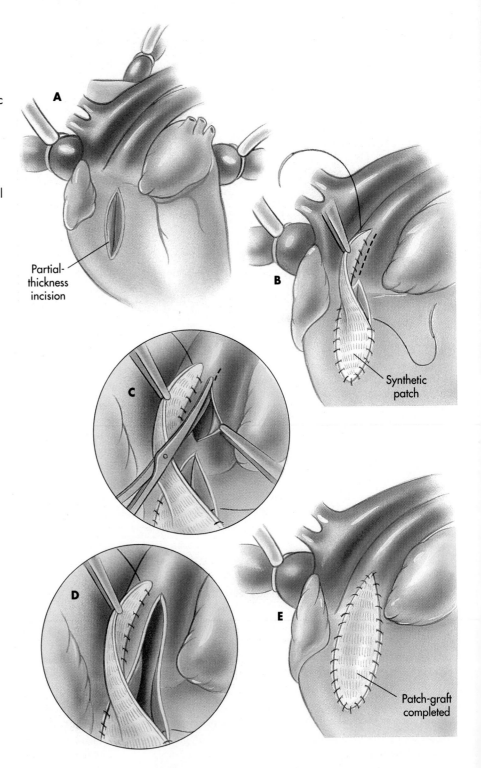

AORTIC STENOSIS

DEFINITIONS

Aortic stenosis is a congenital narrowing of the aortic valve, aorta, or left ventricular outflow tract. The stenosis may be supravalvular, valvular, or subvalvular.

SYNONYMS

Subvalvular aortic stenosis, subaortic stenosis, SAS

GENERAL CONSIDERATIONS AND CLINICALLY RELEVANT PATHOPHYSIOLOGY

Subvalvular aortic stenosis (SAS) is the second most common congenital heart defect of dogs and is the most important defect affecting large-breed dogs. Aortic stenosis (AS) occurs uncommonly in cats. Subvalvular AS accounts for greater than 90% of canine cases and occurs with widely disparate morphology and severity. The typical lesion is a discrete subvalvular fibrous ring that courses across the ventricular septum and reflects onto the anterior mitral valve leaflet. This lesion often is complicated by varying degrees of muscular septal hypertrophy and diffuse fibrosis of the outflow tract. The most severe lesions are associated with an immobile mitral valve leaflet that effectively results in a tunnel-like stenosis. In most cases, SAS is associated with some degree of aortic insufficiency; however, this is usually mild. Concurrent mitral valve insufficiency also occurs.

Subvalvular AS causes pressure overload of the left ventricle. Varying degrees of left ventricular concentric hypertrophy develop depending on severity. Dogs with moderate to severe SAS are at risk for sudden death, presumably the result of myocardial ischemia and malignant ventricular arrhythmias. Dogs with SAS also may develop congestive heart failure, particularly if concurrent mitral insufficiency is present. Lastly, dogs with SAS are at increased risk to develop bacterial endocarditis of the aortic valve due to turbulent blood flow that occurs around the valve.

DIAGNOSIS
Clinical Presentation

Signalment. Newfoundlands, golden retrievers, rottweilers, German shepherds, boxers, and Samoyeds are at increased risk to develop SAS. A genetic basis for SAS has been established in Newfoundland dogs. Phenotypic expression of SAS occurs sometime after birth. The defect may not be clinically apparent until several weeks of age. Subvalvular AS should be considered a progressive lesion until maturity.

History. Dogs with SAS may be asymptomatic or exhibit exercise intolerance, collapse, or syncope. Lack of clinical signs is not an appropriate reason to delay diagnostic evaluation because the first clinical evidence of SAS may be sudden death.

Physical Examination Findings

The predominant physical finding in animals with SAS is a systolic ejection murmur heard best at the left heart base. The murmur radiates well to the right base and thoracic inlet. In moderate to severe cases, femoral pulses are noticeably weak or hypokinetic, unless substantial concurrent aortic insufficiency is present. Electrocardiograms may show a left cranial axis shift or ventricular ectopy, but are usually unremarkable.

Radiography/Echocardiography

Thoracic radiographs may reveal a normal cardiac silhouette or mild left ventricular enlargement. Enlargement of the ascending aorta frequently is evident.

Definitive diagnosis of SAS is obtained by echocardiography. M-mode echocardiography demonstrates variable left ventricular freewall and septal thickening, depending on severity. With moderate to severe disease, left ventricular diameter is small unless substantial concurrent aortic or mitral insufficiency is present. Systolic anterior motion (SAM) of the mitral valve may cause mitral insufficiency. Early closure

TABLE 24-8
Beta-adrenergic Blockers
Propranolol (Inderal)
0.2-2.0 mg/kg PO, BID to TID
Atenolol (Tenormin)
Dogs
6.25-50 mg/dog PO, SID to BID
Cats
6.25-12.5 mg/cat PO, SID to BID

of the aortic valve suggests that dynamic obstruction may be present. Two-dimensional echocardiography provides for direct visualization of the various morphologic components of the lesion. Doppler-measured aortic velocities are increased. The systolic pressure gradient across the aortic valve can be calculated from the peak aortic velocity ($\Delta P = 4 V^2$). Systolic gradients of 25 to 50 mm of Hg are mild, 50 to 75 mm of Hg are moderate, and greater than 75 mm of Hg are severe when measured in unsedated or unanesthetized animals.

Laboratory Findings

Specific laboratory abnormalities are not associated with SAS.

DIFFERENTIAL DIAGNOSIS

Aortic stenosis must be differentiated from other conditions that may cause systolic murmurs (i.e., pulmonic stenosis, ventricular septal defect, tetralogy of Fallot). Physiologic (flow/innocent) systolic murmurs are commonly detected in large-breed dogs but are usually low grade (i.e., I or II) compared with dogs with SAS.

MEDICAL MANAGEMENT

Beta-adrenergic blockage therapy with propranolol or atenolol (Table 24-8) may reduce the risk for sudden death by decreasing myocardial oxygen requirements and suppressing ventricular arrhythmias during exercise. Symptomatic treatment (i.e., furosemide, enalapril) for congestive heart failure is indicated if it occurs. Balloon valvuloplasty may be somewhat beneficial in animals with moderate SAS if facilities for cardiac catheterization are available.

SURGICAL TREATMENT

Surgical intervention should be considered for dogs with substantial left ventricular hypertrophy and systolic gradients above 75 mm of Hg. If surgery is undertaken, it should be done early to minimize degenerative myocardial changes. Surgical options for dogs with SAS include valve dilation and open resection. Open resection during cardiopulmonary bypass is currently the most effective treatment for severe SAS in dogs (Fig. 24-11). Direct visualization of the defect, excision of the discrete fibrous ring, and septal myectomy can be

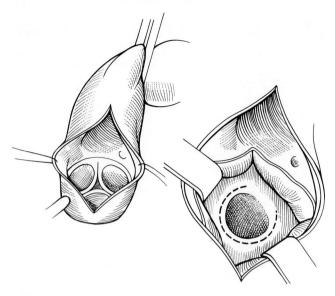

FIG. 24-11
Open resection for subvalvular aortic stenosis is accomplished through an aortotomy during cardiopulmonary bypass. Gently retract the aortic valve leaflets and sharply excise the subvalvular obstruction from the ventricular septum and mitral valve. (Illustration modified from Orton EC: *Small animal thoracic surgery,* Philadelphia, 1995, Williams & Wilkins.)

performed. The latter is indicated if septal hypertrophy is causing dynamic outflow obstruction. Open resection of SAS can be performed in dogs with less than 10% operative mortality by veterinary centers experienced with cardiopulmonary bypass.

Preoperative Management

Arrhythmias should be controlled with appropriate antiarrhythmic drugs (i.e., atenolol, procainamide, tocainamide, sotolol) prior to surgery (see p. 575). Beta-adrenergic blockade should be discontinued 24 hours before surgery by gradually tapering the dose over 3 to 5 days.

Anesthesia

Refer to p. 576 for anesthetic recommendations for cardiac patients.

Surgical Anatomy

The aortic valve consists of right, left, and noncoronary semilunar cusps. The three aortic sinuses are dilations of the aorta on the vessel side of the valve; the right and left coronary arteries leave the right and left sinuses. The aortic bulb is a widening of the base of the ascending aorta formed by the aortic sinuses. The area in which sounds associated with lesions of the aortic valve may be heard best is located at the fourth intercostal space, slightly below a line drawn through the point of the shoulder.

Subvalvular stenosis usually consists of a discrete fibrous ring located 1 to 3 mm below the aortic valve leaflets. The ring generally extends across the septum and reflects onto the anterior mitral valve leaflet. The conduction system (His

bundle) courses through the septum at the juncture of the right and noncoronary aortic leaflets.

Positioning

The animal is positioned in dorsal recumbency to perform a transventricular aortic valve dilation. The entire sternum from proximal to the manubrium to distal to the xiphoid cartilage is prepared for aseptic surgery. Open resection of aortic stenosis is performed through a fourth right intercostal thoracotomy.

SURGICAL TECHNIQUES
Transventricular Aortic Valve Dilation

Perform a median sternotomy (see p. 654). Open the pericardium and suture it to the incision to elevate the apex of the heart. Place a buttressed mattress suture in the left ventricular apex and pass it through a tourniquet. Pass a Cooley valve dilator through a stab incision in the left ventricle and position it in the left ventricular outflow tract by palpating the ascending aorta (Figs. 24-12 and 24-13). Open the valve dilator several times to widen the outflow tract.

SUTURE MATERIALS/SPECIAL INSTRUMENTS

Valve dilation by a transventricular approach is accomplished with a Cooley valve dilator (see Fig. 24-13). Polypropylene (3-0) suture buttressed with Teflon pledgets is used for the transventricular mattress stitch.

POSTOPERATIVE CARE AND ASSESSMENT

Ventilation should be monitored carefully in the early postoperative period. Poor ventilatory efforts may be associated with residual pneumothorax, hemorrhage, anesthetic agents, or pain. Heart rate and rhythm should be monitored postoperatively for 48 to 72 hours, and hemodynamically significant arrhythmias treated. Blood pressure should be measured by direct or indirect means until the animal is fully recovered from anesthesia. Analgesics (local anesthetic techniques and systemic opioids) should be given to decrease postoperative discomfort (see Table 24-6 and p. 581). Urine output should be monitored if hypotension occurred during surgery or postoperatively.

PROGNOSIS

Retrospective analysis of dogs with SAS suggests that those with systolic gradients above 75 mm of Hg have a substantial risk for sudden death in the first several years of life (Kienle, Thomas, Pion, 1994). Valve dilation can be performed at an early age with low operative mortality and without cardiopulmonary bypass. However, there is little evidence that valve dilation results in sustained reduction in the systolic pressure gradient and the long-term benefit of this procedure is questionable. Modest gradient reduction (30% to 40%) has been achieved in approximately 33% of dogs that undergo valve dilation by balloon catheter. It is unclear if valve dilation reduces the risk for sudden death.

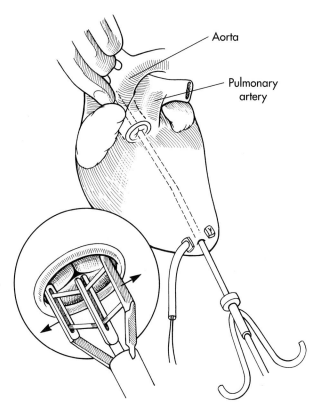

FIG. 24-12
For transventricular dilation of the aortic valve place a pledget-buttressed mattress suture in the left ventricular apex. Pass the suture ends through tubing to form a tourniquet. Make a small stab incision in the left ventricle and pass a dilating instrument across the left ventricular outflow tract while palpating the ascending aorta. Dilate the outflow tract three to five times. (Illustration modified from Orton EC: *Small animal thoracic surgery*, Philadelphia, 1995, Williams & Wilkins.)

Open resection of SAS under cardiopulmonary bypass may result in a 70% to 90% reduction of the systolic pressure gradient that is sustained for at least several years after surgery (Monnet et al, 1996). The procedure reduces, but probably does not eliminate, the risk for sudden death.

References

Kienle RD, Thomas WP, Pion PD: The natural history of canine congenital subaortic stenosis, *J Vet Intern Med* 8:423, 1994.
Monnet E et al: Open resection for subvascular aortic stenosis in dogs, *J Am Vet Med Assoc* 209:1255, 1996.

Suggested Reading

DeLellis LA, Thomas WP, Pion PD: Balloon dilation of congenital subaortic stenosis in the dog, *J Vet Intern Med* 7:153, 1993.
Komtebedde J et al: Resection of subvalvular aortic stenosis: surgical and perioperative management in seven dogs, *Vet Surg* 22:419, 1993.
Linn K, Orton EC: Closed transventricular dilation of discrete subvalvular aortic stenosis in dogs, *Vet Surg* 21:441, 1992.
Wingfield WE, Boon JA, Miller CW: Echocardiographic assessment of congenital aortic stenosis in dogs, *J Am Vet Med Assoc* 183:673, 1983.

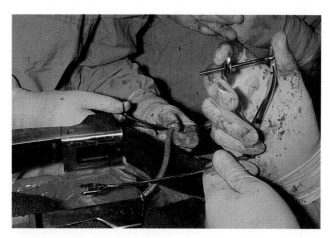

FIG. 24-13
Transventricular dilation of an aortic valve using a Cooley valve dilator.

VENTRICULAR SEPTAL DEFECT

DEFINITIONS

Ventricular septal defect is a congenital defect that results from failure or incomplete development of the membranous or muscular interventricular septum.

SYNONYMS

VSD

GENERAL CONSIDERATIONS AND CLINICALLY RELEVANT PATHOPHYSIOLOGY

Ventricular septal defect (VSD) is the second most common congenital heart defect in cats and accounts for 5% to 10% of congenital heart defects seen in dogs. The etiology of VSD is incompletely understood, but is suspected to have a genetic component. VSD has been demonstrated to be a polygenic trait in keeshonden. Most ventricular septal defects in small animals occur in the membranous septum. Perimembranous defects are located in the membranous septum, medial to the septal tricuspid leaflet, and inferior to the crista supraventricularis. Infundibular or supracristal defects are located in the right outflow tract superior to the crista supraventricularis.

The pathophysiology of VSD depends on the size of the defect and on pulmonary vascular resistance. VSD typically causes a left-to-right shunt. A typical VSD overloads the left heart and, depending on its size and location, may overload the right heart as well. A large VSD can progress to left-sided congestive heart failure. Chronic overcirculation of the lungs can cause progressive pulmonary vascular remodeling leading to severe pulmonary hypertension and right-to-left shunting of blood (Eisenmenger's physiology). Residence at altitude likely accelerates the development of pulmonary hypertension.

Aortic insufficiency is a fairly common secondary abnormality associated with VSD, particularly infundibular VSD.

Aortic insufficiency results from prolapse of an aortic leaflet into the defect. This prolapse is due to the Venturi effect associated with VSD flow and loss of support of the aortic annulus. Aortic insufficiency adds to the left ventricular volume overload and is usually progressive.

DIAGNOSIS
Clinical Presentation

Signalment. No breed predisposition has been clearly determined for VSD; however, English bulldogs may have a higher than expected incidence.

History. Young animals with VSD often are asymptomatic at first presentation. Animals with large VSD may present with signs of left-sided congestive heart failure (i.e., cough and shortness of breath).

Physical Examination Findings

The most prominent physical finding associated with VSD is a systolic murmur with the point of maximal intensity at the right sternum. The murmur usually also is heard well at the left heart base. The murmur is ejection in quality if the defect is small, and regurgitant if the defect is large. A diastolic blowing murmur at the left heart base can give the murmur a continuous quality and suggests the presence of concurrent aortic insufficiency. Animals with right-to-left VSD may have no murmur due to polycythemia.

Radiography/Echocardiography

Thoracic radiographs reveal varying degrees of left or biventricular enlargement depending on the size of the defect. The degree of pulmonary vascular enlargement from overcirculation also depends on the size of the defect and pulmonary vascular resistance. A VSD larger than 5 mm usually can be visualized directly on two-dimensional echocardiography. Color-flow Doppler is particularly useful for detecting small defects. The direction and velocity of shunt flow can be determined by spectral Doppler. A high velocity left-to-right shunt suggests that the VSD is "restrictive" or hemodynamically insignificant and warrants a good prognosis. Large defects are usually associated with lower shunt velocities and suggest the animal is at risk for development of progressive heart failure or pulmonary hypertension. The pulmonary to systemic flow ratio can be calculated from Doppler analysis of aortic and pulmonary flows. Pulmonary to systemic flow ratios (Q_p: Q_s) greater than 2:1 are indicative of a hemodynamically significant VSD.

Laboratory Findings

Polycythemia may be present in dogs with right-to-left shunts.

DIFFERENTIAL DIAGNOSIS

Differential diagnoses include subaortic stenosis, pulmonic stenosis, tetralogy of Fallot, atrial septal defect, and atrioventricular septal defects.

MEDICAL MANAGEMENT

Medical management for VSD (Table 24-9) consists of symptomatic treatment for congestive heart failure. Useful drugs for congestive heart failure include ACE inhibitors (i.e., enalapril), diuretics (i.e., furosemide), and digitalis glycosides (i.e., digoxin). There is no effective medical management for Eisenmenger's physiology. Vasodilator therapy generally will result in increased right-to-left shunting due to preferential dilation of systemic vessels over remodeled pulmonary vessels. Periodic phlebotomy and replacement with crystalloid fluids may be necessary to keep the hematocrit below 60%. Low-dose aspirin therapy is recommended to prevent thromboembolic complications.

SURGICAL TREATMENT

Surgical intervention should be considered for hemodynamically significant VSD. Concurrent aortic insufficiency usually is progressive and also is an indication for surgical intervention. Pulmonary artery banding has been used successfully to palliate dogs and cats with VSD. The goal of pulmonary artery banding is to increase right ventricular systolic pressure, thereby decreasing shunt flow.

Definitive patch closure of VSD can be accomplished with the aid of cardiopulmonary bypass in dogs over 4 kg in body weight. A perimembranous VSD is corrected from the right side via a right atriotomy approach. An infundibular VSD is corrected via a right ventriculotomy from a left thoracotomy or median sternotomy approach.

Preoperative Management

If significant heart failure is present, attempts should be made to control it medically. See also p. 575 for preoperative management of animals with cardiovascular disease.

Anesthesia

Anesthetic management of animals undergoing cardiac surgery is on p. 576.

Surgical Anatomy

The interventricular septum is composed of a dorsal, thin, membranous part and a large, ventral, muscular part. The membranous part is formed by fusion of the atrioventricular cushions. When the cushions fail to fuse, a ventricular septal

TABLE 24-9
Medical Management of Congestive Heart Failure
Enalapril (Vasotec)
0.25-0.5 mg/kg PO, SID to BID
Furosemide (Lasix)
2-4 mg/kg PO, IV, SC, SID to QID as needed
Digoxin (Lanoxin)
0.22 mg/m^2 PO, BID

defect arises. The AV node and its bundle are usually closely associated with the caudal margin of a perimembranous VSD.

Positioning

The animal is positioned in right lateral recumbency for pulmonary artery banding. The entire left thorax is prepared for aseptic surgery.

SURGICAL TECHNIQUES
Pulmonary Artery Banding

Perform a left fourth intercostal thoracotomy. Open the pericardium and suture it to the thoracotomy incision. Separate the pulmonary artery from the aorta using a combination of sharp and blunt dissection. Pass a large cotton or Teflon tape around the pulmonary artery just distal to the pulmonic valve (Fig. 24-14). Tighten the tape to reduce the circumference of the pulmonary artery. Place a purse-string suture in the pulmonary artery wall distal to the ligature and insert a catheter into the pulmonary artery to measure pressures. Constrict the pulmonary artery until the pulmonary artery pressure distal to the band is less than 30 mm Hg. Also, monitor systemic artery pressures, which should increase during the banding. Optimal banding is where the increase in systemic arterial pressures just reaches a plateau.

SUTURE MATERIALS/SPECIAL INSTRUMENTS

Wide cotton or Teflon tape is used for pulmonary artery banding. Polytetrafluoroethylene (PTFE) vascular graft is used for definitive closure of a VSD.

POSTOPERATIVE CARE AND ASSESSMENT

Animals should be closely observed for worsening of heart failure secondary to anesthesia, surgery, or arrhythmias. Hypoxemia or cyanosis suggests that the band may have been placed too tightly. Postoperative pain should be treated with systemic opioids (see Table 24-6 on p. 581) and local anesthetic techniques (see p. 650).

PROGNOSIS

The prognosis for animals with VSD depends on the size of the defect. Animals with small "restrictive" defects may tolerate the defect without ill effects. Large defects (i.e., $Q_p:Q_s$ greater than 2:1) will likely result in the development of progressive heart failure or pulmonary hypertension. Pulmonary artery banding is a reasonably effective procedure for palliation of the consequences of a hemodynamically significant VSD in both dogs and cats. Definitive closure of a VSD under cardiopulmonary bypass is considered curative. Dogs with uncorrected VSD are potentially at increased risk for development of bacterial endocarditis. Aortic insufficiency places an added volume load on the left ventricle and is generally indicative of a poor prognosis.

Suggested Reading

Eyster GE et al: Pulmonary artery banding for ventricular septal defect in dogs and cats, *J Am Vet Med Assoc* 170:434, 1977.
Mann PGH, Stock JE, Sheridan JP: Pulmonary artery banding in the cat: a case report, *J Small Anim Pract* 12:45, 1971.

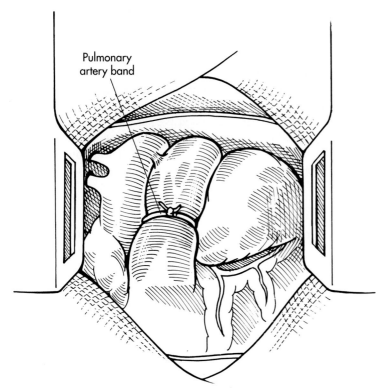

FIG. 24-14
For pulmonary artery banding, pass a tape around the main pulmonary artery. Tighten the tape until pulmonary artery pressure distal to the band is less than 30 mm Hg and systemic artery pressure increases and plateaus. (Illustration modified from Orton EC: *Small animal thoracic surgery*, Philadelphia, 1995, Williams & Wilkins.)

Pulmonary artery band

Sisson D, Luethy M, Thomas WP: Ventricular septal defect accompanied by aortic regurgitation in five dogs, *J Am Anim Hosp Assoc* 27:441, 1991.

Turk JR, Miller JB, Sande RD: Plexogenic pulmonary arteriopathy in a dog with ventricular septal defect and pulmonary hypertension, *J Am Anim Hosp Assoc* 18:608, 1982.

TETRALOGY OF FALLOT

DEFINITION

Tetralogy of Fallot is a complex congenital heart defect that consists of pulmonic stenosis, ventricular septal defect, a dextropositioned overriding aorta, and right ventricular hypertrophy.

SYNONYMS

Tetralogy, T of F

GENERAL CONSIDERATIONS AND CLINICALLY RELEVANT PATHOPHYSIOLOGY

Tetralogy of Fallot (T of F) is the most common congenital heart defect that causes cyanosis in small animals. It occurs in cats and a variety of canine breeds (see below under signalment). Tetralogy of Fallot can be simplified into two physiologically significant defects: pulmonic stenosis and ventricular septal defect (VSD). The pathophysiologic consequences of tetralogy depend on the relative magnitude of these two defects. If a large VSD and hemodynamically insignificant pulmonic stenosis are present, the functional result is a left-to-right shunt and volume overload of the left heart similar to an isolated, large VSD. If severe pulmonic stenosis, suprasystemic right heart pressures, and right-to-left shunt are present, the result is moderate to severe cyanosis, exercise intolerance, and progressive polycythemia. A shortened life span is expected in these animals due to complications of hyperviscosity-induced thromboembolism or sudden death. Animals that have pulmonic stenosis and VSD that are somewhat balanced are functionally similar to those that have a VSD and pulmonary artery banding performed (see p. 593). Animals with predominantly left-to-right shunt are termed acyanotic tetralogy and may function reasonably well as long as the shunt flow is insufficient to cause left heart failure. Progression of pulmonic stenosis due to infundibular hypertrophy is possible and may cause acyanotic animals to become cyanotic as they age.

DIAGNOSIS
Clinical Presentation

Signalment. Breeds most commonly reported to have tetralogy of Fallot include keeshonden, English bulldogs, poodles, schnauzers, terriers, collies, and shelties. In keeshonden, tetralogy is genetically transmitted as part of the spectrum of conotruncal defects.

History. Clinical findings at presentation for a typical tetralogy of Fallot include moderate to severe exercise intolerance, exertional tachypnea, collapse, and syncope.

Physical Examination Findings

Physical findings in animals with T of F include cyanosis unresponsive to supplemental oxygen and systolic murmurs heard well at the left heart base and right sternum. If polycythemia is severe, a murmur may not be heard.

Radiography/Echocardiography/Electrocardiography

Thoracic radiographs typically show evidence of right ventricular enlargement, with or without main pulmonary artery enlargement. Pulmonary vessels are usually small, suggesting pulmonary undercirculation. Electrocardiograms usually show a right axis shift in the frontal plane suggestive of right ventricular hypertrophy.

Two-dimensional echocardiography demonstrates all the elements of tetralogy, including right ventricular hypertrophy, pulmonic stenosis, ventricular septal defect, and overriding aorta. Doppler interrogation of the pulmonic outflow tract and septal defect is useful in determining the direction and magnitude of the shunt.

Laboratory Findings

Polycythemia (i.e., PCV greater than 55%) is often present because of the chronic hypoxemia.

DIFFERENTIAL DIAGNOSIS

Differentials include right-to-left shunting VSD, atrial septal defect, atrioventricular septal defect, complex cyanotic cardiac disease, and patent ductus arteriosus.

MEDICAL MANAGEMENT

Periodic phlebotomy with crystalloid fluid replacement may be necessary to maintain the hematocrit below 60% in animals with severe cyanosis and progressive polycythemia. Extreme caution must be taken to avoid introducing intravenous air during this procedure to avoid systemic vascular air embolism. Low-dose aspirin therapy is also recommended to reduce the risk of thromboembolic complications.

Beta-adrenergic blockage therapy with propranolol or atenolol has been advocated as a palliative treatment for T of F (Table 24-10). Possible beneficial effects include reduced dynamic outflow obstruction, decreased heart rate, increased systemic vascular resistance, and decreased myocardial oxygen demand.

SURGICAL TREATMENT

Surgery should be considered for severely cyanotic animals to lessen clinical signs and prolong life. Animals with a resting arterial oxygen saturation less than 70% should be considered candidates for surgery. Palliative surgeries for tetralogy include isolated correction of the pulmonic stenosis or creation of a systemic-to-pulmonary shunt (e.g., Blalock-Taussig shunt; see below). Correction of the pulmonic stenosis risks overcorrection of the stenosis and an overwhelming left-to-right shunt. For this reason, valve dilation (see p. 586), either surgically or by balloon dilation, is preferred over a more definitive procedure such as a patch-graft (see p. 587). Definitive

TABLE 24-10
Beta-Adrenergic Therapy in Dogs
Propranolol
0.2-2.0 mg/kg PO, BID to TID, or titrate to control heart rate
Atenolol
Dogs
6.25-50 mg/dog, PO, SID to BID
Cats
6.25-12.5 mg/cat, PO, SID to BID

repair of tetralogy can be undertaken in medium- to large-breed dogs with cardiopulmonary bypass. Patch closure of the VSD and patch-grafting of the pulmonary outflow tract are undertaken through a right ventriculotomy approach.

Preoperative Management

Although arrhythmias are uncommon, an ECG should be performed and hemodynamically significant arrhythmias controlled before surgery. Severe polycythemia should be corrected before surgery.

Anesthesia

Recommendations for anesthetic management of animals undergoing cardiac surgery are on p. 576.

Surgical Anatomy

With T of F, the parietal portion of the infundibular septum attaches more cranial and leftward than normal, resulting in a narrowing of the right ventricular outflow tract and dextropositioned overriding of the aorta. The magnitude of this shift determines which type of physiology is associated with the defect. The VSD is usually located high in the infundibular septum, just below the crista supraventricularis, although supracristal septal defects do occur.

Positioning

The animal should be positioned in right lateral recumbency for Blalock-Taussig shunt surgery. The entire left hemithorax is prepared for aseptic surgery.

SURGICAL TECHNIQUES

Several types of systemic-to-pulmonary shunts have been used to palliate tetralogy of Fallot. A modified Blalock-Taussig shunt is accomplished by harvesting the left subclavian artery as a free autogenous graft and placing it between the aorta and main pulmonary artery (Fig. 24-15).

Perform a left fourth intercostal thoracotomy. Harvest an autogenous arterial graft by ligating and dividing the proximal left subclavian artery. Open the pericardium and suture it to the thoracotomy incision. Place tangential vascular clamps on the pulmonary artery and ascending aorta. Make incisions into both vessels by making a longitudinal

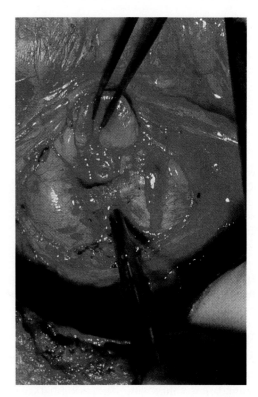

FIG. 24-15
Modified Blalock-Taussig shunt for tetralogy of Fallot.

incision in the vessel wall held within the clamp. Interpose the graft between the aorta and pulmonary artery by end-to-side anastomoses using simple continuous suture patterns. Be sure that the graft is not kinked. Release the clamps and verify hemostasis at the suture sites. The pulmonary artery clamp should be released first.

SUTURE MATERIALS/SPECIAL INSTRUMENTS

Polypropylene (5-0) suture is used for the vascular anastomoses of the Blalock-Taussig shunt. Two tangential vascular clamps are required to control hemorrhage during the surgery.

POSTOPERATIVE CARE AND ASSESSMENT

Postoperative pain should be treated with systemic opioids (see Table 24-6 on p. 581) and local anesthetic techniques (see p. 650). Postoperative care of patients undergoing cardiac surgery is on p. 579.

PROGNOSIS

Animals with reasonably balanced acyanotic tetralogy of Fallot should be followed for progression, but otherwise generally do not require surgical intervention. These animals have a reasonably good prognosis. The prognosis for animals with cyanotic tetralogy depends on the shunt fraction, magnitude of hypoxemia, and degree of polycythemia. Some animals may live several years without surgical therapy despite moderate to severe exercise intolerance. Animals with severe hypoxemia and progressive polycythemia will likely succumb to the effects of the disease or will experience sudden death early in life. Modified Blalock-Taussig shunts are reasonably effective at reducing the magnitude of hypoxemia and palliating the consequences of tetralogy of Fallot.

Suggested Reading

Eyster GE et al: Surgical management of tetralogy of Fallot, *J Sm Anim Pract* 18:387, 1977.

Miller CW et al: Microsurgical management of tetralogy of Fallot in a cat, *J Am Vet Med Assoc* 186:708, 1985.

Ringwald RJ, Bonagura JD: Tetralogy of Fallot in the dog: clinical findings in 13 cases, *J Am Anim Hosp Assoc* 24:33, 1988.

PERICARDIAL EFFUSION AND PERICARDIAL CONSTRICTION

DEFINITIONS

The **pericardium** is a fibroserous envelope that encompasses the heart and great vessels. **Pericardial effusion** is an abnormal accumulation of fluid within the pericardial sac. **Cardiac tamponade** refers to the decompensated phase of cardiac compression resulting from an unchecked rise in intrapericardiac fluid pressure. **Pericardial constriction** results from a restrictive fibrosis of the parietal and/or visceral pericardium that interferes with diastolic function of the heart.

SYNONYMS

For cardiac tamponade—**pericardial tamponade.** For pericardial constriction—**constrictive pericarditis.**

GENERAL CONSIDERATIONS AND CLINICALLY RELEVANT PATHOPHYSIOLOGY

Diseases affecting primarily the pericardium account for approximately 1% of cardiovascular disease. Although primary pericardial disease represents a small percentage of the total number of cardiac diseases in small animals, it is an important cause of right-sided congestive heart failure in dogs. Pericardial diseases of all types are uncommon in cats. Several types of primary and secondary pericardial diseases occur, the most common of which are those resulting in the accumulation of pericardial effusion. Pericardial effusion can be transudative, exudative (inflammatory), or sanguineous. Causes of pericardial transudation include right-sided congestive heart failure, hypoproteinemia, or incarceration of a liver lobe within the pericardial cavity. Transudative pericardial effusions are usually subclinical.

Infectious pericarditis is an uncommon cause of pericardial effusion in dogs and cats, usually producing a purulent or fibrinous exudate. A variety of aerobic and anaerobic bacterial and fungal organisms have been associated with infectious pericarditis. Bacterial pericarditis can arise from bite wounds to the thorax, migrating foreign bodies, or hema-togenous seeding. Coccidioidomycosis is an important cause of pericardial effusion in endemic regions. In cats, feline infectious peritonitis and toxoplasmosis are potential causes of inflammatory effusions.

The most common cause of pericardial effusion in dogs is neoplasia. Neoplasms that produce pericardial effusion in dogs include hemangiosarcoma, chemodectomas, ectopic (heart base) thyroid carcinoma, pericardial mesothelioma, and metastatic carcinoma to the heart. Hemangiosarcomas may be multicentric with simultaneous splenic or hepatic involvement (see also p. 456). Aortic body tumors (chemodectoma, nonchromaffin paraganglioma) sometimes invade the heart base and cause pericardial effusion (see also p. 601). Lymphosarcoma, mesothelioma, and metastatic carcinoma have been implicated in cats with pericardial effusion. Neoplastic pericardial effusions usually are sanguineous.

Idiopathic (benign) pericardial effusion is the second most common cause of pericardial effusion in dogs. This condition has not been reported in cats. The effusion usually appears sanguineous and must be differentiated from neoplastic effusions. Coagulopathies or left atrial rupture secondary to chronic mitral insufficiency are rare causes of acute pericardial hemorrhage.

Pathophysiologic alterations associated with pericardial effusion depend on the rate and volume of fluid accumulation and distensibility or compliance of the pericardium. If effusion accumulates slowly, the pericardium will expand and hypertrophy to accommodate the fluid, intrapericardiac pressure will not increase initially, and cardiac filling will not be compromised. Slow progressive accumulation of pericardial fluid allows compensatory mechanisms to occur. First, fibrous pericardium can stretch and remodel over time to accommodate an increased volume of fluid with only a modest increase in intrapericardiac pressure. Second, neurohumoral mechanisms are evoked that lead to retention of vascular volume and increased diastolic filling pressures within the heart. Although the later compensatory mechanism delays the onset of cardiac tamponade, it leads to signs of progressive right-sided congestive heart failure including jugular venous distention, ascites, peripheral edema, and pleural effusion. Cardiac tamponade eventually does occur despite compensatory mechanisms leading to presentation for acute circulatory collapse.

Conversely, rapid or sudden accumulation of fluid (e.g., pericardial hemorrhage) results in acute *cardiac tamponade.* Rapid fluid accumulation in the pericardial space compresses the ventricles, restricts ventricular filling, and reduces cardiac output. Although significant volumes of fluid are usually required to raise pericardial pressure initially, additional small volumes may markedly increase intrapericardiac pressure and significantly impede ventricular filling. Because of their thin walls and low pressures, the right atrium and ventricle are more vulnerable than the left due to the effects of cardiac compression. Diastolic pressures (i.e., pulmonary wedge pressure, left and right ventricular end-diastolic pressures, and mean right atrial pressure) on both sides of the heart equilibrate.

Pericardial constriction occurs when visceral or parietal pericardial layers, or both, become fused, thickened, densely fibrotic, or inelastic and form a rigid case around the heart. The pericardial space may become totally obliterated or may contain small amounts of fluid. Constrictive pericardial disease may develop asymmetrically so that one ventricle is more affected than the other; however, in most cases both ventricles are affected nearly equally. An audible "pericardial knock" may be heard during early diastolic filling and is attributed to vibrations produced by the sudden deceleration of blood as it strikes the encased nondistensible ventricular wall. As constriction worsens, cardiac output declines even though myocardial systolic function may be maintained. Fluid retention initiated by chronically reduced cardiac output further contributes to venous congestion, which is most commonly manifested as hepatomegaly and ascites accumulation.

DIAGNOSIS
Clinical Presentation

Signalment. Idiopathic benign and neoplastic pericardial effusions are more commonly observed in large- and giant-breed dogs. Hemangiosarcoma of the right atrium is especially common in German shepherds and golden retrievers (see also p. 601). Idiopathic pericardial effusion has been reported most commonly in golden retrievers, German shepherds, and other large-breed dogs. Aortic body tumors are most common in aged brachycephalic dogs. Medium- to large-breed, middle-age dogs are most commonly affected with constrictive pericardial disease; however, the condition is rare.

History. Presenting complaints associated with pericardial effusion include weakness, lethargy, exercise intolerance, and/or collapse. Often, patients present with right-sided congestion, ascites, and/or pleural effusion. The most common owner complaint with constrictive pericarditis is abdominal enlargement. Less frequently, dyspnea, tachypnea, weakness, syncope, and/or weight loss may be noted. Occasionally, there will be a previous history of idiopathic pericardial effusion.

Physical Examination Findings

Clinical findings are related to the consequences of cardiac tamponade and right-sided congestive heart failure. The classic triad of signs of cardiac tamponade (e.g., rapid and weak arterial pulse, distended systemic veins, and diminished heart sounds) are usually present. Jugular venous distention or a positive hepatojugular reflux will be present, but commonly overlooked. Measurement of central venous pressure will document systemic venous hypertension and frequently exceeds 10 ml H_2O (normal = less than 6 ml H_2O). Lung sounds may be diminished if pleural effusion is present. Other auscultatory abnormalities (e.g., gallop rhythms, cardiac murmurs, arrhythmias) are uncommon. Ascites, hepatomegaly, and/or peripheral edema may also be noted.

Although there are no pathognomonic electrocardiographic findings for pericardial disease, there are several electrocardiographic abnormalities that occur. Electrical alternans is a beat-to-beat voltage variation of the QRS or ST-T complexes. It may be recorded in as many as 50% of patients with pericardial effusion. If present electrical alternans is strongly suggestive of pericardial effusion. It is caused by swinging of the heart within large pericardial effusions, rather than alterations in conduction within the heart, and is most likely to occur at heart rates between 90 and 144 beats per minute. Other findings supportive of pericardial effusion on electrocardiograms are diminished QRS voltages and ST segment depression. Sinus tachycardia is the predominant rhythm, although nonsustained ventricular tachycardia may be present.

Radiography/Echocardiography

Thoracic radiography usually demonstrates varying degrees of globoid enlargement (i.e., the cardiac silhouette loses its angles and waists and becomes globe-shaped) of the cardiac silhouette (Fig. 24-16). Radiographic evidence of pulmonary congestion or edema is not an expected finding, and this helps distinguish pericardial effusion from dilated cardiomyopathy. If right-sided congestion has developed, distention of the caudal vena cava, hepatomegaly, ascites, and pleural effusion are usually evident. Heart base tumors may deviate the trachea and produce a mass effect. Abnormal radiographic findings in animals with constrictive pericarditis are subtle; the cardiac silhouette may be rounded. Dilation of the caudal vena cava may be evident.

Fluoroscopy may demonstrate reduced cardiac motion in animals with pericardial effusion. Pneumopericardiography is useful for identifying intrapericardial mass lesions. Angiography will usually show filling defects or tumor vascularity if neoplasia is the cause of the effusion; furthermore, angiography will show increased endocardial-pericardial distance typical of pericardial effusion. Although these modalities are reliable when properly used, echocardiography has supplanted most indications for their use.

Definitive diagnosis of pericardial effusion is obtained readily by echocardiography. The fibrous pericardium is easily identified as a thin echo-dense structure and any degree of separation or echo-free space between the pericardium and

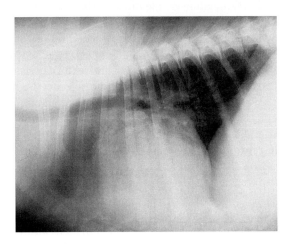

FIG. 24-16
Thoracic radiograph of a dog with idiopathic pericardial effusion. Note the large, globoid heart.

underlying cardiac structures on two-dimensional or M-mode echocardiography is diagnostic of pericardial effusion. Echocardiography is the most reliable procedure for identifying primary cardiac neoplasia, although failure to identify a mass does not rule out neoplasia. Flattening of the left ventricular endocardium during diastole, abnormal diastolic (early notch) and systolic septal motion are often noted in patients with constrictive pericarditis. Differentiation of constrictive pericardial disease and restrictive myopathy may be difficult with echocardiography.

Laboratory Findings

With pericardial effusion, the CBC may indicate inflammation or infection. Increased numbers of circulating nucleated RBCs are suggestive of cardiac or splenic hemangiosarcoma. Cardiac enzymes may be elevated owing to ischemia or myocardial invasion. Other abnormalities may be associated with the primary disease or with CHF. Serum fungal titers (coccidioidomycosis) or ELISA tests for FeLV or FIP (cats) may be positive when pericarditis is related to these infections. Chronic right heart congestion associated with pericardial effusion or constriction can cause splenic dysfunction (functional hyposplenism) and protein-losing enteropathy (intestinal lymphangiectasia). Hyposplenism can result in increased numbers of circulating activated platelets, while protein-losing enteropathy may exacerbate the splenic dysfunction and cause reductions in circulating antithrombin III levels. Both conditions promote a hypercoagulable state and may make affected animals prone to pulmonary thromboembolism.

> ☞ **NOTE** · Pulmonary thromboembolism should be considered likely in dogs with pericardial effusion that exhibit severe, sudden respiratory distress.

Cytologic and microbiologic analysis should be performed on fluid obtained by pericardiocentesis. An inflammatory exudate on cytologic examination suggests infectious pericarditis. The causative organism may be visible on cytologic examination or identified by bacterial or fungal culture. Neoplastic effusions are usually sanguineous (i.e., characterized by large numbers of red blood cells and variable numbers of neutrophils and mononuclear cells). Cytology is unreliable in identifying neoplastic effusions as both false positives and false negatives occur (Sisson, Thomas, Ruehl, 1984). Idiopathic pericardial effusion produces a sanguineous effusion that is difficult to distinguish from neoplastic effusions on fluid analysis alone. Exploratory surgery and histopathology may be necessary to definitively differentiate between neoplastic and idiopathic pericardial effusion.

DIFFERENTIAL DIAGNOSIS

In addition to pericardial effusion, differentials for a globoid-appearing heart on thoracic radiographs include dilated cardiomyopathy and peritoneopericardial diaphragmatic hernia (see p. 685). The latter may be associated with pericardial effusion, particularly when the liver is herniated.

Ultrasonography is used to detect incongruities in the diaphragmatic silhouette and identify abdominal contents within the pericardial sac. Echocardiography differentiates diffuse cardiac enlargement from pericardial effusion. If echocardiography is not available, nonselective angiography can be used.

MEDICAL MANAGEMENT

Pericardiocentesis is the treatment of choice for initial stabilization of dogs and cats with pericardial effusion and cardiac tamponade. When performed properly, pericardiocentesis is associated with minimal complications. It should be attempted in symptomatic animals with suspected pericardial effusion, even if echocardiography is not available to confirm the diagnosis.

> ☞ **NOTE** · If possible, monitor an electrocardiogram during pericardiocentesis because inadvertent cardiac contact usually produces premature ventricular complexes.

Shave and surgically prepare a large area of the right hemithorax (sternum to midthorax, third to eighth rib). Perform a local block with lidocaine and, if necessary, sedate the animal (e.g., oxymorphone, fentanyl; Table 24-11). Be sure to infiltrate the pleura with lidocaine because pleural penetration seems to cause significant discomfort. Place the animal in sternal or lateral recumbency, depending on its demeanor. Pericardiocentesis can be accomplished in the standing animal, but adequate restraint is essential to prevent cardiac puncture or pulmonary laceration. *Determine the puncture site based on heart location on thoracic radiographs.* This is most commonly between the fourth and fifth intercostal spaces at the costochondral junction. *Attach a 14- to 18-gauge needle or catheter to a three-way stopcock, extension tubing, and syringe to allow constant negative pressure to be applied during insertion and drainage. Once the catheter has been inserted through the skin, apply negative pressure. If pleural effusion is present, it will be obtained immediately upon entering the thoracic cavity.* Pleural effusion associated with heart disease is usually a clear to pale yellow color. *Advance the catheter until it contacts the pericardium and a scratching sensation is noticed. Then, advance the catheter slightly to penetrate pericardium. Stop advancing the catheter as soon as fluid is obtained. Withdraw the needle immediately if the epicardium is contacted and cardiac motion is felt through the*

TABLE 24-11
Sedation during Pericardiocentesis in Dogs
Oxymorphone (Numorphan)
0.05-0.1 mg/kg SC, IM, or IV
Fentanyl (Sublimaze)
0.005 IV or 0.01 mg/kg SC, IM

needle. Ultrasound guidance is seldom necessary when performing pericardiocentesis unless the volume of fluid is small or it is compartmentalized.

Pericardiocentesis causes immediate clinical improvement in animals with cardiac tamponade. The pulse slows and strengthens as soon as an adequate volume of fluid has been removed. Pericardial effusion can be differentiated from peripheral blood in that it rarely clots and the PCV is significantly lower than peripheral blood. Approximately 50% of dogs with idiopathic effusion are managed successfully by periodic pericardiocentesis and possibly corticosteroids (oral prednisolone; Table 24-12) without pericardiectomy. In the remainder, repeat centesis is necessary to control clinical signs. Fluid may reaccumulate rapidly (within several days) or may not recur for months or even several years. In patients requiring more than two centeses, subphrenic pericardiectomy is usually indicated. Although anti-inflammatory doses of prednisolone are commonly administered to dogs with idiopathic pericardial effusion, there are no controlled studies to confirm the efficacy of this therapy. Subtotal pericardiectomy is usually curative in dogs with idiopathic pericardial effusion. Recurrent effusion and pericardial constriction are possible late sequelae of idiopathic effusions if pericardiectomy is not performed.

SURGICAL TREATMENT

Although temporary relief of cardiac tamponade is provided by pericardiocentesis, long-term palliation of pericardial effusion often requires pericardiectomy. Removing only a small portion of the pericardium may result in the remaining pericardium adhering to the heart and recurrence of pericardial effusion. Pericardiectomy can be performed through an intercostal thoracotomy (see p. 652) or median sternotomy (see p. 654). It is technically easier to perform a pericardiectomy through a median sternotomy because access to both sides of the heart and both phrenic nerves is provided by this approach. If right atrial hemangiosarcoma is suspected, either a right fifth intercostal thoracotomy or a median sternotomy should be used. Removal of right atrial tumors can be accomplished equally well from either approach (see p. 602). Chemodectomas can arise on either the left or right heart base. Pericardiectomy in these cases should be performed through a thoracotomy on the side where the bulk of the tumor is suspected to be. If cardiac neoplasia is not identified prior to surgery and idiopathic pericardial effusion is suspected, then pericardiectomy should be performed through a right thoracotomy or medial sternotomy so that the right atrium can be examined and resected, if nec-

essary. Although total pericardiectomy can be performed, subphrenic pericardiectomy is usually adequate for animals with pericardial effusion. Total pericardiectomy may be indicated in some animals with neoplasia or infectious processes of the pericardium. Total pericardiectomy is best performed from a median sternotomy approach.

Pericardiectomy is the therapy of choice for constrictive pericarditis. Complications associated with surgery include development of arrhythmias (most notably atrial fibrillation or ventricular tachycardia). The outcome with surgery depends on severity of the underlying disease. If the visceral pericardium (epicardium) is significantly involved, the surgical outcome is less favorable. Epicardial decortication may be necessary.

Preoperative Management

If hemodynamically significant quantities of pericardial effusion are present (i.e., cardiac tamponade as evidenced by jugular vein distention, ascites, and/or pleural effusion), the animal should have pericardiocentesis performed prior to surgery. Metabolic causes of pericardial effusion such as hypoproteinemia should be ruled out. Electrolyte and acid-base abnormalities, which may be associated with high doses of diuretics, should be corrected prior to anesthetic induction.

Anesthesia

Refer to p. 576 for anesthetic management of cardiac patients. Care should be exercised when manipulating the heart because arrhythmias or hypotension may occur.

Surgical Anatomy

The pericardium envelops the heart in a strong flask-shaped sac with extensions that enclose the origins of the ascending aorta, pulmonary artery, distal pulmonary veins, and venae cavae. The adventitia of the great arteries blends with fibrous tissues of the pericardium forming strong attachments. The pericardium is firmly attached to the diaphragm via the pericardiophrenic ligament. Pericardium is composed of two layers: a fibrous outer layer and an inner serous membrane composed of a single layer of mesothelial cells. The inner serous layer forms the epicardium or visceral pericardium. It reflects back on itself to line the outer fibrous layer and together they form the parietal pericardium.

The pericardial cavity is filled with a variable amount of pericardial fluid. This fluid is an ultrafiltrate of serum containing between 1.7 and 3.5 g/dl of protein and having a colloid osmotic pressure approximately 25% that of serum. The volume of pericardial fluid present in normal dogs ranges from 1 to 15 ml. Lymphatic drainage of the pericardium is similar to that of the myocardium with most drainage via epicardial lymphatics, rather than from parietal pericardium. Functions ascribed to the pericardium include the ability to fix the heart anatomically and prevent excessive motion associated with changes in body position, reduction of friction between the heart and surrounding structures, and preventing extension of infection or malignancy from the pleural space.

TABLE 24-12

Oral Prednisone Therapy for Dogs with Idiopathic Pericardial Effusion

Begin at a dose of 1 mg/kg orally every 12 hours; then gradually decrease the dosage over a 2- to 3-week period and discontinue.

Positioning

The animal should be placed in either lateral recumbency for an intercostal thoracotomy or in dorsal recumbency for median sternotomy. A sufficiently large area should be prepared to allow intraoperative placement of a thoracostomy tube.

SURGICAL TECHNIQUES
Subphrenic (Subtotal) Pericardiectomy via Right Thoracotomy

After opening the chest, open the pericardium and submit fluid samples for microbiological examination, fungal culture, and/or cytology, if indicated. Make a T-shaped incision in the pericardium from cardiac base to apex and across the cardiac base ventral to the phrenic nerve (Fig. 24-17, A). Extend the circumferential incision at the car- diac base around the venae cavae taking care not to violate the vessel walls (Fig. 24-17, B). Have an assistant elevate the heart and retract it as the circumferential incision is extended to the opposite side (Fig. 24-17, C). Take care not to injure the contralateral phrenic nerve. Divide the pericardiophrenic ligament with cautery or between ligatures (Fig. 24-17, D). Check the remnants of the pericardium to ensure that there is no hemorrhage. Submit pericardium for histologic analyses. Place a thoracostomy tube prior to thoracic closure.*

Total Pericardiectomy

Using blunt dissection, carefully elevate the phrenic nerves from the pericardial sac. Make a longitudinal incision in the pericardial sac and resect the pericardium as close to

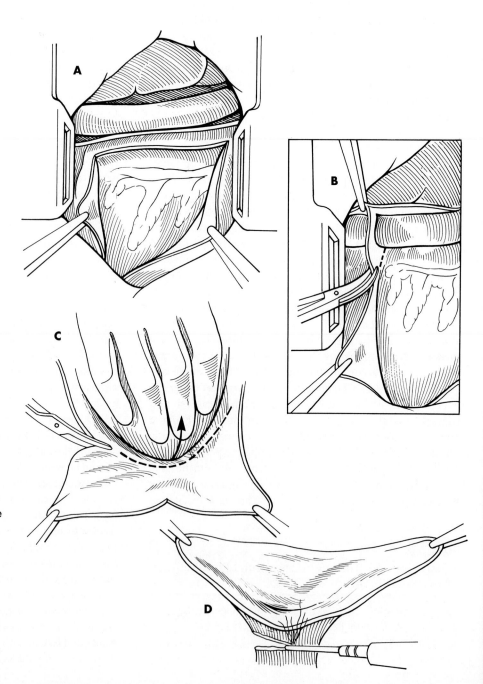

FIG. 24-17
For subtotal pericardiectomy via a right fifth intercostal thoracotomy, **A,** incise the epicardium vertically and horizontally ventral to the right phrenic nerve. **B,** Carefully extend the incision around the venae cavae taking care to identify the vessel wall while making the incision. **C,** Gently retract the heart and extend the incision across the left side, ventral to the left phrenic nerve. **D,** Divide the pericardiophrenic ligament with cautery or between ligatures. (Illustration modified from Orton EC: *Small animal thoracic surgery,* Philadelphia, 1995, Williams & Wilkins.)

the base of the heart as possible. Place a thoracostomy tube prior to thoracic closure.

SUTURE MATERIALS/SPECIAL INSTRUMENTS

Electrocautery is useful for pericardiectomy to decrease intraoperative and postoperative hemorrhage. Inflamed pericardium often has an increased number of blood vessels and significant hemorrhage can occur after pericardiectomy if they are not cauterized or ligated.

POSTOPERATIVE CARE AND ASSESSMENT

The thoracostomy tube should be aspirated every hour initially and the volume of pleural effusion quantitated. After 4 to 6 hours, frequency of drainage may be decreased to every 2 to 4 hours. Once the pleural effusion has decreased to levels consistent with those caused by the thoracostomy tube the tube may be removed. If the patient develops acute respiratory distress without evidence of pleural effusion or significant pulmonary infiltrates suggestive of pulmonary edema, pulmonary thromboembolism should be suspected. Oxygen therapy may be beneficial in such cases. If a definitive diagnosis of pulmonary thromboembolism is made, thrombolytic agents may be used. Postoperative pain should be treated with systemic opioids (see Table 24-6) and local anesthetic techniques (see p. 650).

PROGNOSIS

Pericardiectomy is palliative for neoplastic pericardial effusion and curative for idiopathic pericardial effusion. Long-term palliation after pericardiectomy is possible for dogs with mesothelioma or chemodectoma. Intracavitary cisplatin has shown promise in achieving long-term remission in dogs with mesothelioma (Moore et al, 1991). Chemodectomas are slow-growing tumors and long-term palliation with pericardiectomy and primary mass excision is possible. Median survival for dogs with cardiac hemangiosarcoma is approximately 4 months with pericardiectomy.

References

Moore AS et al: Intracavitary cisplatin chemotherapy experience with six dogs, *J Vet Int Med* 5:227, 1991.

Sisson D, Thomas WP, Ruehl WW: Diagnostic value of pericardial fluid analysis in the dog, *J Am Vet Med Assoc* 51:184, 1984.

Suggested Reading

Berg RJ, Wingfield W: Pericardial effusion in the dog: a review of 42 cases, *J Am Anim Hosp Assoc* 20:721, 1984.

Berg RJ, Wingfield WE, Hoopes PJ: Idiopathic hemorrhagic pericardial effusion in eight dogs, *J Am Vet Med Assoc* 185:988, 1984.

Berry CR et al: Echocardiographic evaluation of cardiac tamponade in dogs before and after pericardiocentesis: four cases (1984–1986), *J Am Vet Med Assoc* 192:1597, 1988.

Bouvy BM, Bjorling DE: Pericardial effusion in dogs and cats. Part 1. Normal pericardium and causes and pathophysiology of pericardial effusion, *Compend Contin Educ Pract Vet* 13:417, 1991.

Bouvy BM, Bjorling DE: Pericardial effusion in dogs and cats. Part II. Diagnostic approach and treatment, *Compend Contin Educ Pract Vet* 13:633, 1991.

de Madron E, Prymak C, Hendricks J: Idiopathic hemorrhagic pericardial effusion with organized thrombi in a dog, *J Am Vet Med Assoc* 191:324, 1987.

Matthiesen DT, Lammerding J: Partial pericardiectomy for idiopathic hemorrhagic pericardial effusion in the dog, *J Am Anim Hosp Assoc* 21:41, 1985.

Rush JE, Keene BW, Fox PR: Pericardial disease in the cat: a retrospective evaluation of 66 cases, *J Am Anim Hosp Assoc* 26:39, 1990.

Thomas WP et al: Constrictive pericardial disease in the dog, *J Am Vet Med Assoc* 184:546, 1984.

Thomas WP, Reed JR, Gomez JA: Diagnostic pneumopericardiography in dogs with spontaneous pericardial effusion, *Vet Rad* 25:2, 1984.

CARDIAC NEOPLASIA

DEFINITIONS

Cardiac neoplasia includes any neoplastic condition involving the heart, great vessels, or pericardium.

SYNONYMS

For hemangiosarcomas—**angiosarcomas, malignant hemangioendotheliomas.** For tumors arising from the chemoreceptor aortic bodies—**chemodectomas, heartbase tumors , aortic body adenomas or carcinomas, or nonchromaffin paragangliomas.**

GENERAL CONSIDERATIONS AND CLINICALLY RELEVANT PATHOPHYSIOLOGY

Cardiac neoplasia is relatively uncommon in small animals. The most important cardiac neoplasms in dogs are right atrial hemangiosarcoma and heart base chemodectoma. A variety of primary intramural and intracavitary neoplasms have been reported in dogs including hemangiosarcoma, fibrosarcoma, chondrosarcoma, rhabdomyosarcoma, ectopic thyroid carcinoma, fibroma, and myxoma. Lymphosarcoma and metastatic neoplasia are the most frequent causes of cardiac neoplasia in cats.

The right atrium is a common primary site for hemangiosarcoma and accounts for 40% to 50% of canine cases of hemangiosarcoma. Other reported primary cardiac sites for hemangiosarcoma include the right ventricular free wall, interventricular septum, and main pulmonary artery. Primary cardiac hemangiosarcoma has not been described in cats, but metastasis of hemangiosarcoma to the heart is reported.

Chemodectomas can arise from the aortic body at the base of the heart (e.g., between aorta and pulmonary artery, between aorta and right atrium, or between pulmonary artery and left atrium) or from the carotid body in the neck. Aortic body chemodectomas account for approximately 80%

of chemodectomas and occur in older dogs. Chemodectomas occur rarely in cats. Residence at altitude and chronic hypoxia are thought to increase the risk for developing these tumors. Chemodectomas can cause pericardial effusion, which probably accounts for the most common clinical presentation of this disease. However, chemodectomas are just as often an incidental finding in older dogs undergoing thoracic radiographs or echocardiography for other reasons. Ectopic thyroid adenomas and carcinomas account for approximately 5% to 10% of all heart base tumors in dogs.

DIAGNOSIS
Clinical Presentation
Signalment. German shepherds and golden retrievers have been identified as having increased risk to develop hemangiosarcoma. Boxers, English bulldogs, and Boston terriers are the most common breeds to develop chemodectomas.

History. Animals with cardiac neoplasia may present for evaluation of dyspnea, cough, syncope, congestive heart failure, or may be asymptomatic.

Physical Examination Findings
The most common clinical presentation for right atrial hemangiosarcoma is acute or chronic cardiac tamponade resulting from intrapericardial hemorrhage (see Pericardial Effusion on p. 596). Animals with chemodectomas may present for evaluation of congestive heart failure, signs of cardiac tamponade, pleural effusion, or may be asymptomatic.

Radiography/Echocardiography
Thoracic radiographs of animals with chemodectomas may show dorsal elevation of the terminal trachea, pleural or pericardial effusion, pulmonary edema, or increased perihilar density. Selective angiography has been used to identify chemodectomas in dogs. Suggestive findings on angiography include identifying tortuous, aberrant vessels at the base of the heart, displacement of the aortic arch, and/or filling defects in the left atria. Angiography is also useful for identifying intracardiac lesions. Echocardiography frequently is useful in identifying masses on the right atrial appendage or at the cardiac base.

Laboratory Findings
Specific laboratory abnormalities are not found with cardiac neoplasia. Cytologic analysis of the sanguineous effusion obtained by pericardiocentesis is *not* useful in differentiating neoplastic from idiopathic pericardial effusion (see p. 598).

DIFFERENTIAL DIAGNOSIS
Cardiac neoplasia must be differentiated from other causes of pericardial effusion (see p. 598), congestive heart failure, or cardiac arrhythmias. Endomyocardial biopsy may be used to make a definitive diagnosis of intracardiac neoplasia. Differentials for radiographic masses near the heart base include hilar lymphadenopathy, left atrial enlargement, aberrant parathyroid or thyroid tissue, and fibrosing pleuritis or pericarditis.

MEDICAL MANAGEMENT
Various chemotherapeutic strategies can be employed for cardiac neoplasia, both as a primary therapy or as an adjunct to surgery. Doxorubicin, cyclophosphamide, and vincristine have been reported as the primary treatment of cardiac hemangiosarcoma (deMadron, Helfand, Stebbins, 1987).

SURGICAL TREATMENT
Pericardiectomy and excision of the right atrial tumor provide palliative relief of signs for atrial hemangiosarcoma. Chemodectomas are highly vascular, slow-growing, and moderately locally invasive. Surgical excision of aortic body chemodectomas is possible depending on size, location, and degree of invasiveness of the tumor. However, many animals with chemodectomas and clinical signs associated with pericardial effusion benefit from pericardiectomy without tumor excision.

Surgical excision of intramural or intracavitary primary cardiac tumors has been attempted rarely in small animals. Surgical excision of well-defined primary cardiac tumors utilizing inflow occlusion or cardiopulmonary bypass is possible in selected cases. However, given the high incidence of malignancy of most primary cardiac tumors, echocardiographic, angiographic, and endomyocardial biopsy findings should be considered carefully in selecting appropriate cases for surgery.

Preoperative Management
Abdominal radiographs or ultrasonography should be performed prior to surgery to detect concurrent intraabdominal neoplasia (e.g., rule out concurrent splenic hemangiosarcoma). If hemodynamically significant quantities of pericardial effusion are present (i.e., cardiac tamponade as evidenced by jugular vein distention, ascites, and/or pleural effusion), the animal should have a pericardial tap performed prior to surgery.

Anesthesia
Refer to p. 576 for anesthetic management of cardiac patients.

Surgical Anatomy
Refer to p. 577 for surgical anatomy of the heart.

Positioning
The animal is positioned in dorsal recumbency for median sternotomy (see p. 654) or in lateral recumbency for intercostal thoracotomy. A sufficiently generous area should be prepped to allow a thoracostomy tube placement intraoperatively.

SURGICAL TECHNIQUES
Right Atrial Hemangiosarcoma
Perform a median sternotomy or right fourth space intercostal thoracotomy. Clamp the atrial appendage with a tangential vascular clamp and excise the appendage (Fig. 24-18). Close the atriotomy incision with a continuous mattress suture pattern. Remove the vascular clamp and oversew the incision with a simple continuous suture pattern. Perform a pericardiectomy if pericardial effusion is present

(see p. 600). Alternatively, the right atrial appendage may be excised with a TA stapling instrument (see p. 655).

Chemodectoma

The surgical approach for removing chemodectomas depends on the suspected location of the tumor. *Sharply dissect the tumor from the walls of the great vessels and atria. Use care to avoid rupturing these structures during dissection. Use electrocautery to decrease hemorrhage during excision of these highly vascular tumors.*

SUTURE MATERIALS/SPECIAL INSTRUMENTS

A tangential vascular clamp is useful for excision of right atrial hemangiosarcoma. Closure of the right atrium can be accomplished with polypropylene (4-0) suture. Electrocautery is useful for excision of chemodectomas.

POSTOPERATIVE CARE AND ASSESSMENT

The animal should be monitored carefully for evidence of hemorrhage (pleural effusion) postoperatively. Arrhythmias are common and animals should be monitored postoperatively for arrhythmias for 36 to 72 hours. Postoperative pain should be treated with systemic opioids (see Table 24-6 on p. 581) and local anesthetic techniques (see p. 650).

PROGNOSIS

The prognosis for right atrial hemangiosarcoma is poor. Micrometastasis is considered present in virtually all cases at the time of diagnosis. Pericardiectomy and excision of the right atrium is palliative. Median survival after surgery is approximately 4 months. Long-term survival of up to several years is possible after surgical removal of an aortic body chemodectoma. In older animals with incidental asymptomatic chemodectoma, the risks of surgical excision should be weighed against the likelihood that the tumor will be slow-growing and can remain asymptomatic for a long period of time.

Reference

de Madron E, Helfand SC, Stebbins KE: Use of chemotherapy for treatment of cardiac hemangiosarcoma in a dog, *J Am Vet Med Assoc* 190:887, 1987.

Suggested Reading

Aronsohn M: Cardiac hemangiosarcoma in the dog: a review of 38 cases, *J Am Vet Med Assoc* 187:922, 1985.

Cantwell HD, Blevins WE, Weirich WE: Angiographic diagnosis of heartbase tumor in the dog, *J Am Anim Hosp Assoc* 18:83, 1982.

Gliatto JM et al: Multiple organ metastasis of an aortic body tumor in a boxer, *J Am Vet Med Assoc* 191:1110, 1987.

Keene BW et al: Primary left ventricular hemangiosarcoma diagnosed by endomyocardial biopsy in a dog, *J Am Vet Med Assoc* 197:1501, 1990.

Swartout MS, Ware WA, Bonagura JD: Intracardiac tumors in two dogs, *J Am Anim Hosp Assoc* 23:533, 1987.

Tilley LP et al: Cardiovascular tumors in the cat, *J Am Anim Hosp Assoc* 17:1009, 1981.

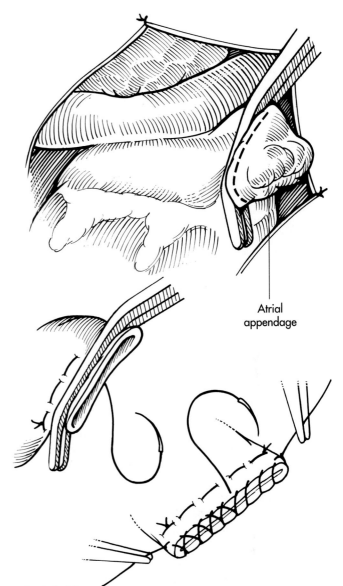

Atrial appendage

FIG. 24-18
To resect a right atrial hemangiosarcoma, place a tangential vascular clamp across the base of the right auricle and excise the tumor and auricle. Place a continuous horizontal mattress suture behind the vascular clamp. Remove the clamp and oversew the incision with a simple continuous suture. (Illustration modified from Orton EC: *Small animal thoracic surgery,* Philadelphia, 1995, Williams & Wilkins.)

Vicini DS, Didier PJ, Ogilvie GK: Cardiac fibrosarcoma in a dog, *J Am Vet Med Assoc* 189:1486, 1986.

Wykes PM, Rouse GP, Orton EC: Removal of five canine cardiac tumors using a stapling instrument, *Vet Surg* 15:103, 1986.

BRADYCARDIA

DEFINITIONS

Bradycardia is a slower-than-normal heart rate. Bradycardia can be physiologic (i.e., **sinus bradycardia**), or can result from a variety of pathologic disorders including **sick sinus**

syndrome, atrial standstill, or **atrioventricular block** with ventricular escape.

GENERAL CONSIDERATIONS AND CLINICALLY RELEVANT PATHOPHYSIOLOGY

Bradycardia can result from extrinsic causes such as exaggerated vagal tone or electrolyte imbalance, or from intrinsic degenerative disorders of the heart. Sinus bradycardia results from a predominance of parasympathetic influence and often is accompanied by other parasympathetically mediated rhythms (i.e., sinus arrhythmia, wandering pacemaker, or low-grade, second-degree atrioventricular block). It is generally considered a physiologic rather than pathologic rhythm.

Atrial standstill occurs when the atria fail to conduct an electrical impulse. The cardiac impulse may arise in the sinus node and be conducted to the atrioventricular (AV) node via internodal pathways in the atria (i.e., sinoventricular rhythm), or an escape rhythm may develop. Transient atrial standstill is caused by hyperkalemia. Persistent atrial standstill occurs as a result of a heritable muscular dystrophy syndrome that involves the cardiac atria, ventricles, and scapulohumeral skeletal muscles.

Frequent and long sinus pauses may result from degeneration and malfunction of the sinus node. Sick sinus syndrome is the clinical result of sinus node malfunction and is characterized by frequent syncopal and near-syncopal episodes. Sick sinus syndrome may also be accompanied by frequent supraventricular tachycardia.

Atrioventricular block results when there is a delay or block of cardiac impulse conduction through the AV node. First-degree AV block is a prolongation of conduction through the AV node and usually results from exaggerated parasympathetic influence on the AV node. Second-degree (incomplete) AV block is characterized by intermittent failure of impulse conduction through the AV node. Low-grade (infrequent) second-degree AV block usually results from exaggerated parasympathetic influence on the AV node. High-grade (frequent) second-degree AV block is more likely the result of intrinsic disease of the AV node. Third-degree (complete) AV block is a complete failure of conduction through the AV node and strongly implies intrinsic degenerative or infiltrative disease of the AV node. Third-degree AV block causes complete AV dissociation and development of a slow ventricular escape rhythm. The result is low and unresponsive cardiac output.

DIAGNOSIS
Clinical Presentation

Signalment. English springer spaniels and Siamese cats are predisposed to persistent atrial standstill. Small-breed dogs, particularly miniature schnauzers, are predisposed to sick sinus syndrome. Third-degree AV block occurs in German shepherds and other large-breed dogs.

History. Clinical signs associated with bradycardia include weakness, exercise intolerance, collapse, and syncope. The relatively short duration of syncopal episodes (usually only a few seconds) and lack of tonic-clonic motor activity or postictal signs help distinguish syncope from neurologic seizures with which it is sometimes confused.

Physical Examination Findings/Electrocardiography

Sinus bradycardia is recognized on the electrocardiogram as a normal but slow rhythm with normal P-QRS-T complexes. It is often accompanied by other vagal-mediated changes (i.e., sinus arrhythmia, wandering pacemaker, and low-grade, second-degree AV block). Sinus bradycardia is abolished by exercise or atropine administration (Table 24-13).

Electrocardiographic abnormalities associated with transient atrial standstill are bradycardia, small or absent P waves, and shortening and widening of the QRS complexes. Diagnostic rule-outs for hyperkalemia include obstructive uropathy, acute renal failure, uroabdomen, acute muscle necrosis, severe acidosis, adrenocortical insufficiency, diabetic ketoacidosis, and iatrogenic potassium intoxication. Electrocardiographic abnormalities associated with persistent atrial standstill are similar (e.g., an absence of P waves and a slow supraventricular or ventricular escape rhythm).

Electrocardiographic findings associated with sick sinus syndrome include intermittent severe bradycardia, sinus pauses that last several seconds, supraventricular escape complexes, and occasionally paroxysmal supraventricular tachycardia. Sick sinus syndrome causes frequent syncopal attacks and places the animal at substantial risk for sudden death. Sick sinus syndrome is usually not responsive to acute administration of atropine.

First-degree AV block (Table 24-14) is recognized by a prolongation of the P-R interval on an electrocardiogram. Second-degree AV block is intermittent failure of impulse conduction through the AV node. It is recognized on an electrocardiogram as a P wave that is not followed by a QRS-T complex. Low-grade, second-degree AV block is characterized by occasional "dropped complexes" after several normal complexes and usually is abolished by atropine. High-grade,

TABLE 24-13
Atropine Response Test
Give 0.02-0.04 mg/kg atropine SC or IM; wait 15-20 minutes then recheck cardiac rhythm.

TABLE 24-14
First–Degree AV Block
Dogs - PR interval > 0.13 sec Cats - PR interval > 0.09 sec

second-degree AV is characterized by more dropped complexes than conducted complexes and usually does not respond to atropine. Third-degree AV block is recognized on an electrocardiogram by complete dissociation of the P waves and QRS-T complexes and the presence of a slow ventricular escape rhythm. Third-degree AV block is not atropine responsive.

Radiography/Echocardiography

Thoracic radiographs are usually normal or show mild to moderate cardiomegaly. With transient atrial standstill, echocardiography shows a lack of atrial motion and little or no flow through the mitral valve during the atrial filling phase. Echocardiography is also used to rule out concurrent valvular or congenital abnormalities.

Laboratory Findings

Hyperkalemia is present with transient atrial standstill; however, with persistent atrial standstill, serum potassium levels are normal. Other specific laboratory abnormalities are not found.

DIFFERENTIAL DIAGNOSIS

Other causes of bradycardia (i.e., hyperkalemia, increased intracranial pressures) should be differentiated from intrinsic conduction system dysfunction.

MEDICAL MANAGEMENT

Therapy for atrial standstill secondary to hyperkalemia should be directed at immediately lowering serum potassium levels and correcting the underlying cause of hyperkalemia. Intravenous fluid therapy should be initiated with 0.9% saline. If the animal has concurrent hyponatremia, 5% dextrose solutions (i.e., D5W) and half-strength saline should be avoided. Severe hyperkalemia may be treated with sodium bicarbonate (Table 24-15). Bicarbonate therapy drives potassium into cells in exchange for hydrogen ions. Alternatively, some clinicians prefer insulin (0.5 to 1.0 units/kg regular insulin intravenously) and dextrose (2 g per unit of insulin) administration. Insulin facilitates cellular uptake of potassium, while dextrose prevents hypoglycemia following insulin administration. If the hyperkalemia appears immediately life-threatening, 10% calcium gluconate given slowly intravenously may protect the heart until other therapy lowers the plasma potassium concentration.

Animals that present with severe life-threatening bradycardia may require emergency therapy to increase heart rate. Short-term anticholinergic therapy with atropine or glycopyrrolate may be attempted, but most clinically relevant bradycardias are not due to parasympathetic mechanisms and will not be responsive to these drugs. Intravenous adrenergic therapy with isoproterenol (Table 24-16) is sometimes effective as a short-term measure for increasing heart rate associated with persistent atrial standstill or third-degree AV block.

The most reliable method for increasing heart rate in animals with unresponsive bradycardia is temporary intravenous pacing. This is accomplished by percutaneous jugular venous placement of a pacing electrode into the right side of the heart under sedation and local anesthesia (see below under anesthesia). The electrode is then connected to an external pulse generator. Long-term oral anticholinergic therapy with propantheline bromide (see Table 24-16) is sometimes advocated for various bradycardias. However, this drug is seldom effective for clinically relevant bradycardias and often is associated with unpleasant side effects. Animals with sick sinus syndrome may require management of supraventricular tachycardia with digoxin, beta-adrenergic blockade, or calcium channel blockade therapy after pacemaker implantation.

SURGICAL TREATMENT

Cardiac pacemaker therapy is indicated for bradycardias that are the result of intrinsic cardiac disease, are not responsive to atropine, and are associated with clinical signs.

Preoperative Management

Most bradycardias are exacerbated by anesthetic drugs. Therefore some accommodation for maintaining an acceptable cardiac rhythm during permanent pacemaker implantation usually is necessary. Preanesthetic medication with an anticholinergic drug (e.g., atropine or glycopyrrolate) is indicated, but rarely sufficient to prevent worsening of bradycardia during anesthesia. Temporary transvenous pacing is the most reliable method of maintaining an adequate heart rate during pacemaker implantation. Constant intravenous infusion of isoproterenol (see Table 24-16) is an alternative, but less reliable, means of maintaining heart rate during

---

TABLE 24-15

Therapy for Hyperkalemia

0.9% saline IV
to dilute potassium

Sodium bicarbonate
1 to 2 mEq/kg IV

Calcium gluconate*
0.5-1 ml/kg over 5 minutes, IV

*Temporary measure to sustain animal while other methods restore the potassium; use with extreme caution.

TABLE 24-16

Drugs Used to Increase Heart Rate in Animals with Unresponsive Bradycardia

Isoproterenol (Isuprel)
0.01 µg/kg/min IV

Propantheline bromide (Pro-Banthine)
0.25-0.5 mg/kg PO, TID to QID

permanent pacemaker implantation. Perioperative antibiotic therapy during pacemaker implantation is indicated to reduce the risk of implant-associated infections.

Anesthesia

Temporary pacemakers can be implanted in dogs under oxymorphone sedation (0.05 to 0.1 mg/kg intravenously) plus diazepam (0.1 to 0.2 mg/kg intravenously) and a local anesthetic block with lidocaine. Once the animal is paced, etomidate (0.5 to 1.5 mg/kg intravenously) can be administered for intubation. Anesthesia should be maintained with isoflurane and oxygen.

Surgical Anatomy

Refer to p. 577 for surgical anatomy of the heart.

Positioning

The animal is placed in dorsal recumbency for transdiaphragmatic pacemaker implantation. The entire abdomen and caudal thorax are prepared for aseptic surgery.

SURGICAL TECHNIQUES

Epicardial pacemaker implantation in small animals is accomplished through a midline celiotomy diaphragmatic incision. The transdiaphragmatic approach has several advantages including avoidance of a thoracotomy and abdominal placement of the generator.

☞ **N O T E ·** The pulse generator does not begin to function until the generator casing is brought into contact with the patient to complete the electrical circuit.

Perform a celiotomy that extends cranially to the level of the xiphoid (Fig. 24-19, A). Make a vertical midline incision in the diaphragm and expose the cardiac apex. Open the pericardium and retract it gently with tissue forceps to expose the apex of the left ventricle (Fig. 24-19, B). Implant a screw-in electrode into the left ventricular apex by turning the electrode tip a specified number of rotations (see in-

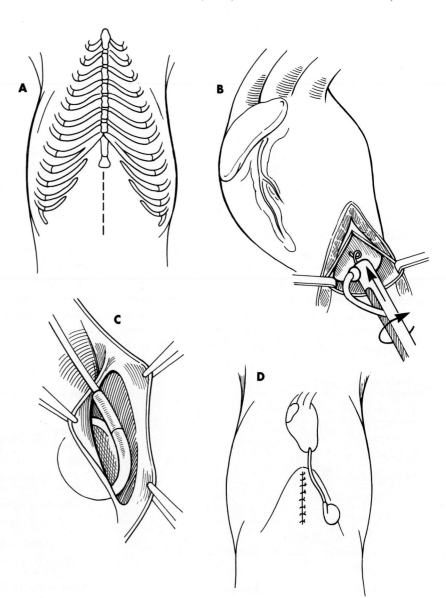

FIG. 24-19
A, Transdiaphragmatic pacemaker implantation may be performed via midline celiotomy. **B,** Incise the diaphragm on its midline and open and retract the pericardium to expose the cardiac apex. **C,** Implant a screw-in electrode into the left ventricular apex by turning the electrode the specified number of rotations. Bring the lead wire through the diaphragmatic incision and connect it to the pulse generator. Place the generator in a pocket created between the transverse abdominis and internal abdominal oblique muscles. **D,** Close the diaphragm and abdomen routinely. (Illustration modified from Orton EC: *Small animal thoracic surgery,* Philadelphia, 1995, Williams & Wilkins.)

struction sheet accompanying pacemaker; usually 2.5 turns) (Fig. 24-20). Bring the lead wire into the abdominal cavity through the diaphragmatic incision and connect it to the pulse generator using a small screwdriver. Place the pulse generator in a pocket created between the transverse abdominis and internal abdominal oblique muscles (Fig. 24-19, C). Avoid using electrocautery once the permanent pacemaker is functioning. Do not suture the pericardium. Close the diaphragm and abdomen in routine fashion (Fig. 24-19, D).

SUTURE MATERIALS/ SPECIAL INSTRUMENTS

Modern cardiac pulse generators are compact, have a long battery life, are programmable after implantation, and generally are capable of a variety of sophisticated pacing modes. A three-letter code identifies the intended site of cardiac sensing, intended site for cardiac pacing, and pacing mode. The most commonly used pacing mode in small animals is VVI, which stands for *ventricular-sensing, ventricular-pacing, inhibited mode.* This means that the pacemaker is intended to pace the cardiac ventricles, but will sense naturally occurring ventricular impulses and inhibit its own output when they occur. This demand function prevents competitive rhythms between the heart and pacemaker should spontaneous intrinsic ventricular activity occur. Most recent-model pulse generators are powered by lithium cells that have a life of 8 to 12 years. Pacemakers that have exceeded their shelf-life for implantation in humans but still have several years of useful battery life left can often be obtained for a fraction of the cost of new pacemakers. Modern pacemakers are programmable by radiofrequency after implantation for several indices (i.e., pacing rate, stimulus voltage, and sensing voltage). Cardiologists or pacemaker technical representatives usually can provide appropriate programmers for setting pulse generator parameters before and after surgery. Dogs are paced at a rate of 70 to 110 bpm, depending on size and nature of the animal. Ideally, the stimulus voltage should be approximately 2 times the mea-sured stimulus capture threshold. A voltage of 4 to 5 V is usually adequate.

Pacemaker electrodes are either *endocardial (transvenous)* or *epicardial.* Endocardial electrodes may be unipolar or bipolar, and are intended for placement in the right ventricle via a jugular vein. Endocardial electrodes may be used for temporary or permanent cardiac pacing. Endocardial electrodes have the advantage of less invasive placement, but require facilities for cardiac catheterization and have a higher incidence of catheter dislodgement. Permanent endocardial electrode placement requires pulse generator implantation in the neck. Epicardial leads are unipolar and require open thoracic surgery for implantation on the epicardial surface. The screw-in epicardial electrode has the advantage of not requiring epicardial sutures and allows a minimal thoracic approach for implantation (Fig. 24-21).

POSTOPERATIVE CARE AND ASSESSMENT

Pacemaker function should be monitored closely for the first 48 hours postoperatively, and thereafter every 3 to 6 months. Recognition of normal pacemaker function is an important aspect of pacemaker management after surgery. Demand (VVI) pacemakers should be monitored both for their ability to pace or capture the heart, and for their ability to sense intrinsic cardiac impulses and inhibit their output when intrinsic rhythms occur. Failure of either of these functions can cause serious problems for the patient. Paced beats are recognized on an electrocardiogram by the presence of a stimulus artifact just prior to the QRS-T. A stimulus artifact will be present on the electrocardiogram regardless of whether the stimulus captures the heart.

Failure to pace is recognized on an electrocardiogram by the presence of a stimulus artifact that is not followed by a QRS-T. Evaluation of paced beats for the presence of a T wave is important since artifacts that mimic the QRS complex may be present and can be misleading. Failure to pace also is recognized by its failure to generate an arterial pulse. Early failure to pace can be caused by an inadequate stimulus

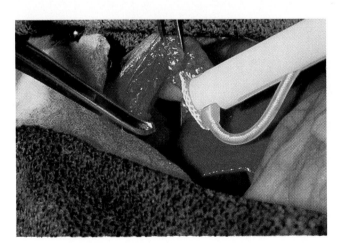

FIG. 24-20
Transdiaphragmatic pericardial electrode placement.

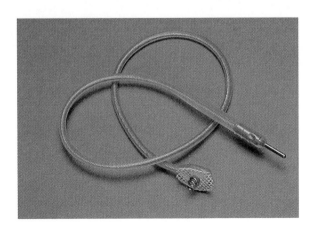

FIG. 24-21
Screw-in epicardial electrode.

voltage or a faulty connection between the electrode and generator. Late failure to pace can be caused by depletion of the generator battery, electrode breakage or dislodgement, or fibrosis leading to increased impedance at the electrode-myocardial interface. Failure to pace may be correctable by adjusting the pacing stimulus voltage of the generator. Radiographs are useful for evaluating for lead breakage, disconnection, or dislodgement.

Failure to sense intrinsic cardiac impulses can lead to competitive rhythms between the heart and pacemaker. Competitive rhythms are harmful because they result in tachycardia and place the patient at risk for ventricular fibrillation. Failure to sense is recognized on the electrocardiogram by the presence of an intrinsic cardiac impulse between two paced impulses with a normal pacing interval. Failure to sense may or may not be accompanied by failure to pace. Failure to sense can be caused by a failing generator battery or by increased impedance at the electrode-myocardial interface. Failure to sense may be correctable by adjusting the sensing voltage threshold of the generator.

Premature ventricular complexes are often observed in the immediate postoperative period after pacemaker implantation. The origin of the ventricular complexes is usually consistent with the site of electrode implantation. Ventricular ectopy usually is self-limiting and not a major problem as long as the pacemaker is sensing the premature complexes. Ventricular tachycardias that exceed 150 bpm should be suppressed with lidocaine therapy.

PROGNOSIS

Animals showing clinical signs of severe exercise intolerance or syncope as a result of bradycardia are at risk for sudden death or development of congestive heart failure. Pacemaker therapy is extremely effective in preventing these consequences and restoring reasonably normal activity to animals with clinically relevant bradycardia.

Suggested Reading

Bonagura JD, Helphrey ML, Muir WW: Complications associated with permanent pacemaker implantation in the dog, *J Am Vet Med Assoc* 182:149, 1983.

Fingeroth JM, Birchard SJ: Transdiaphragmatic approach for permanent cardiac pacemaker implantation in dogs, *Vet Surg* 15:329, 1986.

Fox PR et al: Techniques and complications of pacemaker implantation in four cats, *J Am Vet Med Assoc* 199:1742, 1991.

Fox PR et al: Ventral abdominal, transdiaphragmatic approach for implantation of cardiac pacemakers in the dog, *J Am Vet Med Assoc* 189:1303, 1986.

Klement P, Del-Nido PJ, Wilson GJ: The use of cardiac pacemakers in veterinary practice, *Compend Contin Educ Pract Vet* 6:893, 1984.

Rowland PH, Moise NS, Severson D: Myxoma at the site of a subcutaneous pacemaker in a dog, *J Am Anim Hosp Assoc* 27:649, 1991.

Snyder PS, Atkins CE, Sato T: Syncope in three dogs with cardiac pacemakers, *J Am Anim Hosp Assoc* 27:611, 1991.

Wilbanks RD: Using the abdominal approach for pacemaker placement, *Vet Med* 87:139, 1992.

CHAPTER 25

Surgery of the Upper Respiratory System

GENERAL PRINCIPLES AND TECHNIQUES

DEFINITIONS

Tracheotomy is an incision through the tracheal wall. **Tracheostomy** is creation of a temporary or permanent opening into the trachea to facilitate airflow. **Tracheal resection and anastomosis** is removal of a segment of trachea and reapposition of the divided tracheal ends. **Ventriculocordectomy** is resection of the vocal cords.

SYNONYMS

For ventriculocordectomy—**debarking, devocalization;** for permanent tracheostomy—**tracheostoma**

PREOPERATIVE CONCERNS

Upper airway procedures are performed to remove, repair, or bypass areas of obstruction, injury, or disease (Table 25-1). Affected animals may show signs of mild to severe respiratory distress. Mild or moderately dyspneic patients should initially be examined from a distance to avoid exacerbating the condition. Open-mouth breathing, abducted forelimbs, labored breathing, and restlessness indicate moderate to severe respiratory distress that may require emergency therapy. Minimal restraint should be used in severely dyspneic patients, and they should be allowed to maintain the position

in which they feel most comfortable. Supplemental oxygen may be given via nasal insufflation, tracheostomy tube or catheter, endotracheal intubation, mask, or cage. Corticosteroids, sedation, and/or cooling may relieve distress. Sedation may be beneficial for anxious patients in moderate to severe respiratory distress. Combinations of intravenous drugs are commonly used; oxymorphone or butorphanol in addition to either acepromazine or diazepam are commonly given in dogs (Table 25-2). Alternatively, fentanyl plus droperidol may be used. In cats, acepromazine or diazepam is recommended (Table 25-3). To cool dyspneic animals, a

---

TABLE 25-1

Indications for Upper Respiratory Tract Surgery

- Brachycephalic syndrome
- Devocalization
- Laryngeal collapse
- Laryngotracheal trauma
- Laryngeal paralysis
- Tracheal collapse
- Laryngeal masses
- Tracheal masses
- Nasal tumors or infection

TABLE 25-2

Sedation of Severely Dyspneic Dogs

Oxymorphone (Numorphan)
0.05 mg/kg, max 4 mg IV, IM, or SC

Butorphanol (Torbutrol, Torbugesic)
0.2-0.4 mg/kg IV, IM, or SC

Acepromazine
0.02-0.05 mg/kg, max 1 mg IV, IM, or SC

Diazepam (Valium)
0.2 mg/kg IV

Fetanyl plus droperidol (Innovar-Vet)
1 ml/20-40 kg IV or 1 ml/10-15 kg IM

TABLE 25-3

Sedation of Severely Dyspneic Cats

Acepromazine
0.05 mg/kg, IV, IM, or SC

Diazepam (Valium)*
0.2 mg/kg IV

*Use with caution; may not reliably result in sedation

fan may be directed at the patient, ice packs may be applied to the head, axilla, inguinal area, and extremities, and/or cooled fluids may be administered intravenously.

Diagnosis of upper respiratory disease is based on history and clinical signs, physical examination findings, hematologic and serum biochemical parameters, radiographs, endoscopy, cytology, culture, and/or biopsy. History and clinical signs may include abnormal respiratory noises (e.g., cough, stridor, wheeze), exercise intolerance, hyperthermia, tachypnea, dyspnea, cyanosis, restlessness, and/or collapse. Gagging and regurgitation of secretions are common with nasopharyngeal, laryngeal, and some tracheal abnormalities. Voice change may occur with laryngeal paralysis, and dysphagia may be noted with supraglottic obstructions. Subcutaneous emphysema occurs with penetrating laryngotracheal injuries. Clinical signs may intensify or be precipitated by excitement, stress, eating, drinking, or high ambient temperatures. Laboratory data should be evaluated to determine the presence of underlying metabolic disease and advisability of general anesthesia. Tidal-breathing flow volume loops are helpful in classifying obstructions as fixed or nonfixed. Pulmonary function tests, electromyography, and nerve conduction studies are ancillary tests that may support the presence of pulmonary or neuromuscular disease.

Animals with nasal neoplasia, fungal infection, or foreign bodies may be anemic due to profuse epistaxis. Affected animals should be carefully evaluated for clotting abnormalities by assessing platelet numbers, bleeding from venipuncture sites, or the presence of ecchymoses, petechiation, melena, hematuria, or retinal hemorrhages. If available, coagulative ability may be assessed by activated clotting time, prothrombin time, partial thromboplastin time, and/or mucosal bleeding time. Blood transfusions should be given before surgery if the PCV is less than or equal to 20% (Table 25-4). Bleeding during rhinotomy may be severe, requiring intraoperative blood transfusion and/or carotid artery ligation.

Preoperative antiinflammatory doses of corticosteroids (Table 25-5) may reduce nasopharyngeal and/or upper airway edema secondary to surgical or diagnostic manipulations. They are routinely given when nasopharyngeal and intraluminal laryngeal procedures are performed.

ANESTHETIC CONSIDERATIONS

Patients with upper respiratory obstruction or disruption are extreme anesthetic risks. The periods of greatest danger are during anesthetic induction and recovery (see p. 618 under Postoperative Care). For laryngeal examination, care should be taken to avoid drugs that inhibit laryngeal function. If the animal has already been sedated (see above) an anticholinergic (atropine or glycopyrrolate; Table 25-6) should be given. An opioid (oxymorphone, butorphanol, or buprenorphine) may also be administered to unsedated animals. Propofol may be used for induction because it is noncumulative and may be given in small, incremental doses that maintain laryngeal function (Table 25-7). Diazepam

---

TABLE 25-6

Premedicants for Laryngeal Examination in Dogs

Atropine
0.02-0.04 mg/kg IM, or SC

Glycopyrrolate
0.005-0.011 mg/kg IM, or SC

Oxymorphone (Numorphan)
0.05-0.1 mg/kg IM

Butorphanol (Torbutrol, Torbugesic)
0.2-0.4 mg/kg IM, or SC

Buprenorphine (Buprenex)
5-15 μg/kg IM

TABLE 25-7

Selected Anesthetic Protocols for Use in Animals Undergoing Upper Respiratory Tract Surgery

For Dyspneic, Nonarrhythmic Animals
Induction

Diazepam (0.2 mg/kg IV) followed immediately with thiopental* (10-12 mg/kg IV) or propofol (4-6 mg/kg IV) to effect. Alternatively, give diazepam (0.27 mg/kg IV) plus ketamine (5.5 mg/kg IV) titrated to effect

Maintenance

Isoflurane or halothane

For Very Sick or Arrhythmic Animals
Induction

Diazepam (0.2 mg/kg IV) followed by etomidate* (1-3 mg/kg IV)

Maintenance

Isoflurane or halothane

*For unsedated dogs, oxymorphone (0.05-0.01 mg/kg IV) may be given as part of the induction and the etomidate or barbiturate dose decreased.

TABLE 25-4

Blood Transfusions

ml of Donor Blood Needed

Recipient blood volume* $\times$ $\dfrac{\text{Desired PCV} - \text{actual patient PCV}}{\text{PCV of anticoagulated donor blood}}$

*Total blood volume is estimated at 90 ml/kg for dogs and 70 ml/kg for cats. A rough estimate is that 2.2 ml of blood/kg of body weight will increase the recipient's PCV by 1%.

TABLE 25-5

Preoperative Corticosteroid Administration

Dexamethasone (Azium)
0.5-2 mg/kg IV, IM, SC

plus ketamine are also useful as induction agents because they maintain laryngeal function. Induction doses of thiobarbiturates may impair laryngeal function, making diagnosis of laryngeal paralysis difficult. Oxygen should be supplemented during the exam and oxygen saturation monitored with pulse oximetry (preferable) or by observation of mucous membrane color. The patient should be intubated and anesthesia maintained with inhalant drugs after the examination for further diagnostics or surgery.

General anesthesia is preferred for most upper respiratory procedures as it ensures a patent airway, allows controlled ventilation, facilitates asepsis, and is less stressful for patients. Local anesthesia may allow tracheostomy tube placement when the patient is comatose or cannot tolerate general anesthesia. Dyspneic patients should be preoxygenated with a face mask, if possible. Affected animals being anesthetized (see above for laryngeal exam) may be premedicated with an opioid, but continuous monitoring is necessary. Anticholinergics are indicated for bradycardia. Induction should be rapid (e.g., propofol, thiobarbiturate, or ketamine plus diazepam) and oxygen administered immediately. Mask induction is not recommended. Anesthesia should be maintained with inhalant drugs. Laryngeal or tracheal procedures may necessitate temporary retraction of the endotracheal tube from the surgical site, placing an endotracheal tube distal to the surgical site through a tracheotomy, or using injectable drugs. During surgery the animal should be sighed frequently to renew surfactant. Oxygen saturation and/or blood gases should be monitored from induction until recovery and abnormalities are corrected. Selected anesthetic protocols are provided in Table 25-7.

ANTIBIOTICS

The respiratory tract has a normal bacterial flora; therefore prophylactic antibiotics (e.g., cefazolin; Table 25-8) are frequently given prior to surgery. However, animals with normal immune function undergoing short procedures (e.g., nares resection, laryngeal saccule resection, vocal cordectomy) do not need them. *Streptococcus* spp., *E. coli*, *Pseudomonas* spp., *Klebsiella* spp., and *Bordetella bronchiseptica* are most commonly isolated from normal dogs. In one study, approximately 64% of tracheal cultures were sterile, whereas 95% of pharyngeal cultures were positive (McKiernan, Smith, Kissil, 1984).

Most canine respiratory tract infections are due to gramnegative organisms, many being resistant to commonly used antibiotics. Antimicrobial drug selection should be based on cytologic and culture results of tracheobronchial, pulmonary parenchymal, and/or pleural secretions. Bland aerosol therapy (e.g., sterile 0.9% NaCl) helps loosen secretions and facilitates their clearance in dogs with tracheos-

tomies. Addition of antibiotics to the aerosol is generally unnecessary. Lipid-soluble antibiotics that contain a benzene ring reach highest levels in the normal trachea and bronchus; however, increased permeability associated with inflammation allows numerous antibiotics to achieve high levels during infection. Antibiotics commonly recommended for treatment of respiratory disease include ampicillin, potentiated sulfonamides, cephalosporins, aminoglycosides, and fluoroquinolones (Table 25-9).

SURGICAL ANATOMY

The thyroid cartilage forms the ventral and lateral walls of the larynx (Fig. 25-1). It surrounds the lateral aspect of the cricoid cartilage and articulates with the dorsolateral aspect of the cricoid cartilage (caudal) and thyrohyoid bones (cranial). Ventrally the cricothyroid ligament joins the caudal border of the thyroid cartilage to the cricoid cartilage. The cricoid cartilage is a complete ring that is five times wider dorsally than it is ventrally (see Fig. 25-1). It forms the dorsal wall of the larynx and cranially lies within the wings of the thyroid cartilage. The cricoid cartilage articulates at its cranial dorsolateral margin with the arytenoid cartilage, which is paired (see Fig. 25-1). At the entrance to the glottis there are two cuneiform processes ventrally and two corniculate processes dorsally. The vocal fold attaches to the vocal process of the arytenoid at its ventral aspect. The muscular processes are dorsolateral at the caudal aspect of the arytenoid.

☞ **N O T E** · It is wise to dissect cadaver larynxes before performing laryngoplasty.

The glottis (laryngeal inlet) consists of the vocal folds, vocal processes of the arytenoid cartilages, and rima glottidis (see Fig. 25-1). The vocal folds extend dorsally from the vocal processes of the arytenoids to the thyroid cartilage ventrally. Rostral and lateral to the vocal folds are the laryngeal ventricles or saccules. The laryngeal saccule is a mucosal diverticulum bounded laterally by the thyroid cartilage and medially by the arytenoid cartilage. The vestibular fold (false

TABLE 25-8

Perioperative Antibiotic Therapy

Cefazolin (Ancef or Kefzol)

20 mg/kg IV at induction, repeat once or twice at 4- to 6-hour intervals

TABLE 25-9

Antibiotic Therapy for Treatment of Upper Respiratory Infection

Ampicillin

22 mg/kg IV, IM, SC, or PO, TID

Cefazolin (Ancef, Kefzol)

20 mg/kg IV or IM or TID

Trimethoprim-Sulfadiazine (Tribrissen)

15 mg/kg IM or PO, BID

Amikacin (Amiglyde-V)

10 mg/kg IV, IM, or SC, TID (or 30mg/kg SID)

Enrofloxacin (Baytril)

5-10 mg/kg PO or IV, BID

FIG. 25-1
A, Oral, and **B,** lateral view of laryngeal anatomy.

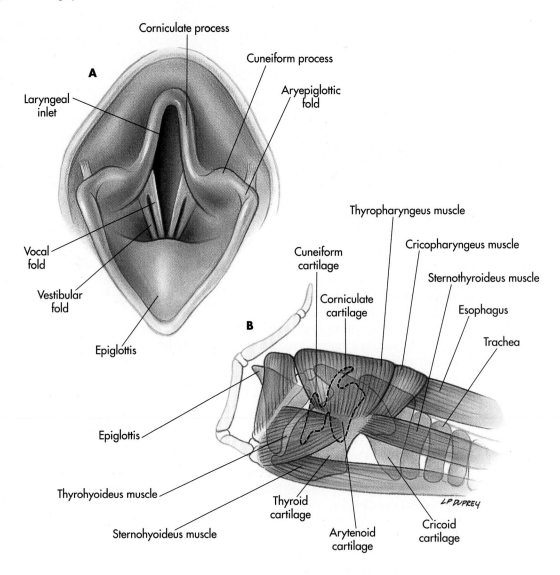

vocal cord) forms the rostral border of the laryngeal saccule and attaches to the cuneiform process.

The intrinsic muscles of the dog's larynx are innervated by somatic efferent axons from the vagus nerve. Some axons leave the vagus in the cranial laryngeal nerve to innervate the cricothyroid muscle; others provide sensory innervation to the mucosa. The recurrent laryngeal nerve, a branch of the vagus, terminates as the caudal laryngeal nerve, which innervates the remaining intrinsic muscles of the larynx. The caudal laryngeal nerve travels along the dorsolateral surface of the trachea and continues over the lateral surface of the cricoarytenoideus dorsalis before deviating to the medial surface of the thyroid cartilage lamina. The cranial laryngeal artery, a branch of the external carotid artery, travels with the cranial laryngeal nerve. It is the main blood supply to the larynx. The cranial laryngeal vein empties into the hyoid venous arch and then the external jugular vein. Lymphatics drain into the retropharyngeal lymph node.

☞ **N O T E ·** Be sure to identify and protect the recurrent laryngeal nerves during cervical surgery to prevent postoperative laryngospasms or paralysis.

The trachea is a semirigid, flexible tube extending from the cricoid cartilage to the mainstem bronchi at about the fourth or fifth thoracic vertebra. Thirty-five to forty-five C-shaped hyaline cartilages, joined by annular ligaments ventrally and laterally and trachealis muscle (dorsal tracheal membrane) dorsally, form the trachea. The tracheal vessels and nerves are found in the lateral pedicles and supply the trachea segmentally. Loose areolar connective tissue surrounds the trachea and forms the lateral pedicles. Vascular branches to the trachea are supplied by the cranial and caudal thyroid arteries and veins, bronchoesophageal arteries and veins, and internal jugular veins. Innervation is by the autonomic nervous system. Sympathetic fibers from the middle cervical ganglion and sympathetic trunk inhibit tracheal muscle contraction and glandular secretions, while parasympathetic fibers from the vagus and recurrent laryngeal nerves cause tracheal muscle contraction and glandular secretions.

SURGICAL TECHNIQUES

Surgical techniques for the management of animals with upper respiratory disease include tracheotomy (see p. 613), tracheostomy (see p. 613), tracheal resection and anastomosis

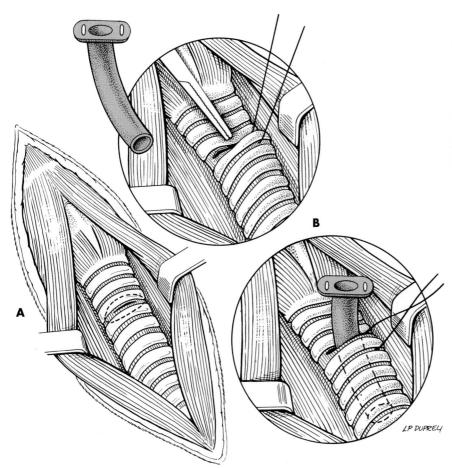

FIG. 25-2
A, For tube tracheostomy, make a transverse incision through the annular ligament. Excise a small ellipse of cartilage from each tracheal cartilage adjacent to the tracheotomy incision to minimize tube irritation *(dotted line)*. **B,** Facilitate tube placement by depressing the proximal cartilages with a hemostat and elevating the distal cartilages with an encircling suture. Insert a tracheostomy tube that does not completely fill the lumen.

LP DUPREY

(see p. 615), ventriculocordectomy (see p. 616), tracheoplasty (see p. 635), arytenoid cartilage lateralization (see p. 630), partial laryngectomy (see p. 631), rhinotomy (see p. 641) and surgery for stenotic nares (see p. 621), elongated soft palates (see p. 623), and everted laryngeal saccules (see p. 626).

Tracheotomy

Tracheotomy is performed to gain access to the tracheal lumen to remove obstructions, collect specimens, or facilitate airflow. The tracheal incision may be closed or allowed to heal by second intention. *Approach the cervical trachea through a ventral cervical midline incision. Extend the incision from the larynx to the sternum as needed to allow adequate exposure. Separate the sternohyoid muscles along their midline and retract them laterally. Dissect the peritracheal connective tissue from the ventral surface of the trachea at the proposed tracheotomy site. Take care to avoid traumatizing the recurrent laryngeal nerves, carotid artery, jugular vein, thyroid vessels, or esophagus. Immobilize the trachea between the thumb and forefinger. Make a horizontal or vertical incision through the wall of the trachea. Place cartilage-encircling sutures around adjacent cartilages to separate the edges and allow lumen inspection or tube insertion. Suction blood, secretions, and debris from the tracheal lumen. Following completion of the procedure, appose tracheal edges with simple interrupted 3-0 or 4-0 polypropylene sutures. To close the tracheal incision, place sutures through the annular ligaments encircling adjacent*

cartilages or through the annular ligaments only. Lavage the surgical site with saline. Appose the sternohyoid muscles with a simple continuous pattern of 3-0 or 4-0 absorbable suture (polydioxanone, polyglyconate, polyglactin, or chromic catgut). Appose subcutaneous tissues and skin routinely.

Tracheostomy

Tracheostomy allows air to enter the trachea distal to the nose, mouth, nasopharynx, and larynx. A tracheotomy is performed, and either a tube is inserted (temporary tracheostomy) or a stoma is created (permanent tracheostomy) to facilitate airflow. A nonreactive tube that is no larger than one half the size of the trachea should be selected. Cuffed or cannulated autoclavable silicone, silver, or nylon tubes are recommended. Polyvinyl chloride and red rubber tubes are irritating and should be avoided. If the animal is being placed on a respirator, a cuffed tube is necessary.

Temporary tracheostomy. Temporary tracheostomy is most commonly performed to provide an alternate airflow route during surgery or as an emergency procedure in severely dyspneic patients. Tube tracheostomies are usually maintained for a short time. *Make a ventral midline incision from the cricoid cartilage extending 2 to 3 cm caudally. Separate the sternohyoid muscles and make a horizontal (transverse) tracheotomy through the annular ligament between the third and fourth or fourth and fifth tracheal cartilages (Fig. 25-2, A). Do not extend the incision around* *more than half the circumference of the trachea. Alternatively, make a vertical tracheotomy across the ventral midline of cartilages 3 through 5. Suction blood and mucus from the lumen, widen the incision, and insert the tracheostomy tube. Facilitate tube placement by encircling a cartilage distal or lateral to the incision with a long stay suture (Fig. 25-2, B). Place tension on this suture to open the incision. Alternately, open a hemostat in the incision or depress the cartilages cranial to the horizontal incision (see Fig. 25-2, B). Resect a small ellipse of cartilage if tube insertion is difficult. Appose the sternohyoid muscles, subcutaneous tissue, and skin cranial and caudal to the tube. Secure the tube by suturing it to the skin or tieing it to gauze that is tied around the neck.*

Permanent tracheostomy. Permanent tracheostomy is the creation of a stoma in the ventral tracheal wall by suturing tracheal mucosa to skin. Tracheostomas are maintained for life or until the stoma is surgically closed. Tracheostomy tubes are not needed to maintain lumen patency following this procedure. Permanent tracheostomies are recommended for animals with upper respiratory obstructions causing moderate to severe respiratory distress that cannot be successfully treated by other methods (e.g., laryngeal col-

lapse, nasal neoplasia). Owners should be warned that these animals must be restricted from swimming and they should be advised that vocalization is diminished or absent following this procedure.

☞ **N O T E** · Inform owners that permanent tracheostomy patients require daily stomal care.

Expose the proximal cervical trachea with a ventral cervical midline incision. Create a tunnel dorsal to the trachea in the area of the third to sixth tracheal cartilages. Using this tunnel, appose the sternohyoid muscles dorsal to the trachea with horizontal mattress sutures to create a muscle sling to reduce tension on the mucosa-to-skin sutures (Fig. 25-3, A). Beginning with the second or third tracheal cartilages, outline a rectangular segment of tracheal wall 3 to 4 cartilage widths long and one third the circumference of the trachea in width. Incise the cartilage and annular ligaments to the depth of the tracheal mucosa (see Fig. 25-3, A). Elevate a cartilage edge with thumb forceps and dissect the cartilage segment from the mucosa. Place one or two prosthetic tracheal rings cranial and caudal to the stoma if the tracheal cartilages

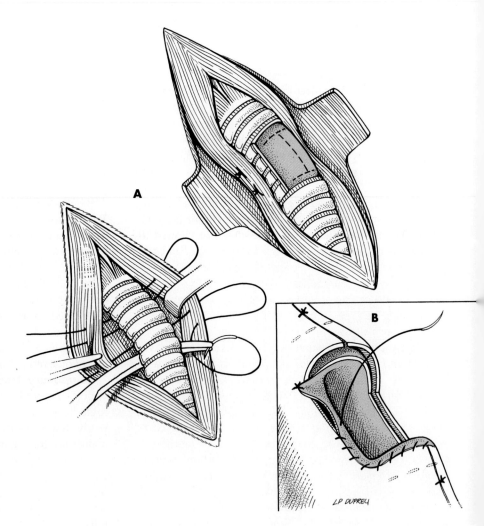

FIG. 25-3
A, For permanent tracheostomy, deviate the trachea ventrally by apposing the sternohyoid muscles with mattress sutures. Excise a rectangular segment of ventral tracheal wall without penetrating mucosa. Note the dotted line where the I-shaped incision is made after removing the cartilage segment. Excise loose skin adjacent to the stoma. **B,** Use intradermal sutures to appose skin to the annular ligaments and peritracheal tissues. Appose tracheal mucosa to skin with three or four interrupted sutures; then, use a simple continuous pattern to complete the closure.

LP DUPREY

show any weakness or tendency to collapse. Excise a similar segment of skin adjacent to the stoma (excise larger segments of skin if the animal has loose skin folds or abundant subcutaneous fat). Suture the skin directly to the peritracheal fascia laterally and the annular ligaments proximal and distal to the stoma with a series of interrupted intradermal sutures (3-0 or 4-0 polydioxanone or polypropylene). Make an I- or H-shaped incision in the mucosa. Fold the mucosa over the cartilage edges and suture it to the edges of the skin with approximating sutures to complete the tracheostoma (Fig. 25-3, B). Use simple interrupted sutures at the corners and a simple continuous pattern to further appose skin and mucosa (4-0 polypropylene) (see Fig. 25-3, B).

Tracheal Resection/Anastomosis

Removal of a tracheal segment may be necessary to treat tracheal tumors, stenosis, or trauma. Depending on the degree of tracheal elasticity and tension, approximately 20% to 60% of the trachea may be resected and direct anastomosis achieved. The split cartilage technique is preferred because it is easier to perform and results in more precise anatomic alignment with less luminal stenosis than many other tech-

niques (Hedlund, 1984). Diseased trachea exceeding the limits of resection and anastomosis may be managed with permanent tracheostomy, intraluminal silicone tubes, grafts, or prostheses with variable success.

Expose the involved trachea through a ventral cervical, midline, lateral thoracotomy (see p. 652), or median sternotomy (see p. 654) approach. Mobilize only enough trachea to allow anastomosis without tension. Preserve as much of the segmental blood and nerve supply to the trachea as possible. Place stay sutures around cartilages cranial and caudal to the resection sites prior to transecting the trachea. Resect the diseased trachea by splitting a healthy cartilage circumferentially at each end or incising annular ligaments adjacent to the intact cartilages (Fig. 25-4, A). Use a No. 11 blade to split the tracheal cartilages at their midpoint. Transect the dorsal tracheal membrane with Metzenbaum scissors. Preplace, and then tie, three or four simple interrupted sutures (3-0 or 4-0 polypropylene) in the dorsal tracheal membrane (Fig. 25-4, B). Retract the endotracheal tube into the proximal trachea during resection and placement of sutures in the dorsal tracheal membrane. Remove blood clots and secretions

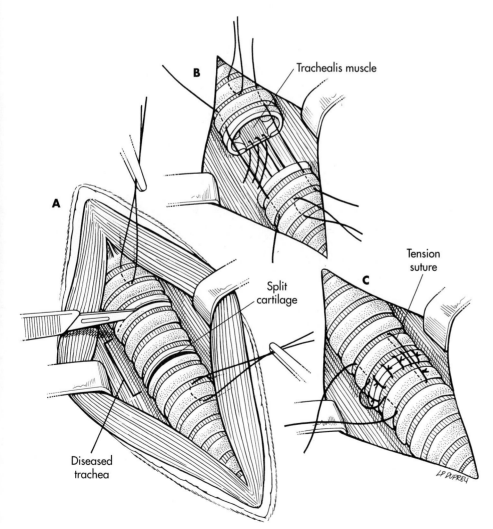

Trachealis muscle

Split cartilage

Tension suture

Diseased trachea

LP DUPREY

FIG. 25-4
A, During tracheal resection and anastomosis, place stay sutures cranial and caudal to the resection sites. Split the cartilages with a No. 11 blade and transect the trachealis muscle with Metzenbaum scissors. **B,** Appose the trachealis muscle with three to four interrupted sutures, then approximate the split cartilages. **C,** Place three or four tension-relieving sutures around cartilages adjacent to the anastomosis.

from the lumen and advance the tube distal to the anastomosis after dorsal tracheal membrane sutures are placed. Complete the anastomosis by apposing the split cartilage halves or adjacent intact cartilages with simple interrupted sutures beginning at the ventral midpoint of the trachea. Space additional sutures 2 to 3 mm apart. Place three or four retention sutures to help relieve tension on the anastomosis. Place and tie these sutures so that they encircle an intact cartilage cranial and caudal to the anastomosis, crossing external to the anastomotic site (Fig. 25-4, C). Lavage the area and appose the sternohyoid muscles with a simple continuous pattern. Close subcutaneous tissues and skin routinely.

If tension-relieving sutures do not adequately relieve tension at the anastomosis, further mobilize the trachea, make partial-thickness incisions through annular ligaments proximal and distal to the anastomosis, or restrict head and neck movement after surgery. Prevent full extension of the neck by placing a suture from the chin to the manubrium or fixing a muzzle to a harness to maintain mild to moderate cervical flexion. Maintain the muzzle for 2 to 3 weeks.

Ventriculocordectomy

Ventriculocordectomy is removal of the vocal cords to alter vocalization, remove masses, or enlarge the ventral glottis. The procedure may be performed using an oral or ventral (laryngotomy) approach. Anesthesia is maintained by using a tube tracheostomy, manipulating the endotracheal tube to the contralateral side of the larynx, or performing the procedure using injectable anesthetic agents. Ventriculocordectomy performed to widen the ventral glottis requires that more vocal fold be resected than for debarking.

☞ **NOTE** · Webbing is a problem after this procedure. Maintaining 1 to 2 mm of mucosa at the dorsal and ventral aspects of the vocal cord may help prevent this complication.

Oral approach. *Position the patient in ventral recumbency with the neck extended. Suspend the maxilla and pull the mandible ventrally to maximally open the mouth. Extend the tongue from the mouth to get maximum exposure of the glottis. Retract the cheeks laterally to improve visualization. Avoid placing padding or hands in the region of the larynx as this may distort the nasopharynx. Remove the central margin of the vocal cord for debarking with a laryngeal or uterine cup biopsy forceps (Fig. 25-5, A). To widen the glottis, use long-handled Metzenbaum scissors and remove as much of the vocal fold extending into the laryngeal lumen as possible (Fig. 25-5, B). With either technique maintain 1 to 2 mm of mucosa at the dorsal and ventral aspects of the vocal cord. Control hemorrhage with pressure. Remove blood clots and secretions with suction or sponges. Allow the incision to heal by second intention.*

☞ **NOTE** · Staging the procedure, by waiting 2 to 3 weeks before removing the contralateral vocal fold, helps prevent glottic stenosis.

Laryngotomy approach. *Position the patient in dorsal recumbency with the neck extended over a rolled towel (Fig. 25-6). Expose the larynx using a ventral midline cervical approach beginning rostral to the basihyoid bone and extending caudally to the proximal trachea. Separate*

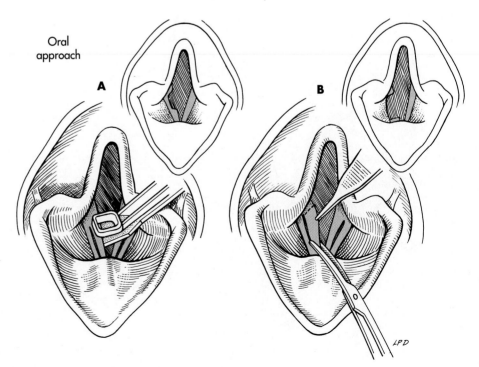

Oral approach

A   **B**

FIG. 25-5
For ventriculocordectomy, either an oral or laryngotomy approach may be used. **A,** For devocalization using an oral approach, remove the central portion of the vocal fold with laryngeal cup forceps or uterine biopsy forceps. **B,** For laryngeal paralysis or devocalization, remove the majority of the vocal fold with Metzenbaum scissors.

and retract the paired sternohyoid muscles. Identify the midline of the thyroid cartilage. Ligate and divide the laryngeal impar vein if necessary. Incise the cricothyroid ligament with a No. 15 or No. 11 blade. Extend the incision along the midline of the thyroid cartilage as needed to expose the vocal folds. Excise the entire vocal fold from the arytenoid cartilage dorsally and the thyroid cartilage ventrally (Fig. 25-6). Close the defect by apposing the mucosa with a simple continuous appositional suture pattern (4-0 polydioxanone) (see Fig. 25-6). Appose the cricothyroid ligament and thyroid cartilage with simple interrupted sutures. Appose the sternohyoid muscles with a simple continuous pattern (3-0 or 4-0 polydioxanone or polyglyconate). Close subcutaneous tissues and skin routinely.

☞ **N O T E** · Be careful to avoid disrupting the blood supply to the larynx and trachea during surgery or necrosis may result.

HEALING OF THE RESPIRATORY TRACT

Laryngeal wounds heal by reepithelialization if mucosal edges are in apposition. Epithelial cells at the wound margins extend and spread over the wound until it is covered. Constant motion associated with breathing and head movement inhibits primary healing. Laryngeal wounds with gaps heal by second intention, first filling with granulation tissue and then reepithelializing. Second intention healing may result in scarring across the glottis. Scarring may be prevented by restricting surgery to one side of the larynx and leaving intact epithelium at the dorsal and ventral commissures.

Tracheal epithelium responds immediately to irritation or disease by increasing mucus production. If the insult continues, cells desquamate and goblet cell hyperplasia occurs to increase the protective mucous layer. Superficial wounds heal by reepithelialization. Healing begins within 2 hours following slough of superficial cells. Intact ciliated columnar cells surrounding the defect flatten, lose their cilia, and migrate over the wound. Mitosis begins about 48 hours after injury in the ciliated columnar and basal epithelial cells. Organization and differentiation begin after 4 days. Squamous cells replace ciliated and goblet cells if injury recurs without healing. Full-thickness tracheal mucosal wounds with a gap between mucosal edges fill with granulation tissue before reepithelialization. Full-thickness wounds may heal with scar tissue protruding into the lumen. Scar tissue narrows the lumen and may interfere with mucus transport. A 20% reduction in lumen diameter reduces mucociliary clearance by 65% (Giordano, Holsclaw, 1976).

☞ **N O T E** · Reduce inflammation by minimal, gentle tissue manipulation and pretreating with corticocosteroids.

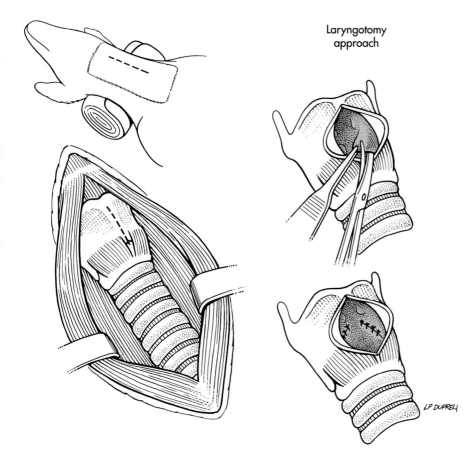

Laryngotomy approach

LP DUFREY

FIG. 25-6
For ventriculocordectomy via a laryngotomy approach, position the patient in dorsal recumbency with the neck extended over a rolled towel. Expose the larynx, identify the midline of the thyroid cartilage, and incise the cricothyroid ligament with a scalpel blade. Expose the vocal folds and excise them. Close the defect by apposing the mucosa with a simple continuous appositional suture pattern.

SUTURE MATERIALS/SPECIAL INSTRUMENTS

An assortment of long-handled instruments are beneficial. Skin hooks, laryngeal or uterine cup biopsy forceps, and tracheal prostheses (see p. 635) are needed for some procedures. Nonreactive, monofilament suture is recommended for surgery of the upper respiratory tract (e.g., polydioxanone or polypropylene).

POSTOPERATIVE CARE AND ASSESSMENT

These patients must be closely monitored during anesthetic recovery for hemorrhage, coughing, gagging, or aspiration. They should be kept intubated as long as possible and reintubated or have a tracheostomy tube placed if respiratory distress occurs following extubation. Supplemental oxygen should be provided if necessary during recovery, and excitement and pain minimized by using postoperative analgesics (Table 25-10). Inserting a nasal oxygen catheter at the conclusion of surgery allows supplemental oxygen to be delivered (Table 25-11). Alternately, the animal may be placed in an oxygen cage. Positioning the patient in sternal recumbency may facilitate respiration. Postoperative corticosteroids (see Table 25-5) may be required to reduce mucosal swelling and edema. Prophylactic antibiotics can be discontinued immediately after surgery. Water may be offered 6 to 12 hours after surgery and if gagging, regurgitation, or vomiting does not occur, soft food made into meatballs may be offered 18 to 24 hours postoperatively. Meatballs should be fed one at a time for 5 to 7 days following nasopharyngeal or laryngeal procedures to slow ingestion. Exercise should be restricted for 4 weeks. A harness rather than a collar should be used for 2 to 4 weeks to avoid incisional, tracheal, or laryngeal trauma.

> ☞ **N O T E** · Clients should be warned that surgery may improve, but seldom cures, upper respiratory problems. Continued medical therapy may be required.

Intensive postoperative care is required after tube tracheostomy. The animal must be observed closely to prevent asphyxiation secondary to tube obstruction or dislodgement. Mucus clearance is inhibited in these animals and mucosal irritation leads to increased mucus production. Tube cleaning may be required every 15 minutes if the trachea is irritated. Sterile technique (i.e., gloves, instruments) should be used to clean tracheostomy tubes. Secretions may be removed by inserting a sterile suctioning cannula into the tube's lumen and distal trachea. When cannulated tubes are used, the inner cannula may be removed and cleaned while the outer tube is suctioned. Injecting sterile saline (1 ml) into the tube a few minutes prior to suctioning helps loosen secretions. A new tube should be used if these techniques do not adequately remove secretions. Tracheostomy tubes may be removed when an adequate airway and spontaneous ventilation are established. Occasionally, occluding the tube and observing the patient while it breathes around the tube are required to determine whether the tube can be removed. This should not be done in animals with cuffed tubes or those that have large tubes that fill the tracheal lumen. After tube removal, the tracheostomy site should be allowed to heal by second intention.

Management of permanent tracheostomies is usually less demanding than tube tracheostomies. Initially, the tracheostoma should be inspected for mucus accumulation every 1 to 3 hours. When mucus begins to occlude the tracheostoma or when respiratory effort increases, the site should be suctioned as described above for tube tracheostomies. Mucus at the stoma may be removed by aspiration or by gently wiping with a sponge or applicator stick. Only a moderate amount of mucus is expected to accumulate during the first 7 to 14 days after surgery unless the animal has severe tracheitis. By 7 days the cleaning interval usually increases to every 4 to 6 hours, and after 30 days twice-daily stomal cleaning is usually sufficient. However, smoke and other noxious stimuli will cause increased mucus production and necessitate more frequent cleaning. Hair should be clipped as needed from around the stoma to prevent hair matting with mucus. Exercise and housing should be restricted to clean areas.

Following tracheal resection and anastomosis, exercise and neck extension should be restricted for 2 to 4 weeks. Animals should be kept quiet and observed for signs of respiratory distress following ventriculocordectomy. Some animals

---

TABLE 25-10

Postoperative Analgesics Following Upper Respiratory Surgery

Oxymorphone (Numorphan)
0.05-0.1 mg/kg IV, IM every 4 hours (as needed)

Butorphanol (Torbutrol, Torbugesic)
0.2-0.4 mg/kg IV, IM, or SC every 2 to 4 hours (as needed)

Buprenorphine (Buprenex)
5-15 μg/kg IV, IM every 6 hours (as needed)

TABLE 25-11

Procedure for Placement of Nasal Catheter for Delivery of Oxygen

- Place a few drops of local anesthetic into the nasal cavity
- Measure the distance to the medial canthus of the eye and mark the catheter
- Advance a lubricated, 5 to 8 French feeding tube through the nostril into the nasopharynx to the premarked site
- Attach the tube to an oxygen source and administer humidified oxygen at 50 ml/kg/min*

*Gastric distention may occur if the flow rate is too high.

will gag and cough. Vocalization should be discouraged for 6 to 8 weeks.

COMPLICATIONS

Acute respiratory obstruction due to mucosal swelling, edema, irritation, and increased mucus production and/or laryngeal or tracheal collapse may occur after upper respiratory surgery and must be relieved promptly (Table 25-12). Infection is a potential problem because the nasopharynx, larynx, and trachea have a resident bacterial flora. Using strict aseptic technique and lavaging contaminated tissues usually prevent infection. Injury to the recurrent laryngeal nerve may cause laryngeal spasms, paresis, or paralysis leading to aspiration pneumonia. Mucostasis may occur following nerve damage. Nerve damage is prevented by gentle tissue handling, appropriate dissection, and careful tissue retraction.

Complications associated with tube tracheostomy include gagging, vomiting, coughing, tube obstruction, tube dislodgement, emphysema, tracheal stenosis, tracheal malacia, and tracheocutaneous or tracheoesophageal fistula. Some animals will occlude their tracheostomy tube when their neck is flexed and when they sleep with bedding. The main complication of permanent tracheostomy is stomal occlusion from accumulated mucus, skin folds, or stenosis. Mucus accumulation, coughing, and gagging may also occur due to tracheal irritation. Tracheostomy tubes and endotracheal tubes causing pressure necrosis of the tracheal mucosa or cartilages may cause strictures.

Complications following tracheal resection and anastomosis may include hemorrhage, voice change, fistula formation, and cartilage malacia. Malacia is uncommon and these other complications are manageable. Dehiscence occurs following tracheal anastomosis if there is too much tension or neck movement following surgery. Subcutaneous emphysema, acute respiratory distress, hemoptysis, and subcutaneous swelling are signs of dehiscence. Excessive anastomotic tension and second-intention healing may lead to tracheal stenosis. Excessive dissection may cause ischemic necrosis of the remaining trachea. Traumatizing the recurrent laryngeal nerves may cause laryngospasms, laryngeal paresis, or laryngeal paralysis.

Following ventriculocordectomy, scar tissue may form within the larynx and trachea leading to obstruction weeks after surgery. Clinical signs of obstruction are not usually ap-

parent until luminal compromise approaches 50%. Scar tissue forms across the larynx from mucosal damage or when there is second-intention healing near the dorsal and ventral commissures. Other complications include edema, hemorrhage, cough, gag, stenosis, and altered vocalization. Mucosal edema may partially obstruct the glottis and can be reduced by pretreating with corticosteroids. Stenosis may occur at the dorsal or ventral commissures of the glottis following ventriculocordectomy if intact mucosa is not preserved in these areas and healing occurs by second intention. Approximating mucosa over the ventriculocordectomy sites also minimizes stenosis. Ventriculocordectomy is expected to alter the normal bark, making it lower pitched and harsher. Resumption of a near-normal bark may occur within months after removal of only the vocal fold margin and second-intention healing.

☞ **N O T E** · Glottic stenosis occurs frequently after bilateral oral vocal cord resection.

SPECIAL AGE CONSIDERATIONS

Tracheal and laryngeal cartilages of very young animals have a high water content. These cartilages may not hold sutures well. Congenital abnormalities involving the respiratory tract should be treated early in the animal's life (within the first year) to avoid progressive respiratory distress and improve their quality of life. Old animals may have ossified, inelastic, brittle cartilages that are difficult to manipulate during surgery.

References

Giordano A, Holsclaw DS: Tracheal resection and mucociliary clearance, *Ann Otol* 85:597, 1976.

Hedlund CS: Tracheal anastomosis in the dog: comparison of two end-to-end techniques, *Vet Surg* 13:135, 1984.

McKiernan BC, Smith AR, Kissil M: Bacterial isolates from the lower trachea of clinically healthy dogs, *J Am Anim Hosp Assoc* 20:139, 1984.

Suggested Reading

Creighton SR, Wilkins RJ: Bacteriologic and cytologic evaluation of animals with lower respiratory tract disease using transtracheal aspiration biopsy, *J Am Anim Hosp Assoc* 10:227, 1974.

Harvey CE, Goldschmidt MH: Healing following short duration transverse incision tracheotomy in the dog, *Vet Surg* 11:77, 1982.

Hedlund CS: Tracheal resection and reconstruction, *Prob Vet Med (Head Neck Surg)* 3:210, 1991.

Hedlund CS et al: A procedure for permanent tracheostomy and its effects on the tracheal mucosa, *Vet Surg* 11:13, 1982.

Hedlund CS et al: Permanent tracheostomy: perioperative and long-term data from 34 cases, *J Am Anim Hosp Assoc* 24:585, 1988.

Meada M, Grillo HC: Effect of tension on tracheal growth after resection and anastomosis in puppies, *J Thorac Cardiovasc Surg* 65:648, 1975.

Venker-van Haagen AJ: Diseases of the larynx, *Vet Clinics of North Am: Small Anim* 22:1155, 1992.

TABLE 25-12

Common Errors in Managing Animals with Upper Respiratory Disease

- Failing to diagnose and treat upper respiratory disease before secondary problems develop (i.e., aspiration pneumonia)
- Failing to recognize laryngeal collapse
- Causing trauma to the recurrent laryngeal nerves
- Failing to intensively monitor the patient after surgery

SPECIFIC DISEASES

STENOTIC NARES

DEFINITIONS

Stenotic nares are nostrils with abnormally narrow openings.

SYNONYMS

Pinched nose

GENERAL CONSIDERATIONS AND CLINICALLY RELEVANT PATHOPHYSIOLOGY

Stenotic nares (congenital malformations of the nasal cartilages) are commonly seen in brachycephalic breeds. The cartilages lack normal rigidity and collapse medially causing partial occlusion of the external nares. Airflow into the nasal cavity is restricted and greater inspiratory effort is necessary, causing mild to severe dyspnea. Concurrent soft palate elongation, everted laryngeal saccules, aryepiglottic collapse, and/or corniculate collapse often contribute to the severity of respiratory distress.

Brachycephalic syndrome refers to the combination of stenotic nares, soft palate elongation, and laryngeal saccule eversion that is commonly seen in brachycephalic dogs (Table 25-13). Concurrent tracheal hypoplasia or advanced laryngeal collapse often contributes to the respiratory distress. Brachycephalic animals exhibit signs of upper airway obstruction due to anatomic and functional abnormalities. They typically have a compressed face with poorly developed nares and a distorted nasopharynx. Their head shape is the result of an inherited developmental defect in the bones of the base of the skull. These bones grow to a normal width, but to a reduced length. The soft tissues of the head are not proportionally reduced and often appear redundant.

DIAGNOSIS
Clinical Presentation

Signalment. Brachycephalic breeds (particularly English bulldogs, Boston terriers, pugs, and Pekingese) are predominantly affected. Dogs are more commonly affected than cats (i.e., Himalayan and Persian). It affects either sex. Stenotic nares are present at birth; however, many animals present for evaluation between 2 to 4 years of age.

TABLE 25-13
Brachycephalic Breeds of Dogs
• English bulldog
• Boston terrier
• Pug
• Pekingese
• Boxer
• Lhasa apso
• Shih tzu
• Shar-pei

History. Patients with upper airway obstruction usually have noisy (stridulous), difficult breathing. Some animals are presented because of frequent retching or gagging up of phlegm. Dogs may have trouble swallowing because the normal occlusion of the airway during deglutition compromises ventilation. Exercise intolerance, cyanosis, restless sleeping ("sleep-disordered breathing"), and collapse are often reported. Excitement, stress, and increased heat and humidity frequently make clinical signs worse.

Physical Examination Findings

Stenotic nares are identified on physical examination. The nares may be mildly, moderately, or severely deviated medially. Signs of increased inspiratory effort include retraction of lip commissures, open-mouth breathing or constant panting, forelimb abduction, and exaggerated use of abdominal muscles. Paradoxical movement of the thorax and abdomen, recruitment of accessory respiratory muscles, inward collapse of the intercostal spaces and thoracic inlet, and orthopneic posture (extended head and neck and reluctance to lie down) may be apparent. The mucous membranes are normal in color with mild or moderate dyspnea, but pale or cyanotic with severe dyspnea. Affected animals are often restless and anxious, especially when restrained. Animals may be hyperthermic due to ineffective cooling. Careful thoracic auscultation is difficult because of referred upper airway noise. Gastrointestinal tract distention may occur secondary to aerophagia associated with open-mouth breathing.

Radiography

Thoracic radiographs should be evaluated to detect underlying cardiac (i.e., cardiomegaly, heart failure) or pulmonary (i.e., pulmonary edema, pneumonia) abnormalities. Lateral radiographs of the nasopharynx, larynx, and trachea are sometimes helpful in assessing concurrent airway abnormalities. The soft palate may be thickened and elongated. Nasopharyngeal, laryngeal, and tracheal masses may be identified. Determining tracheal to thoracic inlet diameter ratios can help assess tracheal size (see p. 633).

Laboratory Findings

Hematology and serum biochemistry values are usually normal. Rarely, blood gas evaluation may reveal hypoxemia and respiratory alkalosis. Oxygen saturation acutely falling below 80% may cause signs of syncope and collapse. Polycythemia may occur if hypoxia is chronic.

DIFFERENTIAL DIAGNOSIS

Stenotic nares generally occur in conjunction with the other respiratory abnormalities that comprise "brachycephalic syndrome" (i.e., elongated soft palate and everted laryngeal saccules). Other abnormalities that may cause upper respiratory obstruction include aryepiglottic collapse, corniculate collapse, tracheal collapse, tracheal hypoplasia, laryngeal paralysis, masses obstructing the glottis, larynx, or trachea, and traumatic disruption of the airway.

MEDICAL TREATMENT

A weight reduction program should be instituted for obese animals. Exercise restriction and elimination of precipitating causes may be beneficial when clinical signs are mild. Sedation (see Table 25-2), corticosteroids (see Table 25-5), supplemental oxygen (see Table 25-11), and cooling may be necessary for moderate to severe respiratory distress.

SURGICAL TREATMENT

Multiple procedures (e.g., stenotic nares resection, resection of elongated soft palate, resection of everted laryngeal saccules) are usually required to alleviate signs of "brachycephalic syndrome." Animals with upper respiratory obstruction are anesthetic and postoperative risks (see p. 618).

Preoperative Management

These animals should be monitored carefully for decompensation and progressive respiratory distress. Emergency therapy (e.g., temporary tracheostomy; see p. 613) may be necessary if dyspnea worsens acutely. Animals undergoing concurrent laryngeal or nasopharyngeal procedures should be treated with antiinflammatory doses of corticosteroids (see Table 25-5).

Anesthesia

Anesthesia or sedation must be done carefully in these animals (see p. 610). Virtually all sedatives and anesthetic agents relax the upper airway dilating muscles, while allowing the diaphragm to continue contracting. This allows the upper airway to collapse and reduces respiratory drive. Airway collapse is worsened by negative inspiratory pressure that draws the pharyngeal walls medially. Anesthesia also relaxes muscles employed by brachycephalics to facilitate breathing (e.g., geniohyoid, genioglossus, sternohyoid). Oxygen saturation can drop rapidly during anesthesia or sedation; it should be monitored during induction, oral examination, anesthesia, and anesthetic recovery. Anesthesia should be induced and the animal intubated as rapidly as possible. General anesthetic recommendations and selected anesthetic protocols for animals with upper respiratory disease are on p. 610.

Surgical Anatomy

The dorsal and ventral lateral nasal cartilages unite laterally to form a cartilage tube, the nostril (Fig. 25-7, *A* and *B*). The nostrils are supported medially and ventrally by the nasal septum and dorsally by the dorsal lateral nasal cartilages. The

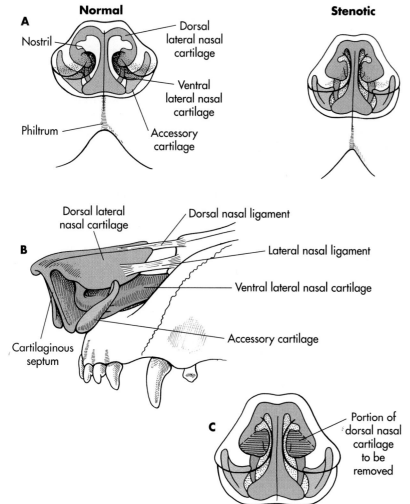

FIG. 25-7
A, Normal vs. stenotic appearance of the nares. **B,** The dorsolateral, ventrolateral, and accessory nasal cartilages form the nostrils. **C,** To widen the nares, resect a portion of the dorsolateral nasal cartilages.

dorsal lateral cartilage also forms the lateral wall of the nostril. The lateral accessory cartilage contributes ventral support to the nostrils.

Positioning

Position the patient in sternal recumbency with the chin resting on a pad. Tape the head to the table to avoid rotation. The planum nasale should be scrubbed with antiseptic soaps and solutions.

SURGICAL TECHNIQUES

Resection of a portion of the dorsal lateral nasal cartilage may be performed to widen the nares (Fig. 25-7, *C*). Other techniques described include resection of horizontal or lateral tissue wedges. *Grasp the margin of the nares with a Brown-Adson thumb forceps. Maintaining this grip, make a V-shaped incision around the forceps with a No. 11 scalpel blade. Make the first incision medially and the second incision laterally. Remove the vertical wedge of tissue. Control hemorrhage with pressure and by reapposing the cut edges. Align the ventral margin of the nares and mucocutaneous junction and place three to four simple interrupted sutures (e.g., polydioxanone, 3-0 or 4-0) to reappose the tissues. Repeat the procedure on the opposite side being careful to excise the same size tissue wedge.*

POSTOPERATIVE CARE AND ASSESSMENT

These animals require constant monitoring during recovery from anesthesia (see p. 618). Nasal insufflation of oxygen (see Table 25-11) may be beneficial. The animal should remain intubated as long as possible—reintubation or placement of a tracheostomy tube may be necessary if respiratory obstruction or severe distress occurs. The surgical site should be cleaned and protected from the animal by using an Elizabethan collar, if necessary. Slight hemorrhage may occur from the surgical sites.

COMPLICATIONS

If the only abnormality the animal has is stenotic nares, complications are minimal. Dehiscence may occur if the patient frequently licks or rubs its nose; healing then occurs by second intention and may cause a pink scar. Respiratory distress may persist if other areas of the airway are obstructed.

> ☞ **N O T E** · Have drugs readily available to induce anesthesia should reintubation be necessary.

PROGNOSIS

Animals with mild stenosis may do well without surgery; however, those with moderate or severe stenosis and other obstructive problems can develop severe respiratory distress. The prognosis following resection of stenotic nares in animals with brachycephalic syndrome is good if advanced laryngeal collapse is not present and the palate and saccules are concurrently resected. Most animals have reduced inspiratory effort and increased exercise tolerance after surgery.

Suggested Reading

Harvey CE: Upper airway obstruction surgery. Part 1. Stenotic nares surgery in brachycephalic dogs, *J Am Anim Hosp Assoc* 18:535, 1982.

Hendricks JC: Brachycephalic airway syndrome, *Vet Clinics North Am: Small Anim Pract* 22:1145, 1992.

Wykes PM: Brachycephalic airway obstructive syndrome, *Prob Vet Med: Head Neck Surg* 3:188, 1991.

ELONGATED SOFT PALATE

DEFINITIONS

An **elongated soft palate** is one that extends more than 1 to 3 mm caudal to the tip of the epiglottis.

SYNONYMS

Soft palate elongation

GENERAL CONSIDERATIONS AND CLINICALLY RELEVANT PATHOPHYSIOLOGY

Elongated soft palate is the most commonly diagnosed respiratory problem in brachycephalic dogs (see Table 25-1). It is a part of the *brachycephalic syndrome* in addition to stenotic nares (see p. 620) and laryngeal saccule eversion (see p. 625). The elongated soft palate, a congenital abnormality, is pulled caudally during inspiration, obstructing the dorsal aspect of the glottis. It is sometimes sucked between the corniculate processes of the arytenoid cartilages, which increases inspiratory effort and causes more turbulent airflow. The laryngeal mucosa becomes inflamed and edematous, further narrowing the airway. The tip of the soft palate is blown into the nasopharynx during expiration. Affected dogs may have trouble swallowing because normal occlusion of the airway during deglutition compromises ventilation. Dysfunctional swallowing may result in aspiration pneumonia.

DIAGNOSIS
Clinical Presentation

Signalment. Elongated soft palate is uncommon except in brachycephalic breeds, especially English bulldogs, Boston terriers, pugs, and Pekingese. It affects either sex. Although the condition is present at birth, many affected animals present for evaluation between 2 to 3 years of age. Older animals often have concurrent, advanced laryngeal collapse (see p. 626).

History. Patients with upper airway obstruction typically have a history of noisy (stridulous), difficult breathing (especially inspiratory). Some may retch or gag phlegm because they have trouble swallowing if normal occlusion of the airway during deglutition compromises ventilation. Exercise intolerance, cyanosis, and collapse are common and may be worsened by excitement, stress, increased heat, and humidity. Restlessness during sleeping (sleep-disordered breathing) may be noted.

Physical Examination Findings

Pharyngeal and laryngeal auscultation reveals prominent snoring obscuring other respiratory sounds. Increased inspiratory effort (i.e., retraction of lip commissures, open mouth breathing or constant panting, forelimb abduction, exaggerated use of abdominal muscles, paradoxical movement of the thorax and abdomen, recruitment of accessory respiratory muscles, inward collapse of the intercostal spaces and thoracic inlet, and orthopneic posture) may be apparent. Animals may be hyperthermic (see also p. 620).

☞ **N O T E** · Always evaluate these animals for the presence of other upper respiratory abnormalities.

It is difficult to visualize the oropharynx and larynx in brachycephalic animals because their tongues are thick and restraint may accentuate respiratory distress. Sedation or general anesthesia is usually necessary (see p. 610 for anesthesia for laryngeal examination). An elongated soft palate overlies the epiglottis by more than a few millimeters (i.e., often more than 1 cm). Dorsally displacing the soft palate will improve visualization of the arytenoid cartilages. The soft palate is often thickened with a roughened and inflamed tip. The arytenoids are frequently inflamed and edematous.

Radiography

Thoracic radiographs are needed to rule out concurrent diseases (i.e., hypoplastic trachea, cardiomegaly). Pharyngeal radiographs may show an abnormally long, thickened soft palate but are usually unnecessary.

Laboratory Findings

Laboratory abnormalities are uncommon (see also p. 620).

DIFFERENTIAL DIAGNOSIS

Concurrent abnormalities (e.g., stenotic nares, laryngeal saccule eversion, aryepiglottic collapse, corniculate collapse, tracheal collapse) are often present. Concurrent tracheal hypoplasia (see p. 633) is usually diagnosed at a young age. Other causes of upper respiratory obstruction may include laryngeal paralysis, masses obstructing the glottis, larynx, or trachea, and traumatic disruption of the airway.

MEDICAL TREATMENT

Medical therapy is recommended to alleviate acute respiratory distress. A weight reduction program should be instituted for obese animals. Exercise restriction and elimination of precipitating causes may be beneficial when clinical signs are mild. Sedation (see Table 25-2), corticosteroids (see Table 25-5), supplemental oxygen (see Table 25-11), and cooling may be necessary when the animal has moderate to severe respiratory distress. Prolonged medical therapy may allow progression of degenerative changes.

SURGICAL TREATMENT

Resection of elongated soft palates is optimally performed when the animal is young (i.e., 4 to 24 months), before laryngeal cartilages degenerate and collapse.

Preoperative Management

Pretreating with antiinflammatory doses of corticosteroids may decrease laryngeal swelling and postoperative obstruction (see Table 25-5). The oral cavity should be gently lavaged with dilute antiseptic solutions and sponges placed around the endotracheal tube at the glottis to prevent fluids from entering the airway. The mucosal surfaces should not be scrubbed, thus avoiding irritation and edema. A tracheostomy tube may be placed before surgery; however, this is usually unnecessary unless other oral procedures are being done concurrently.

Anesthesia

Anesthesia of animals with brachycephalic syndrome is described on p. 621. General anesthetic recommendations for animals with upper respiratory disease are on p. 610.

Surgical Anatomy

The soft palate is a fleshy piece of tissue extending from the hard palate to the tip of the epiglottis which separates the oropharynx from the nasopharynx. The palatine muscle is covered by mucosa, innervated by the pharyngeal plexus (IX and X cranial nerves), and shortens the soft palate during contraction. Palatine glands keep the mucosa moist. Blood supply is via the palatine vessel (see p. 201). The epiglottis is a curved triangular cartilage at the entrance to the larynx. The apex of the epiglottis points to the oropharynx and lies just dorsal to the soft palate. The lingual aspect of the base of the epiglottis is attached to the basihyoid bone. Mucosa attaches the lateral aspects of the epiglottis to the cuneiform process of the arytenoid cartilage forming the aryepiglottic fold (see Fig. 25-1 on p. 612). The epiglottis attaches to the body of the thyroid cartilage.

☞ **N O T E** · Use the tonsillar crypt as a landmark for determining appropriate soft palate length.

The end of the soft palate just covers the tip of the epiglottis in a normal dog. It generally extends no further than the mid to caudal aspect of the tonsillar crypt. The distal end in a normal dog is concave; however, the distal end of an elongated soft palate is frequently sucked into the larynx, giving it a more pointed or pinched appearance.

Positioning

The patient is positioned in sternal recumbency with the mouth fully opened. The maxilla should be suspended from a bar positioned several feet above the surgery table and the mandible secured ventrally with tape. The chin should not be allowed to rest on the table or pads. For maximal visualization, the cheeks should be retracted laterally and the tongue pulled rostrally (Fig. 25-8).

SURGICAL TECHNIQUES

Resection may be done with scissors, carbon dioxide laser, or electrosurgery, although the latter may increase postoperative swelling. Hemorrhage is generally mild to moderate following resection and can be controlled with gentle pressure. The caudal margin of the soft palate should be shortened so that it contacts the tip of the epiglottis. Resection of too little soft palate will not optimally relieve respiratory distress, while resection of too much soft palate results in nasal regurgitation, rhinitis, and sinusitis. *Visually mark the site of proposed resection using the tip of the epiglottis and the caudal or midpoint of the tonsils as landmarks. Handle the soft palate gently and as little as possible to avoid excessive mucosal swelling. Grasp the tip of the soft palate with thumb forceps or Allis tissue forceps. Place stay sutures at the proposed site of resection on the right and left borders of the palate. Place hemostats on these sutures and have an assistant apply lateral traction. Transect across one third to one half the width of the soft palate with curved Metzenbaum scissors. Begin a simple continuous suture pattern (4-0 polydioxanone) at the border of the palate apposing the oropharyngeal and nasopharyngeal mucosa (Fig. 25-9). Continue transecting and suturing until the excess palate has been resected.*

POSTOPERATIVE CARE AND ASSESSMENT

These patients should be closely monitored for respiratory distress postoperatively. Reduced respiratory noise is noted postoperatively in animals without advanced laryngeal collapse. Extubation should be delayed as long as possible and the animal should be kept quiet. Oxygen may be administered by nasal insufflation (see Table 25-11). If severe dyspnea occurs a tracheostomy tube should be placed (see p. 613). Corticosteroids may be administered postoperatively if swelling is severe and respiratory obstruction persists. Intravenous fluids should be maintained until oral intake resumes. Hospital observation is recommended for 24 to 72 hours after surgery. Excessive mucosal swelling may cause asphyxiation. Postoperative coughing and gagging are common. Water may be offered when the animal is fully recovered from anesthesia (6 to 12 hours postoperatively); however, food should be withheld for 18 to 24 hours (see p. 618). Offering food soon after surgery may traumatize swollen tissues, causing swelling, airway obstruction, and/or aspiration.

☞ **N O T E** • A quiet, prolonged anesthetic recovery with nasal oxygen administration reduces the occurrence of postoperative airway obstruction and the need for reinduction and intubation.

PROGNOSIS

The prognosis without surgery is poor because laryngeal collapse and respiratory distress will worsen. The prognosis is good in young patients having elongated soft palate as the primary problem. They breathe with less distress immediately postoperatively. Older animals frequently do not respond as well because their laryngeal cartilages have begun to collapse. If advanced laryngeal collapse has developed, the prognosis is poor unless additional surgery is performed.

Suggested Reading

Bright RM, Wheaton LG: A modified surgical technique for elongated soft palate, *J Am Anim Hosp Assoc* 19:288, 1983.

Clark GN, Sinibaldi KR: Use of a carbon dioxide laser for treatment of elongated soft palate in dogs, *J Am Vet Med Assoc* 204:1779, 1994.

Harvey CE: Upper airway obstruction surgery 2: soft palate resection in brachycephalic dogs, *J Am Anim Hosp Assoc* 18:538, 1982.

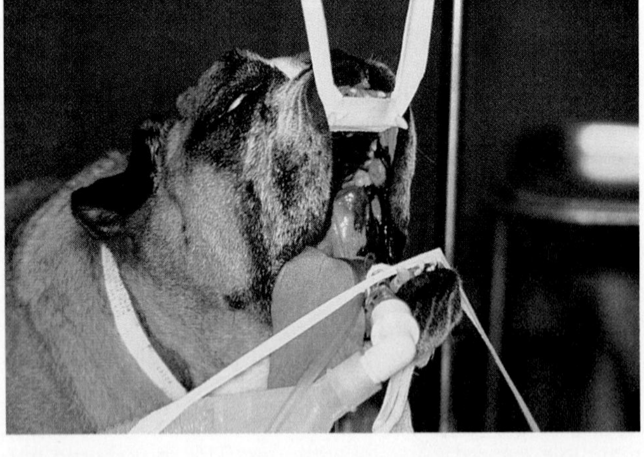

FIG. 25-8
For resection of elongated soft palates, position the patient in ventral recumbency with the maxilla suspended and the mouth widely opened.

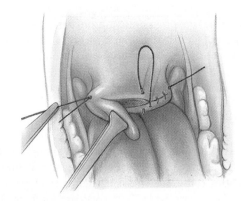

FIG. 25-9
To shorten the soft palate, place stay sutures at the proposed site of resection. Excise one third of the palate, then appose mucosa with sutures. Continue alternating excision and suturing until the resection is complete.

Although clinical signs may be similar, tracheal collapse should not be confused with tracheal stenosis. Tracheal stenosis is an abnormal narrowing of the tracheal lumen due to congenital malformation or trauma. Trauma (e.g., penetrating or blunt wounds, foreign bodies, indwelling tubes) or surgery may cause segmental tracheal stenosis when the wound heals by second intention and excess fibrosis and scarring cause luminal narrowing. Traumatic stenosis is treated by balloon dilation or resection and anastomosis. Congenital stenosis occurs when tracheal cartilages are abnormally small, abnormally shaped, or malpositioned. Tracheal hypoplasia is a form of congenital tracheal stenosis. It is characterized by an abnormally narrow lumen along the entire length of the trachea, rigid tracheal cartilages that are apposed or overlap, and a dorsal tracheal membrane that is narrow or absent. Tracheal hypoplasia primarily affects brachycephalic breeds, especially English bulldogs, who sometimes have other congenital abnormalities (e.g., stenotic nares, elongated soft palate, aortic stenosis, pulmonic stenosis, megaesophagus). It can be associated with continuous respiratory distress, coughing, and recurrent tracheitis, but may be tolerated in the absence of concurrent respiratory or cardiovascular disease. Tracheal hypoplasia can be identified endoscopically or radiographically (Table 25-15). Treatment of tracheal hypoplasia is symptomatic medical therapy (i.e., antibiotics, cough suppressants) and correction of other airway obstructions (e.g., resection of nares, palate, saccules).

DIAGNOSIS
Clinical Presentation

Signalment. Typically, tracheal collapse occurs in toy and miniature-breed dogs; most commonly toy poodles, Yorkshire terriers, Pomeranians, Maltese, and Chihuahuas. Males and females are affected equally. Tracheal collapse in larger dogs is usually associated with trauma, deformity, or intraluminal or extraluminal masses and should not be equated with tracheal collapse in toy breed dogs. Tracheal collapse is classically described as occurring in middle-age or older toy breeds (average 6 to 8 years). However, tracheal collapse is frequently diagnosed in dogs with respiratory problems between 1 and 5 years of age.

History. The onset of clinical signs is often before 1 year of age. Clinical signs often progress with age and include abnormal respiratory noise, dyspnea, exercise intolerance, cyanosis, and syncope. Some dogs never suffer respiratory distress and others die of asphyxiation. Clinical signs are more severe in obese animals. Respiratory noises include wheezing, hacking, coughing, and stridulous breathing. Some dogs do not make abnormal respiratory noises. The cough may be productive or nonproductive but is classically a "goose honk" cough. Coughing often becomes cyclic and paroxysmal. Gagging after coughing may occur in up to 50% of cases. Signs may be elicited or exacerbated by tracheal infections, tracheal compression, exercise, excitement, eating, drinking, or hot, humid weather. Noxious stimuli (i.e., smoke and other respiratory irritants) may also precipitate clinical signs.

☞ **N O T E** · Not all dogs with tracheal collapse have a "goose honk" cough.

Physical Examination Findings

Flaccid tracheal cartilages with prominent lateral borders are occasionally evident on palpation of the cervical trachea. Palpation may elicit paroxysmal coughing. Auscultation may localize abnormal respiratory noises and identify mitral valve disease. A soft end-expiratory snapping together of the tracheal wall may be auscultated in dogs with intrathoracic tracheal collapse. Abnormal heart sounds may be associated with concurrent cardiac disease. Electrocardiography may reveal sinus arrhythmia or evidence of cor pulmonale or left ventricular enlargement. Hepatomegaly, which has been associated with this syndrome in some patients, may result from venous congestion due to cor pulmonale or fatty change.

Laryngoscopy and tracheoscopy should be performed under light anesthesia. Laryngeal paresis, paralysis, or collapse is present in approximately 30% of dogs with tracheal collapse. Approximately 50% of affected dogs show evidence of bronchial compression or collapse. Tracheal conformation should be evaluated as the scope is withdrawn to determine the location and severity of the collapse. The entire trachea is usually collapsed; however, one area of the trachea is often more severely affected and is used for classification purposes. Grade I tracheal collapse is a 25% reduction in lumen diameter with the trachealis muscle being slightly pendulous and the cartilages maintaining a somewhat circular shape. Grade II collapse is a 50% reduction in lumen diameter with the trachealis muscle stretched and pendulous and the cartilages beginning to flatten. Grade III collapse is defined as a 75% reduction in lumen diameter with the trachealis more stretched and pendulous and the cartilages nearly flattened (Fig. 25-14). In grade IV collapse the lumen is essentially obliterated; tracheal cartilages are completely flattened and may invert to contact the trachealis muscle. Tracheal cultures and brushings taken during tracheoscopy are useful in selecting antibiotics.

Radiography/Fluoroscopy

Inspiratory and expiratory lateral radiographs of the neck and thorax are diagnostic in approximately 60% of patients with severe (greater than 50%) tracheal collapse. The cervical trachea is expected to collapse on inspiration and the thoracic

---

TABLE 25-15

Radiographic Diagnosis of Hypoplastic Tracheas

- Ratio of tracheal lumen diameter at the thoracic inlet to the thoracic inlet diameter (TD/TI) less than 0.2
- Ratio of tracheal lumen diameter at the midpoint between the thoracic inlet and carina to width of the third rib (TT/3R) less than 3.0

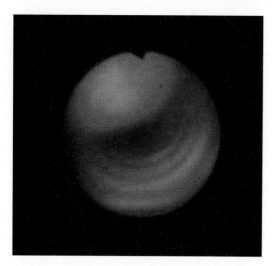

FIG. 25-14
Endoscopic view of a grade III dorsoventral tracheal collapse.

trachea on expiration. Fluoroscopy facilitates evaluation of the dynamic movement of the trachea and mainstem bronchi through all phases of respiration. Thoracic radiographs often reveal cardiomegaly and pulmonary disease.

Laboratory Findings

Hematology and serum biochemistry values are normal unless concurrent systemic disease is present. Positive tracheobronchial cultures are found in more than 50% of animals with tracheal collapse (Buback et al, 1996).

DIFFERENTIAL DIAGNOSIS

Other causes of chronic coughing or respiratory distress include brachycephalic syndrome, tonsillitis, laryngeal collapse, laryngeal paralysis or paresis, bronchitis, tracheobronchitis, allergies, heartworm disease, pulmonary disease, chronic mitral valvular disease, hypoplastic trachea, tracheal stenosis, and tracheal neoplasia.

MEDICAL TREATMENT

Medical therapy is recommended for all animals with mild clinical signs and those with less than 50% collapse. Medical therapy for dogs with tracheal collapse includes antitussives (i.e., butorphanol tartrate, hydrocodone bitartrate; Table 25-16), antibiotics (i.e., ampicillin, cefazolin, clindamycin, enrofloxacin), bronchodilators (i.e., aminophylline, oxtriphylline), and/or corticosteroids (i.e., dexamethasone, prednisone). Sedation with acepromazine (0.05 to 0.2 mg/kg [maximum 1 mg] intravenously, intramuscularly, or subcutaneously, TID) and/or diazepam (0.2 mg/kg intravenously BID) and supplemental oxygen (see Table 25-11) may be required in severely dyspneic patients. Weight reduction should be instituted for obese patients. Exercise restriction is recommended. Affected dogs should be maintained in an environment free of smoke and other respiratory irritants or allergens. Response to medical therapy is usually transient and the disease typically progresses.

TABLE 25-16

Medical Therapy of Tracheal Collapse

Butorphanol Tartrate (Torbutrol)
0.5-1.0 mg/kg PO, BID to TID

Hydrocodone Bitartrate (Hycodan)
0.2 mg/kg PO, TID to QID

Ampicillin
22 mg/kg IV, IM, SC, PO, TID

Cefazolin (Ancef, Kefzol)
20 mg/kg IV, IM, TID

Clindamycin (Antirobe, Cleocin)
11 mg/kg PO, IV, IM, BID

Enrofloxacin (Baytril)
5-10 mg/kg PO or IV, BID

Aminophylline
Dogs—11 mg/kg PO, IM, IV, TID
Cats—5 mg/kg PO, BID

Oxtriphylline Elixir (Choledyl)
15 mg/kg PO, TID

Dexamethasone (Azium)
0.2 mg/kg IV, IM, SC, BID up to 6 mg/kg for emergency treatment

Prednisone
1-2 mg/kg PO, SID to BID

SURGICAL TREATMENT

Surgery is recommended for all dogs with moderate to severe clinical signs, a 50% or greater reduction of the tracheal lumen, and those refractory to medical therapy. Surgery should not be delayed until the animal is in severe respiratory distress. Tracheal collapse is often overlooked in young dogs, which allows degenerative changes to progress, clinical signs to worsen, and secondary problems to develop. Dogs presenting with laryngeal paralysis or collapse, generalized cardiomegaly, and chronic pulmonary disease are poor surgical candidates. Coughing and dyspnea caused by laryngeal, pulmonary, or cardiac disease are not expected to improve without appropriate therapy. Respiratory distress and death may occur in animals with severe laryngeal dysfunction or bronchopulmonary disease. Concurrent mainstem bronchial collapse is present in some dogs. There is presently no technique to support collapsed mainstem bronchi; cervical tracheoplasty may not be beneficial if mainstem bronchial collapse is severe.

The goal of surgery is to support the tracheal cartilages and trachealis muscle, while preserving as much of the segmental blood and nerve supply to the trachea as possible. Many techniques have been described. Currently, the only techniques that meet this goal are placement of individual rings or modified spiral ring prostheses. Generally only the cervical trachea and most proximal portion of the thoracic trachea are supported, even when cervical and thoracic tracheal collapse are present. Tracheoplasty using individual ring prostheses is described below. Patients with concurrent laryngeal paralysis or laryngeal collapse may also require arytenoid lateralization or permanent tracheostomy, respectively.

Preoperative Management

These patients should be observed closely for signs of progressive dyspnea after hospitalization. Surgery should be performed immediately after endoscopy to avoid a second complicated anesthetic recovery. Prophylactic antibiotics (i.e., cefazolin; see Table 25-8) should be given at the time of induction. Corticosteroids may be given to dogs with very small tracheas (i.e., less than 2 to 4 kg) to minimize tracheal mucosal swelling.

Anesthesia

These patients should be preoxygenated and they should be induced and intubated quickly. Manipulation of the endotracheal tube by an assistant is necessary during placement of each ring prosthesis to ensure that sutures have not been placed into the tube. Extubation should be delayed as long as possible after surgery. Laryngeal paralysis may occur secondary to recurrent laryngeal nerve damage (see p. 636). Supplementation of oxygen via nasal insufflation (see Table 25-11 on p. 618) is beneficial, particularly if laryngeal paralysis or severe tracheal inflammation occurs. Anesthesia of animals with brachycephalic syndrome is described on p. 621. General anesthetic recommendations for animals with upper respiratory disease are on p. 610.

Surgical Anatomy

Surgical anatomy of the trachea is discussed on p. 612. The segmental blood and nerve supply to the trachea travels in the lateral pedicles on each side of the trachea. Minimal mobilization of the trachea is necessary to maintain a good blood supply following surgery. The left recurrent laryngeal nerve is located in the lateral pedicle; the right is sometimes located within the carotid sheath.

Positioning

The animal should be positioned in dorsal recumbency with the neck extended and elevated over a pad (to deviate the trachea ventrally). The caudal mandibular area, ventral neck, and cranial thorax should be clipped and prepared for aseptic surgery.

SURGICAL TECHNIQUES

Prosthetic tracheal rings or spirals are made by cutting 3-ml polypropylene syringe cases. To create individual rings, a pipe cutter can be used to divide a syringe case into cylinders 5 to 8 mm wide. Five or more staggered holes should be drilled through each ring for suture placement and the ring should be split ventrally to allow placement. Rough edges of the rings can be smoothened by firing or trimming with a No. 11 blade or file. The rings should be autoclaved prior to implantation. Gas

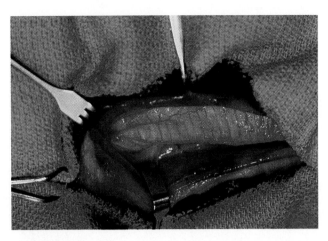

FIG. 25-15
Intraoperative appearance of a grade IV tracheal collapse.

sterilization is possible, but the rings must be aerated at least 72 hours to prevent toxic tissue reactions and tracheal necrosis.

Incise skin and subcutaneous tissues along the ventral cervical midline from the larynx to manubrium. Separate the sternohyoid and sternocephalicus muscles along their midline to expose the cervical trachea. Examine the trachea for evidence of collapse and deformity (Fig. 25-15). Identify and protect the recurrent laryngeal nerves. Place the first tracheal prosthesis one or two cartilages distal to the larynx. Dissect the peritracheal tissues and create a tunnel immediately around the trachea only in the areas of prosthetic ring placement. Guide and position a prosthetic ring through the tunnel and around the trachea with a long curved hemostat (Fig. 25-16, A and B). Position the prosthetic ring with the split on the ventral aspect of the trachea. Chondrotomy is occasionally necessary to allow deformed, rigid cartilages to conform to the prosthesis. *Secure the prosthesis with sutures ventrally, laterally, and dorsally (Fig. 25-16, C). Place three to six sutures (3-0 or 4-0 polypropylene) to secure each prosthesis. Direct sutures around rather than through cartilages and engage the trachealis muscle in at least one suture. Place four to six additional ring prostheses 5 to 8 mm apart along the trachea (Fig. 25-17). Cranial traction on the prostheses around the cervical trachea allows one or two rings to be placed at the thoracic inlet or beyond. Preserve the blood vessels and nerves between the rings. Manipulate the endotracheal tube or trachea after the placement of each prosthesis to be sure the tube cuff has not been engaged by a suture. Lavage the surgical site with sterile saline. Appose the sternohyoid and sternocephalicus muscles with simple continuous sutures (3-0 or 4-0 polydioxanone) and appose subcutaneous tissues and skin routinely.*

POSTOPERATIVE CARE AND ASSESSMENT

These animals should be continuously monitored during recovery. Acute respiratory distress secondary to inflammation,

FIG. 25-16
A, To place prosthetic rings on the trachea, dissect a tunnel around the trachea at each implantation site. **B,** Rotate the prosthesis around the trachea and, **C,** secure it with several sutures.

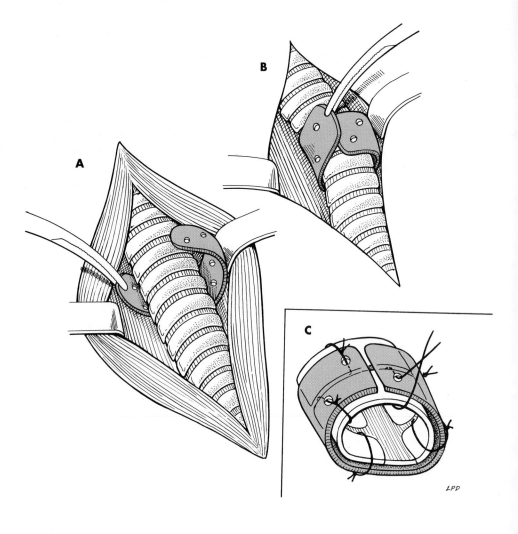

FIG. 25-17
Appearance of trachea after six tracheal ring prostheses have been placed.

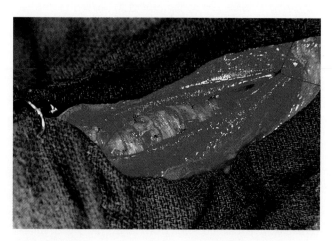

oxygen and an antiinflammatory dose of corticosteroids may be beneficial in animals with edema and inflammation. Antibiotics should be continued for 7 to 10 days if bacterial tracheitis is present. Antitussives, bronchodilators, analgesics, and sedatives may be given as necessary to control coughing and excitement (see Table 25-16). These animals should have strict exercise restriction (cage rest) for 3 to 7 days. Thereafter exercise may be gradually increased. A harness, rather than a collar, should be used for leash walking. Weight reduction is important in obese patients. Tracheoscopy is recommended 1 to 2 months after surgery and later if respiratory signs deteriorate.

Coughing and lack of improvement in clinical signs should be expected for several weeks postoperatively due to tracheitis, peritracheal swelling, and suture irritation. However, clinical improvement (e.g., decreased respiratory noise, less respiratory effort, increased exercise tolerance, fewer tracheobronchial infections) should be noted within 2 to 3 weeks of surgery. Some animals have nearly complete remission of clinical signs after surgery. Others continue to have episodes of coughing or other respiratory noises. Quality of life is improved in most patients, but surgery does not cure the condition.

edema, and/or laryngeal paresis or paralysis may occur postoperatively. Animals with laryngeal paralysis may require surgery to widen the glottis (see p. 629), and those with collapse a permanent tracheostomy (see p. 614) within the first 24 hours to relieve respiratory distress. Nasal insufflation of

COMPLICATIONS

Bruising and mild cervical swelling are expected postoperatively. Infection is a potential problem because the trachea contains bacteria that may be harbored in implants. Tracheal necrosis may occur if too much dissection strips the blood supply away from the trachea or improperly aerated prostheses (gas sterilized) are implanted. Death may result if the trachea is obstructed by severe inflammation or damaged by severe infection or necrosis.

PROGNOSIS

Clinical signs can sometimes be controlled medically if tracheal collapse is not severe, patients do not become obese, and a sedentary lifestyle is practiced. The prognosis is more dependent on concurrent respiratory problems such as laryngeal paralysis or collapse and bronchial disease than on the location or severity of tracheal collapse. Dogs with laryngeal and bronchial disease do not improve clinically as much as those with tracheal collapse alone. Approximately 80% to 90% of dogs with tracheal collapse improve clinically after tracheoplasty.

References

Buback JL, Boothe HW, Hobson HP: Surgical treatment of tracheal collapse: 90 cases (1984–1993), *J Am Vet Med Assoc* 208:380, 1996.

Dallman MJ, McClure RC, Brown EM: Normal and collapsed trachea in the dog: scanning electron microscopy study, *Am J Vet Res* 46:2110, 1985.

Suggested Reading

Coyne BE, et al: Clinical and pathologic effects of a modified technique for application of spiral prostheses to the cervical trachea of dogs, *Vet Surg* 22:269, 1993.

Dallman MJ, McClure RC, Brown EM: Histochemical study of normal and collapsed tracheas in dogs, *Am J Vet Res* 49:2117, 1988.

Hedlund CS: Tracheal collapse, *Prob Vet Med: Head Neck Surg* 3:229, 1991.

Hobson HP: Total ring prosthesis for the surgical correction of collapsed trachea, *J Am Anim Hosp Assoc* 12:822, 1976.

Kirby BM et al: The effect of surgical isolation of the trachea and application of polypropylene spiral prostheses on tracheal blood flow, *Vet Surg* 20:49, 1991.

Tangner CH, Hobson HP: A retrospective study of 20 surgically managed cases of collapsed trachea, *Vet Surg* 11:146, 1982.

White RAS, Williams JM: Tracheal collapse in the dog—is there a role for surgery? A survey of 100 cases, *J Small Anim Pract* 35:191, 1994.

NASAL TUMORS

DEFINITIONS

Nasal tumors are those tumors that arise from the nasal cavity or paranasal sinuses. **Rhinotomy** is an incision into the nasal cavity.

SYNONYMS

Sinonasal tumors

GENERAL CONSIDERATIONS AND CLINICALLY RELEVANT PATHOPHYSIOLOGY

Neoplasms of the nasal cavity and paranasal sinuses are rare in most domestic species; reported prevalence varies from 0.3% to 2.4% of canine tumors. They occur more commonly in dogs than cats. Sinonasal tumors may be classified histologically as epithelial, nonepithelial, or miscellaneous (Table 25-17). Neoplasms of epithelial origin are most common, with adenocarcinomas being the single most frequent histologic diagnosis in dogs. In cats, epithelial tumors and those of lymphoreticular origin are most prevalent. Nonepithelial tumors of skeletal origin (i.e., chondrosarcoma and osteosarcoma) account for approximately one fifth of canine nasal tumors.

The metastatic rate of nasal tumors has generally been considered to be low, with metastasis occurring late in the natural course of these tumors; however, in one survey, 49 of 120 dogs with sinonasal tumors that underwent necropsy had metastasis (Patnaik, 1989). The most common site of metastasis was brain followed in decreasing order of frequency by lymph nodes, lungs, and liver. Esthesioneuroblastomas and neuroendocrine tumors of the nasal cavity are most likely to metastasize to brain, while epithelial tumors usually metastasize to regional lymph nodes and lung. Skeletal tumors in this region have a low incidence of metastasis. Prolonged survival rates in cats with lymphoreticular nasal tumors has been reported following radiotherapy, suggesting that metastasis of these tumors is slow.

TABLE 25-17

Histologic Classification of Sinonasal Neoplasms*

Epithelial

- Squamous cell carcinoma
  Nonkeratinizing
  Keratinizing
- Adenocarcinoma

Nonepithelial

- Skeletal
  Chondrosarcoma
  Osteosarcoma
- Soft tissue
  Lymphosarcoma
  Fibrosarcoma
  Hemangiosarcoma
  Muscular origin
  Fibrous histiocytoma
  Malignant nerve sheath

Miscellaneous

Adenocarcinoid
Esthesioneuroblastoma
Carcinoid
Melanoma

*Modified from Patnaik AK, 1985.

DIAGNOSIS

Clinical Presentation

Signalment. Male dogs and cats seemingly have a higher incidence of sinonasal neoplasms than females, irrespective of histologic diagnosis. Intranasal tumors generally occur in older animals, with a median reported age of approximately 10 years in dogs (Legendre, 1983) and cats (Theon, 1994). However, mean age varies according to histologic diagnosis; the mean age of dogs with chondrosarcomas is less than that of dogs with other tumor types (7 years vs. 9 years). In dogs 1 to 4 years of age, chondrosarcomas are more commonly diagnosed than all other tumor types. Soft tissue tumors involving the nasal cavity have even been reported in 1-year-old dogs (MacEwen, 1977).

History. Most affected dogs present for evaluation of nasal discharge, often with epistaxis. Tumors may cause paroxysmal sneezing (which is violent enough to produce epistaxis). Clinical signs in cats are similar, with most evaluated for sneezing and nasal discharge and occasionally epistaxis. Duration of clinical signs varies, but most animals have them for greater than 1 month and many for greater than 6 months before definitive diagnosis. Initial clinical signs are often intermittent, gradually becoming persistent as the tumor progresses. Infections associated with nasal tumors often respond transiently to antibiotics and other drugs, delaying definitive diagnosis.

Physical Examination Findings

Clinical findings in dogs with nasal tumors include epistaxis, swelling of the facial region (including exophthalmos), nasal discharge, sneezing or snuffling, dyspnea, ocular discharge, and/or bleeding from the oral cavity. Neurologic signs may predominate (seizures, behavior changes, obtundation, paresis, ataxia, circling, visual deficits, and/or proprioceptive deficits). Clinical signs may vary according to histologic type. Seizures are more common in dogs with carcinoids and esthesioneuroblastomas than with tumors of epithelial origin, presumably due to differences in metastatic patterns. Dyspnea may be more typical with epithelial neoplasms and sneezing has been reported most commonly with chondrosarcomas.

Radiography

Thoracic radiography should be performed to evaluate for metastasis. Skull radiographs require general anesthesia in order to obtain satisfactory positioning. Good quality nasal radiographs help define the extent and location of disease and should be performed prior to rhinoscopy, nasal flushes, or surgical biopsies. Lateral, dorsoventral, open-mouth ventrodorsal, and frontal sinus views are suggested. Anesthesia is mandatory. Oblique views may be necessary occasionally to outline lesions that are masked by, or superimposed over, bony structures. The open-mouth ventrodorsal view consistently provides the most information by allowing visualization of the entire turbinate region and reducing superimposition of the mandibles. Radiographs should be evaluated for increased soft tissue density of the nasal cavity or frontal

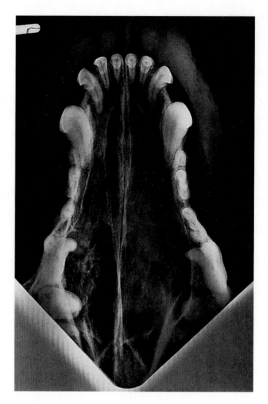

FIG. 25-18
Skull radiograph of an 8-year-old dog with a nasal adenocarcinoma. Note the increased density and loss of turbinate detail in the left nasal cavity.

sinuses, bony lysis, destruction of the normal turbinate pattern, new bone formation, and foreign bodies (Figs. 25-18 and 25-19). Early nasal tumors are often difficult to recognize radiographically because of their similarity to inflammatory changes. Bone destruction usually suggests neoplasia, although severe fungal or bacterial infections may also be responsible. Increased soft tissue density may occur in both neoplastic and inflammatory diseases. Extension into the frontal sinus or the contralateral nasal cavity and destruction of the hard palate indicate an aggressive process. Increased soft tissue density in the frontal sinus, without bony erosion, should not be interpreted as neoplastic extension into the frontal sinus since obstruction of outflow secondary to a nasal tumor often results in fluid accumulation there. Cribriform plate destruction may indicate extension into the brain and a poor prognosis.

☞ **N O T E** · Seeing a fluid density in the frontal sinus does not mean that tumor extends into it. Fluid may accumulate in the frontal sinus because its drainage is obstructed.

Plain and contrast-enhanced x-ray computed tomography (CT) or magnetic resonance imaging helps define the extent of disease in animals with nasal tumors, both for prognosis and for planning radiation therapy. It may also be useful in those patients with minimal neurologic signs, but

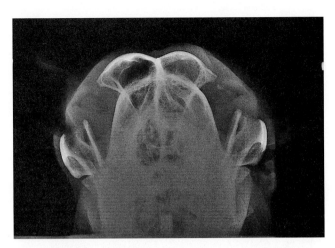

FIG. 25-19
Frontal sinus view of the dog in Fig. 25-18. Note the increased density of the frontal sinus on the right. This may represent neoplasia or fluid accumulation secondary to nasal disease obstructing drainage.

with evidence of destruction of the rostral portion of the calvarium.

Laboratory Findings

Laboratory abnormalities are uncommon. Severe epistaxis may rarely cause anemia. White cell counts are seldom increased, even when a secondary bacterial infection exists. The coagulation system should be assessed (e.g., platelet numbers, bleeding from venipuncture sites, presence of ecchymoses, petechiation, melena, hematuria, or retinal hemorrhages). Cats should be evaluated for feline leukemia virus (FeLV) and feline immunodeficiency virus (FIV) infections.

DIFFERENTIAL DIAGNOSIS

Nasal tumors usually cause unilateral epistaxis or nasal discharge, although bilateral discharge may occasionally be noted. This is in contrast to bacterial and fungal infections, in which the nasal discharge is usually bilateral and purulent (may or may not be bloody). Foreign bodies and bleeding diatheses may also present with unilateral nasal discharge. Diseases or syndromes such as ehrlichiosis, immune-mediated thrombocytopenia, multiple myeloma, systemic hypertension, polycythemia vera, and hyperviscosity syndrome may cause epistaxis and should be ruled out.

MEDICAL MANAGEMENT

Therapy for nasal tumors is directed at control of local disease. Reported treatment options include surgical debulking, surgical debulking combined with radiation therapy, radiation therapy alone, chemotherapy, immunotherapy, and cryosurgery. Radiotherapy appears to be the most effective treatment for nasal tumors. Most studies have investigated orthovoltage (125 to 400 KeV) irradiation, although occasional studies have reported the use of megavoltage (more than 1 KeV) x-irradiation. The optimum dosage and method of delivery have not been determined. Radiotherapy of nasal tumors in cats is as effective as, or more effective than, in dogs (Straw et al, 1986). Whether radiation therapy should be combined with surgical debulking is controversial. One reason for doing so is to improve the clinical status of the dog prior to the radiation therapy. Prior surgery may reduce dyspnea due to nasal cavity obstruction, nasal discharge, and epistaxis during radiation therapy. Cryosurgery or immunotherapy has not appreciably prolonged the survival times of dogs with nasal tumors.

SURGICAL TREATMENT

Surgery, as the sole treatment of dogs with nasal tumors, has not prolonged survival time. The poor response of dogs with nasal tumors to surgery is due to the advanced nature of most tumors at the time of diagnosis, a propensity for these tumors to invade bones that are inaccessible or that cannot be surgically removed, and lack of appreciable encapsulation; each of which makes it almost impossible to completely remove the tumor. However, surgery may palliate clinical signs in some dogs by alleviating obstruction and epistaxis. Permanent tracheostomy (see p. 614) may benefit some dogs that have severe respiratory difficulties and in whom other treatment options are not feasible.

☞ **N O T E** · Have blood available for transfusion because excessive bleeding may occur.

Preoperative Management

Anemic animals may benefit from preoperative blood transfusions (see preoperative concerns; p. 609) and should be preoxygenated. Perioperative antibiotics may be given at anesthetic induction and continued for 12 hours after surgery, but are generally unnecessary and may inhibit bacterial growth from tissue obtained at surgery.

Anesthesia

Selected anesthetic protocols for animals undergoing nasal surgery are provided on p. 610. Biopsy and rhinotomy are performed under general anesthesia. A cuffed endotracheal tube is mandatory for these procedures to prevent aspiration of blood or fluids into the airway. Blood and/or hypertonic saline should be available in the event severe hemorrhage occurs. Placement of two cephalic catheters will allow simultaneous administration of blood and inotropes, if necessary. Evaluation of arterial blood pressure during surgery is warranted and acepromazine should be avoided. The animal should be extubated with the cuff slightly inflated to help remove partially aspirated blood and mucus.

Surgical Anatomy

The nasal cavity extends from the nostrils to the nasopharyngeal meatus and is separated into two halves by the nasal septum (Fig. 25-20). The septum is mostly cartilaginous, but also has bony and membranous portions. The nasal conchae develop from the lateral and dorsal walls of the nasal cavity. The air passages between the conchae are known as

FIG. 25-20
Anatomy of the canine nasal cavity.

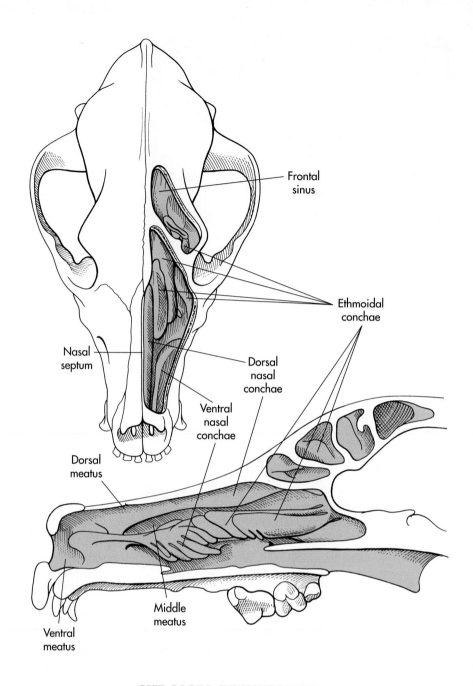

Frontal
sinus

Ethmoidal
conchae

Nasal
septum

Dorsal
nasal
conchae

Ventral
nasal
conchae

Dorsal
meatus

Middle
meatus

Ventral
meatus

meatuses. The paranasal sinuses include a maxillary recess, frontal sinus, and a sphenoidal sinus. The frontal sinus occupies the supraorbital process of the frontal bone (see Fig. 25-20). The two sides are separated by a medium septum and in dogs each side is divided into rostral, medial, and lateral compartments.

Positioning

For a dorsal approach to the nasal cavity the animal is positioned in sternal recumbency with a rolled towel under the neck. The entire head and nasal area should be clipped and prepared for aseptic surgery. For a ventral approach to the nasal cavity the animal is positioned in dorsal recumbency with the mouth tied open maximally (Fig. 25-21). The oral cavity is flushed with sterile saline and the palate swabbed with dilute betadine or chlorhexidine solution.

SURGICAL TECHNIQUES
Biopsy

Definitive diagnosis is made by cytologic or histopathological evaluation of specimens obtained by biopsy or nasal flushing techniques. These procedures require that the animal be anesthetized and intubated with a cuffed endotracheal tube. The cuff should be inflated to prevent aspiration of blood or other materials during the procedure. Visual examination of the palate and posterior nasal area using a flexible fiberoptic endoscope (flexing the scope behind the soft palate) often allows visualization and biopsy of nasal tumors.

Transnostril core biopsies. Transnostril core biopsies may be obtained using the outer protective shield of a Sovereign catheter with the end cut off at a sharp angle or an Alligator forceps. *To prevent inadvertent penetration of the cribriform plate, measure the catheter or forceps with the*

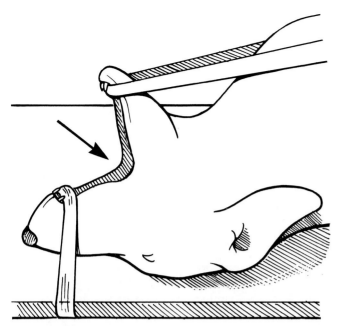

FIG. 25-21
Positioning for a ventral approach to the nasal cavity.

tip placed at the medial canthus of the eye. Do not advance these instruments past this point. Attach the catheter (with the metal stylet removed) to a 12-ml syringe. Discern the location of the lesion from the radiographs and advance the catheter through the tumor several times while applying negative pressure to the syringe. Upon withdrawal of the catheter from the nare, remove the barrel of the syringe and add a small amount of air to the syringe. Use this air to propel the tissue sample forcefully from the syringe hub onto a microscopic slide or into a formalin-filled container. Repeat sampling at various angles until sufficient tissue is obtained. When biopsying masses in the caudal nasal cavity, be sure to adjust the catheter length so as to prevent perforation of the cribriform plate. When using an Alligator forceps, grasp tissue in the area of the lesion and pull it out through the nostril. This latter technique has been the most successful for the author.

Nasal flushes. Nasal flushes may also be performed. The same catheter as described for transnostril core biopsies may be used. Hemorrhage may occur after this procedure, but is generally mild and transient. To prevent inadvertent entry into the calvarium in patients with bony lysis of the cribriform plate, measure the distance from the medial canthus of the eye to the external nare and mark the catheter to correspond to this length. Place gauze sponges above the soft palate and below the external nares to collect fluid and tissues dislodged during flushing. Attach a 35-ml syringe to the catheter and flush 150 to 300 ml of saline into the nasal cavity. Evaluate the gauze sponges for the presence of tissue and debris. Examine the tissues cytologically and save samples for microbiological examination, including fungal and bacterial cultures. If sufficient quantities are obtained, place samples in formalin for histopathology.

Rhinotomy

In cases where the aforementioned techniques do not result in a diagnosis, surgical exploration and biopsy may be necessary. Generally, in such cases the diagnostic and therapeutic procedures (rhinotomy and debulking) are combined. Intraoperative cytology and/or frozen section examination of tissues are helpful. Although rhinotomy may not extend the life of patients with nasal tumors appreciably, it often makes them more comfortable. Some surgeons prefer to perform temporary carotid artery ligation prior to rhinotomy (see p. 203 for technique). If bleeding continues after surgery, the nasal cavity can be packed with sterile gauze. If gauze strips are used (see p. 642 under Special Instruments), the end of the gauze can be exited from the nostril or a dorsal stoma and sutured to the side of the face. The packing is removed 1 or 2 days after surgery. The nasal cavity may be approached through a dorsal or ventral approach. The dorsal approach is most commonly used for nasal tumors; however, the ventral approach can be used to explore the region caudal to the ethmoid turbinates and the ventral aspect of the turbinates.

☞ **N O T E** · Temporary carotid artery ligation may not be safe in cats or anemic or hypovolemic dogs.

Dorsal approach to the nasal cavity and paranasal sinuses. Make a dorsal midline skin incision from the caudal aspect of the nasal planum to the medial canthus of the orbit. Either or both sides of the nasal cavity can be entered through a single midline skin incision. To explore the frontal sinus, extend the incision caudal to a line that connects the zygomatic processes of frontal bone. Incise subcutaneous tissue and periosteum on the midline. Elevate the periosteum and reflect it laterally on either or both sides of the nasal cavity. Use a bone saw to elevate a flap of bone over the proposed site of entry into the nasal cavity (Fig. 25-22, A). Save the bone flap (if healthy) and replace it after the nasal cavity has been explored. Alternately, drill a hole to one side of the nasal septum with a Steinmann pin. Use rongeurs to enlarge the hole and discard the bone fragments. Extend the bone removal bilaterally, if necessary. Gently lavage the nasal passages and remove abnormal tissue. Submit tissues for histologic examination and culture. Use cautery, iced saline, and/or pressure to control hemorrhage. If continued hemorrhage is a problem, pack the nasal cavity with cotton gauze (see below under special instruments). If a bone flap was made, suture it in place with 3-0 or 4-0 wire (do not use wire to replace the bone flap if radiation therapy is planned) placed through predrilled holes in the bone flap and adjacent bone (Fig. 25-22, B). Close periosteum and subcutaneous tissues with absorbable suture material in a simple continuous pattern. Close the skin routinely. If rongeurs were used, close periosteum and subcutaneous tissues, leaving a stoma at the caudal aspect of the incision. Close skin similarly, leaving a stoma (Fig. 25-22, C).

FIG. 25-22
A, For a dorsal approach to the nasal cavity, make a skin incision from the caudal aspect of the nasal planum to the medial canthus of the orbit. Elevate a bone flap or use rongeurs to remove bone. **B,** If a bone flap was made, suture it in place with wire placed through predrilled holes in the bone flap and adjacent bone. **C,** If rongeurs were used to remove bone, close periosteum and subcutaneous tissues leaving a stoma at the caudal aspect of the incision. Close skin similarly, leaving a stoma.

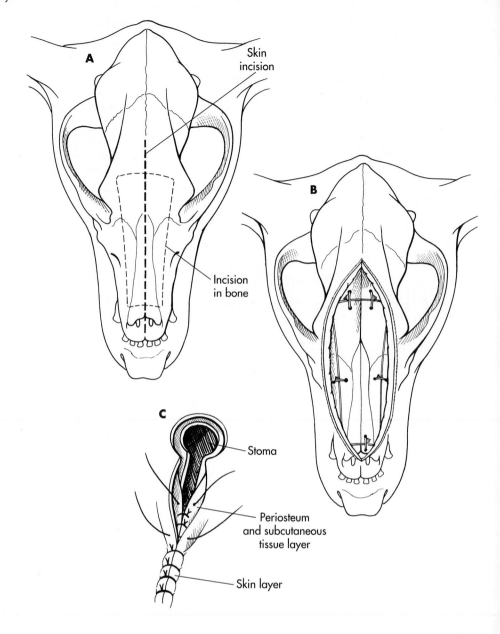

Ventral approach to the nasal cavity. *Make a midline incision in the hard palate. Elevate the mucoperiosteum of the hard palate laterally to the alveolar ridge. Be careful to spare the palatine nerves and vessels as they emerge from the major palatine foramen. Incise the mucoperiosteum and soft palate attachments to the caudal edge of the palatine bone and extend the incision as far caudally as necessary into the soft palate (full-thickness). Retract the edges of the incision with stay sutures. Remove the palatine bone with a power-driven burr or rongeurs and discard it (Fig. 25-23, A). Explore the nasal cavity and remove abnormal tissues. Submit tissues for histologic examination and culture. Close nasal mucosa of the soft palate with absorbable material in a simple continuous or simple interrupted pattern. Then, close submucosa-periosteum of the hard palate with absorbable suture in an interrupted pattern (Fig. 25-23, B). Lastly, close oral mucosa of the hard and soft palate with monofilament nonabsorbable sutures in a simple continuous pattern.*

SUTURE MATERIALS/SPECIAL INSTRUMENTS

Vacuum suction devices and suction tips are extremely helpful during rhinotomy. Without suctioning devices hemorrhage is often severe enough to preclude visualization of abnormal tissues. An oscillating saw is preferred if a bone flap is to be removed, otherwise a Steinmann pin and rongeurs may be used. Sterile gauze packing (e.g., Plain Nu-Gauze packing strip, 2 inches × 5 yards; see Product Appendix) may be used to pack the nose following completion of the procedure.

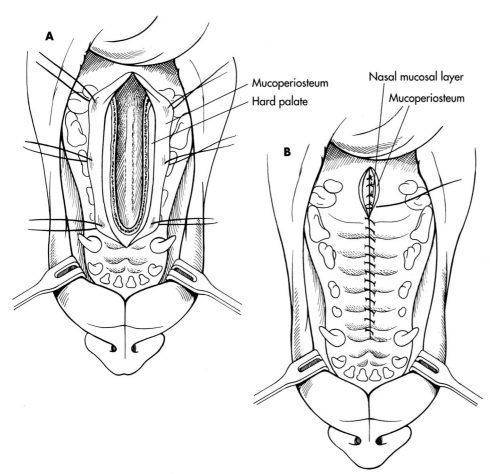

Mucoperiosteum
Hard palate

Nasal mucosal layer
Mucoperiosteum

FIG. 25-23
A, For a ventral approach to the nasal cavity, incise the mucoperiosteum of the hard palate. Remove the palatine bone with a power-driven burr or rongeurs and discard it. **B,** Close the submucosa-periosteum of the hard palate with absorbable suture in an interrupted pattern. Close oral mucosa of the hard and soft palate with monofilament nonabsorbable sutures in a simple continuous pattern.

☞ **NOTE** · Nu-Gauze comes in both plain and betadine-impregnated variety. Use the plain Nu-Gauze to prevent esophageal irritation from swallowing betadine.

POSTOPERATIVE CARE AND ASSESSMENT

The airway should be suctioned to remove blood and fluid before extubation, and the patients should be recovered with their heads down to help decrease aspiration of blood. These animals should be closely monitored for epistaxis following surgery or biopsy.

The hematocrit should be evaluated during and after surgery and transfusions given if the PCV is less than 20% (see above under preoperative considerations). They should be prevented from banging their heads on the cage during recovery. If they appear to be excited or painful during recovery, analgesics may be administered (see Table 25-10). Acepromazine (low dose; Table 25-18) may be given if the patient is normovolemic, not hemorrhaging, does not have a history of seizures, and has been given adequate analgesics. Neurologic function should be assessed postoperatively.

Subcutaneous air may accumulate after a dorsal approach to the nasal cavity if the bone flap is not replaced adequately, or an adequate stoma is not left in the subcutaneous tissues

TABLE 25-18
Postoperative Sedation
Acepromazine
0.05 mg/kg IV or IM, max of 1 mg total dose

and skin for air to exit. Generally, if an adequate stoma is left, subcutaneous air accumulation is not a problem. The stoma will contract and heal within 5 to 10 days. Soft food should be fed for several days after a ventral approach to the nasal passage, and the animal should be prevented from chewing on hard objects for 3 to 4 weeks, until the palate incision is healed.

PROGNOSIS

The prognosis for dogs with nasal tumors is generally poor. In patients not treated and those treated with surgery, chemotherapy, immunotherapy, and cryosurgery, the mean survival time is generally 3 to 5 months. Improvement in this survival period has been accomplished with radiation therapy combined with surgical debulking (see above) with mean reported survival times of 8 to 25 months. The prognosis for carcinomas is better than for sarcomas, and adenocarcinomas appear to have the best overall prognosis. It is unlikely that therapy will result in cure in most dogs, and more successful local control may lead to an increased detection of metastasis. Conversely, the prognosis for cats with lymphoid neoplasia of the nasal cavity appears good.

☞ **N O T E** • Many dogs are euthanized because the owners perceive that their quality of life is poor. Surgery can increase patient comfort and prolong life, despite being noncurative.

One unusual neoplasm associated with a much better long-term prognosis than those previously mentioned is intranasal transmissible venereal tumor (TVT). Clinical signs associated with intranasal TVT are similar to other tumors of this location (epistaxis, sneezing) and the tumor may appear as a space-occupying mass within the nasal cavity. Occasionally bony lysis may be noted. If the tumor is localized, radiation therapy may be curative. Chemotherapy with vincristine is also effective in treating localized or metastatic TVT.

References

Legendre AM, Spaulding K, Krahwinkel DJ: Canine nasal and paranasal sinus tumors, *J Am Anim Hosp Assoc* 19:115, 1983.

MacEwen EG, Withrow SJ, Patnaik AK: Nasal tumors in the dog: retrospective evaluation of diagnosis, prognosis, and treatment, *J Am Vet Med Assoc* 170:45, 1977.

Patnaik AK: Canine sinonasal neoplasms: clinicopathological study of 285 cases, *J Am Anim Hosp Assoc* 25:103, 1989.

Straw RC et al: Use of radiotherapy for the treatment of intranasal tumors in cats: six cases (1980-1985), *J Am Vet Med Assoc* 189:927, 1986.

Theon AP et al: Irradiation of nonlymphoproliferative neoplasms of the nasal cavity and paranasal sinuses in 16 cats, *J Am Vet Med Assoc* 204:78, 1994.

Suggested reading

Adams WM et al: Radiotherapy of malignant nasal tumors in 67 dogs, *J Am Vet Med Assoc* 191:311, 1987.

Gibbs C, Lane JG, Denny HR: Radiological features of intra-nasal lesions in the dog: a review of 100 cases, *J Small Anim Pract* 20:515, 1979.

Rudd RG, Richardson DC: A diagnostic and therapeutic approach to nasal disease in dogs, *Comp Cont Educ Pract Vet* 7:103, 1985.

Thrall DE, Harvey CE: Radiotherapy of malignant nasal tumors in 21 dogs, *J Am Vet Med Assoc* 183:663, 1983.

White R et al: Development of brachytherapy technique for nasal tumors in dogs, *Am J Vet Res* 51:1250, 1990.

Withrow SJ: Cryosurgical therapy for nasal tumors in the dog, *J Am Anim Hosp Assoc* 18:585, 1982.

Withrow SJ et al: Aspiration and punch biopsy techniques for nasal tumors, *J Am Anim Hosp Assoc* 21:551, 1985.

LARYNGEAL AND TRACHEAL TUMORS

DEFINITIONS

Oncocytomas arise from epithelial cells called **oncocytes** that are found in small quantities in various organs (e.g., larynx, thyroid, pituitary, trachea).

GENERAL CONSIDERATIONS AND CLINICALLY RELEVANT PATHOPHYSIOLOGY

Laryngeal and tracheal tumors are rare in dogs and cats. In a 10-year retrospective survey of 56,413 surgical pathology accessions and 7,444 necropsy case reports, laryngeal tumors were identified in 13 dogs and 11 cats (Saik et al, 1986). In another study of 11,774 malignancies only 11 canine and 2 feline laryngeal tumors were identified (Priester, McKay, 1980). Of 289 hematopoietic tumors in cats, 2 tracheal tumors and no laryngeal tumors were identified (Patnaik et al, 1975).

Various tumor types have been identified in the larynx of dogs (Table 25-19). In cats, lymphosarcoma is most commonly identified; squamous cell carcinoma and adenocarcinoma have also been reported. Rhabdomyomas and oncocytomas are laryngeal tumors that appear histologically similar with light microscopy; electron microscopy and immunocytochemistry are necessary to distinguish them. Oncocytomas have been reported in young dogs and warrant special consideration because long-term survival without evidence of metastasis following surgical resection has been reported (Fig. 25-24).

Malignant and benign tracheal tumors have been reported (Table 25-20). Tracheal osteochondromas may occur in dogs less than 1 year of age. These masses probably reflect a malfunction of osteogenesis and are benign. In cats, tracheal squamous cell carcinomas, adenocarcinomas, and lymphosarcomas have been reported. Metastatic thyroid carcinomas, lymphomas, and pharyngeal rhabdomyosarcomas may also involve the larynx and trachea. Incidence of metastasis of laryngeal and tracheal tumors in dogs and cats is unknown.

Filaroides osleri (Oslerus osleri) is a nematode that forms nodules in the canine trachea and mainstem bronchi, which must be differentiated from neoplastic lesions. Definitive diagnosis of filaroidosis is difficult because larvae are intermittently shed in the feces. Diagnosis is best made by finding larvae or adult worms in bronchoscopically obtained biopsy specimens or by identification of the larvae in feces. Anthelmintic therapy and surgical resection have met with varying success.

TABLE 25-19

Laryngeal Tumors

Malignant	
• Squamous cell carcinoma	• Adenocarcinoma
• Lymphoma	• Undifferentiated carcinoma
• Osteosarcoma	
• Fibrosarcoma	**Benign**
• Rhabdomyosarcoma	• Lipoma
• Melanoma	• Oncocytoma
• Mast cell tumor	• Rhabdomyoma
• Other sarcomas	
• Granular cell myoblastoma	

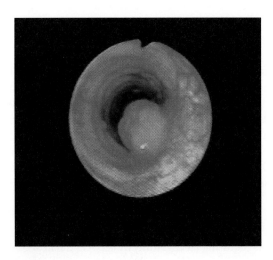

FIG. 25-24
Tracheal oncocytoma in a 7-year-old basset hound that presented for acute respiratory distress.

Laryngeal and tracheal tumors cause luminal obstruction by occupying space or compressing the lumen externally. As lumen size decreases, signs of respiratory distress become apparent (see p. 609). Acute respiratory distress, cyanosis, and/or collapse may occur if excitement, stress, high temperatures, or infections cause mucosal swelling of an already compromised lumen.

DIAGNOSIS
Clinical Presentation

Signalment. Laryngeal and tracheal tumors occur most commonly in middle-age to older animals (i.e., 5 to 15 years). Tumors arising in older animals are more likely to be malignant; however, laryngeal oncocytomas and tracheal osteochondromas may occur in young animals. Benign tracheal osteocartilaginous tumors (osteochondromas) are most common in animals with active osteochondral ossification; they grow with the rest of the musculoskeletal system and may be recognized before a year of age.

History. Animals with laryngeal or tracheal tumors may have an acute or progressive history of upper airway obstruction. Signs may include stridor, dyspnea, cough, decreased exercise tolerance, voice change, hyperthermia, ptyalism, gagging, dysphagia, cyanosis, and/or syncope. Development of a mass in the ventral neck may be reported.

Physical Examination Findings

Physical examination is usually normal unless there are concurrent diseases or abnormalities. Occasionally, extraluminal masses may be palpated along the ventral neck and tracheal palpation may elicit coughing or increased dyspnea. A voice change may be noted in animals with laryngeal masses. Visual examination with a laryngoscope or endoscope allows identification and biopsy of the mass. Most laryngeal and tracheal tumors are inflamed or edematous, pink, fleshy masses protruding into the lumen; however, some laryngeal tumors appear as a diffuse thickening. Definitive diagnosis

TABLE 25-20	
Tracheal Tumors	
Malignant	**Benign**
• Osteosarcoma	• Osteochondroma
• Chondrosarcoma	• Oncocytoma
• Lymphoma	• Leiomyoma
• Mast cell tumor	• Chondroma
• Adenocarcinoma	• Polyps
• Squamous cell carcinoma	

requires histologic or cytologic evaluation of a biopsy specimen. Biopsy may be performed using biopsy forceps or needle biopsy instruments. Biopsy of tracheal tumors is more difficult than laryngeal tumors but can usually be performed using a bronchoscope. Size, consistency, and nature of attachment of the tumor to the tracheal wall should be noted. Enlarged, accessible lymph nodes should be aspirated or biopsied (see p. 444) to help stage the disease. The medial retropharyngeal lymph nodes drain the larynx and proximal trachea but are usually inaccessible.

☞ **NOTE** • Histopathologic identification of tumor type before definite therapy will help determine the extent of surgical resection needed.

Radiography

Cranium and cervical radiographs should be evaluated to determine the location and extent of the tumor. Laryngeal and tracheal masses may appear as soft tissue densities within the airway (Fig. 25-25). Laryngeal distortion and decreased laryngeal space may also be seen. Extraluminal masses may compress the tracheal lumen.

Thoracic radiographs should be evaluated for metastasis and bronchopneumonia. Occasionally, contrast esophograms or esophagoscopy are needed to rule out esophageal involvement.

Laboratory Findings

A complete blood count, serum biochemistry profile, and urinalysis are indicated to evaluate the patient's overall status and evidence of paraneoplastic syndromes. If lymphoma is suspected, a bone marrow aspiration and an FeLV test (in cats) are warranted.

DIFFERENTIAL DIAGNOSIS

Differential diagnoses include obstruction of the larynx caused by elongated soft palate, laryngeal collapse, laryngeal paralysis, nasopharyngeal polyp, foreign bodies, inflammation, cysts, or granulomatous masses (*Filaroides osleri*). Other causes of tracheal obstruction include tracheal collapse or hypoplasia, foreign bodies, congenital malformations, cysts, inflammation, granulomatous masses, or excess respiratory secretions.

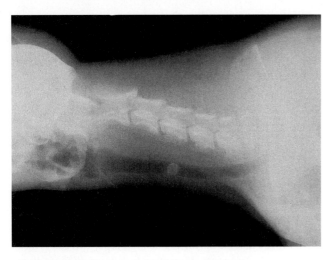

FIG. 25-25
Tracheal osteochondroma in a 6-month-old dog.

MEDICAL MANAGEMENT

Radiation therapy may help treat squamous cell carcinomas, mast cell tumors, and lymphomas, but little information is available. Some tumors (lymphomas, mast cell tumors, adenocarcinomas) respond to chemotherapy. Permanent tracheostomy can palliate signs of respiratory distress during medical therapy.

SURGICAL TREATMENT

Surgical excision may be curative if the tumor is benign, localized, and small. Complete excision of malignant tumors is rarely possible, but excision may provide palliation by alleviating dyspnea. Laryngeal tumors may be resected via partial or total laryngectomy. For removal of tracheal tumors, a tracheal resection and end-to-end anastomosis are required (see p. 615). Twenty percent to sixty percent (i.e., usually six to eight rings) of the trachea may be resected depending on the elasticity of the trachea. Resection of large tumors with a minimum of 1 cm of normal adjacent trachea is not always possible. In cases where resection would be too extensive to achieve end-to-end anastomosis, tracheal replacement or prostheses may be considered, but are rarely successful. Resection of a segment of the tracheal wall without complete transection (i.e., wedge resection) and reapposition of the cut edges is not recommended because it narrows, or kinks, the trachea, which interferes with airflow and mucociliary transport.

Preoperative Management

The animal should be kept calm to prevent progressive dyspnea; sedation may be necessary in some animals (see p. 609). An antiinflammatory dose of corticosteroids may also be administered if dyspnea is severe (see Table 25-5). Before surgery, dyspneic animals should be preoxygenated. An emergency tracheostomy may be necessary in severely dyspneic animals (see p. 613).

Anesthesia

Animals with laryngeal masses may require intubation via a pharyngostomy or tracheotomy incision (see p. 613). Intubation and ventilation of patients with intraluminal tracheal masses may require insertion of a small diameter tube or tracheostomy distal to the obstruction. Specific anesthetic recommendations for animals with respiratory disease are given on p. 610.

Surgical Anatomy

Surgical anatomy of the larynx and trachea is provided on p. 611.

Positioning

Patients requiring laryngotomy or cervical tracheal resection should be positioned in dorsal recumbency with the neck deviated ventrally with a dorsally placed pad or roll (see Fig. 25-6). The entire caudal mandibular area, ventral neck, and cranial thorax should be prepared for aseptic surgery. Partial laryngectomy may be performed with the patient in ventral recumbency with the head suspended and the mouth opened widely, or in dorsal recumbency. Total laryngectomy may be performed with the patient initially positioned in ventral recumbency for oropharyngeal mucosal incision and then repositioned in dorsal recumbency to allow removal of the larynx and permanent tracheostomy.

SURGICAL TECHNIQUES
Partial Laryngectomy

Partial laryngectomy is performed using either an oral or laryngotomy approach (see p. 631). Mucosal closure after tumor resection helps prevent scar tissue formation and is more readily achieved when a laryngotomy approach is used. *Remove the mass with a margin of normal tissue by sharp dissection. If possible, preserve the lateral margin of the corniculate process to allow appropriate epiglottic protection of the glottis. Avoid bilateral disruption of the dorsal and ventral laryngeal commissures to reduce the risk of postoperative glottic stenosis.*

Complete or Total Laryngectomy

Total laryngectomy requires the creation of a permanent tracheostomy. It is a difficult procedure that has infrequently been performed. *Expose the larynx by a ventral midline cervical incision. Transect the right and left sternohyoideus muscles from their insertion on the basihyoid bone. Disarticulate the hyoid apparatus between the keratohyoid and basihyoid articulations with the thyrohyoid bones. Dissect dorsolaterally and excise the thyropharyngeus and cricopharyngeus muscles bilaterally from their insertion on the thyroid cartilage. Incise the pharyngeal mucosa at the base of the epiglottis preserving as much mucosa as possible and still have tumor-free margins. Free the larynx by transecting between the cricoid and first tracheal cartilage or between the first and second tracheal cartilages. Remove additional tissue as necessary to achieve an en bloc resection. Lavage the surgical field. Begin reconstruction by closing the pharyngeal submucosa with a continuous suture pattern (3-0 polydioxanone). This suture line will be under tension. Attach the sternohyoid muscles to the basihyoid bone dorsal to the trachea. Place a Penrose drain if dead space is not completely eliminated. Alternately, incise and appose the pharyngeal mucosa through an oral approach.*

The technique for permanent tracheostomy must be varied when a complete laryngectomy is performed. This procedure is rarely performed and may be challenging. *Either close the end of the proximal trachea with a series of interrupted horizontal sutures and then perform a permanent tracheostomy as described on p. 614 or divert and incorporate the transected proximal trachea to create the tracheostoma. To close the end of the proximal trachea place a series of interrupted horizontal mattress sutures from the annular ligament or tracheal cartilage through the dorsal tracheal membrane. Alternatively, preserve a flap of dorsal tracheal membrane during resection, fold it over the end of the trachea, and secure it with interrupted sutures. To incorporate the proximal trachea in the tracheostoma, create the tracheostoma by first apposing the sternohyoid muscles dorsal to the trachea. Remove the ventral third of four to six tracheal cartilages, taking care to preserve the underlying tracheal mucosa. Elevate the dorsal tracheal membrane, apposing and suturing it directly to the skin proximally (4-0 polypropylene). Excise excess skin surrounding the stoma and place intradermal sutures from the skin to peritracheal tissues to create adhesions and prevent skin flaps. Incise mucosa and suture it laterally and distally to the skin using a simple continuous suture pattern.*

SUTURE MATERIALS/SPECIAL INSTRUMENTS

A laryngoscope, bronchoscope, alligator biopsy instrument, needle biopsy instruments, and endoscopic biopsy forceps are used for laryngeal and tracheal biopsy. Instruments and suture material for laryngeal and tracheal surgery are provided on p. 618.

POSTOPERATIVE CARE AND ASSESSMENT

Postoperatively, these patients should be monitored carefully for signs of airway obstruction (see p. 618). Supplemental oxygen and corticosteroids may be given, if needed. Water should be offered 6 to 12 hours and food 18 to 24 hours postoperatively if gagging, regurgitation, or vomiting do not occur. The animal should be kept quiet and restricted from exercise for 2 to 4 weeks. Endoscopic reevaluation is recommended at 4 to 8 weeks to identify areas of tumor recurrence or stenosis. Stenosis of greater than 20% leads to mucostasis and infection, whereas approximately a 50% decrease in lumen size causes respiratory distress. Periodic physical and radiographic evaluation is recommended to look for metastasis or recurrence.

COMPLICATIONS

Dysphagia, gagging, and pharyngeal dehiscence may occur after complete laryngectomy. Some patients benefit from a gastric feeding tube (see p. 74). Vocalization is absent after laryngectomy. Tracheostomas must be monitored closely to maintain patency and prevent self-trauma (see p. 618). Other complications of laryngectomy include fistula secondary to pharyngeal dehiscence, hypoparathyroidism secondary to ischemia, and tumor recurrence or metastasis.

☞ **N O T E** · Monitor these animals carefully after surgery. Airway obstruction may occur.

Dehiscence may occur following tracheal anastomosis if tension is excessive and head and neck motion are not restricted. To relieve tension, the neck should be kept mildly to moderately ventroflexed by attaching a muzzle to a harness with a lead or placing a suture from the chin to the manubrium for 2 weeks. Subcutaneous emphysema may be evident with dehiscence or anastomotic leakage. Infection and fistula formation are possible. Mild stenosis (less than 10%) is expected with the split cartilage technique where there is minimal anastomotic tension.

PROGNOSIS

Although prognosis is undoubtedly related to histologic type, with some tracheal tumors the prognosis is excellent (e.g., oncocytomas, osteochondromas). Little information is available on the biologic behavior of laryngeal tumors; however, the long-term prognosis is generally poor. Without surgery, complete obstruction of the tracheal or laryngeal lumen and subsequent asphyxiation may occur. Radiation therapy may be a valuable adjuvant following surgery for patients with malignant tumors.

References

Patnaik AK et al: Nonhematopoietic neoplasms in cats, *J Natl Cancer Inst* 54:855, 1975.

Priester WA, McKay FW: The occurrence of tumors in domestic animals, Bethesda, Md, National Cancer Institute, 1980.

Saik JE, et al: Canine and feline laryngeal neoplasia: a 10-year survey, *J Am Anim Hosp Assoc* 22:359, 1986.

Suggested Reading

Carlisle CH, Biery DN, Thrall DE: Tracheal and laryngeal tumors in the dog and cat: literature review and 13 additional patients, *Vet Radiol* 32: 229, 1991.

Hedlund CS: Tracheostomies in the management of canine and feline upper respiratory disease. *Vet Clin North Am Small Anim Pract* 24: 873, 1994.

Henderson RA, Powers RD, Perry L: Development of hypoparathyroidism after excision of laryngeal rhabdomyosarcoma in a dog, *J Am Vet Med Assoc* 198: 639, 1991.

Ogilvie GK, Moore AS: *Managing the veterinary cancer patient,* Trenton, NJ, 1995, Veterinary Learning Systems.

CHAPTER 26

Surgery of the Lower Respiratory System: Lungs and Thoracic Wall

GENERAL PRINCIPLES AND TECHNIQUES

DEFINITIONS

Thoracotomy is surgical incision of the chest wall; it may be performed by incising between the ribs (**intercostal** or **lateral**) or by splitting the sternum (**median sternotomy**). Pulmonary **lobectomy** is removal of a lung lobe (complete) or a portion of a lung lobe (partial). **Pneumonectomy** is removal of all lung tissue on one side of the thoracic cavity.

PREOPERATIVE CONCERNS

Animals with traumatic lesions that impair respiration (e.g., flail chest), or those with acute respiratory impairment (i.e., ruptured bullae, ruptured pulmonary abscess) often require emergency stabilization (e.g., stabilization of rib segments, thoracentesis, oxygen therapy) prior to surgery. Equipment for thoracentesis and chest tube placement should be readily available and clinicians should be familiar with these techniques (see pp. 677 and 678). With large neoplastic lesions, positioning the animal in sternal recumbency, or in lateral recumbency with the affected side down, and providing oxygen (i.e., nasal insufflation or oxygen cage) is often beneficial. Blood gas analysis or evaluation with pulse oximetry is warranted preoperatively in patients undergoing thoracic surgery to detect and define the severity of respiratory impairment. Unexplained abnormalities should be investigated because ventilatory impairment due to nonsurgically correctable disease (i.e., diffuse micrometastasis) will occasionally be identified. Anemia should be corrected before surgery, if possible.

ANESTHETIC CONSIDERATIONS

Pulmonary neoplasia or other space-occupying lesions may prevent normal lung expansion and produce hypoxemia. With pneumonia or emphysematous lesions, ventilation/perfusion disturbances are common. Animals with respiratory dysfunction may have oxygen administered by face mask or nasal insufflation prior to induction to ensure that hemoglobin is optimally saturated and that hypoxemia does not occur during intubation. Sedation with acetylpromazine should be avoided in severely affected patients because of hypotension. Anticholinergics can be used in animals with bradycardia (i.e., heart rate less than 60 bpm). Nitrous oxide should be avoided in patients with respiratory compromise. Opioids may cause severe respiratory depression and should be administered only when oxygen can be provided. Endotracheal intubation must be accomplished rapidly in animals with respiratory dysfunction and anesthesia should be maintained with an inhalation anesthetic (i.e., isoflurane or halothane; Table 26-1). In compromised animals, intubation of a bronchus rather than the trachea may be disastrous; therefore, both sides of the chest cavity should be auscultated to ensure proper endotracheal tube placement. It may be difficult to maintain an adequate depth of anesthesia in animals with severe pulmonary disease with inhalation anesthetics alone; supplementation with opioids may be necessary. All animals with open chest cavities require intermittent positive pressure ventilation (including those with diaphragmatic hernias). High ventilatory pressures should be avoided in patients with chronically collapsed lung lobes, pneumonia, or pulmonary bullae. For specific anesthetic recommendations for animals with flail chest or pectus excavatum (see pp. 660 and 670, respectively).

☞ **N O T E** • Do not use mask or chamber induction in animals with respiratory dysfunction. Use anesthetics that allow for rapid intubation and control of the patient's airway.

Thoracotomy procedures often produce substantial pain and postoperative analgesic therapy is indicated. Placement

TABLE 26-1

Selected Anesthetic Protocols for Use in Animals With Respiratory Dysfunction

For stable (nonarrhythmic, nondyspneic) animals
Premedication

Oxymorphone* (0.05-0.1 mg/kg SC or IM)

Induction

Thiopental (10-12 mg/kg IV) or propofol (4-6 mg/kg IV) or give diazepam (0.27 mg/kg IV) and ketamine (5.5 mg/kg IV) combined and titrated to effect

Maintenance

Isoflurane or halothane

For dyspneic, nonarrhythmic animals
Induction

Diazepam (0.2 mg/kg IV) followed immediately with thiopental (10-12 mg/kg IV)† or propofol (4-6 mg/kg IV) or give diazepam (0.27 mg/kg IV) and ketamine (5.5 mg/kg IV) combined and titrated to effect

Maintenance

Isoflurane or halothane

For very sick or arrhythmic animals
Induction

Diazepam (0.2 mg/kg IV) followed by etomidate (1-3 mg/kg IV)†

Maintenance

Isoflurane

*Use 0.05 mg/kg in cats.
†Can add oxymorphone (0.05-0.1 mg/kg IV) in dogs as part of the induction and decrease the etomidate or barbiturate dose.

TABLE 26-2

Local Anesthesia After Thoracotomy in Dogs*

- Interpleural bupivacaine (2 mg/kg)
  OR
- Intercostal bupivacaine (2 mg/kg)
  OR
- Dose may be split and half given interpleurally and half injected intercostally (see text)

*Bupivacaine has been used in a similar fashion for cats, but at reduced dosages.

TABLE 26-3

Selected Analgesics for Use in Dogs and Cats After Thoracotomy

Oxymorphone (Numorphan)

0.05-0.1 mg/kg IV, IM every 4 hours (as needed)

Butorphanol (Torbutrol, Torbugesic)

0.2-0.4 mg/kg IV, IM, or SC, every 2 to 4 hours (as needed)

Buprenorphine (Buprenex)

5-15 µg/kg IV, IM, every 6 hours (as needed)

of bupivacaine into the thoracic cavity following thoracic closure (interpleural), or performing an intercostal nerve block (i.e., divide bupivacaine and inject dorsally and ventrally in the incised intercostal space and two intercostal spaces cranial and caudal to the incised space) may decrease postoperative pain and promote improved ventilation in the postoperative period (Table 26-2). Patients given bupivacaine interpleurally should be placed with the affected side down for 20 minutes. Injectable analgesics (i.e., oxymorphone, butorphanol, or buprenorphine; Table 26-3) may also be used. Although opioids are respiratory depressants, their analgesic effects often outweigh their negative respiratory effects. If hypoventilation occurs after administration of these drugs, oxygen should be given by nasal insufflation.

Pulmonary edema (reexpansion pulmonary edema; RPE) may develop in some animals with chronically collapsed lung lobes following surgery that allows reexpansion. Although the origin of RPE is unknown and probably multifactorial, it does not appear to be associated with cardiac failure. Beginning usually within a few hours after surgery, the patient typically develops progressively worsening dyspnea and tachypnea. Hypoxemia develops and persists despite intense oxygen therapy. Contrary to the experience in human beings in whom RPE is usually unilateral and therefore not life-threatening, the condition is rapidly fatal in most animals. Reoxygenation of chronically collapsed lungs is thought to release superoxide radicals, which cannot be effectively scavenged, resulting in increased pulmonary capillary permeability and pulmonary edema. Chronically collapsed lung tissue may have decreased mitochondrial superoxide dismutase and cytochrome oxidase activity. Prophylaxis and therapy of patients with RPE are difficult and poorly understood. Reexpansion of chronically collapsed lung tissue should be accomplished slowly (i.e., the thorax may be closed with one or two lung lobes collapsed, allowing them to reexpand slowly) and high ventilation pressures (i.e., greater than 25 cm H_2O pressure) should be avoided. Current recommendations for treating RPE include the use of positive end-expiratory pressure ventilation and drugs that stabilize pulmonary capillary membranes (i.e., methylprednisolone). A number of other pharmaceutical agents are currently being investigated, but conclusive evidence of their beneficial effects is not yet available.

☞ **N O T E** · Avoid high ventilation pressures in patients with chronically collapsed lung lobes.

ANTIBIOTICS

Animals with underlying pulmonary disease or trauma (i.e., pulmonary contusions) are at increased risk to develop pulmonary infections. These patients should be monitored carefully and prophylactic antibiotics (e.g., cefazolin; Table 26-4) provided, or therapeutic antibiotics initiated at the

TABLE 26-4
Perioperative Antibiotic Therapy
Cefazolin
20 mg/kg IV at induction; repeat once or twice at 4- to 6-hour intervals

earliest sign of infection (i.e., leukocytosis and/or fever). Appropriate use of prophylactic antibiotics depends on the length of surgery, type of surgery being performed, animal's immune status, and the underlying disease process. Young, healthy animals undergoing thoracotomy for relatively short procedures (e.g., ligation of a patent ductus arteriosus) generally do not require prophylactic antibiotics. Debilitated animals undergoing thoracotomy for removal of large neoplastic lesions (which may contain focal areas of necrosis) are likely to benefit from prophylactic antibiotic therapy. Prophylactic antibiotics should be given intravenously at induction and generally discontinued within 12 to 24 hours.

SURGICAL ANATOMY

Thoracic cavities of dogs and cats are compressed laterally so that the greatest dimension is dorsoventral. The ribs, sternum, and vertebral column form the thoracic skeleton. The sternum is composed of eight unpaired bones and forms the floor of the thorax (Fig. 26-1). The first and last sternebrae are known as the manubrium and xiphoid, respectively. There are usually 13 pairs of ribs. The 10th, 11th, and 12th ribs do not articulate with the sternum, but instead form the costal arch bilaterally. The cartilaginous portion of the 13th rib terminates free in the musculature. The space between the ribs is known as the intercostal space and is generally 2 to 3 times as wide as the adjacent ribs. Blood supply to the thoracic wall is provided by the intercostal arteries. The intercostal arteries lie caudal to the adjacent rib, in conjunction with a satellite vein and nerve. A typical intercostal nerve begins where the dorsal branch of the thoracic nerve divides and runs distally among the fibers of the internal intercostal muscle. In most intercostal spaces, intercostal vessels and nerves are covered medially only by pleura.

Muscles of the thorax serve not only a structural function, but are also important in respiration. The deepest muscles of the thoracic wall are the intercostal muscles. The fibers of the external intercostal muscle arise on the caudal border of each rib and run caudoventrally to the cranial border of the next rib. This muscle is important primarily in inspiration. The internal intercostal muscles, on the other hand, run from the cranial border of one rib to the caudal border of the preceding rib, primarily functioning to aid expiration. Other inspiratory muscles are the scalenus, serratus dorsalis cranialis, levatores costarum, and diaphragm. Additional expiratory muscles include the rectus abdominis, external abdominal oblique, internal abdominal oblique, transversus abdominis, serratus dorsalis caudalis, transversus costarum, and iliocostalis.

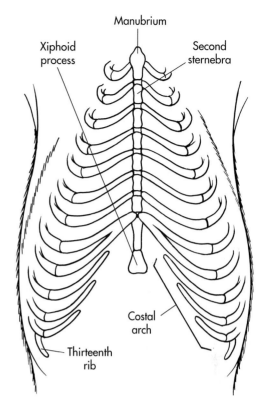

FIG. 26-1
Sternal anatomy.

The lungs of dogs and cats have deep fissures that create distinct lobes allowing the lungs to alter their shape in response to alterations in thoracic cavity shape (i.e., that caused by diaphragmatic movement or flexion or extension of the spine). These fissures also allow individual lobes to be isolated and removed without compromising integrity of the surrounding lobes. The left lung is divided into a cranial lobe with a cranial and caudal part, and a caudal lobe (Fig. 26-2). The right lung is larger than the left and is divided into cranial, middle, caudal, and accessory lobes (see Fig. 26-2). The cardiac notch is a small area overlying the heart where lung tissue is not interposed between the heart and body wall. It is usually located at the ventral aspect of the fourth intercostal space and is larger on the right side.

The pulmonary arteries carry non aerated blood from the right ventricle of the heart to the lungs, while the pulmonary veins return aerated blood from the lungs to the left atrium. The left pulmonary artery lies cranial to the left bronchus, whereas the left pulmonary veins are ventral to it. On the right side, the pulmonary artery lies dorsal and slightly caudal to the right bronchus and the pulmonary veins lie craniodorsal and ventral to it.

SURGICAL TECHNIQUES
Thoracotomy

Thoracotomy may be performed by incising between the ribs or by splitting the sternum. The approach used depends on the exposure needed and underlying disease process. Regardless of the type of thoracotomy performed, a large area

FIG. 26-2

Subdivisions of the canine and feline lung lobes.

Dorsal view

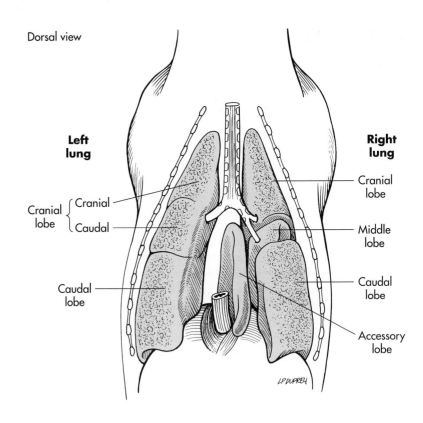

Left lung

Cranial lobe { Cranial / Caudal

Caudal lobe

Right lung

Cranial lobe

Middle lobe

Caudal lobe

Accessory lobe

LP DUPREY

TABLE 26-5

Recommended Intercostal Spaces for Thoracotomy*

	Left	Right
Heart	4,5	4,5
PDA†	4(5)	
PRAA‡	4	
Pulmonic valve	4	
Lungs	4-6	4-6
Cranial lobe	4,5	4,5
Intermediate lobe		5
Caudal lobe	5(6)	5(6)
Esophagus		
Cranial	3,4	
Caudal	7-9	7-9
Cranial vena cava	(4)	4
Caudal vena cava	(6-7)	6-7

Modified from Orton EC: Thoracic wall. Slatter D, ed: *Textbook of small animal surgery*, ed 2. Philadelphia, WB Saunders, 1993.
*( ) indicates alternative surgical site, †=patent ductus arteriosus, ‡=persistent right aortic arch.

should be prepared for aseptic surgery to allow extension of the incision, if needed. Depending on which left lobe is affected, a left lateral thoracotomy at the fourth, fifth, or sixth intercostal space will provide adequate exposure for lobectomy (Table 26-5). A left fourth intercostal space thoracotomy allows exposure of the right ventricular outflow tract, main pulmonary artery, and ductus arteriosus. Bilateral removal of the pericardial sac can be difficult from this approach. A right intercostal thoracotomy provides exposure of the right side of the heart (auricle, atrium, and ventricle), cranial and caudal venae cavae, right lung lobes, and azygous

vein. Median sternotomy affords exposure to both sides of the thoracic cavity. Bilateral, partial lobectomy is easily performed from a median sternotomy; however, complete lobectomy is often difficult. The caudal vena cava, main pulmonary artery, and both sides of the pericardial sac can be isolated and manipulated via this approach. A loose bandage should be placed on the thorax after surgery.

☞ **N O T E** · Count your sponges at the start of the surgical procedure and before closure of the thoracic cavity: do not leave a sponge in the thoracic cavity.

Intercostal thoracotomy. *With the dog in lateral recumbency, select the site for incision. Locate the approximate intercostal space and sharply incise the skin, subcutaneous tissues, and cutaneous trunci muscle. The incision should extend from just below the vertebral bodies to near the sternum. Deepen the incision through the latissimus dorsi muscle with scissors (Fig. 26-3, A), then palpate the first rib by placing a hand cranially under the latissimus dorsi muscle. Count back from the first rib to verify the correct intercostal space.* The ribs cranial to an intercostal incision are more easily retracted than the caudal ribs, so choose the more caudal space if you must choose between two adjacent intercostal spaces. *Transect the scalenus and pectoral muscles with scissors perpendicular to their fibers, then separate the muscle fibers of the serratus ventralis muscle at the selected intercostal space (Fig. 26-3, B). Near the costochondral junction, place one scissor blade under the external intercostal muscle fibers and push the scissors dorsally in the center of the intercostal space to incise the muscle (Fig. 26-3, C). Incise the internal intercostal muscle simi-*

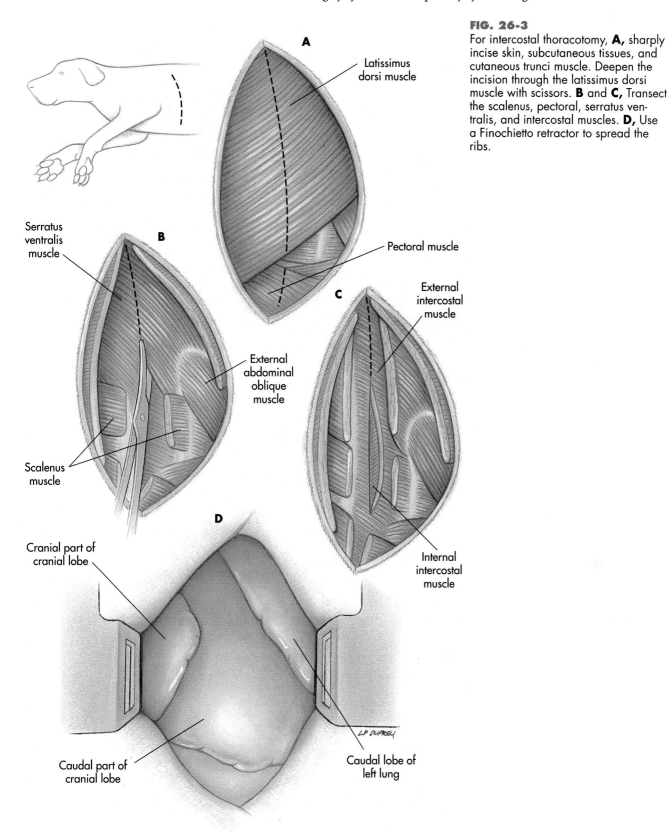

FIG. 26-3
For intercostal thoracotomy, **A,** sharply incise skin, subcutaneous tissues, and cutaneous trunci muscle. Deepen the incision through the latissimus dorsi muscle with scissors. **B** and **C,** Transect the scalenus, pectoral, serratus ventralis, and intercostal muscles. **D,** Use a Finochietto retractor to spread the ribs.

Latissimus dorsi muscle

Serratus ventralis muscle

Pectoral muscle

External intercostal muscle

External abdominal oblique muscle

Scalenus muscle

Internal intercostal muscle

Cranial part of cranial lobe

Caudal part of cranial lobe

Caudal lobe of left lung

LP DUPREY

larly. Notify the anesthetist that you are about to enter the thoracic cavity and, after identifying the lungs and pleura, use closed scissors or a blunt object to penetrate the pleura. This allows air to enter the thorax, causing the lungs to collapse away from the body wall. Extend the incision dorsally and ventrally in order to achieve the desired ex-

posure. Identify and avoid incising the internal thoracic vessels as they course subpleurally near the sternum. Moisten laparotomy sponges and place them on the exposed edges of the chest incision. Use a Finochietto retractor to spread the ribs (Figs. 26-3, D and Fig. 26-4). If further exposure is needed, a rib adjacent to the incision can be removed; however, this is seldom required. If a chest tube is to be placed, do so before closing the thorax. The tube should not exit from the incised intercostal space.

Close the thoracotomy by preplacing four to eight sutures of heavy (3-0 to No. 2, depending on the animal's size) monofilament absorbable or nonabsorbable suture around the ribs adjacent to the incision (Fig. 26-5, A). Approximate the ribs with a towel clamp or rib approximator, or have an assistant cross two sutures to appose the ribs (Fig. 26-5, B), then tie the remaining sutures. Tie all the sutures before you remove the rib approximator or towel clamp. Suture serratus ventralis, scalenus, and pectoralis

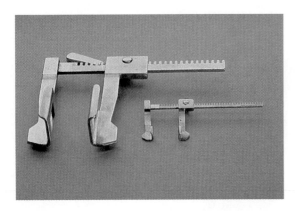

FIG. 26-4
Finochietto retractors.

muscles with a continuous suture of absorbable suture material. Appose the edges of the latissimus dorsi muscle similarly. Remove residual air from the thoracic cavity using the preplaced chest tube (see p. 678) or an over-the-needle catheter (see p. 677). Close subcutaneous tissues and skin in a routine fashion.

Median sternotomy. When performing median sternotomy, two to three sternebrae should be left intact cranially or caudally (depending on where the lesion is located) to decrease postoperative pain and prevent delayed healing caused by sternebral shifting. If exposure of the lungs or heart is necessary (i.e., in dogs with spontaneous pneumothorax or for pericardiectomy) the sternotomy should extend from the xiphoid cartilage cranially to the second or third sternebra. If exposure of the cranial mediastinum is desired, the sternotomy should extend from the manubrium caudally to the sixth or seventh sternebra.

With the dog in dorsal recumbency, incise skin on the midline over the sternum. Expose the sternum by a combination of sharp incision and blunt dissection of the overlying musculature. Transect the sternebrae longitudinally on the midline with a bone saw, chisel and osteotome, or bone cutters (Fig. 26-6). In young animals, heavy scissors may be adequate; however, avoid crushing the bone. Splitting the sternebrae on the midline will facilitate closure. Take care that the underlying lung and heart are not

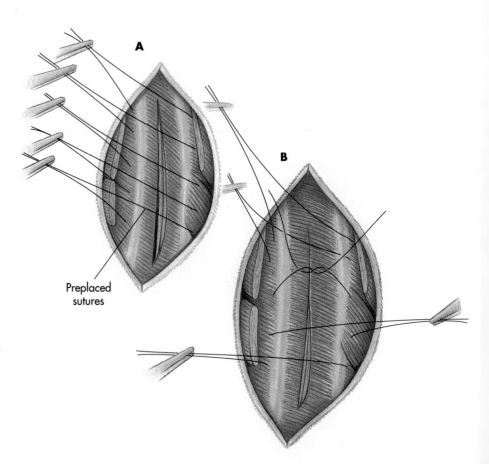

A

B

Preplaced
sutures

FIG. 26-5
A, Close the thoracotomy by preplacing four to eight sutures of heavy monofilament suture around the ribs adjacent to the incision. **B,** Approximate the ribs with a towel clamp or rib approximator, or have an assistant cross two sutures to appose the ribs. Tie the remaining sutures.

damaged while completing the sternotomy. Place moistened laparotomy sponges on the incised edges of the sternebrae and retract the edges with a Finochietto rib retractor. If a chest tube is to be placed, do so before closing the sternotomy. Do not exit the tube from between the sternebrae; exit it from between the ribs or through the diaphragm. Close the sternotomy with wires (dogs larger than approximately 15 kg) or heavy suture (cats and dogs smaller than approximately 15 kg) placed around the sternebrae (Fig. 26-7). Suture subcutaneous tissues with a simple continuous suture of absorbable suture material. Remove residual air from the thoracic cavity and close skin routinely.

Partial Lobectomy

Partial lobectomy may be performed to remove a focal lesion involving the peripheral one half to two thirds of the lung lobe, or for biopsy. Partial lobectomy may be performed via a lateral fourth or fifth space intercostal thoracotomy or median sternotomy. *Identify the lung tissue to be removed and place a pair of crushing forceps across the lobe, proximal to the lesion (Fig. 26-8, A). Place a continuous, overlapping suture pattern of absorbable suture material (2-0 to 4-0) 4 to 6 mm proximal to the forceps (Fig. 26-8, B). A second row of sutures may be placed in a similar manner to the first. Excise the lung between the suture lines and clamps, leaving a 2- to 3-mm margin of tissue distal to the sutures (Fig. 26-8, C). Oversew the lung with a simple continuous suture pattern of absorbable suture (3-0 to 5-0; Fig. 26-8, D). Replace the lung in the thoracic cavity and fill the chest cavity with warmed, sterile saline solution. Inflate the lungs and check the bronchus for air leaks. Remove the fluid before closing the thorax.*

Partial lobectomy may also be performed with stapling devices (e.g., thoracoabdominal [TA] stapler; Fig. 26-9). The stapling equipment comes in various sizes that produce staple lines 30 mm, 55 mm, or 90 mm long. *Select the staple size based on the width of the lung so that the staple line extends across the entire width of the lung to be removed, but does not extend beyond the edges. If air leaks or hemorrhage are noted, place a simple continuous suture pattern of absorbable suture material along the lung margin.* The stapling devices compress tissue to a thickness of either 1.5 mm (3.5-mm-long staples) or 2.0 mm (4.8-mm-long staples). *Avoid stapling excessively thick or fibrotic lung as this may result in large air leaks or hemorrhage. Check the lung for leaks and close as described above.*

Complete Lobectomy

Complete lobectomy is best performed through a lateral thoracotomy. If the lung contains large quantities of purulent material, prevent excessive fluid from draining into the proximal bronchi and trachea by clamping the bronchus near the hilus prior to manipulating the lobe. Similarly, torsed lung lobes should be removed without untwisting the pedicle to prevent release of necrotic material trapped in the lung (see p. 665). Dogs can survive acute loss of up to 50% of their lung volume; however, transient respiratory acidosis and exercise intolerance may occur.

Identify the affected lobe(s) and isolate them from the remaining lobes with moistened sponges (laparotomy or 4x4s depending on the animal's size). Identify the vasculature and bronchus to the lobe (Fig. 26-10, A). Using blunt dissection, isolate the pulmonary artery supplying the affected lobe and pass a ligature of nonabsorbable or absorbable suture material (2-0 to 3-0) around the proximal end of the vessel. Do not compromise the lumen of the parent vessel from which this vessel arises. Place a second ligature in a similar fashion distal to the site where the vessel is to be transected. A transfixing suture may be placed between these sutures, proximal to the transection site, to prevent the first suture from being inadvertently dislodged. Transect the artery between the distal two ligatures. Ligate the pulmonary vein in a similar fashion. Identify the main bronchus supplying the

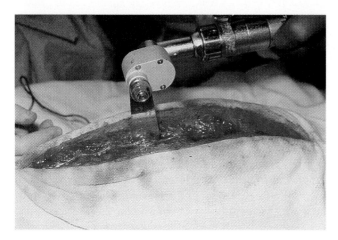

FIG. 26-6
When performing median sternotomy, transect the sternebrae longitudinally on the midline with a bone saw, chisel and osteotome, or bone cutters.

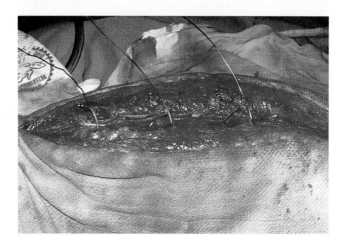

FIG. 26-7
Depending on the animal's size, close a sternotomy with wires or heavy suture placed around the sternebrae.

FIG. 26-8
Partial lobectomy may be performed via an intercostal thoracotomy or median sternotomy. **A,** Identify the lung tissue to be removed and place a pair of crushing forceps proximal to the lesion. **B,** Place a continuous, overlapping suture pattern proximal to the forceps. **C,** Excise the lung between the suture lines and clamps and **D,** oversew the lung with a simple continuous suture pattern of absorbable suture.

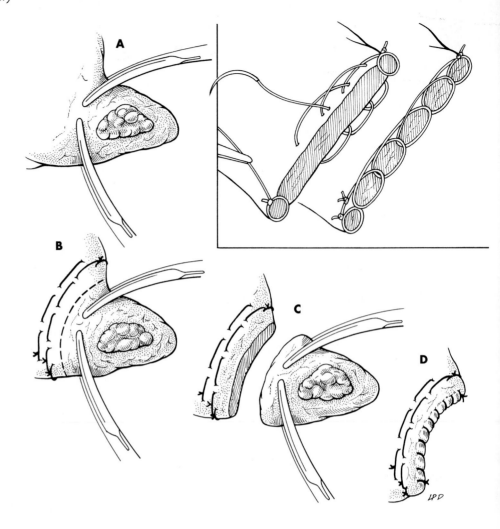

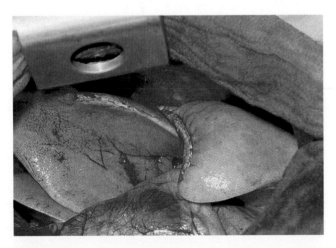

FIG. 26-9
Appearance of lung lobes after partial lobectomy using a stapling device.

lobe and clamp it with a pair of Satinsky or crushing forceps proximal and distal to the selected transection site (Fig. 26-10, B). Sever the bronchus between the clamps and remove the lung. Suture the bronchus proximal to the

remaining clamp with a continuous horizontal mattress suture pattern (Fig. 26-10, C), or in cats and small dogs place a transfixing ligature around the bronchus. Prior to removing the clamp, secure a suture in the bronchus distal to the clamp, and after removing the clamp, oversew the end of the bronchus with a simple continuous suture pattern (see Fig. 26-10, C). Fill the chest cavity with warmed, sterile saline solution. Inflate the lungs and check the bronchus for air leaks. **Observe lungs that have been "packed-off" to make sure they reinflate and are not twisted prior to closure.** *Remove the fluid and close the chest as described above.* Stapling devices may be used for complete lobectomy, but ensure that the bronchus and vessels are adequately ligated by the staples.

HEALING OF THE LUNGS AND STERNUM

Following multiple lobectomies or partial lobectomies of several lobes, expansion of the remaining lung may occur in an attempt to restore normal lung volume. Therefore, exercise intolerance may decrease in some animals with time after pneumonectomy. The healing of median sternotomies has been of concern; however, if several sternebrae are left intact and the closure is performed properly, these incisions

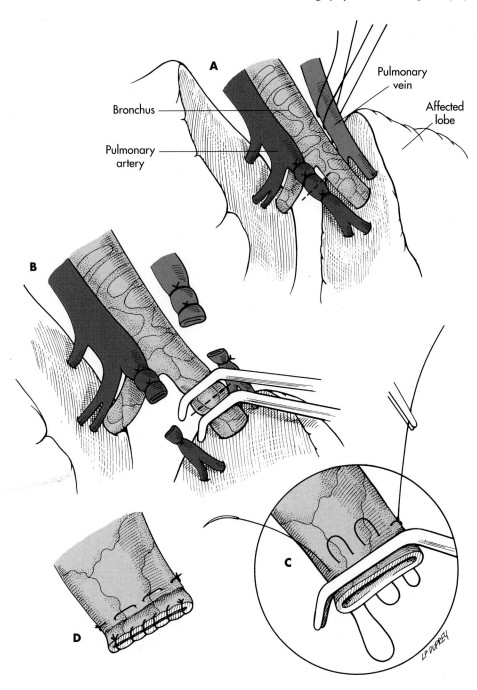

Bronchus

Pulmonary artery

Pulmonary vein

Affected lobe

A

B

C

D

LP DUPREY

FIG. 26-10
For complete lobectomy, **A,** ligate and transect the vasculature to the affected lobe. **B,** Clamp the main bronchus with a pair of Satinsky or crushing forceps and sever the bronchus between the clamps and remove the lung. **C,** Suture the bronchus with a continuous horizontal mattress suture pattern and **D,** oversew the end with a simple continuous suture pattern.

heal readily and without complication, even in animals with pyothorax.

SUTURE MATERIALS/SPECIAL INSTRUMENTS

Absorbable or nonabsorbable suture material can be used for complete lobectomy; however, braided, multifilament, nonabsorbable suture (e.g., silk) should be avoided if infection is present. Finochietto rib retractors, Satinsky clamps (for clamping the bronchus), and right-angled forceps (such as Mixter forceps; a.k.a. gallbladder or gall duct forceps or thoracic forceps) are useful when performing thoracic surgery (Fig. 26-11). A bone saw is recommended for median sternotomy, particularly in medium or large dogs. Vacuum suction devices facilitate removal of the fluid placed in the chest to identify air leaks. Thoracoabdominal staplers (TA) are also useful for lobectomies (see Product Appendix).

POSTOPERATIVE CARE AND ASSESSMENT

Respiration should be monitored closely once the animal begins ventilating on its own. If respiratory excursions are judged to be inadequate, the chest should be evaluated to verify that residual air was removed after chest closure. If there is any doubt, thoracic radiographs should be examined for evidence of pneumothorax (see p. 689). Blood gas

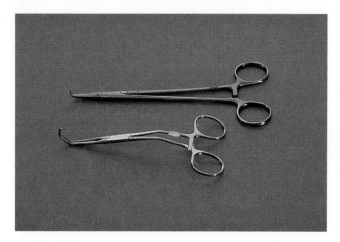

FIG. 26-11
Right-angled forceps (*upper*) and Satinsky clamps (*lower*).

analysis will help evaluate the adequacy of ventilation in these patients. If the animal is hypoxemic, oxygen should be administered by nasal insufflation or placing the animal in an oxygen-enriched environment. Animals with severe or progressive hypoxemia should be evaluated for pulmonary edema. Inadequate ventilation in some animals may be due to pain. Median sternotomy may result in decreased ventilation as compared to intercostal thoracotomy (Albrecht et al, 1995). Administration of analgesics in such patients is needed and should be considered in all patients undergoing thoracotomy procedures (see above under anesthesia). Hypothermia is common following thoracic surgery; warm water bottles and circulating water blankets should be used to rewarm these patients.

☞ **NOTE** • If the animal hypoventilates postoperatively, thoracic radiographs are indicated to rule out pneumothorax, hemothorax, and pulmonary edema.

COMPLICATIONS

The major complication of partial or complete lobectomy is air leakage and/or hemorrhage. Minor air leaks will usually seal, but massive air leaks or severe hemorrhage requires reoperation. Subcutaneous fluid accumulation at the ventral aspect of the thoracotomy incision occasionally occurs but can be avoided by carefully closing the distal musculature (i.e., serratus ventralis and pectoralis). With median sternotomy, adequate closure and leaving several sternebrae intact will prevent delayed healing or nonunions of the sternebrae. Postoperatively, lameness associated with pain and severing the latissimus dorsi muscle is common but usually resolves within 1 to 2 days.

☞ **NOTE** • Monitor these animals closely in the early postoperative period for pneumothorax and/or hemothorax.

SPECIAL AGE CONSIDERATIONS

Uptake of inhalation agents in pediatric patients (i.e., younger than 12 weeks of age) may be more rapid than in adults and the level of anesthesia may fluctuate more readily in these patients; thus extra care should be used when anesthetizing them. Young animals are particularly prone to hypothermia when the chest cavity is opened. Temperature regulation, blood glucose requirements, and fluid and electrolyte replacement should be aggressively managed in these patients. Geriatric patients with compromised pulmonary function and/or decreased cardiovascular capacity may also have abnormal uptake of inhalation anesthetics.

Reference

Albrecht M, Caywood D, Stobie D: The effects of median
    sternotomy or lateral thoracotomy on pulmonary function in
    dogs, *Vet Surg* 24:420, 1995 (abstract).

Suggested Reading

Biller DS, Myer CW: Case examples demonstrating the clinical
    utility of obtaining both right and left lateral thoracic
    radiographs in small animals, *J Am Anim Hosp Assoc* 23:381,
    1987.
Conzemius MG et al: Analgesia in dogs after intercostal thora-
    cotomy: a clinical trial comparing intravenous buprenorphine
    and interpleural bupivacaine, *Vet Surg* 23:291, 1994.
Godshalk CP: Common pitfalls in radiographic interpretation of
    the thorax, *Compend Contin Educ Pract Vet* 16:731, 1994.
LaRue SM, Withrow SJ, Wykes PM: Lung resection using surgical
    staples in dogs and cats, *Vet Surg* 16:238, 1987.
Mattu JS et al: Evaluation of prophylactic use of antibiotics in
    preventing postoperative wound infection following thora-
    cotomy in dogs, *Ind J Anim Sci* 57:1097, 1989.
Pascoe PJ, Dyson DH: Postoperative analgesia following lateral
    thoracotomy: epidural morphine vs. intercostal bupivacaine, *Vet
    Surg* 20:160, 1991.
Popilskis S et al: Epidural vs. intramuscular oxymorphone
    analgesia after thoracotomy in dogs, *Vet Surg* 20:462, 1991.
Rustomjee T, Wagner A, Orton C: Effects of 5 cm of water positive
    end-expiratory pressure on arterial oxygen tension in dogs
    during and after thoracotomy, *Vet Surg* 23:307, 1994.
Sweet DC, Waters DJ: Role of surgery in the management of dogs
    with pathologic conditions of the thorax. II. *Compend Contin
    Educ Pract Vet* 13:1671, 1991.
Waters DJ, Sweet DC: Role of surgery in the management of dogs
    with pathologic conditions of the thorax. I. *Compend Contin
    Educ Pract Vet* 13:1545, 1991.

SPECIFIC DISEASES

THORACIC WALL TRAUMA

DEFINITIONS

Flail chest occurs when several ribs on both sides of the point of impact are fractured such that the fractured segment moves paradoxically with respiration.

GENERAL CONSIDERATIONS AND CLINICALLY RELEVANT PATHOPHYSIOLOGY

Thoracic wall injury may be due to either blunt (i.e., motor vehicular accidents, being kicked by a horse) or penetrating trauma. The most common causes of penetrating injuries of the thorax in dogs are bite wounds and gunshot injuries. Both blunt and penetrating trauma may cause extensive soft tissue damage of the thoracic wall (Fig. 26-12). Although soft tissue damage is rarely the cause of major morbidity or mortality, in some animals it may be the only external evidence of severe thoracic trauma. Occasionally, pain associated with muscular tears may lead to altered respiration because the animal is unwilling to breathe deeply. Unless associated with pulmonary parenchymal damage, alterations in ventilation that lead to hypoxemia seldom occur with chest wall trauma.

Subcutaneous emphysema may occur with both blunt and penetrating trauma, but is usually of little significance. This occurs when air is forced into subcutaneous tissues and dissects along muscular and facial planes. The air may reach the subcutaneous tissues through a disruption of the pleura and intercostal muscles, by direct communication with an external wound, or as an extension of mediastinal emphysema. Treatment of subcutaneous air should be directed at its cause. Similarly, isolated rib fractures are seldom associated with major morbidity. Occasionally rib fractures produce sharp fragments that may injure a major vessel or lacerate the lung. Rib fractures may interfere with ventilation if the animal splints the thorax in an attempt to reduce pain by decreasing motion of the fragments.

Flail chest occurs when several ribs on both sides of the point of impact are fractured such that the intervening rib segments lose their continuity with the remainder of the thorax (Fig. 26-13). Paradoxical movement of the chest wall occurs during respiration due to intrapleural pressure changes; the fractured segment moves inward during inspiration and outward during expiration. Respiratory abnormalities in patients with flail chest may be severe and include decreased vital capacity, reduced functional residual capacity, hypoxemia, decreased compliance, increased airway resistance, and increased work of breathing. These abnormal respiratory parameters were once thought to be due primarily to the movement of the flail segment; however, it is now felt that the underlying lung damage and hypoventilation from chest pain are more important factors in the development of respiratory insufficiency.

DIAGNOSIS

Clinical Presentation

Signalment. Thoracic wall trauma may occur in dogs or cats of any age but it is most common in young animals prone to trauma.

History. A history of trauma may or may not be present. The animal may be presented for evaluation of respiratory distress, reluctance to move due to pain, depression, lethargy, and/or anorexia.

Physical Examination Findings

Animals that have suffered thoracic trauma should be examined for the possibility of delayed-onset cardiac arrhythmias. Cardiac arrhythmias, particularly premature ventricular contractions and ventricular tachycardia, may occur following either blunt or penetrating thoracic trauma, and often occur with little or no external evidence of chest injury. These arrhythmias may not begin until 12 to 72 hours after the trauma and may be associated with myocardial contusion, myocardial ischemia secondary to shock, or neurogenic injuries that result in sympathetic overstimulation. Cardiac contusions are frequently overlooked in injured patients because (1) attention is directed toward visually obvious injuries, (2) there is no external evidence of thoracic trauma, or (3) there is no evidence of thoracic trauma at the initial examination. Therefore, cardiac function should be evaluated frequently in most trauma patients.

Radiography/Ultrasonography

Thoracic radiographs of animals with trauma should be carefully evaluated for the presence of pulmonary hemorrhage/contusions or pneumothorax. Rib fractures are easily missed on thoracic radiographs if careful attention is not paid to the rib contour, particularly if the fractured segment is

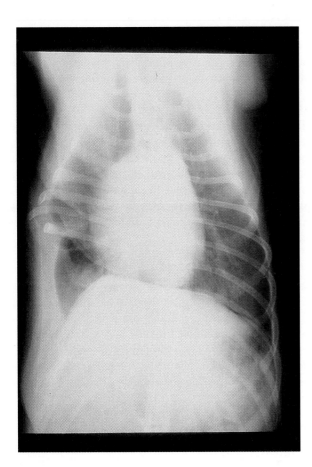

FIG. 26-12
Thoracic radiograph of a dog that was kicked by a horse. Note the large defect between the ribs on the right side of the thorax.

FIG. 26-13
With flail chest, paradoxical move-ment of the chest wall occurs during respiration because of intrapleural pressure changes; **A,** the fractured segment moves inward during inspira-tion and **B,** outward during expiration.

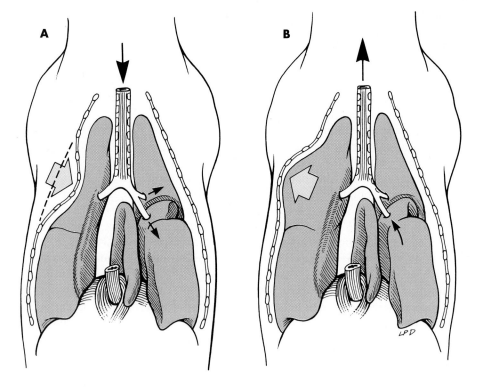

minimally displaced. Both radiographic views should be evalu-ated. Evidence of other bony trauma should be sought by care-fully examining the vertebrae, scapula, and proximal forelimb.

☞ **N O T E** • Evaluate thoracic radiographs of dyspneic animals carefully to differentiate intraparenchymal damage (i.e., contusion/hemorrhage) from pneumothorax.

Laboratory Findings

Laboratory findings are nonspecific. Blood gas analysis may show hypoxemia and respiratory acidosis or alkalosis (result-ing from hyperventilation).

DIFFERENTIAL DIAGNOSIS

Rib fractures may occur secondary to neoplasia or infectious processes; however, these lesions are generally accompanied by lysis or proliferation of the adjacent bone.

MEDICAL MANAGEMENT

Most animals with thoracic wall trauma can be stabilized without surgery. Antibiotic therapy is indicated in patients with marked pulmonary contusion/hemorrhage. Concur-rent pneumothorax should be identified and treated (see p. 687). If the animal is dyspneic, supplemental oxygen should be provided. With flail chest, initially the rib segment can be immobilized by positioning the patient with the af-fected side down. Mechanical ventilation (vs. surgery) is the treatment of choice in humans with pulmonary contusions and flail chest; however, since long-term mechanical ventila-tion may not be possible or practical in many veterinary pa-tients, stabilization of the rib segment is indicated (see be-low). Stabilization may prevent further damage to intratho-racic structures, improve pulmonary ventilation, and de-crease pain associated with movement of fragments.

SURGICAL TREATMENT

Rib fractures seldom require surgical treatment; however, multiple rib fractures may cause a defect in thoracic wall continuity (i.e., concavity) that warrants surgical repair. Ad-ditionally, open stabilization of rib fractures may be indi-cated if there is concurrent intrathoracic trauma that re-quires surgery. Flail chest is generally managed by placing an external splint over the thorax to stabilize the fractured seg-ment (see below).

Preoperative Management

Stabilization of animals with pulmonary contusions should be performed before surgical repair of rib fractures if possi-ble. Shock treatment (i.e., fluids, antibiotics, plus or minus corticosteroids) should be initiated if necessary. Nasal oxy-gen may be beneficial and antibiotics are indicated if pul-monary contusions or hemorrhage is present. If a flail seg-ment is present, placing the animal with the affected side down may be beneficial.

Anesthesia

A splint may be applied to the flail segment of some animals using an intercostal nerve block (see p. 650), rather than gen-eral anesthesia. See anesthetic recommendations on p. 649 for animals with respiratory disease. If general anesthesia is required, refer to the anesthetic protocols and comments on p. 650.

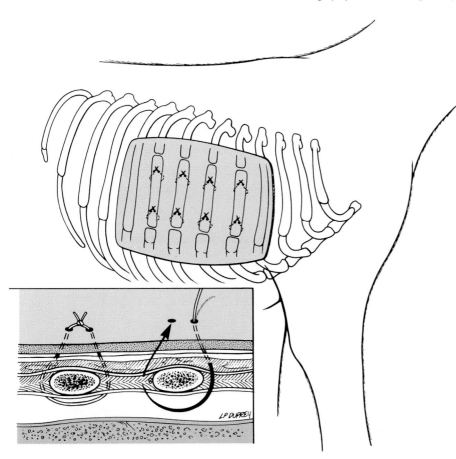

FIG. 26-14
To repair flail chest, secure the affected ribs to a sheet of plastic splinting material. Place sutures circumferentially around the affected ribs and through holes in the splinting material.

Positioning

For rib fractures and flail chest, the lateral thorax encompassing the fractured ribs is clipped and prepared aseptically.

SURGICAL TECHNIQUE
Rib Fractures

Place a small intramuscular pin through the proximal fragment and into the marrow canal. Reduce the fracture and drive the pin into the distal fragment. Exit the pin through the cortex and bend the ends slightly to help prevent migration. Alternately, use cerclage wires or cross pins.

Flail Chest

Secure the affected ribs to a sheet of plastic splinting material (e.g., Orthoplast; see Product Appendix) that has been molded to conform to the thoracic wall (Fig. 26-14). Using a Steinmann pin, place holes in the splinting material large enough to pass the selected suture (see below) through. Place sutures circumferentially around the affected ribs. Pass the suture ends through the predrilled holes and tie securely. Alternately, aluminum rods may be substituted for the plastic splinting material.

SUTURE MATERIALS/SPECIAL INSTRUMENTS

For application of a splint in animals with flail chest use large (2-0 to No. 2; depending on the animal's size) monofilament suture with an attached large, curved needle. A Steinmann pin and pin chuck are also needed. For rib fracture repair, small IM pins and cerclage wire are needed.

POSTOPERATIVE CARE AND ASSESSMENT

Animals with thoracic trauma should be monitored closely in the postoperative period for hypoventilation and/or pneumothorax. Analgesic therapy is warranted in these animals (see p. 649). See p. 657 for additional comments on the postoperative management of animals with respiratory disorders.

PROGNOSIS

The prognosis for animals with thoracic wall trauma generally depends on the amount of concurrent pulmonary or cardiac trauma that is present. Most rib fractures heal without surgery.

Suggested Reading

Bjorling DE, Kolata RJ, DeNovo RC: Flail chest: review, clinical experience and new method of stabilization, *J Amer Anim Hosp Assoc* 18:269, 1982.
Macintire DK, Snider TG: Cardiac arrhythmias associated with multiple trauma in dogs, *J Amer Vet Med Assoc* 184:541, 1984.
Selcer BA et al: The incidence of thoracic trauma in dogs with skeletal injury, *J Small Anim Pract* 28:21, 1987.

PULMONARY NEOPLASIA

DEFINITIONS

Primary pulmonary neoplasms originate in pulmonary tissues and may arise as a solitary mass or rarely may be multicentric.

GENERAL CONSIDERATIONS AND CLINICALLY RELEVANT PATHOPHYSIOLOGY

Primary pulmonary neoplasia is less common than metastatic neoplasia in dogs and cats. The diaphragmatic lobes are most frequently involved, with the right lung lobes more often affected than the left. Classification of primary lung tumors is usually based upon the predominant histologic pattern since specific anatomic localization of tumor origin is not always possible and more than one tumor type may be present. Adenocarcinoma is the most common histologic type found in dogs and cats; squamous cell carcinoma and anaplastic carcinomas are less common (Ogilvie et al, 1989b). Primary pulmonary tumors of connective origin (e.g., osteosarcoma, fibrosarcoma, hemangiosarcoma) are rare. Although most pulmonary tumors are malignant, benign tumors (i.e., papillary adenoma, bronchial adenoma, fibroma, myxochondroma, and plasmacytoma) have been reported. Pulmonary neoplasms are highly aggressive and tend to metastasize early. Most anaplastic carcinomas and squamous cell carcinomas have metastasized at the time of diagnosis, while approximately one half of adenocarcinomas have done so. Metastasis is often to the lung itself and/or regional lymph nodes.

Metastatic pulmonary neoplasia is an important differential diagnosis for nodular lung disease. Tumors with a high likelihood of resulting in pulmonary metastasis include mammary carcinoma, thyroid carcinoma, hemangiosarcoma, osteosarcoma, transitional cell carcinoma, squamous cell carcinoma, and oral and digital melanoma.

DIAGNOSIS
Clinical Presentation

Signalment. The average age of dogs and cats with primary lung tumors is 10 to 11 years and 12 years, respectively (Ogilvie et al, 1989b and Koblick, 1986). Anaplastic carcinomas tend to occur at a slightly younger age (8 to 9 years) than adenocarcinomas. There does not seem to be a sex or breed predilection, although boxers may be overrepresented.

History. Nearly 25% of dogs with pulmonary neoplasia are asymptomatic at the time of diagnosis (i.e., pulmonary neoplasia is an incidental finding when thoracic radiographs are being evaluated for an unrelated problem) (Ogilvie et al, 1989b). If clinical signs are present, the owner may report that they have been apparent for weeks to months.

Physical Examination Findings

The most common clinical finding in dogs with primary pulmonary neoplasia is a nonproductive cough; however, respiratory signs are present in only one third of affected cats. Other signs include hemoptysis, fever, lethargy, exercise intolerance, weight loss, dysphagia, and anorexia. Lameness may be associated with metastasis to bone or skeletal muscle, or to development of hypertrophic osteopathy.

Radiography/Ultrasonography

Thoracic radiographs should be obtained in animals with suspected pulmonary neoplasia (Fig. 26-15). The most common finding with primary pulmonary neoplasia in dogs is a

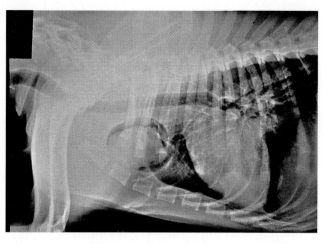

FIG. 26-15
Thoracic radiograph of a 1½-year-old German shepherd dog with a bronchogenic cyst in the left cranial lung lobe. Surgical excision was performed via a median sternotomy approach.

solitary nodular density in the periphery of a dorsocaudal lung lobe. Multiple, miliary lesions are less common (Fig. 26-16). The radiographic pattern may be classified as solitary nodular, multiple nodular, or disseminated-infiltrative. Multiple, discrete lesions within a single lobe or multiple lobes usually represent metastatic neoplasia, rather than multicentric primary neoplasia.

Radiographs should include ventrodorsal and both right and left lateral recumbent views. Lung lesions may go undetected in recumbent lateral radiographs when the affected lung is dependent due to increased opacity of surrounding lung tissue. Thoracic radiographs are relatively insensitive indicators of pulmonary neoplasia because nodules must be at least 1.0 cm in diameter to be reliably recognized. Radiographs should also be evaluated for sternal or hilar lymphadenopathy and/or pleural effusion. It may be difficult to differentiate metastatic pulmonary neoplasia from pulmonary metastasis of a primary pulmonary tumor. Compared with primary lesions, metastatic tumors are generally smaller, more well-circumscribed, and are usually located in the peripheral or middle portions of the lung. Multiple nodules associated with primary lung tumors often consist of 1 large mass and smaller secondary nodules. When multiple nodules are metastases, there are usually several large masses and a variety of smaller lesions. Pulmonary perfusion scans are sensitive, but relatively nonspecific, for thoracic neoplasia. However, a scan may detect lesions at the diaphragmatic border of the lungs that are not readily visualized on thoracic radiographs.

☞ **NOTE** · To improve the likelihood of diagnosing primary or metastatic pulmonary neoplasia, take a V-D and both lateral recumbent views. Always assess radiographs of animals with pulmonary neoplasia for multiple masses, lymphadenopathy, and/or pleural effusion.

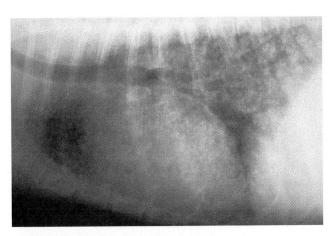

FIG. 26-16
Thoracic radiograph of a dog with pulmonary squamous cell carcinoma. Note the miliary appearance of the pulmonary infiltrate. This tumor could be confused with fungal or heartworm disease radiographically.

Laboratory Findings

Laboratory abnormalities are nonspecific but may include nonregenerative anemia, leukocytosis, and hypercalcemia.

DIFFERENTIAL DIAGNOSIS

Pulmonary neoplasia must be differentiated from abscesses or granulomas (fungal, heartworm). Samples can be collected for cytologic examination by surgical biopsy, percutaneous fine-needle aspiration, transtracheal lavage, and/or bronchoscopy. Fine-needle aspiration cytology may be the most helpful noninvasive diagnostic tool if the needle can be directed into the nodule. Thoracotomy is often necessary for definitive diagnosis of a pulmonary mass.

☞ **N O T E** • Differentiating severe fungal or heartworm disease from miliary neoplasia may be difficult radiographically!

MEDICAL MANAGEMENT

Surgical removal of primary pulmonary neoplasia is the treatment of choice in small animal patients. Chemotherapy is routinely used for some pulmonary neoplasms in human beings; however, there are few reports of its use in similarly affected veterinary patients. Adjunctive chemotherapy may be particularly beneficial in patients with micrometastasis at the time of surgery.

SURGICAL TREATMENT

Wide surgical resection is the treatment of choice for solitary nodules or multiple masses involving a single lobe if there is no evidence of distant metastasis or extrapleural involvement. Surgical resection is occasionally indicated for lung metastasis of a distant primary tumor (e.g., limb osteosarcoma). An intercostal thoracotomy is preferred over median sternotomy since it provides adequate exposure for lobectomy and lymph node biopsy. Partial lobectomy should only be performed when the tumor is located at the periphery of the lung lobe; otherwise, total lobectomy should be performed.

Preoperative Management

Preoperative management of patients with pulmonary neoplasia and dyspnea is similar as for other animals with respiratory diseases (see p. 649). If the mass is large, positioning the animal with the affected side down may improve ventilation.

Anesthesia

See anesthetic management of patients with respiratory abnormalities on p. 649.

Surgical Anatomy

Refer to the anatomical description of the lung lobes on p. 651.

Positioning

Since most neoplasms are removed via an intercostal thoracotomy, the lateral thorax should be prepared for aseptic surgery (see also p. 651).

SURGICAL TECHNIQUE

Perform an intercostal thoracotomy and identify the affected lung lobe. Palpate each lung lobe for additional nodules, and biopsy the hilar lymph node for staging purposes. Perform a partial lobectomy if the tumor is located at the peripheral margin of the lobe; otherwise, perform a complete lobectomy. Submit excised tissue for cytologic and histologic examination. If the neoplasm is cavitary, or there is evidence of prexisting pyothorax, submit cultures of the mass. Place a chest tube prior to thoracic closure if there is evidence of infection, or if pneumothorax or hemorrhage seems likely postoperatively. Remove residual air from the pleural space after closure.

SUTURE MATERIALS/SPECIAL INSTRUMENTS

Avoid nonabsorbable braided suture (e.g., silk) if there is evidence of infection (see also p. 47).

POSTOPERATIVE CARE AND ASSESSMENT

The animal should be monitored postoperatively for dyspnea. Oxygen should be available (see also p. 618). Postoperative analgesics should be given (see p. 658). Evaluation of ventilation by analysis of blood gas parameters or pulse oximetry is useful. Sudden respiratory distress may be associated with hemorrhage or pneumothorax.

PROGNOSIS

The prognosis for primary pulmonary neoplasia is guarded due to the advanced nature of the disease at the time of diagnosis. Over 50% of dogs that have small, solitary lesions (that have not metastasized) and do not have respiratory signs will live for at least a year after surgery (Ogilvie et al, 1989a). Dogs with tumors in the lung periphery or near the base of a lung have better survival times than those whose tumors involve an entire lobe. The most important prognostic factor related to survival in dogs following surgery is whether or not there is lymph node metastasis (Ogilvie et al, 1989a). The prognosis for most cats with primary lung tumors is poor due to the advanced nature of disease at the time of diagnosis and the tumors' aggressive metastatic behavior. Most patients will eventually die or be euthanatized with recurrence of the primary tumor or metastatic disease.

References

Koblik PD: Radiographic appearance of primary lung tumors in cats, *Vet Radiol* 27:66, 1986.

Ogilvie GK et al: Prognostic factors for tumor remission and survival in dogs after surgery for primary lung tumor: 76 cases (1975–1985), *J Am Vet Med Assoc* 195:109, 1989a.

Ogilvie GK et al: Classification of primary lung tumors in dogs: 210 cases (1975–1985), *J Am Vet Med Assoc* 195:106, 1989b.

Suggested Reading

Bell FW: Neoplastic diseases of the thorax, *Vet Clin N Amer* 17:31, 1987.

Lang J et al: Sensitivity of radiographic detection of lung metastases in the dog, *Vet Radiol* 27:74, 1986.

LaRue SM, Withrow SJ, Wykes PM: Lung resection using surgical staples in dogs and cats, *Vet Surg* 16:238, 1987.

Mehlhaff CJ, Mooney S: Primary pulmonary neoplasia in the dog and cat, *Vet Clin N Amer* 14:1061, 1985.

Mehlhaff CJ et al: Surgical treatment of primary pulmonary neoplasia in 15 dogs, *J Am Anim Hosp Assoc* 20:799, 1984.

Miles KG: A review of primary lung tumors in the dog and cat, *Vet Radiol* 29:122, 1988.

Moulton JE, von Tscharner C, Schneider R: Classification of lung carcinomas in the dog and cat, *Vet Pathol* 18:513, 1981.

Pechman RD: Effect of dependency versus nondependency on lung lesion visualization, *Vet Radiol* 28:185, 1987.

PULMONARY ABSCESSES

DEFINITIONS

An **abscess** is a localized collection of pus, which often results in cavitation in the lung.

GENERAL CONSIDERATIONS AND CLINICALLY RELEVANT PATHOPHYSIOLOGY

Pulmonary abscesses are rare, but they may occur as a complication of foreign bodies, neoplasia, bacterial pneumonia, aspiration pneumonia, fungal infections, or parasites. Abscesses secondary to neoplasia may be sterile or infected. The most common organisms cultured from abscesses associated with necrotizing pneumonia in dogs are *Escherichia coli*, *Pseudomonas* spp., and *Klebsiella* spp. Rupture of pulmonary abscesses may result in pyothorax (see p. 698) and/or pneumothorax (see p. 687). In some parts of the country, pulmonary abscesses are common secondary to inhalation or thoracic penetration of plant material (e.g., foxtails) that migrate through the lung.

DIAGNOSIS
Clinical Presentation

Signalment. Pulmonary abscess may occur in dogs or cats of any age, breed, or sex.

History. The animal may present with a persistent low-grade fever, varying degrees of respiratory distress, weight loss, lethargy, and/or anemia. The duration of illness may vary from hours to days or even weeks. Rupture of a pulmonary abscess that causes pneumothorax may result in acute dyspnea.

Physical Examination Findings

Physical examination findings vary depending on whether pneumothorax and/or pleural effusion are present (see pp. 688 and 692). Most animals are febrile and moist rales may be heard over the mass.

Radiography/Ultrasonography

Pulmonary abscesses generally appear as nodular or cavitary radiopaque lesions on thoracic films. The walls of the abscess are poorly defined in general. If pleural effusion is present, thoracentesis may be necessary before a definitive diagnosis can be made. Ultrasound evaluation of thoracic masses may help differentiate noncavitary from cavitary lesions.

Laboratory Findings

Leukocytosis with a degenerative left shift may be present, or the leukogram may be normal. If the infection is chronic, a nonregenerative anemia may be present.

DIFFERENTIAL DIAGNOSIS

Abscesses should be differentiated from other nodular or cavitary pulmonary lesions (i.e., granulomas, *Paragonimus*, neoplasia) by cytology and/or histologic examination of samples obtained by fine-needle aspiration or surgery. Preoperative aspiration of the mass may help differentiate between these lesions and provide samples for culture; however, care should be used to avoid causing pyothorax. Ultrasound is often useful in locating the appropriate site for aspiration. Some nonneoplastic lesions can be managed without surgery (e.g., *Paragonimus*); however, a definitive diagnosis may require surgical biopsy.

MEDICAL MANAGEMENT

Initial therapy is aimed at stabilizing the animal if it is dyspneic. Thoracentesis should be performed if pleural fluid or air is present. Appropriate antibiotics should be given based on results of culture and sensitivity testing. A broad-spectrum antibiotic with a good anaerobic spectrum should be chosen (see p. 699). Antibiotic therapy should be continued for 3 to 6 weeks. If pyothorax is present, chest tubes should be placed and the thorax lavaged (see pyothorax on p. 698). Some animals will respond to medical management and the abscess will resolve. If after several days there is no improvement in clinical signs or lung expansion, or pleural fluid is loculated and does not resolve, surgical intervention is warranted.

SURGICAL TREATMENT

Solitary pulmonary abscesses that do not resolve with medical therapy are best managed by partial or complete lobectomy of the diseased lung performed via an intercostal thoracotomy (see p. 652). A median sternotomy approach (see p. 654) is preferred if multiple opacities are present involving both sides of the thorax.

Preoperative Management

If the animal is dyspneic, thoracentesis should be performed prior to surgery. Antibiotic therapy should be initiated after the mass and/or pleural space have been cultured if not before.

Anesthesia

Refer to comments and anesthetic protocols for animals with respiratory dysfunction on p. 649. See also specific comments regarding the anesthetic management of animals with pneumothorax on p. 690.

Surgical Anatomy

Surgical anatomy of the thorax is described on p. 651.

Positioning

See p. 651 for positioning of animals for intercostal or median thoracotomy.

SURGICAL TECHNIQUE

Identify and remove the diseased lung. Submit the lung for bacterial and/or fungal cultures and for histologic examination. Explore the remainder of the chest cavity for the presence of foreign matter. Palpate all the lung lobes which can be reached to identify other pulmonary lesions. Free remaining lung lobes of adhesions so that all lobes are moveable and remove loculated areas of exudate. Remove sheets of fibrin that cover the lung lobes. Place a chest tube before thoracic closure.

SUTURE MATERIALS/SPECIAL INSTRUMENTS

Braided, multifilament, nonabsorbable suture (e.g., silk) should be avoided in the presence of infection.

POSTOPERATIVE CARE AND ASSESSMENT

Appropriate antibiotics should be continued for 3 to 6 weeks if infection is present. Pyothorax should be treated with thoracic lavage (see p. 700). Postoperative analgesics should be provided (see p. 650).

PROGNOSIS

The prognosis for animals with pulmonary abscesses depends on the underlying cause. With appropriate management, the prognosis of animals with abscesses associated with nonneoplastic disease is good.

Suggested Reading

Crisp MS et al: Pulmonary abscess caused by a *Mycoplasma* sp. in a cat, *J Am Vet Med Assoc* 191:340, 1987.

Forrester SD, Fossum TW, Miller MW: Pneumothorax in a dog with a pulmonary abscess and suspected infective endocarditis, *J Am Vet Med Assoc* 200:351, 1992.

Hesselink JW, van den Tweel JG: Hypertrophic osteopathy in a dog with a chronic lung abscess, *J Am Vet Med Assoc* 196:760, 1990.

Teske E et al: Transthoracic needle aspiration biopsy of the lung in dogs with pulmonic diseases, *J Am Anim Hosp Assoc* 27:289, 1991.

Walter PA: Non-neoplastic surgical diseases of the lung and pleura, *Vet Clin North Am Small Anim Pract* 17:359, 1987.

LUNG LOBE TORSION

DEFINITIONS

Lung lobe torsion (LLT) is a rotation of the lung lobe along its long axis, with twisting of the bronchus and pulmonary vessels at the hilus.

GENERAL CONSIDERATIONS AND CLINICALLY RELEVANT PATHOPHYSIOLOGY

Any mechanism that increases mobility of a lung lobe seems to favor development of a torsion (Table 26-6). Partial collapse of the lung (i.e., with pulmonary disease or trauma) frees it from its normal spatial relationships with the thoracic wall, mediastinum, and adjacent lung lobes. They may enhance mobility. Pleural effusion or pneumothorax, along with subsequent atelectasis of lung lobes, can allow increased movement of a lobe, predisposing to torsion. Although LLT has been reported to cause chylothorax in dogs, it is more likely that the chylothorax caused the LLT. LLT has been reported secondary to previous thoracic surgery, where lung lobes are manipulated and may remain partially collapsed after thoracic closure.

Torsion of a lung lobe results in venous congestion of the affected lobe; however, the arteries remain at least partially patent, allowing blood to enter. As fluid and blood enter the alveoli, lung consolidation occurs and the lobe becomes dark-colored

TABLE 26-6
Possible Causes of LLT
Atelectasis associated with:
• Pneumonia
• Trauma
• Pneumothorax
• Pleural effusion
• Manipulation during surgery
Spontaneous
Surgical manipulation
Not replacing the lobe in its proper relationship after thoracic surgery

and firm, similar in shade to the liver. The shape of the affected lobe is often altered and it may appear displaced from its normal location within the thorax radiographically. Pleural fluid usually accumulates due to continued venous congestion.

☞ **NOTE** · LLT usually causes massive pleural effusion.

DIAGNOSIS
Clinical Presentation

Signalment. Deep-chested, large-breed dogs, especially Afghan hounds, are more commonly affected. LLT in Afghan hounds may be associated with chylothorax (see p. 691). In large breeds, LLT has been reported to occur spontaneously, without previous history of disease or trauma. LLT has also been reported in small breeds but is usually secondary to primary pleural effusion, thoracic surgery, or trauma. LLT is rare in cats. Middle-aged dogs are more commonly affected, but LLT may occur in animals of any age.

History. Affected animals usually have some degree of respiratory distress. Coughing and hemoptysis can also occur, and may be chronic in nature. Some animals may be anorexic and depressed. Frequently there is a previous history of pleural effusion, pneumothorax, pneumonia, and/or trauma.

Physical Examination Findings

Pleural effusion is consistently present in animals with LLT; therefore, findings often include muffled heart and lung sounds. Other findings may include depression, anorexia, coughing, fever, dyspnea, hemoptysis, hematemesis, and/or vomiting.

Radiography/Ultrasonography

Thoracic radiographic changes are variable depending on the volume of pleural fluid, presence or absence of preexisting disease, and duration of the torsion. The most consistent finding is the presence of pleural effusion accompanied by an opacified lung lobe. Initially, air bronchograms will be present in the torsed lobe and can be seen extending toward the abdomen. Air bronchograms eventually disappear as fluid and blood fill the bronchial lumen. The presence of a noninflated, radiopaque lung lobe that persists after removal of pleural fluid should increase suspicion for LLT (Fig. 26-17). Positional radiographs using horizontal beam x-rays (lateral decubitus or upright VD) are often helpful. Pleural fluid secondary to LLT may persist around the affected lobe rather than fall to the dependent side. Failure of the lobe to reinflate in the "up" or nondependent hemithorax is another indication of LLT.

☞ **NOTE** · The right middle lung lobe is the most commonly torsed lobe in dogs.

Laboratory Findings

Laboratory findings with LLT are variable. Fluid analysis may reveal a sterile, inflammatory effusion or chyle, or the fluid may be bloody. Pleural effusion of any etiology, however, can

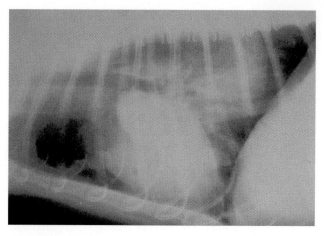

FIG. 26-17
Lateral thoracic radiograph of a dog with a torsion of the right middle lung lobe. Pleural fluid was removed prior to obtaining this radiograph.

initiate a secondary LLT, making results of pleural fluid analysis variable and confusing. The appearance of blood in a previously nonhemorrhagic pleural fluid may indicate occurrence of LLT. An inflammatory leukogram may be present; however, changes in the leukogram may reflect the initial disease process rather than the LLT.

DIFFERENTIAL DIAGNOSIS

Disease such as pneumonia, pulmonary thromboembolism, contusion, neoplasia, atelectasis, hemothorax, diaphragmatic hernia, and pyothorax can mimic radiographic changes seen with LLT. Bronchoscopy may aid diagnosis of LLT once partial or complete occlusion of the affected bronchus is visualized. Bronchial mucosa at the site of obstruction may appear folded and edematous. Demonstration of LLT at surgery provides the definitive diagnosis.

MEDICAL MANAGEMENT

Initial therapy is aimed at stabilizing the animal and alleviating respiratory distress before surgery. Thoracentesis should be performed to remove pleural fluid (see p. 677). Persistent or massive pleural effusion may require placement of a chest tube (see p. 678). Oxygen therapy given by oxygen cage or nasal insufflation is beneficial to some animals. Underlying diseases such as pneumonia should be identified and treated with appropriate antibiotic therapy. Intravenous fluid therapy is beneficial before and during surgery to maintain hydration.

☞ **NOTE** · Spontaneous resolution of LLT is extremely uncommon. This is a surgical condition.

SURGICAL TREATMENT

Spontaneous correction of a torsed lung lobe is uncommon due to swelling of the lobe and rapid formation of adhesions. The treatment of choice for LLT is lobectomy of the affected lobe. Unless LLT is diagnosed very quickly (i.e., immediately after a surgical procedure), damage to the pulmonary parenchyma is generally severe enough that attempts to salvage the lobe are not warranted. Recurrence has been reported following surgical correction where lobectomy was not performed.

Preoperative Management

Prophylactic antibiotics are warranted in animals with LLT. Pleural effusion should be removed prior to anesthetic induction in animals that have compromised ventilation.

Anesthesia

Refer to p. 649 for anesthetic management of animals with respiratory abnormalities.

Positioning

The affected lateral thorax should be prepared for an intercostal thoracotomy (see p. 651).

SURGICAL TECHNIQUE

Clamp the affected pedicle with a noncrushing forceps to prevent release of toxins into the bloodstream, prior to attempting to derotate it. Untwisting the lobe before its removal may help facilitate identification of the vascular structures and bronchus for ligation; however, in some cases, the lobe cannot be easily returned to its normal position due to extensive adhesions. *Check the remaining lobes for position and normal expansion. Culture pulmonary parenchyma following removal of the lobe. Submit excised tissue for histologic examination to help determine underlying causes (i.e., pneumonia, neoplasia). Place a chest tube before closing the thoracic cavity.*

SUTURE MATERIALS/SPECIAL INSTRUMENTS

Avoid braided, multifilament suture because of the risk of infection. Large clamps such as Satinsky clamps (see p. 658) are useful for clamping the bronchus.

POSTOPERATIVE CARE AND ASSESSMENT

Antibiotics should be continued if there is evidence of infection and postoperative analgesics should be provided (see p. 650). The chest tube should be removed when the effusion decreases to less than 2.2. ml/kg/b.w. (see p. 680). Oxygen therapy may be warranted in some patients in the postoperative period, particularly if there is underlying lung disease such as pneumonia. If dyspnea remains after surgery, thoracic radiographs are indicated to rule out LLT in a remaining lobe.

PROGNOSIS

The prognosis is good for most animals with LLT if surgery is performed. Pleural effusion usually resolves within a few days of surgery.

Suggested Readings

Breton L, DiFruscia R, Olivieri M: Successive torsion of the right middle and left cranial lung lobes in a dog, *Can Vet J* 10:386, 1986.

Brown NO, Zontine WJ: Lung lobe torsion in the cat, *J Am Vet Radiol Soc* 17:219, 1976.

Johnston GR et al: Recurring lung lobe torsion in three Afghan hounds, *J Am Vet Med Assoc* 184:842, 1984.

Kerpsack SJ et al: Chylothorax associated with lung lobe torsion and a peritoneopericardial diaphragmatic hernia in a cat, *J Am Anim Hosp Assoc* 30:351, 1994.

Lord P et al: Lung lobe torsion in the dog, *J Am Anim Hosp Assoc* 9:473, 1973.

Railings CA, Lebel JL, Mitchum G: Torsion of the left apical and cardiac pulmonary lobes in a dog, *J Am Vet Med Assoc* 156:726, 1970.

Williams JH, Duncan NM: Chylothorax with concurrent right cardiac lung lobe torsion in an Afghan hound, *J S Afr Vet Assoc* 57:35, 1986.

PECTUS EXCAVATUM

DEFINITIONS

Pectus excavatum (PE) is a deformity of the sternum and costocartilages that results in a dorsal to ventral narrowing of the thorax. **Pectus carinatum** is a protrusion of the sternum that occurs much less frequently than PE.

SYNONYMS

Funnel chest, chondrosternal depression, chonechondrosternon, koilosternia, and **trichterbust**

GENERAL CONSIDERATIONS AND CLINICALLY RELEVANT PATHOPHYSIOLOGY

The cause or causes of PE in animals are unknown (Fig. 26-18). Theories proposed include shortening of the central tendon of the diaphragm, intrauterine pressure abnormalities, and congenital deficiency of the musculature in the cranial portion of

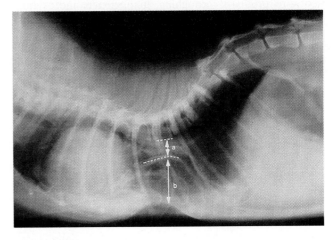

FIG. 26-18
Lateral thoracic radiograph of a cat with severe pectus excavatum. Amount of depression is subjectively assessed based on minimum distance between the vertebral column and dorsal aspect of the sternum (*a*) or the depth of the concavity (*b*). Note that in severe pectus excavatum costocartilages are also deformed. (From Fossum TW et al: Pectus excavatum in 8 dogs and 6 cats, *J Am Anim Hosp Assoc* 25:595, 1989.)

the diaphragm. Abnormal respiratory gradients appear to play a role in the development of this disease in some animals as brachycephalic dogs are most commonly affected, many of which have concurrent hypoplastic tracheas. Pectus excavatum may be associated with "swimmer's syndrome," which is a poorly characterized disease of neonatal dogs in which the limbs tend to splay laterally, impairing ambulation. Abnormalities of the joints of the limbs and the long bones may also occur.

Patients with PE may have abnormalities of both respiratory and cardiovascular function. Circulatory disorders in animals with PE may occur due to abnormal cardiac positioning resulting in kinking of the large veins and disturbance of venous return, compression of the heart predisposing to arrhythmias (particularly the auricles), restriction of ventricular capacity, and decreased respiratory reserve. Cardiac abnormalities are also common (see below under Differential Diagnosis).

☞ **N O T E** · Although the etiology of PE is uncertain, multiple animals in some litters have been affected. Breeding should not be undertaken and affected animals should be neutered.

DIAGNOSIS
Clinical Presentation

Signalment. Pectus excavatum is a congenital abnormality in dogs and cats. In symptomatic animals clinical signs are usually present at birth, or shortly thereafter. PE may occur in any breed, but brachycephalic dogs appear to be predisposed. A sex predisposition has not been identified.

History. Many animals with PE are asymptomatic; however, the defect is often palpable and this may prompt owners to seek veterinary care, despite lack of obvious clinical signs (Fig. 26-19). Symptomatic animals may present for evaluation of exercise intolerance, weight loss, hyperpnea, recurrent pulmonary infections, cyanosis, vomiting, persistent and productive coughing, inappetence, and/or mild

episodes of upper respiratory disease. A correlation between severity of clinical signs and severity of anatomic or physiologic abnormalities has not been observed.

Physical Examination Findings

The sternal deformity is usually palpable. Other physical examination findings may include cardiac murmurs and harsh lung sounds. Dyspnea is variable, but rapid, shallow respirations may be noted.

☞ **N O T E** · Do not assume that cardiac murmurs in animals with PE are due to heart disease. They may be due to abnormal positioning of the heart because of the sternal deformity.

Radiography

Thoracic radiographs show abnormal elevation of the sternum in the caudal thorax. Objective assessment of the deformity may be determined by measuring the frontosagittal and vertebral indices on thoracic radiographs (Table 26-7). Frontosagittal index is calculated by taking the ratio of the width of the chest at the tenth thoracic vertebra, measured on a dorsoventral or ventrodorsal radiograph, and the distance between the center of the ventral surface of the tenth thoracic vertebra and the nearest point on the sternum (Fig. 26-20). Vertebral index is calculated as the ratio of the distance between the center of the dorsal surface of the selected vertebral body to the nearest point on the sternum and the dorsoventral diameter of the center of the same vertebral body (see Fig. 26-20). It has been proposed that the severity of PE be characterized as mild, moderate, or severe based on frontosagittal index and vertebral index (Table 26-8) (Fossum TW, Boudrieau RJ, Hobson HP, 1989). Such determination may aid in the objective assessment of improvement of thoracic diameters following surgery.

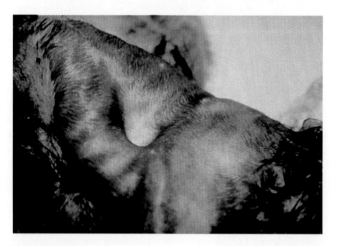

FIG. 26-19
Pectus excavatum in a cat. (From Fossum TW et al: Pectus excavatum in 8 dogs and 6 cats, *J Am Anim Hosp Assoc* 25:595, 1989.)

TABLE 26-7
Normal Frontosagittal and Vertebral Indices

| **Frontosagittal** |
| *Nonbrachycephalic dogs* |
| 0.8 to 1.4 |
| *Brachycephalic dogs* |
| 1.0 to 1.5 |
| *Cats* |
| 0.7 to 1.3 |
| **Vertebral** |
| *Nonbrachycephalic dogs* |
| 11.8 to 19.6 |
| *Brachycephalic dogs* |
| 12.5 to 16.5 |
| *Cats* |
| 12.6 to 18.8 |

TABLE 26-8
Characterization of PE in Dogs and Cats Based on Frontosagittal (FS) and Vertebral (Vert) Indices

PE	Index FS	Vert
Mild	≤2	>9
Moderate	2-3	6-8.99
Severe	>3	<6

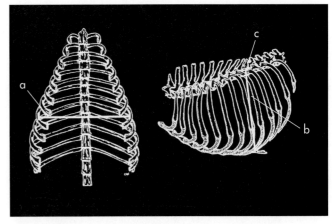

FIG. 26-20
Frontosagittal index is the ratio between the width of the chest at the tenth thoracic vertebra (*a*) and the distance between the center of the ventral surface of the tenth thoracic vertebral body and the nearest point on the sternum (*b*). Vertebral index is the ratio between the distance from the center of the dorsal surface of the tenth vertebral body to the nearest point on the sternum (*b* and *c*) and the dorsal ventral diameter of the vertebral body at the same level (*c*). (From Fossum TW et al: *J Am Anim Hosp Assoc* 25:595, 1989.)

Thoracic radiographs should be evaluated for the evidence of concurrent abnormalities (i.e., tracheal hypoplasia, cardiac abnormalities, pneumonia). Most animals with PE have abnormally positioned hearts (Fig. 26-21), which may cause the heart to appear enlarged radiographically; thus, true cardiac enlargement cannot always be distinguished from apparent enlargement due to abnormal heart position.

Laboratory Findings

Laboratory abnormalities are uncommon.

DIFFERENTIAL DIAGNOSIS

Diagnosis of pectus excavatum is straightforward; however, associated abnormalities may be more difficult to diagnose. Cardiac murmurs are common in patients with PE and appear to be associated with the cardiac malpositioning. These murmurs often disappear following surgical correction of the defect or a change in the patient's position. Systolic murmurs in some patients appear to be related to kinking of the pulmonary artery or to exaggeration of the artery's normal vibrations resulting from its proximity to the chest wall. Animals with PE and innocent systolic murmurs must be differentiated from those that have underlying cardiac defects, such as pulmonic stenosis or atrial septal defects.

MEDICAL MANAGEMENT

Animals with merely a flat chest may contour to a normal or near normal configuration without surgical intervention. However, owners should be encouraged to regularly perform medial-to-lateral compression of the chest on these young animals. Animals with severe elevation of the sternum will not benefit from this technique or from splintage that simply provides medial-to-lateral compression and does not correct the malpositioned sternum. Other medical management includes treatment of respiratory tract infections and if the animal is severely dyspneic, oxygen therapy.

SURGICAL TREATMENT

Application of an external splint to the ventral aspect of the thorax is the most common technique used to correct this defect in animals (Fig. 26-22). Definitive treatment of PE using external splintage is possible because of the young age of affected patients at the time of diagnosis. The costal cartilages and sternum are pliable in these young animals and the thorax can be reshaped by applying traction

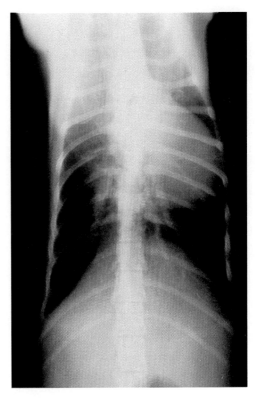

FIG. 26-21
Thoracic radiograph of a dog with pectus excavatum. Note displacement of the heart caused by the sternal abnormality. (From Fossum TW et al: *J Am Anim Hosp Assoc* 25:595, 1989.)

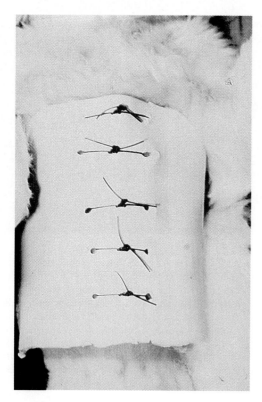

FIG. 26-22
Application of an external splint to the ventral aspect of the thorax in a young dog with pectus excavatum. (From Fossum TW et al: *J Am Vet Med Assoc* 195:91, 1989.)

<table>
<tr><td>TABLE 26-9</td></tr>
</table>

TABLE	26-9

Selected Anesthetic Protocols for Repair of PE in Young Animals That Are Not Dyspneic*

Dogs
Premedication

Atropine (0.02-0.04 mg/kg, SC or IM) or glycopyrollate (0.005-0.01 mg/kg SC or IM) plus oxymorphone (0.05-0.1 mg/kg IM or SC) or butorphanol (0.2-0.4 mg/kg IM or SC)

Induction

Use mask induction with isoflurane after 5 min of preoxygenation

Cats
Premedication

Atropine (0.02-0.04 mg/kg, SC or IM) or glycopyrollate (0.005-0.01 mg/kg SC or IM) plus butorphanol at dose above or buprenorphine (5-15 μg/kg IM or SC)

Induction

Use chamber induction with isoflurane after preoxygenating for 5 min

*See p. 649 if the animal is dyspneic.

to the sternum using sutures that are placed around the sternum and through a rigid splint. Soft tissues that might be abnormal and play a role in the development of this deformity are probably stretched or torn when the sternum is pulled ventrally. Whether surgical correction of the defect should be performed in asymptomatic patients with moderate or severe PE is unknown. Symptomatic patients that do not have associated cardiac abnormalities will benefit from surgery.

Preoperative Management

Respiratory infections should be treated prior to surgery. If the animal is severely dyspneic, oxygen should be provided by nasal insufflation or an oxygen cage until surgery is performed. Prophylactic antibiotic therapy may be given; however, antibiotics are unlikely to prevent skin infections around the splint. Development of intrathoracic infection associated with surgery is uncommon.

Anesthesia

Anesthetic management in these young animals should include attention to airway, ventilation, body temperature, and blood glucose concentration. Animals should be intubated, ventilation should be assisted or controlled, a high inspired fraction of oxygen should be used, intravenously administered fluids should be warm, and fluids should contain glucose if serum glucose concentrations cannot be monitored (Table 26-9). Additionally, the animal should

be insulated from the cool surgical environment. The splint should be formed and fitted before anesthesia to reduce anesthetic duration. Do not use nitrous oxide in these patients because of the risk of pneumothorax. Postoperative analgesia should be provided in puppies with butorphanol, oxymorphone, or buprenorphine and in kittens with butorphanol or buprenorphine (see Table 26-9). Do not use chamber or mask induction if the animal is dyspneic.

Surgical Anatomy

Surgical anatomy of the thorax is described on p. 651.

Positioning

The patient is placed in dorsal recumbency, and the ventral thorax is prepared for aseptic surgery.

SURGICAL TECHNIQUE

Fashion a rectangular piece of moldable splinting material into a U-shape (Fig. 26-23) and mold it to fit the ventral aspect of the thorax. Apply a small amount of adhesive padding to the cranial border and inner surface of the splint, or alternately, pad the splint with cast padding after it has been positioned. Place two parallel rows of four to six holes in the splint with a small Steinmann pin (see Fig. 26-23). Position the holes so that the distance between adjacent holes is slightly greater than the width of the sternum. Pass the selected suture (see below under suture materials) around the sternum by maneuvering the needle blindly off the lateral edge of the sternum. Alternately, pass the needle around the sternebra at a 45-degree angle to incorporate the costocartilage and possibly decrease the

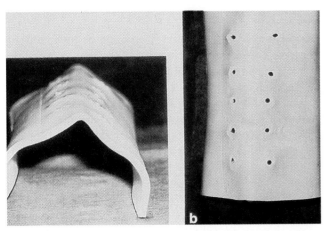

FIG. 26-23
External splint for correction of pectus excavatum. Place two parallel rows of four to six holes in the splint with a small Steinmann pin. (From Fossum TW et al: *J Am Vet Med Assoc* 195:91, 1989.)

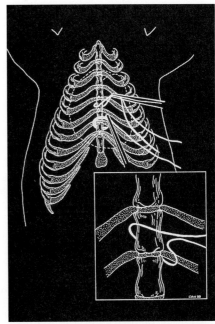

FIG. 26-24
Sutures placed around the sternebrae may be horizontal to the long axis, or at a 45 degree angle (From Fossum TW et al: *J Am Vet Med Assoc* 195:91, 1989.)

chance of the suture pulling through the soft sternebral bone (Fig. 26-24). Sutures must be placed around the sternum and not subcutaneously. Additionally, sutures must be placed in the area of the greatest concavity. If the sutures are placed proximal to the area with the greatest depression the sternum cannot be pulled into a normal position, resulting in less than optimal correction of the defect. *Keep the needle as close as possible to the dorsal aspect of the sternum to avoid piercing the heart or lungs. Leave the suture ends long and tag them. When all sutures have been placed, pass the ends through the predrilled holes in the splint and tie them securely on its ventral aspect (see Fig. 26-22).* Two sutures may be placed and tied to themselves and then these sutures tied together so that the splint can be adjusted without replacement of sutures or use of anesthesia.

SUTURE MATERIALS/SPECIAL INSTRUMENTS

A taper-point needle is recommended; if suture material with a large, swaged-on needle is not available, a large, eyed, taper-point needle should be selected (to prevent bending and possible breakage as it is passed around the sternum). Large (i.e., No. 0–2), monofilament absorbable or nonabsorbable suture material is recommended (i.e., polydioxanone, polyglyconate, or nylon suture).

POSTOPERATIVE CARE AND ASSESSMENT

The animal should be evaluated in the early postoperative period for intrathoracic hemorrhage because piercing of the heart, lung, or internal thoracic vessels as the needle is passed around the sternum is possible. Positioning the animal in dorsal recumbency, paying close attention to the phase of respiration, and keeping the needle as close to the sternum as possible will help prevent such complications. The splint should be left in place 10 to 21 days.

COMPLICATIONS

Suture abscesses, mild superficial dermatitis, and skin abrasions are common, but these are usually minor and heal quickly after splint removal. Adequate padding of the splint may help prevent abrasions. Fatal reexpansion pulmonary edema (see p. 650) has been reported in a kitten after correction of PE (Sonderstrom, Gilson, Gulbas, 1995).

PROGNOSIS

The prognosis is excellent for animals without underlying disease in whom surgery is performed at a young age. Older animals with a less pliable sternum may not respond as favorably to external splintage. Partial sternectomy may benefit such animals (see p. 673).

References

Fossum TW, Boudrieau RJ, Hobson HP: Pectus excavatum in 8 dogs and 6 cats, *J Am Anim Hosp Assoc* 25:595, 1989.
Soderstrom MJ, Gilson SD, Gulbas N: Fatal reexpansion pulmonary edema in a kitten following surgical correction of pectus excavatum, *J Am Anim Hosp Assoc* 31:133, 1995.

Suggested Reading

Boudrieau RJ et al: Pectus excavatum in dogs and cats, *Comp Contin Educ Pract Vet* 12:341, 1990.
Fossum TW et al: Surgical correction of pectus excavatum using external splintage in two dogs and a cat, *J Am Vet Med Assoc* 195:91, 1989.
Grenn HH, Lindo DE: Pectus excavatum (funnel chest) in a feline, *Can Vet Jour* 9:279, 1968.
Pearson JL: Pectus excavatum in the dog, *Vet Med/Small Anim Clin* 68:125, 1973.

Shires PK, Waldon DR, Payne J: Pectus excavatum in three kittens, *J Am Anim Hosp Assoc* 24:203, 1988.

Smallwood JE, Beaver BV: Congenital chondrosternal depression (pectus excavatum) in the cat, *J Am Vet Radiol Soc* 18:141, 1977.

THORACIC WALL NEOPLASIA

DEFINITIONS

Thoracic wall neoplasia may arise from ribs, musculature, or pleura. **Chondrosarcomas** are tumors that arise from cartilage; while **osteosarcomas** arise from bone.

GENERAL CONSIDERATIONS AND CLINICALLY RELEVANT PATHOPHYSIOLOGY

Primary tumors of the rib have a high metastatic rate and are uncommon in dogs or cats. Osteosarcomas are the most common neoplasm of the canine rib, followed by chondrosarcomas; the costochondral junction is the usual site of origin of these tumors. Although also rare, both metastatic and primary tumors of the sternum have been reported in dogs. Primary sternal tumors of dogs include chondrosarcoma and osteosarcoma.

DIAGNOSIS
Clinical Presentation

Signalment. Primary rib tumors generally develop in young and middle-aged dogs. Rib tumors should be considered as a possible differential for masses involving the thoracic wall, even in young dogs.

History. Animals with rib tumors may present for dyspnea or evaluation of a nonpainful thoracic wall mass. Animals with sternal neoplasia often present for evaluation of a palpable sternal mass.

Physical Examination Findings

Most rib tumors cause a localized swelling of the thoracic wall; however, pleural effusion without evidence of a thoracic mass occasionally occurs in dogs with small primary rib tumors and metastatic pulmonary lesions. Other clinical signs of rib tumors are weight loss and dyspnea. Sternal tumors usually cause a localized swelling, but may be associated with dyspnea if they metastasize to the lungs.

Radiography

Rib tumors are generally expansile masses that cause bone destruction. Sternal tumors may also result in lysis of several sternebrae and the adjacent ribs. Thoracic radiographs of animals with neoplasia of the ribs or sternum should be evaluated for pulmonary metastasis, lymph node involvement, and/or pleural effusion.

Laboratory Findings

Laboratory findings are nonspecific. Blood gas analysis may show hypoxemia and respiratory acidosis or alkalosis (because of hyperventilation).

DIFFERENTIAL DIAGNOSIS

Neoplasia of the sternum or ribs should be differentiated from osteomyelitis, fungal infections, or abscesses based on cytologic or histologic findings. A tentative diagnosis of the cell type can usually be made by fine-needle aspiration of the mass. Definitive diagnosis usually requires histologic examination of a biopsy specimen. Although pleural effusion is common in dogs with rib tumors, identification of neoplastic cells in the fluid is uncommon.

MEDICAL MANAGEMENT

Medical management (i.e., thoracentesis if pleural effusion exists, oxygen therapy for dyspnea) of animals with rib or sternal tumors is generally palliative only. Pleuroperitoneal shunts are used in humans with pleural effusion due to terminal neoplasia; however, such use has not been reported in dogs or cats.

SURGICAL TREATMENT

Surgical resection of thoracic wall tumors is the treatment of choice. Full-thickness or "en bloc" resection of three or more ribs for thoracic wall neoplasia requires surgical reconstruction in order to reestablish thoracic wall continuity. Removal of more than six ribs is not recommended. With tumors of the caudal thorax, advancement of the diaphragm cranial to the resected ribs decreases the need for rigid fixation of the thoracic wall. Partial or complete sternectomy may be curative in dogs with primary sternal neoplasia. Although temporary instability of the thorax may occur following large sternal resections, this does not appear to cause any permanent or significant respiratory dysfunction.

Preoperative Management

Thoracentesis should be performed prior to induction in dogs with pleural effusion associated with thoracic wall neoplasia.

Anesthesia

See anesthetics recommendations on p. 649 for animals with respiratory disease.

Positioning

A generous area surrounding the tumor should be prepared for aseptic surgery with thoracic wall or sternal neoplasia.

SURGICAL TECHNIQUE
En Bloc Resection of Thoracic Wall Neoplasia

Remove the thoracic wall containing the neoplasm and a margin of normal tissue, leaving a square or rectangular defect. Cut a piece of polypropylene mesh slightly larger than the defect. Fold over the edges of the mesh and suture the double thickness of mesh to the pleural side of the defect (Fig. 26-25). **Draw the mesh tightly across the defect when suturing it to prevent it from moving paradoxically with respiration.** *If more than four or five ribs are removed, support the ribs with plastic spinal plates or rib grafts. Mobilize and advance thoracic wall musculature over the defect, or if there is insufficient muscle, exteriorize an omental pedicle flap through a paracostal abdominal approach and tunnel it subcutaneously to*

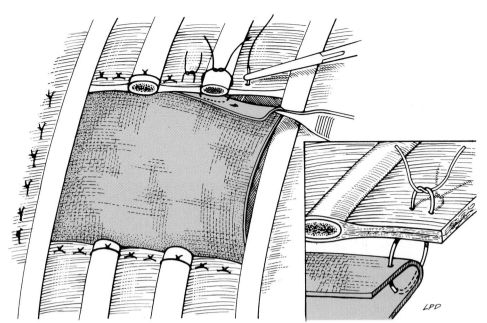

FIG. 26-25
Some thoracic tumors may be removed by en bloc resection of the thoracic wall. Remove the thoracic wall containing the neoplasm and a margin of normal tissue. Fold the edges of a piece of mesh over and suture the double thickness of mesh to the pleural side of the defect.

the defect. Alternatively, exteriorize the omental flap through the diaphragm. Place the omental flap over the mesh and suture skin over the defect. For caudal rib tumors, advancement of the diaphragm may be done following "en bloc" resection of the mass and surrounding tissues. Synthetic reconstruction of the rib cage is rarely necessary.

Partial Sternectomy

Partial sternectomy should only be considered for relatively small, localized sternal neoplasms that do not appear to have intrathoracic involvement.

Sternectomy has been used successfully for extensive sternal osteomyelitis. The entire sternum can be removed in small animals.

Incise through the skin overlying the neoplasm (if skin involvement is suspected, resect the skin). Identify rib articulations on the sternum. Use rongeurs to remove the affected sternebrae and ribs. If possible remove one sternebra caudal and one cranial to the lesion. Assess the thoracic cavity for involvement. Avoid lacerating the internal thoracic arteries—ligate them if necessary. Appose the ribs and intercostal muscles with a large (e.g., No. 1) monofilament suture in an interrupted or horizontal mattress suture pattern. Use a simple continuous suture pattern to appose remnants of the rectus abdominis muscle over the junction of the rib ends. Minimize dead space by apposing skin and underlying tissues with walking sutures. Place a thoracostomy tube and evacuate air from the thoracic cavity. Place a light support wrap over the thorax to protect the incision and thoracostomy tube.

SUTURE MATERIALS/SPECIAL INSTRUMENTS

Reconstruction of thoracic wall defects should be done with monofilament, nonabsorbable suture (i.e., polypropylene or nylon). Polypropylene (Marlex) mesh may be used for thoracic wall reconstruction (see Product Appendix).

POSTOPERATIVE CARE AND ASSESSMENT

Animals with surgically created thoracic wall defects should be monitored closely in the postoperative period for hypoventilation and/or the development of pneumothorax. Analgesic therapy is warranted in these animals (see Table 26-9). See p. 657 for additional comments on the postoperative management of animals with respiratory disorders.

PROGNOSIS

Because of the high rate of pulmonary metastasis, the prognosis for dogs with rib tumors is poor. In one study of 15 dogs with primary rib tumors, greater than 90% died or were euthanatized within 4 months of the diagnosis (Feeney et al, 1982). Too few sternal tumors have been reported to define the prognosis in affected animals.

Reference

Feeney DA et al: Malignant neoplasia of the canine ribs: clinical, radiographic, and pathologic findings, *J Amer Vet Med Assoc* 180:927, 1982.

Suggested Reading

Atwell RB, Seiler R: Primary osteosarcoma of the sternum of a dog, *Aust Vet J* 54:585, 1978.
Bright RM: Reconstruction of thoracic wall defects using Marlex mesh, *J Am Anim Hosp Assoc* 17:15, 1981.
Bright RM, Birchard SJ, Long GG: Repair of thoracic wall defects in the dog with an omental pedicle flap, *J Am Anim Hosp Assoc* 18:277, 1982.
Fossum TW et al: Partial sternectomy for sternal osteomyelitis in the dog, *J Am Anim Hosp Assoc* 25:435, 1989.
Runnels CM, Trampel DW: Full-thickness thoracic and abdominal wall reconstruction in dogs using carbon/polycaprolactone composite, *Vet Surg* 15:363, 1986.

CHAPTER 27

Surgery of the Lower Respiratory System: Pleural Cavity and Diaphragm

GENERAL PRINCIPLES AND TECHNIQUES

DEFINITIONS

The **pleura** is the serous membrane that covers the lung and lines the thoracic cavity. It completely encloses a potential space known as the **pleural cavity.** The **parietal** pleura is the portion of the pleura that lines the walls of the thoracic cavity, while the **visceral** or **pulmonary** pleura invests the lungs and lines their fissures, completely separating the different lobes. **Thoracocentesis** is a surgical puncture of the thoracic wall to remove air (**pneumothorax**) or fluid (**pleural effusion**) from the pleural space. **Pleurodesis** is the creation of adhesions between the visceral and parietal pleura caused by instilling irritating agents into the pleural cavity or mechanically damaging the pleura at surgery.

PREOPERATIVE CONCERNS

Respiratory function should be carefully monitored in patients with pleural cavity or diaphragmatic abnormalities. Qualitative assessments of respiratory function include monitoring respiratory rate and pattern and capillary refill time and color (Tables 27-1 and 27-2). Animals with pleural cavity disease usually exhibit a restrictive respiratory pattern (i.e., rapid, shallow respirations). Arterial blood gas analysis will augment qualitative information concerning the effectiveness of ventilation and gas exchange (Table 27-3). Pulse oximetry is a noninvasive tool that provides information regarding the hemoglobin saturation of blood and thus indirectly provides quantitative information regarding oxygenation. Cardiovascular parameters (i.e., heart rate and rhythm) should also be evaluated (see Table 27-1). An ECG should be performed in all trauma patients. Intravenous fluids should be provided to dehydrated animals or those that are not drinking sufficient fluids to maintain hydration. Care should be taken to avoid causing overhydration and pulmonary edema, which will further compromise respiration. Monitoring central venous pressure may be useful in some patients.

TABLE 27-1

Normal Heart (HR) and Respiratory Rates (RR) in Conscious Dogs and Cats (per minute)

	HR	RR
Dog	70-140	20-40
Cat	145-200	20-40

TABLE 27-2

Normal Capillary Refill Time

<1-2 seconds

TABLE 27-3

Normal pH and Blood Gas Values on Room Air

Value		Range
pH	= 7.4	(7.35-7.45)
PaO_2	= 95 mm Hg	(80-110)
PvO_2	= 40 mm Hg	(35-45)
$PaCO_2$	= 40 mm Hg	(35-45)
$PvCO_2$	= 45 mm Hg	(40-48)
HCO_3	= 24 mEq/L	(22-27)

Animals with pleural effusion or pneumothorax may be extremely dyspneic. In severely dyspneic animals with suspected pleural cavity disease thoracentesis (see below) should be performed before radiographs are made. Removal of even small amounts of pleural effusion or air may significantly improve ventilation, allowing safer manipulation of the patient for radiographic procedures. Most dyspneic animals will allow thoracentesis to be performed with minimal restraint; general anesthetics should be avoided. The animal should be allowed to remain in sternal recumbency and oxygen provided by face mask or nasal insufflation if the animal will tolerate it. A negative tap does not rule out pleural effusion; however, if the animal remains dyspneic after thoracentesis, underlying lung disease (i.e., pneumonia, pulmonary edema, pulmonary contusions, pulmonary neoplasia) or loculated fluid should be suspected. Providing nasal oxygen or placing the animal in an oxygen cage may be beneficial while treatment of the pulmonary disease is initiated.

☞ **NOTE** · Do not attempt to place chest tubes or take radiographs in animals with pleural effusion that are extremely dyspneic—perform thoracentesis first!

Chest tube placement should not be attempted in an animal with severe respiratory distress. Generally, stabilization and improved ventilation can first be accomplished by removing some pleural air or fluid via needle thoracentesis. In critically ill patients, chest tubes can occasionally be placed without the use of general anesthesia: local anesthesia (i.e., local anesthetic infiltration or an intercostal nerve block) is sufficient. However, most animals with pleural cavity disease benefit from intermittent positive pressure ventilation and oxygen supplementation during tube placement. When general anesthesia is used, control of the animal's airway (via endotracheal intubation and positive pressure ventilation) and oxygen therapy should be rapidly achieved (see below). For preoperative concerns of patients with diaphragmatic herniation see p. 684.

ANESTHETIC CONSIDERATIONS

Whenever possible, dogs and cats with respiratory insufficiency should be maintained with inhalation anesthetics (i.e., isoflurane or halothane). Inhalation anesthesia is advantageous because it allows rapid recovery and more precise control of anesthetic depth than maintaining anesthesia with intravenous anesthetics. Respiratory patients should be managed with extreme care until intubation has been accomplished and ventilation can be assisted. Oxygen can be provided by face mask in these patients until an airway has been secured. Intubation should be accomplished as rapidly as possible in patients with pleural effusion or pneumothorax; mask induction is not recommended. Endotracheal intubation and intermittent positive pressure ventilation allow maintenance of an adequate respiratory volume in patients whose lungs may not expand normally due to the presence of pleural cavity or diaphragmatic abnormalities. **Nitrous oxide should not be used in patients with pneumothorax or diaphragmatic hernias because it rapidly diffuses into air-filled spaces (i.e., pleural cavity or gas-filled organs) causing further lung compression or organ enlargement.** Additionally, nitrous oxide is comparatively less soluble in plasma than are oxygen and other inhalation anesthetics. Thus when it is discontinued it rapidly diffuses into the alveoli, which may result in diffusion hypoxia if the patient hypoventilates. For specific anesthetic recommendations for animals with pneumothorax and diaphragmatic hernias see pp. 690 and 684, respectively. See also Chapter 26.

☞ **NOTE** · Do not use mask or chamber induction in patients with respiratory distress—accomplish intubation as rapidly as possible.

ANTIBIOTICS

Needle thoracentesis, if performed with proper aseptic technique, is unlikely to induce infection in patients with normal immune function. Therefore, prophylactic antibiotics generally do not need to be provided when performing this procedure. The use of prophylactic antibiotics in patients with chest tubes is controversial. Studies in human beings have not shown decreased infection rates when patients with chest tubes are given prophylactic antibiotics. However, chest tubes must be maintained and handled with appropriate precautions (e.g., sterile gloves and syringes, chest bandages) to decrease the potential for iatrogenic contamination. Gram-negative bacteria and anaerobes are common isolates in animals with respiratory disease. Therapy of pyothorax should be based on culture and sensitivity test results, if possible, because unpredictable antibiotic sensitivity is common with the microorganisms commonly encountered with this condition. For specific antibiotic recommendations of patients with pyothorax see p. 699.

SURGICAL ANATOMY

Each pleural cavity is only a potential space unless air or fluid collects between the parietal and visceral pleura, preventing normal lung expansion. In the normal animal, only a capillary film of fluid exists to moisten the mesothelial cells that line its surface. Thus, except for this capillary fluid, the visceral pleura is in contact with the pleural lining of the thoracic wall. The pleura of dogs contains smooth muscle fibers and a network of elastic fibers and is more delicate than in other domestic animals. The subserosa is composed of collagen and elastic fibers, which, in the visceral pleura, communicate with the underlying lung. Fluid secreted into the pleural cavity is normally reabsorbed by lymphatics underlying the parietal pleura. Thickening of the pleura (i.e., fibrosing pleuritis) may prevent reabsorption of fluid, resulting in pleural effusion.

Fibers of the diaphragm arise from attachments on the ventral surface of the lumbar vertebrae, ribs, and sternum and radiate toward the tendinous center (Fig. 27-1). The diaphragm is composed of a central tendinous portion and an outer muscular portion. While the costal part of the di-

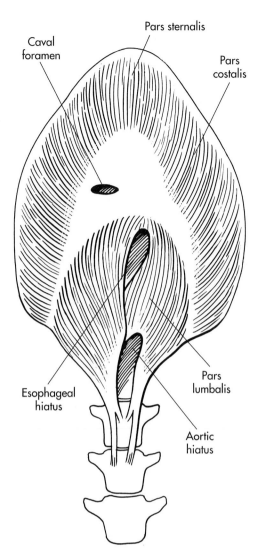

FIG. 27-1
Diaphragmatic anatomy.

phragm attaches to the internal surface of the last few ribs, the central portion extends cranially into the thoracic cavity.

SURGICAL TECHNIQUES

Treatment of pleural cavity disease varies depending on the underlying etiology. For traumatic pneumothorax (see p. 690), intermittent needle thoracentesis may be sufficient in some animals to prevent dyspnea while the lung heals, but chest tubes are occasionally required. However, chest tube placement and continuous drainage of air in animals with spontaneous pneumothorax (see p. 688) that have undergone mechanical pleurodesis are recommended to allow pleurodesis. With some types of pleural effusion (i.e., pyothorax; see p. 698), tube thoracentesis and thoracic lavage are mandatory in the primary treatment of most affected animals.

Needle Thoracentesis

Needle thoracentesis is performed with a small-gauge (No. 19 to No. 23) butterfly needle attached to a three-way stopcock and syringe, or an over-the-needle catheter attached to an

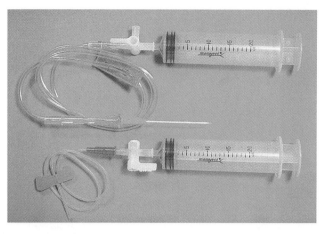

FIG. 27-2
A small-gauge butterfly needle (lower) or an over-the-needle catheter attached to extension tubing (upper), and a three-way stopcock and syringe are used for needle thoracentesis.

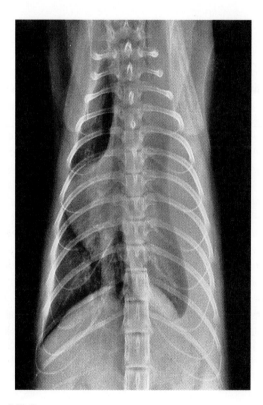

FIG. 27-3
Thoracic radiograph of a cat with unilateral pleural effusion secondary to chronic chylothorax.

extension tubing, three-way stopcock, and syringe (Fig. 27-2). The appropriate site for thoracentesis should be selected based on physical examination or, if available, radiographic findings. Usually, aspiration of either side of the thorax will drain the contralateral hemithorax adequately, because the mediastinum in dogs and cats is thin and permeable to fluids. With some diseases, particularly chylothorax and pyothorax, unilateral effusions may occur due to thickening of the mediastinum associated with chronic inflammation (Fig. 27-3).

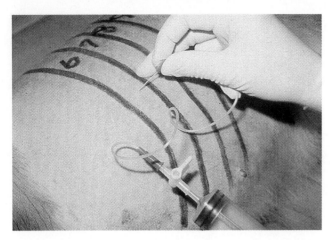

FIG. 27-4
Thoracentesis is performed at the sixth, seventh, or eighth intercostal space, near the level of the costochondral junction.

Perform thoracentesis at the sixth, seventh, or eighth intercostal space, near the level of the costochondral junction (Fig. 27-4). Clip the selected site and perform a local anesthetic block if needed (this is rarely the case). Aseptically prepare the site and introduce the needle into the middle of the selected intercostal space. Be careful to avoid the large vessels associated with the posterior aspect of the rib margins. Advance the needle into the pleural space. Aspirate fluid while the needle is being advanced to allow prompt recognition of the appropriate depth of needle placement. With the bevel of the needle facing inward, orient the needle against the rib cage to prevent damage to the lung surface. Gently aspirate fluid and place 5-ml samples in an EDTA tube and a clot tube for a cell count and biochemical parameters, respectively. Additionally, make six to eight direct smears for cytologic evaluation. Submit samples for aerobic and anaerobic cultures.

Chest Tube Placement

Incorrectly placed or improperly managed chest tubes are extremely dangerous to animals. However, if precautions are taken to ensure that the animal cannot remove the tube prematurely, or against the animal chewing on the tube, a pneumothorax will not occur. Chest tubes simplify the management of some animals with pleural effusion or pneumothorax. The choice of which side to place the chest tube is made by evaluating the radiographs. Occasionally, bilateral chest tubes may be necessary; however, in most dogs and cats the mediastinum is permeable to fluid or air, allowing drainage of both hemithoraxes through a single tube. The exception to this may be in chylothorax or pyothorax (see above).

Components of a tube thoracostomy include a chest tube, an apparatus to connect the tube to a syringe or to a continuous suction bottle, and a device to collect the drained material (syringe or collecting bottle). Commercially available tubes are usually made of polyvinyl chloride or silicone rubber and are less reactive than red rubber feeding tubes. Commercial tubes come with a metal stylet that simplifies tube

TABLE 27-4

Guidelines for Estimating Chest Tube Size

Cats and Dogs < 7 kg	
14-16 Fr	
Dogs 7-15 kg	
18-22 Fr	
Dogs 16-30 kg	
22-28 Fr	
Dogs > 30 kg	
28-36 Fr	

TABLE 27-5

Important Points When Placing a Chest Tube

- When placing additional holes in commercial tubes, make sure that the last hole is through the radiopaque line
- Start the chest tube dorsally rather than midthorax to minimize fluid or air leakage around the tube
- Firmly grasp the tube 1-2 cm above the body wall when inserting the tube
- Clamp the tube before removing the stylet (trocar) to prevent pneumothorax
- Securely fasten all connectors to the tube to prevent inadvertent dislodgement

placement, but may increase the risk of perforating lung tissue when compared with red rubber feeding tubes. The latter are usually inserted using a large hemostat or Carmalt clamp. Commercial chest tubes come in various sizes ranging from 14 to 40 French. The size of the thoracostomy tube should approximate the diameter of the mainstem bronchus; however, smaller tubes may be adequate for removing air, while larger tubes may be required with more viscous effusions (Table 27-4). If a commercial tube is used, attach it via a five-in-one connector (Christmas tree adapter) to either a three-way stopcock or the tubing from a continuous suction device. The ends of red rubber feeding tubes can be cut to accommodate a three-way stopcock; attaching these tubes to a continuous suction device is generally not recommended due to their tendency to collapse (Table 27-5).

Clip and prepare the lateral thorax for aseptic surgery. In order to allow sufficient drainage, place additional holes in the tube by bending the tube and removing a notch with a pair of sterile scissors (Fig. 27-5). Holes should not be greater than one third the circumference of the tube. If using a commercial tube with a radiopaque line, place the last hole through the line in order to allow identification of its position on a thoracic radiograph. Make a small skin incision in the dorsal one third of the lateral thoracic wall at the level of the tenth or eleventh intercostal space. Advance the tube subcutaneously in a cranioventral direction

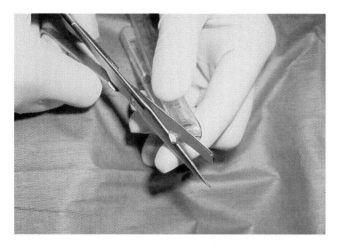

FIG. 27-5
For thoracostomy tube placement, place additional holes in the tube by bending the tube and removing a notch with a pair of sterile scissors.

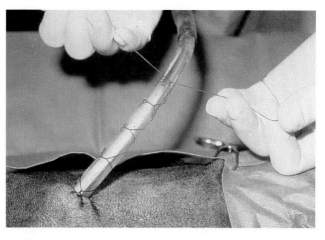

FIG. 27-7
Secure the tube with a Chinese finger-trap or Roman sandal suture.

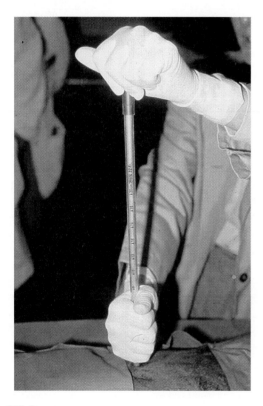

FIG. 27-6
When using a trocar tube, firmly grasp the tube 2 to 4 cm from the body wall with one hand while using the other hand to pop the tube through the intercostal musculature and pleura.

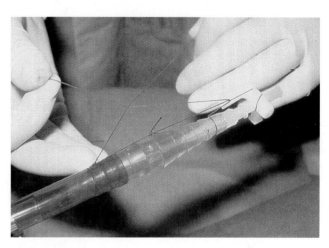

FIG. 27-8
Use suture to secure the tube to the connecting devices so that they will not become inadvertently dislodged.

other thoracic structures. Feed the tube in a cranioventral direction to a predetermined point and before completely removing the trocar, clamp the tube with a hemostat. Place a purse-string suture in the skin around the tube (do not enter the lumen of the tube) and leave both ends of the suture long. Use this suture to perform a "Chinese finger-trap" or "Roman sandal" suture (Fig. 27-7). Connect the chest tube to a three-way stopcock in order to increase the ease of thoracic drainage. Use a five-in-one (Christmas tree) adapter or a female Luer Lok (with small tubes) between the tube and the three-way stopcock to ensure an airtight seal. Use suture to secure the tube to the connecting devices so that they will not become inadvertently dislodged, resulting in a pneumothorax (Fig. 27-8). For added safety when the chest cavity is not being suctioned, clamp the tube where it exits the body wall with a hemostat or C-clamp (Fig. 27-9). Verify appropriate placement of the chest drain radiographically (Fig. 27-10) before covering it with a loose bandage.

for three to four intercostal spaces and introduce the tube through the muscle and pleura using the stylet or a large hemostat. When using a trocar tube, firmly grasp the tube 2 to 4 cm from the body wall with one hand while using the other hand to "pop" the tube through the intercostal musculature and pleura (Fig. 27-6). This will prevent the tube from being inadvertently pushed further into the thorax than anticipated and therefore damaging the lung or

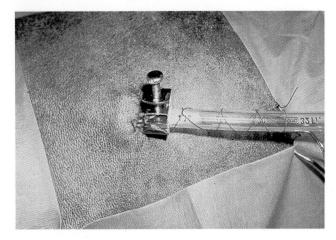

FIG. 27-9
For added safety when the chest cavity is not being suctioned, clamp the tube where it exits the body wall with a hemostat or C-clamp.

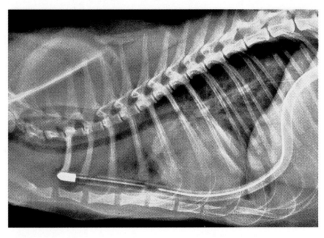

FIG. 27-10
Verify appropriate placement of the chest drain radiographically before covering it with a loose bandage.

FIG. 27-11
Three-bottle system for continuous pleural drainage.

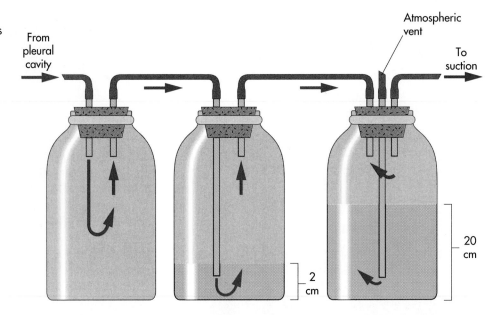

Drainage may be either intermittent or continuous. Generally, intermittent pleural drainage is adequate; however, in some situations (i.e., spontaneous pneumothorax, pleurodesis) continuous suction is preferable. Heimlich valves should only be used in medium to large dogs, because small dogs and cats may not develop sufficient expiratory pressure for effective drainage. Additionally, these valves are prone to malfunction if fluid is aspirated into the apparatus. "Milking" or "stripping" of chest tubes to prevent obstruction of the tube by clots has been recommended in the veterinary literature; however, these techniques generate high intrapleural pressures and may cause pulmonary damage.

Chest Tube Removal

With pleural effusion, remove the tube when the drainage decreases to a volume that is consistent with that caused by the presence of the tube itself (i.e., 2.2 ml/kg body weight/day). The tube can be removed in patients with pneumothorax once negative pressure has been achieved for 12 to 24 hours. Culture the end of the tube following removal if the tube has been present for several days, or if the animal shows signs of infection. Suture the skin incision with one or two simple interrupted sutures.

Continuous Thoracic Suction

If fluid accumulation is so rapid that intermittent drainage is not practical, or if adherence of the visceral pleura to the body wall is desired, continuous suction may be used. Two-bottle and three-bottle systems and commercial suction units are available for veterinary use and are economical and simple to use. A continuous 10-to 15-cm negative pressure on the thorax effectively aspirates pneumothorax, increasing the likelihood of spontaneous sealing of large pulmonary defects. Slightly greater pressures may be necessary (up to 20 cm water) when viscous fluid is being drained.

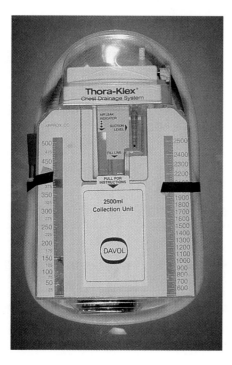

FIG. 27-12
Commercial continuous suction device.

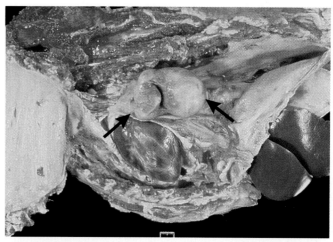

FIG. 27-13
Necropsy specimen of a dog with chronic chylothorax and severe fibrosing pleuritis. Note the small, consolidated lungs (arrows) and the thickened pleura.

Connect the chest tube to a bottle that serves as an under-water seal (filled with 2 to 3 cm of sterile water), which in turn is connected to a suction bottle (also partially filled with water) attached to a suction device (Fig. 27-11). Vary the amount of suction by raising or lowering the level of water in the suction bottle. A rigid plastic vent tube opened to room air serves to allow air to be aspirated into the bottle as the vacuum is applied. A third bottle interposed between the chest tube and the underwater seal bottle serves to collect fluid and prevent the level from rising in the underwater seal bottle as fluid is drained from the chest. The bottle is unnecessary in animals with pneumothorax. Alternatively, a commercial continuous suction device (Fig. 27-12) may be used (see below).

HEALING OF THE PLEURA

Healing or damaged pleura is prone to adhesion formation in some species; however, dogs and cats seem resistant to chemical pleurodesis. They may have greater pleural fibrinolytic capacity than other species (e.g., rabbit or human). Fibrosing pleuritis has been reported in dogs and cats secondary to prolonged exudative or blood-stained effusions. In animals with fibrosis, the pleura is thickened by diffuse fibrous tissue that restricts normal pulmonary expansion (the lungs do not adhere to the body wall in these patients; Fig. 27-13). Exudates are characterized by a high rate of fibrin formation and degradation because chronic inflammation induces changes in mesothelial cell morphologic features that result in increased permeability, mesothelial cell desquamation, and triggering of both pathways of the coagulation cascade. These desquamated mesothelial cells have also been shown to produce type III collagen in cell culture, promoting

fibrosis. Additionally, the chronic presence of pleural fluid might lead to an impairment in the mechanism of fibrin degradation.

SUTURE MATERIALS/SPECIAL INSTRUMENTS

Trocar chest tubes (DekNatel thoracic trocar catheter, Argyle thoracic trocar catheter) and continuous suction devices (DekNatel Pleur-evac chest drainage system, Thora-Seal III three-bottle underwater chest drainage system) (see Fig. 27-12) may be purchased from several commercial sources (see Product Appendix for ordering information).

POSTOPERATIVE CARE AND ASSESSMENT

If dyspnea persists following needle thoracentesis or chest tube placement, oxygen therapy (nasal insufflation or oxygen cage) may be beneficial. Thoracic radiographs should be taken to assess fluid or air removal and/or evaluate chest tube position. Animals with chest tubes should be continually monitored to prevent iatrogenic dislodgement or damage of the tube and/or connectors causing pneumothorax (see below under complications). Care should be exercised when handling tubes to prevent thoracic contamination. Chest tubes should be aspirated gently so that lung tissue is not suctioned into the tube drainage ports.

COMPLICATIONS

Although lung penetration and damage are possible with needle thoracentesis, the risk is minimal if proper technique is used. The major complication associated with chest tubes is pneumothorax following trauma to the tube by the patient (i.e., biting or scratching) or loosening of the connections of the tube to the adapters. The risk of these complications can be minimized by placing a hemostat or C-clamp close to the tube's exit site, by securing the tube to the adapters, and by proper bandaging of the chest and tube (see Figs. 27-8 and

27-9). Constant surveillance of animals with chest tubes is recommended. Other complications associated with chest tube placement are rare but include lung perforation, empyema, laceration of an intercostal vessel, and pulmonary injury due to aspiration of a portion of lung into one of the tube drainage ports. The risk of lung perforation is related to the type of tube placed and underlying pleuropulmonary disease. If needle thoracentesis or ultrasonography suggests that the fluid is severely loculated or extensive adhesions are present, surgical placement of the chest tube may be advisable.

SPECIAL AGE CONSIDERATIONS

Surgical correction of respiratory abnormalities in young animals requires that special attention be paid to the anesthetic requirements of the young (see p. 658). Diaphragmatic hernia repair is commonly performed in young animals (see this page) as they are prone to trauma that may result in such lesions. Peritoneopericardial diaphragmatic hernias are usually diagnosed at a young age (i.e., less than 1 year of age) and concurrent cardiac abnormalities may be present, complicating the anesthetic management of these patients (see p. 685). Geriatric animals may have severe, concurrent underlying pulmonary or cardiac disease that complicates the management of pleural cavity disease in these patients. Careful monitoring is necessary.

Suggested Reading

Arizmendi F, Grimes JE, Relford RL: Isolation of *Chlamydia psittaci* from pleural effusion in a dog, *J Vet Diagnos Invest* 4:460, 1992.

Cantwell HD, Rebar AH, Allen AR: Pleural effusion in the dog; principles for diagnosis, *J Am Anim Hosp Assoc* 19:227, 1983.

Christopher MM: Pleural effusions, *Vet Clin North Am Small Anim Pract* 17:255, 1987.

Clinkenbeard KD: Diagnostic cytology: carcinomas in pleural effusions, *Compend Contin Educ Pract Vet* 14:187, 1992.

Forrester SD: The categories and causes of pleural effusion in cats, *Vet Med* 5:894, 1988.

Forrester SD, Troy GC, Fossum TW: Pleural effusions: pathophysiology and diagnostic considerations, *Compend Contin Educ Pract Vet* 10:121, 1988.

Fossum TW et al: Eosinophilic pleural or peritoneal effusions in dogs and cats: 14 cases (1986–1992), *J Am Vet Med Assoc* 202:1873, 1993.

Grogan DR et al: Complications associated with thoracentesis: a prospective, randomized study comparing three different methods, *Arch Intern Med* 150:873, 1990.

Gruffydd-Jones TJ, Flecknell PA: The prognosis and treatment related to the gross appearance and laboratory characteristics of pathological thoracic fluids in the cat, *J Small Anim Pract* 19:315, 1978.

LeBlanc KA, Tucker WY: Prophylactic antibiotics and closed tube thoracostomy, *Surg Gynecol Obstet* 160:259, 1985.

Lim-Levy F et al: Is milking and stripping chest tubes really necessary? *Ann Thorac Surg* 42:77, 1986.

Meyer DJ, Franks PT: Effusion: classification and cytologic examination, *Compend Contin Educ Pract Vet* 9:123, 1987.

Myer W: Radiography review: pleural effusion, *J Am Vet Radiol Soc* 19:75, 1978.

Rush JE, Hamlin RL: Effects of graded pleural effusion on QRS in the dog, *Am J Vet Res* 46:1887, 1985.

Snyder PS, Sato T, Atkins CE: The utility of thoracic radiographic measurement for the detection of cardiomegaly in cats with pleural effusion, *Vet Radiol* 31:89, 1990.

Steyn PF, Wittum TE: Radiographic, epidemiologic, and clinical aspects of simultaneous pleural and peritoneal effusions in dogs and cats: 48 cases (1982–1991), *J Am Vet Med Assoc* 202:307, 1993.

Stowater JL, Lamb CR: Ultrasonography of noncardiac thoracic diseases in small animals, *J Am Vet Med Assoc* 195:514, 1989.

SPECIFIC DISEASES

TRAUMATIC DIAPHRAGMATIC HERNIAS

DEFINITIONS

Diaphragmatic hernias (DH) occur when continuity of the diaphragm is disrupted such that abdominal organs can migrate into the thoracic cavity.

SYNONYMS

Pleuroperitoneal hernias

GENERAL CONSIDERATIONS AND CLINICALLY RELEVANT PATHOPHYSIOLOGY

DH are commonly recognized by small animal clinicians and may be congenital or occur following trauma. Congenital pleuroperitoneal hernias are seldom diagnosed in small animals because many affected animals die upon, or shortly after, birth. Most DH in dogs and cats are a result of trauma, particularly motor vehicle accidents. The abrupt increase in intraabdominal pressure that accompanies forceful blows to the abdominal wall causes the lungs to rapidly deflate (if the glottis is open), resulting in a large pleuroperitoneal pressure gradient. This pressure gradient causes the diaphragm to tear at its weakest points, generally in the muscular portions. The location and size of the tear(s) depend on the position of the animal at the time of impact and location of the viscera. Traumatic DH are often associated with significant respiratory embarrassment; however, chronic DH in asymptomatic animals are not uncommon.

DIAGNOSIS
Clinical Presentation

Signalment. There is no breed predisposition for traumatic DH; however, a majority of afflicted dogs are young males between 1 and 2 years of age.

History. The duration of DH may range from a few hours to years. In one report 20% were diagnosed greater than 4 weeks after injury (Boudrieau and Muir, 1987). The animals may be presented in shock following the injury (see below). These animals often suffer from associated injuries, such as fractures. With chronic DH, clinical signs are most often referable to either the respiratory or gastrointestinal systems and may include dyspnea, exercise intolerance, anorexia, depression, vomiting, diarrhea, weight loss, and/or pain following ingestion of food.

Physical Examination Findings

Animals with traumatic DH are frequently presented in shock; thus clinical signs may include pale or cyanotic mucous membranes, tachypnea, tachycardia, and/or oliguria. Cardiac arrhythmias are common and are associated with significant morbidity. Other clinical signs are dependent upon which organs herniate and may be attributed to the gastrointestinal, respiratory, or cardiovascular systems. The liver is the most common herniated organ and is often associated with hydrothorax due to entrapment and venous occlusion.

Radiography/Ultrasonography

Definitive diagnosis of pleuroperitoneal DH is via radiography or ultrasonography. Ultrasound examination of the diaphragmatic silhouette is helpful in animals in which the herniation is not obvious radiographically (i.e., hepatic herniation, pleural effusion). If significant pleural effusion is present, thoracentesis may be necessary for diagnostic radiographs. Radiographic signs of DH include loss of the diaphragmatic line, loss of the cardiac silhouette, dorsal or lateral displacement of lung fields, presence of gas or a barium-filled stomach or intestines in the thoracic cavity, and pleural effusion (Figs. 27-14 and 27-15). Positive-contrast celiography may occasionally be needed for the diagnosis. Prewarmed water-soluble contrast agent is injected into the abdominal cavity at a dosage of 1.1 ml/kg (dose is doubled if ascites is present), the patient is gently rolled from side to side or the pelvis is elevated, and films are taken immediately following the injection and manipulation. Criteria used in evaluating these films should include the presence of contrast medium in the pleural cavity, absence of a normal liver lobe outline in the abdomen, and incomplete visualization of the abdominal surface of the diaphragm.

Positive-contrast celiograms should be interpreted cautiously since omental and fibrous adhesions may seal the defect, resulting in false negative films.

☞ **N O T E ·** If hepatic herniation and/or pleural effusion are present, the most helpful diagnostic tool is usually ultrasonography.

Laboratory Findings

Specific laboratory abnormalities are uncommon. Serum alanine aminotransferase and serum alkaline phosphatase values may be elevated in cases of liver herniation.

DIFFERENTIAL DIAGNOSIS

Any disorder that causes respiratory abnormalities (i.e., pleural effusion, pneumothorax, pneumonia, etc.) should be a differential for traumatic DH. The concurrent presence of pleural effusion in many animals with liver herniation may make diagnosis of DH difficult (see above).

MEDICAL MANAGEMENT

If the animal is dyspneic, oxygen should be provided by face mask, nasal insufflation, or an oxygen cage. Positioning the animal in sternal recumbency with the forelimbs elevated may help ventilation. If moderate or severe pleural effusion is present, thoracentesis (see p. 677) should be performed. Fluid therapy and antibiotics should be given if the animal is in shock.

SURGICAL TREATMENT

Traumatic DH have a higher mortality when surgery is performed either less than 24 hours or greater than 1 year following the injury. Surgical repair of DH should be delayed until the patient has been stabilized; however, herniorrhaphy should not be unnecessarily delayed. Animals with

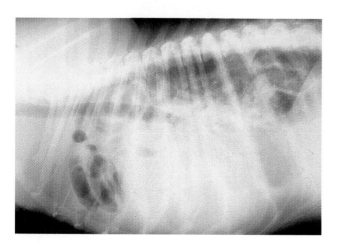

FIG. 27-14
Lateral thoracic radiograph of a dog with a diaphragmatic hernia. Note the air-filled intestinal loops in the thoracic cavity.

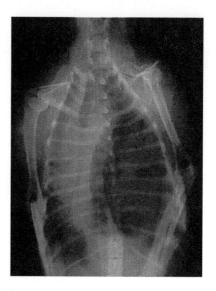

FIG. 27-15
Thoracic radiograph of a dog with a dilated, herniated stomach. (Courtesy H.P. Hobson, Texas A&M University.)

herniation of the stomach should be carefully evaluated for gastric distention and operated on as soon as they can safely be anesthetized because acute gastric distention within the thorax may cause rapid, fatal respiratory impairment.

☞ **N O T E** · Surgery should not be delayed unnecessarily in stable animals. Gastric herniation is a surgical emergency.

Preoperative Management

Prophylactic antibiotics should be given before anesthetic induction in animals with hepatic herniation. Massive release of toxins into the circulation may occur with hepatic strangulation or vascular compromise. Premedicating such patients with steroids may be beneficial. An ECG should be performed on all trauma patients before surgery.

Anesthesia

Chamber or mask induction should be avoided in animals with DH (see p. 676). Before induction, supplementing the inspired oxygen will improve myocardial oxygenation. Because of the animal's already compromised ventilation, drugs with minimal respiratory depressant effects should be used. Injectable anesthetics, which allow rapid intubation, are preferred (see also p. 676). Inhalation anesthetics should be used for anesthetic maintenance. Intermittent positive pressure ventilation should be performed and high inspiratory pressures avoided to help prevent reexpansion pulmonary edema (see p. 650). The lungs should be allowed to slowly expand after surgery. **Nitrous oxide is contraindicated in patients with DH (see p. 676).** Drugs such as methylprednisolone may be beneficial for preventing reexpansion pulmonary edema in animals with chronic DH. See Table 26-1 on p. 650 for examples of selected anesthetic protocols that may be used in animals with diaphragmatic hernias.

Positioning

The animal is placed in dorsal recumbency for a midline abdominal incision. The entire abdomen and caudal one half to two thirds of the thoracic cavity should be prepared for aseptic surgery. Acute ventilatory compromise may occur during positioning; thus these animals should be carefully monitored during this period.

SURGICAL TECHNIQUES

Make a ventral midline abdominal incision; if increased exposure is needed, extend the incision cranially through the sternum. Replace the abdominal organs in the abdominal cavity (if necessary, enlarge the diaphragmatic defect). If adhesions are present, dissect the tissues gently from thoracic structures to prevent pneumothorax or bleeding. With chronic hernias, debride the edge of the defect before closure. Close the diaphragmatic defect with a simple continuous suture pattern. If the diaphragm is avulsed from the ribs, incorporate a rib in the continuous suture for added strength (Fig. 27-16). Remove air from the pleural cavity

following closure of the defect. If continued pneumothorax or effusion is likely, place a chest tube (see p. 678). Explore the entire abdominal cavity for associated injury (i.e., compromise of the vasculature to the intestine, splenic, renal, or bladder trauma) and repair any defects.

☞ **N O T E** · If the diaphragmatic defect is particularly large, synthetic material such as Silastic sheeting can be used to close the defect. This is seldom necessary. An abdominal flap graft has been reported for repair of chronic DH in dogs. The graft is obtained from the peritoneum and transverse abdominal muscle caudal to the diaphragm. The graft is elevated, placed over the defect, and sutured to the diaphragm.

SUTURE MATERIALS/SPECIAL INSTRUMENTS

For diaphragmatic closure use either a nonabsorbable suture material such as polypropylene or an absorbable material such as polydioxanone (PDS) or polyglyconate (Maxon) suture.

POSTOPERATIVE CARE AND ASSESSMENT

Patients should be monitored postoperatively for hypoventilation and oxygen provided, if necessary. Reexpansion pulmonary edema (RPE) is a potential complication associated with rapid lung reexpansion following DH repair

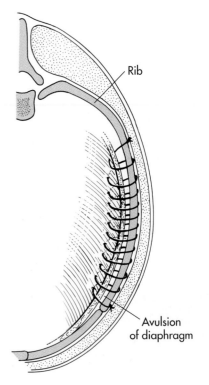

FIG. 27-16
To repair a diaphragm avulsed from the thoracic wall incorporate a rib in the suture line.

(see p. 650). Postoperative analgesics should be provided (see Table 26-3 on p. 650).

PROGNOSIS

If the animal survives the early postoperative period (i.e., 12 to 24 hours) the prognosis is excellent, and recurrence is uncommon with proper technique. Reported mortality rates for animals with traumatic DH have varied from 12% to 48%. Reported survival rates for animals with traumatic DH who are treated surgically are close to 75%.

Reference

Boudrieau RJ, Muir WW: Pathophysiology of traumatic diaphragmatic hernia in dogs, *Compend Contin Educ Pract Vet* 9:379, 1987.

Suggested Reading

Bednarski RM: Diaphragmatic hernia: anesthetic considerations, *Semin Vet Med Surg (Small Anim)* 1:256, 1986.

Cornell KK et al: Extrahepatic biliary obstruction secondary to diaphragmatic hernias in two cats, *J Am Anim Hosp Assoc* 29:502, 1993.

Downs MC, Bjorling DE: Traumatic diaphragmatic hernias: a review of 1674 cases, *Vet Surg* 16:87, 1987.

Fagin B: Using radiography to diagnose traumatic diaphragmatic hernia, *Vet Med* 6:662, 1989.

Helphrey ML: Abdominal flap graft for repair of chronic diaphragmatic hernia in the dog, *J Am Vet Med Assoc* 181:791, 1982.

Mann FA, Aronson E, Keller G: Surgical correction of a true congenital pleuroperitoneal diaphragmatic hernia in a cat, *J Am Anim Hosp Assoc* 27:501, 1991.

Stampley AR, Waldron DR: Reexpansion pulmonary edema after surgery to repair a diaphragmatic hernia in a cat, *J Am Vet Med Assoc* 203:1699, 1994.

Stickle RL: Positive-contrast celiography (peritoneography) for diagnosis of diaphragmatic hernia in dogs and cats, *J Am Vet Med Assoc* 185:295, 1984.

Valentine BA et al: Canine congenital diaphragmatic hernia, *J Vet Intern Med* 2:109, 1988.

Willard MD, Toal RL, Cawley A: Gastric complications associated with correction of chronic diaphragmatic hernia in two dogs, *J Am Vet Med Assoc* 184:1151, 1984.

Wilson GPI, Hayes HMJ: Diaphragmatic hernia in the dog and cat: a 25 year overview, *Semin Vet Med Surg (Small Anim)* 1:318, 1986.

Wilson GPI, Newton CD, Burt JK: A review of 116 diaphragmatic hernias in dogs and cats, *J Am Vet Med Assoc* 159:1142, 1971.

PERITONEOPERICARDIAL DIAPHRAGMATIC HERNIAS

DEFINITIONS

Peritoneopericardial diaphragmatic hernias (PPDH) occur when there is a congenital communication between the abdomen and the pericardial sac.

SYNONYMS

Pericardial diaphragmatic hernias, congenital hernias

GENERAL CONSIDERATIONS AND CLINICALLY RELEVANT PATHOPHYSIOLOGY

PPDH are less commonly recognized by small animal clinicians than are traumatic diaphragmatic hernias. Although they are often associated with respiratory embarrassment, asymptomatic PPDH is common. PPDH may arise in human beings due to trauma (the diaphragm forms one wall of the pericardial sac in human beings); however, they are always congenital in dogs and cats because there is no direct communication between the pericardial and peritoneal cavities after birth. The most widely accepted theory regarding the embryogenesis of this defect is that the hernia arises because of faulty development or prenatal injury of the septum transversum. This could be a result of a teratogen, genetic defect, or prenatal injury.

Cardiac abnormalities and sternal deformities often occur concomitantly with PPDH. The combination of congenital cranial abdominal wall, caudal sternal, diaphragmatic, and pericardial defects has been reported in dogs, often associated with ventricular septal defects or other intracardiac defects (Fig. 27-17). It is not known whether this condition is heritable; however, several breed predispositions have been recognized (see below). Polycystic kidneys have been reported in association with PPDH in cats.

☞ **N O T E** · Cranial abdominal wall defects may be a tip-off that the animal has a PPDH.

DIAGNOSIS
Clinical Presentation

Signalment. Although PPDH are congenital, it is not uncommon for the diagnosis to be made when the animal is middle-aged or older because clinical signs are variable and

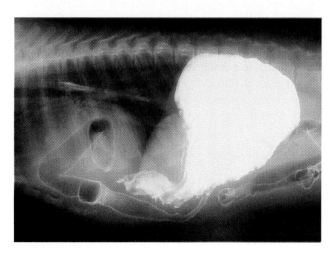

FIG. 27-17
Lateral thoracic radiograph of a dog with a peritoneopericardial diaphragmatic hernia. Note the cranial abdominal hernia.

may be intermittent. Weimaraners and cocker spaniels may be at increased risk.

History. Clinical signs may be referable to the gastrointestinal, cardiac, or respiratory systems and include anorexia, depression, vomiting, diarrhea, weight loss, wheezing, dyspnea, exercise intolerance, and/or pain following ingestion of food. Neurologic signs may occur due to hepatoencephalopathy.

Physical Examination Findings

Physical examination findings in animals with PPDH may include ascites, muffled heart sounds, murmurs due to displacement of the heart by visceral organs or due to intracardiac defects, and concurrent ventral abdominal wall defects. The most commonly herniated organ is the liver, and associated pericardial effusion is common.

Radiography/Ultrasonography

A tentative diagnosis of PPDH may be made based on history, clinical signs, and physical examination, but radiography and/or ultrasonography are essential for a definitive diagnosis. Radiographic signs of PPDH are presented in Table 27-6 (Fig. 27-18). Contrast studies (i.e., nonselective angiogram, barium contrast study) should only be undertaken if a definitive diagnosis cannot be made on plain films (Fig. 27-19) or with ultrasound. A distinct curvilinear radiopacity has been identified between the cardiac silhouette and the diaphragm on a lateral thoracic radiograph in cats with PPDH. This radiographic finding has been termed the *dorsal peritoneopericardial mesothelial remnant* (Berry et al, 1990). Ultrasonography is useful because there is often discontinuity of the diaphragmatic outline. Hepatic herniation is usually evident.

Laboratory Findings

Specific laboratory abnormalities are uncommon.

DIFFERENTIAL DIAGNOSIS

The most common differentials for PPDH are pericardial effusion and cardiomegaly. Ultrasound and echocardiography are useful to distinguish these abnormalities from PPDH.

MEDICAL MANAGEMENT

If the animal is dyspneic, oxygen should be provided by face mask, nasal insufflation, or an oxygen cage. Positioning the animal in sternal recumbency with the forelimbs elevated may help ventilation.

TABLE 27-6
Radiographic Signs of PPDH
• Enlarged cardiac silhouette
• Dorsal elevation of the trachea
• Overlap of the heart and diaphragmatic borders
• Discontinuity of the diaphragm
• Gas-filled structures in the pericardial sac
• Sternal defects
• Dorsal peritoneopericardial mesothelial remnant

SURGICAL TREATMENT

Surgical repair should be performed as early as possible (generally when the animal is between 8 and 16 weeks of age) when it is unlikely that adhesions will be present and the pliable nature of the skin, muscles, sternum, and rib cage facilitates closure of large defects. Early correction of PPDH may prevent acute decompensation and the potential development of acute postoperative pulmonary edema (see below).

PREOPERATIVE MANAGEMENT

Prophylactic antibiotics should be given before anesthetic induction in animals with hepatic herniation. Upon repositioning of the liver into the abdominal cavity of animals with hepatic strangulation or vascular compromise, a massive release of toxins into the bloodstream may occur. Premedicating such patients with steroids may be beneficial.

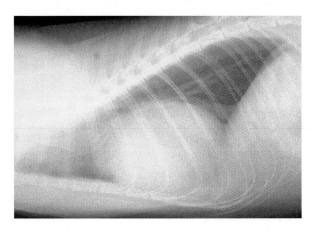

FIG. 27-18
Lateral thoracic radiograph of a cat with peritoneopericardial diaphragmatic hernia. Note the large, globoid appearance of the cardiac silhouette.

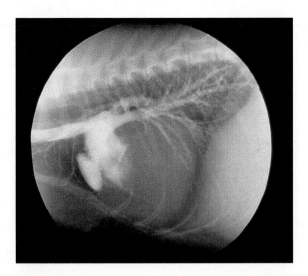

FIG. 27-19
Nonselective angiogram in a cat with a peritoneopericardial diaphragmatic hernia. Note the size of the heart in comparison to the cardiac silhouette. The liver is within the pericardial sac. (Courtesy M. Miller, Texas A&M University.)

ANESTHESIA

Chamber or mask induction should be avoided in animals with PPDH (see p. 676). Before induction, supplementing the inspired oxygen will improve myocardial oxygenation. If the animal's ventilation is already compromised, drugs with minimal respiratory depressant effects should be used. Injectable anesthetics that allow rapid intubation are preferred (see also p. 676). Inhalation anesthetics should be used for anesthetic maintenance. Intermittent positive pressure ventilation should be performed; however, high ventilatory pressures should be avoided to help prevent reexpansion pulmonary edema (see p. 650). The lungs should be allowed to slowly expand after surgery. **Nitrous oxide is contraindicated in patients with diaphragmatic hernia (see p. 676).** Drugs such as methylprednisolone may be beneficial in animals with chronic diaphragmatic hernias. See Table 26-1 on p. 650 for examples of selected anesthetic protocols that may be used in animals with diaphragmatic hernias.

POSITIONING

The animal is placed in dorsal recumbency for a midline abdominal incision. The entire abdomen and caudal two thirds of the thoracic cavity should be prepared for aseptic surgery.

SURGICAL TECHNIQUES

Make a ventral midline abdominal incision. If increased exposure is needed, extend the incision cranially through the sternum. Enlarge the diaphragmatic defect if necessary, and replace the abdominal organs in the abdominal cavity. If adhesions are present, gently dissect the tissues from thoracic structures, resecting or debriding necrotic tissue as necessary. Debride the edges of the defect and close with a simple continuous suture pattern. Do not close the pericardial sac. Remove air from the pericardial sac and/or pleural cavity following closure of the defect. If continued pneumothorax or effusion is likely, place a chest tube (see p. 678). Repair concomitant sternal or abdominal wall defects.

SUTURE MATERIALS/SPECIAL INSTRUMENTS

For diaphragmatic closure use either a nonabsorbable suture material such as polypropylene or an absorbable material such as polydioxanone (PDS) or polyglyconate (Maxon) suture.

POSTOPERATIVE CARE AND ASSESSMENT

These patients should be monitored postoperatively for hypoventilation and oxygen provided, if necessary. Reexpansion pulmonary edema (RPE) is a potential complication associated with rapid lung reexpansion following diaphragmatic hernia repair (see p. 650). Pulmonary hypoplasia may be present in patients with PPDH, contributing to the development of high intrapleural pressures and RPE. Postoperative analgesics should be provided (see Table 27-22).

PROGNOSIS

If the animal survives the early postoperative period (i.e., 12 to 24 hours) the prognosis is excellent and recurrence is uncommon with proper technique. The prognosis is worse in patients with PPDH who have concurrent cardiac abnormalities.

Reference

Berry CR, Koblik PD, Ticer JW: Dorsal peritoneopericardial mesothelial remnant as an aid to the diagnosis of feline congenital peritoneopericardial diaphragmatic hernia, *Vet Radiol* 31:239, 1990.

Suggested Reading

Bednarski RM: Diaphragmatic hernia: anesthetic considerations, *Semin Vet Med Surg (Small Anim)* 1:256, 1986.

Bellah JR et al: Surgical correction of concomitant cranioventral abdominal wall, caudal sternal, diaphragmatic, and pericardial defects in young dogs, *J Am Vet Med Assoc* 195:1722, 1989.

Evans SE, Biery DN: Congenital peritoneopericardial diaphragmatic hernia in the dog and cat: a literature review and 17 additional case histories, *Vet Radiol* 21:108, 1980.

Hay WH, Woodfield JA, Moon MA: Clinical, echocardiographic, and radiographic findings of peritoneopericardial diaphragmatic hernia in two dogs and a cat, *J Am Vet Med Assoc* 195:1245, 1989.

Kerpsack SJ et al: Chylothorax associated with lung lobe torsion and a peritoneopericardial diaphragmatic hernia in a cat, *J Am Anim Hosp Assoc* 30:351, 1994.

Lunney J: Congenital peritoneal pericardial diaphragmatic hernia and portocaval shunt in a cat, *J Am Anim Hosp Assoc* 28:163, 1992.

Schuh JCL: Hepatic nodular myelolipomatosis (myelolipomas) associated with a peritoneopericardial diaphragmatic hernia in a cat, *J Comp Pathol* 97:231, 1987.

Schulman AJ et al: Congenital peritoneopericardial diaphragmatic hernia in a dog, *J Am Anim Hosp Assoc* 21:655, 1985.

Wallace J, Mullen HS, Lesser MA: A technique for surgical correction of peritoneal pericardial diaphragmatic hernia in dogs and cats, *J Am Anim Hosp Assoc* 28:503, 1992.

Willard MD, Aronson E: Peritoneopericardial diaphragmatic hernia in a cat, *J Am Vet Med Assoc* 178:481, 1981.

Wright RP, Wright R, Scott R: Surgical repair of a congenital pericardial diaphragmatic hernia, *Vet Med* 3:618, 1987.

PNEUMOTHORAX

DEFINITIONS

Pneumothorax is an accumulation of air or gas within the pleural space. Traumatic pneumothorax may be classified either as "open" or "closed." An **open pneumothorax** is one in which there is free communication between the pleural space and the external environment. With a **closed pneumothorax,** air accumulates due to leakage from the pulmonary parenchyma, bronchial tree, or esophagus. A **tension pneumothorax** occurs when a flap of tissue acts as a one-way valve so that there is a continuous influx of air into the pleural cavity on inspiration that does not return to the lung on expiration. **Spontaneous pneumothorax** occurs due to air leakage from the lung, but without trauma as a precipitating cause. **Cysts** are closed cavities or sacs lined by epithelium and are usually filled with fluid or semisolid material. **Bullae** are nonepithelialized cavities produced by disruption of intraalveolar septa. A **bleb** is a localized collection of air that is contained within the visceral pleura.

SYNONYMS

For nontraumatic pneumothorax the terms **spontaneous** and **idiopathic** have been used interchangeably.

GENERAL CONSIDERATIONS AND CLINICALLY RELEVANT PATHOPHYSIOLOGY

Traumatic pneumothorax is the most frequent type of pneumothorax in dogs. It most often occurs due to blunt trauma (i.e., vehicular accidents, being kicked by a horse), which causes parenchymal pulmonary damage to the lung and a closed pneumothorax. When the thorax is forcefully compressed against a closed glottis, rupture of the lung or bronchial tree may occur. Alternately, pulmonary parenchyma may be torn due to shearing forces on the lung. Pulmonary trauma occasionally results in subpleural bleb formation, similar to those seen with spontaneous pneumothorax (see below and Fig. 27-20). Open pneumothorax is less common, but is also frequently due to trauma (i.e., gunshot, bite or stab wounds, lacerations secondary to rib fractures). Some penetrating injuries are called "sucking chest wounds" because large defects in the chest wall allow an influx of air into the pleural space when the animal inspires. These large, open chest wounds may allow enough air to enter the pleural space that lung collapse and marked reduction in ventilation occur. There is a rapid equilibration of atmospheric and intrapleural pressure through the defect, interfering with normal mechanical function of the thoracic bellows, which normally provides the necessary pressure gradient for air exchange. Pneumomediastinum may be associated with pneumothorax, tracheal, bronchial, or esophageal defects, or may be due to subcutaneous air migration along fascial planes at the thoracic inlet.

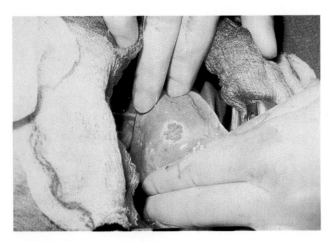

FIG. 27-20
Ruptured subpleural bleb in a dog with spontaneous pneumothorax.

Spontaneous pneumothorax occurs in previously healthy animals without antecedent trauma and may be primary (i.e., an absence of underlying pulmonary disease) or secondary (underlying disease such as pulmonary abscesses, neoplasia, chronic granulomatous infections, pulmonary parasites such as *Paragonimus,* or pneumonia is present). Based on the histologic appearance of the pulmonary lesion, both cysts and bullae have been reported in dogs. Primary spontaneous pneumothorax in dogs may be due to rupture of subpleural blebs—remaining lung tissue may appear normal. These blebs are most commonly located in the apices of the lungs. Secondary spontaneous pneumothorax is more common in dogs than the primary form. In these animals, the subpleural blebs are associated with diffuse emphysema or other pulmonary lesions. It has been shown that volume strain from expansive pressure within the lung increases disproportionately at the apex as height increases. A majority of affected humans are cigarette smokers, suggesting that the underlying pulmonary disease could be a result of interference of the normal function of alpha-1-antitrypsin in inhibiting elastase. It is believed that alpha-1-antitrypsin is inactivated in people who smoke, allowing increased elastase-induced destruction of pulmonary parenchyma.

☞ **N O T E** • Traumatic and spontaneous pneumothorax must be differentiated because the former usually responds to medical management while the latter requires surgery.

DIAGNOSIS
Clinical Presentation

Signalment. Traumatic pneumothorax is most common in young dogs because they are more likely to be hit by cars or to receive other trauma resulting in pulmonary damage. For similar reasons, males may be more commonly affected than females. Traumatic pneumothorax is less common in cats. Spontaneous pneumothorax usually occurs in large and "deep-chested" breeds; however, it may occur in small dogs. Dogs of any age may develop spontaneous pneumothorax: in one study the average age was 6.3 years (range 1 to 13 years) (Holtsinger et al, 1993). Male and female dogs appear to be equally affected.

History. Pneumothorax secondary to trauma usually results in acute dyspnea. The history of trauma is often unknown, making the differentiation between traumatic and spontaneous pneumothorax difficult. Although the history of dogs with spontaneous pneumothorax varies depending on underlying etiology, most animals present with an acute history of dyspnea. Occasionally a chronic cough or fever may be noted. Recurrence of dyspnea in an animal previously treated for pneumothorax suggests spontaneous rather than traumatic pneumothorax.

Physical Examination Findings

Most animals with pneumothorax have bilateral disease and present with an acute onset of severe dyspnea. Other evidence of trauma (i.e., rib fractures, limb fractures, traumatic myocarditis, pulmonary contusions) may be evident in animals with trauma-induced pneumothorax. Most animals with pneumothorax exhibit a restrictive respiratory pattern (i.e., rapid, shallow respirations). If hypoventilation causes hypoxemia they may appear cyanotic, and the heart and lung sounds are often muffled dorsally. Dogs are able to tolerate massive pneumothorax by increasing their chest expansion. Respiration becomes ineffectual in animals with tension pneumothorax as the chest becomes barrel-shaped and fixed in maximal extension. This condition is life-threatening. Subcutaneous emphysema will occasionally be noted in animals with pneumomediastinum and pneumothorax. The air may migrate from the mediastinal space to the thoracic inlet and be noticeable under the skin over the neck and trunk.

☞ **NOTE** · Tension pneumothorax is a life-threatening emergency. It must be recognized and treated promptly.

Radiography/Ultrasonography

Thoracic radiographs should be delayed until after thoracentesis in dyspneic animals (see p. 692). Pneumothorax usually occurs bilaterally in animals since air diffuses through the thin mediastinum. Pneumothorax results in large air-filled spaces within the pleural cavity. The most sensitive view is a horizontal-beam, laterally recumbent thoracic radiograph. On a recumbent lateral thoracic radiograph the lungs collapse and retract from the chest wall and the heart usually appears to be elevated from the sternum (Fig. 27-21). This apparent elevation of the heart is not noticeable on a standing lateral radiograph. Partially collapsed or atelectatic lung lobes appear radiopaque when compared to the air-filled pleural space. The vascular pattern will not extend to the chest wall as the lungs collapse. This may be particularly noticeable in the caudal thorax on a ventrodorsal view.

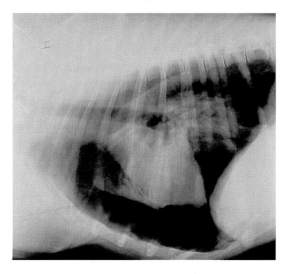

FIG. 27-21
Lateral thoracic radiograph of a dog with pneumothorax. Note the apparent elevation of the heart from the sternum.

Radiographs should be carefully evaluated for underlying pulmonary disease (i.e., abscess, neoplasia) or associated trauma (i.e., rib fractures, pulmonary contusion). Pulmonary blebs found in some animals with spontaneous pneumothorax are seldom visible radiographically. This is probably because the large blebs have ruptured, causing the pneumothorax. In such cases, surgical identification of bullae is necessary. Air-filled bullae may be incidental findings on thoracic radiographs of some animals. Pneumomediastinum is characterized by the ability to visualize thoracic structures (i.e., aorta, thoracic trachea, vena cava, esophagus) that are not usually apparent on thoracic radiographs.

☞ **NOTE** · Remember that bullae are seldom seen in dogs with pneumothorax because they may have already ruptured. Additionally, air in the thoracic cavity may make other (nonruptured) bullae difficult to visualize.

Laboratory Findings

Specific laboratory abnormalities are uncommon in animals with pneumothorax; however, blood gas derangements may occur.

DIFFERENTIAL DIAGNOSIS

Any abnormality that causes respiratory distress (i.e., diaphragmatic hernia, pleural effusion, pulmonary edema) should be considered a differential diagnosis for pneumothorax. Thoracic radiographs usually adequately identify the presence of free pleural air; however, if the diagnosis is uncertain, diagnostic thoracentesis should allow retrieval of air. Because the management of animals with primary and spontaneous pneumothorax differs, once the animal has been stabilized, the cause of pneumothorax should be determined.

MEDICAL MANAGEMENT

Medical management of an animal with pneumothorax consists of initially relieving dyspnea by thoracentesis (see p. 677). If the pleural air accumulates quickly or cannot be effectively managed with needle thoracentesis, a chest tube should be placed (see p. 678). Tube thoracostomy is typically required in animals with spontaneous pneumothorax. Intermittent or continuous pleural drainage may be used, depending on the speed with which air accumulates. Continuous drainage may cause quicker resolution of pneumothorax in animals with large, traumatic defects. Providing an enriched oxygen environment may be beneficial, particularly in animals with concurrent pulmonary trauma (e.g., pulmonary contusion/hemorrhage). Providing analgesics to animals with fractured ribs or severe soft tissue damage may improve ventilation (see p. 649). **Surgical intervention is seldom required in animals with traumatic pneumothorax.** Thoracentesis should be performed as necessary to prevent dyspnea while the pulmonary lesion heals, usually within 3 to 5 days. Recurrence is uncommon. Conversely, animals with spontaneous pneumothorax commonly have recurrent pneumothorax if they are not operated on.

An open chest wound should be covered immediately with any readily available material. A sterile occlusive dressing should be applied as soon as possible and intrapleural air evacuated by thoracentesis or tube thoracostomy.

SURGICAL TREATMENT

Surgical therapy of animals with traumatic pneumothorax is seldom necessary (see above). However, nonsurgical management of spontaneous pneumothorax usually results in a less than satisfactory outcome. Mechanical pleurodesis of the lungs (see below) may decrease the recurrence of pneumothorax in animals operated for spontaneous pneumothorax. Mechanical pleurodesis damages the pleura such that healing results in adherence to the visceral and parietal pleura. Postoperative pneumothorax or pleural effusion must then be prevented as they will result in separation of the parietal and visceral pleura, precluding adhesion formation.

Preoperative Management

An ECG and thoracentesis should be performed prior to anesthetic induction. Preoxygenating these animals is often beneficial (see p. 649). Perioperative antibiotics are seldom warranted and may prevent culturing bacteria from infected pulmonary tissue during surgery.

Anesthesia

Care should be used when anesthetizing and ventilating animals with pneumothorax and/or pulmonary bullae. Intermittent positive pressure ventilation (IPPV) may rupture intact bullae or accelerate air leakage from the damaged lung or bronchial tree. Therefore, do not exceed inspiratory pressures of 10 to 12 cm H_2O pressure in these animals until the chest cavity is opened. The adequacy of ventilatory pressures should then be reevaluated. Because IPPV may induce a tension pneumothorax, immediate treatment of this condition (i.e., needle thoracentesis, chest tube placement) may be necessary and should be anticipated. **The use of nitrous oxide is contraindicated in patients with pneumothorax.** See p. 650 for selected anesthetic protocols for use in animals with respiratory dysfunction.

Surgical Anatomy

Refer to surgical anatomy of the pleural space on p. 676 and the anatomical description of the lungs in dogs and cats on p. 651.

Positioning

See intercostal thoracotomy on p. 652 or median sternotomy on p. 654.

SURGICAL TECHNIQUES

If an underlying pulmonary lesion is readily identified (i.e., pulmonary abscess or neoplasia) and can be localized to one hemithorax, an intercostal thoracotomy (see p. 652) allows lobectomy to be performed more readily than from a median sternotomy approach. However, diffuse, bilateral pulmonary disease with multiple bullae is usually present in dogs with spontaneous pneumothorax. A median sternotomy allows

visualization of all lung lobes, in addition to partial resection of any diseased lobes (see p. 654). Mechanical pleurodesis should be performed in dogs with spontaneous pneumothorax to decrease recurrence (see below).

Identify and remove diseased lung. If the source of the pleural air is not evident, fill the chest with warmed, sterile saline or water and look for air bubbles when the anesthetist ventilates the animal. If multiple, partial lobectomies are necessary, use an automatic stapling device to decrease operative time. Perform pleural abrasion using a dry gauze sponge. Gently abrade the entire surface of the lung and parietal pleura. Before closure, fill the chest cavity with warmed fluid and look for air bubbles when the animal is ventilated to ensure that there are no further air leaks. Place a chest tube and remove residual air before recovering the animal. Postoperatively, if continuous air leakage is present, or pleural effusion develops, place the animal on a continuous suction device (see p. 680).

In animals with an open pneumothorax, definitive closure of large thoracic wall defects may require mobilization of adjacent muscles in order to provide an airtight closure.

SUTURE MATERIALS/SPECIAL INSTRUMENTS

In animals with spontaneous pneumothorax (where multiple pulmonary bullae may be present), stapling devices allow partial lobectomies to be performed rapidly (see p. 655). Continuous suction devices are available commercially or three-bottle systems can be made (see p. 680).

POSTOPERATIVE CARE AND ASSESSMENT

The animal should be observed postoperatively for pain and/or hypoventilation. Nasal insufflation is beneficial in most patients, but is especially indicated in those with diffuse underlying pulmonary diseases or those in which significant portions of the lung were resected. Analgesic therapy should be considered in all animals undergoing thoracotomy (see p. 649).

PROGNOSIS

With appropriate monitoring and care, the prognosis is excellent for animals with traumatic pneumothorax in which therapy is initiated before extreme dyspnea or respiratory arrest. In a recent study of dogs with spontaneous pneumothorax, 100% of those treated with needle thoracentesis alone and 81% of those managed with chest tubes had recurrence of pneumothorax (Holtsinger et al, 1993). The times until recurrence varied from 3 days to 30 months. Three of 12 dogs (25%) undergoing thoracotomy suffered recurrence; only one of these dogs had intraoperative pleural abrasion performed.

Reference

Holtsinger RH et al: Spontaneous pneumothorax in the dog; a retrospective analysis of 21 cases, *J Am Anim Hosp Assoc* 29:195, 1993.

Suggested Reading

Aron DN, Kornegay JN: The clinical significance of traumatic lung cysts and associated pulmonary abnormalities in the dog and cat, *J Am Anim Hosp Assoc* 19:903, 1983.

Barber DL, Hill BL: Traumatically induced bullous lung lesions in the dog: a radiographic report of three cases, *J Am Vet Med Assoc* 169:1085, 1976.

Berkwitt L, Berzon JL: Thoracic trauma, *Vet Clin North Am Small Anim Pract* 15:1031, 1985.

Boudrieau RJ, Fossum TW, Birchard SJ: Surgical correction of primary pneumothorax in a dog, *J Am Vet Med Assoc* 186:75, 1985.

Dallman MJ, Martin RA, Roth L: Pneumothorax as the primary problem in two cases of bronchioloalveolar carcinoma in the dog, *J Am Anim Hosp Assoc* 24:710, 1988.

Holtsinger RH, Ellison GW: Spontaneous pneumothorax, *Comp Cont Educ Pract Vet* 17:197, 1995.

Kramek BA, Caywood DD: Pneumothorax, *Vet Clin North Am Small Anim Pract* 17:285, 1987.

Rochat MC et al: Paragonimiasis in dogs and cats, *Comp Cont Educ Pract Vet* 12:1093, 1990.

Schaer M, Gamble D, Spencer C: Spontaneous pneumothorax associated with bacterial pneumonia in the dog—two case reports, *J Am Anim Hosp Assoc* 17:783, 1981.

Yoshioka MM: Management of spontaneous pneumothorax in twelve dogs, *J Am Anim Hosp Assoc* 18:57, 1982.

CHYLOTHORAX

DEFINITIONS

Chyle is the term used to denote lymphatic fluid arising from the intestine and therefore containing a high quantity of fat. **Chylothorax** is a collection of chyle in the pleural space.

GENERAL CONSIDERATIONS AND CLINICALLY RELEVANT PATHOPHYSIOLOGY

In most animals, abnormal flow or pressures within the thoracic duct (TD) are thought to lead to exudation of chyle from intact, but dilated, thoracic lymphatic vessels (known as thoracic lymphangiectasia; Fig. 27-22). These dilated lymphatic vessels may form in response to increased lymphatic flow (due to increased hepatic lymph formation), decreased lymphatic drainage into the venous system due to high venous pressures, or both factors acting simultaneously to increase lymph flows and decrease drainage. Any disease or process that increases systemic venous pressures (i.e., right heart failure, mediastinal neoplasia, cranial vena cava thrombi, or granulomas) may cause chylothorax (Table 27-7). Trauma is an uncommonly recognized cause of chylothorax in dogs and cats because the TD heals rapidly following injury and within 1 to 2 weeks the effusion resolves without treatment.

Possible causes of chylothorax include anterior mediastinal masses (mediastinal lymphosarcoma, thymoma), heart disease (cardiomyopathy, pericardial effusion, heartworm infection, foreign objects, tetralogy of Fallot, tricuspid dys-

plasia, or cor triatriatum dexter), fungal granulomas, venous thrombi, and congenital abnormalities of the TD. It may occur in association with diffuse lymphatic abnormalities including intestinal lymphangiectasia and generalized lymphangiectasia with subcutaneous chyle leakage. In a majority of animals, despite extensive diagnostic workups, the underlying etiology is undetermined (idiopathic chylothorax). Because the treatment of this disease varies considerably depending on underlying etiology, it is imperative that clinicians identify concurrent disease processes prior to instituting definitive therapy.

DIAGNOSIS
Clinical Presentation

Signalment. Any breed dog or cat may be affected; however, a breed predisposition has been suspected in the Afghan hound for a number of years. Recently, it has been suggested that the Shiba Inu breed may also be predisposed to this disease. Among cats, Oriental breeds (i.e., Siamese and Himalayan) appear to have an increased prevalence. Chylothorax may affect animals of any age; however, in one study

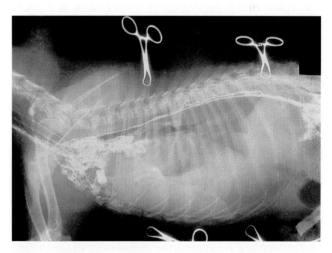

FIG. 27-22
Thoracic lymphangiectasia in a dog with idiopathic chylothorax. Note the dilated, tortuous lymphatics in the cranial mediastinum.

TABLE 27-7

Abnormalities Associated with Chylothorax in Dogs and/or Cats

- Cardiomyopathy
- Mediastinal lymphosarcoma or thymoma
- Cranial vena cava thrombi
- Heartworm disease
- Fungal granulomas
- Pericardial effusion/heart base tumors
- Foreign objects
- Tetralogy of Fallot
- Tricuspid dysplasia
- Cor triatriatum dexter
- Congenital TD abnormalities
- Lymphangioleiomyomatosis

older cats were more likely to develop chylothorax than were young cats (Fossum, 1991). This finding was believed to indicate an association between chylothorax and neoplasia. While Afghan hounds appear to develop this disease when middle-aged, affected Shiba Inus have been less than 1 year old. A sex predisposition has not been identified.

History. Coughing is often the first (and occasionally the only) abnormality noted by owners until the animal becomes dyspneic. Many owners report that they first noticed coughing months prior to presenting the animal for veterinary care; therefore, animals that cough and do not respond to standard treatment of nonspecific respiratory problems should be evaluated for chylothorax. Coughing may be a result of irritation caused by the effusion, or may be related to the underlying disease process (i.e., cardiomyopathy, thoracic neoplasia).

☞ **N O T E ·** Coughing may be the only clinical sign. Chest radiographs are warranted in any animal that presents with a chronic, nonresponsive cough.

Physical Examination Findings

The most common physical examination finding in animals with pleural effusion is dyspnea. The dyspnea may be marked by a forceful inspiration with delayed expiration, making the animal appear to be holding its breath. This respiratory pattern is particularly noticeable in cats. Increased bronchovesicular sounds may be heard dorsally. Lung sounds may be absent ventrally (usually bilaterally, but occasionally unilaterally). Most animals with chylothorax present with a normal body temperature, unless extremely excited or severely depressed. Additional findings in patients with chylothorax may include muffled heart sounds, depression, anorexia, weight loss, pale mucous membranes, arrhythmias, murmurs, and pericardial effusion.

Radiography/Ultrasonography

If the animal is not overtly dyspneic, thoracic radiographs should be taken to confirm the diagnosis of pleural fluid. Taking dorsoventral (rather than ventrodorsal views) and

"standing lateral" radiographic views, minimizing handling, and supplementing oxygen by face mask during the radiographic procedures may help prevent further compromise of respiration. If the animal is not dyspneic and only small amounts of fluid are suspected, ventrodorsal and expiratory views may help delineate the effusion. Radiographic signs associated with pleural effusion include blurring of the cardiac silhouette, interlobar fissure lines, rounding of lung margins at the costophrenic angles, widening of the mediastinum, separation of the lung borders from the thoracic wall, and scalloping of the lung margins at the sternal border (Figs. 27-23 and 27-24). The latter may be the earliest radiographic sign of pleural effusion.

☞ **N O T E ·** Delay thoracic radiographs until after thoracentesis in animals with pleural effusion that are severely dyspneic.

Ultrasonography should be performed before fluid removal because the fluid acts as an "acoustic window" enhancing visualization of thoracic structures. Ultrasonography is used to evaluate cardiac function, valvular lesions and function, congenital cardiac abnormalities, the presence of pericardial effusion, and mediastinal masses. The presence of pleural fluid will often prevent satisfactory radiographic evaluation of the structures of the thoracic cavity. Since adequate visualization of the entire thorax is necessary to rule

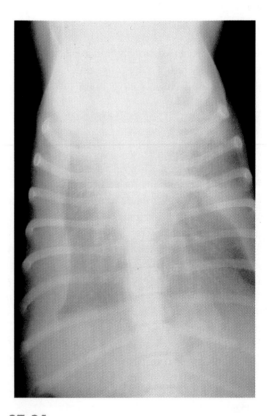

FIG. 27-24
Dorsoventral thoracic radiograph of a dog with pleural effusion. Note the interlobar fissure lines, rounding of lung margins at the costophrenic angles, and separation of the lung borders from the thoracic wall.

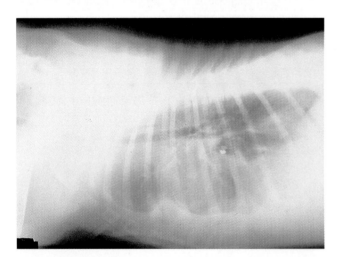

FIG. 27-23
Lateral thoracic radiograph of dog with pleural effusion. Note the scalloped appearance of the sternal border.

out anterior mediastinal masses such as lymphosarcoma or thymoma, radiographs should be repeated following removal of most of the pleural fluid.

Animals that have collapsed lung lobes that do not appear to reexpand following removal of pleural fluid should be suspected of having underlying pulmonary parenchymal or pleural disease, such as fibrosing pleuritis (Fig. 27-25). Although the etiology of the fibrosis is unknown, it apparently can occur subsequent to any prolonged exudative or blood-stained effusion. Diagnosis of fibrosing pleuritis is difficult. The atelectic lobes may be confused with metastatic or primary pulmonary neoplasia, lung lobe torsion, or hilar lymphadenopathy. Radiographic evidence of pulmonary parenchyma that fails to reexpand after removal of pleural fluid should be considered possible evidence of atelectasis with associated fibrosis. Fibrosing pleuritis should also be considered in animals with persistent dyspnea in the face of minimal pleural fluid.

Laboratory Findings

Fluid recovered by thoracentesis should be placed in an EDTA tube for cytologic examination. Placing the fluid in an EDTA tube rather than a "clot-tube" will allow cell counts to be performed. Although chylous effusions are routinely classified as exudates, the physical characteristics of the fluid may be consistent with a modified transudate (Table 27-8). The color varies depending on dietary fat content and the presence of concurrent hemorrhage. The protein content is variable and often inaccurate due to interference of the refractive index by the high lipid content of the fluid. The total

nucleated cell count is usually less than 10,000 and consists primarily of small lymphocytes or neutrophils, with lesser numbers of lipid-laden macrophages.

Chronic chylous effusions may contain low numbers of small lymphocytes due to the inability of the body to compensate for continued lymphocyte loss. Nondegenerative neutrophils may predominate with prolonged loss of lymphocytes or if multiple therapeutic thoracenteses have induced inflammation. Degenerative neutrophils and sepsis are uncommon findings due to the bacteriostatic effect of fatty acids but can occur iatrogenically due to repeated aspirations. To help determine if a pleural effusion is truly chylous, several tests can be performed including comparison of fluid and serum triglyceride levels; Sudan III stain for lipid droplets; and the ether clearance test. The most diagnostic test is comparison of serum and fluid triglyceride levels (Table 27-9). **If the effusion is truly chylous it will contain a higher concentration of triglycerides than simultaneously collected serum.**

DIFFERENTIAL DIAGNOSIS

Any cause of respiratory distress or coughing should be considered a differential diagnosis. Once pleural effusion has been identified, differentials include diseases causing exudative pleural effusion, such as pyothorax. Although chylous effusions have a characteristic appearance, the physical characteristics of chylous effusions and other exudative effusions may be similar. Additionally, the appearance and cell populations of chylous effusions can be altered by diet and chronicity.

Pseudochylous effusion is a term that has been misused in the veterinary literature to describe effusions that look like chyle, but in which a ruptured TD is not found. Given the

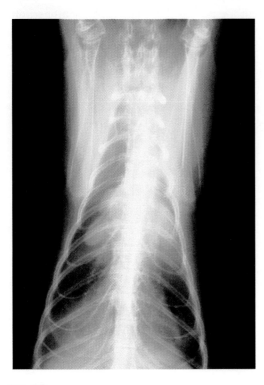

FIG. 27-25
Thoracic radiograph of a cat with fibrosing pleuritis secondary to chronic chylothorax. Note the rounded appearance of the lung lobes.

TABLE 27-8

Characteristics of Chylous Effusions

Characteristic	Cats	Dogs
Color	White or pink, (occasionally red)	Same
Clarity	Opaque, remains opaque when centrifuged	Same
SG*	1.019-1.050	1.022-1.037
TP†	2.6-10.3	2.5-6.2
WBC‡	Avg. 7987	Avg. 6167

*Specific gravity; †total protein in g/dl; ‡total white cells/μl.

TABLE 27-9

Other Characteristics of Chylous Effusions

- Triglyceride content > serum
- Cholesterol content ≤ serum
- Chylomicrons are present
- Predominant cell type may be the lymphocyte or neutrophil
- Sudanophilic fat globules are present
- Clears with ether

known causes of chylothorax in dogs and cats, this term should be reserved for effusions in which the pleural fluid cholesterol is greater than the serum cholesterol concentration and the pleural fluid triglyceride is less than or equal to the serum triglyceride. Pseudochylous effusions are extremely rare in veterinary patients, but may be associated with tuberculosis.

MEDICAL MANAGEMENT

If an underlying disease is diagnosed it should be treated and the chylous effusion managed by intermittent thoracentesis. If the underlying disease is effectively treated the effusion often resolves; however, complete resolution may take several months. Surgical intervention should be considered only in animals with idiopathic chylothorax, or those that do not respond to medical management. Chest tubes should only be placed in those animals with suspected chylothorax secondary to trauma (very rare), with rapid fluid accumulation, or following surgery. Electrolytes should be monitored as hyponatremia and hyperkalemia have also been documented in dogs with chylothorax undergoing multiple thoracentesis. A low-fat diet may decrease the amount of fat in the effusion, which may improve the animal's ability to resorb fluid from the thoracic cavity.

☞ **N O T E** · Animals with traumatic chylothorax heal and resolve the effusion within 2 to 3 weeks, but traumatic chylothorax is extremely rare.

Commercial low-fat diets are preferable to homemade diets; however, if commercial diets are refused, homemade diets are a reasonable alternative (Tables 27-10 and 27-11; the fat content of these diets is about 6% on a dry basis). Medium-chain triglycerides (once thought to be absorbed directly into the portal system, bypassing the TD) are transported via the TD of dogs. Thus, they may be less useful than previously believed. It is unlikely that dietary therapy will cure this disease, but it may help in the management of animals with chronic chylothorax. Clients should be informed that with the idiopathic form of this disease there is no effective treatment that will stop the effusion in all animals. However, the condition may spontaneously resolve in some animals after several weeks or months.

☞ **N O T E** · Do not expect low-fat diets to cure chylothorax, but lower fat chyle may be easier to reabsorb from the pleural space.

Benzopyrone drugs have been used for the treatment of lymphedema in humans for years. Whether these drugs might be effective in decreasing pleural effusion in animals with chylothorax is unknown; however, preliminary findings suggest that greater than 25% of animals treated with Rutin (Table 27-12) had complete resolution of their effusion 2 months after initiation of therapy. Whether the effusion resolved spontaneously in these animals, or was associated with the drug therapy, requires further study.

SURGICAL TREATMENT

Surgical intervention may be warranted in animals that do not have underlying disease and in whom medical management has become impractical or is ineffective. Surgical options in animals that do not have severe fibrosing pleuritis include mesenteric lymphangiography and TD ligation, passive pleuroperitoneal shunting, active pleuroperitoneal or pleurovenous shunting, and pleurodesis (the latter is not recommended by the author). Only TD ligation and active

---

TABLE 27-10

Canine Homemade Low-fat Diet*

Ingredient	Amount
Cooked white rice	2⅔ cups
Stewed chicken	⅓ lb
Dicalcium phosphate†	1¼ tsp
GNC Ca-Mg (250 mg Ca,155 Mg/tab)‡	2 tab
Morton Lite Salt	1 tsp
Zinc (50 mg zinc/tab)§	½ tab
Pet Tab	1 tab
Radiant Valley Natural Selenium (100 mcg Se/tab)¶	1 tab
GNC Copper (2 mg copper/tab)‡	1 tab

Directions: Cook the rice without salt. Boil chicken and skim off fat. Crush tablets to a fine powder. Combine all ingredients and mix well. Refrigerate unused portions
*Calculations based on average published nutrient content of each ingredient indicate this diet meets or exceeds the nutrient requirements for maintenance for adult dogs published by the Association of American Feed Control Officials. This recipe makes about 1½ lbs of food that contains 910 kcals of metabolizable energy.
†Dicalcium phosphate 18.5% phosphorus, 22%-24% calcium, available at farm supply and feed stores.
‡Available at GNC Nutrition Centers.
§Available at most supermarkets.
¶Available at many supermarkets or health food stores.

TABLE 27-11

Feline Homemade Low-fat Diet*

Ingredient	Amount
Cooked white rice	3²/₃ cups
Stewed chicken	½ lb
Dicalcium phosphate[†]	1½ tsp
GNC Ca-Mg (600 mg Ca/tab)[‡]	1½ tab
Morton Lite Salt	1 tsp
Taurine tablets (500 mg taurine/tab)[§]	3 tabs
Zinc (50 mg zinc/tab)[¶]	½ tab
Feline Pet Tab	3 tabs
Radiant Valley Natural Selenium (100 mcg Se/tab)[∥]	½ tab
Nature Made Balanced B-50 Complex[**]	½ tab
GNC Choline (250 mg choline/tab)[‡]	1 tab

Directions: Cook the rice without salt. Boil chicken and skim off fat. Crush tablets to a fine powder. Combine all ingredients and mix well. Refrigerate unused portions.
*Calculations based on average published nutrient content of each ingredient indicate this diet meets or exceeds the nutrient requirements for maintenance for adult cats published by the Association of American Feed Control Officials. This recipe makes about 2¼ lbs of food that contains 1293 kcals of metabolizable energy.
[†]Dicalcium phosphate 18.5% phosphorus, 22%-24% calcium, available at farm supply and feed stores.
[‡]Available at GNC Nutrition Centers.
[§]Taurine tablets can be purchased at most health food stores and cooperatives as 500-mg and 1000-mg tablets.
[¶]Available at many supermarkets.
[∥]Available at many supermarkets or health food stores
[**]Available at many supermarkets.

pleuroperitoneal shunting will be described here. The mechanism by which TD ligation is purported to work is that following TD ligation abdominal lymphaticovenous anastomoses form for the transport of chyle to the venous system. Chyle bypasses the TD and the effusion resolves. Unfortunately, TD ligation results in complete resolution of pleural effusion in only about 50% of animals operated upon (Fossum, 1986; Kerpsack, 1994). The advantage of TD ligation is that, if it is successful, it results in complete resolution of pleural fluid (as compared to palliative procedures such as passive or active pleuroperitoneal shunting). Disadvantages include a long operative time (problematic in debilitated animals), a high incidence of continued or recurrent chylous or nonchylous (from pulmonary lymphatics) effusion, and that mesenteric lymphangiography may be difficult to perform (particularly in cats). Without mesenteric lymphangiography, complete ligation of the TD cannot be assured; however, this technique may not be uniformly successful in verifying complete ligation of the TD. Some small branches of the TD system may be present and yet not fill with dye during lymphangiography.

Preoperative Management

Food is withheld 12 hours before surgery. Cream or oil may be fed 3 to 4 hours prior to surgery to help visualize lymphatics, or alternately, methylene blue may be injected into a lymph node at surgery.

Anesthesia

Refer to p. 650 for selected anesthetic protocols for animals with respiratory disease.

TABLE 27-12

Benzopyrones for Treatment of Chylothorax*

Rutin[†] 50 mg/kg PO, TID
*Efficacy is unproven at this time; clinical studies are needed.
[†]Obtained at health food stores.

Surgical Anatomy

The TD is the cranial continuation of the cisterna chyli and is generally said to begin between the crura of the diaphragm (Fig. 27-26). In cats the TD lies between the aorta and azygous vein on the left side of the mediastinum. In dogs it lies on the right side of the mediastinum until it reaches the fifth or sixth vertebra, then crossing to the left side. The TD terminates in the venous system of the neck (left external jugular vein or jugulo-subclavian angle).

Positioning

If a thoracic approach to the TD is used (see below), the left side (cats) or right side (dogs) of the thorax and abdomen is prepared for aseptic surgery. If a transdiaphragmatic approach is used, the cranial abdomen and caudal chest are prepped.

SURGICAL TECHNIQUES
Mesenteric Lymphangiography

For a thoracic approach, make a paracostal incision (or for a transdiaphragmatic approach make a cranial midline abdominal incision), exteriorize the cecum, and locate an adjacent lymph node.

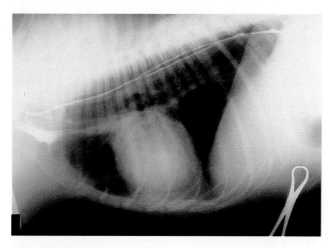

FIG. 27-26
Mesenteric lymphangiogram of a normal dog. Note the multiple branches of the thoracic duct.

☞ **N O T E ·** The TD is difficult to approach transdiaphragmatically in deep-chested dogs. This approach may be used in small dogs and cats, but should be avoided in larger dogs. An intercostal approach to the thoracic duct is preferred in medium and large breeds and can be used in any animal.

If necessary, inject a small volume (0.5 to 1 ml) of methylene blue into the lymph node to increase lymphatic visualization. Avoid repeated doses of methylene blue due to the risk of inducing a Heinz body anemia or renal failure. Find a lymphatic near the node to catheterize by gently dissecting the mesentery. Cannulate the lymphatic with a 20- or 22-gauge over-the-needle catheter and attach a three-way catheter and extension tubing (filled with heparinized saline) to the catheter with a suture (3-0 silk). Place an additional suture around the extension tubing and through a segment of intestine to prevent dislodgement of the catheter. Dilute 1 ml/kg of a water-soluble contrast agent (i.e., Renovist) with 0.5 ml/kg of sterile saline. Inject this mixture into the catheter and take a lateral thoracic radiograph while the last ml is being flushed into the catheter. Use this lymphangiogram to help identify the number and location of branches of the TD that need to be ligated. Repeat the lymphangiogram following TD ligation (see below) to identify branches that were not occluded. Embolization of the TD with cyanoacrylate injected through a mesenteric lymphatic catheter has been reported in dogs. Advantages of TD embolization are that direct visualization of the TD is not required, which negates the need for a thoracotomy or diaphragmatic incision. Disadvantages of this procedure are the same as those for mesenteric lymphangiography and TD ligation (i.e., not all TD branches may fill with the cyanoacrylate mixture and collateralization may occur past the obstruction).

Thoracic Duct Ligation

Perform an intercostal thoracotomy (right side for dogs, left side for cats) at the eighth, ninth, or tenth intercostal space or make an incision in the diaphragm (see note above). Locate the TD and use hemostatic clips and/or silk (2-0 or 3-0) suture to ligate it (see below). Visualization of the TD can be aided by injecting methylene blue into the lymphatic catheter.

Active Pleuroperitoneal or Pleurovenous Shunting

Commercially made shunt catheters (see below for ordering information) are available and can be used to pump pleural fluid into the abdomen (Fig. 27-27) or into a vein (i.e., jugular, azygous, caudal vena cava). Two types of shunts are available: a pleuroperitoneal shunt (Table 27-13) and an ascites (peritoneovenous) shunt (Table 27-14). The latter is meant to pump fluid from the abdomen into a vein and does not require manual pumping (i.e., it acts in an active fashion). This shunt can be placed from the pleural space into a vein (pleurovenous); when used in this manner, manual pumping is required (the shunt will not act in an active fashion). A potential complication of pleurovenous shunt placement is formation of a right atrial and/or ventricular thrombus. This complication may be life-threatening; therefore, pleuroperitoneal shunting is preferred if there is no reason to believe that the animal may not reabsorb the fluid from its abdominal cavity (e.g., presence of diffuse lymphatic disease or cardiac disease). Close observation of these patients for several weeks following pleurovenous shunt placement is necessary and preoperative heparinization and maintenance on heparin, aspirin, or other anticoagulants may be warranted. Both types of catheters are placed under general anesthesia.

Place the pump chamber and tubing in a bowl of sterilized, heparinized saline. Prime the pump by compressing the valve repeatedly until the system is filled with fluid and flow is established. Expel any remaining air bubbles from the tubing or valve. Make a vertical incision over the middle of the sixth, seventh, or eighth rib. Bluntly insert the pleural end of the shunt catheter into the thoracic cavity. For a pleuroperitoneal shunt, create a tunnel under the external abdominal oblique muscle using blunt dissection and pull the pump chamber through the tunnel. Place the efferent (peritoneal) end of the catheter into the abdominal cavity just caudal to the costal arch through a small skin incision and a preplaced purse-string suture in the abdominal musculature. For a pleurovenous shunt, tunnel the efferent (venous) end of the catheter over the shoulder to the ventral cervical region. Make a small incision over the jugular vein and insert the venous end of the catheter into the vein. Using fluoroscopy, place the distal end of the catheter at the caudal aspect of the cranial vena cava, just proximal to the right atrium (the venous end of the catheter may be

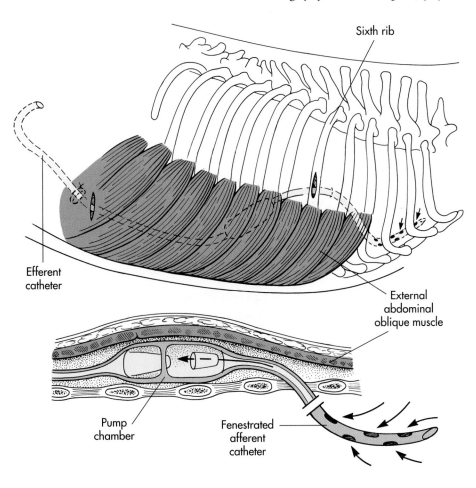

Sixth rib

Efferent catheter

External abdominal oblique muscle

Pump chamber

Fenestrated afferent catheter

FIG. 27-27
To place a pleuroperitoneal shunt, put the afferent end of the catheter into the thoracic cavity and the efferent end into the abdominal cavity. Make sure that the pump chamber overlies a rib so that the chamber can be effectively compressed.

TABLE **27-13**

Pleuroperitoneal Shunt Specifications*

- 27-cm fenestrated pleural end
- Two one-way valves
- 49-cm fenestrated peritoneal catheter
- Each complete pump of the reservoir dome transfers 1.5 ml of fluid

*Denver Biomaterials, Inc.

TABLE **27-14**

Pleurovenous (Peritoneovenous) Shunt Specifications*

- 27-cm fenestrated pleural end
- Single or double one-way valves[†]
- 66-cm fenestrated venous catheter
- Double valve: comes in a standard flow rate (26-40 ml/min at 10-cm head of water) and a low flow rate (< 26 ml/min at 10-cm head of water)

*Denver Biomaterials, Inc.
[†]This shunt comes in a single and double-valve form; the double valve catheter is indicated when placed in a pleurovenous fashion.

---

shortened if necessary). Alternatively, the venous end of the catheter may be placed in the azygous or caudal vena cava through an abdominal incision. Make sure that the pump chamber overlies a rib so that the chamber can be effectively compressed.

SUTURE MATERIALS/SPECIAL INSTRUMENTS

The advantage of using hemoclips is that they can be used as a reference point on subsequent radiographs if further ligation is necessary. However, it is best to also ligate the duct with nonabsorbable suture (i.e., silk) if hemoclips are used. Ordering information for products and supplies (i.e., Butterfly catheter; Methylene blue, USP 1%; Surflo catheter; Renovist

contrast agent; Isobutyl 2-cyanocrylate; and Hemoclips [medium]) for lymphangiography or TD ligation is provided in the Product Appendix. Shunts for active drainage include Denver double-valve peritoneous and pleuroperitoneal shunts (see Product Appendix).

POSTOPERATIVE CARE AND ASSESSMENT

If chylothorax resolves spontaneously or after surgery, periodic reevaluations for several years are warranted to detect recurrence. Fibrosing pleuritis is the most common, serious complication of chronic chylothorax (see p. 693).

Imunosuppression may occur in patients undergoing repeated and frequent thoracentesis because of lymphocyte depletion.

PROGNOSIS

This condition may resolve spontaneously or following surgery. Untreated or chronic chylothorax may result in severe fibrosing pleuritis and persistent dyspnea. Euthanasia is frequently performed in animals that do not respond to surgery or medical management.

References

Fossum TW, Birchard SJ, Jacobs RM: Chylothorax in 34 dogs, *J Am Vet Med Assoc* 188:1315, 1986.

Fossum TW et al: Chylothorax in cats: 37 cases (1969–1989), *J Am Vet Med Assoc* 198:672, 1991.

Kerpsack SJ et al: Evaluation of mesenteric lymphangiography and thoracic duct ligation in cats with chylothorax: 19 cases (1987–1992), *J Am Vet Med Assoc* 205:711, 1994.

Suggested Reading

Birchard SJ, Smeak DD, Fossum TW: Results of thoracic duct ligation in dogs with chylothorax, *J Am Vet Med Assoc* 193:68, 1988.

Fossum TW, Birchard SJ: Lymphangiographic evaluation of experimentally induced chylothorax after ligation of the cranial vena cava in dogs, *Am J Vet Res* 47:967, 1986.

Fossum TW et al: Severe bilateral fibrosing pleuritis associated with chronic chylothorax in 5 cats and 2 dogs, *J Am Vet Med Assoc* 201:317, 1992.

Fossum TW, Jacobs RM, Birchard SJ: Evaluation of cholesterol and triglyceride concentrations in differentiating chylous and nonchylous pleural effusions in dogs and cats, *J Am Vet Med Assoc* 188:49, 1986.

Fossum TW et al: Chylothorax associated with right-sided heart failure in 5 cats, *J Am Vet Med Assoc* 204:84, 1994.

Martin RA et al: Transdiaphragmatic approach to thoracic duct ligation in the cat, *Vet Surg* 17:22, 1988.

Meadows RL, MacWilliams PS: Chylous effusions revisited, *Vet Clin Pathol* 23:54, 1994.

Willard MD et al: Hyponatremia and hyperkalemia associated with idiopathic or experimentally induced chylothorax in four dogs, *J Am Vet Med Assoc* 199:353, 1991.

PYOTHORAX

DEFINITIONS

Pyothorax is a suppurative inflammation of the thoracic cavity with resultant accumulation of pus.

SYNONYMS

Thoracic empyema

GENERAL CONSIDERATIONS AND CLINICALLY RELEVANT PATHOPHYSIOLOGY

The route by which the thoracic cavity becomes infected (i.e., hematogenous spread, migrating foreign objects such as plant awns, penetrating wounds—particularly bite wounds, extension from diskospondylitis, extension from pneumonia, pulmonary neoplasia or abscessation, pulmonary or thoracic wall trauma, esophageal perforation, and postoperative infection) is usually not evident. Immunosuppressive diseases (e.g., FeLV and FIV) should be excluded in animals with pyothorax, but there is no evidence that development of pyothorax requires debilitation or an increased susceptibility to infection.

Multiple organisms are often cultured from animals with pyothorax; there is, however, a high incidence of obligate anaerobic infections as sole pathogens (Table 27-15). Obligate anaerobic infections or gram-positive filamentous organisms (i.e., *Nocardia* and *Actinomyces*) are frequently cultured from dogs with pyothorax (Fig. 27-28), while obligate anaerobes and/or *Pasteurella* spp. are the most common isolates in cats.

DIAGNOSIS
Clinical Presentation

Signalment. There is no breed predisposition, and pyothorax may occur in animals of any age; however, young male cats that fight and receive chest wounds are at increased risk. Similarly, adult, large-breed dogs (particularly hunting dogs) may be affected as they often inhale plant foreign material and suffer penetrating thoracic wounds.

History. A delay of several weeks between the trauma that induced the pyothorax and the onset of clinical signs is

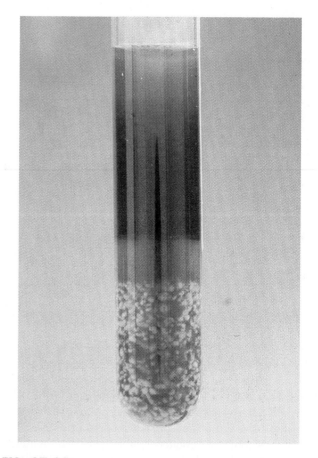

FIG. 27-28
Nocardial pleural effusion.

TABLE 27-15

Morphologic Characteristics of Bacteria Commonly Associated with Pyothorax in Small Animals

Bacteria	Oxygen Requirements	Gram's Stain	Antibiotic Sensitivity
Actinomyces	Facultative anaerobe to strict anaerobe	Gram-positive	**Ampicillin, amoxicillin plus clavulinic acid, penicillin,** cephalosporin, clindamycin, chloramphenicol, erythromycin
Bacteroides	Obligate anaerobe	Gram-negative	Most *Bacteroides* spp.: **ampicillin, amoxicillin plus clavulinic acid,** cephalosporin, clindamycin, chloramphenicol, metronidazole *B. fragilis:* amoxicillin plus clavulanic acid, **clindamycin,** chloramphenicol, metronidazole
Clostridium	Obligate anaerobe	Gram-positive	Most *Clostridium:* ampicillin, amoxicillin plus clavulinic acid, chloramphenicol, metronidazole *Clostridium perfringens:* **ampicillin, amoxicillin plus clavulinic acid,** cefoxitin, clindamycin, chloramphenicol, metronidazole, erythromycin
Fusobacterium	Obligate anaerobe	Gram-negative	**Ampicillin, amoxicillin plus clavulinic acid,** clindamycin, chloramphenicol, metronidazole
Klebsiella	Facultative anaerobe	Gram-negative	**Cephalosporin,** gentamicin, tobramycin, ticarcillin
Nocardia	Aerobe	Gram-positive (partially acid-fast)	**Trimethoprim-sulfa, amikacin**
Pasteurella	Facultative anaerobe	Gram-negative	**Ampicillin, amoxicillin plus clavulinic acid**
Pseudomonas	Aerobe	Gram-negative	**Carbenicillin (IV),** gentamicin, tobramycin, amikacin, **ticarcillin,** cefotaxime, **enrofloxacin**

Bolded type signifies typical drug(s) of choice.

not uncommon. Most animals are presented for evaluation of respiratory distress and/or anorexia.

Physical Examination Findings

Affected animals usually have a restrictive respiratory pattern (i.e., rapid, shallow respirations) and many are febrile. Additional findings in patients with pyothorax may include depression, anorexia, weight loss, dehydration, muffled heart and lung sounds, and pale mucous membranes. The chest wall may seem incompressible in cats with thoracic effusion.

Radiography/Ultrasonography

Thoracic radiographs usually diagnose pleural effusion (see p. 692). The cause of the pyothorax is seldom apparent radiographically; however, increased density in the thoracic cavity following thoracentesis may indicate an abscess or foreign body. Consolidated lung lobes that do not reexpand following fluid removal may be indicative of fibrosing pleuritis (see p. 693) or lung lobe torsion (see p. 665).

Laboratory Findings

Neutrophilia (with or without a degenerative left shift) may be present on a CBC. Fluid analysis is necessary to differentiate pyothorax from other exudative effusions. The fluid can range from amber to red or white in color. Protein content is usually greater than 3.5 g/dl and the fluid appears turbid or opaque due to the high nucleated cell count. Nucleated cells consist primarily of degenerative neutrophils (Fig. 27-29),

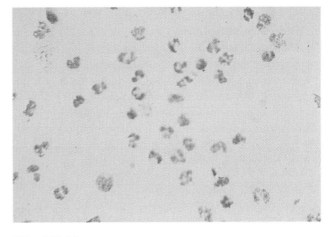

FIG. 27-29
Cytology of pleural fluid from a cat with pyothorax. Note the predominance of degenerative neutrophils.

but nondegenerative neutrophils can predominate, depending on the causative agent. Effusions associated with fungi and higher bacterial agents such as *Actinomyces* and *Nocardia* are often characterized cytologically by nondegenerative neutrophils and macrophages, or may appear hemorrhagic. Macrophages and reactive mesothelial cells are present in purulent effusions in variable numbers depending on the cause and the chronicity of the fluid. Occasionally, fungal elements may be noted in the pleural effusion of animals with fungal disease involving the pulmonary parenchyma. **Positive** cultures may not be obtained in all animals with pyothorax, particularly if anaerobic organisms are present.

DIFFERENTIAL DIAGNOSIS

Any cause of dyspnea should be considered a differential diagnosis (i.e., cardiac disease, pulmonary disease, mediastinal neoplasia, diaphragmatic hernia). Once pleural effusion has been diagnosed, other causes of exudative (i.e., chylothorax, FIP) or transudative (i.e., hypoalbuminemia, congestive heart failure) effusions must also be considered. Foul-smelling fluid suggests anaerobic bacteria.

MEDICAL MANAGEMENT

Although the cause of the effusion is often not discernible, attempts should be made to find and correct, if possible, underlying diseases. Management of these animals needs to be aggressive (Table 27-16). Following diagnosis, a chest tube should be placed. If available, continuous suction devices can be used; however, most animals can be managed with intermittent aspiration. Lavage should be performed two to three times daily. Isotonic fluid, such as saline or lactated Ringer's solution (warmed to room temperature), should be used at a dosage of 20 ml/kg body weight. The fluid remains in the thoracic cavity for 1 hour and is then removed. Addition of antibiotics to the lavage fluid offers no advantage over the use of appropriate systemic antibiotics. If antibiotics are used in the lavage fluid, the systemic dose should be decreased in order to minimize toxicity. The use of proteolytic enzymes is controversial and is no longer recommended by most authors. However, the addition of heparin (1500 units/100 ml of lavage) appears beneficial. Lavage may be required for 5 to 7 days. Systemic antibiotic therapy should be based on results of microbial culture and sensitivity testing (see Table 27-15). Prevalence of anaerobic infections is high (see above) and antibiotics with an anaerobic spectrum (i.e., penicillins or penicillin derivatives, clindamycin, metronidazole) are often used. Antibiotics should be continued for a minimum of 4 to 6 weeks. Recommended antibiotics for *Actinomyces* and nocardial infections are provided in Table 27-17.

SURGICAL TREATMENT

Surgery is indicated in animals that have underlying disease (i.e., lung abscess, lung lobe torsion, foreign body) and in those that do not respond to medical management in 3 to 4 days. If the pyothorax is chronic or localized, or if the patient remains dyspneic in the absence of significant volumes of pleural fluid, fibrosing pleuritis may be present (see p. 693). Decortication may be warranted in such patients.

Preoperative Management

Thoracentesis should be performed before induction if the animal is dyspneic. The animal should be normally hydrated and significant electrolyte and acid-base abnormalities corrected before surgery.

Anesthesia

Refer to anesthetic management of animals with respiratory impairment on p. 649.

Surgical Anatomy

See p. 676 for a description of the pleural space and fluid movement in normal animals.

Positioning

See the description of thoracic procedures beginning on p. 651.

SURGICAL TECHNIQUES

Approach the thorax via an intercostal thoracotomy (see p. 652) if an abnormality can be localized to one hemithorax, or median sternotomy (see p. 654) if localization is not possible. Explore the thoracic cavity for abscesses, foreign bodies, or other abnormalities, and remove affected tissues. If possible, remove fibrin covering the lung tissues. Submit appropriate samples for microbiological examination and culture. Place a chest tube for postoperative lavage. Before closure, lavage the thoracic cavity with warmed, sterile saline solution.

SUTURE MATERIALS/SPECIAL INSTRUMENTS

Braided, nonabsorbable, multifilament suture should not be used for lobectomy or partial lobectomy in these patients. Absorbable suture (i.e., polydioxanone, polyglyconate) is preferred in the presence of infection.

TABLE 27-16

Management of Animals with Pyothorax

1. Perform Gram's stain and culture and sensitivity of fluid and initiate broad-spectrum antibiotic therapy (see text and Table 27-15)
2. Place chest tube(s) and lavage thoracic cavity with 20 ml/kg b.w. warmed, isotonic fluid with heparin added (1500 U heparin/100 ml lavage solution)
3. Alter antibiotic therapy based on culture and sensitivity results and continue antibiotics for 4 to 6 weeks.

TABLE 27-17

Selected Antibiotics*

Actinomyces:
***Ampicillin**[†]*

20-40 mg/kg IM, SC, PO or IV, QID

Nocardia:
***Trimethoprim-sulfadiazine (Tribrissen)**[‡]*

45 mg/kg PO, BID **or**

Amikacin

30 mg/kg IV or SC, SID

*Treat for a minimum of 6 weeks.
[†]May not be effective against L-phase variants.
[‡]Observe for side effects (e.g., anemia, thrombocytopenia, keratoconjunctivitis sicca).

POSTOPERATIVE CARE AND ASSESSMENT

Thoracic lavage should be continued after surgery until the infection resolves (see above). Serum protein and electrolytes (i.e., potassium) should be monitored and fluid therapy continued until the animal is eating and drinking normally. Antibiotic therapy should be continued for 4 to 6 weeks (see above). Refer to the postoperative management of animals undergoing thoracotomy procedures on p. 657 for additional recommendations.

PROGNOSIS

The prognosis for most animals with pyothorax is good if they are managed as described above. Recurrence is common in animals treated with antibiotics only (i.e., without thoracic lavage). Long-standing empyema may resorb leaving a pleural "peel," which is a thick sheet of fibroblasts and inflammatory cells attached to the visceral pleura. This pleural peel may inhibit normal expansion of lung tissue (fibrosing pleuritis; see p. 693). If multiple lung lobes are fibrosed and cannot expand normally, the prognosis may be poor. Decortication is recommended if lung entrapment is suspected. Decortication is best performed once the empyema is mature, but before it adheres to the pleura and becomes vascularized.

Suggested Reading

Holmberg DL: Management of pyothorax, *Vet Clin North Am Small Anim Pract* 9:357, 1979.

Jonas LD: Feline pyothorax: a retrospective study of twenty cases, *J Am Anim Hosp Assoc* 19:865, 1983.

Sherding RG: Pyothorax in the cat, *Compend Contin Educ Pract Vet* 1:247, 1979.

Thompson JC, Gartrell BM, Melville VJ: Successful treatment of feline pyothorax associated with an *Actinomyces* species and *Bacteroides melaninogenicus, N Z Med J* 40:73, 1992.

Turner WD, Breznock EM: Continuous suction drainage for management of canine pyothorax—a retrospective study, *J Am Anim Hosp Assoc* 24:485, 1988.

THYMOMAS AND THYMIC BRANCHIAL CYSTS

DEFINITIONS

Thymomas are tumors that arise from epithelial tissues of the thymus. **Thymic branchial cysts** develop from vestiges of the fetal branchial arch system.

GENERAL CONSIDERATIONS AND CLINICALLY RELEVANT PATHOPHYSIOLOGY

Masses in the mediastinum of dogs and cats are usually neoplastic, although abscesses, granulomas, and cysts are occasionally found. Lymphoma is the most common cranial mediastinal tumor in dogs and cats. Other tumors occasionally found here include thymomas, chemodectomas (aortic and carotid body tumors), and ectopic thyroid and parathyroid tumors. Thymomas are the most common surgically treatable neoplasm of the cranial mediastinum in dogs—most are benign. However, since histological appearance of the tumor correlates poorly with clinical behavior, the terms "invasive" or "noninvasive" are frequently used. Stage I (i.e., noninvasive) thymomas are well circumscribed and do not extend beyond the thymic capsule (Table 27-18). Others may extend beyond the capsule locally or may invade surrounding organs and/or metastasize to other thoracic or extrathoracic structures.

The clinical signs associated with thymomas may be due to occupation of space, a paraneoplastic syndrome, or both. As thymomas enlarge they may cause respiratory distress by compressing the lungs or trachea and/or inducing pleural effusion. Effusions associated with thymomas may be serosanguineous or chylous. Paraneoplastic syndromes are distant effects of a tumor. Nearly 50% of thymomas in dogs are associated with myasthenia gravis (MG). Myasthenia gravis is an autoimmune neuromuscular disorder that is characterized by muscular weakness. The weakness is due to a deficiency of functional acetylcholine receptors in the neuromuscular postsynaptic membrane caused by autoantibodies that bind to and block the receptors. Other paraneoplastic syndromes associated with thymomas are nonthymic cancer and polymyositis. As thymomas enlarge they may compress the cranial vena cava and other cranial thoracic vessels causing edema of the head, neck, and/or forelimbs (cranial vena cava syndrome).

Thymic branchial cysts develop from vestiges of the branchial arch system of the fetus. They may be found in the subcutaneous tissues of the neck or in the thymus. Rupture of these cysts may result in a chronic inflammatory reaction and abscessation.

TABLE 27-18

Proposed Staging Scheme for Thymomas*

Stage	Description
I	Growth completely within intact thymic capsule
II	Pericapsular growth into mediastinal fat tissue, adjacent pleura and/or pericardium
III	Invasion into surrounding organs and/or intrathoracic metastasis
IV	Extrathoracic metastasis
Paraneoplastic syndromes	
P₀	No evidence of paraneoplastic syndrome
P₁	Myasthenia gravis
P₂	Nonthymic malignant tumor

*Modified from Aronson M: Canine thymoma, *Vet Clin North Am Small Anim Pract* 15:755, 1985.

DIAGNOSIS

Clinical Presentation

Signalment. The average age of dogs with thymomas is 8 to 9 years; however, it has been reported in dogs as young as 3 years. Large-breed dogs, particularly German shepherds, golden retrievers, and Labrador retrievers, are more commonly affected than small dogs. A sex predisposition has not been identified. Most cats with thymomas have been greater than 8 years of age. Thymic branchial cysts also occur most commonly in middle-age to older animals; however, one affected dog was 18 months of age (Liu, Patnaik, Burk, 1983).

> 🖙 **N O T E** • Despite the fact that the thymus involutes with age, both thymomas and thymic branchial cysts occur in middle-aged to older dogs.

History. Dogs with thymomas may present for evaluation of dyspnea, coughing, weight loss, lethargy, dysphagia, muscle weakness, vomiting and/or regurgitation, excessive salivation, and/or neck edema. The onset of clinical signs may be acute despite relatively slow tumor enlargement. Lethargy, anorexia, dyspnea, and pleural effusion are common in cats with thymoma. Occasionally, thymomas are fortuitous findings on thoracic radiographs of asymptomatic animals. Clinical findings in dogs and cats with thymic branchial cysts are similar to those in animals with thymomas. Most are presented for evaluation of progressive dyspnea. Lameness and swelling of the head, neck, and forelimbs are also common.

Physical Examination Findings

Clinical findings in dogs with thymomas vary between patients. Respiratory abnormalities caused by pleural effusion or aspiration pneumonia may be the predominant finding. Other animals may present for generalized exertional weakness without evidence of respiratory problems. Occasionally, localized forms of myasthenia are found where the weakness is limited to the esophagus, larynx or pharynx, or facial musculature. The most common clinical findings in dogs and cats with thymic branchial cysts are dyspnea and pleural effusion.

> 🖙 **N O T E** • All dogs with thymomas should be evaluated for myasthenia and megaesophagus.

Radiography/Ultrasonography

Dogs with mediastinal masses may have dorsal elevation of the trachea and caudal displacement of the heart on lateral thoracic radiographs. On the ventrodorsal view the mediastinum may appear widened and the heart may be deviated laterally. Pleural effusion is commonly associated with invasive tumors and pneumothorax is rare. Megaesophagus and/or secondary aspiration pneumonia may be noted on thoracic radiographs. Ultrasonography is often helpful in ruling out extrathoracic metastasis.

Laboratory Findings

Specific laboratory abnormalities are not found with thymoma or branchial cysts. Leukocytosis may be present if the animal has aspiration pneumonia. Pleural effusion associated with thymoma or thymic branchial cysts may contain mature lymphocytes; however, the presence of immature lymphocytes indicates lymphoma. Both lymphoma and thymoma may cause chylous effusions (see p. 691).

DIFFERENTIAL DIAGNOSIS

Differential diagnoses for cranial mediastinal masses include both neoplastic and nonneoplastic disease (Table 27-19). The most important differential is mediastinal lymphoma because treatment for lymphoma does not involve surgery. Therefore, a definitive diagnosis should be made before surgery whenever possible. The presence of hypercalcemia suggests lymphoma, while MG or megaesophagus is suggestive of thymoma. However, hypercalcemia has been reported in conjunction with thymoma in a dog (Harris et al, 1991). A definitive diagnosis of lymphoma may be made by fine-needle aspiration or transthoracic needle biopsy of the mass and/or pleural fluid evaluation. Using ultrasound to locate the site for biopsies may decrease the risk of perforating the cranial vena cava or other vascular structures. If a definitive diagnosis cannot be made preoperatively, a surgical biopsy with intraoperative cytology or analysis of frozen sections is indicated. The histological appearance of thymomas does not correlate well with behavior; therefore, exploratory thoracotomy is often required to determine if the tumor is invasive.

Acquired MG can be diagnosed by the demonstration of circulating antibodies to acetylcholine receptors. Alternately, clinical signs and response to a cholinesterase inhibitor may help diagnose MG. When edrophonium chloride is given intravenously there should be a dramatic, but transient, improvement in voluntary muscle function (Table 27-20). However, the clinician must be aware of possible complications associated with the use of edrophonium (e.g., possible paralysis) and be prepared to deal with them.

TABLE 27-19

Differential Diagnoses for Cranial Mediastinal Masses in Dogs and Cats

- Lymphoma
- Thymoma
- Chemodectoma
- Ectopic thyroid or parathyroid tumor
- Abscess
- Thymic branchial cyst
- Schwannoma
- Teratoma
- Thymic hyperplasia
- Granuloma

TABLE 27-20
Tensilon Test
Edrophonium chloride (Tensilon)*
Dogs 0.1-2.0 mg
Cats 0.5-1.0 mg
*Use with caution (see text).

TABLE 27-21
Drugs Used to Treat Acquired MG in Dogs
Pyridostigmine bromide (Mestinon, Regonol)
0.02-0.04 mg/kg IV, q2hr or 0.5-3.0 mg/kg PO, BID or TID
Prednisone
1-2 mg/kg/day

MEDICAL MANAGEMENT

If aspiration pneumonia is present, the dog should be treated with appropriate antibiotics prior to surgery. Dogs with megaesophagus sometimes benefit from being fed in an upright position. Thoracentesis should be performed to remove pleural effusion and an oxygen-enriched environment provided if the animal is dyspneic. Anticholinesterase (i.e., pyridostigmine bromide) and/or corticosteroid therapy may benefit dogs with megaesophagus and/or weakness secondary to MG (Table 27-21). Fluid therapy and correction of electrolyte abnormalities may be necessary in animals with severe or frequent regurgitation. Radiation therapy may reduce clinical signs in some animals with thymomas.

SURGICAL TREATMENT

Long-term survival without thymectomy (i.e., up to 3 years) has been reported in dogs with thymomas (Aronsohn et al, 1984). However, surgical removal of stage I or stage II thymomas may be indicated. Concurrent MG makes therapy of thymoma more difficult. In humans thymectomy helps resolve MG in many patients despite persistent serum antiacetylcholine receptor autoantibody titers. There have been too few dogs operated with both thymomas and MG to predict the outcome in these patients. Surgical removal of thymic branchial cysts is indicated.

Preoperative Management

Aspiration pneumonia should be resolved before surgery and severe muscle weakness should be treated (see above). Before anesthetic induction, excess pleural fluid should be removed and fluid and electrolyte abnormalities corrected.

Anesthesia

Refer to p. 649 for recommendations for anesthetic management of patients undergoing thoracotomy procedures. Neuromuscular blocking agents (i.e., atracurium, pancuronium) should be avoided in patients with MG. Intubate patients with megaesophagus while positioned sternally, rather than laterally.

Surgical Anatomy

The thymus is derived from the third and fourth pharyngeal pouches adjacent to the primordial cells of the thyroid gland and migrates caudally into the cranial mediastinum. It reaches maximal size in the dog at about 4 or 5 months. The thymus is bordered dorsally by the cranial vena cava and trachea. It is closely associated with many smaller blood vessels (e.g., branches of the brachycephalic trunk and internal thoracic arteries), which often require ligation during thymectomy. The phrenic nerve is closely associated with the dorsal border of the thymus.

Positioning

Depending on surgical approach chosen (see below) either the left thorax or ventral thorax should be prepared for aseptic surgery.

SURGICAL TECHNIQUES

Thymectomy may be performed through a left third or fourth space intercostal thoracotomy if the tumor is small, or a cranial median sternotomy (see pp. 651–655). If the mass is large, a median sternotomy approach allows improved visualization of surrounding structures such as the cranial vena cava. Small encapsulated thymomas can usually be removed without difficulty, but cytoreduction is often all that is possible with large, invasive tumors. Thymomas are often friable and occasionally cystic and they should be handled with care to avoid seeding the thoracic cavity with tumor cells. Thymic branchial cysts appear as multilobulated masses containing numerous cysts on transverse section.

☞ **N O T E ·** If the tumor is adhered to or closely surrounds the cranial vena cava, temporary occlusion of this vessel may facilitate surgery. Permanent ligation of the cranial cava causes chylothorax.

Explore the thoracic cavity for evidence of metastasis. Identify the cranial vena cava and other associated vessels. Locate the phrenic nerve and attempt to preserve it, if possible. Ligate small vessels and bluntly dissect the mass and its capsule from surrounding tissues. Try to maintain the integrity of the thymic capsule where possible. If complete removal of the mass is not possible, remove as much as can safely be excised. Submit tissues for histologic examination. Place a chest tube before thoracic closure.

SUTURE MATERIALS/SPECIAL INSTRUMENTS

Electrocautery is useful when removing thymomas and other vascular neoplasms. See also recommendations for thoracotomy on p. 657.

POSTOPERATIVE CARE AND ASSESSMENT

Animals with thymomas are at great risk to aspirate during the postoperative period; positioning them with their heads elevated may decrease the risk. Additionally, suctioning the pharynx before extubation and extubating with the cuff slightly inflated will decrease the risk of aspiration if there has been passive regurgitation during the surgical procedure. The animal should be observed for hemorrhage and/or pneumothorax postoperatively. Adjuvant radiation therapy may be beneficial in animals with invasive tumors that cannot be completely excised. The animal should be closely observed for development of paraneoplastic disease following therapy. Analgesics should be provided postoperatively in these patients (Table 27-22). With thymomas, the chest tube can generally be removed within 24 hours if hemorrhage or pneumothorax does not occur. Longer-term tube thoracostomy may be necessary in animals with thymic branchial cysts if rupture of a cyst has caused pleuritis.

PROGNOSIS

The prognosis depends on the invasiveness of the tumor, its size at the time of diagnosis, and the presence or absence of paraneoplastic disease. The prognosis for thymic branchial cysts and noninvasive thymomas is good. If paraneoplastic syndromes are present, the prognosis is guarded.

References

Aronsohn MG et al: Clinical and pathologic features of thymoma in 15 dogs, *J Am Vet Med Assoc* 184:1355, 1984.

Harris CL et al: Hypercalcemia in a dog with thymoma, *J Am Anim Hosp Assoc* 27:281, 1991.

Liu S, Patnaik AK, Burk RL: Thymic branchial cysts in the dog and cat, *J Am Vet Med Assoc* 182:1095, 1983.

Suggested Reading

Bellah JR, Stiff ME, Russell RG: Thymoma in the dog: two case reports and review of 20 additional cases, *J Am Vet Med Assoc* 183:306, 1983.

Carpenter JL, Holzworth J: Thymoma in 11 cats, *J Am Vet Med Assoc* 181:248, 1982.

Hitt ME et al: Radiation treatment for thymoma in a dog, *J Am Vet Med Assoc* 190:1187, 1987.

Klebanow ER: Thymoma and acquired myasthenia gravis in the dog: a case report and review of 13 additional cases, *J Am Anim Hosp Assoc* 28:63, 1992.

Poffenbarger E, Klausner JS, Caywood DD: Acquired myasthenia gravis in a dog with thymoma: a case report, *J Am Anim Hosp Assoc* 21:119, 1985.

TABLE 27-22

Postoperative Analgesics

Oxymorphone (Numorphan)
0.05-0.1 mg/kg IV, IM, every 4 hours (as needed)

Butorphanol (Torbutrol, Torbugesic)
0.2-0.4 mg/kg IV, IM, or SC, every 2 to 4 hours (as needed)

Buprenorphine (Buprenex)
5-15 µg/kg IV, IM, every 6 hours (as needed)

CHAPTER 28

Fundamentals of Orthopedic Surgery and Fracture Management

PREOPERATIVE CONCERNS

Orthopedic patients may present for elective surgery (i.e., cranial cruciate ligament injury, hip dysplasia, osteochondritis dissecans), nonelective surgery (i.e., bone fractures, joint luxations), or conditions that require emergency treatment (i.e., open fractures, open joint dislocations). When animals present for elective surgery there is ample time to acquire appropriate preoperative diagnostic evaluation. Younger patients (less than 2 years old) should have selected screening laboratory tests, including PCV, serum total solids, and urinalysis. Fecal analysis and heartworm tests may be indicated, depending on history and geographic location. The need for further laboratory evaluation should be based on signalment, physical examination, and results of initial screening tests. Older patients (2 years or older) with orthopedic disease must be assessed more carefully than younger patients. Just as the physiologic properties of the musculoskeletal system decline with age, other organ systems also deteriorate. Thorough physical examination remains the foundation of preoperative evaluation and should be supplemented with a complete blood count, chemistry profile, and urinalysis. Special diagnostic tests (e.g., coagulation profile) may be indicated, depending on history, signalment, and physical findings.

Patients in need of immediate or emergency surgical care should have a thorough and complete physical evaluation. Serial examinations are important because serious or potentially lethal problems may not become evident for several hours or days after injury. Although organ dysfunction may be evident (or suspected) on initial physical examination, repeated examinations may be necessary to define the severity of injury. Animals that have received an external blow severe enough to disrupt musculoskeletal integrity (i.e., fracture, luxation) often have concurrent external or internal organ system injury. Cardiovascular, pulmonary, urinary, and neurologic systems are most frequently injured. If abnormalities are found, a differential diagnosis and diagnostic plan for each problem should be developed and additional diagnostic tests completed. For example, cardiac arrhythmias and/or femoral pulse abnormalities may be found in patients with traumatic myocarditis necessitating thoracic radiographs and an electrocardiogram to assess treatment options and anesthetic risk. Auscultation may detect pulmonary injury (i.e., lung contusion, pneumothorax), but physical changes may be subtle and missed on physical examination. Because 33% to 42% of fracture patients have some degree of pulmonary injury, preoperative evaluation should include thoracic radiographs (Spackman et al, 1984; Tamas, Paddleford, Krahwinkel, 1985). Some abnormalities may necessitate that surgical repair of the orthopedic disease be delayed (e.g., uroabdomen; see p. 416), whereas others may alter the prognosis such that repairing the orthopedic condition is not justified (i.e., vertebral fracture with loss of deep pain sensation).

Because most orthopedic patients that need immediate or emergency surgical care have sustained trauma, laboratory evaluation is essential. A minimum database should include a complete blood count, chemistry profile, and urinalysis. Additional laboratory tests (i.e., coagulation profile, electrolytes, acid-base balance) may be required to assess differential diagnoses developed on physical examination. Abnormal values should be assessed in light of physical findings, and the need for additional or serial tests should be determined. Serial tests are useful to validate abnormal findings and monitor patient progress. Delaying surgical intervention until abnormal organ function returns to normal is optimal; however, it is often not feasible.

PREOPERATIVE COAPTATION

Unstable injuries should be coapted to reduce further soft tissue injury and increase patient comfort. External splints can be used to provide temporary limb support or as a primary means of fracture stabilization. To avoid complications, external splints must be properly applied and carefully monitored. Most complications associated with external splints are minor (i.e., swelling of the limb distal to the splint, splint slippage, skin abrasions); however, serious complications (i.e., fracture nonunion, loss of a limb because of ischemic necrosis) may occur. Therefore the application of an external splint should not be considered a minor procedure or one that does not require careful observation. The most common temporary supports are Robert Jones bandages and lighter bandages supported with spoon splints or other coaptation materials. Fractures or luxations below the elbow and stifle joint are best managed with a soft padded bandage, with or without additional support using fiberglass casting or metal splints. Fractures above the elbow or stifle joint are more difficult to coapt. A spica splint that crosses the body above the shoulder (or hip) provides the best external coaptation (see below and p. 107).

Robert Jones Bandages

Robert Jones bandages and their modifications are the external splints most commonly used in veterinary patients. These bulky, cotton-gauze wrappings are commonly used before or after surgery for temporary limb splintage. The original Robert Jones bandage used commercially available, 12-inch, rolled cotton that was liberally applied to the limb to a thickness of 4 to 6 inches. Modified Robert Jones bandages use less cotton but still provide compression. The thick cotton layer provides mild compression of soft tissues and immobilizes fractures without causing vascular compromise. Soft tissue and bone immobilization enhances patient comfort and prevents further soft tissue damage from sharp bone fragments. Additionally, Robert Jones bandages help eliminate dead space after surgery. **These bandages extend from the toes to the midfemur or midhumerus and are only useful when applied to injuries below the stifle or elbow joint.**

Prepare the limb by clipping long hair from the midhumerus (midfemur) to the toes and treat any open wounds. Apply adhesive tape stirrups (Table 28-1) to cranial and caudal surfaces of the foot from carpus (tarsus) to 6 inches beyond the toes (Fig. 28-1). Wrap 3 to 6 inches of cotton padding (from a 12-inch roll or cast padding) around the limb from toes to midhumerus (midfemur). Ensure that the nails of the third and fourth digits are visible so that limb swelling can be detected. Then wrap elastic gauze firmly over the cotton to compress it. Apply at least

TABLE 28-1			
Materials Needed for Application of Bandages, Splints, and Casts			
Robert Jones bandage	**Metal spoon splint**	**Spica splint**	**Cast**
Adhesive tape	Metal spoon splint	Adhesive tape	Cast material
Cotton padding	Adhesive tape	Cast padding	Stockinette
Gauze	Cast padding	Gauze	Adhesive tape
Elastic tape or Vetrap	Gauze	Elastic tape or Vetrap	Cast padding
	Elastic tape or Vetrap	Cast material	Gauze
			Elastic tape or Vetrap

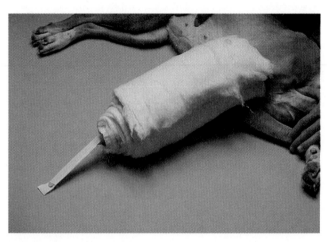

FIG. 28-1
When applying a Robert Jones bandage, place adhesive tape stirrups on the cranial and caudal surfaces of the foot from carpus (tarsus) to 6 inches beyond the toes, then wrap 3 to 6 inches of cotton padding around the limb.

two to three layers of gauze to achieve smooth, even tension. Sufficient compression will cause the bandage to sound like a ripe watermelon when tapped with a finger (Fig. 28-2). Invert the tape stirrups and stick them to the outer layer of gauze. Then apply elastic tape (i.e., Elasticon or Vetrap) to the outer surface of the bandage. See p. 707 for postoperative care.

Metal Spoon Splints

Metal spoon splints (metasplints) are used to provide support to injuries of the distal radius and ulna, carpus or tarsus, metacarpus or metatarsus, and/or phalanges. They are used for ancillary support of internal fixation devices or as a primary means of fixation when the patient fracture-assess-

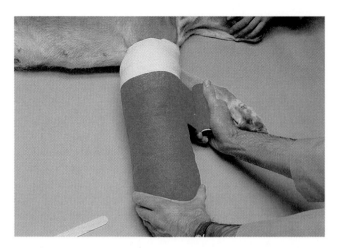

FIG. 28-2
After applying tape stirrups and cotton padding on the limb, wrap elastic gauze firmly over the cotton to compress it. Then apply elastic tape to the outer surface of the bandage.

ment score (see p. 730) indicates minimal stress and rapid healing. Spoon splints are commercially available in aluminum or plastic in a variety of lengths and sizes.

Clip long hair and treat open wounds (see p. 94) before covering them with a sterile dressing. Apply adhesive tape stirrups from the carpus (tarsus) to toes, leaving the ends extending 6 inches beyond the toes. Firmly apply cast padding around the limb in a spiral fashion with a 50% overlap (Fig. 28-3, A). Begin the padding at the toes and extend it proximally 1 inch beyond the proximal aspect of the splint. Apply just enough cotton to prevent skin abrasions and pressure sores, but do not make the bandage so bulky that it will be awkward for the patient. Cover bony prominences with excess padding. Wrap elastic gauze over the cotton to compress it. Place the padded limb in an appropriate-sized splint and secure it to the limb with Vetrap or elastic adhesive tape (Fig. 28-3, B). Invert and stick the stirrups to the final wrapping. See below for postoperative care.

Spica Splints

Spica splints envelop the torso and affected limb and are commonly used as temporary splints to immobilize humeral or femoral fractures or as adjunctive stabilization after internal fixation. They are rarely used as a primary means of stabilization unless the fracture has a simple transverse or short oblique configuration and the fracture-assessment score indicates that rapid bone union will occur.

Clip long hair and treat open wounds (see p. 94) before covering them with a sterile dressing. Place adhesive tape stirrups on the medial and lateral surface of the limb and apply cotton cast padding to the limb and torso. Begin the padding at the paw and wrap it proximally in a spiral fashion, overlapping it 50%. When the inguinal or axillary region is reached, wrap the cotton padding around the ani-

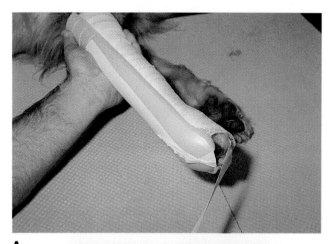

A

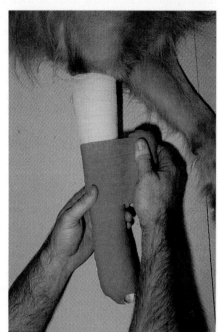

B

FIG. 28-3
A, When placing a spoon splint on a limb, firmly apply cast padding around the limb in a spiral fashion with a 50% overlap. Place the padded limb in an appropriate sized splint and, **B,** secure it to the limb with Vetrap or elastic adhesive tape.

mal's torso several times alternating cranially and caudally to the affected limb. Next wrap elastic gauze over the cast padding (i.e., 50% overlap). Wrap the gauze firmly around the limb to mildly compress the soft tissues. Reinforce the spica bandage with fiberglass casting material to provide additional stabilization of the fracture ends. Fold the casting tape onto itself to provide a lateral splint that is four to six layers thick, extending from toes to dorsal midline. Use Vetrap or elastic adhesive tape to hold the fiberglass cast to the limb and provide an outer covering for the splint.

Postoperative care of coaptation devices. After placement of a Robert Jones bandage, metal spoon splint, or spica splint, the toes should be observed twice a day for swelling. The bandage or splint must be kept clean and dry. If it is wet outside, a plastic bag should be placed over the limb to cover the toes and bandage. The limb should be observed for signs of irritation or discharge, and the bandage or splint should be removed to inspect the limb if either is present.

ANESTHETIC CONSIDERATIONS

Anesthetic protocols should be based on signalment, physical examination findings, and laboratory analysis. Patients presented for correction of elective orthopedic problems (i.e., cruciate reconstruction, OCD) and no preoperative findings suggestive of major organ dysfunction can be managed using a variety of anesthetic techniques (Table 28-2). Patients undergoing correction of acute traumatic injuries or systemic disease should be anesthetized with care. An ECG and thoracic radiographs should be performed in these patients, and hypovolemia should be corrected before surgery.

Assessment of the level of postoperative discomfort and duration of discomfort should be used to determine which analgesic is to be administered before surgery. Clinical and experimental studies clearly indicate that analgesics are most effective when administered before painful stimuli; thus they should be administered initially as part of the preoperative medication. Analgesics are administered for 12 to 24 hours after surgery, depending on procedure and patient evaluation. Butorphanol or buprenorphine is recommended in patients undergoing procedures requiring minimal tissue manipulation (Table 28-3). Buprenorphine provides longer postoperative relief (6 hours) compared with butorphanol

(2 hours) and is more useful when redosing is inconvenient after surgery. In patients undergoing more painful procedures that require significant tissue manipulation (e.g., triple pelvic osteotomy) or in those with traumatic injuries, oxymorphone or morphine is recommended. In the latter patients, opioid epidurals can be administered to supplement systemic opioid analgesia (Table 28-4). Patients undergoing surgery of the rear quarters may be given oxymorphone, buprenorphine, or morphine as an epidural. Animals undergoing surgery of the thoracic limb may be given morphine as an opioid epidural. Systemic opioid premedication must be adjusted to account for epidural administration (calculate total patient dose and divide between systemic and epidural administration).

ANTIBIOTICS

Antimicrobials are commonly used for prophylaxis and treatment of orthopedic infections. There is considerable debate regarding which patients should receive prophylactic antibiotics. Reviews of orthopedic patients have shown that those animals with severe soft tissue and/or bone trauma, multiple fractures, and traumatic surgical procedures are most likely to develop postoperative wound infections. Therefore prophylactic antibiotics should be administered in contaminated cases (open injuries), cases with severe trauma (significant soft tissue bruising and swelling or multiple bone fractures), and cases requiring lengthy operative times (2 hours or longer). Additionally, prophylactic antibiotics are recommended in elective procedures in which postoperative infection would be catastrophic (e.g., hip replacement). See Chapter 10 for general prophylactic antibiotic recommendations.

If prophylactic antibiotics are used, they must be used properly. Timing of antibiotic administration and rational selection of appropriate antibiotics are criteria that must be considered. Effective antimicrobial use is based on two criteria:

1. Which microorganisms are most likely to cause orthopedic wound infections?
2. Which antibiotics are most likely to be effective against potential offending microorganisms?

TABLE 28-2

Suggested Protocols for the Anesthetic Management of Patients with Orthopedic Disease

For stable patients and those presented for elective procedures
Premedication

Glycopyrrolate (0.005-0.011 mg/kg SC or IM) or atropine (0.02-0.04 mg/kg SC or IM) plus
  oxymorphone (0.05-0.1 mg/kg SC or IM) or
  butorphanol (0.2-0.4 mg/kg SC or IM) or
  buprenorphine (5-15 µg/kg IM) and
  acepromazine 0.05 mg/kg, not to exceed 1 mg SC or IM

Induction
Thiopental (10-12 mg/kg IV) or propofol (4-6 mg/kg IV)

Maintenance
Isoflurane or halothane

For unstable animals that have recently had trauma
Induction
Oxymorphone (0.1 mg/kg IV) plus diazepam (0.2 mg/kg IV). Give in incremental dosages. Intubate if possible. If necessary, give etomidate (0.5-1.5 mg/kg IV). Alternatively, mask induction or thiopental or propofol at extremely reduced dosages may be used.

Maintenance
Isoflurane

TABLE 28-3

Systemic Analgesics

Oxymorphone (Numorphan)
0.05-0.1 mg/kg IV, IM, every 4 hr (as needed)

Butorphanol (Torbutrol, Torbugesic)
0.2-0.4 mg/kg IV, IM, or SC, every 2 to 4 hr (as needed)

Buprenorphine (Buprenex)
5-15 µg/kg IV, IM every 6 hr (as needed)

Morphine
0.4 mg/kg SC or IM, every 4 to 6 hr (as needed)

TABLE 28-4

Epidural Anesthesia in the Dog

Drug	Dose	Onset of action	Duration of action
Lidocaine 2%*	1 ml/3.4 kg $(T_5)^\dagger$ 1 ml/4.5 kg $(T_{13}\text{-}L_1)^\dagger$	10 min	1-1.5 hr
Bupivacaine 0.25% or 0.5%* (preservative free)	1 ml/4.5 kg	20-30 min	4.5-6 hr
Fentanyl	0.001 mg/kg	4-10 min	6 hr
Oxymorphone	0.1 mg/kg	15 min‡	10 hr
Morphine (preservative free)	0.1 mg/kg§	23 min	20 hr
Buprenorphine	0.005 mg/kg	30 min‡	12-18 hr

*Avoid head-down position after epidural.
†A block to T_1 leads to intercostal nerve paralysis; a block to C7-C5 leads to phrenic nerve paralysis.
‡Approximate onset of action.
§The dose for epidural morphine in cats is 0.03 mg/kg.

Coagulase-positive *Staphylococcus* spp. and *Escherichia coli* are the predominate aerobic bacteria isolated from surgical wounds in small animal patients. Anaerobic bacteria (e.g., *Bacteroides, Fusobacterium,* and *Clostridium* spp.) are now recognized as important pathogens in orthopedic patients. Knowledge of common offending microorganisms in correlation with results of periodic culture of surgical tables, instrument stands, and surgical lights provides insight into potential bacteria in the surgical environment. Presently, cefazolin is the antibiotic of choice for prophylaxis in small animal orthopedic surgery. Cefazolin levels must be present within tissues at the time bacteria enter the wound to effectively suppress bacterial growth. Thus antibiotics must be administered before surgery rather than after completion of the procedure. However, there is no reason to begin prophylactic antibiotic administration long before surgery. Based on empirical and experimental evidence, antibiotics should be administered intravenously at the time of anesthetic induction, repeated every 2 to 4 hours, and discontinued at completion of surgery. Concentrations of the drug equal to or greater than the MIC needed to prevent proliferation of known pathogens is desirable. The cefazolin MIC for coagulase-positive *Staphylococcus* spp. and *E. coli* is 4 μg/ml. Twenty mg/kg of cefazolin given intravenously 20 minutes before the beginning of surgery and repeated every 2 to 4 hours maintains levels at the surgery site above 4 μg/ml.

Antimicrobial Therapy for Bone Infections

Traditional belief that bone infections are difficult to treat because antibiotics exhibit poor bone penetration has recently been shown to be invalid. Factors known to be important in treatment of bone infection are fracture stability, presence of surgical implants, and ability of bacteria to colonize inanimate biomaterials. Once in place, implants become coated with matrix and serum proteins. One matrix protein (fibronectin) is paramount in the pathogenesis of bone infection because bacteria possess cell membrane receptors for fibronectin that facilitate adhesion of microorganisms to implant surfaces. When bacteria become adherent to biomaterials they produce a biofilm composed of polysaccharides, ions, and nutrients. Biofilm enhances adherence of bacteria and protects the microorganism from host defenses. Antimicrobial agents that readily traverse capillary membranes in both normal and infected bone and that are widely distributed in bone interstitial fluid include β-lactam agents (i.e., penicillins, cephalosporins) and aminoglycosides. Table 28-5 contains a list of commonly used antimicrobial agents. Basic treatment regimens for osteomyelitis are discussed on p. 1027.

BONE HEALING

Fracture healing is the biological process that occurs after cartilage and/or bone disruption, to restore tissue continuity necessary for function. The goals of fracture treatment are to encourage healing, restore function to affected bone and surrounding soft tissues, and obtain a cosmetically acceptable appearance. Each goal should be kept in mind when selecting treatment regimens and fixation devices (see chapters on decision making and fixation systems). Fracture healing varies, depending on biologic (i.e., fracture location in cortical bone, cancellous bone, or physeal cartilage; circulation; and/or concurrent soft tissue injury) and mechanical (stability of bone segments and fragments after fixation device placement) factors that influence the sequence of cellular events occurring in fracture healing.

All physiologic processes occurring within bone, including repair processes during fracture healing, are dependent on an adequate blood supply. Normal circulation to long bones consists of an afferent supply from the principal nutrient artery, proximal and distal metaphyseal arteries, and periosteal arteries that enter bone at areas of heavy fascial attachment. The direction of blood flow through the diaphysis is centrifugal (from medullary canal to periosteum). Under

TABLE 28-5

Commonly Used Antimicrobial Agents for Small Animal Orthopedic Infections*

Agent	Dose (mg/kg)	Route	Interval (hours)
Amikacin[1,2]	10	IV, IM, SC	8
Amoxicillin	22-30	IV, IM, SC, PO	6-8
Amoxicillin-clavulanate	22	PO	6-8
Ampicillin	22	IV, IM, SC, PO	6-8
Cefadroxil	22	PO	8-12
Cefazolin	22	IV, IM, SC	6-8
Cefotamine	20-40	IV, IM, SC	6-8
Cefoxitin	22	IV, IM	6-8
Ceftazidime[3]	25	IV, IM	8-12
Cephalexin	22-30	PO	6-8
Cephalothin	22-30	IV, IM, SC	6-8
Cephapirin	22	IV, IM, SC	6-8
Cephradine	22	IV, IM, SC, PO	6-8
Ciprofloxacin	11	PO	12
Clindamycin[4,5]	11	IV, IM, PO	8-12
Cloxacillin	10-15	IV, IM, PO	6-8
Enrofloxacin	5-11	PO	12
Gentamicin	22	IV, IM, SC	8-12
Oxacillin	22	IV, IM, SC, PO	6-8
Penicillin G (aqueous)	20,000-40,000 IU	IV	6

[1]Nephrotoxic and ototoxic. Renal function must be monitored throughout use.
[2]Limit use to 1 week.
[3]Only effective against *Pseudomonas* spp.
[4]Painful on intramuscular injection; can cause phlebitis if given intravenously.
[5]Parenteral dose every 8 hours; oral dose every 12 hours.
*From Budsberg SC, Kemp DT: Antimicrobial distribution and therapeutics in bone, *Comp Cont Educ Pract Vet* 12:1758-1762, 1990.

normal conditions, medullary pressure probably restricts periosteal blood flow to the outer third of the cortex (Fig. 28-4, *A*). In contrast to mature animals, immature animals have numerous arteries that perforate newly formed appositional bone running longitudinally over the periosteal surface. The metaphysis and epiphysis have separate blood supplies and generally do not communicate across the cartilaginous physis (Fig. 28-4, *B*). The epiphyseal blood supply nourishes the cartilaginous reserve cell zone and growing physeal cells. Interruption of this portion of the circulation results in the death of growing cells and cessation of physeal function. Metaphyseal arteries supply cells involved with endochondral ossification; disruption of metaphyseal blood flow delays endochondral ossification, resulting in widening of the cartilaginous physis. When circulation is reestablished, endochondral ossification resumes. Flat bones with extensive muscle attachment (i.e., pelvis and scapula) have tremendous extraosseous blood supply in addition to that provided by nutrient arteries. Irregular bones (e.g., carpal and tarsal bones) generally have multiple nutrient arteries.

Medullary circulation is disrupted in most long bone fractures. Initially, existing components of the normal vasculature are enhanced to supply the injured area. Additionally, a transient extraosseous vascular supply develops in soft tissues and surrounding fractures to nourish the early periosteal callus (Fig. 28-4, *C*). As bone healing progresses

and stability is restored, medullary blood supply is reestablished. Ultimately, the extraosseous circulation diminishes and normal medullary centrifugal flow dominates (Fig. 28-4, *D*). Closed fracture reduction and application of casts or external fixators causes the least disruption to surrounding soft tissues and newly formed extraosseous blood supply (Fig. 28-5, *A* and *B*), whereas open reduction disturbs developing extraosseous blood vessels and hinders reestablishment of medullary blood flow. Traumatic handling of surrounding soft tissues further impairs the extraosseous circulatory response. Insertion of any type of intramedullary pin disrupts the medullary vasculature; pins that contact endosteal surfaces block medullary afferent flow. Stable implants allow new medullary circulation to develop, which supplies the adjacent endosteal surfaces (Fig. 28-5, *C*). Cerclage wire applied tightly to cortical surfaces does not significantly impair vasculature. Even in immature animals, circumferential wires seemingly do not significantly block periosteal blood flow. Although plate and screw application affords the greatest fracture stability and allows early reformation of medullary circulation, blood supply to outer cortical bone beneath plates is impaired (Fig. 28-5, *D*), causing affected cortices to remodel and become more porous. Newer plate designs (i.e., limited-contact dynamic compression plates) minimize this phenomenon. Because adequate blood supply is essential

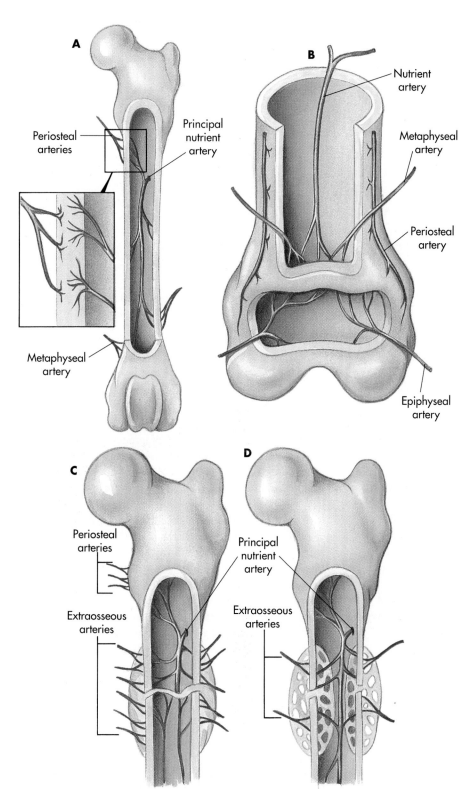

FIG. 28-4
Blood supply to **A,** normal bone, **B,** immature bone, **C,** fractured bone (extraosseous blood supply), and **D,** healing bone.

for bone healing, any circulatory impairment may delay healing. The motion of loose implants, especially cerclage wires, disrupts developing vasculature; excessive fracture motion discourages reestablishment of medullary vasculature. Large bone fragments denuded of soft tissues (and hence blood supply) can be used to anatomically reconstruct fractures; however, these fragments should be rigidly

immobilized to encourage early revascularization. Even with multiple fracture fragments, if the fracture is minimally disturbed and major bone segments are stabilized with a plate or external fixator, fragments will revascularize and incorporate into callus.

Indirect bone healing occurs in fractures with an unstable mechanical environment resulting from the motion of the

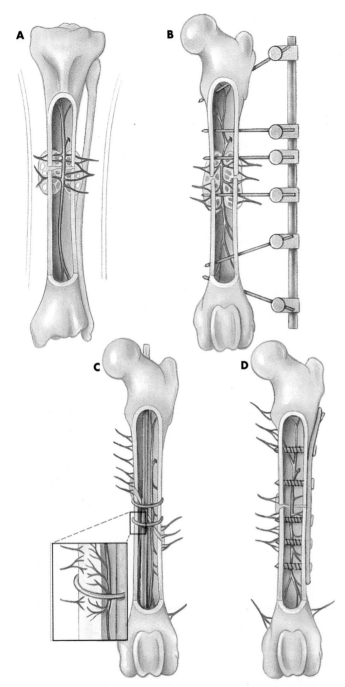

FIG. 28-5
Effect of fixation devices on circulation to fractured bone: **A,** cast, **B,** external fixator, **C,** intramedullary pin and cerclage wires, and **D,** plate and screws. Note that closed fracture reduction and application of casts or external fixators causes the least disruption to surrounding soft tissues and newly formed extraosseous blood supply.

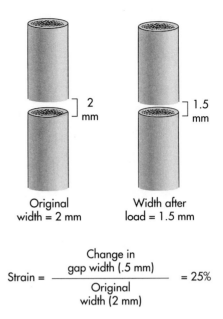

$$\text{Strain} = \frac{\text{Change in gap width (.5 mm)}}{\text{Original width (2 mm)}} = 25\%$$

FIG. 28-6
The ratio between the change in gap width to total gap width is called strain.

adjacent bones. The amount of motion can vary from extremes of untreated (and therefore unrestricted motion) to varying degrees of limited motion achieved with casts, intramedullary pins, external fixators, and/or bone plates. Motion at fracture sites affects the size of gaps between fragments. The ratio between the change in gap width to the total gap width is called *strain* (Fig. 28-6). Because a given tissue's

ability to elongate is limited, excessive strain results in tissue rupture. There are several biologic ways in which strain at fracture sites is decreased. (1) Fragment end resorption increases the width of small gaps subjected to motion, which decreases strain. (2) Strain decreases with increased fracture rigidity as fractures are bridged by less strain-tolerant tissues (Fig. 28-7). (3) Decreased motion occurs at fracture sites when external or periosteal callus is produced because increasing the tissue diameter increases the bone's ability to resist bending. Initially, fracture gaps are bridged by tissues that can withstand motion (i.e., hematoma and granulation tissue); these tissues are sequentially replaced by those that increase the bone's rigidity (i.e., fibrous connective tissue, fibrocartilage, lamellar bone). The orderly sequence of tissue formation in fracture gaps that occurs in indirect bone healing culminates in fibrocartilage mineralization. This mineralization begins at the fragment surfaces and continues toward the gap center, forming trabecular and woven bone. Local resorption of initial bone occurs, followed by vascularization of resorption cavities and replacement with lamellar bone. Continued formation and resorption of lamellar bone at fracture sites results in remodeling of bony callus to cortical bone (see Fig. 28-7).

Direct bone healing (i.e., bone forms directly at fracture sites, without an intermediate cartilage stage) occurs when fixation devices maintain absolute fragment stability. For this to occur the mechanical environment must be such that there is no fracture motion and the fragments are in contact or separated by only small (i.e., 150- to 300-micron) gaps. Direct bone formation, as it occurs in small gaps in the fracture line after rigid fixation, is called *gap healing.* Initially, these gaps are filled with a network of fibrous bone; however, within 7 to 8 weeks this mechanically weak bone union be-

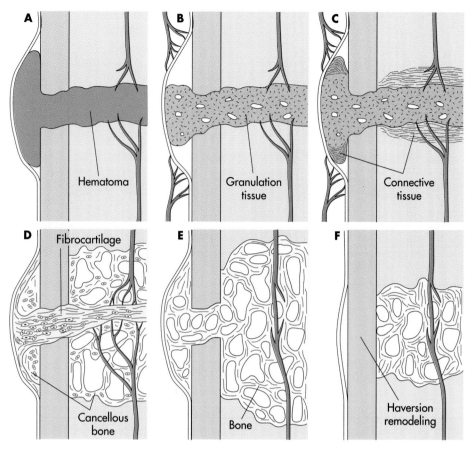

FIG. 28-7
Strain decreases with increased fracture rigidity as fractures are bridged first by more strain tolerant and later by less strain tolerant tissues. **A,** The defect is first filled by a hematoma, which is then replaced by, **B,** granulation tissue. Next, **C,** connective tissue forms. **D,** Fibrocartilage. Fibrocartilage is mineralized, forming cancellous bone and lastly, **E,** bone. **F,** Haversian remodeling occurs to eliminate the callus.

gins to remodel (Fig. 28-8, *A*). The longitudinal reconstruction of fracture sites with haversian remodeling is the second stage of gap healing and provides a strong union between fracture fragments (Fig. 28-8, *B*). Haversian remodeling begins with osteoclastic resorption of bone and formation of resorption cavities that penetrate longitudinally through fragment ends and newly formed bone in fracture gaps. The osteoclasts are followed by vascular loops, mesenchymal cells, and osteoblast precursors. Osteoblasts line resorption cavities and secrete osteoid, which is mineralized to bone. This lamellar bone is arranged along the bone's long axis, through the fragment ends and fracture gaps, and results in a strong union of bone fragments. Where bone fragments are in contact under rigid fixation there is simultaneous union and reconstruction with haversian remodeling (Fig. 28-8, *C*).

Distraction osteogenesis occurs when gradual traction is applied to cortical bone so that sufficient stress is created to stimulate and maintain formation of new bone. This concept is used in external fixation techniques for limb lengthening, treatment of angular deformities, and transportation of cortical bone. To achieve bone formation during slow distraction after corticotomy or osteotomy, medullary and periosteal blood supply must be preserved and major bone fragments must be optimally stabilized. The bone surface is covered with cells that may differentiate into osteoblasts or chondroblasts, depending on the cell's mechanical and biologic environment. Within 3 to 7 days after osteotomy these cells organize and begin to proliferate. The ideal rate of dis-

traction is 1 mm per day divided into two to four distraction periods. Osteoid is laid down in parallel columns that extend from osteotomy surfaces centrally. Normally, lamellar bone develops within these columns; however, if there is sufficient instability at the fracture site, formation of an intermediate cartilaginous phase may occur. After the desired limb length is achieved, the fixator remains in place to allow remodeling of new cortical bone (Fig. 28-9).

Metaphyseal fractures involving trabecular or cancellous bone heal differently than do similar fractures through cortical bone (Fig. 28-10, *A*). Trabecular bone is inherently more stable than cortical bone and does not heal by periosteal callus formation unless there is tremendous instability. Increased osteoblastic activity occurs on either side of these fractures if they have been adequately immobilized (Fig. 28-10, *B*). New bone is deposited on existing trabeculae, and fracture gaps are filled with woven bone. Bridging between trabeculae occurs before union of the cortical shell (Fig. 28-10, *C*). For physeal fracture healing see special age considerations on p. 718.

Radiographic Appearance of Bone Healing

Sequential radiographs allow evaluation of fracture healing. Generally, radiographs should be taken postoperatively to assess fracture alignment and implant position, and they should be repeated every 4 to 6 weeks during healing. Follow-up radiographs should be compared with earlier studies to determine the dynamics of bone healing. Fractures should

FIG. 28-8
Sequence of events in direct bone healing: **A,** In Stage I of gap healing, the gap is filled with fibrous bone. **B,** Then (Stage II) longitudinal reconstruction of bone with haversian remodeling occurs. **C,** Contact bone healing occurs where bone fragments are in contact under rigid fixation; simultaneous union and reconstruction with haversian remodeling occur.

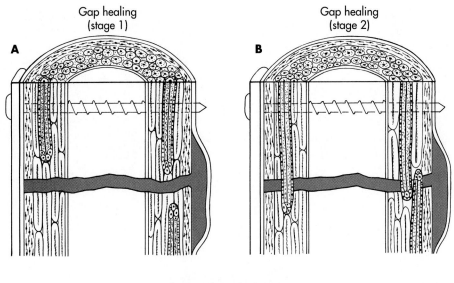

Gap healing (stage 1)

Gap healing (stage 2)

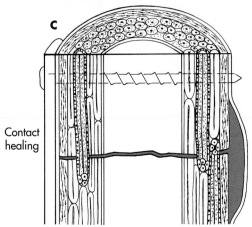

Contact healing

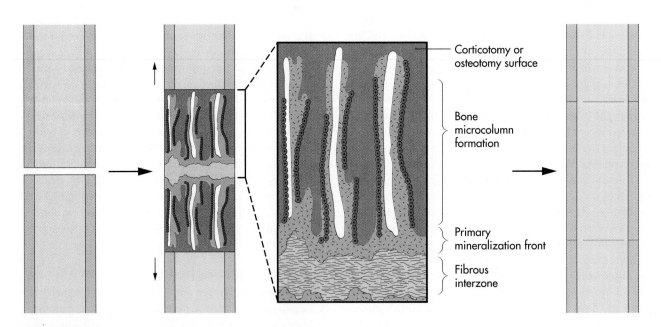

FIG. 28-9
During distraction osteogenesis, osteoid is laid down in parallel columns that extend from osteotomy surfaces centrally. Lamellar bone develops within these columns if the fracture is sufficiently stable.

A Fracture of trabecular bone **B** New trabecular bone formation **C** Healing of cortical shell

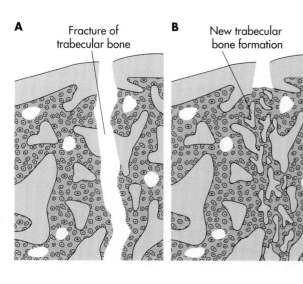 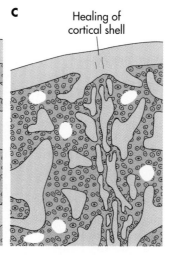

FIG. 28-10
A, Trabecular bone responds to fracture by increasing osteoblastic activity. **B,** New bone is deposited on existing trabeculae and fracture gaps are filled with woven bone. **C,** Bridging between trabeculae occurs before union of the cortical shell.

be evaluated for evidence of bone formation, and implant position should be appraised to detect instability. Development of periosteal callus indicates that indirect bone formation is occurring (see p. 711). Filling of stable fracture lines with bone indicates direct healing. Trabecular bone healing in metaphyseal fractures appears radiographically as the formation of one or two dense bands at the fracture site. Gradual bridging of these bands occurs until finally the cortical shell is completely spanned by bone. Periosteal callus is not usually evident in metaphyseal fractures unless there is tremendous instability of fracture fragments.

Determining when fixation devices are best removed is difficult. This decision is usually made after evaluating radiographs of healing fractures. Knowledge of radiographic appearance of bone healing associated with various fixation systems is mandatory for wise decision making. In general, fixation systems can be removed when there is radiographic evidence of bone bridging the fractures. Fractures stabilized with casts heal by indirect bone formation; radiographically this appears as bridging periosteal and endosteal callus at fracture sites. The large amounts of callus that generally form with this type of fixation serve as an internal support for bone remodeling. An exception to this is with distal radial and ulnar fractures in toy breeds, in which large amounts of callus may not be produced. The cast should be removed once the callus has bridged the fracture.

Bone healing with external fixators may be direct, indirect, or somewhere between these extremes depending on fracture type, mechanical environment afforded by external fixators, and degree of bone reconstruction. In general, fractures stabilized with external fixators have less periosteal callus formation when compared with similar fractures treated with casts. Also, fractures stabilized with external fixators develop more endosteal and uniting callus than periosteal callus. Radiographically, simple fractures that are anatomically reduced and rigidly stabilized with external fixators (e.g., bilateral external fixators with multiple pins) heal with minimal periosteal or endosteal callus. This is radiographically similar to the direct bone union response observed in fractures treated with plates and screws. As fixator stiffness de-

creases, increased callus is usually evident. When simple fractures are not anatomically reduced (e.g., with closed reduction) and/or fixators are not rigid, resorption of bone at fracture lines and callus formation are often evident. This apparently occurs as a normal response of healing bone to high strain when the increased strain is concentrated in a single fracture line. Fixators should be removed after fracture lines have bridged with bone.

The type of bone healing observed in comminuted fractures depends on how well the biologic environment is preserved and on the rigidity of the fixation. Where anatomic reconstruction and rigid fixation of all fragments are difficult or impossible in severely comminuted fractures, preservation of the biologic environment is often best accomplished with closed reduction or limited exposure and rigid fixation (e.g., external fixators or bridging plates). Fractures treated by this method heal with endosteal bone formation and bone bridging between fragments. At 1 month, radiographs show increased mineral density throughout the fracture site with minimal formation of periosteal callus. In most patients, bone formation is evident within 2 months, and remodeling of callus is evident 3 months after fixation. Computer-assisted tomographic images show endosteal bone by 2 weeks and bridging endosteal and interfragmentary bone (which unites the bone fragments) by 12 weeks after fixation. There is minimal evidence of periosteal callus formation.

Fractures stabilized with pins and wires heal by primary bone union if implants have rigidly stabilized fractures (e.g., long oblique fractures managed with intramedullary pins and multiple, appropriately applied cerclage wires). Conversely, if rigid fixation is not achieved with pins and wires, callus formation will be evident radiographically. Pins should be removed once bone has bridged the fracture. Wires are not removed unless they cause problems (i.e., migration, interference with fracture healing).

Fractures that are anatomically reconstructed and rigidly stabilized (e.g., with plates and screws) heal by direct bone union. With direct bone healing, fracture lines disappear and fractures appear devoid of bridging periosteal and endosteal callus. Because the implant is acting as callus to support the fracture during haversian remodeling, implant removal should generally be delayed until 6 to 12 months after surgery to allow adequate time for bone remodeling.

SUTURE MATERIALS/SPECIAL INSTRUMENTS

Special equipment is helpful in fracture repair. Two or more bone-holding forceps are essential in open fracture reduction. Those used most frequently by the authors are Kern bone-holding forceps, point-reduction forceps (Synthes), speed-lock reduction forceps (Synthes), and Richard bone-holding forceps. Hand-held (i.e., Hohmann, Army-Navy) and self-retaining (e.g., Gelpi) retractors are useful with all orthopedic techniques. Periosteal elevators are helpful in reflecting muscle from bone by elevating periosteal attachments. Equipment for fracture stabilization is discussed in the section on fracture fixation systems (see p. 733).

POSTOPERATIVE CARE AND ASSESSMENT

Postoperative instructions for each orthopedic technique are presented in the discussion of various orthopedic conditions. Common to the success of all orthopedic procedures is the use of appropriate physical therapy methods. Passive physical manipulation, heat, and cold are important considerations in rehabilitation of musculoskeletal injuries. Cold therapy is used in the acute phase of injury or during the first 2 to 3 days after surgery. Its beneficial effects are swelling control and analgesia. Cold may be applied using crushed ice in a plastic bag or commercially available freezer packs. The cold packs should be applied to the area for 20 minutes three times a day. Heat therapy in the form of hot compresses is indicated in the chronic phase of healing. Beneficial effects include decreased pain and improved circulation. Heat does not decrease swelling and should not be used in the initial 3 to 4 days after surgery. Heat is most easily applied with moist, hot towels. Caution is necessary to avoid scalding the skin. Towels should be changed frequently to maintain a warm environment for 20 minutes. Heat therapy is also beneficial to relax muscles before beginning passive physical manipulation.

Passive Physiotherapy

Passive physiotherapy is best described as controlled stretching of muscles, tendons, and ligaments. The joint above or below the area in question is gently flexed and extended. Gradually the amount of movement is increased until a near normal range of motion, or one within limits of pain tolerance, is achieved. The joint is flexed and extended for 2 to 3 minutes, then the process is repeated with the other major joints of the limb. Passive therapy is effective in maintaining joint motion and patient comfort but does not enhance muscle tone and strength. For this reason passive therapy should be combined with active physical therapy. Allowing or helping the patient to stand on the operated limb is the simplest form of active physical therapy and should begin during the first postoperative week. Weight bearing may be concentrated on the operated limb by gently raising the uninjured paw from the ground. The patient should be allowed to bear weight on the operated limb for 1 to 2 minutes. The duration of weight bearing is gradually increased until the patient begins to bear weight on the operated limb without coaching. Swimming is also an excellent form of active therapy if ambient temperature allows and a place to swim is accessible because it encourages joint motion and muscle strengthening, without impact loading. Swim therapy is begun with 2- to 3-minute sessions and the duration is gradually increased (depending on patient tolerance). Caution must be used when the patient enters and leaves the water so that he/she does not slip and injure the operated leg. Slow leash walking is encouraged immediately after surgery and should be continued until rehabilitation and healing are complete.

Bandages

Bandages serve many functions postoperatively (i.e., wound protection, application of topical medication, soft tissue compression, increased patient comfort, selective immobilization of soft tissues and joints). Bandages commonly used in veterinary orthopedics for postoperative comfort and soft tissue compression or immobilization are padded soft bandages (see p. 706), Ehmer slings, Velpeau slings, and 90/90 slings.

Ehmer slings. Ehmer slings prevent weight bearing of the pelvic limb (Fig. 28-11). The most common use for Ehmer slings is to support closed or open reduction of hip luxations. *Place a thin layer of cast padding around the metatarsal area and wrap nonadherent gauze (Kling) multiple times over the padding. Maximally flex the stifle and wrap the gauze around the thigh by bringing it medially between the body wall and limb. Pull the gauze firmly and bring it over the front of the knee to maintain flexion. Then wrap the gauze over the lateral surface of the thigh and bring it distally medial to the tarsus and over the padded metatarsal area. Repeat the wrapping three to four times. Finish the bandage by applying elastic adhesive material in the same manner.*

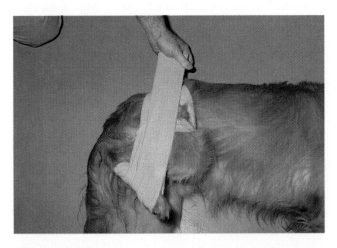

FIG. 28-11
An Ehmer sling being applied to the rear limb of a dog. These slings are used to prevent weight bearing (e.g., after hip luxation).

Velpeau slings. Velpeau slings prevent weight bearing and provide some stability to the proximal forelimb (Fig. 28-12). They are most commonly used to help maintain closed or open reduction of medial shoulder luxations and support scapular fractures. *With the shoulder and elbow flexed and the limb adducted against the body wall, begin by placing two to three layers of padding around the torso and limb. Wrap layers cranial and caudal to the opposite limb to prevent slippage of the incorporated limb. Place an additional layer in a similar manner with gauze (Kling) to add mild compression. Last, place an outer layer of elastic tape or Vetrap to provide support.*

90/90 slings. 90/90 slings are used to provide flexion of the stifle joint and immobilize the pelvic limb after surgery (Fig. 28-13). A common use for 90/90 bandages is after repair of a distal femoral physeal fracture, to prevent quadriceps contracture. *Place the stifle joint and tarsus in 90-degree flexion. Using cast padding, wrap several layers of padding around the metatarsus area. Wrap elastic adhe-sive around the flexed tarsus and stifle joints to maintain 90 degrees of flexion.*

COMPLICATIONS
Nonunions

Fracture nonunions are diagnosed when there is radiographic evidence that bone healing is not occurring or cannot occur. Surgical intervention is necessary in such cases to create an environment conducive to bone healing. Most nonunions are a result of poor decision making and technical failure on the part of surgeons, rather than biologic failures attributable to the patient. The presence of a lucent line through fractures, representing cartilage and fibrous tissue, coupled with callus formation at the fracture site is characteristic of the radiographic appearance of vascular nonunions. This type of nonunion is invariably the result of inadequate fracture stability. The most common cause of vascular nonunions is stabilization of transverse or short oblique femoral fractures with an intramedullary pin and cerclage wires that do not adequately prevent rotational instability. Constant motion at fracture sites prevents cartilage mineralization. Rigid immobilization of fractures with either plates or external fixators usually allows fracture healing to progress.

Hypertrophic nonunions (i.e., vascular nonunions with large amounts of callus) (Fig. 28-14) are treated by removal of loose implants, joint alignment, and placement of a compression plate (see p. 749). Cancellous bone grafts may

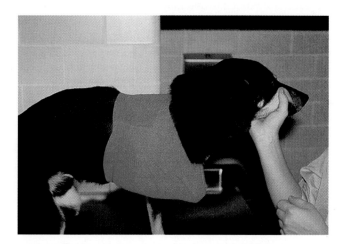

FIG. 28-12
A Velpeau sling applied to the forelimb of a dog with a scapular fracture. The sling was placed to prevent weight bearing while the fracture healed.

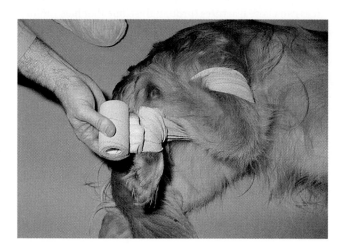

FIG. 28-13
A 90/90 sling applied to the rear limb of a dog with a distal femoral physeal fracture.

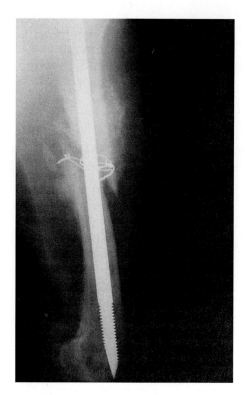

FIG. 28-14
Radiograph of a dog with a hypertrophic nonunion of the femur. Notice the formation of a large periosteal callus that cannot bridge the fracture. The fracture was inadequately stabilized with an intramedullary pin and cerclage wires.

be used; however, the hypertrophic callus usually provides adequate cancellous bone for healing. Swabs for bacterial culture and sensitivity should be obtained when nonunions are treated. If a radiographic or clinical diagnosis of osteomyelitis is made, treatment includes removing any large pieces of necrotic cortical bone. Resultant defects are filled with cancellous bone autografts, which may be placed during the plating procedure or after 5 to 7 days of open wound management. This delay allows formation of healthy granulation tissue beds before grafting. Plate removal is recommended after healing occurs in infected nonunions because plates may serve as a nidus for continued infection.

Atrophic nonunions are biologically inactive pseudoarthroses. Radiographically, there is no evidence of bone reaction at fracture sites, and bone ends appear sclerotic. Histologically, fracture gaps are filled with fibrous tissue and medullary cavities are sealed with cortical bone. This type of nonunion requires surgery to remove fibrous tissues and open medullary canals. Adequate stability is usually achieved with plates and screws, coupled with placement of autogenous cancellous bone grafts. Plate fixation is preferred because prolonged healing is common with this type of nonunion (Fig. 28-15).

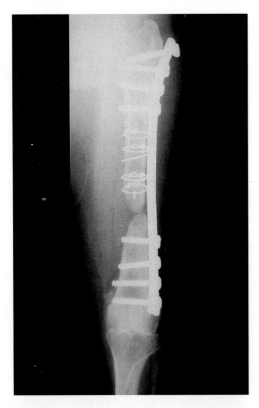

FIG. 28-15
Radiograph of a dog with an atrophic nonunion of the femur. Notice the lack of callus formation at the fracture site. The fracture eventually healed after surgical opening of the medullary canal, shortening of the femur to gain cortical contact, and application of a limited contact dynamic compression plate with a cancellous bone autograft.

Delayed Unions

Fractures that are uniting, albeit more slowly than anticipated, are classified as *delayed unions.* Signs of progressive bone activity (i.e., increasing radiographic density of fracture lines) are visible on sequential radiographs. As long as implants remain intact the animal can be confined and reoperation is not necessary; however, cancellous bone grafts may be added to speed healing. If implants are loose or migrating, they should be removed, fractures should be stabilized appropriately, and cancellous bone autografts should be applied.

Malunions

Malunions are healed fractures in which anatomic bone alignment was not achieved or maintained during healing. Malunions may have a deleterious effect on function. Angular deformities are characterized by loss of correct parallel relationships between joints above and below the fractured bone. Deformities may be classified as valgus, varus, antecurvatum, or recurvatum (Fig. 28-16, *A–D*). When severe, these deformities affect limb function and may precipitate osteoarthritis of adjacent joints. Translational and rotational deformities can also occur (Fig. 28-16, *E–F*). Rotation most commonly occurs with inadequately stabilized femoral fractures and may adversely affect hip function. Shortening of affected bones may also occur. A shortened bone in a single bone system (i.e., femur, humerus) can be compensated for by extension of adjacent joints; however, shortening of a single bone in a paired bone system (i.e., radius/ulna, tibia/fibula) causes incongruity in alignment of adjacent joints. Malunion should be treated with corrective osteotomy if it adversely affects the animal's ability to ambulate.

SPECIAL AGE CONSIDERATIONS

Physeal fractures account for 30% of fractures in immature animals and occur because the physis is weaker than surrounding bone and ligaments (Fig. 28-17, *A,* p. 720). The mechanically weak portion of the physis is the hypertrophic zone because the cells are relatively large in comparison with the amount of matrix (Fig. 28-17, *B*). Avulsion or shearing forces can cause fractures through this zone that heal rapidly by continued growth of physeal cartilage and metaphyseal callus formation. Once fracture gaps are filled, normal endochondral ossification resumes and physeal function continues. However, if damage occurs to growing cells (i.e., reserve and proliferating zones), growth of physeal cartilage does not occur; instead, endochondral ossification proceeds (Fig. 28-17, *C*). Here, bone formation in fracture gaps results in premature physeal closure. Malalignment of the fractured physis (where metaphyseal and epiphyseal bone are in contact) allows trabecular bone healing and physeal bridging. The bone bridge may prevent normal physeal function.

References

Spackman CJA et al: Thoracic wall and pulmonary trauma in dogs sustaining fractures as a result of motor vehicle accidents, *J Am Vet Med Assoc* 185:975, 1984.

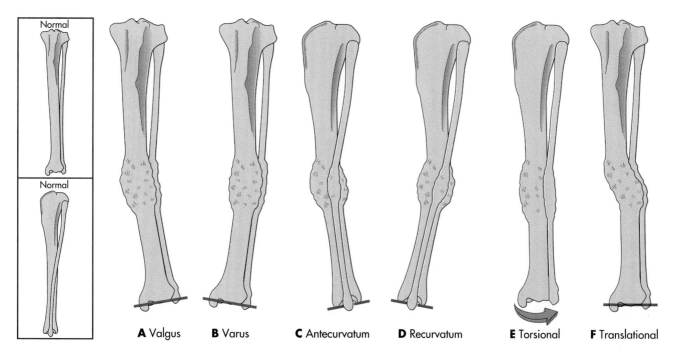

A Valgus **B** Varus **C** Antecurvatum **D** Recurvatum **E** Torsional **F** Translational

FIG. 28-16
Malalignment of bone: **A,** Valgus is lateral, **B,** varus is medial, **C,** antecurvatum is caudal, and **D,** recurvatum is cranial angulation of the distal segment of bone. **E,** Torsion is medial or lateral twisting of the distal segment of bone, while, **F,** translation is displacement of the distal segment of bone with the joint surfaces parallel.

Tamas PM, Paddleford RR, Krahwinkel DJ: Thoracic trauma in dogs and cats presented for limb fractures, *J Am Anim Hosp Assoc* 21:161, 1985.

Suggested Reading

Aron DN, Crowe DT: The 90/90 flexion splint for prevention of stifle joint stiffness with femoral fracture repair, *J Am Anim Hosp Assoc* 23:447, 1987.

Elkins AD, Massimo M, Zembo M: Distraction osteogenesis in the dog using the Ilizarov external ring fixator, *J Am Anim Hosp Assoc* 29:410, 1993.

Johnson JM, Johnson AL, Eurell JA: Histological appearance of naturally occurring canine physeal fratures, *Vet Surg* 23:81, 1994.

Kaderly RE: Delayed union, nonunion, and malunion. In Slatter D, editor: *Textbook of small animal surgery,* ed 2, Philadelphia, 1993, WB Saunders.

Leighton RL: Principles of conservative fracture management: splints and casts, *Semin Vet Med Surg (Small Amin)* 6:39, 1991.

Palmer RH et al: Principles of bone healing and biomechanics of external skeletal fixation, *Vet Clin North Am (Small Anim)* 22:45, 1992.

Perron SM: The concept of biological plating using the limited-contact dynamic compression plate (LC-DCP), *Injury* 22:1, 1992.

Rahn BA: Bone healing: histologic and physiologic concepts. In Sumner-Smith G, editor: *Bone in clinical orthopedics,* Philadelphia, 1982, WB Saunders.

Schatzker J: Concepts of fracture stabilization. In Sumner-Smith G, editor: *Bone in clinical orthopaedics,* Philadelphia, 1982, WB Saunders.

Stevenson S, Olmstead ML, Kowalski J: Bacterial culturing for prediction of postoperative complications following open fracture repair in small animals, *Vet Surg* 15:99, 1986.

Tomlinson J: Complications of fractures repaired with casts and splints, *Vet Clin North Am Small Anim Pract* 21:735, 1991.

Uhthoff HK, Rahn BA: Healing patterns of metaphyseal fractures, *Clin Orthop* 160:95, 1981.

Wilson JW: Vascular supply to normal bones and healing fractures, *Sem Vet Med Surg (Small Anim)* 6:26, 1991.

ORTHOPEDIC EXAMINATION

PROBLEM IDENTIFICATION

Orthopedic surgery includes procedures used to stabilize fractured bones; explore, debride, and stabilize injured joints; replace damaged joints; stabilize spinal column injuries; decompress the spinal cord; resect musculoskeletal tumors; and repair tendon and ligament injuries. Patients with orthopedic problems comprise a significant percentage of the general practice population. Before the most appropriate method for treating a problem can be selected, the orthopedic problem must be identified and assessed. Developing surgical skills and familiarity with specialized instrumentation is necessary for performing most orthopedic procedures. Veterinarians should be aware of their limitations and refer complicated cases when necessary. Knowledge of potential complications and pitfalls helps surgeons take the appropriate steps to prevent these problems.

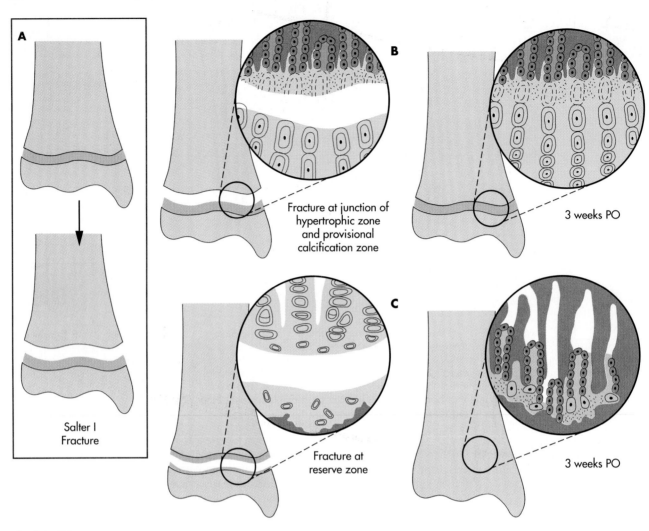

FIG. 28-17
Physeal cartilage healing: **A,** A Salter-Harris Type I physeal fracture occurs through the hypertrophied zone of cartilage. **B,** Such fractures, if reduced accurately, heal by continued formation of cartilage. **C,** If the fracture involves the reserve zone or the germinal cells are damaged, healing occurs by endochondral ossification.

Identifying a fracture as the cause of non–weight-bearing lameness is usually straightforward. The challenging problem is to assess the patient, classify the fracture, and develop plans for fixation that will allow predictable and consistent results. Occasionally, animals will present with nondisplaced fractures that are difficult to detect and require special diagnostic techniques. Most orthopedic cases present for lameness and/or pain; however, identifying the cause of the lameness may be difficult. Accurate historical information, thorough general examination, orthopedic examination, and diagnostic imaging techniques are essential. It is important to realize that the most appropriate therapy is not always surgery.

Signalment and History

Signalment and historical data are helpful for developing an accurate differential diagnosis. Many orthopedic diseases are predictable within certain age groups and breeds (Table 28-6). Information concerning the general condition of the animal (i.e., anorexia, depression or fever, limb affected, multiple limb involvement, degree of pain or lameness, duration, intensity of onset, historical trauma, effect of exercise, time of day of greatest clinical signs, effect of rest, and changes in lameness associated with weather) provides initial clues to form a differential list of potential causes. Additional questioning, physical examination, and radiographic examination will provide data to make a definitive diagnosis.

Physical Examination

The animal's general health should be assessed as part of the physical examination. Baseline examination includes obtaining the animal's temperature, pulse, and respiration. The animal's overall appearance should be noted (e.g., obesity) and thoracic auscultation and abdominal palpation performed. **General health evaluation is important before anesthetizing any animal that has orthopedic disease.** Traumatized animals presenting for fracture evaluation should have thoracic radiographs and serial electrocardiograms performed. Evaluation of the abdominal cavity is done initially with

TABLE 28-6

Differential Diagnoses for Lameness

Signalment	History	Differential Diagnosis
Immature, large dogs Front limb	Acute	Fractured physis* Fractured bone*
	Chronic	OCD shoulder OCD elbow UAP elbow FCP elbow Premature closure of physes Elbow incongruity Retained cartilage cores Panosteitis Hypertrophic osteodystrophy
Immature, large dogs Rear limb	Acute	Fractured physis* Fractured bone*
	Chronic	Hip dysplasia OCD stifle Patellar luxation Avulsion of long digital extensor tendon OCD hock Panosteitis Hypertrophic osteodystrophy
Immature, small dogs Front limb	Acute	Fractured physis Fractured bone
	Chronic	Congenital luxation— shoulder Congenital luxation— elbow Premature closure of physes Atlantoaxial instability
Immature, small dogs Rear limb	Acute	Fractured physis Fractured bone
	Chronic	Avascular necrosis femoral head Patellar luxation*
Adult, large dogs Front limb	Acute	Fractured bone* Luxated shoulder* Luxated elbow*
	Chronic	Degenerative joint disease* Panosteitis Bicipital tenosynovitis Contracture infraspinatus tendon Radius curvus/elbow incongruity Bone/soft tissue neoplasia* Brachial plexus injury* Cervical disk disease Inflammatory joint disease*

TABLE 28-6 cont'd

Differential Diagnoses for Lameness

Signalment	History	Differential Diagnosis
Adult, large dogs Rear limb	Acute	Fractured bone* Luxated hip* Luxated stifle* Cruciate/meniscus syndrome* Ruptured Achilles tendon*
	Chronic	Degenerative joint disease* Panosteitis Patellar luxation Cruciate/meniscus syndrome* Bone/soft tissue neoplasia* Lumbosacral syndrome Thoracolumbar disk disease Inflammatory joint disease*
Adult, small dogs Front limb	Acute	Fractured bone Luxated shoulder Luxated elbow
	Chronic	Degenerative joint disease Luxating shoulder Bone/soft tissue neoplasia Inflammatory joint disease Radius curvus/elbow incongruity Cervical disk disease
Adult, small dogs Rear limb	Acute	Fractured bone Luxated hip Luxated stifle Cruciate/meniscus syndrome
	Chronic	Degenerative joint disease Patellar luxation Cruciate/meniscus syndrome Bone/soft tissue neoplasia Lumbosacral syndrome Thoracolumbar disk disease Inflammatory joint disease

*Denotes potential differential diagnoses in cats.

palpation and evaluation of serum chemistry tests. Abdominocentesis and/or radiographic evaluation of the urinary tract should be performed if clinical signs suggest injury. Traumatized animals with long bone fractures frequently have concurrent soft tissue injuries (e.g., pneumothorax, traumatic myocarditis, diaphragmatic hernia, or ruptured bladder or urethra). It is important to diagnose these injuries before the animal is anesthetized for fracture repair.

Orthopedic Examination

An orthopedic examination begins by observing the animal for signs of lameness while obtaining the history. This is necessary even if the owner has attributed the lameness to a particular limb because the correct limb may not have been identified. **The animal should be allowed to walk around the examination room and observed for obvious lameness and for more subtle signs, such as reducing the weight placed on the affected limb when standing or sitting.** Other observations may include unilateral or bilateral muscle atrophy and abnormal muscle development. Dogs with bilateral hip dysplasia or chronic cruciate ligament rupture can appear underdeveloped or weak in the rear quarters and heavily muscled in the forequarters.

If the lameness has not been localized during the initial observation, the animal should be observed while walking and trotting. It may be necessary to take dogs outside to improved footing. To protect a sore limb, animals quickly shift their weight from the affected limb, making it appear that they are landing heavily on the opposite, or "good," limb. Animals with forelimb lameness will lift their heads after the lame limb strikes the ground in an attempt to remove weight from the affected limb. A short stride occurs when the animal has a decreased range of motion in a diseased joint (e.g., hip dysplasia). External swinging, or paddling, of the affected limb(s) occurs when the animal tries to advance a limb that cannot be adequately flexed. This is commonly observed in dogs with severe degenerative joint disease of the elbows. Animals with bilateral lameness may not limp but often show more subtle signs (e.g., shifting their weight from limb to limb while standing, shortened stride, or bilateral muscle atrophy).

After the lame limb has been identified, the animal should be returned to the examination room and limb palpation and an initial neurologic examination simultaneously performed. **Optimally, the first examination should be done without sedation, to determine the animal's response to pain;** however, this may not be possible in aggressive animals. The examiner should develop a consistent evaluation pattern. One technique is to start at the front of the animal and work toward the rear. Also, starting at the toes of each limb and progressing proximally is useful. It is preferable to begin examining a sound limb to identify the individual's normal response to manipulation and pressure. The initial examination should be done with the animal standing, to assess muscular symmetry, joint enlargement, and proprioceptive responses. As each bone, joint, and soft tissue area is pal-

pated, asymmetry (between limbs), response to pain, swelling, abnormalities in range of motion, instability, and crepitation should be noted. Asymmetry should be assessed before and during individual limb palpation and can indicate tumor, abscess, atrophy, joint swelling, or greenstick fracture. Long bones should be palpated to determine if there is swelling (i.e., fracture, tumor), response to pain while firm pressure is applied (e.g., panosteitis, fracture, tumor), or instability or crepitation (i.e., fracture). Joints should be isolated and moved through a complete range of motion to detect crepitation, pain, or abnormalities in range of motion. Additional tests of hip and stifle instability should be performed if abnormalities are detected in these joints (see pp. 724-727). Muscles and tendons should be palpated to determine if they are normal and intact. After the initial orthopedic examination to localize pain, the animal may be sedated to facilitate closer examination and to perform radiographs (Tables 28-7 and 28-8).

FORELIMB

A complete orthopedic examination of the forelimb includes the following manipulations:

Below carpus. *Examine the paw closely to determine if there is any foreign material present. Spread the toes and nails apart and inspect the webbing and pads. Palpate each digit to determine if the bones are intact and whether there is soft tissue swelling. Extend and flex the phalangeal joints and palpate the corresponding extensor and flexor tendons to see if they relax and tighten appropriately. Test the lateral and medial stability of each joint in extension. Palpate the areas adjacent to the metacarpal pad and over the palmar sesamoids of metacarpophalangeal joints 2 and 5 for sensitivity to pressure. Palpate the metacarpal bones to determine if there is swelling or instability.*

Carpus. *Palpate the dorsal surface of the carpus gently to determine if there is fluctuant swelling associated with joint effusion. This may be a subtle finding in the carpus and is more easily noted when the animal is standing because loading the joint forces the fluid peripherally. Compare the affected limb with the opposite carpus* (NOTE: Bilateral swelling may occur with some diseases, such as rheumatoid arthritis). *Extend and flex the carpus.* Maximum extension of the carpus should be about 180 degrees to 190 degrees; maximum flexion should be 45 degrees. A decreased range of motion may indicate degenerative joint disease. *Note any crepitation. Extend and stress the carpus in the medial to lateral plane to determine if there is joint instability.*

Radius. *Palpate the radius for instability (fracture), swelling (fracture, tumor), and pain response to deep bone palpation (panosteitis).*

Elbow. *Palpate the elbow for fluctuant swelling in the space between the lateral condyle and olecranon and over the medial coronoid process.* This indicates joint effusion that can result from several elbow diseases. Joint effusion may be more easily detected when the animal is standing. Firm, generalized swelling of the elbow often indicates de-

TABLE 28-7

Sedation for Palpation and Radiographs of Dogs

Drug/Combination	Dose	Route	Comments
Acepromazine plus	0.05 mg/kg, max of 1 mg	IV SC IM	Acepromazine is not reversible
Oxymorphone	0.05-0.1 mg/kg	IV SC IM	Animal will require restraint if
or			acepromazine is used alone
Butorphanol	0.2-0.4 mg/kg	IV SC IM	Acepromazine is contraindicated
plus			with seizure history
Atropine or	0.02 mg/kg	IV	Oxymorphone can be reversed
	0.04 mg/kg	SC IM	with 0.02 mg/kg naloxone
Glycopyrrolate	0.005-0.011 mg/kg	IV SC IM	(Narcan) IV
			Auditory hypersensitivity/panting
			with oxymorphone
Xylazine plus	0.2 mg/kg	IV IM	Xylazine can be reversed with 1.0-
			2.0 mg/kg tolazoline, IM or IV
Butorphanol plus	0.2 mg/kg	IV IM	Total dose of xylazine may vary
Atropine or	0.02 mg/kg	IV	with route of administration and
	0.04 mg/kg	SC IM	weight of the patient.
Glycopyrrolate	0.005-0.011 mg/kg	IV SC IM	
Oxymorphone plus	0.05-0.1 mg/kg	IV SC IM	Oxymorphone can be reversed
Diazepam plus	0.1-0.2 mg/kg	IV	with 0.02 mg/kg naloxone
			(Narcan) IV
Atropine or	0.02 mg/kg	IV	Auditory hypersensitivity/panting
	0.04 mg/kg	SC IM	
Glycopyrrolate	0.005-0.011 mg/kg	IV SC IM	

Note: Acepromazine (0.05 mg/kg IM or SC; max of 2 mg) may be used alone for radiographs and palpation; however, it provides minimal restraint.

TABLE 28-8

Sedation for Palpation and Radiographs of Cats

Drug/Combination	Dose	Route*	Comments
Acepromazine plus	0.05 mg/kg	IM	Acepromazine is not reversible
Butorphanol plus	0.2 mg/kg	IM	Animal will require restraint if
Atropine or	0.04 mg/kg	IM	acepromazine is used alone
Glycopyrrolate	0.005-0.011 mg/kg	IM	Acepromazine is contraindicated
			with seizure history
Xylazine plus	0.2 mg/kg	IM	Xylazine can be reversed with 1.0-
Butorphanol plus	0.2 mg/kg	IM	2.0 mg/kg tolazoline, IM or IV
Atropine or	0.04 mg/kg	IM	
Glycopyrrolate	0.005-0.011 mg/kg	IM	
Ketamine	5 mg/kg	IM	Provides little to no muscle
			relaxation

*Other routes of administration may be appropriate for some drugs (e.g., IV if a catheter is in place).

generative joint disease. *Flex and extend the elbow (Figs. 28-18 and 28-19).* Normal extension and flexion are about 165 degrees and 40 degrees to 50 degrees, respectively. The carpus should almost touch the shoulder when the elbow is flexed. Decreased range of motion caused by incomplete flexion of the elbow usually suggests degenerative joint disease, which may occur secondary to a fragmented coronoid process, an ununited anconeal process, or osteochondritis dissecans. *While the elbow is in extension, check the integrity of the collateral ligaments by applying medial and lateral force to the radius and ulna.*

Humerus. *Palpate the humerus for instability (fracture), swelling (fracture, tumor), and pain response to deep palpation (panosteitis). Palpate the bone in areas where it is not covered by muscles, to differentiate panosteitis from muscular pain.*

Shoulder. Swelling from joint effusion is difficult to detect in the shoulder because of the overlying muscles. *Move the shoulder through a range of motion, including hyperextension and hyperflexion while stabilizing the scapula (Fig. 28-20).* Osteochondritis dissecans of the humeral head elicits a pain response when the shoulder is hyperextended.

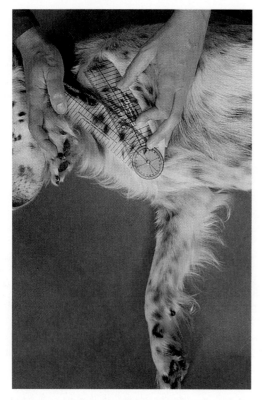

FIG. 28-18
Flex and extend the elbow. Notice the angle of greatest flexion of a normal elbow measured with a goniometer. The carpus should almost touch the shoulder. Compare this to the angle of flexion in a dog with degenerative joint disease (Fig. 28-19).

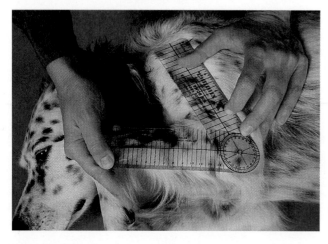

FIG. 28-19
Angle of greatest flexion of an elbow in a dog with degenerative joint disease. Compare this to the angle of flexion in a normal dog (Fig. 28-18).

Hold the acromial process stationary and mobilize the humeral head to detect luxation or subluxation. Many shoulder joints pop or click without significance, but any translation of the humeral head in relationship to the acromion process is abnormal. *Palpate the biceps tendon and apply pressure.* A painful response is indicative of tenosynovitis.

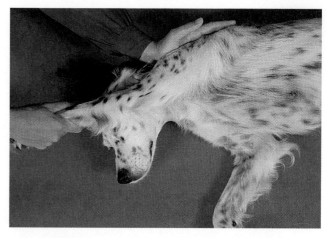

FIG. 28-20
Hyperextend the shoulder while stabilizing the scapula. Pain on hyperextension may indicate osteochondritis dissecans of the humeral head.

Scapula. *Palpate the scapula for instability (fracture) and swelling (fracture, tumor). Palpate the muscle over the scapula and compare it to the opposite side to determine atrophy secondary to disuse or nerve injury. Probe the axillary area for swellings and observe for signs of pain.* This can be indicative of a nerve root tumor.

REAR LIMB

A complete orthopedic examination of the rear limb includes the following manipulations:

Below tarsus. See the procedure for below carpus under the Forelimb section (p. 722).

Hock. *Palpate the tarsal joints for fluctuant swelling indicative of joint effusion.* This may be a subtle finding in the hock and is more easily noted when the animal is standing, because loading the joint forces the fluid peripherally. Firm swelling is suggestive of degenerative joint disease. *Extend and flex the hock.* Normal flexion should be about 45 degrees. Decreased flexion indicates degenerative joint disease, which may be secondary to osteochondritis dissecans. Pain on manipulation of the joint (especially coupled with soft tissue swelling) may indicate a fracture. *Extend, adduct, and abduct the hock and metacarpal bones to demonstrate instability of the collateral ligaments. With the stifle in extension and the hock stressed into flexion, palpate the Achilles tendon (Fig. 28-21).* Rupture of the entire tendon complex allows hock flexion while the stifle is extended. Rupture of the gastrocnemius tendon and common tendon of the biceps femoris, gracilis, and semitendinous muscles, with preservation of the superficial digital flexor, allows partial flexion of the hock while the stifle is extended and causes simultaneous flexion of the digits.

Tibia. *Palpate the tibia for instability (fracture), swelling (fracture, tumor), and pain response to deep bone palpation (panosteitis).*

Stifle. *Perform the initial examination of the stifle with the animal standing. Simultaneously palpate both stifles to detect swelling.* A swollen stifle usually indicates degenerative joint disease. The patellar ligament becomes less distinct with joint effusion and the medial aspect of the stifle enlarges because of capsular thickening and osteophyte formation.

Patella. The remainder of the examination is done with the animal in lateral recumbency. *Extend and flex the stifle while holding one hand over the cranial aspect of the joint to detect crepitation. Next examine the stability of the patella in relationship to the femur. Extend the stifle, internally rotate the foot, and apply digital pressure in an at-* *tempt to displace the patella medially (i.e., medial patellar luxation). Detect lateral patellar luxation by slightly flexing the stifle, externally rotating the foot, and applying digital pressure to attempt to displace the patella laterally (Fig. 28-22).* The patella normally moves slightly medially and laterally, but when it leaves the trochlear groove it is considered to be luxating.

Collateral ligaments. *Test the integrity of the collateral ligaments by holding the stifle in full extension and attempting to open the stifle on the medial and lateral aspects. Test the medial collateral ligament by using one hand to brace the femur while the other hand abducts the tibia.* Normally the medial collateral ligament will not allow joint laxity. *Test the lateral collateral ligament by bracing the femur with one hand and using the other hand to adduct the tibia (Fig. 28-23).* An intact lateral collateral ligament will prevent joint laxity. If the stifle is allowed to flex while the tibia is adducted, it may feel as though there is lateral laxity of the joint. This is a result of anatomic location of the lateral collateral ligament and internal rotation of the tibia and is normal.

Cruciate ligaments. Test the integrity of the cruciate ligaments by trying to elicit a cranial or caudal drawer motion. Drawer movement is caused by the tibia sliding cranially or caudally in relationship to the femur. This motion is not possible when the cruciate ligaments are intact in adult animals. Immature animals may have slight drawer motion, but it stops abruptly as the ligament tightens. *To elicit direct drawer motion, place the index finger and thumb of one hand over the patella and lateral fabellar regions, respectively. Place the index finger of the opposite hand on the tibial tuberosity and, with the thumb positioned caudal to the fibular head, slightly flex the stifle. Stabilize the femur, and gently move the tibia cranial and distal to the femur. Do not allow tibial rotation.* If the muscles are tense, they may prevent this motion. *If this occurs, gently flex and extend the stifle to relax the animal, and repeat the procedure. Test drawer motion with the femur flexed and extended (Fig. 28-24).* Usually, the greatest movement is felt

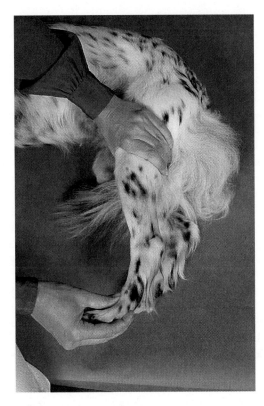

FIG. 28-21
To test integrity of the Achilles tendon complex, attempt to flex the hock with the stifle in extension.

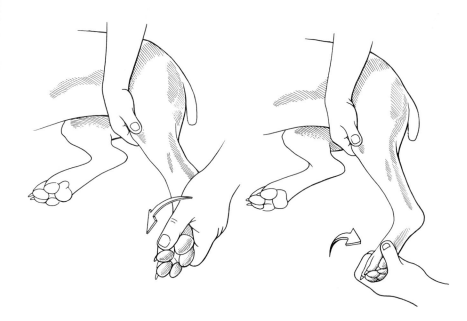

FIG. 28-22
To examine the stifle for medial patella luxation, extend the stifle, internally rotate the foot, and apply medial pressure to the patella with the thumb. To examine the stifle for lateral patella luxation, slightly flex the stifle, externally rotate the foot, and apply lateral pressure to the patella with the fingers.

with the stifle in flexion. *If the patella is luxated, replace it in the trochlear groove before attempting the drawer motion. Perform the tibial compression test to detect indirect drawer motion. Detect forward motion of the tibia by placing the index finger along the patella and the tibial tuberosity. With the leg in a standing position, flex the hock to tense the gastrocnemius muscle.* This compresses the femur and tibia together, causing the tibia to move forward in a cranial cruciate deficient stifle.

The presence and amount of drawer motion depend on the animal's age, size, state of relaxation, and the duration and type of cruciate pathology. There is minimal drawer motion in normal dogs and cats, although very young puppies may have a "lax" stifle. Eliciting drawer motion in larger animals or those that are tense is difficult; sedation or general anesthesia may be necessary. Minimal drawer motion may be noted with chronic cruciate pathology (especially in large dogs) because periarticular fibrosis restricts stifle motion. Minimal or partial drawer motion may also occur with in-

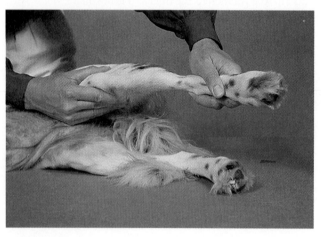

FIG. 28-23
To examine for collateral ligament injury, fully extend the stifle, stabilize the distal femur with one hand, and apply medial and lateral pressure to the tibia with the other hand.

complete tears or stretching of the cranial cruciate ligament. Drawer motion is evident with a torn caudal cruciate ligament. *To identify caudal drawer motion, start with the stifle in a neutral position.* Most caudal ligament ruptures are not discovered until exploration because they are mistaken for cranial ligament injuries.

Meniscus. In most cases, meniscal tears are identified during exploratory arthrotomy. A click or pop may be felt as the stifle is flexed and extended, causing the caudal horn of the medial meniscus to displace.

Femur. *Palpate the femur for instability (fracture), swelling (fracture, tumor), and pain response to deep bone palpation (panosteitis). Take care to isolate bone from muscle during deep palpation.*

Hip. *Extend and flex the hip while a hand is placed over the greater trochanter to detect crepitation.* The femur should extend caudally to a position almost parallel to the pelvis without inducing pain in a normal hip. The stifle should approach the ilium with full flexion. Degenerative joint disease limits the range of motion and may induce pain.

Hip luxation. To detect abnormalities of the hip, use the position of the greater trochanter in relationship to the tuber ischium as a landmark. *In the standing animal, compare the distance from the greater trochanter to the tuber ischium bilaterally.* A unilateral increase in that distance indicates hip luxation. Animals with acute hip luxations are non–weight-bearing and swelling over the greater trochanter may be noted. *Externally rotate the femur while placing the thumb in the space between the greater trochanter; displacement of the thumb should occur (Fig. 28-25, A and B).* With hip luxation, the trochanter rolls over the thumb (Fig. 28-25, C and D).

Hip laxity. Evaluation of hip laxity is best done under sedation. *With the animal in lateral recumbency, perform the Ortolani maneuver to detect hip laxity associated with hip dysplasia. Grasp the stifle with one hand and hold it parallel with the table surface. Place the other hand over the dorsal pelvis and adduct and push the stifle toward the pelvis.*

FIG. 28-24
To examine for cruciate ligament injury, place the thumb of one hand over the lateral fabella and the index finger over the patella. Stabilize the femur with this hand. Place the thumb of the opposite hand caudal to the fibular head with the index finger on the tibial tuberosity. With the stifle first flexed and then extended, attempt to move the tibia cranially and distally to the femur.

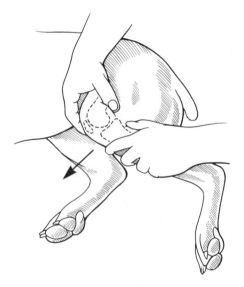
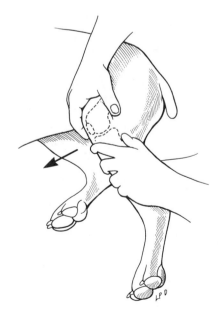

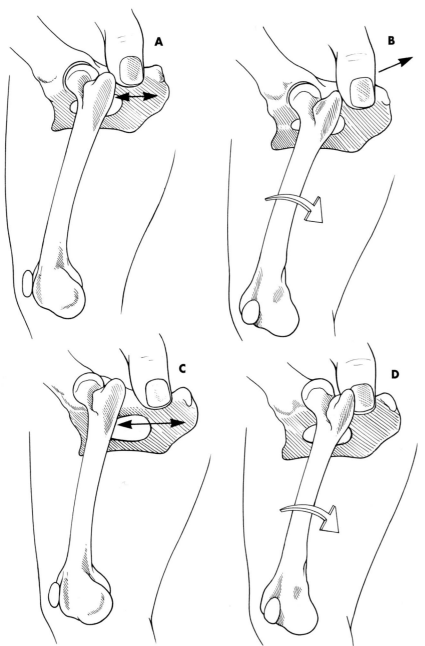

FIG. 28-25
A and **B,** To examine for hip luxation, place the thumb in the space caudal to the greater trochanter and externally rotate the femur. If the coxofemoral joint is intact, the greater trochanter will displace the thumb. **C** and **D,** If the coxofemoral joint is luxated, the greater trochanter will roll over the thumb.

With joint laxity, the hip will subluxate. *Maintain the pressure and abduct the stifle. As the femoral head returns to the acetabulum, use the hand stabilizing the pelvis to detect a click (Fig. 28-26).* This procedure can also be performed with the animal in dorsal recumbency, with the stifles held parallel to each other and perpendicular to the table. *Apply downward pressure on the stifle to subluxate the hip. Maintain pressure and abduct the stifle.* With laxity, a click is noted as the femoral head returns to the acetabulum (Fig. 28-27). The angle of subluxation is the point at which the hip luxates and the angle of reduction is the point at which the femoral head returns to the acetabulum. *Use these calculations to determine the plate angle for pelvic osteotomy (see p. 946).*

Pelvis. *Examine the pelvic region for evidence of fracture (i.e., asymmetry, instability, swelling, crepitation, bruis-* ing, or pain). To detect instability, manipulate the tuber ischia and wings of the ilium. *Radiographic evaluation is superior to physical manipulation for identifying fractures. Perform a rectal examination and note pelvic canal stenosis, pelvic fractures, or prostatic enlargement.*

Neurologic Examination

Because neurologic disorders may mimic orthopedic diseases or they may occur concurrently, every orthopedic examination should include a neurologic examination (see p. 1031). General observations can be made of the animal's mental status during the orthopedic examination. *Evaluate conscious proprioception in all four limbs by gently supporting the animal and individually turning each paw until the dorsal surface of the paw contacts the ground.* Normal

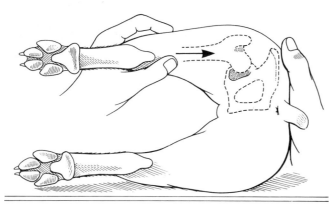

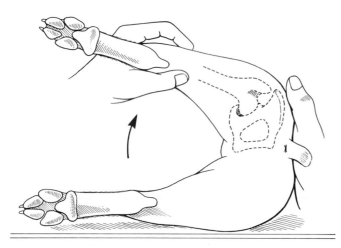

FIG. 28-26
To examine the hip for laxity with the animal positioned in lateral recumbency, place one hand over the back and grasp the stifle with the opposite hand. Hold the femur parallel to the table or in adduction, and subluxate the femoral head by pushing the stifle toward the pelvis. While maintaining pressure, abduct the limb. As the femoral head returns to the acetabulum, a click will be felt.

animals return the paw to the correct position almost immediately. Loss of conscious proprioception usually indicates neurologic disease; however, animals with fractured limbs may be reluctant to move the limb and therefore may appear to have conscious proprioception deficits. *Apply direct pressure on the ventral lumbar musculature to isolate lumbosacral pain.* It is important to differentiate lumbosacral and hip pain because many older dogs with radiographic signs of hip dysplasia are lame as a result of other causes (i.e., lumbosacral instability, cruciate ligament rupture).

Peripheral nerve damage may result concurrently with fractures of the mid to distal humerus (radial nerve) or sacrum (sciatic nerve). *Apply pressure to digits of the affected limb to elicit a response to superficial and deep pain. No response may indicate peripheral nerve damage.*

DIFFERENTIAL DIAGNOSIS AND DIAGNOSTIC IMAGING

A differential diagnosis is developed based on results of history, signalment, and physical examination. Definitive diagnoses may require additional diagnostic tools (e.g., imag-

ing, hematology, serum biochemistry, cytology, or electrodiagnostics).

Radiographs

Quality radiographs are essential for completing an orthopedic examination, refining the differential diagnosis, and arriving at a definitive diagnosis. They are also used to evaluate fracture healing. Appropriate equipment (i.e., 300 mA or greater x-ray machine and processing capabilities) is required to produce radiographs with sufficient contrast and detail. Correct patient positioning is important; chemical restraint is often necessary to allow proper patient manipulation, decrease radiographic study time, and minimize radiation exposure to the operator. Reversible drugs allow temporary patient immobilization (see Tables 28-7 and 28-8); however, patient selection is important. Some animals that are ill or in shock (i.e., after trauma) should not be sedated. To minimize magnification and loss of detail, the area of interest must be placed as close to the x-ray film as possible. Minimizing superimposition of structures overlying the area of interest requires careful patient positioning. For a given site, adequate evaluation usually requires that two views be made at 90 degrees to each other. Additional views (i.e., oblique, flexed, and stress view) may be needed to accurately evaluate the problem. To evaluate fractures and postoperative fracture repairs, radiographs of the long bones must include the joints above and below the bone of interest.

In addition to quality radiographs, detection, knowledge, and correlation of significant radiographic findings with clinical data are essential. Variations in anatomic structure and skeletal conformation between dog breeds may make it difficult to distinguish normal and abnormal. **Remember that animals usually have a normal "control" limb on the opposite side.** Comparing radiographs of the affected and normal limbs helps determine whether the suspect abnormality is a normal structure. Subtle morphologic changes that are bilaterally symmetric are rare. Comparison radiographs are essential for evaluating physeal injuries in immature animals. Early changes in the function of a physis can be detected by measuring the length of the affected bone and comparing it to the length of the unaffected opposite bone. **Always correlate the radiographic findings with clinical information.**

Serial radiographs are necessary to correctly interpret dynamic processes (i.e., fracture healing, inflammatory bone disease). This is especially important when interpreting the significance of bone reaction. Radiographs made 2 to 3 weeks apart may show rapidly accelerated growth with primary bone tumors, or a reparative process with regression in nonneoplastic diseases.

Bone Scintigraphy

Bone scintigraphy is used to evaluate the physiology or activity of bone. Bone-seeking radioisotopes, such as technetium 99m linked to methylene diphosphonate, are administered intravenously. This radiolabeled compound is gradually incorporated into actively metabolizing bone over a period of hours and can be visualized with gamma camera scanning.

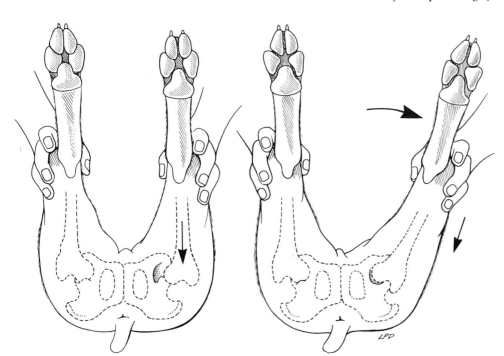

FIG. 28-27
To examine the hip for laxity with the animal positioned in dorsal recumbency, place the hands over the stifles. Hold the femurs parallel to each other and perpendicular to the table. Subluxate the femoral head by pushing the stifle toward the pelvis. While maintaining pressure, abduct the limb. As the femoral head returns to the acetabulum, a click will be felt.

The images obtained represent the distribution of the bone tracer according to current rates of bone turnover and blood flow. Because increased bone turnover occurs before radiographic changes are visible, scintigraphy can identify early bone abnormalities. Scintigraphy is the procedure of choice for obscure lameness in which the origin cannot be pinpointed with physical examination or identified with radiographs because the entire skeleton can be scanned relatively easily. Other indications for scintigraphy in small animals include identification of bone metastasis, acute osteomyelitis, bone sequestration, and evaluation of bone activity in fracture nonunions. Scintigraphy and radiography complement each other because scintigraphy identifies areas of high bone turnover without specifying etiology, whereas radiography often allows lesion interpretion. Therefore radiographs are usually performed after lesions have been identified with scintigraphy.

Computed Tomography

Computed tomography (CT) provides a cross-sectional image of the area of interest. The image is produced by taking multiple radiographs and reconstructing them using a computer. Advantages of CT over conventional radiographs include superior tissue density differentiation and no superimposition of overlying structures. CT also allows images to be reformatted in different planes. Computed tomography is superior to conventional radiography for identifying neoplastic bone margins before tumor resection. It is also used to identify stenosis of the spinal column and lesions of the spinal cord and surrounding soft tissues (when used in conjunction with myelography). Small fragments that may be obscured by surrounding bone on radiographs (i.e., fragmented coronoid processes, bone sequestra) can be detected with CT. Additionally, bone bridging within the physis may be detected and early treatment of growth deformities facilitated.

Magnetic Resonance Imaging

Magnetic resonance imaging is a relatively new modality that provides superior soft tissue definition. When the area of interest is placed within the magnet field, hydrogen atoms align in a single plane. Pulsation of the magnetic field alters atom alignment and causes energy emission. The energy signal is picked up by a radiofrequency receiver, analyzed, and processed by a computer that reconstructs the image. The signal intensity is a complex combination of hydrogen density in the various tissues, the rate at which the hydrogen atoms realign along the magnetic field and lose synchronization with each other's spin, and blood flow. The relative effect of each of these components is altered by varying the pulse sequence. The advantages of MRI include enhanced soft tissue contrast and absence of tissue superimposition over the area of interest. Contrast and definition between soft tissue structures, such as spinal cord, epidural fat, and disk material, is possible without using contrast materials. Magnetic resonance imaging does not provide bone detail because bone has a reduced signal compared to surrounding soft tissues. Magnetic resonance imaging is used to identify central nervous system changes, including spinal cord compression (especially in the lumbosacral spine) and soft tissue components of joints (e.g., cruciate ligament and menisci).

Suggested Reading

Barr ARS, Houlton JEF: Clinical investigation of the lame dog, *J Small Anim Pract* 29:695, 1988.

Brinker WO, Piermattei DL, Flo GL: *Handbook of small animal orthopedics and fracture treatment*, ed 2, Philadelphia, 1990, WB Saunders.

deHaan JJ, Shelton SB, Ackerman N: Magnetic resonance imaging in the diagnosis of degenerative lumbosacral stenosis in four dogs, *Vet Surg* 22:1, 1993.

Lamb CR: The principles and practice of bone scintigraphy in small animals, *Sem Vet Med Surg (Small Anim)* 6:140, 1991.

Lewis DD, McCarthy RJ, Pechman RD: Diagnosis of common developmental orthopedic conditions in canine pediatric patients, *Comp Cont Educ Pract Vet* 14:287, 1992.

Roberts RE: Radiographic examination of the musculoskeletal system, *Vet Clin N Am: Small Anim Pract* 13:19, 1983.

Wheeler SL: Diagnosis of spinal disease in dogs, *J Small Anim Pract* 30:81, 1989.

Wortman JW: Principles of x-ray computed tomography and magnetic resonance imaging, *Sem Vet Med Surg (Small Anim)* 1:176, 1986.

DECISION MAKING IN FRACTURE MANAGEMENT

FRACTURE-ASSESSMENT SCORE

Early progressive consolidation of fractures causes a shift in relative load bearing toward healing bone and away from orthopedic implants. Conversely, slower fracture healing necessitates that implants provide stability longer, increasing the likelihood of implant-related complications. Thus each fracture fixation represents a "timing race" between implant failure and fracture healing. Mistakes often occur because implant selection is based solely on the observation of fracture configuration as seen on a preoperative radiograph or through comparison of the fracture to a surgery textbook diagram.

Implant selection based solely on fracture configuration can lead to significant postoperative complications and/or failures. When this happens, surgeons may become frustrated with orthopedic case management and lose interest in treating these patients. This occurs despite the fact that the problem lies not in the surgeons' abilities but in initial decision making. Choosing an implant system based on fracture configuration ignores important mechanical, biologic, and clinical parameters that affect patient outcome; consideration of these factors allows a fracture-assessment score to be developed to assist in implant selection. The fracture-assessment score ranges from 1 to 10. The lower end of the scale represents mechanical, biologic, and clinical factors that do not favor rapid bone union and return to function, whereas the upper end of the scale represents those factors that favor rapid bone union and return to function.

Mechanical Factors

Mechanical factors influencing bone healing and return to function include the number of limbs injured, patient size and activity, and ability to achieve load-sharing fixation between the bony column and the implant (Fig. 28-28). Because dogs and cats must bear weight with at least three limbs, weight bearing on the implant-bone construct cannot be prevented postoperatively when multiple limbs are injured or when preexisting lameness (e.g., degenerative joint disease of the contralateral stifle secondary to cranial cruciate ligament injury) is present in another limb. Complica-

tions occur more frequently when stresses are applied and implants are heavily loaded immediately after surgery. Large or active patients subject fixations to greater loads and are more prone to have implants loosen prematurely and/or fail. The degree of load sharing between implants and the bony column also influences complication rates. Ideal load sharing occurs when a transverse or short oblique fracture is repaired, because much of the force is transmitted axially through the limb. Loading of the implant is minimized; thus loosening and fatigue failure are less likely. Conversely, when loads are transmitted from bone segment to bone segment through implants rather than through the bony column (i.e., highly comminuted fractures [such as gunshot wounds] that cannot be anatomically reconstructed, segmental bone resections, and limb lengthening procedures), loosening and fatigue failure are more common.

Biologic Factors

Many biologic factors influence the rate of bone healing (Fig. 28-29). The age and general health of the patient are important. A young (i.e., less than 6 months of age), healthy patient is a "healing machine" and requires that fixation devices function for limited times. This is exemplified by a 4-month-old kitten or puppy with a simple transverse femoral fracture treated by closed placement of a single intramedullary pin. Although this fixation is not in accordance with mechanical considerations, the biologic factors are so powerful that uneventful healing generally occurs. However, the same single intramedullary pin placed in a 12-year-old dog with a similar fracture would probably result in implant loosening and subsequent fracture instability because of slower healing.

Other biologic factors to consider are whether the fracture is open or closed and if it occurred secondary to a low- or high-energy injury. A significant degree of soft tissue injury and bony comminution accompanies open, high-energy fractures (e.g., gunshot wounds). This means that a longer time is required for bone union because soft tissues must heal first. The implant-bone construct must have high initial rigidity for neovascularization and healing of fragile tissues to occur. It must also be rigid in order to function as a buttress until biologic callus is formed. With closed or low-energy fractures, less soft tissue damage is present and bone union proceeds more rapidly.

Another factor influencing biologic assessment is whether open reduction is required. If the fracture must be opened, iatrogenic vascular damage occurs. A powerful biologic influence is the surgeon's skill in minimizing soft tissue envelope damage during open reduction. Obtaining desired reduction and stability with minimal soft tissue manipulation and operative time allows greater success than with longer surgeries in which reduction and stability are obtained at the expense of significant soft tissue manipulation. Preservation of the soft tissue envelope with open reduction is exceedingly important. This concept has led to a fracture-management technique termed *bridging osteosynthesis* in which minimal or no manipulation of the soft tissue envelope is done (see p. 757). For example, a comminuted fracture may be repaired

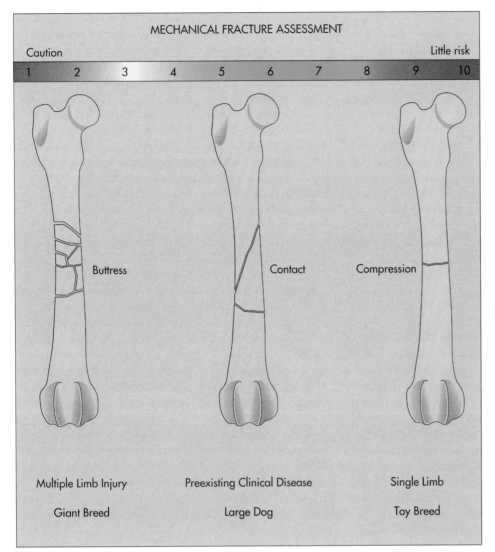

MECHANICAL FRACTURE ASSESSMENT

Caution   Little risk

1   2   3   4   5   6   7   8   9   10

Buttress   Contact   Compression

Multiple Limb Injury   Preexisting Clinical Disease   Single Limb

Giant Breed   Large Dog   Toy Breed

FIG. 28-28
Mechanical factors to be considered when determining patient fracture assessment. Conditions occurring on the left (i.e., buttress function, multiple limb injury) place maximum stress on an implant system and require thoughtful implant choice and application. In contrast, if conditions on the right are present, less stress is applied to the implant system, and the risk of complications is lessened.

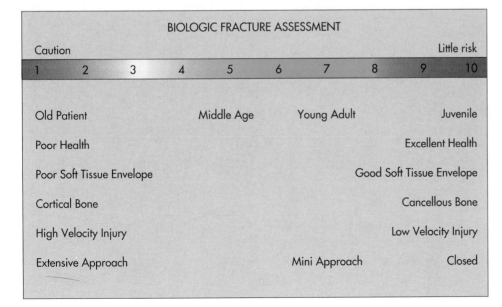

BIOLOGIC FRACTURE ASSESSMENT

Caution   Little risk

1   2   3   4   5   6   7   8   9   10

Old Patient	Middle Age	Young Adult	Juvenile
Poor Health			Excellent Health
Poor Soft Tissue Envelope			Good Soft Tissue Envelope
Cortical Bone			Cancellous Bone
High Velocity Injury			Low Velocity Injury
Extensive Approach		Mini Approach	Closed

FIG. 28-29
Biologic factors to be considered when determining patient fracture assessment. Patient factors listed on the left do not favor rapid healing; thus the implant system must remain in place for prolonged periods. In contrast, patient factors on the right dictate rapid healing and necessitate that the implant function for a short time.

through closed application of an external fixator or through open reduction and bridging of the fracture site with a buttress plate without manipulation of fracture fragments.

Biologic assessment is influenced by the bone injured and injury location because the soft tissue envelope surrounding various long bones differs. Distal radial or distal tibial diaphyseal fractures (i.e., locations with a sparse soft tissue envelope) have delayed unions or other complications more commonly than similar femoral or humeral fractures. Fractures occurring in cancellous metaphyseal or epiphyseal regions heal more rapidly than diaphyseal fractures because cancellous bone has a greater surface area for contact between fracture ends. Additionally, cancellous bone has abundant osteoblasts and other biologic factors that favor bone union. This is fortunate because articular fractures require precise reduction for optimal outcome; the surgical manipulation required for reduction is balanced by the inherent healing potential of the region.

Clinical Factors

Clinical factors (i.e., patient and client factors that affect healing during the postoperative period) also influence patient fracture-assessment scores (Fig. 28-30). Factors to consider include the willingness and ability of clients to attend to their pet's postoperative needs, anticipated patient cooperation following surgery, and postoperative limb function. Consider the client's sincerity and ability to become closely involved with aftercare. Unwilling clients or those unable to commit the time needed to care for stabilization systems requiring moderate or intensive postoperative maintenance (e.g., external coaptation or external skeletal fixations) should not be given this task. This is particularly valid if the biologic assessment dictates an extended time to bone union. Bone plates and screws would be more appropriate in this instance.

A second factor to consider in the clinical assessment is perceived patient cooperation after surgery. Very active, uncontrollable patients are not good candidates for external stabilization systems because high activity levels increase the likelihood of complications with these systems. Hyperactive

patients are not good candidates for external coaptation because casts or splints are difficult to maintain without shifting or sliding. Likewise, external skeletal fixators may be poor choices because these patients may continuously bump the external bar against objects, causing premature transfixation pin loosening.

Anticipated postoperative limb function must also be considered. Rapid return to normal limb function is a goal of fracture management. Therefore patient comfort during healing must be considered when selecting implants. The patient's ability to cope with discomfort and estimated time to bone union must be weighed. When early bone union is not anticipated (i.e., longer than 8 weeks), comfortable implants are preferred, to decrease client concern and prevent fracture disease (i.e., muscle atrophy or tendon contracture). Conversely, when bone union occurs rapidly (i.e., less than 6 weeks), patient comfort is less critical. Breed characteristics and individual variation between animals affect the patient's capacity to withstand discomfort. Although limb function may be good to excellent in a Labrador with an external fixator applied to the femur, an Afghan may have poor function until the implant is removed. Severe muscle atrophy and joint contracture associated with prolonged disuse caused by improper implant selection or ongoing fracture disease secondary to failure of an initial fixation device may prevent a successful outcome even after bone union. Return of limb function is crucial in such cases. Patient comfort that facilitates limb use and allows physical therapy to be performed after surgery is essential. Implant systems vary in degree of comfort, depending on the bone to which the implant is applied and individual patient tolerance. As a general rule, bone plates provide the greatest level of postoperative comfort.

FRACTURE-ASSESSMENT SCORE INTERPRETATION

Fracture-assessment scores are based on a scale of 1 to 10. Successful cases with few complications often have high scores, whereas those that are potentially less successful and have more complications are often at the lower end of the

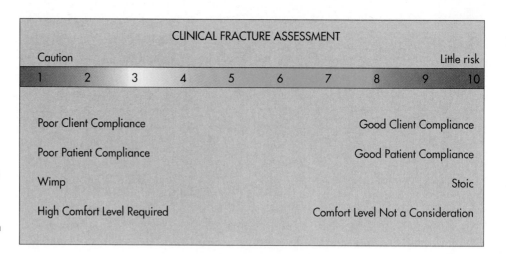

FIG. 28-30
Clinical factors to be considered when determining patient fracture assessment. Clinical factors on the left necessitate a comfortable implant system that requires little postoperative maintenance, whereas any implant system (regardless of postoperative maintenance) is appropriate with clinical factors on the right.

scale. Mechanical assessment considers stress applied to implants and implant-bone interfaces; biologic assessment estimates the length of time implants must be functional (i.e., time to bone union). If the fracture-assessment score falls at the lower end of the scale, the implant will function as a buttress and must carry most, if not all, of the physiologic loads immediately after surgery. The implant must assume this function until bony callus forms. This period will be prolonged for patients with low assessment scores because the time needed for bony callus formation will be lengthy as a result of poor biologic factors. With higher fracture-assessment scores, stress on the fixation system lessens and the time required for bone healing shortens. When the fracture-assessment score falls at the upper end of the scale, implants share the physiologic loads with the bone immediately after surgery, and bone union occurs relatively rapidly.

Low Scores (0 to 3)

Implants bridge fractures and therefore must have sufficient strength to prevent permanent bending or breakage in patients with low fracture-assessment scores. In addition, implants must have sufficient strength to deter excessive motion at the implant-bone interface. Motion at the interface will cause bone resorption, premature implant loosening, and potential migration. Suggested implants (or combinations of implants) with sufficient strength and stiffness to function at the lower end of the fracture-assessment scale are lengthening bone plates (see p. 751), bone plate/IM rod combinations (see p. 751), bone plate/external skeletal fixator combinations (see p. 751), Type II or Type III external skeletal fixators (see p. 741), and external skeletal fixator/IM pin combinations (with or without a tie in; see p. 741). Implants should purchase bone with raised threads to resist axial compression and tension (back-and-forth movement) occurring at implant-bone interfaces. Bone plates fulfill this requirement with the use of the bone screws, but the transfixation pins of external fixators may or may not have raised threads (see p. 735). Raised, threaded transfixation pins or a combination of smooth and raised, threaded transfixation pins should be used with low fracture-assessment scores.

Midscale Scores (4 to 7)

Overlapping biologic and mechanical factors affect healing and implant selection when the fracture-assessment score moves toward midscale. If the implant and bone share the load following surgery, the implant will be subjected to less stress; however, healing may be delayed. Alternatively, the biologic assessment may indicate early callus formation, despite the implant being subjected to high initial loads because it functions to bridge the fracture. In both situations, less implant strength and endurance are required than in patients with low assessment scores because of immediate load sharing and early callus formation. A fracture assessment toward the lower end of center means that the time to union will be long and therefore the implant should purchase the bone in a way that will preserve the implant-bone interface during the healing period. With a fracture assessment toward

the upper end of center, the stress on the implant and the implant-bone interface will be high for a short duration; therefore the interface needs maximum stability until sufficient callus is formed to share the physiologic load. Suggested implants include bone plates, Type I or Type II external skeletal fixators, IM pin/external skeletal fixator combinations (with or without a tie-in), or IM pin/cerclage wire combinations. Connections at implant-bone interfaces should be a thread purchase or combination of thread and friction purchase (depending on assessment of stress occurring at the interface and an estimation of endurance needed at this site).

High Scores (8 to 10)

When the fracture-assessment score is greater than 7 (i.e., mechanical assessment indicates minimal implant stress caused by load sharing and biologic assessment indicates enhanced healing potential), immediate load sharing between the bone-implant construct and rapid bone union is expected. Therefore the strength and stiffness of the implant need not be extreme, nor does the implant need to function for a lengthy time. Suggested implants include Type I external skeletal fixators with smooth transfixation pins, IM pin/cerclage wires, and external coaptation. Implants that hold bone through frictional purchase (i.e., smooth pins and cerclage wire) provide adequate bone purchase.

Suggested Reading

Aron DN, Palmer RH, Johnson AL: Biologic strategies and a balanced concept for repair of highly comminuted long bone fractures, *Comp Cont Educ Pract Vet* 17:35, 1995.

FRACTURE FIXATION SYSTEMS

EXTERNAL COAPTATION

External coaptation may be used to provide patient comfort before surgery and decrease soft tissue damage, or it may be used as the primary repair in some conditions. Descriptions of the commonly used bandages and splints for preoperative coaptation are provided on pp. 706–708. Postoperative bandages and splints are discussed on pp. 716–717.

CASTS
Indications

Full leg casts encircle the limb to rigidly stabilize a fracture. They can be used as a primary means of stabilization or as a supplement to internal fixation devices. As a primary stabilizer, full leg casts are most useful in stable fractures in which the fracture assessment (see p. 730) indicates rapid bone union. The classic casting material is plaster of paris, but with the development of synthetic casting materials its use has declined. Synthetic casts made of fiberglass or polyester fabric impregnated with water-activated polyurethane resin have considerable advantages over plaster casts (i.e., they are lighter, more comfortable, and dry well if they accidentally become wet). Although they are more expensive than plaster of paris, the advantages outweigh the cost. Full leg casts cannot be applied above the midhumerus or midfemur and therefore should only be used for fractures of the distal limb (i.e., radius/ulna and metacarpal/metatarsal fractures). With carpal arthrodesis, full leg casts can also be used to supplement internal fixation devices (i.e., bone plates and screws).

Application

General anesthesia is usually indicated for cast placement to allow closed fracture reduction (see p. 756). *To facilitate reduction, suspend the limb using adhesive stirrups applied to the medial and lateral limb surface (Fig. 28-31, A). If the fractured bone ends cannot be reasonably reduced (i.e., varus-valgus and rotational alignment are maintained with at least 50% contact of major fragment ends), perform surgery. Clip long hair and apply a single layer of cast stockinette onto the limb over the stirrups. Temporarily release the limb to apply the stockinette (alternatively, apply it before reducing the fracture). Extend the stockinette from the toes to 2 inches above the estimated proximal extent of the cast. Fit the stockinette snugly against the limb; do not allow the excess material to fold on itself or wrinkle. Apply cast padding in a spiral fashion to the limb from the toes to the estimated proximal extent of the cast, overlapping the material 50%. Use sufficient cast padding to protect the limb from developing cast sores, but not too much to prevent the cast from resting snugly against and conforming to the limb.* Generally, cast padding should be only two layers thick. *Place extra padding over bony prominences, if desired. Place a layer of gauze over the cast padding, wrapping from the toes proximally. Immerse the casting tape into cold water, squeeze excess water gently from the roll, and apply it to the limb, beginning at the toes. Wrap the cast material in a similar fashion as the cast padding (i.e., 50% overlap). Encompass the toes, but leave the nails of the third and fourth phalanges exposed, to allow limb swelling to be detected. As the cast tape is applied above the elbow or stifle, use firm pressure to compress the larger muscles and conform the cast to the limb. Use two layers of cast tape with 50% overlap (i.e., four layers on cross section) in small and medium dogs and three layers (six on cross section) in larger dogs (i.e., more than 30 kg) (Fig. 28-31, B). Apply the cast tape quickly because it will set in 4 to 6 minutes. Before the cast tape sets, roll the edges of the cast outward by pulling the proximal aspect of the stockinette over the end of the cast. Apply elastic adhesive or Vetrap around the cast and stick the stirrups to this layer. Next fashion a walking bar of aluminum rod into a U shape and tape it to the bottom of the cast so that the animal does not bear weight directly on the cast.* Direct weight bearing may cause the cast material to erode, causing abrasions on the dorsal paw.

An oscillating saw is required for cast removal. Sedation (i.e., oxymorphone 0.05-0.1 mg/kg IV, SC, or IM or fetanyl 0.005-0.01 mg/kg IV, SC, or IM or acepromazine 0.05 mg/kg IV, SC, or IM, not to exceed 1 mg total plus butorphanol 0.02 mg/kg IV, SC, IM) generally facilitates cast removal because the vibration and noise generated by the saw often frighten the animal. *Cut the medial and lateral sides of the cast, separate the two halves, and remove it.* Frequent removal of a cast used for fracture stabilization is not desirable because anatomic fracture reduction may be lost. If skin abrasions or loosening of the cast occurs, replacement may be necessary. If frequent removal is anticipated, bivalve the full cast on initial application. *Use the oscillating saw to cut the medial and lateral walls. Separate the two halves, then tape them securely with three to four layers of adhesive tape. When the underlying skin needs to be treated or the cast needs modification, separate the halves by removing the adhesive tape. Apply new cast padding, replace the halves, and secure them with adhesive tape.*

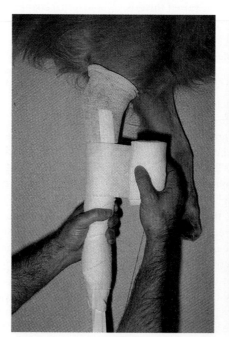
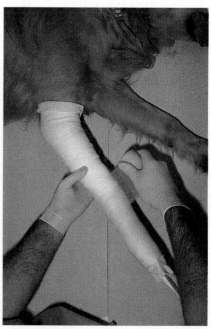

FIG. 28-31
A, When applying a fiberglass cast, place adhesive stirrups on the limb and cover them with a stockinette. Apply cast padding firmly over the stockinette using an overlapping pattern. **B,** Next place four to six layers of casting material on the limb, overlapping each layer 50%.

Postoperative Care

Specific written instructions outlining proper "at-home" cast care should be provided for the client. Casts should be evaluated 24 hours following application and weekly thereafter. Clients should be instructed to observe the toes daily for evidence of swelling (i.e., spreading of the exposed digits), excessive chewing or licking at the cast, or a foul odor. Any of these signs require that the animal be evaluated immediately. The cast should be kept clean and free of moisture. Have the client place a plastic covering over the cast when the animal goes outside. In growing animals the cast may need to be changed every 2 weeks; in adults the cast may last 4 to 6 weeks.

EXTERNAL SKELETAL FIXATORS

Indications

External skeletal fixators are used to stabilize fractures, for joint arthrodesis, and to temporarily immobilize a joint.

Equipment/Supplies

External fixation devices are comprised of three basic units: (1) transfixation pins inserted into bone to hold major fragments, (2) external connectors to support fractured bone, and (3) linkage devices that attach the transfixation pins and external connector. The Kirschner apparatus is the most commonly used external fixator in veterinary orthopedics. It is available in various sizes, but small, medium, and large sizes are most commonly used.

Transfixation pins. Transfixation pins may be categorized by implantation method (e.g., half pin or full pin),

structural design (e.g., threaded or nonthreaded), or their proprietary name (e.g., Kirschner). Half pins are inserted so that they penetrate both cortices but only one skin surface (Fig. 28-32, *A*), whereas full pins penetrate both cortices and skin surfaces (Fig. 28-32, *B*). Nonthreaded transfixation pins have smooth shafts (e.g., Steinmann IM pins) and are often used in external fixators (Fig. 28-33). Threaded pins may be completely threaded, end-threaded, or centrally threaded. Completely threaded pins (i.e., fully threaded Steinmann pins) are seldom used because they are weak and tend to break. Centrally threaded pins are used as full pins with Type II or Type III external fixator frames (see below). The central threads engage bone, and the smooth pin ends extend beyond the skin surface. End-threaded pins are often described according to the number of cortices to be engaged by the threads (i.e., one-cortex or two-cortex end-threaded pins). One-cortex end-threaded pins have threads near the pin tip; therefore, although the pin itself penetrates both cortices, the threads engage only the far cortex. Two-cortex end-threaded pins have sufficient thread length to engage both cortices. Threaded pins can be further described according to thread profile (e.g., negative or positive). Centrally threaded and end-threaded pins in which the core diameter of the threaded section is smaller than the diameter of the smooth section have a negative thread profile. If the core diameter is consistent between smooth and threaded regions, the thread profile is positive. The thread height and thread pitch are specifically designed to engage dense cortical bone (i.e., threaded cortical pins) or spongy cancellous bone (i.e., threaded cancellous pins).

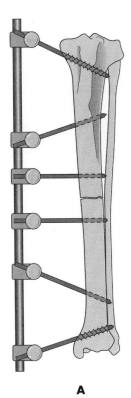
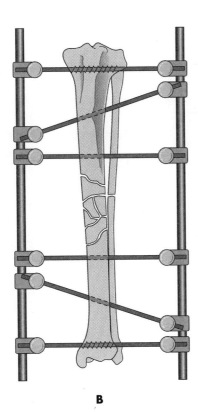

FIG. 28-32
Placement of **A,** half pins and **B,** full pins. Note that half pins are inserted so that they penetrate both cortices but only one skin surface, whereas full pins penetrate both cortices and skin surfaces.

A   **B**

External Connectors. External connectors are made of stainless steel (small and medium Kirschner rods), aluminum (large Kirschner rods), or acrylic (Fig. 28-34). The three sizes of Kirschner metal rods have correspondingly sized pin grippers (linkage devices; see below). The external fixator and linkage devices may be fashioned from acrylic using commercial kits ("acrylic-pin external fixation," or APEF) or from supplies designed to allow "homemade" acrylic splints to be applied. The APEF system contains smooth and enhanced threaded transfixation pins, prepackaged acrylic, and sterilized acrylic column molding tubes. The application kit also contains a reusable temporary alignment frame. Homemade splints use individually purchased materials for construction of frames. The acrylic in homemade splints is polymethylmethacrylate and is derived from dental acrylic or hoof-repair acrylic. The transfixation pins are purchased individually and pediatric anesthesia tubing is used for the column molding tubes.

Linkage devices. The linkage device connects the transfixation pin and external bar. It consists of a single clamp through which the external bar and transfixation pin are placed (Fig. 28-35). The external bar fits through a circular opening at the closed end (base) of the clamp and a hole is drilled in the arms of the U to accept a bolt that holds the transfixation pin. The bolt has a smooth shaft near the head and a threaded section at the tail. A hole is present in the bolt head that accepts the transfixation pin and the threaded tail contains a nut that can be tightened to secure the transfixation pin by squeezing it against the body of the U clamp. This simultaneously secures the external bar by compressing the arms of the U clamp against it.

Application

Because premature loosening of transfixation pins is the most common postoperative complication, external skeletal fixators should be applied in a manner that preserves pin-bone interface stability. Stability of the pin-bone interface is related to pin insertion techniques and the amount of force carried by the transfixation pin. As a general rule, the greater the strength and stiffness of the fixator-bone combination, the more stable the pin-bone interface. If the fracture and pin-bone interface remain stable after surgery, fracture union progresses normally and few fixator-related complications occur. Therefore it is important that factors that significantly influence the strength and stiffness of the external fixator-bone combination (i.e., frame configuration, pin number, pin size, pin placement, pin position, pin design, and bar placement) be understood.

The patient fracture-assessment score (see p. 730) must be considered when choosing an appropriate frame configuration; the lower the fracture-assessment score, the longer the fixator must remain in place and the stronger it must be (and vice versa). It is always better to err on the side of increased strength and stiffness rather than on the side of too little strength and stiffness. An insufficiently strong or durable frame will probably cause complications, whereas an overly rigid frame can always be disassembled to a less rigid frame

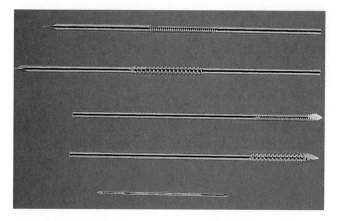

FIG. 28-33
Positive profile transfixation pins used with external skeletal fixation (top to bottom): centrally threaded cortical pin, centrally threaded cancellous pin, end-threaded cortical pin, end-threaded cancellous pin, mandibular transfixation pin.

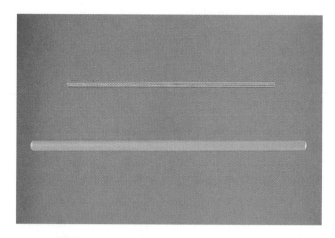

FIG. 28-34
Medium and large external connectors (bars) used with external skeletal fixation.

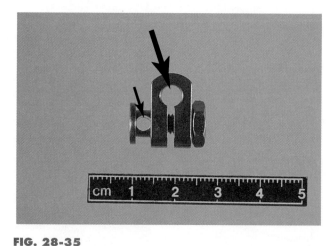

FIG. 28-35
Kirschner type linkage devices (pin gripper, pin clamp). Note the holes for the external connector (*large arrow*) and transfixation pin (*small arrow*).

as healing progresses. Strength and stiffness increase as the size and number of external connecting bars increase. In addition, because bones are subject to bending in two planes (mediolateral and craniocaudal), biplanar fixators are more effective in resisting physiologic bending loads than are fixators with connecting bars aligned in a single plane. There has been much confusion in veterinary medicine about the naming of various external fixator configurations. Recently, ef-

forts have been made to adopt a uniform and descriptive classification system that identifies the number of planes occupied by the frame and the number of sides of the limb from which the fixator protrudes. Using this system, common frames are unilateral-uniplanar (Type Ia), unilateral-biplanar (Type Ib), bilateral-uniplanar (Type II), and bilateral-biplanar (Type III). (Fig. 28-36). Because of an increasing number of bars and planes occupied by the different frame

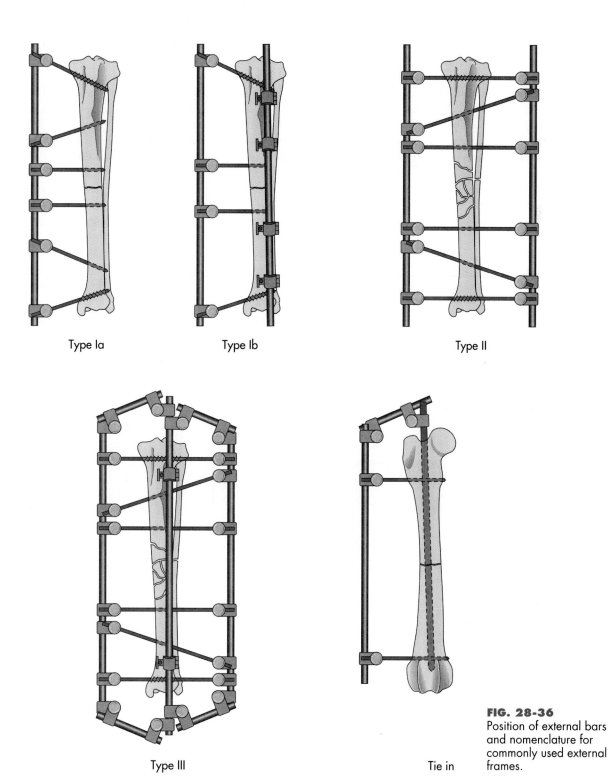

Type Ia   Type Ib   Type II

Type III   Tie in

FIG. 28-36
Position of external bars and nomenclature for commonly used external frames.

configurations, Type Ia, Type Ib, Type II, and Type III external fixators are successively stronger and stiffer. Combining external skeletal fixators with IM pins has gained popularity in recent years. These systems are referred to as *tie-in* configurations (see Fig. 28-36). Other variables that control the strength and stiffness of external fixators are the number, size, and position of transfixation pins placed in each major fragment (Fig. 28-37). The number of transfixation pins in the proximal and distal major fragments influences the fixator stiffness and affects how the physiologic loads are distributed amongst pins. The greater the number of transfixation pins per fragment, the more effective the device is in stabilizing the fracture and maintaining pin-bone interface integrity. This is true for up to four pins per major proximal and distal fragment; beyond this number the increase in mechanical advantage is negligible. The number of pins that should be placed in each fracture segment depends on the fracture-assessment score. Lower fracture-assessment scores require more pins, whereas higher scores require fewer pins. Generally three to four pins should be placed in each major fragment when using Type I frames and two to four transfixation pins should be placed in each major fragment when applying a Type II or Type III frame.

An important variable when choosing a transfixation pin is the size of the pin because pin size affects how much micromotion occurs at the pin-bone interface. The greater the amount of movement between the pin and bone, the greater will be the amount of bone resorption and the more rapidly the pin will loosen. Larger pins are less flexible and therefore allow less micromotion. In general, as large a pin as is feasible should be chosen; however, **the pin diameter should not exceed 20% of the bone diameter.**

Once the number and size of pins have been selected, the method of placement and position of the pins relative to the fracture need to be considered. In canine bone the most effective way to place a transfixation pin is with a power drill, using low revolutions per minute (rpm). However, there are certain situations in which predrilling the transfixation pin site is beneficial (e.g., where the transfixation pin must pass through dense cortical or cancellous bone). Here, the pin site is first drilled with a standard drill bit 0.1 to 1 mm smaller than the transfixation pin's core diameter. The transfixation pin is then placed through the drill hole with a hand chuck or a power drill, using low rpm speed. Specific sites at which predrilling should be performed are covered in the sections on the individual bones.

The site at which each transfixation pin will be placed relative to the fracture is a factor that can positively influence the mechanical performance of external fixators. One pin should be placed 2 cm proximal and one pin placed 2 cm distal to the fracture (see Fig. 28-37). The closer these pins are placed on either side of the fracture, the shorter the distance between connecting clamps on the external bar. Therefore the length of the bar that must sustain the load is shortened, resulting in a stiffer external bar. Generally, the most proximal and distal pins are placed in the respective metaphyses, and remaining pins are spaced evenly in the proximal and distal fragments.

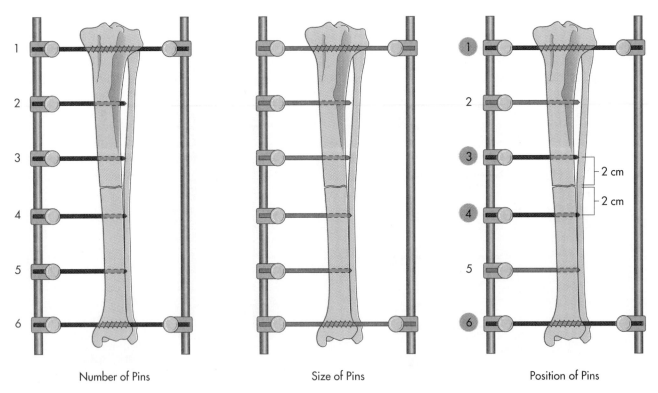

Number of Pins   Size of Pins   Position of Pins

FIG. 28-37
Transfixation pin parameters that can be modified to affect mechanical strength and stiffness of bone-fixator constructs.

Another important consideration in maintaining pin-bone interface stability is pin design (see Fig. 28-33). Numerous studies designed to modify pins to increase the length of time the pin-bone interface will remain stable have been reported. Collectively, these investigations suggest that threaded pins remain stable significantly longer than smooth pins. The type of transfixation pins used in a particular case is dictated by the patient fracture-assessment score. If the fracture-assessment score dictates rapid union (i.e., 4 to 5 weeks) and relatively low loads will be applied to the fixator, smooth transfixation pins will suffice. However, if the fracture-assessment score indicates prolonged union or high loads, threaded pins or a combination of threaded and smooth transfixation pins should be used.

Loosening of a transfixation pin may occur for several reasons, including excessive micromotion at the point of contact between pin and bone, thermal or mechanical damage of the bone at the time of pin insertion, and fatigue failure of the cortex at the point where the pin and bone contact. The principles discussed above serve to minimize micromotion between the pin and bone by maximizing the strength and stiffness of the external fixator. Application of these principles will also help limit fatigue failure of the bone by distributing stresses over a larger area when a greater number of pins and larger pins are used. However, damage to bone and subsequent bone resorption can still occur if the transfixation pins are not inserted properly. Proper methods of pin insertion are discussed below.

A variety of frame configurations and pin designs are available, but there are certain principles of application that are common for all external fixation devices. One of the most important principles is adherence to the practice of aseptic surgery. Proper aseptic technique, including patient preparation, gloving, gowning, draping, and instrument preparation, are just as important, if not more important, in the application of external fixators as for any other fixation method. *Suspend the injured limb from hooks in the ceiling or with an intravenous stand.* Ceiling hooks are preferable because intravenous stands may get in the way during surgery. *Scrub the liberally clipped area with an antiseptic soap. If the fixation is being applied to the radius or tibia, leave the limb suspended during application of the external fixator. If the fixation is being applied to the humerus or femur, release the limb from the suspension after it has been draped (see p. 25). Because the external fixator system is only as strong as the connection of the external frame to the bone, insert the pins carefully. Make a small (1-cm) longitudinal skin incision over the proposed pin site. Use a hemostat to bluntly dissect through the soft tissue from the skin surface to bone to create a soft tissue tunnel that allows free gliding motion of surrounding muscles around the transfixation pin.* The tunnel also prevents the pain and discomfort that can result from impingement of soft tissues against fixation pins. *Create the soft tissue tunnel between large muscle bellies rather than through them and avoid neurovascular structures. Protect the soft tissues comprising the walls of the tunnel from trauma using a*

drill sleeve or retract and stabilize the tissue with a hemostat. This is most important when predrilling a hole in the bone with a twist drill bit or when inserting a threaded transfixation pin because both of these devices will wrap tissue as they are advanced into the bone. Although the optimal technique for pin insertion remains controversial and under investigation, the currently preferred techniques are direct insertion of pins with a slow-speed drill or placement of pins with a hand chuck or slow-speed drill after predrilling the bone with a twist drill bit. The method of insertion is surgeon preference, but each transfixation pin should be drilled into the bone at the point of greatest cross-sectional diameter, and the trochar point should exit the far cortical surface for a distance of 2 to 3 mm.

Once the transfixation pins and external bar(s) are in place, adjust the position of the bar relative to the skin surface. The distance between the external bar and the body affects the length of the transfixation pin from the bar to its point of entrance into the bone. The shorter this distance, the less flexible the transfixation pin and the less micro-movement at the pin-bone interface. *Place the external fixation bar as close to the body as possible without allowing the clamps (pin grippers) or bar to impinge on the skin surface. As a rule of thumb, place the external bar so that one forefinger can be inserted between the clamps and the skin surface (approximately 1 cm).*

Placement of transfixation pins through the currently used Kirschner pin gripper (clamp) requires special consideration. Inserting smooth pins or threaded pins with a "negative" thread profile does not present a problem because the ends of the pins will pass through the hole in the bolt of the pin gripper. However, the insertion of "positive"-profile threaded pins (enhanced threads) can be difficult because the raised threaded section of the pin will not pass through the hole in the pin gripper. This is true for both end-threaded and centrally threaded pins. Nevertheless, enhanced threaded pins dramatically reduce patient morbidity and at least one such pin should be placed in each major bone fragment above and below the fracture in all but the most simple external fixator applications. The easiest positions in which to use enhanced threaded pins are the most proximal and the most distal pin sites because these pins do not require placement through pin grippers (see the discussion on construction of frame designs in the next section). However, if enhanced threaded pins are to be used in intermediate sites between the most proximal and distal positions, the pins must be placed through pin grippers already positioned on the external bar. The method used to insert an enhanced threaded pin through the pin gripper is different for an end-threaded or centrally threaded pin.

When using an end-threaded pin, the nonthreaded end of the pin must first be "backed through" the hole in the pin gripper, and then the threaded end advanced into the soft tissue tunnel (Fig. 28-38). *Remember to protect soft tissues from wrapping up on the threads when advancing the pin*

FIG. 28-38
Reversal technique used for placement of positive profile transfixation pins at an intermediate site. Note the external bar is initially placed away from the skin surface (bone) to allow clearance of the threads. Once the pins are positioned, the external bar is moved closer to the skin surface.

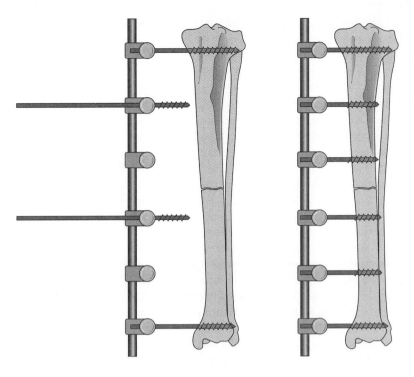

into bone. Because of the length of the threaded section of the pin, the "back through" maneuver requires that the external bar be positioned 4 to 5 cm from the skin surface. *Once all of the pins are in position, slide the external bar down into the recommended position (1 cm from the skin surface).* To facilitate this maneuver, it is preferable to place all pins parallel to each other.

Inserting an enhanced centrally threaded pin at an intermediate site requires a guide system and pilot hole. A centrally threaded pin must pass from one pin gripper, through the bone, and into the pin gripper on the opposite side of the limb. This can be done by visual alignment or, more readily, with a third connecting bar serving as a guide system. Because the enhanced threads will not pass through the pin gripper, the guide system is used to drill a hole through both cortices that will accept the transfixation pin. *First insert the most proximal and distal pins and connect to the medial and lateral external bars. For each centrally threaded transfixation pin, drill a hole through the bone with a twist drill bit 0.1 mm smaller than the core diameter of the transfixation pin. After the hole(s) is(are) drilled, remove one external bar and insert the centrally threaded transfixation pin(s) into the drill hole(s) by hand or with slow rpm power. Replace the external bar.*

An alternative to using the standard pin gripper with raised thread transfixation pins is to use a new design known as a *grooved half clamp.* This technique uses a standard pin gripper in which the base of the U has been cut and a groove has been placed in the face of the clamp to accept the transfixation pin. The half clamp allows insertion of the transfixation pin before placement of the pin gripper (clamp) on the external bar. After the transfixation pin is in place, the pin and bar are captured by sliding the half clamp over the end of

the pin and onto the external bar (Fig. 28-39). This system works equally well for placement of end-threaded or centrally threaded transfixation pins.

Unilateral-uniplanar (Type Ia) fixators. Unilateral-uniplanar fixators (see Fig. 28-36 on p. 737) are usually applied to the medial surface of the radius and tibia and the lateral surface of the femur or humerus. The transfixation pins are referred to as *half pins* because they only penetrate the near skin surface and bone.

Begin by placing a half pin in the metaphyses of the proximal and distal bone fragments. Place the pins in the center of the bone, perpendicular to its long axis and through both cortices. Place an appropriate number of pin grippers on the bar to accommodate placement of subsequent pins (e.g., if three pins are to be inserted in the proximal fragment and three pins in the distal fragment, then slide four empty pin grippers onto the external bar before connecting the pins initially placed in the proximal and distal metaphyses). Reduce the fracture (open or closed) and connect the two pins with an external bar. Place the additional half pins directly through the pin grippers. Remember the difference in placement technique discussed previously for insertion of a smooth or negative-profile threaded pin vs. a positive-threaded profile pin. *Once all of the intermediate pins have been placed, tighten the pin grippers and make a radiograph examination of the limb to assess fracture reduction and pin placement.*

Unilateral-biplanar (Type Ib) fixators. Unilateral-biplanar frame configurations (see Fig. 28-36 on p. 737) are applied most commonly to the radius and tibia. With the radius, one external bar is placed on the craniomedial surface of the bone and a second external bar is placed on the craniolateral bone surface. With the tibia, one external bar is

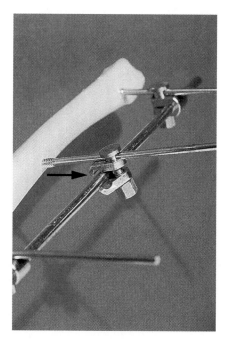

FIG. 28-39
A split external connector (pin clamp) (*arrow*), which can be used in conjunction with positive-profile threaded pins.

placed on the cranial surface of the bone and a second bar is placed on the medial surface. *Begin by placing four half pins (two in each plane) in the metaphysis of each major fragment in a similar fashion as described above. Reduce the fracture (open or closed), place an appropriate number of pin grippers on two external bars, and connect pins in a given plane with external bars. Determine the number of half pins to use, depending on the desired strength and stiffness of the external fixator as determined through the fracture-assessment score. Generally, place four half pins in one plane (craniomedial or medial) and four in the second plane (craniolateral or cranial). Therefore place two empty pin grippers on each connecting bar. Place additional half pins directly through these pin grippers. Once all of the intermediate pins are in place, tighten the pin grippers and make a radiograph examination of the limb.*

Bilateral-uniplanar (Type II) fixators. Because of the adjacent body trunk, bilateral configurations (Type II) (see Fig. 28-36 on p. 737) cannot be placed on the femur or humerus. They are applied only to the radius or tibia and are usually placed in a medial to lateral plane. *First place full pins in the proximal and distal metaphyses so that they lie in the same plane. Place the pins perpendicular to the bone surface and parallel to the adjacent joint line to facilitate restoring axial, varus-valgus, and rotational limb alignment. If necessary, use these pins to apply traction to the limb to aid in fracture reduction. Reduce the fracture, place the appropriate number of empty pin grippers on each external bar to accommodate placement of subsequent intermediate pins, and connect the proximal and distal full pins*

with a medial and lateral connecting bar. Insert intermediate pins as half pins or full pins, using smooth or threaded pins. Determine which pin type to use based on the fracture-assessment score. If intermediate pins are to be positive-profile threaded pins, refer to the special insertion techniques discussed under pin insertion techniques above. Once all of the intermediate pins are in place, tighten the pin grippers and take a radiograph of the limb to assess fracture reduction and pin placement.

Bilateral-biplanar (Type III) fixator. Bilateral-biplanar configurations (see Fig. 28-36 on p. 737) cannot be applied to the femur or humerus because of the position of the body wall. Application of Type III fixators to the radius or tibia requires nothing more than a bilateral-uniplanar frame (Type II) placed in a medial-to-lateral plane, followed by application of a unilateral-uniplanar (Type I) frame placed in a cranial-to-caudal plane. The two frames are then connected to form the tent configuration of Type III external fixator configurations. *Remember to slide empty pin grippers onto the external bar to accept placement of intermediate pins as discussed with construction of Type I and Type II frames. Also plan for the application of half pins or full pins if they are to be enhanced threaded pins.*

External skeletal fixators in combination with IM pins. Humeral and femoral fractures are not commonly stabilized with external skeletal fixators alone because the most stable frames (Type II and Type III) cannot be applied to these bones. To provide the strength and stiffness desired with complicated humeral or femoral fractures, a combination IM pin and Type Ia or Type Ib external fixator is often used (see Fig. 28-36 on p. 737). The transfixation pin design and number of transfixation pins are based on the fracture-assessment score, but normally the number of transfixation pins is limited to one or two pins placed above and below the fracture. The reason more transfixation pins are not used is that the greater the number of pins, the more intense the discomfort associated with pins placed through the large muscle groups.

Begin by reducing the fracture and inserting an IM pin that fills 60% to 75% of the medullary canal. Use cerclage wire to support long oblique fractures, spiral fractures, or comminuted fractures having one or two large fragments. If multiple fragments are present, bridge the comminuted section of bone with the IM pin and external fixator without disturbing soft tissue attachments to small bone fragments. Once the fracture is reduced and the IM pin has been placed, add the external fixator. Use the largest size transfixation pin that does not exceed 20% of the diameter of the bone and will pass adjacent to the IM pin. If you are unsure of the track of the IM pin inside the bone relative to the chosen site for insertion of a transfixation pin, drill the proposed transfixation pin site with a small Kirschner pin. If the IM pin is encountered, select an alternative location; otherwise insert the transfixation pin at this site. If more than two transfixation pins are being placed, insert the intermediate pins through preplaced pin grippers as described above. Connect the transfixation pins to an external bar placed

1 cm from the skin surface. Increasing the number of transfixation pins strengthens the external fixator. However, adding additional fixator pins increases postoperative discomfort. There are two methods that are used to strengthen external fixators without increasing the number of pins. One method is to add more external bars; the addition of a single external bar doubles the strength of the system. Alternatively, the IM pin is left protruding above the skin surface at the exit point proximal to the greater trochanter. The IM pin is then "tied" into the external fixator by connecting the two with an additional short segment of external bar.

Acrylic splints. To apply acrylic splints use a single- or two-stage technique. The advantage of two-stage techniques is that pin placement and fracture reduction can be assessed before hardening of the acrylic. If the single-stage technique is used and postoperative radiographs show fracture reduction or transfixation pin placement to be unsatisfactory, a small section of the acrylic column must be removed before corrective measures can be taken. *With either technique, insert the transfixation pins in the bone fragments following the same principles and guidelines described for construction of standard external fixator frames. Place acrylic column molding tubes over the ends of the transfixation pins 2 cm from the skin surface. If using a single-stage technique, reduce the fracture and pour the acrylic into the columns. Allow the acrylic to cure for 5 to 10 minutes. If a two-stage technique is used, place the tubes over the ends of the transfixation pins but do not add the acrylic. Instead, reduce the fracture and apply a temporary alignment frame consisting of standard Kirschner clamps and external bars that are added to the fixation pins outside of the column molding tubes. Take radiographs to assess pin placement and fracture reduction and, if satisfactory, pour acrylic into the columns and allow it to cure. If alignment needs to be changed after the acrylic has hardened, cut the acrylic column(s) at the fracture line with a saw. Once the appropriate adjustments are made, patch the acrylic column by adding new acrylic to fill the gap. Peel the plastic molding back from each end at the gap and drill several holes in the remaining acrylic to provide a site of attachment for the old and new acrylic. Mold a small amount of new acrylic by hand and place it into the gap, then allow the acrylic to cure (Fig. 28-40).*

Postoperative Care

Postoperative analgesia should be provided (see p. 708). Immediately after surgery, the pin-skin interface should be cleaned with antiseptic solution, using cotton swabs. Sterile gauze sponges should be placed around and between transfixation pins and the limb wrapped with Vetrap or a similar bandage material. After surgery, the pin-skin interface should be cleaned and the bandage changed daily. After approximately 1 week, gauze packing can be discontinued. The pin-skin interface should be cleaned daily until little or no serosanguineous transudate is noted at the surface. Once the interface seals, the daily observations should be continued. After the animal has been released from the hospital it

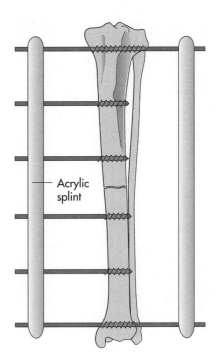

FIG. 28-40
Use of acrylic as external connectors rather than standard metal bars.

should be reevaluated weekly for the first 2 to 3 weeks postoperatively, then once every 2 weeks. The pin-skin interface should be carefully examined and the clamp and skin should be observed for separation. If irritation and/or drainage is present, the involved skin surface should be cleaned and packed with gauze. The fixator should be removed once the bone has healed. The appropriate time to take postoperative radiographs for healing depends on the estimated time to bone union and the patient fracture assessment. The patient should be sedated, the pin-gripper loosened, and the transfixation pin removed with a hand chuck or drill (smooth transfixation pins can also be removed with a pin remover).

INTERNAL FIXATION

INTRAMEDULLARY PINS
Indications and Biomechanical Properties

Intramedullary pins are most often used for fractures of the humerus, femur, and tibia. The biomechanical advantage of intramedullary (IM) pins is their resistance to applied bending loads (Fig. 28-41, *A*). In contrast to other implants (e.g., bone plates, external fixators) pins are equally resistant to bending loads applied from any direction because they are round. Biomechanical disadvantages of IM pins include poor resistance to axial (compressive) or rotational loads and lack of fixation (interlocking) with bone (Fig. 28-41, *B* and *C*). The only resistance to rotation or axial loads provided by an IM pin is friction generated between pin and bone. In general, this friction is not sufficient to prevent rotational move-

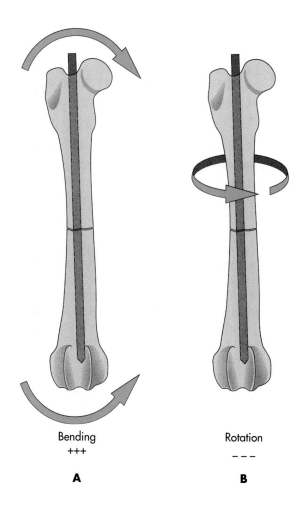

Bending
+++

A

Rotation

– – –

B

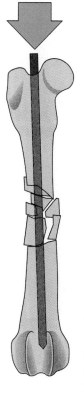

Axial

– – –

C

FIG. 28-41
A, The biomechanical advantage of IM pins is that they are equally resistant to bending loads applied from any direction because they are round. **B** and **C,** Biomechanical disadvantages of IM pins include poor resistance to rotational or axial (compressive) loads and lack of fixation (interlocking) with bone.

ment or axial collapse of a fracture. Contact and friction between pin and epiphyseal cancellous bone vary with the amount of cancellous bone and accuracy of pin placement. The actual pin-bone contact is not substantial because the cross-sectional marrow cavity diameter varies, limiting the amount of friction created between these two surfaces. Because friction created between pin and bone is what prevents premature pin migration, stress associated with unstable fractures results in micromotion at the pin-bone interface, bone resorption, and pin migration. Because of these limitations in mechanical support afforded by single or double (see below) IM pin stabilization, IM pins should be supplemented with other implants (e.g., cerclage wire and external skeletal fixation) to increase rotational and axial support. These implants have their own indications for use and principles of application that should be referred to before they are used in combination with an IM pin (see below).

Some surgeons advocate using multiple IM pins to gain increased axial and rotational support. However, recent clinical and laboratory investigations question the validity of this technique if only two pins are used, because increased rotational support has not been demonstrated. This is true whether the pins are placed in Rush pin fashion or simply stacked into the medullary cavity. Clinical studies have shown a high complication rate when double-pin fixation was used, confirming that this technique does not provide

sufficient mechanical support. A modest increase in rotational support was seen experimentally when multiple pins (i.e., more than two) were stacked into the marrow cavity.

Equipment/Supplies

Intramedullary pins are smooth, round, 316L stainless steel rods that are inserted into the medullary cavity for fracture stabilization. The most common IM pins used in veterinary medicine are Steinmann pins. Steinmann pins are available in sizes ranging from $\frac{1}{16}$ inch to $\frac{1}{4}$ inch and come with a variety of point designs (Fig. 28-42). They can be single-armed (i.e., have one end with a point and one end blunt), or double-armed (i.e., with a point at each end). The most popular point designs are trocar points and chisel points. Chisel points have a two-sided cutting edge that is slightly more effective in cutting through dense cortical bone because it generates less heat than trocar points. Trocar points have a triple cutting edge and cut through cancellous bone easily. Because Steinmann pins are generally used as IM rods and are seated in proximal or distal epiphyseal cancellous bone, trocar points are most commonly used.

IM pins may be smooth or have threads near the end of the pin. The end-threaded Steinmann pin was developed to increase the pin's holding power in cancellous bone. However, use of end-threaded pins is controversial. Proponents argue that the pin must be "screwed out" of the bone on

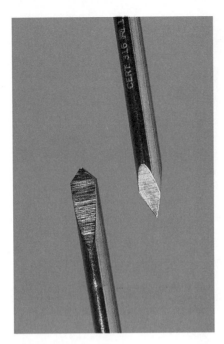

FIG. 28-42
IM pins with chisel (*left*) and trochar (*right*) points.

removal, suggesting that this pin design provides enhanced bone-holding ability when compared with smooth pins. However, some studies have suggested that these pins do not have greater initial holding power because bone merely grows into the threads after surgery (Howard, 1991). Thus, during the critical periods of early postoperative healing, bone holding is not enhanced. Additionally, threaded Steinmann pins have increased potential for premature failure when compared with smooth Steinmann pins. In the manufacturing of the end-threaded Steinmann pin, threads are cut into the tip of a smooth Steinmann pin, causing the pin diameter to be greater in the nonthreaded section of the pin than in the threaded section. This difference in cross-sectional area acts as a stress concentrator that predisposes to premature pin bending or breakage.

Application

Application techniques vary for each fracture type and long bone involved. Specific techniques are described for individual long bones in the discussion of fracture management.

Postoperative Care

Postoperative analgesia should be provided (see p. 708). General postoperative care for fracture management is provided in the section on individual long bones. Generally, postoperative examinations should be done weekly for 2 to 3 weeks following surgery; thereafter, examinations can be done every 2 weeks. Animals with IM pins do not require special postoperative care. Clients may become concerned about a subcutaneous fluid swelling surrounding the pin end. This is a seroma caused by irritation of the pin moving in soft tissues. IM pins should be removed once bone union

has occurred; if a seroma is present, it will resolve following pin removal. *To remove a pin, sedate the patient and clip and aseptically prepare the skin surface overlying the end of the pin. Instill a local anesthetic and make a small skin incision over the palpable end of the pin. Bluntly dissect soft tissues from the pin, grasp it with a pin remover, and extract it from the bone. Place a suture(s) in the skin wound.*

INTERLOCKING INTRAMEDULLARY PINS
Indications and Biomechanical Properties

Interlocking IM pins are one of the most popular implants used for fracture management in human orthopedics. With this technique, screws are placed through the bone and IM pin to provide additional mechanical support (Fig. 28-43). The number of screws interlocked with the IM pin is variable but ranges from a single screw placed proximal and distal to the fracture to as many as three screws proximal and three distal to the fracture. The pin provides bending support while the interlocking screws provide axial and rotational support. This is in contrast to IM Steinmann pins, which only provide bending support; axial and rotational support must be provided through additional implants. A veterinary model of the interlocking pin has been developed and is gaining popularity. It is primarily used for humeral or femoral fractures, but may also be implanted into the tibia.

Equipment/Supplies

Special instrumentation needed to insert an interlocking nail includes a reamer, interlocking nails, interlocking screws, and a guide system for screw placement.

Application

Prepare the marrow cavity for pin placement with an instrument that reams the marrow cavity and establishes an avenue for the pin. Once the pin is in place, attach it to a guiding system to place drill holes in the bone for the interlocking screws. The guide system is mandatory to ensure that the drilled hole intersects the bone at a site where a hole exists in the pin. After the hole has been drilled, place a screw through the cortex to interlock with the IM pin. If the screw is self-tapping, place it directly into the drill hole; if the screw is not self-tapping, tap the drill hole before screw placement. (See pp. 784 and 785 for instructions on placement of IM pins in the femur and humerus, respectively.)

Postoperative Care

Postoperative analgesia should be provided (see p. 708). General postoperative care for fracture management is provided in the section on individual long bones. Generally, postoperative examinations should be done weekly for 2 to 3 weeks following surgery; thereafter, examinations can be done every 2 weeks. The appropriate time to take postoperative radiographs to determine healing depends on the estimated time to bone union, based on the patient fracture assessment. Interlocking IM pins should be removed when the bone has healed. The patient must be placed under general anesthesia. *Clip and aseptically prepare the skin surface*

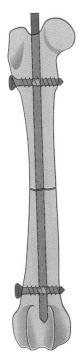

FIG. 28-43
An interlocking IM pin. The interlocking screws provide additional rotational and axial support.

and make small skin incisions over the interlocking screws. Remove the screws and make an incision over the end of the pin. Apply the distraction device and remove the pin.

ORTHOPEDIC WIRE

Orthopedic wire is often referred to as *cerclage wire* or *hemicerclage wire*. It is used in combination with other orthopedic implants to supplement axial, rotational, and bending support of fractures. The term *cerclage wire* is used to denote the use of orthopedic wire placed around the circumference of the bone. *Hemicerclage wire* is the term used to denote wire that is placed through predrilled holes in the bone. Cerclage wire has two distinctions: it is the most commonly used implant and the most commonly *misused* implant in veterinary orthopedics. Misuse of cerclage wire causes a significant percentage of the postoperative complications seen in veterinary patients.

Indications

Cerclage wire is used to provide added stability to long oblique fractures, spiral fractures, and comminuted fractures (Fig. 28-44). The wire may be used with other implants to provide additional stability for a fracture, or it may be used solely to hold fracture fragments in alignment (adaptation) while the other implants provide stability. Making the distinction as to whether cerclage wire will function as a stabilizer or for adaptation preoperatively is important for a successful outcome. For wire to function as a stabilizer it must generate sufficient compression between fracture surfaces to prevent the fragments from moving or collapsing under weight-bearing loads. To accomplish this,

three criteria must be met: (1) the length of the fracture line should be three times the diameter of the marrow cavity, (2) there should be a maximum of three (preferably only two) fracture fragments, and (3) the fracture must be anatomically reduced. When these criteria are met, cerclage wire can provide additional stability by generating sufficient compression between fragments to hold them in place during healing. If more than two or three fragments are present or if the fracture lines are not of sufficient length, cerclage wire can only be used to hold fragments in position; it cannot generate the compression needed to resist weight-bearing loads. The attempt to gain stability with cerclage wire in multifragmented fractures is the most common cause of cerclage wire failure. When multiple fragments are present, movement postoperatively may cause one of the pieces to shift in position, which would allow the entire segment of reconstructed bone to collapse. An analogy to the use of cerclage wire for stabilizing multiple bone fragments is the use of metal rings to hold slats in a wooden barrel. Collapse would occur if one slat (bone fragment) in the barrel were to loosen. A probable outcome when wire is misused is collapse of the fracture, loss of stability, and wire loosening, which further delay healing.

The cruciate hemicerclage wire pattern has been shown to be most effective experimentally in resisting rotation and bending. The degree of support varies, depending on the IM pin size; larger pins afford greater rotational support. Cruciate hemicerclage is recommended only with transverse fractures. If the fracture is oblique and collapses to any degree after surgery, the wire will loosen and not provide the desired support.

Equipment/Supplies

Cerclage wire is made from 316L stainless steel. It may be purchased in a spool or as preformed loop wire and is available in sizes ranging from 22-gauge (0.64 mm) to 18-gauge (1.0 mm). The use of 22- or 20-gauge wire is recommended for cats and small dogs, whereas 18-gauge wire is recommended for larger dogs. Hemicerclage wire should be 18- or 20-gauge monofilament 316L stainless steel. The wire is placed around the bone and secured. A variety of instruments (i.e., single-phase and two-phase tighteners) are available to secure the encircling wire to bone. Some instruments generate tension in the wire while simultaneously securing it with a twist or loop knot; others generate tension in the wire first and then secure it with a twist or loop knot. Although a difference has been noted experimentally in the performance of these two types of instruments, clinical performance seems to be similar as long as the principles of wire application are followed.

Application

Cerclage wire. *Use a wire passer to place the wire around the bone without extensively reflecting soft tissue. Do not entrap tissue between the wire and periosteum. Use a minimum of two wires placed 3 to 4 mm from each end of the fracture line (Fig. 28-45). Place additional wires*

FIG. 28-44
Fracture configurations where cerclage wire is useful for providing mechanical support through interfragmentary compression.

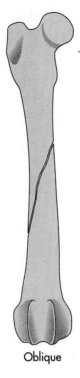

Oblique

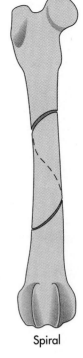

Spiral

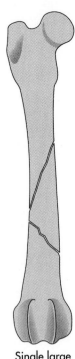

Single large fragment

1 cm apart and within the boundaries of the most proximal and distal wires. To prevent slippage and loosening of the wire, place the wires perpendicular to the bone surface. If the bone changes diameter at the placement site, the wire will tend to slip toward the area of smaller diameter. *To prevent slipping, place a Kirschner wire across the fracture and leave the ends of the Kirschner wire protruding 1 mm beyond the bone surface at both the near and far cortex. Place the cerclage wire around the bone such that the loop rests above the Kirschner pin at the far cortex and below the Kirschner pin at the near cortex (Fig. 28-45). Alternatively, make a small notch in the bone surface with the point of a pin or small file. Place the wire loop within the notch to prevent slippage.*

The instrument used for tightening the wire is not critical; however, the wire must be tight after securing the knot. *Ascertain the degree of tightness by feel and check it by attempting to move the wire with a pair of needle holders. Replace the wire if it is loose. If a twist knot is used, do not bend the twist over because significant tension is lost in the wire loop by this maneuver. Instead, leave the twist in the extended position and cut it near the third twist.* A fibrous cap will rapidly form over the protruding end of the wire, providing protection from soft tissue irritation. *When all of the wires have been placed, recheck the tightness of each wire because loosening of the initial wires may occur with subsequent wire placement.*

Hemicerclage wire. *Drill small holes through the bone 1 cm above and 1 cm below the fracture. Drill the holes so that the wire rests on the tension surface of the bone (e.g.,*

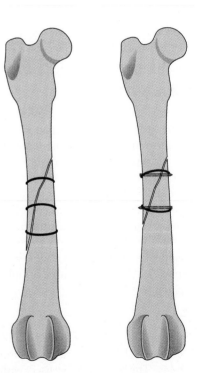

FIG. 28-45
Proper placement of cerclage wire. Wires are placed 3 to 4 mm from fracture ends and at least 1 cm apart.

in the femur, drill the holes near the lateral cortex in a cranial-to-caudal direction). Pass one end of a piece of wire through the hole proximal to the fracture and the other end through the distal hole. Twist the free ends of the wire such that a cruciate pattern is formed on the tension surface of the bone (Fig. 28-46).Cut the ends of the twist knot but do not bend them.

Postoperative Care

Postoperative analgesia should be provided (see p. 708). Wire used for fractures does not require special considerations postoperatively. Wire is generally not removed once the fracture has healed, unless it causes problems.

TENSION BANDS

Indications

Tension is the predominate force when fractures occur at a point where groups of muscles originate or insert in bone (e.g., greater trochanter, olecranon, supraglenoid tuberosity of the humerus). Contraction of the muscle group at these sites generates tension that pulls the bony insertion or origin from its anatomic location. The most effective way to resist tension is through application of a tension band (Fig. 28-47). The purpose of a tension band is to convert distractive tensile forces into compressive forces.

Equipment/Supplies

Equipment needed for placement of a tension band includes small Steinmann pins or Kirschner wire and orthopedic wire.

Application

When using pins and wire to apply a tension band, first reduce the fracture and place two small pins or Kirschner wires across the fracture to maintain reduction. Place the pins perpendicular to the fracture line and parallel to each other. Drill a small hole through the bone 1 to 2 cm below the fracture line such that the wire will rest on the bone's tension surface when tightened (i.e., in the femur, drill the hole from cranial to caudal so that the wire will rest on the lateral or tension surface of the femur). Pass the wire through the drill hole and around the two small pins used to stabilize the fracture. Twist the ends to form a figure-eight from the pins to the drill hole. The twist portion of the wire should be on top of the flat portion of the wire. Wind the twist knot to tighten the arms of the tension band. As the wire is tightened, tension is created that opposes that generated by muscle contraction.

Postoperative Care

Postoperative analgesia should be provided (see p. 708). Special postoperative care is not required for tension bands. If the ends of the pins irritate soft tissues, the pins should be removed. Otherwise, tension bands are not removed once the fracture has healed.

BONE PLATES AND SCREWS

Stabilization of fractures with bone plates and screws is a popular and versatile method of fracture fixation. Modern plating technology began in the early 1960s when a group of Swiss surgeons formed an association for the study of fracture treatment in man. This group, the Swiss Arbeitsgemein-

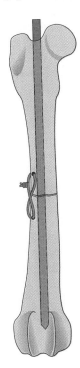

FIG. 28-46
Hemicerclage wire provides bending and rotational support with transverse fractures.

schaft fur Osteosynthesefragen (AO), is referred to as the *Association for the Study of Internal Fixation (ASIF)* in the United States. The group developed (and continues to develop) recommendations for application of orthopedic devices that have led to increased success and fewer complications associated with fracture management. In the 1970s an arm of the AO group, the AO-Vet, was established to specifically document and address problems associated with fracture management in animals. Arising from this group, specialized instrumentation and bone plates were designed to treat animal injuries. To achieve consistent and predictable results with bone plating, a thorough understanding of the principles and techniques of application is essential. Although there are several companies marketing varied designs of equipment, the AO/ASIF system will be used to describe the principles of application in this text.

Indications

Bone plates and screws offer a versatile method of fracture stabilization. They can be used to stabilize any long bone fracture and are often used for fractures of the axial skeleton. Bone plates and screws are particularly useful when postoperative comfort and early limb use are desired (e.g., fractures involving joint surfaces, patients with fracture disease).

Equipment/Supplies

Cortical and cancellous bone screws are made of 316L stainless steel or titanium and may or may not be self-tapping. A non−self-tapping screw requires that threads be cut into bone with a tap; a self-tapping screw has a cutting tip to cut threads into bone and flutes to accept bone debris. Which of these types of screws is best is controversial, but currently the most commonly used ASIF screws are non–self-tapping. Cortical screws are fully threaded and designed for use in compact cortical bone. The pitch of the screw (number of threads per inch) is greater than that of a cancellous screw (Fig. 28-48). This allows a greater number of threads to engage the matrix of the relatively narrow-diameter cortical bone. Cancellous screws are either completely or partially threaded and are used primarily in the epiphysis or metaphysis. The thread height (difference between the core diameter and outer screw diameter) of cancellous screws is greater than the thread height of cortical screws, which allows deep purchase into the soft spongy epiphyseal or metaphyseal bone. Cortical and cancellous screws are named for their outside diameter (e.g., 3.5-mm cortical screws are designated as such because the outer screw diameter is 3.5 mm). Cancellous and cortical screws are available in a variety of sizes ranging from 1.5 to 6.5 mm.

Bone screws are used either to anchor bone plates to bone or to hold bone fragments in place. When used to anchor a bone plate to bone, the screw is called a *plate screw*. The screws used to hold bone fragments in anatomic position and prevent them from collapsing into the marrow cavity are called *position screws*. Position screws can be inserted through a plate hole or placed in bone independent of the plate. Lag screws (also termed *compression screws*) are used to apply compression between fragments. Whether a screw is used as a plate screw, a position screw, or a lag screw, appropriate instrumentation must be used to implant the screw correctly. Each different screw size has a drill bit corresponding to the inner core diameter (shaft) of the screw, a drill bit corresponding to the outer diameter of the screw, and a tap corresponding to the threads of the screw. The manufacturer (ASIF) provides a chart to assist in choosing the appropriate instrumentation for each screw size. Additional instrumentation includes a depth gauge to measure the length of screw desired and a countersink to cut a circular groove in the cortex to accept the head of the screw. The countersink is only used when a lag screw is inserted into the cortex independent of the bone plate.

ASIF bone plates are made of 316L stainless steel or titanium; however, because titanium plates and screws are more expensive than stainless steel, the latter are more commonly used. Bone plates are designated in several different ways, including plate length, screw size that the plate hole will accept, plate and screw hole configuration, and function. For example, a 10-hole, 3.5-mm broad dynamic compression plate (DCP) may be used in a buttress function in which the plate length is designated by the number of plate holes (e.g., 10). Each of the different plate sizes is available in wide range of

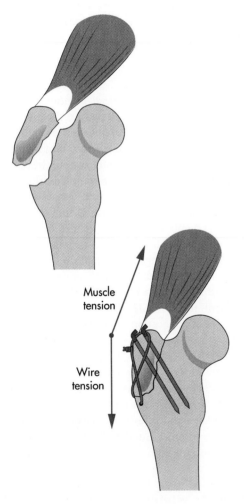

FIG. 28-47
Placement and mechanical principle of a tension band. Tightening the wire exerts a force that counters the force of muscle contraction and compresses the fracture surface.

Muscle tension

Wire tension

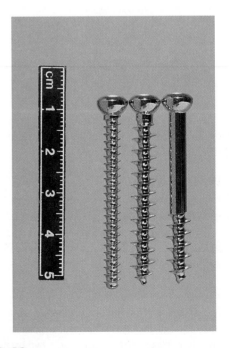

FIG. 28-48
Types of bone screws (left to right): cortical, fully threaded cancellous, partially threaded cancellous.

lengths. The 3.5-mm broad plates range in length from 4 to 22 holes and the 2.7-mm plates range in length from 4 to 12 holes. The plate size is determined by the cortical screw that the plate holes will accept. A 3.5-mm broad plate is so named because the plate holes will accept 3.5-mm cortical bone screws. Similarly, 2.7-mm bone plates accept 2.7-mm cortical bone screws and 4.5-mm bone plates accept 4.5-mm cortical bone screws.

Plate hole configuration is also used to designate the type of plate. A plate hole can be round (e.g., veterinary cuttable plate) or oblong (e.g., dynamic compression plate). A bone plate with oblong holes is referred to as a *dynamic compression plate (DCP)* because compression can be applied to the bone through the dynamic action of the screw being tightened (Fig. 28-49). The configuration of the oblong hole is based on a spherical gliding principle modeled after a ball rolling down an inclined plane. The conical shape of the screw head is representative of the ball and the oblong plate hole is representative of the inclined plane. With the plate hole being inclined, the screw head will slide toward the center of the oblong hole as the screw is tightened. When the screw slides toward the center of the plate hole, horizontal movement of bone beneath the plate occurs. If this is done on each side of the fracture line, the bone is pushed together from both sides, resulting in compression at the fracture line. Proper screw placement is ensured by using drill guides that center the drill hole in either a loading or neutral position. In the loading position, approximately 1 mm of compression is achieved for each screw tightened, whereas in the neutral position approximately 0.1 mm of compression is achieved.

In addition to plate hole design, bone plate configuration is also used to designate the plate type. The 3.5- and 4.5-mm bone plates are available as standard plates and broad plates. The broad plates are wider, which gives them increased strength and stiffness, an important feature when bone plates are used in large and giant dogs. Titanium plates are designed as limited-contact plates (LCP plates). They are manufactured so that there is limited contact between the plate and bone, to minimize interruption of blood flow. This is accomplished by undercutting the bottom surface of the plate between the screw holes. The screw holes are based on the dynamic compression principle, but differ in that the oblong screw hole is inclined from both ends of the screw hole toward the center, allowing compression to be applied in either direction. Specialized bone plates (e.g., reconstruction plates, angled plates, and condylar screw plates) are available for selected orthopedic conditions.

Bone plates specifically designed for use in small animals (e.g., veterinary cuttable plate, canine acetabular plate, and canine distal radial plate) are advantageous for specific injuries. Veterinary cuttable plates (VCP) are available in two sizes, designated by the size screw that the plate hole will accept. The 2.0/2.7 VCP can be used with either a 2.0- or 2.7-mm cortical screw, while the 1.5/2.0 VCP can be used with either a 2.0- or a 1.5-mm cortical screw. The VCP is popular because it is available in varying lengths up to 50 screw holes (300 mm). The plate can be cut so that it has the desired number of holes. VCP are often used in a stacked configuration to bridge comminuted fractures in smaller patients. Stacking two plates onto each other increases the strength and stiffness of the fixation as compared with using a single plate. The canine acetabular plate is manufactured to conform to the dorsolateral surface of the canine acetabulum and is available in two sizes. This plate is particularly useful in large and giant breeds of dogs because it is strong and stiff. The canine distal radial plate is made for distal radial and ulnar fractures in small breeds. Typically, this fracture has a very short distal segment that makes it difficult to place an

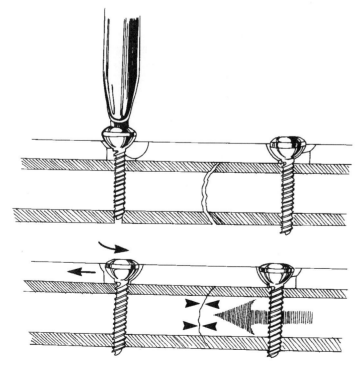

FIG. 28-49
To obtain static compression of a fracture line using a load guide, first fix one of the bone segments to the plate with a screw(s) in the neutral position. Reduce the other bone segment, and use the load guide to eccentrically place a screw in the plate hole. The load screw engages the edge of the plate hole first. As the screw is tightened and slides along the glide slope, it moves the plate and attached opposite bone segment closer to its position. If the gap between the segments is less than 1 mm, compression occurs as the fracture surfaces are forced together. (From Olmstead ML: *Small animal orthopedics*, St Louis, 1995, Mosby.)

adequate number of plate screws. The canine distal radial plate has a T configuration, with the horizontal bar conforming to the epiphysis/metaphysis of the distal radius. The shape and size of the plate allow adequate plate screws to be placed in the short metaphyseal segment.

Although bone plates are designated as to their intended function (i.e., compression plates, neutralization plates, or buttress plates), depending upon how they are applied to the bone, it is important to realize that the plate configuration (DCP plate, veterinary cuttable plate, broad plate) does not change. A 3.5-mm broad DCP plate may serve as a compression plate, neutralization plate, or buttress plate, depending on how it is applied to the bone (Fig. 28-50). A bone plate serves as a compression plate when compression is applied to the fracture line through proper application of the plate and screws. **A DCP plate may only function as a compression plate if the fracture line is transverse or short oblique (no greater than 45 degrees).** If the fracture line is greater than 45 degrees or is comminuted, the plate cannot be used to compress the fracture lines. A neutralization plate is one that neutralizes physiologic forces acting on a section of bone that has been repaired with screws and/or wire. Indications for a neutralization plate include comminuted fractures in which the section of fragmented diaphysis can be reconstructed with bone screws or cerclage wire and oblique fractures in which the fracture line exceeds 45 degrees.

A buttress plate is one that bridges a fragmented section of bone or holds a collapsed epiphysis in position. The most frequent application of a buttress plate is with fragmented diaphyseal fractures in which surgical reduction and stabilization of the bone fragments are not technically feasible. Careful assessment of preoperative radiographs is needed to determine whether a neutralization or buttress plate is indicated. A neutralization plate-bone construct is mechanically more stable and prone to fewer complications than is a buttress plate-bone construct. Because of the inherent stability of a neutralization construct, this plate function should be used when possible. However, if reduction and stabilization of bone fragments is not technically feasible or if significant soft tissue devitalization of the bone fragments would occur, a buttress plate should be considered.

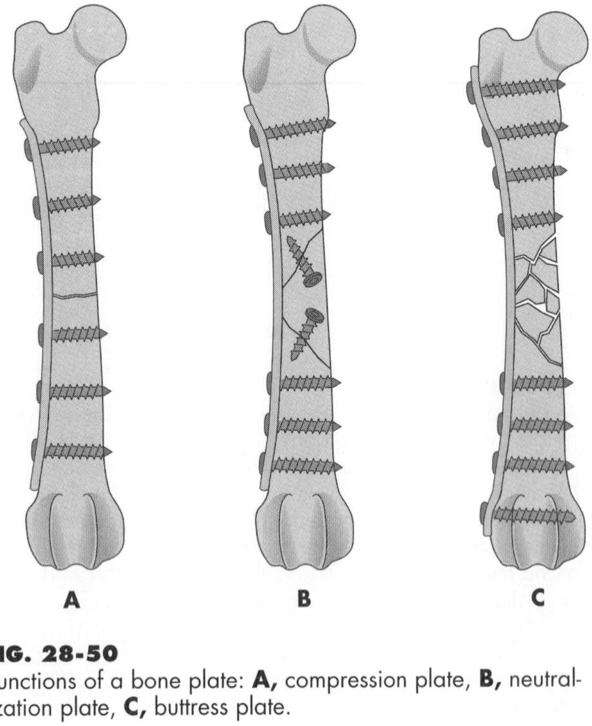

Plate size (2.0 mm, 2.7 mm, 3.5 mm, 4.5 mm) needed varies, depending on patient weight and bone dimensions. ASIF/AO have developed charts that can be used to select a suitable plate, relative to body weight. The plate length should be sufficient to prevent premature loosening of plate screws and subsequent loosening of the plate from the bone surface. The minimum length of plate should allow purchase of six cortices (three screws if both cortices are purchased by each screw) in the main bone fragment above the fracture and six cortices in the main fragment below the fracture. This number of screws will ensure adequate distribution of stress among the plate screws. **However, the minimum of six cortices on each side of the fracture is often exceeded to ensure that the plate spans the diaphyseal length.**

The surface on which the plate is located influences the degree of stability obtained. In general, all long bones are subject to bending forces because physiologic loads are applied eccentrically to the bone center. When a bone is subject to this type of loading, a bend will occur that causes compression on the concave surface of the bone and tension on the convex surface. It is the tension that must be prevented because it will cause a fracture line to pull apart. This is accomplished by laying the plate on the tension surface and thereby allowing the plate to absorb the tensile stress that would separate the fracture.

Application

Plates

Compression plates (Fig. 28-51). It is important to properly contour the plate relative to the bone surface. *To apply a plate as a compression plate, contour it so that the plate remains slightly offset (1 to 2 mm) from the surface of the bone at the fracture line.* If the plate is contoured to conform accurately to the bone surface, asymmetric loading of the fracture line will occur. This is because the compression generated through the plate is applied to the bone eccentrically (it is greatest on the surface on which the plate rests). The net result is compression of the fracture line beneath the plate and widening of the fracture near the far cortex. Because there is a gap in the far cortex, the plate supports all of the applied loads without any significant contribution from the bony column. The gap in the far cortex is prevented through proper contouring of the bone plate relative to the bone surface. When the plate screws on each side of the fracture line are tightened, each main bone fragment is pulled up against the plate, compressing the far cortex. *Insert the two plate screws nearest the fracture first. Place both screws in a loaded position and tighten them to achieve compression of the fracture line. Insert subsequent plate screws in holes*

FIG. 28-50
Functions of a bone plate: **A,** compression plate, **B,** neutralization plate, **C,** buttress plate.

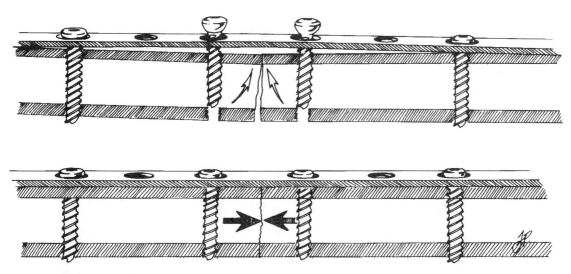

FIG. 28-51
Prestress a plate by slightly overbending it at the fracture site during contouring. This creates a 1- to 2-mm gap between the plate and bone when the first screws are inserted in the ends of the plate. When the screws next to the fracture line are inserted the bone is pulled up to the plate, creating static compression along the fracture line. The fracture segments need to be anatomically reduced for compression to occur. (From Olmstead ML: *Small animal orthopedics,* St Louis, 1995, Mosby.)

in an alternating fashion on either side of the fracture, working toward the plate ends. Adequate compression of the fracture is generally achieved with loading of the first two screws. *If you desire greater compression, place an additional screw on each side of the fracture in the loaded position (insert the remaining screws in a neutral position).*

Neutralization plates (Fig. 28-52). *First reduce and stabilize the fracture with a series of lag screws, multiple cerclage wires, or a combination of both. Because the screws and/or wire are not sufficiently strong to resist physiologic forces generated by weight bearing, use a bone plate to bridge the area and neutralize those forces that would act to collapse the fracture. As with a compression plate, apply a neutralization plate to the tension surface of the bone but contour it to the anatomic surface of the bone.* Separation of the fracture line beneath the plate will not occur because the fracture lines have already been compressed with lag screws or cerclage wire. The recommended number of cortices (six) engaged on each side of the fracture is the same as for a compression plate. However, with a neutralization plate, *insert all screws in the neutral position, beginning from the end of the plate and working toward the center. If a plate screw cannot be inserted because it lies over a fracture line, leave the hole empty. If the plate hole lies over a lag screw placed through the bone, leave the hole empty or insert a screw that purchases only the near cortex.*

Buttress plates (Fig. 28-53). *Apply a buttress plate to the tension surface of the bone and contour it to the anatomic shape of the bone. Use a radiograph of the intact bone of the opposite leg as a template to help contour the plate if the affected bone is severely comminuted.* All the applied loads will be carried by the plate and screws during the early postoperative period, causing greater stress to be

placed on the bone screws than occurs with compression or neutralization plates in which the applied loads are shared with the bone. *Therefore purchase a minimum of eight cortices, rather than six. Similarly, use a stronger and stiffer plate because it too will be subject to substantial loads until bone is deposited within the fracture gap to form a bony column. For optimal strength and stiffness use a broad plate, lengthening plate, or stacked VCP plates, rather than a standard plate. Alternatively, support the plate with ancillary implants (IM pins or external skeletal fixators) that share the applied loads during the early healing period. With a plate/IM pin combination, insert an IM pin approximately 50% the diameter of the marrow cavity, being careful to maintain the rotational alignment and axial length of the bone. Contour a plate of appropriate length and apply it to the tension surface of the bone. Insert the most proximal and distal plate screws so that they avoid the IM pin and engage both near and far cortices. Insert the plate screws near the center of the plate so that they engage only the near cortex (monocortical screws; Fig. 28-54). With a plate/external skeletal fixator combination, contour the plate and apply it to the tension surface of the bone. Insert the transfixation pins proximal and distal to the plate and connect them with an external bar.* With either system, methods to enhance the formation of callus are as important as the mechanical properties of the plate-bone construct. *Use autogenous cancellous bone and avoid manipulating the fragmented section of bone (bridging osteosynthesis; see Fig. 28-53).*

Screws. A precise order of maneuvers is followed when inserting a plate screw, position screw, or lag screw. *When inserting a plate screw in the diaphysis, drill a thread hole through the near (cis) and far (trans) cortices, using the*

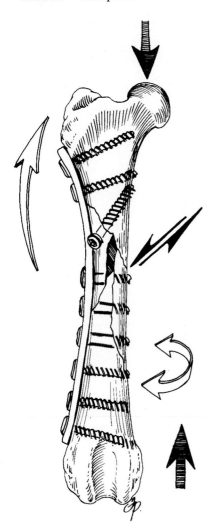

FIG. 28-52
Neutralization plates transmit loads from one end of the bone to the other, while protecting the reconstructed fracture from bending, torsion, and axial loads (*arrows*). The load transmission surfaces of the bone must be anatomically reconstructed and securely stabilized (usually with lag screws). (From Olmstead ML: *Small animal orthopedics*, St Louis, 1995, Mosby.)

appropriate drill guide. To create a thread hole where the screw purchases bone when tapped, use a drill bit corresponding to the inner core diameter of the screw. To insert a 3.5-mm plate screw, use a drill bit that corresponds to the inner core diameter (shaft) of the screw (2.5 mm) and a tap that corresponds to the outer thread diameter of the screw (3.5 mm). Determine the length of screw needed with the depth gauge and cut threads into the near and far cortices with a tap (Fig. 28-55). Use a tap sleeve when cutting threads, to maintain axial alignment relative to the thread hole and to prevent soft tissue from winding around the tap threads. Remove the tap and flush the hole with sterile saline to eliminate bone debris and lubricate the hole. Insert a cortical screw and use fingers only on the screwdriver to tighten it. In spongy metaphyseal or epiphyseal bone, use a cancellous bone screw as a plate screw and place in a similar fashion.

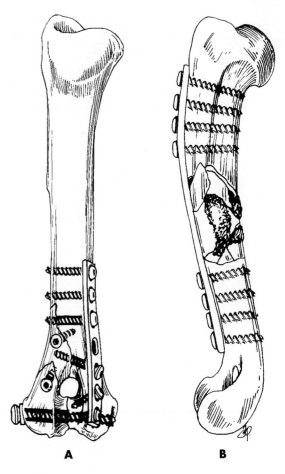

FIG. 28-53
Buttress plates, **A,** maintain joint integrity or, **B,** span a non-reconstructible fracture gap. (From Olmstead ML: *Small animal orthopedics*, St Louis, 1995, Mosby.)

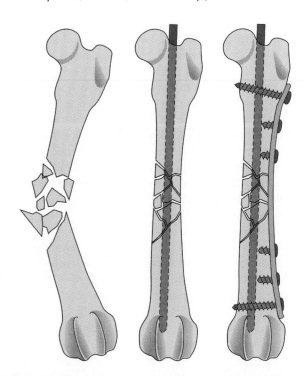

FIG. 28-54
Stabilization of a comminuted fracture with a plate/rod combination.

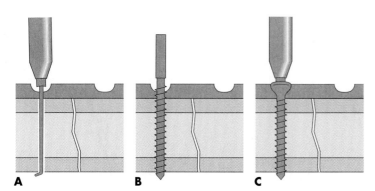

FIG. 28-55
To place a plate screw, drill the thread hole, **A,** measure the screw length, **B,** tap threads in the cis and trans cortex, and **C,** insert the screw.

A lag screw functions to compress a fracture line between two bony fragments. It may be inserted through a plate hole or directly into bone, independent of the bone plate. The optimal position of a lag screw is one that bisects the angle formed between a line perpendicular to the fracture surface and one perpendicular to the long axis of the bone. The drill hole in the near cortex must be a glide hole (a hole equal in diameter to the outside diameter of the screw), whereas the drill hole in the far cortex must be a thread hole (a hole equal in diameter to the inner core diameter or shaft of the screw). *To insert a lag screw, use a drill bit that corresponds to the outer diameter of the screw to create a glide hole through which the screw will pass without purchasing bone (Fig. 28-56). When creating the glide hole, drill the bone using a drill guide to maintain alignment and protect soft tissues. Insert a drill sleeve into the glide hole in preparation for creating the thread hole in the far cortex (the drill sleeve insert centers the thread hole in the far cortex relative to the glide hole, which prevents stripping the thread hole on screw insertion). After the glide hole and thread hole are made, use a countersink to prepare a site for the screw head in the cortex and use a depth gauge to determine the appropriate length screw to use. Tap the thread hole through a tap sleeve to maintain alignment and protect soft tissues. Insert the appropriate length screw and tighten it with your fingers only on the screwdriver.* The threads of the screw will glide through the hole in the near cortex (glide hole) and purchase the bone in the far cortex (thread hole). As the screw is tightened, the screw head contacts the near cortex. As the threads purchase the far cortex, the fracture line is compressed. A lag screw can be placed through a plate hole by following the same procedure. However, because the screw head rests against the bone plate, it is not necessary to countersink the near cortex. Fully threaded cancellous screws can also be inserted as lag screws, either through the plate or independent of the plate, by following the same procedures. The only difference in placement is the instrumentation needed to match the screw size.

Partially threaded cancellous bone screws can also be used as lag screws. In fact, because of ease of application, partially threaded cancellous bone screws are used more commonly as lag screws than are fully threaded cancellous bone screws. *With partially threaded screws, drill the near and far cortices as thread holes (Fig. 28-57). Use a depth gauge to de-* *termine the appropriate length screw and tap both cortices before inserting the screw.* Because the screw is only partially threaded, there are no threads to engage the bone on the near side of the fracture and bone is purchased only in the far cortex. As the screw head contacts bone and the screw is tightened, compression is achieved. It is critical that the smooth shaft of the screw crosses the fracture line; if threads are present at the fracture line, compression cannot be achieved.

Either a cortical screw or fully threaded cancellous screw can function as a position screw. A position screw is used to hold two bone fragments in anatomic alignment when compression would cause one fragment to collapse into the marrow cavity. *Hold the fragments in position with bone-holding forceps and drill a thread hole through the cortex of each fragment with a drill bit corresponding the inner core diameter (shaft) of the screw (Fig. 28-58). Use a depth gauge to determine the appropriate length screw and cut threads in both cortices with the appropriate tap. Insert the screw, using bone-holding forceps to hold the fragments in position and prevent distraction at the fracture line. Gently tighten the screws ("finger-tight") until the screw head rests adjacent to the near cortex (or bone plate).* The screw holds the fragments in position when the bone-holding forceps are removed.

Postoperative Care

Bone plates and screws require minimal postoperative maintenance. Postoperative analgesia should be provided (see p. 708). General postoperative care for fracture management is provided in the section on individual long bones. Generally, postoperative examinations should be done weekly for 2 to 3 weeks following surgery; thereafter, examinations can be done every 2 weeks. The appropriate time to take postoperative radiographs to determine healing depends on the estimated time to bone union, based upon the patient fracture assessment. If plates are removed, removal should be done 3 to 4 months following radiographic bone union. When bone plates are applied to long bone fractures in younger patients, they should be removed. Removal is also recommended when plates have been applied in areas with limited soft tissue covering (e.g., radius, tibia) because in these locations, cold conduction may cause discomfort. Plate removal should be performed aseptically with the patient under general anesthesia. *Incise the skin overlying the plate screws and*

FIG. 28-56

A, To insert a cortex screw with lag function, drill a glide hole in the near bone segment with a drill bit the diameter of the outside screw thread. Use the drill guide to protect soft tissues and align the drill bit. **B,** Place an insert sleeve through the glide hole until the far bone segment is engaged. Drill a thread hole with a drill bit the same diameter as the core of the screw. The drill sleeve keeps the thread hole centered relative to the glide hole. **C,** Use a countersink to cut a bevel in the cortical bone at the entrance of the glide hole. This increases the contact area between the bone and screw and decreases the amount of the screw head exposed. This step is not needed if the lag screw is placed through a plate hole. **D,** Determine the length of screw to be inserted with a depth gauge. **E,** Use a tap to cut threads for the screw in the far bone segment. This step is unnecessary if self-tapping screws are used. **F,** Insert the screw and tighten it to create interfragmentary compression. (From Olmstead ML: *Small animal orthopedics,* St Louis, 1995, Mosby.)

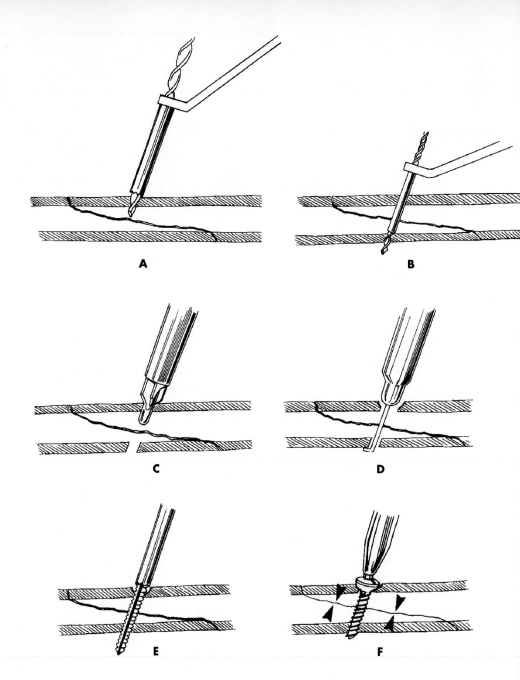

A

B

C

D

E

F

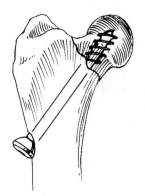

FIG. 28-57

Application of interfragmentary compression with a partially threaded cancellous bone screw. Note that the screw threads have crossed the fracture line, and the smooth shaft of the screw lies within the fracture plane. (From Olmstead ML: *Small animal orthopedics,* St Louis, 1995, Mosby.)

bluntly dissect through soft tissues to the head of the screw. Once all plate screws are removed, lift the plate from the bone surface at one end and extract it.

References

Howard PE: Principles of intramedullary pin and wire fixation, *Semin Vet Med Surg (Small Anim)* 6:52, 1991.

Suggested Reading

Aron DN, Crowe DT: The 90/90 flexion splint for prevention of stifle joint stiffness with femoral fracture repair, *J Am Anim Hosp Assoc* 23:447, 1987.

Aron DN, Dewey C: Experimental and clinical experience with an IM pin external skeletal fixator tie-in configuration, *Vet Comp Orthop Traum* 4:86, 1991.

FIG. 28-58
Screws with position function purchase bone on both sides of the fracture line. This type of screw is used when compression of the fragments would cause one segment to collapse into the medullary cavity. (From Olmstead ML: *Small animal orthopedics,* St Louis, 1995, Mosby.)

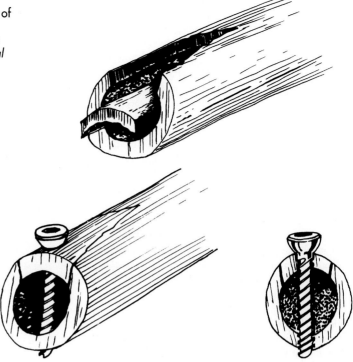

Aron DN, Palmer RH, Johnson AL: Biologic strategies and a balanced concept for repair of highly comminuted long bone fractures, *Comp Cont Educ Pract Vet* 17:35, 1995.

Aron DN, Toombs JP: Updated principles of external skeletal fixation, *Comp Cont Educ Pract Vet* :845, 1984.

Blass CE et al: Static and dynamic cerclage wire analysis, *Vet Surg* 15:181, 1986.

Brinker WO, Hohn RB, Prieur WD, editors: *Manual of internal fixation in small animals,* Berlin, 1984, Springer-Verlag.

Brinker WO, Verstraete MC, Soutas-Little RW: Stiffness studies on various configurations and types of external fixators, *J Am Anim Hosp Assoc* 21:801, 1985.

Bruecker KA, Schwarz PD, Polher O: A comparison of porous coated titanium screws versus smooth titanium screws with titanium bone plates in an unstable fracture model in dogs, *Vet Surg* 17:30, 1988.

Dallman MJ et al: Rotational strength of double-pinning techniques in repair of transverse fractures in femurs of dogs, *Am J Vet Res* 51:123, 1990.

Dueland RT et al: Preliminary results: biomechanical analysis of canine femoral, solid intramedullary pins, and interlocking intramedullary pins, *Vet Surg* 20:334, 1991.

Egger EL et al: Type I biplanar configuration of external skeletal fixation: application technique in nine dogs and one cat, *J Am Anim Med Assoc* 187:262, 1985.

Egger EL, Woo S: Effects of destabilizing rigid external fixation on healing of unstable canine osteotomies, *Trans Orthop Res Soc* 13:302, 1988.

Fanton JEW, Blass CE, Withrow SJ: Sciatic nerve injury as a complication of intramedullary pin fixation of femoral fractures, *J Am Anim Hosp Assoc* 19:687, 1983.

Foland MA, Egger FL: Application of type III external fixators: a review of 23 clinical fractures in 20 dogs and 2 cats, *J Am Anim Hosp Assoc* 27:193, 1991.

Foland MA, Schwarz PD, Salman MD: The adjunctive use of half pin (type I) external skeletal fixators in combination with intramedullary pins for femoral fracture fixation, *Vet Comp Orthop Traum* 4:77, 1991.

Fox SM: Using the Kirschner external fixation splint: a guide for the uninitiated, *Vet Med* 81:214, 1986.

Goodship AE, Kenwright J: The influence of induced micromovement upon the healing of experimental tibial fractures, *J Bone Joint Surg* 67B:650, 1985.

Leighton RL: Principles of conservative fracture management: splints and casts, *Semin Vet Med Surg (Small Anim)* 6:39, 1991.

Lesser AS: Complications from improper intramedullary pin placement in tibial fractures, *Mod Vet Pract* 65:940, 1984.

McPherron MA, Schwarz PD, Histand MB: Mechanical evaluation of half-pin (type 1) external skeletal fixation in combination with a single intramedullary pin, *Vet Surg* 21:178, 1992.

Olmstead ML: Complications of fractures repaired with plates and screws, *Vet Clin North Am Small Anim Pract* 21:669, 1991.

Orton EC et al: Comparison of porous titanium-surfaced and standard smooth-surfaced bone plates and screws in an unstable fracture model in dogs, *Am J Vet Res* 47:677, 1986.

Palmer RH, Aron DN: Ellis pin complications in seven dogs, *Vet Surg* 19:440, 1990.

Palmer RH, Aron DN, Purinton PT: Relationship of femoral intramedullary pins to the sciatic nerve and gluteal muscles after retrograde and normograde insertion, *Vet Surg* 17:65, 1988.

Roush JK, Wilson JW: Effects of plates luting on cortical vascularity and development of cortical porosity in canine femurs, *Vet Surg* 19:208, 1990.

Schatzker J: Concepts of fracture stabilization. In Sumner-Smith G, editor: *Bone in clinical orthopaedics,* Philadelphia, 1982, WB Saunders.

Schrader SC: Complications associated with the use of Steinmann intramedullary pins and cerclage wires for fixation of long-bone fractures, *Vet Clin North Am Small Anim Pract* 21:687, 1991.

Stevenson S, Olmstead ML, Kowalski J: Bacterial culturing for prediction of postoperative complications following open fracture repair in small animals, *Vet Surg* 15:99, 1986.

Swaim SF et al: Evaluation of the dermal effects of cast padding in coaptation casts on dogs, *Am J Vet Res* 53:1266, 1992.

Tomlinson J: Complications of fractures repaired with casts and splints, *Vet Clin North Am Small Anim Pract* 21:735, 1991.

Toombs JP: Principles of external skeletal fixation using the Kirschner-Ehmer splint, *Semin Vet Med Surg (Small Anim)* 6:68, 1991.

Toombs JP, Aron DN, Basinger RR: Angled connecting bars for transarticular application of Kirschner-Ehmer external fixation splints, *J Am Anim Hosp Assoc* 25:213, 1989.

Turner AS et al: Improved plate fixation of unstable fractures due to bone cement around the screw heads, *Vet Surg* 20:349, 1991.

Walter MC et al: Treatment of severely comminuted diaphyseal fractures in the dog, using standard bone plates and autogenous cancellous bone graft to span fracture gaps: 11 cases (1979–1983), *J Am Vet Med Assoc* 189:457, 1986.

Willer RL, Egger EL, Histand MB: A comparison of stainless steel versus acrylic for the connecting bar of external skeletal fixators, *J Am Anim Hosp Assoc* 27:541, 1991.

FRACTURE REDUCTION

Reduction is the process of reconstructing fractured bones to their normal anatomic configuration and/or restoring normal limb alignment. Normal limb alignment is achieved by restoring normal limb length, maintaining spatial orientation of the limb, and restoring alignment of joints adjacent to fractured bones (Fig. 28-59). Fracture fragments need not necessarily be anatomically reconstructed during restoration of normal limb alignment. After bones fracture, several natural processes occur that serve to increase fracture stability in preparation for healing. In response to injury, muscles that attach to proximal and distal bone ends and span fractures contract. This contraction causes fractured diaphyseal segments to override each other, resulting in a shorter lever arm action on the fracture site and increased stability. Fractured limbs are painful and animals tend to minimize using them, which favors fracture stability. Techniques used to reduce fractures or align limbs must overcome these physiologic processes.

The initial decision when planning fracture treatment is to determine whether to use closed or open reduction (Table 28-9). Closed reduction refers to reducing fractures or aligning limbs without surgically exposing fractured bones. Advantages of closed reduction include: (1) preservation of soft tissues and blood supply, which speeds healing; (2) decreased possibility of inducing infection; and (3) reduced operating time. The main disadvantage of closed reduction is the difficulty of gaining accurate fracture reduction without visualizing fracture segments and fragments. Open reduction refers to using a surgical approach to expose fractured bone segments and fragments so they can be anatomically reconstructed and held in position with implants. Advantages of open reduction

include: (1) visualization and direct contact with bone fragments facilitates anatomic fracture reconstruction; (2) direct placement of implants (i.e., cerclage wire, lag screws, plates) is possible; (3) bone reconstruction allows bone and implants to share loads, which results in stronger fracture fixation; and (4) cancellous bone grafts can be used to enhance bone healing (see p. 760). Disadvantages of open reduction include increased surgical trauma to soft tissues and blood supply and greater opportunity to introduce bacterial contamination. The advantages and disadvantages of each method must be considered before selecting the reduction method.

CLOSED REDUCTION

Fractures that are appropriately treated with closed reduction include greenstick and nondisplaced fractures of bones distal to the elbow and stifle. These fractures may be managed with limb realignment and fracture immobilization with casts or external fixators (see pp. 733–742). Simple, easily palpable, femoral or humeral fractures in young animals can be treated with closed reduction and intramedullary pin placement (i.e., introduction of an intramedullary pin normograde through the proximal segment, closed reduction, and seating of the intramedullary pin into the distal segment). Severely comminuted fractures (particularly tibial and radial fractures) that are difficult or impossible to anatomically reconstruct are also appropriately treated with closed reduction, limb alignment, and rigid stabilization with external fixators (see Table 28-9). When closed reduction is used, anatomic fracture reconstruction is seldom possible. Instead, goals for closed reduction are to restore bone length and limb alignment. Careful attention must be paid to eliminating rotation and angular deformity of distal segments. True lateral and craniocaudal radiographic projections of proximal and distal joints allow the postoperative radiographs to be scrutinized to determine if joint surfaces above and below fractured bones are parallel to each other and in correct rotational alignment.

OPEN REDUCTION

Fractures that can be anatomically reconstructed (i.e., most simple displaced fractures or those with large fragments and long oblique fracture lines) or those that are displaced and

---

TABLE 28-9

Indications for Open or Closed Reduction

Open reduction
- Articular fractures
- Simple fractures that can be anatomically reconstructed
- Complex fractures of long bones

Closed reduction
- Greenstick/nondisplaced fractures of long bones below the elbow and stifle
- Simple fractures for closed pinning
- Complex/comminuted diaphyseal fractures of long bones

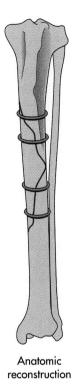
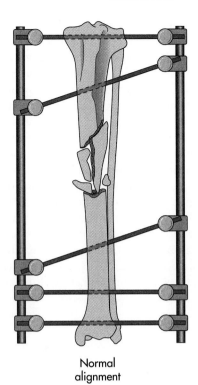

Anatomic
reconstruction

Normal
alignment

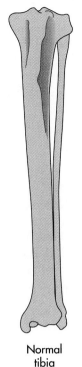

Normal
tibia

FIG. 28-59
Anatomic reconstruction of cortex is achieved by replacing all fracture fragments and holding them securely. Normal alignment of the limb is achieved by aligning adjacent joints, restoring normal bone length, and ensuring rotation of the distal bone segment does not occur.

involve joint surfaces are appropriately managed with open reduction. Bone columns and/or articular surfaces are restored and stabilized (see Fig. 28-59). Surgical approaches for exposing bones for fracture repair are found in subsequent chapters pertaining to individual bones. General principles include: (1) follow normal separations between muscles, (2) obtain adequate exposure of fractured bones, (3) handle soft tissues gently and preserve soft tissue attachments to bone fragments, and (4) avoid trauma to major nerves and vessels.

Biologic environment at fracture sites plays an important role in modulating fracture healing. Surgical techniques and implants that compromise surrounding soft tissues and interfere with vasculature to injured bone delay bone union. Realignment of joint surfaces, rather than anatomic fracture reconstruction, minimal to no soft tissue dissection, and optimal stability that results in moderate strain levels and bone formation are hallmarks of biologically oriented techniques or biologic fracture fixation. Concepts developed by Perron and co-workers ("It is better to trade some stability to achieve optimal biologic response" and "Single fractures concentrate tissue strain but multiple fractures distribute and thus reduce tissue strain") have been validated by the clinical success of this approach (Fig. 28-60). Because the animal's own bone rather than a cortical allograft is used, biologic fracture repair is preferred for treatment of severely comminuted middiaphyseal fractures (especially open fractures).

An important goal of biologic fracture fixation of comminuted fractures is to cause minimal disruption of soft tissues. Radial and tibial fractures can be treated with closed re-

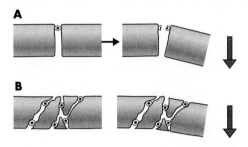

FIG. 28-60
A, Deflection of a single fracture line causes displacement of the bone and results in high strain at the fracture line. **B,** Deflection of multiple fracture lines allows the same amount of displacement to be distributed between fragments, resulting in lower strain at each fracture line.

duction and external fixators; however, comminuted femoral or humeral fractures are more difficult to reduce and external fixators are less suitable for these bones (see p. 741). When internal implants are chosen as the fixation method, an "open but do not touch" philosophy is used. A standard approach exposes major bone segments, the bone is distracted to length, and a precontoured, buttress plate (see p. 751) is applied. The fracture fragments are not disturbed. The same criteria used to evaluate successful closed reduction of fractures are used after this type of fixation.

ANESTHESIA

Maintenance on inhalant anesthesia is preferred over barbiturate anesthesia to obtain adequate muscle relaxation for fracture reduction. Balanced anesthesia techniques provide even greater muscle relaxation. Epidural anesthesia (with lidocaine or bupivacaine; see Chapter 12 and Table 28-4) in combination with general anesthesia provides profound relaxation of rear limb muscles, easing fracture reduction of the pelvis, femur, and tibia. The duration of action depends on the drug used but is usually 1 to 2 hours. Morphine can be added to the epidural injection, providing postoperative pain relief for up to 20 hours. See p. 708 for additional information regarding anesthetic techniques for fracture patients.

SURGICAL TECHNIQUES FOR FRACTURE REDUCTION

The major difficulty in achieving reduction is counteracting muscle contraction that has caused bone segments to override. Slow manual distraction of segments using bone-holding forceps will eventually fatigue muscles and allow reduction. Transverse fractures can be reduced by applying traction, countertraction, and bending forces. The bone ends should be lifted from the incision and brought into contact. Force is slowly applied to replace the bones in a normal position (Fig. 28-61). A lever can also be used to reduce transverse fractures (Fig. 28-62). Long oblique fractures can be difficult to reduce because the fracture line configuration makes bending or levering techniques difficult and overriding may occur even after reduction. Two self-retaining reduction forceps can be used to slowly force distraction of segments until reduction is achieved (Fig. 28-63). Rough handling of bone with any of these techniques can cause additional fragmentation. The bone should be inspected for fissure fracture lines. Weak bone segments should be supported by cerclage wires before attempting reduction (Fig. 28-64). Fractures with more than two pieces that can be completely reconstructed are first treated by securing loose fragments to one segment with lag screws or cerclage wire.

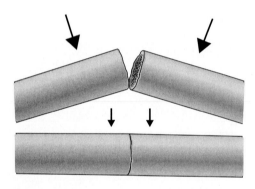

FIG. 28-61
To reduce a transverse fracture, lift the bone segments from surrounding soft tissues until the fracture surfaces are apposed. While maintaining contact, slowly replace the segments into a normal position.

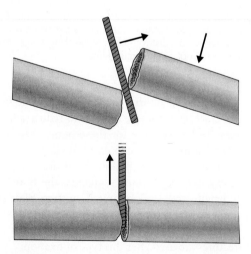

FIG. 28-62
To reduce overriding bone segments of a transverse fracture, carefully place a lever (small periosteal elevator or scalpel blade handle) between the overriding bone segments. Use the lever to gently apply pressure and help distract and reduce the bone segments.

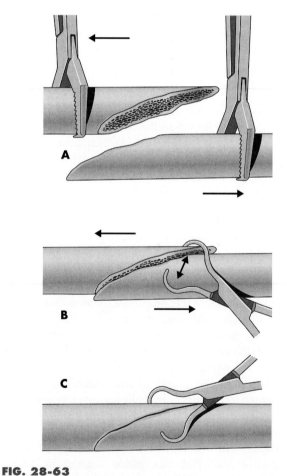

FIG. 28-63
A, Manually return the bone segments of a long oblique fracture to close approximation with bone-holding forceps. **B,** Place pointed reduction forceps at an angle to the fracture line. **C,** As the pointed reduction forceps are gently closed, the bone ends are distracted. The pointed reduction forceps should be manipulated to aid reduction and secured perpendicular to the fracture line. Multiple attempts may be necessary before reduction is achieved and held with pointed reduction forceps.

The two-piece fracture is then carefully distracted and aligned for definitive fixation (Fig. 28-65).

Fracture distractors are instruments that can be attached to the proximal and distal metaphyses of fractured bones or to intact bones adjacent to the fracture by means of fixation pins. This device facilitates fragment distraction and the offset position of the distractor allows access to fractures for fragment reconstruction and plate application (Fig. 28-66). Distractors can also be used during closed reduction and fracture stabilization with external fixation. The fracture distractor is attached to proximal and distal fixation pins and used to lengthen the bone before the rest of the fixator frame is constructed (see Fig. 29-111 on p. 872).

Intramedullary pins can also be used to distract fractures. The pin is driven normograde through the proximal bone

segment to the fracture site. It is then centered into the distal segment and driven distally until it engages metaphyseal bone. The proximal segment is steadied with bone-holding forceps while the pin is advanced distally until appropriate distraction is achieved (Fig. 28-67).

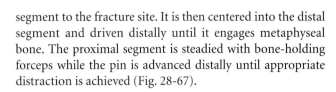

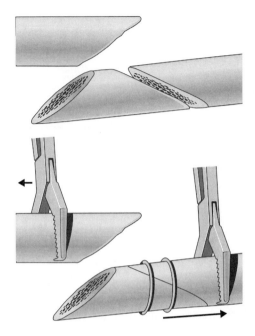

FIG. 28-65
Anatomic reconstruction of a fracture with a large butterfly fragment is achieved by first reducing the fragment and securing it to one segment of bone. This creates a two-piece fracture to be reduced and stabilized.

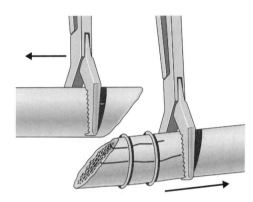

FIG. 28-64
The bone segment ends are secured with cerclage wire if fissure fractures are present.

FIG. 28-66
When using a fracture distractor, the device is attached to pins placed in the metaphyses perpendicular to the long bone. The distractor is engaged by twisting the circular knob and distracting the distal arm of the distractor and distal segment.

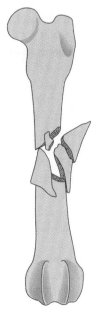

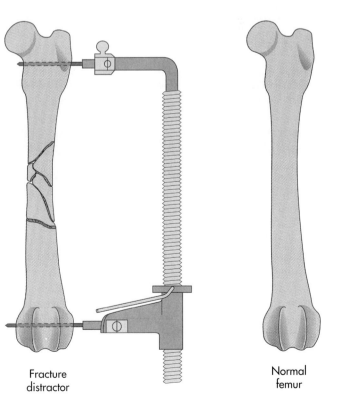

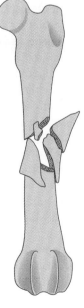

Fractured
femur

Fracture
distractor

Normal
femur

FIG. 28-67
When using an IM pin to distract fractures, the proximal segment is stabilized with a bone-holding forceps and an IM pin is used to push the distal segment of bone away from the proximal segment.

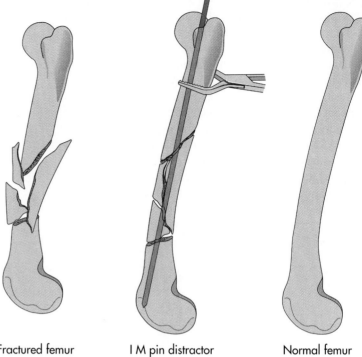

Fractured femur   I M pin distractor   Normal femur

The animal's own weight can be used to advantage by suspending the fractured limb from a secure ceiling bolt. The animal is draped and the surgical procedure performed with the limb suspended. Temporarily lowering the operating table causes the animal's weight to distract the fracture. This method can be used during both closed and open reduction of fractures. When the fracture is secured in the appropriate position, the operating table is raised to remove the traction force from the limb.

Suggested Reading

Brinker WO, Piermattei DL, Flo GL: *Handbook of small animal orthopedics and fracture treatment,* Philadelphia, 1990, WB Saunders.

BONE GRAFTING

Bone grafting, the technique of transplanting cancellous or cortical bone, has been used in veterinary medicine for many years. Bone grafts are named to indicate their structure and source. Autogenous cancellous bone grafting is a vital component of fracture management that helps fractures heal before implants loosen or fail. Cortical bone allografts are occasionally used to treat long bone fractures with severe cortical bone loss or to replace bone removed in limb-sparing techniques. Corticocancellous grafts contain cortical and cancellous bone (e.g., rib or ilial wing); osteochondral grafts also contain articular cartilage (e.g., proximal femur). Vascularized grafts are harvested with their blood supply and implanted using microvascular anastomosis techniques that preserve the bone's blood supply.

Bones transplanted from one site to another in the same animal are autografts. Such grafts are histocompatible with host immune systems and will not initiate rejection responses. Bones transplanted from one animal to another of the same species are allografts. Cellular antigens of these grafts may be recognized as foreign by host immune systems, resulting in graft rejection. Alloimplants are bone treated by freezing, freeze-drying, autoclaving, chemical preservation, or irradiation so that they are devoid of cellular activity. Allografts reinforced with cancellous autografts are composite grafts. Bones transplanted from one animal to another of a different species are xenografts. Bone substitutes of β-tricalcium phosphate ceramics are available as extenders for cancellous bone grafts.

Bone grafts can be sources of osteoprogenitor cells (osteogenesis), either providing cells directly or inducing formation of osteoprogenitor cells from surrounding tissues (osteoinduction). Bone grafts provide varying degrees of mechanical support, ranging from forming space-occupying trellises for host bone invasion (osteoconduction) to supplying weight-bearing struts within fractures. The type of bone graft chosen to augment fracture repair is determined by the function required to optimize fracture healing. Cancellous autografts are highly cellular, but mechanically weak. Therefore they provide superior osteoinductive capabilities but do not provide substantial fracture support. In contrast, cortical alloimplants provide excellent mechanical support but in most cases are acellular and stimulate little osteogenic response. Partial decalcification of cortical allografts allows release of bone morphogenetic protein to induce osteoprogenitor cells. However, partial decalcification weakens cortical bone and decreases its ability to support fractures. Autogenous cancellous bone grafts are used when rapid bone formation is desired, to assist healing when optimal healing is not anticipated (i.e., cortical defects after fracture repair, adult and elderly animals with fractures, delayed unions, nonunions, osteotomies, joint arthrodesis, and cystic defects), or to promote bone formation in infected fractures.

CANCELLOUS BONE GRAFTS

Cancellous bone may be harvested from any long bone metaphysis; however, the proximal humerus, the proximal tibia, and the ilial wing are most commonly used because they are accessible and contain large amounts of cancellous bone. The graft is usually harvested after fracture stabilization; however, it may be harvested before the primary orthopedic procedure if there is concern that the donor site may be contaminated with tumor cells or infection is present at the recipient site. Alternatively, a separate surgical team and instrumentation may be used to harvest the graft. The graft site is selected because of accessibility when the animal is positioned for fracture repair.

Proximal Humerus

Prepare the graft site for aseptic surgery. Perform a craniolateral approach to the proximal humerus by incising through skin and subcutaneous tissues. Retract the acromial head of the deltoid muscle caudally and expose the flat aspect of the craniolateral metaphysis, just distal to the greater tubercle. Make a round hole in the bone cortex, using an intramedullary pin or drill bit (Fig. 28-68, A). A round hole is made through the cortex to minimize formation of a stress riser that could contribute to fracture through the cortical defect. After penetrating bone cortex, insert a bone curette and harvest cancellous bone (Fig. 28-68, B). Place the cancellous bone directly into the recipient bed or store it in a blood-soaked sponge or stainless steel cup (Fig. 28-68, C and D). Add blood to the graft if it is placed in a cup, to keep it moist. The blood will clot and form a moldable composite with the graft, which facilitates handling. Do not store cancellous bone grafts in saline or treat them with antibiotics because this may kill cells. Secure stored grafts on the instrument table to avoid inadvertent disposal. Flush the fracture site and loosely pack all defects and fracture lines with graft material. Close subcutaneous tissues around the graft to hold them in position. Close subcutaneous tissues and skin of the graft site routinely.

Proximal Tibia

Make a craniomedial skin incision over the medial surface of the proximal tibia. After incising subcutaneous tissues, harvest cancellous bone as described above.

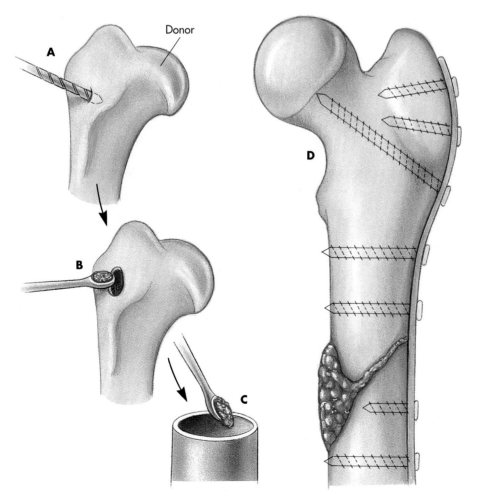

FIG. 28-68
A, To obtain cancellous bone from the humerus, make a round hole through the near cortex. **B,** Use a bone curette to harvest cancellous bone. **C,** Place the bone into a stainless steel cup with whole blood for short-term storage. **D,** Loosely pack the cancellous bone in the fracture gap or along fracture lines.

Ilial Wing

Make a skin incision over the craniodorsal iliac spine. Incise subcutaneous tissues and expose the dorsal surface of the ilial wing. Elevate gluteal musculature from the lateral surface and harvest cancellous bone as described above. Alternatively, obtain a corticocancellous graft by using rongeurs to remove a cortical wedge from the ilial wing. Macerate the wedge with rongeurs (Fig. 28-69) and place it into the recipient site.

Revascularization of cancellous bone autografts begins as early as 2 days after grafting and is usually completed within 2 weeks (Fig. 28-70, *A* and *B*). Transplanted osteogenic cells or differentiated mesenchymal cells become active osteoblasts, secreting osteoid on transplanted trabecular bone (Fig. 28-70, *C*). This osteoid is mineralized and forms new host bone in fracture sites (Fig. 28-70, *D*). This new bone also incorporates the graft into host bone. Eventually the necrotic cores of trabecular bone are resorbed by osteoclasts and grafts are totally replaced by host bone. Trabecular new bone is remodeled into cortical bone in response to the mechanical environment (Fig. 28-70, *E*). This healing response can be monitored radiographically by observing filling of the defect with cancellous bone, followed by cortical reconstruction. The donor site is initially filled with hematoma that is later replaced with fibrous connective tissue. Osteoblasts migrate to the area and deposit osteoid. Mineralization occurs and new trabecular bone is formed within defects. This process takes approximately 12 weeks; additional cancellous bone should not be harvested from the same area before this time.

There are few complications associated with autogenous cancellous bone-grafting techniques. Donor site pain is seldom clinically evident. Seroma formation or wound dehiscence may occur at donor sites. Infection or seeding of tumor to donor sites occurs rarely and can be prevented by proper sequencing of bone graft harvesting. Fractures through the donor site have been reported infrequently. Complications at the recipient site (e.g., failure of grafts to stimulate bone formation) are difficult to recognize.

CORTICAL BONE AUTOGRAFTS

Cortical autografts are harvested from areas where cortical bone can be removed without adversely affecting function (i.e., ribs, ilial wing, distal ulna, and fibula). The most common use of a cortical autograft is transplantation of a rib to form a segmental strut for mandibular fractures. Cortical autograft harvest is done during fracture repair and the graft is incorporated into the fracture site as a segmental graft (i.e., it is placed between fracture segments) or as a sliding onlay graft (i.e., it is placed over the fracture site). Cortical autografts are usually held in place with the same implant used to stabilize the fracture.

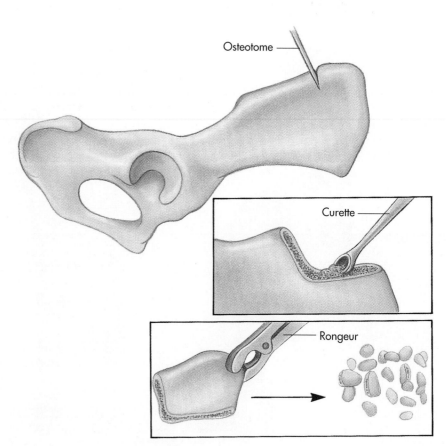

FIG. 28-69
To obtain cancellous bone from the wing of the ilium, use an osteotome to remove a wedge from the dorsal cranial ilial wing. Use a bone curette to harvest cancellous bone. Use rongeurs to fragment the osteotomized wedge of corticocancellous bone.

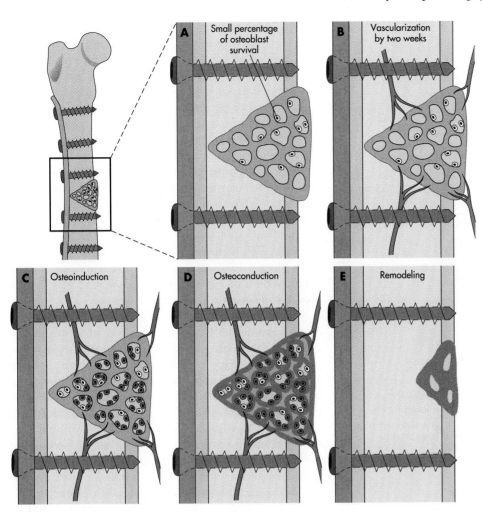

FIG. 28-70
Stages of cancellous bone incorporation into a healing fracture: **A,** graft placement, **B,** vascularization of the graft, **C,** osteoinduction, **D,** osteoconduction, **E,** remodeling.

CORTICAL BONE ALLOGRAFTS

Cortical bone can be harvested and transplanted immediately as a fresh allograft or it can be harvested and banked to provide a ready source of cortical alloimplants. Harvesting must be done under aseptic conditions unless the bone is sterilized following collection.

Euthanize the donor animal and prepare the femur, tibia, and/or humerus for aseptic surgery. Make surgical approaches to the bone diaphyses, elevate soft tissues, and isolate the bones. Use an oscillating bone saw to resect the diaphyses, then clean the marrow canals and flush them with saline. Immediately transplant the bones into the fracture site or store them for future use. To bank bones, double-package them in presterilized containers and store at 0° C for up to 6 to 12 months. Radiograph them so you will have a record of bone sizes available in the bank. Before use, culture one of the harvested bones to check sterility of the harvesting technique. Alternatively, cleanly harvest cortical bones and double-wrap them in semipermeable packaging material. Sterilize them with ethylene oxide. Following sterilization, aerate the bones to eliminate toxic residues and store at 0° C for up to 6 to 12 months.

With the advent of biologic fracture-repair techniques (see p. 757) that incorporate fragments into comminuted fractures, cortical bone allografts are now more commonly used for limb-sparing procedures than for fracture repair. The principles of using cortical bone allografts are similar, regardless of their intended purpose. Plate and screw fixation is needed to ensure stability of host-graft interfaces for prolonged periods while fractures heal and grafts remodel. Therefore adequate host bone must be present to allow placement of three bone screws proximal and distal to grafts. Radiographs of the contralateral matching bone are used to determine graft size and length, and to serve as a model for precontouring plates. The required graft length is determined by measuring the lengths of intact segments of fractured bone on a lateral radiograph and subtracting this measurement from the length of the contralateral bone (Fig. 28-71).

Adherence to aseptic technique is essential for successful cortical allograft use. *Prepare the affected limb and cancellous bone autograft site for aseptic surgery. Approach the fracture, remove fragments, and resect bone segments proximally and distally to uninjured bone. Use an oscillating bone saw to cut the bones perpendicular to their long*

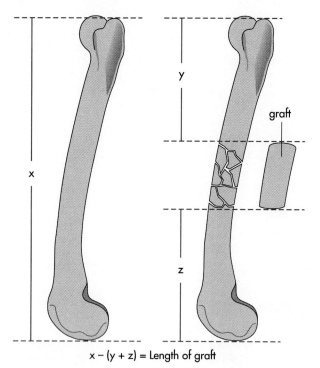

FIG. 28-71
To determine the proper length for the cortical allograft, measure the length of the normal bone from a lateral radiograph (*x*). Measure the length of the intact proximal and distal segments of the fractured bone from a lateral radiograph (*y* and *z*). Use the formula $x - (y + z)$ to determine graft length.

axes. Cut the graft to an appropriate length in a similar manner (i.e., perpendicular to its long axis) in order to allow 360-degree contact of graft and host bone. Determine the appropriate number and length of cortical bone screws for the graft length and secure the graft to the center of the precontoured plate. Place the graft-plate composite in the fracture gap and reduce bone segments to the plate. Secure the plate to host bone segments using cortical bone screws. To achieve compression of host-graft interfaces, insert those screws that are immediately proximal and distal to the graft into the host bone in a loaded fashion. Insert the remaining screws in a neutral position (Fig. 28-72). Flush the fracture with sterile saline. Then harvest a cancellous bone autograft and place it at host-graft interfaces. Obtain samples for microbiologic culture and close the skin and subcutaneous tissues routinely. Document allograft and metal implant positioning with postoperative radiographs.

Fracture healing with cortical allografts or alloimplants consists of filling host-graft interfaces with bone, followed by graft vascularization, graft resorption, and graft replacement with host bone (Fig. 28-73). Host-graft interfaces heal within 1 to 3 months; however, graft remodeling takes months to years (depending on graft length) and may never be completed. The process of remodeling can be monitored radiographically. Host-graft interfaces initially fill with the cancellous bone. As resorption and remodeling proceed from host-graft interfaces toward the graft center, grafts change from cortical structures to porous, cancellous bone. Eventually the cancellous bone remodels into cortical bone. It is often difficult to determine when plate removal should be done based on radiographic appearances because the amount of graft that has been remodeled may be difficult to ascertain. Because premature plate removal may predispose

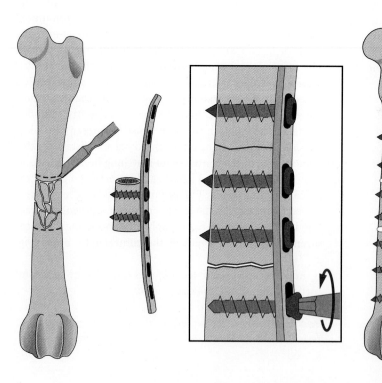

FIG. 28-72
To stabilize a cortical bone allograft, cut the bone segments perpendicular to the long axis of the bone and remove the fragments. Secure the graft to a precontoured plate. Reduce the graft plate segment into the fracture and compress the host-graft interfaces by loading the screws above and below the interfaces. Add cancellous bone autograft around the host-graft interfaces.

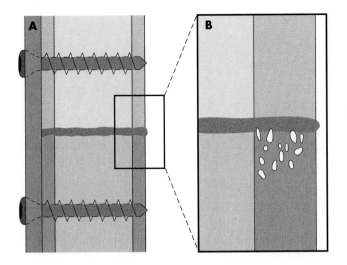

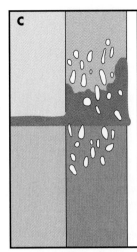

FIG. 28-73
During incorporation of cortical allografts or alloimplants into a healing fracture, **A,** the host-graft interface is stabilized, and, **B,** is filled with fibrous bone while bone remodeling units become active. **C,** The graft is vascularized and portions of it resorb and are replaced with host bone.

grafts to fracture, plate removal should not be done until definitive radiographic evidence of remodeling of the entire graft is noted. Generally, unless complications occur, plate removal is not recommended.

Complications associated with cortical allografts include infection, graft rejection, failure of fracture repair, and graft fracture. Graft infection usually results from graft or fracture site contamination, coupled with instability. This results in a large, sequestered piece of foreign material that must be debrided when fracture stabilization is performed. Cancellous bone autografts may be used to fill resultant fracture gaps. Signs of graft rejection (i.e., failure of graft and host bone to unite, graft resorption without replacement) are rarely noted clinically. Plate fracture may be observed when reduction and fixation of host-graft interfaces provide inadequate reconstruction of the bone column. Grafts may also fracture after plate removal.

Suggested Reading

Hanson PD, Markel MD: Bone and cartilage transplantation, *Vet Comp Ortho Trauma* 5:163, 1992.

Johnson AL: Principles of bone grafting, *Sem Vet Med Surg (Small Anim)* 6:90, 1991.

CHAPTER 29

Management of Specific Fractures

MAXILLARY AND MANDIBULAR FRACTURES

DEFINITIONS

Maxillary and **mandibular fractures** may occur secondary to trauma, severe periodontitis, or neoplasia. **Periodontitis** is an inflammatory reaction of the tissues surrounding a tooth that usually results from the extension of gingival inflammation into the periodontium.

GENERAL CONSIDERATIONS AND CLINICALLY RELEVANT PATHOPHYSIOLOGY

Maxillary and mandibular fractures are usually caused by head trauma and concurrent injuries (i.e., upper airway obstruction, central nervous system trauma, pneumothorax, pulmonary contusions, and/or traumatic myocarditis) are often present. These abnormalities may be acutely life-threatening and require prompt diagnosis and treatment. Definitive fracture repair must often be delayed until the animal has been appropriately stabilized. Mandibular fractures occasionally occur as a result of bone loss associated with severe periodontitis. Teeth extraction should be performed with care in older patients with severe periodontitis to avoid this complication. With severe periodontitis, bone healing may be impaired. Diseased teeth must be extracted prior to fracture stabilization in these patients. Pathologic fractures may also occur secondary to mandibular neoplasia (see p. 220). Histopathologic examination of bone from animals with mandibular fractures is warranted, unless fractures are clearly due to trauma. Mandibular fractures associated with neoplasia are treated by mandibulectomy, rather than definitive fracture repair (see p. 204).

The teeth occupy a large portion of the mandible and are integral components of normal mandibular structure (Fig. 29-1). Teeth involved in fractures should not be removed unless they are loose. This is especially important with fractures involving the caudal mandibular body because the large premolar and molar teeth occupy a substantial portion of this bone and are essential contributors to fracture stability. Periodic evaluation of these teeth for evidence of infection or loosening is necessary postoperatively to determine whether irreversible damage has occurred that requires endodontic therapy or extraction. The anatomy and location of tooth roots must be considered when implants are applied to the mandible. Damage to tooth roots from pins, wires, drill bits and screws may cause sufficient damage that extraction becomes necessary after fracture healing.

DIAGNOSIS
Clinical Presentation

Signalment. Traumatic mandibular or maxillary fractures may occur in any age dog; however, young dogs are at greater risk. Pathologic fractures of the mandible are particularly common in geriatric small and toy breed dogs (i.e., poodles) that have not had regular dental prophylaxis and are fed soft food and/or table scraps.

History. There is usually a history of trauma (e.g., being hit by a car or kicked by a horse) in animals with traumatic oral fractures. Mandibular symphyseal fractures and fractures of the hard palate may occur in cats that fall from great heights ("high-rise syndrome"). Tooth extraction may be associated with pathologic fractures of dogs with severe periodontitis.

Physical Examination Findings

Animals with mandibular fractures may drool excessively, exhibit pain on opening of the mouth, and are often reluctant to eat. Saliva may be blood tinged; however, profuse bleeding is uncommon. Crepitation and instability can often be palpated during careful oral examination; however, thorough inspection of these structures for mucosal wounds and crepitation often requires general anesthesia. Mandibular symphyseal fractures allow one hemimandible to be moved separately from the other. Less instability is usually present with maxillary fractures than mandibular fractures. The teeth should be examined carefully for evidence of trauma. Fractures associated with marked bony lysis or proliferation should be biopsied.

FIG. 29-1
Skull anatomy. Note that the tooth roots occupy a large portion of the mandible. Normal relationship of the maxillary and mandibular dental arcades are illustrated.

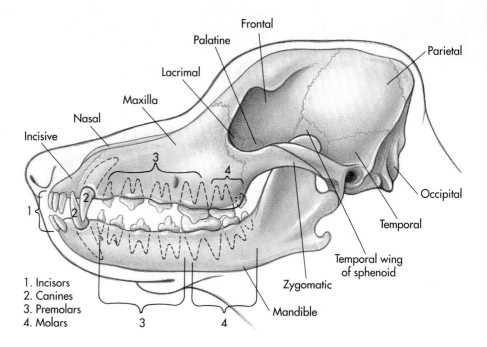

1. Incisors
2. Canines
3. Premolars
4. Molars

☞ **N O T E** · Teeth fractured above the gumline are treated with endodontic therapy. Teeth fractured below the gumline should be extracted.

Radiography

Radiographs of the mandible and maxilla generally require that animals be anesthetized or heavily sedated. Thorough radiographic examination of the skull usually requires five radiographic views (i.e., dorsoventral, lateral, right and left oblique, and intraoral projections). Because skull radiographs are often difficult to interpret due to the presence of multiple, overlying structures, comparison with a normal skull is often helpful. Symmetry between the two sides should be assessed. Computed tomography can help identify fractures in the caudal mandibular body, vertical ramus, and mandibular condyle which may be difficult to detect radiographically.

Laboratory Findings

Specific laboratory abnormalities are not present with mandibular or maxillary fractures due to any cause. Traumatized animals should have sufficient blood work done to determine if contraindications to anesthesia exist.

DIFFERENTIAL DIAGNOSIS

Animals presenting with mandibular or maxillary fractures should be evaluated to determine whether fractures are the result of trauma or underlying pathology (i.e., periodontitis, neoplasia, or metabolic disease; see above).

MEDICAL OR CONSERVATIVE MANAGEMENT

A tape muzzle may be applied to support the mandible if there is minimal displacement of fracture fragments (usually fractures of the ramus) and dental occlusion is adequate and if the fracture-assessment score is favorable and dictates early union. A muzzle can be made from two pieces of tape placed with the sticky sides together and fashioned into a circle that fits over the dog's nose. A similarly made piece of tape extends from the circle around the head and behind the ears. The muzzle should allow the dog to open its mouth enough to lap water and eat gruel. To allow adequate healing, muzzles should remain in place 6 weeks. Dogs with mandibular plus maxillary fractures may not tolerate tape muzzles because the muzzle may pressure the maxillary fracture. Because of the cat's short nose, tape muzzles are difficult to apply and maintain. Similarly, it may be difficult to maintain a tape muzzle in brachycephalic breeds.

SURGICAL TREATMENT

The appropriate method of treating mandibular and maxillary fractures is determined based on fracture-assessment score (see p. 730) and fracture location. Conservative treatment with a tape muzzle may be appropriate for some fractures (see above). Fixation systems applicable for mandibular fractures are orthopedic wire plus Kirschner wires, plates and screws, and external fixators (both standard and acrylic frames). Many maxillary fractures are nondisplaced and require only conservative therapy; however, segmental maxillary fractures or depressed fracture lines may require repositioning and stabilization. Mandibular or maxillary fractures that alter normal occlusion should be reduced and stabilized. Many animals learn to compensate for malocclusion; however, temporomandibular arthritis, impaired mastication, abnormal tooth wear, plaque and tartar accumulation, and periodontitis are possible sequelae. Mild malocclusion with interference of teeth can be treated by remodeling the teeth involved to allow clearance. Maxillary fractures that result in nasal malpositioning or instability should be reduced and stabilized. Interfragmentary wires are most often used to sta-

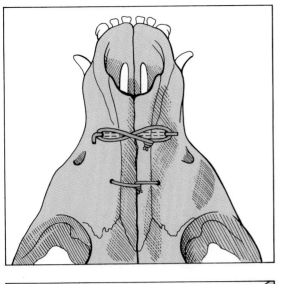

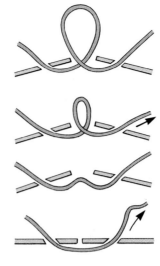

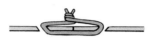

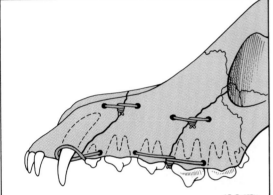

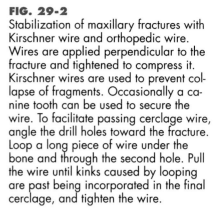

FIG. 29-2
Stabilization of maxillary fractures with Kirschner wire and orthopedic wire. Wires are applied perpendicular to the fracture and tightened to compress it. Kirschner wires are used to prevent collapse of fragments. Occasionally a canine tooth can be used to secure the wire. To facilitate passing cerclage wire, angle the drill holes toward the fracture. Loop a long piece of wire under the bone and through the second hole. Pull the wire until kinks caused by looping are past being incorporated in the final cerclage, and tighten the wire.

bilize maxillary fractures (Fig. 29-2); Kirschner wires are incorporated into many of these maxillary fixation techniques.

Application of Interdental Wires

Interdental wires are placed around teeth adjacent to fracture lines. The wires must be positioned securely in the bone around the tooth's neck to prevent them from sliding off the crown. They are placed through guide holes that are drilled between the teeth and through the superficial cortical bone surface. The wire is passed through the guide holes, circling the teeth, and tightened. The ends of the wire should be bent into the mucosa (Fig. 29-3).

Application of Interfragmentary Wires

Interfragmentary wires are ideal for stabilizing relatively simple, reconstructible mandibular and maxillary fractures. Large-gauge wire (18 to 22 gauge), properly applied, provides adequate fracture support (Table 29-1); however, wires may be difficult to position and tighten unless certain application guidelines are followed. Use the largest gauge wire that can be manipulated. Kirschner wire is used to place drill holes in the bone, 5 to 10 mm from the fracture line (Fig. 29-4, *A*). These holes should be positioned so that the wire will be perpendicular to the fracture line when it is tightened. The drill holes

TABLE 29-1

Comparable Wire Sizes

Gauge	Mm	Inches
	1.25	.049
18	1.00	.040
20	0.80	.035
		.032
		.030
22	0.60	.028
24		.020

should be sloped toward the fracture line because this results in obtuse angles on the bone side opposite to where the wire knot will be tightened. This positioning allows the wire to slide into position easily and enhances tightening efforts. Long segments of wire should be used to facilitate wire passage and allow manipulation of any wire kinks away from the area of wire that is to be tightened (Fig. 29-4, *B*). The wire may be tightened using either a twist knot or a tension loop (see p. 745). It

FIG. 29-3
Interdental wires are placed through holes drilled in the maxillary or mandibular bone to prevent the wire from slipping.

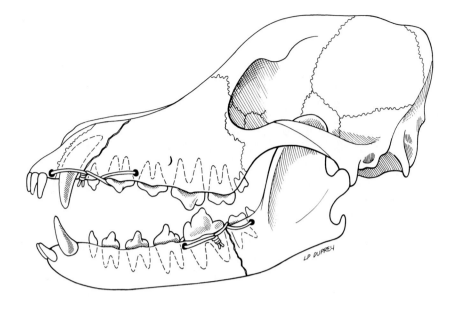

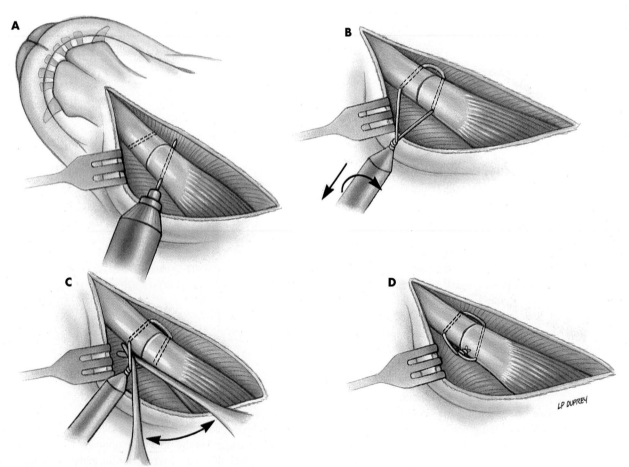

FIG. 29-4
A, To place an interfragmentary wire on the mandible, angle the drill holes toward the fracture. **B,** Place the wire and begin the twist while placing traction on the wire. **C,** To ensure that the wire is in contact with the far cortex, place a forceps between the twist and the near cortex and lever the wire away from the near cortex. **D,** Finish tightening the wire, cut the twist, and bend it into the bone.

should be twisted in such a manner that even tension is applied to both strands. A periosteal elevator or large tissue forceps may be used to lever the orthopedic wire under the twist and eliminate slack (Fig. 29-4, *C*). When the wire is tightened, it should be bent perpendicular to the wire surface and away from the gingival margin. The wire is cut and the ends twisted and bent into the bone surface (Fig. 29-4, *D*).

Optimally, wires should be located near the oral margin to neutralize forces that tend to disrupt fractures. Because this margin also contains the teeth, care must be used to position drill holes between teeth or tooth roots. When multiple wires are used, all holes are drilled and wires positioned prior to any wires being tightened. Wires are tightened beginning at the caudal fracture line and working toward the symphysis. If bending or slippage is encountered with oblique or transverse fractures, Kirschner wires with figure-eight–patterned orthopedic wire may be used. The Kirschner wire helps prevent sliding or bending while the orthopedic wire is tightened.

Application of Bone Plates and Screws

Bone plates can be used to stabilize simple or complex mandibular fractures (see p. 747). Plates are applied to the ventrolateral mandibular surface. Care must be taken to correctly contour the plate because the mandible aligns with the plate as the screws are tightened; malalignment results in malocclusion. Screws must be positioned to avoid tooth roots (Fig. 29-5).

Application of External Skeletal Fixators

Kirschner fixators. Kirschner external fixators (see p. 735) can be used to stabilize mandibular body fractures if there is sufficient bone to hold fixation pins. Fixation pins

are placed percutaneously through the mandibular body, avoiding tooth roots. Type I fixators are applied to the ventrolateral mandibular surface with at least two pins inserted on either side of the fracture line. Positive profile end-threaded pins should be used to increase the fixator's holding power. For bilateral mandibular body fractures, a Type II fixator may be constructed using bilateral and unilateral fixation pins. A connecting bar is placed on either side of the dog's jaw (Fig. 29-6).

Acrylic fixators. Dental acrylic, used to replace clamps and connecting bars, is a versatile rigid fixation for mandibular fractures, especially severely comminuted fractures. After pins have been placed in appropriate locations in the mandible (use fixation pins of appropriate size for the bone, located in different places), the ends are bent parallel to the skin (Fig. 29-7, *A*). The animal's mouth should be closed to evaluate dental occlusion and reduce fractures. If necessary, Kirschner clamps and a connecting bar may be placed to temporarily hold the fracture in reduction while the acrylic is being mixed and molded (Fig. 29-7, *B*). Soft tissues should be protected by laying wet sponges beneath the pins. After the acrylic is mixed it is molded over the bent pins to form a connecting bar (Fig. 29-7, *C*). Alternatively, plastic tubing may be impaled over the pins (do not bend them) and used as a mold for the liquid phase acrylic. The acrylic splint can be curved around the rostral portion of the mandible.

☞ **N O T E** · Acrylic bars are versatile because they can accommodate various sizes of fixation pins placed in multiple planes.

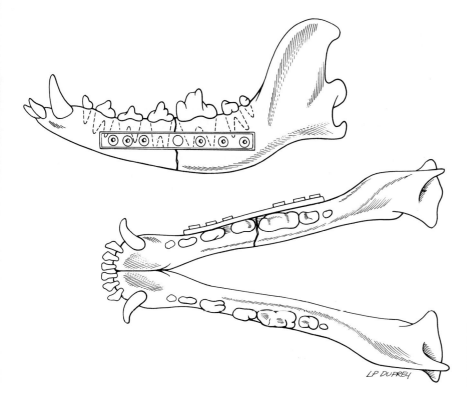

FIG. 29-5
Compression plates are applied to the lateral mandibular surface to stabilize transverse fractures. Avoid penetrating the tooth roots with screws.

LP DUPREY

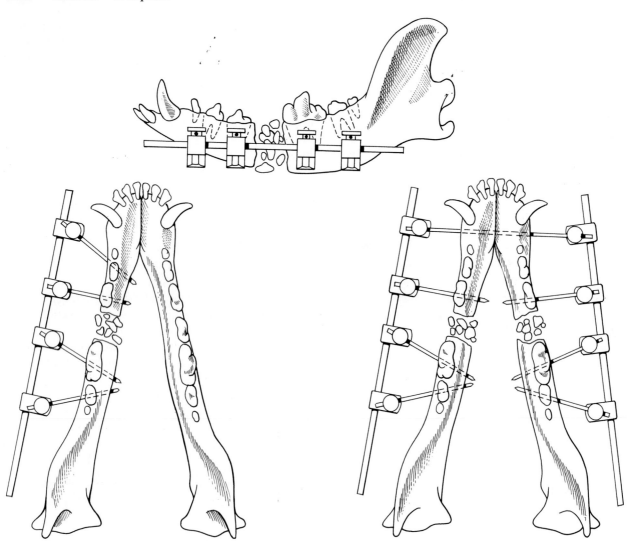

FIG. 29-6
When placing a Type I or Type II external fixator to stabilize comminuted mandibular fractures, use positive-profile end-threaded pins if the fracture-assessment score indicates prolonged healing. Avoid penetrating tooth roots with fixation pins.

Animals with mandibular fractures that have high (8-10) fracture-assessment scores (i.e., simple fractures in young animals; see p. 733) may be treated with tape muzzles, interdental wiring, or interfragmentary wiring techniques depending on fracture location. Interfragmentary wire is usually sufficient to stabilize simple, bilateral, mandibular fractures if they can be anatomically reconstructed and fracture-assessment scores indicate rapid healing (Table 29-2). If fracture-assessment scores are between 4 and 7 (e.g., larger or older dogs with longer healing times) and bilateral fractures are present that can be anatomically reconstructed, interfragmentary wires, external fixation, or bone plates and screws may be used for fracture fixation. A cancellous bone autograft can be used to promote rapid bone union in these patients.

If fracture-assessment scores are low (0-3) and/or comminution, bone loss, or severe soft tissue damage are present, fractures are best treated with closed reduction and external fixator application. Mandibular alignment is determined by observing dental occlusion. Whenever there is potential for healing times to be prolonged, external fixators should be constructed using several positive-profile threaded pins (see p. 735). Plate-and-screw fixation can be used to stabilize mandibular fractures with cortical bone loss; however, the plate must be carefully contoured to the fractured bone. If open reduction is performed in patients with low fracture-assessment scores, autogenous cancellous bone grafts should be used to facilitate healing. Dogs with severely comminuted fractures of the vertical ramus are best treated with a tape muzzle, relying on the heavy masseter muscle to maintain fragment alignment. In some cases, interarcade wiring (mandibular-maxillary wires) can be used to maintain mandibular and maxillary alignment. Although interarcade wiring is well tolerated by most cats, dogs may be more difficult to manage postoperatively.

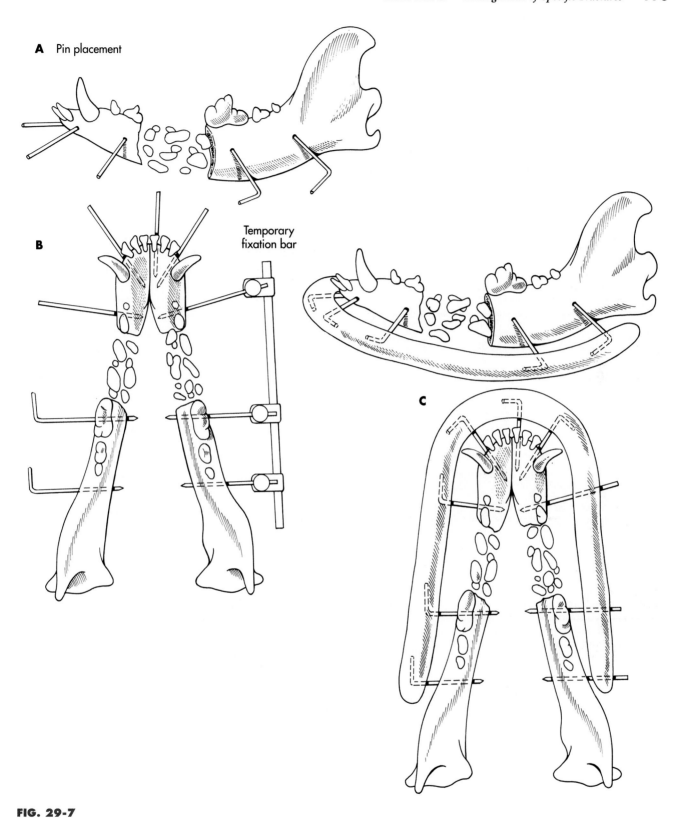

A Pin placement

B

Temporary
fixation bar

C

FIG. 29-7
An acrylic splint may be used to accommodate fixation pins of various sizes, placed
in multiple planes. **A,** Place the fixation pins where there is adequate bone. Use positive-
profile end-threaded pins when the fracture-assessment score indicates prolonged healing.
B, Use a temporary fixation bar to maintain mandibular alignment. **C,** Bend the fixation
pins and apply the acrylic over them while it has a doughy consistency.

Preoperative Management

After the status of the animal has been determined, mandibular fractures in most dogs may be gently reduced and temporarily held in position with a tape muzzle until a definitive stabilizing procedure can be performed. However, mandibular fractures in cats and brachycephalic dogs cannot be easily stabilized with tape muzzles and are often not treated until surgery. Because the oral cavity contains numerous bacteria, prophylactic antibiotics are recommended. Infections are rare, however, because the vasculature supplying this area is well developed and plentiful. If infection is likely and open reduction is performed, bacterial cultures can be submitted during surgery.

TABLE 29-2

Implant Use According to Fracture-Assessment Score (FAS)

FAS 0 to 3
- Closed reduction and external fixator application
- Plate-and-screw fixation
- Tape muzzle for vertical ramus

FAS 4 to 7
- Interfragmentary wires
- Bone plates and screws
- External skeletal fixation

FAS 8 to 10
- Tape muzzle
- Interdental wiring
- Interfragmentary wiring
- Cerclage wires (symphyseal fractures)

Anesthesia

Anatomic reconstruction or realignment of mandibular cortices is mandatory in order to provide proper dental occlusion in many patients. Simple mandibular fractures can be anatomically reconstructed using bone cortex as a guide. However, with complex fractures or those where cortical bone loss has occurred, dental occlusion must be used to guide mandibular realignment. Because mandibular and maxillary teeth closely interdigitate, precise alignment of upper and lower arcades is necessary. If precise dental occlusion cannot be determined with the endotracheal tube in place, it should be repositioned through a pharyngotomy incision (Fig. 29-8). This allows the mouth to be completely closed during surgery which facilitates determination of adequate dental occlusion. After surgery the endotracheal tube is removed and the pharyngotomy incision is allowed to granulate closed.

Surgical Anatomy

The bones of the maxilla and mandibular body are easily palpated and surgically approached through skin and subcutaneous tissue (Fig. 29-9). The maxillary nerve (branch of the trigeminal nerve that innervates cutaneous muscles of the head, nasal and oral cavities, and muscles of mastication) passes rostrally through the alar canal and can be injured with maxillary fractures. The mandibular alveolar nerve, which is sensory to the teeth of the mandible, passes through the mandibular canal along with the mandibular alveolar artery. These structures are frequently damaged with mandibular fractures, although clinical signs are seldom evident. Tooth roots must be avoided when placing implants in the maxilla or mandible. The approach to the ramus and temporomandibular joint involves dissection and elevation of

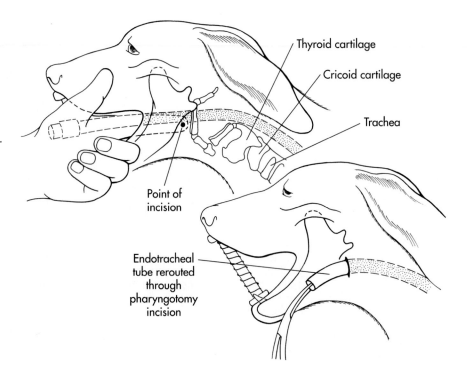

FIG. 29-8
To place an endotracheal tube via a pharyngotomy incision, insert an index finger into the oral cavity and locate the pharyngeal area immediately cranial to the hyoid bones. Incise skin, subcutaneous tissues, and mucous membrane to create a passage for the endotracheal tube. Place a forceps through the surgically created passage to grasp the endotracheal tube (with connector removed) and reroute it.

Thyroid cartilage

Cricoid cartilage

Trachea

Point of incision

Endotracheal tube rerouted through pharyngotomy incision

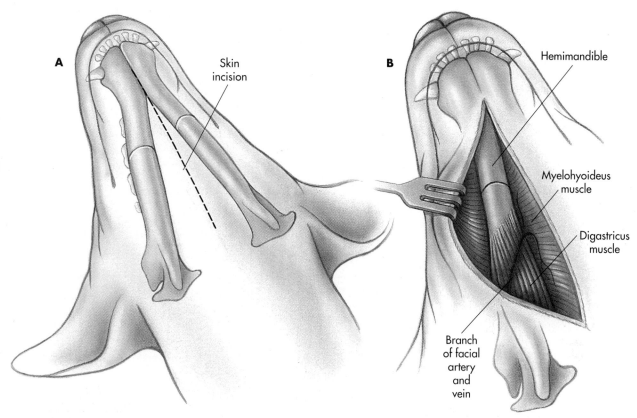

FIG. 29-9
A, For a ventral approach to the mandible, make a ventral midline incision in the skin be-tween the mandibles. **B,** Elevate soft tissues from the mandibles to expose the fracture(s), but maintain the digastricus muscle attachment.

the masseter muscle (Fig. 29-10). The parotid duct and gland and facial nerve are dorsal and superficial to the masseter muscle, and should be avoided.

> ☞ **N O T E** · The shape of the mandibular canal and the presence of major vessels and nerves preclude intramedullary (IM) pin fixation of mandibular fractures.

Positioning

Animals are positioned in ventral recumbency for treatment of maxillary fractures and dorsal recumbency for treatment of mandibular fractures. If an autogenous cancellous bone graft is required, animals may be positioned in dorsal recum-bency with forelimbs tied caudally. The skin over the proxi-mal humerus is prepared for aseptic surgery. This position-ing allows simultaneous access to the proximal humeral metaphysis and oral cavity. Because this is an uncommon limb position for obtaining a bone graft, care must be taken to orient oneself prior to the procedure.

SURGICAL TECHNIQUES
Open Reduction of Mandibular Fractures

With bilateral mandibular fractures, make a ventral midline incision in the skin between the mandibles. Move this inci-sion in either direction to expose both mandibles. If only one mandible is involved, make a ventral skin incision di-rectly over that mandible. Elevate soft tissues from the mandibles to expose the fracture(s). Maintain the digastri-cus muscle attachment (see Fig. 29-9). Reduce and stabi-lize the fracture (see below). If there is a segmental fracture of the mandibular body, stabilize the caudal fracture first. Because there is little musculature around the mandibular body, reduction is usually easily accomplished. Open reduc-tion of the mandibular cortex will realign the teeth. *Evaluate the oral cavity for open wounds. If large wounds are pre-sent, close the mucosa partially to decrease their size. Do not completely close contaminated wounds so that postop-erative drainage may be allowed. Place a Penrose drain if infection is present or likely.*

Open Reduction of Fractures of the Vertical Ramus and Temporomandibular Joint

Make a skin incision over the ventrolateral border of the caudal mandibular body and separate the platysma mus-cle to expose the digastricus muscle. Elevate the masseter muscle from the ramus to expose its lateral mandibular surface and angular and coronoid processes (see Fig. 29-10). Reduce the fracture and stabilize it (see below). Repair large, open wounds of the oral cavity as de-scribed above.

FIG. 29-10
A, For a lateral approach to the ramus of the mandible, make a skin incision over the ventrolateral border of the caudal mandibular body and separate the platysma muscle to expose the masseter muscle. **B** and **C,** Incise and elevate the masseter muscle from the ramus to expose its lateral mandibular surface and angular and coronoid processes.

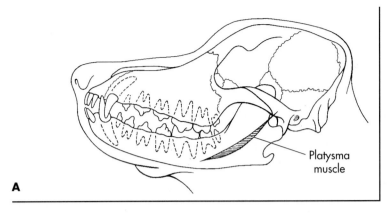

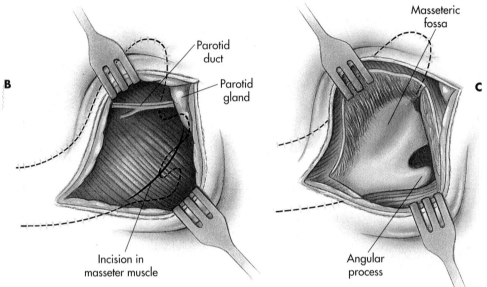

Open Reduction of Maxillary Fractures

Make a skin incision over the fracture(s) and gently elevate the soft tissues from the bone. Reduce the fracture and stabilize it. Repair large, open wounds to the oral cavity as described above.

Stabilization of Mandibular Symphyseal Fractures

Symphyseal fractures are best treated with cerclage wire. A single wire is effective treatment for symphyseal fractures. Symphyseal cerclage wires encircle the mandible caudal to the canine teeth. The wire can be removed once the fracture has healed (generally 6 to 8 weeks) by cutting it with wire scissors where it is exposed behind the canine teeth.

Make a small nick in the skin overlying the ventral aspect of the symphysis. Insert a 16- or 18-gauge hypodermic needle through this nick and along one lateral mandibular surface (under the subcutaneous tissues). Exit the needle in the oral cavity caudal to the canine tooth and thread an 18- or 20-gauge wire through the needle. Reposition the needle on the opposite side of the mandible and curve the wire across and behind the canine teeth and reinsert it through the hypodermic needle. Exit the wire from the skin incision

at the original insertion point. Once the fracture is reduced, tighten the wire. Leave the ends of the wire exposed through the skin incision and bend them to decrease the possibility of injury to the owner (Fig. 29-11).

Stabilization of Mandibular Transverse Fractures

Transverse fractures should be realigned and compressed. One or two interfragmentary wires applied perpendicular to the fracture line will result in compression (Fig. 29-12, A-C). Alternatively, if the patient's fracture warrants more rigid fixation, an external fixator or compression bone plate can be used.

Stabilization of Oblique Fracture Lines

Oblique fractures may override when parallel wires are tightened so that alternative wire patterns may be required. Caudal-to-rostral oblique fracture lines can be stabilized with two wires placed at right angles to each other. More than one wire may be placed through a single drill hole. Medial-to-lateral oblique fracture lines should be stabilized with two wires placed perpendicular to each other in two perpendicular planes. In both cases the second wire prevents overriding of the fracture as the wires

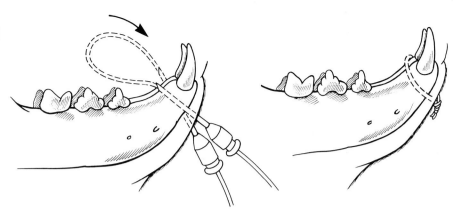

FIG. 29-11
To stabilize mandibular symphyseal fractures, use a 16- or 18-gauge hypodermic needle to place the cerclage wire.

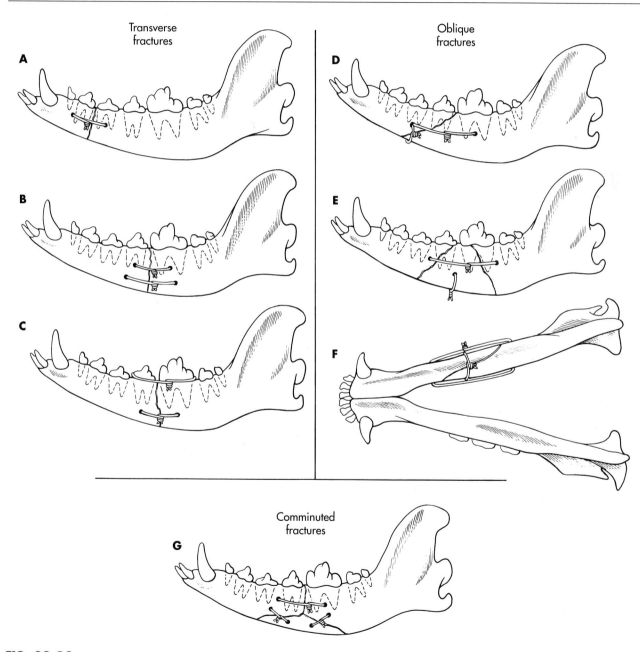

Transverse fractures

Oblique fractures

Comminuted fractures

FIG. 29-12
Interfragmentary wire may be used to stabilize mandibular fractures. **A-C,** For transverse fractures, wires may be placed perpendicular to the fracture line. **D,** Stabilize caudal to rostral, long, oblique fracture lines with two wires placed at right angles to each other. The wire around the ventral mandibular border prevents the caudal segment from displacing rostrally when the interfragmentary wire is tightened. **E** and **F,** To stabilize long, oblique, slab fractures, place wire through both bone segments and around the ventral mandibular border to prevent overriding of bone segments. **G,** Secure large butterfly fragments with interfragmentary wires.

are tightened (Fig. 29-12, *D-F*). Butterfly fragments can be incorporated into the fixation if they are large and relatively stable (Fig. 29-12, *G*).

Stabilization of Comminuted Fractures

Comminuted fractures that have long fracture lines and can be anatomically reconstructed can be stabilized with interfragmentary wires. Comminuted fractures that cannot be reconstructed can be bridged with a bone plate or external fixator. Careful attention must be paid to ensure dental occlusion is appropriate (see discussion on application of plates and acrylic fixators on p. 771).

SUTURE MATERIALS/SPECIAL INSTRUMENTS

A low-rpm power drill is helpful for placing fixation pins. A pin chuck or power drill is used to drill holes in the bone for wires and to place Kirschner wires. Polymethylmethacrylate or dental acrylic may be used to form the acrylic splint. Bone plating equipment is needed for plates.

POSTOPERATIVE CARE AND ASSESSMENT

Postoperative radiographs should be evaluated for implant position. Occlusion of the teeth, however, takes precedence over accurate fragment reduction. Dental occlusion is more readily determined on physical examination than with radiographs. Occasionally a tape muzzle can be used postoperatively to support the fixation. When muzzles are used (either as a primary fixation or support for internal fixation), the skin on the ventral surface of the mandible may become irritated. If this occurs, the skin should be carefully cleaned and treated with a soothing ointment. External fixators should be evaluated postoperatively to ensure that the clamps or acrylic is not too close to the skin. The animal should be fed soft food until the fracture heals—chew toys should be avoided. Owners should be instructed not to allow the animal to chew on rocks or sticks or play tug-of-war. Clients should be instructed to clean the skin beneath a tape muzzle daily and to clean the area around external fixation pins. The animal should be reevaluated 10 days postoperatively and sutures removed. Radiographs should be obtained after 6 weeks to evaluate healing and they should be repeated every 6 weeks thereafter until healing is complete. Intraoral wires, external fixators, and plates should be removed when fractures are healed; interfragmentary wires are not removed unless they cause problems.

PROGNOSIS

The prognosis for healing of mandibular and maxillary fractures is generally excellent if proper techniques of fracture management are observed. Osteomyelitis (see p. 1027) and bone sequestration should be treated by sequestrectomy, removal of loose implants, mandibular stabilization (if necessary), cancellous bone autografts, culture/sensitivity, and appropriate antibiotics. Nonunions are treated with appropriate stabilization and cancellous bone autografts. Partial

mandibulectomy (see p. 204) is an option for treatment of chronic nonunion of the mandible.

☞ **NOTE ·** Mandibular and maxillary fractures generally heal without a large callus.

Suggested Reading

Davidson JR, Bauer MS: Fractures of the mandible and maxilla, *Vet Clin of N Am (Small Anim)* 22:109, 1992.

Lewis DD et al: Maxillary-mandibular wiring for the management of caudal mandibular fractures in two cats, *J Small Anim Pract* 32: 253, 1991.

Lantz GC, Salisbury SK: Partial mandibulectomy for treatment of mandibular fractures in dogs: eight cases (1981–1984), *J Am Vet Med Assoc* 191:243, 1987.

Manfra-Marretta S, Schrader SC, Matthiesen DT: Problems associated with the management and treatment of jaw fractures, *Prob Vet Med* 2:220, 1990.

Roush JK, Wilson JW: Healing of mandibular body osteotomies after plate and intramedullary pin fixation, *Vet Surg* 18:190, 1989.

Rudy RL, Boudrieau RJ: Maxillofacial and mandibular fractures, *Sem Vet Med Surg (Small Anim)* 7:3, 1992.

Umphlet RC, Johnson AL: Mandibular fractures of the dog: a retrospective study of 157 fractures, *Vet Surg* 19:272, 1990.

Umphlet RC, Johnson AL: Mandibular fractures of the cat: a retrospective study, *Vet Surg* 17:333, 1988.

SCAPULAR FRACTURES

DEFINITIONS

Scapular fractures may occur through the body, spine, acromion, neck, supraglenoid tubercle, and/or glenoid cavity.

GENERAL CONSIDERATIONS AND CLINICALLY RELEVANT PATHOPHYSIOLOGY

Scapular fractures are relatively uncommon in dogs and cats because the large muscles surrounding the scapula protect it from direct injury. Common concurrent injuries include pulmonary contusions, pneumothorax, rib fractures, traumatic cardiomyopathy, and nerve injury (i.e., suprascapular nerve). Thus, cardiorespiratory parameters and neurologic function of the limb should be determined preoperatively in animals presenting with scapular fractures.

Scapular fractures are classified according to location (e.g., body, spine, acromion, neck, supraglenoid tubercle, glenoid cavity). Scapular body and spine fractures are frequently minimally displaced and require only conservative therapy. However, transverse fractures of the scapular body and spine may allow the scapula to fold on itself, resulting in a poor cosmetic appearance if the fractures are not reduced and stabilized. Avulsions of the supraglenoid tuberosity occur in immature dogs and are physeal separations. Fractures of the scapular neck and glenoid cavity may affect scapulohumeral joint function and thus should be anatomically reduced and stabilized with internal fixation methods.

DIAGNOSIS
Clinical Presentation

Signalment. Traumatic scapular fractures may occur in any age animal; however, young animals are at increased risk.

History. Affected animals usually have a history of trauma.

Physical Examination Findings

Most affected animals present with a non–weight-bearing lameness. Swelling may occur over the scapula and crepitation may be obvious when this region is palpated.

Radiographs

Radiographs of the scapula should include lateral and caudal-cranial views. To avoid superimposing scapulae, the contralateral forelimb should be extended during the lateral projection. A distal-proximal or axial projection provides a skyline view of the scapular spine and cranial and caudal scapular borders. Because of the manipulation necessary for diagnostic radiographs, some animals may require sedation.

Laboratory Findings

Specific laboratory abnormalities are not present with scapular fractures. Traumatized animals undergoing surgery should have sufficient blood work done to determine the optimal anesthesia regimen.

DIFFERENTIAL DIAGNOSIS

Animals presenting with forelimb lameness attributable to scapular fractures should be carefully evaluated for concurrent nerve damage before surgery. Fractures are generally evident radiographically. Special attention should be given to identifying concurrent thoracic injuries.

MEDICAL OR CONSERVATIVE MANAGEMENT

Conservative treatment with a Velpeau sling (see p. 717) and/or limited exercise is appropriate for most closed, minimally displaced fractures of the scapular body and spine. However, fractures of the articular surface must be treated with open reduction, anatomic alignment, and rigid fixation (see below). Velpeau slings should be left on for 2 to 3 weeks or until there is radiographic evidence that the fracture has bridged with bone.

SURGICAL TREATMENT

Fixation systems applicable for scapular fractures include orthopedic wire, plates and screws, and Kirschner wires. The most appropriate fixation method should be determined based on fracture-assessment score and fracture location.

Application of Orthopedic Wire

Orthopedic wire may be used as interfragmentary wire for fractures of the scapular spine and body (Figs. 29-13 and 29-14) or in conjunction with Kirschner wires as a tension band for avulsions of the supraglenoid tuberosity (Fig. 29-15, *A-B*). Large-gauge wire (18- to 22-gauge) is used for interfragmentary fixation, while smaller gauge (20- to 24-gauge) wire is used in a figure-eight pattern. Large-gauge wire may be difficult to position and tighten unless application guidelines are followed (see p. 745 for principles of interfragmentary wire application).

☞ **NOTE** · Portions of the scapula are thin, and large-gauge wire may pull through when tightened.

Application of Kirschner Wires

Kirschner wires can be used as crossed pins to stabilize transverse fractures of the scapular neck (Fig. 29-16, *A-B*). Multiple Kirschner wires, placed at diverging angles while the fracture lines are held in reduction with reduction forceps, can be used to stabilize moderately comminuted neck and glenoid fractures. Kirschner wires are also used with figure-eight orthopedic wire for tension band fixation of avulsion fractures or repair of acromial osteotomies.

Application of Bone Plates and Screws

Small, semitubular plates can be inverted and used to stabilize fractures of the scapular spine and body (see Fig. 29-13), and small (2.7- and 2.0-mm) angle and T plates can be used to stabilize neck fractures (Fig. 29-16, *C*). With neck fractures, plates are placed under the suprascapular nerve and the nerve must be protected from trauma while the plate is positioned. Cancellous and cortical bone screws can be used as lag screws for stabilizing avulsion fractures of the supraglenoid tuberosity and T fractures of the neck (see Figs. 29-15, *C* and 29-16, *D*).

☞ **NOTE** · Articular fractures are best treated with anatomic reconstruction and lag screw compression.

Preoperative Management

The overall health of the animal should be determined prior to surgery. Thoracic radiography and electrocardiographic analysis are warranted prior to anesthetic induction.

Anesthesia

Refer to p. 708 for anesthetic management of patients with fractures.

Surgical Anatomy

Palpable landmarks are the spine and acromial process of the scapula, and the cranial, dorsal, and caudal borders of the scapula. The body and spine of the scapula are easily approached with dissection and elevation of muscle. The neck of the scapula is surrounded by muscles and tendons

FIG. 29-13
A and **B,** Transverse fractures of the scapular body may cause unsightly folding deformities. **C,** Orthopedic wire may be used to repair these fractures in patients with a high fracture-assessment score. **D** The same fracture in a patient with a low fracture-assessment score may require stabilization with a semitubular plate.

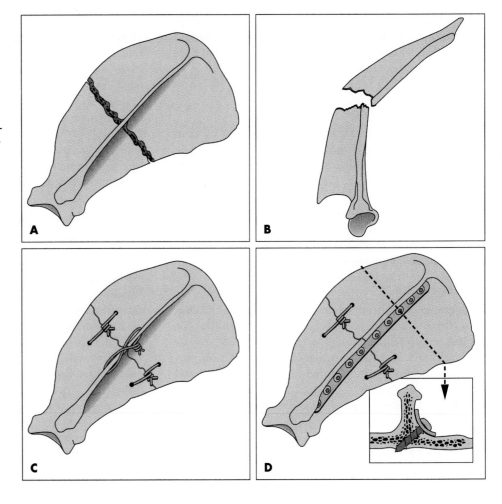

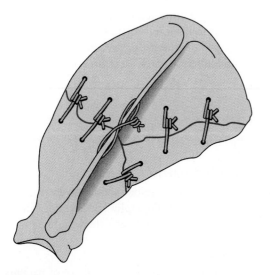

FIG. 29-14
Comminuted fractures of the scapular body can be reconstructed with orthopedic wire in patients with high fracture-assessment scores.

that support the scapulohumeral joint (Fig. 29-17, *A*). Osteotomy of the acromial process allows reflection of a portion of the deltoideus muscle and visualization of the

joint. The suprascapular nerve and artery course over the scapular notch and under the acromial process, and care should be taken to avoid these structures (Fig. 29-17, *B*). The axillary artery and nerve are located immediately caudal to the joint, but are not usually visualized with routine approaches.

Positioning

The animal is placed in lateral recumbency with the affected side up. The entire scapular region should be prepared for aseptic surgery. The most accessible site for a cancellous bone graft is the ipsilateral proximal humerus. If a bone graft is needed (i.e., comminuted fractures with a fracture-assessment score less than 3), the prepped area should encompass the proximal humerus (see p. 760).

SURGICAL TECHNIQUES

Approaches to the scapulohumeral joint are described on pp. 905-907. Excision arthroplasty and shoulder arthrodesis are discussed on pp. 911-913.

Approach to the Scapular Spine and Body

Make a lateral skin incision extending the length of the spine distally to the shoulder joint. Transect the omotransversarius muscle from the spine and reflect it cranially (Fig.

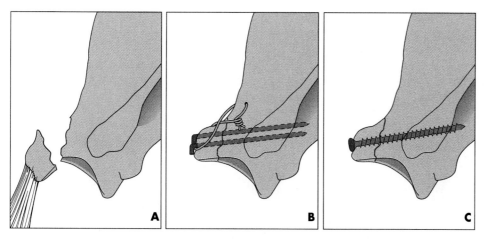

FIG. 29-15
To overcome the pull of the biceps brachii muscle, **A,** avulsions of the supraglenoid tuberosity are treated with **B,** a tension band wire in patients with a high fracture-assessment score or **C,** a lag screw in patients with a low fracture-assessment score.

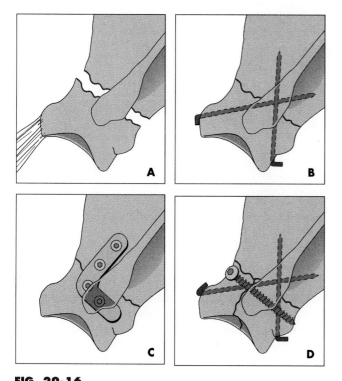

FIG. 29-16
A, Transverse fractures of the scapular neck are best treated with internal fixation. **B,** Crossed Kirschner wires can be used in patients with high fracture-assessment scores; **C,** angle plates may be used in those with low fracture-assessment scores. **D,** Articular fractures must be anatomically reconstructed and stabilized with a lag screw. The T fracture is then stabilized with Kirschner wires (as shown) or a plate.

29-18, A). Incise trapezius and scapular parts of the deltoideus muscles from the spine and reflect them caudally. Incise the supraspinatus and infraspinatus muscular attachments to the spine and elevate these muscles from the scapular body (Fig. 29-18, B).

Approach to the Scapular Neck and Glenoid Cavity

Make a lateral skin incision from the middle portion of the scapular spine and extend it distally to the shoulder joint. Expose the acromion process by incising attachments of the omotransversarius, trapezius, and scapular head of the deltoideus muscles to the scapula. Osteotomize the acromial process and reflect it distally with the acromial head of the deltoideus muscle. Reflect the supraspinatus and infraspinatus muscles away from the scapular spine and neck. Take care to identify and protect the suprascapular nerve. If needed for complete joint exposure, tenotomize the infraspinatus muscle. Incise the joint capsule to observe the articular surface during reduction of fractures involving the glenoid cavity. For additional exposure, osteotomize the greater tubercle of the humerus and reflect the supraspinatus muscle. Close the joint capsule with interrupted sutures of 3-0 absorbable suture material. Reappose the infraspinatus tendon with a tendon suture (i.e., three-loop pulley suture, Bunnell, or locking loop; see p. 1003). and support it with interrupted 0 or 2-0 nonabsorbable sutures. Repair the osteotomies with tension band wire (see Fig. 29-17). Suture deep fascia, subcutaneous tissues, and skin separately.

Stabilization of Scapular Body and Spine Fractures

If the fracture-assessment score (see p. 730) indicates rapid healing (fracture-assessment score of 8 to 10), conservative therapy is indicated for scapular body and spine fractures; however, if these fractures are grossly displaced or result in folding of the body, open reduction and stabilization with interfragmentary wiring may be preferred (see Fig. 29-13). If the fracture assessment score is between 4 and 7 (i.e., older or larger dogs where healing may be delayed) displaced fractures of the scapular body and spine should be treated with open reduction and plate and screw fixation. Fracture-assessment

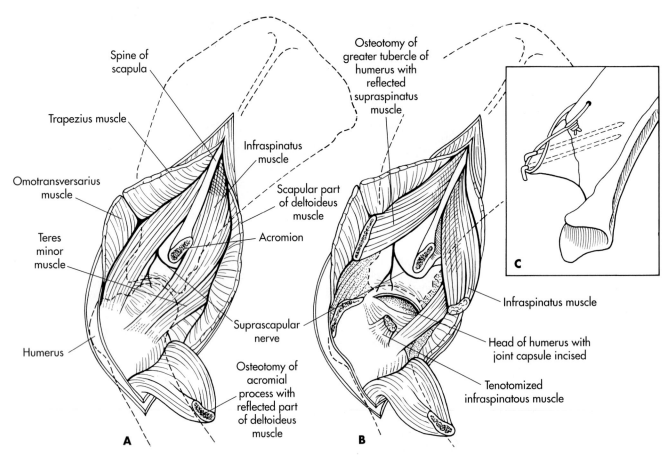

FIG. 29-17
A, For a lateral approach to the scapular neck, make a lateral skin incision from the mid-portion of the scapular spine distally to the shoulder joint. Incise scapular attachments of the omotransversarius, trapezius, and scapular head of the deltoideus muscles. Osteotomize the acromial process and reflect it distally with the acromial head of the deltoideus muscle. **B,** For additional exposure, tenotomize the infraspinatus muscle and if necessary osteotomize the greater tubercle of the humerus. Incise the joint capsule to observe the articular surface during reduction of fractures involving the glenoid cavity. **C,** Repair the osteotomy(s) of the acromial process (and greater tubercle) with a tension band wire.

TABLE 29-3

Implant Use for Fractures of the Scapular Body and Spine According to Fracture-Assessment Score (FAS)

FAS 0 to 3
- Conservative therapy if severe angulation not present
- Bone plate

FAS 4 to 7
- Interfragmentary wires
- Bone plates and screws

FAS 8 to 10
- Conservative therapy
- Open reduction with interfragmentary wiring

---

scores less than 3 indicate prolonged healing. Severely comminuted fractures of the scapular body and spine that cannot be reconstructed should be treated conservatively if severe angulation of the joint is not present (Table 29-3). However, if the animal has multiple limb trauma or must bear weight on the limb, bridging the scapula with a bone plate may be indicated.

Articular fractures must be anatomically reconstructed. Animals with a patient fracture assessment of 8 to 10 may be stabilized with Kirschner wires or a tension band wire, but those with lower patient fracture assessments will benefit from plate or screw fixation (Table 29-4).

Stabilization of Avulsion Fractures of the Supraglenoid Tuberosity and Fractures of the Scapular Neck and Articular Surface

Avulsion fractures of the supraglenoid tuberosity should be treated with open reduction and placement of a lag screw or tension band wire. Simple fractures of the scapular neck and articular surface should undergo open reduction and stabilization with crossed Kirschner wires, lag screws, or a small plate. Severely comminuted fractures involving the neck and glenoid must be reconstructed and buttressed with a small plate. Cancellous bone autografts are indicated in conjunction with open reduction to promote healing in these patients.

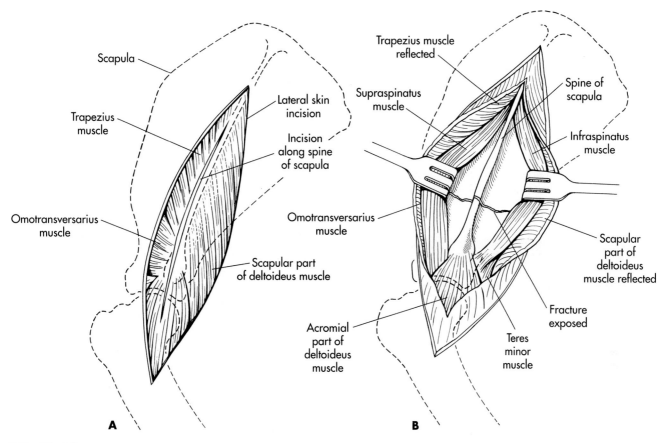

FIG. 29-18
A, For a lateral approach to the scapula, make a lateral skin incision extending the length of the spine distally to the shoulder joint. **B,** Incise the omotransversarius, trapezius, and scapular parts of the deltoideus muscles from the spine. Elevate the supraspinatus and infraspinatus muscles from the scapular body to expose the fracture.

SUTURE MATERIALS/SPECIAL INSTRUMENTS

Army-Navy and/or Myerding retractors are useful for retracting muscles. A high-speed drill is necessary for application of a plate and can be used to drill holes for placement of orthopedic wire or Kirschner wires. Plating equipment is needed for lag screw and plate placement.

POSTOPERATIVE CARE AND ASSESSMENT

Postoperative radiographs should be taken to evaluate fracture reduction and implant position. Radiographs should be repeated every 4 to 6 weeks until fractures are healed. If there is concern about implant stability during full weight bearing, a Velpeau sling (see p. 717) may be applied postoperatively; however, early return to function is preferred for joint fractures. After fractures are healed, implant removal may be considered, but removal is usually unnecessary. Limited activity is advised until radiographic signs of fracture bridging with bone are visible. Owners should be instructed to confine animals to a small area (preferably a cage) if activity cannot be supervised. If a Velpeau sling is applied, it should be kept clean and dry and the owner should observe it daily for evidence of slippage or irritation.

TABLE 29-4
Implant Use for Articular Fractures According to Fracture-Assessment Score (FAS)
FAS 0 to 3
• Lag screws • Bone plate
FAS 4 to 7
• Lag screws • Bone plate
FAS 8 to 10
• Kirschner wires • Tension band wire

PROGNOSIS

Most scapular fractures heal without complication. Potential complications of scapular fracture repair include iatrogenic infection (with open reduction), malunion, delayed union, and secondary degenerative joint disease after articular fracture. Kirschner wires can migrate if the fracture is unstable. The prognosis for normal limb function is excellent unless malunion leads to scapulohumeral joint incongruity and secondary degenerative joint disease. Nonunions are uncommon after repair of scapular fractures because of the large muscle mass and good blood supply of this region.

Suggested Reading

Brinker WO, Piermattei DL, Flo GL: *Handbook of small animal orthopedics and fracture treatment,* ed 2, Philadelphia, 1990, WB Saunders.

Harari J, Dunning D: Fractures of the scapula in dogs: a retrospective review of 12 cases, *Vet Comp Ortho Trauma* 6:105, 1993.

Roush JK, Lord PF: Clinical application of a distoproximal (axial) radiographic view of the scapula, *J Am Anim Hosp Assoc* 26:129, 1990.

HUMERAL FRACTURES

HUMERAL DIAPHYSEAL AND SUPRACONDYLAR FRACTURES

DEFINITIONS

Humeral diaphyseal fractures result in disruption of the continuity of the diaphyseal cortical bone. An intramedullary pin that is placed into the humerus in a **normograde** fashion is inserted from the greater tubercle across the fracture line and seated in the medial epicondyle. A pin that is placed in the humerus in a **retrograde** fashion is inserted at the fracture line, driven proximally to exit the greater tubercle, and then (following fracture reduction) driven across the fracture and into the distal fragment.

GENERAL CONSIDERATIONS AND CLINICALLY RELEVANT PATHOPHYSIOLOGY

High-velocity injuries (e.g., motor vehicle accidents, gunshot injuries, blunt trauma) are a common cause of humeral fractures in veterinary patients. When evaluating a patient subjected to a high-velocity injury it is important to not focus on the obvious fracture, but to complete a thorough examination of all body systems to rule out any concurrent injury. Common injuries associated with fractures of the humerus include chest wall trauma, pneumothorax, and/or pulmonary contusion. Radiographs should be taken to assess the degree of thoracic injury prior to anesthesia. The radial nerve courses from medial to lateral in the musculospiral groove of the distal humerus. Radial nerve injury may occur with fractures involving the distal humerus; therefore a careful assessment of the animal's neurologic status is essential. Reflexes and proprioception may be difficult to assess due to muscle trauma and tissue swelling associated with the fracture. However, superficial pain sensation should be easily elicited on the dorsum of the paw if the radial nerve is functional.

DIAGNOSIS
Clinical Presentation

Signalment. Any age, sex, or breed of dog or cat may be affected.

History. Motor vehicle accidents cause the majority of humeral fractures. Other modes of injury include gunshots and falls.

Physical Examination Findings

Patients with humeral diaphyseal fractures are usually non-weight bearing and exhibit varying degrees of limb swelling. Pain and crepitus may be elicited upon limb manipulation. Affected animals often drag the limb when walking and may not lift the paw when proprioception is checked. This may cause the examiner to assume that neurologic injury is present. However, similar findings may occur because of the orthopedic injury alone if pain and swelling make the patient reluctant to move the limb when proprioception is evaluated.

Radiography

The majority of these animals are painful and require sedation for proper positioning to obtain quality radiographs. Craniocaudal and lateral radiographs are necessary to assess the extent of bone and soft tissue injury. Radiographs can be taken under anesthesia just prior to surgery, but this decreases the time available for planning the surgical procedure. If the fracture is comminuted and bone plate fixation is contemplated, radiographs of the contralateral limb are useful for assessment of bone length and shape. These radiographs assist in proper contouring of the bone plate.

Laboratory Findings

Consistent laboratory abnormalities are not present.

DIFFERENTIAL DIAGNOSIS

Differential diagnoses include shoulder or elbow luxation, severe soft tissue contusion, and pathologic fractures secondary to neoplasia.

MEDICAL OR CONSERVATIVE MANAGEMENT

Medical or conservative management is not indicated. Casts or splints are not indicated for repair of humeral fractures because the scapulohumeral joint cannot be effectively immobilized.

SURGICAL TREATMENT

Intramedullary pins, intramedullary pins plus external skeletal fixation, external skeletal fixators alone, and bone plates may be used to repair humeral fractures. Techniques for applying each implant system are given below.

Application of Intramedullary (IM) Pins

Canine humerus. Two methods may be used to place an IM pin in the distal humerus: the first is to wedge the pin into the most narrow part of the marrow cavity (isthmus), and the second is to guide the pin through the epicondyloid ridge to seat into the medial epicondyle (Fig. 29-19). Pin size is dependent on which of the two methods is chosen to seat the pin distally. If the pin is to be seated at the isthmus of the marrow cavity just proximal to the supracondylar foramen, a pin of the correct diameter to wedge into the isthmus can

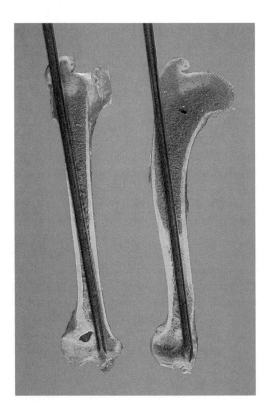

FIG. 29-19
To "seat" an intramedullary pin in the distal humerus, wedge the pin into the most narrow part of the marrow cavity (isthmus) or guide the pin through the epicondyloid ridge to seat into the medial epicondyle.

be determined at surgery or from the preoperative radiographs. Similarly, if the pin is to be seated into the medial epicondyle, an estimation of space through the epicondyloid ridge can be made at surgery or by evaluating the preoperative radiograph.

☞ **N O T E** · Estimate pin size from the preoperative radiograph.

An IM pin may be placed in a retrograde or normograde manner in the humerus (Fig. 29-20). There are no advantages of one method over the other. Generally, if open reduction is performed, retrograde placement is used; if the fracture is to be stabilized through closed pinning, normograde placement is used. When retrograding an IM pin in the humerus, the pin is driven in a proximal direction from the fracture surface toward the shoulder joint. To ensure that the pin exits at the proper site proximally, the shaft of the pin should be pressed against the medial and caudal surface of the marrow cavity. This forces the point of the pin to glide along the craniolateral cortex and exit craniolateral to the shoulder joint. This also "presets" the pin in the proximal fragment so that the distal pin point is directed toward the caudomedial cortex when the fracture is reduced and the pin is driven into the distal fragment. In order to wedge the pin above the supratrochlear foramen, a pin close to the diameter of the isthmus is driven to the level of the lateral epicondyloid ridge. This can be estimated with a reference pin

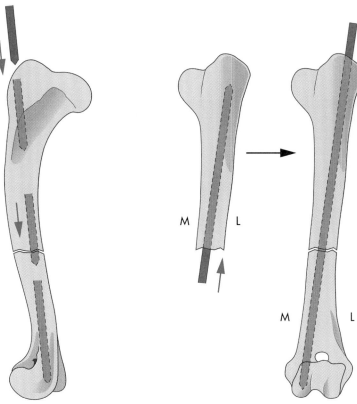

Normograde   Retrograde

FIG. 29-20
Humeral pins may be placed in a normograde or retrograde fashion.

of equal length placed sagittal to the pin within the marrow cavity. To seat the pin into the medial epicondylar ridge, a pin equal in diameter to the width of the epicondylar ridge is driven to the level of the medial epicondyle. This can also be estimated with a reference pin of equal length to the IM pin.

☞ **N O T E** · To properly align the pin, press the shaft against the caudomedial cortex. This causes the pin to exit craniolateral to the shoulder joint.

Normograde placement of an IM pin is generally performed with closed reduction. The pin is driven from proximal to distal beginning at the craniolateral aspect of the greater tubercle. The proximal fragment can be palpated through the skin surface and held to determine the direction of the marrow cavity. A small skin incision is made at the point of pin entry over the greater tubercle and the pin is driven in line with the marrow cavity to exit at the fracture surface. The pin point can be palpated as it exits the marrow cavity of the proximal fragment and driven to extend 3 to 5 mm beyond the fracture surface. The distal fragment is toggled over the end of the pin point, aligned for proper reduction, and the pin is then driven distally. The same two methods for distal seatage and choice of pin size apply for normograde placement as discussed previously for retrograde placement.

Feline humerus. Retrograde and normograde placement follow the same guidelines as discussed for dogs. Normograde placement is easier in cats because the marrow cavity has a uniform diameter, there is less curvature to the bone, and there is less soft tissue envelope covering the bone than there is in dogs. Care must be taken to not enter the supratrochlear foramen because of the presence of the median nerve in this area.

Application of IM Pins with External Skeletal Fixation

Combining the bending support of an IM pin with axial and rotational support from an external fixator is useful to control all weight-bearing forces. An IM pin that occupies 50% to 60% of the medullary cavity is first inserted in a normograde or retrograde manner. An appropriate number of transfixation pins and the external frame are then applied. The frame, number, and type of transfixation pins vary with the rigidity of fixation desired and the length of time the fixator must remain in place (see p. 736). A single external bar with one transfixation pin placed proximal to the fracture and one placed distal to the fracture is commonly used for moderately stable fractures that are expected to heal in a relatively short time period (i.e., less than 6 weeks). The proximal transfixation pin is placed craniolaterally, approximately 3 cm distal to the greater tubercle. A small Kirschner wire can be used as a "feeler" pin to identify the proper angle of insertion for the transfixation pin to avoid intersecting the IM pin (see p. 741). Predrilling the condyles is recommended because this area is composed of dense cancellous bone. The distal transfixation pin is inserted laterally across the humeral condyles and should be centered within the

condyles. The lateral epicondyle is palpated and the pin is inserted 1 to 2 mm cranial and distal to the epicondylar prominence. The transfixation pin is exited medially from the bone near the medial epicondylar prominence. For unstable fractures additional transfixation pins may be added, but alternative strategies can also be used to enhance rigidity of the fixation while minimizing postoperative discomfort. Placement of an additional external bar and/or connecting the IM pin to the external fixator frame to make a "tie-in" configuration increases the strength of the fixation system without adding to patient morbidity through placement of additional pins (Fig. 29-21). A Type Ib external skeletal fixator can be constructed by placing an additional transfixation pin proximally at a 60- to 90-degree angle to the transfixation pin already in place. The external bars are then constructed to form a triangular shape. If more transfixation pins are desired, intermediate half pins may be placed to achieve additional strength and stiffness (refer to p. 739 for guidelines on pin number, design, and position). If one or more transfixation pins are placed in the distal third of the humerus, care must be taken when making the soft tissue tunnel and placing the transfixation pins so as to avoid radial nerve injury.

Application of External Skeletal Fixation

The use of external skeletal fixation as the sole means of stabilization for complex fractures of the humerus has recently gained popularity (Fig. 29-22). When external fixators are applied to the humerus, stress on transfixation pins

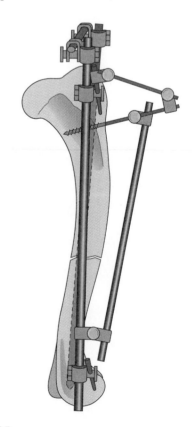

FIG. 29-21
To increase the strength of the fixation system, connect the IM pin to an external fixator frame to make a tie-in configuration.

is high due to the long distance from the external bar to their entrance into the bone and the inability to use stronger bilateral frames. Thoughtful preoperative planning and strict adherence to principles of application are necessary to avoid fixator-related complications and unacceptable patient morbidity. Open reduction is recommended to achieve adequate spatial alignment of the humerus. Achieving spatial alignment can be assisted through placement of a temporary IM pin through the intact proximal segment of intact bone, across the area of comminution, and into the distal segment of intact bone. In keeping with the concept of bridging osteosynthesis, bone fragments in the area of comminution should not be reduced or manipulated. The most proximal and distal transfixation pins should be placed as half-pins into their respective metaphyseal-epiphyseal junctions. There is usually no problem bypassing the IM pin but a "feeler" Kirschner wire can be used to find an appropriate site for the transfixation pin (see p. 741). The external bar is connected to the proximal and distal transfixation pin to maintain spatial alignment of the humerus before the temporary IM pin is removed. The remaining transfixation pins are placed and connected to the external bar. Care must be exercised when placing transfixation pins in the distal third of the humerus so as to not injure the radial nerve. The number and type of transfixation pins depend upon the rigidity and duration of function needed for the external skeletal fixator. It is better to err on the side of being too rigid than to have a fixator that is not rigid enough. The former can be destabilized as the fracture heals, but the latter may result in premature fixation failure and high morbidity.

Application of Bone Plates and Screws

Bone plates provide needed stability and allow early return to function when used for complex or stable humeral fractures. Bone plates are generally used when the time to bone union will be lengthy or when postoperative comfort is desirable. Factors that influence plate size are its intended function (i.e., compression, neutralization, or buttress plate) and patient size. The plate may be placed on the craniolateral, caudolateral, caudomedial, or medial surfaces of the humerus (Fig. 29-23). Although craniolateral plate application is easiest with proximal and midshaft humeral fractures, it is also commonly used with distal fractures. Medial and caudomedial placement is easiest with distal fractures. A minimum of three plate screws (six cortices) proximal to the fracture and three plate screws distal to the fracture is recommended with compression or neutralization plates while a minimum of four plate screws (eight cortices) proximal and distal to the fracture is recommended for buttress plates. Compression plates may be used with transverse or short oblique fractures.

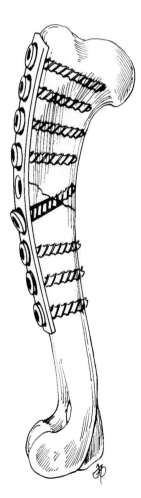

FIG. 29-23
A bone plate applied to the cranial (illustrated), medial, or lateral humeral surfaces may also be used to stabilize humeral diaphyseal fractures. (From Olmstead ML: *Small animal orthopedics*, St Louis, 1995, Mosby.)

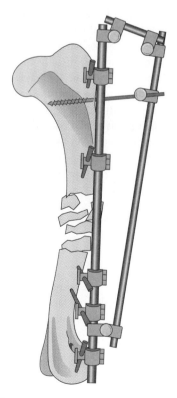

FIG. 29-22
An external skeletal fixator *(Type Ib shown here)* may be used as the sole means of stabilizing a comminuted fracture.

The plate should be contoured to 1 mm offset from the bone surface at the fracture site to achieve compression of the transcortex. Neutralization plates are used with long oblique fractures or comminuted fractures where the bone fragments can be reduced and stabilized with compression screws or cerclage wire. The plate is contoured to the anatomic surface of the bone. Buttress plates are used with comminuted fractures where bone fragments cannot be reduced anatomically or in cases in which attempted reduction and stabilization of the fragments would cause excessive soft tissue trauma. The plate is contoured to reflect the anatomy of the humerus; this is most easily accomplished by contouring the plate to a craniocaudal radiograph of the contralateral limb. Spatial alignment of the bone is assisted by insertion of an IM pin. The pin may be retrograded or normograded through the proximal intact segment of bone, passed through the fragmented section of bone, and seated into the medial condyle. When placing the pin into the medial condyle, do not prevent the fragment from displacing distally. This allows the pin to distract the proximal and distal segments and helps to regain humeral length. In keeping with the concept of bridging osteosynthesis, the bone fragments in the comminuted area should not be disturbed. Once spatial alignment of the humerus is achieved, the bone plate can be attached to the bone with plate screws. Leaving the alignment pin in place will provide a plate/pin buttress of the fracture. The diameter of the alignment pin should equal approximately 50% the diameter of the marrow cavity to allow screws to be placed. Bicortical screws should be used proximally and distally when possible and monocortical screws used centrally. The plate/pin combination increases the strength and fatigue life of the fixation and thereby protects the plate from premature breakage (Fig. 29-24). The plate/pin system can be destabilized between 6 and 8 weeks by removing the IM pin. Alternately, if the alignment pin is removed, bicortical plate screws (screws that engage both cortices) may be used. A cancellous bone graft can be harvested and placed in the fracture zone if soft tissues are not excessively disrupted.

Preoperative Management

Before surgery, a spica splint (see p. 707) can be applied to increase patient comfort and protect soft tissues from further injury induced by bone fragments. Because these fractures occur secondary to trauma, all affected animals should be examined for concurrent injury and stabilized if necessary prior to surgery. Analgesics should be provided to animals that appear to be in pain.

Anesthesia

Anesthetic management of animals with fractures is discussed on p. 708.

Surgical Anatomy

Most often a craniolateral exposure is used to approach the humeral diaphysis. The radial nerve must be identified and protected during fracture reduction and stabilization. The radial nerve lies superficial to the brachialis muscle and deep to the lateral head of the triceps. The canine humerus has a

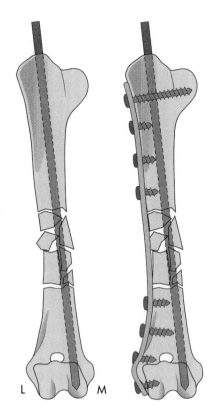

FIG. 29-24
Application of a plate/rod combination for stabilization of a comminuted humeral fracture. The intramedullary pin reduces cyclic bending stress in the bone plate.

normal cranial to caudal curvature that positions the long axis of the marrow cavity cranial to the shoulder joint. This facilitates pin placement by assuring that an IM pin will exit cranial to the joint. However, distally the supratrochlear foramen is in direct line with the long axis of the marrow cavity, which makes distal placement of the IM pin into the cancellous bone more difficult. The anatomy of the feline humerus is similar to that of the canine. However, there is less cranial to caudal curvature and the diameter of the marrow cavity is more uniform. In cats, care must be taken to avoid entering the supratrochlear foramen due to the presence of the median nerve.

☞ **N O T E** • Be sure to identify and protect the radial nerve during surgical approaches to the humerus.

Positioning

The animal is positioned in lateral recumbency with the affected leg up. A "hanging leg" prep facilitates limb manipulation during surgery. The limb should be prepped from the dorsal midline to the carpus.

SURGICAL TECHNIQUE

The fixation system chosen depends on the patient fracture-assessment rating and other factors discussed in the section on Decision Making in Fracture Management (see p. 730). Readers are encouraged to review this section before choosing a fixation system.

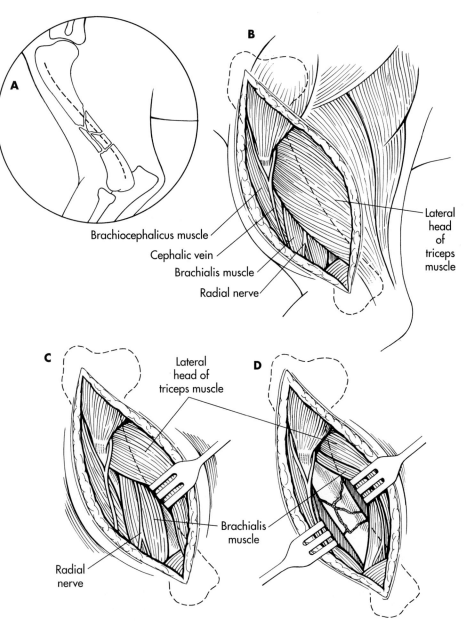

FIG. 29-25
A, To expose the midhumeral diaphysis, make a skin incision from the cranial border of the tubercle of the humerus to the lateral epicondyle distally. **B,** Incise subcutaneous fat and brachial fascia along the same line, being careful to isolate and protect the cephalic vein. **C,** Visualize the radial nerve when incising fascia along the cranial border of the triceps overlying the brachialis muscle. **D,** Make an incision through the periosteal insertion of the superficial pectoral and brachiocephalicus muscles at their insertion on the humeral shaft.

Surgical Approach to the Humeral Diaphysis

The proximal and central humeral diaphysis is most easily exposed through a craniolateral approach.

Make a skin incision from the cranial border of the tubercle of the humerus to the lateral epicondyle distally (Fig. 29-25, A). The incision should follow the normal curvature of the humerus. Incise the subcutaneous fat and brachial fascia along the same line, being careful to isolate and protect the cephalic vein (Fig. 29-25, B). The cephalic vein may be ligated if necessary to achieve the desired exposure. Incise the brachial fascia along the border of the brachiocephalicus muscle and the lateral head of the triceps. Use caution when incising the fascia along the cranial border of the triceps overlying the brachialis muscle until the radial nerve is visualized (Fig. 29-25, C). Once the nerve is isolated, make an incision through the periosteal insertion of the superficial pectoral and brachiocephalicus muscles at their insertion on the humeral shaft (Fig. 29-25, D). Reflect these two muscles cranially and the brachialis muscle caudally to expose the proximal and central humeral shaft. To gain further exposure of the distal humeral shaft reflect the brachialis muscle cranially and the lateral triceps muscle caudally. Release the origin of the extensor carpi radialis muscle from the ridge of the lateral epicondyle for maximum exposure. To close, suture the brachiocephalicus muscle and superficial pectoral muscles to the fascia of the brachialis muscle. Suture the subcutaneous tissue and skin using standard methods.

The distal one third of the humerus is also accessible through a medial exposure and is the choice of some surgeons when a bone plate is used as the fixation method. *Make an incision from the greater tubercle proximally to the medial epicondyle distally. Incise the deep brachial*

FIG. 29-26
A, To expose the medial surface of the distal third of the humerus, incise deep brachial fascia along the caudal border of the brachiocephalicus muscle. **B,** At the distal aspect be careful to preserve and isolate the median, musculocutaneous, and ulnar nerves and brachial artery and vein. **C,** Reflect the biceps brachii and neurovascular structures caudally, and the superficial pectoral muscle cranially.

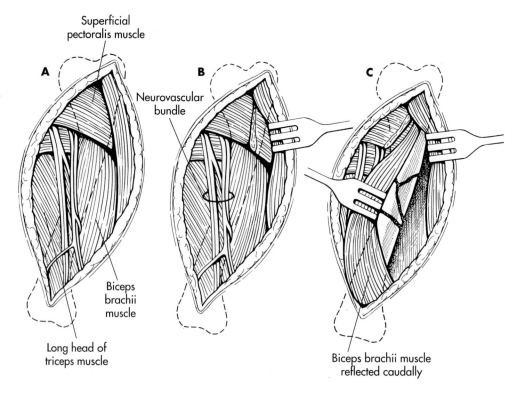

fascia along the caudal border of the brachiocephalicus muscle (Fig. 29-26, A). Take care distally to preserve and isolate the neurovascular structures (i.e., median, musculocutaneous, and ulnar nerves and brachial artery and vein) (Fig. 29-26, B). Reflect the brachiocephalicus muscle cranially and incise through the insertion of the superficial pectoral muscle. For exposure of the midportion of the humerus, reflect the superficial pectoral muscle cranially and the biceps brachii and neurovascular structures caudally (Fig. 29-26, C). For exposure of the distal humerus, reflect the biceps brachii, neurovascular structures, and superficial pectoral muscle cranially. To close, suture the superficial pectoral to the brachiocephalicus fascia. Suture the remaining deep fascia, subcutaneous tissue, and skin in a routine fashion.

Stabilization of Midshaft Transverse or Short Oblique Fractures

From a mechanical perspective, this fracture configuration allows load sharing between the bone and implant following surgery. Factors that negatively affect healing include multiple limb injuries or if the patient is large and active. From a biologic perspective, the patient fracture assessment dictates whether the time to union will be lengthy or of short duration. With a long duration to healing the implant needs to remain functional for 8 or more weeks. In these cases, implants that purchase bone with threads are desirable; with shorter healing periods implants that have frictional hold are adequate.

Stabilization of a transverse or short oblique fracture requires rotational and bending support. This can be achieved with bone plates, an IM pin with cruciate hemicerclage wire, an IM pin with an external fixator, or an external fixator alone. The final implant choice should be determined by the

fracture location and patient fracture-assessment (Fig. 29-27). Fixation systems that are useful with a low patient fracture assessment (i.e., 0 to 3) include a bone plate and screws inserted to function as a compression plate, and a 6-pin Type Ib external skeletal fixator with raised threaded transfixation pins "tied in" with an IM pin (Table 29-5). With a moderate patient fracture assessment (i.e., 4 to 7), a compression plate, an IM pin "tied in" with a 3-pin, a Type Ib external skeletal fixator, or an IM pin and cruciate hemicerclage wire combined with an external fixator for additional support would be functional. The transfixation pins can be a combination of smooth, negative-profile, and raised threaded pins depending on the length of time the fixator must stay in place. Transverse or short oblique fractures are common in puppies and kittens because they are often stepped on by their owners. These patients have a high patient fracture-assessment (i.e., 8 to 10) and can be stabilized with an IM pin/cruciate hemicerclage wire or an IM pin, 2-pin Type Ia external skeletal fixator. In small patients who are less than 4 to 5 months of age, a single IM pin placed closed in a normograde fashion can be used. Rapid formation of biologic callus will provide mechanical support (Fig. 29-28).

Stabilization of Midshaft Long Oblique Fractures or Comminuted Fractures With a Large Butterfly Fragment

From a mechanical perspective, these fractures can be reduced and interfragmentary compression applied with cerclage wire or lag screws. Once the interfragmentary fracture lines are reduced and compressed, the bone is able to share the loads with the implant postoperatively. Factors that negatively affect healing include the presence of multiple in-

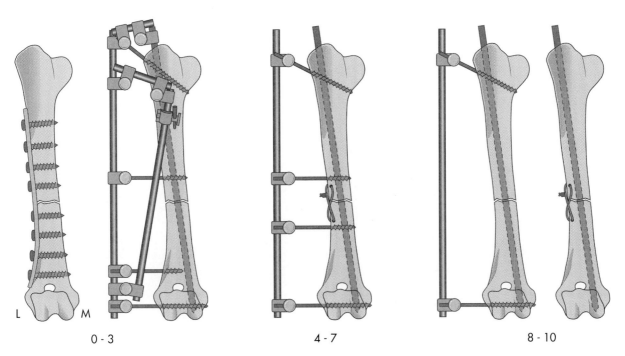

0 - 3   4 - 7   8 - 10

FIG. 29-27
Recommended methods of stabilizing transverse or short oblique fractures. If the patient fracture-assessment score is 0 to 3, a compression plate or external skeletal fixator plus IM pin (tie-in configuration) may be used. If the patient fracture-assessment score is 4 to 7, an external skeletal fixator in conjunction with IM pin and cerclage wire may be used. With patient fracture-assessment scores of 8 to 10, an external skeletal fixator plus IM pin or an IM pin plus cerclage wire provides necessary stability.

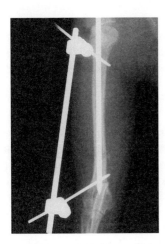

FIG. 29-28
Craniocaudal radiograph showing positioning of a single intramedullary pin for stabilization of a transverse humeral fracture in a young dog.

TABLE 29-5

Implant Use According to Fracture-Assessment Score (FAS) for Midshaft Transverse or Short Oblique Humeral Fractures

FAS 0 to 3
- Compression plate
- 6-pin Type Ib external skeletal fixator tied to an IM pin

FAS 4 to 7
- Compression plate
- 3-pin, Type Ib external skeletal fixator tied to an IM pin
- IM pin and cruciate hemicerclage wire plus an external skeletal fixator

FAS 8 to 10
- IM pin/cruciate hemicerclage wire
- IM pin, 2-pin Type Ia external skeletal fixator combination
- Single IM pin

---

juries, a large, active patient, and the necessity for open reduction and tissue manipulation to reduce and apply interfragmentary compression.

If a long duration to healing is expected, the implant needs to remain functional for 8 or more weeks; those implants that purchase bone with threads are desirable. With shorter healing periods, implants that have frictional hold (smooth pins and wire) are adequate.

Stabilization of this fracture configuration requires axial, rotational, and bending support. This can be achieved with bone plates, IM pins/cerclage wire/external fixator combinations, and IM pin and cerclage wire (Fig. 29-29). Fixation systems that are useful with a low patient fracture assessment (i.e., 0 to 3) are neutralization plates (Table 29-6). Interfragmentary compression is first achieved with wire or compression screws to reconstruct the cylinder of bone and the area

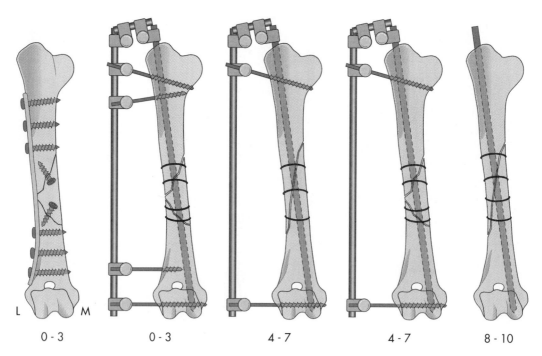

| 0 - 3 | 0 - 3 | 4 - 7 | 4 - 7 | 8 - 10 |

FIG. 29-29
Recommended methods for stabilizing long oblique fractures or simple comminuted fractures (single large fragment). If the patient fracture-assessment score is 0 to 3, a neutralization plate or 4-pin external skeletal fixator plus IM pin (tie-in configuration) and cerclage wires may be used. If the patient fracture-assessment score is 4 to 7, a 2-pin external skeletal fixator in conjunction with IM pin (tie-in configuration) and cerclage wire may be used. With patient fracture-assessment scores of 8 to 10, an IM pin plus cerclage wire provides necessary stability.

TABLE 29-6

Implant Use According to Fracture-Assessment Score (FAS) for Long Oblique Simple Comminuted Midshaft Humeral Fractures

FAS 0 to 3
- Neutralization plate plus wire, compression screws
- IM pin, cerclage wire and external skeletal fixator (tie-in configuration)

FAS 4 to 7
- Neutralization plate
- IM pin plus cerclage wire combined with a 2-pin, Type Ia external skeletal fixator

FAS 8 to 10
- IM pin plus cerclage wire

---

then bridged with a bone plate. Alternatively, an IM pin can be inserted initially and interfragmentary compression applied with cerclage wire. Additional support is then supplied by an external skeletal fixator, with or without a tie-in to the IM pin. With a moderate patient fracture assessment (i.e., 4 to 7), a neutralization plate, or an IM pin plus cerclage wire for interfragmentary compression combined with a 2-pin, Type Ia external skeletal fixator may be used. The transfixation pins should have a raised thread or have a negative thread

profile. With a high patient fracture assessment (i.e., 8 to 10) an IM pin combined with cerclage wire for interfragmentary compression is a useful method to stabilize the fracture (Fig. 29-30).

Stabilization of Midshaft Comminuted Fractures With Multiple Fragments

From a mechanical perspective these fractures cannot be reduced without significant soft tissue manipulation and there is no load sharing between the implant and bone until biologic callus forms to provide support. Therefore very high stresses will be imposed on the implant and its connection to the bone. If the biologic assessment is favorable, the imposed stresses will be of short duration and the likelihood of implant failure is lessened. However, if the biologic assessment is not favorable, imposed stresses will act on the implant for an extended period and implant failure is more likely. Enhancing the biologic response by not attempting to reduce the fragments (bridging osteosynthesis) and/or inserting an autogenous cancellous bone graft when appropriate is recommended. From a mechanical perspective, these types of fractures need rigid axial, rotational, and bending support.

Stabilization can be achieved with a bone plate/pin combination, Type Ib or Ia external skeletal fixator/pin tie-in combination, a bone plate alone (lengthening plate, broad plate), or an interlocking nail (Fig. 29-31). Patients with low fracture assessments (i.e., 0 to 3) are best managed with a bone plate/pin combination, a rigid Type Ib external skeletal

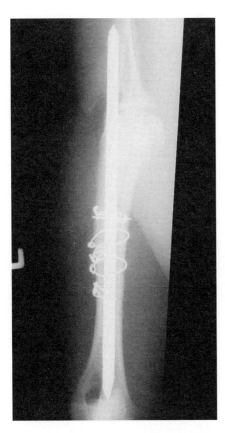

FIG. 29-30
Postoperative radiograph showing stabilization of a simple comminuted humeral fracture with an intramedullary pin and cerclage wires.

TABLE 29-7

Implant Use According to Fracture-Assessment Score (FAS) for Comminuted Midshaft Humeral Fractures

FAS 0 to 3
- Bone plate/pin combination
- Rigid Type Ib external skeletal fixator tied in to an IM pin
- Type Ib external skeletal fixator

FAS 4 to 7
- Buttress plate (lengthening plate or broad plate)
- External skeletal fixator, with or without a tie-in to an IM pin
- Interlocking nail

FAS 8 to 10
- IM pin with or without a tie-in to a Type Ia or Type Ib external skeletal fixator

Stabilization of Supracondylar Fractures

Supracondylar fractures are commonly transverse or short oblique fractures. Occasionally a comminuted fracture with multiple small fragments will be seen. However, when comminution is present the length of bone involved is usually limited to a small area. The fracture can be bridged with an implant to serve as a buttress or the fracture can be collapsed to resemble a load sharing transverse or short oblique fracture. If the zone of comminution is lengthy and limb length must be preserved, reconstruction of the bony column or bridging the area of comminution with an appropriate implant system serving as a buttress is recommended.

Stabilization of supracondylar fractures depends upon the fracture configuration and patient fracture assessment (Fig. 29-33). Transverse or short oblique fractures require rotational and bending support, whereas comminuted fractures require axial, rotational, and bending support. In patients with a low fracture assessment (i.e., 0 to 3), a caudolateral plate combined with a caudomedial plate or caudolateral plate combined with a medial IM pin is preferred. The function of the plate will be a compression plate with transverse fractures and a buttress plate with highly fragmented fractures. A neutralization plate combined with lag screws for intrafragmentary compression is used with long oblique fractures or comminuted fractures where reconstruction of the bony column is feasible. In patients with a moderate fracture assessment (i.e., 4 to 7), a medial plate, caudolateral plate, or an IM pin supported with an external skeletal fixator are suggested. The external skeletal fixator frame, number of pins, and pin design are dependent upon the fracture assessment. If the external skeletal fixator must remain in place for an extended period, a biplanar frame with enhanced threaded pins should be used. The IM pin may be tied in with the external skeletal fixator to increase rigidity and reduce morbidity. With a high assessment (i.e., 8 to 10), a medial and lateral IM pin provide the needed stability to allow for fracture union.

fixator "tied in" to an IM pin, or a Type Ib external skeletal fixator (Table 29-7). The transfixation pins should have a raised thread and at least three pins should be applied above and two pins below the area of comminution. It is always better to err on the side of too much rigidity than too little rigidity since the fixator can be destabilized postoperatively. A patient with a moderate fracture assessment (i.e., 4 to 7) can be managed with a bone plate functioning as a buttress plate (lengthening plate or broad plate). The plate can be applied to the cranial, medial, or lateral surface dependent upon the location of the fracture and surgeon preference. An external skeletal fixator, with or without a tie-in to the IM pin, or an interlocking nail may also be used. The choice of frame, number of pins, and pin design for the external skeletal fixator depend on the fracture assessment. The only time a patient with this type of fracture would have a high fracture-assessment rating (i.e., 8 to 10) would be when the biologic assessment is extremely favorable (e.g., a 4- to 5-month-old animal with a low-velocity, closed, single limb injury). These animals could be managed using bridging osteosynthesis with an intramedullary pin with or without a tie-in to a Type Ia or Type Ib external skeletal fixator. The transfixation pins can be smooth pins or have a negative thread profile depending on the amount of time the fixator needs to remain in place (Fig. 29-32).

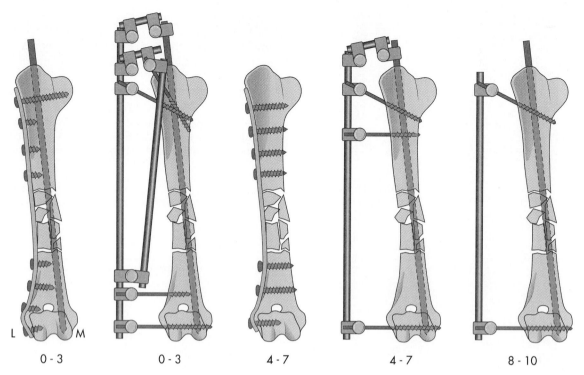

L M

0 - 3   0 - 3   4 - 7   4 - 7   8 - 10

FIG. 29-31
Recommended methods for stabilizing complex comminuted humeral fractures (multiple fragments). If the patient fracture-assessment score is 0 to 3, a plate/rod combination or 4-pin external skeletal fixator plus IM pin (tie-in configuration) may be used. If the patient fracture-assessment score is 4 to 7, a buttress plate or 3-pin external skeletal fixator in conjunction with IM pin (tie-in configuration) may be used. With patient fracture-assessment scores of 8 to 10, a 2-pin external skeletal fixator plus IM pin provides necessary stability.

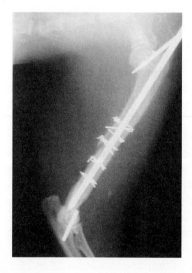

FIG. 29-32
Postoperative radiograph showing stabilization of a complex comminuted fracture with an IM pin and external skeletal fixator in a patient with a favorable fracture-assessment score (8 to 10).

SUTURE MATERIALS/SPECIAL INSTRUMENTS

Special instrumentation other than those necessary for application of the fixation device are not needed.

POSTOPERATIVE CARE AND ASSESSMENT

After surgery activity should be controlled to leash walking until there is radiographic evidence of fracture healing. Time to bone union depends upon the patient fracture assessment. Passive flexion and extension of the elbow should be performed to maintain range of motion. IM pins and external skeletal fixations should be removed when healing occurs; bone plates are not to be removed unless a problem is associated with their presence.

PROGNOSIS

The prognosis depends on the fracture assessment; patients with poor assessment are more prone to have complications. Poor implant choice relative to the fracture assessment is the most common reason for fixation failure. The most common complication seen in companion animals is premature loosening of the implant (i.e., loosening and migration of IM pins, external skeletal fixator transfixation pins, and cerclage wires). Fatigue breakage of bone plates or plate screw pullout can occur when principles of bone plating are not followed or when an inaccurate assessment of the length of time to bone union is made. Plate failure is most often noted when reduction and stabilization of the zone of comminution with cerclage wire are unsuccessful. This may devascularize bone fragments and create small fracture gaps that

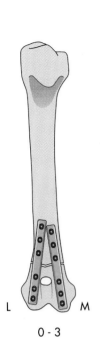 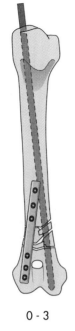 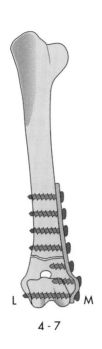 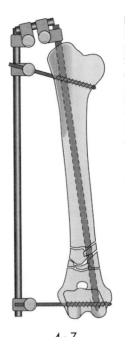

L M   L   L M

0 - 3   0 - 3   4 - 7   4 - 7

FIG. 29-33
Recommended methods for stabilizing supracondylar fractures. If the patient fracture-assessment score is 0 to 3, two plates or a plate/rod combination may be used. If the patient fracture-assessment score is 4 to 7, a medial compression plate or 2-pin external skeletal fixator plus IM pin (tie-in configuration) may be used. If the fracture-assessment score is 8 to 10, medial and lateral IM pins may be used (not illustrated).

concentrate strain. These factors delay healing and result in long-term cyclic stress on the bone plate.

If failure of the initial implant system has occurred, the recommended treatment is application of a bone plate serving as a compression plate or neutralization plate if the fracture configuration allows or application of a plate/rod construct if a zone of comminution must be bridged. These systems serve to stabilize the fracture while at the same time providing patient comfort that allows limb use and early physical therapy.

Suggested Reading

Anderson SM, Lippincott CL, Schulman AJ: Longitudinal myotomy of the flexor carpi radialis: a new approach to the medial aspect of the elbow joint, *J Am Anim Hosp Assoc* 25:499, 1989.

Aron DN, Palmer RH, Johnson AL: Biologic strategies and a balanced concept for repair of highly comminuted long bone fractures, *Compend Cont Educ Pract Vet* 17:35, 1995.

Bardet JF, Hohn RB, Olmstead ML: Fractures of the humerus in dogs and cats: a retrospective study of 130 cases, *Vet Surg* 12:73, 1983.

Brinker WO, Hohn RB, Prieur WD: *Manual of internal fixation in small animals,* New York, 1984, Springer-Verlag.

Brinker WO, Piermattei DL, Flo GL: *Handbook of small animal orthopedics and fracture treatment,* ed 2, Philadelphia, 1990, Saunders.

Harari J et al: Medial plating for the repair of middle and distal diaphyseal fractures of the humerus in dogs, *Vet Surg* 15:45, 1986.

Martinez SA et al: Effects of a fixed compression load on the osteogenic effect of autogenous cancellous bone grafts in dogs, *Am J Vet Res* 53:2381, 1992.

Matthiesson DT: Fractures of the humerus, *Vet Clin North Am* 22:121, 1992.

Mclaughlin RM, Cockshutt JR, Kuzma AB: Stacked veterinary cuttable plates for treatment of comminuted diaphyseal fractures in cats, *Vet Compara Ortho Trauma* 5:22, 1992.

Montgomery RD, Milton JL, Mann FA: Medial approach to the humeral diaphysis, *J Am Anim Hosp Assoc* 24:433, 1988.

Piermattei DL, Greely RG: *An atlas of surgical approaches to the bones of the dog and cat,* ed 2, Philadelphia, 1980, Saunders.

Vannini R, Olmstead ML, Smeak DD: An epidemiological study of 151 distal humeral fractures in dogs and cats, *J Am Anim Hosp Assoc* 24:531, 1988.

HUMERAL EPIPHYSEAL AND METAPHYSEAL FRACTURES

DEFINITIONS

Epiphyseal and/or **metaphyseal fractures** may occur at the proximal or distal ends of the humerus.

SYNONYMS

Slippage of the proximal or distal growth plate, elbow fracture

GENERAL CONSIDERATIONS AND CLINICALLY RELEVANT PATHOPHYSIOLOGY

Fractures of the proximal humeral metaphysis and/or epiphysis are uncommon, but occasionally occur in young animals through the proximal humeral growth plate. Fractures through the growth plate may result from minimal external force and exhibit only slight displacement. Careful scrutiny of the lateral radiograph and comparison to a radiograph of the contralateral limb may be needed to correctly diagnose these fractures.

Fractures of the distal epiphysis (elbow) are common. Lateral condylar fractures predominate over medial condylar fractures for two reasons. First, the radial head articulates with the lateral condyle causing weight-bearing forces to be transmitted primarily through the lateral condyle. Second, the anatomic position of the lateral condyle is eccentric to the bony column, causing weight-bearing forces to be transmitted through the weaker epicondyloid ridge to the humeral diaphysis. Fractures of the lateral condyle are frequently diagnosed in young, toy breed dogs that fall or jump from furniture or the owner's arms with the elbow extended. When the animal lands, high loads are transmitted through the radial head-lateral condyle axis resulting in separation of the lateral condyle. The fracture line passes between the lateral and medial condyle, crosses the growth plate, and exits through the metaphysis. Because the growth plate is involved, the fracture is classified as a Salter fracture. Careful evaluation of the craniocaudal radiograph is essential since minimal displacement of the intercondylar fracture can occur. Adult animals also sustain lateral condylar fractures through the mechanism described above. In spaniel breeds these fractures may occur as a result of incomplete ossification between the medial and lateral condyles. Hairline fractures through the cancellous bone of the epicondyloid ridge or the intercondylar cancellous bone may cause forelimb lameness before the fracture is apparent radiographically.

☞ **N O T E** · Evaluate radiographs carefully to avoid missing intercondylar fractures that are minimally displaced.

Isolated medial condylar fractures are not common but do occur in both immature and mature patients; T or Y fractures of the elbow are more common, however. This fracture configuration represents a separation between the medial and lateral condyles in conjunction with a transverse (T) or oblique (Y) fracture through both medial and lateral epicondyloid ridges.

DIAGNOSIS
Clinical Presentation

Signalment. Lateral condylar fractures are frequently diagnosed in young, toy breed dogs; however, Salter fractures may occur in any juvenile dog or cat of any breed or sex that has open growth plates. Adult animals of any breed or sex may sustain a proximal epiphyseal or distal epiphyseal (elbow) fracture. Spaniel breeds appear to predispose to lateral condylar fractures (see above).

History. Salter fractures usually occur following a fall, but may also be caused by automobile accidents. Elbow fractures or proximal humeral fractures in adult animals are usually associated with vehicular trauma.

Physical Examination Findings

Most affected animals present with a non–weight-bearing lameness. Swelling of the affected limb is usually obvious if the fracture is secondary to an automobile accident. Pain and crepitus can be elicited with limb manipulation.

Radiography

Craniocaudal and medial to lateral radiographs are usually sufficient to make a diagnosis. In spaniels, if a fracture of the intercondylar articular surface is suspected but not evident, oblique radiographic views of the elbow are recommended. Hairline fractures through cancellous bone of the epicondyloid ridge or intercondylar cancellous bone may cause a slight periosteal reaction over the epicondylar ridge, before the fracture line becomes evident radiographically.

Laboratory Findings

Consistent laboratory abnormalities are not present.

DIFFERENTIAL DIAGNOSIS

Differential diagnoses include ligament injury of the shoulder or elbow, scapular fractures, and proximal radius and/or ulna fractures.

MEDICAL OR CONSERVATIVE MANAGEMENT

Fractures involving or in close proximity to the joint should not be managed with conservative treatment.

SURGICAL TREATMENT

Treatment of humeral metaphyseal and epiphyseal fractures depends on the animal's age, overall health, and fracture configuration. The fracture-assessment score (see p. 730) is used to help determine the rigidity of stabilization needed for the fracture to heal.

Preoperative Management

Patients that have sustained trauma should be stabilized prior to anesthesia and fracture treatment. Analgesics may be indicated to increase patient comfort.

Anesthesia

Anesthetic considerations for patients with fractures is provided on p. 708.

Surgical Anatomy

Depending on the severity of injury, the normal anatomy and surgical landmarks of this region may be distorted by soft tissue bruising and swelling. Starting the surgical dissection in an area with less swelling or bruising and using bony landmarks is helpful. Proximally, the lateral tuberosity and acromion of the scapula are readily palpable; distally, the medial and lateral epicondyles are easy to identify. The cephalic vein courses within the subcutaneous tissue along the craniolateral surface of the limb. The radial nerve lies beneath the lateral head of the triceps near the distal third of the humerus. This nerve must be identified as it courses superficial to the brachialis muscle before the brachialis muscle is reflected from the humeral diaphysis. To visualize the nerve, dissection should be initiated adjacent to the cranial edge of the lateral head of the triceps, near the lateral epicondyle. The tissue plane between the brachiocephalicus and triceps muscles must be carefully dissected to avoid injury to this nerve.

☞ **N O T E** • To make identification of landmarks easier, begin the surgical dissection proximal or distal to the area of bruising.

Positioning

The patient is positioned in lateral recumbency for all lateral approaches and for olecranon osteotomy. A hanging leg prep will facilitate manipulation of the limb during surgery. The region from just dorsal to the scapula proximally to the carpus distally should be clipped and prepped for aseptic surgery.

SURGICAL TECHNIQUES
Surgical Approach to the Proximal Epiphysis

Make an incision over the craniolateral region of the proximal humerus (Fig. 29-34, A). Begin the incision 2 to 3 cm proximal to the greater tubercle and extend it distally to a point near the midshaft of the humerus. Incise through the subcutaneous tissue along the same line to expose deep fascia along the lateral border of the brachiocephalicus muscle and insertion of the deltoid muscle (Fig. 29-34, B). Elevate and reflect the brachiocephalicus muscle from the cranial surface of the bone. Elevate the deltoid muscle and retract it caudally to expose the insertions of the teres minor and infraspinatus muscles. Make an incision through the insertions of these two muscles to expose the lateral surface of the proximal humerus (Fig. 29-34, C). If increased exposure of the craniomedial surface of the proximal humerus is needed, release the insertion of the superficial pectoral muscle deep to brachiocephalicus muscle. To close, suture the fascia of the superficial pectoral muscle to the fascia of the deltoid muscle. Appose the fascia of the brachiocephalicus muscle, then suture subcutaneous tissue and skin.

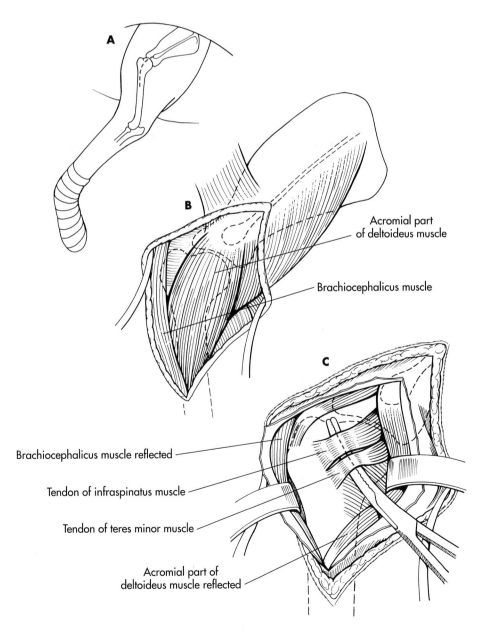

Acromial part of deltoideus muscle

Brachiocephalicus muscle

Brachiocephalicus muscle reflected

Tendon of infraspinatus muscle

Tendon of teres minor muscle

Acromial part of deltoideus muscle reflected

FIG. 29-34
A, To expose the proximal humerus, make an incision over the craniolateral region of the proximal humerus. **B,** Expose deep fascia along the lateral border of the brachiocephalicus muscle and insertion of the deltoid muscle. **C,** Make an incision through the insertions of the infraspinatus and teres minor muscles to expose the lateral surface of the proximal humerus.

FIG. 29-35
A, To expose the distal humeral condyles, make a lateral incision over the distal third of the humerus, extending 4 to 5 cm distal to the ulnar joint. **B,** Incise the intermuscular septum between the extensor carpi radialis and common digital extensor muscles and continue the incision proximally through the periosteal origin of the extensor carpi radialis muscle. **C,** Retract the muscle cranially to expose the joint capsule and underlying lateral condyle. **D,** For further exposure of the epicondyle, incise through the anconeus muscle at its origin on the epicondylar ridge.

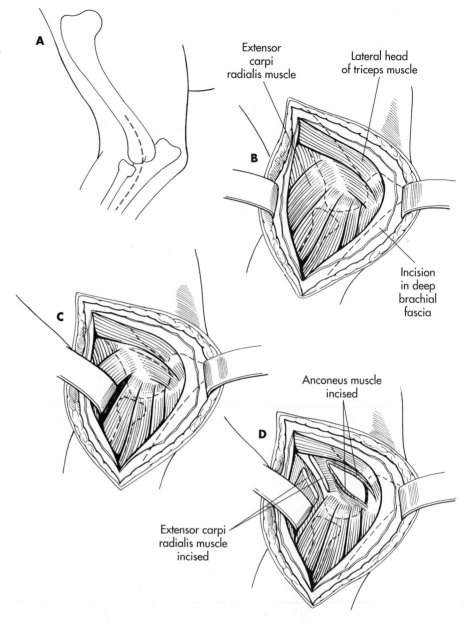

Surgical Approach to the Lateral Condyle and Epicondyle

Make a lateral incision beginning over the distal third of the humerus and extending to a point 4 to 5 cm distal to the joint line overlying the ulna (Fig. 29-35, A). Incise the subcutaneous tissue to expose the deep brachial fascia. Incise the deep fascia along the cranial border of the lateral triceps muscle and continue this incision across the joint line over the extensors. Incise the intermuscular septum between the extensor carpi radialis and the common digital extensor muscle and continue the incision proximally through the periosteal origin of the extensor carpi radialis muscle (Fig. 29-35, B). Retract the muscle cranially to expose the joint capsule and underlying lateral condyle (Fig. 29-35, C). For further exposure of the epicondyle, incise through the anconeus muscle at its origin on the epicondylar ridge (Fig. 29-35, D). Incise the joint capsule with an

L-shape incision to visualize the lateral humeral condyle. To close the incision, suture the joint capsule with interrupted sutures and close the intermuscular septum with a continuous suture pattern. Suture the origins of the external carpi radialis and anconeus muscles together with interrupted sutures and then suture subcutaneous tissue and skin.

Surgical Approach to the Elbow Via Olecranon Osteotomy

Make an incision from the distal third of the humerus to the proximal third of the ulna. Center the incision at the level of the olecranon process over the caudolateral region of the leg. Undermine the subcutaneous tissue such that the caudal skin margin can be reflected over the olecranon process to expose the medial epicondyle. Laterally, free the cranial border of the lateral head of the triceps near its tendinous insertion at the olecranon (Fig. 29-36, A). Next, flex the elbow

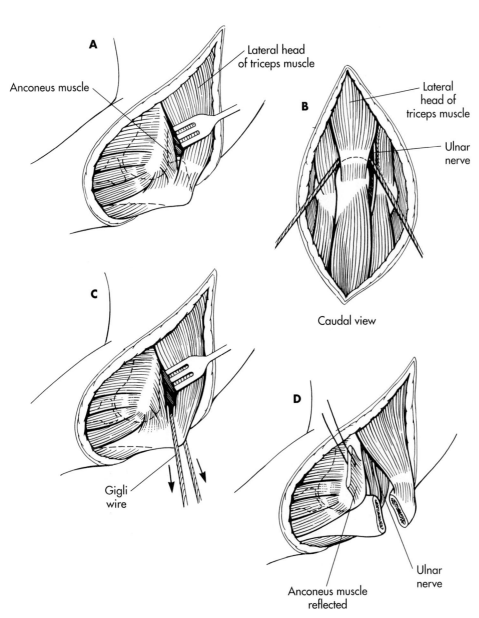

A, Anconeus muscle, Lateral head of triceps muscle

B, Lateral head of triceps muscle, Ulnar nerve, Caudal view

C, Gigli wire

D, Anconeus muscle reflected, Ulnar nerve

FIG. 29-36
A, For osteotomy of the olecranon, free the cranial border of the lateral head of the triceps near its tendinous insertion at the olecranon. **B,** Pass a Gigli wire through a lateral fascial incision to exit through a medial fascial incision. **C,** Pull the wire caudally next to the olecranon beneath the tendon of the triceps. **D,** Incise and retract the anconeus muscle from the lateral and medial epicondylar ridges.

and palpate the ulnar nerve as it courses in the deep fascia along the cranial edge of the medial head of the triceps. The nerve should be isolated and protected during the osteotomy procedure. Incise the fascia along the cranial border of the medial head of the triceps near its insertion at the olecranon. Pass a Gigli wire through the lateral fascial incision so that it exits through the medial fascial incision (Fig. 29-36, B). Pull the wire caudally next to the olecranon beneath the tendon of the triceps (Fig. 29-36, C). Make sure the ulnar nerve is free from the wire and then osteotomize the olecranon process with the Gigli wire. Incise and retract the anconeus muscle from the lateral and medial epicondylar ridges (Fig. 29-36, D), then reflect the olecranon process and triceps muscle proximally to visualize the caudal surface of the elbow joint. For closure, reduce and stabilize the olecranon process with a tension band wire. Suture the border of the triceps to the deep fascia on the medial and lateral sides of the leg and close the subcutaneous tissue and skin.

Surgical Approach to the Elbow Joint Through Osteotomy of the Proximal Ulnar Diaphysis

Begin the incision 6 to 7 cm above the olecranon in the space between the lateral epicondyle and the olecranon process (Fig. 29-37, A). Extend the incision distally along the caudolateral border of the proximal olecranon. Incise the subcutaneous tissue along the same line to expose the deep fascia. Make two incisions in the deep fascia to expose the shaft of the ulna. Make the first incision distally between the ulna and ulnaris lateralis; extend this incision proximally through the insertion of the anconeus muscle on the lateral surface of the olecranon process (Fig. 29-37, B). On the medial surface of the ulna, incise between the flexor carpi ulnaris and bone. Reflect and retract the medial and lateral muscles and place Hohmann retractors in the interosseous space between the radius and ulna to protect soft tissues. Perform an oblique osteotomy of the ulna with

FIG. 29-37
A, For a proximal ulnar diaphyseal osteotomy, begin the incision 6 to 7 cm
above the olecranon in the space between
the lateral epicondyle and olecranon
process. Extend the incision distally along
the caudolateral border of the proximal
olecranon. **B,** Make two incisions in the
deep fascia to expose the shaft of the
ulna. Make the first incision distally between the ulna and ulnaris lateralis; extend
this incision proximally through the insertion of the anconeus muscle on the lateral
surface of the olecranon process. **C,** Perform an oblique osteotomy of the ulna with
a power saw.

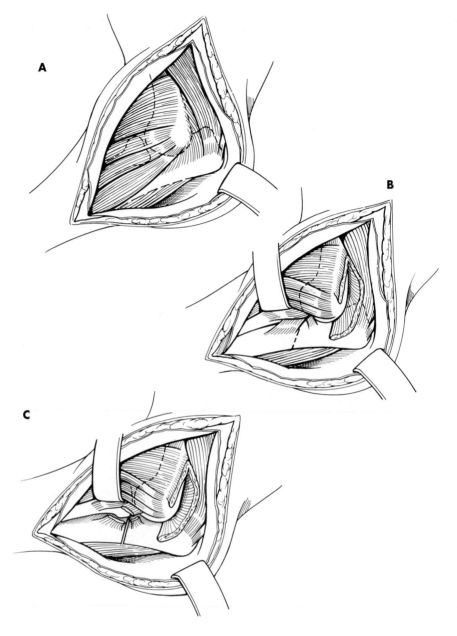

*a power saw (Fig. 29-37, C). The cranial cortex of the ulna
can be cut with an osteotome. On the lateral surface at the
joint line, incise the ulnar collateral ligament and annular
ligament to allow medial rotation of the proximal ulnar segment. This will allow visualization of the elbow joint. To
close, reduce and stabilize the osteotomy with an IM pin
and figure-eight wire. Do not suture the annular or collateral ligaments. Suture the fascia of the lateral and medial
musculature with an interrupted pattern. Suture subcutaneous tissue and skin routinely.*

Stabilization of Proximal Epiphyseal and Metaphyseal Fractures

Patients with gunshot injuries or injuries resulting from
high-velocity motor vehicle accidents generally have comminuted fractures and significant soft tissue injury. Implant
choices in such patients with a low fracture assessment (i.e.,

0 to 3) include a buttress plate, buttress plate/rod construct,
buttress plate/external skeletal fixator (ESF) construct, or
Type Ib external skeletal fixator, with or without an IM pin
tie-in. These fractures may lack intact bone stock proximally
in which to place screws, transfixation pins, or in which to
seat an IM pin. If this is the case, the combination of implant systems (plate/rod, ESF/rod, ESF/plate) allows greater
versatility. Low fracture assessment indicates a lengthy time
to union and dictates that transfixation pins used with ESF
be raised threaded or combined with smooth pins. Comminuted fractures with a moderate fracture assessment (i.e.,
4 to 7) can be repaired using a buttress plate or a Type Ia or
Type Ib ESF, with or without an IM pin tie-in. Patients with
a low or moderate fracture assessment and a simple fracture
pattern (i.e., transverse, oblique) are best treated using a
compression plate or neutralization plate (Fig. 29-38). Alternatively, an IM pin combined with cerclage wire and sup-

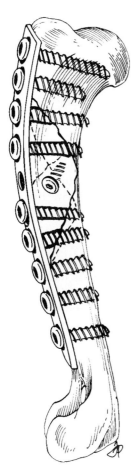

FIG. 29-38
Reduction and stabilization of a comminuted fracture with a single, large fragment using interfragmentary compression screws and a neutralization plate. (From Olmstead ML: *Small animal orthopedics,* St Louis, 1995, Mosby.)

ported with a Type Ia ESF can be used. Physeal fractures of the proximal humerus in juvenile patients with favorable fracture-assessment scores (i.e., 8 to 10) may be closed reduced and stabilized with diverging Kirschner wires or small Steinmann pins if adequate reduction can be achieved. The pins should enter the bone proximally at the greater tubercle and be driven distocaudally to cross the fracture line and seat in the caudal metaphysis. If closed reduction is not possible, open reduction and pin stabilization should be performed.

Lateral or Medial Condyle Fractures

In adults, stabilization is best attained with an intercondylar compression screw combined with a pin bridging the fracture of the epicondyloid crest (Table 29-8). In older patients, or those with injury or disease of another limb, a compression plate placed across the epicondyloid crest should be used. Intercondylar compression can be achieved in one of three ways. A partially threaded cancellous bone screw can be placed such that the smooth shaft of the screw crosses the fracture line and the threads only purchase bone across the fracture plane, a cortical screw can be placed us-

TABLE 29-8
Implant Use According to Fracture-Assessment Score (FAS) for Humeral Condylar Fractures
FAS 4 to 10
• Compression screw plus pin
FAS 0 to 3
• Compression plate plus screw

ing a glide hole drilled in the lateral condyle and a thread hole drilled in the medial condyle, or a position screw can be placed after the fracture is reduced and compressed with bone holding forceps.

If a partially threaded cancellous screw or a position screw is used, the fracture is reduced and held in position with bone-holding forceps and Kirschner pins are placed perpendicular to the fracture surface. Take care to not place the Kirschner pins where they will interfere with the bone screw. Drill the thread hole for the screw and measure and tap it. Start the thread hole at a point 1 to 2 mm cranial and distal to the lateral epicondyle and exit it near the medial epicondyle. Remove the Kirschner pins or leave them in place if they are not interfering with normal function of the elbow joint. If a cortical screw is to be used as a compression screw, drill the glide hole prior to reducing the fracture. The glide hole may be drilled from the fracture surface to exit at the lateral epicondyle or, alternatively, from the lateral epicondyle to exit at the fracture surface. Reduce the fracture and hold it in position with bone-holding forceps and Kirschner pins placed perpendicular to the fracture surface. Take care to not place the Kirschner pins where they will interfere with the bone screw. Place an appropriately-sized drill sleeve in the glide hole and drill, measure, then tap the thread hole to accept the appropriate screw. As before, the Kirschner pins can be left in place or removed. Additional rotational support can be achieved by placement of a small pin or caudal bone plate across the lateral epicondyloid crest (Fig. 29-39).

Fracture assessment in immature toy breeds of dogs with lateral condylar fractures is extremely favorable for rapid bone union. Stabilization can be accomplished by intercondylar compression achieved with a bone screw and a small pin crossing the epicondyloid crest for rotational support. Alternatively, stabilization can be accomplished with small pins placed at diverging angles. If the latter method is chosen, patient selection is critical: these patients are often hyperactive and difficult for the owners to confine. This, coupled with the soft cancellous bone of a young dog, makes premature pin migration and displacement of the fracture surface a factor to consider. With either method of stabilization, implant application can be attempted through closed reduction. Implant position is identical to that described previously for adult patients. If postoperative radiographs

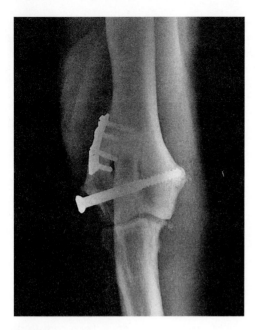

FIG. 29-39
Postoperative radiograph showing stabilization of a lateral condylar fracture with a transcondylar screw and plate.

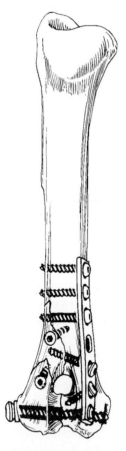

FIG. 29-40
Stabilization of a Y fracture of the elbow with a transcondylar lag screw supplemented with a buttress plate applied to the caudal or lateral aspect of the distal humerus. (From Olmstead ML: *Small animal orthopedics*, St Louis, 1995, Mosby.)

show that anatomic alignment is not satisfactory, open reduction and implant insertion is indicated. Alternatively, open reduction and stabilization can be used as the primary method of treatment.

T or Y Fractures of the Elbow

These fractures most commonly occur due to a motor vehicle accident or a fall from a significant height. The intercondylar fracture is accompanied by a transverse, oblique, or comminuted fracture through the medial and lateral epicondyloid crests. Open reduction is necessary for accurate alignment of the intercondylar fracture. The method of stabilization depends upon the patient fracture assessment. Those with a low assessment (i.e., 0 to 3) require an implant system rigid enough to resist major weight-bearing loads and able to maintain that rigidity for an extended period of time. A compression screw is recommended for the intercondylar fracture; the condyles can be affixed to the humerus with a plate/rod combination or medial and/or lateral plates (Fig. 29-40). When a plate/rod system is used, the IM pin is placed in the medial position and the bone plate placed caudolaterally. As well, the condyles may be affixed to the shaft of the humerus by using a plate applied to the caudomedial epicondyloid crest with a second plate applied to the caudolateral epicondyloid crest. Elbow fractures in patients with an intermediate fracture assessment (i.e., 4 to 7) can be managed with an intercondylar compression screw with the condyles affixed to the humeral diaphysis with a medially applied bone plate or two IM pins. One pin passes through the medial epicondyloid crest, across the fracture plane, and into the proximal segment of the humerus. The pin will exit the bone near the greater tubercle. A second pin is placed through the lateral epicondyloid crest and across the fracture to exit the metaphysis of the proximal segment of the humerus. Elbow fractures in patients with a favorable fracture assessment (i.e., 8 to 10) can be managed with an intercondylar compression screw and two pins placed as described above. Small diverging pins can be substituted for the compression screw if the patient is young and not overly active.

SUTURE MATERIALS/SPECIAL INSTRUMENTS

Helpful instruments for fracture repair include a battery- or air-driven drill and self-retaining retractors. Each implant system has special requirements for application.

POSTOPERATIVE CARE AND ASSESSMENT

Daily monitoring of the surgical wound and general well-being of the patient is required. Activity should be restricted to leash walking until the fracture has healed. Radiographs to assess healing should be made if complications arise or when the fracture is expected to have healed based on the estimated time to union. Physical therapy (i.e., gentle flexion and extension of the joints above and below the fracture and muscle massage) enhances use of the limb and maintains flexibility.

This should be done once or twice daily. Communication with the client to inquire about patient progress and to reinforce activity constraints should be done on a weekly basis.

PROGNOSIS

Epiphyseal fractures of the humerus generally heal without complication. This is particularly true in young patients because of their favorable healing potential. Nevertheless, implants can loosen or break. Either complication is often due to poor implant choice relative to the fracture-assessment score (see p. 730). Loosening and migration of IM pins, ESF transfixation pins, and/or cerclage wire are examples of what can occur with poor preoperative decision making. With improper decisions, the implant and its connections to bone may be subject to high stress causing micromotion at the implant-bone interface. Alternatively, if healing is prolonged, the implant may be subjected to moderate stresses for extended periods. In either case, bone resorption and implant loosening eventually result. Fatigue breakage of implants can occur. This is most often noted in patients treated with bone plates when unsuccessful reduction and stabilization of a zone of comminution with cerclage wire (or lag screws) cause devascularized bone fragments and small fracture gaps. The small gaps are unfavorable for healing and concentrate stress over a small section of the bone plate resulting in delayed healing and long-term cyclic stress on the bone plate. If the initial implant system fails, application of a compression bone plate or a plate/rod construct is recommended. These systems serve to stabilize the fracture and increase patient comfort, which in turn optimizes limb use and allows physical therapy to begin.

Suggested Reading

Anderson SM, Lippincott CL, Schulman AJ: Longitudinal myotomy of the flexor carpi radialis: a new approach to the medial aspect of the elbow joint, *J Am Anim Hosp Assoc* 25:499, 1989.

Cockett PA, Clayton-Jones DG: The repair of humeral condylar fractures in the dog: a review of seventy-nine cases, *J Sm An Pract* 26:493, 1985.

Kaderly RE, Lamothe M: Incomplete humeral condylar fracture due to minor trauma in a mature cocker spaniel, *J Am Anim Hosp Assoc* 28:361, 1992.

Marcellin-Little DJ et al: Incomplete ossification of the humeral condyle in spaniels, *Vet Surg* 23:475, 1994.

Mattiesson DT, Walter M: Surgical management of distal humeral fractures, *Compend Cont Educ Pract Vet* 6:1027, 1984.

Piermattei DL, Greely RG: *An atlas of surgical approaches to the bones of the dog and cat*, ed 2, Philadelphia, 1980, Saunders.

Tomlinson JL, Constantinescu GM: Fixations of lateral humeral condylar fractures with multiple Kirschner wires, In Bojrab MG, editor: *Current techniques in small animal surgery*, ed 3, Philadelphia. London, 1990, Lea & Febiger.

Turner TM, Hohn RB: Craniolateral approach to the canine elbow for repair of condylar fractures or joint exploration, *J Am Vet Med Assoc* 176:1264, 1980.

Vannini R, Olmstead ML, Smeak DD: Humeral condylar fractures caused by minor trauma in 20 adult dogs, *J Am Anim Hosp Assoc* 24:355, 1988.

Vannini R, Smeak DD, Olmstead ML: Evaluation of surgical repair of 135 distal humeral fractures in dogs and cats, *J Am Anim Hosp Assoc* 24:537, 1988.

RADIAL AND ULNAR FRACTURES

RADIAL AND ULNAR DIAPHYSEAL FRACTURES

DEFINITIONS

Radial and **ulnar diaphyseal fractures** are a result of trauma to the forelimb. **Open fractures** (wounds through the skin over the bone) may occur because of the sparse soft tissue coverage.

GENERAL CONSIDERATIONS AND CLINICALLY RELEVANT PATHOPHYSIOLOGY

Fractures of the radius and ulna make up 8.5% to 18% of all fractures in dogs and cats (Rudd, Whitehair, 1992). Diaphyseal fractures are most common and usually involve the middle to distal diaphysis of both bones. Usually these fractures are secondary to trauma; consequently, the animal should be closely evaluated to detect concurrent injuries (e.g., pulmonary contusions, pneumothorax, rib fractures, and/or traumatic myocarditis). Because of the minimal soft tissue coverage of the bone, open fractures are common.

DIAGNOSIS
Clinical Presentation

Signalment. Any age, breed, or sex of dog or cat may be affected. Young animals sustain vehicular trauma more frequently.

History. Affected animals usually present with a non-weight-bearing lameness after trauma. Occasionally, owners are unaware that trauma occurred.

Physical Examination Findings

Because of the traumatic nature of this injury the entire animal must be assessed to detect abnormalities of other body systems. Palpation of the limb reveals swelling, pain, and crepitation. The fracture may be open. Affected animals often appear to have abnormal proprioceptive responses due to a reluctance to move the limb.

Radiography

Craniocaudal and lateral radiographs of the affected radius and ulna (which include the proximal and distal joints) are required to assess the extent of bone and soft tissue injury. Fractious or extremely painful animals may require sedation for radiography after it has been determined that contraindications (i.e., shock, hypotension, severe dyspnea) for administration of sedatives do not exist. Thoracic radiography should be performed to evaluate pulmonary changes.

Laboratory Findings

Complete blood count and serum chemistry evaluation should be done to evaluate the status of the animal for anesthesia and determine if concurrent injury or damage of the renal or hepatobiliary systems exists.

DIFFERENTIAL DIAGNOSIS

Animals presenting with radial and ulnar fractures should be evaluated to determine whether fractures are the result of trauma or underlying pathology (i.e., neoplasia or metabolic disease).

MEDICAL OR CONSERVATIVE MANAGEMENT

Medical treatment of animals with radial and ulnar fractures may include analgesics (see p. 708) and antibiotics to treat open fractures. Conservative management of radial and ulnar diaphyseal fractures consists of splints and casts and is reserved for closed nondisplaced or greenstick fractures in immature animals. Cast fixation is appropriate for these fractures because the joint above and below the fractured bone (i.e., elbow and carpus) can be immobilized, and they heal rapidly.

SURGICAL TREATMENT

The decision to perform an open or a closed reduction of radial and ulnar diaphyseal fractures is made based upon fracture configuration and fracture-assessment score (Table 29-9). Simple or moderately comminuted fractures with large fragments that can be anatomically reconstructed to establish the bone column are candidates for open reduction and stabilization with internal fixation, external skeletal fixation, or a combination of techniques. Severely comminuted fractures that cannot be completely reconstructed are candidates for closed reduction and external skeletal fixation or open reduction and application of a buttress plate and cancellous bone autograft (see p. 760). Whether the fracture is open or closed is less important than the potential of the fracture to be anatomically reconstructed. Advantages and disadvantages of open and closed reduction need to be weighed to determine the best approach for each individual fracture. The ulna is usually supported indirectly by radial stabilization; however, stabilization of the ulna is indicated when doing so will add support to a comminuted radial fracture, when

additional support is needed for a large dog, and when anatomic reduction of radius and ulna is essential to future performance of an athlete. Fixation systems applicable to fractures of the radial and ulnar diaphysis are casts, intramedullary pins (ulna), external skeletal fixation, and plates and screws.

Application of Casts

Casts can be applied as the sole method of fixation for stable fractures in young dogs or cats when the fracture will maintain adequate reduction and heal quickly (see p. 734 for technique of cast application). The cast is applied so that it immobilizes the carpus and elbow. Although manipulation of the fracture is rarely possible during casting, the limb should be positioned with slight carpal flexion and varus angulation (Fig. 29-41). The cast can be applied over extra cast padding, cut longitudinally along the medial and lateral surfaces, and taped in position to form a "bivalve cast" that can be changed

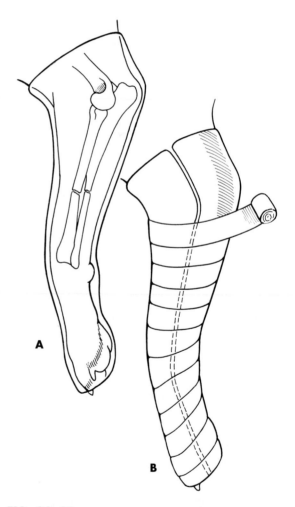

FIG. 29-41
Casts are used to stabilize closed, nondisplaced radial/ulna fractures in patients with fracture-assessment scores between 8 and 10. **A,** A full cylinder cast, which immobilizes the elbow and carpus, is placed with the limb positioned in slight carpal flexion and varus angulation. **B,** The cast can be bivalved by placing the cast material over multiple layers of padding, cutting it on the lateral and medial aspects, and securing it with elastic tape.

TABLE 29-9

Decision Making for Open or Closed Reduction

Open Reduction
- Displaced fractures
- Simple fractures
- Comminuted fractures necessitating a cancellous bone graft

Closed Reduction
- Nondisplaced fractures
- Comminuted fractures that cannot be anatomically reconstructed

periodically. This type of cast does not offer as rigid a fixation as a cylinder cast, but is useful as additional support with pin or plate fixation and is easily changed to allow wound treatment.

Application of Intramedullary (IM) Pins

IM pins are difficult to use in the radius because of the narrow configuration of the radial medullary canal and necessity of invading the carpal joint to position the pin. Complications associated with IM pin placement in the radius include angulation, distraction, rotation, osteomyelitis, delayed union, nonunion, and degenerative joint disease of the elbow and carpus. These complications were reported to occur in 80% of animals with radial diaphyseal fractures treated with IM pins in one study (Lappin et al, 1983).

An IM pin can be used to align the ulna, stabilize a simple ulnar fracture, and add support to the primary fixation of a comminuted radial fracture (i.e., external fixator or plate). Refer to p. 742 for techniques for IM pins. The IM pin should be introduced into the medullary canal from the proximal surface of the olecranon and driven in an antegrade manner to the fracture surface. Care should be taken to parallel the lateral cortex of the ulna to maintain the pin within the medullary canal. Once the fracture is aligned, the pin should be driven distally as far as possible without penetrating the cortex. The pin is cut below the level of the skin, over the proximal ulna.

Application of External Skeletal Fixators

Type Ia or Ib frames. External skeletal fixation (see p. 735) is particularly useful for treating a wide variety of radial diaphyseal fractures. The stiffness of the fixator can be increased in animals with low fracture-assessment scores by adding fixation pins and using bilateral and biplanar frames. Radial fractures are frequently open, making use of external fixation attractive for avoiding invasion of the fracture site with metal implants. With open fractures, implant removal is desirable after fracture healing and easily accomplished with external fixation. A Type Ia (unilateral external fixation splint) is usually applied to the cranial medial surface of the radius (Fig. 29-42, *A* and *B*). Applying it to this location avoids penetration of the major muscle masses with the fixation pins and decreases the morbidity associated with the pins. When a Type Ib fixation splint is applied, every effort should be made to locate the fixation pins in areas of bone that have minimal muscle coverage (Fig. 29-42, *C*).

☞ **N O T E** · Construct the fixator to suit the patient and the fracture. A lower fracture-assessment score requires a stiffer fixator.

Type II frames. Penetration of major muscle masses is unavoidable with Type II or bilateral fixation splints; they are often favored because of their increased stiffness, however. The fixation splint should span the length of the bone with the most proximal and distal pins placed in the metaphyses and the central pins placed about 1 to 2 cm from the fracture line. Additional pins can be placed when there is adequate bone. Apply smaller fixation pins to the medial or lateral surface of the radius to avoid splitting the bone. Type II frames with transfixation pins that are clamped on both bars are placed in the following manner (see p. 736 for general principles of external fixation application). The initial transfixation pins should be placed in the proximal and distal metaphyses of the radius. These pins should be centered in the bone on the medial to lateral plane and parallel to the respective joint surfaces. The fracture is reduced by distracting the transfixation pins manually, using the weight of the animal in the hanging limb position, or with a fracture distractor placed on the concave side of the fracture (see p. 757 for fracture reduction). Open reduction through a limited approach may be used to facilitate reconstruction of the bone column in simple fractures.

Severely comminuted fractures are usually reduced in a closed manner. The medial and lateral connecting bars containing the predetermined number of clamps are applied to the transfixation pins. A third connecting bar is secured with three clamps to the transfixation pins on one side of the limb. The remaining transfixation pins are placed using the guide bar to ensure proper alignment of the pins with the clamps. At least two pins (preferably three) should be placed proximal and distal to the fracture. If the anterior curve of the radius precludes the placement of bilateral transfixation pins, unilateral pins can be applied to the diaphysis of the radius (Fig. 29-43). If additional rigidity is necessary a Type III fixation splint should be constructed at this time. Postoperative radiographs should be taken to ensure that appropriate fracture reduction, pin placement, and joint alignment were achieved. Valgus or varus deformities can be corrected by loosening the clamps and distracting the appropriate side of the limb (see p. 872). Mild rotation can be corrected by reversing the position of the clamps on the appropriate side of the pins in the distal fragment. Every effort should be made to achieve correct alignment of the limb before the procedure is completed.

Methylmethacrylate fixators. External fixation with fixation pins and methylmethacrylate connecting bars is a versatile alternative to the standard external fixation system (see p. 736). Fixation pins of any size can be directed at angles which optimize the purchase of good quality bone, without regard for clamp compatibility or uniplanar pin placement. This technique is useful to rigidly stabilize distal diaphyseal fractures in toy-breed dogs.

Application of Bone Plates and Screws

Bone plates are an excellent method of stabilizing radial and ulnar diaphyseal fractures. Plates are usually applied to the wide, flat, cranial surface of the radius—they are equally effective when applied to the medial surface of the distal radius to stabilize transverse distal diaphyseal fractures (see p. 750 for plating techniques). A wide exposure of the fracture and intact bone is needed for fracture reconstruction and plate application. Plates are applied as compression plates to transverse fractures. Long oblique or spiral fractures should be reconstructed and the fracture lines compressed with lag screws. The reconstructed fracture is protected with a neutralization plate. Comminuted diaphyseal fractures that cannot be reconstructed can be treated by

FIG. 29-42
Type Ia and Ib external fixators are used to treat radial fractures in patients with high and moderate fracture-assessment scores. **A,** Sequence for placement of a Type I external fixator on the cranial craniomedial surface of the radius: (1) Place unilateral fixation pins in the proximal and distal metaphyses, entering the pins from the craniomedial aspect of the limb. (2) Add the connecting bar and appropriate number of pin-gripping clamps. (3) Place the remainder of the fixation pins through the clamps and into the bone diaphysis. **B,** Anatomic reconstruction of a long oblique fracture with cerclage wire restores the bone column and allows load-sharing with the external fixator. **C,** A Type Ib fixator is applied to patients with moderate fracture-assessment scores.

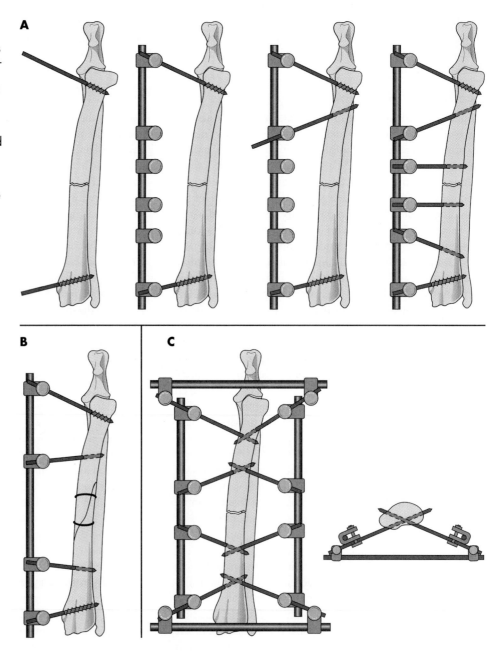

distracting the fracture, realigning the limb, and bridging the fracture with a buttress plate (Fig. 29-44). If open reduction of the fractured radius is performed, consideration should be given to harvesting autogenous cancellous bone to enhance bone healing. The most accessible site for cancellous bone harvest is the ipsilateral proximal humerus (see p. 760). The ipsilateral ilium and tibia can also be prepared for cancellous bone harvest.

SURGICAL TREATMENT
Preoperative Management

There may be extensive damage and/or loss of tissues in the area of the fracture. Open wounds should be managed initially by carefully clipping surrounding hair, cleaning the wound, and taking a swab for bacterial culture and suscep-

tibility testing. The antebrachium should be temporarily stabilized with a Robert Jones bandage (see p. 706) to immobilize fragments, decrease or prevent soft tissue swelling, protect or prevent open wounds, and increase patient comfort until surgery can be performed. Concurrent injuries should be managed before anesthetic induction for fracture fixation.

Anesthesia

Anesthetic management of animals with fractures is discussed on p. 708.

Surgical Anatomy

The craniomedial surface of the radius and the caudal lateral surface of the ulna are not covered by muscle and can be eas-

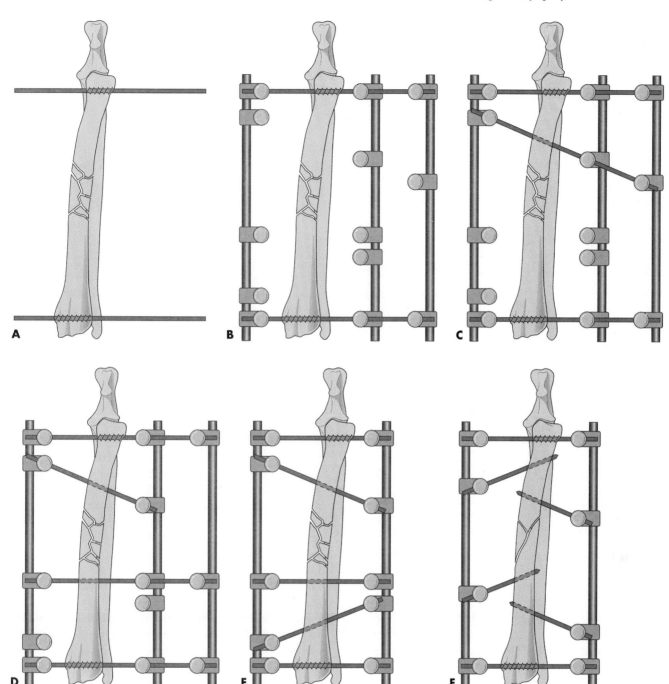

FIG. 29-43

Type II external fixators are used to treat radial fractures in patients with moderate and low fracture-assessment scores. The sequence for placement of a Type II external fixator on the radius is as follows: **A,** Place transfixation pins in the proximal and distal metaphyses of the bone parallel to their respective joint surface; **B,** secure the medial and lateral connecting bars containing the predetermined number of clamps to the transfixation pins; secure a third connecting bar with three clamps to the transfixation pins on one side of the limb; **C** and **D,** place the remaining transfixation pins using the guide bar to ensure proper alignment of the pins with the clamps; cut each pin before moving the guide clamp to the next position; **E,** cut the excess pin and tighten the clamps. **F,** Because of the anterior curve of the radius, unilateral pins may be used to fill out the Type II frame.

FIG. 29-44
Radial/ulnar fractures in patients with moderate and low fracture-assessment scores can be treated with plate fixation to ensure adequate stabilization for fracture healing. **A,** Transverse fractures are treated with a compression plate, which can be placed on the cranial or medial surface of the distal radius; **B,** long oblique fractures are treated with interfragmentary lag screws and a neutralization plate; **C,** comminuted fractures are treated with a buttress plate. An intramedullary pin can be placed in the ulna to provide additional support.

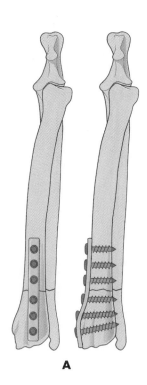

A

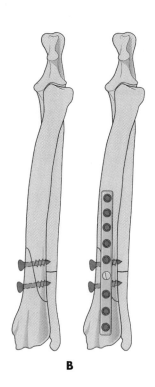

B

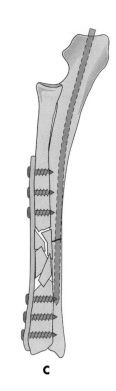

C

ily palpated to serve as landmarks for location of the incision. Extensor muscles are located cranial and flexor muscles caudal to the radius and can be retracted to expose the bone. The cephalic vein crosses the medial portion of the distal radius. The lateral radial head is palpable beneath the extensor muscles of the forearm.

Positioning

The limb should be prepped from shoulder to carpus. If cancellous bone graft harvest is anticipated, a donor site (e.g., proximal humerus) should also be prepared. If closed reduction or limited open reduction with external skeletal fixation is chosen, positioning the animal with the affected leg suspended from the ceiling facilitates visualization of correct joint alignment (p. 760). If open reduction is performed the animal is also positioned in dorsal recumbency and the limb is draped out.

SURGICAL TECHNIQUE
Craniomedial Approach to the Radius

Palpate the radius directly under the skin and subcutaneous tissue on the craniomedial surface of the limb. Make an incision through skin and subcutaneous tissue to expose the radial diaphysis. Extend the incision distally and elevate the extensor tendons to expose the cranial surface of the distal metaphysis of the radius (Fig. 29-45).

Approaches to the Proximal and Distal Ulna

See pp. 812 and 821 for approaches to the proximal and distal ulna, respectively.

Stabilization of Midshaft Transverse or Short Oblique Radial Fractures

From a mechanical perspective, this fracture configuration allows load sharing between the bone and implant following surgery. Factors that negatively affect healing include multiple limb injuries and a large and active patient. From a biologic perspective, patient fracture assessment dictates whether the time until union will be lengthy or short. With prolonged healing the implant needs to remain functional for 8 or more weeks. In these cases, implants that purchase bone with threads are desirable; frictional hold implants are adequate for shorter healing periods.

Stabilization of a transverse or short oblique fracture requires rotational and bending support. This can be achieved with bone plates, an external fixator, or a cast. The final implant choice should be determined by the fracture location and patient fracture assessment. Useful fixation systems in toy-breed dogs (in which the complication rate is high with these fractures) and in animals with a low fracture assessment (i.e., 0 to 3) include a bone plate and screws inserted to function as a compression plate, or a Type II or III external skeletal fixator with raised threaded transfixation pins. With a moderate fracture assessment (i.e., 4 to 7), a compression plate, Type II external skeletal fixator, or Type Ia or Ib external skeletal fixator would serve. The transfixation pins can be a combination of smooth, negative-profile, and raised-threaded pins depending on the length of time the fixator must stay in place. Transverse or short oblique fractures in patients with a high patient fracture assessment (i.e., 8 to 10) can be stabilized with a 4- to 6-pin Type Ia external skeletal fixator or cast.

Medial
view

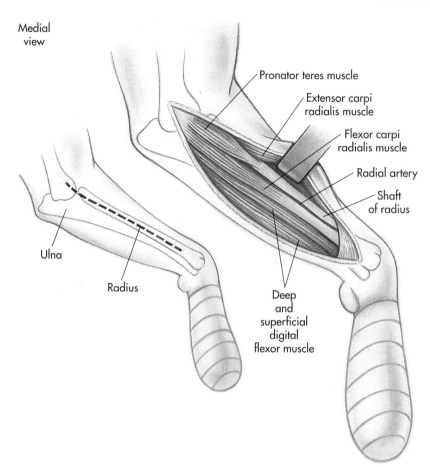

Pronator teres muscle

Extensor carpi
radialis muscle

Flexor carpi
radialis muscle

Radial artery

Shaft
of radius

Ulna

Radius

Deep
and
superficial
digital
flexor muscle

FIG. 29-45
For a craniomedial approach to the radial
diaphysis, make an incision through skin and
subcutaneous tissues to expose the radial
diaphysis. Retract the extensor carpi radialis
muscle laterally to expose the diaphysis.

Stabilization of Midshaft Long Oblique Radial Fractures or Comminuted Fractures With a Large Butterfly Fragment

From a mechanical perspective, these fractures can be reduced and interfragmentary compression applied with cerclage wire or lag screws. Once the interfragmentary fracture lines are reduced and compressed, the bone and implant can bear weight postoperatively. Factors that negatively affect healing include the presence of multiple injuries, a large, active patient, and the necessity for open reduction and tissue manipulation to reduce and apply interfragmentary compression. If a prolonged healing period is expected, the implant needs to remain functional for 8 or more weeks; those implants that purchase bone with threads are desirable. With shorter healing periods, implants which have frictional hold (smooth pins and wire) are adequate.

Stabilization of this fracture configuration requires axial, rotational, and bending support. This can be achieved with bone plates or cerclage wire/external fixator combinations. Fixation systems that are useful with a low patient fracture assessment (i.e., 0 to 3) are neutralization plates or rigid external skeletal fixators. Interfragmentary compression is first achieved with wire or compression screws to reconstruct the cylinder of bone and the area then bridged with a bone plate. Alternatively, interfragmentary compression can be applied with cerclage wire and additional support supplied by an external skeletal fixator. With a moderate fracture assessment

(i.e., 4 to 7), lag screws or cerclage wire for interfragmentary compression combined with a neutralization plate or Type Ia, Ib, or II external skeletal fixator may be used. Transfixation pins should have a raised thread or have a negative thread profile. With a high patient fracture assessment (i.e., 8 to 10) cerclage wire for interfragmentary compression combined with a Type Ia external skeletal fixator is a useful method to stabilize the fracture.

Stabilization of Midshaft Comminuted Radial Fractures With Multiple Fragments

From a mechanical perspective these fractures cannot be reduced without significant soft tissue manipulation and no load sharing between the implant and bone occurs until biologic callus forms to provide support. Very high stresses will therefore be imposed on the implant and its connection to the bone. If the biologic assessment is favorable, the imposed stresses will be of short duration and the likelihood of implant failure is lessened. However, if the biologic assessment is not favorable, imposed stresses will act on the implant for an extended period and implant failure becomes more likely. Enhancing the biologic response by not attempting to reduce the fragments (closed reduction and bridging osteosynthesis) and inserting an autogenous cancellous bone graft (when appropriate) is recommended. From a mechanical perspective, these types of fractures need rigid axial, rotational, and bending support.

Stabilization of patients with low fracture-assessment scores (i.e., 0 to 3) is best achieved with a bone plate used in a buttress fashion, or Type II or III external skeletal fixation. The transfixation pins should have a raised thread and at least three pins should be applied above and two pins below the area of comminution (or vice versa). It is always better to err on the side of too much rigidity rather than too little since the fixator can be destabilized postoperatively. A patient with a moderate fracture assessment (i.e., 4 to 7) can be managed with a bone plate functioning as a buttress plate. A Type II or Ib external skeletal fixator may also be used. The choice of frame, number of pins, and pin design for the external skeletal fixator depend on the fracture assessment. The only time a patient with this type of fracture would have a high fracture assessment rating (i.e., 8 to 10) would be when the biologic assessment is extremely favorable (e.g., a 4- to 5-month-old animal with a low velocity, closed, single limb injury). These animals could be managed using bridging osteosynthesis with a Type II or Type Ib external skeletal fixator. The transfixation pins can be smooth or have a negative thread profile depending on the amount of time the fixator needs to remain in place.

SUTURE MATERIALS/SPECIAL INSTRUMENTS

Equipment necessary for pin and wire placement includes retractors, bone-holding forceps, reduction forceps, Jacob pin chuck, IM pins, Kirschner wires, and orthopedic wire. Additional equipment needed for external fixation includes a low-rpm power drill and external fixation clamps and bars or acrylic. Plating equipment and a high-speed drill are necessary for application of plates and screws.

POSTOPERATIVE CARE AND ASSESSMENT

Postoperative radiographs should be made to document fracture reduction or alignment and implant position. Casts require intensive management by owners and frequent evaluations by the veterinarian. Abrasions and wounds caused by pressure from the cast are a common occurrence. Treatment involves removal of the cast or replacement with a bivalve cast, and wound treatment. Early destabilization of the fracture to treat wounds can cause delayed unions and nonunions. After internal fixation a soft, padded bandage should be applied for a few days to control swelling and support soft tissues.

After open reduction with external skeletal fixation, the incision should be covered but the fixation splint may be left exposed. Open wounds should be treated daily with wet-to-dry dressings until a granulation bed has formed. Wounds are then covered with a nonadhesive pad and the bandage changed as needed. Daily hydrotherapy aids in cleaning open wounds, reduces postoperative swelling, and cleans pin sites. The animal should be released to the owner with instructions to limit exercise, avoid fixator snares, and administer daily hydrotherapy with a hand held shower massage. Checkups should be scheduled at 2 weeks for suture removal and fixator evaluation, and every 4 or 6 weeks for radiographic evaluation. Although a rigidly stabilized fracture site is optimal for initial bone formation, subsequent bone remodeling is enhanced by increasing the load through the fractured bone. Removal of one half of a Type Ib external fixation splint or selected transfixation pins from a Type I or Type II splint decreases rigidity of the fixator allowing more load on the remodeling bone, while still protecting the healing fracture. Destabilization is usually done at 6 to 8 weeks after surgery, depending on the fracture-assessment. There should be some radiographic evidence of bone formation and bridging of the fracture site before destabilization is done. The external fixation splint can be removed completely when there is radiographic evidence of bone bridging of the fracture lines. A support bandage or a splint may be used to protect the healing bone for a few weeks after fixator removal.

After placement of a plate on a diaphyseal fracture the limb should be supported for a few days with a soft padded bandage to reduce swelling. The animal will usually be fully weight bearing within 2 to 3 weeks.

Confinement is recommended until there are radiographic signs of bone union. Although long-term plate application does not appear to have an effect on radial cortical bone density, plate removal is usually recommended after bone union because tissue irritation and cold sensitivity have been associated with the minimal soft tissue coverage over the plate.

PROGNOSIS

Complications with radial fractures include malunion, delayed union, and nonunion in animals treated with external coaptation (Table 29-10). These are common in toy breed dogs sustaining fractures of the distal radial and ulnar diaphyses that have been inadequately stabilized. Treatment involves open reduction and application of a bone plate and cancellous bone autograft. Complications after open reduction include osteomyelitis, implant migration and irritation of soft tissues, malunion, delayed union, and nonunion. Complications encountered with external fixation of the radius include pin loosening and pin tract drainage. Usually neither of these problems is severe enough to warrant pin removal until the fracture has healed. Rarely, severe hemorrhage occurs from the medial exit hole of a proximal pin after the pin has eroded through an artery. Removal of the pin, and in some cases, ligation of the vessel is necessary to control hemorrhage.

TABLE 29-10

Common Errors

- IM pin placement through the carpus causes degenerative joint disease and loss of function
- Inadequate rotational stabilization for transverse or short oblique fractures causes delayed union or nonunion, especially in toy-breed dogs
- Premature removal of fixation from slowly healing distal radial fractures contributes to the formation of nonunions
- Valgus deformities after comminuted fracture fixation occur because of malalignment with the external fixator

References

Lappin MR et al: Fractures of the radius and ulna in the dog, *J Am Anim Hosp Assoc* 19:643, 1983.

Rudd RG, Whitehair JG: Fractures of the radius and ulna, *Vet Clin N Am: Small Anim Pract* 22:135, 1992.

Suggested Reading

Aron DN, Toombs JP, Hollingsworth SC: Primary treatment of severe fractures by external skeletal fixation: threaded pins compared with smooth pins, *J Am Anim Hosp Assoc* 22:659, 1986.

Glennon JC et al: The effect of long-term bone plate application for fixation of radial fractures in the dog, *Vet Surg* 23:40, 1994.

Johnson AL, Kneller SK, Weigel RM: Radial and tibial fracture repair with external skeletal fixation: effects of fracture type, reduction, and complications on healing, *Vet Surg* 18:367, 1989.

Marti JM, Miller A: Delimitation of safe corridors for the insertion of external fixator pins in the dog, II. Forelimb, *J Small Anim Pract* 35:78, 1994.

Tomlinson JL, Constantinescu GM: Acrylic external skeletal fixation of fractures, *Compend Cont Educ Pract Vet* Pr13:235, 1991.

Wallace MK et al: Mechanical evaluation of three methods of plating distal radial osteotomies, *Vet Surg* 21:99, 1992.

Waters DJ, Breur GJ, Toombs JP: Treatment of common forelimb fractures in miniature and toy breed dogs, *J Am Anim Hosp Assoc* 29:442, 1993.

RADIAL AND ULNAR METAPHYSEAL AND EPIPHYSEAL FRACTURES

DEFINITIONS

Metaphyseal and **epiphyseal fractures** occur in trabecular bone. **Articular fractures** disrupt the joint surface. A **Monteggia fracture** is a fracture of the ulna coupled with a dislocation of the radial head.

GENERAL CONSIDERATIONS AND CLINICALLY RELEVANT PATHOPHYSIOLOGY

Fracture of the proximal ulna may occur singularly or in combination with luxation of the radial head (i.e., Monteggia fracture). The fracture may involve the articular surface of the trochlear notch. The pull of the triceps muscle displaces the proximal segment of the ulna and must be neutralized by internal fixation to achieve bone union.

Fractures of the proximal radius are rare because the radial head is well protected by surrounding musculature. Fractures of the distal radius may be extraarticular or intraarticular. Intraarticular fractures usually disrupt the medial epicondyle and result in loss of ligamentous support for the carpus. The ligamentous attachment on the epicondyle causes displacement of the fragment that must be neutralized with internal fixation. Fractures of the styloid process of the ulna cause similar disruptions to the lateral aspect of the carpus.

DIAGNOSIS
Clinical Presentation

Signalment. Any age, breed, or sex of dog or cat may be affected. Young animals more frequently sustain vehicular trauma.

History. Affected animals usually present with a non-weight bearing lameness after trauma. Occasionally, owners are unaware that trauma occurred.

Physical Examination Findings

Because of the traumatic nature of this injury, the entire animal must be assessed to detect abnormalities of other body systems. Palpation of the limb reveals swelling, pain, crepitation, and apparent instability of the adjacent joint. Degloving injuries of the carpus (see p. 938) may be associated with fractures of the distal radius. Although there are no major nerves in the immediate area, dogs often have abnormal proprioceptive responses due to reluctance to move the limb.

Radiography

Craniocaudal and lateral radiographs of the affected radius and ulna (which include the proximal and distal joints) are required to assess the extent of bone and soft tissue injury. Animals that are fractious or in extreme pain may require sedation for radiography after it has been determined that contraindications (i.e., shock, hypotension, severe dyspnea) for administration of sedatives do not exist. Thoracic radiography should be performed to evaluate pulmonary changes.

Laboratory Findings

Complete blood count and serum chemistry evaluation should be done to evaluate the advisability of anesthesia and to determine if concurrent injury or damage of the renal or hepatobiliary systems exist.

DIFFERENTIAL DIAGNOSIS

Animals presenting with distal radial fractures should be evaluated to determine whether fractures are due to trauma or underlying pathology (i.e., neoplasia or metabolic disease). Joint luxations can be differentiated from fractures radiographically.

MEDICAL OR CONSERVATIVE MANAGEMENT

Medical treatment of animals with radial and ulnar metaphyseal and epiphyseal fractures may include analgesics (see p. 708) and antibiotics to treat open fractures.

SURGICAL TREATMENT

Fixation systems applicable to proximal ulnar fractures include tension band wire techniques and plates and screws.

Application of Bone Plates and Screws

Bone plates are an excellent method of stabilizing proximal ulnar fractures (see p. 750 for plating techniques). The plate is applied to the caudal surface to function as a tension band plate (Fig. 29-46, *A*). In some comminuted fractures the plate

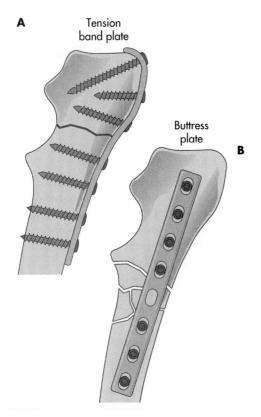

A
Tension
band plate

Buttress
plate

B

FIG. 29-46
A, Transverse articular fractures should be anatomically reduced and stabilized with a compression plate in patients with moderate or low fracture-assessment scores. **B,** Severely comminuted fractures are bridged with a buttress plate.

is applied to the lateral surface of the proximal ulna and functions as a buttress plate (Fig. 29-46, *B*).

Preoperative Management

There may be extensive damage and/or loss of tissues in the area of the fracture. Open wounds should be managed initially by carefully clipping surrounding hair, cleaning the wound, and sampling deep tissues for microbial culture and susceptibility testing. The antebrachium should be temporarily stabilized with a Robert Jones bandage (see p. 706) to immobilize fragments, decrease or prevent soft tissue swelling, protect or prevent open wounds, and increase patient comfort until surgery can be performed. Concurrent injuries should be managed prior to anesthetic induction for fracture fixation.

Anesthesia

Refer to p. 708 for anesthetic management of animals with fractures.

Surgical Anatomy

Landmarks for the approach to the proximal ulna are the olecranon and the palpable caudal border of the ulna. The articular surface of the trochlear notch can be exposed surgically by muscle elevation. The ulnar nerve courses over the medial aspect of the elbow, caudal to the medial epicondyle.

The antebrachial carpal joint is supported by the short radial collateral ligaments, which arise from the medial styloid process of the radius, the dorsal radiocarpal ligament arising from the dorsal surface of the distal radius, and the short ulnar collateral and radioulnar ligaments arising from the ulnar styloid process. The extensor tendons lie cranial to the antebrachial carpal joint and may need to be retracted to expose the joint surface.

Positioning

The limb should be prepped from shoulder to carpus. If cancellous bone graft harvest is anticipated, a donor site should also be prepped. The animal is positioned in lateral recumbency and the limb draped out for proximal radial and ulnar fractures. Placing the animal in dorsal recumbency allows more flexibility in visualizing distal radial and ulnar fractures.

☞ **N O T E ·** Avoid the ulnar nerve during surgical approaches to the ulna.

SURGICAL TECHNIQUE
Caudal Approach to the Ulna

Palpate the caudal border of the ulna directly under the skin and subcutaneous tissue on the caudal surface of the limb. Make an incision through skin and subcutaneous tissues along the ulnar diaphysis (Fig. 29-47, A). Elevate the flexor carpi ulnaris and deep digital flexor muscles medially and the ulnaris lateralis muscle laterally to expose the bone surface (Fig. 29-47, B). Reflect the origin of the flexor carpi ulnaris muscle to expose the trochlear notch (Fig. 29-47, C).

Approaches to the Proximal and Distal Radius and Ulna

See p. 816 under radial physeal fractures for approaches to the proximal radius. See pp. 808 and 821 for approaches to the distal radius and ulna, and extend the approach distally.

Stabilization of Proximal Radial and Ulna Fractures

If the fracture-assessment score is between 8 and 10 (see p. 733), pins and wires are usually sufficient to stabilize the fracture. Extraarticular fractures of the proximal and distal radius can often be stabilized with crossed Kirschner wires or small intramedullary pins (see radial physeal fractures on p. 815) in animals with fracture-assessment scores of 4 to 7. Severely comminuted, open fractures of the proximal ulna or fractures in dogs with anticipated prolonged healing times (fracture-assessment scores between 0 and 3; see p. 733) should be stabilized with plates and screws (i.e., buttress plate). Articular fractures must be anatomically reduced and stabilized with tension band wires or lag screws to restore joint continuity and function and limit development of degenerative joint disease.

To place a tension band wire, reduce the fracture (i.e., proximal ulna, styloid process of the ulna, or medial epicondyle

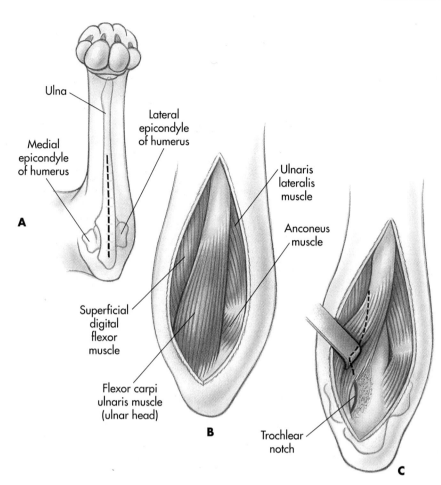

A

B

C

Ulna

Medial epicondyle of humerus

Lateral epicondyle of humerus

Ulnaris lateralis muscle

Anconeus muscle

Superficial digital flexor muscle

Flexor carpi ulnaris muscle (ulnar head)

Trochlear notch

FIG. 29-47
A, For a caudal approach to the proximal ulna, make an incision through skin and subcutaneous tissues over the caudal proximal ulna. **B,** Elevate the flexor carpi ulnaris and deep digital flexor muscles to expose the bone surface. **C,** Reflect the origin of the flexor carpi ulnaris muscle to expose the trochlear notch.

of the radius) and start two Kirschner wires in the fragment. Drive the wires across the fracture line to lodge in the major bone segment. Place a transverse drill hole in the major bone segment, pass a figure-eight wire through the hole and around the Kirschner wires, and tighten (Fig. 29-48).

Stabilization of Distal Radial and Ulnar Fractures

Distal radial and ulna fractures can be stabilized with a lag screw or tension band wire (Table 29-11) (Fig. 29-49, *A* and *B*). *To place a lag screw, reduce the fracture and hold it in place with a Kirschner wire. Drill a gliding hole (equal to the diameter of the threads on the screw) in the epicondylar fragment (see p. 753 for lag screw technique). Insert a drill sleeve into the gliding hole and drill a smaller hole (equal to the core diameter of the screw) across the radius. Measure and tap the hole and select and place the appropriate length screw in it. Compression of the fracture should occur.* The Kirschner wire may be left to provide rotational stability.

SUTURE MATERIALS/SPECIAL INSTRUMENTS

Plating equipment is necessary for plate and lag screws. Other equipment needed for the procedures described here includes a high-speed power drill, Kirschner wires, IM pins, orthopedic wire, and reduction forceps.

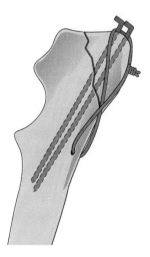

FIG. 29-48
Fractures (or osteotomies) of the olecranon can be treated with a tension band wire technique.

POSTOPERATIVE CARE AND ASSESSMENT

Postoperative radiographs should be made to document fracture reduction or alignment and implant position. After internal fixation, a soft padded bandage should be applied for a few days to control swelling and support soft tissues.

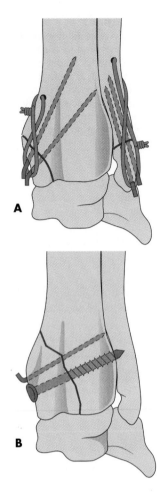

FIG. 29-49
A, Fractures of the styloid processes can be stabilized with tension band wire in patients with high and moderate fracture-assessment scores. Intraarticular fractures must be anatomically reduced and rigidly stabilized. **B,** Lag screws are used in patients with moderate and low fracture-assessment scores. A Kirschner wire is used as an antirotational implant.

Physical therapy (i.e., performing range of motion exercises for 10 to 15 minutes, two to three times a day) is indicated to help restore joint function. Open wounds are treated daily with wet to dry dressings until a granulation bed has formed. The wounds are then covered with a nonadhesive pad and the bandage changed as needed. Daily hydrotherapy aids in cleaning open wounds and reducing postoperative swelling. The animal should be released to the owner with instructions to limit exercise until radiographic evidence of bone healing is apparent. Rechecks should be scheduled at 2 weeks for suture removal and every 4 or 6 weeks for radiographic evaluation. Implant removal may be necessary after bone healing if the implants interfere with or irritate soft tissues.

PROGNOSIS

The prognosis for bone healing depends on the mechanical and biological factors present in each animal and the stability of the fixation (Table 29-12). In general, trabecular bone heals quickly with minimal callus formation (see p. 713), although comminuted proximal ulnar fractures may require

TABLE 29-11
Implant Use According to Fracture-Assessment Score (FAS) for Distal and Ulnar Fractures
FAS 0 to 3
• Lag screw
FAS 4 to 7
• Lag screw
• Tension band wire
FAS 8 to 10
• Tension band wire

TABLE 29-12
Common Errors
• Failure to anatomically reduce a joint surface results in degenerative joint disease and loss of function.
• Using only one fixation pin for tension band wire gives inadequate rotational stabilization and can result in nonunion.

long healing periods. Degenerative joint disease (DJD) may occur after articular fractures. DJD can be severe if anatomic reduction and rigid fixation of the fracture are not achieved. DJD is initially treated with conservative management including rest, judicious exercise, and nonsteroidal antiinflammatory drugs. Arthrodesis may be used to treat dogs with progressive instability, lameness, and pain that is unresponsive to medical management. Delayed union and nonunion can occur if the fracture is not adequately stabilized. The constant tensile stress exerted on the fracture line from the pull of the triceps muscle or collateral ligaments can cause nonunion. Treatment consists of rigid fixation with a tension band or lag screw and autogenous cancellous bone graft.

Suggested Reading

Clark DM: Treatment of open comminuted intra-articular fractures of the proximal ulna in dogs, *J Am Anim Hosp Assoc* 23:331, 1987.
Schwarz PD: Ulnar fracture and dislocation of the proximal radial epiphysis (Monteggia lesion) in the dog and cat: a review of 28 cases, *J Am Vet Med Assoc* 185:190, 1984.
Bellah JR: Use of a double hook plate for treatment of a distal radial fracture in a dog, *Vet Surg* 16:278, 1987.

RADIAL AND ULNAR PHYSEAL FRACTURES

DEFINITIONS

Physeal fractures may occur through the cartilaginous growth plates of the proximal or distal radius or ulna in immature animals.

SYNONYMS

Epiphyseal plate fractures, slipped physis

GENERAL CONSIDERATIONS AND CLINICALLY RELEVANT PATHOPHYSIOLOGY

The cartilaginous physis is weaker than surrounding bone and ligaments, making it more susceptible to injury. The weakest portion of the physis is the junction of the zone of hypertrophying cells with the zone of ossification. The zone of hypertrophying cells has a large cell-to-matrix ratio, which results in a relatively weak structure. Additionally, stress concentration is created when two areas of different mechanical properties (i.e., the weak hypertrophying zone and the stronger zone of ossification) are located adjacent to each other. Consequently, when a physis is fractured the separation should occur through the zone of hypertrophying cells. A fracture in this location does not affect proliferating cells and will not compromise potential growth. However, when severe trauma causes physeal fractures, the fracture line can occur anywhere within the physis and damage growing cells. Trauma resulting in compression of the zone of proliferating cells and destruction of the chondrocytes causes premature physeal closure. This commonly occurs following trauma to the V-shaped distal ulnar physis in dogs where trauma that would normally result in physeal separation instead compresses the zone of growing cells.

Fractures of the proximal and distal radial physis are usually radiographically classified as Salter-Harris Type I and II (Table 29-13). Occult Type V fractures of the radial physes can occur and are diagnosed after closure of the physis and alteration of forelimb growth have occurred. The most common fracture of the distal ulnar physis is the Salter-Harris Type V. This fracture is caused by trauma and may be associated with a radial fracture. Because they are nondisplaced and confined to the cartilage, these fractures are not visible radiographically until 2 to 3 weeks after trauma when premature closure of the physis is observed (see also p. 818).

DIAGNOSIS
Clinical Presentation

Signalment. These fractures occur in immature dogs or cats with open physes.

History. Affected animals usually present with a non–weight-bearing lameness after trauma. Occasionally owners are unaware that trauma occurred.

Physical Examination Findings

Because of the traumatic nature of this injury, the entire animal must be assessed to detect abnormalities of other body systems. Palpation of the limb reveals swelling, pain, crepitation, and apparent instability of the adjacent joint. Dogs often appear to have abnormal proprioceptive responses due to reluctance to move the limb.

Radiography

Craniocaudal and lateral radiographs of the affected radius and ulna, which include the proximal and distal joints, are required to diagnose Salter I to Salter IV fractures. Fractious

TABLE 29-13
Salter-Harris Classification
• Type I fractures involve only the cartilaginous physis.
• Type II fractures involve the physis and metaphyseal bone.
• Type III fractures involve the physis and epiphyseal bone.
• Type IV fractures involve metaphyseal and epiphyseal bone and cross the physis.
• Type V fractures crush the physis.

or extremely painful animals may require sedation for radiography after it has been determined that contraindications (i.e., shock, hypotension, severe dyspnea) for administration of sedatives do not exist. Thoracic radiography should be performed to evaluate pulmonary changes. Radiographs made at the time of injury do not give information about Salter V fractures (i.e., crushing injuries to the physis) or damage to the physeal blood supply. It is therefore difficult to give an accurate prognosis for growth at the time of injury.

☞ **N O T E ·** Compare radiographs of the contralateral bone to detect subtle changes in the physis.

Laboratory Findings

Complete blood count and serum chemistry evaluation should be done to evaluate the status of the animal for anesthesia and determine if there is damage to the renal or hepatobiliary systems.

DIFFERENTIAL DIAGNOSIS

Physeal fractures can be differentiated from joint luxations or soft tissue trauma radiographically.

MEDICAL MANAGEMENT

Medical treatment of animals with radial and ulnar physeal fractures may include analgesics (see p. 708) and antibiotics to treat open fractures.

SURGICAL TREATMENT

Most physeal fractures are classified as having fracture-assessment scores between 8 and 10 (see p. 733) as affected animals are young and physeal fractures heal quickly. Therefore, the implant system chosen need not function for a long time.

Application of Casts

Casts can be applied as the sole method of fixation for nondisplaced physeal fractures (see p. 733 for technique of cast application). Apply the cast so that it immobilizes the carpus and elbow. The limb should be positioned with slight carpal flexion and varus (inward) angulation.

Application of Crossed Kirschner Wires or IM Pins

Physeal fractures should be reduced carefully so as to avoid crushing or injuring the physeal cartilage. For proximal radial physeal fractures, a Kirschner wire can be driven from the lateral surface of the proximal radial epiphysis across the physis, into the radial metaphyses, and through the medial cortex. A second wire is then driven from the lateral proximal radial metaphysis across the fracture into the epiphysis (Fig. 29-50, *A*). Care should be taken to avoid penetrating the articular surface. For distal physeal fractures, a Kirschner wire is driven from the medial styloid process across the physis, into the radial metaphyses, and through the lateral cortex. The second wire is driven from the lateral aspect of the distal radial epiphysis, across the fracture into the metaphysis, and through the medial cortex (Fig. 29-50, *B*), avoiding the articular surface.

☞ **N O T E** • Use smooth implants when crossing the physis.

Preoperative Management

The antebrachium should be temporarily stabilized with a Robert Jones bandage (see p. 706) to immobilize the fragments, decrease or prevent soft tissue swelling, protect or prevent open wounds, and increase patient comfort until surgery can be performed. Concurrent injuries should be managed prior to anesthetic induction for fracture fixation.

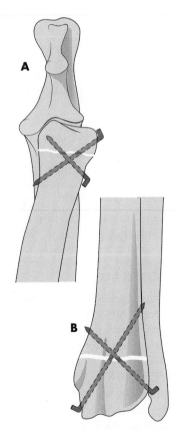

FIG. 29-50
A, For proximal radial physeal fractures, Kirschner wires can be driven from the lateral surface of the proximal radial epiphysis and from the lateral proximal radial metaphysis.
B, For distal physeal fractures, Kirschner wires can be driven from the medial styloid process and from the lateral aspect of the distal radial epiphysis.

Anesthesia

Anesthetic management of animals with fractures is discussed on p. 708. Small dogs and cats may require pediatric anesthetic techniques.

Surgical Anatomy

The lateral radial head is palpable beneath the extensor muscles of the forearm. The radial nerve lies deep to the extensor carpi radialis muscle. The cranial medial surface of the distal radius can be easily palpated to serve as a landmark for location of the incision. Extensor tendons are located cranial and flexor tendons caudal to the distal radius. The cephalic vein crosses the medial portion of the distal radius.

Positioning

The limb should be prepped from shoulder to carpus. The animal is positioned in lateral recumbency with the limb draped out for proximal radial physeal fractures. Placing the animal in dorsal recumbency allows more flexibility in visualizing distal radial and ulnar physeal fractures.

SURGICAL TECHNIQUES
Approach to the Proximal Radial Physis

Make a skin incision over the lateral humeral condyle, extending over the proximal third of the radius (Fig. 29-51, A). Continue the incision through subcutaneous tissues and brachial and antebrachial fascia (Fig. 29-51, B). Identify and separate the lateral digital extensor and ulnaris lateralis muscles to expose the proximal radius (Fig. 29-51, C). Close the wound by suturing fascia, subcutaneous tissues, and skin in separate layers.

Approach to the Distal Radial Physis

Use the craniomedial approach to the radius described on p. 808 to expose the distal radial physis.

Approach to the Distal Ulnar Physis

See approach for ulnar ostectomy described on p. 821 to expose the distal ulnar physis.

Stabilization of Nondisplaced Physeal Fractures

Fractures of the radial physes and distal ulnar physis that are nondisplaced can be treated with a cast. The limb is cast from the toes to above the elbow with the carpus held in slight flexion and varus (inward angulation) until the cast hardens.

Stabilization of Displaced Physeal Fractures

Kirschner wires or small Steinmann pins are used as crossed pins to stabilize physeal fractures that require open reduction (see above for technique).

SUTURE MATERIALS/SPECIAL INSTRUMENTS

Necessary equipment includes Kirschner wires, small IM pins, Jacobs pin chuck, and reduction forceps.

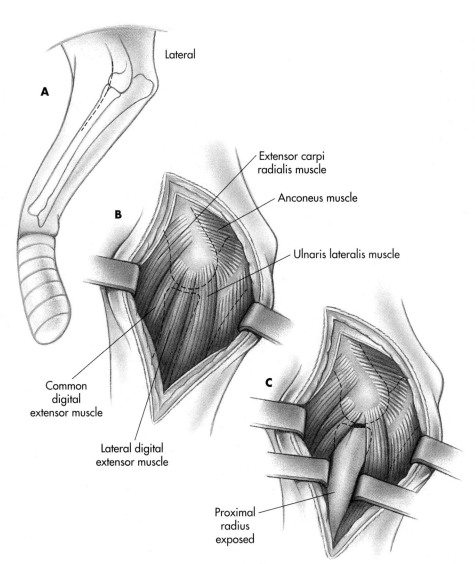

FIG. 29-51
A, For a lateral approach to the radial head, make a skin incision over the lateral humeral condyle, extending over the proximal third of the radius. **B** and **C,** Identify and separate the lateral digital extensor and ulnaris lateralis muscles to expose the proximal radius.

Lateral

A

Extensor carpi radialis muscle

Anconeus muscle

B

Ulnaris lateralis muscle

C

Common digital extensor muscle

Lateral digital extensor muscle

Proximal radius exposed

POSTOPERATIVE CARE AND ASSESSMENT

Postoperative radiographs should be made to document fracture reduction and implant position. After internal fixation, a soft padded bandage should be applied for a few days to control swelling and support soft tissues. Physical therapy (i.e., performing range of motion exercises for 10 to 15 minutes, two to three times a day) is indicated to help restore joint function. The animal should be released to the owner with instructions to limit exercise for 4 to 6 weeks. Rechecks should be scheduled at 2 weeks for suture removal and at 4 to 6 weeks for radiographic evaluation of fracture healing. Radiographs of the injured bone and the contralateral bone can be made and compared for length as early as 2 to 3 weeks following the injury to determine physeal function. Cartilage physes that heal in a manner allowing continued function appear radiographically as a lucent line. Additionally, increased bone length should be apparent. If the physeal line appears as a bone density, endochondral ossification has occurred and continued physeal function is likely. Implant removal is indicated after physeal healing to allow bone growth (if the physis is functional after the trauma).

PROGNOSIS

Although the prognosis for fracture healing with physeal fractures is excellent, the prognosis for continued function or growth of the physis depends on the severity of damage sustained by the zone of proliferating cells. The prognosis is good for future physeal growth after a fracture that separates the cartilaginous physis at the zone of hypertrophying cells, whereas the prognosis is poor for future physeal growth following trauma that crushes the physis. Unfortunately, most traumatically induced physeal fractures sustain damage to the growing cells and have a guarded prognosis for growth. Bridging of bone across the physis may occur in fractures that cross the growth plate, causing abnormal bone growth. Damage to one physis of a paired bone system like the radius and ulna can cause shortened limbs, angular deformities, rotational deformities, and disruption of normal joint anatomy resulting in degenerative joint disease.

The most common complication associated with radial and ulnar physeal fractures is premature physeal closure causing growth deformities. The severity of the deformity depends on the animal's age when physeal closure occurs and location and extent of the physeal closure. Younger animals with greater growth potential have more severe sequelae. Premature closure of the distal ulnar physis interferes with the normal development of the radius by acting as a restraint. This results not only in a shortened ulna but also in shortening, rotation, and angulation of the radius. Additionally, asynchronous growth of the paired bones results in incongruity of the elbow and carpal joints leading to degenerative joint disease. Asymmetrical or partial closure of the distal radial physis results in angular deformity of the bone and may affect the anatomy of adjacent joints, again resulting in degenerative joint disease.

Suggested Reading

Johnson JM, Johnson AL, Eurell JA: Histological appearance of naturally occurring canine physeal fractures, *Vet Surg* 23:81, 1994.

Manfra SM, Schrader SC: Physeal injuries in the dog: a review of 35 cases, *J Am Vet Med Assoc* 182:708, 1983.

Salter RB: Salter-Harris classification of epiphyseal plate injuries. In Uhthoff HK, Wiley JJ, editors: *Behavior of the growth plate.* New York, 1988, Raven.

RADIAL AND ULNAR GROWTH DEFORMITIES

DEFINITIONS

Growth deformities are abnormal conformation of the limb after premature closure of a physis. **Corrective osteotomy** is a planned osteotomy of the bone followed by restoration of normal alignment of the bone and rigid fixation. **Ostectomy** is the removal of a portion of bone.

SYNONYMS

Radius curvus, angular limb deformity, premature closure of the radial or ulnar physes

GENERAL CONSIDERATIONS AND CLINICALLY RELEVANT PATHOPHYSIOLOGY

Growth deformities of the forelimb occur frequently because of the paired bone system and unique shape of the distal ulnar physis. Synchronous growth of the radius and ulna in the dog is essential for the development of a normal forelimb. The radius receives 40% of its length from the proximal physis and 60% from the distal physis, whereas 85% of the ulnar length comes from the distal physis; the proximal physis contributes only 15%. In most dogs, growth accelerates rapidly during the fourth to sixth months and tapers off in the ninth or tenth month. This period varies depending on the breed of dog (smaller dogs mature faster than larger dogs).

The cone-shaped distal ulnar physis is frequently injured during forelimb trauma. These injuries are considered a Salter-Harris Type V crushing injury and result in complete physeal closure. Sequelae include shortening of the ulna with cranial bowing, valgus angulation, external rotation, and

shortening of the radius. Varying amounts of elbow and carpal incongruity can occur (Fig. 29-52, *A*). The proximal and distal radial physes can also close prematurely causing forelimb growth deformities. Symmetrical, complete closure of the proximal or distal radial physis results in a shortened but straight radius, elbow incongruity, and a varus angulation of the carpus (Fig. 29-52, *B*). The limb deformity seen with asymmetrical or partial physeal closure of the distal radius varies depending on the location of the closure. The most common deformity is a caudolateral closure of the physis resulting in valgus deformity of the carpus (Fig. 29-52, *C*). The normal anatomy of the carpus may be disrupted.

Retained cartilage core is caused by retarded endochondral ossification at the distal ulnar physis and may lead to slower growth of the physis and ulnar shortening. This causes shortening, cranial bowing, external rotation, and valgus angulation of the radius. Histologic examination of the affected physis shows normal reserve and proliferative zones with a thickened hypertrophic zone in the center of the physis. The matrix septa in the abnormally thickened hypertrophic zone do not appear to calcify normally, and vascularization does not occur. Therefore, bone production and remodeling are delayed.

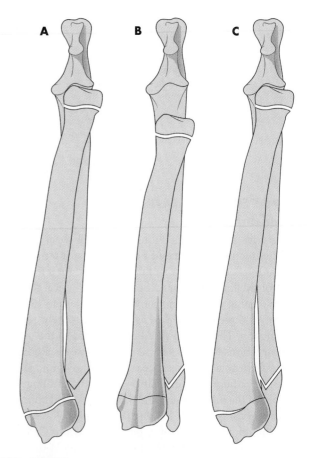

FIG. 29-52
A, Premature closure of the distal ulnar physis causes shortening, cranial bowing, external rotation, and valgus angulation of the radius. **B,** Complete premature closure of the distal (or proximal) radial physis causes shortening of the radius and subluxation of the radial humeral joint. **C,** Partial distal radial physeal closure causes angular deformity of the radius.

Several theories have been proposed regarding the etiology of retained cartilage cores. The condition appears primarily in large, fast-growing dogs and some speculate that nutrition may play a role in the development. This is a difficult hypothesis to prove because dietary oversupplementation of many of these dogs may be done as a response to the condition. These dogs should be fed the recommended calcium-to-phosphorus ratio and the amount of food decreased to slow the dog's overall growth. Loss of vascularization to the central metaphysis can also result in retained cartilage cores. Another theory suggests that the condition is part of generalized osteochondrosis. Finally, the syndrome may result from an abnormality of the chondrocytes, which can no longer control the progress of calcification of the cartilaginous septa.

DIAGNOSIS
Clinical Presentation

Signalment. Young dogs are affected. Growth deformities are rare in cats.

History. There may be a history of fracture of the radius and ulna, or an obscure history of trauma.

Physical Examination Findings

Initially, dogs with premature closure of the physes show minimal deformity of the forelimb. As the deformity progresses, premature closure of the distal ulnar physis causes lameness, cranial bowing of the forelimb, and valgus deformity of the carpus. The dog may extend its elbow to compensate for the short radius. Dogs with symmetrical closure of the radial physes may show minimal angular deformity but suffer pain on palpation of the elbow. Dogs with asymmetrical closure of the distal radial physis may show an angular deformity. The direction of the deformity is dependent on the location of the initial partial closure of the physis. Retained cartilage core may be indistinguishable from traumatic premature closure of the distal ulnar physis by physical examination.

Radiography

Radiographic examination is necessary to definitively diagnose the cause of deformity in animals with premature closure of the radius or ulna. Craniocaudal and lateral radiographs should be made of the affected forelimb. Each radiograph should include the radius, ulna, elbow, and carpus. The normal functioning physis is radiolucent. A physis that has slowed or ceased functioning will still be radiolucent until endochondral ossification of the physis is complete. The physis appears as bone density after ossification. Radiographs of the opposite normal limb are made to obtain a control for determining normal radial and ulnar length and normal forelimb anatomy. In early cases of premature closure of the distal ulnar physis, a discrepancy in ulnar lengths may be determined before there are obvious radiographic signs of physeal closure or forelimb deformity. Bone length and angular limb deformity should be measured from the radiographs to establish a preoperative standard against which the results of treat-

ment may be compared. Radiographic examination of retained cartilage core reveals a radiolucent cartilage core in the center of the distal ulnar physis extending into the metaphysis.

☞ **N O T E** • Always radiograph the contralateral radius and ulna for comparison. Make length measurements from lateral radiographs.

Laboratory Findings

These animals are usually young and healthy. There are no consistent laboratory findings associated with growth deformities after premature physeal closure.

DIFFERENTIAL DIAGNOSIS

Growth deformities caused by premature physeal closure must be differentiated from poor conformation and laxity or contracture of supporting soft tissue structures such as ligaments and tendons. Diagnosis of premature closure of the radial or ulnar physes is made with physical and radiographic examinations of the forelimb.

MEDICAL MANAGEMENT

There is no medical therapy for growth deformities after premature physeal closure. Antibiotics may be used prophylactically to protect the ostectomy or osteotomy site during surgery (see Chapter 10) if the surgery is expected to exceed 2 hours.

Treatment of the retained cartilage cores depends on the severity of the clinical signs. Dogs with mild deformities may respond to dietary limitations. Dogs treated conservatively in this manner should be monitored weekly to determine if the deformities are correcting or progressing. If the deformities progress, an ulnar ostectomy and autogenous fat graft should be done to remove the restraint on radial growth.

SURGICAL TREATMENT

Destruction of the growing cells and closure of the physis are irreversible phenomena. Treatment is therefore directed at reducing the severity of, or correcting the sequelae to, physeal closure (Table 29-14). Animals with forelimb

---

TABLE 29-14

Important Considerations for Treating Growth Deformities

- Growth deformities of the radius and ulna require surgical intervention.
- Allow as much natural growth of the limb as possible by using ostectomy techniques in growing animals.
- An osteotomy procedure to correct angular and rotational deformity is usually required after ostectomy techniques allow growth in length.
- Growth deformities in mature animals are treated with a corrective osteotomy if the deformity has an adverse effect on limb function.
- The prognosis for normal appearance and function of the affected limb is always guarded.

growth deformities are initially classified according to potential for growth in either the radius or the ulna. Animals with radiographically lucent physes may have growth potential and are treated with ostectomies and fat grafting to allow as much growth of the limb to occur as possible. Those that have all their physes closed are treated with corrective osteotomy.

The objective of corrective osteotomy is to return the limb to normal function. Indications for a corrective osteotomy are: (1) correcting excessive angulation of the bone(s), (2) creating an angulation in the bone to realign joint surfaces, (3) establishing adequate length of the bone(s), (4) correcting torsional deformity, and (5) improving articular configuration. Corrective osteotomy requires careful preoperative planning including comparison of the radiographs of the affected limb and the contralateral limb (serving as an internal control) for position and relationship of adjacent joints, point of greatest curvature of the bone, degree of rotation, and length of the bone. The radiographs can be traced and templates used for planning the osteotomy and visualizing the correction. The type of osteotomy chosen depends on the animal's age and type of deformity. Lengthening osteotomies are chosen when a short bone or limb is the primary problem. Continuous distraction can be used to increase the overall length of the limb in order to match the opposite limb. Oblique osteotomy is used to treat angular deformities of the limb. Derotational osteotomy is used to correct rotational deformity. Correction of angular deformity and rotational deformity can be done with an oblique osteotomy stabilized with external skeletal fixation. Corrective osteotomies are most frequently performed on the radius and ulna; however, the principles can be applied to any long bone. Treatment of tibial deformities is similar to treatment of radial deformities. When treating femoral or humeral deformities, plate fixation may be more appropriate.

Goals of treatment in immature dogs with premature closure of the distal ulnar physis are to allow unrestricted growth of the normal physes of the radius and ulna, which results in maximal limb growth, and in some cases corrects the angular deformity. An ulnar ostectomy is used to release the constraint placed on the radius by the ulna and is coupled with the placement of a free autogenous fat graft to prevent union of the ulnar segments. The goal of treatment of partial premature closure of the distal radial physis in immature dogs is to allow unrestricted growth of the normal portion of the distal radial physis. Tomographic examination of the distal radial physis may be indicated to accurately define the area of the physis that is closed and bridged with bone. The animal is treated by resecting the bone bridged area of the physis, followed by placement of a free autogenous fat graft in the defect to prevent reestablishment of the bone bridge. The goal of treatment of complete premature closure of the proximal or distal radial physis in immature dogs is to allow unrestricted growth of the normal radial and ulnar physes and to restore and maintain elbow congruency by performing a radial ostectomy and free autogenous fat graft. The goal of treating complete premature clo-

sure of the distal ulnar and radial physes in immature dogs is to gain length to match the opposite normal limb. These dogs are treated with transverse osteotomy and continuous distraction. This procedure is complex and requires constant postoperative monitoring by both veterinarians and clients. Goals of treatment of premature closure of the distal ulnar physis in mature dogs are to correct angular and rotational deformities, while preserving as much limb length as possible during the corrective osteotomy procedure. An oblique radial and ulnar osteotomy with repositioning of the distal radial segment is used. Preoperative radiographs are evaluated to determine the location of the point of greatest radial curvature and to evaluate the anatomy of the adjacent elbow and carpus. The goal of treatment of premature closure of the proximal or distal radial physis in mature dogs is to improve limb function by reestablishing normal radial length and elbow congruency. A transverse lengthening osteotomy is performed. An alternative approach used to treat elbow incongruity caused by premature closure of the radial physes in dogs with minimal limb length discrepancies is transverse ostectomy of the proximal ulna above the interosseous ligament.

> ☞ **N O T E** • Ostectomies release restraint so functional physes can grow normally. The animal must have growth potential for an effective ostectomy.

Preoperative Management

Preoperative management of the dog consists of obtaining a CBC and chemistry profile to confirm that the dog is healthy. Preoperative counseling to the owners is imperative. Owners must understand the goals and expectations of the surgeon, the limitations of the procedures, and the potential for complicated aftercare and further procedures.

Anesthesia

Anesthetic management of animals with fractures is discussed on p. 708.

Surgical Anatomy

Surgical anatomy of the radius is discussed on p. 816. The distal ulna in the immature dog is large and easily palpated on the lateral aspect of the limb. The flexor tendons of the carpus border the distal ulna. In immature dogs there is a thick layer of periosteum that must be identified and resected during ostectomies. The interosseous artery lies between the radius and ulna and is often encountered when performing an ostectomy.

Positioning

For premature closure of the distal ulnar physis both the affected forelimb and the ipsilateral flank are prepared for aseptic surgery. The animal is positioned in lateral recumbency. For oblique osteotomy and possible cancellous bone graft harvest, the forelimb is prepped from the dorsal border of the scapula to below the carpus and the dog is positioned in dorsal recumbency with the affected limb suspended securely from the ceiling (see p. 24).

SURGICAL TECHNIQUE
Ulnar Ostectomy and Free Autogenous Fat Graft

Make a lateral skin incision extending over the mid- to distal ulna (Fig. 29-53, A). Incise subcutaneous tissues and identify and separate the lateral digital extensor muscle from the extensor carpi ulnaris muscle to expose the ulna distal metaphysis. Isolate 1 to 2 cm of the ulna metaphysis immediately proximal to the physis by elevating surrounding musculature and fascia. The ostectomy must be below the interosseous ligament to maintain elbow stability. *Ensure that all of the periosteum, with its osteogenic potential, remains with the segment of bone to be resected.* Failure to remove all periosteum causes premature bone bridging of the ostectomy. *Resect a 1- to 2-cm segment of ulna with bone cutters or an oscillating bone saw cooled with a saline flush. Remove the segment of bone and associated periosteum (Fig. 29-53, B). If the interosseous artery is cut, achieve hemostasis by clamping the*

vessel if possible, or applying pressure for 5 minutes. To harvest the fat graft, make a 2- to 3-cm skin incision in the ipsilateral flank to expose the subcutaneous fat (Fig. 29-53, C). Using sharp dissection, free a large, single piece of fat and place it in the ostectomy gap (Fig. 29-53, D). Close the flank wound by suturing subcutaneous tissues and skin. Close the limb wound over the fat graft by suturing adjacent soft tissues. Close subcutaneous tissue and skin separately.

Partial Physeal Resection

Surgically expose the closed and bridged portion of the distal radial physis. Determine the limitations of the bone bridge by exploring the area with a hypodermic needle (Fig. 29-54, A). The cartilage of the normal physis is easily penetrated by a needle as opposed to the resistance felt when the bone bridge or adjacent metaphyseal or epiphyseal bone is probed. *Remove the bone bridge with a curette or a high-speed burr (Fig. 29-54, B). Curettage is complete when normal physeal cartilage is observed or probed with the needle. Harvest free autogenous fat from the flank as described above and place it within the*

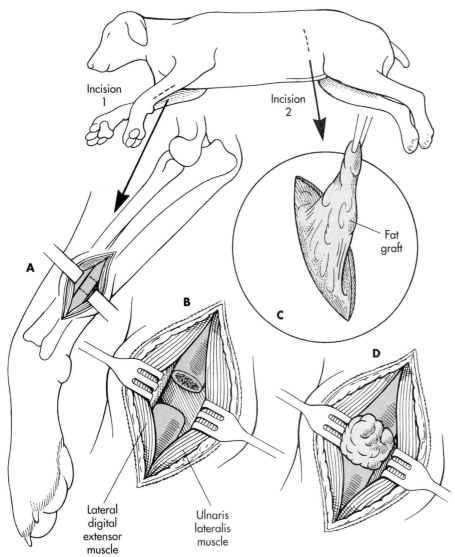

Incision 1

Incision 2

Fat graft

A

B

C

D

Lateral digital extensor muscle

Ulnaris lateralis muscle

FIG. 29-53
A, For ulnar ostectomy with a free autogenous fat graft, prepare two sites for surgery *(incision 1 and incision 2)*. Make a lateral skin incision extending over the mid- to distal ulna. Separate the lateral digital extensor muscle from the ulnaris lateralis muscle to expose the ulna's distal metaphysis.
B, Resect a 1- to 2-cm segment of ulna. **C,** Make a 2- to 3-cm skin incision in the ipsilateral flank area to expose subcutaneous fat. **D,** Free a large single piece of fat and place it in the ostectomy gap.

FIG. 29-54
A, During resection of a partial physeal closure/fat graft, determine the limitations of the bone bridge by exploring the area with a hypodermic needle. **B,** Remove the bone bridge with a curette or a high-speed burr and **C,** harvest free autogenous fat from the flank and place it within the physeal defect.

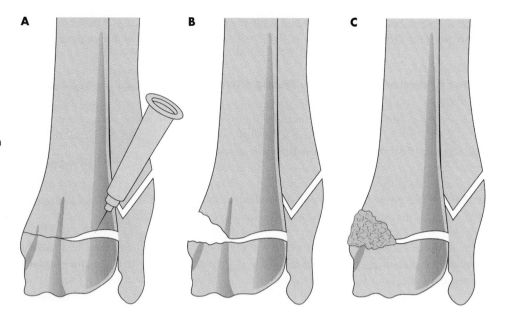

physeal defect (Fig. 29-54, C). Close soft tissue and skin over the transplanted fat.

Radial Ostectomy and Free Autogenous Fat Graft

Expose the middiaphysis of the radius using a craniomedial approach (see p. 808). Isolate 1 to 2 cm of the radial diaphysis by elevating surrounding musculature and fascia. Ensure that all periosteum, with its osteogenic potential, remains with the segment of bone to be resected. Resect a 1- to 2-cm segment of the radius with bone cutters or an oscillating bone saw cooled with a saline flush. Remove the segment of bone and associated periosteum (Fig. 29-55, A). If the interosseous artery is cut, achieve hemostasis by clamping the vessel if possible, or applying pressure for 5 minutes. Harvest a free autogenous fat graft from the flank and place it in the defect to prevent bone union (Fig. 29-55, B). Close the wound over the fat graft.

Transverse Radial Osteotomy With Continuous Distraction

Place a centrally threaded positive profile fixation pin through the proximal radius from the lateral aspect so that the pin parallels the proximal radial articular surface and is within the lateral transverse plane of the proximal radius. Place an identical pin through the distal radius from the lateral aspect. The pin should parallel the distal radial articular surface and be within the lateral transverse plane of the distal radius. Make a lateral approach to the distal ulna and resect a 1- to 2-cm segment of bone with bone cutters or an oscillating saw cooled with a saline flush. Then make a craniomedial approach to expose the mid-diaphysis of the radius. Perform a mid-diaphyseal radial osteotomy with an osteotome or an oscillating saw. If there is an angular deformity of the radius, make an oblique osteotomy at the point of greatest curvature of the radius that parallels the distal articular surface. Realign the radius and ulna using

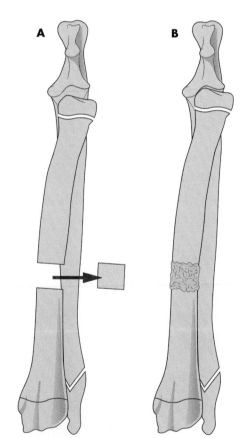

FIG. 29-55
A, To perform a radial ostectomy and fat graft, resect a 1- to 2-cm segment of the radius. **B,** Harvest a free autogenous fat graft from the flank and place it in the defect to prevent bone union.

the proximal and distal transfixation pins as guides to eliminate any angular or rotational deformity. Place threaded or turnbuckle distraction bars (see Product Appendix) with single fixation clamps on the lateral and medial aspect of the limb. Drive additional fixation pins through single

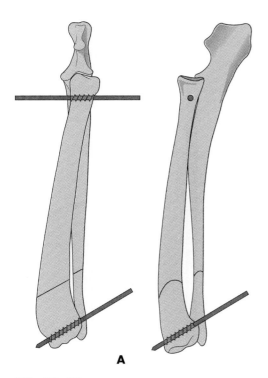
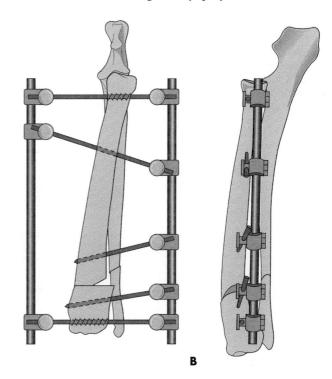

FIG. 29-56
A, For oblique osteotomy, place centrally threaded positive profile fixation pins through the proximal and distal radial metaphyses, parallel to their respective joint surfaces and within the respective lateral transverse planes of the proximal and distal radius. **B,** Plan and perform an osteotomy across the greatest curvature of the radius, parallel to the distal articular surface. Perform an osteotomy of the distal ulna also. Realign the radius and ulna using the proximal and distal transfixation pins as guide pins to eliminate angular or rotational deformities. Stabilize the radius with a Type II external fixator.

clamps placed on the medial and lateral bars. At least one additional pin should be placed in each radial segment. Harvest an autogenous fat graft from the flank and place it in the ulnar ostectomy gap. Close the wound to hold the fat in place. Close the radial incision by suturing the subcutaneous tissue and skin separately. Tighten the clamps and cut the fixation pins to the correct length.

☞ **N O T E** • Continuous distraction requires an owner committed to intensive aftercare and frequent reevaluations.

Oblique Osteotomy

Place a centrally threaded positive-profile fixation pin through the proximal radius from the lateral aspect (Fig. 29-56, A). The pin should parallel the proximal radial articular surface and be within the lateral transverse plane of the proximal radius. Place an identical pin through the distal radius from the lateral aspect. The pin should parallel the distal radial articular surface and be within the lateral transverse plane of the distal radius. The transfixation pins serve as landmarks: pay special attention to correct placement. *Make a lateral approach to the distal ulna and cut the bone with an osteotome or oscillating saw. Make a craniomedial approach to the distal radius at its point of greatest curva-*

ture. Perform an oblique osteotomy of the radius with an osteotome or an oscillating bone saw, directing the osteotomy line parallel to the distal radial articular surface in both the craniocaudal and mediolateral planes. Lower the operating table so that the weight of the animal distracts the distal radius and helps to align the proximal and distal joint surfaces parallel to each other. Realign the radius and ulna using the proximal and distal transfixation pins to eliminate any angular or rotational deformity. Place a connecting bar with single fixation clamps on the lateral and medial aspect of the limb (Fig. 29-56, B). Drive additional fixation pins through single clamps placed on the medial and lateral bars. At least one additional pin should be placed in each radial segment. Harvest an autogenous cancellous bone graft from the proximal humerus and place it at the radial osteotomy site. Close the wounds by suturing the subcutaneous tissue and skin separately. Tighten the clamps and cut the fixation pins to the desired length.*

Transverse Lengthening Osteotomy

Place a centrally threaded positive-profile fixation pin through the proximal radius from the lateral aspect (Fig. 29-57, A). The pin should parallel the proximal radial articular surface and be within the lateral transverse plane of the proximal radius. Place an identical pin through the distal radius from the lateral aspect. The pin should parallel

FIG. 29-57
A, For a radial lengthening osteotomy, place centrally threaded positive-profile fixation pins through the proximal and distal radial metaphyses, parallel to their respective joint surfaces and within the respective lateral transverse planes of the proximal and distal radius. **B,** Perform a transverse osteotomy of the mid-radial diaphysis. Distract the proximal and distal radial segments until the radial head contacts the capitulum of the humerus; then, stabilize the radius with a Type II external fixator.

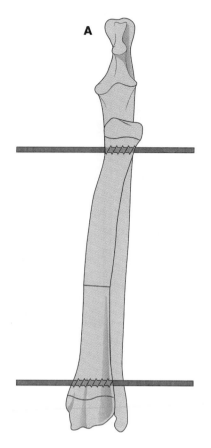

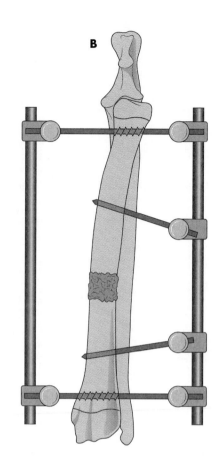

the distal radial articular surface and be within the lateral transverse plane of the distal radius. Use a craniomedial approach to expose the mid-diaphysis of the radius. Cut the radius with an osteotome or an oscillating saw. Distract the proximal and distal segments of the radius until the head of the radius has contacted the capitulum of the humerus. Place a connecting bar with single fixation clamps on the lateral and medial aspect of the limb (Fig. 29-57, B). Drive additional fixation pins through single clamps placed on the medial and lateral bars. At least one additional pin should be placed in each radial segment. Harvest an autogenous cancellous bone graft from the proximal humerus and place it at the radial osteotomy site.

☞ **N O T E** · When using a plate to stabilize the osteotomy, approach the lateral aspect of the elbow to visualize joint congruity before the plate is secured.

Close the wounds by suturing the subcutaneous tissue and skin separately. Tighten the clamps and cut fixation pins to the desired length.

Obtain postoperative radiographs to document the position of the radial head and location of fixation pins. Some correction of the radial segment location can be made at this time by adjusting the external fixator. *If the radial head does not appear to contact the humeral capitulum, place a transverse bilateral fixation pin through the olecranon proximal to the most proximal transverse pin in the radius. Loosen*

the external fixator clamps proximal to the radial osteotomy. Connect the ulnar pin and proximal radial pin bilaterally with elastic bands, placing tension on the proximal radius and pulling it toward the humerus.

Proximal Ulnar Ostectomy

Proximal ulnar ostectomy is described on p. 935 under treatment of elbow subluxation in dogs with premature closure of the radial physes. This technique is indicated if shortening of the leg will not affect limb function.

SUTURE MATERIALS/SPECIAL INSTRUMENTS

Instruments needed include an osteotome and mallet, or oscillating saw. Equipment needed for external fixation includes a low-rpm power drill, fixation pins, external fixation clamps, and connecting bars, or acrylic.

POSTOPERATIVE CARE AND ASSESSMENT

After ulnar ostectomy postoperative radiographs are made to document the location and length of the ostectomy gap. A soft padded bandage or splint may be used to protect the limb for 2 weeks if bilateral procedures are done. Owners should be instructed to limit activity and to return for monthly reexaminations. Radiographs should be taken monthly and compared to immediate postoperative radiographs for radial growth, correction of angular deformity, and ostectomy gap patency. Restoration of normal elbow configuration due to release of the proximal ulna may be noted. Reevaluations can be discontinued when the animal is skeletally mature.

☞ **N O T E** • If ostectomies prematurely bridge with bone, a second ostectomy may be needed.

Postoperative radiographs should be made to document complete resection of the bone bridge and placement of the fat graft after partial physeal resection. A soft padded bandage is used to protect the limb postoperatively. Owners should be instructed to limit exercise and to return monthly for reevaluation. Radiographs should be made monthly and compared to the postoperative radiographs for radial length, correction of angular deformity, and patency of the resected area. A goniometer can be used to determine angular limb deformity and the results compared to preoperative findings. Reevaluations can be discontinued when the animal reaches skeletal maturity.

Postoperative radiographs should be made after radial ostectomy to document the location and length of the ostectomy. Release of tension on the proximal and distal radius will usually allow adjacent joints to reestablish normal position. Postoperatively the limb may require a soft padded bandage or splint support as the radius is the primary weight-bearing bone in the distal forelimb. A second surgical procedure to reunite the radial segments by bridging the ostectomy gap with autogenous cancellous bone graft may be indicated when the dog has reached maturity.

After transverse radial osteotomy with continuous distraction, postoperative radiographs should be made to document the correction obtained and position of the fixation pins. The radial joint surfaces must be parallel and the cranial surfaces of the proximal and distal radial segments located in the same transverse plane. If they are not, a measure of correction may be obtained by readjusting the external fixator. Distraction is started on the fifth day after surgery. The optimal rate of distraction to obtain membranous bone formation is 1 mm per day. Smaller increments are preferable and owners should be instructed to distract ½ mm BID or ¼ mm QID. Animals should be evaluated weekly during this phase. Distraction may need to be increased to match the growth rate of the contralateral limb or to prevent premature bone union. After limb distraction is completed the fixator is left in place to allow the osteotomy to heal. Postoperative management of the external fixator and the reevaluation schedule is the same as that described for fractures of the radius (see p. 810).

☞ **N O T E** • Good aftercare by the owner is essential for maintaining an external fixator.

After oblique osteotomy, postoperative radiographs should be made to document the correction obtained and position of fixation pins. The radial joint surfaces must be parallel and the cranial surfaces of the proximal and distal radial segments located in the same transverse plane. If they are not, some correction may be obtained by readjusting the external fixator (see p. 872). Postoperative management of the external fixator and reevaluations are the same as described for radial fractures on p. 810.

After transverse lengthening radial osteotomy and placement of the external fixation pins in the ulna, the limb should be radiographed within 24 to 48 hours. Once the articulation is correct, the elastic bands and ulnar pin can be removed and the proximal clamps tightened. Postoperative management of the external fixator and reevaluation schedule are the same as that described for fractures of the radius on p. 810.

PROGNOSIS

Prognosis for normal appearance and function is guarded in immature animals after ulnar ostectomy. Much of the outcome depends on the growth potential of the radial physes. With favorable conditions, an animal may achieve normal limb length and some correction of valgus angulation; however, rotational deformities are not corrected by this procedure. Owners must be informed of the possibility that additional surgical procedures may be necessary for complete treatment. Ulnar union while the animal is still growing is an indication for reoperation. A corrective radial and ulnar osteotomy may be indicated if the angular deformity has not corrected itself once the dog has reached maturity.

The prognosis is guarded after partial physeal resection until there is radiographic evidence of physeal function. Owners must be informed of the possibility that additional surgical procedures may be necessary. Reestablishment of the bone bridge or worsening of the angular deformity may be an indication for reoperation. A corrective radial and ulnar osteotomy may be indicated if the angular deformity has not corrected when the dog has reached maturity.

Prognosis for normal appearance and function is guarded after radial ostectomy. Much of the outcome depends on the growth potential of the distal ulnar physes. With favorable conditions limb length will increase. Owners must be informed of the possibility that additional surgical procedures may be necessary. Healing of the ostectomy occurs when the periosteum has not been adequately resected. A second ostectomy may be indicated if the animal still has growth potential in the distal ulnar physis.

Prognosis after transverse osteotomy with continuous distraction is guarded because of the complexity of the technique and potential complications (i.e., pin track drainage, pin loosening, and premature loss of stability of the fixator). Premature healing of the osteotomy stops progressive lengthening of the radius.

After oblique osteotomy and transverse lengthening osteotomy the prognosis is good for bone union at the osteotomy site. Function of the limb depends on the amount of correction achieved and presence of degenerative joint disease. Complications are those that occur with external fixation of radial fractures (see p. 810).

Prognosis after ulnar ostectomy to treat radial head subluxation is good for bone union at the ostectomy site. Pin removal may be required if the implant irritates the soft tissues. Limb function depends on the amount of correction achieved and presence of degenerative joint disease.

Suggested Reading

Forell EB, Schwarz PD: Use of external skeletal fixation for treatment of angular deformity secondary to premature distal ulnar physeal closure, *J Am Anim Hosp Assoc* 29:460, 1993.

Gilson SD, Piermattei DL, Schwarz PD: Treatment of humeroulnar subluxation with a dynamic proximal ulnar osteotomy: a review of 13 cases, *Vet Surg* 18:114, 1989.

Henney LHS, Gambardella PC: Premature closure of the ulnar physis in the dog: a retrospective clinical study, *J Am Anim Hosp Assoc* 25:573, 1989.

Henney LHS, Gambardella PC: Partial ulnar ostectomy for treatment of premature closure of the proximal and distal radial physes in the dog, *J Am Anim Hosp Assoc* 26:183, 1990.

Johnson AL: Correction of radial and ulnar growth deformities resulting from premature physeal closure. In Bojrab MF, editor: *Current techniques in small animal surgery,* Philadelphia, 1990, Lea and Febiger.

Johnson AL: Osteotomies. In Olmstead ML, editor: *Small animal orthopedics,* St. Louis, 1995, Mosby.

VanDeWater AL, Olmstead ML: Premature closure of the distal radial physis in the dog: a review of 11 cases, *Vet Surg* 12:7, 1983.

Yanoff SR et al: Distraction osteogenesis using modified external fixation devices in five dogs, *Vet Surg* 21:480, 1992.

CARPAL AND TARSAL FRACTURES

DEFINITIONS

Carpal and **tarsal fractures** may cause a loss of weight-bearing support if integrity of these bones is disrupted. A **plantigrade** stance occurs when the foot is positioned such that the plantar surface of the calcaneus contacts the ground. A **valgus** position of the foot is an outward deviation; a **varus** position is an inward deviation.

SYNONYMS

Fractures of the wrist joint or **hock joint; fractures of the fibular tarsal bone (calcaneus); fractures of the tibial tarsal bone (talus)**

GENERAL CONSIDERATIONS AND CLINICALLY RELEVANT PATHOPHYSIOLOGY

Although carpal or tarsal fractures are rare in companion animals, such fractures are often disabling because the carpal-tarsal joints serve a major weight bearing function. If injuries involving these joints are not treated, joint incongruity and subsequent development of osteoarthritis often lead to severe lameness. Fractures of the distal row of carpal bones may occur as compression fractures in conjunction with carpal hyperextension injuries. Radial carpal bone fractures are the most frequently diagnosed injury involving fracture of the carpal bones in pet animals. Accessory carpal bone fractures occur in racing greyhounds and

sled dogs, but are rare in companion animals. Most accessory carpal bone fractures occur in the right leg because of the counterclockwise direction of racing. Accessory carpal bone fractures are considered avulsion injuries since they occur at tendinous or ligamentous insertions and are classified according to site of injury on the accessory carpal bone. Readers are referred to the suggested reading list for additional information relative to this injury in these breeds.

The most common tarsal fracture in companion animals is a transverse fracture of the calcaneus (Fig. 29-58). Distraction of the fracture by the pull of the gastrocnemius muscle prevents bone contact between fragments and interferes with healing; treatment methods must therefore resist the tensile forces attempting to separate bone fragments. Occasionally, comminuted fractures of the articular surface of the talus occur. As with all articular fractures, anatomic reduction and rigid fixation are needed for optimal outcome. Reconstruction may be difficult due to the small size of the trochlea and degree of comminution. If reconstruction is not feasible, primary arthrodesis may be performed (see p. 992). Racing greyhounds often incur fractures of the central tarsal bone; however, this injury is rarely seen in companion animals. Central tarsal fractures are graded according to fracture type and degree of fragment displacement. Once the buttress effect of the central tarsal bone is lost, fractures of the fourth tarsal bone and/or calcaneus may occur. Repair requires accurate placement of one or more small compression screws. Readers are referred in the suggested reading list for detailed information on treatment methods.

DIAGNOSIS
Clinical Presentation

Signalment. Any age, breed, or sex of dog or cat may be affected. Racing greyhounds most commonly develop fractures of the central tarsal bone and accessory carpal bones.

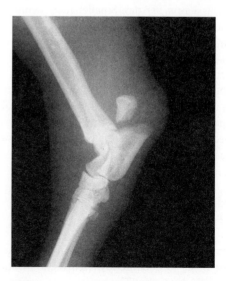

FIG. 29-58
Lateral radiograph of a dog with a transverse fracture of the calcaneus.

History. Affected animals usually present for an acute onset of non–weight-bearing lameness, or if the calcaneus is fractured they may be partially weight bearing with a plantigrade stance.

Physical Examination Findings

Patients with fractures of the carpus or tarsus usually have a non–weight-bearing lameness; attempts to place weight on the limb cause the carpus/tarsus to collapse in a plantigrade stance. If the calcaneus is fractured, the animal may walk plantigrade on the limb or may be non-weight bearing. Pain, swelling, and crepitus are present in the affected limb. Varus or valgus deviation of the foot is usually present.

Radiography

Standard craniocaudal and medial to lateral radiographs are usually sufficient to make the diagnosis. Oblique radiographs of the tarsocrural joint help delineate fractures of the articular surface of the tibial tarsal bone.

Laboratory Findings

Consistent laboratory abnormalities are not present.

DIFFERENTIAL DIAGNOSIS

Fractures of the carpus/tarsus must be differentiated from ligamentous injury, which may occur concurrently with fractures. Standard radiographs are sufficient to make this observation. Calcaneal fractures must be differentiated from lacerations or rupture of the Achilles tendon. Acute lacerations are accompanied by an open wound and soft tissue swelling is limited to an area proximal to the calcaneal tuberosity, whereas fractures of the calcaneus exhibit swelling caudal to the tarsus and crepitation may be elicited on palpation.

MEDICAL MANAGEMENT OR CONSERVATIVE TREATMENT

Anatomic reduction and rigid fixation are needed for optimal outcome in animals with intraarticular fractures of the carpus or tarsus; conservative treatment with casts or splints is not effective. External coaptation is also not appropriate for calcaneal fractures because bandaging or splint application is ineffective in countering tensile forces produced by the Achilles muscle/tendon unit.

SURGICAL TREATMENT

The radial carpal bone is a major weight-bearing structure. Congruity of the articular surface between it and the distal radius is necessary for optimal long-term function. Small chip fragments that cannot be stabilized should be removed; large fragments, however, should be anatomically reduced and rigidly stabilized with compression screws or a combination of compression screws and Kirschner wires. With calcaneal fractures, pull of the gastrocnemius muscle must be resisted with a tension band (see p. 828). Fractures of the talus bone must be anatomically reduced and rigidly stabilized for optimal outcome. If preoperative assessment indicates that is not feasible, arthrodesis of the tarsocrural joint should be considered (see p. 992).

Preoperative Management

Patients with comminuted fractures of the carpus/tarsus may present with open wounds. These wounds should be cleaned and protected from further damage and contamination with a sterile bandage until surgery can be performed.

Anesthesia

See p. 708 for anesthetic management of animals with fractures. Racing greyhounds should be anesthetized with care. Avoid thiamylal and thiopental; methohexital (an ultra–short-acting barbiturate), a combination of ketamine and Valium, or propofol may be used in these patients.

Surgical Anatomy

The carpus is composed of the proximal and distal row of carpal bones. The radial carpal bone articulates primarily with the radius and serves as the major weight-bearing area in the joint. It is the most common carpal bone fractured in companion animals.

The calcaneus is the largest of the tarsal bones. The distal half of the bone has two facets and two processes that articulate with the talus to form a stable joint. Proximally, the tuber calcanei forms a sturdy prominence to accommodate insertion of the Achilles tendon (see p. 1004). The talus is the second largest of the tarsal bones. It articulates proximally with the tibia and fibula and distally with the central tarsal bone. The tarsus is divided into medial and lateral trochlea that articulate with the tibia proximally and a body that articulates with the central tarsal bone distally. The sides of the trochlea articulate with the medial and lateral malleoli respectively.

Positioning

For carpal fractures the animal is placed in dorsal recumbency. The limb should be clipped and prepared for aseptic surgery from the elbow to the digits. A hanging limb prep facilitates limb manipulation during surgery. Animals are placed in lateral recumbency with the affected limb uppermost for calcaneal fractures and in lateral recumbency with the injured leg adjacent to the operating table for fractures of the talus. With the latter injuries, the limb should be clipped and surgically prepped from the stifle joint to digits.

SURGICAL TECHNIQUES
Stabilization of Radial Carpal Bone Fractures

Make a craniomedial incision beginning 3 to 4 cm proximal to the radiocarpal joint (see p. 940). Extend the incision distally to the midmetacarpus and incise subcutaneous tissues along the same line. Continue deep dissection medial to the extensor carpi radialis tendon to expose the joint capsule. Incise joint capsule and identify the fracture plane through the radial carpal bone. Reduce the fracture and stabilize fragments with one or more compression screws (Fig. 29-59). Close the joint capsule and subcutaneous tissue with absorbable suture and close skin with nonabsorbable suture.

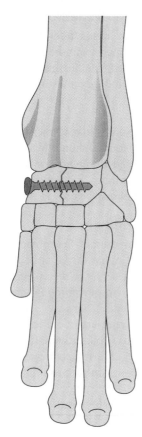

FIG. 29-59
Reduction of a radial carpal bone fracture with a compression screw.

Stabilization of Calcaneal Fractures

Make an incision along the lateral surface of the calcaneus. Begin the incision along the common calcanean tendon, just proximal to the tuber calcanei. Continue the incision distally to the level of the tarsometatarsal joint. Incise superficial and deep fascia overlying the caudal border of the calcaneus. Identify the lateral aspect of the superficial digital flexor tendon and make an incision parallel to this border. Retract the tendon medially to expose the caudal surface of the calcaneus. Reduce the fracture fragments and place two small pins or Kirschner wires to maintain reduction. Drill a hole from lateral to medial in the distal fragment to accept orthopedic wire. Proximally, pass the wire around the ends of the pins or through a second predrilled hole positioned through the body of the calcaneus proximal to the fracture. Tighten the wire to complete the tension band procedure (Fig. 29-60). Replace the superficial digital flexor tendon and suture surrounding deep fascia with absorbable suture to maintain the position of the tendon. Next suture superficial fascia and skin using standard techniques.

Stabilization of Talus Bone Fractures

Exposure of the trochlea and visualization of the fracture is best accomplished with an osteotomy of the medial malleolus. *Center the skin incision over the medial malleolus. Begin 5 cm proximal to the malleolus and carry the incision*

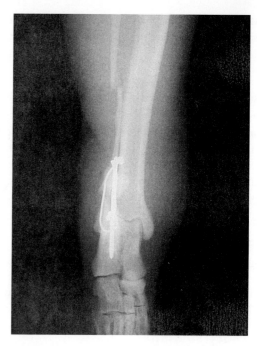

FIG. 29-60
Radiograph showing repair of a calcaneal fracture with a Kirschner wire and tension band.

distally to the tarsometatarsal joint. Incise through superficial and deep fascia to identify the long component of the medial collateral ligament. Make a transverse, caudal to cranial incision through joint capsule overlying the distal tibia to allow visualization of landmarks for completion of an osteotomy of the medial malleolus. Retract the malleolus and attached ligaments to expose the talus. Reduce fracture fragments and stabilize each with a lag screw (see p. 753) or Kirschner wire. Once fracture reduction and stabilization are satisfactory, reduce and stabilize the medial malleolus with a tension band (see p. 813). Suture superficial and deep fascia with absorbable suture and close skin with nonabsorbable sutures.

SUTURE MATERIALS/SPECIAL INSTRUMENTS

Necessary equipment includes Kirschner wire, small intramedullary Steinmann pins, orthopedic wire, and instrumentation needed for insertion of lag screws. An air-driven or battery-operated drill is often helpful.

POSTOPERATIVE CARE AND ASSESSMENT

Controlled activity on a leash is mandatory until healing is complete. Short leash walks should be used initially to help maintain strength and joint mobility. The distance walked can be gradually increased. Passive flexion and extension of the carpus/tarsus can be performed to maintain joint motion, enhance patient comfort, and improve synovial nutrient presentation to the articular cartilage. Pins used in application of the tension band for stabilization of calcaneal fractures may irritate soft tissues and should be removed following healing. Screws used for reconstruction of radial carpal bone/talus are not removed unless they cause a problem.

PROGNOSIS

Prognosis with calcaneal fractures is excellent for return to normal activity. Return to function with carpus/tarsus fractures is fair to good, depending on the degree of articular cartilage damage present and whether the articular surface can be reconstructed.

Suggested Reading

Boudrieau RJ, Dee JF, Dee LG: Central tarsal bone fractures in the racing greyhound: a review of 114 cases, *J Am Vet Med Assoc* 184:1486, 1984.

Boudrieau RJ, Dee JF, Dee LG: Treatment of central tarsal bone fractures in the racing greyhound, *J Am Vet Med Assoc* 184:1492, 1984.

Brinker WO, Piermattei DL, Flo GL: *Handbook of small animal orthopedics and fracture treatment,* ed 2, Philadelphia, 1990, Saunders.

Ercegan MG, Somber T: Detailed anatomy of the antebrachiocarpal joint in dogs, *Anatom Rec* 233:329, 1992.

Johnson KA, Dee JF, Piermattei DL: Screw fixation of accessory carpal bone fractures in racing greyhounds: 12 cases (1981–1986), *J Am Vet Med Assoc* 194:1618, 1989.

Moore RW: Orthopedics of the forelimb-carpus and digits. In Slatter DH, editor: *Small animal surgery,* vol 2, Philadelphia, 1985, Saunders.

Ost PC et al: Fractures of the calcaneus in racing greyhounds, *Vet Surg* 16:53, 1994.

Vaughan LC: Disorders of the carpus in the dog I, *Br Vet J* 141:332, 1985.

Vaughan LC: Disorders of the carpus in the dog II, *Br Vet J* 141:435, 1985.

Vaughan LC: Disorders of the tarsus in the dog I, *Br Vet J* 143:388, 1987.

Vaughan LC: Disorders of the tarsus in the dog II, *Br Vet J* 143:498, 1987.

METACARPAL, METATARSAL, PHALANGEAL, AND SESAMOID BONE FRACTURES AND LUXATIONS

DEFINITIONS

Sesamoid bones are small round or oblong bones found adjacent to joints.

GENERAL CONSIDERATIONS AND CLINICALLY RELEVANT PATHOPHYSIOLOGY

Metacarpal and metatarsal bone fractures are common in dogs and cats. They may occur from a direct blow or force to the paw or else arise when the paw is caught in a trap. Metacarpal and metatarsal fractures are classified according to location (e.g., base or proximal end of the bone, shaft or diaphysis, and head or distal end of the bone). Avulsion frac-

tures of the base occur most commonly on the second and fifth bones because of their ligamentous insertions. Phalangeal fractures occur similarly in dogs and cats; however, fragments are often smaller and more difficult to secure. There are two palmar or plantar sesamoid bones per metacarpal or metatarsal phalangeal joint, numbered 1 through 8 beginning on the medial side. Sesamoid fractures occur after excessive tension on the digital flexor tendons. Sesamoid bones 2 and 7 of either the forelimb or rear limb are most commonly affected. Luxations of the metacarpophalangeal joints or interphalangeal joints occur most commonly in working dogs or racing greyhounds. Early surgical repair yields better results than closed reduction and splintage as chronic instability leads to degenerative joint disease and less than optimal function.

DIAGNOSIS
Clinical Presentation

Signalment. Any age, breed, or sex of dog or cat may be affected. Racing greyhounds develop stress fractures of the second metacarpal and/or third metatarsal bones of the right foot and luxations of the distal interphalangeal joints. Sesamoid fractures are most common in large-breed dogs.

History. There is generally a history of trauma. Dogs with sesamoid fractures may have a previous history of acute lameness that subsided, but recurs with exercise.

Physical Examination Findings

Animals with metacarpal, metatarsal, or phalangeal fractures present with a non–weight-bearing lameness of the affected limb. Soft tissues surrounding the fracture are swollen, crepitation can be palpated, and deformity of the paw may be noted. The animal will be in pain when the area is palpated. Dogs with sesamoid fractures, especially chronic fractures, usually have a weight-bearing lameness. Mild swelling may be evident and affected animals are painful on deep palpation over the bone. Dogs with joint luxations present with lameness, swelling over the affected joint, medial or lateral deviation of the digit, joint instability, and pain on palpation.

☞ **N O T E** • Most fractures in the paw cause non–weight-bearing lameness, but sesamoid fractures cause less obvious lameness.

Radiographs

Radiographs should include lateral and caudal-cranial views extending from the carpus or tarsus to the ends of the digits. Oblique views, with the digits spread, may be necessary to isolate individual bones. Stress radiographs taken while the distal digit is displaced may be needed to show joint instability.

Laboratory Findings

Specific laboratory abnormalities are not present with these fractures or luxations. Traumatized animals should have sufficient blood work done to assess the risk of anesthesia and surgery.

DIFFERENTIAL DIAGNOSIS

Animals presenting with fractures of the metacarpal, metatarsal, and/or phalangeal bones should be carefully evaluated for concurrent ligamentous injury in the carpus, tarsus, and distal joints of the paw. Radiographs help to differentiate between fractures and luxations caused by ligamentous injury.

MEDICAL OR CONSERVATIVE MANAGEMENT

Conservative treatment with a fiberglass bivalve cast or metasplint (see p. 706) is appropriate for treating closed, nondisplaced metacarpal and metatarsal diaphyseal fractures affecting one or two bones (especially the second and fifth bones). This treatment is also appropriate for most phalangeal fractures and acute sesamoid bone fractures. The cast or splint should not be removed until there is radiographic evidence that the fracture has bridged with bone (usually 4 to 8 weeks). Chronic sesamoid fractures causing lameness do not usually respond to conservative therapy. Acute luxations can be treated conservatively with a cast or splint, but are best treated surgically in working or racing dogs. Chronic luxations causing lameness do not respond to conservative care and are usually treated with arthrodesis or amputation.

☞ **NOTE·** Casts and splints are inappropriate treatment when three or four metacarpal or metatarsal bones are fractured.

SURGICAL TREATMENT

Metacarpal or metatarsal fractures occurring in athletic or racing dogs usually require anatomic reduction and rigid stabilization (plates and screws) for optimal return to racing form (Fig. 29-61). Avulsed fragments from the base of the second and fifth metacarpals/metatarsals generally require open reduction and internal fixation because their ligamentous insertions cause fragment distraction (Fig. 29-62). Fracture of the shaft of one or two metacarpal or metatarsal bones can be treated with external coaptation because the unaffected bones form an internal splint to prevent deformity (Table 29-15). Fractures affecting three or four metacarpal or metatarsal bones require internal fixation for optimal results (Fig. 29-63; see also Fig. 29-61).

Fractures of the phalanges occur less frequently, but are handled similarly to metacarpal and metatarsal bone fractures. Fractures of the proximal sesamoid bones of the metacarpophalangeal joints and metatarsal phalangeal joints cause chronic lameness and are generally treated by removing the fragments.

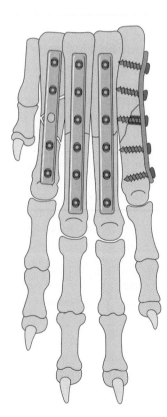

FIG. 29-61
Plate fixation of metacarpal/metatarsal fractures. Plate fixation is used when the fracture-assessment score is low or athletic function is desired. A bridging buttress plate has been used to span and support a comminuted fracture *(digit 2)*, compression plates have been applied to transverse fractures *(digits 3 & 4)*, and lag screw compression of an oblique fracture line was protected by a neutralization plate *(digit 5)*.

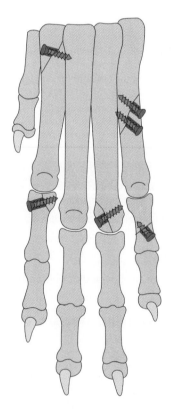

FIG. 29-62
Lag screw fixation for avulsion fractures. Lag screws are used to counteract the pull of adjacent ligaments or compress oblique fractures.

Acute luxations are treated surgically with open reduction and suturing of the joint capsule and collateral ligaments. Failure of the initial surgical stabilization or chronic joint luxations are best treated with amputation (second or fifth toe) or arthrodesis (middle weight-bearing third and fourth digits) (Table 29-16).

Fixation systems applicable for metacarpal, metatarsal, and phalangeal fractures include orthopedic wire, intramedullary (IM) pins, external fixation, and plates and screws. The most appropriate fixation method should be determined based on fracture-assessment score and fracture location (Table 29-17). If the fracture-assessment score (see p. 730) indicates rapid healing (fracture-assessment score of 8 to 10), conservative therapy is indicated; however, if three or four bones are affected resulting in gross displacement or folding of the paw, open reduction and stabilization with IM pins should be considered. If athletic function is desired, accurate reduction and plate and screw fixation should be considered. Non-displaced avulsion fractures of the base or head of these bones can be treated with a splint or cast, but some displacement of the fracture usually occurs during the healing process. Open reduction and placement of a lag screw or tension band wire offers the best chance for return to normal function. If the fracture-assessment score (see p. 730) is between 4 and 7 (i.e., older or larger dogs where healing may be delayed, displaced comminuted fractures of the diaphysis of three or four metacarpal or metatarsal bones, or animals with multiple limb fractures) consideration should be given to treating the fractures with open reduction and plate and screw fixations. Fracture-assessment scores less than 4 indicate prolonged healing. Severely comminuted fractures or open fractures with degloving injuries can be treated with bridging plates or external fixation with small pins and acrylic (see p. 742 and Fig. 29-64). Cancellous bone autografts are indicated in conjunction with open reduction to promote healing in these patients.

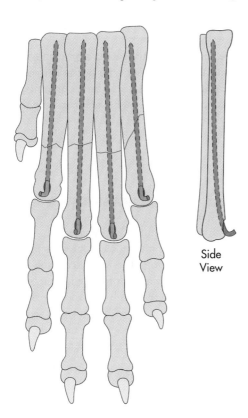

FIG. 29-63
Intramedullary pinning technique used to treat multiple transverse or short oblique fractures in patients with high fracture-assessment scores. A slot is developed in the distal metaphysis and the pin is directed through the slot (proximally across the fracture line) and is seated in the proximal metaphysis of the metacarpal or metatarsal bone.

Side View

TABLE 29-15

Important Considerations for Treating Metacarpal/Metatarsal Fractures

- Fractures of one or two metacarpal or metatarsal bones can be treated with a splint or cast.
- Fractures of three or four metacarpal or metatarsal bones should be treated with internal fixation.
- Avulsion fractures should be treated with a lag screw.
- A splint or bivalve cast should be applied after internal fixation until there is radiographic evidence of bone healing.

TABLE 29-16

Important Considerations in Treating Luxations

- Acute luxations in working or racing dogs are best treated with open reduction and suturing the joint capsule and collateral ligaments.
- Chronic luxations of the second or fifth toe can be treated with amputation.
- Arthrodesis of metacarpophalangeal and interphalangeal joints can result in good function and pain relief.

TABLE 29-17

Implant Use According to Fracture-Assessment Score (FAS)

FAS 0 to 3
- Bridging plates*
- External fixators*
- Lag screws for avulsion fractures

FAS 4 to 7
- Bone plates and screws*
- IM pins*
- Lag screws for avulsion fractures

FAS 8 to 10
- Splint or cast*
- IM pins*
- Tension band wire for avulsion fractures

*Choice depends on number of bones fractured, comminution, displacement, number of limbs injured, and desired function of animal (see text).

FIG. 29-64
Fixation pins are placed in two planes and connected with acrylic bars for rigid stabilization of comminuted fractures. This fixation does not interfere with open wound treatment.

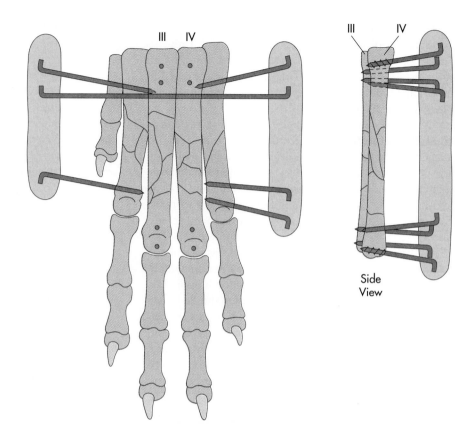

III   IV

III   IV

Side View

Preoperative Management

The paw should be temporarily stabilized with a soft padded bandage and metasplint (see p. 706) to immobilize fragments, decrease or prevent soft tissue swelling, protect or prevent open wounds, and increase patient comfort until surgery can be performed. Open wounds should be initially managed by carefully clipping surrounding hair, cleaning the wound, obtaining a sample for microbial culture and sensitivity testing, and administering broad-spectrum bactericidal antibiotics. Concurrent injuries should be managed prior to anesthetic induction for fracture fixation.

Anesthesia

Refer to p. 708 for anesthetic management of patients with fractures.

Surgical Anatomy

The primary weight-bearing bones are the third and fourth digits. The superficial dorsal metacarpal or metatarsal artery courses over the dorsal aspect of the paw. The extensor tendons course down the dorsal aspect of each digit. The flexor tendons and superficial and deep metacarpal or metatarsal artery and vein lie on the palmar or plantar aspect of the digits. Each joint has a medial and lateral collateral ligament. The paired proximal sesamoid bones are located caudal to the metacarpophalangeal or metatarsophalangeal joints and have firm ligamentous attachments. There is minimal soft tissue coverage, and the bones and joints can be easily palpated. Skin incisions are generally made on the dorsal surface

of the paw, directly over the fracture or luxation. The extensor tendons and ligaments of the dorsal surface of the paw need to be retracted to expose the bones or joints. Ventral approaches to the digits are only made to expose the proximal sesamoid bones.

> ☞ **N O T E** · A tourniquet may help control hemorrhage from the paw.

Positioning

The entire distal limb should be prepared for aseptic surgery. The animal is placed in dorsal recumbency with the affected paw isolated for draping. The most accessible site for harvesting a cancellous bone graft for the forelimb is the proximal humerus; for the rear limb it is the proximal tibia (see p. 760 for bone grafting techniques). These areas should be prepared and draped if a bone graft is needed (i.e., comminuted fractures with a fracture-assessment score less than 4).

SURGICAL TECHNIQUES
Stabilization of Transverse Metacarpal or Metatarsal Fractures

Multiple, simple transverse (or very short oblique) metacarpal bone fractures can be repaired with IM pins. *Incise skin over the dorsal surface of the third and fourth bones. Incise subcutaneous tissues and elevate and retract extensor tendons to expose the fractures. Introduce the pin into the distal, dorsal surface of the bone to avoid the joint (use a high-speed burr to develop a slot in the bone). Blunt the tip of the pin to prevent it from penetrating the intact opposite cortex. Drive the pin through the slot and proximally across the fracture line and seat it in the proximal bone segment. Bend the distal end of the pin to prevent migration and simplify removal. Repeat the procedure for at least the third and fourth metacarpal or metatarsal bone (and preferably all four bones; see Fig. 29-63). Protect the fixation with a splint or cast for 4 to 6 weeks.*

If more rigid fixation is required in animals with low patient fracture assessment (i.e., large dogs with multiple limb injury), bone plates can be applied as compression plates.

Stabilization of Avulsion Fractures and Oblique Diaphyseal Fractures

Avulsion fractures of the base or head and intraarticular fractures of the metacarpal, metatarsal, or phalangeal bones can be repaired using lag screws (see p. 753). Lag screws are placed after anatomic reconstruction of these fractures and counteract the pull of attached ligaments (see Fig. 29-62). Orthopedic wire with Kirschner wires can be used as tension band wire (see p. 746) in avulsion fractures in animals with patient fracture assessment of 8 to 10. Simple, oblique fractures of the diaphyses can often be reconstructed with lag screws and the repair supported with a splint or bivalve cast. The screws only minimally interfere with function. If diaphyseal fractures require additional support, bone plates can be applied as neutralization plates.

☞ **NOTE** • Use anatomic reconstruction with lag screws for best results in athletic dogs.

Stabilization of Comminuted Diaphyseal Fractures

Severely comminuted fractures of the diaphyses of the metacarpal and metatarsal bones can be repaired with small, dynamic compression plates (2.7 mm or 2.0 mm) or veterinary cuttable plates (see p. 749), which bridge the comminuted portions of the fracture. Fragments should be left undisturbed and the plate attached to the proximal and distal segments. Plates should be applied to two to four bones (depending on fracture configuration and number of bones fractured). A splint or cast should be used to support the fixation after surgery. Alternatively, multiple Kirschner wires or IM pins can be inserted through the proximal and distal segments of the bones and connected with acrylic to form an external fixator (see Fig. 29-64). This type of fixation is also useful for treating open fractures.

☞ **NOTE** • Acrylic fixator bars are versatile: they can accommodate various size pins placed in multiple planes.

Sesamoid Bone Excision

Incise the skin adjacent to the large central pad directly over the ventral aspect of the affected joint. Continue the incision through subcutaneous tissues and identify the fractured sesamoid. Sharply dissect the sesamoid fragments from their ligamentous attachments. If the fragment is less than one third of the sesamoid bone, remove only the fragment. If the fragment is larger, remove the entire sesamoid bone. Suture subcutaneous tissues and skin separately.

Suture Repair of Luxations

Incise skin and subcutaneous tissue dorsally over the affected joint to expose the torn joint capsule and collateral ligaments. Use multiple absorbable horizontal mattress sutures to repair the joint capsule and ligament. Continue to imbricate (tighten the joint capsule with mattress sutures) the capsular tissues until the joint is stable. Repair the capsule bilaterally if necessary. Also inspect the extensor tendon retinaculum for tears and stabilize it with interrupted sutures. Suture subcutaneous tissues and skin.

Digit Amputation

Make an elliptical skin incision paralleling the long axis of and around the digit, starting proximodorsally and ending distally on the palmar or plantar surface (Fig. 29-65). Preserve the pad if amputating at the interphalangeal joints. Disarticulate the joint with sharp dissection. Remove the sesamoid bones (metacarpophalangeal or metatarsophalangeal joint amputation). Resect the distal end of the proximal remaining bone. Make a transverse osteotomy line for the interphalangeal joints and third and fourth metacarpal

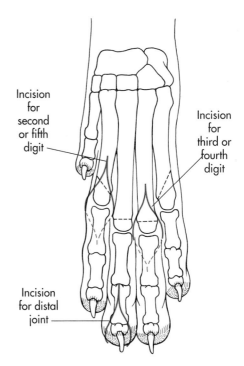

FIG. 29-65
Suggested skin incision lines and osteotomy lines for proximal and distal digit amputation.

or metatarsal bones, but bevel the osteotomy distally toward the midline for the second and fifth metacarpal or metatarsal bones. Suture soft tissues and skin taking care to obtain a cosmetic closure.

Arthrodesis

Expose the joint using the approach described for suturing joint luxations. Open the joint capsule and remove the articular cartilage with rongeurs. Conform the surfaces to get good contact at a functional angle (determined by observing adjacent toes). Temporarily hold the bones in position by driving small K-wires from the dorsal surface of each bone across the joint surface. Contour a small plate (2.0 mm) to the dorsal surface of the bones. Attach the plate using at least one lag screw across the joint surface (Fig. 29-66, A). Alternatively, stabilize the arthrodesis with the small K-wires and a tension band wire (Fig. 29-66, B) in small dogs or cats in which rapid healing is anticipated.

SUTURE MATERIALS/SPECIAL INSTRUMENTS

Equipment that should be available for management of fractures or luxations of the distal extremity includes IM pins, Kirschner wires, orthopedic wire, Jacobs pin chuck, wire tightener, plating equipment, hoof or dental acrylic, and rongeurs, bone cutters, or an osteotome. A tourniquet applied to the distal limb is useful for controlling hemorrhage during surgery, but should only be maintained for 1 hour.

POSTOPERATIVE CARE AND ASSESSMENT

Postoperative radiographs should be made to evaluate fracture reduction and implant position, reduction of luxations, and

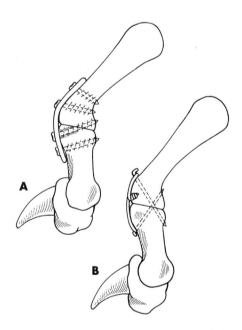

FIG. 29-66
A, Arthrodesis of the proximal interphalangeal joint with a plate and lag screw or **B,** Kirschner wires and a tension band wire.

alignment of arthrodeses. Radiographs should be repeated every 4 to 6 weeks until the fracture(s) or the arthrodesis is healed. The foot should be supported in a splint or bivalve cast until there is radiographic evidence of bone healing (even after internal fixation). After digit amputation, the paw should be supported in a soft bandage for 1 to 2 weeks. After fracture healing has occurred IM pins, plates, and external fixators should be removed, but orthopedic wire and screws may be left in place as long as no implant-associated complications arise. Limited activity is advised until radiographic signs of fracture bridging with bone are visible. Owners should be instructed to confine animals to a small area (preferably a cage). The cast or splint should be kept clean and dry and the owner should observe it daily for evidence of slippage or irritation.

PROGNOSIS

Most metacarpal and metatarsal fractures heal without complication. Fractures of the diaphyses of three or four metacarpal or metatarsal bones treated with a metasplint may develop delayed union or malunion and frequently become nonunions. Other potential complications include iatrogenic infection (with open reduction) and secondary degenerative joint disease after articular fracture. In most cases however, the prognosis for normal limb function after fracture healing or removal of fractured sesamoid bones is good.

Prognosis for function after surgical repair of joint luxations is dependent on the stability of the repair. Unstable joints will develop progressive degenerative joint disease and cause lameness. Function after amputation of the second and fifth digit is usually good. The more distal the amputation, the better the prognosis. Function after arthrodesis is generally good.

Suggested Reading

Brinker WO, Piermattei DL, Flo GL: *Handbook of small animal orthopedics and fracture treatment*, ed 2, Philadelphia, 1990, Saunders.

PELVIC FRACTURES

ACETABULAR FRACTURES

DEFINITIONS

Acetabular fractures occur through the articular surface and medial fossa of the acetabulum.

SYNONYMS

Hip joint fractures

GENERAL CONSIDERATIONS AND CLINICALLY RELEVANT PATHOPHYSIOLOGY

The hip joint transfers weight from the rear limb through the pelvis to the spine. Loss of normal articular contour between the femoral head and acetabulum occurs if a displaced ac-

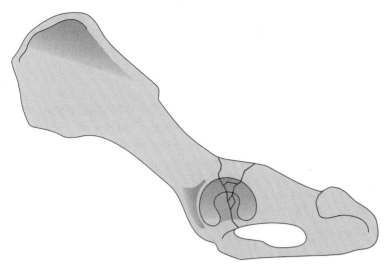

FIG. 29-67
Central transacetabular fracture with comminution arising from the medial fossa.

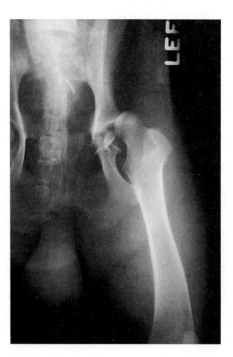

FIG. 29-68
Ventrodorsal radiograph of a central transacetabular fracture with comminution arising from the medial fossa.

etabular fracture is left to heal without surgical reduction and stabilization. The end result is secondary degenerative joint disease that may cause pain and lameness.

Fractures of the acetabulum are classified according to involvement of the articular surface and may be cranial transacetabular, central transacetabular, caudal transacetabular, or comminuted transacetabular. Central transacetabular fractures are most common, followed by comminuted transacetabular fractures (Figs. 29-67 and 29-68).

DIAGNOSIS
Clinical Presentation

Signalment. Any age, breed, or sex of dog or cat may be affected; acetabular fractures are rare in cats, however.

History. Acetabular fractures commonly occur as a result of motor vehicle accidents, but may be associated with other forms of blunt trauma or a fall.

Physical Examination Findings

Affected animals generally present for evaluation of a non–weight-bearing lameness. Some patients bear weight on the affected limb if fracture displacement is minimal. Pain can generally be elicited upon manipulation of the hip joint; however, crepitation may or may not be present.

Radiography

Ventrodorsal and lateral radiographs should be taken to assess the fracture plane. Medial to lateral radiographs or oblique radiographs often help delineate the fracture. The radiographic appearance of an acetabular fracture may be misleading in that the fracture may appear to be comminuted when there is actually a single fracture line through the articular surface. The bone fragments in these cases arise from the medial-ventral fossa of the acetabulum and are not from the weight-bearing articular surface of the acetabulum.

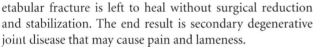

N O T E · Caution: Central transacetabular fractures may be mistaken for comminuted articular fractures.

Laboratory Findings

Consistent laboratory abnormalities are not present.

DIFFERENTIAL DIAGNOSIS

Differential diagnoses include capital physeal fractures, coxofemoral luxations, proximal femoral fractures, and ipsilateral ilial or ischial fracture.

MEDICAL OR CONSERVATIVE MANAGEMENT

To maintain joint congruity and the normal distribution of stress over the articular surface, reduction and stabilization of acetabular fractures are recommended in all cases. If the client cannot afford surgery, conservative treatment may be considered; however, it may result in less than optimal limb function. Conservative treatment for acetabular fractures is similar to that described for ilial fractures on p. 839.

SURGICAL TREATMENT
Preoperative Management

Urination and bowel movements should be monitored before surgery. Respirations should be monitored and chest radiographs are indicated. An ECG is useful to determine cardiac rhythm, particularly if peripheral pulses appear weak or irregular. Analgesics should be considered in patients that appear to be in pain.

Anesthesia

Special anesthetic considerations for patients with orthopedic disease are included on p. 708.

Surgical Anatomy

The hip joint is a ball-and-socket joint comprising the femoral head and acetabulum. The normal conformation, surrounding musculature, suctionlike effect of the synovial fluid, and ligament of the femoral head act to stabilize the joint. The articular surface is on the dorsolateral face of the acetabulum, while the medial face is occupied by the round ligament. The fibrous joint capsule originates from the lateral acetabular rim and inserts onto the femoral neck. Stabilizing musculature surrounding the hip includes the gluteal musculature, internal and external rotators, and the iliopsoas medially.

The sciatic nerve courses dorsomedial to the acetabulum. Fractures cause the caudal acetabular segment to become displaced medial and cranial to the cranial segment. The sciatic nerve may be positioned directly dorsal or dorsolateral to the caudal acetabular segment. Caution must be exercised when exposing and reducing the caudal segment to avoid damaging this nerve. Soft tissue bruising and swelling often distort the normal anatomy. Dissection adjacent to the greater trochanter facilitates correct tissue identification and reflection. The insertion of the deep gluteal muscle at the greater trochanter can be used as a landmark for dissection.

Positioning

The animal is positioned in lateral recumbency with the dorsum raised 30 degrees from the operating table. The hip should be prepped from the dorsal midline to the tarsus. A hanging leg preparation facilitates manipulation of the limb during surgery.

SURGICAL TECHNIQUE

Make a skin incision centered over the cranial border of the greater trochanter. Begin the incision 3 to 4 cm proximal to the dorsal ridge of the greater trochanter and curve it distally 3 to 4 cm following the cranial border of the femur. Incise the superficial leaf of the fascia lata at the cranial border of the biceps femoris muscle and retract the muscle caudally (Fig. 29-69, A). Incise the deep leaf of the fascia lata and carry the incision proximally through the insertion of the tensor fasciae latae muscle at the greater trochanter and along the cranial border of the superficial gluteal muscle. Incise through the insertion of the superficial gluteal muscle at the third trochanter. Reflect the superficial gluteal muscle proximally and the biceps femoris caudally to find and visualize the course of the sciatic nerve (Fig. 29-69, B). Perform an osteotomy of the greater trochanter with an osteotome and mallet (Fig. 29-69, C). Position the osteotome just proximal to the insertion of the superficial gluteal muscle at the third trochanter. Angle the osteotome 45 degrees to the long axis of the femur to remove the trochanter with the insertions of the deep gluteal and mid-

dle gluteal muscles (Fig. 29-69, D). Reflect the gluteal muscles and greater trochanter from the joint capsule with a periosteal elevator. Visualize the insertions of the gemellus muscle and tendon of the internal obturator and preplace a suture through the two near the trochanteric fossa. Incise both structures together at the trochanteric fossa and elevate the gemellus muscle from the caudolateral surface of the acetabulum with a periosteal elevator (Fig. 29-69, E and F). Use the suture to retract the muscle proximally and caudally. When reducing the fracture, pay particular attention to the alignment of the articular surface (which is facilitated by incising the joint capsule) (Fig. 29-69, G). To achieve maximum rigidity, use a bone plate and screws (Fig. 29-69, H). Specially designed canine acetabular plates, metacarpal plates, and mandibular reconstruction plates have all been used successfully to repair acetabular fractures. *Place plates on the dorsolateral surface of the acetabulum. Attempt to place two plate screws in the caudal fragment and three plate screws in the cranial fragment (Fig. 29-70). After reduction and stabilization, suture the gemelli and internal obturator tendon to their point of insertion. Reduce and stabilize the greater trochanter with two Kirschner wires and a tension band wire. Place interrupted sutures in the insertion of the superficial gluteal muscle and a continuous suture in the insertion of the tensor fasciae latae muscle and deep leaf of the fascia lata. Use a continuous suture in the superficial leaf of the fasciae latae and the subcutaneous tissue. Suture skin with an interrupted suture pattern.*

SUTURE MATERIALS/SPECIAL INSTRUMENTS

Equipment is needed for application of an acetabular bone plate (see p. 747) and an osteotome and mallet are necessary to perform a trochanteric osteotomy. Small pins and wire are used to stabilize the trochanteric osteotomy with a tension band.

POSTOPERATIVE CARE AND ASSESSMENT

Limit activity to leash walking until there is evidence that the fracture is healed radiographically. Healing generally occurs between 4 and 8 weeks, depending on the biologic fracture assessment. Implants are not routinely removed. Occasionally, the tension band wire and Kirschner wires will need to be removed due to soft tissue irritation.

PROGNOSIS

The prognosis is good to excellent if the fracture is anatomically reduced and appropriately stabilized. Of 55 patients with acetabular fractures treated surgically, 44 returned to normal limb function and 7 had occasional lameness (Anson et al, 1987; Hulse, 1983). The remainder had unsatisfactory limb function associated with sciatic nerve injury and/or osteoarthrosis. It was previously believed that fractures involving the caudal third of the articular surface of the acetabulum did not require surgery. This concept has been refuted

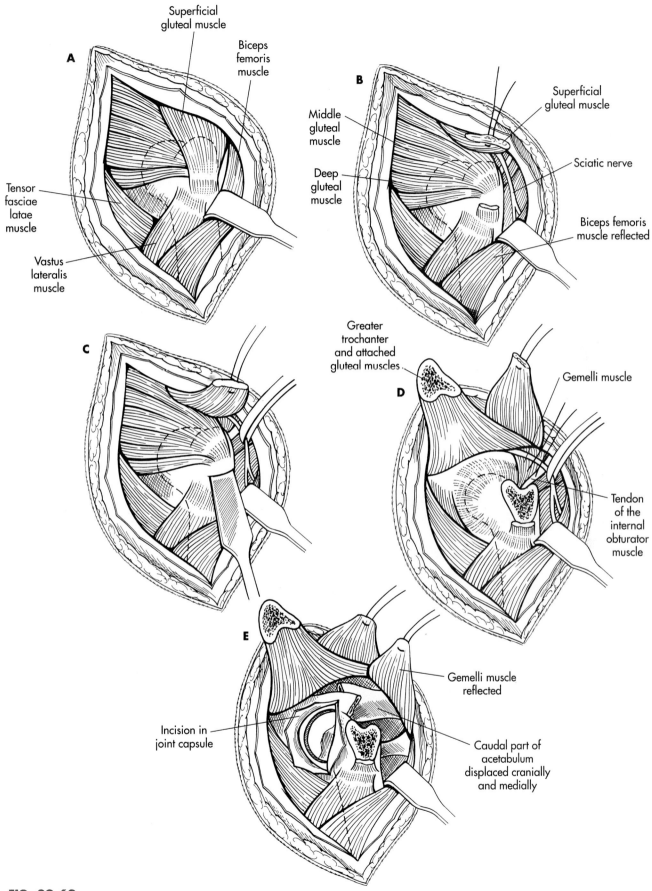

A

Superficial
gluteal muscle

Biceps
femoris
muscle

Tensor
fasciae
latae
muscle

Vastus
lateralis
muscle

B

Middle
gluteal
muscle

Deep
gluteal
muscle

Superficial
gluteal muscle

Sciatic nerve

Biceps femoris
muscle reflected

C

D

Greater
trochanter
and attached
gluteal muscles

Gemelli muscle

Tendon
of the
internal
obturator
muscle

E

Incision in
joint capsule

Gemelli muscle
reflected

Caudal part of
acetabulum
displaced cranially
and medially

FIG. 29-69
For legend, see p. 838.

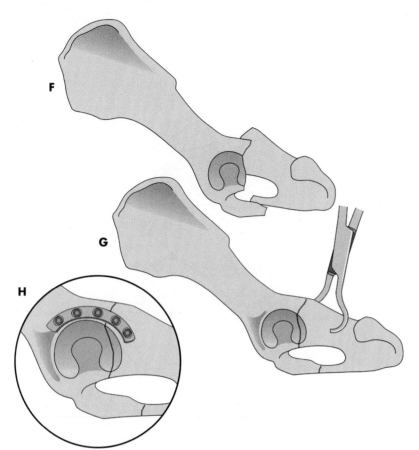

FIG. 29-69, CONT'D.
A, To expose the hip joint through osteotomy of the greater trochanter, retract the biceps femoris muscle caudally and **B,** reflect the superficial gluteal muscle to expose the third trochanter. **C** and **D,** Osteotomize the greater trochanter and reflect the attached musculature dorsally. **E** and **F,** Incise and reflect the gemelli and internal obturator muscles. Incise the joint capsule. Note that the caudal fragment of the fracture is displaced craniomedially. **G,** Reduce the fracture with bone-holding forceps placed across the lesser ischiatic notch and **H,** stabilize it with a bone plate and screws.

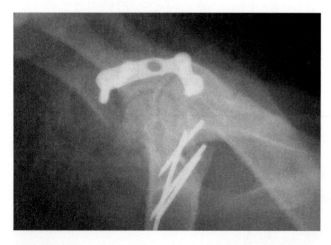

FIG. 29-70
Postoperative radiograph showing reduction and placement of a bone plate and screws to stabilize an acetabular fracture.

with a long-term clinical study that showed the majority of these patients exhibit pain and show radiographic evidence of osteoarthrosis when treated conservatively (Boudrieau, Kleine, 1988). Therefore it is recommended that all acetabular fractures, regardless of location, be surgically reconstructed.

References

Anson LW et al: Follow-up evaluation of acetabular fractures repaired with AO/ASIF acetabular plates, *Vet Surg* 16:80, 1987.

Boudrieau RJ, Kleine LJ: Nonsurgically managed caudal acetabular fractures in dogs: 15 cases (1979–1984), *J Am Vet Med Assoc* 193:701, 1988.

Hulse DA: Acetabular fractures. In Bojrab MJ, editor: *Current techniques in small animal surgery,* ed 2, Philadelphia, 1983, Lea & Febiger.

Suggested Reading

Betts CW: Pelvic fractures. In Slatter D, editor: *Textbook of small animal surgery,* ed 2, Philadelphia, 1993, Saunders.

Brinker WO, Piermattei DL, Flo GL: *Handbook of small animal orthopedics and fracture treatment,* ed 2, Philadelphia, 1990, Saunders.

Brinker WO, Braden TD: Pelvic fractures. In Brinker WO, Hohn RB, Prieur WD, editors: *Manual of internal fixation in small animals,* Berlin, 1984, Springer-Verlag.

DeCamp CE: Principles of pelvic fracture management, *Semin Vet Med Surg (Small Amin)* 7:63, 1992.

Denny HR: Pelvic fractures in the dog: a review of 123 cases, *J Small Anim Pract* 19:151, 1978.

Olmstead ML: Surgical repair of acetabular fractures. In Bojrab MJ, editor: *Current techniques in small animal surgery,* ed 3, Philadelphia, 1990, Lea and Febiger.

Ost PC, Kaderly RE: Use of reconstruction plates for the repair of segmental ilial fractures involving acetabular comminution in the dog, *Vet Surg* 15:129, 1986.

ILIAL, ISCHIAL, AND PUBIC FRACTURES

DEFINITIONS

Fractures may occur through the body or wing of the ilium. Fractures of the ischium and pubis may occur through the ischial body, floor, or pubis.

GENERAL CONSIDERATIONS AND CLINICALLY RELEVANT PATHOPHYSIOLOGY

The pelvis is a boxlike structure and for displacement of bone fragments to occur the hemipelvis must be fractured at three different sites. Commonly the ilium, ischium, and pubis are fractured simultaneously, resulting in loss of weight transfer from the affected limb to the spine, instability, and pain. Because soft tissue injury may accompany obvious bony injury, careful patient assessment is necessary. Bladder and/or urethral rupture may occur concurrent with pelvic fractures, particularly if the bladder is full at the time of impact (see p. 496). Muscle separation or avulsion of the bony insertion of the rectus abdominal muscle and herniation of abdominal viscera may also occur (see p. 184). Herniation of abdominal viscera may result in strangulation and necrosis of tissue if early diagnosis and treatment are not initiated. Impaired sensory and motor functions of the lumbosacral plexus or sciatic nerve can result from an ilial fracture.

☞ **N O T E** · Because concurrent injuries such as bladder and/or urethral tears, hernias, and peripheral nerve injuries are common in these patients, be sure to perform a complete physical examination.

Isolated ischial or pubic fractures are rare. When ischial and/or pubic fractures occur in combination with other pelvic fractures, reduction and stabilization of the primary weight-bearing segment usually results in acceptable reduction and stabilization of the pubis and ischium. The most common reason for surgical intervention of a pubic or ischial fracture is associated soft tissue herniation. Herniation of abdominal viscera can occur by separation of the pubic symphysis, cranial pubic ligament avulsion, or (rarely) herniation may occur caudal to the acetabulum.

DIAGNOSIS
Clinical Presentation

Signalment. Any breed, age, or sex of dog or cat may be affected.

History. Vehicular accidents are the usual cause of such injuries, but gunshot injuries, dog fights, and blunt trauma may also result in pelvic fractures.

Physical Examination Findings

Affected animals usually present with a non-weight bearing lameness; however, if little displacement and soft tissue injury has occurred they may be partially weight bearing. Severe bruising is common in patients sustaining pelvic fractures; however, if ventral abdominal bruising is severe or progresses, urethral trauma should be suspected. The integrity of abdominal musculature should be carefully assessed and function of the sciatic nerve determined before surgery.

Radiography

Ventrodorsal and lateral radiographs should be taken to assess the degree of injury to the hemipelvis and delineate fracture planes (Fig. 29-71). Additional diagnostics may be needed to confirm the presence or absence of soft tissue injury (i.e., cystogram, urethrogram).

Laboratory Findings

Consistent laboratory abnormalities are not found. Bladder or urethral rupture may result in azotemia and hyperkalemia (see p. 496).

DIFFERENTIAL DIAGNOSIS

Differential diagnoses include fracture/separation of the sacroiliac joint, acetabular fracture, and coxofemoral luxation.

MEDICAL OR CONSERVATIVE MANAGEMENT

Conservative treatment is indicated with ilial fractures that are minimally displaced and relatively stable. Conservative treatment may also be considered in patients if the owners are unable to afford surgery. The pelvic girdle is unstable when fractured and excessive weight bearing may cause further medial displacement of the hemipelvis, resulting in continued pain and further compromise of the pelvic canal.

Conservative treatment is appropriate for isolated ischial and/or pubic fractures. If they occur in combination with other pelvic fractures, reduction and stabilization of the primary weight-bearing segment (i.e., ilium, acetabulum) results in acceptable reduction and stabilization of the pubis and ischium.

Conservative therapy should include enforced rest for the initial 3 weeks following injury. After 3 weeks, supervised activity on a leash should be encouraged followed by controlled activity for an additional 4 weeks (with the amount of exercise gradually increased). Nonsteroidal antiinflammatory drugs can be used to control inflammation and pain (see p. 890), but the animal must be observed for adverse side effects (i.e., vomiting, melena). The animal should be maintained on well-padded bedding that is changed frequently to prevent decubital ulcers and urine scalding. Bowel movements should be monitored and stool softeners given if necessary. Warm-water sponge baths may be used to decrease odor and improve patient comfort. Physical therapy (i.e., passive flexion and extension of the hip, stifle, and tarsal joints) should be performed to prevent joint and muscle contracture. Passive movement can be replaced by more active therapy (i.e., swimming or walking up a grade) as healing progresses.

☞ **N O T E** · Limb manipulation may be painful in these animals. Be sure that owners are not bitten when performing physical therapy.

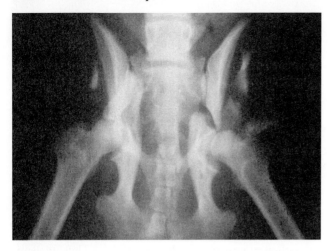

FIG. 29-71
Ventrodorsal radiograph of a dog with bilateral ilial fractures. Note comminution of the ilial body.

SURGICAL TREATMENT

Surgery is indicated with ilial fractures when nerve entrapment is suspected or when there is moderate to severe displacement and instability. Animals that have sustained bilateral pelvic limb injury benefit from surgery because they are able to walk more quickly and require less intensive postoperative care. Bone plates are usually applied to the ilial body; however, many ilial fractures have a long oblique configuration and are readily stabilized with compression screws.

☞ **N O T E** · Inform owners that although many fractures heal adequately with conservative therapy, surgery will shorten the rehabilitation time.

Surgery is indicated with ischial fractures when associated soft-tissue herniation is present, or to reestablish integrity of the pelvic girdle in intact female dogs or cats that are to be bred. Surgery is indicated with pubic fractures when associated soft-tissue herniation is present.

Preoperative Management

Urination and bowel movements should be monitored prior to surgery (see above). Respirations should be monitored and chest radiographs are indicated. An electrocardiogram is useful to determine cardiac rhythm, particularly if peripheral pulses appear weak or irregular. Analgesics should be considered in patients that appear to be in pain.

Anesthesia

See p. 708 for a discussion of anesthetic management of patients with orthopedic trauma.

Surgical Anatomy

The ilium is formed by the ilial wing and ilial body. The ilial wing is located cranially and is recognized by the palpable ilial crest dorsally. The bone curves medially to allow for the middle and deep gluteal muscles and in this area the bone is thin and may not hold implants well. The sacroiliac joint is located medially. The body of the ilium is rectangular and located between the wing of the ilium cranially and acetabulum caudally. The ilial body holds implants well due to its cortical dimensions. The sciatic nerve is located medial to the body, along its dorsal longitudinal plane. Reestablishment of ilial integrity is required for weight transfer from the limb to axial skeleton. With ilial fractures the caudal fragment is often displaced medially and cranially to the wing of the ilium. For orientation purposes it is often helpful to identify the ventral border of the ilial wing. The deep gluteal muscle is usually torn and lies between the two fragments. Because the sciatic nerve may be sandwiched between the dorsal borders of the two fragments, fragment manipulation should be done carefully.

☞ **N O T E** · Use caution when dissecting near the dorsal ilial border (or when placing bone holding forceps over the dorsal border) to prevent injury to the sciatic nerve.

The ischium is formed by the lesser ischiatic notch cranially, ischial floor medially, and ischial tuberosity caudally. Caution must be exercised with surgical dissection of the ischial notch due to the presence of the sciatic nerve. Identification of the nerve is necessary for exposure and implant application. The sciatic nerve is protected once the insertion of the external rotators is incised and reflected.

Herniation of soft tissue is the most common indication for repair of pubic fractures. Often the surgical area is bruised and swollen, making identification of normal anatomical landmarks difficult. The key for surgical dissection is to begin cranial to the injury where the ventral midline is visible. Surgical dissection can be continued caudally along the midline to expose the fractured pubis. The obturator foramen is located caudal to the cranial pubic brim. Hernia repair is discussed on p. 186.

☞ **N O T E** · If dissection is carried out near the obturator foramen, caution must be used with lateral surgical dissection because the obturator nerve passes through the foramen in this region.

Positioning

For ilial and ischial fractures, the patient is positioned in lateral recumbency. The surgical site should be prepped from the dorsal midline to the stifle joint and from a point 10 cm cranial to the ilial crest to the tailhead caudally. Animals with pubic fractures should be positioned in dorsal recumbency and the ventral midline prepped from the umbilicus to the perineal region.

SURGICAL TECHNIQUES
Approach to the Ilial Body

Make an incision from the cranial extent of the iliac crest to 1 to 2 cm beyond the greater trochanter caudally. Center the incision over the ventral third of the ilial wing. Incise subcutaneous tissues and gluteal fat along the same line to visualize the intermuscular septum lying between the middle gluteal muscle and long head of the tensor fasciae latae muscle (Fig. 29-72, A). Visualize the intermuscular septum between the superficial gluteal and short part of the tensor fasciae latae caudally. Continue the incision to separate the tensor fasciae latae muscle and middle gluteal muscle cranially and the tensor fasciae latae and superficial gluteal muscle caudally. Sharply dissect cranially to separate the middle gluteal muscle and long head of the tensor fascia lata muscle (Fig. 29-72, B). Palpate the ventral border of the ilium and make an incision at the border through the middle gluteal muscle. Isolate and ligate the iliolumbar vessel and reflect the deep and middle gluteal muscles from the lateral surface of the ilium (Fig. 29-72, C).

If additional exposure is needed, incise the branch of the cranial gluteal nerve that innervates the tensor fasciae latae muscle.

☞ **N O T E** · For increased exposure so that compression screws may be inserted, incise through the origin of the iliacus muscle along the ventral border of the body of the ilium.

Stabilization of the Ilium With a Bone Plate

Reduce the fracture by placing bone-holding forceps over the dorsal edge of the caudal ilial fragment and retracting it caudally. Be careful not to injure the sciatic nerve when

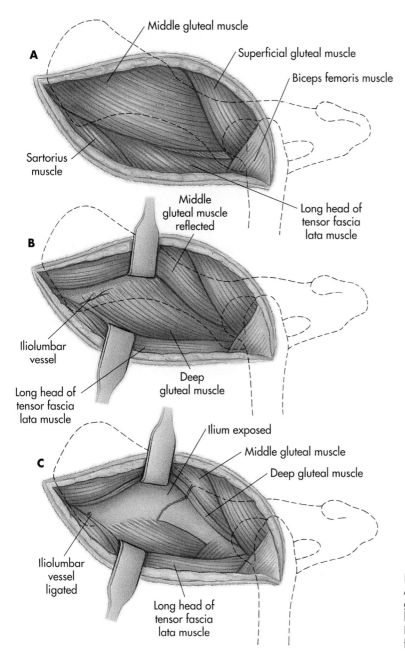

FIG. 29-72
A, To expose the ilium, dissect between the middle gluteal muscle and long head of tensor fasciae latae muscle and **B,** separate these muscles. **C,** Elevate the deep gluteal muscle to expose the fracture.

FIG. 29-73
Application of a bone plate and screws to the ilial wing. Note how application of the bone plate can assist fracture reduction.

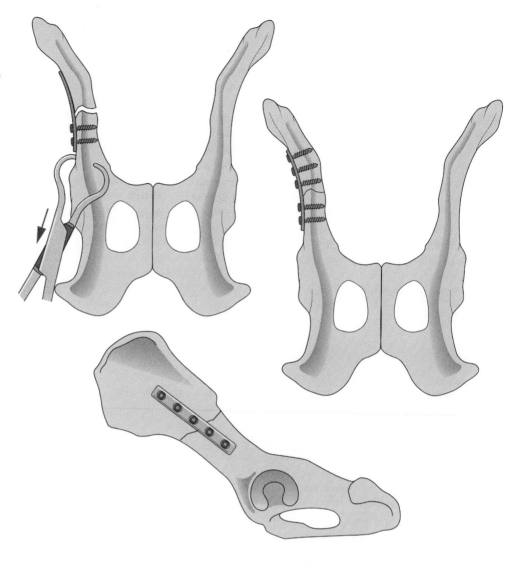

manipulating the fracture fragments. Contour a plate to fit the normal curvature of the lateral surface of the bone. Use a ventrodorsal radiograph of the opposite ilium as a guide for plate contouring preoperatively. Reduce the fragment with bone-holding forceps and attach the plate to the caudal fragment first to allow the contour of the plate to assist in reduction of the cranial fragment. Then place screws in the cranial fragment. Caudal distraction of the ilial fragment is readily achieved, but lateral distraction of the caudal fragment can be difficult. Use the contour of the plate to aid in mediolateral reduction of the fracture. As the screws in the cranial fragment are tightened, the shape of the precontoured plate helps bring the caudal fragment into position. *Place at least three plate screws in the cranial fragment and two in the caudal fragment (Fig. 29-73). To close the incision, place sutures between the fascia of the middle gluteal muscle and tensor fasciae latae muscle cranially and the superficial gluteal muscle and tensor fasciae latae caudally. Approximate deep gluteal fat, subcutaneous tissue, and skin routinely.*

Stabilization of the Ilium with Compression Screws

Reduce the fracture as described above and temporarily stabilize it with bone-holding forceps. Rotate the hemipelvis to visualize the ventral surface of the body of the ilium and insert two small Kirschner pins from ventral to proximal. To achieve additional stability place two compression screws in a ventral to proximal direction (Fig. 29-74).

Approach to and Stabilization of Ischial Fractures

Make a skin incision adjacent to the caudal border of the greater trochanter. Reflect the biceps femoris muscle caudally to expose the sciatic nerve and external rotators as they insert into the trochanteric fossa (see above discussion of surgical anatomy). Incise and reflect the insertions of the external rotators caudally to expose the ischial body. Reduce and stabilize the fragments with a small bone plate and screws or a tension band (Fig. 29-75).

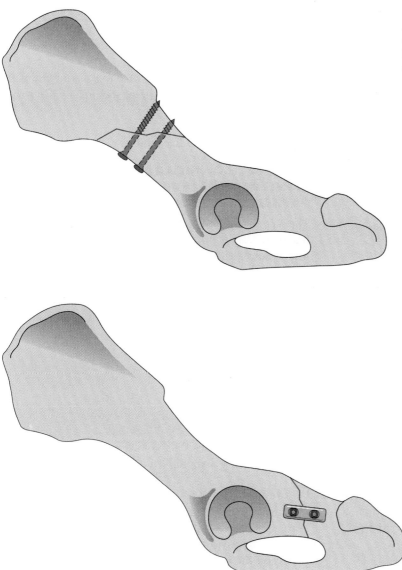

FIG. 29-74
Stabilization of an oblique fracture of the ilial wing with compression screws. The screws have been inserted in a ventral to dorsal direction, across the fracture line.

FIG. 29-75
Stabilization of an ischial fracture with a bone plate and screws.

Approach to and Stabilization of Pubic Fractures

Make a skin incision along the ventral midline (in the male dog adjacent to the penile sheath). Visualize the midline cranial to the pubic brim and incise through the tissues overlying the pubic symphysis. If herniated tissues are present, be careful to avoid inadvertently incising vital structures. Replace the herniated tissues into the abdominal cavity (see p. 186). Use a periosteal elevator to reflect adductor muscles from the pubis. Reduce the fragments and drill holes in adjacent fragments for placement of orthopedic wire (Fig. 29-76). Place and tighten the wire to stabilize the fragments.

SUTURE MATERIALS/SPECIAL INSTRUMENTS

Instruments for implantation of bone plates and/or screws are needed. Bone-holding forceps and self-retaining retrac-

tors are beneficial. For pubic fractures, the symphysis can be stabilized with 20-gauge orthopedic wire in small- and medium-sized dogs and 18-gauge wire in larger dogs.

POSTOPERATIVE CARE AND ASSESSMENT

Activity should be restricted to leash walks until evidence of radiographic healing is present. Radiographs should be taken to assess healing 6 to 8 weeks after surgery. Implants need not be removed unless they are determined to be causing pain or lameness.

PROGNOSIS

A number of clinical studies have evaluated surgical stabilization with bone plates and screws or screws alone. These studies have confirmed that the prognosis is excellent for return to normal function with most ilial fractures after surgery. Factors that warrant a more guarded prognosis

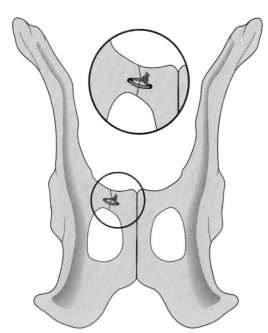

FIG. 29-76
Pubic fractures may be stabilized with orthopedic wire. The wire serves to align the bone fragments.

include ipsilateral acetabular fractures with potential development of osteoarthrosis. There are no recent studies comparing surgical and nonsurgical treatment of ilial fractures. The prognosis for isolated pubic and ischial fractures is excellent for return to normal function. If other pelvic fractures are present, the prognosis depends on how these fractures heal, rather than the pubic or ischial fractures.

Suggested Reading

Betts CW: Pelvic fractures. In Slatter D, editor: *Textbook of small animal surgery,* ed 2, Philadelphia, 1993, Saunders.

Brinker WO, Braden TD: Pelvic fractures. In Brinker WO, Hohn RB, Prieur WD, editors: *Manual of internal fixation in small animals,* Berlin, 1984, Springer-Verlag.

Brinker WO, Piermattei DL, Flo GL: *Handbook of small animal orthopedics and fracture treatment,* ed 2, Philadelphia, 1990, Saunders.

DeCamp CE: Principles of pelvic fracture management, *Semin Vet Med Surg (Small Anim)* 7:63, 1992.

Denny HR: Pelvic fractures in the dog: a review of 123 cases, *J Small Anim Pract* 19:151, 1978.

Ost PC, Kaderly RE: Use of reconstruction plates for the repair of segmental ilial fractures involving acetabular comminution in the dog, *Vet Surg* 15:129, 1986.

Tarvin GB, Lenehan TM: Management of sacroiliac dislocations and ilial fractures. In Bojrab MJ, editor: *Current techniques in small animal surgery,* ed 3, Philadelphia, 1990, Lea and Febiger.

VanGundy TE: Fixation for iliac fractures, *Vet Med Report* 2:303, 1990.

SACROILIAC LUXATIONS/FRACTURES

DEFINITIONS

Sacroiliac luxation results when there is disruption of the articulation between the wing of the sacrum and ilial wing.

SYNONYMS

Separation of the sacroiliac joint

GENERAL CONSIDERATIONS AND CLINICALLY RELEVANT PATHOPHYSIOLOGY

The sacroiliac joint is commonly injured when the pelvis is fractured. Displacement of the pelvic girdle following a fracture requires either bilateral separation of the sacroiliac joints or fracture of the pelvic bones at three sites. Commonly, one of these points of fracture is a separation of the sacroiliac articulation. The femoral and sciatic nerves are in close proximity to the sacroiliac joint and concurrent nerve damage may occur. Preoperative attention to neurologic status is necessary before treatment.

DIAGNOSIS
Clinical Presentation

Signalment. Any age, breed, or sex of dog or cat may be affected.

History. Sacroiliac luxations/fractures are most commonly secondary to motor vehicle accidents.

Physical Examination Findings

Patients are usually non-weight bearing or minimally weight bearing on the affected limb. However, if there is contralateral long bone or pelvic injury, the animal may be required to bear weight on the limb with sacroiliac luxation. Swelling, pain, and crepitus are often not apparent. When the patient is sedated, dorsoventral movement of the ilium can be detected.

Radiography

Ventrodorsal and lateral radiographs must be taken to assess the degree of injury to the hemipelvis and delineate fracture planes. The width of the pelvic canal should be ascertained.

Laboratory Findings

Consistent laboratory abnormalities are not present.

DIFFERENTIAL DIAGNOSIS

Differential diagnoses include fracture of the hemipelvis (i.e., ilium and acetabulum) and sacral fractures. These fractures can usually be differentiated with appropriate radiographs.

MEDICAL OR CONSERVATIVE MANAGEMENT

Most patients function normally with asymmetric cranial-caudal positioning of the hip joints. Conservative treatment is indicated when there is little patient discomfort and minimal displacement of the hemipelvis, or when financial limitations preclude surgery. The majority of patients treated conservatively for a sacroiliac luxation regain normal function. However, lameness may persist for up to 12 weeks. Surgical reduction is indicated if there is significant narrowing of the pelvic outlet, which could lead to constipation or obstipation. Conservative treatment of sacroiliac fractures is similar to that described for ilial fractures on p. 839.

SURGICAL TREATMENT

Surgical stabilization of a sacroiliac fracture-separation can be accomplished with bone screws or small intramedullary pins; however, the majority of veterinary orthopedic surgeons prefer the former.

Preoperative Management

These patients should be adequately stabilized prior to fracture treatment. The neurologic status of the patient must be determined preoperatively. Because urinary trauma may be associated with pelvic fractures, function of the lower urinary tract should be determined prior to surgical repair of the sacroiliac fracture.

Anesthesia

See p. 708 for anesthetic considerations of patients with orthopedic disease.

Surgical Anatomy

The sacroiliac joint has two distinct components: a semilunar, crescent-shaped synovial joint and a fibrocartilaginous synchondrosis. The joint's strength is derived from dorsal and ventral ligaments as well as the fibrocartilaginous synchondrosis (Fig. 29-77).

Positioning

The animal should be positioned in lateral recumbency with the dorsal midline raised 45 degrees from the table. The prepped area should extend from the dorsal midline to the stifle joint and from a point 10 cm cranial to the ilial crest to the tailhead caudally.

SURGICAL TECHNIQUE
Surgical Approach

Make a skin incision beginning over the dorsal iliac crest and continue it caudally parallel to the spine to a point even with the hip joint (Fig. 29-78). Incise subcutaneous tissues and pelvic fat along the same line to expose the iliac crest. Incise through the periosteal origin of the middle gluteal muscle on the lateral ridge of the iliac crest. Make a second incision through the deep gluteal fascia and periosteal origin of the sacrospinalis muscle on the medial ridge of the iliac crest. The incisions merge caudally, where it may be necessary to incise through fibers of the superficial gluteal muscle. The supporting ligamentous tissues between the sacrum and ilium are usually separated with the impact of the original trauma. Therefore, incision

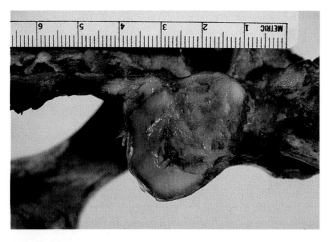

FIG. 29-77
Lateral surface of the sacroiliac joint. Note the C-shaped zone of articular cartilage (arrows).

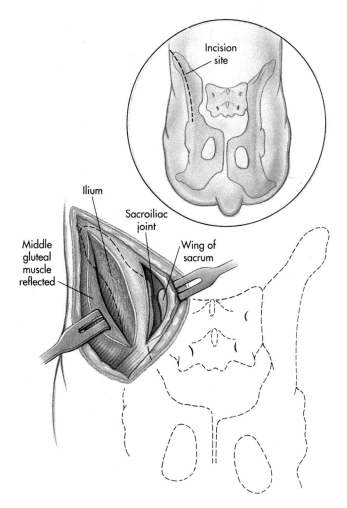

FIG. 29-78
To expose the sacroiliac joint via a dorsal exposure, make an incision over the iliac crest. Reflect the gluteal muscles laterally and the sacrococcygeus dorsalis lateralis muscle medially.

of the lumbar fascia allows lateral reflection of the ilium and exposure of the sacroiliac joint. *Elevate the middle gluteal muscle from the lateral surface of the ilium to further expose the ilium for placement of implants. To close the incision, suture fascia of the middle gluteal and sacrospinalis muscles with an absorbable suture in an interrupted pattern. Next suture subcutaneous tissues and skin using standard methods.*

Stabilization Using a Screw

Once the joint is exposed, position a blunt Hohmann retractor between the ilium and ventral bony shelf of the sacrum. Reflect the ilium ventrally with the retractor. This maneuver exposes the crescent-shaped articular cartilage and fibrocartilaginous joint surfaces of the sacrum. To position a screw properly in the sacrum, direct visualization of the lateral surface of the sacral wing is preferred. *Use the appropriately sized drill bit to drill a thread hole 2 mm cranial and 2 mm proximal to the center of the crescent-shaped articular cartilage. The depth of the thread hole in the sacral body should be such that the screw tip will extend to the midline of the sacral body. Determine the proper location of the glide hole in the ilium by palpating the articular prominence on the medial surface of the ilial wing. Drill the glide hole at the predetermined position with the appropriately sized drill bit.* A glide hole is not needed if a partially threaded cancellous screw is used. *Advance the proper length cancellous screw through the glide hole until the tip appears on the medial surface of the ilium. Bring the ilium caudally in alignment with the articular surface of the sacroiliac joint. Visually guide the screw tip into the prepared thread hole in the sacrum and tighten the screw (Fig. 29-79).*

SUTURE MATERIALS/SPECIAL INSTRUMENTS

Instruments required for placement of a compression screw are recommended. A Hohmann retractor and drill sleeve will increase the ease of implant insertion.

POSTOPERATIVE CARE AND ASSESSMENT

Activity should be restricted to leash walking for 3 weeks; then activity can be gradually increased over the ensuing 3 weeks. Implants do not need to be removed unless they cause a problem.

PROGNOSIS

The prognosis for return to normal activity is excellent after surgical stabilization of sacroiliac luxations/fractures. Long-term clinical studies of animals that received surgical stabilization found that normal limb function returned in an average of 6 weeks (DeCamp, Braden, 1985; Denny, 1978). Without surgery, longer rehabilitation times can be expected. Factors that influence the prognosis include accuracy of implant placement and depth of the implant. Screws placed in the body of the sacrum that exceed in depth 60%

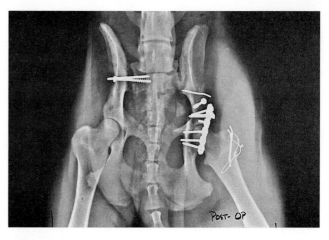

FIG. 29-79
Postoperative radiograph showing proper placement of a bone screw to stabilize a sacroiliac luxation.

the width of the sacrum are less likely to have screw loosening than those that are placed more shallowly.

References

DeCamp CE, Braden TD: Sacroiliac fracture-separations in the dog: a study of 92 cases, *Vet Surg* 14:127, 1985.
Denny HR: Pelvic fractures in the dog: a review of 123 cases, *J Small Anim Pract* 19:151, 1978.

Suggested Reading

Betts CW: Pelvic fractures. In Slatter D, editor: *Textbook of small animal surgery,* ed 2, Philadelphia, 1993, Saunders.
Brinker WO, Braden TD: Pelvic fractures. In Brinker WO, Hohn RB, Prieur WD, editors: *Manual of internal fixation in small animals,* Berlin, 1984, Springer-Verlag.
Brinker WO, Piermattei DL, Flo GL: *Handbook of small animal orthopedics and fracture treatment,* ed 2, Philadelphia, 1990, Saunders.
DeCamp CE: Principles of pelvic fracture management, *Semin Vet Med Surg (Small Anim)* 7:63, 1992.
DeCamp CE, Braden TD: The anatomy of the canine sacrum for lag screw fixation of the sacroiliac joint, *Vet Surg* 14:131, 1985.
Radasch RM et al: Static strength evaluation of sacroiliac fracture-separation repairs, *Vet Surg* 19:155, 1990.
Tarvin GB, Lenehan TM: Management of sacroiliac dislocations and ilial fractures. In Bojrab MJ, editor: *Current techniques in small animal surgery,* ed 3, Philadelphia, 1990, Lea and Febiger.

FEMORAL FRACTURES

FEMORAL CAPITAL PHYSEAL FRACTURES

DEFINITIONS

Femoral capital physeal fractures occur through the capital physeal growth plate between the femoral epiphysis and neck.

SYNONYMS

Slipped capital epiphysis

GENERAL CONSIDERATIONS AND CLINICALLY RELEVANT PATHOPHYSIOLOGY

Because the injury occurs through cartilage of the growth plate, femoral capital physeal injuries may occur without significant trauma. The femoral neck is usually externally rotated and displaced craniodorsally, such that it lies adjacent to the ilial wing. Occasionally, the physis of the greater trochanter is also fractured, causing the femoral shaft to be displaced more dorsally than expected.

DIAGNOSIS
Clinical Presentation

Signalment. Most affected animals are less than 10 months of age. Young, male dogs are more likely to sustain trauma resulting in this type of fracture. This probably is a reflection of their tendency to roam.

History. Most animals are presented for evaluation of an acute non-weight bearing lameness. The trauma may or may not be witnessed by the owner.

Physical Examination Findings

Affected animals usually exhibit a non–weight-bearing lameness with pain and crepitation on manipulation of the hip joint. Some animals present weight bearing and do not have detectable crepitus referable to the hip joint. These animals usually have minimal displacement of the femoral head.

Radiography

Standard ventrodorsal and medial to lateral projections are required to confirm the diagnosis (Fig. 29-80). A capital epiphysis with minimal displacement may be difficult to detect with standard radiograph projections. A ventrodorsal view with the limbs in a "frog" position may help confirm the diagnosis in such cases. Sedation is often required for proper positioning (see Table 28-7). If there is a concurrent greater trochanter physeal fracture the cap of the greater trochanter will be superimposed over the shaft of the femur and will appear as a half-moon radiodense object on a ventrodorsal radiograph. On a lateral projection, the cap of the trochanter will appear as a radiodense fragment caudal to the femur.

Laboratory Findings

Consistent laboratory abnormalities are not present.

DIFFERENTIAL DIAGNOSIS

Differential diagnoses include severe coxofemoral joint sprain, femoral neck fracture, and acetabular fractures.

MEDICAL OR CONSERVATIVE MANAGEMENT

Surgical intervention is required to prevent severe degenerative joint disease and lameness.

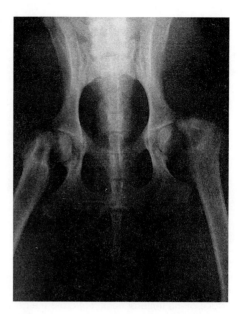

FIG. 29-80
Ventrodorsal radiograph of a young dog with bilateral capital physeal fractures.

SURGICAL TREATMENT

Anatomic reduction is critical for optimal outcome with capital physeal fractures. The fracture may be stabilized with either a compression screw or three triangulated Kirschner pins. One fixation system does not appear to have advantages over another. Biologically, these fractures heal rapidly since they occur in cancellous bone of young animals. Mechanically, prevention of movement of the capital epiphysis is assisted by the transverse nature of the fracture, shape of the fracture surfaces, and friction of cancellous bone resting on cancellous bone. If the physis of the greater trochanter is separated, it must also be anatomically reduced and stabilized with Kirschner wires or a tension band (depending on the weight of the patient; see p. 746).

Preoperative Management

Because these fractures occur secondary to trauma, all affected animals should be examined for concurrent injury and stabilized if necessary prior to surgery.

Anesthesia

See p. 708 for a discussion of anesthetic management of animals with fractures.

Surgical Anatomy

The proximal capital physis lies between the femoral epiphysis and femoral neck and acts as a barrier for passage of blood vessels from the femoral neck to the femoral epiphysis (Fig. 29-81). The blood supply to the femoral epiphysis is through a series of cervical ascending vessels lying outside the femoral neck that cross the physis and then penetrate the epiphysis. The physis functions to provide femoral neck length until the animal is approximately 8 months of age.

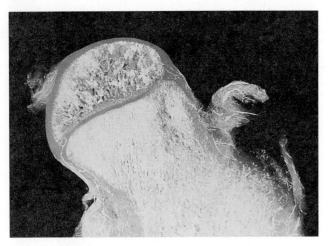

FIG. 29-81
Photomicrograph of a barium-injected normal coxofemoral joint from a young dog. Note vessels along the superior and inferior surface of the femoral neck that cross the growth plate to supply the femoral epiphysis.

Positioning

The animal is positioned in lateral recumbency with the affected limb up. The limb should be clipped from dorsal midline to midtibia (bilaterally) and draped from a hanging position (see p. 25) to allow maximal manipulation during surgery.

SURGICAL TECHNIQUES
Surgical Approach

Incise the skin 5 cm proximal to the greater trochanter. Curve the incision distally adjacent to the cranial ridge of the trochanter, and extend it distally for 5 cm over the proximal femur (Fig. 29-82, A). Incise subcutaneous tissues and the juncture at the superficial leaf of the fascia lata and cranial border of the biceps femoris muscle. Incise the deep leaf of the tensor fasciae latae between the tensor fasciae latae muscle and deep border of the biceps femoris muscle and superficial gluteal muscle. Reflect the tensor fasciae latae muscle cranially and the superficial gluteal and biceps femoris muscles caudally (Fig. 29-82,

FIG. 29-82
A, To perform a craniolateral exposure of the hip joint, incise skin 5 cm proximal to the greater trochanter. Curve the incision distally adjacent to the cranial ridge of the trochanter, and extend it distally for 5 cm over the proximal femur. **B,** Reflect the tensor fascia lata muscle cranially and superficial gluteal and biceps femoris muscles caudally. **C,** Incise the deep gluteal tendon for one third to one half of its width at its point of insertion into the greater trochanter. Incise the joint capsule and the origin of the vastus lateralis muscle to expose the hip joint.

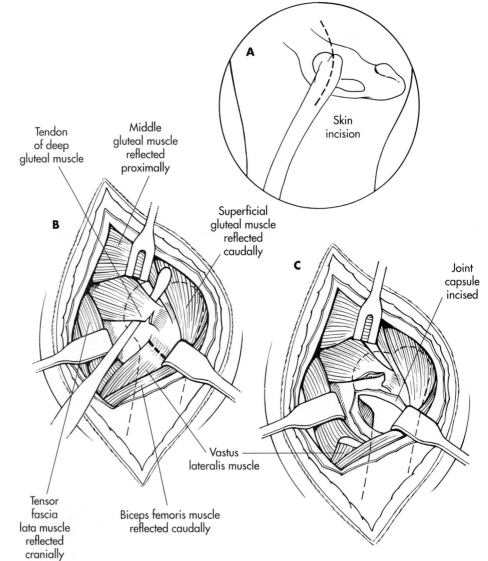

Tendon of deep gluteal muscle

Middle gluteal muscle reflected proximally

Superficial gluteal muscle reflected caudally

Skin incision

Joint capsule incised

Vastus lateralis muscle

Tensor fascia lata muscle reflected cranially

Biceps femoris muscle reflected caudally

B). Visualize the tendinous insertion of the deep gluteal muscle by retracting the middle gluteal muscle proximally. Place a periosteal elevator beneath the deep gluteal muscle near its insertion and separate the deep gluteal muscle from the joint capsule using a sweeping motion with the elevator. Incise the deep gluteal tendon for one third to one half of its width at its point of insertion onto the greater trochanter (Fig. 29-82, C). Leave 1 to 2 mm of tendon on the trochanter for closure but make the incision through the tendon close to the bone. The joint capsule is commonly lacerated exposing the fracture surface of the femoral neck. If this is the case, enlarge the opening in the joint capsule with an incision from the rim of the acetabulum laterally through the point of origin of the vastus lateralis. If the joint capsule is intact, incise it parallel to the long axis of the femoral neck near its proximal ridge. Continue the joint capsule incision laterally through the point of origin of the vastus lateralis muscle on the cranial face of the proximal femur. It is important to keep this cut at the proximal point of origin just under the cut edge of the deep gluteal tendon. *Reflect the vastus lateralis distally to expose the hip joint.*

Fracture Reduction

Reduction of the fracture is facilitated by proceeding in a stepwise manner. The femoral epiphysis remains in the acetabulum due to its attachment to the round ligament. The femoral neck is displaced cranial and dorsal to the acetabulum, is anteverted, and lies adjacent to the surface of the ilium. *To reduce the fracture, first bring the femoral neck distally so it lies cranial and level with the acetabulum. Next, derotate the femur to correct for the abnormal anteversion and third, slide the fracture surface of the femoral neck caudally into the matching surface of the femoral epiphysis (Fig. 29-83).*

Application of a Compression Screw

Initially, place two Kirschner pins in the femoral neck in a lateral to medial direction so that they lie parallel to one another. Position them so that one pin lies in the superior

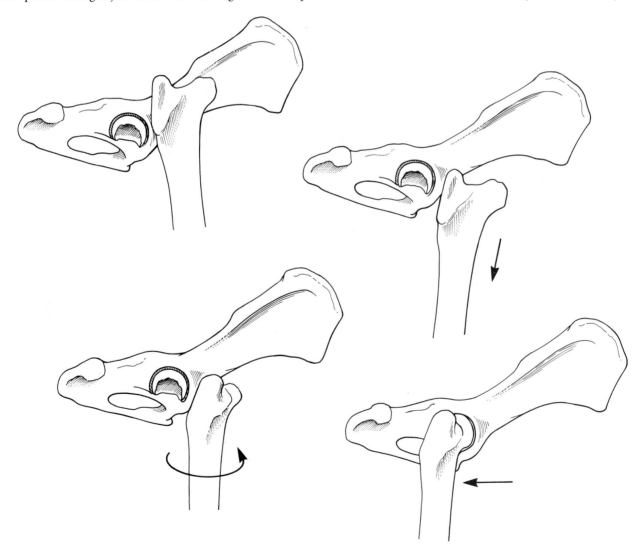

FIG. 29-83
To reduce a capital physeal fracture, bring the femoral neck ventral until it is level with the hip joint. Then derotate the femur and slide it caudally.

FIG. 29-84
A, To stabilize a femoral capital physeal fracture with a compression screw, place two Kirschner wires (one superior and one inferior) in the femoral neck, perpendicular to the fracture surface. Drill a glide hole between the Kirschner wires.
B, Reduce the fracture and advance the Kirschner wires into the femoral epiphysis. Drill the thread hole in the epiphysis, measure to determine screw length, and tap threads in the epiphysis. **C,** Insert the compression screw.

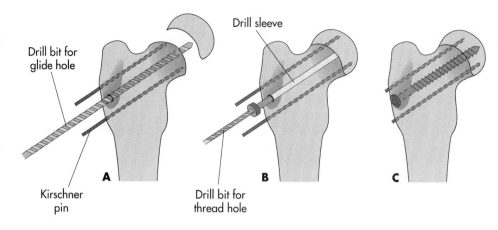

section of the femoral neck and one pin lies in the inferior section of the femoral neck. Drill a glide hole between the two pins to emerge at the center of the fracture surface (Fig. 29-84, A). Angle the Kirschner pins and glide hole to correct for normal anteversion of the femoral neck. Reduce the fracture and drive the Kirschner pins into the femoral epiphysis. Place a drill insert into the glide hole for accurate drilling of the thread hole (Fig. 29-84, B). The thread hole can penetrate the femoral epiphysis. Countersink the glide hole and determine the appropriate screw length by measuring the distance from the lateral surface of the greater trochanter to the femoral epiphyseal articular surface. Choose a screw that is 2 mm shorter than that measured with the depth gauge. Tap the thread hole and insert the screw (Fig. 29-84, C). Remove one or both Kirschner pins and close the wound routinely (Fig. 29-85).

Application of Triangulated Kirschner Pins

With this technique, three Kirschner pins are placed through the femoral neck (Fig. 29-86). The pins are placed parallel to one another and positioned in the femoral neck so that they lie in a triangle. The points of the pins should just be visible at the fracture surface of the femoral neck. The fracture is reduced and the pins driven into the femoral epiphysis. One problem often encountered with this technique is pins that have penetrated the articular cartilage aren't visible to the surgeon at the time of surgery. The femoral head is a dome structure so the length of pin placed in the periphery will be different from the length of pin placed in the center of the dome. *To determine the proper length of pins, place the first pin in the periphery of the femoral epiphysis so that it penetrates the articular cartilage where it is visible. Estimate the length of this pin that would not penetrate the articular cartilage and use it as a gauge for the remaining pins. Drive the remaining pins into the femoral epiphysis and place the joint through a normal range of motion to ensure that a pin has not penetrated the articular surface. Close the wound routinely.*

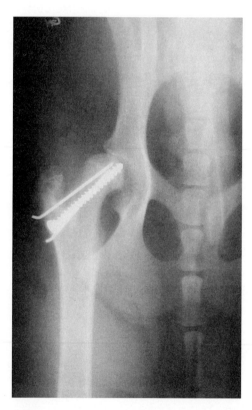

FIG. 29-85
Postoperative radiograph of a femoral capital physeal fracture after stabilization with a compression screw and two Kirschner wires.

SUTURE MATERIALS/SPECIAL INSTRUMENTS

A battery- or air-driven drill is helpful for inserting the implants. If a screw is used, instrumentation for proper insertion of a lag screw is required.

POSTOPERATIVE CARE AND ASSESSMENT

Restrict activity to leash walking until radiographic healing has occurred, which will generally be complete in 5 to 6

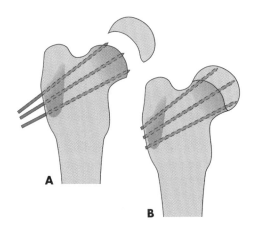

FIG. 29-86
A, To stabilize a femoral capital physeal fracture with Kirschner wires, place three wires through the femoral neck to the fracture surface. Triangulate the Kirschner wires. **B,** Reduce the fracture and advance the wires into the epiphysis.

weeks. Ventrodorsal and medial-to-lateral radiographs should be taken to assess healing. Implants should not be removed unless clinical problems arise.

PROGNOSIS

The prognosis for long-term, pain-free function is good if the fracture is adequately reduced and appropriately stabilized. However, in animals less than 5 months of age, a shortened femoral neck may result from closure of the capital physis. A shortened femoral neck may cause hip joint subluxation and increase the potential for development of degenerative joint disease. If the fracture is not appropriately reduced and/or implants penetrate the articular cartilage, significant degenerative changes may develop necessitating additional surgical treatment.

Suggested Reading

Daly WR: Femoral head and neck fractures in the dog and cat: a review of 115 cases, *Vet Surg* 7:29, 1978.

DeCamp CE, Probst CW, Thomas MW: Internal fixation of femoral capital physeal injuries in dogs: 40 cases (1979–1987), *J Am Vet Med Assoc* 194:1750, 1989.

Gibson KL, vanEe RT, Pechman RD: Femoral capital physeal fractures in dogs: 34 cases (1979–1989), *J Am Vet Med Assoc* 198:886, 1991.

Hulse DH et al: Revascularization of femoral capital physeal fractures following surgical fixation, *J Vet Orthop* 2:50, 1981.

Miller A, Anderson TJ: Complications of articular lag screw fixation of femoral capital epiphyseal separations, *J Sm Anim Pract* 34:9, 1993.

Olsson SE, Poulos PW, Ljunggren G: Coxa plana-vara and femoral capital fractures in the dog, *J Am Anim Hosp Assoc* 21:563, 1985.

Rivera LA et al: Arterial supply to the canine hip joint, *J Vet Orthop* 1:20, 1979.

Vernon FF, Olmstead ML: Femoral head fracture resulting in epiphyseal fragmentation: results of repair in five dogs, *Vet Surg* 12:123, 1983.

FEMORAL NECK FRACTURES

DEFINITIONS

Femoral neck fractures occur at the base of the neck where it joins the metaphysis of the proximal femur.

SYNONYMS

Basilar fractures of the femoral neck

GENERAL CONSIDERATIONS AND CLINICALLY RELEVANT PATHOPHYSIOLOGY

The fracture configuration is generally that of a single basilar fracture plane, but comminution of the femoral neck can occur. Mechanically, these are highly unstable fractures because the length of the moment arm acting at the fracture is long (entire femoral neck length) and the plane of the fracture is along lines of maximal shear stress. Compression of the fracture surface is needed to resist the high shear stress. The fracture plane is extracapsular, preserving blood flow to the fracture zone following injury.

DIAGNOSIS
Clinical Presentation

Signalment. Any age, breed, or sex of dog or cat may be affected. This condition occurs more commonly in mature patients after the femoral capital physeal growth plate has closed.

History. Most injuries are due to a motor vehicle accidents, but this injury can occur following a fall.

Physical Examination Findings

Most affected animals present for evaluation of a non–weight-bearing lameness. Pain and crepitation are evident upon manipulation of the hip joint.

Radiography

Femoral neck fractures do not require special radiographic views for detection. If only a lateral view of the hip joint is taken, however, the diagnosis may be missed (Fig. 29-87).

Laboratory Findings

Consistent laboratory abnormalities are not present.

DIFFERENTIAL DIAGNOSIS

Differential diagnoses include coxofemoral luxation, acetabular fractures, proximal femoral fractures, and capital physeal fracture in young patients.

MEDICAL OR CONSERVATIVE MANAGEMENT

Medical or conservative management is not a treatment option. Surgical intervention is required.

SURGICAL TREATMENT

Fractures with a single fracture plane are best treated with a compression screw or triangulation of Kirschner wires. If irreparable comminution is present, total hip replacement and femoral head ostectomy are treatment options. If financial restraints preclude fracture repair, a femoral head ostectomy may be performed.

Preoperative Management

Because these fractures occur secondary to trauma, all affected animals should be examined for concurrent injury and stabilized if necessary before surgery.

Anesthesia

Anesthetic management of animals with orthopedic disease is discussed on p. 708.

Surgical Anatomy

The femoral neck/femoral shaft junction in the frontal plane is known as the angle of inclination. This angle is normally 135 degrees and should be approximated when surgical reduction is performed. The normal angle of anteversion is 15 to 20 degrees. This angle must also be taken into consideration when inserting screws or pins into the femoral neck.

Normal anatomy of the hip joint is described on p. 835. A craniolateral approach is performed for exposure of these fractures (see Fig. 29-82). Care must be taken to ensure adequate ventral reflection of the vastus lateralis to visualize the fracture surface. The femoral shaft is located craniodorsal to the femoral neck (which remains in the acetabulum). Adequate longitudinal incision of the joint capsule is necessary for accurate reduction. A greater trochanteric osteotomy may be required (see Fig. 29-69), if visualization is not adequate for anatomic reduction and placement of implants.

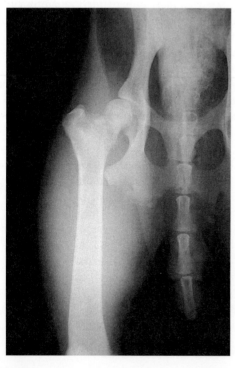

FIG. 29-87
Ventrodorsal radiograph of a femoral neck fracture in a dog.

Positioning

The animal is positioned in lateral recumbency with the affected leg up. A hanging leg preparation will facilitate manipulation of the limb during surgery.

SURGICAL TECHNIQUES

A craniolateral approach to the hip joint (as described for capital physeal fractures) is most commonly used (see p. 848). If alignment of the fracture is difficult, a trochanteric osteotomy can be performed to improve accessibility (see p. 836). This injury is best stabilized with a compression screw except when the biological assessment is extremely favorable. In the latter patients, Kirschner wires may be used.

Application of a Partially Threaded Cancellous Compression Screw

Place two Kirschner pins so they lie at the most proximal and distal level of the fracture surface (Fig. 29-88, A). Drive the pins from medial to lateral, beginning at the fracture surface or from the lateral surface medially to exit at the fracture surface. Reduce the fracture and drive the Kirschner pins into the femoral epiphysis. Take care to avoid penetrating the articular surface. Drill a thread hole through the femoral epiphysis with the appropriate size drill bit parallel to and centered between the Kirschner pins. Measure the length of screw needed and tap the thread hole. Insert a partially threaded cancellous screw 2 mm shorter than the length measured so that all the threads cross the fracture plane and are seated into the femoral head. Leave one or both pins in place to serve as antirotational devices.

Application of Triangulated Kirschner Pins

Insert three Kirschner pins from the fracture surface parallel to one another to form a triangle (Fig. 29-88, B). Retrograde the pins to exit the bone near the third trochanter. Alternatively, normograde the pins so that they enter the bone at the third trochanter and exit at the fracture site. Reduce the fracture and drive the pins into the femoral epiphysis. Take care not to penetrate the articular surface.

SUTURE MATERIALS/SPECIAL INSTRUMENTS

Appropriate surgical instrumentation for application of Kirschner pins or compression screws is needed.

POSTOPERATIVE CARE AND ASSESSMENT

Activity should be controlled to leash walking until there is radiographic evidence of healing. Fracture healing may take 5 to 10 weeks and is dependent upon biologic fracture assessment (see p. 730). Implants should not be removed unless they cause a problem.

PROGNOSIS

Inappropriate reduction and/or poor implant choice are the most common problems reported with femoral neck frac-

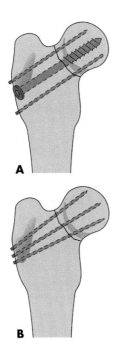

FIG. 29-88
Femoral neck fracture repair with **A,** a compression screw centered between two Kirschner wires or **B,** triangulated Kirschner wires.

tures. Significant bending and shear stress across the fracture plane places extreme bending loads on implants. The most common implant error is the use of a single pin or two pins when the fracture assessment indicates a fairly lengthy healing time. In such cases, micromotion at the pin-bone interface arising from the high physiologic stress may cause pins to loosen too early. The best way to avoid or treat this problem is to use a compression screw and antirotational pin or two compression screws except where the biologic assessment indicates rapid healing will occur.

Suggested Reading

Daly WR: Femoral head and neck fractures in the dog and cat: a review of 115 cases, *Vet Surg* 7:29, 1978.

Milton JL: Fractures of the femur. In Slatter DH, editor: *Textbook of small animal surgery*, ed 2, Philadelphia, 1993, Saunders.

Nunamaker DM: Repair of femoral head and neck fractures by interfragmentary compression, *J Am Vet Med Assoc* 163:569, 1973.

FEMORAL DIAPHYSEAL FRACTURES

DEFINITIONS

The femoral **diaphysis** (shaft) is the midportion of the bone that curves craniocaudally in dogs and lies between the articular extremities. An intramedullary pin that is placed into the femur in a **normograde** fashion is inserted from the trochanteric fossa across the fracture line and seated in the femoral condyles. A pin that is placed in the femur in a **retrograde** fashion is inserted at the fracture line, driven proximally to exit the trochanteric fossa, and then (following fracture reduction) driven across the fracture and into the distal fragment.

GENERAL CONSIDERATIONS AND CLINICALLY RELEVANT PATHOPHYSIOLOGY

Femoral fractures are usually caused by trauma. Occasionally a patient will present with an acute femur fracture without discernible or historical trauma; fractures in these patients may be secondary to preexisting bone pathology. Primary or metastatic bone tumors are the most common cause of pathologic fractures. When preexisting disease is present, radiographs made at the time of injury show cortical lysis and/or new bone formation in the area of the fracture.

High-velocity injuries are the most common type of trauma causing femoral fractures in veterinary patients. The majority of these are automobile accidents, but gunshot injuries and blunt trauma are also common. A thorough physical examination is necessary to rule out concurrent injury (e.g., thoracic trauma, coxofemoral luxations, and pelvic girdle injuries) in these patients. Careful thoracic auscultation and percussion help detect cardiac or airway abnormalities. Abnormal heart rhythm or pulse deficits are indicative of traumatic myocarditis, while lack of normal air movement on auscultation may indicate pulmonary contusion, pneumothorax, or diaphragmatic hernia. Thoracic radiographs and a lead II ECG are useful and should be done on a routine basis as part of the anesthetic preoperative database for patients sustaining high-velocity injuries.

Coxofemoral luxations (see p. 949) may occur concurrently with femoral fractures. Diagnosis is often made when radiographs are taken to evaluate the femur since swelling in the limb often precludes palpation of bony landmarks used for assessing femoral head position relative to the hip joint. Concurrent fractures or luxations must be considered when choosing the appropriate implant for fracture stabilization. Observation of pelvic girdle symmetry and gentle rectal palpation help determine the presence of pelvic fractures. Additional radiographs centered on the pelvis are indicated if abnormalities are found. If fractures of the pelvis are found, careful assessment of urinary tract integrity is recommended.

DIAGNOSIS
Clinical Presentation

Signalment. Any age, breed, or sex of dog or cat may be affected. However, young male dogs are most apt to receive trauma resulting in femoral fractures.

History. Trauma may or may not have been observed. Often the animal is found with a non–weight-bearing lameness.

Physical Examination Findings

Patients with femoral diaphyseal fractures are usually non–weight bearing and have varying degrees of limb swelling.

Pain and crepitus can often be elicited with limb manipulation. Proprioception may appear to be abnormal because the animal may not lift its paw when placed on its dorsum. The animal's reluctance to move the limb may be due to pain.

Radiography

Both craniocaudal and lateral radiographs of the femur are necessary to assess the extent of bone and soft tissue injury. The majority of affected animals suffer pain when the limb is manipulated and require sedation for proper positioning so quality radiographs may be obtained. Alternatively, radiographs can be taken under anesthesia just prior to surgery; however, this reduces the amount of time available for planning surgical repair. If bone plate fixation is contemplated, radiographs of the contralateral limb are useful to assess bone length and shape. These radiographs can be used to more precisely contour the bone plate before surgery, reducing operative time.

Laboratory Findings

Consistent laboratory abnormalities are not present. Animals sustaining fractures secondary to trauma should have sufficient blood work done to determine appropriate anesthetic regimens and concurrent diseases (see Chapter 5).

DIFFERENTIAL DIAGNOSIS

Femoral fractures should be differentiated from muscle contusion, coxofemoral luxation, fractures of the pelvic girdle, and ligamentous injury to the stifle.

MEDICAL OR CONSERVATIVE MANAGEMENT

The fracture must be stabilized to allow adequate healing. Casts or splints are not recommended for femoral fractures because it is difficult to adequately stabilize the femur using these methods. However, animals that have stable or incomplete fractures and an excellent biologic assessment (see p. 730) may heal despite lack of rigid fixation. Analgesics (see p. 708) may be administered to increase patient comfort prior to definitive treatment.

SURGICAL TREATMENT

Femoral fractures may be stabilized using a variety of techniques. General application guidelines for various fracture fixation systems used to repair femoral diaphyseal fractures are given below.

Application of Intramedullary (IM) Pins

Generally, an IM pin should equal 70% to 80% of the diameter of the marrow cavity. Because an IM pin traverses the entire length of bone, it must pass through the entire length of marrow cavity. The femoral diameter and curvature dictate the size of pin that can be used (see below under surgical anatomy). An IM pin can be normograded or retrograded for placement in the femur (see definitions above). The advantage of normograde placement is that the pin can be placed laterally, adjacent to the greater trochanter (Fig. 29-89). This

positions the pin so that it passes through less soft tissue than when it is placed in a retrograde fashion and also assures that the pin is positioned lateral to the sciatic nerve. The disadvantage of normograde placement is that it is difficult to identify the correct entry point into the bone because insertion of the pin into the trochanteric fossa is generally done blindly. To normograde an IM pin, a small skin incision is made at the point of pin entry over the bony prominence of the greater trochanter. Palpation of the greater trochanter may be difficult if the limb is swollen secondary to trauma of the soft tissues. If this is the case, limited surgical exposure may be needed to locate the greater trochanter prominence. After the greater trochanter is located either by palpation or direct exposure, the point of the pin is pushed through soft tissues until it contacts the most proximal trochanteric ridge. The pin point is walked off the medial edge of the greater trochanter until it falls into the trochanteric fossa. From this point, the pin is driven through the proximal metaphyseal cancellous bone in a slightly caudomedial direction. As the pin point emerges from the marrow cavity at the fracture site the fracture is overreduced and the pin is driven into the distal fragment.

> ☞ **N O T E** · Normograde placement of the pin is advantageous because it allows the pin to be inserted more laterally than with retrograde placement. To help identify the correct entry point for the pin, you may wish to perform a limited surgical exposure of the greater trochanter.

The advantage of retrograde pin placement in the femur is that the site of insertion of the pin at the fracture can be visualized (Fig. 29-90). The disadvantage of retrograde placement is that controlling the pin's point of exit at the trochanteric fossa is difficult as it may exit too far medially causing soft tissue irritation and the increased likelihood of sciatic palsy. So that the pin will exit more laterally in the trochanteric fossa with retrograde placement, use a pin that is approximately 70% the diameter of the isthmus. As the pin is being retrograded (driven through the proximal fragment) the shaft of the pin should be forced against the caudomedial cortex of the proximal fragment. This compels the tip of the pin to glide along the cranial lateral cortex of the proximal fragment and exit more laterally in the trochanteric fossa. This maneuver is more effective with midshaft and proximal femoral fractures; the more distal the fracture, the more difficult it is to control retrograde placement. Once the pin has exited through the trochanteric fossa, the fracture is overreduced and the pin seated in the distal fragment.

> ☞ **N O T E** · During retrograde pin placement use a slightly smaller pin to enhance control of the exit point. Force the shaft of the pin against the caudomedial cortex.

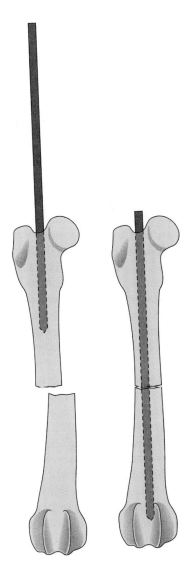

FIG. 29-89
For normograde placement of an intramedullary pin in the femur, insert the pin so that it enters the bone proximally in the craniolateral trochanteric fossa. Direct it caudally to glide along the caudal cortex and seat it in the caudocentral aspect of the condyle.

Whether the IM pin is normograded or retrograded, overreduction of the fracture is preferred (Fig. 29-91). Over-reduction of the distal fragment helps compensate for the normal craniocaudal femoral curvature and allows the pin to be seated better in the distal extremity. Overreduction is accomplished by bringing the distal fragment forward using the cranial cortex as a fulcrum point. If the fracture has a simple transverse or oblique configuration, the cranial cortex of both fragments is in contact and this point of contact becomes the fulcrum for overreduction. If the fracture is comminuted, the cranial cortex of the fragment can be used as a reference point to overreduce the fracture. To estimate the appropriate pin length, a second pin of equal length to that being placed in the marrow cavity can be used for a point of reference. The pin in the marrow cavity is driven distally until it is well seated in the cancellous bone of the femoral

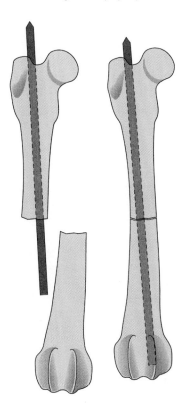

FIG. 29-90
For retrograde placement of an intramedullary pin in the femur, insert the pin into the marrow cavity at the fracture surface. Force the shaft of the pin against the caudomedial cortex. Reduce the fracture and drive the pin distally to seat in the caudocentral aspect of the femoral condyle.

condyles. The reference pin is then compared to the pin placed in the marrow cavity by approximating the position of the proximal tips of both pins and laying the reference pin over soft tissues outside the limb. When the distal tip of the reference pin is near the level of the proximal pole of the patella, the surgical wound is closed and radiographs taken to verify proper placement of the IM pin. In cats, normograde or retrograde placement can be used and overreduction of the distal fragment is not necessary (see discussion on surgical anatomy on p. 857).

☞ **N O T E** • Always have a reference pin available that is the same length as the IM pin being inserted.

Application of IM Pin Plus External Skeletal Fixation

Combining the bending support of an IM pin with the axial and rotational support provided by an external fixator is useful to control physiologic forces acting on fractures during healing. An IM pin that occupies 50% to 60% of the medullary cavity is first inserted in a normograde or retrograde manner. This is followed by insertion of an appropriate number of transfixation pins. The number and type of transfixation pins vary with the rigidity of fixation desired and the length of time the fixator must remain in place.

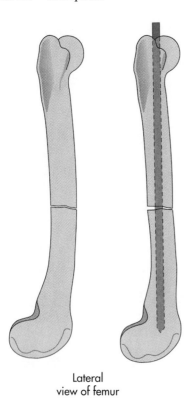

Lateral
view of femur

FIG. 29-91
Overreduction of the distal fragment for proper placement of an intramedullary pin into the condyles.

However, transfixation pins that pass through the large muscles of the thigh cause patient discomfort. Therefore, it is advisable to use as few transfixation pins as possible. Pins should also be placed through zones where they will penetrate the least soft tissue. A single external bar with one transfixation pin placed proximal to the fracture and one placed distal to the fracture is a common configuration for moderately stable fractures. The proximal transfixation pin is placed laterally at the level of the third trochanter. A small Kirschner wire is used as a "feeler" pin to identify a proper angle of insertion for the transfixation pin that avoids intersecting the IM pin (see p. 741 for insertion of transfixation pins). The distal transfixation pin is inserted laterally 2 to 3 cm proximal to the femoral condyles. The fabella is usually palpable and can be used as a landmark for this pin (use a small Kirschner wire as a feeler pin to avoid intersection with the IM pin). For unstable fractures additional transfixation pins may be added. If a third transfixation pin is desired, proximal placement causes less discomfort than distal placement. The third pin is placed craniolateral at the level of the third trochanter at a 60-degree angle to the first transfixation pin. A feeler pin is again used to avoid the IM pin. The two proximal and one distal pins are connected, forming a triangle external frame that enhances the strength of the fixation system.

Alternative strategies are also effective to enhance rigidity of the fixation while minimizing the number of transfixation pins. For example, placement of an additional external bar and/or connecting the IM pin to the external fixator frame to make a tie-in configuration increases the fixation system strength without adding to patient morbidity through placement of additional transfixation pins.

> ☞ **NOTE ·** Transfixation pins placed very distally cause discomfort. Add additional pins proximally if necessary.

Application of External Skeletal Fixation

The use of external skeletal fixation as the sole means of stabilization for complex femoral fractures has gained popularity in recent years. When applied to the femur, stress on transfixation pins is high because of the long distance from the external bar to the point where the transfixation pin enters the bone (because of the muscle mass in this area) and an inability to use stronger bilateral frames. Thoughtful preoperative planning and strict adherence to application principles are necessary to avoid fixator-related complications and unacceptable patient morbidity. Open reduction is recommended to achieve adequate spatial alignment of the femur. Achieving spatial alignment is assisted through placement of a temporary IM pin through the intact proximal segment of bone, across the fracture site, and into the distal segment of intact bone. In keeping with the concept of bridging osteosynthesis, bone fragments in the area of comminution are not reduced or manipulated (see p. 757). The most proximal and distal transfixation pins are placed as half-pins into their respective metaphyseal-epiphyseal junctions. There is usually no problem bypassing the IM pin but a feeler Kirschner wire can be used to find an appropriate site for the transfixation pin. The external bar is connected to the proximal and distal transfixation pin to maintain spatial alignment of the femur and the temporary IM pin is removed. The remaining transfixation pins are now placed and connected to the external bar. The number and type of transfixation pins used depend upon rigidity and duration of function needed for the external skeletal fixator. It is better to initially err on the side of being too rigid than to have a fixator that is not rigid enough. Overly rigid fixators can be destabilized as the fracture heals, whereas inadequate rigid fixators result in premature fixation failure and high morbidity.

> ☞ **NOTE ·** Multiple transfixation pins increase morbidity and may reduce postoperative limb function.

Application of Bone Plates and Screws

Bone plates are ideally suited for complex or stable fractures of the femur when prolonged healing (bone union) is anticipated or when optimal postoperative limb function is desirable. Plate size depends upon patient size and plate function. The plate may serve as a compression plate, neutralization plate, or buttress plate. Independent of function, the plate is placed on the craniolateral tension surface of the femur. A minimum of three plate screws (six cortices) proximal and three plate screws distal to the fracture is recommended with compression or neutralization plates, while a minimum of four plate screws (eight cortices) proximal and distal to the fracture is recommended for buttress plates. A compression plate is used with transverse or short oblique fractures. A neutralization plate is used with long oblique fractures or comminuted fractures where the bone fragments can be reduced and stabilized with compression screws or cerclage wire. A buttress plate is used with comminuted fractures where the bone fragments cannot be reduced anatomically or where attempted reduction and stabilization of the fragments would cause excessive soft tissue trauma. The plate is contoured to reflect the femoral anatomy; this is most easily accomplished by contouring the plate to a craniocaudal radiograph of the contralateral limb. Spatial alignment of the bone is assisted by insertion of an IM pin. The pin may be retrograded or normograded through the proximal intact segment of bone, passed through the fragmented section of bone, and seated into the distal intact segment of bone. Passing the pin into the distal intact segment of bone without tightly restricting movement of the distal fragment allows the pin to distract the proximal and distal segments to regain femoral length. In keeping with the concept of bridging osteosynthesis, the bone fragments in the comminuted area are not disturbed. Once spatial alignment of the femur is achieved, the bone plate is attached to the bone with plate screws at the most proximal and distal plate holes. If the alignment pin is removed, bicortical plate screws (screws that engage both cortices) are used. Alternatively, the alignment pin can be left in place to achieve a plate/pin buttress of the fracture. In this case, bicortical screws are used proximally and distally while monocortical screws are used centrally. The plate/pin combination increases the strength and fatigue life of the fixation and thereby protects the plate from premature breakage. The plate/pin system can be destabilized between 6 and 8 weeks by removing the IM pin. A cancellous bone graft (see p. 760) can be harvested and placed in the fracture zone.

Preoperative Management

The patient should be stabilized prior to fracture treatment. Fractures of the femur are not usually immobilized preoperatively due to the difficulty in applying coaptation splints. Contraction of thigh muscles helps immobilize bone fragments but patients should be confined to a small area until surgery. Analgesics are administered as required (see p. 708).

Anesthesia

Patients that have sustained significant soft tissue injury and bony comminution or those patients requiring extensive exposure and soft tissue manipulation will benefit from a preoperative epidural agent (see Table 28-4).

Surgical Anatomy

The shape of the femur dictates the pin size that can be used. The diameter of the femur marrow cavity varies along its length, being more narrow proximally than distally. The narrowest area of the marrow cavity is called the isthmus. In the femur it is located within the proximal third of bone, just distal to the third trochanter. The diameter of the marrow cavity at the isthmus must be considered when choosing an appropriate IM pin and can be estimated from preoperative radiographs. Another factor that governs pin size is the curvature of the femur. The canine femur is normally curved in a cranial to caudal direction; the curvature is most accentuated in the distal third of the femur. The amount of curvature varies between breeds, but the greater the curvature and more distal the fracture, the smaller the pin that must be used to properly seat within the femoral condyles. The curvature of the femur can be compensated for to some extent through proper implantation technique but the normal curvature remains a limiting factor when choosing the pin to be inserted. The cross-sectional diameter of the feline femur is uniform from proximal to distal and has little or no cranial to caudal bend.

☞ **N O T E** • The anatomy of the canine and feline femur differs. The cat femur is straighter, with little cranial to caudal bend.

Normal anatomy of the femur and surrounding tissues may be less apparent when fractures are present. Soft-tissue swelling and bruising vary depending on the velocity of the injury. The vastus lateralis often appears swollen and bruised when the fascia lata is incised. Cranial retraction may be accomplished by gentle release of the muscle from the femoral caudolateral surface. Hematomas and serum are frequently encountered, which may make the fractured bones difficult to identify. Proximal and distal fracture segments can be identified using a combination of gentle retraction and probing. It is often useful to begin dissection proximal or distal to the fracture site in an area of more normal anatomy. The dissection is then carried into the fracture zone.

Positioning

Position the patient in lateral recumbency. It is advantageous to use a hanging leg prep to allow maximum manipulation of the limb during surgery. The leg is prepped from the dorsal midline to the tarsal joint.

SURGICAL TECHNIQUES
Surgical Approach to the Femoral Diaphysis

Make an incision along the craniolateral border of the thigh (Fig. 29-92, A). Be careful to ensure that the incision is made slightly more cranial than lateral since the exposure plane will be at the cranial border of the biceps. The length of the incision is dependent upon the type of implant used for stabilization and fracture configuration. In general, inserting a bone plate or comminuted fracture patterns require a longer incision (Fig. 29-92, B). *Incise the superficial leaf of the fascia lata along the cranial border of the biceps femoris muscle for the length of the incision.*

Retract the biceps femoris caudally to expose the vastus lateralis muscle (Fig. 29-92, C). Incise the fascial septum of the vastus lateralis as it inserts at the caudal lateral border of the femur. Reflect the vastus lateralis from the surface of the femur to expose the femoral diaphysis (Fig. 29-92, D). Carefully manipulate soft tissues and fracture hematoma to allow fracture reduction and application of a fixation system.

The fixation system chosen depends upon the patient fracture assessment and other factors discussed in the section on Decision Making in Fracture Management (see p. 730). Readers are encouraged to review this section before choosing a fixation system.

Stabilization of Midshaft Transverse or Short Oblique Fractures

From a mechanical perspective, this fracture configuration allows load sharing between bone and implant following surgery. Less optimal healing might occur if multiple limb injuries are present or if the patient is large and active. From a biologic perspective, patient fracture assessment is used to determine whether the time to union will be lengthy or short. With prolonged healing times, the implant must re-

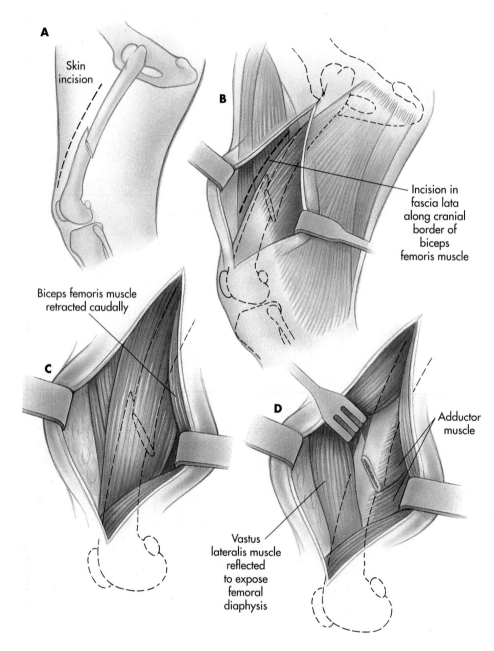

FIG. 29-92
A, To expose the femoral diaphysis, make an incision along the craniolateral border of the thigh. **B,** Incise the superficial leaf of the fascia lata along the cranial border of the biceps femoris muscle for the length of the incision. **C,** Retract the biceps femoris caudally to expose the vastus lateralis muscle. **D,** Reflect the vastus lateralis from the surface of the femur to expose the femoral diaphysis.

main functional for 8 or more weeks. In these cases, implants that purchase the bone with threads are desirable, whereas with shorter healing periods, implants that have frictional hold (IM pins and wire) are adequate.

Stabilization of transverse or short oblique fractures requires rotational and bending support. This can be achieved with bone plates, an IM pin with cruciate hemicerclage wire, an IM pin with an external fixator, or an external fixator alone (Fig. 29-93). Examples of implants that can be used to treat patients with a low fracture assessment (e.g., 0 to 3) are a bone plate and screws applied to function as a compression plate (Fig. 29-94), a 6 pin Type Ia or Type Ib external skeletal fixator with raised threaded transfixation pins, or an IM pin tied in with an external skeletal fixator having raised thread transfixation pins.

Examples of implants that can be used to treat patients with a moderate fracture assessment (e.g., 4 to 7) are bone plate and screws or an IM pin combined with or tied in with an external skeletal fixator. If an external skeletal fixator is used, the transfixation pins can be negative thread profile, raised thread profile, or a combination of each depending on the length of time one wishes to keep the fixator in place. Examples of implants that can be used in patients with a high fracture assessment (e.g., 8 to 10) are an IM pin with a cruciate hemicerclage wire, or an IM pin with two-pin external skeletal fixator. If an external skeletal fixator is chosen, the transfixation pins can be smooth pins or negative thread profile pins. In small patients who are less than 4 to 5 months of age, a single intramedullary pin placed closed in a normograde fashion can be used since rapid formation of biologic callus will provide mechanical support.

Stabilization of Midshaft Long Oblique Fractures or Comminuted Fractures With One or Two Large Butterfly Fragments

From a mechanical perspective, these fractures can be reduced and interfragmentary compression applied with cerclage wire or lag screws. Once the interfragmentary fracture lines are reduced and compressed, the bone is able to share loads with the implant postoperatively, removing undue stress on the implant and its attachment site. Mechanical factors that negatively influence healing include the presence of multiple limb injuries and/or a large active patient. Biologic assessment is used to determine whether the time to union will be lengthy or short. A potential requirement in treating this type of fracture is that open reduction may be necessary to apply interfragmentary compression. Stabilization of this type of fracture requires axial, rotational, and bending support. This can be achieved with bone plates, IM pins, cerclage wires, and external skeletal fixator combinations, or IM pins plus cerclage wires (Fig. 29-95).

Useful fixation systems in patients with low fracture-assessment score (e.g., 0 to 3) are interfragmentary compression with lag screws combined with neutralization plates to protect the reconstruction (Fig. 29-96). A fixation system useful in patients with moderate fracture-assessment scores (e.g., 4 to 7) is an IM pin combined with cerclage wire for interfragmentary compression. The pin and wire can be supported with an external skeletal fixator, or in cases where the biologic assessment is favorable, the pin and wire may be used alone. If an external skeletal fixator is applied for additional support, transfixation pins should be raised thread or have negative thread profiles. A useful fixation system in patients with high

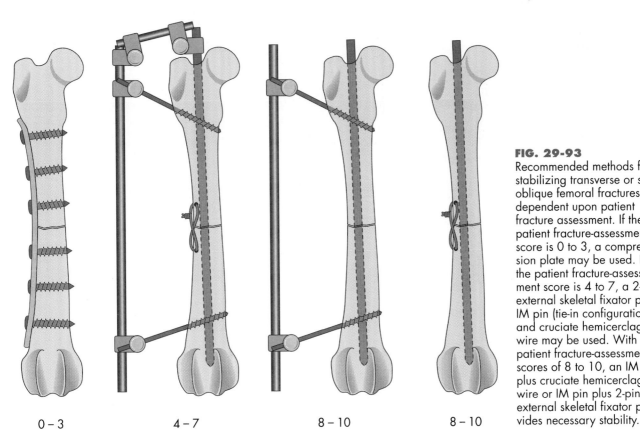

FIG. 29-93
Recommended methods for stabilizing transverse or short oblique femoral fractures dependent upon patient fracture assessment. If the patient fracture-assessment score is 0 to 3, a compression plate may be used. If the patient fracture-assessment score is 4 to 7, a 2-pin external skeletal fixator plus IM pin (tie-in configuration) and cruciate hemicerclage wire may be used. With patient fracture-assessment scores of 8 to 10, an IM pin plus cruciate hemicerclage wire or IM pin plus 2-pin external skeletal fixator provides necessary stability.

0 – 3   4 – 7   8 – 10   8 – 10

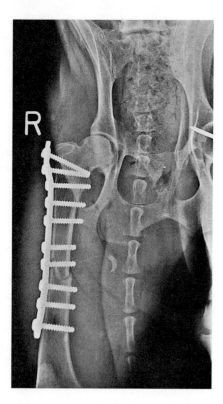

FIG. 29-94
Postoperative radiograph of a middiaphyseal femoral fracture stabilized with a compression plate.

fracture-assessment score (e.g., 8 to 10) is an IM pin combined with cerclage wire to compress the fracture lines.

Stabilization of Midshaft Comminuted Fractures With Multiple Fragments

From a mechanical perspective, it is difficult to reduce and rigidly stabilize all small fragments in comminuted fractures. Even when reduction is attempted, it seldom can be accomplished without causing significant soft tissue disruption. The implant must carry all the load until biologic callus forms to provide additional mechanical support, subjecting the implant to high stress levels. If the biologic assessment is favorable, the imposed stresses will be of short duration and implant failure is less likely. However, if the biologic assessment is not favorable, stresses acting on the implant for extended periods will often cause implant failure. Enhancing the biologic response by applying the concept of bridging osteosynthesis (see p. 730) and inserting an autogenous cancellous bone graft (see p. 760) is recommended.

From a mechanical perspective, these fractures need rigid axial, rotational, and bending support. This can be achieved with a bone plate/pin combination, a Type Ib or Ia external skeletal fixator/pin tie-in combination, a bone plate alone (lengthening plate, broad plate; see p. 749), or an interlocking nail (Fig. 29-97). Patients with low fracture-assessment scores (e.g., 0 to 3) are best managed with bone plate/pin combinations or rigid Type Ib external skeletal fixators tied in to an IM pin (Fig. 29-98). The transfixation pins should

FIG. 29-95
Recommended methods for stabilizing long oblique fractures or simple comminuted fractures (single large fragment) dependent upon patient fracture assessment. If the patient fracture-assessment score is 0 to 3, a neutralization plate or 2-pin external skeletal fixator plus IM pin (tie-in configuration) and cerclage wires may be used. If the patient fracture-assessment score is 4 to 7, an external skeletal fixator plus IM pin (tie-in configuration) and cerclage wire may be used. With patient fracture-assessment scores of 8 to 10, an IM pin plus cerclage wire provides necessary stability.

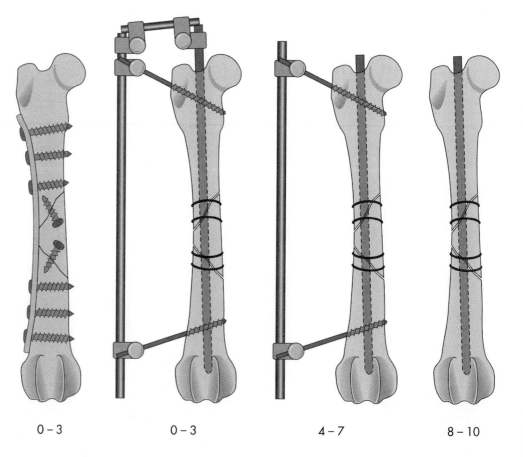

0 – 3   0 – 3   4 – 7   8 – 10

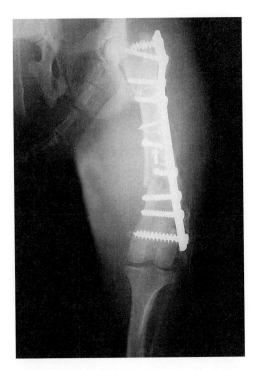

FIG. 29-96
Postoperative radiograph of a femoral fracture repaired with interfragmentary compression screws and a neutralization plate.

have a raised thread and at least two pins should be applied above and one pin below the area of comminution. It is always better to err on the side of too much rigidity rather than too little rigidity since the fixator can be destabilized postoperatively. Patients with moderate fracture-assessment scores (e.g., 4 to 7) are best managed with bone plates functioning as a buttress plate, Type Ia or Ib external skeletal fixators (with or without a tie-in to an IM pin), or an interlocking nail. Lengthening plates, broad plates, or in small patients stacked veterinary cuttable plates must be used. If an external skeletal fixator is applied, transfixation pins should be raised thread pins or combined with negative-thread profile pins. A patient with this fracture having a high fracture-assessment score (e.g., 8 to 10) must have an extremely favorable biologic assessment (i.e., young patients [4 to 5 months of age] having closed comminuted fractures with no other injuries). An appropriate method of treatment would be to bridge the area of comminution (bridging osteosynthesis) with an IM pin tie-in to a 2 pin, Type Ia external skeletal fixator (Fig. 29-99). Transfixation pins can be smooth or have a negative thread profile depending on the amount of time the fixator is to remain in place.

Stabilization of Intertrochanteric Fractures

Intertrochanteric fractures are often complex and involve the femoral neck, greater trochanter, and proximal femoral

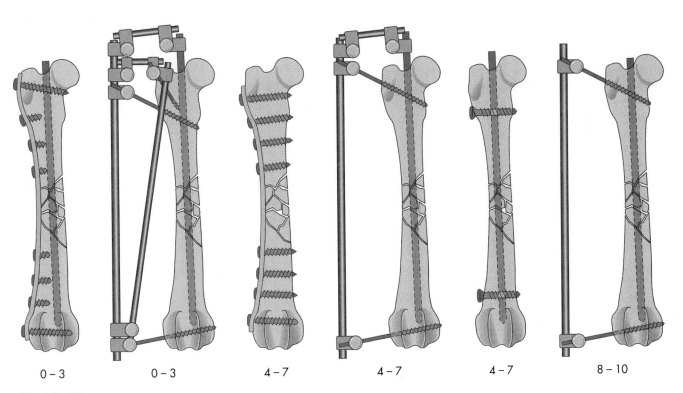

| 0 – 3 | 0 – 3 | 4 – 7 | 4 – 7 | 4 – 7 | 8 – 10 |

FIG. 29-97
Illustration of recommended methods for stabilizing complex comminuted fractures (multiple fragments) dependent upon patient fracture assessment. If the patient fracture-assessment score is 0 to 3, a plate/rod combination or biplanar external skeletal fixator plus IM pin (tie-in configuration) may be used. If the patient fracture-assessment score is 4 to 7, a buttress plate, external skeletal fixator plus IM pin (tie-in configuration), or an interlocking nail may be used. With patient fracture-assessment scores of 8 to 10, an external skeletal fixator plus IM pin provides necessary stability.

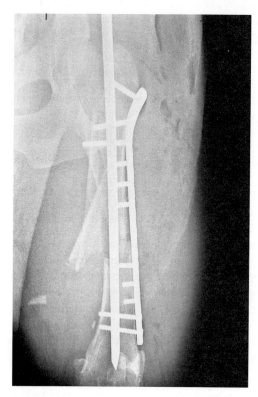

FIG. 29-98
Postoperative radiograph of a femoral fracture in a dog with a patient fracture-assessment score of 2 stabilized with a plate/rod combination serving as a buttress.

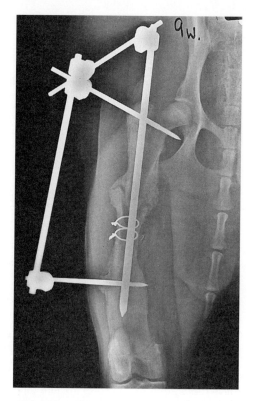

FIG. 29-99
Postoperative radiograph of a femoral fracture stabilized with an intramedullary pin and an external skeletal fixator serving as a buttress. The patient fracture-assessment score was 6.

metaphysis. The method of fixation may vary dependent upon the fracture-assessment score but includes compression screw stabilization of the femoral neck with some method of fixation applied to the proximal femur. The exception is the immature patient with a favorable biologic assessment. In these patients, multiple small pins can be used in the femoral neck and femoral metaphysis. In adult patients, IM pins are not used because the screw traverses the proximal metaphysis and does not allow placement of an IM pin. The preferred method of stabilization in adult patients is a bone plate. If the metaphyseal fracture is a transverse or short oblique fracture, the plate functions as a compression plate. If the area of comminution is reconstructed with cerclage wire and/or compression screws, the reconstruction can be protected with a neutralization plate. Alternatively, the area of comminution can be bridged with a buttress plate or a plate/rod combination, without manipulating the fracture fragments. The compression screw used for stabilization of the femoral neck fracture can be placed through a plate hole or offset caudally to the plate (Fig. 29-100).

SUTURE MATERIALS/SPECIAL INSTRUMENTS

Helpful instruments for fracture repair include a battery- or air-driven drill and self-retaining retractors. Each implant system has special requirements for application (see Chapter 28).

POSTOPERATIVE CARE AND ASSESSMENT

Daily monitoring of the surgical wound and general well-being of the patient are required. Activity should be restricted to leash walking until the fracture has healed. Radiographs to assess healing should be made depending on the estimated time to union. Physical therapy to maintain joint motion and enhance use of the limb is advisable. Gentle flexion and extension of joints above and below the fracture in conjunction with gentle muscle massage are helpful. Communication with the client to inquire about patient progress and to reinforce activity constraints should be done weekly.

PROGNOSIS

Femoral fractures generally heal without complication unless the implant loosens prematurely. Premature loosening (i.e., loosening and migration of IM pins, external skeletal fixator transfixation pins, and/or cerclage wire) is often the result of poor implant choice relative to the fracture-assessment score (see p. 730). When inappropriate or improper implants or techniques are chosen, the implant and its bony connection are subjected to excessive stress, which promotes micromotion at the implant-bone interface. Alternatively, the stress may be moderate, but may occur over a time period beyond which that implant may reasonably be expected to remain stable. In either case, the result is bone

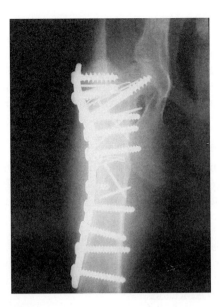

FIG. 29-100
Postoperative radiograph of a femoral fracture stabilized with a compression screw through the femoral neck, interfragmentary compression screws, and a bone plate serving as a neutralization plate. The patient fracture-assessment score was 2.

resorption and eventual implant loosening. Fatigue breakage of implants can occur. This is most often noted with bone plates when reduction and stabilization of a zone of comminution with cerclage wire or lag screws are unsuccessful causing devascularized bone fragments and small fracture gaps. The small gaps are unfavorable for healing and concentrate stress over a small section of the bone plate. The result is delayed healing and long-term cyclic stress on the bone plate. If failure of the initial implant system has occurred, the recommended treatment is application of a compression bone plate or a plate/rod construct. These systems serve to stabilize the fracture and provide patient comfort necessary to allow physical therapy and optimal limb use.

Suggested Reading

Aron DN, Crowe DT: The 90-90 flexion splint for prevention of stifle joint stiffness with femoral fracture repair, *J Am Anim Hosp Assoc* 23:447, 1987.

Aron DN, Palmer RH, Johnson AL: Biologic strategies and a balanced concept for repair of highly comminuted long bone fractures, *Compend Cont Educ Pract Vet* 17:35, 1995.

Brinker WO, Piermattei DL, Flo GL: *Handbook of small animal orthopedics and fracture treatment*, ed 2, Philadelphia, 1990, Saunders.

Fanton JW, Blass CE, Withrow SJ: Sciatic nerve injury as a complication of intramedullary pin fixation of femoral fractures, *J Am Anim Hosp Assoc* 19:687, 1983.

McPherron MA, Schwarz PD, Histand MB: Mechanical evaluation of half-pin (type 1) external skeletal fixation in combination with a single intramedullary pin, *Vet Surg* 21:178, 1992.

Milton JL: Fractures of the femur. In Slatter D, editor: *Textbook of small animal surgery,* ed 2, Philadelphia, 1993, Saunders.

Palmer RH, Aron DN, Purinton PT: Relationship of femoral intramedullary pins to the sciatic nerve and gluteal muscles after retrograde and normograde insertion, *Vet Surg* 17:65, 1988.

DISTAL FEMORAL PHYSEAL FRACTURES

DEFINITIONS

Distal femoral physeal fractures are those that occur through the distal femoral growth plate.

SYNONYMS

Slippage of the distal femoral growth plate

GENERAL CONSIDERATIONS AND CLINICALLY RELEVANT PATHOPHYSIOLOGY

Distal femoral physeal fractures are often classified according to the Salter-Harris scheme for physeal fractures (see Table 29-13). The majority of these injuries are Salter II physeal fractures. A combination of a Salter II and Salter IV fractures occurs with crushing of the trochlea and cancellous bone.

DIAGNOSIS
Clinical Presentation

Signalment. These fractures occur in dogs or cats less than 9 months of age. Any breed or sex of dog or cat may be affected.

History. These fractures most commonly occur after motor vehicle accidents. However, minor trauma such as a fall may be sufficient to separate the growth plate.

Physical Examination Findings

Affected animals present with a non–weight-bearing lameness. Swelling of the stifle region is usually apparent. Pain and crepitus can be elicited on stifle manipulation.

Radiography

Standard craniocaudal and lateral to medial radiographs should be performed. The femoral shaft is displaced cranially and distally and may be superimposed over the femoral condyles (Fig. 29-101). If the displacement is slight, the fracture may be missed when a single craniocaudal radiograph is taken. Additional oblique and skyline projections are useful to evaluate the articular surface of the trochlea and femoral condyles if fissures or fractures of these structures are suspected.

☞ **N O T E** · Superimposition may be such that the fracture could be missed with a single radiograph. Always take two views.

Laboratory Findings

Consistent laboratory abnormalities are not present.

DIFFERENTIAL DIAGNOSIS

Distal femoral fractures should be differentiated from femoral diaphyseal fractures and acute ligamentous injury of the stifle joint.

MEDICAL OR CONSERVATIVE MANAGEMENT

When financial restraint precludes surgery and minimal separation of fracture surfaces is present, external splintage (see p. 707) in flexion or in a normal standing angle may be done.

SURGICAL TREATMENT

Surgical repair of distal femoral fractures depends on the configuration of the fracture. Techniques for fixation of the various fracture configurations are given below.

Preoperative Management

Patients that have sustained trauma should be stabilized prior to anesthesia and fracture treatment. Analgesics should be given to increase patient comfort.

Anesthesia

Anesthetic considerations for patients with fractures are provided on p. 708. Because these animals are young, special care must be used to ensure that hypothermia and hypoglycemia do not occur during surgery.

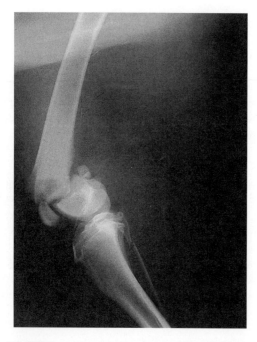

FIG. 29-101
Radiographs of a Salter II fracture through the distal femoral physis.

Surgical Anatomy

The distal femoral growth plate is shaped like a "w" and lies at the joint capsule reflection. The configuration of the growth plate and cancellous bone surface provide a degree of inherent stability for the fracture. The position of the growth plate necessitates an arthrotomy incision to facilitate exposure.

Positioning

The patient is positioned in lateral recumbency with the affected leg up or in dorsal recumbency. The leg is prepped from the dorsal midline to the tarsal joint.

SURGICAL TECHNIQUES
Surgical Approach

The most recognizable structure is often the palpable distal end of the femoral shaft and this point serves as the center of the incision. *Make an incision on the craniolateral surface of the stifle joint centered over the palpable femoral shaft. Begin the incision 4 to 5 cm proximal to the center point and extend it 4 to 5 cm distally. Incise the subcutaneous tissue along the line and identify the fascia lata and patella tendon. Make a parapatellar arthrotomy through the distal fascia lata and joint capsule. Make the incision along the caudal border of the vastus lateralis muscle through the intermuscular septum of the fascia lata. Most often the distal femoral metaphysis lies cranial and lateral to the femoral condyles and will be exposed as the incision is made through the joint capsule and fascia lata (Fig. 29-102). Reflect the quadriceps muscles, patella, and patella tendon medially to expose the articular surface of the femoral condyles. To reduce the fracture lever the condyles cranially and distally with a "spoon" Hohmann retractor placed between the fracture fragments.*

Stabilization of Salter I or Salter II Fractures With Steinmann Pins

With Salter I or Salter II fractures, Steinmann pins may be used alone or in combination with small Kirschner pins. They may be placed either as IM pins or cross pins (Figure 29-103). When Steinmann pins are used as IM pins they should be retrograded such that they enter the bone at the distal end of the femoral shaft. Insert one pin in the lateral metaphysis in line with the caudolateral cortex and the other in the medial metaphysis in line with the caudomedial cortex. Use small-diameter pins so they can bend with the curvature of the femoral canal as they pass proximally. Exit the pins through the bone and skin at the hip joint. Overreduce the fracture and drive the lateral pin into the lateral condyle and the medial pin into the medial condyle. When a single pin is used, retrograde the pin from the center of the fracture surface. Overreduce the fracture and insert the pin into the condyle. When placing Steinmann pins as cross pins, position them so that they enter the epiphysis and drive them prox-

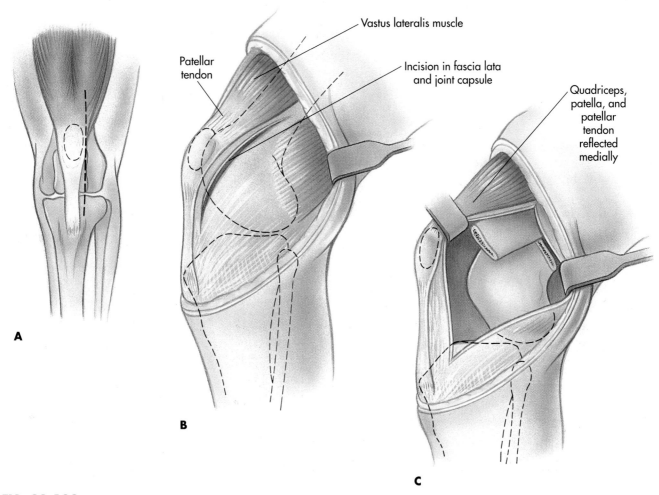

Vastus lateralis muscle

Patellar tendon

Incision in fascia lata and joint capsule

Quadriceps, patella, and patellar tendon reflected medially

A

B

C

FIG. 29-102
A, To expose the distal femur, make an incision on the craniolateral surface of the stifle joint centered over the palpable femoral shaft. **B,** Make a parapatellar arthrotomy through the distal fascia lata and joint capsule. **C,** Reflect the quadriceps muscles, patella, and patella tendon medially to expose the articular surface of the femoral condyles.

imally to a point where they are just visible at the fracture surface. Overreduce the fracture and drive the pins into the femoral condyles. Suture joint capsule using an interrupted suture pattern. Close subcutaneous tissues and skin routinely.

Stabilization of Salter III or Salter IV Fractures With Steinmann Pins or Bone Plates and Screws

Reduce the femoral condyles and apply compression with a partially threaded cancellous bone screw placed across the fracture (Fig. 29-104). In patients less than 4 months of age, diverging Kirschner pins may be used instead of a compression screw. After condylar reduction and stabilization, insert two small Steinmann pins as described for stabilization of Salter I and II fractures.

Stabilization of Comminuted Distal Femoral Physeal Fractures

Comminuted distal femoral physeal fractures often involve the trochlea and articular surface of the femoral condyles. Visualization of the fracture planes is necessary to achieve the anatomic reduction and rigid fixation required with articular fractures. Surgical exposure is best accomplished through a combination of the standard approach described with osteotomy of the tibial crest (see p. 980) and a medial arthrotomy. Proximal reflection of the patella tendon, patella, and quadriceps muscle group allows excellent visualization.

Reconstruct the articular surface using a combination of partially threaded cancellous screws serving as compression screws and Kirschner pins. Once the articular fractures

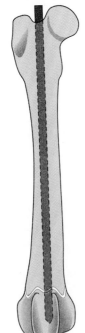

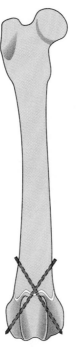

FIG. 29-103
Stabilization of distal femoral physeal fractures may be done with multiple pins placed in rush pin fashion, a single intramedullary pin, or cross pins.

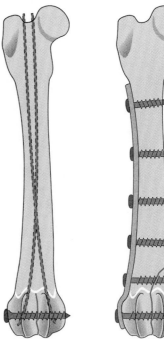

FIG. 29-104
Stabilization of Salter III or Salter IV fractures may be done with a compression screw plus intramedullary pin combination or a compression screw with a buttress plate.

have been reconstructed, reduce the femoral condyles and stabilize them with Steinmann pins or a reconstruction plate. Steinmann pins are more commonly used, but in large- and medium-sized dogs nearing maturity use a reconstruction plate. Contour the reconstruction plate to the lateral surface of the distal femur and femoral condyles.

SUTURE MATERIALS/SPECIAL INSTRUMENTS

Absorbable suture material should be used to close the joint capsule and subcutaneous tissues. Instruments that facilitate fracture reduction include Hohmann retractors and pointed reduction forceps. Small intramedullary Steinmann pins and an assortment of Kirschner wires are needed. Bone plates are useful in larger patients for comminuted fractures.

POSTOPERATIVE CARE AND ASSESSMENT

Patients with moderate to severe trauma of the distal quadriceps benefit by placement of a 90/90 bandage for 7 days (see Fig. 28-13). Gentle flexion and extension of the joint enhance healing and maintain a functional range of motion. Activity should be restricted to leash exercise until healing has occurred (generally 4 to 5 weeks). The pins should be removed once healing has occurred. Plates used to reconstruct comminuted distal femoral physeal fractures that lie within the joint should also be removed once the fracture has healed.

☞ **NOTE** • Using a 90/90 bandage will reduce the incidence of quadriceps contracture.

PROGNOSIS

Because these fractures occur in patients with favorable biologic assessment, bone union usually occurs within 3 to 5 weeks. Although growth retardation or premature closure of the distal femoral growth plate is likely, the prognosis for normal limb use is excellent with Salter I or Salter II fractures. The exception is in the large- or giant-breed dogs when the injury occurs at 3 to 5 months of age, when considerable growth potential is still present. Salter III, Salter IV, and comminuted Salter fractures have a good prognosis if anatomic reduction is achieved. However, due to the trauma incurred by the articular cartilage the client should be advised as to the potential development of secondary degenerative joint disease.

Suggested Reading

Carmichael S, Wheeler SJ, Vaughan LC: Single condylar fractures of the distal femur in the dog, *J Small Anim Pract* 30:500, 1989.

Hardie EM, Chambers JN: Factors influencing the outcome of distal femoral physeal fracture fixation: a retrospective study, *J Am Anim Hosp Assoc* 20:927, 1984.

Parker RB, Bloomberg MS: Modified intramedullary pin technique for repair of distal femoral physeal fractures in the dog and cat, *J Am Vet Med Assoc* 184:1259, 1984.

Shires PK, Hulse DA: Internal fixation of physeal fractures using the distal femur as an example, *Compend Cont Educ Pract Vet* 11:854, 1980.

Wagner SD et al: Effect of distal femoral growth plate fusion on femoral-tibial length, *Vet Surg* 16:435, 1987.

Whitney WO, Schrader SC: Dynamic intramedullary crosspinning technique for repair of distal femoral fractures in dogs and cats: 71 cases (1981–1985), *J Am Vet Med Assoc* 191:1133, 1987.

PATELLAR FRACTURES

DEFINITIONS

Patellar fractures arise when there is a loss of bony and articular continuity between the superior and inferior poles of the patella.

SYNONYMS

Fractured kneecap

GENERAL CONSIDERATIONS AND CLINICALLY RELEVANT PATHOPHYSIOLOGY

Fractures of the patella may occur secondary to direct or indirect trauma, but are uncommon. Direct trauma results from an external blow to the cranial surface of the patella. The resulting fracture may be a transverse separation midway between the superior and inferior poles, fragmentation of the superior or inferior pole, or comminution of the patellar body. Indirect trauma is due to forceful contraction of the quadriceps muscle group, which causes excessive tensile forces to be applied across the body of the patella. These forces result in a transverse fracture midway between the superior and inferior poles. Transverse or comminuted fractures through the patellar body are disabling injuries because they cause loss of quadriceps function and resultant inability to bear weight on the affected limb. Without treatment, the superior and inferior fragments of the patella separate due to countering forces of the quadriceps muscle and patella tendon. A fibrous union develops between the fragments that affords some stability, but the support is insufficient to allow normal function. Additionally, loss of articular surface congruity results in degenerative arthritis of the patella-femoral articulation. Small fragments at the superior or inferior poles of the patella may not be disabling if integrity of the insertion of the quadriceps muscle group is maintained.

DIAGNOSIS
Clinical Presentation

Signalment. Any age, breed, or sex of dog may be affected. Breeds known to be afflicted with congenital myotonia and sporting breeds are most prone to transverse fractures due to forceful contraction of the quadriceps.

History. Animals with patellar fractures due to trauma are usually evaluated because of a non–weight-bearing lameness. The trauma itself is seldom witnessed by owners. Indirect trauma usually occurs when the animal is undergoing strenuous activity and acutely becomes non-weight bearing.

Physical Examination Findings

Animals are usually non-weight bearing on the affected limb. Palpation shows pain and swelling over the cranial surface of the stifle. Crepitation is usually not noted because the fragments separate. Palpation may detect a void in the quadriceps-patella-tendon mechanism.

Radiography

Standard craniocaudal and medial to lateral radiographs should be taken (Fig. 29-105).

Laboratory Findings

Consistent laboratory abnormalities are not present.

DIFFERENTIAL DIAGNOSIS

Patellar fractures should be differentiated from lacerations or rupture of the patella tendon resulting in quadriceps insufficiency. This differentiation is made based on the radiographic appearance of the patella.

MEDICAL MANAGEMENT

Conservative management (i.e., rest and passive physical therapy) is not indicated if a transverse or comminuted fracture has separated the superior and inferior poles of the patella. Fibrous union may occur but the stability afforded is insufficient to allow normal activity. Small fragments near the superior or inferior pole may be managed conservatively if they do not interfere with motion of the patella-femoral joint.

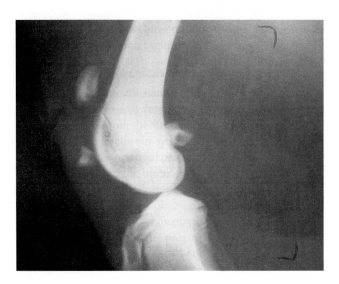

FIG. 29-105
Lateral radiograph of a dog with a transverse patella fracture.

SURGICAL TREATMENT
Preoperative Management

The animal should be confined to a cage until surgery is performed.

Anesthesia

Refer to p. 708 for anesthetic management of animals with orthopedic disease.

Surgical Anatomy

The patella is the largest sesamoid in the body and is embedded within the tendons of the quadriceps muscle group. The undersurface tracks within the trochlear groove of the femur and is formed of hyaline articular cartilage. The function of the patella is twofold: (1) to maintain straight line stability during contraction of the quadriceps muscle group, and (2) to provide mechanical efficiency for the quadriceps muscle group. During surgery care must be used to preserve the insertion of the quadriceps muscle insertion and patella tendon.

Positioning

The patient is positioned in ventral recumbency. The limb should be clipped and surgically prepped from the greater trochanter proximally to the tarsus distally. A hanging-leg preparation facilitates manipulation of the limb during surgery.

SURGICAL TECHNIQUE

Make a craniolateral skin incision 1 cm lateral to the patella. Begin the incision 5 cm proximal to the patella and extend it distally to the tibial crest. Incise subcutaneous tissues overlying the patella and patella tendon to expose the fragment ends. Place the limb in extension to reduce the fracture and then stabilize the fragments with a tension band placed over the cranial surface of the patella (Fig. 29-106). If possible, drill small holes through the bone at the superior and inferior poles for wire placement; if this is not feasible because of patient size or comminution, place the wire deep within the fibrous tissue adjacent to the superior and inferior poles of the patella. Visualize the articular surface of the patella to ensure anatomic reduction after tightening the wire.

SUTURE MATERIALS/SPECIAL INSTRUMENTS

Self-retaining retractors are useful to reflect adjacent tissues. Orthopedic wire, small pins, and an air-driven or battery-operated drill is needed for placement of the tension band.

POSTOPERATIVE CARE AND ASSESSMENT

Limit activity to leash walking until radiographic union is apparent. Strict adherence to limited activity is mandatory since forceful contraction of the quadriceps will disrupt the repair. Time to union varies with biologic assessment of the

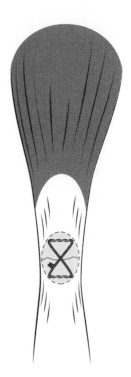

FIG. 29-106
Stabilization of a transverse patellar fracture using a tension band wire.

patient (see p. 730), but is generally between 6 and 12 weeks.

PROGNOSIS

Return to athletic function is dependent upon adequate healing and reduction of fragments. Prognosis is good to excellent if postoperative instructions are followed closely and integrity of the patella-femoral joint is maintained.

Suggested Reading

Curtis MJ: Internal fixation for fractures of the patella. A comparison of two methods, *J Bone Joint Surg* 72B:280, 1990.
Harari JS, Person M, Berardi C: Fractures of the patella in dogs and cats, *Compend Cont Educ Pract Vet* 12:1557, 1990.
Hulse DA, Shires PK: The stifle joint. In Slatter DH, editor: *Textbook of small animal surgery,* ed 1, Philadelphia, 1985, WB Saunders.

TIBIAL AND FIBULAR FRACTURES

TIBIAL AND FIBULAR DIAPHYSEAL FRACTURES

DEFINITIONS

Tibial and **fibular diaphyseal fractures** occur as a result of trauma to the rear limb. **Open fractures** (i.e., with wounds through skin overlying the bone) may occur because of the sparse soft tissue coverage.

GENERAL CONSIDERATIONS AND CLINICALLY RELEVANT PATHOPHYSIOLOGY

Fractures of the tibia in dogs and cats are primarily the result of trauma (i.e., motor vehicle trauma, gunshots, fights with other animals, and falls). Although the fibula is usually fractured as well, it is seldom stabilized unless stability of the stifle or hock is threatened. In several studies, tibial fractures accounted for approximately 20% of documented fractures (Boone et al, 1986; Johnson, Kneller, Weigel, 1989). Underlying pathology (i.e., skeletal tumors) may predispose to fracture. The tibia is subject to a number of mechanical forces and fractures observed can be avulsion, transverse, oblique, spiral, comminuted, or severely comminuted. The paucity of soft tissues around the tibia contributes to the frequency of open fractures.

Because tibial fractures are most commonly caused by trauma, the entire animal must be evaluated to detect concurrent injuries (i.e., pulmonary contusions, pneumothorax, rib fractures, and traumatic myocarditis). Concurrent injuries to the limb may include extensive soft tissue damage and loss.

DIAGNOSIS
Clinical Presentation

Signalment. Any age, breed, or sex of dog or cat may be affected. Young animals more commonly sustain vehicular trauma.

History. Affected animals usually present with a non–weight-bearing lameness after trauma. Occasionally owners are unaware that trauma occurred.

Physical Examination Findings

Affected animals are usually non-weight bearing on the affected limb and have palpable swelling, crepitation, and pain at the fracture site.

Radiography

The extent of bone and soft tissue damage should be assessed on craniocaudal and lateral radiographs that include joints proximal and distal to the affected tibia. Fractious or animals in extreme pain may require sedation for radiography after it has been determined that contraindications (i.e., shock, hypotension, severe dyspnea) for administration of sedatives do not exist. Thoracic radiography should be performed to evaluate pulmonary changes.

Laboratory Findings

Complete blood count and serum chemistry evaluation should be done to evaluate the status of the animal for anesthesia and determine if concurrent injury or damage to the renal or hepatobiliary systems exists.

DIFFERENTIAL DIAGNOSIS

Diagnosis of tibial fractures is based on physical and radiographic examination. Animals presenting with tibial and fibular fractures should be evaluated to determine whether fractures are the result of trauma or underlying pathology (i.e., neoplasia or metabolic disease).

MEDICAL MANAGEMENT

Medical treatment of animals with tibial and fibular fractures may include analgesics (see p. 708) and antibiotics to treat open fractures (see p. 708). Conservative management of tibial and fibular diaphyseal fractures consists of splints and casts and is reserved for closed, nondisplaced, or greenstick fractures in immature animals (see fracture-assessment score on p. 730). Cast fixation may be appropriate for these fractures because the joint above and below the fractured bone (stifle and hock) can be immobilized and the fracture should heal rapidly.

> ☞ **N O T E** · Consider whether the animal will be able to bear weight on the opposite limb when applying a cast.

SURGICAL TREATMENT

The decision to do an open or a closed reduction depends in part on fracture configuration (see Table 29-9). Simple or moderately comminuted fractures with large fragments that can be anatomically reconstructed to establish the bone column are candidates for open reduction and stabilization with internal fixation, external fixation, or a combination of techniques. Severely comminuted fractures that cannot be completely reconstructed are candidates for closed reduction and external fixation or open reduction and application of a buttress plate. Whether the fracture is open or closed is not as important as the potential of the fracture to be anatomically reconstructed. Advantages and disadvantages of open and closed reduction need to be weighed to determine the best approach for each individual fracture. Reduction and fixation techniques applicable to tibial diaphyseal fractures include: (1) closed reduction with external coaptation (cast) or an external fixation splint, or (2) open reduction with internal fixation using pins and orthopedic wire, an external fixation splint, or plate and screws. Selection of the reduction method and fixation technique depends on fracture type and location, signalment, fracture-assessment score, presence of additional skeletal injuries, and the surgeon's familiarity with the various types of fixation equipment.

Application of Casts

Casts can be applied as the sole method of fixation for stable fractures in young dogs or cats when the fracture will maintain adequate reduction and heal quickly. Greenstick or incomplete fractures of the tibia require minimal reduction. Casts that are applied over a padded bandage, cut on the lateral and medial sides, and taped together are occasionally used to support internal fixation. Bivalve casts do not offer as rigid a fixation as cylinder casts, but provide additional support with pin or plate fixation and are easily changed to allow wound treatment. The cast should be

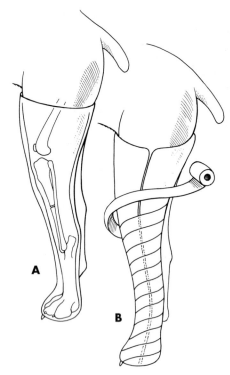

FIG. 29-107
Casts may be used to stabilize closed, nondisplaced tibial/fibular fractures in patients with fracture-assessment scores between 8 and 10. **A,** A full cylinder cast, which immobilizes the stifle and hock, is placed with the limb in slight extension and varus angulation. **B,** The cast can be bivalved by placing cast material over multiple layers of padding, cutting it on the lateral and medial aspects, and securing the two halves around the limb with elastic tape.

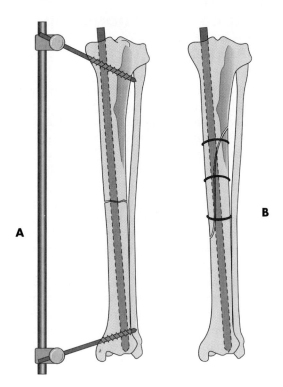

FIG. 29-108
Simple tibial fractures in patients with fracture-assessment scores between 8 and 10 can be treated with **A,** an intramedullary pin and unilateral external skeletal fixator or **B,** an intramedullary pin plus cerclage wires.

☞ **NOTE** · Pins must be placed in a normograde manner starting at the proximal tibia. Always manipulate the hock to ensure the pin does not interfere with the joint.

applied so that it immobilizes the stifle and hock (Fig. 29-107). Casts are applied with the limb positioned in slight extension with varus angulation.

Application of IM Pins

Intramedullary pins can be used to stabilize tibial fractures. Transverse or short oblique fractures treated with an IM pin require a concurrent unilateral external fixation splint to control rotation (Fig. 29-108, *A*). Spiral or oblique fractures, where the length of the fracture line is two to three times the diaphyseal diameter, can be treated with an IM pin and multiple cerclage wires (Fig. 29-108, *B*). Correct placement of the IM pin is important to avoid interfering with the stifle joint. The pin is inserted through skin on the medial aspect of the proximal end of the tibia so that it penetrates the bone at a point midway between the tibial tubercle and the medial tibial condyle on the medial ridge of the tibial plateau (Fig. 29-109). The pin diameter should allow the pin to traverse the curve of the medullary canal without disrupting fracture reduction. If an external skeletal fixator is used in conjunction with the IM pin, a pin small enough should be used so that fixation pins can be placed through the tibial metaphysis.

Application of External Skeletal Fixation

External skeletal fixation is particularly useful for treating a wide variety of tibial diaphyseal fractures. The stiffness of a fixator can be increased in animals with low fracture-assessment scores (see p. 730) by adding fixation pins and using bilateral and biplanar frames. Because fractures of the tibia are frequently open, the use of external fixation is attractive in order to avoid invading the fracture site with metal implants. Another advantage is that removal of external fixation devices is easily accomplished. Implant removal is desirable because of the lack of soft tissue covering and frequency of open fractures. Type Ia or unilateral external fixation splints are usually applied to the cranial medial surface of the tibia (Fig. 29-110, *A-C*). This location avoids penetration of the major muscle masses with fixation pins and thus decreases morbidity. When Type Ib fixation splints are applied, every effort should be made to locate the fixation pins in areas of the bone which have minimal muscle coverage. Penetration of major muscle masses is unavoidable with Type II or bilateral fixation splints, but they are often favored because of their increased stiffness. Fixation splints should span the length of the bone with the most proximal and distal pins

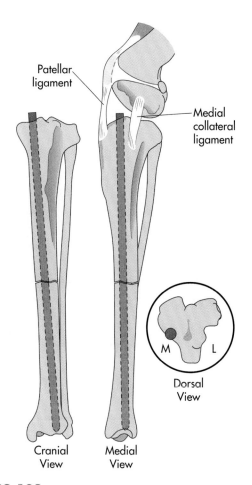

Patellar ligament

Medial collateral ligament

M   L

Dorsal View

Cranial View

Medial View

FIG. 29-109
Illustration showing the correct antegrade placement of an intramedullary pin in the tibia. The pin is inserted through skin on the medial aspect of the proximal tibia so that it penetrates bone at a point midway between the tibial tubercle and the medial tibial condyle on the medial ridge of the tibial plateau.

placed in the metaphyses and the central pins placed 1 to 2 cm from the fracture line. Additional pins can be placed when there is adequate bone (Fig. 29-111, *A-F*).

Type Ia and Ib frames. For placement of Type Ia frames, the fracture is reduced using closed reduction or limited open reduction to reestablish the bone column and obtain alignment (see above). A unilateral fixation pin is placed from the medial aspect of the proximal tibial metaphysis through the lateral cortex. If a threaded pin is used, a hole should be predrilled with a power drill prior to inserting the pin. The procedure is repeated to place a pin in the distal metaphysis. The connecting bar and an appropriate number of pin gripping clamps are added, then the rest of the smooth fixation pins are placed through the clamps and into the diaphysis of the bone (see Fig. 29-110 and p. 736 for external fixator techniques). Type Ib frames are placed cranially and medially on the tibia.

☞ **N O T E** · Positive-profile thread pins increase the stability of the fixator.

Type II frames. For placement of Type II frames with transfixation pins that are clamped on both bars, place the initial transfixation pins in the proximal and distal metaphyses of the bone. These pins should be centered in the bone on the medial to lateral plane and parallel to their respective joint surface. The fracture is then reduced by distracting the transfixation pins manually, using the weight of the animal in the hanging-limb position, or with a fracture distractor placed on the concave side of the fracture (see discussion on fracture reduction on p. 757). A limited open approach may be performed to facilitate reduction of simple fractures where the bone column can be reconstructed.

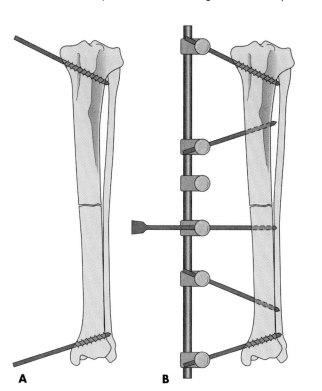

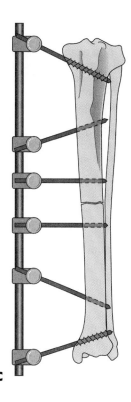

A   B   C

FIG. 29-110
Type I external skeletal fixators are used to treat fractures in patients with high fracture-assessment scores. Sequence for placement of a Type Ia external fixator on the cranial medial surface of the tibia: **A,** Place unilateral fixation pins in the proximal and distal metaphyses. The pins should enter from the cranial medial aspect of the limb. **B,** Add the connecting bar and appropriate number of pin-gripping clamps. Place the remainder of the fixation pins through the clamps and into the bone diaphysis. **C,** Cut the excess pin and tighten the clamps.

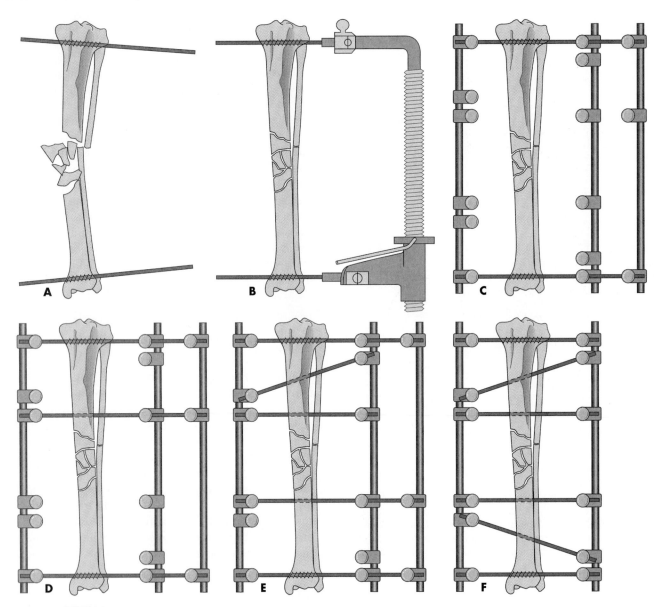

FIG. 29-111
Type II external skeletal fixators are used to treat tibial fractures in patients with moderate and low fracture-assessment scores. Sequence for placement of Type II external skeletal fixators on the tibia: **A,** Place transfixation pins in the proximal and distal metaphyses of the bone, parallel to their respective joint surfaces. **B,** Reduce the fracture. If a fracture distractor is used, place it on the concave side of the fracture. **C,** Secure the medial and lateral connecting bars containing the predetermined number of clamps to the transfixation pins. Secure a third connecting bar with three clamps to the transfixation pins on one side of the limb. **D** and **E,** Place the remaining transfixation pins using the guide bar to ensure proper alignment of the pins with the clamps. Cut each pin before moving the guide clamp to the next position. **F,** Cut the excess pin and tighten the clamps.

Comminuted fractures can be reduced in a closed manner by distraction. The medial and lateral connecting bars containing the predetermined number of clamps are secured to the transfixation pins. A third connecting bar with three clamps is secured to the transfixation pins on one side of the limb. Remaining transfixation pins are placed using the guide bar to ensure proper alignment of the pins with the clamps. At least two pins (preferably three) should be placed proximal and distal to the fracture (see Fig. 29-111). If additional stiffness of the Type III fixation splint is needed, it should be constructed at this time (see p. 735 for external fixator techniques).

Radiographs should be critically assessed to determine if the proximal and distal joint surfaces are parallel to each other. Corrections can be made to the angulation of the limb by loosening the distal clamps and repositioning the distal segment of the bone (Fig. 29-112, *A* and *B*). Also evaluate radiographs to determine if there is rotational malposition.

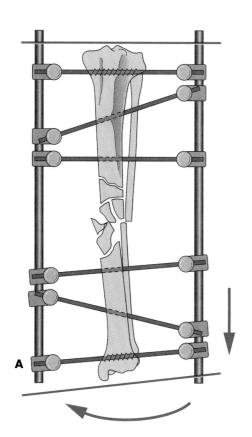

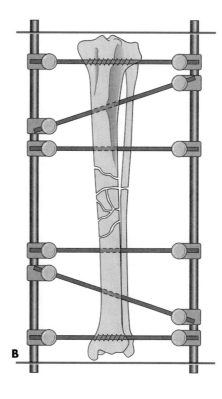

FIG. 29-112
A, To correct a valgus angulation of the tibia, loosen the clamps distal to the fracture and reposition the distal segment of bone by moving the clamps distally on the lateral bar and proximally on the medial bar until the joints are parallel. Reverse the procedure to correct a varus angulation. **B,** When the joints are aligned, tighten the clamps.

When a true lateral and craniocaudal view is made of the proximal joint, there should also be a true lateral and craniocaudal view of the distal joint visible on the film. Limited corrections to rotational alignment can be made by removing one connecting bar, rotating the distal clamps, and replacing the bar. After all adjustments have been made, the clamps should be tightened.

☞ **N O T E** · Do not manipulate the fragments at the comminuted fracture site.

Application of Bone Plates and Screws

Bone plates are an excellent method of stabilizing tibial diaphyseal fractures (Fig. 29-113, *A*). The plate is usually applied to the wide, flat, medial surface of the tibia. A wide exposure of the fracture and intact bone is needed for fracture reconstruction and plate application. Care must be taken to make the skin incision cranial to the position of the plate to avoid the implant irritating healing tissues. The plate is applied as a compression plate to transverse fractures. Long oblique or spiral fractures are reconstructed and the fracture lines compressed with lag screws (Fig. 29-113, *B*). The reconstructed fracture is protected with a neutralization plate. Comminuted fractures that cannot be reconstructed can be treated by distracting the fracture, realigning the limb, and applying the plate in a bridging manner (attaching it to the intact bone without disturbing fragments) (Fig. 29-113, *C*). A plate/rod combination can also be used for comminuted fractures (see p. 751). When planning the plate for a com-

minuted fracture, the plate should be contoured to match the craniocaudal radiographic view of the contralateral tibia.

☞ **N O T E** · Careful contouring of the plate to match the normal configuration of the tibia is essential. Failure to reproduce the normal curve of the tibia will result in valgus angulation of the limb.

If open reduction of the fractured tibia is performed, consideration should be given to harvesting autogenous cancellous bone to enhance bone healing (see p. 760). The most accessible site for cancellous bone harvest is the ipsilateral proximal humerus. The ipsilateral ilium and tibia and the contralateral tibia can also be prepared for cancellous bone harvest.

Preoperative Management

Open wounds should be managed initially by carefully clipping surrounding hair, cleaning the wound, and obtaining a swab for bacterial culture and susceptibility testing. Cultures of open wounds should be obtained prior to administration of antibiotics. The limb should be temporarily stabilized with a Robert Jones bandage to immobilize the fragments, decrease or prevent soft tissue swelling, protect or prevent open wounds, and increase patient comfort until surgery can be performed (see p. 706). Concurrent injuries should be managed prior to anesthetizing the animal for fracture fixation. Prophylactic antibiotics are indicated when surgery time is apt to exceed 2 hours.

FIG. 29-113
Fractures in patients with moderate and low fracture-assessment scores can be treated with plate fixation to ensure adequate stabilization for fracture healing. Illustrations showing treatment of **A,** a transverse fracture with a compression plate, **B,** a long oblique fracture with interfragmentary lag screws and a neutralization plate, and **C,** a comminuted fracture with a buttress or bridging plate.

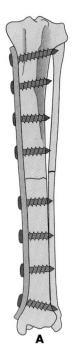
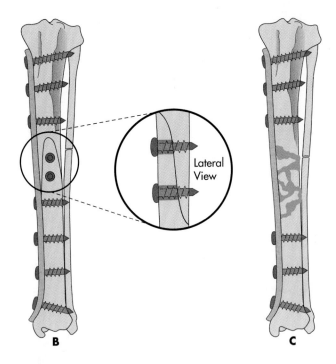

A   B   C

Lateral View

Anesthesia

Anesthetic management of animals with fractures is discussed on p. 708.

Surgical Anatomy

The craniomedial surface of the tibia is not covered by muscle and can be easily palpated to serve as a landmark for location of the incision. Extensor muscles located on the lateral surface of the tibia and flexor muscles located caudal to the tibia can be retracted to expose the bone. The medial saphenous vein crosses the medial portion of the distal tibia.

Positioning

The leg should be prepped from the hip to below the hock. If cancellous bone graft harvest is anticipated, a donor site should also be prepped. For closed reduction or limited open reduction and external skeletal fixation, the animal should be positioned with the affected leg suspended from the ceiling to improve visualization of correct joint alignment (see p. 760). If open reduction is performed, the animal should be positioned in dorsal recumbency and the limb draped out and released to expose the medial surface.

SURGICAL TECHNIQUES
Craniomedial Approach to the Tibia

Make a craniomedial skin incision parallel to the tibial crest, which extends the entire length of the tibia (Fig. 29-114, A). Continue dissection through the fascia, avoiding the medial saphenous vein and nerve crossing the middle to distal third of the tibial diaphysis (Fig. 29-114, B).

Stabilization of Midshaft Transverse or Short Oblique Fractures

From a mechanical perspective, this fracture configuration allows load sharing between the bone and implant after surgery. Factors that affect healing negatively include multi-

ple limb injuries or if the patient is large and active. From a biologic perspective, the patient fracture assessment dictates whether the time to union will be lengthy or of short duration. When a prolonged healing period is expected the implant needs to remain functional for 8 or more weeks. In these cases, implants that purchase bone with threads are desirable; with shorter healing periods implants that have frictional hold are adequate.

Stabilization of a transverse or short oblique fracture requires rotational and bending support. This can be achieved with bone plates, an IM pin with an external fixator, or an external fixator alone. The final implant choice should be determined by the fracture location and patient fracture assessment. Fixation systems that are useful with a low patient fracture assessment (i.e., 0 to 3) include a bone plate and screws inserted to function as a compression plate, and Type II external skeletal fixator with raised threaded transfixation pins (see Figs. 29-111 and 29-113). With a moderate patient fracture assessment (i.e., 4 to 7), a compression plate, Type II external skeletal fixator or an IM pin and 2-pin, Type Ia external fixator would be functional. The transfixation pins can be a combination of smooth, negative profile, and raised threaded pins depending on the length of time the fixator must stay in place. Transverse or short oblique fractures in patients with a high patient fracture assessment (i.e., 8 to 10) can be stabilized with a cast, Type Ia 4- to 6-pin external fixator, or IM pin, 2-pin Type Ia external skeletal fixator.

Stabilization of Midshaft Long Oblique Fractures or Comminuted Fractures With a Large Butterfly Fragment

From a mechanical perspective, these fractures can be reduced and interfragmentary compression applied with cerclage wire or lag screws. Once the interfragmentary fracture lines are reduced and compressed, the bone is able to share the loads with the implant postoperatively. Factors that negatively

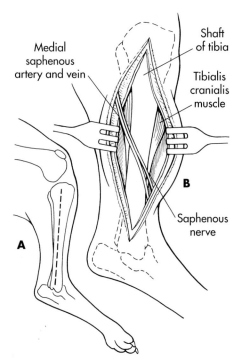

Medial
saphenous
artery and vein

Shaft
of tibia

Tibialis
cranialis
muscle

B

Saphenous
nerve

A

FIG. 29-114
A, To approach the craniomedial aspect of the tibia, make a craniomedial skin incision. Extend the incision the length of the tibia if a plate is being applied. **B,** Dissect through fascia, avoiding the medial saphenous vein and nerve crossing the middle to distal third of the tibial diaphysis.

affect healing include the presence of multiple injuries, a large, active patient, and the necessity for open reduction and tissue manipulation to reduce and apply interfragmentary compression. If a prolonged healing period is expected, the implant needs to remain functional for 8 or more weeks and those implants that purchase bone with threads are desirable. With shorter healing periods, implants that have frictional hold (smooth pins and wire) are adequate.

Stabilization of this fracture configuration requires axial, rotational, and bending support. This can be achieved with bone plates, IM pins, cerclage wire/external fixator combinations, and IM pin and cerclage wires. Useful fixation systems in cases with a low patient fracture assessment (i.e., 0 to 3) are neutralization plates (see Fig. 29-113). Interfragmentary compression is first achieved with wire or compression screws to reconstruct the cylinder of bone—the area is then bridged with a bone plate. Alternatively, an IM pin can be inserted initially and interfragmentary compression applied with cerclage wire. Additional support is then supplied by an external skeletal fixator with threaded fixation pins. With a moderate patient fracture assessment (i.e., 4 to 7), a neutralization plate, or an IM pin plus cerclage wire for interfragmentary compression combined with a 2-pin, Type Ia external skeletal fixator may be used. The fixation pins should have a raised thread or have a negative thread profile. With a high patient fracture assessment (i.e., 8 to 10) an IM pin combined with cerclage wire for interfragmentary compression is a useful method to stabilize the fracture (see Fig. 29-108).

Stabilization of Midshaft Comminuted Fractures With Multiple Fragments

From a mechanical perspective these fractures cannot be reduced without significant soft tissue manipulation and there is no load-sharing between the implant and bone until biologic callus forms to provide support. Therefore, very high stresses will be imposed on the implant and its connection to the bone. If the biologic assessment is favorable, the imposed stresses will be of short duration and the likelihood of implant failure is lessened. However, if the biologic assessment is not favorable, imposed stresses will act on the implant for an extended period and implant failure is more likely. Enhancing the biologic response by not attempting to reduce the fragments (closed reduction and bridging osteosynthesis) or inserting an autogenous cancellous bone graft if open reduction is used is recommended. From a mechanical perspective, these types of fractures need rigid axial, rotational, and bending support.

Stabilization can be achieved with a buttress plate, Type II or III external skeletal fixator, or a bone plate/pin combination. Patients with low fracture assessments (i.e., 0 to 3) are best managed with a bone plate/pin combination or rigid Type II or III external skeletal fixator. The transfixation pins should have a raised thread and at least two pins should be applied above and two pins below the area of comminution. It is always better to err on the side of too much rigidity rather than too little rigidity since the fixator can be destabilized postoperatively. A patient with a moderate fracture assessment (i.e., 4 to 7) can be managed with a bone plate functioning as a buttress plate (lengthening plate or broad plate) (see Fig. 29-113). A Type II external fixator applied with closed reduction can be used.

The choice of number of pins and pin design for the external skeletal fixator depends on the fracture assessment. The only time a patient with this type of fracture would have a high fracture-assessment rating (i.e., 8 to 10) would be when the biologic assessment is extremely favorable (e.g., a 4- to 5-month-old animal with a low-velocity, closed, single limb injury). These animals could be managed using bridging osteosynthesis with a Type II external skeletal fixator. The transfixation pins can be smooth pins or have a negative thread profile depending on the amount of time the fixator needs to remain in place.

SUTURE MATERIALS/SPECIAL INSTRUMENTS

Equipment necessary for pin and wire placement includes retractors, bone-holding forceps, reduction forceps, Jacob pin chuck, IM pins, Kirschner wires, and orthopedic wire. Additional equipment needed for external fixation includes a low-rpm power drill and external fixation clamps and bars. Plating equipment and a high-speed drill are necessary for application of plates and screws.

POSTOPERATIVE CARE AND ASSESSMENT

Postoperative care is the same as that described for radial diaphyseal fractures on p. 810. External fixation devices can be removed when there is radiographic evidence of bridging callus. IM pins are removed after the fracture has healed.

Plates are generally removed after the fracture has healed because tissue irritation and cold sensitivity may occur due to the minimal soft tissue coverage over the plate.

PROGNOSIS

Complications with tibial fractures after open reduction include osteomyelitis, implant migration resulting in soft tissue irritation, malunion, delayed union, and nonunion. Complications encountered with external fixation of the tibia include pin loosening and pin tract drainage. Usually neither of these problems is severe enough to warrant removal or replacement of the pin prior to fracture healing.

References

Boone EG et al: Fractures of the tibial diaphysis in dogs and cats, *J Am Vet Med Assoc* 188:41, 1986.

Johnson AL, Kneller SK, Weigel RM: Radial and tibial fracture repair with external skeletal fixation: effects of fracture type, reduction, and complications on healing, *Vet Surg* 18:367, 1989.

Suggested Reading

Aron DN, Toombs JP, Hollingsworth SC: Primary treatment of severe fractures by external skeletal fixation: threaded pins compared with smooth pins, *J Am Anim Hosp Assoc* 22:659, 1986.

Marti JM, Miller A: Delimitation of safe corridors for the insertion of external fixator pins in the dog. I. Hindlimb, *J Small Anim Pract* 35:16, 1994.

Richardson EF, Thacher CW: Tibial fractures in cats, *Compend Cont Educ Pract Vet* 15:383, 1993.

TIBIAL AND FIBULAR METAPHYSEAL AND EPIPHYSEAL FRACTURES

DEFINITIONS

Metaphyseal and **epiphyseal fractures** occur in trabecular bone. **Articular fractures** disrupt the joint surface.

GENERAL CONSIDERATIONS AND CLINICALLY RELEVANT PATHOPHYSIOLOGY

Fractures of the proximal tibial metaphysis and epiphysis are infrequent in mature dogs and cats. When they do occur they are usually transverse or short oblique in nature. Fractures of the distal tibia in mature animals usually involve the malleoli, either as fractures of the malleoli or as erosion injuries that remove the malleoli. Loss of malleolar stability results in loss of collateral ligament function and talocrural instability. Accurate alignment of malleolar fractures and rigid fixation of the fragment are necessary to achieve joint stability and decrease subsequent development of degenerative joint disease.

DIAGNOSIS
Clinical Presentation

Signalment. Any age, breed, or sex of dog or cat may be affected. Young animals more frequently sustain vehicular trauma.

History. Affected animals usually present with a nonweight bearing lameness after trauma. Occasionally owners are unaware that trauma occurred.

Physical Examination Findings

Because of the traumatic nature of this injury, the entire animal must be assessed to detect abnormalities of other body systems. Palpation of the limb reveals swelling, pain, crepitation, and apparent instability of the adjacent joint. There may be a degloving injury of the tarsus (see p. 987) associated with fracture of the distal tibia. Although there are no major nerves in the immediate area, dogs often appear to have abnormal proprioceptive responses due to reluctance to move the limb.

Radiography

The extent of bone and of soft tissue damage should be assessed on craniocaudal and lateral radiographs that include joints proximal and distal to the affected tibia. Fractious or extremely painful animals may require sedation for radiography after it has been determined that contraindications (i.e., shock, hypotension, severe dyspnea) for administration of sedatives do not exist. Thoracic radiography should be performed to evaluate pulmonary changes.

Laboratory Findings

Complete blood count and serum chemistry evaluation should be done to evaluate the status of the animal for anesthesia and to determine if concurrent injury to the renal or hepatobiliary systems exists.

DIFFERENTIAL DIAGNOSIS

Animals presenting with proximal or distal tibial fractures should be evaluated to determine whether fractures are due to trauma or underlying pathology (i.e., neoplasia or metabolic disease). Joint luxations can be differentiated from fractures radiographically.

MEDICAL MANAGEMENT

Medical treatment of animals with tibial and fibular metaphyseal and epiphyseal fractures may include analgesics (see p. 708) and administration of antibiotics to treat open fractures.

SURGICAL TREATMENT
Application of an IM Pin and Figure-Eight Kirschner Wire for Transverse or Short Oblique Proximal Tibial Fractures

Proximal tibial fractures may be reduced and stabilized with IM pins as described for diaphyseal fractures of the tibia on p. 810. *If the fracture is not rotationally stable, angle a Kirschner wire across the fracture line. Place a figure-eight orthopedic wire around both ends of the Kirschner wire to provide compression to the fracture line (Fig. 29-115, A).*

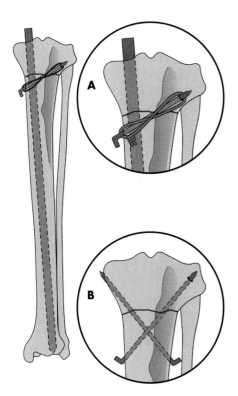

FIG. 29-115
Simple fractures of the proximal tibial metaphysis may be stabilized with an intramedullary pin. **A,** A Kirschner wire and figure-eight orthopedic wire may be added for rotational stability. **B,** Crossed Kirschner wires can also be used.

Application of Crossed Kirschner Wires or IM Pins for Transverse or Short Oblique Proximal or Distal Tibial Fractures

Reduce the fracture and drive a Kirschner wire from the lateral surface of the tibial epiphysis, across the fracture into the tibial metaphysis, and exit the medial cortex. Drive a second wire from the medial tibial epiphysis, across the fracture into the metaphysis, and exit the lateral cortex. Take care to avoid penetrating the articular surface. Alternatively, drive the Kirschner wires from the metaphysis to the epiphysis (Fig. 29-115, B). This technique can also be used for transverse fractures of the distal tibial metaphysis.

Preoperative Management

There may be extensive damage and/or loss of tissues in the area of the fracture. Open wounds should be managed initially by carefully clipping surrounding hair, cleaning the wound, and taking a culture for microbial sensitivity testing from deep tissues. The tibia should be temporarily stabilized with a Robert Jones bandage (see p. 706) to immobilize fragments, decrease or prevent soft tissue swelling, protect or prevent open wounds, and increase patient comfort until surgery can be performed. Concurrent injuries should be managed prior to anesthetic induction for fracture fixation.

Anesthesia

Anesthetic management of animals with fractures is discussed on p. 708.

Surgical Anatomy

The medial aspect of the proximal tibia is covered only with skin and subcutaneous tissue and can easily be palpated and approached. The saphenous nerve lies caudal to the medial surface of the proximal tibia. The lateral aspect of the tibia and fibula is covered by the cranial tibial muscle and the tendon of the long digital extensor muscle is visible. The lateral collateral ligament attaches from the lateral femoral condyle to the fibular head and stabilizes the stifle. The peroneal nerve and popliteal artery lie caudal to the fibular head.

The medial malleolus of the distal tibia and lateral malleolus of the fibula extend distal to the articulating surfaces of the distal tibia and talus. The long and short parts of the medial collateral ligaments arise from the medial malleolus. The long and short parts of the lateral collateral ligaments arise from the lateral malleolus. These ligaments are essential for hock stability. Tendons of the cranial tibial and long digital extensor muscles cross the cranial surface of the distal tibia. The medial saphenous vein crosses the medial surface of the distal tibia.

Positioning

The limb should be prepped from the hip to below the hock. If cancellous bone graft harvest is anticipated, a donor site should be prepped (i.e., ipsilateral proximal tibia or proximal humerus). The animal should be positioned in lateral or dorsal recumbency and the limb draped out for proximal tibial and fibular fractures. The animal is positioned in dorsal recumbency for treatment of distal tibial and fibular fractures.

SURGICAL TECHNIQUES
Surgical Approach to the Proximal Tibia

The craniomedial approach to the tibia described on p. 874 is extended proximally to include the metaphysis. The lateral approach to the stifle (see p. 961) is used to expose the fibular head for stabilization.

Surgical Approach to the Distal Tibia

The craniomedial approach to the tibia described on p. 874 is extended distally to expose the medial malleolus. The lateral malleolus is approached via a lateral skin incision over the malleolus and blunt and sharp dissection of surrounding tissues to expose the bone.

Stabilization of Proximal Tibial and Fibular Metaphyseal Fractures

Fractures of the proximal tibial metaphysis may be stabilized with a cast if the fracture can be reduced closed, is stable, and will heal rapidly (fracture-assessment score of 8 to 10). Refer to p. 733 for general casting techniques and p. 869 for application of a cast to the tibia. If open reduction is necessary, stabilization can be achieved with an IM pin and adjunct wire fixation. Crossed Kirschner wires or cancellous lag screws may also be used, although additional external support may be required (see Fig. 29-115). Fractures of the proximal fibula require stabilization if stability of the stifle is impaired due to disruption of the lateral collateral ligament (Fig. 29-116). The fibular head and attached lateral collateral ligament may be secured to the tibia with a bone screw and Teflon washer.

Stabilization of Malleolar Fractures

Fractures of the malleoli are usually treated with open reduction and internal fixation with a tension band wiring technique; however, a cancellous screw functioning as a lag screw can also be used if the fracture-assessment score is low (Fig. 29-117). Additional external fixation or coaptation is used as necessary to support the internal fixation device.

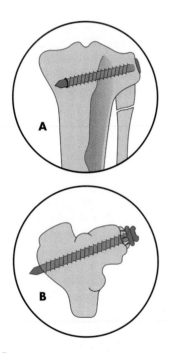

FIG. 29-116
Fractures of the proximal fibula resulting in stifle instability may be stabilized with a lag screw placed through the fibular head and secured to the tibia. **A,** Cranial view. **B,** Dorsal view.

Application of a tension band. *Reduce the fracture (i.e., medial malleolus of the tibia or lateral malleolus of the fibula) and start two Kirschner wires in the fragment. Drive the wires across the fracture line to lodge in the major bone segment. Place a transverse drill hole in the major bone segment and pass a figure-eight wire through the hole, around the Kirschner wire, and tighten it.*

Application of lag screws. *For the medial malleolus, reduce the fracture and drill a gliding hole (equal to the diameter of the threads on the screw) in the malleolar fragment. Place an insert drill sleeve into the gliding hole and drill a smaller hole (equal to the core diameter of the screw) across the tibia. Measure, tap, and select and place the appropriate length screw. Compression of the fracture should occur (see Fig. 29-117 and p. 753 for lag screw techniques). When stabilizing the proximal or distal fibula to the tibia, the fibula is treated as the fragment by drilling the gliding hole through the fibula and the tapped hole in the tibia.*

SUTURE MATERIALS/SPECIAL INSTRUMENTS

Instruments needed include a high-speed power drill, equipment for lag screws, Kirschner wires, IM pins, orthopedic wire, and reduction forceps.

POSTOPERATIVE CARE AND ASSESSMENT

Postoperative radiographs should be made to document fracture reduction or alignment and implant position. After internal fixation, a soft padded bandage should be applied for a few days to control swelling and support soft tissues. Physical therapy (i.e., performing range of motion exercises for 10 to 15 minutes, two to three times a day) is indicated to help restore joint function. Open wounds are treated daily with wet to dry dressings until a granulation bed has formed. The wound(s) should then be covered with a nonadhesive pad and the bandage changed as needed. Daily hydrotherapy aids in cleaning open wounds and reducing postoperative swelling. The animal should be released to the owner with instructions to limit exercise until radiographic evidence of bone healing is apparent. Rechecks should be scheduled at 2 weeks for suture

FIG. 29-117
A and **B,** Fractures of the tibial and fibular malleoli may be repaired with a lag screw. **C,** In patients with high fracture-assessment scores, tension band wires may be used.

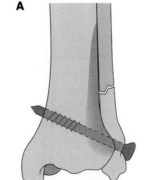
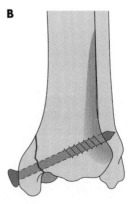
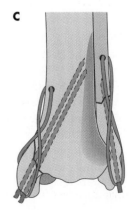

removal and monthly or every 6 weeks for radiographic evaluation. Implant removal may be necessary after bone healing if implants interfere with or irritate soft tissues.

PROGNOSIS

Metaphyseal fractures usually heal quickly because of the large amounts of cancellous bone surrounding the fracture. Possible complications include malunion, which may cause incongruities in joint and limb alignment. Fractures that involve the articular surface predispose the joint to development of degenerative joint disease. Malalignment of articular fractures routinely causes degenerative joint disease.

Suggested Reading

Boone EG et al: Distal tibial fractures in dogs and cats, *J Am Vet Med Assoc* 188:36, 1986.

TIBIAL AND FIBULAR PHYSEAL FRACTURES

DEFINITIONS

Physeal fractures may occur through the cartilaginous growth plate of the proximal or distal tibia or tibial tuberosity in immature animals.

SYNONYMS

Epiphyseal plate fractures, slipped physis

GENERAL CONSIDERATIONS AND CLINICALLY RELEVANT PATHOPHYSIOLOGY

The cartilaginous physis is weaker than surrounding bone and ligaments, making it more susceptible to injury (see also p. 815). Salter-Harris classification is used to categorize physeal fractures on the basis of radiographic and histologic appearance (Table 29-18). Type III and IV fractures are intraarticular. Tibial physeal fractures may or may not be displaced. Proximal tibial physeal fractures are usually Salter Type I or II fractures, although rarely Salter III or IV fractures occur. With Salter I or II fractures, the epiphysis may be displaced caudolateral to the tibial diaphysis and there may be additional injury to collateral ligaments. Open reduction and internal fixation is usually required for treatment. Distal tibial physeal fractures are also usually Salter Type I or II fractures.

DIAGNOSIS
Clinical Presentation

Signalment. These fractures occur in immature dogs or cats with open physes.

History. Affected animals usually present with a non–weight-bearing lameness after trauma. Occasionally owners are unaware that trauma occurred.

Physical Examination Findings

Because of the traumatic nature of this injury, the entire animal must be assessed to detect abnormalities of other body

TABLE 29-18
Salter-Harris Fracture Classification

Type I
Involves only the cartilaginous physis

Type II
Involves physis and metaphyseal bone

Type III
Involves physis and epiphyseal bone

Type IV
Involves metaphyseal and epiphyseal bone and crosses the physis

Type V
Physis is crushed

systems. Palpation of the limb reveals swelling, pain, crepitation, and apparent instability of the adjacent joint. Dogs often appear to have abnormal proprioceptive responses due to reluctance to move the limb.

Radiography

Craniocaudal and lateral radiographs of the affected tibia and fibula (which include the proximal and distal joints) are required to diagnose Salter I to Salter IV fractures. With minimally displaced fractures, it may be difficult to determine if the normally radiolucent physis is really fractured. Comparing radiographs of the opposite limb is often beneficial, particularly with tibial tuberosity avulsions. Fractious or animals in extreme pain may require sedation for radiography after it has been determined that contraindications (i.e., shock, hypotension, severe dyspnea) for administration of sedatives do not exist. Thoracic radiography should be performed to evaluate pulmonary changes.

Radiographs made at the time of injury do not provide information about crushing injuries to the physis or damage to the physeal blood supply. Therefore it is difficult to give an accurate prognosis for growth at the time of injury with these fractures.

Laboratory Findings

Complete blood count and serum chemistry evaluation should be done to evaluate the status of the animal for anesthesia and determine if concurrent injury or damage of the renal or hepatobiliary systems exist.

DIFFERENTIAL DIAGNOSIS

Physeal fractures can be differentiated from joint luxations or soft tissue trauma radiographically.

MEDICAL MANAGEMENT

Medical treatment of animals with tibial physeal fractures may include analgesics (see p. 708) and antibiotics to treat open fractures (see Chapter 10).

SURGICAL TREATMENT

Fractures through and adjacent to the tibial physes can be treated with external coaptation or internal fixation. External coaptation devices will not affect physeal function; however, internal fixation may. Plates and screws or external skeletal fixation devices that span the physis prevent normal function by indirectly applying pressure on the physis. Pins and screws that directly cross the physis have the potential to damage the portion of the physis invaded. Threads of a pin or screw placed across the physis will not allow continued growth; however, a smooth IM pin or Kirschner wire crossing the physis allows proliferating cartilage to slide along the pin. Pins placed perpendicular to the physis allow growth more readily than pins placed obliquely and anchored in cortical bone (i.e., cross-pinning technique). The growth potential of individual animals also dictates the fixation used. The growth of an animal that is close to skeletal maturity will not be adversely affected by fixation inhibiting physeal function, whereas immature animals often develop some deformity.

Application of Casts

Cast should be applied to the tibia so that they reach from the toes to above the stifle (see p. 733 for casting techniques). The limb should be held in slight extension with the hock in slight varus while the cast hardens (Fig. 29-118).

☞ **NOTE** · Be careful to avoid angular deformities when casting the limb. Placing the animal in lateral recumbency with the affected limb down during casting aids in attaining a varus position of the limb.

Application of Crossed Kirschner Wires or IM Pins

Crossed Kirschner wires or IM pins may be used to stabilize tibial physeal fractures. Care should be used when reducing the fragments to avoid traumatizing the physis. One Kirschner wire is driven from the lateral surface of the tibial epiphysis across the physis, into the tibial metaphysis, and through the medial cortex. The second wire is driven from the medial tibial epiphysis across the physis, into the metaphysis, and through the lateral cortex. Care should be used to avoid penetrating the articular surface. This technique can also be used for physeal fractures of the distal tibia even though the Kirschner wire or pin driven from the lateral aspect of the tibia penetrates the fibular malleolus (Fig. 29-119).

☞ **NOTE** · Use smooth implants when crossing the physis.

Application of a tension band wire. Tension band wire may be used to stabilize tibial tubercle physeal fractures. The tibial tubercle is reduced and two Kirschner wires are started in the fragment. The wires are driven across the physis to lodge in the proximal tibia and the repair checked to see if stabilization is sufficient to prevent avulsion of the fracture. If not, a tension band wire should be used even though it may prevent physeal growth. To place a tension band wire, drill a transverse hole in the major bone segment and pass a figure-eight wire through the hole and around the Kirschner wire. Then, tighten the wire (Fig. 29-120) (see p. 747 for tension band wire techniques).

Preoperative Management

The rear limb should be temporarily stabilized with a Robert Jones bandage (see p. 706) to immobilize fragments, decrease or prevent soft tissue swelling, protect or prevent open

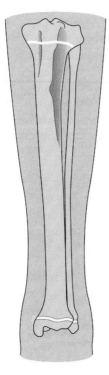

FIG. 29-118
Nondisplaced tibial physeal fractures can be stabilized with a cast.

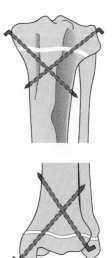

FIG. 29-119
Displaced tibial physeal fractures may be treated with open reduction and placement of crossed Kirschner wires.

wounds, and increase patient comfort until surgery can be performed. Concurrent injuries should be managed prior to anesthetic induction for fracture fixation.

Anesthesia

Anesthetic management of animals with fractures is discussed on p. 708.

Surgical Anatomy

Surgical anatomy of the tibia and fibula are provided on p. 877.

Positioning

The limb should be prepped from hip to below the hock. The animal is positioned in dorsal recumbency and the limb draped out for physeal fractures of the tibia.

SURGICAL TECHNIQUE
Surgical Approach to the Craniomedial Tibia

A proximal extension of the craniomedial approach to the tibia described on p. 874 is used for proximal tibial physeal fractures and tibial tuberosity avulsions.

Surgical Approach to the Distal Physis

Distal physeal fractures can be approached with a distal extension of the craniomedial approach to the tibia or with a cranial skin incision and retraction of the extensor tendons.

Stabilization of Nondisplaced Fractures

Most physeal fractures have a fracture-assessment score between 8 and 10 (see p. 733) because affected animals are

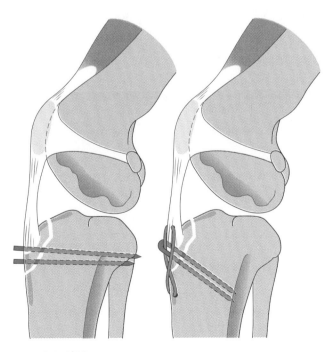

FIG. 29-120
Avulsions of the tibial tuberosity may be reduced and stabilized with two Kirschner wires. If displacement of the fragment occurs when the stifle is flexed, a figure-eight orthopedic wire may be added.

young and physeal fractures heal quickly. Therefore, the implant system chosen does not need to function for a long time. Nondisplaced physeal fractures may be treated with closed reduction and a cast that immobilizes the stifle and the hock (see Fig. 29-119).

Stabilization of Displaced Fractures

Displaced fractures require a surgical approach and gentle reduction to restore physeal alignment. Internal fixation of choice for proximal physeal fracture in immature dogs is Kirschner wires or small IM pins. Minimally displaced distal tibial fractures may be closed reduced and stabilized with a cast. Kirschner wires or small Steinmann pins can also be used as crossed pins to stabilize fractures that require open reduction.

Stabilization of Avulsion Fractures of the Tibial Tubercle

Fractures through the physis of the tibial tubercle result in proximal displacement of the tubercle and must be reduced and stabilized in order to restore quadriceps muscle function and stifle extension. Open reduction is usually necessary to anatomically reduce the tubercle, although occasionally closed reduction achieved by sufficiently extending the stifle realigns it. The limb can then be cast in extension for 2 to 3 weeks. Fixation following open reduction consists of two Kirschner wires or a tension band wire.

SUTURE MATERIALS/SPECIAL INSTRUMENTS

Kirschner wires, IM pins, orthopedic wire, and reduction forceps are needed.

POSTOPERATIVE CARE AND ASSESSMENT

Postoperative radiographs should be made to document fracture reduction and implant position. After internal fixation, a soft padded bandage should be applied for a few days to control swelling and support soft tissues. Physical therapy (i.e., performing range of motion exercises for 10 to 15 minutes, two to three times a day) is indicated to help restore joint function. The animal should be released to the owner with instructions to limit exercise for 4 to 6 weeks. Rechecks should be scheduled at 2 weeks for suture removal and at 4 to 6 weeks for radiographic evaluation of fracture healing. Radiographs of the injured bone and the contralateral bone can be made and compared for length as early as 2 to 3 weeks after the injury to determine physeal function. Cartilage physes that heal in a manner that allows continued function appear radiographically as a lucent line and increased bone length should be apparent. If the physeal line appears as a bone density, endochondral ossification has occurred and continued physeal function is unlikely. Implant removal is indicated after physeal healing to allow bone growth (if the physis is functional after the trauma). Early removal of tension band wires used to stabilize the tibial tubercle is indicated to encourage physeal function (i.e., 3 to 4 weeks postoperatively).

PROGNOSIS

Although the prognosis for healing of a physeal fracture is excellent, the prognosis for continued function or growth of the physis depends on the amount of damage sustained by the zone of proliferating cells. The prognosis is good for future physeal growth after a fracture that separates the cartilaginous physis at the zone of hypertrophying cells, whereas the prognosis is poor for future physeal growth following trauma that crushes the physis. Unfortunately, most traumatically induced physeal fractures sustain damage to the growing cells and have a guarded prognosis for growth. Although the tibia and fibula are a paired bone system, premature closure of the proximal or distal tibial physis usually results in a short (but straight) limb for which the animal compensates by extending the stifle. Premature closure of the tibial tuberosity physis can alter the conformation of the proximal tibia and result in impaired function and degenerative joint disease of the stifle.

Suggested Reading

Johnson JM, Johnson AL, Eurell JA: Histological appearance of naturally occurring canine physeal fractures, *Vet Surg* 23:81, 1994.

Manfra SM, Schrader SC: Physeal injuries in the dog: a review of 35 cases, *J Am Vet Med Assoc* 182:708, 1983.

Salter RB: Salter-Harris classification of epiphyseal plate injuries. In Uhthoff HK, Wiley JJ, editors: *Behavior of the growth plate*, New York, 1988, Raven.

CHAPTER 30

Management of Joint Disease

GENERAL PRINCIPLES, TECHNIQUES, AND NONSURGICAL JOINT DISEASE

DEFINITIONS

Arthropathies are diseases that affect joints. **Polyarthritis** is inflammation that simultaneously affects several joints. **Osteoarthritis** is noninflammatory degenerative joint disease characterized by degeneration of articular cartilage, hypertrophy of marginal bone, and synovial membrane changes. **Synovial joints** (e.g., shoulder joint, hip, stifle) are lined with synovial membrane and allow for relatively free movement. Components of **fibrous joints** (i.e., skull, tooth sockets) and **cartilaginous joints** (i.e., mandibular symphysis, growth plates) are connected with fibrous tissue or cartilage, respectively; hence these joints allow for little or no movement.

GENERAL CONSIDERATIONS

Diagnosis and treatment of joint disorders is an important aspect of veterinary orthopedic practice. Many joint diseases are managed medically rather than surgically. Basic knowledge of nonsurgical joint diseases is necessary to differentiate surgical and nonsurgical joint disease and prescribe appropriate therapy (Table 30-1). Knowledge of normal joint structure and function, joint response to injury, and treatment of joint diseases also is essential to selection of appropriate treatment regimens and accurate prognostication.

The common arthropathies of dogs and cats are generally categorized according to whether they are inflammatory or noninflammatory (Table 30-2). Inflammatory arthropathies are further classified as infectious or noninfectious. Noninfectious arthropathies may be erosive or nonerosive. The common noninflammatory arthropathies in dogs and cats are degenerative joint disease and those resulting from trauma or neoplasia. Numerous etiologic agents have been associated with infectious arthropathies in dogs and cats including bacteria, spirochetes (*Borrelia burgdorferi*), rickettsia (*Ehrlichia* spp., *Rickettsia rickettsii*), mycoplasmas, fungi, caliciviruses (cats), bacterial L-forms (cats), and protozoa.

Nonerosive, noninfectious arthropathies include idiopathic immune-mediated nonerosive polyarthritis, chronic inflammatory-induced polyarthritis, plasmacytic-lymphocytic synovitis, and arthritis associated with systemic disease such as systemic lupus erythematosus. Erosive or deforming arthropathies include rheumatoid arthritis, feline chronic progressive polyarthritis, erosive polyarthritis of greyhounds, and periosteal proliferative arthropathy. The most commonly diagnosed arthropathies are discussed in this chapter (see below). Further information regarding arthropathies may be found in most medicine texts.

MEDICAL MANAGEMENT OF JOINT DISEASE

Medical management of specific arthropathies is provided below. Some nonsteroidal antiinflammatory drugs (salicylates, fenoprofen, ibuprofen) inhibit net proteoglycan synthesis in normal articular cartilage. This negative effect appears to be directly related to drug concentrations in synovial fluid. Because increased concentrations of drug penetrate damaged cartilage, antiinflammatory drugs exert a greater effect in osteoarthritic joints than in normal joints. The combination of aspirin and limb immobilization further decreases matrix proteoglycan content and synthesis. However, salicylates and other nonsteroidal antiinflammatory drugs act as analgesics and antiinflammatory agents to reduce pain and encourage joint motion. Although increased motion may be deleterious to healing cartilage in dogs with degenerative joint disease, the advantages of increased muscle activity and joint support appear to outweigh the disadvantages. The antiinflammatory effects of these drugs provide additional benefits in animals with degenerative joint disease by decreasing the synovitis associated with this disease. Some nonsteroidal antiinflammatory drugs that do not appear to have negative effects on proteoglycan synthesis are piroxicam, naproxen, and diclofenac.

Corticosteroids depress chondrocyte metabolism and alter the matrix composition by decreasing proteoglycan and collagen synthesis. Because of the adverse systemic effects of long-term corticosteroid administration and their deleterious

TABLE 30-1

Initial Screening to Classify Arthropathies for Additional Diagnostics (Culture, Serology, Biopsy)

Synovial fluid findings	Radiographic findings			
	Normal	Proliferative bone lesions	Soft tissue changes	Erosive bone lesions
Normal	Normal			
Phagocytic mononuclear cells		Degenerative joint disease		
Nondegenerative neutrophils	SLE*	Feline chronic progressive polyarthropathy Plasmacytic-lymphocytic synovitis (after cruciate rupture)	Idiopathic immune-mediated nonerosive polyarthritis Chronic inflammatory-induced polyarthritis, SLE*	Rheumatoid arthritis Feline chronic progressive polyarthropathy
Degenerative neutrophils, organisms		Chronic bacterial arthritis	Acute bacterial arthritis Rickettsial or spirochete polyarthritis	Chronic bacterial arthritis

*Systemic lupus erythematosus.

TABLE 30-2

Classification of Arthropathies in Dogs and Cats

Inflammatory
Infectious
Bacteria
Rickettsia
Spirochetes
Fungi
Mycoplasma
Protozoa

Noninfectious
Erosive
    Rheumatoid arthritis
    Feline chronic progressive polyarthritis
    Erosive polyarthritis of greyhounds
    Periosteal proliferative arthropathy
Nonerosive
    Idiopathic immune-mediated polyarthritis
    Chronic inflammatory-induced polyarthritis
    Plasmacytic-lymphocytic synovitis
    Systemic lupus erythematosus

Noninflammatory

Degenerative joint disease
Trauma
Neoplasia

effects on cartilage, they are seldom indicated for treatment of cartilage injury or degenerative joint disease. Administration of polysulfated glycosaminoglycans induces articular cartilage matrix synthesis and decreases matrix degradation. These effects appear to be more beneficial in prophylaxis than in treatment of ongoing osteoarthritis.

ANTIBIOTICS

Antibiotics should be administered for infectious arthritis (see p. 891) and prophylactically for surgical procedures. In general, antibiotics should be selected for treatment of bacterial septic arthritis on the basis of identification of the or-ganism and its sensitivity to the antibiotic. Broad-spectrum, bactericidal antibiotics should be administered until the results of culture and sensitivity test are obtained. If bacterial L-forms are suspected, tetracycline (22 mg/kg PO, BID) is the antibiotic of choice. Antibiotics are administered for 4 to 6 weeks, or at least 2 weeks after cessation of clinical signs.

Prophylactic administration of antibiotics is done to prevent surgical infections, especially in joint-replacement procedures, but it is not a substitute for aseptic technique. A broad-spectrum, bactericidal antibiotic such as cefazolin (20 mg/kg, IV) is administered after an intravenous line has been placed and anesthesia induced. This dose can be repeated every 2 to 3 hours during surgery. Antibiotics can be discontinued after surgery or may be continued until culture results are obtained. If cultures are negative, antibiotics should be discontinued; if results are positive, antibiotics may be continued or changed in response to results of susceptibility testing.

SURGICAL ANATOMY

Synovial joints permit motion while providing stability for load transfer between bones (Table 30-3). Synovial joint cavities are surrounded by joint capsules made up of an outer layer of fibrous connective tissue, lined with a synovial membrane. Nerves, blood vessels, and lymphatic vessels are located between synovial membranes and fibrous capsules. Synovial fluid is formed as a dialysate of plasma from the rich vascular supply of synovial membranes. This fluid filters through the vascular endothelium and synovial interstitium to provide lubrication for the joint and nutrition for the articular cartilage. The synovial membrane is composed of synovial A and B cells and dendritic cells. Mucoproteins, such as hyaluronic acid, are added to the fluid by synovial B cells; synovial A cells function as phagocytes and secrete interleukin-1 and prostaglandin E. The articulating joint surfaces are covered with 1 to 5 mm of a dense, white connective tissue (usually hyaline cartilage). This articular cartilage facilitates the gliding motion of the joint, distributes mechanical loads, and prevents or minimizes injury to underlying

TABLE 30-3

Joint Classification

Fibrous joints

Syndesmosis (e.g., temporohyoid joints)
Sutures (e.g., skull)
Gomphosis (e.g., tooth sockets)

Cartilaginous joints

Hyaline cartilage or synchondrosis (growth plates)
Fibrocartilage or amphiarthrosis (e.g., mandibular
   symphysis)

Synovial joints

Articular hyaline cartilage (e.g., shoulder joint)

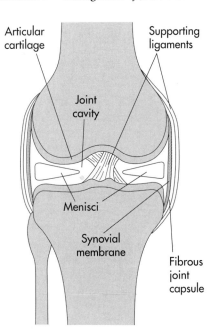

FIG. 30-1
Structure of a synovial joint.

subchondral bone. Additionally, some synovial joints (e.g., stifle joint) have intraarticular ligaments, menisci, and fat pads (Fig. 30-1) that further facilitate joint function and stress reduction during weight bearing. External joint support is provided by surrounding ligaments and tendons.

Loss of joint stability occurs after ligament rupture (i.e., ruptured cranial cruciate ligament) or secondary to developmental or anatomical abnormalities such as canine hip dysplasia. Abnormal joint motion places abnormal physiologic loads on portions of the articular cartilage. These loads can cause the cartilage matrix to fracture or fissure, disrupting the collagen fibril network and causing cell death. The tissue response to cartilage loss is similar to that which occurs during healing of cartilage defects (see p. 886). Subchondral bone sclerosis, osteophyte formation, periarticular soft tissue fibrosis, and synovial membrane inflammation are all definitive signs of degenerative joint disease, and all are physiologic responses to joint instability.

Hyaline cartilage is a dense, white connective tissue made up of chrondocytes (10%) dispersed within an extracellular matrix (90%). Seventy percent of articular cartilage's weight is fluid. Because articular cartilage is avascular and devoid of nerve endings, it relies on synovial fluid for nutrition. Chondrocytes produce matrix and are most numerous and active during cartilage formation; their numbers and metabolic activity decrease with age. The noncellular matrix is composed of collagen, proteoglycans, and noncollagenous proteins. Collagen fibrils embedded in the matrix form a supporting scaffold for cartilage. Proteoglycans are primarily glycosaminoglycan chains (e.g., chondroitin sulfate, keratin sulfate, hyaluronic acid) that repel each other and help to give form to the cartilage. Interaction between chondrocytes and matrix is facilitated by the presence of noncollagenous proteins. This macromolecular conglomerate serves to organize and hold water in the extracellular matrix of articular cartilage.

Adult articular cartilage is categorized into four distinct zones based on cellular morphology and spatial arrangement. The superficial zone has a thin, cell-free matrix that provides the gliding surface of articular cartilage. Deep to this layer are thin, elongated chondrocytes oriented parallel to the articular surface. The transitional zone is wider than the superficial zone and is made of spherical chondrocytes and matrix with large collagen fibrils. The deep zone is the largest zone and contains small chondrocytes that are arranged in short columns perpendicular to the joint surface. The deep zone has the highest proteoglycan content and the least water of the cartilage zones. The zone of calcified cartilage is separated from the preceding zones by the "tidemark," which is visible when articular cartilage is stained with hematoxylin and eosin. The zone of calcified cartilage anchors cartilage to subchondral bone (Fig. 30-2).

Articular cartilage functions as a gliding surface to facilitate joint movement and as a shock absorber to buffer forces applied to long bones during locomotion. The dynamic fluid mechanics of cartilage provide these capabilities. Fluid movement through cartilage plays a fundamental role in (1) augmenting transport of nutrients into and waste products out of cartilage, (2) controlling cartilage deformation, and (3) lubricating joint surfaces during exudation and imbibition of fluid associated with cartilage deformation during weight bearing. Interstitial fluid containing water, metabolites, and small proteins is filtered from synovial fluid and absorbed into the cartilage matrix. This fluid nourishes cartilage cells and adds bulk and resilience to the matrix. As the cartilage deforms with weight bearing, some of this fluid is extruded into the joint, carrying waste products and lubricating joint surfaces. When the load is removed and the cartilage expands, interstitial fluid is reabsorbed by the matrix.

SURGICAL TECHNIQUES
Synovial Fluid Collection

Joint taps to obtain synovial fluid are an essential technique for obtaining information to differentiate arthropathies. Sedation is helpful, especially if the animal is fractious (see p. 723). Equipment needed includes sterile gloves, 25-gauge needles, 22-gauge 1½-inch needles (for shoulder, elbow and

FIG. 30-2
Histologic structure of adult articular cartilage.

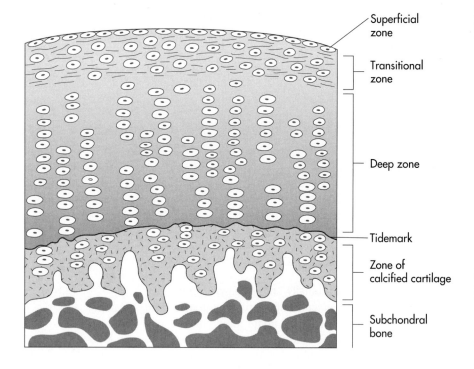

Superficial zone
Transitional zone
Deep zone
Tidemark
Zone of calcified cartilage
Subchondral bone

stifle joints in larger dogs), 3-inch needles (for the hip joint), and 3-cc syringes. Only a small amount of fluid is needed to determine viscosity, estimated cell count, differential cell count, and culture. The hip joint can be very difficult to tap; if no joints are swollen, tap the carpus and/or stifle.

Synovial fluid aspirates commonly show no bacterial growth when cultured directly on blood agar plates. More reliable results are obtained if the synovial fluid sample is incubated for 24 hours in blood culture medium before culturing onto blood agar plates.

Select the joint(s) that are swollen for initial taps. Clip the appropriate area over the joint and prepare the site for an aseptic procedure (Fig. 30-3). Use a gloved hand to palpate landmarks. Insert a needle attached to a syringe into the joint. Apply gentle suction to the syringe. After the fluid has been collected, release the negative pressure on the syringe and withdraw the needle. If blood appears in the syringe, withdraw the syringe immediately; contamination with blood can alter cell counts. If only a few drops of fluid are obtained (common in small dogs and cats), spray the material directly onto a slide and examine it cytologically. Estimate viscosity as the fluid drops from the needle to the slide. Normal joint fluid is viscous and forms a long string. Place a drop of fluid on a slide and make a smear for an estimated complete cell count and a differential cell count. Culture fluid for bacterial and mycoplasmal growth.

HEALING OF CARTILAGE DEFECTS AND RESPONSE OF CARTILAGE TO TREATMENT

Loss of proteoglycans from matrix occurs with infection, inflammation, and joint immobilization, or when cartilage is exposed during surgery or as a result of traumatic disruption of synovial membranes. With reversible damage, chondrocytes may replace the lost matrix components once the insult is removed. However, irreversible damage may occur. Lacerations or abrasions of the cartilage surface destroy chondrocytes and disrupt the matrix. With superficial lacerations (those that do not penetrate to subchondral bone) a standard inflammatory response does not occur because inflammatory cells from marrow and blood vessels cannot gain access to the joint (Fig. 30-4, *A*). Chondrocytes near the injury respond by proliferating and synthesizing new matrix; however, this response is usually inadequate to heal the injury. Although superficial lacerations do not appear to heal, they seldom progress. When a full-thickness cartilage defect occurs, marrow cells capable of participating in an inflammatory response gain access to the defect (Fig. 30-4, *B*). The size of the defect affects healing; small (1 mm diameter) defects heal more completely than large defects. The defect is initially filled with a fibrin clot, which is replaced within 5 days by fibroblast-like cells and collagen fibers. After 2 weeks, metaplasia of these fibroblast-like cells into chondrocytes occurs. These chondrocytes do not function normally, as is indicated by lower concentrations of proteoglycans in the reparative tissue at 6 months after injury. The reparative tissue is also thinner than articular cartilage and is prone to fibrillation and erosive changes.

Joint Stabilization

In animals with acute joint instability (i.e., traumatic joint luxations, acute cruciate ligament injuries), joint stabilization that re-creates normal anatomical relationships and permits normal joint function promotes cartilage repair if irreversible damage is not present and if cartilage was normal before injury. Dogs with cranial cruciate ligament injuries are often presented for treatment after initial changes leading to degenerative joint disease have occurred. In addition, most surgical techniques for treatment of ruptured cranial

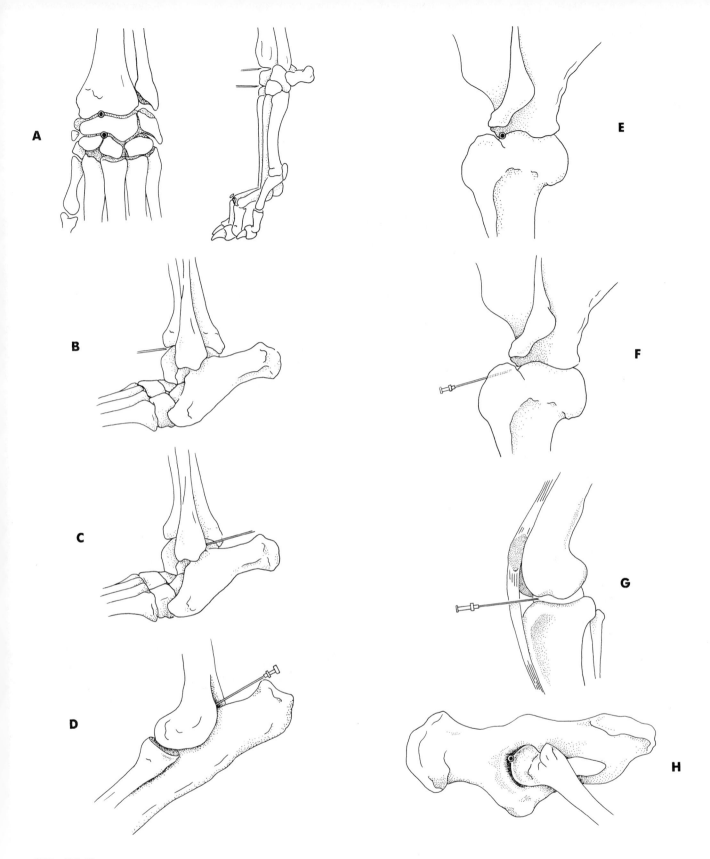

FIG. 30-3
Synovial fluid collection. Recommended sites for arthrocentesis in dogs and cats. **A,** *Carpus:* Partially flex the joint. Palpate and enter the craniomedial aspect of the middle carpal or radiocarpal space. **B,** *Hock (anterior approach):* Palpate the space between the tibia and tibiotarsal bone on the craniolateral surface of the hock; insert the needle in the shallow palpable space. **C,** *Hock (lateral approach):* Partially flex the joint and insert the needle under the lateral malleolus of the fibula. **D,** *Elbow:* Insert the needle just medial to the lateral epicondylar ridge, proximal to the olecranon process. Advance parallel to the olecranon process into the olecranon fossa. **E,** *Shoulder: (lateral approach):* Insert the needle just distal to acromion process, direct medial to greater tubercle, ventral to supraglenoid tubercle of the scapula. **F,** *Shoulder: (cranial approach):* Insert the needle just medial to greater tubercle, ventral to supraglenoid tubercle of the scapula. **G,** *Stifle:* Insert the needle just lateral to the straight patellar ligament distal to the patella. **H,** *Coxofemoral:* Abduct and medially rotate the limb. Insert the needle dorsal to the greater trochanter, angle ventrally and caudally. From Nelson RW, Couto CO: *Essentials of small animal internal medicine,* St. Louis, 1992, Mosby.

FIG. 30-4
Healing of **A,** superficial and **B,**
deep lacerations of articular
cartilage.

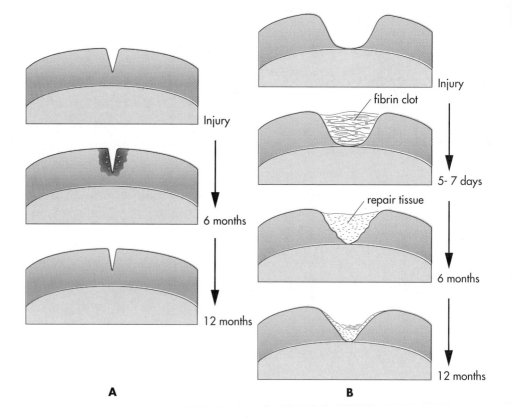

FIG. 30-4
Healing of **A,** superficial and **B,**
deep lacerations of articular
cartilage.

Injury

fibrin clot

Injury

5- 7 days

repair tissue

6 months

6 months

12 months

12 months

A

B

cruciate ligament injury do not restore normal anatomical relationships or allow normal joint function. Therefore, many animals develop progressive degenerative joint disease despite surgical treatment.

Joint Immobilization

Prolonged immobilization of synovial joints causes progressive proteoglycan loss and depression of proteoglycan synthesis, which leads to cartilage softening. When limited activity is allowed, cartilage restoration occurs; however, forced activity after immobility may further damage softened cartilage. Rigid joint immobilization (i.e., that obtained with a transarticular external fixator) results in more severe cartilage degeneration than does less rigid immobilization (i.e., with a cast).

Continuous Passive Motion

Experimentally, early motion and weight bearing are beneficial for repair of full-thickness cartilage defects. Continuous passive motion also appears to accelerate repair of full-thickness cartilage defects, which results in repair tissue that more closely approximates hyaline cartilage.

SELECTED NONSURGICAL DISEASES OF JOINTS

DEGENERATIVE JOINT DISEASE

Degenerative joint disease (DJD) is a noninflammatory, noninfectious degeneration of articular cartilage accompa-

---

TABLE 30-4

Important Considerations in Degenerative Joint Disease

In most instances of DJD in dogs, there is a primary joint problem (e.g., hip dysplasia, fragmented coronoid process, or ruptured cruciate ligament) that was the inciting cause. The underlying disease must be diagnosed and treated appropriately.

DJD is usually progressive, regardless of treatment.

The diagnosis of DJD is based on radiographic evaluation, but treatment is based on clinical signs.

Medical management of DJD includes weight control, exercise or physical therapy to maintain joint mobility and muscle mass, rest during acute clinical signs, and medication.

---

nied by bone formation at the synovial margins and by fibrosis of periarticular soft tissues. DJD may be classified as primary or secondary, depending on etiology. Primary DJD is a disorder of aging in which cartilage degeneration occurs for unknown reasons. Secondary DJD occurs in response to abnormalities that cause joint instability (e.g., cranial cruciate ligament rupture) or abnormal loading of articular cartilage (i.e., developmental or anatomical abnormalities such as hip dysplasia), or in response to other recognizable joint disease (e.g., infection, immune-mediated inflammation). Secondary DJD is more common than primary DJD in dogs and cats (Table 30-4). Abnormal joint motion increases the physiologic loads placed on some portions of normal articular

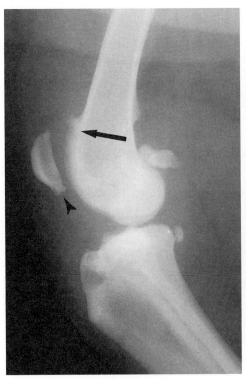
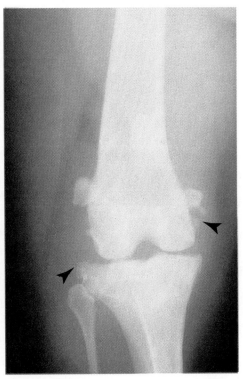

A   **B**

FIG. 30-5
A, Lateral radiograph of a dog with degenerative joint disease. Note the periarticular osteophytes along the trochlear ridges (arrow) and patella (arrowhead). Joint effusion is causing displacement of the fat pad and caudal distension of the joint capsule. **B,** On a
craniocaudal view periarticular osteophytes (*arrowheads*) are evident off the lateral aspect
of the tibial plateau and distal to the medial fabella. Increased prominence of periarticular
soft tissues is present medially and laterally.

cartilage, initiating molecular changes that lead to DJD. Normal stress on abnormal cartilage (i.e., injured by genetic or
metabolic cartilage disorders, inflammation, or immune responses) can initiate the same changes. Disruption of the
collagen fibril network and cell death trigger tissue responses
associated with DJD. Cytokines and active metallopro-
teinases contribute to the degradation of chondrocytes and
cartilage matrix. Articular fibrillation, cartilage loss, subchondral bone sclerosis, osteophyte formation, periarticular
soft tissue fibrosis, and synovial membrane inflammation are
observed in joints affected with DJD.

Conditions associated with DJD include joint fractures,
osteochondritis dissecans, congenital or chronic joint luxations, inflammatory joint disease, septic arthritis, and neuropathies. Additional causes in the forelimbs include fragmented coronoid processes, ununited anconeal processes,
and premature physeal closure. In the rear limbs, hip dysplasia, aseptic necrosis of the femoral head, patella luxation, and
cruciate ligament ruptures may also cause DJD. The signalment varies, depending on the underlying etiology precipitating DJD. The presenting clinical sign of DJD is lameness,
which may be acute or chronic and persistent or intermittent. Unilateral lameness is usually evident when the affected
animal stands or ambulates. Bilateral conditions, such as hip

dysplasia, often appear as unilateral lameness if one joint is
more severely affected than another. Acutely affected joints
may be swollen because of joint effusion, but swelling is
more commonly caused by periarticular fibrosis in chronic
disease. Decreased range of motion, palpable crepitus during
motion, and joint instability are common. Joint palpation
may elicit pain.

The severity of radiographically detected changes depends on chronicity. Radiographic signs observed include
subchondral bone sclerosis, articular and periarticular osteophyte formation, joint-space narrowing, joint effusion, and
increased prominence of periarticular soft tissues (Fig.
30-5). Laboratory abnormalities associated with systemic
disease are seldom present. Rheumatoid factor, systemic lupus erythematosus (SLE) preparations, and antinuclear antibody (ANA) test results are usually normal. Synovial fluid
analysis may reveal decreased synovial fluid viscosity, increased synovial fluid volumes, and increased numbers of
mononuclear phagocytic cells (6000 to 9000 WBC/μl).

Because DJD in small animals usually develops secondary
to other orthopedic problems, the underlying problem
should be corrected, if possible. Surgical therapy, plus medical
treatment, is often necessary to reduce or eliminate clinical
signs. However, correction of the inciting problem, although

necessary to reestablish function, does not usually eliminate degenerative changes that are already present and may not prevent progression of degenerative changes. Correction of the primary problem is not possible, or indicated, in some animals. Many animals with radiographic signs of DJD are asymptomatic, and these animals may or may not develop lameness as they age. Owners should be apprised of the animal's condition; however, they should be reassured that the animal may function normally with minimal or no treatment. In many cases, inflammatory synovitis is responsible for clinical signs of pain and lameness associated with DJD. Because exercise will exacerbate and prolong this inflammation, cage confinement for 2 to 3 days, plus judicious use of antiinflammatory drugs, may be necessary to break the cycle and return the animal to controlled levels of activity.

☞ **NOTE** • Asymptomatic dogs do not need treatment just because they have radiographic signs of DJD.

Many dogs exhibiting clinical signs of DJD are obese. Obesity may be a causative or inciting factor in the development of DJD, or it may be a response to chronic pain. Dogs that are reluctant to exercise may gain weight if food intake is not regulated. Weight loss or weight control for the dog with DJD should be stressed to the owners. Weight loss can be associated with decreased pain and increased function in animals with chronic DJD. Once the inflammatory phase of the disease is controlled, moderate (not severe enough to cause lameness), regular exercise is important to maintain joint mobility, muscle strength, and joint support. Swimming appears to maintain muscle strength without increasing joint loads.

Nonsteroidal antiinflammatory drugs (NSAIDs) are often used to decrease joint inflammation associated with DJD and to provide pain relief. Because their analgesic effects may encourage premature limb use, confinement should be recommended during acute exacerbations of clinical signs. Aspirin helps decrease synovial inflammation and provides some pain relief (Table 30-5). It is the initial drug of choice in dogs with DJD because it is effective, inexpensive, has few side effects, and is readily available. Carprofen is effective for treating DJD, without producing gastrointestinal side effects. It has recently been approved for use in dogs. Many other NSAIDs are available for human use. Extrapolating dosages from other species may be dangerous because the drug may not be tolerated by dogs or cats. Side effects of NSAIDs include damage to the gastrointestinal tract and reduction of the glomerular filtration rate. Administering the drug with food and using Ascriptin (a buffered aspirin combination of aspirin with an aluminum-magnesium antacid) can help prevent erosion/ulceration. Misoprostol (Table 30-6) can also be used to help prevent gastrointestinal erosion/ulceration caused by NSAIDs in patients that have problems despite these precautions. Gastric mucosal sensitivity to aspirin may be manifested by anorexia, vomiting, diarrhea, or melena. If any of these signs are noted, aspirin use should be modified or discontinued to prevent gastric ulceration.

TABLE 30-5
Antiinflammatory Drugs for Treatment of Degenerative Joint Disease in Dogs

Aspirin

25 mg/kg (1 regular-strength aspirin per 25 lbs of body weight, not to exceed 3 tablets per dose) PO with food, BID or TID

Buffered aspirin (Ascriptin)

25 mg/kg, PO with food, BID or TID

Phenylbutazone (Butazolidin)

15 mg/kg PO, BID or TID, not to exceed 800 mg/day

Meclofenamic acid (Arquel)

1.1 mg/kg PO SID after eating, for 5 days, then decrease dose

Naproxen (Naprosyn, Anaprox)

2.2 mg/kg PO with food, SID or EOD not approved for use in dogs

Carprofen (Rimadyl)

2.2 mg/kg PO, BID

However, severe ulceration can occur in animals without obvious clinical signs.

Phenylbutazone (Butazolidin) is an analgesic, antiinflammatory drug that may be used in dogs with DJD (see Table 30-5). Chronic administration of phenylbutazone may cause bone marrow depression (i.e., aplastic anemia, thrombocytopenia), especially in cats, and gastrointestinal perforation. Animals receiving this drug for more than 2 weeks should be carefully monitored. Meclofenamic acid (Arquel) is a NSAID that has been effective in the treatment of DJD in dogs. Acute diarrhea may be noted in a small percentage of dogs. When this occurs, meclofenamic acid treatment should be discontinued and the diarrhea managed with intestinal protectorants and food withdrawal for 24 hours. Corticosteroids have antiinflammatory effects on joint tissues. They have been shown to depress chondrocyte metabolism and alter cartilage matrix, which results in decreased proteoglycan and collagen synthesis. Because of this and the adverse systemic effects of long-term corticosteroid administration, they should be used in animals with DJD only as a last resort. If they are used, they should be administered infrequently and the animal should be restricted from exercising for several weeks after treatment to protect the cartilage. Always counsel owners about the side effects of NSAIDs and steroids. **These drugs should not be given together.**

Surgical treatment of the underlying disease may be indicated to control signs of DJD (e.g., stabilization of stifles with cranial cruciate ligament ruptures). Removal of damaged tissue (e.g., torn menisci) may be necessary to control signs of DJD in stifles with ruptured cranial cruciate ligaments. Associated severe synovitis may require a total synovectomy to

TABLE 30-6

Protectant Against NSAID-Induced Gastrointestinal Erosion

Misoprostol (Cytotec)
Dogs: 2-5 µg/kg PO, BID or TID

TABLE 30-7

Clinical Signs of Septic Arthritis

Acute

Single-limb lameness
Severe lameness, may carry the limb
Joint swollen, painful, and warm

Chronic

Single-limb lameness or multiple-limb lameness with subacute endocarditis
Weight-bearing lameness
Joint swelling

help break the inflammatory cycle. Uncontrollable pain and loss of limb function associated with DJD warrant surgical intervention. Several surgical procedures are available to salvage limb function. Femoral head and neck ostectomy (see p. 947) and glenoid cavity resection (see p. 913) have been described in veterinary patients. After resection of bone and interposition of soft tissues over the cut surface, a fibrous tissue joint or pseudoarthrosis is allowed to form. Function varies after these procedures. Although the joint mechanics are not normal, in many cases limb function is satisfactory. Replacement of an arthritic joint with a prosthesis offers improved chances for normal limb function and superior pain relief. Currently, total hip replacement is the only joint replacement routinely available in small animal patients. Arthrodesis (surgical fusion of the joint) can relieve pain and allow good function of the limb when used to treat carpal instability. Amputation is a salvage procedure that should be considered only in selected patients: those that are non–weight-bearing and have unilateral disease causing unrelenting pain that has been unresponsive to other therapies. Most animals with DJD can function sufficiently to serve as household pets if given appropriate medical and surgical therapy. However, prognosis is inversely related to owner expectations. Affected animals will not usually function as competitive athletes. Complete recovery, without recurrence of clinical signs, is unusual.

SEPTIC (BACTERIAL) ARTHRITIS

Septic arthritis (infective arthritis, suppurative arthritis) is an infection of joints caused by bacterial organisms and may be initiated after hematogenous spread of infection from respiratory, digestive, umbilical, or valvular infections. More frequently, septic arthritis results from direct bacterial inoculation of joints from penetrating trauma, surgical procedures, or intraarticular injections. Bacterial contamination of synovium causes inflammation and promotes extravasation of fibrin, clotting factors, polymorphonuclear leukocytes, and proteinaceous serous fluid into the joint. Fibrin deposition on articular cartilage surfaces inhibits synovial fluid penetration. Leukocytes phagocytize bacteria and release lysosomal enzymes that break down cartilage matrix and expose collagen fibrils to further enzymatic destruction. Enzymatic destruction of the matrix and collagen fibrils, loss of normal synovial fluid nutrition, and mechanical trauma on diseased cartilage combine to cause eventual loss of the cartilaginous joint surface. Eventually the infective process invades subchondral bone, which results in bacterial osteomyelitis. Ankylosis of the joint is the final outcome.

The severity of pathological changes occurring in affected joints depends on the chronicity of infection. Early changes include hyperemia, edema, synovial inflammation, and a purulent-appearing joint fluid. Both hyperplasia and hypertrophy of synovial cells occur. Cartilage fibrillation and granulation-tissue production within the joint soon ensue, and eventually there is loss of articular cartilage. The articular surface fills with granulation and fibrous tissue and, finally, these tissues calcify, causing the joint to ankylose. The diagnosis of septic arthritis is made on the basis of synovial fluid analysis, radiographic changes, and positive bacterial cultures.

Animals with septic arthritis after joint inoculation usually exhibit a marked, unilateral lameness (Table 30-7). The onset of clinical signs may be acute or gradual. Penetrating wounds, surgical intervention, or joint injection are often historical findings. Dogs with septic arthritis from septicemia (e.g., bacterial endocarditis) have multiple limb involvement and no history of joint intervention. Animals with acute onset of signs are often severely lame or non–weight-bearing on the affected limb. The affected joint may be swollen, painful, warm, crepitate, drain purulent material, and have reduced range of motion. Systemic signs (pyrexia, lethargy, and anorexia) are present in a small percentage of animals with septic arthritis. With low-grade chronic infections the signs may be more subtle (i.e., only lameness and joint swelling). Dogs with bacterial infection from bacterial endocarditis typically have multiple joint involvement, lameness, pyrexia, lethargy, anorexia, and/or cardiac murmurs.

Early radiographic signs of septic arthritis are joint effusion and soft tissue swelling (Fig. 30-6). Later changes include bone lysis, periosteal new bone formation, joint surface irregularities, subchondral bone sclerosis, and joint subluxation. Echocardiography demonstrating valvular lesions helps confirm a diagnosis of bacterial endocarditis even in dogs without heart murmurs. Complete blood counts may indicate an inflammatory response in acute stages of septic arthritis. Chronic disease is essentially walled off within the joint and is seldom associated with significant changes in hemograms or serum biochemistry profiles. Joint fluid obtained via arthrocentesis may provide a definitive diagnosis. Purulent joint fluid with increased numbers (40,000

FIG. 30-6
Radiograph of a coxofemoral joint with septic arthritis. There is extensive periosteal new bone formation along the right ilial body and medial aspect of the right acetabulum and ischium. The subchondral margins of the right acetabulum and femoral head are irregular and difficult to identify. (From Olmstead ML: Small animal orthopedics, St. Louis, 1995, Mosby.)

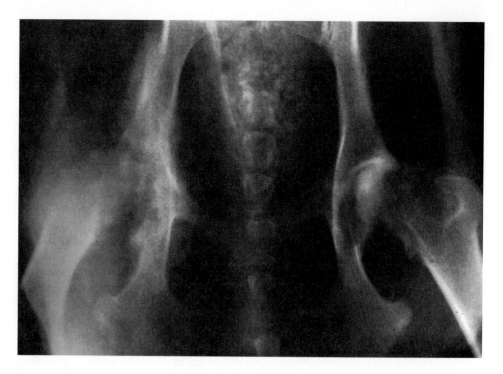

cells/μl to more than 100,000 cells/μl) of polymorphonuclear leukocytes (especially if they are degenerating) and bacteria is indicative of a septic arthritis. Positive bacterial culture and sensitivity results confirm the diagnosis and allow appropriate antibiotic selection. Results of bacterial culture of synovial fluid from septic joints are negative approximately 50% of the time (Meric, 1992). Blood culture media may be used to facilitate bacterial growth from synovial fluid. Bacterial culture of surgically retrieved synovial samples may be necessary to identify bacterial agents.

Other infectious agents causing arthropathies (e.g., spirochetes, rickettsiae, fungi, bacterial L-forms that cannot be cultured by routine techniques, mycoplasmas, and protozoa) must be differentiated from bacterial causes. Noninfectious causes of arthropathy, including DJD, also must be differentiated from infectious causes. Samples of joint fluid and synovium for bacterial culture and sensitivity should be obtained to identify causative organisms and determine appropriate antibiotic therapy. Broad-spectrum antibiotics (i.e., ampicillin, amoxicillin plus clavulanic acid or cephalosporins; see Table 28-5 on p. 710 for dose) should be administered immediately after samples for culture are obtained, and antibiotic therapy should be adjusted as necessary, once results of microbial sensitivity tests are obtained. If bacterial L-forms are considered a likely cause, tetracycline (22 mg/kg PO, BID) or doxycycline are the drugs of choice. Antibiotics are administered for 4 to 6 weeks, and at least 2 weeks after cessation of clinical signs.

The goal of surgical treatment is to rapidly control infections and remove purulent material and fibrin from joints to minimize cartilage destruction. Immediate joint exploration, including debridement of fibrin and granulation tissue and sterile saline lavage, is indicated for postoperative joint infections, septic joints where treatment was delayed for 72 hours or longer, joints that have not responded to 72 hours of appropriate medical therapy, and penetrating joint wounds. Surgery is not indicated in dogs with inflammatory joint disease secondary to bacterial endocarditis. General anesthesia is recommended for exploration of the joint and placement of ingress-egress drains. After arthrotomy and joint lavage, a system of ingress and egress drains can be installed so that joint lavage can be performed 2 to 3 times daily. Alternatively, the joint incision can be left open for daily lavage. Lavage fluid should consist of saline or a balanced electrolyte solution, either of which has minimal effects on joint tissues. Povidone-iodine at a concentration of 0.1% has minimal adverse effects on synovium. However, stronger concentrations of povidone-iodine and chlorhexidine cause a chemical synovitis and should be avoided.

☞ **NOTE** · Acute septic arthritis is a surgical emergency.

Postoperative care for animals with septic arthritis consists of oral antibiotics, daily wound management until joint drainage is no longer purulent, and passive range of motion. Oral antibiotics should be continued for 4 to 6 weeks. The limb can be protected in a bandage or splint for 4 weeks to allow cartilage healing to occur before the stress of full weight bearing. The animal can be slowly returned to normal activity after the bandage is removed. The prognosis for normal joint function varies and is dependent on the amount of cartilage destruction that has occurred. In a reported series of 57 dogs with septic arthritis, 32 dogs had a complete recovery, 18 had slight lameness, and 7 had severe lameness after treatment (Bennett, Taylor, 1988). Salvage procedures for chronically painful joints include arthrodesis or amputation (see p. 1017). The prognosis for animals with bacterial endocarditis is poor because of impending cardiac failure.

RICKETTSIAL POLYARTHRITIS

Polyarthritis may be caused by rickettsiae (e.g., *Rickettsia rickettsii* or *Ehrlichia canis*), which are usually transmitted by arthropods. *R. rickettsii*, the causative agent of Rocky Mountain spotted fever, is transmitted by ticks of the *Dermacentor* genus and is endemic in wooded areas of the central and eastern United States. *E. canis* has been observed in much of the United States, but especially in the southeastern portions. Rocky Mountain spotted fever often has an acute onset of symptoms including multiple-limb lameness, joint pain, fever, petechial hemorrhages, lymphadenopathy, neurologic signs, facial edema, and edema of the extremities. Clinical signs associated with ehrlichiosis may be acute or chronic and include fever, anorexia, lymphadenopathy, weight loss, lameness, joint pain, petechiation, and neurologic signs.

Diagnosis of rickettsial polyarthritis is based on serologic testing for the causative agent and on finding other evidence of the disease during historical, physical, and clinicopathological evaluation. Titers to the causative agents may not increase for 2 to 3 weeks after exposure, and paired samples may be necessary for diagnosis. Radiographic changes indicating rickettsial polyarthritis include joint effusion and periarticular soft tissue swelling. Surfaces of bones and cartilage usually appear normal. Thrombocytopenia is frequently present, and increased numbers of nondegenerate polymorphonuclear leukocytes are observed upon joint fluid analysis.

Treatment of rickettsial polyarthritis usually involves doxycycline, tetracycline, or chloramphenicol administration for 3 weeks (Table 30-8). Limiting exposure to ticks by using airicide sprays and removing ticks daily from dogs is important to prevent future infections. Surgical therapy is not indicated for rickettsial polyarthritis. The prognosis for dogs with Rocky Mountain spotted fever varies, depending on clinical signs. Animals treated early in the disease process usually have a good prognosis. Dogs not treated until late in the disease may develop generalized central nervous system signs, uveitis, necrosis of affected tissues, and chronic, progressive polyarthritis. Dogs treated for *Ehrlichia* infections generally respond well to appropriate medical therapy.

LYME DISEASE

Polyarthritis can also be caused by tick-borne spirochetes (spiral bacteria) such as *Borrelia burgdorferi*, which causes Lyme disease. *B. burgdorferi* infection should be suspected in dogs with transient or recurrent arthritis if they have been exposed to ticks or inhabit areas in which ticks are endemic. The disease can be transmitted by larval, nymphal, and adult *Ixodes dammini* ticks. Several hours of feeding are necessary to transmit the spirochete. Septicemia then occurs, allowing spread of the spirochete to target organs. Any dog that has the potential for contact with vectors of the disease may be infected; however, there is little evidence that cats exhibit clinical diseases associated with these agents. The history for dogs with Lyme disease can include transient lameness of one or more limbs. Clinical signs may be intermittent, with animals appearing normal between acute exacerbations; episodes may include multiple-limb lameness, fever, lymphadenopa-

TABLE 30-8
Treatment of Rickettsial Polyarthritis
Doxycycline (Vibramycin)
10 mg/kg PO, SID
Tetracycline (Panmycin, Achromycin)
22 mg/kg PO, BID
Chloramphenicol (Chloromycetin)
50 mg/kg PO, TID (Warning to owners: Do not eat or drink while handling this product. Do not touch eyes. Wash hands after use.)

thy, and anorexia. Glomerulonephritis, renal tubular damage, or cardiac abnormalities (atrioventricular block and myocarditis) may occur in chronically infected dogs.

Radiographs of joints, abdomen, and thorax are usually normal during the acute phase of Lyme disease. Synovial fluid from affected joints of animals with Lyme disease is less viscous and contains increased numbers of nondegenerate neutrophils compared with normal synovial fluid. Phasecontrast or dark-field microscopy may allow visualization or organisms in synovial fluid. Attempts to culture *B. burgdorferi* from synovial fluid are usually unsuccessful. Synovial biopsy typically shows invasion of the synovial lining with plasmocytes and lymphocytes. Exposure to *B. burgdorferi* can be demonstrated with serologic antibody-detection tests using indirect immunofluorescent antibody (IA) or enzymelinked immunosorbent assay (ELISA) procedures; however, positive titers do not diagnose active infection; they may simply reflect prior exposure. An extremely high titer or dramatic increase in a convalescent titer, coupled with clinical signs and a response to antibiotic therapy, suggests a diagnosis of Lyme borreliosis; however, it is very difficult to definitely diagnose borreliosis. Differential diagnoses include other inflammatory, nonerosive, and erosive arthropathies (e.g., septic arthritis, rheumatoid arthritis, DJD).

☞ **N O T E** · Positive serological findings reflect exposure to the organism, not necessarily active infection.

Doxycycline is also effective for treating Lyme disease (Table 30-9). Tetracycline, ampicillin, cephalosporin, erythromycin, and chloramphenicol also have been used. Surgery is generally not indicated; however, some animals with chronic Lyme disease and severe villous synovitis may benefit from subtotal synovectomy. Dogs treated promptly for acute infections of *B. burgdorferi* have an excellent prognosis. The prognosis for dogs with chronic infections is uncertain.

NONEROSIVE IDIOPATHIC IMMUNE-MEDIATED POLYARTHRITIS

Idiopathic nonerosive inflammatory arthropathies have no identifiable cause and are diagnosed by ruling out all other

---

TABLE 30-9

Treatment of Lyme Disease

Doxycycline (Vibramycin)
10 mg/kg PO, SID

Tetracycline (Panmycin, Achromycin)
22 mg/kg PO, BID

Ampicillin
22 mg/kg PO, TID or QID

Cefadroxil (Cefa-Tab)
22 mg/kg PO, BID

Erythromycin
10-20 mg/kg PO, BID or TID

Chloramphenicol (Chloromycetin)
50 mg/kg PO, TID (Warning to owners: Do not eat or drink while handling this product. Do not touch eyes. Wash hands after use.)

TABLE 30-10

Treatment of Idiopathic Immune-Mediated Polyarthritis

Prednisone
2 to 4 mg/kg/day for 2 weeks; then 1 to 2 mg/kg/day for 2 weeks; if animal is clinically normal at this time and synovial inflammation has subsided, decrease dose to 1 to 2 mg/kg EOD* for 4 weeks

Azathioprine (Imuran)
Dogs
2 mg/kg/day PO for 2 to 3 weeks; then 2 mg/kg, EOD* if clinical signs resolve

Cyclophosphamide (Cytoxan)
50 mg/m^2
Give up to 4 consecutive days each week for up to 4 months
*Every other day.

causes of polyarthritis: septic arthritis, rickettsial arthritis, rheumatoid arthritis, other inflammatory nonerosive polyarthropathies, and DJD. The term canine idiopathic polyarthritis is sometimes used synonymously for this condition. The etiology is unknown but presumed to be associated with immune complex formation. The synovium is thickened, congested, and edematous and may contain fibrin deposits. Cartilage and bone are relatively unaffected; however, occasionally there may be superficial fibrillation of the articular cartilage.

This history of lameness in affected animals may be acute or chronic. Stiffness, difficulty rising, pyrexia, anorexia, and/or lethargy may be present. Although more than one joint usually is involved, single-limb lameness is common. Affected animals may have difficulty rising and walking. Joint palpation may reveal pain, effusion, or loss of range of motion. Cervical pain and vertebral hypersensitivity may reflect intervertebral involvement. Other systemic abnormalities (dermatitis, glomerulonephritis, uveitis) may occur.

Idiopathic immune-mediated nonerosive polyarthritis is diagnosed by synovial fluid analysis, by joint radiographs that do not show erosive or proliferative bone lesions, and by eliminating other known causes. A therapeutic trial of antibiotics is sometimes used to eliminate infectious causes. Radiographs of affected joints usually reveal either no abnormalities or synovial fluid effusion and periarticular soft tissue swelling. Synovial fluid is thin and turbid, and the mucin clot test is usually normal. Nucleated cell counts are markedly elevated with predominately nondegenerate neutrophils. Most dogs test negative for antinuclear antibody (ANA) and rheumatoid factor. Synovial biopsy usually reveals hypertrophy of the synovial lining plus polymorphonuclear or mononuclear cell infiltration. Microbial organisms are not observed and bacterial cultures are negative.

Glucocorticoids are the initial treatment of choice (Table 30-10). The dosage should be titrated to the lowest amount that will prevent clinical signs; however, many animals require life long therapy. Cyclophosphamide or azathioprine can be administered if clinical signs persist despite prednisone therapy. These drugs can cause myelosuppression, and a complete blood count (CBC) and platelet count should be monitored every 2 weeks. Cyclophosphamide may also cause a sterile cystitis, and azathioprine may cause hepatopathy or pancreatitis. Although the prognosis for achieving remission of clinical signs is good, adverse side effects associated with long-term corticosteroid therapy may develop.

CHRONIC INFLAMMATORY-INDUCED POLYARTHRITIS

Nonerosive inflammatory polyarthritis may occur secondary to any chronic inflammatory disorder or persistent antigenic stimulus. Another disease (e.g., chronic infection, gastroenteritis, ulcerative colitis, neoplasia) or drug therapy (e.g., sulfamethoxazole-trimethroprim or sulfadiazine-trimethoprim) incites immune complex formation, which mediates the arthritis. The synovium becomes thickened, congested, edematous, and may contain fibrin deposits. Occasionally there may be superficial fibrillation or articular cartilage, but cartilage and bone are usually unaffected. Affected animals may have a history of either acute or chronic lameness, stiffness, difficulty rising, pyrexia, anorexia, and/or lethargy. Other clinical signs may be associated with the inciting disease. Joint palpation may elicit pain and detect effusion or decreased range of motion.

This condition must be differentiated from septic arthritis, rheumatoid arthritis, idiopathic inflammatory nonerosive polyarthropathy, and DJD. Chronic inflammatory-induced polyarthritis is diagnosed on the basis of results of synovial fluid analysis and identification of the inciting disease. Radiographs of affected joints usually reveal either no abnormalities or synovial fluid effusion and periarticular soft tissue swelling. Thoracic and abdominal radiographs should be taken and may reveal the inciting disease. Synovial fluid is typically thin and turbid, while the mucin clot test is usually normal. Nucleated cell counts are markedly elevated, with nondegenerate neutrophils being the predominate cell type. Most dogs do not have ANA or rheumatoid factor. Synovial biopsy reveals hypertrophy of the synovial lining, with polymorphonuclear or mononuclear cell infiltration. In spite of chronic infection elsewhere in the body, the joints are usually sterile.

Treatment should be directed at eliminating the underlying disease. Antibiotics, selected after culture and sensitivity testing, are indicated for infections. Glucocorticoids, administered orally, may be given short term to control the synovitis in severe cases.

PLASMACYTIC-LYMPHOCYTIC SYNOVITIS

Plasmacytic-lymphocytic synovitis (lymphoplasmacytic synovitis) is an immune-mediated arthropathy associated with plasmacytic and lymphocytic infiltration of the synovium. It often affects stifle joints, leading to cruciate ligament degeneration and rupture, joint instability, and DJD. The synovium is thickened, congested, and edematous and may contain fibrin deposits. Affected dogs generally present with unilateral or bilateral rear limb lameness of either acute onset or chronic duration. The presenting history is similar to that of cranial cruciate ligament rupture and a cranial drawer sign is usually present once cruciate ligament rupture has occurred. The stifles are generally enlarged because of joint effusion and chronic periarticular soft tissue fibrosis. Suspect joints should be biopsied during surgery for cranial cruciate rupture.

Cruciate ligament rupture in dogs with plasmacytic-lymphocytic synovitis must be differentiated from ruptures associated with trauma (see p. 957). Radiographs of the stifles reveal joint effusion and varying signs of DJD, depending on chronicity of the cranial cruciate ligament rupture. CBC and serum chemistries are usually normal. Synovial fluid is usually thin and turbid with an increased nucleated cell count comprised primarily of lymphocytes and plasma cells. Synovial biopsy reveals villus hyperplasia and infiltration of the synovium and cruciate ligament with lymphocytes and plasmacytes.

Surgical therapy to stabilize the cranial cruciate ligament is indicated in these patients. Some animals may also benefit from subtotal synovectomy. Medical treatment for plasmacytic-lymphocytic synovitis is the same as for idiopathic immune-mediated polyarthritis (see Table 30-10). The prognosis is generally good for achieving remission of clinical signs.

SYSTEMIC LUPUS ERYTHEMATOSUS-INDUCED POLYARTHRITIS

Systemic lupus erythematosus (SLE) is a multisystemic disease caused by autoantibodies against tissue protein and DNA. Circulating immune complexes of antigen and au-

toantibodies pass through endothelial cell junctions and are trapped in basement membranes, causing inflammation and eventual organ dysfunction. The synovium is typically thickened and discolored, but cartilage and bone are relatively unaffected. Other lesions associated with this systemic disease may include glomerulonephritis, myositis, scaly crusting cutaneous lesions, hemolytic anemia, or thrombocytopenia. Affected animals may be brought for examination because of generalized stiffness, shifting leg lameness, pyrexia, anorexia, or lethargy. Effusion may cause swollen joints, especially carpi and tarsi. Other physical findings depend on the body systems affected.

This condition must be differentiated from rheumatoid arthritis, idiopathic inflammatory nonerosive polyarthropathy, septic arthritis, and DJD. Radiographs of affected joints usually reveal either no abnormalities or synovial fluid effusion and periarticular soft tissue swelling. Synovial fluid is usually thin and turbid, while the mucin clot test is normal. Nucleated cell counts are markedly elevated with predominately nondegenerate neutrophils. Lupus erythematosus (LE) cells are rarely present in the joint fluid. Antinuclear antibody test results should be positive, and rheumatoid factor is usually normal. The ANA test is sensitive but nonspecific for SLE, and a positive result must be combined with other criteria for a positive diagnosis. The ANA test results should be positive at high dilutions (see each lab for what constitutes a high dilution). Anemia, a positive Coombs' test, leukopenia, thrombocytopoenia, and proteinuria may be present. Synovial biopsy typically reveals hypertrophy and hyperplasia of the synovial lining, with an inflammatory infiltrate of polymorphonuclear cells, macrophages, lymphocytes, and plasma cells. Immunofluorescence studies may show IgG- and IgM-producing plasma cells. Microbial organisms are not observed histologically and bacterial cultures are negative. There should be involvement of more than one body system and a positive ANA for a diagnosis of SLE. If serologic tests are normal but there is involvement of two or more body systems, SLE should be suspected.

Glucocorticoids are the initial treatment of choice for SLE-induced polyarthritis (see Table 30-10). The drugs may be stopped in some cases because of long periods of remission, but in other cases they must be maintained for the animal's entire life. Cyclophosphamide or azathioprine can be administered to dogs with clinical signs that persist in spite of prednisone therapy. These drugs can cause myelosuppression; therefore, a CBC and platelet count should be monitored every 2 weeks initially. Cyclophosphamide may also cause a sterile cystitis, and azathioprine may cause hepatopathy or pancreatitis. The prognosis is generally good for control of the polyarthritis; however, abnormalities in other organs (e.g., glomerulonephritis) may progress.

RHEUMATOID ARTHRITIS

Erosive, noninfectious inflammatory joint disease (i.e., rheumatoid arthritis) is characterized by chronic, bilaterally symmetrical, erosive destruction of the joints. The etiology of rheumatoid arthritis is unknown but it is considered an immune-mediated arthropathy. The antigens are altered host immunoglobulins (IgG and IgM), which are known as "rheumatoid factors." Resultant immune complexes are deposited in the synovium, initiating an inflammatory response that is followed by synovial cell proliferation, villus hypertrophy, pannus formation over the cartilage surface, cartilage and subchondral bone destruction, joint swelling, and rupture of the collateral ligaments. The outcome is a nonfunctional joint. The synovial membrane is generally discolored, edematous, congested, and thickened and may contain fibrin deposits. Pannus of granulation tissue originates at the periphery of the joint and covers portions of the articular cartilage, which may fibrillate and ulcerate. Most affected dogs have a history of stiffness after rest, limping, or difficulty walking. Joints are generally enlarged with periarticular soft tissue swelling and joint effusion. The distal joints (i.e., carpi and tarsi) may be unstable, with obvious deformity and angulation.

Differential diagnoses include arthritis, inflammatory nonerosive polyarthropathies, and DJD. Radiographs of the joints show a generalized loss of mineralization, radiolucent foci, and irregular joint margins. Bone proliferation can also be present. Soft tissue swelling and joint effusion may be evident (Fig. 30-7). Synovial fluid is often yellow, turbid, and increased in volume. The mucin clot may be poor and friable. Nucleated cell counts are markedly elevated with predominately degenerate neutrophils. Between 20% and 70% of affected dogs show positive test results for rheumatoid factor; most show normal ANA levels (Meric, 1992). In the Rose-Waaler agglutination test for rheumatoid factor, a differential titer of 1:8 and above is positive. (Note: appropriate controls need to be run with sheep RBCs.) In latex agglutination tests, agglutination denotes a positive test at serum dilutions specified by the producer of the test. Synovial biopsy generally shows villus hypertrophy, proliferation of synovial cells, and lymphocyte and plasma cell infiltration. Immunofluorescent studies demonstrate complexes of IgG or IgM in synovial lining cells, blood vessel walls, and in the extracellular tissues. Microbial organisms are not observed on histologic samples, and bacterial cultures are negative.

Classical rheumatoid arthritis requires the presence of destructive lesions seen radiographically, a positive rheumatoid factor, characteristic histopathologic changes in the synovial membrane, plus four additional criteria listed in Table 30-11. Rheumatoid arthritis is usually diagnosed when 5 of the 11 criteria are present and joint signs have been present for at least 6 weeks. Subcutaneous nodules are rare in dogs.

A combination of immunosuppressive drugs (prednisone, azathioprine or cyclophosphamide, gold salts) is typically needed to achieve remission of clinical signs (Table 30-12). Therapy is usually initiated with prednisone and then additional imunosuppressive drugs (i.e., azathioprine and/or cyclophosphamide) are added. Cyclophosphamide usage has major risks to the dog and the person administering the drug. After each month of treatment the dog should be reevaluated and the synovial fluid analyzed. After the first month, the dose of prednisone is reduced to 1 to 2 mg/kg every 48 hours and the azathioprine or cyclophosphamide is continued. If inflammation persists, gold salts may be added to the therapy. Gold salts can be toxic, and hematology should be monitored at least

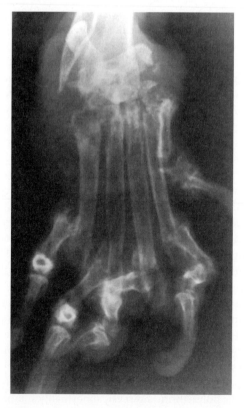

FIG. 30-7
Radiograph of the carpus of a dog with advanced abnormalities associated with rheumatoid arthritis. Note the erosion of subchondral bone and articular cartilage. Carpal instability, metacarpal-phalangeal luxation, and severe deformity of the digits are present. (From Olmstead ML: Small animal orthopedics, St. Louis, 1995, Mosby.)

TABLE 30-11
Characteristics of Rheumatoid Arthritis
Stiffness after rest
Pain in at least one joint
Swelling in at least one joint
Swelling of at least one other joint within 3 months
Symmetrical joint swelling
Subcutaneous nodules over bony prominence, extensor surfaces, or in juxta-articular regions
Destructive radiographic lesions
Positive rheumatoid factor
Poor mucin precipitate from synovial fluid
Characteristic histopathologic changes in the synovial membrane
Characteristic histopathologic changes in subcutaneous nodules

TABLE 30-12

Therapy of Rheumatoid Arthritis

Prednisone

2 to 4 mg/kg/day PO for 2 weeks; then 1 to 2 mg/kg/day PO for 2 weeks; then 1 to 2 mg/kg EOD*

Azathioprine (Imuran)

Dogs

2 mg/kg/day PO for 2 to 3 weeks; then 2 mg/kg/EOD* if clinical signs resolve

Cyclophosphamide (Cytoxan)

50 mg/m²
Give up to 4 consecutive days each week for up to 4 months

Aurothioglucose (gold salts)

1 mg/kg IM once a week for 10 weeks or until remission occurs

*Every other day.

every 2 weeks. Joints that have lost all collateral ligament support may benefit from arthrodesis. However, the high concentrations of immunosuppressive drugs also inhibit body defenses against infection and may delay bone healing. Rheumatoid arthritis is progressive, and dogs rarely if ever make a full recovery. Lameness and stiffness usually persist in spite of treatment.

FELINE CHRONIC PROGRESSIVE POLYARTHRITIS

Feline chronic progressive polyarthritis is an immune-mediated disease of male cats and is associated with progressive periosteal-proliferative and erosive polyarthritis. Female cats are seemingly unaffected. The etiology may involve exposure to the feline syncytium-forming virus (FeSFV) and feline leukemia virus (FeLV); however, the disease cannot be experimentally induced by these viruses. The periosteal-proliferative form of the disease results in osteoporosis and periosteal new bone formation around the joint. Periarticular erosions and collapse of the joint space with fibrous ankylosis occur with time. The erosive form of the disease causes joint changes similar to canine rheumatoid arthritis. Synovium is infiltrated with lymphocytes and plasma cells. Clinical signs include lameness, reluctance to move, depression, anorexia, weight loss, and occasionally, deformity of affected joints. Examination of the cat may reveal pyrexia, depression, lymphadenopathy, and multiple joint involvement. Joint palpation causes pain. The joints are sometimes swollen and may be deformed in animals with the erosive form of the disease.

Differential diagnoses for this condition include septic arthritis, DJD, and hypervitaminosis A. Changes noted on radiographs of affected joints include proliferative new bone formation on the periphery of the joints, generalized

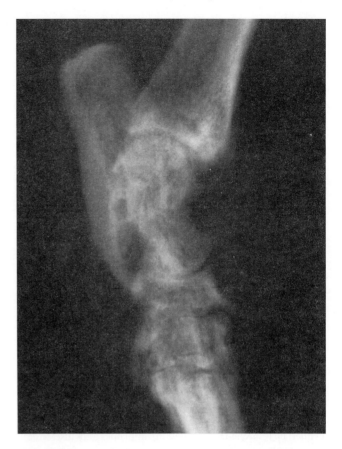

FIG. 30-8
Radiograph of the tarsus of a cat with the periosteal proliferative form of feline progressive arthritis. There is proliferative new bone formation on the periphery of the joints, generalized loss of density of subchondral bone, and loss of the joint space. Radiolucent foci are visible throughout the tarsal bones. (From Olmstead ML: Small animal orthopedics, St. Louis, 1995, Mosby.)

loss of density of the subchondral bone, and the loss of the joint space. Radiolucent foci in the subchondral bone and irregular joint margins may also occur. Periarticular soft tissue swelling and joint effusion may be noted (Fig. 30-8). Results of tests for FeSFV and feline leukemia virus (FeLV) may be positive. Although only small amounts of synovial fluid can be obtained, it is thin with an increased nucleated cell count of predominately nondegenerate neutrophils. Bacterial and fungal cultures of synovial fluid and synovial membrane are negative.

Treatment involves immunosuppressive drugs and usually begins with prednisone (Table 30-13). Therapy is often needed for the lifetime of the cat. Other immunosuppressive drugs such as cyclophosphamide or azathioprine may aid in long-term control; however, cats are very sensitive to the myelosuppressive effects of these drugs, and hematologic parameters should be assessed frequently. The prognosis is good for remission of signs, but guarded for complete control of the disease. Other FeLV related disorders may occur in cats that test positive.

TABLE 30-13

Treatment of Feline Chronic Progressive Polyarthritis

Prednisone

4 to 6 mg/kg/day PO; if cat improves after 2 weeks, decrease dose to 2 mg/kg/day; then place on maintenance therapy (1-2 mg/kg EOD*)

Cyclophosphamide (Imuran)

6.25-12.5 mg/cat PO, given up to 4 consecutive days of each week for up to 4 months

Azathioprine (Cytoxan)

0.3 mg/kg PO, EOD*

*Every other day, watch for neutropenia.

References

Bennett D, Taylor DJ: Bacterial infective arthritis in the dog, *J Small Anim Pract* 29:207, 1988.

Meric SM: Joint disorders. In Nelson RW, Couto CG, editors: *Essentials of small animal internal medicine,* St. Louis, 1992, Mosby.

Suggested Reading

Behrens F, Kraft EL, Oegema TR: Biochemical changes in articular cartilage after joint immobilization by casting or external fixation, *J Ortho Res* 7:335, 1989.

Bennett D: Immune-based erosive inflammatory joint disease of the dog: canine rheumatoid arthritis. 1. Clinical, radiological and laboratory investigations, *J Small Anim Pract* 28:779, 1987.

Bennett D: Immune-based erosive inflammatory joint disease of the dog: canine rheumatoid arthritis. 2. Pathological investigations, *J Small Anim Pract* 28:799, 1987.

Bennett D: Immune-based non-erosive inflammatory joint disease of the dog: canine rheumatoid arthritis. 1. Canine systemic lupus erythematosus, *J Small Anim Pract* 28:871, 1987.

Bennett D: Immune-based non-erosive inflammatory joint disease of the dog: canine rheumatoid arthritis. 3. Canine idiopathic polyarthritis, *J Small Anim Pract* 28:909, 1987.

Bennett D, Kelly DF: Immune-based non-erosive inflammatory joint disease of the dog: canine rheumatoid arthritis. 2. Polyarthritis/polymyositis syndrome, *J Small Anim Pract* 28:891, 1987.

Bennett D, May C: Joint diseases of dogs and cats. In Ettinger SJ, Feldman EC, editors: *Textbook of veterinary internal medicine,* Philadelphia, 1995, WB Saunders.

Bennett D, Taylor DJ: Bacterial endocarditis and inflammatory joint disease in the dog, *J Small Anim Pract* 28:347, 1987.

Brandt KD, Slowman-Kovacs S: Nonsteroidal antiinflammatory drugs in treatment of osteoarthritis, *Clin Orthop Rel Res* 213:84, 1986.

Clark, DM: The biochemistry of degenerative joint disease and its treatment, *Comp Cont Educ Pract Vet* 13:275, 1991.

Cowell RL et al: Ehrlichiosis and polyarthritis in three dogs, *J Small Anim Pract* 192:1093, 1988.

Giger U et al: Sulfadiazine-induced allergy in six Doberman pinschers, *J Small Anim Pract* 186:479, 1985.

Kornblatt AN, Urband PH, Steere AC: Arthritis caused by *Borrelia burgdorferi* in dogs, *J Am Vet Med Assoc* 186:960, 1985.

Lipowitz AJ: Degenerative joint disease. In Slatter D, editor: *Textbook of small animal surgery,* ed 2, Philadelphia, 1993, WB Saunders.

Magnarelli LA et al: Clinical and serologic studies of canine borreliosis, *J Am Vet Med Assoc* 191:1089, 1987.

Montgomery RD et al: Comparison of aerobic culturette, synovial membrane biopsy, and blood culture medium in detection of canine bacterial arthritis, *Vet Surg* 18:300, 1989.

Mow VC, Holmes MH, Lai WM: Fluid transport and mechanical properties of articular cartilage: a review, *J Biomechanics* 17:377, 1984.

Pederson NC et al: Joint diseases of dogs and cats. In Ettinger SJ, editor: *Textbook of internal medicine,* Philadelphia, 1988, WB Saunders.

Woo SL-Y, Buckwalter JA, editors: *Injury and repair of the musculoskeletal soft tissues,* Savannah, Ga., 1987, American Academy of Orthopedic Surgeons.

Woodard JC et al: Erosive polyarthritis in two greyhounds, *J Am Vet Med Assoc* 198:873, 1991.

TEMPOROMANDIBULAR JOINT

TEMPOROMANDIBULAR JOINT LUXATION

DEFINITIONS

Temporomandibular joint luxation results when the mandibular condyles separate from articular surfaces of the temporal bone and mandibular fossae.

SYNONYMS

Temporomandibular joint dislocation

GENERAL CONSIDERATIONS AND CLINICALLY RELEVANT PATHOPHYSIOLOGY

Temporomandibular joint luxation occurs as a result of head trauma; however, luxation of these joints is uncommon because they are protected by heavy temporal muscles. Luxation may occur unilaterally or bilaterally and may be associated with mandibular fractures. Although mandibular condyles can displace cranial or caudal to the mandibular fossa, craniodorsal displacement is most common.

DIAGNOSIS
Clinical Presentation

Signalment. This condition occurs in both dogs and cats. Animals of either sex or any age may be affected.

History. There is usually a history of recent trauma.

Physical Examination Findings

Animals usually present with an open mouth, which they appear reluctant to close. The direction of the luxation can often be determined by evaluating jaw position. Unilateral craniodorsal luxations cause the mandible to shift toward the opposite side of the mouth, whereas bilateral craniodorsal luxations cause the entire mandible to protrude forward, and caudal condylar luxations cause the mandible to shift caudally and toward the side of the luxation. Thorough inspection of the mandible and maxilla for oral wounds, visible fractures, and palpable crepitation of the caudal mandible should be performed under anesthesia before closed reduction. Radiographs are warranted in animals in which fracture is suspected.

Radiography

Definitive diagnosis is made from skull radiographs taken with the animal anesthetized or heavily sedated. Five radiographic views are standard for complete evaluation of the skull (see p. 768). The most reliable radiographic sign is an increase in joint space width; this finding is usually most evident on a dorsoventral projection. Radiographs should be carefully assessed to determine whether there are concurrent mandibular or maxillary fractures that warrant open reduction and stabilization.

Laboratory Findings

Specific laboratory abnormalities are not present. Because this condition results from trauma, sufficient blood work should be obtained to evaluate the risk of anesthesia in affected animals.

DIFFERENTIAL DIAGNOSIS

Differential diagnoses include mandibular or maxillary fractures (see p. 767) and temporomandibular joint dysplasia (see p. 900), which may show similar clinical signs.

MEDICAL OR CONSERVATIVE MANAGEMENT

The luxation usually can be reduced without surgical intervention, but general anesthesia is required. A wooden dowel rod is placed transversely between the mandibular and maxillary molars and used as a fulcrum to distract the condyles distally while the rostral mandible and maxilla are squeezed together. The mandible is manipulated cranially or caudally to move the condyle into place. After the joint is reduced, it should be carefully palpated to determine stability. Unstable joints can be supported with tape muzzles (see p. 768) or interarcade wiring (see p. 772) for 7 to 14 days until fibrosis occurs. If it is impossible to reduce or maintain joint reduction, open reduction and stabilization should be performed.

SURGICAL TREATMENT

Reduction of temporomandibular joint luxations should be attempted as soon as the animal can undergo general anesthesia. Closed reduction (see above) is frequently successful and is the initial procedure of choice if concurrent fractures are not present; however, open reduction may be necessary if luxations are unstable after closed reduction.

Preoperative Management

Animals should be evaluated for concurrent trauma and treated appropriately. Thoracic radiographs and electrocardiograms are indicated in animals that have sustained trauma.

Anesthesia

General anesthesia is necessary for closed or open reduction of temporomandibular luxations (see p. 708). Endotracheal tubes may interfere with closed reduction techniques and with evaluation of occlusion. The endotracheal tube can be temporarily removed during closed reduction procedures or rerouted through a pharyngotomy incision for longer procedures (see p. 774).

Surgical Anatomy

See p. 774 for a description of surgical anatomy of the mandible. Landmarks for approaching the temporomandibular joint are the ventral border of the zygomatic arch and the temporomandibular joint (palpated while the mandible is manipulated). The masseter muscle is elevated off the zygomatic arch to expose the joint. The parotid duct and gland and facial nerve are located dorsally and superficially to the masseter muscle and should be avoided. The temporomandibular joint is composed of a mandibular condyle, articular disk (meniscus), mandibular fossa of the temporal bone, mandibular ligament, and joint capsule. The articular disk divides the joint into the dorsal (meniscotemporal) compartment and ventral (meniscomandibular) compartment.

Positioning

The patient is positioned in lateral recumbency for a unilateral approach and in ventral recumbency for bilateral approaches.

SURGICAL TECHNIQUES

Make a skin incision following the ventral border of the caudal zygomatic arch and centered over the temporomandibular joint. Be sure to avoid the parotid duct and gland and facial nerve. *Elevate the caudal periosteal insertion of the masseter muscle from the zygomatic arch to expose the joint capsule. Incise the joint capsule and mandibular ligament to expose the articular surfaces. Irrigate the joint and remove any bone fragments or debris that may have interfered with reduction. Replace the mandibular condyle in the fossa. To hold the condyle in position, suture the joint capsule and mandibular ligament. Suture the masseter muscle to the fascia on the dorsal edge of the zygomatic arch. Close platysma muscle and skin in separate layers (see Fig. 30-10).*

SUTURE MATERIALS/SPECIAL INSTRUMENTS

The joint capsule should be sutured with absorbable suture material (polydioxanone, polyglyconate). A periosteal elevator is needed to elevate the masseter muscle and expose the joint capsule.

POSTOPERATIVE CARE AND ASSESSMENT

Postoperative radiographs should be evaluated to document that the mandibular condyles are normally positioned. If the joints are stable the animal should be allowed to eat only soft food for 2 to 3 weeks. Unstable joints in dogs can be supported with a tape muzzle (see p. 768) for 1 to 2 weeks; muzzles are difficult to maintain in cats, and interarcade wiring may be necessary (see p. 772). Liquid diets should be fed to these animals until muzzles or interarcade wires are removed; then, soft food is recommended for an additional 1 to 2 weeks.

☞ **NOTE** · Consider interarcade wiring in cats if the joints appear unstable after reduction.

PROGNOSIS

Prognosis is generally good for normal function if luxations can be reduced and joints made stable. Complications include failure to reduce the joint, repeated luxation, and joint arthrodesis. A mandibular condylectomy (see p. 901) is recommended for joints that remain or become unstable, painful, fibrotic, or stiff after surgery.

Suggested Reading

Egger EL: Skull and mandibular fractures. In Slatter D, editor: *Textbook of small animal surgery*, Philadelphia, 1993, WB Saunders.

TEMPOROMANDIBULAR JOINT DYSPLASIA

DEFINITIONS

Temporomandibular joint dysplasia is a disease characterized by the jaws locking in an open position.

SYNONYMS

Open-mouth jaw locking, temporomandibular subluxation, congenital temporomandibular luxation/subluxation

GENERAL CONSIDERATIONS AND CLINICALLY RELEVANT PATHOPHYSIOLOGY

Temporomandibular joint dysplasia is a disease of unknown etiology affecting young, adult dogs. Deformation of the mandibular condyloid processes and mandibular fossa allow subluxation and recurrent locking of the mandible in an open-mouthed position. In some affected animals the mandibular fossae are shallow and condyloid processes are more obliquely situated than normal, and this combination allows joint subluxation. Joint instability leads to osteoarthrosis, pain, and locking of the jaw in an open position. Instability, coupled with mandibular symphyseal laxity, allows independent movement of the mandibles, which may result in malpositioning of coronoid processes lateral to the zygomatic arch, further promoting open-mouth locking. Open-mouth locking occurs in some dogs without evidence of coronoid process malpositioning.

DIAGNOSIS
Clinical Presentation

Signalment. The syndrome of open-mouth locking caused by coronoid process malpositioning has been reported in basset hounds, Irish setters, and a Saint Bernard. Pain and occasional open-mouth locking without malposition of the coronoid process occur in retriever and boxer breeds (Bennett, Prymack, 1986). Clinical signs usually are first noted when the dogs are young adults.

History. Owners usually describe repeated incidents of open-mouth locking after yawning. Usually the joints spontaneously reduce, but owners occasionally will seek veterinary care because manual reduction of the jaws is not possible. Some animals exhibit pain on oral manipulation and are reluctant to eat. There is no history of trauma in these animals.

Physical Examination Findings

Animals are usually presented with the jaws locked in an open-mouth position. If the coronoid process is locked outside of the zygomatic arch, a bulge in the subcutaneous tissues overlying the zygomatic arch on the affected side can be visualized and palpated. Affected animals may exhibit pain on temporomandibular joint palpation.

Radiography

A standard skull series with the mouth open and closed is used to evaluate the temporomandibular joints and position of the coronoid process. Changes consistent with temporomandibular joint dysplasia include increased or irregular joint spaces on a lateral projection, shallow mandibular fossae, and secondary osteoarthritis. On ventral dorsal projections, the condyles may be more oblique than normal and the coronoid process may be positioned lateral to the zygomatic arch when the mouth is opened.

☞ **NOTE** · Compare the radiographs with those of a normal skull if the diagnosis is in doubt.

Laboratory Findings

Specific laboratory abnormalities are not seen.

DIFFERENTIAL DIAGNOSIS

Differential diagnoses include traumatic luxation of the temporomandibular joint, mandibular fractures, and lodged oral foreign bodies.

MEDICAL OR CONSERVATIVE MANAGEMENT

Manual reduction may be possible by opening the mouth widely and manipulating the mandible away from the locked side. If the dog resists this manipulation, general anesthesia may be required.

SURGICAL TREATMENT

Repeated episodes can occur, and definitive treatment in such animals requires either partial resection of the zygomatic arch, if the coronoid process locks outside of the zygomatic

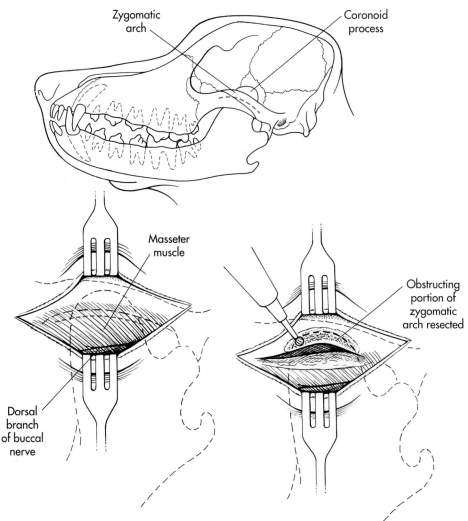

Zygomatic arch

Coronoid process

Masseter muscle

Dorsal branch of buccal nerve

Obstructing portion of zygomatic arch resected

FIG. 30-9
To expose the zygomatic arch, make an incision in skin and subcutaneous tissues overlying the ventral border of the rostral portion of the zygomatic arch. Elevate fascial attachments to the arch and resect the obstructing portion of the arch with a rongeur or high speed burr.

arch, or mandibular condylectomy, if displacement of the coronoid process does not occur outside the zygomatic arch.

Preoperative Management
These animals are usually young and healthy and require minimal preoperative care.

Anesthesia
A variety of anesthetic regimens can be used (see p. 708).

Surgical Anatomy
Refer to the description of surgical anatomy of the mandible on p. 774. Surgical anatomy of the temporomandibular joint is described on p. 899.

Positioning
The patient is positioned in lateral recumbency with the affected side up for resection of the zygomatic arch and for mandibular condylectomy.

SURGICAL TECHNIQUES
Partial Resection of the Zygomatic Arch
Make an incision in the skin and subcutaneous tissues overlying the ventral border of the rostral portion of the zygo-

matic arch. Elevate the fascial attachments to the arch while preserving the dorsal buccal branch of the facial nerve. Open the mouth widely to induce coronoid process displacement in order to identify the portion of the arch that obstructs replacement of the process. Resect the obstructing portion of the arch with a rongeur or high-speed burr (Fig. 30-9). Before closure, ensure that the coronoid process is normally positioned. Close the subcutaneous tissues and skin separately.

Mandibular Condylectomy
Make a skin incision along the ventral border of the caudal zygomatic arch, centered over the temporomandibular joint. Elevate the caudal periosteal insertion of the masseter muscle from the zygomatic arch to expose the joint capsule. Identify the joint by palpating it while an assistant moves the mandible. Incise the joint capsule between the meniscus and condyle and elevate the capsule. Identify the condylectomy site at the base of the condylar neck (at the level of the mandibular notch) (Fig. 30-10). First, resect the lateral portion of the condyle with a rongeur, then make a cut along the osteotomy line with a high-speed burr. Fracture the remaining portion of the condyle with an osteotome, but leave the meniscus intact. Close the masseter fascia, subcutaneous tissues, and skin separately.

FIG. 30-10
A and **B,** To expose the temporomandibular joint, make a skin incision along the ventral border of the caudal zygomatic arch, centered over the temporomandibular joint. **C,** Elevate the caudal periosteal insertion of the masseter muscle from the zygomatic arch to expose the joint capsule. Incise joint capsule between the meniscus and condyle and elevate it. **D,** Identify the condylectomy site at the base of the condylar neck.

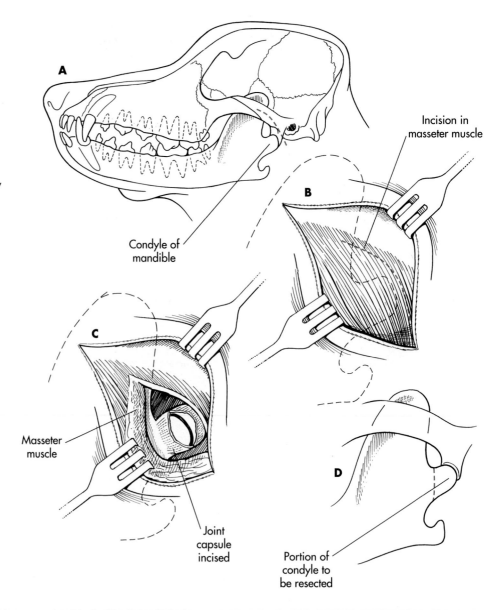

Condyle of mandible

Incision in masseter muscle

Masseter muscle

Joint capsule incised

Portion of condyle to be resected

SUTURE MATERIALS/SPECIAL INSTRUMENTS

A rongeur or high-speed burr is necessary for zygomatic arch removal. Fascial attachments of the masseter muscle should be elevated with a periosteal elevator. Instruments that facilitate mandibular condylectomy include a periosteal elevator and retractors. Rongeurs, high-speed burrs, and an osteotome and mallet are used to remove the condyle.

POSTOPERATIVE CARE AND ASSESSMENT

Dogs treated with zygomatic arch resection or condylectomy should be released to the owners with instructions to return for suture removal in 10 to 14 days. Limitation of exercise or dietary restrictions are not necessary.

PROGNOSIS

If the opposite temporomandibular joint is affected, recurrence of jaw locking may be noted after unilateral mandibu-

lar condylectomy or zygomatic arch resection; however, most animals have normal jaw function after surgery. Potential complications of these procedures include seroma formation and iatrogenic infection.

Reference

Bennett D, Prymack C: Excision arthroplasty as a treatment for temporomandibular dysplasia, *J Small Anim Pract* 27:361, 1986.

Suggested Reading

Robins G, Grandage J: Temporomandibular joint dysplasia and open-mouth jaw locking in the dog, *J Am Vet Med Assoc* 171:1072, 1977.
Tomlinson J, Presnell KR: Mandibular condylectomy: effects in normal dogs, *Vet Surg* 12:148, 1983.

SCAPULOHUMERAL JOINT

OSTEOCHONDRITIS DISSECANS OF THE PROXIMAL HUMERUS

DEFINITIONS

Osteochondritis dissecans is a manifestation of a general syndrome called osteochondrosis in which a flap of cartilage is lifted from the articular surface. **Osteochondrosis** is a disturbance in endochondral ossification that leads to cartilage retention. Detached pieces of articular cartilage are often referred to as **joint mice.**

SYNONYMS

Osteochondrosis, OCD

GENERAL CONSIDERATIONS AND CLINICALLY RELEVANT PATHOPHYSIOLOGY

Osteochondrosis (OCD) occurs commonly in the shoulders, elbows, stifles, and hocks of immature, large- and giant-breed dogs. Despite unilateral lameness, this condition is often bilateral. In the shoulder it is usually evidenced as a cartilage flap found on the midline or lateral aspect of the dorsocaudal humeral head. In some cases, the subchondral bone defect occupies half of the area of the humeral head. The abnormal cartilage may fissure and cause protrusion of a loose flap of cartilage into the joint, or the cartilage may completely detach from the underlying bone and become lodged in the caudoventral joint pouch.

☞ **N O T E** • This condition is often bilateral. Both shoulders should be radiographed and evaluated for OCD, even if the animal exhibits unilateral lameness.

Osteochondrosis begins with a failure of endochondral ossification in either the physis or articular epiphyseal complex that is responsible for long-bone epiphyseal formation. The etiology of OCD is unknown but genetics, rapid growth, overnutrition, trauma, ischemia, and hormonal factors have all received speculative consideration as contributing factors. Failure of endochondral ossification leads to cartilage thickening. Because developing cartilage is nourished initially by synovial fluid and later by vascularization through subchondral bone, increased cartilage thickness may result in malnourished, necrotic chondrocytes. Loss of chondrocytes deep in the cartilage layer leads to formation of a cleft at the junction of calcified and noncalcified tissues. Subsequently, normal activity may lead to development of vertical fissures in the cartilage that eventually communicate with the joint, forming a cartilage flap (Fig. 30-11). This communication allows cartilage degradation products to reach the synovial fluid and induce joint inflammation. OCD does not apparently cause clinical signs until a loose cartilage flap forms. Free cartilage flaps can lodge in joints and may increase in size with calcification until they become radiographically visible joint mice. Alternatively,

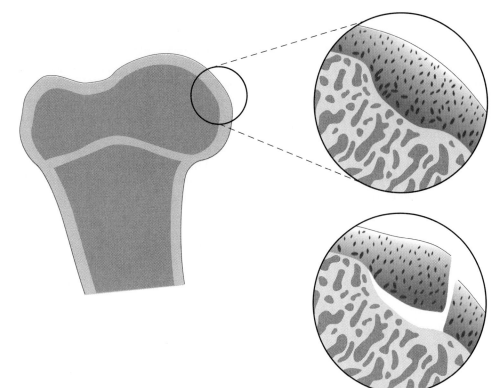

FIG. 30-11
Failure of endochondral ossification leads to cartilage thickening. Loss of chondrocytes deep in the cartilage layer produces a cleft and causes development of vertical fissures in the cartilage. These fissures eventually communicate with the joint, forming a cartilage flap.

the cartilage flaps can be gradually resorbed. Degenerative joint disease is often the final outcome.

> ☞ **N O T E** · OCD has a hereditary component, and owners should be counseled against breeding these dogs.

DIAGNOSIS
Clinical Presentation

Signalment. Large- and giant-breed dogs are commonly affected; this disease is rarely diagnosed in cats or small dogs. Males are more commonly affected than females. Clinical signs often develop between 4 and 8 months of age; however, some dogs may not be presented for veterinary evaluation until they are mature or middle-aged.

History. Affected animals are usually presented for examination because of unilateral forelimb lameness. Owners usually report a gradual onset of lameness that improves after rest and worsens after exercise. Owners may occasionally associate the onset of lameness with trauma.

Physical Examination Findings

The shoulder should be palpated and moved through a complete range of motion. Crepitation or palpable swelling of the joint is seldom evident, but affected animals usually exhibit pain when the shoulder is moved into extreme extension (i.e., moving the humerus forward with one hand while the other hand is positioned as a fulcrum on the cranial aspect of the shoulder; see p. 723). Extreme flexion of the shoulder may also cause pain.

> ☞ **N O T E** · Be careful not to elicit pain when holding the elbow to extend the shoulders.

Radiography

Diagnosis of OCD is based on typical radiographic findings evident on lateral projections of the shoulder joints; craniocaudal projections do not contribute to the diagnosis. Both shoulders should be radiographed because this condition is often bilateral, despite apparent lameness in only one limb. The dog should be positioned in lateral recumbency with the shoulder of interest down and the head elevated to prevent superimposition of the humeral head over the cervical spine (Fig. 30-12). The uppermost forelimb is retracted caudally and the down forelimb is extended cranially. Slight external rotation of the humerus may help silhouette the affected portion of the humeral head. Sedation may be required for quality radiographs. Multiple views made while the humerus is rotated into different positions may be necessary to locate the lesion.

The earliest radiographic sign of OCD is flattening of the subchondral bone of the caudal humeral head. As the disease progresses, a saucer-shaped radiolucent area in the caudal humeral head may be visualized (Fig. 30-13). Calcification of the flap may allow visualization of the flap either in situ or

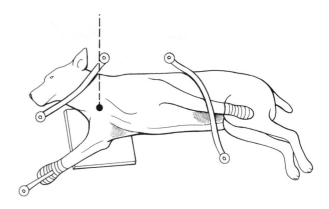

FIG. 30-12
Proper position for shoulder radiograph.

within the joint if it has detached from the underlying bone. In chronic cases, large calcified joint mice are often observed in the caudoventral joint pouch.

Contrast arthrography using 1.5 to 4 ml of a 25% solution of meglumine-sodium diatrizoate with an admixture of 0.2 mg of epinephrine can be used to determine the presence and location of cartilage flaps. Accuracy of arthrography in delineating loose cartilage flaps is approximately 88% (van Brée, 1993). Most dogs with loose cartilage flaps overlying a subchondral bone defect are lame, whereas those identified with thick articular cartilage over the flattened subchondral bone usually are not lame.

Laboratory Findings

Analysis of synovial fluid in animals with OCD reflects underlying inflammation and development of degenerative joint disease. Other specific laboratory abnormalities are not present.

DIFFERENTIAL DIAGNOSIS

Forelimb lameness in large immature dogs can be caused by many diseases: osteochondritis dissecans, ununited anconeal process, or fragmented coronoid process of the elbow, panosteitis, premature closure of physes, elbow incongruity, retained cartilage cores, and hypertropic osteodystrophy. Forelimb lameness attributable to the shoulder or scapulohumeral joint must be differentiated from injuries associated with trauma or septic arthritis, usually by evaluation of the animal's history and the results of radiographic and synovial fluid analysis.

MEDICAL OR CONSERVATIVE MANAGEMENT

Conservative therapy may benefit some dogs with OCD of the shoulder; however, animals that are likely to respond to conservative therapy are difficult to distinguish from those that will not. A therapeutic trial of exercise restriction (brief leash walks only) for a minimum of 6 weeks can be attempted. Buffered aspirin can be administered two or three times a day (Table 30-14), but care should be used in prescribing analgesics to these animals because pain relief may

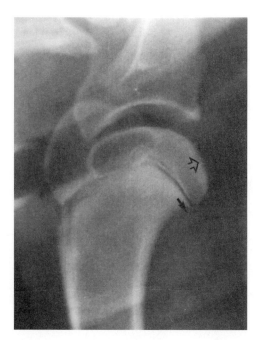

FIG. 30-13
Radiograph of a shoulder with osteochondritis dissecans of the caudal humeral head. Note the flattening and irregularity of the subchondral bone of the caudal aspect of the humeral head (*open arrow*). A portion of the cartilage flap is located in the caudal cul-de-sac of the joint where it has become mineralized (*closed arrow*). (From Olmstead ML: Small animal orthopedics, St. Louis, 1995, Mosby.)

make it difficult to enforce exercise restriction. If lameness resolves, surgery may not be indicated; however, if lameness persists more than 6 weeks, surgical removal of the flap is indicated.

SURGICAL TREATMENT

Surgical treatment involves exploratory arthrotomy and removal of the cartilage flap. It is indicated in dogs with persistent lameness that are unresponsive to conservative treatment. The goals of surgery are to remove the cartilage flap from the humeral head and curette the edges of the bony defect to ensure removal of all affected cartilage. Subchondral bone that appears pale and sclerotic should also be curetted. The joint should be carefully explored and flushed extensively in order to identify and remove any pieces of dislodged cartilage.

A technique using arthroscopy has been described for exploration of the shoulder joint and removal of cartilage flaps (Van Ryssen, van Bree, Missinne, 1993). A triangulation technique allows visualization of the joint and insertion and manipulation of instruments. Postoperative recovery is good. Surgical exposure of the scapulohumeral joint may be performed by using one of several different approaches, depending on the location of the defect and any detached cartilage flaps. Infraspinatus tenotomy affords excellent exposure of the humeral head and access to both the cranial and caudal joint compartments. However,

TABLE 30-14

Analgesic Therapy in Dogs with Osteochondritis Dissecans (OCD) of the Scapulohumeral Joint

Buffered aspirin (Ascriptin)

25 mg/kg (1 regular-strength buffered aspirin per 25 lbs of body weight, not to exceed 3 tablets per dose) PO with food, BID or TID

because the infraspinatus tendon is cut and the joint is subluxated during the procedure, this approach is more traumatic than approaches that do not involve tenotomy. Longer postoperative recovery periods should be expected than with other techniques. A caudal approach to the joint affords good exposure of the humeral head and excellent access to the caudal ventral joint compartment without tenotomy; however, it does not allow the cranial aspect of the joint to be explored.

☞ **N O T E** · Animals with unilateral lameness that have bilateral radiographic lesions should have surgery performed on the lame leg. The other leg may require surgery if lameness subsequently develops in that limb.

Preoperative Management

The overall health of the animal should be determined prior to surgery. A complete physical examination should be performed to determine whether other joints are similarly affected.

Anesthesia

These animals are usually young and healthy, and a variety of anesthetic regimens can be used (see p. 708).

Surgical Anatomy

Important anatomical landmarks used to identify the location of the scapulohumeral joint are the acromion process of the scapular spine, greater tubercle, and acromial head of the deltoid muscle. The omobrachial vein is located superficially over the acromial head of the deltoid muscle. The caudal circumflex humeral artery and vein and axillary nerve are encountered and must be protected during the caudal approach to the shoulder.

Positioning

The dog is positioned in lateral recumbency with the affected limb up. The limb should be prepared from the dorsal midline to below the elbow.

SURGICAL TECHNIQUES
Infraspinatus Tenotomy for Exposure of the Scapulohumeral Joint

Make an incision in skin and subcutaneous tissues from just proximal to the acromial process to the proximal humerus

FIG. 30-14

A, For a craniolateral approach to the shoulder, make an incision in skin and subcutaneous tissues from just proximal to the acromial process to the proximal humerus. **B,** Incise the deep fascia along the cranial margin of the acromial portion of the deltoideus muscle and retract the muscle caudally. **C,** Isolate the infraspinatus tendon, place a stay suture in its proximal portion, and incise the tendon. **D,** Incise the joint capsule midway between the glenoid rim and humeral head.

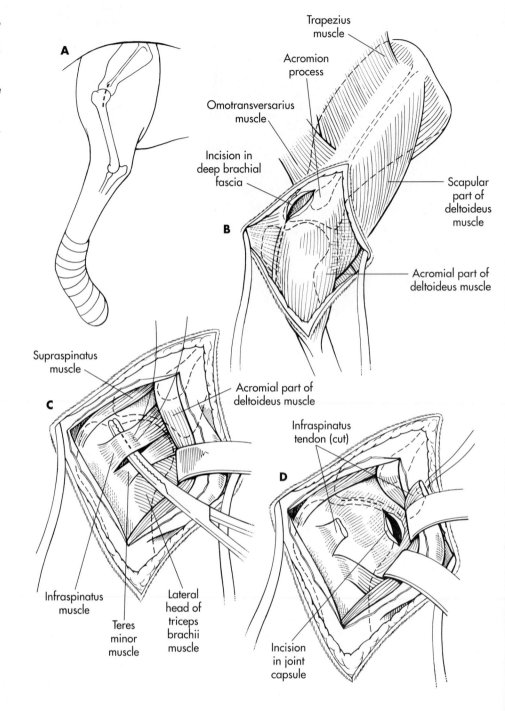

(Fig. 30-14, A). Curve the incision over the joint along the palpable cranial margin of the deltoid muscle's acromial head. Incise the deep fascia along the cranial margin of the acromial portion of the deltoid muscle and retract the muscle caudally (Fig. 30-14, B). Isolate the infraspinatus tendon and place a stay suture in its proximal portion. Incise the tendon 5 mm from its insertion on the humerus and retract it caudally (Fig. 30-14, C). Incise the joint capsule midway between the glenoid rim and humeral head (Fig. 30-14, D). Internally rotate the humerus until the head sub-

luxates, exposing the caudal surface of the humeral head (Fig. 30-14, E). Remove the cartilage flap from the humeral head and curette the edges of the bony defect to ensure removal of all affected cartilage (Fig. 30-14, F). Flush all parts of the joint thoroughly to remove any cartilage debris or joint mice. Close the joint capsule with 3-0 absorbable sutures in a simple interrupted pattern. Reappose the infraspinatus tendon with an absorbable suture in a Bunnell or locking-loop pattern (see p. 1003). Close muscular fascia, subcutaneous tissues, and skin separately.

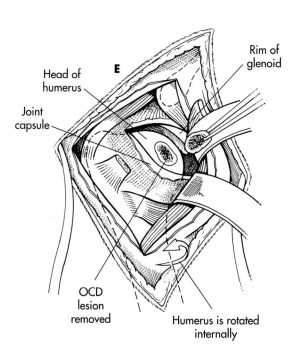

Head of humerus

Joint capsule

OCD lesion removed

Humerus is rotated internally

Rim of glenoid

E

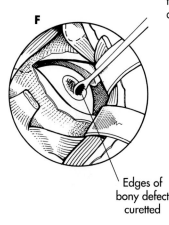

F

Edges of bony defect curetted

FIG. 30-14 CONT.
E, Internally rotate the humerus until the head subluxates and remove the cartilage flap. **F,** Curette the edges of the bony defect to ensure removal of all affected cartilage.

Caudal Approach to the Scapulohumeral Joint

Make an incision in skin, subcutaneous tissues, and deep fascia that extends from the midscapular spine to mid-humeral diaphysis (Fig. 30-15, A, p. 908). Incise the intermuscular septum between the caudal border of the scapular portion of the deltoid muscle and the long head of the triceps muscle, and separate the muscles (Fig. 30-15, B). Use blunt dissection to free the deltoid muscle and expose the caudal circumflex artery and vein, muscular branch of the axillary nerve, and teres minor muscle (Fig. 30-15, C). Elevate and retract the teres minor muscle cranially, exposing the axillary nerve and joint capsule (Fig. 30-15, D). Place a Penrose drain around the nerve and gently retract it caudally. Incise the joint capsule 5 mm from and parallel to the glenoid rim to expose the humeral head (Fig. 30-15, E). To expose OCD lesions of the humeral head, internally rotate the humerus and flex the shoulder. Explore the joint and remove the cartilage as described above. Close joint capsule with interrupted sutures of 3-0 absorbable suture material. Then suture the intermuscular septum, deep fascia, subcutaneous tissues, and skin as separate layers.

POSTOPERATIVE CARE AND ASSESSMENT

The animal usually can be released to the owner within 1 or 2 days after surgery. The client should be instructed to limit the animal's activity for 1 month to allow soft-tissue healing. The dog can then be returned gradually to full activity. The incision site should be observed for seroma formation, which will usually resolve without therapy.

SUTURE MATERIALS/SPECIAL INSTRUMENTS

Army-Navy retractors are used to retract soft tissues and improve visualization of the humeral head. A bone curette is used to remove damaged articular cartilage from the humeral head.

PROGNOSIS

The prognosis for normal limb function with osteochondritis dissecans of the shoulder is good. Dogs who respond to medical therapy generally return to full function; however, many asymptomatic dogs have radiographic evidence of OCD. After surgery, most dogs become sound within 4 to 8 weeks. In one study of 44 shoulders treated surgically to remove cartilaginous flaps, 75% had excellent function and 22.5% had good function on long-term evaluation (Rudd, Whitehair, Margolis, 1990). Despite the absence of lameness in these dogs, degenerative joint disease may develop and owners should be forewarned of this.

References

Rudd RG, Whitehair JG, Margolis JH: Results of management of osteochondritis dissecans of the humeral head in dogs: 44 cases (1982–1987), *J Am Anim Hosp Assoc* 26:173, 1990.

van Bree H: Comparison of the diagnostic accuracy of positive contrast arthrography and arthrotomy in evaluation of osteochondrosis lesions in the scapulohumeral joint in dogs, *J Am Vet Med Assoc* 203:84, 1993.

Van Ryssen B, van Bree H, Missinne S: Successful arthroscopic treatment of shoulder osteochondrosis in the dog, *J Small Anim Pract* 34:521, 1993.

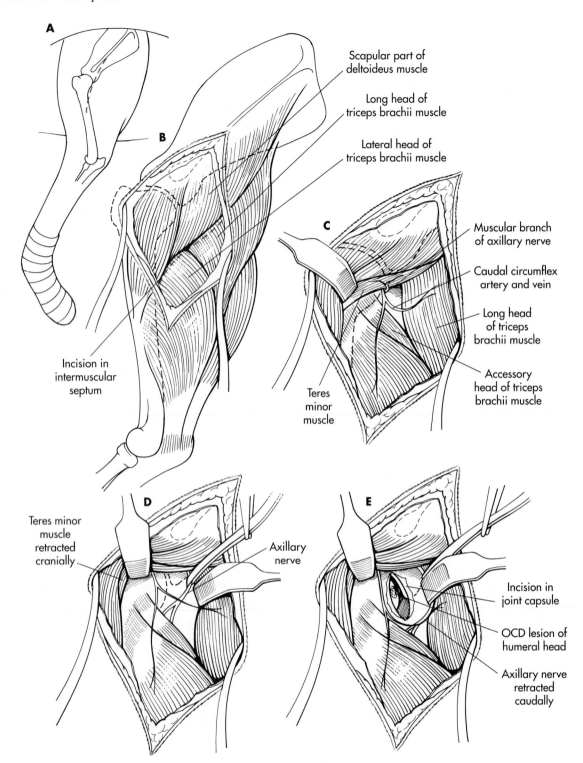

Scapular part of
deltoideus muscle

Long head of
triceps brachii muscle

Lateral head of
triceps brachii muscle

Muscular branch
of axillary nerve

Caudal circumflex
artery and vein

Long head
of triceps
brachii muscle

Accessory
head of triceps
brachii muscle

Teres
minor
muscle

Incision in
intermuscular
septum

Teres minor
muscle
retracted
cranially

Axillary
nerve

Incision in
joint capsule

OCD lesion of
humeral head

Axillary nerve
retracted
caudally

FIG. 30-15
A, For a caudal approach to the shoulder, make an incision in skin, subcutaneous tissues,
and deep fascia that extends from the midscapular spine to midhumeral diaphysis. **B,** Incise
the intermuscular septum between the caudal border of the scapular portion of the
deltoideus muscle and the long head of the triceps muscle. **C,** Elevate and retract the teres
minor muscle cranially, exposing the axillary nerve and joint capsule. **D,** Place a Penrose
drain around the nerve and gently retract it caudally. **E,** Incise the joint capsule 5 mm from
and parallel to the glenoid rim to expose the humeral head.

Suggested Reading

McLaughlin R, Roush JK: A comparison of two surgical approaches to the scapulohumeral joint in dogs, *Vet Surg* 24:207, 1995.

Olsson S-E: General and etiologic factors in canine osteochondrosis, *Veterinary Quarterly* 9:286, 1987.

Olsson S-E: Pathophysiology, morphology, and clinical signs of osteochondrosis in the dog. In Bojrab MJ, editor: *Disease mechanisms in small animal surgery,* ed 2, Philadelphia, 1993, Lea & Febiger.

Probst CW, Flo GL: Comparison of two caudolateral approaches to the scapulohumeral joint for treatment of osteochondritis dissecans in dogs, *J Am Vet Med Assoc* 191:1101, 1987.

Tomlinson J et al: Caudal approach to the shoulder joint in the dog, *Vet Surg* 15:294, 1986.

van Bree H: Evaluation of the prognostic value of positive-contrast shoulder arthrography for bilateral osteochondrosis lesions in dogs, *Am J Vet Res* 51:1121, 1990.

SCAPULOHUMERAL JOINT LUXATIONS

DEFINITIONS

Scapulohumeral joint luxations occur when there is sufficient loss of supporting structures of the joint to cause separation of the humerus from the scapula.

SYNONYMS

Dislocated shoulder, shoulder luxation

GENERAL CONSIDERATIONS AND CLINICALLY RELEVANT PATHOPHYSIOLOGY

Scapulohumeral luxations may be caused by trauma or may be congenital in origin. The scapulohumeral joint is supported by joint capsule, glenohumeral ligaments, and surrounding tendons (supraspinatus, infraspinatus, teres minor, and subscapularis). When these structures are torn or deficient, humeral head luxation may occur. Scapulohumeral luxations are named for the direction in which the humeral head deviates. Medial or lateral deviations are most common; cranial and caudal luxations are rare.

Traumatic luxations are usually the result of shoulder injury. Traumatic lateral humeral luxations occur after glenohumeral ligament and infraspinatus tendon rupture, while traumatic medial humeral luxations are associated with tearing of the medial glenohumeral ligament and subscapularis tendon. Concurrent thoracic trauma (i.e., pneumothorax, hemothorax, pulmonary contusions, or fractured ribs) is common. Congenital or development laxity of the capsule and ligaments may result in medial instability and medial luxation of the humeral head. The glenoid cavity may be sufficiently deformed or hypoplastic to prevent reduction of the humeral head. This condition often occurs bilaterally in affected animals.

☞ **N O T E** · Be sure to differentiate traumatic from congenital luxations because treatment and prognosis are different.

DIAGNOSIS
Clinical Presentation

Signalment. Traumatic luxations may occur in any age or breed of dog; they are rare in cats. Congenital, medial luxations usually occur in small and miniature dog breeds such as toy poodles and Shetland sheepdogs; lameness usually appears when the animal is young.

History. A history or evidence of trauma is usually present in dogs with traumatic luxations. Chronic forelimb lameness that first becomes evident at a young age and without a history of trauma is suggestive of congenital luxation.

Physical Examination

With traumatic luxations, affected animals may be non–weight-bearing and the limb is often carried in a flexed position. With lateral luxations, the foot is internally rotated and the greater tubercle is palpable lateral to its normal position, whereas with medial luxations the foot is externally rotated and the greater tubercle is palpated medial to its normal location. Pain and crepitation are evidenced with shoulder manipulation.

Dogs with chronic, congenital medial luxations are often lame. The joint is easily luxated and reduced, but manipulation does not usually cause pain. If the glenoid cavity is deformed, reduction of the humeral head may be impossible. Some small dogs with chronic medial luxations show only mild intermittent lameness and minimal degenerative joint disease.

Radiography

Lateral and craniocaudal radiographs of the shoulder are evaluated to confirm the diagnosis (Fig. 30-16). With traumatic luxations, special attention should be given to identifying concurrent scapular fractures or thoracic injuries.

Laboratory Findings

Specific laboratory abnormalities are not present with traumatic or congenital luxations. Traumatized animals undergoing surgery should have sufficient blood work done to determine optimal anesthetic regimens. Analysis of synovial fluid from affected animals may reflect associated inflammation and development of degenerative joint disease.

DIFFERENTIAL DIAGNOSIS

Degenerative joint disease and contracture of infraspinatus or supraspinatus tendons must be differentiated from luxations on the basis of physical findings and results of radiography.

MEDICAL OR CONSERVATIVE MANAGEMENT

Dogs with chronic medial luxations, only mild intermittent lameness, and minimal degenerative joint disease may be managed with exercise restriction and administration of

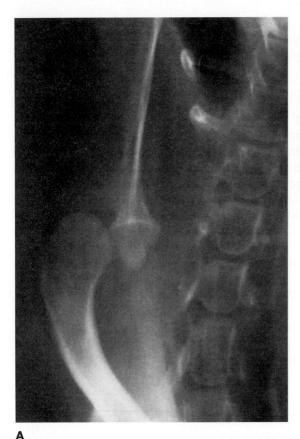

A

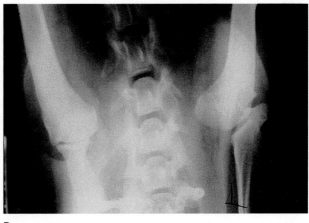

B

FIG. 30-16
Ventrodorsal radiographs illustrating **A,** lateral and **B,** medial luxation of the humeral head. (*A* from Olmstead ML: *Small animal orthopedics,* St. Louis, 1995, Mosby.)

aspirin during acute excerbations. Closed reduction can be attempted for traumatic luxations that are presented soon after injury, provided they are not associated with humeral or scapular fractures. General anesthesia is required for closed reduction. Lateral luxations are reduced with the leg held in extension. Medial pressure is applied to the humeral head, and lateral pressure is applied to the medial surface of the scapula (Fig. 30-17). The humeral head should remain in place when it is gently moved through a normal range of motion. If the luxation appears stable, a lateral spica splint should be applied for 10 to 14 days (see p. 707). Medial luxations caused by trauma are reduced in the opposite manner and are immobilized by placing the limb in a Velpeau sling (see p. 717).

SURGICAL TREATMENT

If a traumatic luxation is unstable enough after closed reduction that reluxation occurs, or if the luxation is chronic, open reduction and stabilization with capsulorrhaphy or tendon transposition are required. Surgery is warranted in animals with congenital luxations that cause severe or persistent lameness. In cases of severe joint dysplasia or degenerative joint disease, open reduction and stabilization are unsuccessful, and salvage procedures (glenoid excision or arthrodesis) must be performed.

Surgical arthrodesis of the shoulder is reserved for animals with chronic intractable luxations, comminuted fractures of the humeral head or glenoid, or severe degenerative joint disease that precludes primary fixation. This is consid-

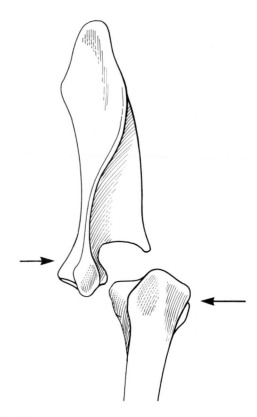

FIG. 30-17
To close reduce a lateral luxation, apply medial pressure to the humeral head and lateral pressure to the medial surface of the scapula.

ered a salvage procedure and should be done only as a last resort and only when other joints are normal. Because scapular mobility compensates for loss of motion in the scapulohumeral joint, most animals have good limb function after shoulder arthrodesis.

Excision arthroplasty is a salvage procedure that causes a pseudoarthrosis to form between the scapula and humerus, which allows limited scapulohumeral joint motion. This procedure does not require implantation of orthopedic hardware (plates, screws), and most dogs are pain free and bear weight on the limb at a walk or run. However, gait abnormalities and mild or moderate atrophy of shoulder muscles are usually noted after surgery.

Preoperative Management

The overall health of the animal should be determined before surgery. Thoracic radiography and electrocardiographic analysis are warranted in animals with traumatic luxations.

Anesthesia

General anesthesia is required for closed or open reduction. A variety of anesthetic regimens can be used in young, healthy animals (see p. 708). Special care should be exercised in anesthetizing older animals or those with concurrent injuries.

Surgical Anatomy

Important landmarks used to identify the location of the scapulohumeral joint are the acromion process of the scapular spine, greater tubercle, and acromial head of the deltoid muscle. Anatomical landmarks for positioning the skin incision include the acromion of the scapula, greater tubercle of the humerus, and pectoral muscles. The suprascapular nerve is present over the cranial lateral surface of the scapula and the caudal circumflex humeral artery and axillary nerve are present on the caudolateral aspect of the shoulder and should be avoided.

Positioning

For either medial or lateral luxations the animal is positioned in dorsal recumbency with the affected leg draped. The prepared area should extend from the dorsal and ventral midlines to below the elbow.

SURGICAL TECHNIQUES
Surgical Stabilization of Medial Luxations

An approach to the craniomedial shoulder joint is used to expose the luxated joint. It may be helpful to reduce the joint before the approach is made to reestablish normal anatomical relationships. *Beginning at the medial aspect of the acromion, incise skin and subcutaneous tissue over the greater tubercle and continue the incision medially to the midhumeral diaphysis (Fig. 30-18, A). Incise the fascia along the lateral border of the brachiocephalicus muscle and retract the muscle medially. Incise the insertions of the superficial and deep pectoral muscles from the humerus and retract them medially (Fig. 30-18, B). Carefully incise the fascial attachment between the deep pectoral muscle*

and supraspinatus muscle to avoid causing trauma to the suprascapular nerve (Fig. 30-18, C). Retract the supraspinatus muscle laterally. Transect the tendon of the coracobrachialis muscle to expose the subscapularis muscular tendon (Fig. 30-18, D). If the joint capsule is not torn, incise it to inspect the joint and assess the condition of the humeral head and medial labrum of the glenoid (Fig. 30-18, E). If the labrum is worn, the prognosis for successful stabilization of the shoulder is poor. The tendon of the coracobrachialis muscle may be torn and retracted with traumatic luxations. *Reduce the joint and imbricate the capsule and subscapularis tendon with nonabsorbable mattress sutures. If this does not sufficiently stabilize the joint, incise the transverse humeral ligament over the biceps tendon. Make a small incision in the joint capsule under the biceps tendon to free it and move the tendon medially. Secure it to the humerus with a bone screw and spiked washer (Fig. 30-18, F). To prevent external rotation of the humeral head during healing, place a rotational suture of heavy nonabsorbable material from the medial labrum of the glenoid through a bone tunnel in the greater tubercle. For closure, suture the joint capsule, and then suture pectoral muscles to deltoid fascia. Suture subcutaneous tissues and skin separately.*

Surgical Stabilization of Lateral Luxations

Transposition of the biceps brachii tendon is performed to stabilize lateral luxations. An approach to the cranial region of the shoulder joint is used to expose the luxated joint (also used to approach cranial luxations of the shoulder). It may be helpful to reduce the joint before the approach is made to reestablish normal anatomical relationships. *Incise skin and subcutaneous tissues and deepen the incision through the pectoral muscles as described above for medial luxations (Fig. 30-19, A). Perform an osteotomy of the greater tubercle that includes the supraspinatus muscular insertion (Fig. 30-19, B). If the joint capsule is not torn, incise it to inspect the joint and assess the condition of the humeral head and lateral labrum of the glenoid (Fig. 30-19, C).* If the labrum is worn, the prognosis for successful stabilization of the shoulder is poor. *Reduce the joint and imbricate the capsule with nonabsorbable mattress sutures. If sufficient stabilization is not achieved, incise the transverse humeral ligament over the biceps tendon. Make a small incision in the joint capsule under the biceps tendon to free it and move the tendon laterally across the osteotomy site. While the tendon is held in place, reduce and stabilize the osteotomy with Kirschner wires and a tension-band wire or lag screw (Fig. 30-19, D). Suture the biceps tendon to the deltoid fascia. Close as described above.*

Shoulder Arthrodesis

Perform a combined craniolateral and cranial approach to the shoulder with osteotomy of the acromial process (see p. 782) and greater tubercle (see above). Detach the biceps tendon from the supraglenoid tubercle. Using an oscillating saw or osteotome, perform ostectomies of the glenoid process and humeral head, which parallel each other when

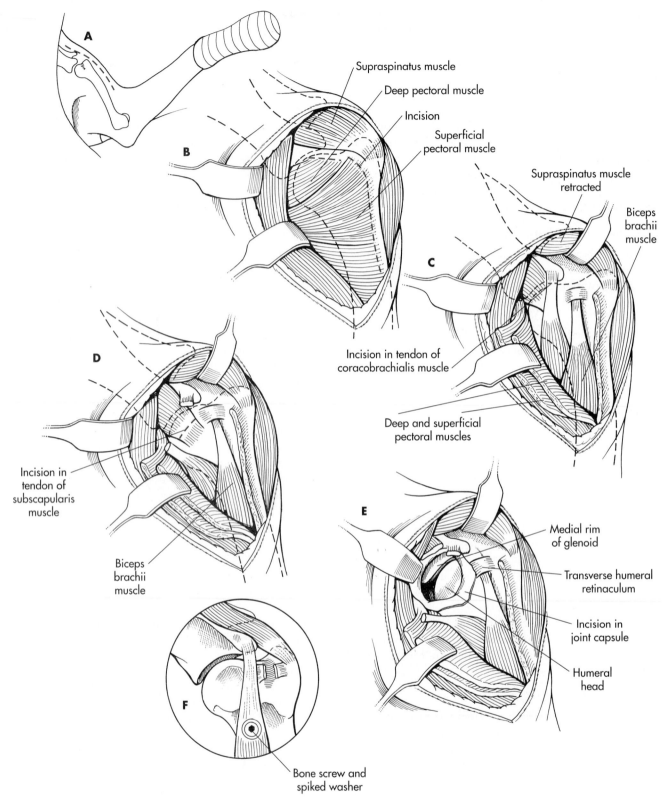

FIG. 30-18
A, To treat medial shoulder luxations, perform a craniomedial approach with biceps tendon transposition. Incise skin and subcutaneous tissue over the greater tubercle and continue the incision medially to the midhumeral diaphysis. **B,** Incise the fascia along the lateral border of the brachiocephalicus muscle. **C,** Incise the insertions of the superficial and deep pectoral muscles from the humerus and retract them medially. Retract the supraspinatus muscle laterally. **D,** Transect the tendon of the coracobrachialis muscle to expose the subscapularis muscular tendon. Incise the tendon of the suprascapularis muscle. **E,** Incise joint capsule to inspect the joint. **F,** To transpose the biceps tendon, incise the transverse humeral ligament. Make a small incision in the joint capsule under the biceps tendon to free it and move the tendon medially. Secure it to the humerus with a bone screw and spiked washer.

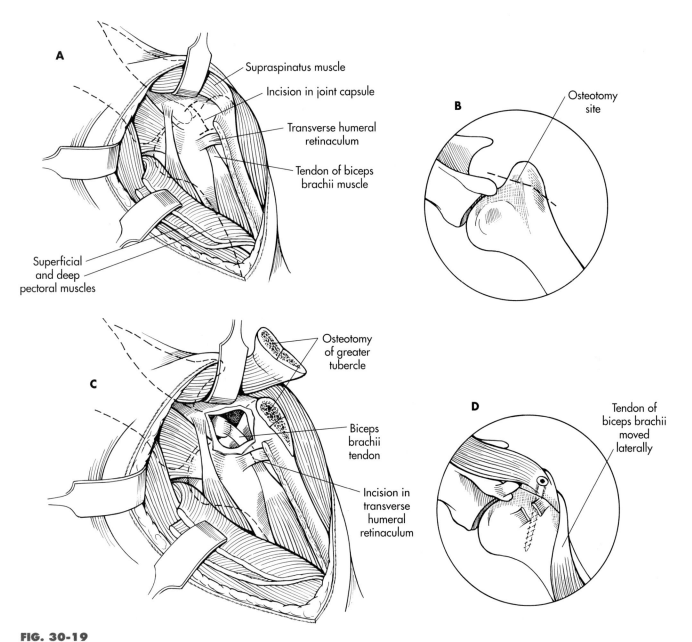

FIG. 30-19
To treat lateral shoulder luxations, perform a cranial approach with biceps tendon transposition. **A,** Expose the joint. **B,** Perform an osteotomy of the greater tubercle, including the infraspinatus muscular insertion. **C,** Incise the joint capsule and the transverse humeral ligament over the biceps tendon. **D,** Free the biceps tendon and move it laterally across the osteotomy site. Hold the tendon in place and reduce and stabilize the osteotomy with Kirschner wires and a tension band wire or a lag screw.

the humerus is held at an angle of 105° to the scapula. Take care to preserve the suprascapular nerve and caudal circumflex humeral artery. Oppose the flat surfaces and temporarily stabilize the bones with a Kirschner wire driven through the cranial aspect of the humerus and into the glenoid. Contour an 8- or 10-hole plate to fit from the dorsocranial junction of the spine and scapula, over the cranial aspect of the humerus (Fig. 30-20). Be sure that the plate does not impinge on the suprascapular nerve. If necessary, contour the cranial humerus with rongeurs to obtain a better fit for the plate.

Insert one of the screws across the opposed ostectomy lines as a lag screw. Remove the Kirschner wire and attach the biceps tendon to the surrounding fascia, or attach it to the humerus with a bone screw and spiked washer. Secure the greater tubercle to the humerus lateral to the plate with Kirschner wires or bone screws. Suture the soft tissues and close skin routinely.

Excision Arthroplasty

Perform a craniolateral approach to the shoulder with osteotomy of the acromial process (see Fig. 29-17). Detach the

FIG. 30-20
A, For shoulder arthrodesis, osteotomize the greater tubercle and acromial process. Make the ostectomy lines for the glenoid and humeral head parallel to each other when the humerus is held at 105 degrees with the scapula. **B,** Compress the bone surfaces with a contoured compression plate. Place a lag screw across the fracture line. A cancellous bone autograft may be added.

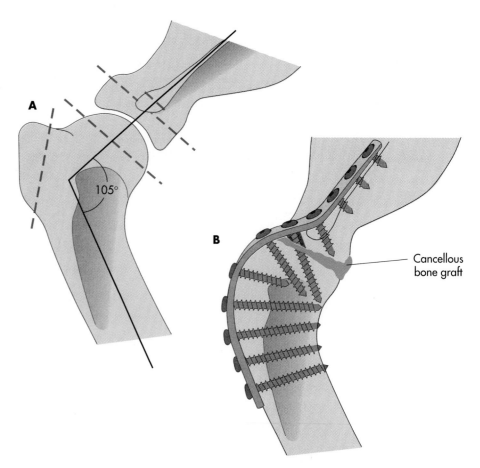

Cancellous bone graft

biceps tendon from the supraglenoid tubercle and incise the joint capsule. Using an oscillating saw or osteotome, perform an ostectomy of the glenoid (Fig. 30-21). Be careful to preserve the suprascapular nerve and caudal circumflex humeral artery when performing the excision. *Bevel the glenoid so that the lateral edge is longer than the medial edge.* Part of the humeral head can be ostectomized to create a vascular surface to promote pseudoarthrosis. *Pull the teres minor muscle over the glenoid ostectomy site and suture it to the medial joint capsule and biceps tendon to provide soft-tissue interposition between bone surfaces. Pull the acromial process proximally until the deltoid muscle is taut. Wire the process to the scapular spine (see p. 781), then close soft tissues.*

SUTURE MATERIALS/SPECIAL INSTRUMENTS

Stabilization techniques for scapulohumeral luxations require retractors, a periosteal elevator, osteotome and mallet, Kirschner wires, orthopedic wire, wire driver, wire twister, bone screw and spiked washer, drill, drill bit, tap, depth gauge, and screwdriver. Plating equipment is required for arthrodesis. Excision arthroplasty requires instruments similar to those for luxations.

POSTOPERATIVE CARE AND ASSESSMENT

Postoperative radiography is performed to document the position of the humeral head and any implants used. After lateral luxations, the limb should be supported in a spica splint (see p. 707) for 10 to 14 days; after medial luxations it should be supported in a Velpeau sling (see p. 717) for a similar period of time. Owners should be cautioned to limit activity and protect the bandage. After the bandage is removed, activity should be limited for an additional 3 to 4 weeks.

After shoulder arthrodesis, postoperative radiographs should be made to evaluate implant position and serve as a comparison for subsequent evaluations. A spica splint is applied until there are radiographic signs of bone union, in 6 to 12 weeks. Once bone union is evident, the splint can be removed and the animal gradually returned to full activity.

After excision arthroplasty, postoperative radiographs are assessed to document alignment of the scapula and humeral head. Early postoperative use of the limb should be encouraged. The animal should be walked on a leash and physical therapy (range-of-motion exercises) should be performed, beginning 1 or 2 days after surgery. Once sutures have been removed (10 to 14 days after surgery), activity should be encouraged to promote rapid pseudoarthrosis formation. Lameness is often evident for 4 to 8 weeks after surgery.

PROGNOSIS

After closed reduction, the prognosis is good for maintenance of reduction and return of limb function if joints are stable during forelimb manipulation. However, the progno-

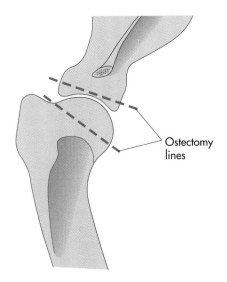

FIG. 30-21
Ostectomy lines for glenoid excision.

sis is guarded if joints appear unstable; open reduction and joint stabilization should be considered in such cases. The major complication associated with surgical repair of scapulohumeral joint luxations is reluxation of the humeral head. With traumatic luxations, most dogs regain normal limb usage; however, some degenerative joint disease may occur and require periodic treatment with analgesics. The prognosis is guarded for dogs with congenital or developmental medial luxations. When it is not possible to maintain reduction of scapulohumeral joints, a salvage procedure may be indicated (i.e., shoulder arthrodesis, excision arthroplasty, or amputation).

Suggested Reading

Bone DL: Chronic luxations, *Vet Clin North Am (Small Anim Pract)* 17:923, 1987.

Fowler, JD, Presnell KR, Holmberg DL: Scapulohumeral arthrodesis: results in seven dogs, *J Am Anim Hosp Assoc* 24:667, 1988.

Franczuszki D, Parkes LJ: Glenoid excision as a treatment in chronic shoulder disabilities: surgical technique and clinical results, *J Am Anim Hosp Assoc* 24:637, 1988.

Vasseur PB: Luxation of the scapulohumeral joint. In Slatter D, editor: *Textbook of small animal surgery,* ed 2, Philadelphia, 1993, WB Saunders.

SCAPULAR LUXATIONS

DEFINITIONS

Scapular luxations are characterized by upward displacement of the scapula after rupture of supporting musculature.

SYNONYMS

Scapular dislocation

GENERAL CONSIDERATIONS AND CLINICALLY RELEVANT PATHOPHYSIOLOGY

Scapular luxations are rare, but they occasionally occur with trauma that causes the serratus ventralis, rhomboideus, and trapezius muscular insertions to be torn from their scapular attachments. This allows upward displacement of the scapula during weight bearing. Concurrent injuries such as rib fractures, pneumothorax, or pulmonary contusions are common and may require immediate treatment.

DIAGNOSIS
Clinical Presentation

Signalment. This condition occurs more often in cats than dogs; animals of either sex or any age may be affected.
History. Typically, there is a recent history of trauma.

Physical Examination Findings

Marked dorsal displacement of the scapula is observed as the animal bears weight on the affected limb. Adduction of the limb induces lateral scapular displacement. The symmetry of scapular location and prominence should be compared with the normal limb.

Radiography

Radiographs are made of the thorax and observed for signs of thoracic trauma such as fractured ribs, pulmonary contusions, or pneumothorax. Usually the scapula is not fractured but may appear displaced.

Laboratory Findings

Specific laboratory abnormalities are not present. Traumatized animals undergoing surgery should have sufficient blood work done to determine optimal anesthetic regimens.

DIFFERENTIAL DIAGNOSIS

This condition must be differentiated from scapular fractures (see p. 778).

MEDICAL OR CONSERVATIVE MANAGEMENT

Surgical stabilization of the scapula is usually required for a good cosmetic and functional result; however, closed reduction with placement of a Velpeau bandage (see p. 717) has been reported to be successful in cats with acute luxations.

SURGICAL TREATMENT

Although the torn muscles' bellies can occasionally be identified and reattached to the scapula, this repair is usually insufficient to allow weight bearing. Generally, the scapula is held in its normal position by wire suture that is placed around an adjacent rib and through holes drilled in the caudal scapular border.

Preoperative Management

Thoracic radiographs and electrocardiographic analysis are warranted to determine the presence of concurrent thoracic or cardiovascular trauma in acute injuries. Prophylactic antibiotic therapy is usually unnecessary.

Anesthesia

If the animal is healthy and there are no significant concurrent injuries, a number of anesthetic regimens can be used safely (see p. 708); however, if there is evidence of concurrent thoracic or cardiovascular injury, anesthesia should be induced and monitored with care. Equipment should be available for ventilating the animal if the chest is opened inadvertently.

Surgical Anatomy

Refer to p. 779 for a detailed discussion of the anatomy of the scapula. Important surgical landmarks for surgical repair of scapular luxations are the dorsocaudal scapular border and the fifth, sixth, or seventh ribs.

Positioning

The animal is positioned in lateral recumbency with the affected side up. The entire scapular region (from midcervical region to midthorax) should be prepared for aseptic surgery.

SURGICAL TECHNIQUES

After repositioning the scapula to its normal position, incise through skin and subcutaneous tissues along the dorsal caudal scapular margin to expose the caudal scapular border. Identify the torn edges of the muscles, if possible. Elevate a small portion of the teres major muscle from the caudal scapular border and identify the underlying rib. Elevate periosteum from the rib surface, using care to avoid penetrating the parietal pleura. Use a wire passer to position a piece of wire around the rib. Use 18- to 20-gauge wire to secure the scapula to the rib. Drill two holes in the caudal scapular border adjacent to the exposed rib and pass the free ends of the wire through these holes in a medial-to-lateral direction. Tighten the wire by twisting the ends to secure the scapula to the rib. If you have identified the torn muscle edges, reattach them prior to closing subcutaneous tissues and skin.

SUTURE MATERIALS/SPECIAL INSTRUMENTS

Necessary equipment includes 18- or 20-gauge wire, wire passer, periosteal elevator, and Steinmann pin and hand chuck. Absorbable (polydioxanone or polyglyconate) or nonabsorbable (polypropylene or nylon) suture material can be used to reattach the muscles to their scapular insertions.

POSTOPERATIVE CARE AND ASSESSMENT

Respiratory rate and effort should be carefully observed postoperatively to determine if the animal is able to ventilate normally. Ventilatory difficulties may indicate a pneumothorax if the pleura was inadvertently penetrated during wire passage. Thoracic radiographs should be taken and thoracentesis performed in such patients. A spica splint (see p. 707) should be applied to immobilize the limb for 3 weeks after surgery (the bandage may need to be changed every 5 to 7 days). Owners should be instructed to confine the animal until bandage removal; normal exercise may be resumed at 6 weeks.

PROGNOSIS

Chronic luxations will not resolve without surgical intervention. Potential complications of surgery include fixation failure, iatrogenic infection, and eventual wire fatigue and breakage with migration; however, complications are rare. Most animals bear weight normally on affected limbs after surgery.

Suggested Reading

Leighton RL: *Small animal orthopedics,* St. Louis, 1994, Mosby.

BICIPITAL TENOSYNOVITIS

DEFINITIONS

Bicipital tenosynovitis is an inflammation of the biceps brachii tendon and its surrounding synovial sheath.

SYNONYMS

Bicipital tendinitis, mineralization of biceps tendon

GENERAL CONSIDERATIONS AND CLINICALLY RELEVANT PATHOPHYSIOLOGY

The etiology of bicipital tenosynovitis is either direct or indirect trauma to the bicipital tendon. Repetitive injury or overuse may be an inciting factor. Chronic inflammation causing synovial hyperplasia and dystrophic mineralization of the tendon may occur. The tendon may be partially or completely ruptured. Proliferative fibrous connective tissue and adhesions between the tendon and sheath limit motion and cause pain. Osteophytes may form in the intertubercular groove. It has been hypothesized that mineralization of the supraspinatus tendon causes a secondary mechanical tenosynovitis and lameness that are refractory to steroid injection but responsive to curettage of the mineralization.

DIAGNOSIS
Clinical Presentation

Signalment. Affected dogs are usually medium- to large-sized, and middle-aged or older. There is no predisposition in either sex. Working, active dogs and sedentary dogs may be affected.

History. Intermittent or progressive forelimb lameness, which worsens after exercise, is common. The owner may relate the lameness to trauma, but usually there is slow onset of clinical signs.

Physical Examination Findings

Lameness of one forelimb is usually evident. The animal usually will stand on the limb but is lame during gaiting. Pain may be evident during palpation of the bicipital tendon, especially with concurrent flexion and extension of the shoulder. In some cases the condition is present bilaterally. Atrophy of the supraspinatus and infraspinatus muscle may be palpable.

Radiography

Radiographic views should include standard lateral projections of both shoulders. A cranial-caudal projection of the humerus with the shoulder flexed can be used to identify the bicipital groove. Calcification of the biceps tendon and osteophytes in the intertubercular groove may be evident. Arthrography (see p. 904) can be used to outline the tendon and reveal irregularities and filling defects suggestive of synovial hyperplasia, tendon rupture, and joint mice.

Laboratory Findings

Results of hematologic and serum biochemical analyses reflect the general health of the dog. Results of arthrocentesis are typically normal or may suggest mild inflammation and degenerative joint disease, with higher concentrations of monocytes and macrophages in the joint fluid. Evidence of sepsis is a contraindication to arthrography or intraarticular corticosteroid therapy.

DIFFERENTIAL DIAGNOSIS

Bicipital tenosynovitis must be differentiated from osteoarthritis of the shoulder, early osteosarcoma or other bone tumors of the proximal humeral metaphysis, cervical disk disease, or neurofibroma of the brachial plexus.

MEDICAL MANAGEMENT

Medical therapy is generally used initially to treat dogs with bicipital tenosynovitis. Methylprednisolone acetate (10 to 40 mg) can be infiltrated into the bicipital tendon sheath or, alternatively, injected into the scapulohumeral joint. This treatment is followed by confinement for 6 weeks. Afterwards, gradually increasing exercise is indicated to strengthen surrounding musculature. Oral administration of corticosteroids does not appear to be effective.

SURGICAL TREATMENT

Bicipital tendon tenodesis (surgically moving the bicipital tendon from the intertubercular groove) is used to eliminate movement of the biceps tendon in the inflamed tendon sheath. This procedure is indicated in dogs with ruptured bicipital tendons and chronic bicipital tenosynovitis if they have not responded to medical therapy.

Preoperative Management

Most affected animals are middle-aged or older, and concurrent medical problems should be identified before surgery.

Anesthesia

Anesthetic management of dogs with orthopedic disease is discussed on p. 708. Postoperative analgesics are discussed on p. 708.

Surgical Anatomy

Surgical anatomy of the shoulder is discussed on p. 905. The bicipital tendon arises from the supraglenoid tubercle and crosses the cranial portion of the scapulohumeral joint. The tendon courses through the intertubercular groove of the humerus and is held in position by the transverse humeral ligament. The tendon is surrounded by a synovial sheath that communicates with the scapulohumeral joint.

Positioning

The dog is positioned in dorsal recumbency with the affected leg draped. The prepared area should extend from the dorsal and ventral midlines to below the elbow.

SURGICAL TECHNIQUES

An approach to the cranial region of the shoulder joint is used to expose the bicipital tendon and bicipital groove (see p. 912). *Incise the transverse humeral ligament and joint capsule to expose the tendon and intertubercular groove. Transect the tendon near the supraglenoid tubercle. Reattach the tendon to the humerus distal to the groove with a bone screw and spiked Teflon washer. Alternatively, redirect the tendon through a bone tunnel created in the humerus and suture it to the supraspinatus muscle.*

SUTURE MATERIALS/SPECIAL INSTRUMENTS

Equipment for placing a screw and spiked washer is needed.

POSTOPERATIVE CARE AND ASSESSMENT

The limb should be supported in a Velpeau sling (see p. 717) after surgery for 2 to 3 weeks. The animal should be closely confined for 6 weeks, after which gradual resumption of normal activity should be encouraged.

PROGNOSIS

Results of medical treatment range from excellent to poor. Results of surgical treatment are generally good to excellent. The time required for dogs to regain optimal function ranges from 2 to 9 months.

Suggested Reading

Brinker WO, Piermattei DL, Flo GL: *Handbook of small animal orthopedics and fracture treatment,* ed 2, Philadelphia, 1990, WB Saunders.

Kriegleder H: Mineralization of the supraspinatus tendon: clinical observations in seven dogs, *Vet Comp Ortho Trauma* 8:91, 1995.

Stobie D et al: Chronic bicipital tenosynovitis in dogs: 29 cases (1985–1992), *J Am Vet Med Assoc* 207:201, 1995.

ELBOW JOINT

OSTEOCHONDRITIS DISSECANS OF THE DISTAL HUMERUS

DEFINITIONS

Osteochondrosis is a disturbance in endochondral ossification that leads to retention of cartilage; it occurs commonly in the shoulder, elbow, stifle, and hock of immature, large dogs. **Osteochondritis dissecans** occurs when fissure formation in the abnormal cartilage leads to development of a flap of cartilage. A loose flap of cartilage in the joint is a **joint mouse.**

SYNONYMS

Osteochondrosis, OCD

GENERAL CONSIDERATIONS AND CLINICALLY RELEVANT PATHOPHYSIOLOGY

Osteochondrosis (OCD) begins with a failure of endochondral ossification in either the physis or the articular epiphyseal complex, which is responsible for formation of metaphyseal bone. Osteochondrosis has been implicated in the pathophysiology of osteochondritis dissecans, fragmented coronoid process, and ununited anconeal process of the elbow. The etiology is unknown, but genetic factors, rapid growth, overnutrition, trauma, ischemia, and hormonal factors are possible causes (Table 30-15). Failure of endochondral ossification leads to cartilage thickening. Because developing cartilage is nourished initially by synovial fluid and later by vascularization through subchondral bone, in-

TABLE 30-15

Important Considerations for Treatment of OCD,* FCP,[†] and UAP[‡]

All three of these diseases appear to be manifestations of OCD.

There is strong evidence for a hereditary component in the etiology of FCP and OCD.

Loss of elbow range of motion is evidence of DJD[§]; in immature, large dogs this finding usually indicates the presence of one of these three diseases.

Careful attention to positioning for radiographs is essential for diagnosis of subtle lesions.

Both elbows should be radiographed.

Surgical removal of bone and cartilage pieces usually results in improved limb function if the dog is treated before extensive secondary DJD develops.

Surgical treatment does not appear to alter the progression of DJD, and medical therapy is often necessary.

*Osteochondrosis.
[†]Fragmented coronoid process.
[‡]Ununited anconeal process.
[§]Degenerative joint disease.

creased cartilage thickness may result in malnourished, necrotic chondrocytes. Chondrocyte loss deep in the cartilage layer leads to formation of a cleft at the junction of calcified and noncalcified tissues. Subsequent trauma caused by normal activity can lead to development of vertical fissures in the cartilage; eventually the fissures communicate with the joint, and a cartilage flap is formed. This communication allows cartilage degradation products to reach the synovial fluid, where they may cause joint inflammation. OCD does not cause apparent clinical signs until a loose flap of cartilage develops. This loose body of cartilage does not ossify. Degenerative joint disease (DJD) of the elbow is the final outcome.

With OCD of the distal humerus, a flap of cartilage covering a defect in the surface of the trochlear ridge of the medial humeral condyle is usually observed. Opposing joint cartilage of the coronoid process may be eroded. Histologic examination of the lesion confirms that the flap consists of cartilage, subchondral bone trabeculae in the defect are thickened, and bone marrow fibrosis is present.

DIAGNOSIS
Clinical Presentation

Signalment. Affected dogs are usually large (Labrador retrievers, golden retrievers). The usual age of onset of lameness is 5 to 7 months.

History. Forelimb lameness, which worsens after exercise, may be acute or chronic. Owners frequently complain that the dog is stiff in the morning or after rest. There may be a coincidental history of trauma. Some owners delay seeking veterinary help initially because the lameness is mild and they believe the animal will "grow out of it."

Physical Examination Findings

Lameness of one forelimb is usually evident. The gait may be stiff or stilted if forelimb steps are shortened because of bilateral lameness. Pain may be elicited on elbow extension and on lateral rotation of the forearm. Palpation of the elbows should include an evaluation of range of motion. A decrease in the animal's ability to flex the elbow is indicative of secondary DJD. Crepitation during elbow flexion and extension, joint effusion, and periarticular swelling may be noted if DJD is present. It is important that the shoulder not be inadvertently flexed and extended during elbow manipulation to avoid confusing shoulder pain and elbow pain.

Radiography

Radiographic views should include a standard lateral of the elbow, a flexed lateral to expose the anconeal process, and a cranial-caudal view made while the elbow is flexed 30 degrees and slightly rotated medially (Fig. 30-22). Radiographs of both elbows should be made because bilateral disease is common. Oblique views may be necessary to demonstrate the lesion on the humeral condyle. Definitive radiographic diagnosis of OCD is made when a radiolucent concavity is observed on the distal trochlear ridge of the medial humeral condyle (Fig. 30-23). Radiographic signs of secondary DJD are similar to those seen with fragmented coronoid process (see p. 923).

> 👉 **N O T E** • It may be necessary to sedate the dog for quality radiographs.

Laboratory Findings

Results of hematologic and serum biochemical analyses are normal in most affected animals. Results of arthrocentesis may include decreased synovial fluid viscosity, increased fluid volume, and increased numbers (up to 6000 to 9000 WBC/μl) of mononuclear phagocytic cells.

DIFFERENTIAL DIAGNOSIS

OCD must be differentiated from fragmented coronoid process (FCP), ununited anconeal process (UAP), combined UAP and FCP, and other diseases of young, growing dogs that affect the forelimb (OCD of the shoulder, panosteitis) and may produce similar clinical signs. These diseases are usually differentiated radiographically.

MEDICAL MANAGEMENT

Dogs that have radiographic abnormalities but no symptoms do not require treatment. Medical therapy (confinement and aspirin administration; see Table 30-14) is generally used to treat occasional lameness. After lameness has subsided or resolved, exercise should be gradually increased to strengthen surrounding musculature. Weight control is also important in the management of this disease.

SURGICAL TREATMENT

Surgical removal of the cartilage flap is recommended in young animals when the disease is diagnosed before the onset of DJD, and can also be helpful in treating animals with chronic moderate to severe lameness.

Preoperative Management

Most affected animals are young and require minimal preoperative workup before surgery.

Anesthesia

These animals are usually young and healthy and a variety of anesthetic regimens can be used (see p. 708).

Surgical Anatomy

Landmarks for the surgical incision include the medial epicondyle, epicondyloid crest, and proximal radius. The median nerve and brachial artery and vein course cranially to the medial epicondyle. The ulnar nerve courses caudally to

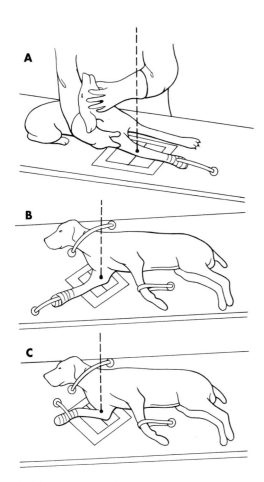

FIG. 30-22
A, For a craniocaudal radiograph of the elbow, position the dog in sternal recumbency with the elbow flexed 30 degrees and slightly medially rotated. Position the dog in lateral recumbency with the elbow against the cassette for **B,** standard lateral and **C,** flexed lateral views.

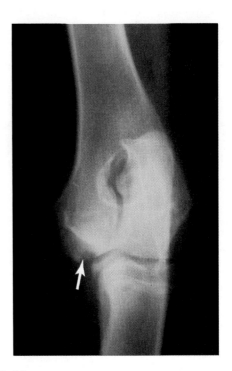

FIG. 30-23
Radiograph of an elbow with OCD of the medial portion of the humeral condyle. There is a radiolucent defect in the humeral condyle directly above the medial ulnar coronoid process (*arrow*).

the medial epicondyle, over the anconeus muscle. The median nerve and brachial artery and vein are visible in the surgical field and must be identified and protected.

Positioning

The limb is prepared from shoulder to elbow. The dog is positioned in dorsal recumbency with the affected limb suspended for draping. The limb is then released to allow access to the medial surface of the elbow.

SURGICAL TECHNIQUES

Exposure of the medial portion of the elbow joint can be obtained with several techniques. Tenotomy of the pronator teres muscle and incising the medial collateral ligament offer good exposure at the expense of the supporting structures. A muscle-splitting technique preserves the joint's supporting tendons and ligaments but limits exposure.

Osteotomy of the medial epicondyle provides the most extensive exposure, but it requires implantation of a lag screw or wire to replace the epicondyle. Regardless of technique used for exposure, the medial condyle of the humerus is examined and the flap of cartilage removed. Curettage is done only to remove fragments of cartilage from the edges of the lesion. The joint is flushed repeatedly to remove any small fragments. The coronoid process is inspected and removed if fragmented (see p. 923).

Transection of the Pronator Teres Muscle

Make an incision on the medial surface of the joint, starting at the medial epicondylar crest and extending distally over the medial epicondyle to the proximal radius (Fig. 30-24, A). Incise subcutaneous tissues along the same line. Identify the pronator teres muscle, median nerve, and brachial artery and vein (Fig. 30-24, B). Gently retract the nerve

Medial View

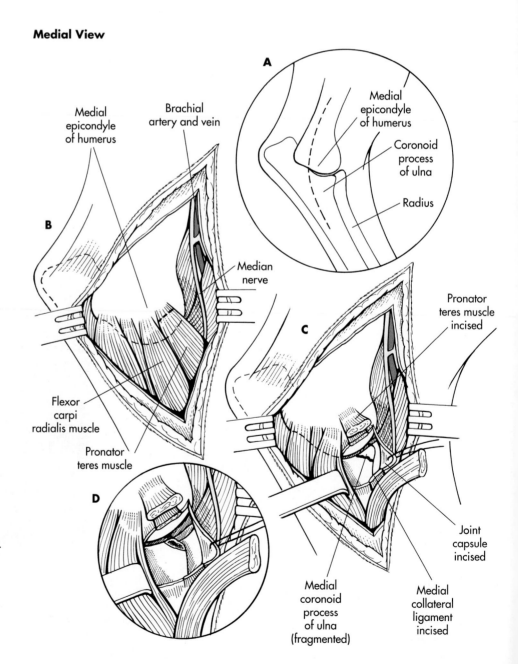

FIG. 30-24
A, To expose the medial aspect of the elbow joint via transection of the pronator teres muscle, make a skin incision on the medial surface of the joint, starting at the medial epicondylar crest and extending distally over the medial epicondyle. **B,** Gently retract the median nerve and brachial artery and vein cranially. **C,** Transect the pronator teres tendon and make an incision parallel to the humeral condyle through the joint capsule and collateral ligament to expose the fragmented coronoid process. **D,** Remove the fragment.

and vessels cranially. Transect the pronator teres tendon and retract the muscle distally, exposing the joint capsule and collateral ligament (Fig. 30-24, C). Make an incision parallel to the humeral condyle through the joint capsule and collateral ligament to expose the joint (Fig. 30-24, D). Curette the edges of the lesion and flush the joint. Close the joint capsule with interrupted absorbable sutures. Place several nonabsorbable sutures in the collateral ligament. Reattach the pronator teres tendon with a Bunnell or locking-loop nonabsorbable suture (see p. 1003). Suture fascia, subcutaneous tissue, and skin in separate layers.

Muscle Splitting

Incise skin and subcutaneous tissues as described above. Identify the demarcation between the flexor carpi radialis and superficial digital flexor muscles, and separate and retract them. Expose the joint capsule and incise it parallel to the muscle-splitting incision to expose the medial humeral condyle and coronoid process (Fig. 30-25). Curette the lesion and flush the joint. Suture the joint capsule with interrupted absorbable sutures. Suture fascia, subcutaneous tissue, and skin in separate layers.

Epicondyle Osteotomy

Incise skin and subcutaneous tissues as described above. Expose the epicondyle and plan the osteotomy to include the origin of the pronator teres and flexor carpi radialis muscles (Fig. 30-26, A, p. 922). If the proposed method of epicondylar reattachment is a lag screw, drill the hole before cutting the epicondyle. Make three cuts with an osteotome (Fig. 30-26, B). First, make proximal and caudal cuts perpendicular to the epicondyle to a depth of 5 mm. Then, make a cranial cut parallel to the surface of the

condyle and connect it with the previous cuts to produce a segment of bone. Take care to avoid damaging the articular surface when making your cuts. Retract the bone piece distally to expose the joint. Curette the lesion and flush the joint. Reattach the bone piece with a lag screw or tension-band wire (Fig. 30-26, C). Close the wound as described above. Obtain postoperative radiographs to document location of the implants.

SUTURE MATERIALS/SPECIAL INSTRUMENTS

An Oschner forceps is useful for grasping the flap. A bone curette is needed to curette the defect. For epicondylar osteotomy, necessary instruments include an osteotome and mallet, instrumentation for bone screws, Jacobs pin chuck, or high-speed drill, Kirschner wires, and orthopedic wire.

POSTOPERATIVE CARE AND ASSESSMENT

Immediate postoperative radiographs should be made if implants are used. The limb should be bandaged after surgery for up to 2 weeks to provide soft-tissue support and the animal should be confined for 4 weeks (Table 30-16). Gradual return to normal activity is recommended. Repeat radiographs are recommended 6 weeks after surgery if an osteotomy is performed. Implant removal may be necessary.

PROGNOSIS

Dogs treated conservatively for OCD of the distal humerus will usually have continued intermittent lameness and progressive DJD. In one study evaluating 30 dogs treated conservatively for elbow disease (OCD and/or FCP), 20 dogs were

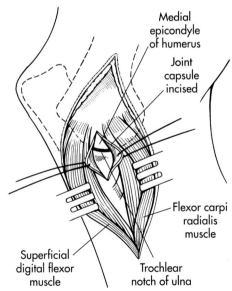

FIG. 30-25
To expose the medial aspect of the elbow joint via a muscle splitting approach, identify the demarcation between the flexor carpi radialis and superficial digital muscles, and separate and retract them. Expose the joint capsule and incise it parallel to the muscle splitting incision to expose the coronoid process.

TABLE 30-16
Important Information for Clients of Dogs with Osteochondrosis
There is strong evidence for a hereditary component in the etiology of FCP* and OCD.†
Bilateral elbow radiographs should be made because of the frequency of bilateral disease; however, unless the animal shows clinical signs, surgery of the opposite limb is not performed.
Surgical removal of the bone and cartilage pieces usually results in improved function of the limb if the dog is treated before there are extensive secondary degenerative changes in the joint.
After surgery the dog is confined and exercise is limited to short walks on a leash for 2 to 4 weeks.
Surgical treatment does not appear to alter the progression of DJD,‡ and the dog may require medical therapy after surgery.
Dogs usually function well as pets with DJD of the elbow, but they may not be appropriate as working or competitive sporting dogs.

*Fragmented coronoid process.
†Osteochondrosis.
‡Degenerative joint disease.

FIG. 30-26
To expose the medial aspect of the elbow joint via an epicondyle osteotomy, drill a hole for the lag screw prior to cutting the epicondyle. Make proximal and caudal cuts perpendicular to the epicondyle to a depth of 5 mm. Make a cranial cut parallel to the surface of the condyle and connect it with the previous cuts to produce a segment of bone. Take care to avoid the articular surface. **B,** Retract the bone piece distally to expose the joint. **C,** Reattach the bone piece with a lag screw or tension-band wire.

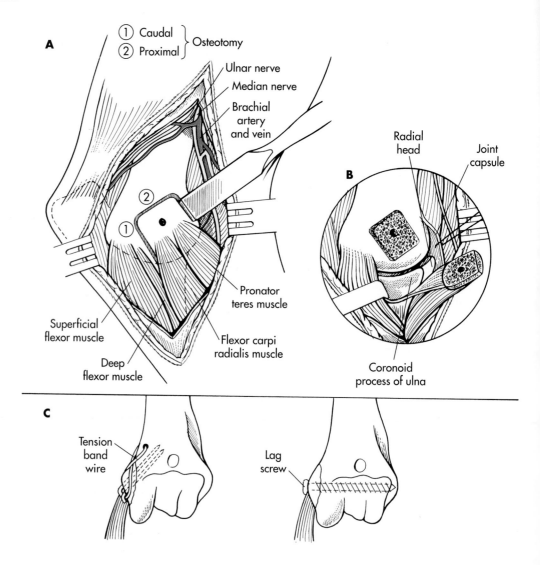

followed, and 70% of these were considered to be free from observable lameness (Mason et al, 1980). In other reports, dogs treated conservatively have had chronic lameness. Dogs treated surgically for OCD of the distal humerus usually have improved limb function; however, lameness may be evident after exercise. DJD is usually present and requires medical treatment (see above), but most dogs are functional pets and are only intermittently lame. Potential surgical complications include iatrogenic infection and implant irritation of the soft tissues.

☞ **N O T E ·** Counsel owners about the probability of progressive DJD in these dogs, even after surgery.

References

Mason TA et al: Osteochondrosis of the elbow joint in young dogs, *J Small Anim Pract* 21:641, 1980.

Suggested Reading

Boudrieau RJ, Hohn RB, Bardet JF: Osteochondritis dissecans of the elbow in the dog, *J Am Anim Hosp Assoc* 19:627, 1983.

Denny HR, Gibbs C: The surgical treatment of osteochondritis dissecans and ununited coronoid process in the canine elbow joint, *J Small Anim Pract* 21:323, 1980.

Guthrie S, Pidduck HG: Heritability of elbow osteochondrosis within a closed population of dogs, *J Small Anim Pract* 31:93, 1990.

Guthrie S, Plummer JM, Vaughn LC: Aetiopathogenesis of canine elbow osteochondrosis: a study of loose fragments removed at arthrotomy, *Res Vet Science* 52:284, 1992.

Houlton JEF: Osteochondrosis of the shoulder and elbow joints in dogs, *J Small Anim Pract* 25:399, 1985.

Olsson S-E: The early diagnosis of fragmented coronoid process and osteochondritis dissecans of the canine elbow joint, *J Am Anim Hosp Assoc* 19:616, 1983.

Piermattei DL: *An atlas of surgical approaches to the bones and joints of the dog and cat,* ed 3, Philadelphia, 1993, WB Saunders.

Probst CW et al: A simple medial approach to the canine elbow for treatment of fragmented coronoid process and osteochondritis dissecans, *J Am Anim Hosp Assoc* 25:331, 1989.

Studdert VP et al: Clinical features and heritability of osteochondrosis of the elbow in Labrador retrievers, *J Small Anim Pract* 32:557, 1991.

FRAGMENTED CORONOID PROCESS

DEFINITIONS

Fragmented coronoid process is a separation of the medial coronoid process from the ulna that results in lameness and degenerative joint disease.

SYNONYMS

Ununited coronoid process, fractured coronoid process, elbow dysplasia, FCP

GENERAL CONSIDERATIONS AND CLINICALLY RELEVANT PATHOPHYSIOLOGY

The etiology of this condition is unknown; however, two theories have been proposed. (1) Fragmented coronoid process (FCP) may result from an osteochondrosis (OCD) lesion where disruption of endochondral ossification of the coronoid process leaves it vulnerable to cartilage degeneration, necrosis, and fissure formation. (2) Developmental elbow incongruity has also been implicated in the pathophysiology of FCP. Uneven growth of the radius and ulna (causing the ulna to be longer than the radius) may result in an increase of weight-bearing forces on the medial coronoid process, which precipitates fragmentation. Fragmentation of the coronoid process results in a separate piece of cartilage and trabecular bone, which is attached to the annular ligament with fibrous tissue. Separation occurs through calcified trabeculae that are then covered, in part, with a thin layer of fibrous tissue. The end result is joint instability and development of degenerative joint disease (DJD). Cartilage of the opposing medial humeral condyle may be eroded by the loose coronoid fragment. Increasing amounts of periarticular osteophytes and soft-tissue fibrosis develop over time.

DIAGNOSIS
Clinical Presentation

Signalment. Large dogs (Labrador retrievers, Rottweillers, Bernese mountain dogs, Newfoundlands, golden retrievers, German shepherds, and chows) are usually affected. The disease process starts when the animal is immature, with clinical signs first becoming apparent at 5 to 7 months of age. However, the dog may not be presented for evaluation until it is 1 to 2 years of age and has DJD.

History. Forelimb lameness, which worsens after exercise, may be acute or chronic. Owners frequently complain that the dog is stiff in the morning or after rest. There may be a coincidental history of trauma. Some owners delay seeking veterinary help initially because the lameness is mild and they believe the animal will "grow out of it."

Physical Examination Findings

Lameness of one forelimb is usually evident. The gait may appear stiff or stilted if bilateral lameness is present because the animal may walk with shortened steps. Palpation of the elbows should include an evaluation of range of motion. De- creased ability to flex the elbow is indicative of DJD and may be one of the earliest signs of FCP. Crepitation during elbow flexion and extension may be felt if DJD is present. Joint effusion and periarticular soft-tissue swelling may be palpable. Manipulation of the joint is often painful, particularly when the medial coronoid process is palpated. It is important that the shoulder not be inadvertently flexed and extended during elbow manipulation to avoid mistaking shoulder pain for elbow pain.

Radiography

Many times the diagnosis is made on the basis of radiographic signs of degenerative joint disease. Radiographic views should include a standard lateral of the elbow, flexed lateral to expose the anconeal process, and cranial-caudal view made with the elbow flexed 30 degrees and slightly rotated medially (see Fig. 30-22). Radiographs of both elbows should be made because bilateral disease is common. Blunting, visible fragments, and osteophytes associated with the coronoid process may be visible (Fig. 30-27). The FCP cannot always be observed, and the diagnosis may be made by inference from the presence of DJD. The earliest radiographic sign that an animal with DJD may have FCP as an underlying cause is the presence of osteophytes on the anconeal process. Later signs include subchondral bone sclerosis, articular and periarticular osteophyte formation, joint space narrowing, joint effusion, and an increase in periarticular soft tissues.

Linear tomography and computed tomography (CT scan) may be helpful for identifying FCP. In one study, CT scans were more accurate for identifying FCP than plain radiographs, arthrography, or xeroradiography (Carpenter et al, 1993).

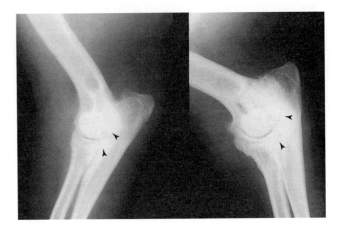

FIG. 30-27
Preoperative radiographs (*left*) of a dog with a fragmented coronoid process and degenerative joint disease. There is subchondral bone sclerosis caudal and distal to the trochlear notch of the ulna (*arrows*). Radiographs of the same dog, 8 years after surgical removal of the fragmented coronoid process (*right*). Note the progression of degenerative changes (*arrowheads*).

Laboratory Findings

Results of hematologic and serum biochemical analyses are normal in most affected animals. Results of arthrocentesis may include decreased synovial fluid viscosity, increased fluid volume, and increased numbers (up to 6000 to 9000 WBC/μl) of mononuclear phagocytic cells.

DIFFERENTIAL DIAGNOSIS

Other conditions affecting the elbow of immature dogs (OCD, UAP, combined UAP and FCP, and subluxation resulting from premature physeal closure) may produce similar clinical signs and must be differentiated from FCP. Other diseases affecting the forelimb of young growing dogs (OCD of the shoulder, panosteitis) should also be differentiated from FCP. These conditions usually can be differentiated radiographically.

MEDICAL MANAGEMENT

Dogs with mild clinical signs and radiographic evidence of advanced DJD should be treated for DJD. Many dogs with radiographic signs of DJD are asymptomatic and remain so for several years. Although owners should be apprised of the problem, they should also be reassured that the dog may function quite well as a pet with minimal treatment. When the dog is lame, confinement to a cage or run for 2 to 3 weeks, coupled with antiinflammatory drug therapy (i.e., aspirin; see Table 30-14), may be required for analgesia and for control of synovial inflammation. After the inflammatory phase of the disease is controlled, moderate regular exercise is important for maintaining muscle strength; however, exercise should be increased slowly to avoid causing lameness before muscle support has been established.

SURGICAL TREATMENT

Affected animals are candidates for surgery when they are persistently lame and have mild degenerative changes. Occasionally, animals with advanced DJD and persistent lameness not amenable to medical therapy may benefit from joint exploration and removal of a loose fragment. However, surgical treatment does not halt the progression of DJD, and continued medical therapy may be required in these patients. In one study there did not appear to be any correlation between severity of lameness before treatment, severity of radiographic signs, and type of lesion found at surgery. Surgical treatment did not appear to decrease the incidence of lameness when compared with medical therapy; however, dogs with chronic, moderate-to-severe lameness had a better prognosis if treated surgically (Read et al, 1990).

☞ **N O T E** • Although radiography may reveal bilateral disease, perform surgery only on the lame leg.

Preoperative Management

Most affected animals are young and require minimal preoperative workup before surgery.

Anesthesia

These dogs are usually young and generally healthy, and a variety of anesthetic regimens may be used (see p. 708).

Surgical Anatomy

Surgical anatomy of the elbow joint is provided on p. 919.

Positioning

The limb is prepared from shoulder to carpus. The dog is positioned in dorsal recumbency with the affected limb suspended for draping. The limb is then released to allow access to the medial surface of the elbow.

SURGICAL TECHNIQUES

Exposure of the medial coronoid process can be obtained with one of several techniques. Tenotomy of the pronator teres muscle and incising the medial collateral ligament offer good exposure, but at the expense of the supporting structures. A muscle-splitting technique has been proposed that preserves the joint's supporting tendons and ligaments but limits exposure. Osteotomy of the medial epicondyle provides the best exposure, but it requires implantation of a lag screw or wire to replace the epicondyle.

Transection of the Pronator Teres Muscle

Make an incision on the medial surface of the joint, starting at the medial epicondylar crest and extending distally over the medial epicondyle to the proximal radius. Protect the median nerve and brachial artery. Make an incision to the humeral condyle through the joint capsule and collateral ligament to expose the joint (see Fig. 30-24). Identify the coronoid process and any lesions on the medial humeral condyle. Remove the coronoid fragment. In removal of the coronoid fragment, the line of cleavage of the fragment may not be readily visible and may require prying with an elevator to allow identification. *Use rongeurs to remove the base of the medial coronoid process so that it matches the level of the radial head. This eliminates excessive forces on the medial coronoid process that are present when incongruities in radial and ulnar length exist. Close the wound by suturing the joint capsule with simple interrupted absorbable sutures. Place several nonabsorbable sutures in the collateral ligament. Reattach the pronator teres tendon with a Bunnell or locking-loop nonabsorbable suture (see p. 1003). Suture fascia, subcutaneous tissue, and skin in separate layers.* In chronic cases, osteophytes may obscure the line of cleavage and must be removed with a rongeur to allow fragment identification.

Muscle Splitting

Incise skin and subcutaneous tissues as described above. Identify the demarcation between the flexor carpi radialis and superficial digital muscles, and separate and retract them. Expose the joint capsule and incise it parallel to the muscle-splitting incision to expose the coronoid process (see Fig. 30-25). Remove the fragmented coronoid as described above. Suture the joint capsule with interrupted ab-

sorbable sutures. Suture fascia, subcutaneous tissue, and skin in separate layers.

Epicondyle Osteotomy

Incise skin and subcutaneous tissues as described above. Expose the epicondyle and perform an osteotomy (see Fig. 30-26). Predrill the hole for the lag screw before making the osteotomy. Remove the fragmented coronoid as described above. Reattach the bone piece with a lag screw or tension-band wire. Close the wound as described above.

SUTURE MATERIALS/SPECIAL INSTRUMENTS

An Oschner forceps is useful for grasping the flap. For epicondylar osteotomy, necessary instruments include an osteotome and mallet, instrument for bone screws, Jacobs pin chuck or high-speed drill, Kirschner wires, and orthopedic wire.

POSTOPERATIVE CARE AND ASSESSMENT

Immediate postoperative radiographs should be made if implants are used. The limb should be bandaged after surgery for 2 weeks to provide soft-tissue support, and the animal should be confined for 4 weeks. Gradual return to full activity is recommended. Repeat radiographs are recommended 6 weeks after surgery if an osteotomy is performed. Implant removal may be necessary.

PROGNOSIS

The prognosis for return to full function is guarded because of progressive DJD, which develops regardless of treatment method; however, most dogs function as pets and are only intermittently lame. Recurrent lameness can be treated with antiinflammatory drugs and analgesics (see above). Potential surgical complications include iatrogenic infection and soft-tissue irritation by implants.

☞ **N O T E** • Be sure to warn owners that most affected dogs will have progressive DJD, despite surgery.

References

Carpenter LG et al: Comparison of radiologic imaging techniques for diagnosis of fragmented medial coronoid process of the cubital joint in dogs, *J Am Vet Med Assoc* 203:78, 1993.

Read RA et al: Fragmentation of the medial coronoid process of the ulna in dogs: a study of 109 cases, *J Small Anim Pract* 31:330, 1990.

Suggested Reading

Grondalen J, Lingaas F: Arthrosis in the elbow of young rapidly growing dogs: a genetic investigation, *J Small Anim Pract* 32:460, 1991.

Huibregtse BA et al: The effect of treatment of fragmented coronoid process on the development of osteoarthritis of the elbow, *J Am Anim Hosp Assoc* 30:190, 1994.

Wind AP: Elbow incongruity and developmental elbow disease in the dog: part I, *J Am Anim Hosp Assoc* 22:711, 9186.

Wind AP, Packard ME: Elbow incongruity and developmental elbow disease in the dog: part II, *J Am Anim Hosp Assoc* 22:725, 1986.

Wind AP: Elbow dysplasia. In Slatter D, editor: *Textbook of small animal surgery*, ed 2, Philadelphia, 1993, WB Saunders.

UNUNITED ANCONEAL PROCESS

DEFINITIONS

Ununited anconeal process is a disease of large, growing dogs in which the anconeal process does not form a bony union with the proximal ulnar metaphysis.

SYNONYMS

Elbow dysplasia, UAP

GENERAL CONSIDERATIONS AND CLINICALLY RELEVANT PATHOPHYSIOLOGY

The anconeal process arises as a secondary center of ossification in the elbow at 11 to 12 weeks of age. It does not fuse to the ulna until 4 to 5 months of age; therefore, the diagnosis of ununited anconeal process (UAP) cannot be made before this age. Ununited anconeal process may be a manifestation of osteochondrosis (OCD) (see Table 30-15). Failure of timely endochondral ossification of the attachment of the anconeal process to the ulna leads to thickened cartilage, necrosis, and fissures. The stress of weight bearing on this abnormal cartilage can cause failure of ulna unification. Other possible etiological factors include heredity, hormonal influences, nutrition, and acute or chronic trauma.

In chondrodystrophic breeds (i.e., basset hounds), uneven growth of the radius and ulna is theorized to cause increased pressure or trauma to the anconeal process. Premature closure of the distal ulnar physis with shortening of the ulna results in distal subluxation of the ulnar trochlear notch. Pressure of the trochlear notch against the humeral condyles may cause a shearing stress on the anconeal process resulting in a fracture. A similar etiology may be a factor in UAP in nonchondrodystrophic breeds.

The ununited anconeal process may be free within the joint, but in most cases it is attached to the ulna with fibrous tissue. Ununited or fractured anconeal processes are unstable and result in secondary degenerative joint disease (DJD). Pathologic changes include joint effusion, chondromalacia, periarticular fibrosis, and osteophyte formation.

DIAGNOSIS
Clinical Presentation

Signalment. Large- to giant-breed male dogs are most commonly affected. The usual age of presentation is 6 to 12 months. Some older animals may be seen for lameness caused by secondary DJD.

History. The history is generally of intermittent lameness, of one or both forelimbs, that worsens after exercise. Owners frequently complain that the dog is stiff in the morning or after rest.

Physical Examination Findings

Lameness of one forelimb is usually evident. The gait may be stiff or stilted because elbow range of motion is decreased. This causes the elbow to circumduct laterally during the swing phase of the gait. The dog may sit and stand with the paw externally rotated. If DJD is present, there may be crepitation during elbow flexion and extension. Joint effusion and periarticular soft tissue swelling may be palpable. The animal may experience pain during joint manipulation, particularly during palpation over the anconeal process. It is important that the shoulder not be inadvertently flexed and extended during elbow manipulation to avoid mistaking shoulder pain for elbow pain.

Radiography

Radiographic views include a standard lateral of the elbow, a flexed lateral to expose the anconeal process, and a cranial-caudal view of the elbow made while the elbow is flexed 30 degrees and slightly rotated medially (see Fig. 30-22). Radiographs of both elbows should be made because bilateral disease occurs in 20% to 35% of cases (Thacher, 1985). UAP is visible as a lucent, indistinct line separating the anconeal process from the ulna. It is best visualized on the flexed lateral view (Fig. 30-28). Concurrent fragmented medial coronoid process (FCP) can occur. Signs of DJD may include subchondral bone sclerosis, articular and periarticular osteophyte formation, joint space narrowing, joint effusion, and an increase in periarticular soft tissues.

☞ **NOTE** · Be sure the animal is old enough for physeal closure before diagnosing UAP.

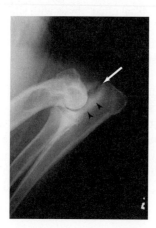

FIG. 30-28
A flexed lateral radiograph of an elbow with an ununited anconeal process. There is a lucent, irregular line between the anconeal process and the olecranon (*white arrow*), with subchondral bone sclerosis of the olecranon (*arrowheads*).

Laboratory Findings

Results of hematologic and serum biochemical analyses are normal in most affected animals. Results of arthrocentesis may include decreased synovial fluid viscosity, increased fluid volume, and increased numbers (up to 6000 to 9000 WBC/μl) of mononuclear phagocytic cells.

DIFFERENTIAL DIAGNOSIS

Differential diagnoses include OCD, FCP, combined UAP and FCP, and other diseases of young, growing dogs that affect the forelimb (i.e., OCD of the shoulder and panosteitis). These diseases can usually be differentiated radiographically.

MEDICAL MANAGEMENT

Dogs that are less than 5 or 6 months old when seen with suspected UAP may be treated with confinement and limited exercise. Follow-up radiographs should be made monthly to document either fusion of the anconeal process or UAP.

Medical therapy is generally used to treat older dogs with established DJD. Surgical removal of the anconeal process after extensive development of DJD does not stop the progression of osteoarthritis. Lame animals may be treated with confinement and aspirin (see Table 30-15). After the lameness has subsided, exercise should be gradually increased to strengthen surrounding musculature. Weight control is an important component of conservative therapy in UAP.

SURGICAL TREATMENT

Surgical removal of the anconeal process is recommended if UAP is diagnosed before the onset of extensive DJD. However, ulnar osteotomy to relieve pressure on the anconeal process may allow spontaneous healing of the fragment to the ulna. This procedure was first proposed for treatment of chondrodystrophic dogs, but more recently it has been applied to other dogs with UAP.

Preoperative Management

Most affected animals are young and require minimal preoperative workup before surgery.

Anesthesia

These animals are usually young, and a variety of anesthetic regimens can be used (see p. 708).

Surgical Anatomy

Landmarks for the skin incision when performing a lateral approach for removal of an ununited anconeal process include the lateral humeral epicondyle, epicondylar crest, and proximal radius. The deep branch of the radial nerve runs under the proximal-cranial border of the extensor carpi radialis muscle. The superficial branch of the radial nerve lies between the lateral head of the triceps and the brachialis muscle and can be visualized in the proximal portion of the incision. Landmarks for the combined medial approach are the medial epicondyle, epicondylar crest, and proximal radius. The median nerve and brachial artery and vein course cranial to the medial epicondyle and run under the pronator teres muscle. These structures must be identified and protected. The ulnar nerve courses caudal to the medial epicondyle, over the anconeus muscle, and is visualized during the medial approach to the anconeal process. The landmark for ulnar osteotomy is the caudal border of the ulna, which is easily palpated.

Positioning

For a lateral approach to the elbow, the animal is positioned in lateral recumbency, whereas for a medial approach and for ulnar osteotomy the animal is positioned in dorsal recumbency. The limb should be suspended for draping to facilitate limb manipulation during surgery.

SURGICAL TECHNIQUES
Removal of the Anconeal Process: Lateral Approach

Make an incision in the skin, starting proximal to the lateral humeral epicondyle. Curve the incision to follow the epicondylar crest and end it over the proximal portion of the radius. Incise subcutaneous tissues to expose the cranial border of the lateral head of the triceps muscle. Retract the cranial border of the triceps muscle caudally to expose the anconeus muscle. Incise the anconeus muscle and joint capsule along the epicondylar crest and retract them caudally to expose the anconeal process (Fig. 30-29). Grasp the process with towel forceps or an Oschner forceps and remove it. Fibrous tissue attachments to the ulna may have to be incised before the anconeal process can be mobilized. If necessary, smooth the remaining bone surface with a file. Flush the joint. Suture the joint capsule and anconeus muscle to the extensor carpi radialis muscle. Suture subcutaneous tissues and skin in separate layers.

Removal of the Anconeal Process and Medial Coronoid Process: Combined Medial Approach

Expose the medial coronoid process using one of the techniques described on p. 920. After closing the craniomedial compartment of the elbow, approach the caudomedial compartment by retracting the ulnar nerve cranially and exposing the cranial border of the medial head of the triceps muscle. Retract the triceps muscle caudally to expose the caudal border of the medial epicondylar crest and origin of the anconeus muscle. Incise the anconeus muscle and joint capsule parallel to the medial epicondylar crest, leaving 2 to 4 mm of tissue attached to the crest for closure (Fig. 30-30). Remove the anconeal process. Suture the anconeus muscle and joint capsule in one layer to close the joint.

Ulnar Osteotomy

Make a skin incision along the caudal border of the ulna, beginning medial to the tuber olecranon and ending at the middiaphysis of the ulna. Incise subcutaneous tissues and fascia along the same line. Incise attachments of the flexor carpi ulnaris and ulnaris lateralis along the medial and lateral borders of the ulna and elevate the muscles to expose the joint capsule. Incise the joint capsule on both sides of the ulna to expose the distal trochlear notch area (see p. 813). Make an oblique osteotomy of the ulna distal to

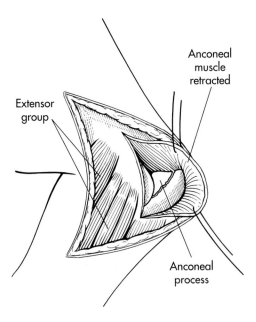

FIG. 30-29
For a lateral approach to the caudal compartment on the elbow, make a skin incision starting proximal to the lateral humeral epicondyle and curving to follow the epicondylar crest. End the incision over the proximal portion of the radius. Incise the anconeus muscle and joint capsule along the epicondylar crest and retract them caudally to expose the anconeal process.

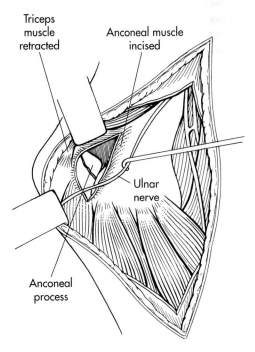

FIG. 30-30
For a medial approach to the caudal compartment of the elbow, retract the ulnar nerve cranially and triceps muscle caudally to expose the caudal border of the medial epicondylar crest and origin of the anconeus muscle. Incise the anconeus muscle and joint capsule parallel to the medial epicondylar crest to expose the anconeal process.

the trochlear notch, running from cranial-distal to caudal-proximal with an oscillating saw or Gigli wire. A gap should occur at the osteotomy site. If necessary, elevate the interosseous ligament to free the proximal ulna so it can move into position. Drive a small, smooth pin or Kirschner wire from the tuber olecranon down the medullary canal, across the fracture gap, and into the medullary canal of the distal ulna (see p. 935). The smooth pin and direction of the oblique osteotomy allow the forces of the surrounding musculature to exert a dynamic effect on the proximal ulna and slide it into position with the humerus, without causing angular distraction of the proximal ulna. *Suture the joint capsule. Suture flexor carpi ulnaris fascia to the ulnaris lateralis fascia over the caudal border of the ulna. Suture subcutaneous tissue and skin separately.*

SUTURE MATERIALS/SPECIAL INSTRUMENTS

An Oschner forceps is useful for extracting the ununited anconeal process. Rongeurs and bone files are used to smooth the area. A Gigli wire or oscillating saw and intramedullary pins are needed for ulnar osteotomy.

POSTOPERATIVE CARE AND ASSESSMENT

Immediate postoperative radiographs should be made if implants are used. The limb should be bandaged after surgery for 2 weeks to provide soft-tissue support, and the animal should be confined for 4 weeks. Repeat radiographs are recommended 6 weeks after surgery if an osteotomy is performed. Implant removal may be necessary.

PROGNOSIS

The prognosis for dogs with UAP is guarded for normal limb function because secondary DJD will occur. The prognosis for limb function is good in most dogs that are less than 1 year old when treated surgically by removal of the anconeal process. However, despite treatment, loss of range of motion, crepitation, and progressive DJD occurs. Potential surgical complications include iatrogenic infection and irritation of the soft tissues by implants.

☞ **N O T E** · Be sure to warn owners that progressive DJD is common in affected dogs, despite surgery.

Suggested Reading

Gilson SD, Piermattei DL, Schwarz PD: Treatment of humeroulnar subluxation with a dynamic proximal ulnar osteotomy, *Vet Surg* 18:114, 1989.

Guthrie S: Some radiographic and clinical aspects of ununited anconeal process, *Vet Record* 124:661, 1989.

Piermattei DL: *An atlas of surgical approaches to the bones and joints of the dog and cat*, ed 3, Philadelphia, 1993, WB Saunders.

Roy RG, Wallace LJ, Johnston GR: A retrospective long-term evaluation of ununited anconeal process excision on the canine elbow, *Vet Comp Orthop Trauma* 7:94, 1994.

Sjöstrom L, Kosstrom H, Kollberg M: Ununited anconeal process in the dog: pathogenesis and treatment by osteotomy of the ulna, *Vet Comp Orthop Trauma* 8:170, 1995.

Thacher C: Ununited anconeal process. In Slatter D, editor: *Textbook of small animal surgery*, Philadelphia, 1985, WB Saunders.

Wind AP: Elbow dysplasia. In Slatter D, editor: *Textbook of small animal surgery*, ed 2, Philadelphia, 1993, WB Saunders.

TRAUMATIC ELBOW LUXATION

DEFINITIONS

Traumatic elbow luxation is usually associated with disruption of the elbow joint because of lateral displacement of the radius and ulna with respect to the humerus.

SYNONYMS

Dislocated elbow

GENERAL CONSIDERATIONS AND CLINICALLY RELEVANT PATHOPHYSIOLOGY

Trauma to the elbow that results in rupture or avulsion of one or both collateral ligaments allows luxation of the radius and ulna (Table 30-17). The radius and ulna usually luxate laterally because the large medial condyle of the humerus generally prevents medial luxation. The bone to which the collateral ligaments attach may be avulsed, or rupture of the ligaments may occur. In severe injuries, the origins of the extensor or flexor muscles may be ruptured or avulsed from the humeral condyle as well. Damage to the cartilage may occur at the time of injury. Chronic luxation results in chondromalacia, articular cartilage destruction, and secondary degenerative joint disease (DJD).

DIAGNOSIS
Clinical Presentation

Signalment. Any age or breed of dog may be affected, but traumatic elbow luxations are rare in cats. Immature animals tend to have physeal fractures rather than traumatic luxations.

TABLE 30-17

Important Considerations in Traumatic Elbow Luxation

Closed reduction of the elbow should be attempted as soon as possible.
Stability of the elbow should be carefully evaluated after reduction.
The elbow's response to trauma is DJD* and decreased range of motion.
Prognosis is good if the elbow is quickly reduced and stabilized.

*Degenerative joint disease.

History. The history usually includes trauma such as vehicular or dogfight encounter. The animal usually is acutely
lame on the affected limb.

Physical Examination Findings

Affected dogs are unable to bear weight on the affected limb,
and the elbow is carried in a flexed position. The forelimb is
abducted and externally rotated. Palpation of the elbow reveals a prominent radial head, indistinct lateral humeral-
condyle, and lateral displacement of the olecranon. Most animals are in pain and resist elbow extension.

Radiography

Lateral displacement of the radius and ulna is apparent on a
cranial-caudal view of the elbow (Fig. 30-31). The lateral
view shows an uneven joint space between the humeral
condyle and radius and ulna. Avulsion fractures of the medial or lateral condyle of the humerus may be evident. Because of the traumatic etiology, thoracic radiographs before
surgery are usually indicated.

Laboratory Findings

Significant laboratory abnormalities are not associated with
elbow luxation but may be associated with the trauma that
caused the injury.

DIFFERENTIAL DIAGNOSIS

Traumatic elbow luxations must be differentiated from elbow fractures.

MEDICAL MANAGEMENT

Most luxated elbows can be reduced by closed manipulation
if treated within the first few days after injury. However, dogs
with avulsion fractures may be candidates for open reduction
and stabilization of the fractured bone in order to provide
greater immediate stability. Closed reduction may be facilitated by suspending the limb from an intravenous-drip stand
for 5 to 10 minutes to allow muscle relaxation; the dog is then
placed in lateral recumbency with the affected limb up. The
objective during manual reduction is to hook the anconeal
process between the condyles. *To reduce the elbow, determine the position of the anconeal process in relation to the
humeral condyles (Fig. 30-32, A). Flex the elbow to about
100 degrees and inwardly rotate the antebrachium (Fig.
30-32, B). After the anconeal process hooks over the lateral
condyle, extend the elbow slightly. Abduct and inwardly rotate the antebrachium while placing medial pressure over
the head of the radius to force it under the humeral capitulum and into the reduced position (Fig. 30-32, C). After the
elbow is reduced, evaluate stability provided by the collateral ligaments by flexing the elbow and paw to 90 degrees
and rotating the paw medially and laterally.* If the lateral
collateral ligament is intact, the paw can be rotated medially
to about 70 degrees (vs 140 degrees if it is ruptured). If the
medial collateral ligament is intact, the paw can be rotated
laterally to 45 degrees; rupture allows the paw to be rotated
laterally to about 90 degrees.

After the elbow has been reduced, radiographs should be
taken to document the location of the radius and ulna and to
evaluate joint stability. Mild subluxation, or widening of the
joint space, usually responds to immobilization. Marked
subluxation is an indication for open reduction and internal
stabilization. If reduction is achieved, the limb should be positioned with the elbow in extension and suppported with a
soft, padded bandage and spica splint for 2 weeks (see
p. 707). After bandage removal, range-of-motion exercises
should be performed daily. Exercise should be limited for 3
to 4 weeks after bandage removal. Complications of closed
reduction may include reluxation and DJD.

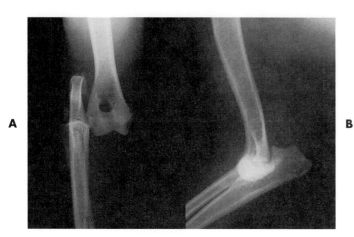

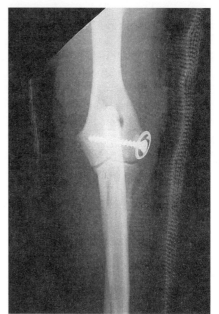

FIG. 30-31
A, Craniocaudal and **B,** lateral radiographs of a luxated
elbow in a dog. The radius and ulna are luxated laterally.
On the lateral view, there is loss of the humeroradial joint
space. **C,** Open reduction and stabilization of the collateral
ligament with a screw and Teflon washer was performed.

FIG. 30-32
A, To close reduce a laterally luxated elbow **B,** flex the elbow and inwardly rotate the ante-brachium to hook the anconeal process into the olecranon fossa. **C,** Then extend the elbow slightly and abduct and inwardly rotate the antebrachium while placing pressure on the radial head.

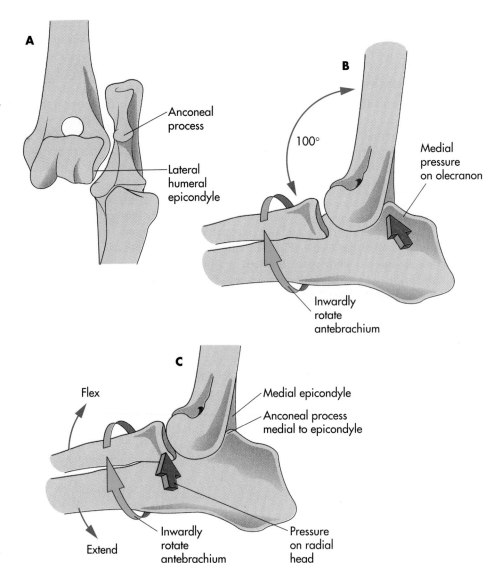

SURGICAL TREATMENT

Open reduction of a luxated elbow is indicated when it is impossible to achieve closed reduction. This is most common when the luxation is chronic. Open reduction should also be considered when the elbow is unstable after closed reduction, or when stabilization of an avulsion fracture will improve joint stability. Elbow arthrodesis should be considered when there is severe damage to the cartilage from the trauma of luxation. It is also performed when fixation of articular fractures of the elbow is unsuccessful and when there is chronic DJD that is unresponsive to medical management. Elbow arthrodesis limits the dog's function because a normal range of motion in this joint is essential for a normal gait. It is a salvage procedure that is done as a last resort and as an alternative to amputation.

☞ **N O T E** · Excessive instability of the joint indicates the need for open stabilization of surrounding joint tissues. If the joint is stable despite collateral ligament damage, immobilization will allow periarticular fibrosis and some degree of stability; however, this may not provide sufficient stability for large, active dogs.

Preoperative Management

The extent of the preoperative workup is dependent on the animal's overall health. Laboratory evaluation, thoracic radiographs, and an electrocardiogram (ECG) evaluation may be indicated before anesthetizing traumatized animals. Stabilization of the trauma patient is more important than reduction of the elbow. However, as soon as the patient is stabilized, reduction should be attempted.

Anesthesia

General anesthesia is necessary for closed reduction to achieve the profound muscle relaxation necessary for manipulation of the elbow into position. Neuromuscular blockage may be necessary in some cases. Special care should be exercised in anesthetizing older animals or those with concurrent injuries.

Surgical Anatomy

Anatomical landmarks for open reduction of elbow luxations are the radial head, olecranon and anconeal processes, and lateral humeral condyle. The deep branch of the radial nerve runs under the proximal-cranial border of the exten-

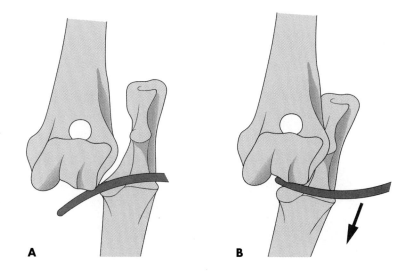

FIG. 30-33
A and **B,** Open reduction of the elbow may be accomplished using a blunt, curved instrument as a lever. **C** and **D,** Or perform an olecranon osteotomy to eliminate the pull of the triceps muscle during reduction.

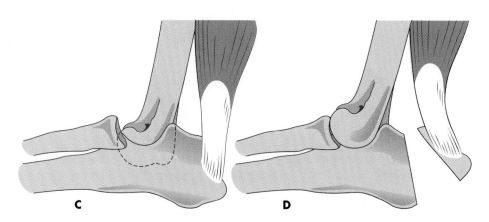

sor carpi radialis muscle. The superficial branch of the radial nerve lies between the lateral head of the triceps and the brachialis muscle and may be exposed in the cranial portion of the incision. It must be identified and protected during surgery. The median nerve and brachial artery and vein course cranially to the medial epicondyle, and the ulnar nerve courses caudally to the medial epicondyle, over the anconeus muscle. These structures must be visualized and protected if a medial approach is made to repair the medial collateral ligament.

Positioning

The dog is positioned in lateral recumbency with the affected leg up. The leg should be prepared from shoulder to carpus.

SURGICAL TECHNIQUES
Open Reduction of Elbow Luxations

Make a lateral approach to the caudal compartment of the elbow (see p. 927). Reduce the elbow as described for closed reduction, above. Protect the articular cartilage during reduction. If muscle contraction and subsequent overriding are severe, use a blunt instrument to gently lever the radial head into position (Fig. 30-33, A and B). If reduction is not achieved, perform an olecranon osteotomy to eliminate the pull of the triceps muscle (Fig. 30-33, C and D), or use a fracture distractor with pins placed in the humeral di-

aphysis and proximal ulna (see p. 759). After reduction, flush the joint and assess stability. Stability may be enhanced by primary repair of the lateral collateral ligament. Identify the ends of the ligaments and appose them with nonabsorbable sutures in a locking-loop or Bunnell pattern (see p. 1003). If the ligament has torn from its attachment to the bone, secure it to the bone with a screw and spiked Teflon washer. If the collateral ligament is beyond repair, replace it with two screws and a figure-eight wire or heavy (No. 1 or No. 2) nonabsorbable suture (Fig. 30-34, A and B). Reduce avulsion fractures of the humeral condyle and secure them with a lag screw or tension-band wire technique (Fig. 30-34, C and D). Suture torn muscles. Suture fascia, subcutaneous tissue, and skin in separate layers. If additional stability is necessary, expose the medial surface of the elbow (see p. 927) and repair or replace the medial collateral ligament.

Elbow Arthrodesis

Predetermine the angle of arthrodesis by measuring the standing angle of the opposite elbow. Make a caudolateral approach to the joint (see p. 927) and osteotomize the olecranon (Fig. 30-35, A). Expose the joint by incising the lateral collateral ligament and elevating the origins of the extensor muscles. Remove the cartilage from the distal humerus, radial head, and trochlear notch with a

FIG. 30-34
A and **B,** To stabilize the elbow, replace collateral ligaments by using two screws and a figure-eight wire. **C** and **D,** To secure an avulsed fragment, use a lag screw with a spiked Teflon washer.

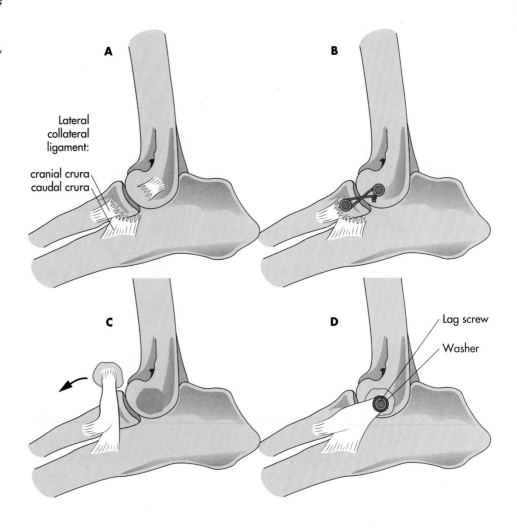

Lateral collateral ligament:

cranial crura
caudal crura

Lag screw

Washer

high-speed burr. Follow the contours of the joint. Temporarily stabilize the elbow in the correct position with a pin placed through the humerus and into the ulna. Contour a plate to fit onto the caudal surface of the humerus, over the joint, and onto the caudal surface of the ulna. Place at least three screws in the humerus and three in the ulna. Use additional screws as lag screws to gain compression where they cross the arthrodesis site (Fig. 30-35, B). Check limb alignment, rotation, and angulation before securing fixation. Harvest and place a cancellous bone graft at the arthrodesis site. The most accessible site for cancellous bone harvest is the ipsilateral proximal humerus (see p. 761). Reattach the olecranon to the ulna on either side of the plate with a tension-band wire (see p. 747).

SUTURE MATERIALS/SPECIAL INSTRUMENTS

Instruments needed for open reduction of the elbow include an osteotome and mallet, pin chuck, Kirschner wires, orthopedic wire, and bone screws and instrumentation for their insertion. A fracture distractor may be helpful in some cases. For arthrodesis a high-speed drill, burrs, and plating equipment are necessary.

POSTOPERATIVE CARE AND ASSESSMENT

After open reduction, postoperative radiographs should be made to document the location of the radius and ulna and evaluate implant position. After surgery the limb should be positioned with the elbow in extension and supported with a soft, padded bandage for several days. If questionable stability was achieved, a spica splint can be applied to the limb for 2 weeks. After bandage removal, joint flexion and extension should be performed daily, but exercise should be limited for 3 to 4 weeks. Potential surgical complications include recurrent luxation, infection, decreased range of motion of the elbow, irritation or migration of implants, and secondary DJD.

After arthrodesis, radiographs of the elbow should be taken to evaluate implant position and limb alignment. A soft, padded bandage should be applied for a few days after surgery. If there is concern about the stability of the implants, a spica splint can be applied for 6 weeks or until there is radiographic evidence of bone healing. Activity should be limited until the arthrodesis has healed. Complications of arthrodesis include iatrogenic infection, delayed union or nonunion, implant migration, implant irritation to soft tis-

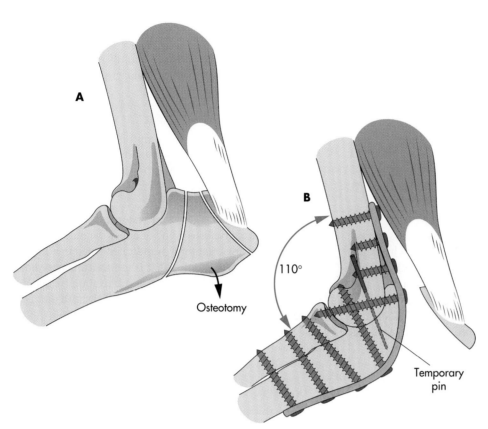

FIG. 30-35
A, To arthrodese the elbow, make two osteotomies and remove a portion of the proximal ulna. Temporarily stabilize the elbow in the correct position with a pin placed through the ulna and into the humerus. **B,** Contour a plate to fit onto the caudal surface of the humerus and onto the caudal surface of the ulna. Place at least three screws in the humerus and three in the ulna. Use additional screws as lag screws to gain compression across the arthrodesis site.

110°

Osteotomy

Temporary
pin

sues, fracture of the bone at either end of the plate, and increased degenerative changes in the limb's distal joints, which are forced to compensate for the loss of elbow range of motion.

PROGNOSIS

The prognosis after a stable closed reduction is good for normal limb function; however, there will be variable development of DJD and limited range of motion. The prognosis after an unstable closed reduction is fair for normal limb function. Smaller, less active dogs have a better prognosis because the periarticular fibrosis that occurs is likely to be adequate to maintain the elbow in position, whereas it may not be adequate in large or active dogs. DJD and limited range of motion are also more likely to occur in large animals. The prognosis after surgical reduction and stabilization of the elbow is dependent on chronicity of the luxation and severity of joint damage. Most dogs have good limb function after surgery. Smaller, less active dogs have a better prognosis than do larger, more active dogs. Varying degrees of DJD and limited range of joint motion commonly develop after surgery.

Suggested Reading

Billings LA et al: Clinical results after reduction of traumatic elbow luxation in nine dogs and one cat, *J Am Anim Hosp Assoc* 28:137, 1992.

Komtebedde J, Vasseur PB. Elbow luxation. In Slatter D, editor: *Textbook of small animal surgery*, ed 2, Philadelphia, 1993, WB Saunders.

ELBOW LUXATION/SUBLUXATION CAUSED BY PREMATURE CLOSURE OF THE DISTAL ULNAR OR RADIAL PHYSES

DEFINITIONS

Elbow luxation or subluxation may be associated with **asynchronous radial or ulnar growth** caused by premature closure of one of the distal physes. An **osteotomy** is a cut made through bone. An **ostectomy** is removal of a section of bone.

SYNONYMS

Elbow incongruity

GENERAL CONSIDERATIONS AND CLINICALLY RELEVANT PATHOPHYSIOLOGY

Two syndromes are grouped under elbow subluxation or incongruity. One syndrome is observed as a part of the pathophysiology of premature closure of the distal ulnar or radial physes after trauma in immature dogs (see p. 818). The other occurs in chondrodystrophic breeds and is caused by asynchronous growth of the radius and ulna with no apparent injury to the growth plate (Table 30-18). This asynchronous growth results in incongruity of the elbow joint because either the radius or ulna is inappropriately short. Untreated, elbow incongruity causes instability of the joint and development of secondary degenerative joint disease (DJD).

TABLE 30-18

Important Considerations in Elbow Incongruity

Elbow incongruity is the most likely cause of elbow pain and lameness in dogs with asynchronous radial and ulnar growth.
Elbow incongruity leads to secondary DJD.*
Ulnar osteotomy or ostectomy is designed to allow dynamic reduction of the elbow.

*Degenerative joint disease.

When the ulna is too short, the trochlear notch is pulled distally and the anconeal process impinges on the humeral trochlea. In some dogs this may be associated with an ununited anconeal process (UAP). When the radius is too short, the radial head is pulled distally and does not articulate with the humeral capitulum. The trochlea of the humerus then rests directly on the coronoid process of the ulna, which transmits all of the force of weight bearing.

DIAGNOSIS
Clinical Presentation

Signalment. This condition occurs in immature dogs with open physes. Any breed of dog affected with premature closure of the physes after trauma may present with subluxation of the elbow. Bassett hounds and other chondrodystrophic dogs are more frequently affected with asynchronous growth of the radius and ulna that is not attributable to trauma. The animal may be presented for examination at the onset of the problem or as an older animal with established secondary DJD.

History. Affected animals often have a history of intermittent lameness. Owners may relate the lameness to trauma.

Physical Examination Findings

Affected dogs exhibit varying degrees of lameness. A gross deformity of the limb may be present, depending on the physeal plate affected and the relationship of the injury to the animal's growth. Even if there is no limb deformity, the animal is usually lame and sensitive to joint manipulation because of the elbow incongruence. Crepitation and limited range of motion may be present during elbow manipulation.

Radiography

Radiographs of the radius and ulna should include the carpus and elbow to determine the exact configuration and cause of the elbow incongruity. Radiographs of the contralateral forelimb can often be used to compare the affected limb with a normal one; however, bilateral disease may be present.

Laboratory Findings

Specific laboratory abnormalities are not found with this condition.

DIFFERENTIAL DIAGNOSIS

Differential diagnoses in large dogs include fragmented coronoid process, UAP, or osteochondrosis. Other conditions that may show similar clinical signs in small dogs include trauma and DJD.

MEDICAL MANAGEMENT

Medical treatment is aimed at symptomatic treatment of the resultant DJD, but it has no effect on the primary problem of joint malarticulation (see Table 30-5).

SURGICAL TREATMENT

Surgical treatment is directed at restoring elbow congruity by doing a corrective osteotomy of either the radius or ulna. Ulnar-lengthening osteotomy is indicated when the cause of elbow incongruity is an ulna that is too short. Ulnar-shortening ostectomy is performed when subluxation (widening) of the humeroradial joint is caused by radial shortening. Because this procedure results in shortening of the limb, the animal should be evaluated to determine whether limb shortening would be detrimental. If so, a lengthening osteotomy of the radius should be performed (see p. 822).

Preoperative Management

Affected animals are young and require minimal preoperative workup prior to surgery.

Anesthesia

These animals are usually young and generally healthy, and a variety of anesthetic regimens can be used (see p. 708).

Surgical Anatomy

Landmarks for ulnar-lengthening osteotomy include the caudal border of the ulna, which is palpable, and the trochlear notch, which can be exposed surgically by muscle elevation and must be avoided when the osteotomy is performed.

Positioning

The dog is positioned in dorsal recumbency with the affected leg suspended for draping. The leg is prepared from shoulder to carpus.

SURGICAL TECHNIQUES
Ulnar-lengthening Osteotomy

Make a skin incision along the caudal border of the ulna, beginning medial to the tuber olecranon and ending at the ulnar middiaphysis. Incise subcutaneous tissue and fascia along the same line. Incise the attachments of the flexor carpi ulnaris and ulnaris lateralis along the medial and lateral borders of the ulna and elevate the muscles to expose the joint capsule. Incise the joint capsule on both sides of the ulna to expose the distal trochlear notch area (see p. 813). Make an oblique osteotomy of the ulna distal to the trochlear notch, running from cranial-distal to caudal-proximal, with an oscillating saw or Gigli wire (Fig. 30-36). A gap should form at the osteotomy site. If necessary, elevate

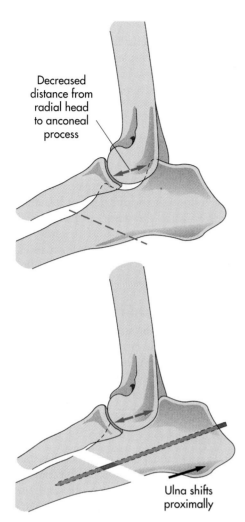

FIG. 30-36
For an ulnar-lengthening osteotomy, make an oblique osteotomy of the ulna distal to the coronoid process. Stabilize the ulna with a small intramedullary pin.

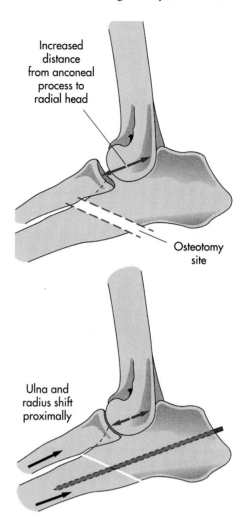

FIG. 30-37
For an ulnar shortening ostectomy, make two oblique osteotomies of the ulna distal to the coronoid process. Remove a length of bone sufficient to allow reduction of the radial head. Stabilize the ulna with a small intramedullary pin.

the interosseous ligament to free the proximal ulna so that it can move into position. Drive a small, smooth pin or Kirschner wire from the tuber olecranon down the medullary canal, across the fracture gap, and into the medullary canal of the distal ulna. The smooth pin and the oblique direction of the osteotomy allow the forces of the surrounding musculature to exert a dynamic effect on the proximal ulna and slide it into position with the humerus, without causing angular distraction of the proximal ulna. *Suture the joint capsule. Suture the flexor carpi ulnaris fascia to the ulnaris lateralis fascia over the caudal border of the ulna. Suture the subcutaneous tissue and skin separately.*

Ulnar-shortening ostectomy

Shortening the ulna allows the radial head to come into contact with the humeral capitulum. *Approach the ulna as described earlier for the ulnar-lengthening osteotomy. Using an oscillating saw or Gigli wire, resect a segment of ulna that is greater*

in length than the measured distance from the radial head to the humeral capitulum. Drive a small, smooth pin or Kirschner wire from the tuber olecranon down the medullary canal, across the fracture gap, and into the medullary canal of the distal ulna (Fig. 30-37). The smooth pin allows the forces of the surrounding musculature to exert a dynamic effect on the proximal ulna, causing it to collapse into the ostectomy site.

SUTURE MATERIALS/SPECIAL INSTRUMENTS

Instruments needed include a Gigli wire or oscillating saw, Steinmann pins, and a pin chuck or power drill for pin insertion.

POSTOPERATIVE CARE AND ASSESSMENT

Postoperative radiographs should be taken to evaluate the position of the ulna. Obvious changes in position may not be evident until several days after surgery. A soft padded bandage should be applied to the limb postoperatively. Early motion of the elbow is important for dynamic reduction of the subluxated elbow; therefore, leash activity should be encouraged. Serial radiographs should be made until ostectomy healing has occurred. Implant removal can be done after bone healing.

☞ **N O T E** · Radiographs taken 48 to 72 hours after surgery will demonstrate the effect of motion on ulnar position.

PROGNOSIS

Without surgery, the abnormal anatomy of the elbow will cause DJD and lameness. If surgery is performed before DJD is established, the prognosis is good for relatively normal limb function, although some DJD will usually occur. After DJD is established, periodic treatment with analgesics and antiinflammatory drugs may be necessary (see Table 30-5). Potential surgical complications include iatrogenic infection, implant migration, delayed union or nonunion of the osteotomy, and implant irritation of soft tissues. If the IM pin irritates the triceps tendon, it should be removed.

Suggested Reading

Gilson SD, Piermattei DL, Schwarz PD: Treatment of humeroulnar subluxation with a dynamic proximal ulnar osteotomy, *Vet Surg* 18:114, 1989.

CONGENITAL ELBOW LUXATION

DEFINITIONS

Congenital elbow luxation results in lateral rotation of the proximal ulna and subluxation or luxation of the humeroulnar joint.

SYNONYMS

Congenital elbow luxation, **congenital elbow malformation**

GENERAL CONSIDERATIONS AND CLINICALLY RELEVANT PATHOPHYSIOLOGY

The etiology of congenital elbow luxation is unknown. The bone malpositioning occurs at a young age, and because the bones do not articulate normally, congruent joint surfaces do not form. At approximately 3 months of age, secondary remodeling occurs and degenerative changes begin to develop. Pathology varies with chronicity of the condition. The olecranon is rotated lateral to the distal humerus, and the trochlear notch does not contact the humeral condyles. There may be (1) hypoplasia and remodeling of the trochlea and trochlear notch; (2) hypoplasia of the medial humeral condyle, with

stretching of the medial collateral ligament and joint capsule; (3) hyperplasia of the lateral humeral condyle, with contracture of the lateral joint capsule and lateral collateral ligament; (4) contracture and displacement of the triceps muscle; and (5) degenerative changes of the articular cartilage.

DIAGNOSIS
Clinical Presentation

Signalment. Small breeds of dogs are affected: pugs, Yorkshire terriers, Boston terriers, miniature poodles, Pomeranians, Chihuahuas, cocker spaniels, and English bulldogs. The condition can be unilateral or bilateral and is usually recognized when the puppy begins to walk at 3 to 6 weeks of age.

History. There is a history of inability to extend the front leg(s) and difficulty with walking because of the crouching position.

Physical Examination Findings

Affected puppies carry the affected forelimb in flexion. If the condition is bilateral, the puppy supports weight on the caudomedial aspect of the forelimbs. The elbows cannot be extended. The olecranon is located on the lateral aspect of the limb and may be mistaken for the lateral humeral condyle. The condition is usually not painful.

Radiography

Lateral and craniocaudal radiographs of the elbow show lateral displacement and rotation of the olecranon, with varying degrees of contact between the ulna and humerus (Fig. 30-38). Usually the radial head is in contact with the humerus, although this may change as the animal matures. Secondary degenerative joint disease (DJD) is apparent in chronic cases.

Laboratory Findings

Abnormal laboratory findings are uncommon.

DIFFERENTIAL DIAGNOSIS

Differential diagnoses include hemimelia (congenital segmental deficiency of the radius or ulna), ectrodactyly (congenital splitting of the limb), and previous fracture and malunion of the limb.

MEDICAL MANAGEMENT

Conservative therapy (splints and bandages) does not alter the course of disease. Joint reduction and stabilization should be done as soon as possible, before secondary degenerative changes and joint remodeling occur (usually before the animal is 4 months of age). The type of reduction technique used depends on the pathology present. Closed reduction can be successful if the joint can be manipulated into position. Closed reduction is indicated in dogs that have only mild changes in bone and soft tissue. The olecranon should be rotated medially into position and secured by placing a transarticular pin from the caudal aspect of the olecranon,

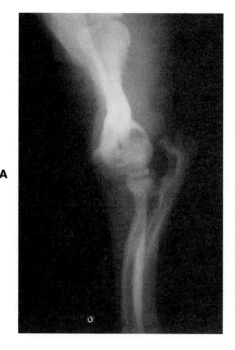
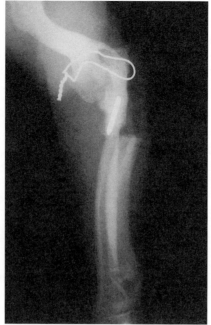

FIG. 30-38
A, Preoperative craniocaudal radiograph of the forelimb of a dog with congenital elbow luxation. **B,** Craniocaudal radiograph of the forelimb after reduction of the elbow and translocation of the olecranon.

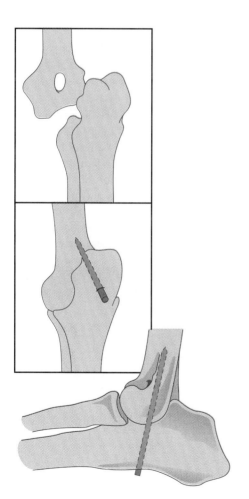

FIG. 30-39
A transarticular pin can be placed to hold the ulna in position after manual reduction of a congenitally luxated elbow.

TABLE 30-19
Important Considerations in Congenital Elbow Luxation
Immediate surgical treatment provides the best outcome.
Repositioning the ulna results in improved limb function because the pull of the triceps muscle is redirected.
Limited range of motion and DJD* occur even with surgery.
*Degenerative joint disease.

through the olecranon, and into the humerus. The pin is left in place for 10 to 14 days (Fig. 30-39).

SURGICAL TREATMENT

Open reduction and corrective osteotomy are used when the joint cannot be manually replaced (Table 30-19). Techniques for open reduction and stabilization vary, depending on the degree of pathology present. Techniques used include lateral release of soft tissues (including joint capsule and anconeus muscle), medial support of the olecranon using capsular imbrication and stay sutures, olecranon or ulnar osteotomy and transposition to reconstruct the joint, and redirect the pull of the triceps muscle to allow joint extension. The osteotomy is stabilized with Kirschner wires and, if necessary, a tension-band wire (see Fig. 30-38, *B*).

Preoperative Management

Affected animals are young and require minimal preoperative workup before surgery.

Anesthesia

General anesthesia is required for both closed and open reduction. Pediatric anesthesia techniques should be used. Anesthetic management of animals with orthopedic disease is discussed on p. 708.

Surgical Anatomy

Anatomical landmarks are the olecranon and the medial and lateral humeral condyles. The ulnar nerve is present on the medial aspect of the surgical site and should be identified and protected.

Positioning

The dog is placed in dorsal recumbency with the affected limb prepared from shoulder to carpus.

SURGICAL TECHNIQUES

Make an incision on the lateral surface of the joint, starting on the lateral epicondylar crest and extending distally over the lateral epicondyle to the proximal radius, as described on p. 798. Incise subcutaneous tissues and retract the skin medially to expose both medial and lateral surfaces of the elbow. Incise soft tissues on the lateral aspect of the humeroulnar joint (including the anconeus muscle and joint capsule) to expose the joint and reposition the ulna. If repositioning is possible, stabilize the ulna by imbricating the medial joint capsule, and placing a large (No. 0 to No. 2) nonabsorbable suture from the proximal ulna to the humeral condyle through tunnels drilled in the bone with the needle or a small Kirschner wire. Perform an olecranon osteotomy and transpose the osteotomized bone to a position on the ulna that best redirects the pull of the triceps muscle to extend the joint. Stabilize the osteotomy with Kirschner wires and possibly a tension-band wire (see p. 747). Reposition the skin to the lateral aspect of the elbow and close subcutaneous tissues and skin with interrupted sutures.

SUTURE MATERIALS/SPECIAL INSTRUMENTS

Instruments needed for open reduction include a general surgery pack, pin chuck, Kirschner wires, and orthopedic wire.

POSTOPERATIVE CARE AND ASSESSMENT

Postoperative radiographs should be made to evaluate the location of the ulna with respect to the humerus and position of any implants. The limb should be bandaged to support the fixation for 2 to 3 weeks. Splint the elbow in a functional position. Activity should be restricted to leash walking for 4 to 6 weeks. The Kirschner wires should be removed when the osteotomy has healed.

PROGNOSIS

Without surgery, the dog may learn to compensate for the loss of normal forelimb function by using the rear limbs for support and locomotion; however, ambulation will always be abnormal. The prognosis is good for return of satisfactory function after surgery, but poor for development of a normal joint. Potential surgical complications include loss of joint reduction, iatrogenic infection, implant migration, and irritation of soft tissues.

Suggested Reading

Milton JL, Montgomery RD: Congenital elbow dislocations, *Vet Clin North Am: Small Anim Pract* 17:873, 1987.

CARPAL LUXATION/SUBLUXATION

DEFINITIONS

Carpal luxation/subluxation results from loss of collateral and/or palmar ligamentous support of the antebrachial, middle carpal, and/or metacarpal joints. **Pancarpal arthrodesis** involves fusion of all three carpal joints, while **partial arthrodesis** is a selective fusion of one or more of the carpal joints.

SYNONYMS

Carpal hyperextension injury

GENERAL CONSIDERATIONS AND CLINICALLY RELEVANT PATHOPHYSIOLOGY

Carpal hyperextension injuries are divided into three categories (Fig. 30-40). Type I injuries are subluxations or luxations of the radiocarpal joint. Type II injuries result in subluxation of the middle carpal and carpometacarpal joints and are associated with disruption of the accessory carpal ligaments, palmar fibrocartilage, and palmar ligaments of the middle carpal and carpometacarpal joints. Dorsal displacement of the free end of the accessory carpal and ulnar carpal bones occurs. Type III injuries are disruptions of the

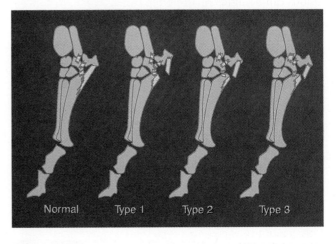

FIG. 30-40
Ligamentous injury associated with various hyperextension injuries of the carpus.

accessory carpal ligaments, carpometacarpal ligaments, and palmar fibrocartilage. In these injuries, subluxation of the carpometacarpal joint occurs without disruption and displacement of the accessory carpal and ulnar carpal bones.

DIAGNOSIS
Clinical Presentation

Signalment. Any age or breed and either sex of dog or cat may be affected.

History. Affected animals usually have a non–weight-bearing lameness. Because the animal is not using the limb, the extent of hyperextension may not be apparent initially.

Physical Examination Findings

With acute injuries, there are clear indications of swelling, pain, and instability. In Type I injuries, the animal usually remains unable to bear weight until definitive treatment is performed. With Type II or III injuries, the animal may begin to bear minimal weight on the limb after the injury. However, as increased weight is placed on the limb, collapse and hyperextension of the carpus become evident.

Radiography

Standard craniocaudal and medial-to-lateral radiographs are needed to determine the presence of bone fractures or joint malalignment. However, to accurately assess carpal integrity, stress radiographs should be taken (Fig. 30-41). Stress radiographs may be obtained by performing a standing lateral radiograph while the animal is bearing weight on the limb. If the animal refuses to place weight on the limb, it should be positioned in lateral recumbency with stress applied to the foot.

Laboratory Findings

There are no consistent laboratory abnormalities.

DIFFERENTIAL DIAGNOSIS

Differential diagnoses include acute sprains, distal radial fractures, and fractures of the metacarpal bones. These conditions can be differentiated from carpal luxation/subluxation radiographically by use of standard and stress views.

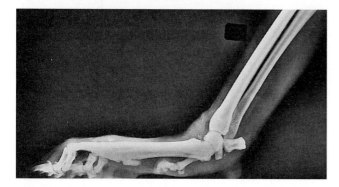

FIG. 30-41
Stress radiograph of a dog with a Type II carpal hyperextension injury. Stress radiographs should be performed to help classify hyperextension injuries.

MEDICAL MANAGEMENT

Medical, or conservative, management of carpal hyperextension injuries is often unrewarding. External coaptation may be tried in younger patients, but gradual hyperextension often occurs as weight bearing returns.

SURGICAL TREATMENT

Carpal hyperextension injuries are best treated with either pancarpal arthrodesis or partial arthrodesis via a cranial approach to the joint. Type I injuries should be treated with a pancarpal arthrodesis. A pancarpal arthrodesis or a partial carpal arthrodesis may be used to manage Type II injuries; however, the former fuses the radiocarpal articulation unnecessarily, while the latter maintains movement of the radiocarpal articulation. With Type II injuries, integrity of the accessory carpal moment arm, which resists the moment generated by the ground reaction force, is lost. Therefore, a partial arthrodesis that does not reestablish the accessory carpal moment arm may eventually fail because of breakdown of the radiocarpal joint. A partial arthrodesis for a Type II injury should include fusion of the middle carpal and carpometacarpal joints, with selective fusion of the accessory carpal–ulnar carpal articulation. Stabilization of Type I injuries may be accomplished by placement of a bone plate on the cranial surface. Stabilization of Type II injuries may be accomplished with a bone plate, cross pins, or placement of longitudinal metacarpal pins. Placement of multiple cross pins may be easiest and provides adequate fixation when combined with external coaptation. The articular cartilage should be removed, cancellous bone placed in the fusion site, and the site stabilized with cross pins.

With Type III injuries, the carpometacarpal joint and middle carpal joint should be fused. Although the accessory carpal ligaments may be compromised, the ligaments between the base of the accessory carpal bone, ulnar carpal bone, and fifth metacarpal bone are intact, thus preserving integrity of the accessory carpal moment arm. The articular cartilage should be removed, cancellous bone placed in the fusion site, and the site stabilized with cross pins as described for Type II injuries.

Preoperative Management

An external coaptation splint or bandage should be applied to protect the limb until definitive surgical treatment is undertaken. The animal should be kept in a cage until surgery, and activity should be strictly limited to prevent further joint damage.

Anesthesia

Anesthetic management of animals with fractures is presented on p. 708.

Surgical Anatomy

The carpus consists of seven bones arranged in two rows. The radial carpal and ulnar carpal bones make up the proximal row, while the first, second, third, and fourth carpal bones make up the distal row. The accessory carpal bone lies caudally and articulates with the ulnar carpal bone. The radial carpal bone and ulnar carpal bone articulate with the radius and styloid process of the ulna to form the radiocarpal joint. This joint has the greatest amount of movement; the middle carpal joint, formed by the articulation of the proximal and distal rows of carpal bones, accounts for 10% to 15% of carpal motion. Very little motion occurs in the carpometacarpal and intercarpal joints.

Collateral ligamentous support arises from the short radial collateral ligament medially and from the short ulnar collateral ligament laterally. Additionally, sleeves of collagenous tissue that house tendons provide medial and lateral collateral support. Palmar support is from the flexor retinaculum proximally and palmar fibrocartilage distally. Multiple small ligaments cross the intercarpal articulations between carpal bones to provide additional collateral and palmar support. Two accessory ligaments originate from the free end of the accessory carpal bone and insert onto the palmar surface of the fourth and fifth metacarpal bones. The caudal position of the free end of the accessory carpal bone, in conjunction with the accessory carpal ligaments, serves to act as a moment arm to balance the vertical force produced when the paw strikes the ground.

Positioning

The animal should be positioned in dorsal recumbency. A hanging-leg preparation allows maximal manipulation of the limb during surgery (see p. 25). The leg should be clipped and prepared from the distal humeral region to the tips of the toes.

SURGICAL TECHNIQUES

Considerable collagenous and bony tissue proliferation often occurs with carpal luxation/subluxation. Increased vascularity, which accompanies the fibrous proliferation, can make surgical dissection difficult. Use of a tourniquet is helpful. The joint is approached dorsally where proliferative tissue is pronounced. Sharp dissection through scar tissue and joint capsule creates the least trauma.

Approach to the Carpal Bones

Make a skin incision over the midline of the dorsal surface of the carpus, extending from 4 cm proximal to the radiocarpal joint line to 4 cm distal to the carpometacarpal joint line (Fig. 30-42, A). Incise subcutaneous tissues, proliferative fibrous tissue, and joint capsule overlying the radiocarpal, middle carpal, and carpometacarpal joints (Fig. 30-42, B). The proliferative fibrous tissue will be confluent with the joint capsule proximally and distally. *Reflect the synovial joint capsule incision from the cranial face of the carpal bones both medially and laterally using sharp dissection. Place Gelpi retractors to maintain exposure of the joint surfaces and position a small Hohmann retractor between joint surfaces to help visualize the articular cartilage of each joint. Use a low-speed power burr to remove articular cartilage from the surface of the carpal bones in each joint. Attempt to preserve the tendon of the extensor carpi radialis muscle as it crosses the craniolateral aspect of the joint. Harvest a cancellous bone graft and insert the graft within the denuded surfaces of each joint. Stabilize the arthrodesis with an implant as discussed below.*

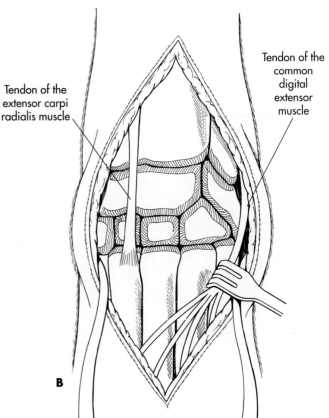

Tendon of the common digital extensor muscle

Tendon of the extensor carpi radialis muscle

B

FIG. 30-42
A, To approach the dorsal surface of the carpus, make a skin incision over the midline, extending from 4 cm proximal to the radiocarpal joint line to 4 cm distal to the carpometacarpal joint line. **B,** Incise subcutaneous tissues, proliferative fibrous tissue, and joint capsule overlying the radiocarpal, middle carpal, and carpometacarpal joints.

A

Pancarpal Arthrodesis

Expose the joint surfaces of the radiocarpal, middle carpal, and carpometacarpal articulations and remove articular cartilage as described above. Use a small Kirschner wire to drill multiple holes through the distal radial epiphysis into the marrow cavity to aid vascularization of the fusion. Stabilize the fusion with a bone plate applied as a compression plate to the dorsal surface of the radius. Apply the plate so that the proximal three plate screws enter the distal radius and the distal three plate screws enter the third metacarpal bone. Place one intermediate plate screw in the radial carpal bone and the others where bone stock is available. Because the plate is not positioned on the tension surface of the joint, it should be supported with small Steinmann pins and/or external coaptation. If pins are selected, place one pin from medial to lateral, entering the bone near the head of the second metacarpal and exiting through the distal ulna. Place a second pin from lateral to medial, entering the bone near the head of the fifth metacarpal and exiting through the distal radius (Fig. 30-43).

Partial Carpal Arthrodesis Used for Type II Injuries

Expose the joint surfaces of the carpal and metacarpal joints and remove articular cartilage as described above. Harvest and insert a cancellous bone graft. Stabilize the fusion by placing a pin from medial to lateral, entering the bone near the head of the second metacarpal and pene-

trating the radial carpal bone. Place a second pin from lateral to medial, entering the bone near the head of the fifth metacarpal and penetrating the ulnar carpal bone.

Partial Carpal Arthrodesis Used for Type III Injuries

Expose the joint surfaces of the carpal and metacarpal joints and remove articular cartilage as described above. Harvest and insert a cancellous bone graft. Stabilize the fusion by placing a pin from medial to lateral, entering the bone near the head of the second metacarpal and penetrating the radial carpal bone. Place a second pin from lateral to medial, entering the bone near the head of the fifth metacarpal and penetrating the ulnar carpal bone. Fuse the accessory carpal–ulnar carpal articulation by removing articular cartilage between joint surfaces of the accessory carpal bone and ulnar carpal bone, placing a cancellous bone graft, and stabilizing it with a compression screw. Make an incision lateral to the base of the accessory carpal bone. Incise subcutaneous tissues and deep fascia adjacent to the lateral accessory carpal ligament. (The medial and lateral accessory carpal ligaments will be torn.) Continue the incision lateral to the abductor digiti quinti muscle to the joint capsule. Incise the joint capsule to expose and remove articular cartilage from the ulnar carpal and accessory carpal bones. Insert a cancellous bone graft and stabilize the fusion with a compression screw and wire. Insert the compression screw from the cranial face of the ulnar carpal bone into the accessory carpal bone. Place a wire from the base of the accessory carpal bone through the head of the fifth metacarpal bone (Fig. 30-44).

☞ **N O T E** • Be sure to remove articular cartilage and rigidly stabilize the joint or arthrodesis will not occur.

SUTURE MATERIALS/SPECIAL INSTRUMENTS

Instruments for arthrodesis should include a battery- or air-driven power drill, a selection of raised end-threaded cortical pins, bone curette, and bone plates and screws.

POSTOPERATIVE CARE AND ASSESSMENT

A coaptation splint should be applied postoperatively to support the internal fixation. Healing of an arthrodesis takes 12 to 16 weeks. The external splint should be worn for 6 to 8 weeks, then the splint removed and the internal fixation allowed to support the arthrodesis until radiographic evidence of fusion is apparent. Activity should be strictly controlled until union has occurred.

PROGNOSIS

Pancarpal and partial carpal arthrodeses result in excellent limb function in 80% of patients treated with Type I, Type II, or Type III hyperextension injuries (Denny, Barr, 1991;

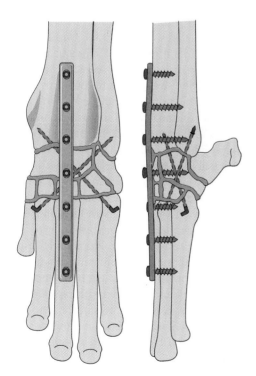

FIG. 30-43
Pancarpal arthrodesis for stabilization of Type I carpal hyperextension injuries. Note cranial application of a bone plate and caudal placement of cross pins. The plate should be contoured 5 to 10 degrees.

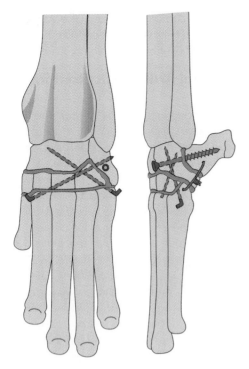

FIG. 30-44
Partial carpal arthrodesis with selective fusion of the accessory-ulnar articulation. Note that the pins do not cross the radiocarpal joint.

Parker, Brown, Wind, 1981). The remainder are substantially improved after surgery but may have varying degrees of limb dysfunction (lameness) after exercise. A small percentage exhibit continued, slight, weight-bearing lameness, but limb function is vastly improved relative to preoperative function.

References

Denny HR, Barr ARS: Partial carpal and pancarpal arthrodesis in the dog: a review of 50 cases, *J Sm Anim Pract* 32:329, 1991.

Parker RB, Brown SG, Wind AP: Pancarpal arthrodesis in the dog: a review of forty-five cases, *Am Col Vet Surg* 10:35, 1981.

Suggested Reading

Boudrieau RJ et al: Pancarpal arthrodesis using absorbable pins for skeletal fixation in four dogs, *Vet Surg* 21:384, 1992.

Ercegan MG, Somber T: Detailed anatomy of the antebrachiocarpal joint in dogs, *Anatom Rec* 233:329, 1992.

Johnson KA: A radiographic study of the effects of autologous cancellous bone grafts on bone healing after carpal arthrodesis in the dog, *Am Col Vet Rad* 22:177, 1981.

Moore RW, Withrow SJ: Arthrodesis, *Comp Cont Educ Pract Vet* 3:319, 1981.

Slocum B, Devine T: Partial carpal fusion in the dog, *J Am Vet Med Assoc* 180:1204, 1982.

Vaughan LC: Disorders of the carpus in the dog. I. *Br Vet J* 141:332, 1985.

Vaughan LC: Disorders of the carpus in the dog. II. *Br Vet J* 141:435, 1985.

COXOFEMORAL JOINT

HIP DYSPLASIA

DEFINITIONS

Hip dysplasia is an abnormal development of the coxofemoral joint characterized by subluxation or complete luxation of the femoral head in younger patients and mild to severe degenerative joint disease in older patients. **Luxation** of the coxofemoral joint is a complete separation between the femoral head and acetabulum, while **subluxation** is a partial or incomplete separation. **Angle of inclination** is the angle formed between the long axis of the femoral neck and the femoral diaphysis in the frontal plane. **Angle of anteversion** is the angle formed between the long axis of the femoral neck and the transcondylar axis.

GENERAL CONSIDERATIONS AND CLINICALLY RELEVANT PATHOPHYSIOLOGY

Causes of hip dysplasia are multifactorial; both hereditary and environmental factors play a part in development of abnormal bone and soft tissue. Rapid weight gain and growth through excessive nutritional intake may cause a disparity of development of supporting soft tissues, leading to hip dysplasia. Factors that cause synovial inflammation (mild, repeated trauma and/or viral or bacterial synovitis) may also be important. Synovitis leads to increased joint fluid volume, which abolishes joint stability derived from the suction-like action produced by a thin layer of normal synovial fluid between articular surfaces. These factors contribute to the development of hip joint laxity and subsequent subluxation, which are responsible for early clinical signs and joint changes. Subluxation stretches the fibrous joint capsule, producing pain and lameness. Acetabular cancellous bone is easily deformed by continual dorsal subluxation of the femoral head. The piston-like action of the femoral head dynamically subluxating from the acetabulum with each step causes tilting of the acetabular articular surface from a normal horizontal plane to a more vertical plane. It also decreases the surface area of articulation, which concentrates the stress of weight bearing over a small area in the hip joint. Fractures of the acetabular trabecular cancellous bone may occur and exacerbate the pain and lameness. Physiologic responses to joint laxity (subluxation) are proliferative fibroplasia of the joint capsule and increased trabecular bone thickness. These changes relieve the pain associated with capsular sprain and trabecular fractures. However, the surface area of articulation is still decreased, which results in potential premature wear of articular cartilage, exposure of subchondral pain fibers, and lameness.

☞ **NOTE** · Hip dysplasia is painful because wear of articular cartilage exposes pain fibers in subchondral bone.

DIAGNOSIS
Clinical Presentation

Signalment. The incidence of hip dysplasia is greatest in Saint Bernards and German shepherds, but most sporting breeds are affected. History and clinical signs vary with the patient's age. Two populations of animals are affected: (1) patients 5 to 10 months of age, and (2) patients with chronic degenerative joint disease. Hip dysplasia is rare in cats.

History. Symptoms in young patients include difficulty rising after rest, exercise intolerance, and intermittent or continual lameness. As animals mature they may develop additional signs attributable to hip joint pain. Progressive degenerative joint disease in these patients causes difficulty in rising, exercise intolerance, lameness following exercise, pelvic musculature atrophy, and/or a waddling gait attributed to abnormal movement of the rear limbs. Frequently, patients are seen for evaluation of lameness that has suddenly worsened during or after increased activity or injury.

Physical Examination Findings

Juvenile patients with lameness are first seen between 5 and 10 months of age. Physical findings in these patients include pain during external rotation and abduction of the hip joint, poorly developed pelvic musculature, and exercise intolerance. Hip examination performed under general anesthesia shows increased laxity of the hip joints as evidenced by abnormal angles of reduction and subluxation (Figs. 30-45 and 30-46). Some affected animals are presented for evaluation of an acute, unilateral, non–weight-bearing lameness. These animals have usually torn the round ligament in the affected hip joint and severely sprained the fibrous joint capsule, allowing complete subluxation of the femoral head. Many juvenile dogs spontaneously improve with increasing age after conservative management (see p. 944). Physical examination findings in older animals include pain during extension of the hip joint, reduced range of motion, atrophy of the pelvic musculature, and exercise intolerance. There is generally no detectable joint laxity because of the proliferative fibrous response, but crepitus may be detected on joint manipulation. It is important to note that clinical signs do not always correlate with radiographic findings. A correct diagnosis of hip dysplasia as the cause of clinical problems is based on age, breed, history, physical findings, and radiographic changes.

Radiography

The Orthopedic Foundation for Animals has established seven grades for categorizing radiographic congruity between the femoral head and acetabulum. Hips determined to be "normal" radiographically may be further classified as excellent, good, fair, or near normal; animals with dysplasia are categorized as mild, moderate, or severe (Fig. 30-47). Stress radiographs can be used to detect breed susceptibility to hip dysplasia as early as 4 months. Stress radiographs require

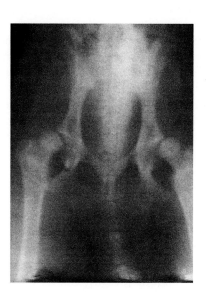

FIG. 30-46
Angle of subluxation is the measured point where the femoral head slips out of the acetabulum when the limb is adducted.

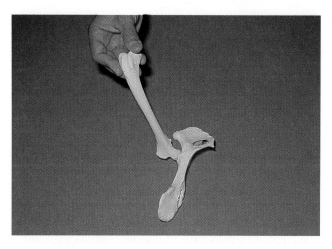

FIG. 30-47
Ventrodorsal radiograph of a dog with severe hip dysplasia. Early osteophyte formation and subluxation of the femoral head from the acetabulum are evident.

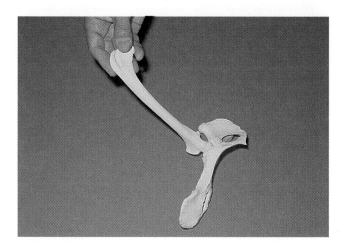

FIG. 30-45
Angle of reduction is the measured point where the femoral head slips back into the acetabulum when the limb is abducted.

that the dog be under deep sedation or light anesthesia to eliminate muscle tension. Radiographic views are taken with the hips in both a neutral stance position and distracted (obtained by levering a custom-designed distractor between the legs). A distraction index is calculated from these views and is used to predict the likelihood of developing degenerative joint disease secondary to hip laxity. Individual logistic regression curves that predict the risk of developing degenerative joint disease are being developed for different breeds because it appears that some breeds are more "laxity tolerant" than others. Speciality centers have been certified nationally to determine a patient's distraction index.

☞ **N O T E** · Clinical signs often do not correlate with radiographic findings. Some dogs with moderate or severe dysplasia are asymptomatic.

Laboratory Findings

Consistent laboratory abnormalities are not present.

DIFFERENTIAL DIAGNOSIS

A number of neurologic and orthopedic problems cause similar clinical signs. In younger dogs, lameness caused by panosteitis, osteochondrosis, physeal separation, hypertrophic osteodystrophy, and partial or complete cranial cruciate ligament injury must be differentiated from hip dysplasia. In older patients it is necessary to rule out neurologic (cauda equina) and orthopedic (rupture of the cranial cruciate ligament, polyarthritis, bone neoplasia) conditions before attributing clinical signs to hip dysplasia.

MEDICAL OR CONSERVATIVE MANAGEMENT

Treatment depends upon the patient's age, degree of discomfort, physical and radiographic findings, and client expectations and finances. Conservative and surgical options are available for younger and mature animals experiencing hip pain secondary to hip dysplasia. Although early surgical intervention increases the prognosis for long-term acceptable clinical function, approximately 60% of young patients treated conservatively return to acceptable clinical function with maturity (Barr, Denny, Gibbs, 1987). The remainder require further medical or surgical management at some point in life. Surgery is indicated when conservative treatment is not effective, when athletic performance is desired, or in young patients when the owner wishes to slow the progression of degenerative joint disease and enhance the probability of good long-term limb function.

Pain relief and clinical improvement associated with conservative treatment are derived from fibrous proliferation of the joint capsule, which strengthens the capsule and prevents further capsular sprain. Concurrently, increased thickness of the cancellous trabeculae in the subchondral bone strengthens the bony trabeculae and prevents fractures. However, these patients are still afflicted with hip dysplasia and have a decreased surface area of hip joint articulation. Clinical signs that develop as the animal matures are attributable to articular cartilage wear and progressive degenerative joint disease. Conservative treatment is divided into short- and long-term phases. Initially, these patients should be treated for an acute sprain. Complete rest is mandatory and must be enforced for 10 to 14 days. Often the animal improves in 3 to 4 days and owners may allow excessive activity, which predisposes to recurring injury, pain, and prolonged recovery. Adjunct physical therapy is helpful during this period in maintaining range of motion and providing comfort. Moist heat applied over the joint is beneficial, but care should be exercised to avoid burning the skin. (Apply the heat to yourself for 2 to 3 minutes to make sure it is safe.) Once the joint and muscles are warm, passive movement of all joints in the affected limb(s) should be done. Initially, small movements should be performed, but the range of motion should gradually be increased to the maximum tolerated by the patient. Massage (in conjunction with moist heat) is also encouraged to maintain flexibility. Antiinflammatory drugs are indicated to relieve pain and make the administration of physical therapy more admissible. However, antiinflammatory drugs are likely to make the patient more comfortable, which may make the enforcement of rest more difficult. Clients must be advised to continue the rest period even if the patient appears to have returned to normal function.

☞ **N O T E** · Be sure to stress to the owner of an animal with an acute injury that they must enforce rest, even if the animal feels like exercising.

There are a number of nonsteroidal antiinflammatory drugs (NSAIDs) available over the counter and through prescriptions. NSAIDs most commonly used in veterinary medicine are aspirin and phenylbutazone (Table 30-20). NSAIDs

---

TABLE 30-20

Nonsteroidal Antiinflammatory Drugs* Used in Dogs with Hip Dysplasia

Buffered aspirin (Ascriptin)
25 mg/kg PO, BID or TID

Phenylbutazone (Butazolidin)
15 mg/kg PO, TID, not to exceed 800 mg/day

Naproxen (Naprosyn, Anaprox)
2.2 mg/kg/day PO, SID or EOD; not approved for use in dogs

Piroxicam
10 mg/day PO

Carprofen (Rimadyl)
2.2 mg/kg, PO, BID

*Give with food.

available for use in humans (but not approved for dogs) include ibuprofen, naproxen, and piroxicam. It is important to note that these drugs are used in lower doses in dogs than in people. **Caution must be used with these products since the pharmacokinetics are largely unknown in dogs and overdosage may cause severe gastrointestinal ulceration.** Clients should be advised to avoid giving their pets NSAIDs without the recommendation of a veterinarian. NSAIDs that cause less gastrointestinal injury (e.g., etodolac, carprofen) are currently being investigated. These drugs do not inhibit gastric prostaglandin and are less likely to disrupt the mucosal protective barrier. Etodolac is approved for use in humans, and caprofen has recently been approved for use in dogs. When administering NSAIDs, begin with the lowest possible therapeutic dosage and administer with small amounts of food. Cytoprotective therapy, such as concurrent administration of sucralfate or the prostaglandin analog misoprostol (1 to 3 μg/kg PO, TID), can be used to help prevent gastrointestinal ulcers. Although some NSAIDs do not significantly alter cartilage metabolism, most NSAIDs interfere with chondrocyte glycosaminoglycan synthesis and therefore should be used continuously for only a short time. Polysulfated glycosaminoglycans (PSGAGs) are frequently used to treat inflammation associated with chronic degenerative joint disease. In vitro laboratory experiments indicate PSGAGs are effective in inhibiting the expression of metalloproteases in synovial fluid. Clinical trials suggest some clinical improvement in patients treated with PSGAGs; however, statistically significant differences between treated and untreated dogs have not been found.

☞ **N O T E** · Administer NSAIDs at the lowest effective dose, with food, and consider giving cytoprotective drugs concurrently.

Long-term conservative treatment for pain associated with degenerative joint disease includes weight control, exercise, and administration of antiinflammatory drugs. The animal should be weighed weekly and calorie intake determined. Feeding bulk diets low in fat and protein may be beneficial. Exercise (e.g., swimming and long walks) is important to maintain an appropriate weight. High-intensity activity should be allowed only for short durations after an adequate warm-up period. Antiinflammatory drugs should be administered only as needed and should not take the place of weight control and a moderate exercise program. Food additives (i.e., cosequin) may be useful to control pain. These preparations contain chondroprotective agents that are thought to decrease inflammatory agents within the joint.

☞ **N O T E** · Stress to owners that weight control is an important part of managing chronic hip dysplasia. If pain associated with hip dysplasia prevents their animal from exercising normally, they should reduce the animal's caloric intake to prevent weight gain.

SURGICAL TREATMENT

The four surgical procedures commonly used for treatment of hip dysplasia are pelvic osteotomy, femoral osteotomy, total hip prosthesis, and femoral head ostectomy. Pelvic osteotomy is useful in younger patients to axially rotate and lateralize the acetabulum in an effort to increase dorsal coverage of the femoral head. This procedure is indicated in patients leading athletic lives (i.e., working breeds) or where the client wishes to arrest or slow the progress of osteoarthritis. The most favorable prognosis is in patients with (1) radiographic evidence of minimal degenerative changes in conjunction with (2) an angle of reduction less than 45 degrees and (3) an angle of subluxation less than 10 degrees. Of the procedures described, Slocum osteotomy is the most effective method of obtaining axial rotation and acetabular lateralization (Slocum, Devine, 1987; Slocum, Slocum, 1992). With this procedure the amount of axial rotation is set by previously determined angles of reduction (maximum amount of rotation) and subluxation (minimum degree of rotation). The angle of acetabular rotation that is commonly used is slightly less than the measured angle of reduction (see Figs. 30-45, 30-46, 28-26, and 28-27).

Proximal femoral varus osteotomy, derotational osteotomy, or a combination of the two also results in increased joint stability. Varus osteotomy involves intertrochanteric osteotomy with removal of a wedge-shaped piece of bone. Removal of the correctly sized (predetermined) wedge of bone decreases the angle of inclination and elevates the height of the greater trochanter. Realignment of both the femoral neck angle and the mechanical force of the gluteal muscles results in a more stable hip. Large femoral anteversion angles have been reported in dogs with hip dysplasia. If present, a derotational femoral osteotomy may be combined with varus osteotomy to increase hip joint stability (Braden, Prieur, 1992).

A total hip prosthesis is replacement of a degenerative hip joint with a prosthetic acetabular cup and femoral component (Fig. 30-48). The procedure is most commonly used in mature patients where conservative treatment is not effective. The success rate is usually good to excellent but depends on the surgeon's experience with the procedure. Therefore, total hip replacement should be performed only by experienced surgeons trained in this procedure.

Femoral head and neck excision limits bony contact between the femoral head and acetabulum and allows formation of a fibrous false joint (Fig. 30-49). This procedure can be used in younger patients and older animals where conservative treatment has failed and financial constraints preclude alternative methods of surgical intervention. Because fibrous pseudoarthrosis is an unstable joint, clinical function postoperatively is unpredictable. For this reason most surgeons consider femoral head and neck excision to be a salvage procedure. However, many patients with painful arthritic hips undergoing femoral head and neck excision have improved limb function and quality of life postoperatively.

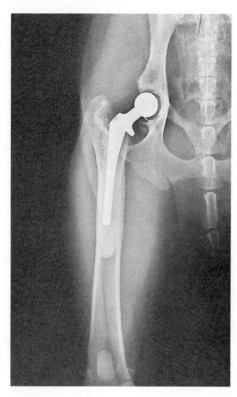

FIG. 30-48
Radiograph of a dog after total hip replacement. Note the radiopaque cement mantel surrounding the femoral and acetabular prostheses.

Preoperative Management

A complete orthopedic and neurologic examination should be performed to correctly attribute the clinical problem to hip dysplasia. Intraoperative systemic antibiotics should be administered when pelvic osteotomy or total hip replacement is performed.

Anesthesia

Epidural administration of analgesics preoperatively is useful for lowering anesthetic dose requirement and for reducing postoperative discomfort.

Surgical Anatomy

Surgical anatomy of the hip joint is discussed on p. 835. Special anatomic considerations for femoral head ostectomy are important to note in patients with hip dysplasia. In those patients with atrophied hip musculature, the joint capsule is obvious as soon as the deep gluteal muscle is reflected. If subluxation of the hip joint is moderate or severe, the joint capsule usually appears thickened and "bulges" outward. In mature patients, thickening of the joint capsule is even more pronounced. To obtain adequate exposure of the femoral head and neck, the vastus lateralis muscle must be released and reflected ventrally. The femoral head and neck are often short and deformed. To perform a femoral head and neck ostectomy in these patients, the juncture of the femoral neck and femoral shaft must be clearly visualized. In young pa-

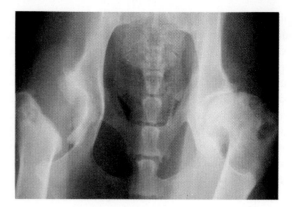

FIG. 30-49
Radiograph of a dog after femoral head ostectomy. Note complete removal of the femoral neck.

tients, the round ligament may be intact and must be severed; the ligament is usually absent in older patients.

☞ **N O T E** · Before performing pelvic osteotomy, review the relationship between the gluteal musculature and iliacus muscle, position of the sciatic nerve, and course of the internal pudendal artery and nerve (see p. 834).

Positioning

The patient is positioned in lateral recumbency for pelvic osteotomy. Clip and prepare the leg for aseptic surgery from the midline of the tarsal joint on both medial and lateral limb surfaces. For femoral head and neck excision the patient is positioned in lateral recumbency and the area from the dorsal midline to the stifle is clipped and prepared for aseptic surgery. It is desirable to drape the patient in a manner that allows manipulation of the limb during surgery (see p. 24).

SURGICAL TECHNIQUES
Pelvic Osteotomy

Pelvic osteotomy requires that an incision be made through the pubic brim, ischial floor, and ilial body. Recent studies show the optimal position for pubic osteotomy is adjacent to the medial walls of the acetabulum. *With the patient in lateral recumbency, abduct the leg while maintaining the femur perpendicular to the acetabulum. Locate the origin of the pectineus muscle and center a 6-cm skin incision over this point. Incise subcutaneous tissues to further isolate the origin of the pectineus muscle at the ilieopectineal eminence. Release the origin of the pectineus muscle to expose the cranial brim of the pubis. Reflect the periosteum from the cranial, lateral, and caudal pubic surfaces. To protect soft tissues during the osteotomy, place spoon Hohmann retractors cranial to the pubis and within the obturator foramen caudally. Perform a pubic osteotomy adjacent to the medial wall of the acetabulum (Fig. 30-50). Alternatively ostectomize a portion of the pubis. Suture soft tissues and skin using standard methods.*

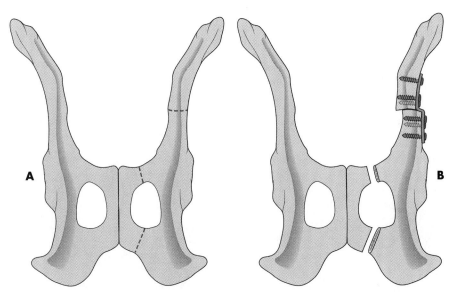

FIG. 30-50
A, Position of osteotomies for completion of a triple pelvic osteotomy (TPO) and **B,** ilial osteotomy stabilization with a bone plate. Note axial rotation and lateralization of the hemipelvis.

Next perform an osteotomy of the ischial floor. Make a skin incision midway between the medial prominence of the ischium and lateral tuberosity. Make the incision in the vertical plane, beginning 4 cm proximal to the ischial floor and extending 3 cm distally. Incise subcutaneous tissues and deep fascia. Make a 3-cm incision through the periosteal insertion of the internal obturator muscle at the dorsal crest of the ischial floor. Elevate the internal obturator muscle cranially to the obturator foramen. Then, incise the periosteal origin of the external obturator muscle at the ventral crest of the ischial floor and reflect the muscle from the ventral surface of the ischium cranially to the obturator foramen. Place two spoon Hohmann retractors to protect the soft tissue; insert one into the obturator foramen dorsally and one into the foramen ventrally. Direct an osteotome caudal to cranial in line with the center of the Hohmann retractors; this will center the osteotomy line into the obturator foramen. **Close the incision after the osteotomy of the ilium is completed.** *At that time, drill two small holes on either side of the osteotomy adjacent to each other. Place orthopedic wire through the holes and twist them in a figure-eight fashion to stabilize the osteotomy. Suture the fascia of the internal obturator muscle to that of the external obturator muscle, then close subcutaneous tissue and skin using standard methods.*

Next perform an osteotomy of the ilium to allow axial rotation of the acetabulum. Make an incision from the cranial extent of the iliac crest caudally 1 to 2 cm beyond the greater trochanter. Center the incision over the ventral third of the ilial wing. Incise subcutaneous tissues and gluteal fat along the same line to visualize the intermuscular septum between the superficial gluteal muscle and the short part of the tensor fascia lata muscle. Incise the muscular septum to separate the tensor fascia lata muscle and middle gluteal muscle cranially and tensor fascia lata and superficial gluteal muscles caudally. Cranially, use sharp dissection to separate the middle gluteal muscle and long head of the tensor fascia lata muscle. Palpate the ventral border of the ilium and make an incision to the bone near the ventral insertion of the middle and deep gluteal muscles. Isolate and ligate iliolumbar vessels and reflect the deep gluteal muscle from the lateral surface of the ilium. Incise the origin of iliacus muscle at the ventral border of the ilium and reflect the muscle from the ventral surface. Elevate periosteum from the medial surface of the ilium with a periosteal elevator. Place two spoon Hohmann retractors to protect soft tissue during the osteotomy: place one medial to the ilium to reflect the iliacus muscle and one over the dorsal crest of the ilium to retract the gluteal muscle mass. Judge the cranial position of the osteotomy by placing the osteotomy plate such that the most caudal plate hole is 1 to 2 cm cranial to the acetabulum. Perform the ilial osteotomy with a power saw on a line perpendicular to the long axis of the hemipelvis. Lateralize the caudal segment with bone-holding forceps and secure an appropriate osteotomy plate to this segment. Next reduce the osteotomy and apply plate screws in the cranial segment. To close the incision, place sutures between the fascia of the middle gluteal muscle and that of the tensor fascia lata muscle cranially and between the superficial gluteal muscle and tensor fascia lata caudally. Approximate deep gluteal fat, subcutaneous tissue, and skin, using standard methods.

Femoral Head and Neck Ostectomy

Make a craniolateral approach to the hip joint and luxate the hip (see p. 848). If the round ligament is intact, incise it. Incising the round ligament is facilitated by placing lateral traction on the greater trochanter with bone-holding forceps and subluxating the femoral head. This allows curved scissors to be placed into the joint to cut the ligament. Perform the osteotomy by externally rotating the limb to where the joint line of the stifle is parallel to the operating table. Identify the line of osteotomy perpendicular to the operating table at the junction of the femoral neck and femoral

FIG. 30-51
To expose the femoral head for ostectomy, make a craniolateral skin incision centered over the hip joint. **A,** Retract the biceps femoris muscle caudally and tensor fascia lata muscle cranially. **B,** Incise the vastus lateralis muscle and reflect it ventrally. **C,** Incise joint capsule and perform the osteotomy by externally rotating the limb to where the joint line of the stifle is parallel to the operating table. Identify the line of osteotomy perpendicular to the operating table at the junction of the femoral neck and femoral metaphysis.

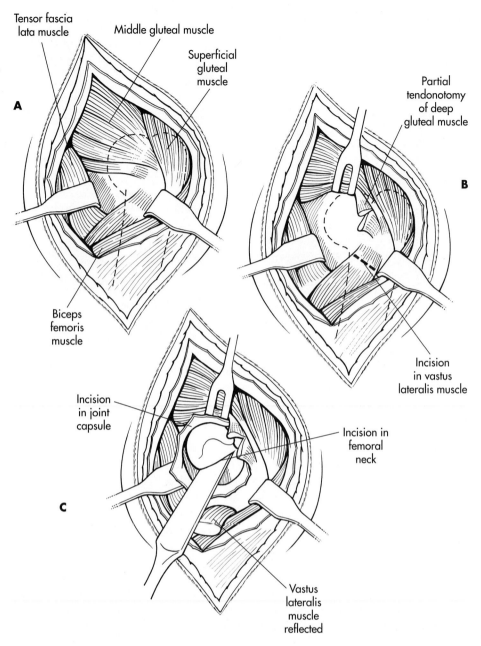

metaphysis (Fig. 30-51). To ensure accuracy of the bony cut, the surgeon can predrill a series of three or more holes along the line of the osteotomy. Use an osteotome and mallet to complete the cut. Ventral reflection of the vastus lateralis muscle facilitates proper placement of an osteotome during this procedure. Once the femoral neck and head are removed, palpate the cut surface of the femoral neck for irregularities. The most common finding is a shelf of femoral neck left on the caudal surface of the femur. Remove edges with rongeurs. Suture the joint capsule over the acetabulum, if possible. Alternatively, fashion a proximally based biceps femoris muscle pedicle and pass it from caudal to cranial across the excision site. Clinical studies indicate improved postoperative function when soft tissue is interposed between the cut surface of the femoral neck and acetabulum (Lippincott, 1992). To close, reposition the vastus lateralis and deep gluteal muscles with absorbable suture using a simple interrupted pattern. Suture fascia lata with absorbable suture using a simple continuous pattern. Suture skin with nonabsorbable suture using a simple interrupted pattern.

SUTURE MATERIALS/SPECIAL INSTRUMENTS

An oscillating saw, osteotome and mallet, self-retaining retractors, Hohmann retractors, and instrumentation for insertion of bone plate and screws are necessary for pelvic osteotomy. Femoral head ostectomy requires an osteotome and mallet.

POSTOPERATIVE CARE AND ASSESSMENT

After pelvic osteotomy the patient should be restricted to leash exercise until radiographic evidence of healing of the osteotomies is complete, generally in 6 weeks. The duration of exercise (leash walks) should be gradually increased according to the patient's tolerance. Passive flexion and extension of the hip should be performed to help maintain hip motion. If the contralateral side is to have surgical treatment, the second surgery should be performed when discomfort associated with the first surgery is tolerated by the dog. Reported complications include implant failure, loss of limb abduction, and pelvic outlet narrowing. However, the incidence of complications is low, and reports of long-term clinical function are good to excellent. Early active use of the limb is also beneficial after femoral head ostectomy. Passive flexion and extension of the hip joint should be performed two to three times daily. Frequent leash walking should be begun immediately after surgery. After suture removal, running and swimming should be encouraged. Good return of active limb function is dependent upon the length of time the hip joint pathology was present and upon severity of the degenerative changes. Patients with chronic disease (muscle atrophy and proliferative degenerative joint disease) are slower to return to function than patients with acute lameness.

PROGNOSIS

The prognosis after pelvic osteotomy is largely determined by case selection. Best results are obtained in patients with acceptable physical findings (see above) and few or no degenerative changes. Long-term function is good to excellent. Although degenerative changes are radiographically evident after this procedure, they are less than what would be expected without surgery. Long-term function is good after varus osteotomy, and, as is the case with pelvic osteotomy, degenerative changes progress radiographically but are less than what would be expected without surgery. Total hip replacement results in excellent return to normal function. Results after femoral head ostectomy vary. The prognosis is highly dependent upon patient size and postoperative physical therapy. In large patients, 50% of animals have good or excellent function (Duff, Campbell, 1977). The remainder have varying degrees of lameness, but function is usually improved when compared with preoperative status. Medium and small patients usually have good or excellent limb function.

References

Barr ARS, Denny HR, Gibbs C: Clinical hip dysplasia in growing dogs: the long-term results of conservative management, *J Sm Anim Pract* 28:243, 1987.

Braden TD, Prieur WD: Three-plane intertrochanteric osteotomy for treatment of early stage hip dysplasia, *Vet Clin North Am Small Anim Pract* 22:623, 1992.

Duff R, Campbell JR: Long term results of excision arthroplasty of the canine hip, *Vet Rec* 101:181, 1977.

Lippincott CL: Femoral head and neck excision in the management of canine hip dysplasia, *Vet Clin North Am Small Anim Pract* 22:721, 1992.

Slocum B, Devine T: Pelvic osteotomy in the dog as a treatment for hip dysplasia, *Semin Vet Med Surg* 2:107, 1987.

Slocum B, Slocum TD: Pelvic osteotomy for axial rotation of the acetabular segment in dogs with hip dysplasia, *Vet Clin North Am Small Anim Pract* 22:645, 1992.

Suggested Reading

Hauptman JH: Orthopedics of the hind limb: the hip joint. In Slatter DH, editor: *Textbook of small animal surgery,* ed 2, Philadelphia, 1993, WB Saunders.

Hauptman JH et al: The angle of inclination of the canine femoral head and neck, *Vet Surg* 8:74, 1979.

Hosgood G, Lewis DD: Retrospective evaluation of fixation complications of 49 pelvic osteotomies in 36 dogs, *J Sm Anim Pract* 34:123, 1993.

Johnston SA: Conservative and medical management of hip dysplasia, *Vet Clin North Am* 22:595, 1992.

Kealy RD et al: Effects of limited food consumption on the incidence of hip dysplasia in growing dogs, *J Am Vet Med Assoc* 201:857, 1992.

Lust G, Rendano VT, Summers BA: Canine hip dysplasia: concepts and diagnosis, *J Am Vet Med Assoc* 187:638, 1985.

McLaughlin RM Jr et al: Force plate analysis of triple pelvic osteotomy for the treatment of canine hip dysplasia, *Vet Surg* 20:291, 1991.

Olmstead ML: Total hip replacement, *Semin Vet Med Surg Small Anim* 23:131, 1987.

Olmstead ML: The canine cemented modular total hip prosthesis, *J Am Anim Hosp Assoc* 31:109, 1995.

Slocum B, Devine TM: Dorsal acetabular rim radiographic view for evaluation of the canine hip, *J Am Anim Hosp Assoc* 26:289, 1990.

Smith GK, Biery DN, Gregor TP: New concepts of coxofemoral joint stability and the development of a clinical stress-radiographic method for quantitating hip joint laxity in the dog, *J Am Vet Med Assoc* 196:59, 1990.

Trevor PB et al: Evaluation of compatible osteoconductive polymer as an orthopedic implant in dogs, *J Am Vet Med Assoc* 200:1651, 1992.

COXOFEMORAL LUXATIONS

DEFINITIONS

Coxofemoral luxations are traumatic displacements of the femoral head from the acetabulum.

SYNONYMS

Hip luxation

GENERAL CONSIDERATIONS AND CLINICALLY RELEVANT PATHOPHYSIOLOGY

Coxofemoral luxation typically results in dorsal displacement of the femoral head relative to the acetabulum. The majority of affected animals have sustained trauma such as motor vehicle accidents. Ventrocaudal displacements, where the femoral head may lodge within the obturator foramen, occur less frequently. This type of luxation is often a result of a fall. The amount of soft tissue damage surrounding the hip joint is dependent on the trauma incurred. The round ligament of the femoral head always fails completely; it may be an interstitial rupture or an avulsion of the ligament from the fovea capitis. The fibrous joint capsule must also be completely torn to permit dislocation of the femoral head. The tear in the joint capsule may be a small rent through which the femoral head is dislodged or complete fraying of the entire capsule may occur.

Treatment of hip luxation should be performed as quickly as possible to prevent continued damage of the soft tissues surrounding the hip joint and degeneration of articular cartilage. Articular cartilage derives its nutrients from synovial fluid, which is pumped into the matrix during normal articular movement. Therefore, early reduction allows rapid return of the articular cartilage's nutrient source. Because coxofemoral luxations are always associated with trauma, as many as half of these patients have a major injury in addition to the hip luxation. A careful physical examination should be performed before anesthesia and treatment of the luxated hip to identify concurrent trauma.

☞ **N O T E** · Early reduction of luxated hips is essential. Do not delay in treating these animals.

DIAGNOSIS
Clinical Presentation

Signalment. Any age or breed and either sex of dog or cat may be affected.

History. Affected animals usually exhibit a unilateral non–weight-bearing lameness. The traumatic episode may or may not be witnessed by the owner.

Physical Examination Findings

Animals with hip luxation are presented for evaluation of a non–weight-bearing lameness associated with trauma.

When the femur is displaced craniodorsally, the limb is carried adducted, with the stifle externally rotated (Fig. 30-52). When it is displaced caudoventrally, the limb is carried abducted, with the stifle internally rotated. Manipulation of the limb causes crepitus or pain. There is a palpable lack of symmetry between the tuber ischii and greater trochanter on the affected side when compared with the normal limb. With craniodorsal displacement, the greater trochanter is dorsal to an imaginary line drawn from the crest of the ilium to the tuber ischii and the distance between the tuber ischii and greater trochanter is larger than that in the normal limb (Fig. 30-53). With a ventrocaudal luxation, the greater trochanter is displaced ventrally and the space between the tuber ischii and greater trochanter may be narrowed.

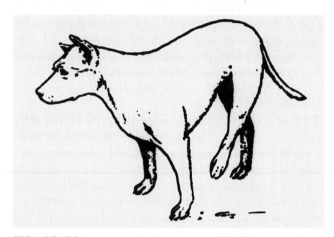

FIG. 30-52
Typical carriage of the limb in a patient with a craniodorsal coxofemoral luxation. Note the position of the paw beneath the body and external rotation of the stifle.

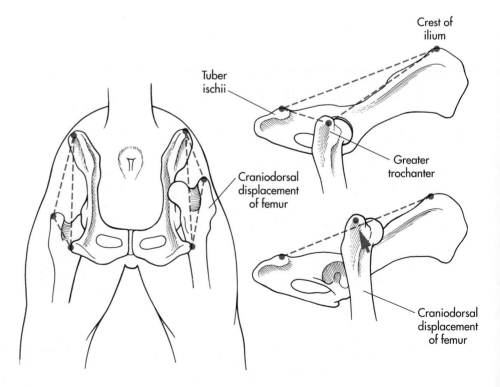

FIG. 30-53
With craniodorsal displacement of the femur, the greater trochanter is dorsal to an imaginary line drawn from the crest of the ilium to the tuber ischii and the distance between the tuber ischii and greater trochanter is increased relative to the normal limb.

Radiography

The diagnosis of hip luxation should be confirmed with ventrodorsal and lateral radiographs (Fig. 30-54). Before a treatment method is chosen, radiographs should be carefully evaluated for evidence of avulsion of the fovea capitis, associated hip joint fractures, and the presence of degenerative changes secondary to poor joint conformation.

Laboratory Findings

Consistent laboratory abnormalities are not present.

DIFFERENTIAL DIAGNOSIS

Differentials include acute subluxation of the hip joint secondary to hip dysplasia, femoral capital physeal fracture, femoral neck fracture, and acetabular fracture.

MEDICAL OR CONSERVATIVE MANAGEMENT

Coxofemoral luxation may be managed with open surgical manipulation or with closed manipulation to replace the femoral head within the acetabulum. Closed reduction should be attempted before performing open reduction in most animals, unless there is radiographic evidence of severe hip dysplasia or a fracture. The animal should be anesthetized for a closed reduction.

Closed Reduction of Craniodorsal Luxations

Place the patient in lateral recumbency under general anesthesia. Grasp the affected limb with one hand near the tarsal joint and place the other hand under the limb against the body wall to provide resistance (Fig. 30-55, A). Externally rotate the limb and pull it caudally to position the femoral head over the acetabulum (Fig. 30-55, B). When the femoral head lies lateral to the acetabulum, internally rotate the limb to seat the femoral head within the acetabulum (Fig. 30-55, C). Apply medial pressure to the greater trochanter while flexing and extending the joint to help expel debris from the acetabular cup. Place the limb in an Ehmer bandage (see p. 716). Limit the animal to controlled activity on a leash until the bandage is removed in 4 to 7 days. After bandage removal, limit activity to controlled leash activity for an additional 2 weeks.

Closed Reduction of Caudoventral Luxations

Place the patient in lateral recumbency with the limb held perpendicular to the spine. Grasp the limb at the tarsal joint with one hand and place the other hand under the limb medial to the hip joint (Fig. 30-56, A). Place traction on the limb while simultaneously abducting the leg to pull the femoral head beyond the medial rim of the acetabulum (Fig. 30-56, B). Once the femoral head has cleared the acetabular rim, exert lateral pressure to position the femoral head lateral to the acetabulum. Push proximally and allow the femoral head to fall into the acetabulum (Fig. 30-56, C). After reduction, place the patient in hobbles to prevent

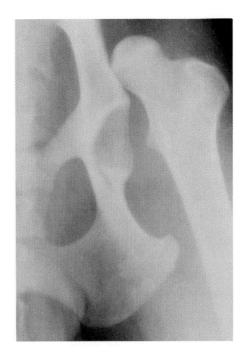

FIG. 30-54
Ventrodorsal radiograph of an animal with a craniodorsal coxofemoral luxation.

abduction of the limb. Limit activity to controlled activity on a leash until the bandage is removed in 4 to 7 days. Limit activity to leash walking for an additional 2 weeks after the hobbles have been removed.

SURGICAL TREATMENT

Open reduction is indicated when avulsion of the fovea capitis is present or when closed reduction has failed to maintain hip reduction. The hip joint should be explored to assess the soft-tissue injury and likelihood of maintaining reduction with a reconstructive procedure. If stability of the hip joint can be achieved through a reconstructive procedure, there are a number of techniques from which to choose. If there is not a reasonable chance of maintaining long-term reduction after a stabilization procedure, an alternate procedure such as a femoral head ostectomy (see p. 947) or total hip replacement must be considered.

Preoperative Management

These animals should be thoroughly examined for evidence of concurrent trauma. Surgery may need to be delayed until the animal has been adequately stabilized.

Anesthesia

See p. 708 for anesthetic considerations for patients with orthopedic disease.

Surgical Anatomy

Normal anatomy of the hip is described on p. 836. With hip luxations the anatomy may appear abnormal and tissues may be difficult to identify. The muscles surrounding the joint are

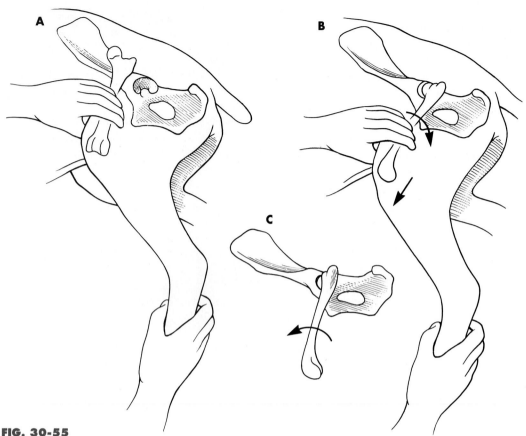

FIG. 30-55
A, To reduce craniodorsal hip luxations, grasp the affected limb near the tarsus with one hand and place the other hand under the limb against the body wall to provide resistance. **B,** Externally rotate the limb and pull it caudally to position the femoral head over the acetabulum. **C,** When the femoral head lies lateral to the acetabulum, internally rotate the limb to seat the femoral head within the acetabulum.

often bruised and swollen. The cranial edge of the greater trochanter may be used to help identify the correct plane of surgical dissection. The prominent tendinous insertion of the deep gluteal muscle can also be used for orientation. When the hip is luxated the femoral head usually lies beneath the deep gluteal muscle. The proximal femur is usually displaced craniodorsally and may obscure visualization of the acetabulum.

Positioning

The patient is positioned in lateral recumbency with the affected limb up. The limb is suspended for surgical preparation to allow limb manipulation during surgery.

SURGICAL TECHNIQUES

Surgical stabilization of hip luxations may be accomplished by capsular reconstruction if the joint capsule is intact. If the joint capsule is not intact or if added stability is needed, joint reconstruction and/or translocation of the greater trochanter may be performed.

Exploration of the Hip Joint

Perform a craniolateral exposure to the hip joint (see p. 848); if additional exposure is necessary, perform a trochanteric osteotomy (see p. 836). Reflect the deep *gluteal muscle and visualize the femoral head craniodorsal to the hip joint. Visualize and remove remnants of the round ligament and debris from the femoral head and acetabulum; this allows the femoral head to completely seat within the acetabulum. Once the hip is reduced, assess stability by viewing the acetabular coverage of the femoral head and placing the hip joint through a complete range of motion. Perform the chosen stabilization technique (see below).*

☞ **NOTE** • A Hohmann retractor placed within or just caudal to the acetabulum and used to lever the femur caudally will improve visualization of the acetabulum.

Capsule Reconstruction

It is not uncommon for the joint capsule to be intact except for a small rent, through which the femoral head has luxated, or an area where the capsule has torn loose from its insertion site at the femoral neck. In both situations, if after replacing the femoral head the acetabular coverage is adequate and the joint stable through a range of motion, primary suturing of the capsule can be used as the sole reconstructive procedure.

☞ **N O T E ·** Reconstruction of the joint capsule as the sole means of stabilization requires that the dorsal joint capsule be identifiable and conformation of the hip joint be normal or near normal.

Suture the joint capsule with nonabsorbable monofilament material using an interrupted pattern (Fig. 30-57). If the capsule has torn from its insertion site, drill small holes in the femoral neck through which the suture can pass, *or reattach the capsule with screws and spiked washers.*

Translocation of the Greater Trochanter

If the joint capsule is injured beyond repair but the gluteal musculature is not compromised, a trochanteric osteotomy can be performed to translocate the greater trochanter distally and slightly caudally. Relocation of the greater trochanter enables contraction of the gluteal muscles to abduct and internally rotate the femoral head.

Perform a trochanteric osteotomy (see p. 836) and reflect the gluteal musculature proximally. Once the hip has been cleaned of debris and reduced, place the limb in abduction. Use an ostetotome and mallet to create a new surface caudal and distal to the point where the greater trochanter normally seats (Fig. 30-58). Replace the greater trochanter at its new attachment site and secure it in position with a tension band (see p. 747).

Joint Reconstruction

The joint capsule can be shredded beyond where primary suturing is possible and the gluteal muscle mass is compromised, making stabilization with a trochanteric transposition impossible. In these cases, a prosthetic capsule or transacetabular pin can be used to maintain reduction during the healing of the fibrous joint capsule. A prosthetic capsule is made of suture material inserted in the craniodorsal acetabular rim and trochanteric fossa (Fig. 30-59). *Place two screws with flat metal washers in the dorsal rim of the acetabulum. Insert one screw at the 10 o'clock position and one at the 1 o'clock position. Place a third screw and washer in the trochanteric fossa (alternatively, drill a hole through the femoral neck in the trochanteric fossa to accept suture). Pass heavy nonabsorbable suture in a figure-eight pattern between the acetabular screws and trochanteric fossa.*

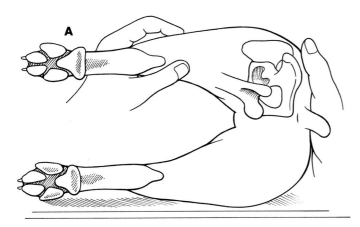

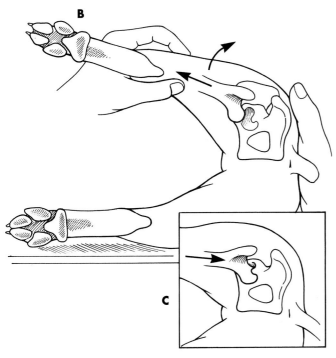

FIG. 30-56
A, For ventral hip luxations, place the patient in lateral recumbency with the limb held perpendicular to the spine. Grasp the limb at the tarsal joint with one hand and place the other hand under the limb medial to the hip joint. **B,** Place traction on the limb while simultaneously abducting the leg to pull the femoral head beyond the medial rim of the acetabulum. **C,** Once the femoral head has cleared the acetabular rim, exert lateral pressure medial to the hip joint to position the femoral head lateral to the acetabulum. Push proximally and allow the femoral head to fall into the acetabulum.

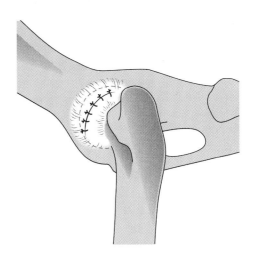

FIG. 30-57
Hip joint capsule reconstruction. Coxofemoral joint stabilization via capsulorrhaphy. Interrupted sutures have been placed to appose the joint capsule.

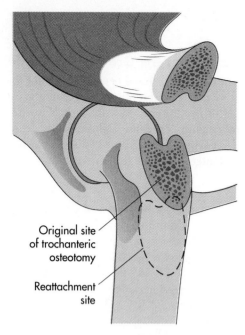

FIG. 30-58

To stabilize the coxofemoral joint by translocating the greater trochanter, prepare a new site distal and slightly caudal to the normal anatomic position. Stabilize the greater trochanter in this position with small pins and orthopedic wire (tension band).

☞ **N O T E** · When placing a transacetabular pin, use care to avoid driving the pin too far into the pelvic canal. The depth of the medial wall of the acetabulum is only 3 to 4 mm.

A transacetabular pin is placed through the femoral neck into the medial wall of the acetabulum (Fig. 30-60). *Predrill a hole, slightly smaller than the diameter of the pin to be used, from the third trochanter and through the femoral head to exit from the femoral head where the round ligament inserts. Insert the smooth pin through the drill hole until the pin point is visible just beneath the articular surface of the femoral head. Reduce the luxation and place the limb in abduction and slight internal rotation. While exerting medial pressure on the greater trochanter, drill the pin into the acetabular fossa. Bend the pin at the third trochanter to prevent medial migration. Place the patient in an Ehmer bandage until the transacetabular pin is removed (generally 4 to 7 days).*

Placement of an Elastic External Fixator

If there is a concurrent injury that prevents weight bearing in another limb, or if immediate weight bearing after hip reduction is desired, the Ehmer bandage cannot be properly placed for postoperative support. An alternate method of assisting postoperative maintenance of hip reduction is the application of an elastic external fixator (Fig. 30-61). *Reduce the hip through either closed reduction or open reduction.*

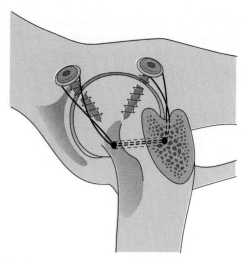

FIG. 30-59

Coxofemoral joint stabilization by placement of a prosthetic capsule. Note strategic placement of bone screws in the dorsolateral acetabulum. Suture material is passed from the screws through a pre-drilled tunnel in the dorsal femoral neck and tightened. The presence of suture in this position prevents craniodorsal reluxation.

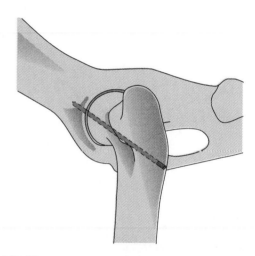

FIG. 30-60

Stabilization of the coxofemoral joint by placement of a transacetabular pin. The site for pin placement is through the center of the femoral neck. The pin should exit the femoral head at the fovea, cross the joint space, and enter the nonarticular wall of the medial acetabular fossa.

Make a small incision overlying the greater trochanter and prepare a tunnel through the soft tissue to the trochanteric fossa. Protect the soft tissue while inserting an end-threaded pin into the marrow cavity of the femur. The pin need not extend beyond the proximal one third of the femur. Insert a second end-threaded pin from proximal to distal across the body of the ilium 2 cm cranial to the acebatulum. Connect the pins outside the skin margins with a heavy elastic band. You may wish to place a Kirschner clamp on the pin as it exits the skin surface to help prevent the elastic band from

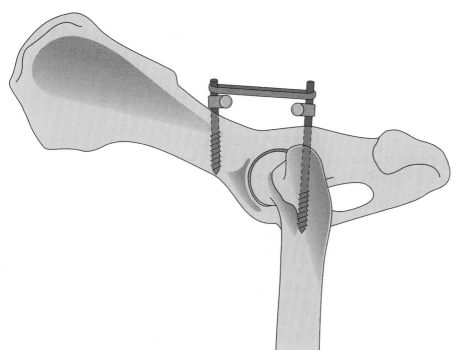

FIG. 30-61
An elastic external fixator may be used to stabilize the coxofemoral joint. Note the position of the external skeletal fixator transfixation pins cranial to the acetabulum and through the trochanteric fossa. The ends of the pin exit the skin dorsal to the hip and are connected by an elastic band.

placing pressure on the skin and potentially causing necrosis. Postoperatively, maintain the skin-to-pin interface with daily cleansing and application of an antiseptic. Remove the pins in 10 to 14 days.

SUTURE MATERIALS/SPECIAL INSTRUMENTS

Either No. 1 or No. 2 nonabsorbable suture is used for capsule reconstruction. An osteotome, mallet, pins, and wire are needed for translocation of the greater trochanter. Prosthetic capsule reconstruction requires screws and stainless steel washers. A small Steinmann pin is used for transacetabular pin reconstruction. An elastic external fixator requires end-threaded pins, Kirschner clamps, and an elastic band (bicycle tubing or a heavy rubber band).

POSTOPERATIVE CARE AND ASSESSMENT

Patients are usually placed in an Ehmer bandage to assist hip reduction in the early postoperative period. The bandage is removed 4 to 7 days after reduction. Leash activity is required for an additional 3 weeks, and the animal is gradually returned to full activity over a 2-week period. Reexamination 3 days after removal of the Ehmer bandage and before resumption of unsupervised activity is advised.

PROGNOSIS

Success rates for maintaining reduction and regaining good to excellent limb function with closed reduction are about 50%. The success rate is lower in patients with poor conformation of the hip joint secondary to hip dysplasia or previous trauma. Clinical studies indicate that the success of surgical intervention following failure of closed reduction is not different from the success rate in patients undergoing surgical reduction as a primary treatment. Therefore, it is reasonable to attempt closed reduction in patients with a hip luxation. Success rates for maintaining reduction with good to excellent limb function following open reduction is approximately 85% to 90% (Bone, Walker, Cantwell, 1984; Basher, Walter, Newton, 1986). The results do not appear to favor any one reconstruction technique.

References

Basher WP, Walter MC, Newton CD: Coxofemoral luxation in the dog and cat, *Vet Surg* 15:356, 1986.
Bone DL, Walker M, Cantwell HD: Traumatic coxofemoral luxation in dogs; results of repair, *Vet Surg* 13:263, 1984.

Suggested Reading

Bennett D, Duff SR; Transarticular pinning as a treatment for hip luxation in the dog and cat, *J Small Anim Pract* 21:373, 1980.
Braden TD, Johnson ME: Technique and indications of a prosthetic capsule for repair of recurrent and chronic coxofemoral luxations, *Vet Comp Orth Tram* 1:26, 1988.
Hunt CA, Henry WB: Transarticular pinning for repair of hip dislocation in the dog: a retrospective study of 40 cases, *J Am Vet Med Assoc* 187:828, 1985.
Johnson ME, Braden TD: A retrospective study of prosthetic capsule technique for treatment of problem cases of dislocated hips, *Vet Surg* 16:346, 1987.
Katcherian G: Pelvic osteotomy and distal transfer of the greater trochanter for luxation of the hip, *Canine Pract* 15:7, 1990.

LEGG-PERTHES

DEFINITIONS

Legg-Perthes disease is a noninflammatory aseptic necrosis of the femoral head occurring in young patients before closure of the capital femoral physis.

SYNONYMS

Osteochondritis dissecans of the femoral head, avascular necrosis of the femoral head

GENERAL CONSIDERATIONS AND CLINICALLY RELEVANT PATHOPHYSIOLOGY

Legg-Perthes results in collapse of the femoral epiphysis because of an interruption of blood flow. The reason for the loss of blood flow is not positively known, but several theories have been proposed. The vascular supply to the femoral head in young animals with open proximal femoral physes is derived solely from epiphyseal vessels. Metaphyseal vessels do not cross the physis to contribute to femoral head vascularity. Epiphyseal vessels course extraosseously along the surface of the femoral neck, cross the growth plate, and penetrate bone to supply nourishment to the femoral epiphysis. Synovitis or sustained abnormal limb position may cause sufficient increased intraarticular pressure to collapse the fragile veins and inhibit blood flow. An autosomal recessive gene has been proposed as a genetic cause for development of aseptic necrosis of the femoral head. After cell death occurs, the reparative processes begin. The bone substance is weakened mechanically during the revascularization period, and normal physiologic weight-bearing forces may cause collapse and fragmentation of the femoral epiphysis (Fig. 30-62). When this happens, incongruency of the femoral

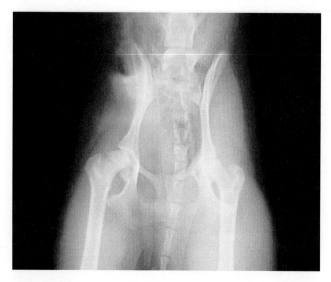

FIG. 30-62
Radiograph of a young dog with Legg-Perthes disease. The femoral head appears moth-eaten and is misshapen.

epiphysis and acetabulum results in degenerative joint disease. Fragmentation (fractures) of the femoral epiphysis and osteoarthrosis cause pain and resulting lameness.

> ☞ **N O T E** · Because this condition has been linked to an autosomal recessive gene, be sure to advise owners to have affected animals neutered.

DIAGNOSIS
Clinical Presentation

Signalment. Legg-Perthes is diagnosed in young, small-breed dogs (i.e., under 10 kg). Peak incidence of onset is 6 to 10 months, and males and females are equally affected. This condition occurs bilaterally in 12% to 17% of affected animals (Lee, Fry, 1969). Cats apparently are not affected.

History. Affected animals usually are presented for evaluation of a slow-onset, weight-bearing lameness that worsens over a 6 to 8-week period. Lameness may progress to non–weight-bearing status. Some clients report acute onset of clinical lameness. In these patients, sudden collapse of the epiphysis may cause acute exacerbation of an already present, but imperceptible, lameness. Other clinical signs can include irritability, reduced appetite, and chewing at the skin over the affected hip.

Physical Examination Findings

Manipulation of the hip joint consistently elicits pain in affected animals. Limited range of motion, muscle atrophy, and crepitus may be present with advanced disease.

Radiography

Radiographs show deformity of the femoral head, shortening of the femoral neck, and foci of decreased bone density within the femoral epiphysis (see Fig. 30-62).

Laboratory Findings

Consistent laboratory abnormalities are not present.

DIFFERENTIAL DIAGNOSIS

Differential diagnoses include physeal trauma and medial patella luxation. Small dogs may have concurrent bilateral, medial patella luxation (see p. 976), and care must be taken to examine the stifle joint carefully to diagnose this condition.

MEDICAL OR CONSERVATIVE MANAGEMENT

The diagnosis is often made after collapse and fragmentation have resulted in joint incongruity and degenerative joint disease. Conservative treatment with antiinflammatory medication may provide pain relief, but definitive treatment requires surgical intervention.

SURGICAL TREATMENT
Preoperative Management

Limit activity until definitive surgical treatment is done. Antiinflammatory medications may be administered for pain relief.

Anesthesia

Anesthetic management of animals with orthopedic disease is provided on p. 708.

Surgical Anatomy

The anatomy of the coxofemoral joint is discussed on p. 835. In animals with Legg-Perthes diseases the joint capsule appears thickened and more vascular than normal. The femoral head and neck often appear misshapen. The bone may be soft and may fragment when the head and neck are excised, requiring that rongeurs be used to remove small fragments.

Positioning

The animal is positioned in lateral recumbency with the affected leg up. A hanging-limb preparation may be used to facilitate manipulation of the limb during surgery. The leg should be prepared from the dorsal midline to midtibia.

SURGICAL TECHNIQUES

Excision of the femoral head and neck is the treatment of choice. See p. 947 for a description of the technique.

SUTURE MATERIALS/SPECIAL INSTRUMENTS

Instruments necessary to remove the femoral head and neck in small dogs include an osteotome and mallet, bone cutters, or rongeurs.

POSTOPERATIVE CARE AND ASSESSMENT

The animal should be encouraged to use the limb immediately after surgery. Passive flexion and extension of the hip joint should be performed twice daily as soon as the animal will tolerate it. Physical therapy should be initiated with small movements and the range of motion gradually increased over 5 to 10 minutes.

PROGNOSIS

The prognosis for normal limb use is good to excellent after femoral head and neck excision because of the small size of affected dogs. Continued lameness should be expected in animals that do not have surgery performed.

References

Lee R, Fry PD: Some observations on the occurrence of Legg-Calve-Perthes disease (coxa plana) in the dog and an evaluation of excision arthroplasty as a method of treatment, *J Small Anim Pract* 19:309, 1969.

Suggested Reading

Gambardella P: Legg-Calve-Perthes disease in dogs. In Bojrab MJ, editor: *Pathophysiology in small animal surgery*, Philadelphia, 1981, Lea & Febiger.

Gibson KL, Lewis DD, Pechman RD: Use of external coaptation for the treatment of avascular necrosis of the femoral head in the dog, *J Am Vet Med Assoc* 197:868, 1990.

Lippincott CL: A summary of 300 surgical cases performed over an 8-year period: excision arthroplasty of the femoral head and neck with a caudal pass of the biceps femoris muscle sling, *Vet Surg* 16:96, 1987.

Roperto F, Papparella S, Crovace A: Legg-Calve-Perthes disease in dogs: histological and ultrastructural investigations, *J Am Anim Hosp Assoc* 28:156, 1992.

Vasseur PB: Mode of inheritance of Perthes' disease in Manchester terriers, *Clin Orthop* 157:287, 1989.

Warren DV, Dingwall JS: Legg-Perthes disease in the dog: a review, *Can Vet J* 13:135, 1972.

STIFLE

CRANIAL CRUCIATE LIGAMENT RUPTURE

DEFINITIONS

Cranial cruciate ligament injuries are complete or partial tears. **Cranial drawer** is a term used to describe excessive craniocaudal movement of the tibia relative to the femur as a result of cruciate ligament injury.

SYNONYMS

Football player's knee, deranged knee

GENERAL CONSIDERATIONS AND CLINICALLY RELEVANT PATHOPHYSIOLOGY

The cranial cruciate ligament (CCL) is divided into craniomedial and caudolateral bands, which have different insertion points on the tibial plateau. The craniomedial band is taut during all phases of flexion and extension; the caudolateral band is taut in extension but becomes lax in flexion. The CCL also functions to limit internal rotation of the tibia; as the stifle is flexed, the cranial and caudal cruciate ligaments twist on each other, limiting the degree of internal rotation of the tibia relative to the femur. Interaction of the cranial and caudal cruciate ligaments during flexion also serves to provide a limited degree of varus-valgus support to the flexed stifle joint. Mechanoreceptors and afferent nerve endings have been identified within the interfiber layers of the cranial cruciate ligament. Innervation of the ligament serves as a proprioceptive feedback mechanism to prevent excessive flexion or extension of the stifle joint. This protective action is accomplished through stimulation or relaxation of muscle groups that lend support to the joint.

☞ **N O T E ·** The craniomedial band of the cranial cruciate ligament is the primary check against craniocaudal drawer motion.

The mechanism of CCL injury is primarily a reflection of its function as a constraint to joint motion. Injury is most commonly associated with violent internal rotation of the leg. When this occurs, the cruciate ligaments twist and become tightly wound on themselves. As internal rotation progresses, the cranial cruciate ligament is subject to injury from the caudomedial edge of the lateral femoral condyle as the condyle rotates against the ligament. Another mechanism of CCL injury is hyperextension of the stifle. When the stifle joint is hyperextended, the roof of the intercondylar notch may act as a knife and transect the cranial cruciate ligament. Although ligament injury can be purely traumatic, other factors may be involved in the pathogenesis of cruciate disease (e.g., structural and histologic changes that occur in the ligament as the animal ages, abnormal conformation). Histologically, a loss of fiber-bundle organization and metaplastic changes of the cellular elements occur. Biomechanically, this correlates with a loss of structural and material strength and stiffness. Abnormal conformation may play a role in development of CCL injuries. Certain breeds (rottweiler and chow chow) appear to have a greater standing angle of the stifle joint than other breeds, and this may predispose to complete or partial tearing of the craniomedial band of the CCL from the roof of the intercondylar notch. Anticollagen antibodies and immune complexes have been detected in synovial fluid and sera of dogs with CCL rupture. The significance of this finding is unknown.

DIAGNOSIS
Clinical Presentation

Signalment. Either sex and any age or breed of dog may be affected. CCL injury is rare in cats. Recent studies suggest that younger, more active breeds of dogs may be predisposed to CCL rupture (Bennett et al, 1988).

History. Acute injury, chronic injury, and partial tears are three clinical presentations associated with cranial cruciate ligament injury. Patients with acute tears are seen for sudden non–weight-bearing or partial–weight-bearing lameness. Lameness usually resolves within 3 to 6 weeks after injury without treatment, particularly in patients weighing less than 10 kg. Retrospective studies of dogs weighing less than 10 kg indicate that they typically have adequate clinical function with conservative treatment (Vasseur, 1984). However, in dogs larger than 10 kg, lameness improves but they never return to preinjury activity without evidence of recurring lameness. Chronic lameness is associated with development of degenerative joint disease. Partial cranial cruciate ligament tears are difficult to diagnose in the early stages of injury. Initially, affected animals have a mild weight-bearing lameness associated with exercise, and until degenerative changes develop, the lameness resolves with rest. Later, however, as the ligament continues to tear and the stifle becomes increasingly unstable, degenerative changes worsen and lameness becomes more pronounced and does not resolve with rest.

Physical Examination Findings

Animals with acute tears are often apprehensive during examination of the stifle joint, but pain is usually mild or absent. Instability can be difficult to elicit because of patient apprehension and resulting muscle contraction. Joint effu-

sion may be palpable adjacent to the patella tendon. Patients with chronic tears may have thigh muscle atrophy (compared with the normal limb) and crepitus may be evident when the stifle is flexed and extended. When the joint is extended from a flexed position, a clicking or popping may be heard and felt; this is commonly associated with a meniscal tear. However, the absence of joint noise does not eliminate the possibility of meniscal injury. An enlargement along the medial joint surface can often be palpated and is caused by osteophyte formation along the trochlear ridges. Craniocaudal instability can be difficult to elicit, particularly in large or apprehensive patients with chronic tears caused by proliferation of the fibrous joint capsule.

With partial tears, early instability is difficult to detect because a portion of the ligament is intact and inhibits craniocaudal movement. Tearing of the caudolateral band alone will not produce instability because the intact craniomedial band is taut in both flexion and extension. If an isolated injury to the craniomedial band occurs (caudolateral band remains intact), the joint is stable in extension since the caudolateral band remains taut; however, instability will be present in flexion since the caudolateral band normally becomes lax during flexion. Initially, pain, synovial effusion, and crepitus are absent, but signs of instability and degenerative joint disease eventually become evident.

☞ **N O T E** · Always compare the limb that has the suspected injury with the opposite limb if the instability is questionable.

Cranial drawer movement is diagnostic of cruciate ligament injury. The cranial drawer test is performed with the patient in lateral recumbency. Lack of adequate patient relaxation is the single most common cause of failure to elicit cranial drawer movement. Therefore if there is high suspicion that the lameness is caused by cruciate ligament injury, general anesthesia or heavy sedation is necessary to negate the influence of muscle tension (see p. 723). Once the dog is in lateral position, the examiner stands to the patient's rear and positions the thumb and forefinger on one hand on the femur (Fig. 30-63). The thumb is placed directly behind the fabella and the forefinger over the patella. The remaining fingers are wrapped around the thigh. The other hand is placed on the tibia, with the thumb directly behind the fibular head and the forefinger over the tibial crest. The three remaining fingers are wrapped around the tibial shaft. The femur is stabilized with the one hand while the second hand moves the tibia forward and back in a direction parallel to the transverse plane of the tibial plateau. The pressure to move the tibia forward should be applied through the thumb behind the fibular head. The tibia must be held in neutral position, as determined by the position of the fingers on the patella and tibial tuberosity, and not be allowed to internally rotate. If this occurs, internal rotation of the joint may appear as cranial drawer movement. The examiner must test for signs of instability with the stifle joint in extension, normal stand-

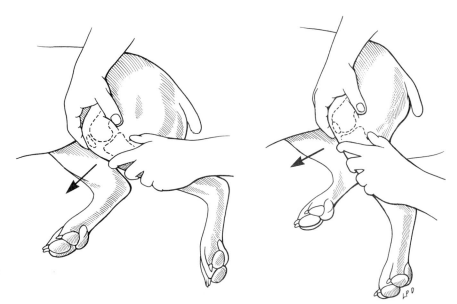

FIG. 30-63
To examine for cruciate ligament injury, place the thumb of one hand over the lateral fabella and the index finger over the patella. Stabilize the femur with this hand. Place the thumb of the opposite hand caudal to the fibular head with the index finger on the tibial tuberosity. With the stifle flexed and then extended, attempt to move the tibia cranially and distally to the femur.

ing angle, and 90 degrees of flexion. If the degree of movement is questionable, comparison with the opposite limb is helpful. A positive test is craniocaudal movement beyond the 0 to 2 mm found in normal stifle joints. In younger patients, craniocaudal translation may be as great as 4 to 5 mm, but ligament rupture is confirmed by the absence of an abrupt stop at the cranial extent of movement. Because most isolated cruciate ligament tears involve the cranial cruciate ligament, craniocaudal instability is usually associated with injury of this ligament. If a partial tear is present, the cranial drawer sign may reveal only 2 to 3 mm of instability when the test is done with the stifle flexed and no instability with the stifle in extension. Following completion of the cranial drawer test, the stifle should be flexed and extended through a range of normal movement. With the leg in extension, collateral stability should be assessed.

☞ **N O T E** · Juvenile dogs have increased joint laxity (4 to 5 mm) but maintain a distinct end point when the tibia is moved cranially.

Radiography

With acute tears, radiographs are helpful in ruling out other causes of stifle joint lameness. Radiographic findings in patients with chronic ligament tears include ostophyte formation along the trochlear ridge, caudal surface of the tibial plateau, and inferior pole of the patella (Fig. 30-64). Thickening of the medial fibrous joint capsule and subchondral sclerosis are also evident.

Laboratory Findings

If joint palpation and radiographs are inconclusive, joint centesis and synovial fluid examination are helpful. In cases of partial ligament tear, centesis is particularly helpful in identifying stifle joint involvement as the cause of the lame-

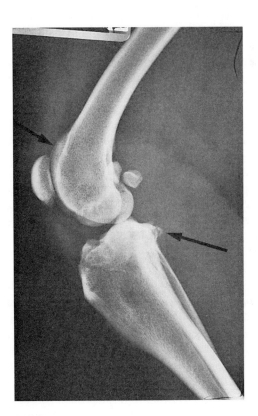

FIG. 30-64
Lateral radiograph of a dog with a chronic cruciate ligament rupture. Note the osteophyte formation along the trochlear ridge and caudal tibial plateau (*arrows*).

ness. Increased amounts of joint fluid and a two- to three-fold increase in cell numbers (6000 to 9000/µl) are indicative of secondary degenerative joint disease (see also p. 889).

DIFFERENTIAL DIAGNOSIS

Differential diagnoses include mild joint sprains or muscle strains, patella luxation, caudal cruciate ligament injury, primary meniscal injury, long digital extensor tendon avulsion, and primary or secondary arthritis.

MEDICAL OR CONSERVATIVE MANAGEMENT

Conservative treatment is best tolerated in patients weighing less than 10 kg; however, surgical stabilization is recommended in patients of any size to ensure optimal function. Lameness often resolves within 6 weeks in small patients managed conservatively (i.e., rest and antiinflammatory drugs). These patients appear to function normally on the injured leg; however, instability persists and secondary degenerative joint disease frequently develops. Despite the fact that the animal appears to function adequately after the initial injury, body weight is often merely shifted to the uninjured leg. Abnormal stress, coupled with the increasing mechanical weakness of the cruciate ligament associated with aging, may lead to rupture of the cruciate ligament in the opposite stifle joint within 12 to 18 months. Because these patients are then nonambulatory, they are often incorrectly diagnosed as having an acute neurologic problem. An accurate history and physical examination should alert the clinician to the fact that bilateral cruciate ligament injury, rather than neurologic disease, is the problem. Treatment of patients with bilateral cruciate ligament ruptures is less successful than in animals with only one injured stifle joint. For this reason, surgical reconstruction is recommended in all patients with cranial cruciate ligament injury.

☞ **NOTE** · Injury of the contralateral cruciate occurs in 40% of patients. The percentage increases (60%) if radiographic changes are visible in the uninjured joint.

SURGICAL TREATMENT

Surgical therapy is divided into reconstruction techniques and primary repair with augmentation. Primary repairs are not used commonly and should always be supplemented with a reconstructive technique. The reconstruction method chosen for an individual patient is a matter of surgeon's preference because retrospective studies have shown the success rate to be near 90% regardless of technique (Denny, Barr, 1987; Elkins et al, 1991). Intracapsular and extracapsular reconstruction of the cranial cruciate ligament are techniques that share equal popularity among veterinary surgeons. Intracapsular reconstructions consist of passing autogenous tissue through the joint using the "over-the-top" method or passing the tissue through predrilled holes in the femur and/or tibia. Extracapsular reconstructions involve the placement of sutures outside the joint or redirection of the lateral collateral ligament. It is often useful to combine intracapsular and extracapsular reconstructions in large- and giant-breed dogs.

Regardless of technique used to stabilize the stifle, the meniscus should be inspected for tears or other evidence of trauma. Damage to the caudal body of the medial meniscus

is seen in 50% to 75% of patients with a torn cranial cruciate ligament (Hulse, Shires. 1985). The majority of these patients have a "bucket-handle" tear, which needs to be excised.

Preoperative Management

Patients with torn cranial cruciate ligaments should have activity limited before surgery, to prevent further damage to the articular cartilage caused by instability.

Anesthesia

General anesthetic recommendations for orthopedic patients are discussed on p. 708. Opioid epidural administration will decrease postoperative discomfort (see p. 708).

Surgical Anatomy

Knowledge of the origin and insertion of normal ligamentous structures in the stifle joint is important when considering surgery to repair a cruciate ligament rupture. The CCL originates from the inside (medial) surface of the lateral femoral condyle (Fig. 30-65). The ligament is a complex arrangement of longitudinally oriented collagen fiber bundles that function to prevent excessive cranial translation of the tibia relative to the femur. The ligament fibers course distal and medial, spiral 90 degrees, and insert onto the craniomedial surface of the tibial plateau beneath the intermeniscal ligament. The medial and lateral menisci are fibrocartilaginous disks that have a semilunar shape. The medial meniscus is often injured with cruciate ligament damage. If an extracapsular reconstruction is chosen as a method of treatment,

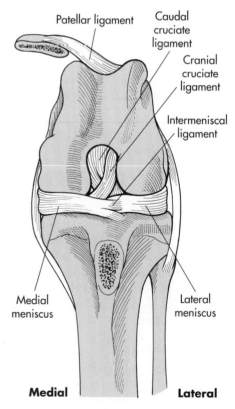

FIG. 30-65
Orientation of cruciate ligaments and menisci.

the location of the peroneal nerve must be identified to avoid inadvertently damaging it.

Positioning

The patient may be positioned in dorsal or lateral recumbency. The limb should be prepared in a suspended position to allow maximal manipulation during surgery. The leg should be clipped and prepared for aseptic surgery from the hip to the tarsus.

SURGICAL TECHNIQUES
Lateral Approach to the Stifle Joint

Make a craniolateral skin incision centered over the patella (Fig. 30-66, A). Begin the incision 5 cm proximal to the patella and continue it distally 5 cm below the tibial crest. Incise subcutaneous tissues along the same line to visualize the septum between the superficial leaf of the fascia lata and the biceps femoris muscle proximally and the lateral retinaculum distally. Make an incision through the fascia lata proximally and carry the incision through the fascia lata and lateral retinaculum distally (Figure 30-66, B). Make an incision through the joint capsule, beginning 1 cm distal to the patella. Continue the incision proximally, along a line adjacent to the patellar tendon, to the inferior pole of the patella. Then incise along the border of the vastus lateralis muscle toward the fabella (Fig. 30-66, C). Displace the patella medially to expose the cranial surface of the joint.

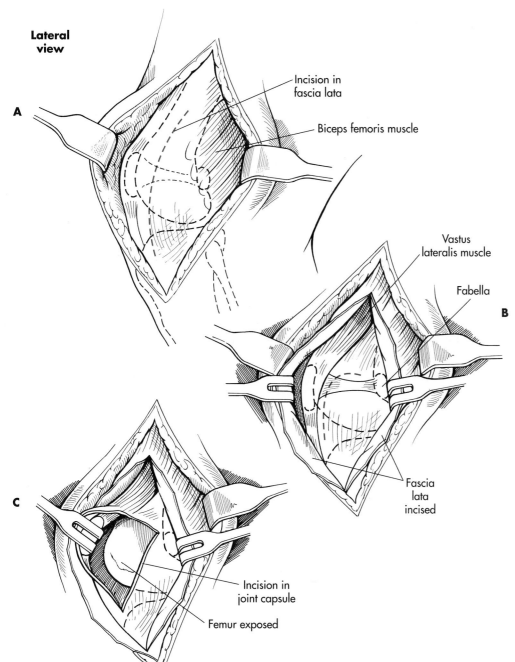

Lateral view

A

Incision in fascia lata

Biceps femoris muscle

Vastus lateralis muscle

Fabella

B

Fascia lata incised

C

Incision in joint capsule

Femur exposed

FIG. 30-66
A, For a lateral approach to the stifle joint, make a craniolateral skin incision centered over the patella. Incise subcutaneous tissues along the same line to visualize the septum between the superficial leaf of the fascia lata and biceps femoris muscle proximally and lateral retinaculum distally. **B,** Make an incision through the fascia lata proximally and carry the incision through the fascia lata and lateral retinaculum distally. **C,** Incise joint capsule and continue the incision proximally adjacent to the patellar tendon. Then incise along the border of the vastus lateralis toward the fabella. Displace the patella medially to expose the cranial surface of the joint.

Medial View

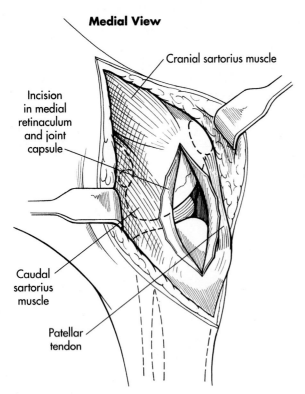

Cranial sartorius muscle

Incision
in medial
retinaculum
and joint
capsule

Caudal
sartorius
muscle

Patellar
tendon

FIG. 30-67
For a medial approach to the stifle joint, make a craniomedial incision centered over the patella. Incise subcutaneous tissues along the same line to expose the parapatellar medial retinaculum. Make an incision through the medial retinaculum and joint capsule adjacent to the medial ridge of the patellar tendon.

Medial Approach to the Stifle Joint

Make a craniomedial incision centered over the patella (Fig. 30-67). Begin the incision 5 cm proximal to the patella and continue distally 5 cm below the tibial crest. Incise subcutaneous tissues along the same line to expose the parapatellar medial retinaculum. Make an incision through the medial retinaculum and joint capsule adjacent to the medial ridge of the patellar tendon. Continue the incision proximally and distally to equal the extent of the subcutaneous tissue incision.

Intracapsular Repair

A popular intracapsular reconstruction is the placement of an autogenous tissue graft through the joint to mimic the course of the cranial cruciate ligament. The technique described here uses the lateral one third of the patella tendon and distal fascia lata. The tissue is placed through a tibial tunnel, through the joint, and over the top of the lateral condyle. Alternately, the graft may be placed through a tibial and femoral tunnel.

Perform a lateral approach to the stifle joint as described above. Free the superficial surface of the patella tendon from all loose connective tissue and flex the limb to tighten the patella tendon and lateral retinacular tissue. Make an incision beginning at the lateral edge of the distal pole of the patella and extend it through the lateral one third of the patella tendon and retinaculum to the tibial crest distally. The landmark for the most distal extent of the incision is the palpable tuberosity cranial to the groove of the long digital extensor muscle. *Place a periosteal elevator in the incision and separate the patella tendon and fascia lata from the joint capsule. As the graft is freed from the joint capsule near the patella, use the lateral edge of the elevator to reflect the graft from the lateral patella surface. Use scissors to incise the fascia lata along the medial edge of the cranial sartorius muscle. Carry the incision through the fascia lata proximally the full length of the skin incision. When the proximal extent of the incision is reached, incise the fascia lata caudally to the cranial border of the biceps femoris muscle. Continue the incision distally along the cranial edge of the biceps muscle to the tibial plateau (Fig. 30-68, A).* When bringing the fascial incision distally, it is extremely important to maintain equal width of the fascial graft along its entire length. *Incise the joint capsule from the distal pole of the patella to the tibial crest. At the level of the patella, direct the capsule incision proximally and caudally along the border of the vastus lateralis muscle to the region of the lateral fabella. Luxate the patella medially to expose the cranial view of the stifle. Remove remnants of the torn cruciate ligament with a scalpel and examine the internal structures of the joint. To visualize the caudomedial compartment of the joint, place the tip of a Hohmann retractor on the caudal tibial spine and force the body of the retractor against the distal femoral trochlea. Place caudal pressure on the retractor handle to force the tibia forward and down, exposing the medial meniscus. Inspect the meniscus for damage. If it is torn, grasp the torn section of meniscus with a forceps and excise the medial and lateral attachments. Widen the roof and lateral wall of the intercondylar notch to ensure adequate space for the graft (notchoplasty).* Notchoplasty ensures that the walls of the intercondylar notch will not impinge on the graft. *Next, free the insertion of the fascial graft from the tibial plateau with a small osteotome and mallet. Place an osteotome behind the tibial tuberosity just cranial to the muscular groove of the long digital extensor muscle. Free the graft from this site by removing a small section of bone. Cranially, use the osteotome to free the patella tendon part of the graft from the craniolateral tibial crest. Remove a thin layer of bone with the tendon to free this section of the graft. Use a periosteal elevator to reflect the cranial tibialis muscle from the craniolateral face of the proximal tibia. Drill a tunnel, large enough to accept the graft, from the cranial surface of the tibia to the insertion of the cranial cruciate ligament inside the joint (Fig. 30-68, B). Place a wire loop through the tunnel from inside the joint to exit laterally. Pull the graft through the tunnel into the joint with the aid of the wire loop.* When placing the graft be sure that the bone is seated well inside the tunnel. *Then pass the graft through the joint by passing it "over the top" of the lateral condyle or by passing it through a drill hole in the femur. To perform the over-the-top maneuver,*

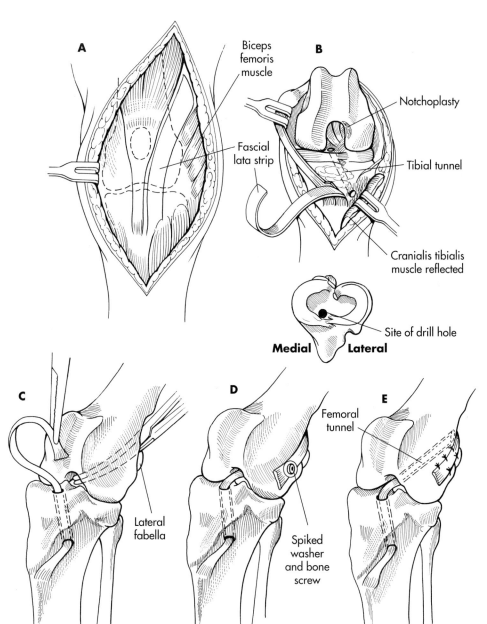

A, Biceps femoris muscle

Fascial lata strip

B, Notchoplasty

Tibial tunnel

Cranialis tibialis muscle reflected

Site of drill hole

Medial **Lateral**

C, Lateral fabella

D, Femoral tunnel

Spiked washer and bone screw

E,

FIG. 30-68
A, For an intracapsular reconstruction using distal fascia lata and patella tendon, perform a lateral approach to the stifle joint. Isolate a graft from the lateral patellar tendon and retinaculum. **B,** Drill a tunnel that is large enough to accept the graft from the cranial surface of the tibia to the insertion of the cranial cruciate ligament inside the joint. **C,** Place the graft through the tibial tunnel and **D,** over the top of the lateral condyle. **E,** Alternately, place the graft through a tunnel drilled in the femoral condyles.

pass a curved forceps over the top of the fabella from caudal to cranial. Glide the forceps next to the lateral condyle and penetrate the caudal joint capsule. Grasp the free end of the graft and pull it through the joint (Fig. 30-68, C). To place the graft through a tunnel drilled in the femoral condyles, drill a tunnel of sufficient diameter to accept the graft. The tunnel must enter the joint at a point that is caudal and inferior to the point where the normal cruciate ligament originated from the inside surface of the lateral femoral condyle. *Make an incision through the femoral fabellar ligament and pass the graft through the ligament. Secure the fascial graft to the lateral femoral condyle with a spiked polyacetyl washer and bone screw, or suture it to the femoral fabellar ligament, fibrous joint capsule, and patella tendon (Fig. 30-68, D and E). When the graft is being secured to the femoral condyle, do not attempt to elim-*

inate all the cranial drawer; this would place excessive tension within the graft. As a rule, all but 2 to 3 mm of cranial drawer should be eliminated while the leg is positioned in normal standing angle. *Suture the fibrous joint capsule, cut edge of fascia lata, and subcutaneous tissues with absorbable suture using a simple interrupted pattern. Suture skin with nonabsorbable suture in a simple interrupted pattern.*

Lateral Retinacular Stabilization

Perform a lateral approach to the stifle joint, open the joint, and inspect the meniscus for tears or damage. Remove the damaged meniscus, if present, and close the arthrotomy with absorbable suture using a simple interrupted pattern. Alternately, perform a medial approach to the stifle joint (see above) and displace the patella laterally, remove remnants of the cranial cruciate ligament, and inspect the internal structures of the stifle.

Treat meniscal tears as discussed on p. 975. Replace the patella in the trochlear groove and suture the arthrotomy with absorbable suture using an interrupted pattern. Reflect the skin laterally and make an incision through the distal fascia lata. Elevate the biceps femoris muscle from the lateral surface of the joint capsule to expose the gastrocnemius muscle. Pass monofilament polyester sutures or monofilament wire through the femoral-fabellar ligament

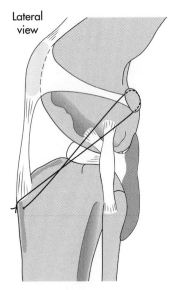

FIG. 30-69

An extracapsular reconstruction using heavy nonabsorbable suture(s). The suture(s) passes through deep fascia surrounding the fabella and through a predrilled hole in the tibial crest. Tying the suture(s) eliminates the cranial drawer.

and around the fabella. Next, pass the suture or wire through a predrilled hole through the tibial crest. Flex the stifle to 90 degrees or to a normal standing angle and hold the tibia caudally to remove drawer motion and tie the sutures (or twist the wire) until it engages the joint capsule (Fig. 30-69). In addition to the stabilizing suture, place a series of imbricating sutures through the fibrous joint capsule with nonabsorbable suture. Place each suture through the fibrous capsule caudal to the arthrotomy line, cross superficial to the arthrotomy, and penetrate the fibrous capsule cranial to the arthrotomy. Preplace individual sutures and do not tie until all sutures in the series are in place. Close as described above. The extracapsular sutures can be augmented with tissue advancements. Commonly, advancement of the biceps femoris muscle by suturing the cranial edge of the biceps fascia incision to the patella tendon will aid in restricting cranial drawer.

Fibular Head Advancement

Static advancement of the lateral collateral ligament is a useful technique for elimination of instability in the cranial cruciate–deficient stifle joint. This is accomplished by advancing the fibular head, which is the point of insertion of the lateral collateral ligament.

Perform a lateral approach to the stifle joint and arthrotomy as described above and inspect the meniscus for tears or damage. Remove the damaged meniscus, if present, and close the arthrotomy with absorbable suture using a simple interrupted pattern. Reflect the fascia lata caudally. To facilitate reflection of the fascia lata, make a craniocaudal transverse incision of the fascia lata 2 to 3 cm distal to the joint line. Free the fibular head cranially and caudally from the tibial epiphysis with sharp dissec-

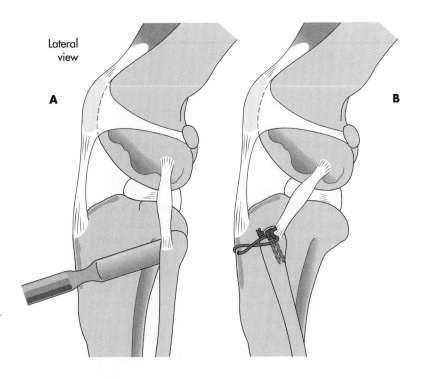

FIG. 30-70

A, For fibular head advancement, free the fibular head cranially and caudally from the tibial epiphysis with sharp dissection and elevation. **B,** Advance the fibular head and stabilize it with a small Steinmann pin and tension band wire.

tion and elevation (Fig. 30-70, A). Make an incision along the cranial and caudal edges of the lateral collateral ligament to allow cranial transposition of the ligament-bone complex. While being careful not to injure the popliteal tendon or lateral meniscus, free the deep surface of the ligament from its origin at the femoral epicondyle to its insertion at the fibular head. This is most easily accomplished with a small periosteal elevator. Incise the fibularis longus muscle and lateral digital extensor muscle at the joint line and reflect them craniodistally to allow cranial redirection of the fibular head. Externally rotate the tibia and advance the fibular head and collateral ligament cranially using bone-holding forceps. Stabilize the fibular head with a small Steinmann pin and tension-band wire (Fig. 30-70, B). Suture extensor muscles and fascia lata with absorbable suture using a simple interrupted pattern. Repair subcutaneous tissues and skin incisions as previously described.

☞ **N O T E** · Use extreme care to identify and protect the peroneal nerve throughout this procedure.

Primary Repair with Augmentation

Primary repair with augmentation is reserved for a small percentage of patients that have experienced failure of the cruciate ligament at the point of insertion on the tibial plateau or failure from the origin of the ligament on the femur. This mode of ligament failure may occur following trauma to the stifle joint in patients less than 1 year old. The most frequent site of failure is the point of insertion of the ligament on the tibial plateau. Surgical exposure is the same as described for intracapsular or extracapsular reconstruction. A reconstructive procedure is always used in addition to primary repair.

Perform either a medial or lateral approach to the stifle joint as described above. Once the arthrotomy is made, identify the cranial cruciate ligament. A small piece of cancellous bone often remains attached at the site of failure. Pass nonabsorbable suture through the ligament using a locking-loop pattern (see p. 1003). Make two small parallel drill holes from the medial tibial metaphysis to exit within the joint at the insertion point of the cranial cruciate ligament. Place wire loops through the holes and pass the free ends of the suture through the wire. Pull the wire through the predrilled holes to exit laterally. Perform a reconstructive procedure to augment the primary repair. Once the reconstruction is completed, tie the sutures from the ligament outside the joint (Fig. 30-71). Close the surgical wound using the technique described above.

SUTURE MATERIALS/SPECIAL INSTRUMENTS

Hohmann retractors are useful for inspecting the medial meniscus. With intracapsular repairs, instruments to drill holes in the tibia, a periosteal elevator, and osteotome are also needed. For extracapsular repairs, nonabsorbable suture (usually No. 2 to No. 5 polyester or nylon, depending upon the weight of the patient) or orthopedic wire (18- to 20-gauge) is used. Steinmann pins and wire are used to secure the fibula in a fibular head advancement.

POSTOPERATIVE CARE AND ASSESSMENT

After extracapsular repairs, patient activity is limited to exercise on a leash for 6 weeks. If wire is used, it will ultimately break, but this usually occurs after periarticular fibrous tissue has formed to help stabilize the joint. Occasionally, lameness will result when the wire breaks, but it usually resolves with 2 weeks of rest and administration of nonsteroidal antiinflammatory drugs (see Table 30-5). Following fibular head advancement, the limb is placed in a soft, padded bandage for 10 to 14 days. Then, exercise is limited to leash walking for an additional 3 weeks.

For intracapsular repairs a soft bandage is maintained for 2 weeks. Activity is restricted to a leash for a minimum of 12 weeks. Leash walking is encouraged, gradually increasing the time and distance of walks. Flexion and extension of the joint are encouraged to maintain range of motion. If a screw and washer are used, they should be removed 2 to 3 months postoperatively.

PROGNOSIS

Long-term function for patients having undergone a reconstructive procedure is good, and success has not been

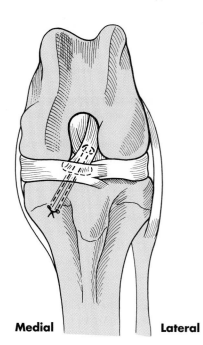

Medial   **Lateral**

FIG. 30-71
For a primary repair of an avulsed cranial cruciate ligament place a suture through the avulsed piece of bone and ligament. Pass the free ends of the suture through parallel tunnels and tie them outside the joint.

influenced by the method of reconstruction. Factors that do affect long-term outcome are the dog's size, activity, and intended use. Larger, active patients (particularly if athletic performance is expected) have a poorer prognosis for acceptable long-term function. A significant percentage of patients injure the ligament in the opposite knee within 3 years. If this occurs in a large athletic dog, the prognosis for long-term performance is fair.

References

Bennett D et al: A reappraisal of anterior cruciate ligament disease in the dog, *J Sm Anim Pract* 29:275, 1988.

Denny HR, Barr ARS: A further evaluation of the 'over-the-top' technique for anterior cruciate ligament replacement in the dog, *J Sm Anim Pract* 28:681, 1987.

Elkins AD et al: A retrospective study evaluating the degree of degenerative joint disease in the stifle joint of dogs following surgical repair of anterior cruciate ligament rupture, *J Am Anim Hosp Assoc* 27:533, 1991.

Hulse DA, Shires PK: The stifle joint. In Slatter DH, editor: *Textbook of small animal surgery,* Philadelphia, 1985, WB Saunders.

Vasseur PB: Clinical results following non-operative management for rupture of the cranial cruciate ligament in dogs, *Vet Surg* 13:243, 1984.

Suggested Reading

Bennett D, May C: An 'over-the-top with tibial tunnel' technique for repair of cranial cruciate ligament rupture in the dog, *J Sm Anim Pract* 32:103, 1991.

Doverspike M et al: Contralateral cranial cruciate ligament rupture: incidence in 114 dogs, *J Am Anim Hosp Assoc* 29:167, 1993.

Dulish ML: Suture reaction following extra-articular stifle stabilization in the dog: a retrospective study of 161 stifles, *J Am Anim Hosp Assoc* 17:569, 1981.

Fallon RK, Tomlinson JL: Prognostic indicators in 80 consecutive cases of cranial cruciate ligament rupture: a prospective study, *Vet Surg* 15:118, 1986.

Gambardella PC et al: Lateral suture technique for management of anterior cruciate ligament rupture in dogs: a retrospective study, *J Am Anim Hosp Assoc* 17:33, 1981.

Johnson SG et al: Material and structural biochemical properties of cranial cruciate reconstruction autografts in the canine, *Vet Surg* 18:58, 1989.

Niebaurer GW et al: Antibiodies to canine collagen types I and II in dogs with spontaneous cruciate ligament rupture and osteoarthritis, *Arthritis Rheum* 30:319, 1987.

Olmstead ML: The use of orthopedic wire as a lateral suture for stifle stabilization, *Vet Clin N Am Sm Anim Pract* 23:735, 1993.

Scavelli TD et al: Partial rupture of the cranial cruciate ligament of the stifle in dogs: 25 cases (1982–1988), *J Am Vet Med Assoc* 196:1135, 1990.

Smith GK, Torg JS: Fibular head transposition for repair of cruciate deficient stifle in the dog, *J Am Vet Med Assoc* 187:375, 1985.

Vasseur PB, Berry CR: Progression of stifle osteoarthrosis following reconstruction of the cranial cruciate ligament in 21 dogs, *J Am Anim Hosp Assoc* 28:129, 1992.

Vasseur PB et al: Correlative biomechanical and histological study of the cranial cruciate ligament in dogs, *Am J Vet Res* 9:1842, 1985.

CAUDAL CRUCIATE LIGAMENT INJURY

DEFINITIONS

Caudal cruciate ligamentous tears may be complete or partial, with resultant instability causing progressive degenerative joint disease.

GENERAL CONSIDERATIONS AND CLINICALLY RELEVANT PATHOPHYSIOLOGY

The caudal cruciate ligament can be functionally separated into two components; the larger cranial portion is taut in flexion and lax in extension, whereas the smaller caudal section is taut in extension and lax in flexion. The cranial and caudal bands function to prevent caudal translation (sliding) of the tibia during flexion. The caudal cruciate ligament also functions in concert with the cranial cruciate ligament to provide rotational stability in flexion and varus-valgus stability in extension.

Isolated caudal cruciate ligament tears are rare in small animals because (1) the caudal cruciate ligament is positioned in the joint such that loads commonly causing ligament injury are directed toward the cranial cruciate ligament, (2) the caudal cruciate ligament is stronger than the cranial cruciate ligament, and (3) the types of accidents that might cause caudal cruciate ligament rupture are seldom encountered. Nevertheless, isolated ruptures of the caudal cruciate ligament do occur and are generally caused by a cranial-to-caudal blow directed against the proximal tibia. This type of injury is most commonly associated with an automobile accident or falling on the limb while the stifle joint is flexed. Caudal cruciate ligament injuries are more commonly associated with severe derangement of the stifle joint. In these patients, combinations of primary (cranial cruciate ligament, caudal cruciate ligament, medial collateral ligament) and secondary (joint capsule, muscle tendon units, meniscocapsular ligaments) joint restraints are ruptured following a severe traumatic episode such as an automobile accident.

DIAGNOSIS
Clinical Presentation

Signalment. Dogs or cats of either sex and any breed or age may be affected. Isolated tears are more frequently encountered in large breeds of dogs. In cats, tears of caudal cruciate and medial collateral ligaments commonly occur concurrently.

History. Patients with an isolated caudal cruciate ligament rupture will initially have a non–weight-bearing lameness. The lameness will progressively improve, but the patient seldom regains athletic status. The animal may have a normal gait at a walk but will be lame when undergoing strenuous activity because the caudal cruciate ligament functions to stabilize the joint primarily when it is flexed. During walking, flexion occurs in the swing phase of the gait; during running and turning, the knee is more flexed in the stance (weight-bearing) phase of the gait.

☞ **N O T E** · Nonathletic dogs usually function normally with caudal cruciate tears.

Physical Examination Findings

Diagnosis of isolated caudal cruciate ligament tears is based on the presence of cranial-caudal instability. Often it is difficult to differentiate craniocaudal movement caused by cranial cruciate ligament rupture from that caused by caudal cruciate ligament injury. The following points may help make this differentiation:

- When the joint is held in extension, the degree of palpable instability is less with caudal cruciate ligament tears than with cranial cruciate ligament tears.
- With the patient in dorsal recumbency and the limb positioned such that the stifle is flexed and the tibia is parallel to the ground, the tibial tuberosity forms a distinct prominence cranial to the patella. If a caudal cruciate ligament injury is present, the weight of the limb causes a caudal "sag" of the tibia, resulting in loss of the tuberosity prominence.
- When the tibia is moved forward, there is a distinct endpoint to the cranial movement when the caudal cruciate ligament is ruptured.
- With the tibia in an extended position, there will be a distinct caudal subluxation of the tibia when the stifle joint is flexed and internally rotated if the caudal cruciate ligament is torn.

Caudal cruciate ligament tears that are part of a multiple ligament injury are diagnosed by the presence of severe instability (see p. 972).

Radiography

Radiographs are often helpful in the diagnosis of caudal cruciate ligament injuries (Fig. 30-72). Small bone densities may be apparent on the lateral projection just behind and distal to the femoral condyles. With a lateral radiographic projection, the tibial plateau is seen to be caudally displaced relative to the femoral condyles.

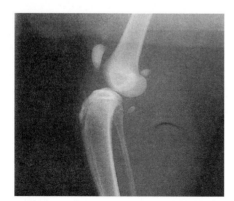

FIG. 30-72
Lateral radiograph of the stifle of a cat with cranial and caudal cruciate ligament tears.

Laboratory Findings

There are no consistent laboratory abnormalities.

DIFFERENTIAL DIAGNOSIS

Differential diagnoses include cranial cruciate ligament injury (see above) and multiple-ligament injury.

MEDICAL OR CONSERVATIVE MANAGEMENT

Long-term evaluation of dogs having reconstruction of isolated caudal cruciate ligament tears shows the prognosis to be good, and independent of treatment method. Experimental studies question the need of caudal cruciate reconstruction, but clinical experience dictates reconstruction is warranted in larger breeds of dogs and in athletic dogs. Conservative management (activity restricted to leash walking for 8 weeks) of isolated caudal cruciate tears is an option for smaller dogs or cats and for dogs leading inactive lives.

SURGICAL TREATMENT

Joints with cruciate ligament injury are repaired by one of several extracapsular reconstruction techniques: suture stabilization, redirection of the medial collateral ligament, or popliteal tendon tenodesis. Suture stabilization consists of imbrication of the caudomedial joint capsule and placement of a medial or lateral stabilizing suture. Redirection repair uses existing autogenous tissue such as the medial collateral ligament.

Preoperative Management

These animals should be evaluated for evidence of other ligamentous or bony trauma.

Anesthesia

Opioid epidural administration can be used to reduce anesthetic requirement and provide increased postoperative comfort (see p. 708).

Surgical Anatomy

The caudal cruciate ligament originates from the intercondyloid fossa of the craniolateral (inside) surface of the medial condyle (see Fig. 30-65). From the point of origin, the ligament courses distally to insert into the popliteal notch of the tibia.

Positioning

The animal is positioned in lateral recumbency with the affected limb up or in dorsal recumbency.

SURGICAL TECHNIQUES
Suture Stabilization

Make a standard craniomedial approach to the stifle joint (see p. 962) and explore internal structures. Drill a hole in the caudomedial corner of the tibial epiphysis. Place a stabilizing suture from the proximal patella tendon through the predrilled hole (Fig. 30-73). On the lateral side, imbricate the caudal joint capsule and place a stabilizing suture from the proximal patella tendon through a predrilled hole in the fibular head.

Use of Autogenous Tissue

Make a standard craniomedial approach to the stifle joint (see p. 962). Incise through the insertion of the caudal sar- *torius muscle and medial fascia along the tibial metaphysis. Reflect the muscle and fascia caudally to expose the medial collateral ligament. Free the body of the ligament with a periosteal elevator and direct the ligament caudally to course in the same sagittal plane as the caudal cruciate ligament. Secure the ligament in this position with a bone screw and spiked washer (Fig. 30-74).*

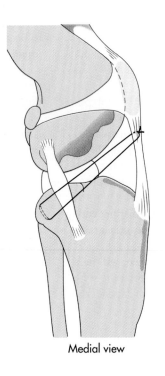
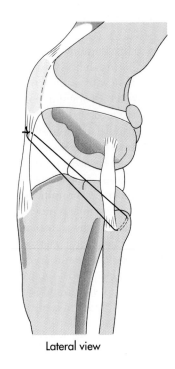

Medial view   Lateral view

FIG. 30-73
For caudal cruciate ligament tears, extracapsular sutures are placed from the patella tendon just distal to the patella to the caudal tibia (medially) and fibular head (laterally).

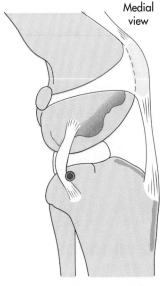

Medial view

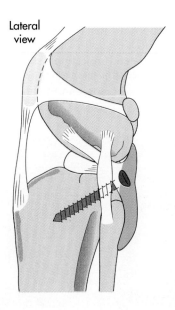

Lateral view

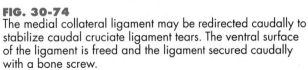

FIG. 30-74
The medial collateral ligament may be redirected caudally to stabilize caudal cruciate ligament tears. The ventral surface of the ligament is freed and the ligament secured caudally with a bone screw.

FIG. 30-75
Tenodesis of the popliteal tendon may be performed to stabilize caudal cruciate ligament tears. Entrap the popliteal tendon with a screw as it passes caudal and proximal to the fibular head.

Entrapment (Tenodesis) of the Popliteal Tendon

Make a lateral approach to the stifle joint (see p. 962) and reflect the fascia lata to isolate the popliteal tendon as it passes beneath the lateral collateral ligament (Fig. 30-75). Entrap the popliteal tendon with a screw and Teflon or polyacetyl washer as it passes caudal and proximal to the fibular head.

SUTURE MATERIALS/SPECIAL INSTRUMENTS

A screw is used to secure the medial collateral ligament or popliteal tendon to bone. For the suture stabilization technique, heavy (No. 2) nonabsorbable suture material is necessary.

POSTOPERATIVE CARE AND ASSESSMENT

Exercise should be restricted to leash walking for 8 weeks; then the animal should be gradually returned to unsupervised activity over a 4-week period. Passive flexion and extension of the stifle joint should be performed postoperatively to maintain range of motion.

PROGNOSIS

The prognosis is good to excellent for return to normal limb function in most animals after surgery or conservative treatment (see comments above).

Suggested Reading

Arnoczky SP, Marshall JL: The cruciate ligaments of the canine stifle: an anatomical and functional analysis, *Am J Vet Res* 38:1807, 1977.

DeAngelis MP, Betts CW: Posterior cruciate ligament rupture, *J Am Anim Hosp Assoc* 9:447, 1973.

Egger E: Caudal cruciate ligament repair. In Bojrab MJ, editor: *Current techniques in small animal surgery*, ed 3, Philadelphia, 1990, Lea & Febiger.

Johnson AL, Olmstead ML: Caudal cruciate ligament rupture: a retrospective analysis of 14 dogs, *Vet Surg* 16:202, 1987.

COLLATERAL LIGAMENT INJURY

DEFINITIONS

Collateral ligament injuries are either complete or partial tears of the medial or lateral collateral ligaments.

GENERAL CONSIDERATIONS AND CLINICALLY RELEVANT PATHOPHYSIOLOGY

As the medial collateral ligament crosses the medial joint surface, it forms a strong attachment to the joint capsule and medial meniscus. This attachment is important in stabilizing the medial meniscus, but it predisposes the caudal body of the meniscus to injury from the medial femoral condyle when cranial cruciate ligament rupture is present. The medial and lateral collateral ligaments function in concert to limit varus-valgus motion of the stifle joint. This is most important when the stifle joint is extended and both the medial and lateral collateral ligaments are taut. As the stifle joint flexes, the medial collateral ligament remains tight but the lateral collateral ligament relaxes to allow internal tibial rotation. This motion permits the foot to turn inward beneath the body during ambulation. As the stifle joint extends, the lateral collateral ligament becomes taut once again to assist in external rotation of the tibia. This motion aligns the foot into proper position for weight bearing.

Isolated medial or lateral collateral ligament tears are rare in small animals. The majority of injuries that involve the medial or lateral collateral ligaments occur in conjunction with injury to other primary and secondary restraints of the stifle joint. These multiple-ligament injuries are often the result of severe trauma directed to the stifle joint and involve injury to a myriad of stifle joint ligaments.

DIAGNOSIS
Clinical Presentation

Signalment. Any age or breed and either sex of dog or cat may be affected.

History. Frequently, the injury is not witnessed by clients. They often report that the animal was normal earlier in the day and then developed a non–weight-bearing lameness. This injury may occur while the animal is exercising (without evidence of trauma) or during a traumatic incident, such as a vehicular accident, in which the animal has sustained major injuries.

Physical Examination Findings

Diagnosis of collateral ligament injury, whether an isolated ligament tear or part of a complex injury, is based upon palpation. It is important to remember that the stifle joint must be extended to be examined for collateral restraint injury. The valgus stress test is used to evaluate the integrity of the medial collateral ligament. With the patient in lateral recumbency, one hand is used to stabilize the femur while the other hand grasps the distal tibia and applies an upward force (abduction). If the medial joint restraints (medial collateral ligament, joint capsule, peripheral meniscal ligaments) are torn, opening of the medial joint line will be apparent (Fig. 30-76). The varus stress test is used to evaluate the integrity of the lateral collateral ligament. One hand stabilizes the femur while the other hand grasps the distal tibia and applies an inward force (adduction). If the lateral joint restraints are torn, opening of the lateral joint will be apparent. Isolated tears show minimal opening, whereas obvious opening occurs with more extensive injuries (lateral collateral ligament, joint capsule, peripheral meniscal ligaments).

☞ **N O T E** • Be sure to hold the stifle joint in extension when assessing the medial and lateral restraints.

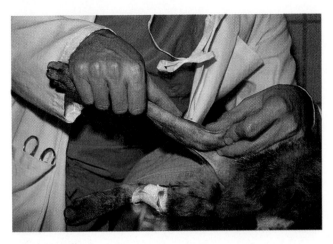

FIG. 30-76
Medial collateral ligament injury in a cat. Note the appearance of the stifle when a valgus stress is applied. The foot displaces upward and the medial joint line opens.

Radiography

Radiographs should be taken to assess the presence or absence of bone chips associated with ligament damage. Craniocaudal and medial-to-lateral radiographs are indicated to confirm the presence or absence of bony avulsions. Stress radiographs are useful for demonstrating increased medial or lateral joint space (Fig. 30-77).

Laboratory Findings

Consistent laboratory findings are not present. Laboratory evaluation is dependent upon signalment and physical findings in animals that have sustained trauma.

DIFFERENTIAL DIAGNOSIS

Differentials include muscle strains or cranial or caudal cruciate ligament tears and nondisplaced physeal fractures in immature animals.

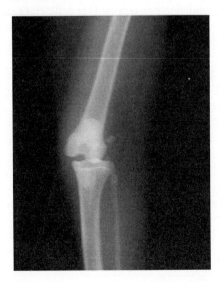

FIG. 30-77
Stress radiograph of a cat with medial collateral ligament injury. Note the severity of joint opening when a valgus stress is applied to the joint.

MEDICAL OR CONSERVATIVE MANAGEMENT

The decision to use conservative or surgical treatment for isolated collateral ligament injury is based upon the degree of injury to the ligament and secondary joint restraints (joint capsule, peripheral meniscal ligaments). This assessment is based on palpation and radiographs. Minimal swelling and only slight opening of the joint space when the joint is placed under stress are indications for conservative treatment: fiberglass cast applied for 2 weeks, followed by controlled activity for 6 additional weeks. This recommendation is supported by in vivo experiments showing that animals with selectively transected collateral ligaments heal well when treated with only immobilization (Vasseur, 1981).

SURGICAL TREATMENT

Moderate to severe swelling and significant opening of the joint space when the joint is placed under stress indicate significant injury to the collateral restraints. In these patients, surgery is recommended. Treatment includes reconstruction of the collateral ligament, meniscocapsular ligaments, and joint capsule. Primary repair of the collateral ligament is undertaken if the point of failure is the origin or insertion of the ligament or an intrasubstance tear with large segments of the ligament intact. Occasionally, there may be a small fragment of bone present on the end of the ligament that can be incorporated into the repair.

☞ **N O T E** • Be sure to repair *all* injured restraints.

Preoperative Management

To avoid additional damage to the articular cartilage or menisci, limit activity to leash walking until definitive surgical treatment can be done. Nonsteroidal antiinflammatory drugs can be given to control acute discomfort.

Anesthesia

Opioid epidural administration may help to control pain in animals with severely deranged joints.

Surgical Anatomy

Knowledge of origin and insertion points of the collateral ligaments is important. The medial collateral ligament originates from the medial femoral epicondyle and courses distally to insert onto the proximal tibial metaphysis (Fig. 30-78). As the ligament crosses the medial joint line, it forms a strong attachment to the joint capsule and medial meniscus. The lateral collateral ligament originates from an oval area on the lateral femoral epicondyle; it then courses distally to insert onto the fibular head. The medial collateral ligament lies deep to the caudal sartorius muscle, while the lateral collateral ligament lies deep to the fascia lata. The peroneal (fibular) nerve is a branch of the sciatic nerve. It obliquely crosses the distal aspect to the stifle joint, where it lies superficial to the gastrocnemius muscle and sends an articular branch to the lateral collateral ligament. Care

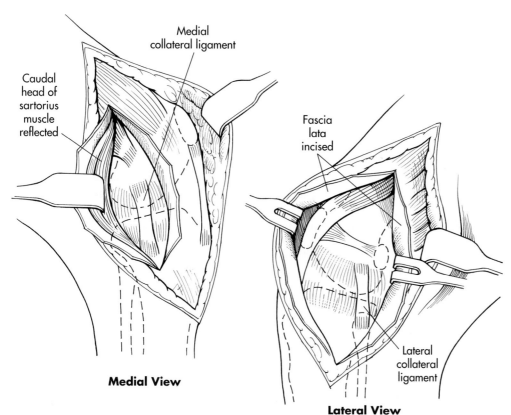

Medial View

Lateral View

FIG. 30-78
Medial and lateral views of the stifle illustrating soft-tissue structures surrounding the collateral ligaments.

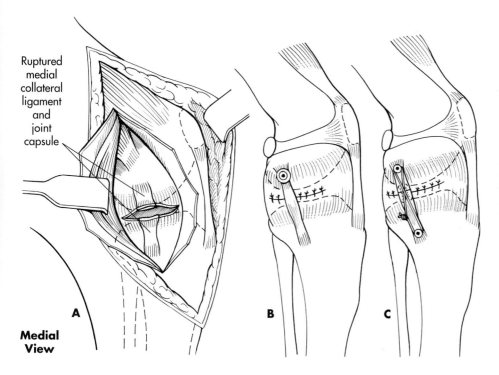

FIG. 30-79
A, To repair a medial restraint injury, incise the insertion of the caudal head of the sartorius muscle and deep fascia along the craniomedial border of the proximal tibia. **B,** Replace the collateral ligament to its anatomical site and secure with a screw and polyacetyl spiked washer. **C,** If the ligament injury is an intrasubstance tear, perform primary repair by suturing the ligament ends with a locking-loop suture pattern. Supplement the primary repair with screws and figure-eight support.

should be used when dissecting near the lateral collateral ligament to preserve this nerve.

Positioning

Position the patient in lateral recumbency with the affected leg up to repair a lateral collateral ligament injury. For medial collateral ligament injuries, position the animal in lateral recumbency with the affected leg down. If multiple ligament tears are present, the animal can be positioned in dorsal recumbency to facilitate exposing both sides of the limb. Suspend the limb and prepare it for aseptic surgery (see p. 24).

SURGICAL TECHNIQUES
Medial Collateral Ligament

Make a medial parapatellar incision. Use a medial approach to expose the medial collateral ligament (see p. 962). Incise the insertion of the caudal head of the sartorius muscle and deep fascia along the craniomedial border of the proximal tibia (Fig. 30-79, A, p. 971). Retract the muscle and fascia caudally to expose the collateral ligament and medial joint capsule. Replace the ligament to its anatomical site and secure it with a screw and polyacetyl spiked washer (Fig. 30-79, B). If the ligament injury is an intrasubstance tear, perform primary repair by suturing the ligament ends; use a locking-loop suture pattern with small nonabsorbable suture (see p. 1003). Supplement the primary repair with screws and figure-eight support (Fig. 30-79, C). *Following repair of the collateral ligament, carefully reconstruct the meniscocapsular ligaments and joint capsule using interrupted sutures of small nonabsorbable suture material (polypropylene or nylon).*

Lateral Collateral Ligament

Use a craniolateral approach to expose the lateral collateral ligament (see p. 961). Make a proximal-to-distal parapatellar incision through the fascia lata. Continue the incision distally 4 cm below the tibial crest, parallel to the joint line. Use caution in isolating the peroneal nerve and protect it carefully during surgery (see Surgical Anatomy discussion on p. 970). *Reflect the fascia lata caudally to expose the collateral ligament and lateral joint capsule. Repair the ligament as described above.*

SUTURE MATERIALS/SPECIAL INSTRUMENTS

Bone screws, polyacetyl spiked washers, and heavy, nonabsorbable suture are needed for collateral ligament repair.

POSTOPERATIVE CARE AND ASSESSMENT

The limb is placed in a soft, padded bandage for 10 days. The animal should be restricted to leash walking only for 8 weeks. Passive flexion and extension of the stifle should be performed for 10 minutes, twice a day.

PROGNOSIS

Prognosis for isolated collateral ligament tears is good to excellent. If multiple ligaments are torn, prognosis is fair.

Reference

Vasseur PB, Arnoczky SP: Collateral ligaments of the canine stifle joint: anatomic and functional analysis, *Am J Vet Res* 42:1133, 1981.

Suggested Reading

Aron DN, Robello GT: Use of sutures in repairing ligaments and tendons, *Vet Med Report* 3:88, 1991.

Berg RJ, Egger EL: In vitro comparison of the three loop pulley and locking loop suture patterns for repair of canine weightbearing tendons and collateral ligaments, *Vet Surg* 15:107, 1986.

MULTIPLE LIGAMENT INJURIES

DEFINITIONS

Multiple ligament injuries are those where the cranial or caudal cruciate ligaments and other sustaining restraints of the stifle joint are simultaneously damaged. **Varus angulation** is an inward rotation of the leg (toward the midline of the body), while **valgus angulation** is an outward rotation (away from the midline of the body).

SYNONYMS

Deranged stifle joint

GENERAL CONSIDERATIONS AND CLINICALLY RELEVANT PATHOPHYSIOLOGY

Multiple ligament injuries most commonly result from automobile accidents; they rarely occur when the foot is caught as the animal jumps a fence. A common triad of injuries includes cranial and caudal cruciate ligament tears, failure of the primary and secondary medial restraints, and peripheral medial meniscal tears. Varus angulation of the limb with a medial stress indicates lateral restraint injury, while valgus angulation of the limb (with a lateral stress applied to the foot) indicates medial restraint injury.

DIAGNOSIS
Clinical Presentation

Signalment. Either sex and any age or breed of dog or cat may be affected.

History. The animal is usually presented for evaluation of an acute, non–weight-bearing lameness. The trauma may or may not have been observed.

Physical Examination Findings

Combined cranial and caudal cruciate tears are characterized by marked craniocaudal movement of the tibia relative to the femur. Concurrent damage to the collateral ligament and joint capsule complexes can usually be determined by palpation. With the leg in extension, a varus stress applied to the distal tibia causes opening of the lateral joint line if the lateral restraints are injured, while a valgus stress causes opening of the medial joint line if the medial restraints are injured.

Radiography

Radiographs show subluxation of the stifle joint. Careful assessment of both craniocaudal and mediolateral radiographs may show small bone chips at the origin or insertion of ligaments.

Laboratory Findings

Consistent laboratory abnormalities are not present.

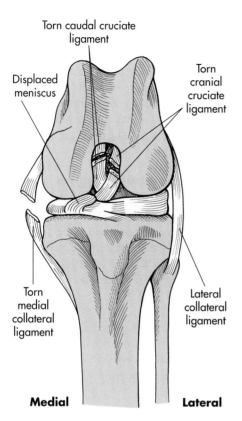

FIG. 30-80
Structures commonly injured with multiple ligament derangement of the stifle joint. Note loss of cranial and caudal cruciate ligaments and disruption of medial restraints.

DIFFERENTIAL DIAGNOSIS

Distal femoral and proximal tibial metaphyseal fractures may show similar clinical signs and should be differentiated from ligamentous injuries.

MEDICAL OR CONSERVATIVE MANAGEMENT

Multiple ligamentous injuries require surgical intervention. Conservative treatment with external coaptation (splints or casts) is not effective in maintaining alignment of the stifle joint and will lead to severe degenerative joint disease.

SURGICAL TREATMENT

Surgical treatment involves careful reconstruction of the cranial and caudal cruciate ligaments, collateral restraints, and menisci. Repair of the collateral ligament complex is performed first and is followed by reconstruction of the cruciate ligaments. Specific repair and reconstruction techniques are dependent upon the preference of the surgeon and are described in the discussion of each individual ligament.

Preoperative Management

A soft, padded bandage should be applied and activity limited until surgery can be done, to prevent damage to the articular surfaces of the joint.

Anesthesia

There are no special considerations. Epidural opioid administration reduces both the amount of anesthesia required and the postoperative discomfort.

Surgical Anatomy

Normal anatomy of the stifle joint is described on pp. 960 and 975. With multiple ligamentous injury, moderate to severe swelling and bruising of soft tissues surrounding the joint will be present. Knowledge of the normal origins and insertions of the collateral ligaments, meniscocapsular ligaments, and ligaments within the joint is required. Torn collateral ligaments are difficult to identify because they are often encased in edematous connective tissue. Menisci are often displaced from their normal positions and folded cranially or caudally (Fig. 30-80).

Positioning

The patient is positioned in dorsal recumbency with the affected limb up. The leg is prepared from the dorsal midline to the tarsal joint. A hanging-limb preparation facilitates manipulation of the leg during surgery.

SURGICAL TECHNIQUES

Cruciate ligament repair is discussed on pp. 960 and 967, collateral ligament repair on p. 970, and meniscal injuries on p. 975.

SUTURE MATERIALS/SPECIAL INSTRUMENTS

See methods of reconstruction for specific primary or secondary restraints (p. 972).

POSTOPERATIVE CARE AND ASSESSMENT

Postoperatively, the limb should be placed in a support bandage for 3 to 4 weeks and activity should be limited to leash walks only for 8 weeks. The support bandage should be placed before the patient recovers from anesthesia to allow accurate positioning of the bandage with the leg in extension. The bandage provides comfort in the early postoperative period by immobilizing soft tissues and preventing extension and flexion of the stifle joint. It should be changed weekly, or more often if necessary. Bandage changes usually require that the animal be sedated with a narcotic-tranquilizer combination to increase patient comfort and allow accurate positioning. Once the bandage is removed, passive flexion and extension of the stifle should be performed to maintain an adequate range of motion.

PROGNOSIS

The prognosis is good for return to nonathletic performance. Subsequent to extensive ligamentous injury, loss of flexion tighter than 110 degrees and mild to moderate instability are common after surgery. This instability and loss of normal range of motion limit athletic performance. Severe lameness should be expected in animals that are managed without surgery.

Suggested Reading

Aron DN: Traumatic dislocation of the stifle joint: treatment of 12 dogs and one cat, *J Am Anim Hosp Assoc* 23:41, 1987.

Hulse DA, Shires P: Multiple ligament injury of the stifle joint in the dog, *J Am Anim Hosp Assoc* 22:105, 1986.

Welches CD, Scavelli TD: Transarticular pinning to repair luxation of the stifle joint in dogs and cats: a retrospective study of 10 cases, *J Am Anim Hosp Assoc* 26:207, 1990.

MENISCAL INJURY

DEFINITIONS

Excessive crushing or shearing forces associated with stifle injury may result in **meniscocapsular detachment** or separation in the substance of the meniscus.

SYNONYMS

Torn cartilage

GENERAL CONSIDERATIONS AND CLINICALLY RELEVANT PATHOPHYSIOLOGY

The menisci are important intraarticular structures. They function in load transmission and energy absorption, help provide rotational and varus-valgus stability, lubricate the joint, and render joint surfaces congruent. Isolated meniscal injuries are uncommon in dogs, although isolated meniscal tears involving the midbody of the lateral meniscus occasionally occur during a fall where the leg is twisted. Most meniscal tears causing lameness in dogs, however, occur in conjunction with cranial cruciate ligament ruptures; the incidence may be as high as 75% of all meniscal tears. These tears usually involve the caudal body of the medial meniscus because the craniocaudal instability associated with cranial cruciate ligament rupture displaces the medial femoral condyle caudally during stifle joint flexion. The caudal body of the medial meniscus becomes wedged between the femur and tibia and is crushed upon weight bearing and joint extension. The most common type of injury is a "bucket-handle" tear. This is a transverse tear in the caudal body of the medial meniscus that extends from medial to lateral in a transverse direction. The free portion of the meniscus is frequently folded forward (Fig. 30-81). Peripheral meniscal tears are the second most frequent type of meniscal injury. These injuries are associated with a severe traumatic episode that results in multiple ligament injuries. Rupture of the medial meniscocapsular ligaments commonly occurs, allowing the entire meniscal body to fold forward.

☞ **N O T E** · Isolated meniscal tears are uncommon. They usually occur in conjunction with cruciate ligament injury. Isolated lateral meniscal tears occur in the caudal horn.

DIAGNOSIS
Clinical Presentation

Signalment. Dogs of either sex and any age or breed may be affected. Meniscal tears are rare in cats.

History. Meniscal injury is usually associated with instability of the stifle caused by cranial cruciate ligament rupture (see p. 957). If a long-standing lameness suddenly worsens in a dog with cranial cruciate ligament injury, tearing of the meniscus should be suspected.

Physical Examination Findings

The client may report hearing a popping sound when the dog walks, or a popping sound may be noted when the stifle is examined. This is caused by movement of the "free" section of the bucket-handle tear. Not all patients with meniscal tears have an audible or palpable click. Close inspection of the medial and lateral menisci at surgery provides a definitive diagnosis.

Radiography

Standard craniocaudal and medial-to-lateral radiographs should be taken for diagnostic evaluation of lameness attributed to the stifle joint; however, radiographic findings do not correlate with meniscal injury.

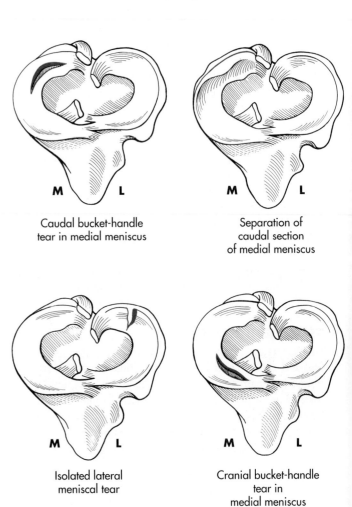

Caudal bucket-handle tear in medial meniscus

Separation of caudal section of medial meniscus

Isolated lateral meniscal tear

Cranial bucket-handle tear in medial meniscus

FIG. 30-81
Meniscal tears in dogs. Bucket-handle tears occur most commonly.

Laboratory Findings

No consistent hematologic abnormalities are present. Joint fluid analysis may be helpful in diagnosis of partial cruciate tears; patients with meniscal tears may have cell counts that are slightly higher than those in patients with ligament tears alone.

DIFFERENTIAL DIAGNOSIS

Cruciate ligament injury should be suspected in any animal with a meniscal tear. Sprain of the medial restraints should be differentiated from meniscal injury.

MEDICAL OR CONSERVATIVE MANAGEMENT

Conservative treatment is not an option if meniscal injury is noted on physical examination because continued back-and-forth sliding of the torn meniscus accelerates degenerative joint disease.

SURGICAL TREATMENT

Methods of treatment include partial meniscectomy, primary repair of peripheral meniscal injuries, and total meniscectomy. A partial meniscectomy involves removal of the torn section of the meniscus. Experimentally, partial meniscectomy carries less morbidity than does a total meniscectomy and is the treatment of choice for bucket-handle tears of the medial meniscus. Primary repair of a torn meniscal body is advocated by some human orthopedic surgeons. However, because of the low morbidity associated with partial meniscectomy and difficulty in suturing meniscal body tears in dogs, primary repair should be reserved for peripheral tears of the meniscocapsular ligaments. Tearing of the peripheral meniscocapsular ligaments usually occurs after significant trauma and subsequent injury to both primary and secondary restraints of the stifle joint. The medial meniscus is more commonly involved in conjunction with injury of the me-

dial collateral restraints. Meticulous repair with interrupted sutures using an absorbable suture will allow meniscocapsular tissue to heal. Total meniscectomy should be considered only when the peripheral rim of the meniscus is damaged to a point where primary suturing of the meniscocapsular tissue is not possible.

Preoperative Management

Until definitive treatment is performed, activity should be limited to prevent further damage to the meniscus and articular surfaces of the joint.

Anesthesia

See p. 708 for anesthetic considerations in animals with orthopedic disease.

Surgical Anatomy

The lateral and medial menisci are two semilunar fibrocartilage discs interposed between the femur and tibia (Fig. 30-82). They are positioned in the joint with the open side of the C facing the midline and are held in place by cranial meniscotibial ligaments, caudal meniscotibial ligaments, and meniscocapsular ligaments. The lateral meniscus has an additional ligament that inserts into the caudal intercondyloid fossa of the femoral condyles. This ligament and loose meniscocapsular ligaments of the lateral meniscus render the lateral meniscus more mobile than the medial meniscus. Clinically, the lack of mobility of the medial meniscus predisposes it to injury.

Positioning

The animal is placed in lateral recumbency with the affected limb up. The limb is prepared for aseptic surgery from the dorsal midline to the tarsal joint. Preparing the limb in a hanging-leg position facilitates manipulation of the limb during surgery.

SURGICAL TECHNIQUES
Partial Meniscectomy

Partial meniscectomy requires that the torn meniscus be adequately exposed. Exposure is facilitated with suction and by levering the tibial plateau down and forward. *Lever the tibia forward by placing the tip of a small Hohmann retractor behind the caudal edge of the tibial plateau and forcing the body of the retractor against the nonarticular portion of the trochlear groove (Fig. 30-83). Once the damaged section of meniscus is visualized, remove it with a No. 11 scalpel blade. Incise the most medial attachment of the bucket handle first, then incise the most lateral attachment. After removal of the torn section of meniscus, inspect the remaining meniscus for additional tears.*

SUTURE MATERIALS/SPECIAL INSTRUMENTS

Suction is desirable to evacuate fluid and blood from the caudomedial compartment. A small Hohmann retractor is useful for levering the tibia down and forward to allow visualization of the caudal horn of the medial meniscus.

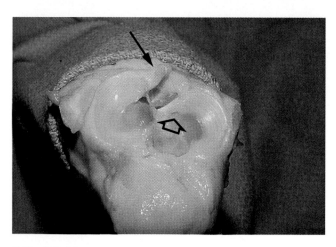

FIG. 30-82
Appearance of menisci and surrounding soft tissue in a cadaver specimen. Note the C-shaped appearance and tibial insertion of the medial meniscus (*open arrow*). The lateral meniscus is larger and inserts into the caudal femur (*closed arrow*).

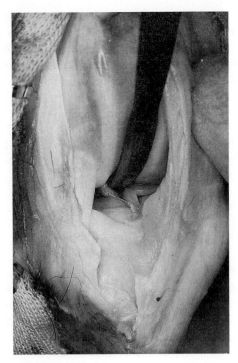

FIG. 30-83
To improve visualization of the caudomedial compartment (where most meniscal tears occur), place a small Hohmann retractor to force the tibia forward and down.

POSTOPERATIVE CARE AND ASSESSMENT

Postoperative management should follow recommendations given for reconstruction of the cranial cruciate ligament (see p. 965).

PROGNOSIS

Prognosis for recovery in animals with cranial cruciate ligament injury is discussed on p. 965. Total meniscectomy may promote degenerative joint disease and should be avoided; however, partial meniscectomy or primary repair of the damaged meniscus lessens the degree of degenerative joint disease and makes the prognosis for return to normal function more favorable.

Suggested Reading

Arnoczky SP, Warrn RF: The microvasculature of the meniscus and its response to injury: an experimental study in the dog, *Am J Sports Med* 11:131, 1983.

Cox JS et al: The degenerative effect of partial and total resection of the medial meniscus in dogs' knees, *Clin Orthop* 109:178, 1975.

Hulse DA, Shires PK: The meniscus: anatomy, function and treatment, *Comp Cont Educ Pract Vet* 5:765, 1983.

Smith K: Meniscectomy. In Bojrab MJ, editor: *Current techniques in small animal surgery*, Philadelphia, 1975, Lea & Febiger.

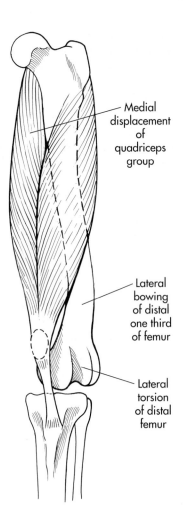

FIG. 30-84
Soft tissue and skeletal abnormalities associated with medial patella luxation include medial displacement of the quadriceps apparatus, lateral bowing of the distal one third of the femur, and lateral torsion of the distal femur.

MEDIAL PATELLAR LUXATION

DEFINITIONS

Medial patellar luxation is a displacement of the patella from the trochlear sulcus.

SYNONYMS

Slipped knee cap

GENERAL CONSIDERATIONS AND CLINICALLY RELEVANT PATHOPHYSIOLOGY

Medial patellar luxation is a common cause of lameness in small-breed dogs. The majority of patients with patellar luxation have associated musculoskeletal abnormalities: medial displacement of the quadriceps muscle group, lateral torsion of the distal femur, a lateral bowing of the distal one third of the femur, femoral epiphyseal dysplasia, rotational instability of the stifle joint, or tibial deformity (Fig. 30-84). The extent of anatomic derangement is dependent on the severity of patella luxation and the amount of growth plate activity. Skeletal deformities in affected animals arise secondary to changes occurring within the metaphyseal growth plates. There exists a large potential for axial and torsional growth in cartilage columns of the metaphyseal growth plates of young animals. The growth plate is composed of actively dividing cells that rapidly yield to physiologic forces by either increasing or decreasing their growth rate. Existing bone responds to increased force through bone deposition or resorption; therefore, remodeling of existing bone occurs more slowly.

Torsional and angular deformities of the skeleton associated with patella luxations are secondary to abnormal pressures exerted on the growth plate by displacement of the quadriceps muscle group. These abnormal pressures lead to alterations in growth. An abnormal torsional force leads to a deflection of the cartilage columns of the growth plate in a spiral pattern. Therefore, a lateral or a medial torsion of the femur may result, depending on the direction of the deforming force. The torsional force with medial luxation is in a lateral direction, resulting in a lateral torsion of the distal femur. Abnormal compression, or tension forces (axial forces), also affects the growth of the cartilage columns. Increased medial axial force leads to bowing of the distal one third of the femur in dogs with medial patellar luxation. This abnormal bowing is secondary to shortening of the longitudinal length of the medial cortex relative to the lateral cortex; the shortening is caused by increased pressure parallel to the growth plate, which retards growth. Decreased pressure parallel to the growth plate allows accelerated growth. The pressure need not be extreme, and mild forces originating from postural abnormalities, gravitational forces, or muscle forces are sufficient to affect the growth plate.

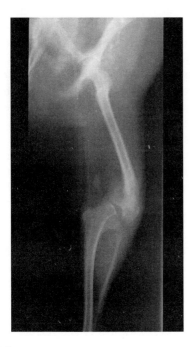

FIG. 30-85
Radiographic appearance of severe skeletal abnormalities associated with medial patellar luxation in a dog.

There is medial malalignment of the quadriceps muscles in dogs with medial patella luxation; it produces sufficient pressure on the growth plate to retard growth. At the same time, there is less pressure on the lateral aspect of the growth plate, which allows accelerated growth. Decreased length of the medial cortex relative to the increased length of the lateral cortex results in the lateral bowing of the distal femur. Abnormal growth continues as long as the quadriceps is displaced medially and the growth plates are active. Therefore, the degree of lateral bowing depends on the severity of patellar luxation and the patient's age at the onset of luxation. With mild luxations, the quadriceps is rarely displaced medially and has minimal abnormal effect on the growth plate. However, with severe luxations the quadriceps is medially displaced at all times, and maximal effect on the growth plate results in severe lateral bowing of the distal femur in young patients (Fig. 30-85). Tibial deformities seen with patella luxations are the result of abnormal forces acting on the proximal and distal growth plates of the tibia. Tibial deformities described with medial patella luxation include medial displacement of the tibial tuberosity, medial bowing (varus deformity) of the proximal tibia, and lateral torsion of the distal tibia.

The articular cartilage is the "growth plate" for the epiphysis and responds to increased or decreased pressure in the same manner as the metaphyseal growth plate: increased pressure retards growth, whereas decreased pressure accelerates growth. Abnormal development of the trochlear groove is present in dogs with medial patella luxation. The degree of abnormality varies from a near-normal trochlea to an absent trochlear groove. The articulation of the patella within the trochlear groove exerts a physiologic pressure on the articular cartilage that retards cartilage growth. Continued pressure by the patella is responsible for the development of normal depth of the trochlear groove. If the physiologic pressure exerted by the patella is not present on the trochlear articular cartilage, the trochlea fails to gain proper depth. Immature patients with mild luxations show minimal loss of depth to the trochlear groove because the patella is normally positioned during development. However, immature patients with severe luxations have an absent trochlear groove because the normal pressure responsible for groove development is not present. The degree of skeletal pathology associated with patella luxation varies considerably between the mildest and severest forms; therefore, a system for classifying canine patella luxation has been developed (Table 30-21).

DIAGNOSIS
Clinical Presentation

Signalment. Dogs of any age or breed and either sex may have medial patellar luxations, but small- and toy-breed dogs are most frequently affected. Medial patellar luxations are more common than lateral patellar luxations in large-breed dogs; however, large dogs have a higher percentage of lateral luxations than small dogs.

History. Most affected animals have an intermittent weight-bearing lameness. Owners may report the dog occasionally holds the leg in a flexed position for one or two steps.

TABLE 30-21

Grades of Patella Luxation

Grade I

The patella can be luxated, but spontaneous luxation of the patella during normal joint motion rarely occurs. Manual luxation of the patella may be accomplished during physical examination, but the patella reduces when pressure is released. Flexion and extension of the joint are normal.

Grade II

Angular and torsional deformities of the femur may be present to a mild degree. The patella may be manually displaced with lateral pressure or may luxate with flexion of the stifle joint. The patella remains luxated until it is reduced by the examiner or is spontaneously reduced when the animal extends and derotates its tibia.

Grade III

The patella remains luxated medially most of the time, but may be manually reduced with the stifle in extension. However, after manual reduction, flexion and extension of the stifle result in reluxation of the patella. There is a medial displacement of the quadriceps muscle group. Abnormalities of the supporting soft tissues of the stifle joint and deformities of the femur and tibia may be present.

Grade IV

There may be an 80- to 90-degree medial rotation of the proximal tibial plateau. The patella is permanently luxated and cannot be manually repositioned. The femoral trochlear groove is shallow or absent, and there is medial displacement of the quadriceps muscle group. Abnormalities of the supporting soft tissues of the stifle joint and deformities of the femur and tibia are marked.

Physical Examination Findings

The diagnosis of medial patellar luxation is based upon finding or eliciting medial patellar luxation during physical examination. Physical findings are variable and dependent upon the severity of luxation. Patients with grade I luxations generally exhibit no lameness and the diagnosis is made as an incidental finding on physical examination. Patients with grade II luxations exhibit occasional "skipping" when walking or running. On occasion, these patients will stretch the lateral retinacular structures and develop a non–weight-bearing lameness. Lameness in patients with grade III patella luxation varies from an occasional skip to a weight-bearing lameness. Patients with grade IV luxations walk with the rear quarters in a crouched position because of the inability to fully extend their stifle joints. The patella is hypoplastic and may be found displaced medially alongside the femoral condyle.

Radiography

With grade III or grade IV luxations, standard craniocaudal and medial-to-lateral radiographs show the patella to be displaced medially, whereas with grade I or II luxations the patella may be within the trochlear sulcus or may be displaced medially.

Laboratory Findings

Consistent laboratory findings are not present.

DIFFERENTIAL DIAGNOSIS

Differential diagnoses include avascular necrosis of the femoral head, coxofemoral luxation, ligamentous sprain of the stifle, and muscle strain. Careful examination of the hip joint is essential because some patients with patellar luxation also have avascular necrosis of the femoral head (see p. 956).

MEDICAL OR CONSERVATIVE MANAGEMENT

Treatment of medial patella luxation may be conservative or surgical. The choice of treatment method depends on the clinical history, physical findings, and patient's age. Surgery is seldom warranted in asymptomatic older patients, whereas young animals or those that are lame usually benefit from surgery. Clients should be advised to observe the animal for development of clinical signs attributable to medial patellar luxation.

SURGICAL TREATMENT

Surgery is advised in symptomatic and asymptomatic immature or young adult patients because intermittent patellar luxation may prematurely wear the articular cartilage of the patella. Surgery is indicated at any age in patients exhibiting lameness and is strongly advised in those with active growth plates because skeletal deformity may worsen rapidly. Surgical techniques used in actively growing animals should be those that will not adversely affect skeletal growth.

There are numerous surgical techniques aimed at restraining the patella within the trochlear groove. Tibial tuberosity transposition, medial restraint release, lateral restraint reinforcement, trochlear groove deepening, femoral osteotomy, and tibial osteotomy have all been advocated for correction of patella luxation. Generally, a combination of techniques is required. The techniques used depend on the severity of luxation, presence of skeletal deformities, and surgeon preference. The specific abnormalities associated with the luxation must be recognized and used to determine which technique(s) is most appropriate in a given stifle. Tibial crest transposition is an effective method of treatment for grades II, III, and IV patella luxations. Reinforcement of the lateral retinaculum is accomplished with suture placement and imbrication of the fibrous joint capsule, placement of a fascia lata graft from the fabella to the parapatellar fibrocartilage, or excision of redundant retinaculum. None of the reinforcement techniques alone is adequate to permanently prevent reluxation. If the mechanical forces pulling the patella out of the trochlear groove have not been neutralized, the reinforced retinaculum eventually stretches. If the medial and lateral trochlear ridges do not constrain the patella, the trochlear groove must be deepened. Deepening of the trochlear groove is usually necessary in patients with grades III and IV luxations; it may be

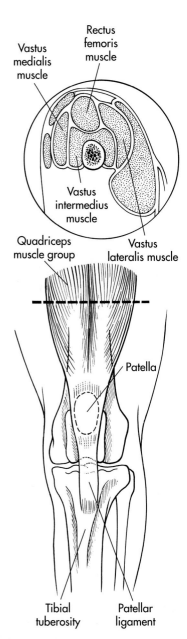

FIG. 30-86
Anatomical diagram of normal soft-tissue and skeletal structures associated with the quadriceps extensor mechanism.

achieved with a trochlear wedge recession or a trochlear resection. A trochlear wedge recession is technically more demanding but preserves the articular cartilage, while the simpler trochlear resection destroys articular cartilage.

Osteotomy of the femur is only used in patients with severe skeletal deformity in which it is determined that it is not possible to maintain patellar reduction with the previously described techniques. Deformities usually seen are varus bowing of the distal femur and medial torsional deformity of the proximal tibia. The goal of surgery is to realign the stifle joint in the frontal plane where the transverse axis of the femoral condyles is perpendicular to the longitudinal axis of the femoral diaphysis. This requires accurate preoperative measurement and wedge osteotomy of the femur. Transposition of the tibial crest,

lateral retinacular reinforcement, medial restraint release, and deepening of the trochlear groove are also required for success. These techniques require special equipment and training; as such, they should be performed by a trained specialist.

Preoperative Management

Perioperative antibiotics are not indicated for repair of patellar luxations unless the animal is immunocompromised or has concurrent disease that may increase the risk of infection.

Anesthesia

See p. 708 for anesthetic management of animals with orthopedic disease.

Surgical Anatomy

The extensor mechanism of the stifle joint is composed of the quadriceps muscle groups, patella, trochlear groove, straight patellar ligament, and tibial tuberosity (Fig. 30-86). The quadriceps muscle group is formed by the rectus femoris, vastus lateralis, vastus intermedius, and vastus medialis. The vastus medialis and vastus lateralis muscles are fixed to the patella by the medial and lateral parapatellar fibrocartilage. The fibrocartilage rides on the ridges of the femoral trochlea and, along with the medial and lateral retinacula, aids in patellar stability. The medial and lateral retinacula are groups of collagen fibers that course from the fabella to blend with the medial and lateral parapatellar fibrocartilages, respectively. The quadriceps muscle group functions to extend the stifle joint and, along with the entire extensor mechanism, aids in stability of the stifle joint. The quadriceps muscle group converges on the patella and then continues distally as the straight patellar tendon.

The patella is a sesamoid bone embedded in the tendon of the quadriceps muscle. The inner articular surface is smooth and curved so as to fully articulate with the trochlea. The normal gliding articulation of the patella and trochlea is necessary for maintaining the nutritional requirements of the trochlear and patellar articular surfaces. Lack of normal articulation, as shown experimentally through patellectomy, results in degeneration of the trochlear articular cartilage. The patella is also an essential component of the functional mechanism of the extensor apparatus. The patella maintains even tension when the stifle is extended and also acts as a lever arm increasing the mechanical advantage of the quadriceps muscle group. An increase in contractile force of 15% to 30% is necessary in human beings when patellectomy has removed the mechanical advantage of the patella.

The tibial tuberosity is located cranial and distal to the tibial condyles. Its location and prominence are important for the mechanical advantage of the extensor mechanism. The alignment of the quadriceps, patella, trochlea, patellar tendon, and tibial tuberosity must be normal for proper function. Malalignment of one or more of these structures may lead to patellar luxation.

Special anatomic considerations in patients with medial patellar luxation must be noted. When the patella is positioned medially, the patella tendon must be identified before making a parapatellar incision to enter the joint. The lateral capsule is stretched and thin, while the medial capsule is contracted and thickened. Thickening and contraction of the medial capsule will be apparent if medial release is performed. Insertions of the cranial head of the sartorius muscle and the vastus medialis muscle should be identified. The medial ridge of the trochlear sulcus and ventral surface of the patella may be worn.

Positioning

The animal is positioned in lateral or dorsal recumbency and the leg is prepared from the dorsal midline to the tarsal joint.

SURGICAL TECHNIQUES
Tibial Tuberosity Transposition

Make a craniolateral skin incision 4 cm proximal to the patella and extend the incision 2 cm below the tibial tuberosity. Incise subcutaneous tissues along the same line. Make a lateral parapatellar incision through the fascia lata and carry the incision distally onto the tibial tuberosity below the joint line. Reflect the cranialis tibialis muscle from the lateral tibial tuberosity and tibial plateau to the level of the long digital extensor tendon (Fig. 30-87, A). Use sharp dissection to gain access to the deep surface of the patellar tendon for placement of an osteotome. Beginning at the level of the patella, make a medial parapatellar incision through the fascia and distally through the periosteum of the tibial tuberosity. Position an osteotome beneath the patellar tendon 3 to 5 cm caudal to the cranial point of the tibial tuberosity (Fig. 30-87, B). Use a mallet to complete the osteotomy in a proximal to distal direction. Do not transect the distal periosteal attachment. The degree of lateral movement of the tibial tuberosity is subjective but is based on the longitudinal realignment of the tuberosity relative to the trochlear groove. *Once the site of relocation is chosen, remove a thin layer of cortical bone with a rasp or osteotome. Lever the tibial tuberosity into position and stabilize it with one or two small Kirschner wires directed caudally and slightly proximally*

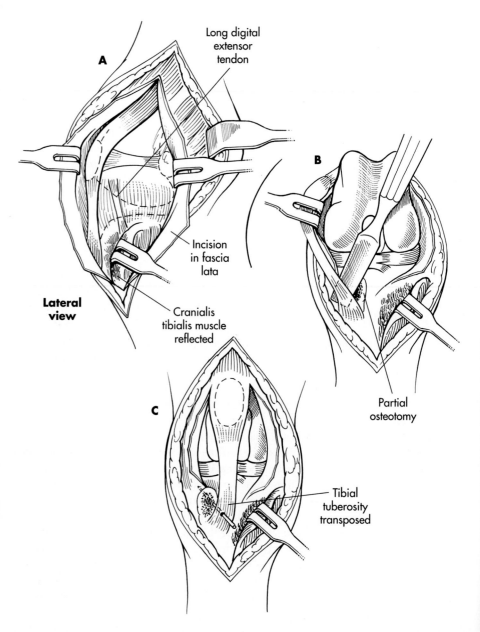

FIG. 30-87
A, For medial patellar luxations, transpose the tibial crest laterally. Make a lateral parapatellar incision through the fascia lata and carry the incision distally onto the tibial tuberosity below the joint line. Reflect the cranialis tibialis muscle from the lateral tibial tuberosity and tibial plateau to the level of the long digital extensor tendon. **B,** Position an osteotome beneath the patellar tendon and partially ostectomize the tibial crest. Do not transect the distal periosteal attachment. **C,** Stabilize the tibial tuberosity in its new location with one or two small Kirschner wires.

(Fig. 30-87, C). Engage the caudal cortex, but do not exit the pin from the tibia caudally; if the pin protrudes too far from the caudal cortex of the tibia, persistent lameness will result. Suture the arthrotomy with absorbable suture material using a simple interrupted pattern. Appose subcutaneous tissues with a continuous pattern using absorbable suture and then suture the skin with nonabsorbable suture material.

Lateral Reinforcement

For suture reinforcement, place a polyester suture through the femoral-fabellar ligament and lateral parapatellar fibrocartilage (Fig. 30-88). Next, place a series of imbrication sutures through the fibrous joint capsule and lateral edge of the patella tendon. With the leg in slight flexion, tie the femoral-fabellar suture and imbrication sutures.

To transpose the fascia lata, isolate a section of fascia lata equal in width to the patella and twice the length of the distance from the patella to the fabella. Free the graft proximally and leave it attached to the proximal pole of the patella distally. Pass the free end of the graft deep to the femoral-fabellar ligament and back to the lateral parapatellar fibrocartilage. Suture the graft to itself and the femoral-fabellar ligament with the leg in slight flexion.

If the patella is out of position most of the time, the retinaculum opposite the side of the luxation will be stretched; with medial luxations, there is redundant lateral retinaculum. *Once the patella is reduced, excise the excess retinaculum and joint capsule allowing tight closure of the arthrotomy (see above).*

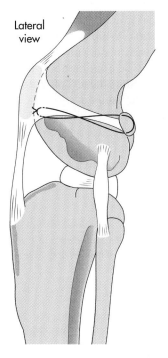

Lateral
view

FIG. 30-88
Lateral reinforcement of the retinaculum may be performed by placing a polyester suture through the femoral-fabellar ligament and lateral parapatellar fibrocartilage.

Release of the Medial Joint Capsule

The medial joint capsule is thicker than normal and contracted in patients with grade III or IV patella luxations. In these patients the medial joint capsule and retinaculum must be released to allow lateral placement of the patella. *Using a scalpel, make a medial parapatellar incision through the medial fascia and joint capsule. Begin the incision at the level of the proximal pole of the patella and extend it distally to the tibial crest. Allow the incision to separate and do not suture the cut edges when surgery is completed. Rather, suture medial subcutaneous tissue to the cranial cut edge of the incision. If dynamic contraction of the cranial sartorius muscle and vastus medialis muscle directs the patella medially, release the insertions of these muscles at the proximal patella. Redirect the insertions and suture them to the vastus intermedius muscle.*

Deepening of the Trochlear Groove

Trochlear wedge recession. Trochlear wedge recession deepens the trochlear groove to restrain the patella and maintain the integrity the patellofemoral articulation. In larger patients, an oscillating saw is often used, but in smaller breeds and toy breeds a fine-toothed hand-held saw or the cutting edge of a No. 20 scalpel blade and mallet may be used to make the cuts in the trochlea. *Cut into the articular cartilage of the trochlea, making a diamond-shaped outline.* Be sure that the width of the cut is sufficient at its midpoint to accommodate the width of the patella. *Remove an osteochondral wedge of bone and cartilage by following the outline previously made (Fig. 30-89). Make the osteotomy so that the two oblique planes that form the free wedge intersect distally at the intercondylar notch and proximally at the dorsal edge of the trochlear articular cartilage. Remove the osteochondral wedge and deepen the recession in the trochlea by removing additional bone from one or both sides of the newly created femoral groove.* The osteochondral wedge remains in place because of the net compressive force of the patella and friction between the cancellous surfaces of the two cut edges. If necessary, remodel the free osteochondral wedge with rongeurs to allow the wedge to seat deeply into the new femoral groove. The wedge can also be rotated 180 degrees when it is returned to the femoral groove if doing so will aid in heightening the medial ridge. *Replace the free osteochondral wedge when the depth is sufficient to house 50% of the height of the patella. Close the arthrotomy as described for lateral approach to the stifle joint (see p. 963).*

Trochlear resection. Trochlear resection is a method of deepening the trochlear groove through removal of articular cartilage and subchondral cancellous bone. The advantage of this technique is its simplicity. The disadvantage is that it removes the articular cartilage of the trochlea and allows articulation of the patella on the rough cancellous surface, which results in wearing of patellar articular cartilage. Nevertheless, the trochlear groove eventually fills with a combination of fibrous tissue and fibrocartilage and the patients appear to have acceptable limb function. *Measure the width of the articular surface of the patella and use this measurement to*

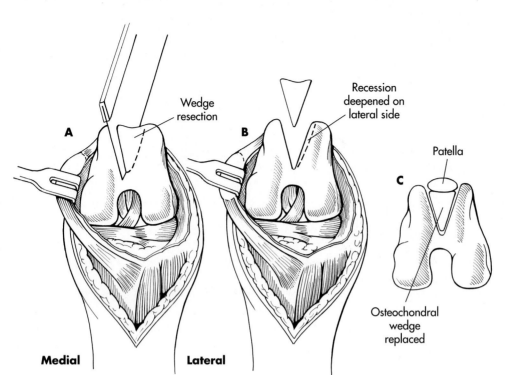

FIG. 30-89
A, For trochlear wedge recession, resect an osteochondral wedge from the patellar groove, and **B,** remove bone from the sides of incised groove to deepen the sulcus. **C,** Then replace the osteochondral wedge.

Wedge resection

Recession deepened on lateral side

Patella

Osteochondral wedge replaced

Medial   **Lateral**

determine the proper width of the trochlear resection. Remove articular cartilage and bone with a bone rasp, power burr, or rongeurs (Fig. 30-90). Make the length of the trochlear resection extend to the proximal margin of articular cartilage and distally to the cartilage margin just above the intercondylar notch. The depth of the groove should be such as to accommodate 50% of the height of the patella and allow the parapatellar fibrocartilage to articulate with the newly formed medial and lateral trochlear ridges. Make the medial and lateral trochlear ridges parallel to each other and the base of the groove perpendicular to each trochlear ridge.

☞ **N O T E ·** With medial luxations, it is often best to take more bone from the lateral side of the groove, thus preserving as much of the medial ridge as possible.

SUTURE MATERIALS/SPECIAL INSTRUMENTS

An osteotome and mallet, Kirschner pins, and a hand chuck or drill are needed to secure the tibial crest when tibial tuberosity transposition is performed. A fine-toothed saw (No. 12 X-acto saw, available at most hobby shops) is used for trochlear wedge recession.

POSTOPERATIVE CARE AND ASSESSMENT

The limb is placed in a soft, padded bandage for 3 days. Then leash walking only is allowed for 6 weeks before returning the animal to normal activity.

PROGNOSIS

The clinical results of surgical correction of medial patella luxation depend on the dog's gait, and on physical and radiographic findings. Recurrent luxation after surgery is present in 48% of joints evaluated (Willhauer, Vasseur, 1987). However, the majority are grade I luxations that do not affect clinical function. In one study, 48 of 52 stifle joints functioned well enough that lameness was not apparent during examination nor was clinical dysfunction reported by clients (Willhauer, Vasseur, 1987). The majority of patients with recurrent luxations exhibited reluxation only on physical examination when manual force was used to displace the patella. This study did not correlate reluxation with the method(s) of surgical correction so it was not possible to determine whether a particular corrective measure was more or less successful. Overall, the prognosis for patients undergoing surgical correction of a patella luxation is excellent for return to normal limb function.

Reference

Willhauer C, Vasseur P: Clinical results of surgical correction of medial luxation of the patella in dogs, *Vet Surg* 16:31, 1987.

Suggested Reading

Arkin AM: The effects of pressure on epiphyseal growth: a mechanism of plasticity of growing bone, *J Bone Joint Surg* 5:38, 1956.

Boone EG, Hohn RB, Weisbrode SE: Trochlear recession wedge technique for patellar luxation: an experimental study, *J Am Anim Hosp Assoc* 19:735, 1983.

FIG. 30-90
For trochlear resection, remove articular cartilage and bone with a bone rasp, power burr, or rongeurs to a depth where the patella rides within the new sulcus. Make the medial and lateral trochlear ridges parallel to each other and the base of the groove perpendicular to each trochlear ridge.

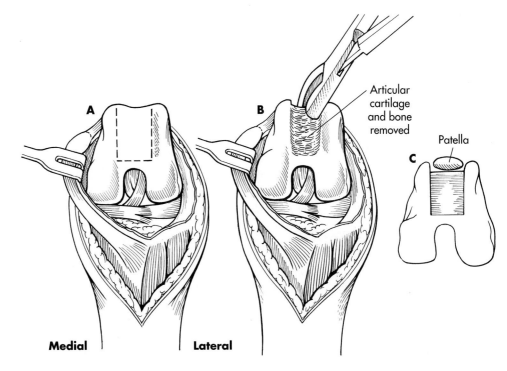

Butterworth SJ: Congenital medial patellar luxation in the dog, *Vet Ann* 33:193, 1993.

Hulse D, Miller D, Roberts D: Resurfacing canine trochleoplasties with free autogenous periosteal grafts, *Vet Surg* 15:284, 1986.

Moore J, Banks W: Repair of full thickness defects in the femoral trochlea of dogs after trochlear arthroplasty, *Am J Vet Res* 50:1406, 1989.

Priester WA: Sex, size, and breed as risk factors in canine patellar dislocation, *J Am Vet Med Assoc* 160:740, 1972.

Putnam RW: Patellar luxation in the dog. Thesis presented to the faculty of graduate studies, Guelph, Ontario, Canada, January 1968, University of Guelph.

LATERAL PATELLAR LUXATION

DEFINITIONS

Lateral patellar luxation is an intermittent or permanent displacement of the patella from the trochlear sulcus. **Anteversion** is excessive external rotation of the proximal femur relative to the distal femur. **Coxa valga** is an abnormal increase in the angle formed by the femoral neck and shaft in the frontal plane.

SYNONYMS

Slipped knee cap

GENERAL CONSIDERATIONS AND CLINICALLY RELEVANT PATHOPHYSIOLOGY

Lateral patella luxation is seen most frequently in large breeds of dogs but does occur in small and toy breeds of dogs. The cause is unknown but is thought to be related to anteversion or coxa valga of the coxofemoral joint, which shift the line of force produced by the pull of the quadriceps lateral to the longitudinal axis of the trochlear groove. This abnormally directed lateral force pulls the patella from the trochlear sulcus. Abnormal force placed on the growth plates of immature patients causes skeletal abnormalities that are mirror images of those seen with medial patella luxation. For further discussion of the pathophysiology of patella luxation see p. 976.

DIAGNOSIS
Clinical Presentation

Signalment. Dogs of either sex and of any age or breed may be affected. Lateral patella luxations are more frequently seen in large breeds of dogs than in small and toy breeds. Medial patella luxations, however, are more common than the lateral luxations in dogs of all sizes. Lateral patellar luxation has not been described in cats.

History. Affected animals most commonly are seen for evaluation of an intermittent, weight-bearing lameness. Owners may report that the animal occasionally holds the leg in a flexed position for one or two steps.

Physical Examination Findings

Physical findings are variable and dependent upon the severity of luxation. Diagnosis is determined by finding or eliciting lateral luxation of the patella and eliminating other causes of rear limb lameness (see below). Patients with grade I luxations generally exhibit no lameness, and the diagnosis is made as an incidental finding on physical examination. Patients with grade II luxations exhibit occasional "skipping" when walking or running. On occasion these patients will stretch the medial retinacular structures and appear for the first visit exhibiting a non–weight-bearing lameness. Lameness in patients with a grade III patella luxation varies from an occasional skip to a weight-bearing lameness. Patients with grade IV luxations walk with the rear quarters in a crouched position because of inability to extend the stifle joints fully.

Radiography

With grade III or IV luxations, standard craniocaudal and medial-to-lateral radiographs consistently show the patella to be displaced laterally. With grades I or II, the patella may be within the trochlear sulcus at the time of radiographs or may be displaced laterally.

Laboratory Findings

Consistent laboratory findings are not present.

DIFFERENTIAL DIAGNOSIS

Differential diagnoses include hip dysplasia, osteochondritis of the stifle or tarsal joints, panosteitis, hypertrophic osteodystrophy, capital physeal injury, cranial cruciate ligament rupture, and muscle strain. It is important to note that many patients with lateral patella luxation also have evidence of hip dysplasia. Both conditions may contribute to the lameness and require appropriate treatment for the dog to become sound.

MEDICAL OR CONSERVATIVE MANAGEMENT

Treatment of lateral patella luxation may be conservative or surgical. The choice of treatment method depends on the patient's age, clinical history, and physical findings. Older patients that are not lame and have patella luxation diagnosed as an incidental finding do not warrant surgical intervention. Rather, the client should be instructed to observe for clinical signs associated with patella luxation.

SURGICAL TREATMENT

Goals and methods of treatment for lateral patella luxation are similar to those described for medial patella luxation on p. 978. The surgical technique used in animals with lateral patellar luxations is similar to that described for osteotomy of the tibial tuberosity in animals with medial patellar luxations (see p. 980), except that the tuberosity is repositioned and stabilized medially (Fig. 30-91). The medial retinaculum is reinforced with suture reconstruction, fascial lata transposition, and/or excision of redundant joint capsule. The lateral restraints are released to help neutralize lateral forces acting on the patella. Methods for deepening the trochlear groove are the same as described for medial patella luxation. Osteotomies of the femur and tibia may be required to correct severe angular and/or torsional deformities. Corrective osteotomies are best performed by a specialist with the necessary equipment and training to perform these complex procedures.

Preoperative Management

Perioperative antibiotics are not indicated for repair of lateral patellar luxations unless the animal is immunocompromised or has concurrent disease that may increase the risk of infection.

Anesthesia

See p. 708 for a discussion of the anesthetic management of patients with orthopedic disease.

Surgical Anatomy

See p. 979 for normal anatomy of the stifle joint. In patients with lateral patellar luxation, abnormal wear of the lateral trochlear ridge may be evident. The patella and patella ten-

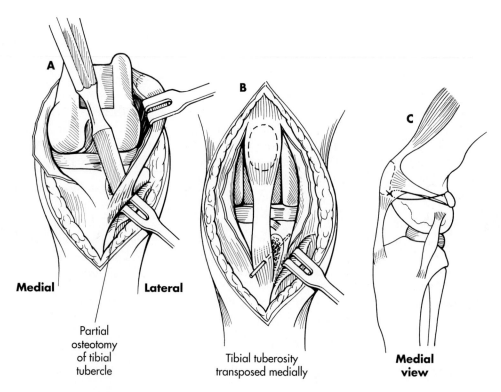

FIG. 30-91
For lateral patellar luxations, transpose the tibial crest medially. **A,** Make a parapatellar incision through the fascia lata and carry the incision distally onto the tibial tuberosity below the joint line. Position an osteotome beneath the patellar tendon and partially ostectomize the tibial crest. Do not transect the distal periosteal attachment. **B,** Stabilize the tibial tuberosity in its new location with one or two small Kirschner wires. **C,** Reinforce the medial retinaculum with suture placed from the fabella to the parapatellar fibrocartilage.

Medial   **Lateral**

Partial osteotomy of tibial tubercle

Tibial tuberosity transposed medially

Medial view

don lie lateral to the trochlear sulcus in these patients. The patella tendon must be identified before making a parapatellar incision to enter the joint. The medial retinaculum appears stretched in these patients, while the lateral retinaculum appears contracted. Release of the lateral retinaculum (with incision into the joint) reveals a thickened joint capsule.

Positioning

The patient is positioned in lateral recumbency with the affected leg up or in dorsal recumbency. The leg should be prepared from the dorsal midline to the tarsal joint. A hanging-leg preparation facilitates manipulation of the leg during surgery.

SURGICAL TECHNIQUES

A description of the surgical technique for correction of patellar luxation is given above and on p. 980.

SUTURE MATERIALS/SPECIAL INSTRUMENTS

Instruments needed for tibial tuberosity transposition are an osteotome and mallet, Kirschner pins to secure the tibial crest transposition, and a hand chuck or drill. A fine-toothed saw is needed for trochlear wedge recession.

POSTOPERATIVE CARE AND ASSESSMENT

The limb is placed in a soft, padded bandage for 3 days, after which the animal is limited to leash activity for 6 weeks.

PROGNOSIS

The prognosis is less optimal in large dogs with lateral patellar luxations than it is in smaller dogs with medial patella luxations; however, the prognosis is good for a return to functional activity.

Suggested Reading

Olmstead ML: Lateral luxation of the patella. In Bojrab MJ, editor: *Disease mechanisms in small animal surgery,* ed 2, Philadelphia, 1993, Lea & Febiger.

Vasseur PB: The stifle joint. In Slatter DH, editor: *Textbook of small animal surgery,* ed 2, Philadelphia, 1993, WB Saunders.

OSTEOCHONDRITIS DISSECANS OF THE STIFLE

DEFINITIONS

Osteochondritis issecans is a disturbance in endochondral ossification leading to retention of cartilage; it occasionally occurs in the stifle of immature, large dogs.

SYNONYMS

Osteochondrosis, OCD

GENERAL CONSIDERATIONS AND CLINICALLY RELEVANT PATHOPHYSIOLOGY

Osteochondritis dissecans (OCD) begins with a failure of endochondral ossification in either the physis or articular epiphyseal complex, which is responsible for the formation of metaphyseal bone. This condition occurs more commonly in the shoulder, elbow, and hock. The pathogenesis of OCD is discussed on p. 918. With OCD of the stifle, a piece of cartilage and subchondral bone is usually observed that involves the medial surface of the lateral femoral condyle (most frequently affected) or the medial femoral condyle.

DIAGNOSIS
Clinical Presentation

Signalment. Affected dogs are usually large (e.g., retrievers) and young, the average age at onset of lameness being 5 to 7 months. Both males and females are affected.

History. Rear limb lameness, which worsens after exercise, may be acute or chronic and mild or severe. Owners frequently complain that the dog is stiff in the morning or after rest. Owners are generally concerned that the dog may have hip dysplasia.

Physical Examination Findings

Lameness of one rear limb is usually evident. There may be stifle joint effusion and crepitation, especially if degenerative joint disease (DJD) is progressing. In immature dogs, a very slight cranial drawer may be noted, especially if there is muscle atrophy. However, when the cranial drawer is tested in animals with stifle OCD, there should be an abrupt halt to drawer motion, indicating that the cranial cruciate ligament is intact (see p. 958).

Radiography

Radiographic views should include a standard lateral view of the stifle. Radiographs of both stifles should be made to identify bilateral disease. Definitive radiographic diagnosis of OCD is made when a radiolucent concavity is observed on the medial or lateral femoral condyle (Fig. 30-92). More subtle radiographic signs include flattening of the articular surface and subchondral sclerosis. Radiographic signs of secondary DJD are usually visualized (see p. 923).

Laboratory Findings

Results of hematologic and serum biochemical analyses are normal in most affected animals. Results of arthrocentesis may include decreased synovial fluid viscosity, increased fluid volume, and increased numbers (up to 6000 to 9000 WBC/μl) of mononuclear phagocytic cells.

DIFFERENTIAL DIAGNOSIS

OCD must be differentiated from other diseases of young growing dogs that affect the rear limb and may cause similar clinical signs of lameness (hip dysplasia and panosteitis). Cranial cruciate ligament rupture is ruled out by physical examination and the presence of radiographic evidence of OCD.

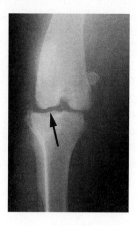

FIG. 30-92
Radiograph of a stifle with osteochondritis dissecans of the lateral femoral condyle. There is a radiolucent defect on the distal surface of the lateral femoral condyle (*arrow*).

MEDICAL MANAGEMENT

Medical therapy is generally used to treat older dogs with established DJD. Lame animals should be treated with confinement and administration of NSAIDs (see Table 30-15). After the lameness has subsided, exercise is gradually increased to strengthen surrounding musculature. Weight control is also important in the management of DJD.

SURGICAL TREATMENT

Surgical removal of the cartilage flap allows the defect to heal by outgrowth of fibrocartilage from underlying subchondral bone. Surgery may be useful in young animals, when the disease is diagnosed before the onset of DJD, and in lame animals that are unresponsive to medical therapy. However, surgical management does not usually alter the progression of DJD.

Preoperative Management

Most affected animals are young and otherwise healthy. Therefore, only minimal preoperative workup (complete blood count and serum chemistries) is usually necessary before surgery.

Anesthesia

Anesthetic management of young animals undergoing elective surgery for hip disease typically consists of inducing anesthesia with thiobarbiturates or other injectable agents and maintaining anesthesia with inhalants (halothane, isoflurane) in oxygen (see p. 708). Postoperative analgesia may be indicated (see p. 708).

Surgical Anatomy

Surgical anatomy of the stifle is discussed on p. 960. Either a standard medial or lateral parapatellar approach can be used to expose the lesion.

Positioning

The dog is positioned in dorsal recumbency with the affected limb suspended for draping. The limb is then released to allow access to the medial or lateral surface of the stifle.

SURGICAL TECHNIQUES

The surgical approach selected depends on the preference of the surgeon (see p. 961 for lateral parapatellar approach and p. 962 for medial parapatellar approach). Regardless of technique used for exposure, the appropriate femoral condyle should be examined and the flap of cartilage removed. Curettage is done only to remove fragments of cartilage from the edges of the lesion. The joint should be repeatedly flushed to remove any small fragments before closure.

SUTURE MATERIALS/SPECIAL INSTRUMENTS

Ochsner forceps are helpful in grasping the cartilage fragment. A bone curette is needed to curette the edges of the lesion.

POSTOPERATIVE CARE AND ASSESSMENT

The limb should be bandaged after surgery for 3 to 5 days to provide soft tissue support. The animal should be confined to leash walks only for 4 to 6 weeks and then allowed gradual resumption of normal activity.

PROGNOSIS

Dogs treated conservatively for OCD of the stifle usually have continued intermittent lameness and progressive DJD. Those treated surgically for OCD of the stifle may have improved limb function, but lameness may be evident after exercise. DJD is usually present even after surgery and requires occasional medical treatment (see above). Most dogs are functional pets and are only intermittently lame. Rarely, infection of the surgical site may occur after surgery.

Suggested Reading

Denny HR, Gibbs C: Osteochondritis dissecans of the canine stifle joint, *J Small Anim Pract* 20:317, 1980.
Olsson SE: General and aetiologic factors in canine osteochondrosis, *The Vet Quarterly* 9:268, 1987.
Olsson SE: Pathophysiology, morphology, and clinical signs of osteochondrosis in the dog. In Bojrab MJ, editor, *Disease mechanisms in small animal surgery*, Philadelphia, 1993, Lea & Febiger.

TARSUS

LIGAMENTOUS INJURY OF THE TARSUS

DEFINITIONS

Ligamentous injury to the tarsal joint may result from injury within or surrounding the tarsocrural, proximal intertarsal, distal intertarsal, or tarsometatarsal joints. **Luxation** is a complete separation between one of the above joint surfaces, while **subluxation** is a partial or incomplete separation. The term **varus** denotes an inward deviation of the limb, while **valgus** denotes an outward deviation.

SYNONYMS

Tarsal joint luxation, tarsocrural luxation

GENERAL CONSIDERATIONS AND CLINICALLY RELEVANT PATHOPHYSIOLOGY

Ligamentous injuries of the tarsus usually result from severe trauma such as vehicular accidents. Most injuries are open abrasions with moderate to severe loss of soft tissue and/or bone. Shearing injuries usually involve the tarsocrural joint. They typically occur when the limb is caught beneath a tire and are associated with severe abrasion of the soft tissues and malleoli. Shear injuries can involve the lateral or medial surface of the tarsus, but the medial surface is more commonly injured. Subluxation results from injury of the medial or lateral collateral ligament complex or fracture of the medial or lateral malleolus. Luxation generally results from injury of both the medial and the lateral collateral ligament complexes, fracture of both malleoli, or fracture of one malleolus with injury to the contralateral collateral ligament complex. A number of intertarsal injuries have been recognized as resulting from disruption of various ligament complexes between tarsal bones. Proximal intertarsal subluxation, proximal intertarsal luxation, and tarsometatarsal luxation are most common.

DIAGNOSIS
Clinical Presentation

Signalment. Any age or breed and either sex of dog or cat may be affected.

History. Most animals are presented for evaluation of a non–weight-bearing lameness. Some animals have an associated open wound over the tarsus.

Physical Examination Findings

Complete tarsocrural joint luxation is obvious; the animal is non–weight-bearing and the paw deviates at an unnatural angle. Pain, swelling, and crepitus are present. Subluxations may be more difficult to diagnose, particularly if only one part of the medial or lateral ligament complex is injured. Animals with complete subluxations are unable to bear weight, and the paw deviates to the direction opposite the ligamentous damage (i.e., if the subluxation is medial the paw deviates laterally). If partial tears of the collateral complex are suspected, varus and valgus forces should be applied to the joint while it is extended and flexed. Laxity in extension denotes injury to the long components of the collateral ligament complex, while laxity in flexion only denotes injury to the short component of the collateral ligament complex.

☞ **N O T E** • Always place the joint in extension to evaluate medial or lateral restraint injury.

With shearing injuries that cause luxation or subluxation, soft-tissue abrasion and bone loss are present. Often the bone surface and articular cartilage are exposed. With intertarsal luxations and tarsometatarsal subluxation, animals usually are in pain and unable to bear weight on the affected limb, and the involved area is swollen. Abnormal rotation and deviation of the foot are present.

Radiography

Standard craniocaudal and medial-to-lateral radiographs are often sufficient for complete evaluation (Fig. 30-93). If instability is suspected but not confirmed, standing lateral and varus-valgus stress films are useful (Fig. 30-94).

Laboratory Findings

Consistent laboratory abnormalities are not present.

DIFFERENTIAL DIAGNOSIS

Differential diagnoses include mild sprain, fractures of one or more tarsal bones, osteochondritis dissecans of the talus, and arthritis. These conditions can be differentiated from tarsal luxation or subluxation by radiography.

MEDICAL MANAGEMENT

Medical, or nonsurgical, management is not rewarding with these injuries. Surgery is needed to restore functional integrity of the joint.

SURGICAL TREATMENT

Each patient needs a thorough neurologic and vascular evaluation to determine the feasibility of treatment. With tarsocrural luxation or subluxation, objectives of treatment are to reestablish joint stability to achieve pain-free weight bearing. Reconstruction of the short and long collateral ligament components is recommended for optimal results. With severe ligamentous injuries of the tarsus, partial or complete fusion and limb amputation are alternatives to joint reconstruction. With shearing injuries, the objective of management is to achieve a pain-free, functional patient. If the cartilage and bone damage is limited to the malleolus, reconstruction can be attempted. However, if damage to the cartilage and bone is severe, amputation or tarsal arthrodesis should be considered.

Proximal intertarsal subluxation with plantar instability (Fig. 30-95) occurs when excessive dorsal flexion causes disruption of the plantar ligament complex between the calcaneus and fourth tarsal bones. Treatment is by selective fusion of the joint surfaces between the calcaneus and fourth tarsal bones.

Proximal intertarsal subluxation can occur with dorsal instability. This injury results from hyperextension-caused damage to the dorsal ligaments and dorsal joint capsule between the talus and central tarsal bone. Treatment in most cases is best accomplished with rigid coaptation. If this is not successful, selective fusion of the talocentral joint can be performed.

Proximal intertarsal luxation occurs when excessive dorsal flexion causes disruption of the plantar ligament

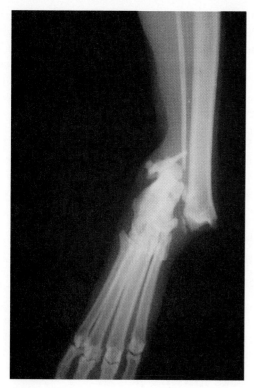

FIG. 30-93
Craniocaudal radiograph of a luxated tarsal joint. Note fracture of the lateral malleolus and medial displacement of the tibia.

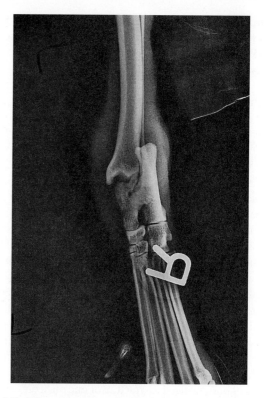

FIG. 30-94
Varus stress radiograph of the tarsus. Widening of the medial joint space indicates damage to the medial collateral ligament and joint capsule.

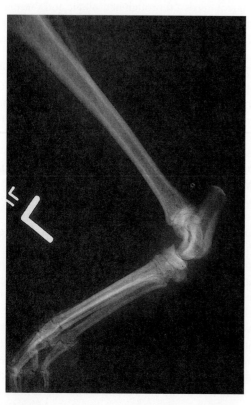

FIG. 30-95
Lateral radiograph of the tarsus of dog with proximal intertarsal subluxation.

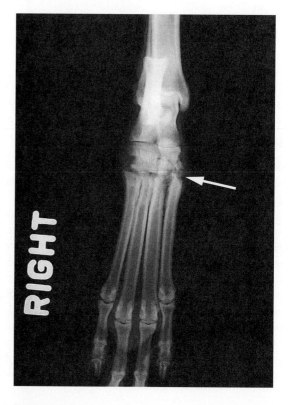

FIG. 30-96
Craniocaudal radiograph of dog with tarsometatarsal subluxation. Note fragmentation of second tarsal bone (*arrow*).

complex, both between the calcaneus and fourth tarsal bones and between the talus and the central tarsal bone. Treatment is by selective fusion of the proximal intertarsal joint.

Tarsometatarsal luxation (Fig. 30-96) occurs when excessive dorsal flexion causes disruption of the plantar ligaments and fibrocartilage. The luxation occurs between the distal row of tarsal bones and metatarsal bones. Treatment is best accomplished with selective fusion of the distal intertarsal joint (tarsometatarsal joint). Occasionally, the luxation occurs laterally between the fourth tarsal bone and adjacent metatarsal bones, with the medial separation occurring between the second and third tarsal bones and the central tarsal bone. In these patients, selective fusion of the joint space between the fourth tarsal and adjacent metatarsal bones is accomplished with a bone plate secured to the fourth tarsal bone and fifth metatarsal bone. Medially, a small bone plate is secured to the central tarsal bone proximally and the second tarsal and second metatarsal bones distally.

Preoperative Management

Open wounds should be cleaned and a sterile dressing applied before surgery (see under shearing injuries, p. 990). Those with open wounds should be started on therapeutic antibiotics (see p. 708). A bandage should be applied to support the limb and the animal confined to a small space to prevent further joint damage until definitive surgery can be performed.

Anesthesia

Anesthetic management of animals with joint disease is provided on p. 708.

Surgical Anatomy

The tarsus consists of the tibia, fibula, and proximal tarsal, distal tarsal, and metatarsal bones (Fig. 30-97). These bones form the tarsocrural, intertarsal, and tarsometatarsal joints. The tarsocrural joint is formed by the fibula and cochlea of

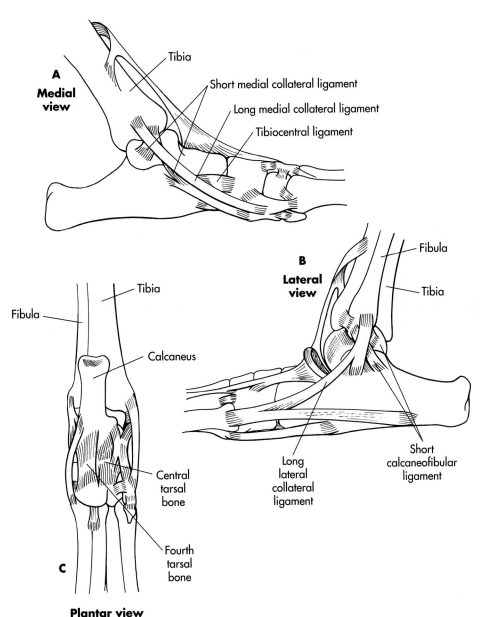

FIG. 30-97
A, Medial, **B,** lateral, and **C,** plantar views of ligamentous structures that provide stability to the tarsal joint.

the tibia proximally and the talus and calcaneus distally. The intertarsal joints are formed by articulations between the tarsal bones, and the tarsometatarsal joints are formed by the articulations between the distal tarsal and metatarsal bones. The tarsal joints are supported by a complex arrangement of ligaments. The major ligaments providing medial support of the tarsocrural joint are the long medial collateral ligament, short medial collateral ligament, and tibiocentral ligament (Fig. 30-97, *A*). Lateral support is provided by the long lateral collateral ligament and short calcaneofibular ligament (Fig. 30-97, *B*). Knowledge of the anatomic points of origin and insertion of each ligament is important for reconstruction of medial and lateral ligament injuries. Most of the stability of the intertarsal and tarsometatarsal joints is provided by a complex network of plantar ligaments, tarsal fibrocartilage, and joint capsule. Plantar ligaments originate from the calcaneus and attach to the central and fourth tarsal bones, before inserting on the metatarsal bones (Fig. 30-97, *C*).

Positioning

The limb is clipped from the coxofemoral joint to the digits so that the paw can be included in the sterile field. This allows direct manipulation and visual orientation of the paw during reconstruction. A hanging-leg prep facilitates manipulation of the limb during surgery (see p. 25).

SURGICAL TECHNIQUES
Tarsocrural Luxation or Subluxation

Depending on which side is injured, make a curved incision centered over the medial or lateral malleolus. Begin the incision 4 cm above the joint line and continue distally to a point 4 cm below the tarsometatarsal joint line. Incise subcutaneous tissues and deep fascia along the same line. Remnants of the collateral ligament complex and joint capsule are exposed and the articular surface is visible once the deep fascia is incised. *Reduce and align the joint surfaces.*

Suture the joint capsule and injured ligaments with small-sized, nonabsorbable suture. Protect the repair with nonabsorbable, heavy (No. 2 to No. 5, depending on the animal's size) figure-eight sutures strategically placed to mimic the short and long components of the collateral ligament complex. Drill bone tunnels in the malleolus where the ligament complex originates. Next, drill tunnels where the short and long components of the collateral ligament complex insert. Place two strands of nonabsorbable polyester suture through the predrilled holes in the malleolus. Pass one end of the suture strand through the tunnel drilled to mimic the insertion of the short component and pass the end of the other strand through the tunnel drilled to mimic the insertion of the long component of the collateral ligament complex. Place the sutures in a figure-eight pattern and tie them such that the suture placed as the short component is tied with the joint in 90 degrees of flexion (Fig. 30-98). Tie the suture placed to simulate the long component with the joint in a normal standing angle.

Shearing Injuries

When the animal is first seen, cover the wound with a sterile dressing and temporarily immobilize the limb with an external splint. Once the animal is stable enough to be anesthetized, debride the wound. Liberally flush the wound with 0.05% chlorhexidene. Fill the wound with sterile KY jelly and clip the surrounding area. Transfer the patient to the operating room and debride obvious necrotic tissue and remove foreign material. If the medial surface is abraded, perform ligament reconstruction by inserting bone screws in the malleolus and talus to mimic the origin and insertion of the medial collateral ligament complex (Fig. 30-99). If the lateral surface is abraded, place bone screws in the malleolus and calcaneus to mimic the origin and insertion of the lateral collateral ligament complex (Fig. 30-100). Place figure-eight, heavy, nonabsorbable su-

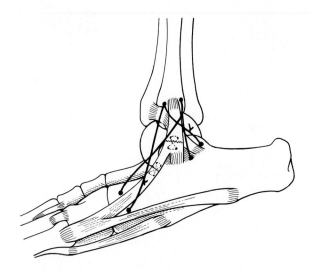

FIG. 30-98
Primary repair of collateral ligaments are supported with heavy suture to stimulate long and short components of the collateral ligament complex.

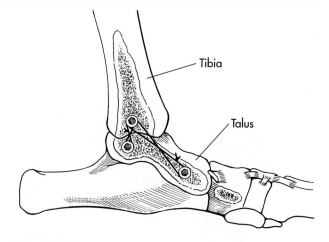

FIG. 30-99
Reconstruction of the medial collateral restraint complex with screws and suture material. Note proper placement of the proximal and distal talar screws to mimic insertion points of the short and long components of the restraint complex, respectively.

ture between the screws. Tie the suture used to mimic the short component of the ligament complex with the joint at 90 degrees, and tie the suture used to mimic the long component of the ligament complex with the tarsus in a normal standing angle. If malleolar fracture is present, rather than ligament injury, reduce and stabilize the fracture with a tension-band technique. *Immobilize the reconstruction for 2 to 4 weeks with a transarticular external skeletal fixator. Place one full pin 6 to 7 cm proximal to the malleolus and one full pin through the metatarsal bones, just below the tarsometatarsal joint line. Contour medial and lateral external bars to an angle simulating the standing angle of the tarsal joint. Place a half pin 2 to 3 cm above the malleolus and a second half pin through the central and fourth tarsal bones. Tighten the pin clamps.*

> ☞ **NOTE** · After placement of the medial and lateral bars, resistance to craniocaudal bending can be improved by adding an additional external bar.

Proximal Intertarsal Subluxation with Plantar Instability

Expose the joint through a caudolateral incision. Remove articular cartilage from the articular surface of the calcaneus and fourth tarsal bones with a curette or pneumatic burr. Place a Steinmann pin from the proximal calcaneus down the calcaneal shaft to the point where the tip of the pin can be seen exiting where the cartilage was removed. Harvest a cancellous bone graft and pack it into the space between the calcaneus and fourth tarsal bone. Reduce the joint and drive the pin across it to seat in the body of the fourth tarsal bone. Drill a transverse hole across the distal

quadrant of the fourth tarsal bone and drill a second transverse hole in the proximal quadrant of the calcaneus. Place orthopedic wire through the drill holes in a figure-eight pattern to complete a tension-band wire (Fig. 30-101). Use 20-gauge orthopedic wire for small and medium-sized dogs and cats and 18-gauge for large dogs.

Proximal Intertarsal Luxation

Make a lateral incision beginning at the proximal end of the calcaneus and extending distally 3 to 4 cm below the tarsometatarsal joint line. Remove articular cartilage from the joint surfaces and insert a cancellous bone graft. Apply a compression plate to the lateral surface of the calcaneus, fourth tarsal bone, and fifth metatarsal bone (Fig. 30-102).

Tarsometatarsal Luxation

Expose the articular surfaces of the joint through a cranial incision. Reflect extensor tendons laterally to gain adequate exposure. Remove articular cartilage and insert a cancellous bone graft. Reduce the joint and stabilize with cross pins. Place one pin so that it enters the base of the fifth metatarsal bone, crosses the joint, and is seated in the central tarsal bone. Place the second pin so that it enters the base of the second metatarsal bone, crosses the joint, and is seated in the fourth tarsal bone. If the luxation occurs laterally, between the fourth tarsal bone and adjacent metatarsal bones, with the medial separation occurring between the second and third tarsal bones and central tarsal

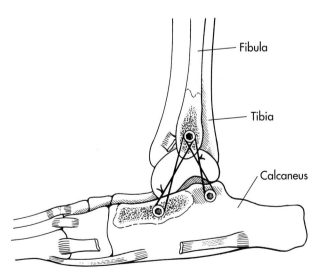

FIG. 30-100
Reconstruction of the lateral collateral restraint complex with screws and suture material. Note proper placement of the proximal and distal talar screws to mimic insertion points of the short and long components of the restraint complex, respectively.

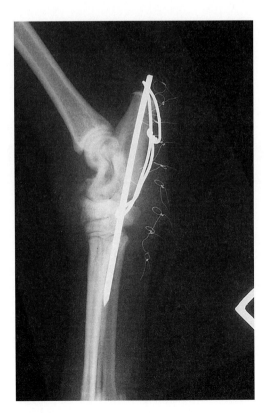

FIG. 30-101
Lateral radiographs showing stabilization of proximal plantar instability with a pin and tension band.

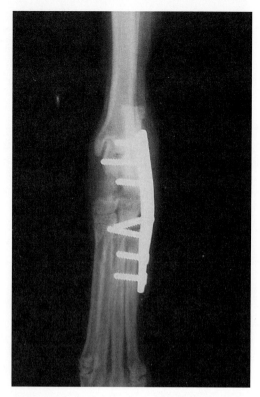

FIG. 30-102
Craniocaudal radiograph showing stabilization of proximal plantar instability with a bone plate placed on the lateral surface of the calcaneus and fifth metatarsal bones.

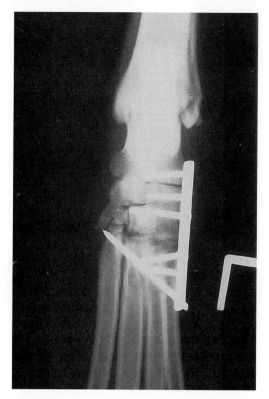

FIG. 30-103
Craniocaudal radiograph showing stabilization of tarsometatarsal instability with a bone plate placed on the lateral surface of the calcaneus and fifth metatarsal bones.

bone, expose the tarsometatarsal joint with two incisions. Make a lateral incision extending 5 cm proximal and distal to the tarsometatarsal joint line. Make a similar incision medially. Remove articular cartilage from all exposed joint surfaces and insert a cancellous bone graft. Stabilize the fusion with small bone plates. Laterally secure a plate to the fourth tarsal and fifth metatarsal bones (Fig. 30-103). Medially, secure a small bone plate to the central tarsal bone proximally and to the second tarsal and second metatarsal bone distally.

Tarsocrural Joint Arthrodesis

Tarsocrural joint arthrodesis is indicated when there is severe injury of the tibial cochlea and condyles of the talus that precludes maintaining a long-term, pain-free articulation. Arthrodesis is also indicated when painful degenerative joint disease is not responsive to conservative measures. In conjunction with tarsocrural joint fusions, the proximal intertarsal and distal tarsometatarsal joints are also fused.

Determine the normal standing angle of the opposite limb before surgery and use it to approximate the fusion angle during arthrodesis of the injured limb. Make an incision over the cranial surface of the joint. Begin the incision over the distal one third of the tibia and extend it distally mid-

way down the metatarsal bones. Enter the tarsocrural joint to expose the articular surfaces. With a power saw, remove the articular surface of the distal tibia by cutting perpendicular to the long axis of the bone. Cut the trochlea of the talus to achieve the appropriate fusion angle when the cut surfaces rest flush with each other. Use the normal standing angle of the opposite limb to approximate the fusion angle. Maintain reduction of the cut surfaces with small Kirschner pins and pack a cancellous bone graft around the joint. Open the joint capsule of the proximal intertarsal and tarsometatarsal joints to expose the articular surfaces. Remove the cartilage with a pneumatic burr and insert a cancellous bone graft. Stabilize the joints with a bone plate applied to the cranial surface. Bend the plate to conform to the established fusion angle and secure it proximally by placing three screws in the distal tibia, two to four screws in the tarsal bones, and three screws in the third metatarsal bone. Alternatively, if a lengthening plate is used to bridge the tarsus, attach the plate to the distal tibia and metatarsus with three or four screws in each bone (Fig. 30-104).

SUTURE MATERIALS/SPECIAL INSTRUMENTS

Nonabsorbable suture is generally used throughout the pro-

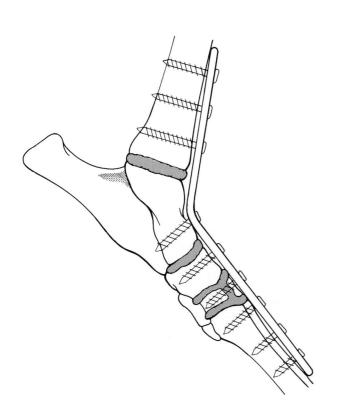

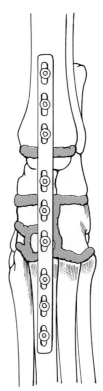

FIG. 30-104
Dorsal placement of a plate for tarsocrural arthrodesis. Because the plate is on the compression surface of the bone, it is subject to failure. A lengthening plate should be used, if possible.

cedures described above. A power drill, bone plate and screws, and a curette or air drill to remove articular cartilage are necessary for arthrodesis.

POSTOPERATIVE CARE AND ASSESSMENT

After repair of tarsocrural luxations or subluxations the tarsus should be placed in a normal standing angle and immobilized with rigid external coaptation or a transarticular external skeletal fixator for 3 weeks. During this time, activity should be limited to leash walking and the coaptation bandage checked frequently. After the splint is removed, passive flexion and extension of the joint can be initiated and activity slowly increased over the next 6 weeks. If a shearing injury is present, treat the wound as an open wound with daily changes of a sterile adherent dressing and liberal flushing with 0.05% chlorhexidene (see p. 94). Once healthy granulation tissue is formed, apply a nonadherent sterile dressing. After arthrodesis, protect the repair with external coaptation or an external skeletal fixator for 4 to 6 weeks and restrict activity until there is radiographic evidence of bone union.

PROGNOSIS

Adequate limb function can be expected in most patients with tarsal injuries after appropriate surgical intervention; however, the prognosis depends on the severity of ligamentous injury, cartilage damage, and the joint involved. Continued lameness should be expected in animals with subluxations or luxations that are not adequately stabilized.

Suggested Reading

Aron DN: Prosthetic ligament replacement for severe tarsocrural joint instability, *J Am Anim Hosp Assoc* 23:41, 1987.

Aron DN, Purinton PT: Collateral ligaments of the tarsocrural joint: an anatomical and functional study, *Vet Surg* 14:173, 1985.

Aron DN, Purinton PT: Replacement of the collateral ligaments of the canine tarsocrural joint: a proposed technique, *Vet Surg* 14:178, 1985.

Doverspike M, Vasseur PB: Clinical findings and complications after talocrural arthrodesis in dogs: experience with six cases, *J Am Anim Hosp Assoc* 27:553, 1991.

OSTEOCHONDRITIS DISSECANS OF THE TARSUS

DEFINITIONS

Osteochondritis dissecans is a disturbance in endochondral ossification that leads to cartilage retention; it occurs in the hocks of immature, large-breed dogs.

SYNONYMS

Osteochondrosis, OCD

GENERAL CONSIDERATIONS AND CLINICALLY RELEVANT PATHOPHYSIOLOGY

Osteochondritis dissecans (OCD) begins with a failure of endochondral ossification in either the physis or articular epiphyseal complex, which is responsible for the formation of epiphyseal bone. This condition also occurs commonly in the shoulder, elbow, and stifle. The pathogenesis of OCD is discussed on p. 918. With OCD of the talus, a large piece of cartilage and subchondral bone is usually observed involving the medial (most frequently affected) or lateral trochlear ridge. Histologically, the flap consists of cartilage, subchondral bone trabeculae in the defect are thickened, and bone marrow fibrosis is noted.

DIAGNOSIS
Clinical Presentation

Signalment. Affected dogs are usually large; rottweilers are most frequently affected. The average age of onset of lameness is 5 to 7 months, and the condition affects both males and females.

☞ **N O T E** · There is evidence of a hereditary component in the etiology based on the predilection of rottweilers to develop this condition.

History. Rear limb lameness, which worsens after exercise, may be acute or chronic. Owners, who frequently report that the dog is stiff in the morning or after rest, are generally concerned that the dog may have hip dysplasia.

Physical Examination Findings

Lameness of one rear limb is usually evident. The dog may hyperextend the hocks and have a stiff or stilted gait because of bilateral lameness. Pain may be elicited on hock flexion. Palpation of the hocks should include an evaluation of range of motion. A decrease in the animal's ability to flex the hock is indicative of secondary degenerative joint disease (DJD). Crepitation during hock flexion and extension, joint effusion, and periarticular swelling may be noted if DJD is present.

Radiography

Radiographic views should include a standard lateral of the hock, flexed lateral to expose the proximal portion of the talus, a cranial-caudal view of the hock (made while the hock is extended, to visualize the proximal portion of the trochlear ridges), and a cranial-caudal view (made with the hock flexed, to visualize the cranial portion of the trochlear ridges and to visualize the lateral condylar ridge without superimposition of the calcaneus) (Fig. 30-105). Radiographs of both hocks should be made because bilateral disease is common. Definitive radiographic diagnosis of OCD is made when a radiolucent concavity is observed on the medial or lateral trochlear ridge (Fig. 30-106). Radiographic signs of secondary DJD will usually be visualized (see p. 923).

☞ **N O T E** · Both hocks should be radiographed because of the frequency of bilateral disease; however, unless the animal is clinical, surgery of the opposite limb may not be necessary.

Laboratory Findings

Results of hematologic and serum biochemical analyses are normal in most affected animals. Results of arthrocentesis may include decreased synovial fluid viscosity, increased fluid volume, and increase numbers (up to 6000 to 9000 WBC/μl) of mononuclear phagocytic cells.

DIFFERENTIAL DIAGNOSIS

OCD must be differentiated from other diseases of young growing dogs that affect the rear limbs and may cause similar clinical signs of lameness (i.e., hip dysplasia and panosteitis). Decreased range of motion and swelling in the hock usually identify hock disease as a potential cause of lameness.

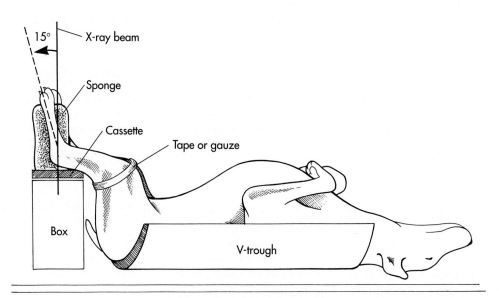

FIG. 30-105
Positioning for a craniocaudal view of the flexed hock, which allows visualization of the lateral condylar ridge, without superimposition of the calcaneus.

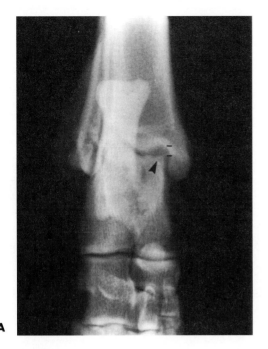

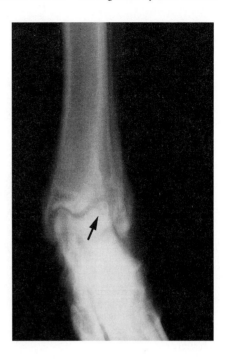

FIG. 30-106
Radiographs of hocks with osteochondritis dissecans. **A,** Standard craniocaudal view with a lesion on the medial trochlear ridge of the talus. There is a flattening of the medial trochlear ridge, and the joint space is widened (*arrow*). **B,** Flexed craniocaudal view with a lesion on the lateral trochlear ridge of the talus. A subchondral fissure is visible at the base of the lateral trochlear ridge.(From Olmstead ML: *Small animal orthopedics,* St. Louis, 1995, Mosby.)

MEDICAL MANAGEMENT

Medical therapy is generally used to treat older dogs with established DJD. Lame animals are treated with confinement and administration of NSAIDs (see Table 30-5). After the lameness has subsided, gradually increasing exercise is indicated to strengthen surrounding musculature. Weight control is also important in the management of DJD.

SURGICAL TREATMENT

Surgical removal of the cartilage flap allows the defect to heal by outgrowth of fibrocartilage from underlying subchondral bone. Surgery may be useful in young animals when the disease is diagnosed before the onset of DJD, and in lame animals that are unresponsive to medical therapy. However, surgical management does not usually alter the progression of DJD.

Preoperative Management

Most affected animals are young and otherwise healthy. Therefore minimal preoperative workup (complete blood count and serum chemistries) is usually necessary before surgery.

Anesthesia

Anesthetic management of young animals undergoing surgery for orthopedic disease is described on p. 708. Postoperative analgesics may be indicated (see p. 708).

Surgical Anatomy

Surgical anatomy of the hock is discussed on p. 989. Approaches to the lateral and medial trochlear ridge that do not involve osteotomy of the epicondyle or collateral ligament transection appear to result in less postoperative morbidity and faster return to function than do osteotomy approaches.

Positioning

The dog is positioned in dorsal recumbency with the affected limb suspended for draping. The limb is then released to allow access to the medial or lateral surface of the hock.

SURGICAL TECHNIQUES

The surgical approach selected depends on the location of the lesion. Lesions of the medial trochlear ridge are visualized using a dorsomedial and/or plantaromedial surgical approach, while lesions of the lateral trochlear ridge are visualized using a dorsolateral and/or plantarolateral surgical approach. Regardless of technique used for exposure, the appropriate trochlear ridge is examined and the flap of cartilage removed. Curettage is done only to remove fragments of cartilage from the edges of the lesion. The joint should be repeatedly flushed to remove any small fragments before closure.

Dorsomedial Approach to the Tarsus

Extend the hock and palpate the dorsal portion of the medial trochlear ridge. Make a skin incision starting proximal to the trochlear ridge and extending distally over the trochlear ridge. Incise subcutaneous tissues along the same line. Identify the tendon of the tibialis cranialis muscle, saphenous nerve, cranial tibial artery and vein, and dorsal

Dorsomedial approach

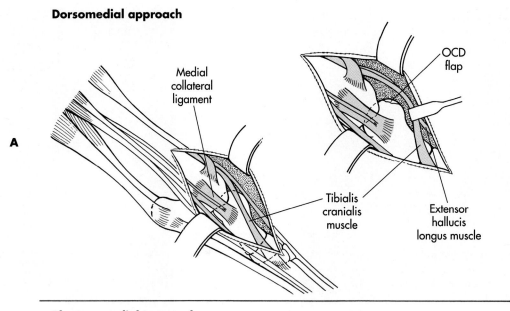

Plantaromedial approach

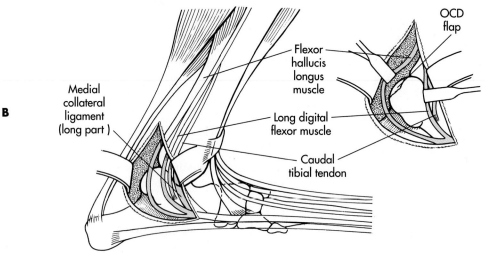

FIG. 30-107
A, For a dorsomedial approach to the hock, make a skin incision starting proximal to the trochlear ridge and extending distally over it. Incise subcutaneous tissues along the same line. Identify the tendon of the tibialis cranialis muscle, saphenous nerve, cranial tibial artery and vein, and dorsal branches of the saphenous artery and vein and retract them laterally. Incise deep fascia and joint capsule along the midline of the palpable portion of the medial trochlear ridge. Extend the incision proximally into the periosteum of the distal tibia. **B,** For a plantaromedial approach to the hock, incise skin and subcutaneous tissues caudal to the medial malleolus over the trochlear ridge. Identify the tendon of the long digital flexor muscle and distal attachment of the caudal tibial tendon and retract them cranially. Identify the tendon of the flexor hallucis longus muscle, tibial nerve, plantar branches of the medial saphenous vein and saphenous artery, and superficial plantar metatarsal vein and retract them laterally. Incise deep fascia and joint capsule longitudinally along the midline of the palpable portion of the medial trochlear ridge.

branches of the saphenous artery and vein and retract them laterally. Incise the deep fascia and joint capsule along the midline of the palpable portion of the medial trochlear ridge. Extend the incision proximally into the periosteum of the distal tibia (Fig. 30-107, A). Visualize the cranial and distal part of the medial trochlear ridge. Extend the hock to increase the amount of visible trochlear ridge. Identify and remove the cartilage flap. Curette the edges of the lesion and flush the joint. Close the wound by suturing fascia and joint capsule with simple interrupted absorbable sutures. Suture subcutaneous tissues and skin in separate layers.

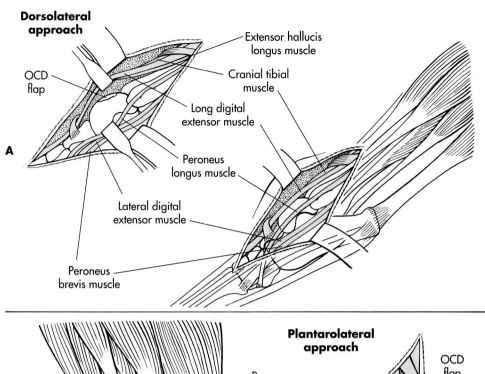

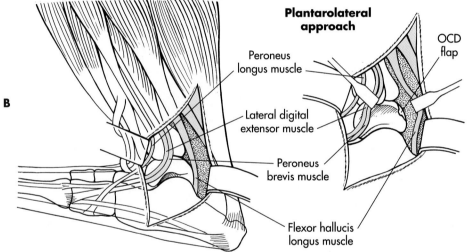

FIG. 30-108
A, For a dorsolateral approach to the hock make a skin incision starting proximal to the trochlear ridge and extending distally over it. Incise subcutaneous tissues along the same line. Identify the tendons of the long digital extensor muscle, cranial tibial muscle and extensor hallucis longus muscle, dorsal branch of the lateral saphenous vein, and superficial peroneal nerve and retract them medially. Identify the tendons of the peroneus longus, lateral digital extensor muscle, and peroneus brevis muscle and retract them in a plantar direction. Incise deep fascia and joint capsule longitudinally along the midline of the palpable portion of the lateral trochlear ridge. **B,** For a plantarolateral approach to the hock, make a skin incision starting proximal to the trochlear ridge and extending distally over the trochlear ridge. Incise subcutaneous tissues along the same line. Identify and retract tendons of the peroneus brevis, lateral digital extensor, and peroneus longus muscles dorsally. Retract the tendon of the flexor hallucis longus in a medial direction. Incise deep fascia and joint capsule longitudinally along the midline of the palpable portion of the trochlear ridge.

Plantaromedial Approach to the Tarsus

Flex the hock and palpate the proximal or plantar aspect of the medial trochlear ridge. Incise skin and subcutaneous tissues caudal to the medial malleolus over the trochlear ridge. Identify the tendon of the long digital flexor muscle and the distal attachment of the caudal tibial tendon and retract them cranially. Identify the tendon of the flexor hallucis longus muscle, tibial nerve, plantar branches of the medial saphenous vein and saphenous artery, and superficial plantar metatarsal vein and retract them laterally. Incise the deep fascia and joint capsule longitudinally along the midline of the palpable portion of the medial trochlear ridge (Fig. 30-107, B). Identify and remove the cartilage flap. Flex the hock to increase the amount of medial trochlear ridge visible. Curette the edges of the lesion and flush the joint. Close the wound by suturing fascia and joint capsule with simple interrupted absorbable sutures. Suture subcutaneous tissues and skin in separate layers.

Dorsolateral Approach to the Tarsus

Extend the hock and palpate the cranial portion of the lateral trochlear ridge. Make a skin incision starting proximal to the trochlear ridge and extending distally over the trochlear ridge. Incise subcutaneous tissues along the same line. Identify the tendons of the long digital extensor muscle, cranial tibial muscle, and extensor hallucis longus muscle, the dorsal branch of the lateral saphenous vein, and the superficial peroneal nerve and retract them medially. Identify the tendons of the peroneus longus, lateral digital extensor, and peroneus brevis muscles and retract them in a plantar direction. Incise the deep fascia and joint capsule longitudinally along the midline of the palpable portion of the lateral trochlear ridge (Fig. 30-108, A). Visualize the cranial and distal part of the lateral trochlear ridge. Extend the hock to increase the amount of visible trochlear ridge. Identify and remove the cartilage flap. Curette the edges of the lesion and flush the joint. Close the wound by suturing fascia and joint capsule with simple interrupted absorbable sutures. Suture subcutaneous tissues and skin in separate layers.

Plantarolateral Approach to the Tarsus

Flex the hock and palpate the proximal aspect of the lateral trochlear ridge. Incise skin and subcutaneous tissues plantar to the lateral malleolus over the trochlear ridge. Retract the tendons of the peroneus brevis muscle, lateral digital extensor muscle, and peroneus longus muscle dorsally.

It is difficult to retract the tendons of the peroneus brevis, lateral digital extensor, and peroneus longus muscles very far because they are firmly embedded in deep fascia over the lateral malleolus. *Retract the plantar branch of the lateral saphenous vein and a branch of the caudal cutaneous sural nerve in a plantar direction, and the tendon of the flexor hallucis longus in a medial direction. Incise the deep fascia and joint capsule longitudinally along the midline of the palpable portion of the lateral trochlear ridge (Fig. 30-108, B). Identify and remove the cartilage flap. Flex the hock to increase the amount of lateral trochlear ridge visible. Curette the edges of the lesion and flush the joint. Close the wound by suturing fascia and joint capsule with simple interrupted absorbable sutures. Suture subcutaneous tissues and skin in separate layers.*

SUTURE MATERIALS/SPECIAL INSTRUMENTS

Ochsner forceps are helpful in grasping the cartilage fragment. A bone curette is needed to curette the edges of the lesion.

POSTOPERATIVE CARE AND ASSESSMENT

The limb should be bandaged after surgery for 3 to 5 days to provide soft tissue support. The animal should be confined to leash walks only for 4 to 6 weeks.

PROGNOSIS

Dogs treated conservatively for OCD of the hock usually have continued intermittent lameness and progressive DJD. Those treated surgically for OCD of the hock may have improved limb function, but lameness may be evident after exercise. DJD is usually present even after surgery and requires medical treatment (see above); however, most dogs are functional pets and are lame only intermittently. Rarely, infection of the surgical site may occur after surgery.

☞ **N O T E ·** Advise owners that surgical treatment does not appear to alter the progression of DJD, and affected dogs may require medical therapy after surgery.

Suggested Reading

Beale BS, Goring RL: Exposure of the medial and lateral trochlear ridges of the talus in the dog. I. Dorsomedial and plantaromedial surgical approaches to the medial trochlear ridge, *J Am Anim Hosp Assoc* 26:13, 1990.

Beale BS et al: A prospective evaluation of four surgical approaches to the talus of the dog used in the treatment of osteochondritis dissecans, *J Am Anim Hosp Assoc* 27:221, 1991.

Goring RL, Beale BS: Exposure of the medial and lateral trochlear ridges of the talus in the dog. II. Dorsolateral and plantarolateral surgical approaches to the lateral trochlear ridge, *J Am Anim Hosp Assoc* 26:19, 1990.

Smith MM, Vasseur PB, Morgan JP: Clinical evaluation of dogs after surgical and nonsurgical management of osteochondritis dissecans of the talus, *J Am Vet Med Assoc* 187:31, 1985.

Mason TA, Lavelle RB: Osteochondritis dissecans of the tibial tarsal bone in dogs, *J Small Anim Pract* 20:423, 1979.

Miyabayashi T et al: Use of a flexed dorsoplantar radiographic view of the talocrural joint to evaluate lameness in two dogs, *J Am Vet Med Assoc* 199:598, 1991.

CHAPTER 31

Management of Muscle and Tendon Injury or Disease

MUSCLE CONTUSION AND STRAINS

DEFINITIONS

A **contusion** is a bruise of the muscle with varying degrees of hemorrhage and fiber disruption. A **strain** is a longitudinal stretching or tearing of muscle fibers or groups of fibers. Contusions and strains result in disruption of the normal architecture of the muscle-tendon unit secondary to interstitial edema, hemorrhage, or overstretching.

SYNONYMS

Pulled muscle

GENERAL CONSIDERATIONS AND CLINICALLY RELEVANT PATHOPHYSIOLOGY

Muscle contusions are the result of external trauma. An external blow causes disruption of fibril continuity, disruption of the vascular compartment, and subsequent hemorrhage into the interstitial space. Muscle strains are the result of overstretching or overuse. These injuries are not commonly recognized in animals but do occur.

Muscles may span one or more joints and when contracted cause a specific joint movement to occur. For example, the biceps originates from the supraglenoid tuberosity of the scapula and inserts onto the medial tuberosity of the radial head. Contraction causes extension of the shoulder joint and flexion of the elbow. An injured muscle can cause considerable pain during normal body motion. Muscle has the intrinsic ability to heal by regeneration of myofibrils if the sarcolemmal cells survive and the endomysial connective tissue sheath is not destroyed. With mild contusions and strains, the cells and endomysial sheath are not destroyed, and their preservation allows for complete healing. However, if the contusion is severe and causes extensive cell death and hemorrhage, which preclude muscle regeneration, healing occurs with fibrous interposition between the muscle ends.

DIAGNOSIS
Clinical Presentation

Signalment. Any age, breed, or sex of dog or cat may be affected; however, muscle contusion and strain are most commonly diagnosed in athletic dogs (e.g., racing greyhounds, field trial dogs). They are rarely diagnosed in cats.

History. Contusion and strain injuries frequently occur during strenuous activity. The animal may be brought to the examining room for evaluation of a noticeable limp or a complete inability to bear weight. The trauma frequently is unobserved by the client. In cases with mild strains, owners may relate that the animal became reluctant to move 12 to 24 hours after strenuous exercise.

Physical Examination Findings

Clinical signs depend upon the severity and chronicity of injury. With mild contusions the animal may exhibit minimal lameness and the source of pain may be difficult to find on examination. With more severe contusions, pain and swelling are present. The majority of severe contusions occur in conjunction with fractures and, although the focus is on the fractured bone, the injury to the muscle also should be evaluated during surgery. Severe muscle strains are recognized by swelling and pain of the affected muscle unit (Fig. 31-1). Chronic muscle strains occasionally are recognized in dogs (e.g., bicipital tenosynovitis).

Radiography

Standard craniocaudal and medial-to-lateral radiographs are necessary to rule out bone injury. Acute injuries may show soft-tissue swelling. Ultrasonography may show interstitial fluid accumulation.

FIG. 31-1
Muscle fibril disruption and interstitial hemorrhage. Blood accumulates between the disrupted fibers.

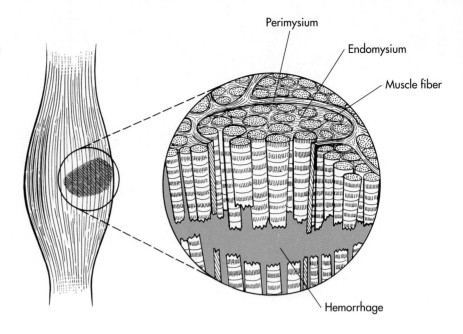

Perimysium
Endomysium
Muscle fiber
Hemorrhage

Laboratory Findings

Consistent laboratory abnormalities are not found.

DIFFERENTIAL DIAGNOSIS

Muscle contusions and strains must be differentiated from joint sprains, fractures, polymyopathies, and polyarthropathies. Physical examination often differentiates muscle injury from joint sprains. Gentle palpation of muscle contusions causes pain and identifies swelling, whereas the pain associated with sprains is elicited on manipulation of the involved joint. Arthrocentesis (see p. 885) helps differentiate joint sprain or arthropathy from muscle injury.

MEDICAL MANAGEMENT

The primary treatment for muscle contusions and strains is rest. Enforced rest with controlled activity is necessary for a minimum of 3 weeks. If the injury is recurrent or severe, longer periods of enforced rest may be necessary. If the muscle is not allowed to heal adequately, repeated injury is likely. With acute injuries, that is, those in the initial 24 hours, cold compresses can be applied to the affected muscle for 15 minutes, three or four times a day. If the injury is more than 24 hours old, topical heat application is recommended, but care should be taken to ensure that the patient is not burned. Nonsteroidal antiinflammatory drugs can be administered for the initial 3 to 4 days, but restricted activity must be continued even if lameness and pain disappear. When a severe contusion is recognized during surgical stabilization of a fracture, decompression of the muscle compartment can be achieved through incision of the epimysium (see p. 1001).

> ☞ **N O T E** • Warn owners that the animal may feel like exercising before it should be allowed to, particularly if it has been given nonsteroidal antiinflammatories.

SURGICAL TREATMENT

Surgical treatment is necessary only if interstitial fluid accumulation causes sufficient pressure to compromise blood flow.

Preoperative Management

Surgical intervention should be undertaken as soon as possible. The animal should be confined prior to surgery to prevent further damage to the muscle.

Anesthesia

Anesthetic considerations for animals with orthopedic disease are given on p. 708.

Surgical Anatomy

Skeletal muscle is made of long cylindrical fibers encased within connective tissue sheaths (Fig. 31-2). Each individual fiber is enclosed within a sheath called the endomysium. Each fiber bundle is also enclosed within a sheath (perimysium), as is the entire muscle (epimysium). The connective tissue sheaths house blood vessels and nerve fibers that serve to integrate muscle contraction of individual fibers. Muscles are attached to bone by cordlike tendons or flat aponeuroses. The fascial compartment overlying the muscle group appears tight and congested with contusions, and the underlying muscle appears severely bruised and often protrudes from the incision through the fascial compartment.

Positioning

The animal should be positioned so that the affected muscle group can be exposed. A generous area should be clipped and prepared for aseptic surgery to allow the incision to be extended beyond the boundaries of the affected muscle if necessary.

SURGICAL TECHNIQUE

Make an incision through the skin and subcutaneous tissues overlying the muscle to be exposed. Once the muscle

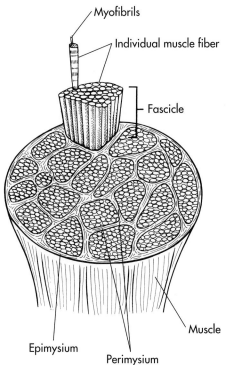

FIG. 31-2
Normal muscle anatomy. Note how the individual muscle fibrils combine to form muscle fibers. Groups of muscle fibers form fascicles, which are surrounded by the perimysium. Groups of fascicles form the muscle, which is covered by a thin fascial layer (epimysium).

group is identified, make an incision through the fascia to decompress the muscle compartment. Suture subcutaneous tissues and skin using standard methods.

SUTURE MATERIALS/SPECIAL INSTRUMENTS

Self-retaining retractors are useful for retracting soft tissues from the area of interest.

POSTOPERATIVE CARE AND ASSESSMENT

The wound should be monitored for swelling and/or drainage for 7 to 10 days after surgery. Suture removal can be performed when the skin incision has healed.

PROGNOSIS

Return to normal function should be expected with most contusions and muscle strains; however, repeat injury is likely if adequate rest is not provided.

Suggested Reading

Brinker WO, Piermattei DL, Flo GL: *Handbook of small animal orthopedics and fracture treatment,* ed 2, Philadelphia, 1990, WB Saunders.
Farrow CS: Sprain, strain and contusion, *Vet Clin North Am* 8:169, 1979.

Woo SL-Y, Buckwalter JA: Symposium on Injury and Repair of the Musculoskeletal Soft Tissues, Savannah, Ga, 1987, American Academy of Orthopaedic Surgeons.

MUSCLE-TENDON UNIT LACERATION

DEFINITIONS

Lacerations are tears within the muscle-tendon unit.

GENERAL CONSIDERATIONS AND CLINICALLY RELEVANT PATHOPHYSIOLOGY

Lacerations are usually the result of penetration of the muscle-tendon unit by a sharp object. These injuries most commonly involve the tendons near the carpometacarpal and tarsometatarsal joints, but they may involve muscle units in other parts of the body.

DIAGNOSIS
Clinical Presentation

Signalment. Any age, breed, or sex of dog or cat may be affected.

History. The animal usually has an open wound and a non–weight-bearing lameness.

Physical Examination Findings

After acute penetration of a muscle-tendon unit by a foreign object, the animal frequently has a non–weight-bearing lameness. The extent of internal damage can be assessed only through visual exploration of the wound. Once the patient has been stabilized, it should be anesthetized so that the wound can be explored. This usually needs to be done under a general anesthetic. Failure to explore the wound can result in lacerations being undiagnosed until the patient attempts to bear weight. The greater the time span from injury to repair, the more difficult the apposition of the severed tendon ends.

Radiography

Standard craniocaudal and medial-to-lateral radiographs should be taken to determine whether foreign bodies are present and whether there are concurrent fractures.

Laboratory Findings

Consistent laboratory abnormalities are not present.

DIFFERENTIAL DIAGNOSIS

Muscle-tendon lacerations must be differentiated from superficial lacerations and muscle strain (see p. 1000).

MEDICAL MANAGEMENT

Lacerations that involve a tendon should be managed with surgery; medical management is not indicated.

SURGICAL TREATMENT

Lacerations of the muscle require appositional sutures supported with deeper stent sutures. If the laceration has occurred through tendon, delicate manipulation and apposition with small-diameter suture are recommended.

Preoperative Management

The wound should be cleaned and a sterile bandage applied until definitive treatment is performed. Exercise should be restricted prior to surgery.

Anesthesia

Anesthetic management of animals with orthopedic disease is given on p. 708.

Surgical Anatomy

Tendons are longitudinally oriented bundles of collagen fibers that are surrounded by loose connective tissue sheaths. Blood vessels and nerves also reside within the tendon sheaths. The entire tendon is surrounded by the epitenon, which is enveloped by an outer connective tissue sheath called the paratenon. Tendons crossing joint surfaces are often encased in a tendon sheath to facilitate movement during joint motion.

> ☞ **N O T E** · The cut ends of the tendon (or muscle) are often retracted and will appear frayed. Tendon ends may retract within a tendon sheath and require longitudinal incision to identify the severed ends.

Positioning

The animal should be positioned so that the tendon and muscle can be fully exposed. A generous area should be clipped and prepared for aseptic surgery to allow the incision to be extended above and below the injury if necessary.

SURGICAL TECHNIQUE
Muscle Laceration

Thoroughly debride the wound edges to fresh, bleeding muscle tissue (Fig. 31-3). Debride carefully to avoid excess removal of tissue, which will make apposition of the severed ends difficult. Place interrupted sutures in the outer muscle sheath around the circumference of the muscle. Support the appositional sutures with heavy stent sutures placed in a cruciate pattern.

Tendon Laceration

Delicately manipulate and debride the tendon ends. With small, flat tendons, use small-diameter, nonabsorbable material placed in a series as interrupted vertical mattress or cruciate sutures. For larger tendons, select the largest suture diameter that will readily pass through the tendon atraumatically. A locking-loop suture pattern is recommended (Fig. 31-4). Place each loop of the pattern in a slightly different plane (i.e., a near-far, middle-middle, and far-near pattern). Alternatively, use a three-loop pulley, Bunnell-

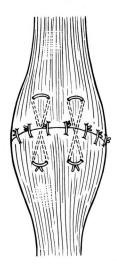

FIG. 31-3
Repair of muscle laceration with appositional sutures supported by tension stent sutures.

Mayer, or far-near, near-far suture pattern. Using adjoining fascia to support the tendon appositional sutures.

SUTURE MATERIALS/SPECIAL INSTRUMENTS

Nonabsorbable or absorbable suture material may be used to repair muscle, provided the material maintains its mechanical strength for 3 to 4 weeks. Nonabsorbable suture material is recommended for tendon repair. Swaged-on needles are helpful in limiting tissue trauma during suturing. Self-retaining retractors are useful for holding surrounding tissues away from the working area.

HEALING OF TENDONS AND MUSCLES

Healing of tendons follows a pattern similar to that for other connective tissues. The inflammatory phase is characterized initially by presence of neutrophils and later by presence of mononuclear cells. The tendon injury is rarely isolated but exists in a zone with other wounded tissue. Unsuccessful attempts to isolate tendon healing from surrounding tissue has lead to the concept of one wound, one scar. This implies that successful healing is dependent upon activation of undifferentiated mesenchymal cells, which migrate into the wound. Mesenchymal cells produce the collagen and matrix that lend strength to the entire wound. The resultant scar unites the tendon ends, which remodel with collagen fibers oriented parallel to lines of stress. Strength is regained through the one-wound, one-scar principle, but function is regained through active and passive use of the limb postoperatively.

POSTOPERATIVE CARE AND ASSESSMENT

After tendon repair, the limb should be immobilized for 3 weeks by use of rigid external coaptation (see p. 733). When the splint is removed the limb should be semirigidly immobilized for an additional 3 weeks with a heavy padded bandage. Activity should be limited to leash walks. Physical

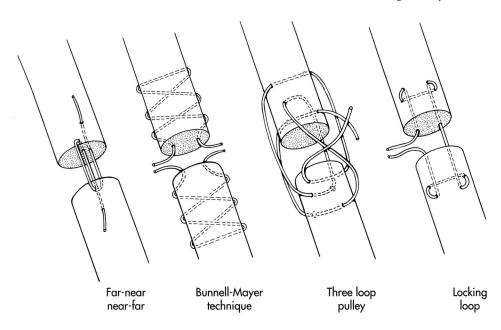

FIG. 31-4
Suture patterns used to appose tendon ends.

Far-near near-far   Bunnell-Mayer technique   Three loop pulley   Locking loop

therapy (passive flexion and extension of the limb) should be done for an additional 4 weeks once the bandage has been removed. Then the animal should be gradually returned to normal activity. Premature weight bearing will result in failure of the tendon to heal.

PROGNOSIS

Return to normal function is expected if postoperative recommendations are followed. Failure generally is associated with the animal's being allowed to exercise prior to complete tendon healing.

Suggested Reading

Aron DN, Robello GT: Use of sutures in repairing ligaments and tendons, *Vet Med Report* 3:88, 1991.

Berg RJ, Egger EL: In vitro comparison of the three loop pulley and locking loop suture patterns for repair of canine weightbearing tendons and collateral ligaments, *Vet Surg* 15:107, 1986.

Brinker WO, Piermattei DL, Flo GL: *Handbook of small animal orthopedics and fracture treatment*, ed 2, Philadelphia, 1990, WB Saunders.

Egger EL, Berg RJ: Comparison of the locking loop and three loop pulley suture patterns for anastomosis of canine tendon and ligament, *Vet Surg* 14:53, 1985.

Morshead D, Leeds EB: Kirschner-Ehmer apparatus immobilization following Achilles tendon repair in six dogs, *Vet Surg* 13:11, 1984.

Tomlinson J, Moore R: Locking loop tendon suture use in repair of five calcanean tendons, *Vet Surg* 11:105, 1982.

Van Bree H: Avulsion of the insertion of the gastrocnemius tendon in three dogs, *J Sm Anim Pract* 27:759, 1986.

Vanghan LC: Tendon injury in the dog, *Vet Ann* 27:324, 1987.

Woo SL-Y, Buckwalter JA: Symposium on Injury and Repair of the Musculoskeletal Soft Tissues, Savannah, Ga, 1987, American Academy of Orthopaedic Surgeons.

MUSCLE-TENDON UNIT RUPTURE

DEFINITIONS

Rupture of the muscle-tendon unit is a complete or partial loss of integrity of the muscle-tendon unit caused by extreme overstretching.

SYNONYMS

Torn muscle

GENERAL CONSIDERATIONS AND CLINICALLY RELEVANT PATHOPHYSIOLOGY

Muscle ruptures are the result of a powerful contraction occurring during forced hyperextension of the muscle-tendon unit. This type of injury is seen most often in sporting breeds of dogs and performance athletes (such as racing greyhounds). The injury most commonly encountered is partial or complete rupture of the Achilles tendon. Injury of the Achilles mechanism may arise from an acute traumatic episode or from chronic progressive stretching of the tendon. Acute injuries are often secondary to a fall or a penetrating wound. Conversely, chronic injuries are often secondary to overuse that causes chronic stretching and deterioration of the tendon. Chronic injuries more commonly occur in sporting breeds (e.g., field trial dogs, bird hunting dogs) and are often bilateral.

DIAGNOSIS
Clinical Presentation

    Signalment. Any age, breed, or sex of dog or cat may be affected. Athletic dogs are most commonly affected.

    History. Affected animals usually exhibit a weight-bearing lameness after strenuous activity.

Physical Examination Findings

Tarsal hyperflexion is frequently noted in affected animals. If the injury is secondary to an acute traumatic episode, the animal will be unable to bear weight, and flaccidity of the Achilles tendon will be noted upon passive dorsal flexion of the tarsus when the stifle is extended. If the injury is secondary to a chronic stretching of the Achilles tendon, the patient will be weight bearing but will walk plantigrade because of hyperflexion of the tarsus. Patients with chronic Achilles tendon injuries show varying degrees of tarsal hyperflexion, depending on the length of time the injury has been present. If the entire tendon complex is involved, the tarsus and digits hyperflex; if the tendon of the superficial flexor muscle is not involved, the tarsus will hyperflex and the digits will flex. Postural changes associated with a palpable swelling of the Achilles tendon confirm the diagnosis. Occasionally the injury occurs at the myotendinous juncture. Postural changes and careful palpation of the muscle-tendon unit confirm the diagnosis.

Radiography

Ultrasonography is helpful in determining the extent of tendon fiber disruption. Standard craniocaudal and medial-to-lateral radiographs are indicated to determine the presence or absence of bone avulsion from the tuber calcaneus.

Laboratory Findings

Consistent laboratory abnormalities are not found.

DIFFERENTIAL DIAGNOSIS

Sciatic nerve injury and congenital tarsal hyperflexion must be differentiated from tendon rupture. Gentle palpation of the muscle-tendon unit will reveal loss of continuity and/or an area of swelling with tendon rupture, whereas patients with congenital tarsal hyperflexion lack these findings. When nerve injury is present, neurological examination will show sciatic reflexes to be absent or decreased.

MEDICAL MANAGEMENT

Surgical repair of completely ruptured tendons should be performed; medical management is not indicated. With partial ruptures, external coaptation may be tried, but the results are usually unsatisfactory.

SURGICAL TREATMENT
Preoperative Management

Activity should be limited until definitive treatment is begun. If an open wound is present (i.e., laceration of the Achilles tendon), it should be cleaned and covered with a sterile dressing.

Anesthesia

Anesthetic management of animals with orthopedic disease is discussed on p. 708.

Surgical Anatomy

The Achilles tendon unit is composed of tendons arising from the gastrocnemius and superficial digital flexor muscles, and a common tendon from the semitendinosus muscle, gracilis muscle, and biceps femoris muscles. The common tendon of the gastrocnemius muscle is the major component of the Achilles tendon. With acute injuries it is possible to identify each component of the Achilles complex and suture each individually. However, with chronic injuries the tendon ends retract, leaving a void to be filled with fibrous tissue. Identification of each component is not possible. The complex (fibrous scar and Achilles tendon) is treated as a single structure.

Positioning

Position the patient in lateral recumbency. A hanging-leg preparation will facilitate manipulation of the limb during surgery. For Achilles tendon injuries, clip and prepare the limb for surgery from proximal to the stifle joint to the phalanges distally.

SURGICAL TECHNIQUE
Achilles Tendon Rupture

Make an incision over the site of injury on the caudolateral surface of the limb. If the injury is acute, identify the three tendons composing the Achilles complex and suture each tendon separately with an interrupted far-near, near-far pattern (see Fig. 31-4) using nonabsorbable, small-diameter (3-0 to 4-0, depending the animal's size) monofilament suture. If the injury is chronic, identification of individual tendon units is not possible; continue surgical dissection to expose the circumference of the thickened fibrous band. Then, sequentially remove sections of scar tissue from the center of the mass. Remove enough tissue so that tension is present in the Achilles complex when the stifle joint is in a normal standing position and the tarsus is slightly extended. Be careful to not remove too much of the proliferative fibrous tissue. If excess fibrous tissue is excised, apposition of the cut ends will be difficult. Suture the cut ends with a three-loop pulley pattern (see Fig. 31-4) or maintain apposition with tendon plating. For tendon plating, appose the cut ends of the tendon with nonabsorbable monofilament suture. Use 3-0 suture for small dogs and cats, 2-0 for medium-sized dogs, and 0 for large dogs. Support the anastomosis by placing a small bone plate adjacent to the tendon (Fig. 31-5). Place interrupted sutures through the plate holes into the body of the tendon. Use large-diameter, nonabsorbable monofilament suture.

Whether the injury is acute or chronic, support of the tendon anastomosis is critical for a favorable outcome. Support is provided by immobilization of the tarsal joint in slight extension. *Place a raised, threaded transfixation pin threaded through the free end of the calcaneus into the distal tibia. Cut through the pin shaft to leave the pin just below the skin surface. Provide additional support with a fiberglass cast.*

SUTURE MATERIALS/SPECIAL INSTRUMENTS

Nonabsorbable suture material is recommended for tendon repair. Swaged-on needles are helpful in limiting tissue trauma during suturing. Self-retaining retractors are useful

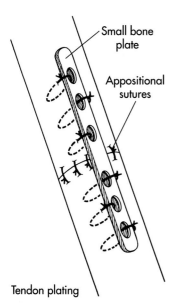

Small bone plate

Appositional sutures

Tendon plating

FIG. 31-5
Tendon anastomosis supported with a small bone plate. The plate serves to neutralize forces acting on the anastomosis.

for holding surrounding tissues away from the working area. An air-driven or battery-operated drill is useful if a bone screw or transfixation pin is to be inserted.

POSTOPERATIVE CARE AND ASSESSMENT

The cast and transfixation pin are left in place for 3 weeks, after which both may be removed. The limb should then be supported in a padded bandage to prevent full dorsal flexion of the tarsus. Activity should be limited to leash walking for 10 weeks. If tendon plating is performed, the plate should be removed 8 to 10 weeks after surgery.

PROGNOSIS

Prognosis for return to strenuous athletic activity is unlikely. However, most patients are able to resume normal pet activity.

Suggested Reading

Aron DN, Robello GT: Use of sutures in repairing ligaments and tendons, *Vet Med Report* 3:88, 1991.

Berg RJ, Egger EL: In vitro comparison of the three loop pulley and locking loop suture patterns for repair of canine weightbearing tendons and collateral ligaments, *Vet Surg* 15:107, 1986.

Egger EL, Berg RJ: Comparison of the locking loop and three loop pulley suture patterns for anastomosis of canine tendon and ligament, *Vet Surg* 14:53, 1985.

Lin GT et al: Biomechanical studies of running suture for flexor tendon repair in dogs, *J Hand Surg* 13:553, 1988.

Morshead D, Leeds EB: Kirschner-Ehmer apparatus immobilization following Achilles tendon repair in six dogs, *Vet Surg* 13:11, 1984.

Tomlinson J, Moore R: Locking loop tendon suture use in repair of five calcanean tendons, *Vet Surg* 11:105, 1982.

Van Bree H: Avulsion of the insertion of the gastrocnemius tendon in three dogs, *J Sm Anim Pract* 27:759, 1986.

Vanghan LC: Tendon injury in the dog, *Vet Ann* 27:324, 1987.

MUSCLE CONTRACTURE AND FIBROSIS

DEFINITIONS

Muscle contracture may occur when there is replacement of normal muscle-tendon unit architecture with fibrous tissue resulting in functional shortening of the muscle or tendon. This shortening may cause abnormal motion in adjacent joints.

GENERAL CONSIDERATIONS AND CLINICALLY RELEVANT PATHOPHYSIOLOGY

Muscle contracture is most commonly recognized in the infraspinatus and quadriceps muscle-tendon units. Quadriceps muscle contracture occurs most commonly following distal femoral fractures in young dogs; however, congenital contracture of the quadriceps muscle has been reported. Inadequate fracture stabilization, excessive tissue trauma during surgery, or prolonged limb immobilization with the stifle in extension may singly, or in combination, contribute to quadriceps contracture. Joint stiffness develops as a result of fibrous adhesions between the quadriceps and fracture callus. With time, adhesions form between the joint capsule and distal femur, limiting limb use and causing the quadriceps muscle to atrophy. The etiology of congenital quadriceps contracture and why contracture occurs most commonly in young dogs is unknown.

Infraspinatus muscle contracture occurs most frequently in hunting dogs after irreversible muscle fiber injury. The cause is unknown, but it appears to be a primary muscle disorder rather than secondary to neurologic or immune-mediated causes. Histological findings—degeneration, atrophy, and fibroplasia within damaged areas of the muscle—are compatible with severe strain.

DIAGNOSIS
Clinical Presentation

Signalment. Any age, breed, or sex of dog may develop quadriceps muscle contracture; however, it most commonly occurs in immature patients following distal femoral fracture. Contracture of the infraspinatus muscle usually occurs in young, adult, sporting breeds of dogs. Cats rarely develop quadriceps contracture, and infraspinatus muscle contracture has not been reported in this species.

History. Animals with quadriceps muscle contracture usually are seen for evaluation of lameness 3 to 5 weeks after having sustained femoral trauma. Frequently, internal reduction and stabilization of a distal femoral fracture or application of an external splint for stabilization of a femoral fracture has been performed. Usually there is a history of acute lameness following strenuous activity in the 3 weeks prior to evaluation for infraspinatus muscle contracture (see p. 1006).

Physical Examination Findings

The stifle joint of animals with quadriceps muscle contracture has a limited range of motion (Fig. 31-6). Initially the joint can be fully extended but can be flexed only 20 to 30 degrees. Gradually the amount of flexion decreases to less than 10 degrees. Contracture may be such that the stifle joint appears hyperextended. Cranial thigh muscles are generally atrophied and palpate as a thickened cord.

Animals with infraspinatus muscle contracture initially have a weight-bearing forelimb lameness (Fig. 31-7). Soft tissue swelling in the region of the shoulder joint may be noted. The lameness usually resolves and is absent for 3 to 4 weeks, but then mild lameness and a gait abnormality develop. The characteristic gait abnormality is secondary to progressive fibrosis and contracture of the infraspinatus muscle. As the muscle shortens from contracture, external rotation of the shoulder occurs, causing elbow abduction and outward rotation of the paw.

Radiography

Standard radiographs do not show abnormalities of the muscle-tendon unit but will help differentiate fracture or neoplasia as the cause of lameness.

Laboratory Findings

Consistent laboratory abnormalities are not present.

DIFFERENTIAL DIAGNOSIS

The diagnosis of quadriceps or infraspinatus muscle contracture usually can be made from historical and physical examination findings.

MEDICAL MANAGEMENT

Medical or conservative (nonsurgical) management is not effective with either condition.

SURGICAL TREATMENT

Treatment of quadriceps contracture is aimed at restoring limb function. Release of fibrous thickening and adhesions between the joint capsule and femur and between the quadriceps muscle and femur is necessary. If a functional range of motion is not achieved following adhesion release, lengthening of the quadriceps muscle-tendon unit is required. Lengthening may be accomplished by a Z-plasty, or release of the origin of each muscle. Recurrence of the contracture, with resultant loss of stifle joint motion, occurs if preventive rehabilitation measures are not taken after surgery. An effective method by which to maintain a functional range of motion in the stifle is to apply a transarticular fixator postoperatively, which maintains passive flexion of the stifle joint but allows active or passive extension (see p. 1007). Alternatively, if sufficient flexion is obtained at surgery, a 90/90 bandage can be used (see p. 717). For infraspinatus contracture, treatment is directed at releasing the fibrotic, myotendinous infraspinatus muscle as it crosses the shoulder joint.

Preoperative Management

These animals otherwise are generally healthy, and minimal preoperative care is necessary.

Anesthesia

See p. 708 for anesthetic management of animals with orthopedic disease.

Surgical Anatomy

The quadriceps muscle-tendon unit is composed of the vastus medialis, vastus intermedius, rectus femoris, and vastus lateralis muscles. These muscles all atrophy in patients with quadriceps muscle contracture. Proximally, the

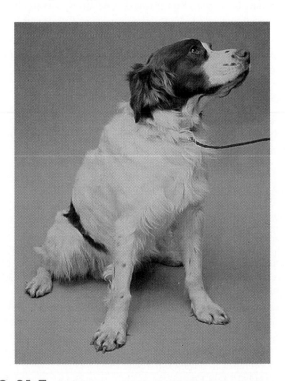

FIG. 31-7
Dog with infraspinatus muscle contracture. Note external rotation of the shoulder and internal displacement of the elbow.

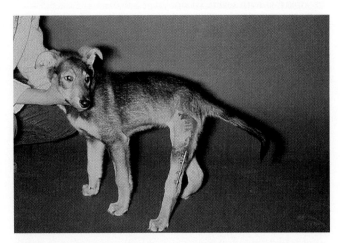

FIG. 31-6
Dog with quadriceps muscle contracture. Note hyperextension of the femur.

rectus femoris muscle palpates as a thickened cord. At surgery all four muscles of the quadriceps appear small and pale in color. In patients with distal femoral fractures, the atrophied muscles lie superficial to, and are intertwined with, proliferative fibrous tissue. Normal range of motion in the stifle joint is from 180 degrees (full extension) to 30 degrees (full flexion).

The infraspinatus muscle-tendon unit is a cuff muscle of the shoulder joint. The muscle lies next to the scapula, just caudal to the spine. The tendon crosses the joint craniolaterally to insert onto the lateral tuberosity of the proximal humerus. At surgery the tendon appears thickened and, because of fibrinous tissue invasion, has an off-white color rather than the white, glistening appearance typical of normal tendons. The muscle is atrophied and appears pale relative to normal, healthy muscle.

Positioning

For quadriceps contracture, clip the limb from the dorsal midline to the tarsus and position the patient in lateral recumbency. A hanging-leg preparation facilitates manipulation of the limb during surgery. For infraspinatus muscle contracture, clip the shoulder from the dorsal midline to the elbow and position the patient in lateral recumbency.

SURGICAL TECHNIQUE
Quadriceps Contracture

Expose the stifle joint and distal femur through a liberal craniolateral incision (see p. 961). Elevate and release adhesions between the quadriceps muscle group and femur with sharp dissection. Release adhesions between the fibrous joint capsule and femoral condyles. Luxate the patella medially and flex the joint to its full extent. If a functional range of motion (greater than 40 degrees) is not achieved after releasing the adhesions, perform a quadriceps muscle-tendon-unit lengthening procedure.

Z-plasty. *Make a longitudinal incision through the center of the muscle-tendon unit beginning 8 to 10 cm proximal to the patella. Extend the incision distally to a point 3 cm proximal to the patella. At the proximal extent of the longitudinal incision, make a transverse incision laterally through the muscle and fibrous tissue. At the distal extent of the longitudinal incision, make a transverse incision medially through the muscle and fibrous tissue. Flex the stifle and allow the cut edges of the longitudinal incision to slide on each other. When a functional range of flexion is achieved, place interrupted sutures across the longitudinal incision to maintain the desired length of the quadriceps muscle-tendon unit.*

Muscle release. *Extend the lateral incision to expose the proximal femur. At the level of the third trochanter, elevate the quadriceps from the medial, lateral, and caudal surfaces of the femur. Incise through the origins of each muscle group to release the quadriceps and allow distal sliding of the muscle group. Release the vastus intermedius near its point of origin on the ilium. Close the surgical wound using standard methods.*

Transarticular fixator. *Insert a half pin just below the third trochanter of the femur using an end-threaded transfixation pin and insert a full pin through the tibia 4 cm above the tarsus using a centrally threaded transfixation pin. Maximally flex the stifle joint and maintain this position with a heavy rubber band connecting the proximal and distal transfixation pins. Fashion a bandage and connect it to the distal transfixation pin to maintain a functional angle of the tarsus.*

Infraspinatus Muscle Contracture

Perform a craniolateral approach to the shoulder joint (see p. 905). Isolate the circumference of the infraspinatus muscle with sharp dissection. Transect the fibrotic muscle and any fibrous bands restricting movement of the joint. Once the fibrous contracture is incised, the limb will assume a normal position and a normal range of motion of the shoulder will be possible.

SUTURE MATERIALS/SPECIAL INSTRUMENTS

Self-retaining retractors and a periosteal elevator assist tissue retraction and reflection. Instruments for placement of pins are necessary if a transarticular fixator is placed postoperatively.

POSTOPERATIVE CARE AND ASSESSMENT

After application of a transarticular fixator for quadriceps muscle contracture the pin-to-skin interfaces must be cleaned daily (see p. 742). Passive flexion and extension of the stifle joint and tarsus should be begun as soon as the patient will allow limb manipulation. Joint movement should be repeated 20 to 30 times, at least 3 times daily; increased frequency of manipulation will improve rehabilitation. The external fixator should be maintained for 3 to 5 weeks. After it is removed, physical therapy should be continued for an additional 5 weeks. If a 90/90 bandage (see p. 717) is applied, it should be maintained for 3 weeks. After bandage removal, passive flexion and extension of the joint should be performed as described above. Special postoperative care is not required after surgery for infraspinatus muscle contracture. These animals usually will begin to use the limb within a few days after surgery.

PROGNOSIS

The prognosis after surgery for quadriceps muscle contracture depends on the degree of degenerative joint changes present and on whether a functional range of motion is obtained at surgery. The prognosis is fair for functional limb use, but contracture may recur following surgery. A normal range of motion is seldom achieved, and most animals are able to flex the stifle only 45 to 90 degrees. The prognosis for infraspinatus muscle contracture is excellent and return to preinjury function is expected after surgery.

Suggested Reading

Anderson SM, Lippincott CL, Schulman AJ: Longitudinal myotomy of the flexor carpi radialis: a new approach to the medial aspect of the elbow joint, *J Am Anim Hosp Assoc* 2 5:499, 1989.

Bardet JF: Quadriceps contracture and fracture disease, *Vet Clin North Am Small Anim Pract* 17:957, 1987.

Bardet JF, Hohn RB: Quadriceps contracture in dogs, *J Am Vet Med Assoc* 183:680, 1983.

Benett RA: Contracture of the infraspinatus muscle in dogs: a review of 12 cases, *J Am Anim Hosp Assoc* 22:481, 1986.

Lin GT et al: Biomechanical studies of running suture for flexor tendon repair in dogs, *J Hand Surg* 13:553, 1988.

CHAPTER 32

Other Diseases of Bones and Joints

HYPERTROPHIC OSTEOPATHY

DEFINITIONS

Hypertrophic osteopathy is a diffuse periosteal reaction resulting in new bone formation around the metacarpal, metatarsal, and long bones.

SYNONYMS

Pulmonary osteoarthropathy, hypertrophic pulmonary osteoarthropathy, hypertrophic pulmonary osteopathy

GENERAL CONSIDERATIONS AND CLINICALLY RELEVANT PATHOPHYSIOLOGY

Hypertrophic osteopathy is a condition affecting all four limbs. It appears to be a paraneoplastic syndrome associated with other primary disease processes (e.g., neoplasia, including primary lung tumors, metastatic lung tumors, esophageal carcinoma, and rhabdomyosarcoma of the bladder; granulomatous lesions; bacterial endocarditis; and heartworm disease). The precise pathophysiology of this disease is unknown. It has been suggested that alterations in pulmonary function lead to increased peripheral blood flow, resulting in connective tissue congestion. The increased peripheral blood flow is considered to be neurally mediated. The periosteum responds by forming new bone on the cortical surfaces of the metacarpal, metatarsal, and long bones. This new bone may appear nodular. Histologically, it is made of bands of new cortical bone that contain small, fibrous marrow spaces.

DIAGNOSIS
Clinical Presentation

Signalment. Any breed or size of dog may be affected; however, because it is most commonly associated with neoplasia, hypertrophic osteopathy is usually seen in older animals. This condition has been reported in a cat.

History. Dogs usually present because of lethargy, reluctance to move, and swelling of the distal extremities. The onset of clinical signs may be acute or gradual.

Physical Examination Findings

Affected limbs are warm and swollen. Because this condition is secondary to a primary disease process located elsewhere in the body, an effort should be made to determine the underlying etiology. Thorough physical examination is an essential component of the evaluation of affected animals.

Radiography

Radiographs of the limbs reveal irregular periosteal new bone formation, which is initially seen on phalanges, metacarpal, and metatarsal bones (Fig. 32-1). As the disease

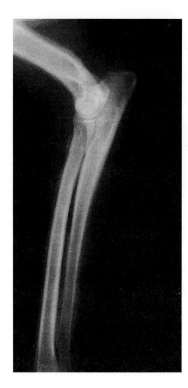

FIG. 32-1
Radiograph of a forelimb of a dog with hypertrophic osteopathy. Note periosteal new bone along the radius, ulna, and humerus.

progresses, periosteal new bone occurs on more proximal bones (i.e., radius/ulna and tibia/fibula). Articular surfaces of long bones appear normal.

Thoracic radiographs should be taken to determine if underlying pulmonary or mediastinal neoplasia or infection is present (e.g., primary or metastatic neoplasia, granulomatous lesions, bacterial endocarditis, or heartworm disease). Radiographic and ultrasonographic evaluation of the abdomen should also be done to identify underlying abdominal disease.

Laboratory Findings

Results of laboratory analysis usually reflect the underlying disease. Thrombocytosis may occur in some dogs; however, the etiology is only poorly understood.

MEDICAL MANAGEMENT

Treatment is aimed at the underlying disease process. Remission of the exostosis may occur after resection of the primary lesion.

PROGNOSIS

The prognosis depends on the possibility for complete resolution of the underlying disease process. If the primary disease can be resolved, the secondary hypertrophic osteopathy often resolves. Although clinical signs often disappear within 1 to 2 weeks after treatment, bone lesions may take months to remodel.

Suggested Reading

Brodey RS. Hypertrophic osteoarthropathy in the dog: a clinicopathologic survey of 60 cases, *J Am Vet Med Assoc* 159:1242, 1971.

Manley PA, Romich JA. Miscellaneous orthopedic diseases. In Slatter D, editor: *textbook of small animal surgery,* Philadelphia, 1993, WB Saunders.

PANOSTEITIS

DEFINITIONS

Panosteitis is a disease of young dogs causing lameness, bone pain, endosteal bone production, and occasionally subperiosteal bone production.

SYNONYMS

Enostosis, eosinophilic panosteitis, juvenile osteomyelitis, osteomyelitis of young German shepherd dogs

GENERAL CONSIDERATIONS AND CLINICALLY RELEVANT PATHOPHYSIOLOGY

Panosteitis is a disease of unknown etiology associated with endosteal and periosteal new bone formation. Although some periosteal new bone is often evident, the predominant change is endosteal bone formation as the marrow is invaded

by bone trabeculae. The marrow remains highly cellular with varying degrees of fibrosis and there is no evidence of chronic inflammation, acute infection, or malignancy.

DIAGNOSIS
Clinical Presentation

Signalment. Panosteitis predominantly affects male (80%), large-breed dogs. Young dogs (less than 2 years of age) are most commonly affected; however, older dogs have occasionally been diagnosed with clinical signs of this disease.

History. The hallmarks of panosteitis are shifting leg lameness associated with pain on deep bone palpation. Although initial episodes of panosteitis may present as acute lameness in a single limb, typically there is a history of chronic, intermittent, shifting leg lameness.

☞ **N O T E** · *Owners often believe these dogs have hip dysplasia or OCD.*

Physical Examination

Affected dogs are commonly lame in only a single limb. Firm palpation of affected long bones usually elicits a pain response.

Radiography

Radiographic signs of panosteitis are progressive. During early stages of the disease radiographs of affected limbs are often normal. Clinical signs may precede radiographic abnormalities by as many as 10 days. If clinical signs are consistent with panosteitis, but radiographs are normal, radiographs should be repeated in 7 to 10 days. Nuclear scintigraphy is a better indicator of early bone changes than radiographs. The earliest radiographic signs are a widening of the nutrient foramen and blurring and accentuation of trabecular patterns, followed by appearance of radiodense, patchy, or mottled bone within medullary canals (Fig. 32-2). Eventually, remodeling of medullary canals occurs and cortical thickening remains as the only residual finding.

Laboratory Findings

Consistent laboratory abnormalities are not present.

DIFFERENTIAL DIAGNOSIS

Panosteitis must be differentiated from other orthopedic diseases of large, immature dogs (i.e., osteochondritis dissecans, fragmented coronoid process, and ununited anconeal process in forelimbs; hip dysplasia and osteochondritis of rear limbs). Where radiographic evidence of panosteitis and other orthopedic diseases is present concurrently, panosteitis is usually assumed to be the cause of acute clinical signs.

☞ **N O T E** · *Panosteitis has the best prognosis of all "growing dog diseases."*

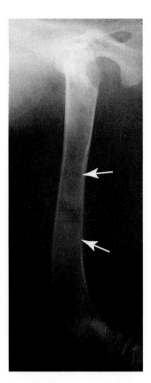

FIG. 32-2
Lateral radiograph of the femur of an immature dog with panosteitis. Note the areas of increased density within the medullary canal (*arrows*).

MEDICAL TREATMENT

The disease is self-limiting so treatment should be to control pain. Nonsteroidal, antiinflammatory drugs (i.e., aspirin or Ascriptin; Table 32-1) are usually administered during acute episodes of lameness. They are the drugs of choice because of their effectiveness, low price, availability, and minimal side effects. Gastric mucosal sensitivity to aspirin may cause vomiting, diarrhea, and/or melena. If these signs are noted, aspirin use should be discontinued to prevent gastric ulceration. Ascriptin (a combination of aspirin and Maalox) or buffered aspirin should be given after feeding to decrease the potential for adverse side effects or carprofen may be used (see Table 30-5).

SURGICAL TREATMENT

Surgical treatment of panosteitis is not indicated.

PROGNOSIS

The disease is self-limiting and most animals eventually have normal function of affected limbs without evidence of pain. However, the disease may continue to affect different limbs causing pain and lameness until the dog reaches maturity. Clinical signs rarely persist after maturity.

☞ **NOTE** • Advise owners that panosteitis will probably recur but it usually resolves by the time the dog is 2 years of age.

TABLE 32-1
Antiinflammatory Drugs for Treatment of Panosteitis

Aspirin*
25 mg/kg (1 regular strength aspirin per 25 lbs of body weight; not to exceed 3 tablets PO, BID or TID)

Ascriptin*
25 mg/kg PO, BID or TID

Phenylbutazone (Butazolidin)
1–5 mg/kg PO, BID or TID; dosage should not exceed 800 mg/day
*Give with food

Suggested Reading

Bohning RH et al: Clinical and radiographic survey of canine panosteitis, *J Am Vet Med Assoc* 156:870, 1970.

Stead AC, Stead MC, Galloway F: Panosteitis in dogs, *J Small Anim Pract* 24:623, 1983.

Turnier JC, Silverman S: A case study of canine panosteitis: comparison of radiographic and radioisotopic studies, *Am J Vet Res* 39:1550, 1978.

CRANIOMANDIBULAR OSTEOPATHY

DEFINITIONS

Craniomandibular osteopathy is a proliferative bone disease of immature dogs involving the occipital bones, tympanic bullae, and mandibular rami.

SYNONYMS

Mandibular periostitis, lion's jaw

GENERAL CONSIDERATIONS AND CLINICALLY RELEVANT PATHOPHYSIOLOGY

The etiology of craniomandibular osteopathy is unknown. It is most frequently recognized in West Highland white terriers, cairn terriers, and Scottish terriers—there is speculation that these breeds are genetically predisposed to this condition. An autosomal recessive inheritance pattern was suggested by a study of affected West Highland white terriers (Padgett, Mostosky, 1986).

Proliferation of new, coarse, trabecular bone occurs adjacent to the mandibular rami, occipital bones, and tympanic bullae in affected animals. This new bone formation results in irregular enlargement of the mandibles and tympanic bullae. Existing lamellar bone is resorbed by osteoclasis and replaced with new bone that expands beyond the periosteal borders. Osteoclastic destruction of the original lamellar bone is accompanied by invasion of inflammatory cells (i.e., neutrophils, lymphocytes, and plasma cells). Normal bone marrow is lost as it is replaced with a vascular fibrous stroma. This proliferative stage of the disease occurs when the dog is approximately 5 to 7 months old and is accompanied by intermittent fever, discomfort when eating, and pain when the mouth is forced open. Owners should be warned that multiple relapses may occur; however, bone proliferation decreases as dogs reach maturity and physes close.

DIAGNOSIS
Clinical Presentation

Signalment. Although young West Highland white terriers, cairn terriers, or Scottish terriers are most commonly affected, this disease has been sporadically reported in other breeds. Clinical signs are usually first noted when the dog is 5 to 7 months of age.

History. Owners often note that the animal is reluctant to eat and has trouble chewing food. Pain is often evident when the mouth is opened. Occasionally, swelling of the mandibular rami is present.

Physical Examination Findings

Affected dogs present with bilaterally enlarged mandibles and tympanic bullae. In severe cases, fusion of these structures may occur preventing the jaws from being fully opened. Pain on opening of the mouth and intermittent fever (104° F for 3 to 4 days) may also be observed.

Radiography

Skull radiographs reveal increased irregular bone density of the caudal mandibles and tympanic bullae. As dogs reach maturity, edges of the new bone become smooth and affected areas shrink.

Laboratory Findings

Specific laboratory abnormalities are not seen. Blood cultures are negative.

DIFFERENTIAL DIAGNOSIS

Craniomandibular osteopathy must be differentiated from infectious processes (i.e., abscesses or osteomyelitis) that may cause similar signs.

MEDICAL MANAGEMENT

Analgesics (Table 32-2) should be given to control pain until the animal reaches maturity. Severely debilitated animals that cannot open their mouths enough to eat solid foods require oral fluid nourishment. Although antibiotics and corticosteroids are often administered during febrile episodes, they will not alter disease progression.

SURGICAL TREATMENT

Surgical therapy is not indicated. Surgical resection of bone bridging the mandible and tympanic bullae in dogs with severely restricted jaw motion has been unsuccessful. Affected dogs should not be used for breeding purposes.

PROGNOSIS

The prognosis is guarded until the extent of bone production is known (i.e., at maturity). Excessive bone production, lead-

TABLE 32-2

Analgesics

Buffered acetylsalicylic acid* (aspirin) or Aspirin Maalox† (Ascriptin)

25 mg/kg PO‡, BID–TID

*Analgesic, antiinflammatory
†Protects mucosa
‡Give with food

---

ing to mandibular and tympanic bullae fusion, can restrict mandibular motion sufficiently to prevent dogs from eating. These animals are often euthanized.

☞ **N O T E ·** Warn owners that multiple relapses may occur until maturity.

Reference

Padgett GA, Mostosky UV: The mode of inheritance of craniomandibular osteopathy in West Highland white terrier dogs, *Am J Med Genet* 25:9, 1986.

Suggested Reading

Riser WH: Canine craniomandibular osteopathy. In Bojrab MJ, ed: *Disease mechanisms in small animal surgery,* ed 2, Philadelphia, 1993, Lea & Febiger.

HYPERTROPHIC OSTEODYSTROPHY

DEFINITIONS

Hypertrophic osteodystrophy is a disease that causes disruption of metaphyseal trabeculae in long bones of young, rapidly growing dogs.

SYNONYMS

Skeletal scurvy, canine scurvy, Moeller-Barlow disease, osteodystrophy Types I and II, hypovitaminosis C, metaphyseal osteopathy, metaphyseal dysplasia

GENERAL CONSIDERATIONS AND CLINICALLY RELEVANT PATHOPHYSIOLOGY

The etiology of hypertrophic osteodystrophy (HOD) is unknown. Proposed etiologies include vitamin C deficiency, oversupplementation of dietary calcium, and infectious organisms. The pathogenesis is obscure, but an apparent disturbance of metaphyseal blood supply leads to changes in the physis and adjacent metaphyseal bone, resulting in delayed ossification of the physeal hypertrophic zone. The acute phase of this disease lasts about 7 to 10 days. Affected animals show signs ranging from mild lameness to anorexia, pyrexia, lethargy, severe lameness, refusal to rise, and generalized weight loss. Clinical signs may wax and wane.

☞ **N O T E** · These animals may be very ill and require intense supportive care.

Grossly, the metaphyseal regions of long bones are widened with perimetaphyseal soft tissue swelling. A line of separation of metaphyseal trabeculae is present parallel to the growth plate. Histologically, microfractures of the trabeculae are evident and are surrounded by inflammatory cells and necrosis. Failure of bone deposition on the calcified cartilage lattice of metaphyseal bone is evident.

DIAGNOSIS

Clinical Presentation

Signalment. This disease affects young, rapidly growing, large-breed dogs. Clinical signs are usually first noted at 3 to 4 months of age; however, they may occur as early as 2 months. Relapses may occur as late as 8 months of age.

History. An acute onset of lameness is often reported and puppies may be so severely affected that they refuse to walk. Inappetence and lethargy are commonly reported by owners. A history of recent diarrhea may precede the onset of lameness.

Physical Examination Findings

Findings on physical examination range from mild lameness to severe lameness affecting all four limbs. More severely affected animals are often unable to stand or walk. Long bone metaphyses are swollen, warm, and painful on palpation. Swelling is often present in all four limbs; however, forelimb swelling may be more obvious (especially in distal radial metaphyses). Severely affected dogs may be depressed, anorexic, and pyrexic (up to 106° F).

Radiography

Radiographs of affected long bones reveal an irregular radiolucent zone in the metaphysis, parallel and proximal to the physis. This gives the appearance of a double physeal line. Flaring of the metaphysis with increased bone density occurs due to periosteal proliferation. This reaction subsides with time, but may leave a permanently widened metaphysis (Fig. 32-3).

Laboratory Findings

Laboratory abnormalities are not usually found; however, hypocalcemia has been noted in a few affected dogs. The significance of this finding is unknown.

DIFFERENTIAL DIAGNOSIS

This condition should be differentiated from septic arthritis (see p. 891) and panosteitis (see p. 1010).

MEDICAL MANAGEMENT

Analgesics should be administered to control pain (see Table 32-1). Occasionally, severely debilitated animals require fluid support. Corticosteroids, antibiotics, and vitamin C have

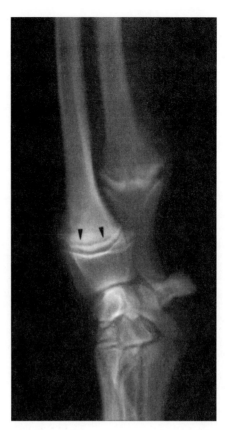

FIG. 32-3
Radiograph of the distal radius and ulna of a dog with hypertrophic osteodystrophy. There is a double physeal line at the growth plate of the distal radius (*arrows*). Similar changes are present on the distal ulna. (From Olmstead ML: *Small animal orthopedics*, St Louis, 1995, Mosby.)

been administered but have not proven effective in shortening the course or severity of this disease.

PROGNOSIS

Most animals recover fully within 7 to 10 days of the onset of clinical signs; however, multiple relapses may occur. Occasionally, severe debilitation or multiple, severe relapses cause owners to request that affected animals be euthanized. Interference with normal physeal development may result in permanent deformity of long bones.

☞ **N O T E** · Warn owners that multiple relapses may occur.

Suggested Reading

Bellah JR: Hypertrophic osteodystrophy. In Bojrab MJ, editor: *Disease mechanisms in small animal surgery,* ed 2, Philadelphia, 1993, Lea & Febiger.

Grondalen J: Metaphyseal osteopathy (hypertrophic osteodystrophy) in growing dogs: a clinical study, *J Small Anim Pract* 17:721, 1976.

Woodard JC: Canine hypertrophic osteodystrophy, a study of the spontaneous disease in littermates, *Vet Pathol* 19:337, 1982.

BONE NEOPLASIA

DEFINITIONS

Primary bone neoplasia arises from cells located within the bone structure. Soft tissue tumors that spread to bone (**metastatic bone tumors**) may occur in either the **appendicular** skeleton (i.e., long bones) or **axial** skeleton (skull, vertebrae, ribs, and pelvis).

GENERAL CONSIDERATIONS AND CLINICALLY RELEVANT PATHOPHYSIOLOGY

Primary tumors of bone include osteosarcoma, chondrosarcoma, fibrosarcoma, hemangiosarcoma, giant cell tumor, liposarcoma, periosteal osteosarcoma, periosteal fibrosarcoma, osteomas, multilobular osteoma, multilobular chondroma, osteochondroma, and chondroma. The accu-

TABLE 32-3

Malignant Bone Neoplasia in Dogs

Tumor	Incidence	Metastasis	Treatment	Prognosis
Osteosarcoma of the appendicular skeleton	75% of all bone tumors	High rate of early metastasis to lungs and soft tissues. Bone metastasis is a late complication.	Amputation and chemotherapy with cisplatin and/or doxorubicin Limb–sparing in selected cases Palliative radiation therapy for painful bone lesions	Mean survival time with amputation alone is 12 to 16 weeks, median survival time with limb sparing or amputation plus cisplatin and doxorubicin is about 300 to 400 days
Osteosarcoma of the axial skeleton	Less common than appendicular tumors	Highly metastatic, local recurrence except for mandible, which is slower to metastasize	Local resection of tumor (i.e., mandible, rib) Cisplatin, local radiation as adjunct to surgery to reduce local recurrence	Median survival time is 22 weeks, 1 year survival is 26.3%, rate of tumor recurrence is 66.7%
Fibrosarcoma	<5% of bone tumors	Slower to metastasize than osteosarcoma	Amputation (chemotherapy not of proven benefit) Limb sparing in select cases	Poor prognosis (but complete excision of low-grade tumors without metastases may be curative)
Chondrosarcoma	5%-10% of bone tumors	Slow to metastasize	Amputation (chemotherapy not of proven benefit)	May be good after amputation or resection of lesion
Hemangiosarcoma	<5% of bone tumors	May be multicentric, often involve spleen and right atrium, highly metastatic	Amputation (chemotherapy not of proven benefit) Limb sparing in select cases	Poor prognosis because of multiple organ involvement, mean survival time less than 5 months
Giant cell tumor	Rare	Metastasis to lymph nodes, lung, and bones	Amputation	Poor prognosis
Liposarcoma	Rare	Metastasis to lung, liver, and lymph nodes	Amputation or local resection	Poor prognosis
Fracture-associated sarcoma	Uncommon, associated with fractures in which healing has been complicated; represents 5% of osteosarcomas	Metastasis has occurred in 14% of reported cases	Amputation Limb-sparing techniques Chemotherapy	Same as osteosarcoma

TABLE 32-4

Malignant Bone Neoplasia in Cats

Tumor	Incidence	Metastasis	Treatment	Prognosis
Osteosarcoma	Most common primary bone tumor in cats (70%-80%)	Metastasis is uncommon	Amputation, radiation therapy, or excision of skull tumors	Median survival time is 24-50 months; greater than 50% of cats are alive at 64 months
Fibrosarcoma	Rare, more often due to secondary invasion of bone from soft tissue	Incidence is unknown	Amputation	Long disease-free intervals reported (e.g., 10 to 18 months)
Chondrosarcoma	4% of bone tumors, reported in the scapula	Incidence is unknown	Amputation	Prognosis guarded
Squamous cell carcinoma	Local bone invasion, occurs in oral cavity and digits	See section on oral tumors (p. 222)	Amputation, mandibulectomy, maxillectomy, +/− radiation therapy, see section on oral tumors (p. 222)	See section on oral tumors (p. 222)
Multiple cartilaginous exotosis	Uncommon, usually FeLV positive	Multiple sites common, scapula, vertebra, mandible	Palliative removal of painful lesions	Guarded

rate diagnosis of a primary bone tumor requires that an established protocol be followed (i.e., history taking, physical examination, hematologic and serum biochemical evaluation, radiographic examination, and biopsy for histologic evaluation). Primary tumors of the appendicular skeleton most commonly arise in the distal radial metaphysis, proximal humerus, proximal or distal femur, and proximal or distal tibia. Benign bone tumors (i.e., osteoma, ossifying fibroma, multilobular osteomas and chondromas, osteochondromas, enchondromas, and chondromas) are generally slow growing. Depending on tumor accessibility, complete surgical excision of benign bone tumors is usually curative.

☞ **N O T E** • Primary bone tumors can be malignant or benign and must be accurately diagnosed for appropriate treatment.

Osteosarcoma is the most common primary bone neoplasm; 75% of osteosarcomas originate in the appendicular skeleton (Straw, 1996) (Tables 32-3 and 32-4). Metastasis is common and usually occurs early in the course of disease. Although fewer than 5% of affected dogs have radiographically detectable thoracic metastases at presentation, 90% die or are euthanized within 1 year of diagnosis because of complications associated with pulmonary metastasis (Straw 1996). Improved chances for survival are possible with amputation or limb-sparing procedures combined with chemotherapy (e.g., cisplatin).

☞ **N O T E** • Osteosarcomas arise most commonly in the metaphyses of the proximal humerus, distal radius, and distal femur.

Osteosarcoma is also the most common tumor of the axial skeleton. Of 116 axial osteosarcomas evaluated, the most common sites of occurrence were mandible (31), maxilla (26), spine (17), cranium (14), ribs (12), nasal cavity and paranasal sinuses (10), and pelvis (6) (Heyman et al, 1992). Because osteosarcoma is the most frequently diagnosed bone tumor, it is used as the model for evaluation, diagnosis, treatment and prognosis of bone tumors in this section. Although the workup needed to diagnose neoplasia is similar for all bone tumors, treatment and prognosis vary depending on tumor type (see Tables 32-3 and 32-4).

Histologically, osteosarcoma is composed of anaplastic mesenchymal cells that produce osteoid. Histologic subgroups include osteoblastic, fibroblastic, osteoclastic, poorly differentiated, and telangiectatic osteosarcoma. An inflammatory component is frequently present in fracture-associated sarcoma (sarcomas that arise in the diaphysis of a long bone at the site of a previous fracture), reflecting altered healing patterns and chronic inflammation associated with these tumors.

DIAGNOSIS
Clinical Presentation

Signalment. Large- and giant-breed dogs have the greatest incidence of appendicular bone neoplasia. The median age of dogs with osteosarcoma is 7 years (Straw, 1996). Males are more commonly affected than females. Primary bone tumors of the axial skeleton are most common in medium-sized and large-breed dogs. The median age of affected animals is 8.7 years and females are more frequently affected than males (Heyman et al, 1992). Osteosarcoma is the most common feline primary bone tumor, primarily affecting older (i.e., 10 years mean age) cats.

History. Dogs with primary bone neoplasia affecting the appendicular skeleton are usually presented for evaluation of lameness and/or localized limb swelling. Owners often believe that a recent history of mild trauma has caused the lameness. Pathologic fracture may be associated with acute signs of lameness. Dogs with primary bone tumors of the axial skeleton usually present for evaluation of pain, reluctance to eat or walk, visible swelling, and/or bleeding from tumor surfaces. Clinical signs may be acute or chronic and progressive.

Physical Examination Findings

Dogs affected with appendicular tumors are often lame. The limb may be enlarged and firm; rarely are cutaneous fistulae present. Systemic signs of illness (i.e., fever, anorexia, weight loss) are uncommon in acute stages of disease. Tumors of the axial skeleton are often palpable as firm swellings. Tumors affecting the vertebral column may cause acute signs of lameness or paralysis (see p. 1096). Respiratory abnormalities associated with pulmonary metastasis may be noted in some animals.

☞ **NOTE** · Lameness is often the first sign of appendicular bone tumors.

Radiography

Radiographs of affected bones and thorax should be evaluated. Radiographic signs of osteosarcoma include cortical lysis, periosteal bone proliferation, and soft-tissue swelling (Fig. 32-4). Thoracic radiographs should include a dorsoventral or ventrodorsal view and both lateral views (i.e., right and left lateral views). These radiographs should be carefully evaluated for evidence of tumor metastasis. Although radiographic signs associated with osteosarcoma cannot be differentiated from those associated with fungal osteomyelitis, coupling radiographic signs with signalment and history can help determine whether neoplasia should be considered probable, or not.

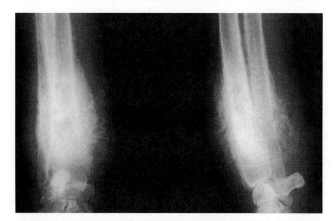

FIG. 32-4
Radiographs of a distal radius of a dog with osteosarcoma. Note the cortical lysis, periosteal proliferation, and soft-tissue swelling.

☞ **NOTE** · Right and left lateral thoracic radiographs are essential to look for metastases.

Laboratory Findings

Specific laboratory abnormalities are not consistent hallmarks of primary or metastatic bone neoplasia; however, the bone isoenzyme of serum alkaline phosphatase may be greatly elevated in dogs with osteosarcoma.

DIFFERENTIAL DIAGNOSIS

Suspected primary neoplastic lesions must be differentiated from bacterial osteomyelitis, fungal osteomyelitis, metastatic bone tumor (i.e., prostatic carcinoma), direct extension of soft tissue tumors (i.e., nail bed carcinomas), hypertrophic pulmonary osteopathy, bone infarcts, hypervitaminosis A, periosteal response to trauma, and aneurysmal bone cysts.

Definitive diagnosis of bone neoplasia necessitates histologic evaluation of samples obtained by biopsy or excision. Successful identification of a tumor requires that biopsy samples are obtained accurately and that a pathologist accustomed to interpreting bone samples performs the histologic evaluation. Multiple samples should be obtained to increase diagnostic accuracy. Closed trephine biopsy (see p. 1017) from the center of radiographic lesions is more accurate than biopsy of transitional zones between tumor and normal bone. The latter biopsies are more frequently interpreted as reactive bone. Radiographs made after biopsy can be used to confirm biopsy location.

MEDICAL OR CONSERVATIVE MANAGEMENT

Multiple modality treatment (e.g., amputation and chemotherapy) has extended the life span of dogs with osteosarcoma to a median of 43 weeks with a 40% one year survival (Shapiro et al, 1988). Adjunctive chemotherapy usually involves administration of cisplatin immediately after amputation at a dose of 70 mg/m^2 body surface area. Cisplatin therapy is continued every 3 weeks until six treatments have been performed. Adverse side effects of cisplatin therapy (i.e., renal damage, nausea, vomiting, loss of appetite, and bone marrow suppression) are potentially life-threatening and necessitate that animals be carefully monitored during treatment. CBC, platelet count, BUN, serum creatinine, and urine specific gravity should be assessed frequently. Readers are referred to a medicine text for additional information regarding medical treatment of osteosarcoma.

SURGICAL TREATMENT

Treatment of appendicular bone tumors involves limb amputation (see p. 1017) or tumor resection combined with limb salvage techniques and cisplatin chemotherapy (see p. 1021). Maxillary and mandibular tumors are treated by mandibulectomy (see p. 204) or maxillectomy (see p. 203), plus appropriate chemotherapy or radiation therapy. Spinal tumors can occasionally be treated with en bloc resection but the procedure is difficult. Tumors of the ribs are treated with en bloc resection.

☞ **NOTE** · Be aware that after amputation, dogs with severe concurrent orthopedic disease may have difficulty ambulating.

Preoperative Management

Thorough physical examinations should be performed to identify concurrent problems that might interfere with anesthesia. Limb amputation involves loss of a large amount of tissue, fluid, electrolytes, and red blood cells. Animals should be well hydrated before surgery and adequate fluids should be administered during surgery. Broad-spectrum antibiotics should be administered perioperatively during mandibulectomy, maxillectomy, and limb-sparing techniques. Antibiotics are not necessary during limb amputations unless there is concurrent infection or possible contamination.

☞ **NOTE** · Perioperative fluid management is essential during limb amputation.

Anesthesia

Bone biopsy, amputation, and limb-sparing techniques are performed under general anesthesia (see p. 708 for suggested protocols).

Surgical Anatomy

Surgical anatomy varies with tumor location. Refer to the appropriate bone for an anatomic description.

Positioning

For bone biopsy the animal is usually positioned in lateral recumbency with the affected leg uppermost. A wide area around the proposed biopsy site is clipped and prepped for aseptic surgery. For scapulectomy, forelimb amputation, and rear limb amputation the animal is positioned in lateral recumbency with the affected leg uppermost. The front or rear leg is prepped from the dorsal and ventral midline to the foot. For limb-sparing of the forelimb, the animal is positioned and prepped similarly to forelimb amputation.

SURGICAL TECHNIQUES
Bone Biopsy

Either a Michele trephine or Jamshidi needle can be used to obtain a bone biopsy. Advantages of Michele trephines are that a larger sample of bone is obtained; however, there may be an increased risk of fracture through the biopsy site (Table 32-5). Jamshidi needles secure a smaller sample that may decrease the risk of pathologic fracture after biopsy. Accurate diagnoses can be obtained with either technique in greater than 80% of cases (Powers et al, 1988).

Make a small skin incision over the center of the lesion. Locate the skin incision so that biopsy tracts that may be seeded with tumor during the biopsy can be removed during the definitive treatment procedure (position the biopsy tract so that it does not interfere with skin flaps developed

to cover the amputated bone end, should amputation be necessary). Push the trephine or needle through soft tissues to the bone cortex. Remove the stylet and advance the trephine or cannula through the bone. Remove the cannula and push the specimen out by inserting the probe into it. Repeat the procedure to obtain multiple specimens (Fig. 32-5).

Amputation

Occasionally, tumors involve only the scapula and total or partial scapulectomy can be performed. This procedure spares the limb and allows fair to excellent limb function. Forelimb amputation may be performed by removing the scapula or, alternately, the limb can be removed by resecting the distal humerus. Scapular removal (forequarter amputation) is often preferred because it eliminates the need to cut through bone and is cosmetic because the potential for unsightly muscular atrophy around the scapular spine is eliminated. Midhumeral amputation involves transection of only three tendinous insertions of muscles. The technique can be used for dogs or cats with neoplasia involving bones of the distal extremities (distal to the elbow). Retention of the scapula may afford some thoracic protection.

TABLE 32-5

Important Considerations for Bone Biopsy

- Obtain samples from the radiologic center of tumors.
- Obtain multiple samples.
- Take radiographs after biopsy to confirm biopsy site.
- Using Jamshidi needles may reduce the risk of pathologic fracture.
- Have pathologists experienced in evaluating bone biopsies perform histology.

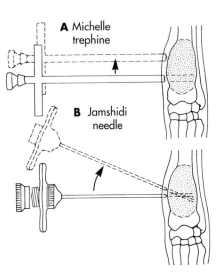

FIG. 32-5
Bone biopsy may be performed with, **A,** a Michele trephine or, **B,** Jamshidi needle.

Rear limb amputation may be performed at the mid-femoral diaphysis, or by disarticulating the coxofemoral joint. When tumors affect the femur, the coxofemoral joint should be disarticulated and the entire femur removed. This procedure is more difficult than midfemoral amputation. After amputation, the entire tumor should be resubmitted for histologic evaluation to confirm the diagnosis.

Scapulectomy. *Make a skin incision from several centimeters dorsal to the dorsal border of the scapula, over the scapular spine, to the middle third of the humerus (Fig. 32-6, A). Transect superficial muscles (i.e., omotransversarius m., trapezius m.) as close to their origin on the lateral surface of the scapula as the tumor will allow. Expose* the medial scapular surface by transecting the rhomboideus m. and elevating the serratus m. from the scapula (Fig. 32-6, B and C). Protect the brachial plexus and axillary artery and vein during dissection. Transect the suprascapular and subscapular nerves. Transect the teres major and long head of the triceps muscles from their origins on the caudal border of the scapula (Fig. 32-6, D). Transect the coracobrachialis tendon, teres minor, infraspinatus, supraspinatus, and subscapularis muscles close to their humeral origin (Fig. 32-6, E). Incise the joint capsule. Osteotomize the supraglenoid tubercle and remove the scapula (Fig. 32-6, F). To close the wound, suture the tendon origin of the biceps brachii muscle to the joint capsule.

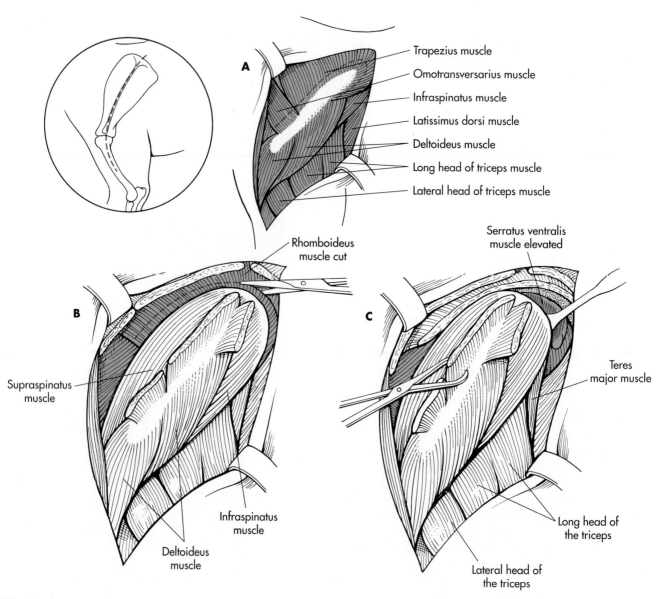

A, Trapezius muscle
Omotransversarius muscle
Infraspinatus muscle
Latissimus dorsi muscle
Deltoideus muscle
Long head of triceps muscle
Lateral head of triceps muscle

Rhomboideus muscle cut

Serratus ventralis muscle elevated

B, Supraspinatus muscle
Infraspinatus muscle
Deltoideus muscle

C, Teres major muscle
Long head of the triceps
Lateral head of the triceps

FIG. 32-6

A, For scapulectomy, make a skin incision several centimeters dorsal to the dorsal border of the scapula, over the scapular spine, to the middle third of the humerus. **B,** Transect the omotransversarius, trapezius, and rhomboideus muscles. **C,** Elevate the serratus ventralis muscle from the scapula.

Attach the free muscle flaps to adjacent musculature. Suture subcutaneous tissue and skin. Perform partial scapulectomy similarly, but osteotomize the scapula proximal to the scapular notch.

Forequarter amputation. *Make a skin incision from the dorsal border of the scapula, over the scapular spine, to the proximal third of the humerus (Fig. 32-7, A). Continue the skin incision around the forelimb at this level. Transect the trapezius and omotransversarius muscles at their insertions on the scapular spine. Transect the rhomboideus muscle from its attachment on the dorsal border of the scapula and retract the scapula laterally to expose its medial surface (Fig. 32-7, B). Next, elevate the serratus ventralis muscle from the medial surface of the scapula (Fig. 32-7, C). Continue to retract the scapula to expose the brachial plexus and axillary artery and vein. Ligate the axillary artery and vein with a three-clamp and transfixation suture technique (Fig. 32-8). Transect the brachial plexus. Transect the brachiocephalicus muscle, deep and superficial pectoral muscles, and latissimus dorsi muscle near their humeral insertions (Fig. 32-7, D and E). Remove the fore-*

limb. To close the wound, approximate the muscle bellies to cover the brachial plexus and vessels and suture subcutaneous tissues and skin (Fig. 32-7, F).

Midhumeral amputation. *Make a skin incision around the forelimb at the level of the distal third of the humerus (Fig. 32-9, A). The lateral portion of the skin incision should extend further distally than the medial portion of the skin incision. Dissect subcutaneous tissues in the same plane. Abduct the limb and separate the biceps brachii muscle and medial head of the triceps muscle to expose the brachial artery and vein and median, ulnar, and musculocutaneous nerves (Fig. 32-9, B). Ligate the artery and vein with a three-clamp and transfixation suture technique (see Fig. 32-8). Transect the nerves, then transect the triceps tendon and reflect the muscles proximally to expose the humerus. Transect the biceps brachii and brachialis muscles at their insertions on the radius and ulna (Fig. 32-9, C). Ligate the cephalic vein and transect the radial nerve. Elevate the brachiocephalicus muscle from the humerus. Osteotomize the humerus with an oscillating saw, Gigli wire, or osteotome and remove the distal forelimb*

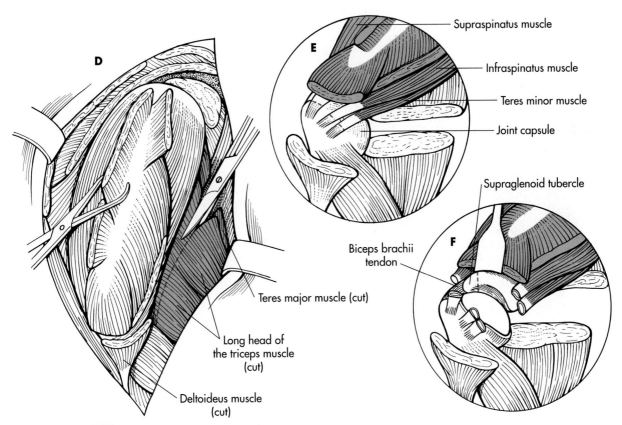

FIG. 32-6 CONT'D
D, Transect the acromial and spinous heads of the deltoideus muscle close to the scapula.
E, Transect the teres major and long head of the triceps muscles from the caudal border of the scapula. Transect the tendons of the teres minor, infraspinatus, supraspinatus, coracobrachialis (not pictured), and subscapularis (not pictured) muscles close to their humeral origins. **F,** Incise joint capsule, osteotomize the glenoid tubercle, and remove the scapula.

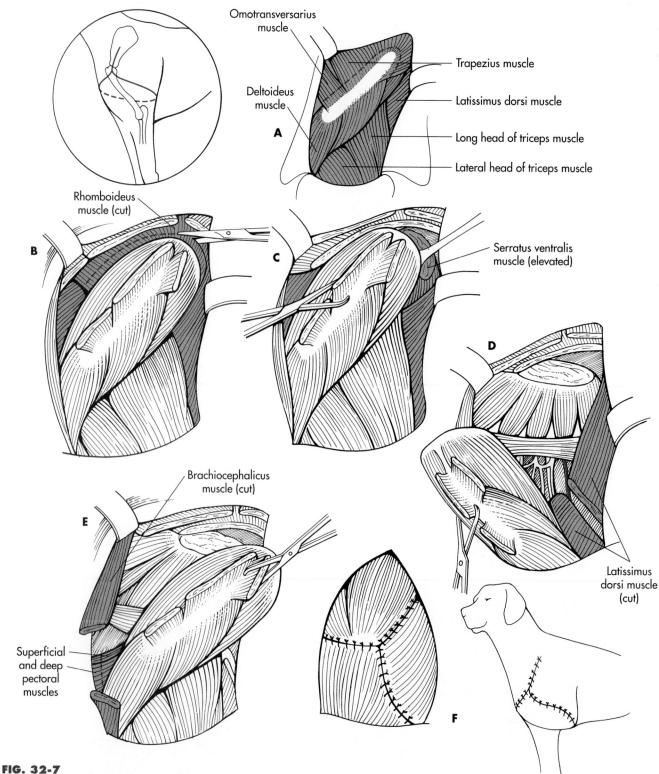

FIG. 32-7
A, For forequarter amputation, make a skin incision from the dorsal border of the scapula, over the scapular spine, to the proximal third of the humerus. Continue the skin incision around the forelimb at this level. Transect the trapezius and omotransversarius muscles at their insertions on the scapular spine. **B,** Transect the rhomboideus muscle from its attachment on the dorsal border of the scapula. **C,** Elevate the serratus ventralis muscle from the medial surface of the scapula. **D,** Retract the scapula laterally to expose the axillary artery and vein for ligation. Transect the brachial plexus. Transect the latissimus dorsi muscle near its humeral insertion. **E,** Transect the brachiocephalicus and deep and superficial pectoral muscles near their humeral insertions and remove the forelimb. **F,** To close the wound, approximate the muscle bellies to cover the brachial plexus and vessels and suture subcutaneous tissues and skin.

(Fig. 32-9, C). Close the wound by suturing the triceps tendon around the humeral stump to the biceps and brachialis muscles. Suture subcutaneous tissues and skin.

Coxofemoral disarticulation. *Make a skin incision around the rear limb at the level of the middle third of the femur (Fig. 32-10, A). The lateral aspect of the skin incision should extend further distally than the medial aspect. On the medial side, open the femoral triangle by incising between the pectineus muscle and caudal belly of the sartorius muscle to expose and ligate the femoral artery and vein (Fig. 32-10, B) using a three-clamp technique (see Fig. 32-8). Transect sartorius, pectineus, gracilis, and adductor muscles approximately 2 cm from the inguinal crease (Fig. 32-10, C). Isolate the medial circumflex femoral vessels over the iliopsoas muscle and ligate them. Transect the iliopsoas muscle at its insertion on the lesser trochanter and reflect it cranially to expose the joint capsule (Fig. 32-10, D). Incise the joint capsule and cut the ligament of the head of the femur (Fig. 32-10, E). On the lateral side, transect biceps femoris muscle and tensor fascia lata at midfemoral level and reflect them proximally to expose the greater trochanter and sciatic nerve (Fig. 32-10, F). Sever the sciatic nerve distal to its muscular branches to the semimembranosus, semitendinosus, and biceps femoris muscles. Transect the gluteal muscles insertions close to the greater trochanter (Fig. 32-10, G). Transect semimembranosus and semitendinosus muscles at the level of the proximal third of the femur. Sever the external rotator muscles and quadratus femoris muscle at their attachments around*

the trochanteric fossa. Elevate the rectus femoris muscle from its origin on the pelvis. Incise the joint capsule circumferentially and remove the limb. Close the wound by flapping the biceps femoris muscle medially and suturing it to the gracilis and semitendinosus muscles. Flap the tensor fascia lata caudally and suture it to the sartorius muscle. Suture subcutaneous tissues and skin.

Midfemoral amputation. *Make a skin incision around the rear limb at the level of the distal third of the femur (Fig. 32-11, A). The lateral aspect of the skin incision should extend further distally than the medial aspect. On the medial side, transect the gracilis muscle and the caudal belly of the sartorius at the midfemoral level (Fig. 32-11, B). Isolate and ligate the femoral vessels (see Fig. 32-8). Transect the pectineus muscle through its musculotendinous junction (Fig. 32-11, C). Transect the cranial belly of the sartorius muscle. Transect the quadriceps muscle proximally to the patella (Fig. 32-11, D). Transect the biceps femoris muscle at the same level as the quadriceps muscle. Isolate and cut the sciatic nerve at the level of the third trochanter. Transect the caudal muscles, including the semimembranosus, semitendinosus, and adductor muscles at midfemoral level (Fig. 32-11, E). Elevate the insertion of the adductor muscle from the linea aspera of the femur (Fig. 32-11,F). Cut the femur at the junction of the proximal and middle thirds of the diaphysis and remove the limb. Close the wound by flapping the quadriceps muscle caudally to cover the femoral stump and suturing it to the adductor muscle. Flap the biceps muscle medially and suture it to the gracilis and semitendinosus muscles. Muscles should be apposed to completely protect the distal end of the femur. Suture subcutaneous tissues and skin.*

Limb-sparing Techniques

Some dogs with preexisting orthopedic and neurologic disease will not ambulate adequately after amputation. Additionally, some owners will not permit amputation. Limb-sparing techniques that involve en bloc resection of the tumor and replacement with a bone allograft can be used in selected cases. The most suitable candidates for limb-sparing are dogs with osteosarcoma of the distal radius that affects less than 50% of the bone (Straw, Withrow, Powers, 1990).

Position the dog in lateral recumbency. Dissect around the pseudocapsule of the tumor. Osteotomize the bone 2 to 3 cm proximal to the radiographic margin of the tumor. Transect the extensor carpi radialis muscle and remove it with the tumor (along with any other muscles or tendons that are involved). The distal margin of resection is the joint surface. Incise the joint capsule and dissect the tumor free. Remove the articular cartilage of the carpal bones in preparation for carpal arthrodesis. Replace the resected bone with a cortical allograft stabilized with a long, dynamic compression plate (see p. 750). Make sure that the plate is of sufficient length that at least four screws can be positioned in

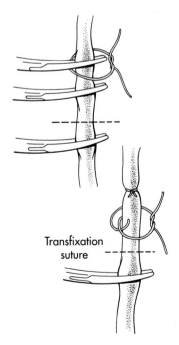

Transfixation suture

FIG. 32-8
A three-forceps and transfixation suture technique. Place three forceps on the artery and ligate it in the crushed area of the proximal forceps. Place a transfixation ligature distal to the first ligation and cut the vessel between the middle and distal clamps.

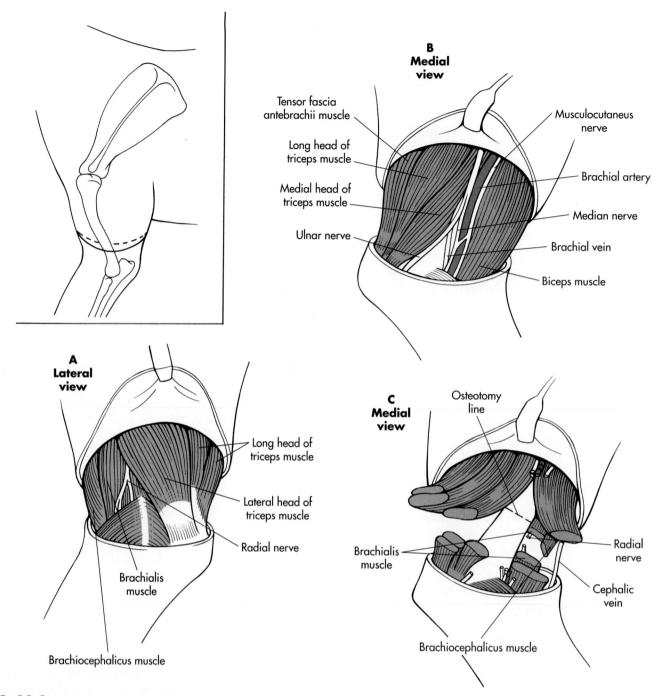

FIG. 32-9
A, For a midhumeral amputation, make a skin incision around the forelimb at the level of the distal third of the humerus. **B,** Abduct the limb and separate the biceps brachii muscle and medial head of the triceps muscle to expose the brachial artery and vein for ligation and median, ulnar, and musculocutaneous nerves for transection. **C,** Transect the triceps tendon, cut the biceps brachii and brachialis muscles at their insertions on the radius and ulna, and elevate the brachiocephalicus muscle from the humerus. Ligate the cephalic vein and transect the radial nerve. Osteotomize the humerus and remove the limb.

the proximal radius and three positioned distal to the graft. Harvest autogenous cancellous bone and place it at the host-graft interface and at the arthrodesis site (Fig. 32-12). If desired, insert a closed suction drain adjacent to the graft before closing the wound. Close subcutaneous tissues and skin routinely.

SUTURE MATERIALS/SPECIAL INSTRUMENTS

A Michele trephine or Jamshidi needle is needed for bone biopsy. An osteotome and mallet, oscillating saw, or Gigli wire is used to sever the bone when performing a midhumeral or midfemoral amputation. Nonabsorbable (poly-

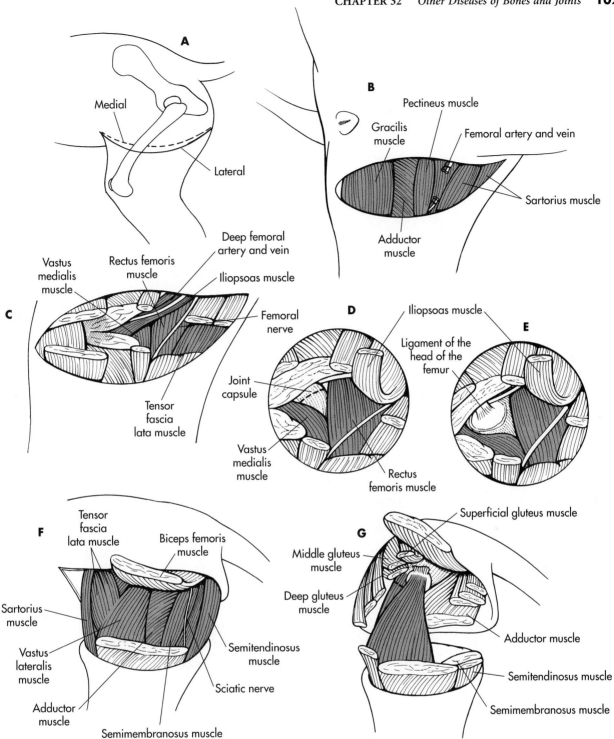

FIG. 32-10
A, For coxofemoral disarticulation, make a skin incision around the rear limb at the level of the middle third of the femur. **B,** On the medial side, open the femoral triangle by incising between the pectineus muscle and caudal belly of the sartorius muscle to expose and ligate the deep femoral artery and vein. **C,** Transect sartorius, pectineus, gracilis, and adductor muscles approximately 2 cm from the inguinal crease. **D** and **E,** Transect the iliopsoas muscle at its insertion on the lesser trochanter and reflect it cranially to expose the joint capsule. Incise the joint capsule and cut the ligament of the head of the femur. **F,** On the lateral side, transect biceps femoris muscle and tensor fascia lata at midfemoral level. **G,** Sever the sciatic nerve distal to its muscular branches to the semimembranosus, semitendinosus, and biceps femoris muscles. Transect the gluteal muscle insertions close to the greater trochanter. Transect the semimembranosus and semitendinosus muscles at the level of proximal third of the femur. Sever the external rotator muscles and quadratus femoris muscle at their attachments around the trochanteric fossa. Elevate the rectus femoris muscle from its origin on the pelvis. Remove the limb.

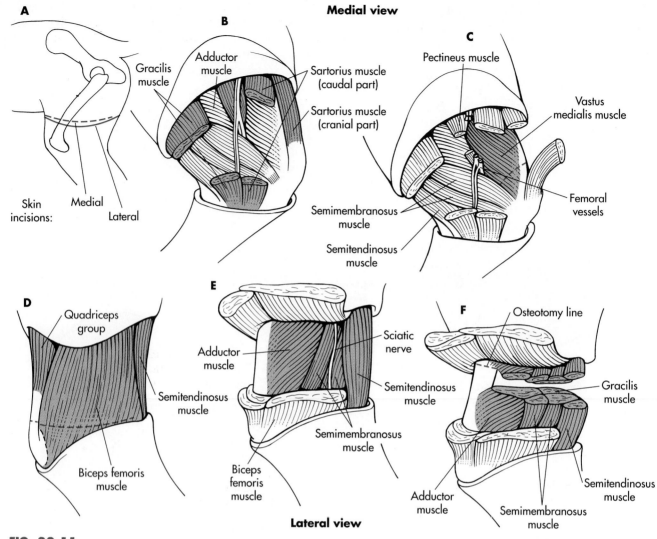

FIG. 32-11
A, For midfemoral amputation, make a skin incision around the rear limb at the level of the distal third of the femur. **B,** On the medial side, transect the gracilis muscle and the caudal belly of the sartorius at the midfemoral level. **C,** Isolate and ligate the femoral vessels. Transect the pectineus muscle through its musculotendinous junction. Transect the cranial belly of the sartorius muscle. **D,** Transect the quadriceps muscle proximally to the patella. **E,** Transect the biceps femoris muscle at the same level as the quadriceps muscle. Isolate and cut the sciatic nerve at the level of the third trochanter. Transect the semimembranosus, semitendinosus, and adductor muscles at midfemoral level. **F,** Elevate the insertion of the adductor muscle from the linea aspera of the femur. Cut the femur at the junction of the proximal and middle thirds of the diaphysis and remove the limb.

propylene or nylon) or strong synthetic absorbable (polydioxanone or polyglyconate) suture should be used for vessel ligation during amputation. Plating equipment is needed for limb sparing.

POSTOPERATIVE CARE AND ASSESSMENT

Postoperative care after biopsy is minimal. Pressure bandages may be needed if there is excessive bleeding. After amputation, the surgical site should be observed for swelling, redness, and/or discharge. If hemorrhage or seroma formation is noted, pressure may be applied to the surgical site by applying a circumferential bandage around the thorax or pelvis. Mobility should be encouraged after surgery so that the animal can learn to walk on three legs; however, some animals require initial support to prevent falling (especially on slick surfaces). Most animals are quick to learn to ambulate on three limbs; however, some dogs may require coaxing and encouragement. Pain relief is often evident after amputation of limbs with large neoplastic lesions. Sequential thoracic radiographs are indicated after surgery to detect metastasis. Potential complications of amputation include seroma formation, bleeding, infection, and suture line dehiscence.

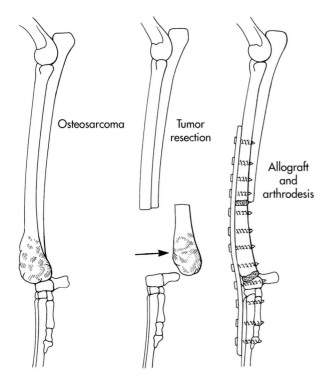

FIG. 32-12
A limb-sparing procedure for distal radial osteosarcoma. Resect the affected bone and soft tissues. Replace the bone with a cortical allograft and stabilize it with a compression plate. Perform an arthrodesis of the carpus concurrently.

☞ **N O T E ·** Many owners are reluctant to accept amputation and must be advised of the animal's ability to adapt to walking on three legs.

Postoperative care after limb-sparing includes care of the closed suction drainage system (if used) and removal of the drain when drainage subsides (usually 1 day after surgery). The leg should be supported in a padded bandage to control postoperative swelling. The incision must be protected from self-mutilation with bandages and/or an Elizabethan collar. Decreased exercise is recommended for 3 to 4 weeks; however, controlled exercise or physical therapy may be necessary to prevent flexure contracture of the digits.

PROGNOSIS

Dogs treated for osteosarcoma with amputation alone have a median survival time of 5 months, with a 10% 1-year survival. Dogs treated with amputation and cisplatin have median survival times of 9 months and 38% to 43% 1-year survival. Euthanasia is usually requested by owners when pulmonary metastases cause clinical signs of depression, anorexia, and/or respiratory distress.

Limb-sparing procedures in conjunction with cisplatin treatment have resulted in good or adequate limb function in approximately 80% of treated dogs. There does not appear to be a difference in survival rates between dogs treated with amputation in conjunction with chemotherapy and those

treated with limb-sparing procedures in conjunction with chemotherapy. Complications associated with limb-sparing include local tumor recurrence (up to 40%), implant failure (8%), and allograft infection (49%)(Straw, Withrow, Powers, 1990). Infection can require allograft removal or amputation.

References

Heyman SJ et al: Canine axial skeletal osteosarcoma: a retrospective study of 116 cases (1986–1989), *Vet Surg* 21:304, 1992.
Powers BE et al: Jamshidi needle biopsy for diagnosis of bone lesions in small animals, *J Am Vet Med Assoc* 193:205, 1988.
Shapiro W et al: Use of cisplatin for treatment of appendicular osteosarcoma in dogs, *J Am Vet Med Assoc* 192:507, 1988.
Straw RC: Tumors of the musculoskeletal system. In Withrow SJ, MacEwen EG, editors: *Small animal clinical oncology,* ed 2, Philadelphis, 1996, WB Saunders.
Straw RC, Withrow SJ, Powers BE: Management of canine appendicular osteosarcoma, *Vet Clin of N Am Small Anim Prac* 20:1141, 1990.

Suggested Reading

Bone DL, Aberman HA: Forelimb amputation in the dog using humeral osteotomy, *J Am Anim Hosp Assoc* 24:525, 1988.
Kirpensteijn J et al: Partial and total scapulectomy in the dog, *J Am Anim Hosp Assoc* 30:313, 1994.
Ogilvie GK, Moore AS: Management of bone tumors. In *Managing the veterinary cancer patient: a practice manual,* Trenton, NJ, 1995, Veterinary Learning Systems.
Slocum B: Amputation of the canine pelvic limb. In Bojrab, MJ, ed: *Current techniques in small animal surgery,* ed 1, Philadelphia, 1975, Lea & Febiger.
Stevenson S: Fracture associated sarcomas, *Vet Clin of North Am* 21:859, 1991.
Withrow ST, MacEwen EG: *Small animal clinical oncology,* ed 2, Philadelphia, 1996, WB Saunders.

JOINT NEOPLASIA

DEFINITIONS

Primary joint neoplasms are tumors that arise from synovial linings of diarthrodial joints, tendon sheaths, and/or bursae. The tumors of practical importance are those arising from synovioblastic tissue, called **synovial sarcomas.**

SYNONYMS

Malignant synovioma, synovial cell sarcoma

GENERAL CONSIDERATIONS AND CLINICALLY RELEVANT PATHOPHYSIOLOGY

Synovial cell sarcomas are rare tumors arising from synovioblastic mesenchyme in deep connective tissues around joints. Joints above the carpus and tarsus are more commonly affected than distal joints. Biological behavior of these tumors range from slow growth to aggressive invasion of adjacent tissues. Metastasis occurs to regional lymph nodes, lungs, and other locations including bone. Histopathologic examination of synovial sarcomas reveals synovioblastic and fibrosarcomatous cells in varying proportions. The matrix is composed of collagen and reticulin fibers.

DIAGNOSIS
Clinical Presentation

Signalment. Synovial sarcomas occur most commonly in large, middle-age dogs. There is a 3:2 male-to-female ratio. A breed predisposition has not been identified.

History. Dogs and cats are usually evaluated because of lameness. A mass near a joint may be occasionally noticed by owners. Masses may grow slowly for a period of time; rapid growth may then occur.

Physical Examination Findings

Masses vary in size, but are usually firm with some fluctuant areas. They are generally nonpainful. The degree of lameness appears to correlate with the amount of bone involvement.

Radiography

Radiographs of involved joints should be made to evaluate the extent of bone and soft-tissue involvement. There may be evidence of lobulated soft-tissue masses in the joint region. Bone changes (i.e., lysis of subchondral bone and cortex, new bone production) are often noted on either side of the joint (Fig. 32-13). This contrasts with the appearance of primary bone tumors, which seldom appear to "cross a joint." Thoracic radiographs should be taken to evaluate for pulmonary metastasis.

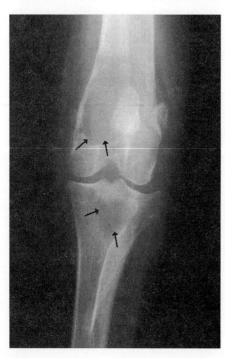

FIG. 32-13
Radiograph of a stifle joint with synovial sarcoma. There is bone lysis in the distal femur and proximal tibia (*arrows*) giving the appearance that the tumor has crossed the joint.

Laboratory Findings

Consistent laboratory abnormalities are not present.

DIFFERENTIAL DIAGNOSIS

Neoplastic joint lesions must be differentiated from synovial cysts, which are well-circumscribed masses attached to joint capsule, tendon sheath, or bursa (see below). Synovial cell sarcomas must also be differentiated from fungal and infectious joint diseases (i.e., septic arthritis, erosive arthritis, villonodular synovitis) and other tumors (i.e., fibrosarcoma, hemangiopericytoma, malignant fibrous histiocytomas, giant cell tumors of soft tissue, and primary bone tumors). A definitive diagnosis requires that the lesion be biopsied; however, if massive bone destruction is present and precludes therapy other than amputation, excisional biopsy (limb amputation) rather than incisional biopsy might be warranted. Fine-needle aspiration can reveal the presence of malignant cells, but will not allow visualization of tumor architecture necessary for definitive diagnosis of tumor type in many cases.

SURGICAL TREATMENT

Amputation appears to be the most effective treatment for this tumor (see p. 1017). Local excision is not recommended because of the high recurrence rate. Concurrent chemotherapy may be beneficial. Synovial cell sarcoma regressed in one animal after treatment with doxorubicin and cyclophosphamide (Tilmant et al, 1986).

POSTOPERATIVE CARE AND ASSESSMENT

Refer to p. 1024 for recommendations for the postoperative care of animals following amputation. Periodic examination of affected animals is recommended for early detection of local recurrence or metastasis.

PROGNOSIS

The prognosis is guarded after limb amputation. Although these tumors have historically been considered to be slow-growing tumors that metastasize late in the course of disease, a recent study has suggested that metastasis is common following amputation. Twenty of 37 cases reported in the literature developed metastasis at some time during the clinical course of disease (McGlennon, Houlton, Gorman, 1988).

References

McGlennon NJ, Houlton JEF, Gorman NT: Synovial sarcoma in the dog—a review, *J Small Anim Pract* 29:139, 1988.
Tilmant LL et al: Chemotherapy of synovial cell sarcoma in a dog, *J Am Vet Med Assoc* 188:530, 1986.

SYNOVIAL CYSTS

DEFINITIONS

Synovial cysts are benign, well-circumscribed masses attached to joint capsule, tendon sheath, or bursa.

GENERAL CONSIDERATIONS AND CLINICALLY RELEVANT PATHOPHYSIOLOGY

Synovial cysts are usually reported as incidental findings and rarely cause clinical signs other than localized enlargement of the joint or surrounding tissues. The pathogenesis in human beings is believed to involve inflammation of the synovial membrane. A well-circumscribed cystic lesion forms when synovial membrane herniates through the joint capsule, or a bursa connected to a joint enlarges. Diagnosis is based on histological evaluation of tissues. The cyst consists of a synovial cell lining supported by a zone of collagen. Typically, inflammatory cells are not present.

DIAGNOSIS
Clinical Presentation

Signalment. The age of affected animals at presentation has ranged from 5 to 16 years. There does not appear to be a sex or breed predilection.

History. Animals are presented for evaluation of a mass near a joint (typically carpus, elbow, or tarsus). Lameness is seldom evident.

Physical Examination Findings

Masses are usually small, well-circumscribed, and firmly attached to deeper tissues.

Radiography

These lesions are not associated with bone lysis or proliferation. Soft-tissue swelling may be noted in the joint or in surrounding soft tissues.

Laboratory Findings

Consistent laboratory abnormalities are not found.

DIFFERENTIAL DIAGNOSIS

Soft-tissue tumors and tumor-like lesions (i.e., hemangiopericytoma, lipoma, sebaceous adenoma, fibroma, synovial sarcoma, histiocytoma, mast cell tumor, epidermal and follicular cysts, calcinosis circumscripta, and local villonodular synovitis) must be differentiated from synovial cysts. These lesions are generally differentiated histologically.

SURGICAL TREATMENT

Excision of the cyst is recommended. The cyst should be carefully freed from surrounding soft tissues by dissection and removed. Drainage of the cyst, without removal of the synovial lining, will result in recurrence.

PROGNOSIS

Recurrence has not been reported after complete surgical excision.

Suggested Reading

Prymak C, Goldschmidt MH: Synovial cysts in five dogs and one cat, *J Am Anim Hosp Assoc* 27:151, 1991.

OSTEOMYELITIS

DEFINITIONS

Osteomyelitis is inflammation of bone marrow, cortex, and possibly periosteum. **Acute osteomyelitis** is characterized by systemic illness, pain, and soft-tissue swelling without visible radiographic alterations in bone. **Chronic osteomyelitis** exists when acute and systemic clinical signs have subsided, but infection manifested by draining sinuses, recurrent cellulitis, abscess formation, and progressive destructive and proliferative osseous changes is present. **Sequestra** are fragments of necrosed bone that have become separated from surrounding tissue.

SYNONYMS

Bone infection

GENERAL CONSIDERATIONS AND CLINICALLY RELEVANT PATHOPHYSIOLOGY

Most bone infections in dogs and cats are bacterial in origin. Many of these are monomicrobial infections, with β-lactamase producing *S. intermedius* or *S. aureus* predominating. Polymicrobial infections are also common and may harbor mixtures of *Streptococcus* spp., *Proteus* spp., *E. coli*, *Klebsiella* spp., and *Pseudomonas* spp. Anaerobic bacteria are recognized as an important cause of osteomyelitis, being present in up to 70% of bone infections (Caywood, Wallace, Braden, 1978). Anaerobes may exist alone as the sole causative agent, or more commonly, as one organism in polymicrobial infections. Anaerobes isolated from bone infections include *Actinomyces* spp., *Clostridium* spp., *Peptostreptococcus* spp., *Bacteroides* spp., and *Fusobacterium* spp. Characteristics of anaerobic infections include fetid odor, sequestration of bone fragments, and evidence of bacteria with differing morphology on Gram-stained smears.

☞ **N O T E ·** Treatment failures may result from lack of identification and inappropriate treatment of anaerobic bacteria.

Bacterial osteomyelitis is frequently classified as either hematogenous or posttraumatic; however, it should be recognized that the division between the two is often indistinct as hematogenous seeding of fractures by infectious agents occurs and may induce osteomyelitis. Nevertheless, studies indicate that a common source of bacterial inoculation is surgical site contamination during open fracture reduction. Although the type and quantity of bacteria inoculated are important factors in development of bone infections, bacteria alone will not necessarily cause osteomyelitis. Other important factors in the pathogenesis of posttraumatic osteomyelitis are (1) extent of soft-tissue damage and alteration of blood supply; (2) formation of a biofilm (glycocalyx); (3) and stability of fracture repair. The first of these, tissue damage, may be caused by the injury or may occur during the surgical procedure. The presence of damaged soft tissue and devitalized bone serves as an excellent culture medium for bacteria. Bacterial proliferation is also potentiated by foreign materials in the wound (e.g., synthetic suture materials, implants). Glycocalyx is a combination of bacterial slime and host cellular debris that shrouds bacterial colonies and facilitates bacterial adhesion. The biofilm also protects bacteria from phagocytosis, host antibodies, and antibiotic effectiveness. Osteomyelitis is worsened by fracture instability. Continual motion impairs revascularization of spaces between fractured bone ends, which in turn prevents host defense mechanisms from gaining access to the area.

Mycotic bone infections are acquired through hematogenous dissemination of inhaled spores. Offending organisms are endemic in some geographic locations and include *Coccidioides immitis, Blastomyces dematiditis, Histoplasma capsulatum,* and *Cryptococcus neoformans.* Although viral osteomyelitis is thought to be uncommon, newer evidence suggests that some canine bone diseases may be viral in origin. Sequences of RNA homologous with canine distemper viral RNA have been detected in osteoblasts of dogs with metaphyseal osteopathy (hypertrophic osteopathy). It has also been suggested that panosteitis is associated with viral infections. Other causes of osteomyelitis include parasites, foreign bodies, and corrosion of metallic implants.

DIAGNOSIS

The diagnosis of osteomyelitis is often suspected based upon history, clinical signs, and radiographic findings.

Clinical Presentation

Signalment. Any age, breed, or sex of dog or cat may be affected.

History. Historical findings may include recent open reduction and stabilization of a fracture, bite wounds, open traumatic wounds, or habitation of an endemic fungal region.

Physical Examination Findings

Clinical features of osteomyelitis vary depending on stage of the disease. The initial response of bone to infection is inflammation; soft tissues in the area become hot, reddened, swollen, and painful (Fig. 32-14). The animal is often pyrexic, depressed, and partially or totally anorexic. Distinguishing between acute osteomyelitis and inflammation associated with surgical intervention is frequently difficult. Persistence of an elevated temperature for longer than 48 hours postoperatively or a neutrophilic left shift increases the likelihood that infection is present rather than only manifestations of surgically induced trauma. However, lack of either of these findings does not exclude the possibility of infection. Animals with chronic osteomyelitis usually present for evaluation of draining tracts and/or lameness; pyrexia, anorexia, and other clinical signs associated with systemic disease are frequently lacking. Accordingly, hematologic abnormalities are usually mild or absent.

Radiography

Specific radiographic findings vary depending on the stage of disease, site of infection, and pathogenicity of infective organism. Soft-tissue swelling is the first sign of acute osteomyelitis and may be observed as early as 24 hours postinfection. Radiographic changes in bone generally are not present before 2 weeks postinfection. Early radiographic bone changes include a periosteal shadow with deposition of new bone in a lamellar pattern oriented perpendicular to the long axis of the bone. Lamellated periosteal reactions are typically observed in association with osteomyelitis, whereas solid periosteal new bone formation is not typically associated with infection (Fig. 32-15). As the infection progresses, lysis of the medullary cavity becomes apparent. Sequestra may develop and as involucra (new bone formation around a sequestrum) form, sclerosis and lysis become interspersed throughout cortical and medullary bone at the site of infection. Radiographically, sequestered bone appears more dense than surrounding bone.

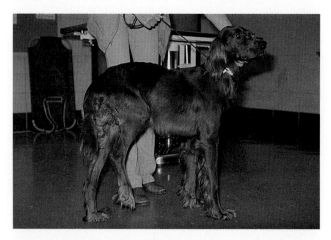

FIG. 32-14
A dog with femoral osteomyelitis. Note the draining tract on the caudolateral aspect of the thigh.

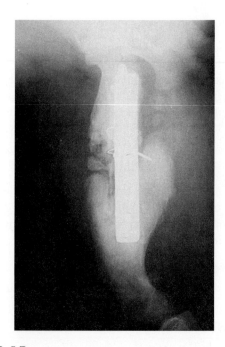

FIG. 32-15
Radiograph of a dog with acute osteomyelitis following open reduction and stabilization of a femoral fracture. Extensive periosteal reaction and involucrum formation are present.

Occasionally, when an animal presents with draining tracts and skeletal lesions that are not confluent, fistulography may be beneficial in confirming that the draining tracts lead to the bone lesion. Fistulography is performed by retrograde filling of each draining sinus with a water-soluble contrast agent. The concentration and volumes of contrast agents used varies; however, they should be diluted (approximately 25% to 60% is recommended) in order to not obscure identification of associated foreign bodies. Unfortunately, incomplete filling of sinuses and false-negative results are common.

Laboratory Findings

With acute osteomyelitis, systemic evidence of infection is often present and indicated by an elevated white blood cell count with a neutrophilic left shift. Results of laboratory analysis in dogs with chronic osteomyelitis are usually normal.

DIFFERENTIAL DIAGNOSIS

Microbiologic culturing is the definitive test for osteomyelitis and is essential in determining the organism('s) in vitro susceptibility to antimicrobial drugs. Sample collection of specimens for culture should not be obtained from draining tracts. Organisms cultured from draining tracts correlate with the pathogen isolated at surgery in fewer than 50% of patients. Preferably, aerobic and anaerobic cultures should be obtained from bone at the time of surgical intervention. Alternately, collection of culture samples via fine-needle aspiration of material directly surrounding the involved bones may be of value. In cases of suspected fungal osteomyelitis, fungal cultures, titers, and histologic evaluation of biopsies may be diagnostic.

☞ **N O T E** · Collect samples for bacterial culture from deep fine-needle aspirates. Do not culture draining tracts.

MEDICAL OR CONSERVATIVE MANAGEMENT

Medical management consisting of antibiotic therapy and application of warm packs may be effective in patients with hematogenous osteomyelitis or those having postoperative osteomyelitis. Medical therapy may be used when the affected area exhibits signs of inflammation but sequestra, necrotic tissue, or pockets of exudate should not be present. Additionally, if the patient has postoperative osteomyelitis, implant and bone stability must be present. Appropriate antibiotic therapy is determined by culture and sensitivity and is continued for a period of at least 28 days.

SURGICAL TREATMENT

If sequestra or pockets of exudate are present, drainage and debridement of necrotic tissue are necessary. The fracture must be stable and appropriate antimicrobial therapy should be instituted based upon culture and susceptibility testing. Treatment of chronic osteomyelitis entails maintaining or providing fracture stability, removal of loose implants and sequestered bone, cancellous bone grafting of bony deficits, and appropriate antimicrobial therapy.

Preoperative Management

In patients with acute osteomyelitis, antibiotic therapy should be initiated immediately with bactericidal agents that have a broad spectrum of activity against aerobic and anaerobic bacteria. Definitive antimicrobial therapy is determined through culture and susceptibility testing. Antimicrobial therapy of animals with chronic osteomyelitis is based upon culture and sensitivity testing of the offending organisms at surgery. Perioperative antibiotics should not be administered to these patients until intraoperative cultures have been obtained.

Anesthesia

Most animals with osteomyelitis are otherwise healthy and a variety of anesthetic regimens can be used (see p. 708). If preoperative blood work suggests organ dysfunction (i.e., renal, hepatic) refer to the appropriate chapter in this textbook for specific anesthetic recommendations.

Surgical Anatomy

Refer to the appropriate chapter for anatomy of the involved bone.

Positioning

Refer to the appropriate chapter for exposure of the bone involved.

SURGICAL TECHNIQUE
Acute Osteomyelitis

Open infected wounds and debride necrotic tissues. If a fracture is present, stabilize bone fragments with an appropriate implant system (bone plates and screws or external skeletal fixators are usually preferred).

☞ **N O T E** · Stabilization of fractures is the key to successful treatment of osteomyelitis. Bone union will occur in the presence of infection if fragments are stable.

If previous surgery was performed and the fracture remains stable, leave the original implants in place. If the implants have loosened, choose another fixation system to provide rigid fixation. Establish drainage by treating the surgical site as an open wound. Irrigate the wound with 0.05% chlorhexidine and then pack it with sterile gauze soaked with 0.05% chlorhexidine. Cover wounds with a sterile outer dressing that will absorb drainage products accumulated between bandage changes. Once the infection is eliminated, suture the wound.

Chronic Osteomyelitis

Determine the degree of fracture stability by palpation and radiographic assessment. If fractures and original implants are stable, leave them in place. However, if implants are loose and fractures have not healed, remove the loose implants and rigidly stabilize the fracture. Identify and remove sequestered bone through radiographic imaging and surgery. At surgery, sequestered bone is recognized by a yellowish discoloration and has no soft tissue attachments. Do not try to stabilize sequestered bone fragments; instead, remove them and place an autogenous cancellous bone graft in areas devoid of bone. Establish drainage as described above.

SUTURE MATERIALS/SPECIAL INSTRUMENTS

Aerobic and anaerobic culturettes should be available. Other instruments which are needed include those necessary for the insertion of the selected implant, bone curettes, self-retaining retractors, and a selection of absorbable suture material. Nonabsorbable suture material should generally be avoided in infected tissues.

POSTOPERATIVE CARE AND ASSESSMENT

In patients with acute osteomyelitis antibiotic therapy should be continued for 3 to 4 weeks. With chronic osteomyelitis, antibiotics should be administered for 4 to 6 weeks. If the wound is managed in an open fashion, the area should be irrigated with 0.05% dilute chlorhexidine twice daily and packed with a chlorhexidine-soaked sponge. Using umbilical tape secured to the skin on either side of the incision that can be tied over the gauze packing facilitates frequent changing of the packing materials. The limb should be bandaged until the wound is closed to decrease the likelihood of iatrogenic infection. If a fracture is present, postoperative care is dictated by the fracture configuration and stabilization procedure used. Generally, activity should be restricted to leash walks until the fracture has healed. Affected animals should be observed daily for signs of recurring fever, pain, swelling, and/or draining tracts.

PROGNOSIS

If all bone sequestra are removed and fractures are adequately stabilized, the prognosis for resolving infection and returning the patient to normal activity is good. Removal of all implants following bone union may be necessary to completely resolve the infection.

Suggested Reading

Bardett JF, Hohn RB, Basinger R: Open drainage and delayed autogenous cancellous bone grafting for treatment of chronic osteomyelitis in dogs and cats, *J Am Vet Med Assoc* 183:312, 1983.

Bissonnette KW: Modified Papineau technique for infected limb salvage cases, *Vet Surg* 19:58, 1990.

Budsberg SC, Kemp DT: Antimicrobial distribution and therapeutics in bone, *Compend Cont Educ Pract Vet* 12:1758, 1990.

Caywood DD, Wallace LJ, Braden TD: Osteomyelitis in the dog: a review of 67 cases, *J Am Vet Med Assoc* 172:943, 1978.

Fossum TW, Hulse DA: Osteomyelitis, *Semin Vet Med Surg Small Anim* 7:85, 1992.

Hodgin EC et al: Anaerobic bacterial infections causing osteomyelitis/arthritis in a dog, *J Am Vet Med Assoc* 201:886, 1992.

Johnson KA: Osteomyelitis in dogs and cats, *J Am Vet Med Assoc* 205:1882, 1994.

Lee AH et al: Wound healing over denuded bone, *J Am Anim Hosp Assoc* 23:75, 1987.

Lenehan TM, Smith GK: Management of infected tibial nonunions with sequestration in the dog, *Vet Surg* 13:115, 1984.

Rudd RG: A rational approach to the diagnosis and treatment of osteomyelitis, *Compend Cont Educ Pract Vet* 8:225, 1986.

Stead AC: Osteomyelitis in the dog and cat, *J Sm Anim Pract* 25:1, 1984.

Stevenson S, Olmstead ML, Kowalski J: Bacterial culturing for prediction of postoperative complications following open fracture repair in small animals, *Vet Surg* 15:99, 1986.

Varshney AC et al: Evaluation of therapeutic regimens in osteomyelitis: a clinical and radiological study in dogs, *Indian J Vet Surg* 10:107, 1989.

Walker RD et al: Anaerobic bacteria associated with osteomyelitis in domestic animals, *J Am Vet Med Assoc* 182:814, 1983.

CHAPTER 33

Fundamentals of Neurosurgery

GENERAL PRINCIPLES AND TECHNIQUES

DEFINITIONS

Neurology and neurosurgery have a unique set of terms, the definition of which may vary from one neurologist to another. It is important to establish consistent definitions to ensure accurate communication. **Plegia** and **paralysis** are a *complete* loss of sensory and motor function to the affected extremity, while **paresis** is *partial* loss of sensation, plus complete or partial loss of motor function to the affected extremity. Terms used to describe anatomic variations of affected extremities include **tetraparesis** (tetraplegia), all four limbs affected; **paraparesis** (paraplegia), both pelvic limbs affected; **hemiparesis** (hemiplegia), front and hind limbs on one side affected; and **monoparesis** (monoplegia), one limb affected.

PROBLEM IDENTIFICATION

A proper systematic examination of animals suspected of having neurologic disorders includes signalment, history, physical examination, and neurologic examination. Signalment (i.e., age, sex, breed, use of animal), correlated with anatomic localization of the lesion, often helps refine differential diagnoses and indicate appropriate diagnostic procedures.

Use the history to characterize the disorder as acute or chronic, progressive or static, and persistent or intermittent. Previous illnesses, vaccination history, and systems evaluation (i.e., gastrointestinal, cardiovascular, urogenital) should be considered. Owners should be questioned regarding behavioral changes, seizures, head tilt, circling, or other signs of cranial nerve abnormalities. Careful historical evaluation for the presence or absence of pain and/or paresis can assist in determining differential diagnoses (Table 33-1). If there is pain, determine its location (i.e., cervical, thoracolumbar, lumbosacral, extremity), duration (acute vs. chronic), progression (progressive vs. static), persistence (persistent vs. intermittent), and character (sharp vs. dull). It is also important to determine whether affected patients are mono-, para-, hemi-, or tetraparetic and whether the paresis is acute or chronic, progressive or static, and persistent or intermittent. Use of a graph illustrating the patterns of disease may be helpful when obtaining a history. Frequently, historical data suggest the lesion's location within the spinal canal (i.e., extradural, intradural-extramedullary, intramedullary). Typically, patients with extradural spinal lesions have an acute onset of persistent and sometimes progressive pain and paresis (Table 33-2). Patients with intradural-extramedullary spinal lesions generally have histories of chronic, dull pain with slowly progressive paresis. Those with intramedullary spinal lesions generally have an acute onset of sudden pain and paresis; the pain is short-lived and the paresis is persistent, but not progressive. These are general guidelines, but there are some cases that do not fit the classic pattern.

PHYSICAL EXAMINATION

A complete general physical examination should be performed in patients with possible neurologic disease. Some metabolic, cardiovascular, and musculoskeletal disorders mimic the clinical appearance of neurologic disorders (e.g., Addison's disease, toxic pyometra, cardiovascular insufficiency, bilateral cruciate ruptures). The animal should be observed as it moves around the exam room while obtaining the history from the owner. Visual difficulties may be more apparent when the animal is placed in new surroundings. Proprioceptive loss may also be evident, especially on a slippery floor. Purposeful movements should be noted; does the animal voluntarily try to move its legs? Certain components of the neurologic examination are included in a general physical examination, including mental status, gait, posture, evidence of trauma, facial expression, and breathing patterns. Movement of the traumatized patient should be minimized until the presence of a spinal fracture can be eliminated. A thorough physical examination may help establish the presence or absence of neurologic disease.

NEUROLOGIC EXAMINATION

The neurologic examination is an extension of the general physical examination and is performed after signalment,

TABLE 33-1

Etiology of Spinal Lesions Based on History of Pain and/or Paresis

Acute/Static	Acute/Progressive	Chronic/Progressive
Vascular	Degenerative	Degenerative
Fibrocartilaginous emboli	IVD—type I	IVD—type I and II
Infarction	Inflammatory	Cauda equina
Trauma	Diskospondylitis	Wobbler syndrome
Fracture/luxation	Vertebral osteomyelitis	Degenerative myelopathy
Degenerative	Trauma	Inflammatory
IVD—type I	Fracture/luxation	Diskospondylitis
	Anomalous	Vertebral osteomyelitis
	Atlantoaxial instability	Neoplastic
	Neoplastic	Meningeal tumors
	Spinal cord tumors	Spinal cord tumors
	Vertebral tumors	

TABLE 33-2

Etiology of Spinal Lesions Based on Lesion Location

Extradural	Intradural-Extramedullary	Intramedullary
Intervertebral disk extrusion	Meningeal neoplasia	Vascular insult
Vertebral fracture/luxation	Meningioma	Fibrocartilaginous embolus
Extradural neoplasia	Neurofibroma	Parenchymal neoplasia
Wobbler syndrome		
Atlantoaxial instability		
Diskospondylitis		
Vertebral osteomyelitis		

history, and a general physical examination have been completed. The neurologic examination should establish the presence of neurologic disease and determine its neuro-anatomic location. A consistent and methodical approach is necessary to prevent oversight of any abnormalities. A standardized neurologic examination form will keep the examination consistent. Serial neurologic examinations are used to assess patient status (i.e., improving, static, deteriorating). The neurologic examination should be performed in a distraction-free area with good footing. Sedatives, narcotics, and/or tranquilizers should not be administered prior to examination. However, it is important that the animal be relaxed. Begin the examination by evaluating the patient's mental status, posture, and gait.

Mental status. Allow the animal to move round the examination room. Mental status may be defined as (1) alert (normal); (2) depressed (conscious, but inactive); (3) unresponsive to environment; (4) stuporous (sleeps when undisturbed; will not respond to harmless stimuli such as noise but will awaken with a painful stimulus); or (5) comatose (cannot be aroused, even with painful stimulus).

Animals with brain lesions that are unresponsive to their environment usually have diffuse cerebral cortical disease. Those that are stuporous generally have diffuse cerebral disorders or brain stem compression, while comatose animals have complete disconnection of the reticular formation and cerebral cortex.

Posture. Posture is evaluated while the animal is free to move about the exam area and can be further assessed by moving the animal into different positions to observe its ability to regain normal posture. Abnormalities include head tilt, abnormal truncal posture, improper positioning of limbs (proprioceptive deficits), decreased muscle tone in a limb (flaccidity), or increased muscle tone (spasticity). Continuous head tilts are often associated with vestibular abnormalities. Abnormal truncal posture may be associated with congenital or acquired spinal cord lesions.

Gait. Evaluation of an animal's gait requires an area with good footing. The animal is observed from the side, moving toward and away from the examiner, in tight circles, and backing up. Neurologic organization of gait and posture is complicated, involving brain, spinal cord, and peripheral nerves. Proprioception (position sense) is the ability to recognize the location of the limbs in relation to the rest of the body. Deficits cause knuckling, misplacement of the foot, and/or scuffing of the toenails and may be associated with lesions at any level of the spinal cord. Paresis is a deficit of voluntary movements; it can be monoparesis, paraparesis, tetraparesis, or hemiparesis (see above). It is caused by disruption of the voluntary motor pathways, which extend from the cerebral cortex through the brain stem and out to the peripheral nerves. Circling in tight circles is usually caused by caudal brain stem lesions; head tilt in association with circling usually indicates involvement of the vestibular system. Ataxia is lack of coordination without paretic, spastic, or involuntary movements (although these may be seen in association with ataxia). Ataxia can be caused by lesions at any level, but usually involves cerebellar, vestibular, or spinal cord lesions. Dysmetria is characterized by movements that are too long (hypermetria) or too short (hypometria) and are usually caused by cerebellar lesions.

Palpation. Careful palpation of the musculoskeletal and integumentary systems while comparing one side with the other is done to check for symmetry. Examiners should look for worn toenails, deep and cutaneous masses, deviation of normal contour, abnormal motion, or crepitation, and also evaluate muscular size, tone, and strength.

Postural Reactions

Postural reactions are complex responses that maintain an animal's normal upright position. Abnormal postural reactions do not provide precise localizing information, but may indicate neurologic disease.

Proprioceptive positioning. Proprioceptive positioning (knuckling) is performed by flexing the paw so the dorsal surface is on the floor (Fig. 33-1). The animal should immediately return the paw to a normal position. Delayed or absent correction of the knuckled paw indicates neurologic disease. Worn dorsal toenails, skin abrasions, or calluses on the dorsum of the foot may signify long-standing proprioceptive deficits.

Purposeful movement. Purposeful movement is an animal's conscious attempt to move the legs. It is most applicable to weakly ambulatory and nonambulatory animals that drag their legs as they pull themselves along. The legs should be watched for movement, including hip flexion and pushing off with the feet. Assessment of purposeful movements in nonambulatory paraparetic animals can be done by grasping the base of the tail with one hand, lifting the animal, and walking it around. If the legs hang down, purposeful movements are not present, which implies severe—but not necessarily irreversible—spinal cord injury.

Wheelbarrowing. Wheelbarrowing is performed by having the animal bear weight on the thoracic limbs while it is being supported under the abdomen. Normal animals walk forward with coordinated movements of both thoracic limbs. Slow initiation of movement may be due to a cervical spinal cord, brain stem, or cerebral cortical lesion. Exaggerated movements (dysmetria) may indicate cervical spinal cord, lower brain stem, or cerebellar abnormalities.

Hopping. Hopping is tested with the animal positioned as for wheelbarrowing, except one thoracic or pelvic limb is lifted from the ground. The entire weight of the animal is supported on one limb as the patient is moved medially and laterally (Fig. 33-2). Poor initiation of hopping suggests proprioceptive deficits, whereas poor movement suggests motor deficits. Asymmetry may help lateralize a lesion. Generally, testing thoracic limbs yields more reliable information than pelvic limbs.

Extensor postural thrust. Extensor postural thrust is performed by supporting the animal under the thorax while lowering it to the floor. When the pelvic limbs touch the floor they should move caudally in symmetric walking movements to achieve a position of support. Patient assessment is the same as for wheelbarrowing.

Hemistanding/Hemiwalking. Hemistanding and hemiwalking are performed by elevating the front and rear limbs of one side so that all the animal's weight is supported

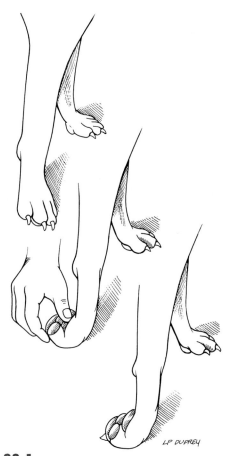

FIG. 33-1
Proprioceptive positioning—the animal should return the paw to a normal position.

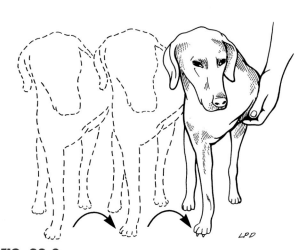

FIG. 33-2
The hopping postural reaction.

by the opposite limbs. Lateral walking movements are then evaluated. Patient assessment is the same as for wheelbarrowing.

Placing. Placing reactions are evaluated first without vision (tactile placing) and then with vision (visual placing). During tactile placing, the examiner supports the animal under the thorax and covers its eyes with one hand. The distal thoracic limbs (at or below the carpi) are brought in contact with the edge of a table. The normal response is immediate placement of the feet on the table surface in a position that will support weight. Visual placing is tested by allowing the animal to see the table surface. Normal animals reach for the surface before the carpus touches the table. Visual placing requires normal visual pathways to the cerebral cortex, communication from the visual cortex to the motor cortex, and motor pathways to the forelimb peripheral nerves. A lesion of any portion of the pathway may cause a deficit in the placing reaction. Normal tactile placing with absent visual placing indicates a lesion in the visual system, whereas normal visual placing with abnormal tactile placing suggests a sensory pathway lesion. Cortical lesions produce a deficit in the contralateral (opposite) limb. Lesions below the midbrain usually produce an ipsilateral (same side as lesion) deficit.

Spinal Reflexes

Spinal reflexes (myotactic reflexes) test the integrity of sensory and motor components of the reflex arc and the influence of descending motor pathways on the reflex. Three kinds of responses may be seen: (1) absence or depressed reflex, indicating complete or partial loss of either the sensory or motor nerves responsible for the reflex (lower motor neuron); (2) normal reflex, indicating sensory and motor nerves are intact; and (3) exaggerated reflex, indicating an abnormality in the descending pathways from the brain and spinal cord that normally inhibit the reflex (upper motor neuron).

A list of lower motor neuron (LMN) and upper motor neuron (UMN) signs is given in Table 33-3. In general, the thoracic limb has fewer reliable localizing spinal reflexes than the pelvic limb.

Pelvic limb
Patellar reflex. Patellar reflex (Table 33-4) is the most reliable pelvic limb reflex. It is performed with the animal in lateral recumbency. The uppermost leg is supported by the hock, with the stifle slightly flexed. When the straight patellar ligament is struck briskly with a reflex hammer (Fig. 33-3), the response is a single, quick extension of the stifle. Absence or depression of the patellar reflex (hypopatellar reflex) and decreased muscle tone (flaccidity) indicate a lesion of the sensory or motor component of the reflex arc (LMN). Unilateral loss of the reflex suggests a femoral nerve lesion, while bilateral loss suggests a segmental spinal cord lesion involving spinal cord segments L4-L6. Exaggerated reflexes (hyperpatellar reflex) and increased muscle tone (spasticity) suggest a lesion cranial to the L4 spinal cord segment (UMN).

Withdrawal reflex. Pelvic limb withdrawal reflex (see Table 33-4) is performed with the animal in lateral recumbency. The least harmful stimulus possible is applied to the foot; the normal response is flexion of the entire limb (Fig. 33-4). This reflex primarily involves spinal cord segments L6-S1 and the sciatic nerve. Absence or depression of the reflex indicates lesion of these spinal cord segments or nerves (LMN). Unilateral absence of the reflex is most likely the result of a peripheral nerve lesion, whereas bilateral absence or depression is more likely the result of a spinal cord lesion. An exaggerated withdrawal reflex indicates a lesion cranial to spinal cord segment L6 (UMN).

Thoracic limb
Triceps reflex. Triceps reflex (see Table 33-4) is performed with the animal in lateral recumbency. The limb is supported under the elbow; flexion of the elbow and carpus

---

TABLE 33-3

Comparison of Common Neurologic Findings in UMN and LMN Disease

Spinal Reflexes	LMN	UMN
Patellar	Absent or depressed	Normal or exaggerated
Triceps	Absent or depressed	Normal or exaggerated
Biceps	Absent or depressed	Normal or exaggerated
Pelvic limb withdrawal	Absent or depressed	Normal or exaggerated
Thoracic limb withdrawal	Absent or depressed	Normal or exaggerated
Crossed extensor	Absent or depressed	Normal or exaggerated
Anal sphincter	Absent or depressed	Normal or exaggerated
Tail wagging	Absent or depressed	Normal or exaggerated
Strength	Poor	Variable but stronger than with LMN
Muscle tone	Flaccid	Spastic
Muscle fasciculation	Present	Absent
Muscle atrophy	Early, neurogenic	Late, disuse
Clonus	Absent	Present
Bladder expression	Easy	Difficult
Root signature	Present	Absent

TABLE 33-4
Spinal Reflexes

Patellar reflex
- Absent or depressed reflex
  Unilateral—femoral nerve
  Bilateral—lesion at spinal cord segments L4-L6
- Exaggerated reflex
  Bilateral—lesion cranial to spinal cord segment L4

Withdrawal reflex—pelvic limb
- Absent or depressed reflex
  Unilateral—sciatic nerve
  Bilateral—lesion at spinal cord segments L6-S1
- Exaggerated reflex
  Bilateral—lesion cranial to spinal cord segment L6

Triceps reflex
- Absent or depressed reflex
  Lesion in spinal cord segments C7-T1
  Not always reliable
- Exaggerated reflex
  Bilateral—lesion cranial to spinal cord segment C7

Biceps reflex
- Absent or depressed reflex
  Lesion in spinal cord segments C6-C8
  Not always reliable
- Exaggerated reflex
  Bilateral—lesion cranial to spinal cord segment C8

Withdrawal reflex—thoracic limb
- Absent or depressed reflex
  Lesion in spinal cord segments C6-T1
- Exaggerated reflex
  Unilateral—peripheral nerves
  Bilateral—lesion cranial to spinal cord segment C6

Anal sphincter reflex
- Absent or depressed reflex
  Lesion in spinal cord segments S1-S3
- Normal or exaggerated reflex
  Lesion cranial to spinal cord segment S1

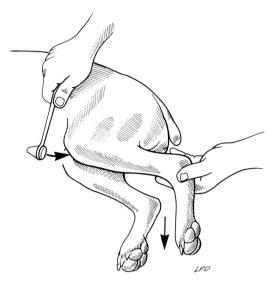

FIG. 33-3
The patellar reflex is initiated by striking the straight patellar ligament with a reflex hammer.

Withdrawal reflex. Thoracic limb withdrawal reflex (see Table 33-4) is performed in a similar manner as the pelvic limb withdrawal reflex. This reflex primarily involves spinal cord segments C6-T1. Absent or depressed reflexes indicate a lesion of these spinal cord segments or of the peripheral nerves (LMN). Exaggerated reflexes indicate a lesion cranial to spinal cord segment C6 (UMN).

Other reflexes
Anal sphincter reflex. The perineal or anal sphincter reflex (see Table 33-4) is elicited by gentle perineal stimulation with a needle or forceps. A normal response is contraction of the anal sphincter muscle. Sensory and motor innervation occurs through the pudendal nerve and spinal cord segments S1 to S3. The anal sphincter reflex is the best indication of functional integrity of sacral spinal cord segments and sacral nerve roots. Evaluation of this reflex is important in animals with urinary bladder dysfunction. It may be absent, depressed, or normal. Absence or depression of the reflex (failure of the anus to contract or dilate) indicates a sacral spinal cord or pudendal nerve lesion (LMN).

Bladder expression. The two general components of urinary bladder innervation are autonomic (hypogastric and pelvic) and somatic (pudendal) nerves. Simplistically, clinical observations of bladder dysfunction can be attributed to spinal cord injury based on the pudendal nerve (S2-3). The pudendal nerve innervates urethral striated muscle and helps maintain urinary continence. A lesion above the S2-3 spinal cord segments causes spasm of bladder outflow, making the bladder difficult to express (UMN). A lesion involving S2-3 spinal cord segments causes lack of sphincter tone and an easily expressible bladder (LMN).

Crossed extensor reflex. The crossed extensor reflex may be observed when withdrawal reflexes are elicited. With the animal in lateral recumbency and legs relaxed, the toes of

is maintained. The triceps tendon is struck with a reflex hammer just proximal to the olecranon (Fig. 33-5). Normal response is slight extension of the elbow. The triceps muscle is innervated by the radial nerve, which originates from spinal cord segments C7-T1. The triceps reflex is difficult to elicit in normal animals; thus absent or depressed reflexes may not indicate an abnormality. However, an exaggerated reflex indicates a lesion cranial to C7 (UMN).

Biceps reflex. To perform the biceps reflex (see Table 33-4), the index finger of the examiner's hand that is holding the animal's elbow is placed on the biceps tendon cranial and proximal to the elbow. The elbow is slightly extended and the finger is struck with the reflex hammer. Normal response is slight flexion of the elbow. This reflex is difficult to elicit in the normal animal. Absent or decreased reflexes suggest a lesion involving spinal cord segments C6-T8 (LMN), but may be normal in some animals. An exaggerated reflex indicates a lesion cranial to spinal cord segment C6 (UMN).

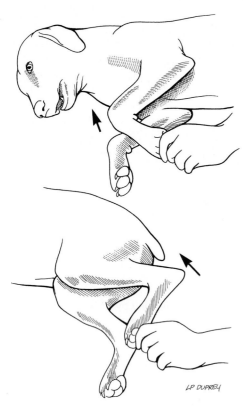

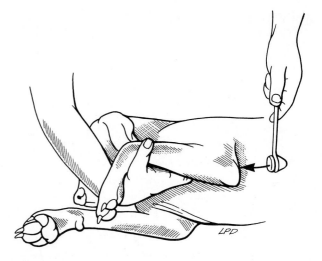

FIG. 33-5
The triceps reflex is initiated by striking the triceps tendon just proximal to the olecranon.

FIG. 33-4
The withdrawal reflex (thoracic and pelvic limbs) occurs when a noxious stimuli is applied to the foot. The entire limb should flex.

the down limb (thoracic or pelvic) are gently pinched, eliciting a withdrawal reflex (Fig. 33-6). An abnormal response is extension of the upper limb. The stimulus must be gentle; excessive stimulus causes the animal to attempt to right itself, negating any findings. The crossed extensor reflex results from a lesion that affects descending inhibitory pathways of the spinal cord (UMN). This reflex is frequently associated with severity or chronicity, but does not constitute a poor prognosis.

Tail wag reflex. The significance of tail wagging in patients with spinal cord injuries is often misinterpreted. Animals with a completely transected spinal cord above the sacral and caudal spinal cord segments *can* wag their tails. This *reflex wag* is often observed when expressing the bladder or eliciting the anal sphincter reflex. Tail wagging may also be a conscious response to pleasurable stimuli such as petting the head, calling the animal's name, or seeing the owner. This conscious response implies that some spinal cord pathways are intact. It is important to distinguish between spontaneous (reflex) and conscious tail wagging.

Panniculus reflex. Panniculus reflex (cutaneous trunci reflex) is elicited by pinprick stimulus to the skin over the back, beginning in the region of the fifth lumbar vertebra and continuing cranially. Normal response is twitching of the cutaneous trunci muscle on both sides of the dorsal midline, at the point of stimulation and cranial. Absence of a re-

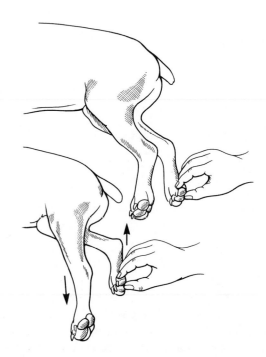

FIG. 33-6
A crossed extensor reflex suggests a lesion afflicting descending inhibitory pathways of the spinal cord (UMN).

sponse occurs one or two segments caudal to the spinal cord lesion. This reflex must be interpreted with some caution; it may be unreliable with the exception of brachial plexus avulsion injuries, where it is consistently absent only on the side of the avulsion (ipsilateral).

Clonus. Clonus refers to a sustained after-contraction or quivering that may be seen or felt when performing spinal reflexes, especially patellar and crossed extensor reflexes. The hand supporting the extremity being tested may feel this reaction; this reflex is often not visual. Presence of clonus implies a chronic condition.

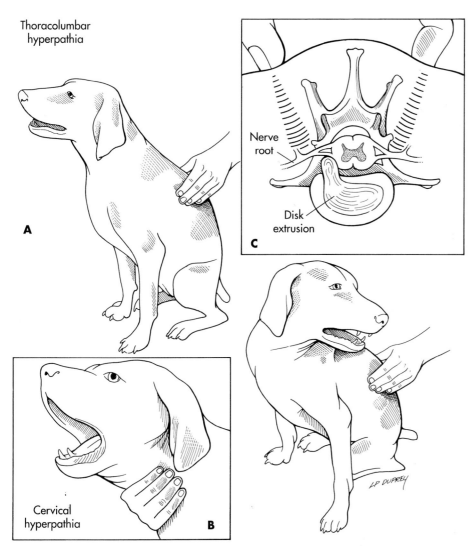

Thoracolumbar hyperpathia

Nerve root

Disk extrusion

Cervical hyperpathia

A

B

C

LP DUPREY

FIG. 33-7
Thoracolumbar and cervical hyperpathia; digital pressure placed over the, **A,** thoracolumbar paraspinal or, **B,** cervical paraspinal muscles at the site of an extradural lesion results in pain and a behavioral response from the patient. **C,** Pressure placed on epaxial muscles is transferred to the entrapped nerve root, causing nerve root compression and ischemia; the result is pain and a behavioral response.

Sensory Evaluation

Presence or absence of deep pain perception is the most important prognostic test of the neurologic examination, and is a reliable indicator of spinal cord integrity. As a general rule, sensory evaluation should be done *last*. It is performed by applying painful stimuli to each limb and the tail. A significant *behavioral response* (e.g., animal attempts to vocalize, turns to look or bite, or attempts to get away from the examiner) indicates the presence of sensation. **Withdrawal of a limb is *not* a behavioral response.** Progressively stronger painful stimuli (e.g., hemostatic forceps) are used to assess presence or absence of deep pain perception. As a general rule, loss of function after spinal cord injury develops as follows: (1) loss of proprioception, (2) loss of voluntary motor function, (3) loss of superficial pain sensation, and (4) loss of deep pain sensation. Therefore, an animal with spinal cord compression that has lost proprioception and voluntary motor function, but still has superficial and deep pain sensation (paresis) has less severe spinal cord damage than one that has lost all four functions (plegia, paralysis). Loss of deep pain indicates a severely damaged spinal cord and a poor prognosis. As an animal recovers from spinal cord injury, sensation returns first, followed by motor function and lastly proprioception. Because of the prognostic importance of sensory examination, an evaluation of the animal by a second, unbiased examiner or a repeat of the examination in 1 or 2 hours is critical.

Hyperpathia. Hyperpathia is noted when pressure applied to spinous processes and paraspinal muscles of the thoracic and lumbar region and transverse processes and paraspinal muscles of the cervical region results in pain and a *behavioral response* (see above)(Fig. 33-7). Pain perception occurs at the level of spinal cord involvement, making hyperpathia an accurate localizing feature of the neurologic examination.

Sensory level. Sensory level is determined by pinprick stimulus applied to the skin over the back, beginning in the region of the 7th lumbar vertebrae and continuing cranially. The junction between an area of depressed *behavioral response* and one of normal *behavioral response* is the sensory level (Fig. 33-8). Pain perception occurs one or two segments caudal to the level of spinal cord involvement.

FIG. 33-8
A, Sensory level is the junction between an area of depressed or absent sensation and area of normal sensation. **B,** Because thoracolumbar nerve roots course caudoventrally, the sensory level is one or two vertebral bodies caudal to the spinal cord lesion.

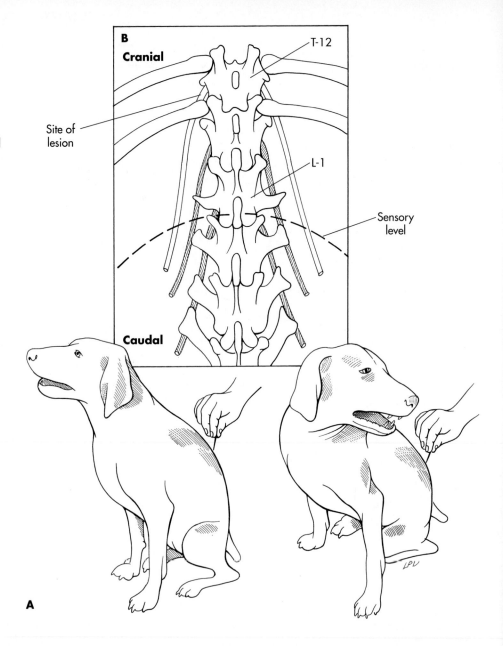

Cranial Nerve Examination

Examination of cranial nerves is important, especially when a brain lesion is suspected.

Olfactory nerve. The olfactory nerve is sensory for conscious perception of smell. Rhinitis, tumors of the nasal passages, and diseases of the cribriform plate are the most common causes for loss of olfaction.

Optic nerve. The optic nerve is the sensory pathway for vision and pupillary light reflexes. It is examined by means of three major tests: menace response (elicited by making a threatening gesture with the hand at each eye); visual placing reaction (see p. 1034); and ophthalmoscopic examination. Abnormalities include loss of vision, dilated pupils, and loss of pupillary light response (direct and consensual) when light is shined in the affected eye.

Oculomotor nerve. The oculomotor nerve contains parasympathetic motor fibers for pupillary constriction. It is motor to the extraocular eye muscles and levator muscle of the upper eyelid. After shining a light into each eye, pupils are observed for size and symmetry. Both pupils should constrict symmetrically when a light is shined into either eye (consensual response). Abnormalities include loss of pupillary light response on the affected side (even if light is shined in the opposite eye), fixed lateral deviation (strabismus) of the eye, and dilated pupil.

Trochlear nerve. Lesions of the trochlear nerve cause lateral rotation of the eye.

Abducent nerve. Lesions of the abducent nerve cause medial strabismus, loss of gaze, and inability to retract the globe.

Trigeminal nerve. The trigeminal nerve innervates muscles of mastication and is sensory to the face. Motor function is tested by assessing muscle mass and jaw tone of the masticatory muscles. Sensory function is assessed by checking pain perception of the face, eyelids, cornea, and nasal mucosa. Bilateral motor paralysis produces a "dropped jaw" and muscle atrophy; unilateral paralysis results in decreased jaw tone and strength.

Facial nerve. The facial nerve is motor to the muscles of facial expression and sensory to the palate and rostral two thirds of the tongue. Facial paralysis generally causes facial asymmetry (e.g., lips, eyelids, and ears may droop) and loss of ability to blink or retract the lips.

Vestibulocochlear nerve. The vestibulocochlear nerve has two divisions: vestibular (which provides information about the orientation of the head with respect to gravity) and cochlear (which means hearing). Abnormalities associated with nerve dysfunction include ataxia, head tilt, circling, nystagmus, and loss of hearing.

Glossopharyngeal and vagus nerves. Swallowing is controlled by glossopharyngeal and vagus nerves. The swallowing reflex is elicited by gentle external pressure on the hyoid region. The gag reflex is elicited by insertion of the finger into the caudal pharynx. The glossopharyngeal nerve is motor to pharyngeal muscles, and the vagus nerve is motor to pharyngeal and laryngeal muscles. The vagus nerve is sensory to the caudal pharynx and larynx. Abnormalities caused by glossopharyngeal and vagus nerve dysfunction include loss of the gag reflex, dysphagia, and laryngeal paralysis.

Hypoglossal nerve. The hypoglossal nerve is motor to muscles of the tongue. Abnormalities can be observed by wetting the animal's nose and observing its ability to extend the tongue. Strength of tongue retraction, tongue deviation, and presence or absence of atrophy should be evaluated.

LESION LOCALIZATION

Once the neurologic examination has been completed, an attempt is made to determine a single neuroanatomic location that explains all abnormal findings. The lesion is initially categorized as being located above or below the foramen magnum. Lesions suspected of being above the foramen magnum are further localized to one of five locations in the brain: cerebral cortex, diencephalon (thalamus and hypothalamus), brain stem (pons, medulla oblongata), vestibular, or cerebellum. Table 33-5 lists characteristic abnormal neurologic findings that aid in localizing brain lesions.

Lesions suspected of being below the foramen magnum are further localized to one of five locations in the spinal cord: cranial cervical (C1-C5), caudal cervical (C6-T2), thoracolumbar (T3-L3), lumbosacral (L4-S3). and sacral (S1-S3) (Fig. 33-9). The ability to predict the expected UMN and/or LMN signs with lesions at various levels of the spinal cord improves accurate lesion localization. This may be confusing, however, because a single spinal lesion can be LMN and UMN to various nerve and muscle groups simultaneously. Fig. 33-9 illustrates locations of various spinal cord injuries, and the expected UMN and LMN reactions to the front and hind limbs. In the unusual circumstance that an animal has two spinal cord lesions, it

TABLE 33-5
Abnormal Neurologic Findings that Help Localize Brain Lesions

Cerebral cortex

Altered mental status
Ipsilateral circling, pacing, head pressing
Contralateral postural and proprioceptive deficits
Contralateral cortical blindness (normal pupils and pupillary light reflexes)
Contralateral UMN hemiparesis
Seizures

Diencephalon (thalamus and hypothalamus)

Altered mental status: aggression, disorientation, hyperexcitability, coma
Contralateral postural and proprioceptive deficits
Bilateral visual deficits
Abnormalities of eating, drinking, sleeping, and temperature (hypothalamus)
Muscle tone, segmental reflexes, and sensation are unaltered

Brain stem (pontomedullary)

Mental status may be unaltered, to severe depression and coma
Ipsilateral UMN hemiparesis or tetraparesis; may circle if ambulatory
Cranial nerve deficits involving cranial nerves V through XII
  Trigeminal—motor and sensory
  Abducent—medial strabismus
  Facial—facial paralysis
  Vestibulocochlear—central vestibular signs; hearing loss
  Glossopharyngeal/vagus—dysphagia, reduced gag reflex, laryngeal dysfunction
  Hypoglossal—abnormal tongue movement

Vestibular

Disoriented or unaltered mental status
Ipsilateral head tilt, circling, rolling, falling, asymmetric ataxia, incoordination
Nystagmus (spontaneous or positional) with fast phase away from the side of the lesion
Ipsilateral ventrolateral strabismus
Must differentiate central from peripheral vestibular disease

Cerebellum

Unaltered mental status
Ataxic gait, wide-based stance, dysmetria, head tremor, intention tremor, truncal ataxia
Visual but may have ipsilateral loss of menace response
Hypermetric postural reactions, goose stepping gait
Muscle tone, segmental reflexes, and sensation are unaltered

is important to predict the expected UMN and LMN signs. Notice also that if an animal has both an UMN and a LMN lesion to a specific site (e.g., sites 3 and 4, Fig. 33-9), LMN reflex changes predominate. Lesion localization of spinal cord disorders based on neurologic examination findings should not be limited to spinal cord segments (within the spinal canal). It is important to be able to localize spinal cord segment abnormalities within a vertebral body (Table 33-6 and Fig. 33-10). Once the neuroanatomic location of the lesion has been identified and signalment, history, and physical examination findings reviewed, differential diagnoses and appropriate diagnostic plans can be formulated.

DIFFERENTIAL DIAGNOSIS OF SPINAL DISORDERS AND DIAGNOSTIC METHODS

Establishing a list of differential diagnoses requires incorporation of historical as well as physical and neurologic examination findings. The minimum data required for a diagnostic plan includes hematology, serum chemistry, and urinalysis. These data may vary depending on a differential diagnosis including an electrocardiogram, echocardiogram, additional laboratory data, and/or chest and abdominal radiographs. Patients suspected of having an intracranial lesion may require additional serum chemistry

TABLE 33-6

Location of Spinal Cord Segments Within Vertebral Bodies

General Location	Spinal Cord Segments	Vertebral bodies
Craniocervical	C1-C5	C1-C4
Caudocervical	C6-T2	C5-T1
Thoracolumbar	T3-L3	T2-L3
Lumbosacral	L4-S3	L4-L6
Sacral	S1-S3	L5
	L4	L3-4 interspace
	L5-L6	L4
	L7	L4-5 interspace
Spinal cord ends		L5-6 interspace

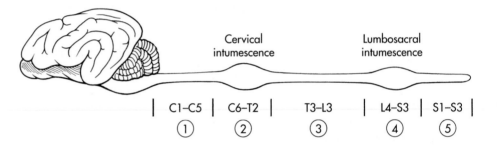

Site number	Spinal cord segments	Expected neurologic response
1 craniocervical	C1-C5:	UMN to the front limbs UMN to the rear limbs
2 caudocervical	C6-T2:	LMN to the front limbs UMN to the rear limbs
3 thoracolumbar	T3-L3:	Normal to the front limbs UMN to the rear limbs
4 lumbosacral	L4-S3:	Normal to the front limbs LMN to the rear limbs
5 sacral	S1-S3:	Normal to the front limbs Normal to the rear limbs LMN to the tail and anus

The expected reflex response to multiple lesions of the spinal cord

Lesion location	Expected neurologic response
Site 1 and 2	LMN front; UMN rear
Site 1 and 3	UMN front; UMN rear
Site 1 and 4	UMN front; LMN rear
Site 1 and 5	UMN front; UMN rear; LMN tail and anus
Site 2 and 3	LMN front; UMN rear
Site 2 and 4	LMN front; LMN rear
Site 2 and 5	LMN front; UMN rear; LMN tail and anus
Site 3 and 4	LMN rear; UMN tail and anus
Site 3 and 5	UMN rear; LMN tail and anus
Site 4 and 5	LMN rear; LMN tail and anus

FIG. 33-9
Expected UMN and LMN reflex abnormalities caused by lesions located in various segments of the spinal cord.

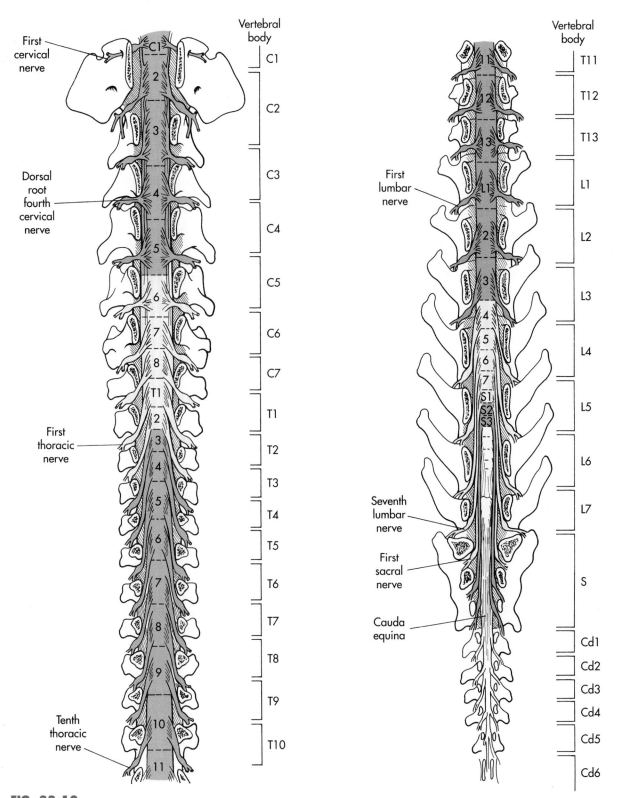

First cervical nerve

Dorsal root fourth cervical nerve

First thoracic nerve

Tenth thoracic nerve

First lumbar nerve

Seventh lumbar nerve

First sacral nerve

Cauda equina

Vertebral body

C1
C2
C3
C4
C5
C6
C7
T1
T2
T3
T4
T5
T6
T7
T8
T9
T10

Vertebral body

T11
T12
T13
L1
L2
L3
L4
L5
L6
L7
S
Cd1
Cd2
Cd3
Cd4
Cd5
Cd6

FIG. 33-10
Laminectomized spine showing the relationship of spinal cord segments with vertebral bodies. (Modified from Evans HE, editor: *Miller's anatomy of the dog,* ed 3, Philadelphia, 1993, WB Saunders.)

tests, cerebral spinal fluid analysis, electroencephalography, skull radiographs, computed tomography (CT scan), and/or magnetic resonance imaging (MRI). Those suspected of having a spinal lesion may require a spinal series of survey radiographs, myelography, electromyography, CT scan, and/or MRI. These diagnostic tests should localize an intracranial or spinal lesion (extradural, intradural-extramedullary, or intramedullary), help determine the most effective treatment (medical or surgical), and may suggest an etiology (Tables 33-2 and 33-7). The selection of diagnostic tests depends upon historical data (i.e., pattern of disease progression: acute/static, acute/progressive, chronic/progressive), neurologic examination findings (i.e., lesion located above or below the foramen magnum), and initial minimum data.

IMAGING THE SPINE

Accurate localization of most spinal disorders can be accomplished with conventional radiographs (spinal radiographs and myelography). The spinal cord, surrounded by CSF, is encased in an osseous spine composed of individual vertebrae connected by complex ligamentous structures (i.e., annulus fibrosus, nucleus pulposus, and diarthrodial facet joints). Each section of the spine (i.e., cervical, thoracic, lumbar, sacral, and coccygeal) is anatomically unique. The complexity of the spine demands that careful attention be given to proper radiographic technique, positioning, and interpretation. When spinal radiographs are taken, the following

---

TABLE 33-7

Differential Diagnosis of Spinal Cord Disorders Based on DAMNIT-V Scheme

D—Degenerative

Intervertebral disk disease
Wobbler syndrome
Cauda equina syndrome
Degenerative myelopathy

A—Anomalous

Atlantoaxial instability

M—Metabolic

N—Neoplastic

Spine
Spinal cord
Meninges

I—Inflammatory/Infections

Diskospondylitis
Vertebral osteomyelitis

T—Traumatic

Vertebral fracture/luxation

V—Vascular

Fibrocartilaginous embolism
Spinal cord infarction

---

guidelines should be followed: (1) general anesthesia should be used; (2) symmetric positioning with care to support the spine during repositioning is required; (3) lateral and ventrodorsal projections of each section of the spine should be obtained; (4) high-quality radiographic film should be used; (5) each section of the spine should be radiographed separately; and (6) high-contrast radiographic technique (less than 60 kVp) with narrow collimation is necessary. Knowledge of normal anatomic variations for each section of the spine is mandatory and accurate interpretation must be based on minimum data, historical, physical, and neurologic examination findings.

Survey Radiographs

Survey radiographs allow accurate lesion localization if vertebrae or their ligamentous attachments are directly involved (i.e. congenital anomalies, vertebral fracture/luxation, vertebral body neoplasia, diskospondylitis, vertebral body osteomyelitis, extruded calcified intervertebral disk). Radiographic signs of spinal disease consist of changes in shape, size, alignment, and density (Fig. 33-11). Survey radiographs do not allow direct view of the spinal cord. Lesion localization in patients with spinal disorders that do not cause visible changes in the vertebrae (i.e., fibrocartilaginous emboli, neoplasia of the spinal cord or meninges, intervertebral disk extrusion, cauda equina syndrome, wobbler syndrome) requires myelography, CT scan, or MRI.

Stress Radiography

Stress radiography may be used in the definitive diagnosis of spinal disorders. It is performed by placing various sections of the vertebral column in gentle dorsal hyperextension, ventral flexion, and/or linear traction. The end result is to exacerbate or relieve compressive lesions. This information may be important in establishing lesion location and planning therapy. Stress radiography is most commonly used in the diagnosis of atlantoaxial instability (Fig. 33-12), cervical vertebral instability, and lumbosacral instability. **Perform stress radiography carefully, so as not to exacerbate the patient's neurologic deficits.**

Myelography

Myelography requires subarachnoid injection of contrast media (lumbar or cisternal) to outline the spinal cord. It is indicated when (1) a visible lesion is not identified on survey radiographs; (2) multiple lesions compatible with the neurologic examination are observed; or (3) a lesion is visualized that is not compatible with the neurologic examination. Contrast agents used in myelographic procedures should be radiopaque, water soluble, miscible with CSF, nontoxic, and rapidly absorbed from the subarachnoid space. The most commonly used myelographic contrast agents are iopamidol (Isovue) and iohexol (Omnipaque). Appropriate doses and concentrations for each contrast agent are given in Table 33-8. Myelography is performed with the patient under general anesthesia. Lumbar (L4-5 or L5-6) or cisternal puncture can be performed; advantages

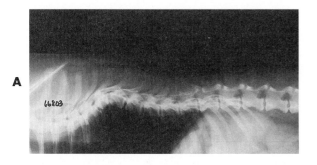
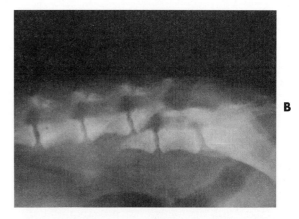
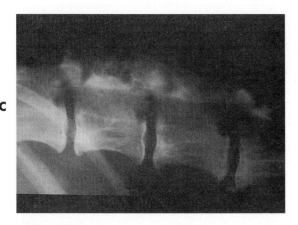
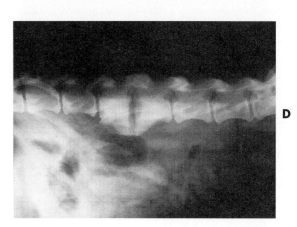

FIG. 33-11
A, Lateral radiography of a dog with a T6-T7 congenital malformation. Notice the elongated dorsal spinous processes, collapse of the intervertebral space, and narrowing of the spinal canal. **B,** Lateral radiograph of a dog with an L6 spinal fracture. Notice the oblique vertebral body and laminar fracture with cranial displacement and overriding. **C,** Lateral radiograph of a dog with L2 laminar neoplasia. Notice the osteoproduction of the dorsal lamina. **D,** Lateral radiograph of a dog with L3-L4 diskospondylitis. Notice the lysis of the vertebral endplates, spondylosis, and increased bone density of the L3 and L4 vertebral body.

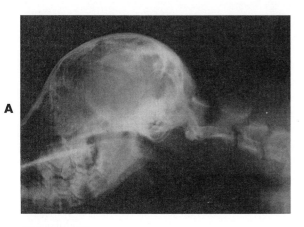
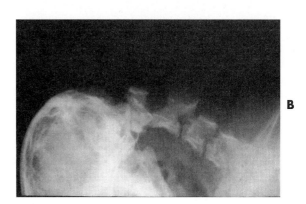

FIG. 33-12
A, Radiograph of a dog with atlantoaxial instability. The head and neck are in normal functional position. **B,** Ventral flexion of the head and neck reveals an increased space between dorsal lamina of C1 and dorsal spinous process of C2, indicating instability.

TABLE 33-8

Contrast Agents Commonly Used in Myelography

Contrast Agents	Dosage Range	Concentration Range	Midrange Dose	Midrange Concentration
Iopamidol (Isovue)	0.25-0.45 ml/kg	180-300 mgI/ml	0.33 mg/kg	240 mgI/ml
Iohexol (Omnipaque)	0.25-0.45 ml/kg	180-300 mgI/ml	0.33 mg/kg	240 mgI/ml

TABLE 33-9

Advantages and Disadvantages of Cisternal vs. Lumbar Myelography

Cisternal Tap	Lumbar Tap (L4-5 or L5-6)
Advantages	**Advantages**
Easier to perform	Flows forward under pressure to outline lesions
Excellent view of cervical spine	
Disadvantages	**Disadvantages**
Distribution of contrast depends on gravity and CSF flow	More difficult to perform
Contrast may not pass by compressive lesions	Needle often penetrates spinal cord
Contrast may migrate into the brain	More likely to deposit contrast epidurally

and disadvantages of each technique are listed in Table 33-9. The skin over the selected site is clipped and prepared for surgery.

Complications associated with myelography using iohexol or iopamidol are infrequent (less than 10%) and include exacerbation of neurologic abnormalities, seizures, cardiopulmonary alterations, and death. Seizures are more common in patients over 29 kg and patients requiring more than one injection of contrast medium to obtain diagnostic radiographs. Anesthetic agent, duration of anesthesia, type of fluid administration, and whether or not surgery is performed immediately after myelography are not factors associated with complications of myelography. Iopamidol and iohexol are the contrast media of choice in dogs.

Cisternal puncture for myelography or CSF analysis. *Position the patient in lateral recumbency. Palpate the wings of the atlas with the thumb and middle finger, and palpate the occiput with the index finger, making a triangle (Fig. 33-13). Gently flex the head and place a 20- to 22-gauge, 1½- to 2½-inch spinal needle with stylet in the center of the triangle. Place the bevel of the spinal needle in the direction of desired flow of contrast medium. As the needle is advanced a "pop" is felt as it penetrates the dura and enters the subarachnoid space. Return of CSF confirms proper location of the spinal needle. Slowly withdraw a volume of CSF for analysis, followed by injection of contrast. Elevate the head for 2 to 4 minutes to enhance flow of contrast caudally through all sections of the spine.*

Lumbar puncture for myelography or CSF analysis. A successful lumbar puncture requires practice and a lumbar spine skeleton for constant referral to anatomic structures. Fluoroscopy also simplifies accurate

needle placement. Lumbar myelography typically results in the most diagnostic myelogram. *Position the patient in lateral recumbency. Flex the spine, palpate the caudal dorsal spinous process of L5 or L6 (L5 in a L4-5 puncture and L6 in a L5-6 puncture), and place a 20- to 22-gauge, 2½- to 3½-inch spinal needle with stylet at its caudal aspect. Place the needle at a 45-degree angle caudally, and slowly advance cranioventrally and toward the midline in the direction of the L4-5 or L5-6 interspace (Fig. 33-14). A characteristic "pop" will be felt as the needle penetrates ligamentum flavum and dura. At this point withdraw the stylet to examine for flow of CSF. If CSF is visible remove some for analysis, then slowly inject the calculated dose of contrast. If CSF is not visible, advance the needle through the spinal cord until it contacts the floor of the spinal canal; occasionally, a tail twitch or leg jerk will result. Withdraw the needle slightly until the flow of CSF is visible. Place the bevel of the spinal needle in the direction of desired flow of contrast and slowly inject the calculated dose.*

Lesions identified by myelography are classified as extradural, intradural-extramedullary, and intramedullary. Each classification has a list of possible etiologies (see Table 33-2) and characteristic appearance on myelography. Extradural lesions cause the "contrast column" (subarachnoid space) to be elevated away from the spinal canal on at least one projection (ventrodorsal or lateral) depending upon location of the extradural mass (Fig. 33-15, *A*). On the opposite view, the contrast column may appear narrower due to spinal cord swelling (Fig. 33-15, *B* and *C*). Intradural-extramedullary lesions cause the contrast column to become wider on one projection; this widening may resemble a "golf tee" in appearance (Fig. 33-16). From the opposite view the contrast column may

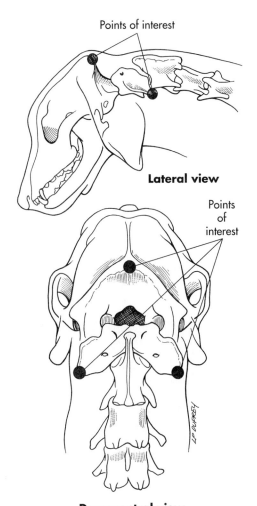

FIG. 33-13
The right and left wings of the atlas and occipital protuberances form a triangle; cisternal puncture is performed by placing a spinal needle in the center of this palpable triangle.

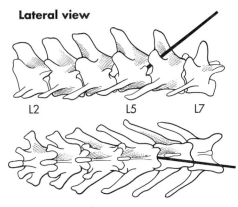

FIG. 33-14
Lumbar spinal puncture is performed at L4-L5 or L5-L6. The needle is placed at a 45-degree angle caudally, advanced to the L4-L5 or L5-L6 midline, and passed through the ligamentum flavum and into the dura.

appear narrower due to spinal cord swelling. Intramedullary lesions cause the contrast column to become narrower on ventrodorsal and lateral projections due to generalized spinal cord swelling (Fig. 33-17).

Stress Myelography. Stress myelography may allow accurate spinal lesion location and help determine treatment. It is most commonly used in the diagnosis of Wobbler syndrome. Stress myelography is performed by placing segments of the vertebral column in dorsal hyperextension, ventral flexion, and linear traction, thus exacerbating or relieving compressive lesions (Fig. 33-18). It is important that stress myelography be performed carefully so as not to exacerbate the patient's neurologic deficits.

Other Spinal Imaging Techniques

Diskography. Diskography is the intradiskal injection of a nonionic contrast medium into the nucleus pulposus and recording the image with radiography. It is most commonly used in the diagnosis of cauda equina syndrome. The technique is performed by placing a spinal needle into the nucleus pulposus of the affected disk and injecting 0.1-0.3 ml of contrast medium (normal disks cause back pressure after 0.1 ml). Radiographic abnormalities include extravasation of contrast medium, indicating disk protrusion, or an irregular contrast pattern within the nucleus pulposus and injection of greater than 0.1 ml volume of contrast medium, indicating disk degeneration (Fig. 33-19). Significant complications have not been reported with diskography. Diskography is contraindicated in patients with diskospondylitis of the disk to be injected.

Epidurography. Epidurography is the injection of a non-ionic contrast medium into the caudal epidural space and recording the image with radiography. It is most commonly used in the diagnosis of cauda equina syndrome. The technique is performed by inserting a 20- to 22-gauge spinal needle between the dorsal lamina of the caudal (coccygeal) vertebra 3-4 or 4-5 and injecting 0.15 mg/kg of contrast medium. Lateral and ventrodorsal views are taken; additional contrast at the rate of 0.1 mg/kg can be injected if necessary. A lateral view of the lumbosacral spine in hyperextension may accentuate a subtle lesion. Significant complications have not been reported with epidurography. Radiographic abnormalities include elevation or compression of the contrast column by the spinal lesion (Fig. 33-20).

Computed tomography and magnetic resonance imaging. Although adequate diagnostic imaging of the spine can usually be accomplished using conventional radiography, computed tomography (CT) and magnetic resonance imaging (MRI) are capable of detecting subtle changes conventional radiography cannot reveal.

Computed tomography provides a three-dimensional image of structures and increased contrast resolution, enabling differentiation of soft-tissue structures that cannot be differentiated on routine radiographic studies. CT is valuable in diagnosing the cause of spinal stenosis (soft tissue or osseous), intervertebral foraminal masses (neoplasia, intervertebral disk

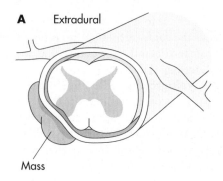

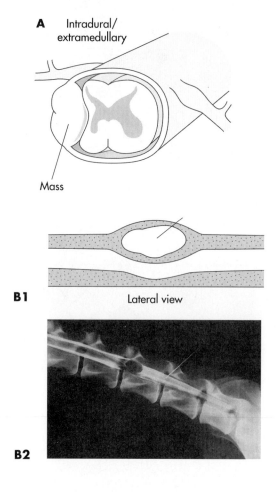

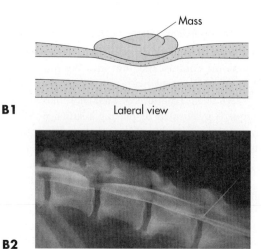

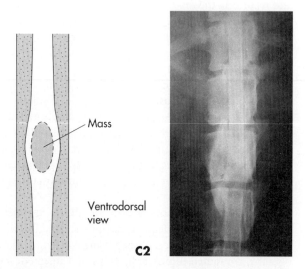

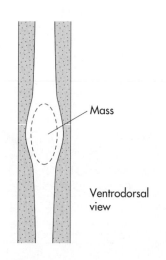

FIG. 33-15

Illustrations and examples of myelographic findings with extradural spinal cord compression. **A,** Schematic showing cross-sectional location of an extradural mass. **B1,** Illustration and **B2,** myelogram showing L2-L3 extradural spinal cord compression (lateral view). **C1,** Illustration and **C2,** myelogram showing L2-L3 extradural spinal cord compression (ventrodorsal view).

FIG. 33-16

Illustrations and examples of myelographic findings with an intradural-extramedullary lesion. **A,** Schematic showing cross-sectional location of an intradural-extramedullary meningioma. **B1,** Illustration and **B2,** myelogram of a lumbar meningioma causing intradural-extramedullary spinal cord compression (lateral view). **C,** Illustration of an intradural-extramedullary compressive lesion on a ventrodorsal view.

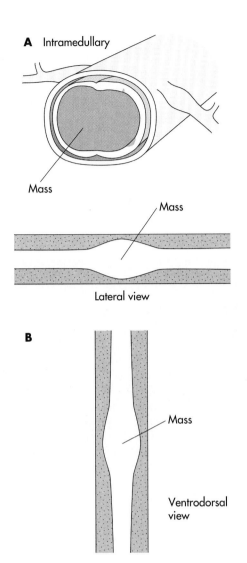

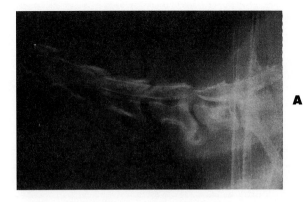

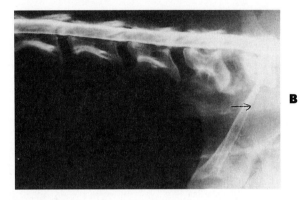

FIG. 33-18
A, C6-C7 mass. **B,** Linear traction results in relief of the extradural compression.

FIG. 33-17
Illustrations of myelographic findings with an intramedullary lesion. **A,** Schematic showing cross-sectional location of an intramedullary lesion. **B,** Illustration of myelographic findings with an intramedullary lesion.

[IVD], bony proliferation), and helps define the extent and invasiveness of a lesion (i.e., infection, neoplasia, trauma). However, this procedure is costly and not readily available for use in veterinary medicine.

Magnetic resonance imaging of the spine results in enhanced soft-tissue contrast that enables direct visualization of the spinal cord, epidural space, intervertebral disks, and ligaments of the spine. MRI is most useful in the diagnosis of lumbosacral stenosis and intramedullary tumors. The disadvantages of MRI are cost, inaccessibility, and poor resolution of dense or cortical bone.

IMAGING THE SKULL AND BRAIN

Diagnostic imaging of the skull and brain is indicated when the neurologic examination localizes a lesion above the foramen magnum. Due to the advent of refined diagnostic imaging tools such as the CT scan (survey and contrast enhanced) and MRI, there has been a marked improvement in identification and localization of intracranial lesions.

Survey radiographs of the skull may help assess patients with trauma to the calvarium, middle ear infection, neoplasms invading or causing mineralization of the calvarium, or any lesion causing direct involvement of the osseous structures of the skull. When skull radiographs are taken the following guidelines should be considered: (1) use general anesthesia; (2) position the patient carefully to display bilateral symmetry; (3) take lateral and ventrodorsal projections; and (4) use high-quality radiographic film. Knowledge of normal anatomic variation of the skull and results of minimum database, historical, physical, and neurologic examinations are necessary to allow accurate interpretation. Survey radiographs may be normal in patients with significant neurologic deficits secondary to intracranial disorders (e.g., hematoma, neoplasia, abscess, hydrocephalus, and inflammatory disorders).

CT provides excellent detail of bone and soft tissue, and allows identification and precise localization of most intracranial lesions (Fig. 33-21). Intravenous contrast medium can be used in conjunction with CT to enhance identification of specific soft-tissue structures (e.g., intracranial neoplasia).

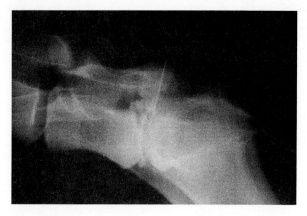

FIG. 33-19
Lateral diskogram of a dog with cauda equina syndrome. Notice the irregular contrast pattern within the L7-S1 nucleus pulposus and extravasation of contrast into the lumbosacral spinal canal.

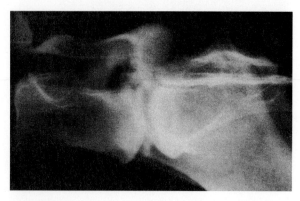

FIG. 33-20
Combination diskogram and epidurogram in a dog with cauda equina syndrome. Notice that the contrast column of the epidurogram is compressed at the lumbosacral junction.

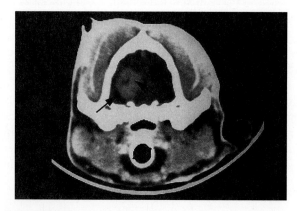

FIG. 33-21
Contrast-enhanced CT scan of a patient with intracranial neoplasia. Note the radiodense mass in the right cerebral hemisphere (*arrows*).

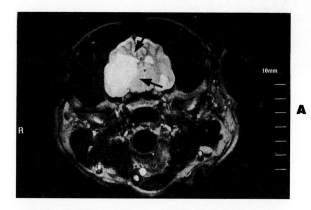

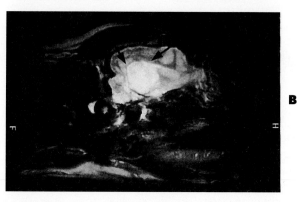

FIG. 33-22
MRI image of a patient with intracranial neoplasia; **A,** cross section and, **B,** sagittal section reveal a radiodense mass in the right cerebral hemisphere (*arrows*).

CT images can be used to determine the extent of a lesion and whether or not the calvarium has been invaded. This procedure is also valuable for planning approaches to the cranial vault; however, it is expensive and not readily available.

MRI is noninvasive, does not require the use of contrast media, and does not expose the patient to radiation. Advantages of MRI over CT are improved anatomic detail of soft-tissue structures and absence of image degradation due to the thick canine calvarium (Fig. 33-22). MRI may be more sensitive than CT in diagnosing and localizing brain abnormalities in dogs and cats. The greatest limitations of MRI, as with CT, are the high cost of equipment and maintenance and the lack of availability.

Suggested Reading

Withrow, SJ: Localization and diagnosis of spinal cord lesions in small animals. Part I. *Compend Contin Educ Pract Vet* 2:464, 1980.

Withrow, SJ: Localization and diagnosis of spinal cord lesions in small animals. Part II. Case examples, *Compend Contin Educ Pract Vet* 2:599, 1980.

Surgery of the Cervical Spine

GENERAL PRINCIPLES AND TECHNIQUES

DEFINITIONS

Dorsal laminectomy is removal of dorsal spinous processes, lamina, and portions of the pedicles to expose the dorsal aspect of the spinal cord and nerve roots. **Hemilaminectomy** and **dorsolateral hemilaminectomy** refer to unilateral removal of the lateral and dorsolateral lamina, respectively, in addition to removal of the pedicles and articular facets. **Foramenotomy** refers to the removal of the roof of the intervertebral foramen; **facetectomy** is the complete excision of the cranial and caudal articular facets. Unilateral facetectomy and foramenotomy are commonly performed with dorsolateral hemilaminectomy to expose nerve roots. **Ventral slot** refers to the creation of a bony defect in the ventral aspect of a cervical intervertebral space to gain entrance and visualization of the ventral spinal canal. The ventral slot provides limited access to the intervertebral foramen. **Fenestration** is the creation of a window or fenestra in the lateral or ventral annulus fibrosus to remove nucleus pulposus from the intervertebral space. **Tetraparesis** is the loss of conscious proprioception and variable motor weakness of all four limbs; **tetraplegia** is the loss of conscious proprioception, motor function, and the ability to perceive superficial and deep pain in all four limbs.

PREOPERATIVE CONCERNS

Neurologic function and ambulation should be carefully assessed in patients that require cervical spinal cord surgery. Weakly ambulatory or nonambulatory tetraparetic patients often have subclinical respiratory compromise and require ventilatory support during surgery. Tetraplegic patients usually develop respiratory difficulties as a result of lack of diaphragmatic and intercostal muscle function. Respiratory arrest and subsequent death are more common in patients undergoing dorsal decompressive laminectomy than in those undergoing ventral decompressive procedures (i.e., ventral slot, ventral stabilization). This is probably because dorsal decompressive procedures are more complicated and often require extensive manipulation of the cervical spinal cord.

Preoperative care of patients with unstable cervical fractures, luxations, or subluxations (i.e., palpable crepitus, instability) includes cage rest and serial neurologic examinations. A neck brace should be used to prevent movement of the cervical spine. Weakly ambulatory or nonambulatory tetraparetic patients should be secured to a rigid surface (i.e., board or Plexiglas) until diagnostics have been performed and treatment initiated.

Spinal surgery generally requires that the spinal cord and/or nerve roots be carefully retracted to treat the underlying disorder (e.g., removal of disk material or neoplastic lesions, fracture stabilization). Preoperative administration of corticosteroids may provide some protection to these structures during surgery; however, they should be used cautiously because they may predispose to gastrointestinal ulceration/perforation (see p. 1066). Ulceration/perforation seems to be associated with the combination of spinal cord trauma, stress of hospitalization or spinal surgery, and steroid administration; the cause remains unknown, however.

During cervical fracture reduction, hemorrhage as a result of laceration of one or both vertebral venous sinuses may be fatal. Blood should be available for transfusion and techniques to control venous sinus hemorrhage should be employed promptly (as shown in Table 34-1). These techniques should be practiced by the surgeon and assistant surgeon before performing a ventral slot procedure.

ANESTHETIC CONSIDERATIONS

Animals undergoing cervical spinal surgery should have two cephalic catheters placed to allow rapid fluid administration should venous sinus hemorrhage occur. Blood for transfusion and mechanical ventilatory support should be available; mechanical ventilation or intermittent positive-pressure ventilation is necessary in tetraparetic patients. A balanced electrolyte solution should be administered intravenously during surgery. Intraoperative measurement of direct arterial blood pressure is recommended. Administration of hypertonic saline (4-5 ml/kg intravenously) and/or positive

TABLE 34-1
Techniques for Controlling Venous Sinus Hemorrhage
Before procedure begins: 1. Cut several pieces of Gelfoam into 5 mm × 5 mm pledgets and place them in saline. 2. Cut 1 or 2 pieces of Cottonoid sponge ~ 1 cm × 3-4 cm and place them in saline. 3. Have two Brown-Adson thumb forceps readily available. **Once venous sinus hemorrhage begins:** NOTE: This sequence of events should be practiced by the surgeon and assistant surgeon before performing a ventral slot procedure. 1. Use suction to locate the point of hemorrhage (assistant surgeon). 2. Once the source of hemorrhage is located, quickly remove the suction device and place a Gelfoam pledget at the site (surgeon). 3. Place a Cottonoid sponge over the Gelfoam pledget (surgeon). 4. Gently place the suction tip on top of the Cottonoid sponge to evacuate blood from the surgical site and draw it through the Gelfoam pledget (assistant surgeon). 5. Continue suctioning; apply gentle pressure with the suction tip to the Cottonoid sponge until hemorrhage subsides. 6. After hemorrhage is under control, gently remove the Cottonoid sponge; leave the Gelfoam pledget to encourage hemostasis. NOTE: Do not apply suction directly on the Gelfoam pledget as it will disappear into the suction device.

TABLE 34-2
Perioperative Drug Therapy for Hypotension
Dobutamine 2-10 µg/kg/min IV
Dopamine 2-10 µg/kg/min IV

TABLE 34-3
Selected Anesthetic Protocols for Dogs Undergoing Spinal Surgery
Premedication Methylprednisolone sodium succinate (30 mg/kg IV) or dexamethasone (1.5 mg/kg IV) plus oxymorphone (0.05-0.1 mg/kg SC or IM), or butorphanol (0.2-0.4 mg/kg SC or IM), or buprenorphine (5-15 µg/kg IM) **Induction** Thiopental (10-12 mg/kg IV) or propofol (4-6 mg/kg IV) **Maintenance** Isoflurane or halothane

TABLE 34-4
Criteria for Use of Antibiotics in Neurosurgery Patients
Prophylactic antibiotics: • Geriatric patients (i.e., > 7 years old) • Debilitated patients • Clean, open wounds associated with the surgery site • Estimated surgical time > 90 min • "Break" in aseptic surgical technique **Therapeutic antibiotics:** • Nonspinal infection that cannot be treated before surgery (e.g., severe dental disease, pyoderma, open appendicular fracture/luxation) • Spinal infection requiring surgical intervention (e.g., diskospondylitis, vertebral osteomyelitis) • Contaminated open wounds associated with the surgical site (e.g., open vertebral fracture/luxation)

inotropes (i.e., dobutamine or dopamine; Table 34-2) may be necessary if bleeding is severe or hypotension profound. A syndrome characterized by paradoxical bradycardia associated with hypotension ("acute sympathetic blockade") can occur intraoperatively in dogs with acute cervical spinal cord trauma. No effective treatment has yet been described. Animals undergoing surgery of the cervical spinal cord should be premedicated with corticosteroids (methylprednisolone sodium succinate or dexamethasone phosphate) (Table 34-3). Dogs may also be premedicated with an anticholinergic plus oxymorphone, butorphanol, or buprenorphine and induced with a thiobarbiturate or propofol. Isoflurane or halothane is preferred for anesthetic maintenance. Acepromazine should be avoided because of the risk of hypotension. Acepromazine is also contraindicated in animals undergoing myelography because it may promote seizures.

☞ **NOTE** · Manipulate the neck carefully in these patients during anesthetic induction and positioning for surgery or radiographs, especially if instability is present.

ANTIBIOTICS

Use of therapeutic or prophylactic antibiotics in cervical surgery is based on criteria listed in Table 34-4. Antibiotics selected for prophylaxis should be effective against common causes of postoperative infection (i.e., coagulase-positive

Staphylococcus, E. coli). Cefazolin (Table 34-5) is the antibiotic of choice for antimicrobial prophylaxis in patients undergoing neurologic surgery because of its low toxicity and excellent in vitro activity against these bacteria.

Selection of an appropriate antibiotic for therapeutic use (i.e., treatment extending for 7 to 10 days after surgery) should be based on the most probable pathogen. Selection is best determined by culture and susceptibility testing; however, empirical antibiotic selection can be based on published studies of similar cases or on data accumulated from practice records. The most common cause of postoperative wound infection in neurologic surgery is *Staphylococcus* spp.; therefore, antibiotics of choice include cefazolin, amoxicillin-clavulanate, enrofloxacin, or cephalothin (Table 34-6).

Perioperative Antibiotic Therapy

Cefazolin (Ancef or Kefzol)
20 mg/kg IV at induction, repeat at 4- to 6- hr intervals for
24 hrs

**Antibiotics Used in Animals Undergoing Spinal
Surgery**

Cefazolin (Ancef, Kefzol)
20 mg/kg IV or IM TID

Amoxicillin plus clavulonate (Clavamox)
Dogs—12.5-25 mg/kg PO BID
Cats—62.5 mg PO BID

Enrofloxacin (Baytril)
2.5-10 mg/kg; PO bid

Cephalothin (Keflin)
20 mg/kg IV or IM TID to QID

SURGICAL ANATOMY

There are seven cervical vertebrae. Knowledge of anatomic variation of cervical vertebrae enables localization of affected laminae. The anatomy of a typical vertebra consists of a body, a vertebral arch (which is composed of right and left pedicles and laminae), and various processes (i.e., transverse, spinous, articular, accessory, and mammillary). The first cervical vertebra (atlas) articulates with the skull and axis. The dorsal surface of the body of the atlas contains a depression (fovea of the dens) that articulates with the dens of C2. The dens is a cranioventral peglike projection from the cranial aspect of the vertebral body. The wings of the atlas are large, lateral projections that are easily palpated. The axis (C2) has a bladelike dorsal spinous process that overhangs the cranial and caudal articular surfaces of the vertebral body.

For dorsal laminectomy, the dorsal spine of C2 is a distinguishing landmark, often overshadowing a short, rudimentary C3 dorsal spinous process. It is the most prominent of the dorsal cervical spinous processes (Fig. 34-1). C3 through C5 differ slightly and are difficult to differentiate. C6 and C7 have fairly prominent dorsal spinous processes that slope cranially. The dorsal spinous process of T1 is prominent, easy to palpate, and allows identification of the adjacent (but much shorter) cranially facing dorsal spinous process of C7.

For ventral procedures, landmarks that can be used to identify the affected intervertebral space are the prominent transverse processes (wings) of C6 and the prominent ventral spinous process of C1. The prominent ventral annulus of the C5-C6 intervertebral space lies on the midline at the most cranial aspect of the transverse process of C6 (Fig. 34-2, *A* and *B*). The prominent ventral spinous process of C1 is palpable just cranial to the C1-C2 intervertebral space (Fig. 34-3).

SURGICAL TECHNIQUES

Patients with surgical disorders of the cervical spine may be treated by ventral decompression via ventral slot, fenestration, dorsal laminectomy, dorsolateral hemilaminectomy, or cervical stabilization via a dorsal or ventral approach. Patients with cervical disk extrusion or cervical vertebral instability should be positioned with the neck in linear traction. This manipulation may enhance visualization of herniated disk material by widening the intervertebral space or it may decompress the spinal cord during surgery in animals with cervical vertebral instability. Patients with atlantoaxial instability or cervical fracture/luxation should be positioned so as to reduce the subluxation or fracture (e.g., linear traction, gentle flexion, or extension) and encourage decompression of spinal cord and nerve roots. Patients requiring dorsal or dorsolateral decompression are positioned with the neck gently flexed to open the articular facets and interarcuate spaces facilitating laminectomy, foramenotomy, and facetectomy.

☞ **N O T E** • Pay special attention to how the patient is positioned for surgery because proper positioning of the cervical spine is critical.

Ventral Slot

Ventral slots are used to gain entrance and visualization of the ventral cervical spinal canal for decompression of patients with cervical disk protrusion (Fig. 34-4). They provide limited access to the intervertebral foramen. Ventral slots are often combined with stabilization procedures in animals with cervical vertebral instability (see p. 1078). Surgical exposure of the ventral aspect of the cervical spine without creating a slot is used for cervical disk fenestration and some cervical stabilization techniques (i.e., atlantoaxial instability, fracture/luxation). Ventral slots may be combined with fenestration. Ventral slot procedures require minimal dissection through normal tissue planes and minimal disruption of normal anatomic structures. They provide adequate visualization of the spinal canal and access to the intervertebral foramina. Minimal manipulation of the spinal cord is necessary and recovery is generally rapid with few complications. Operative time is less than that required for dorsal exposure of the cervical spine.

During the procedure, bipolar cautery, bone wax, Gelfoam pledgets, Cottonoid sponges, and suction are used to ensure the meticulous hemostasis necessary to adequately visualize and control venous sinus hemorrhage. Bipolar cautery helps control hemorrhage in soft tissues surrounding the bony defect. Bone hemorrhage may be encountered as the cancellous layer of the vertebral body is drilled. If bleeding is excessive, bone wax may be pressed into the bleeding surface to provide adequate hemostasis. Once the spinal canal is reached, inadvertent damage to the vertebral venous sinuses must be avoided while obtaining appropriate exposure. If a venous sinus is lacerated, suction, Gelfoam pledgets, and Cottonoid sponges are used to control hemorrhage (see Table 34-1). Once severe hemorrhage from a

FIG. 34-1
Distinguishing anatomic landmarks of the cervical spine.

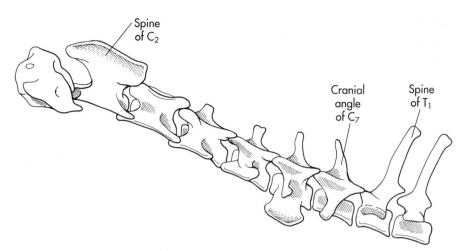

A **Ventral**

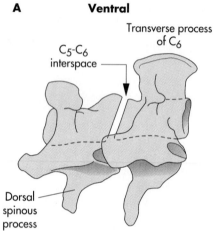

Cranial

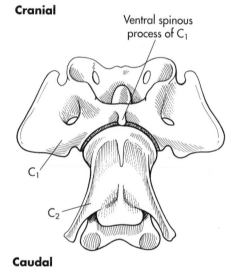

FIG. 34-3
Prominent ventral spinous processes of C1.

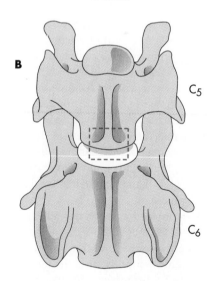

Dorsal

FIG. 34-2
A, Relationship of intervertebral space C5-C6 to the prominent transverse processes of C6. **B,** Notice the prominent ventral median ridge of cervical vertebral bodies.

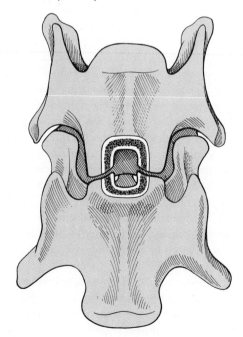

FIG. 34-4
Proper size and location of a completed ventral slot.

lacerated venous sinus has occurred it is best to avoid further manipulation in the spinal canal because continued hemorrhage prevents adequate visualization. If hemorrhage can be lateralized and adequately controlled, it may be possible to manipulate within the spinal canal from the opposite side of the slot.

Clip and prepare the neck from midmandible to caudal to the manubrium sterni for aseptic surgery. Position the animal in dorsal recumbency with the chest in a "V" trough. Tape the front legs caudally and tie the head cranially. Apply mild linear neck traction to help stabilize the cervical spine and slightly distract the intervertebral spaces (Fig. 34-5). Make a midline ventral incision from the caudal aspect of the thyroid cartilage to the manubrium sterni (determine the exact length of the incision by the location of the involved intervertebral space or spaces). Separate the paired sternohyoid and sternomastoid muscles on their midline. Identify the esophagus and trachea and digitally retract them to the left. Locate the carotid sheaths bilaterally and digitally retract them. Determine the location of the affected intervertebral space by palpating the prominent transverse processes (wings) of C6. Locate the prominent ventral annulus of the C5-C6 intervertebral space just midline of the most cranial aspect of the transverse process of C6 (see Fig. 34-2). Alternatively, identify the affected intervertebral space by palpating the prominent ventral spinous process of C1 (thus identifying the C1-C2 intervertebral space) and counting caudally (see Fig. 34-3).

Once the involved intervertebral space has been located, bluntly separate the longus colli muscles along their median raphe and cut their tendinous insertions on the ventral spinous processes of affected vertebrae. Subperiosteally elevate longus colli muscle from the ventral surface of affected vertebral bodies or directly adjacent to involved

intervertebral space(s). Insert Gelpi retractors to hold the longus colli muscles apart (Fig. 34-6) but take care to protect the carotid sheath and esophagus from inadvertent damage. Meticulously control hemorrhage to prevent pooling of blood in the slot to be created. Remove the ventral spinous process of affected vertebral bodies with rongeurs. Excise the ventral annulus fibrosus with a No. 11 scalpel blade. ***Remember that intervertebral spaces of cervical vertebrae have a slight caudal-to-cranial angle that must be compensated for when making this cut*** *(Fig. 34-7). Remove the entire ventral annulus fibrosus and any disk material present with a disk rongeur or dental scraper. Use a high-speed pneumatic drill with assorted sizes of carbide and diamond head burrs to create a midline rectangular defect in the bodies of the two vertebrae at the level of the affected intervertebral space. Be sure to remain on midline throughout the procedure to avoid lacerating the laterally located vertebral artery and vertebral venous sinuses (Fig. 34-8). Use frequent irrigation with physiologic saline solution to dissipate heat, prevent burning bone, and keep tissues moist. Do not perform irrigation during drilling because visualization of slot depth is difficult when the drill aerosolizes saline. Extend the slot no further laterally than three quarters of the width of the intervertebral space (Fig. 34-9). Because of the caudal-to-cranial angle of the cervical intervertebral spaces, center the slot slightly toward the cranial vertebral body (Fig. 34-10). This ensures the slot will be centered directly over the intervertebral space when the spinal canal is reached. To prevent inadvertent laceration of vertebral*

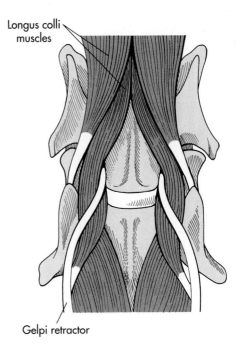

FIG. 34-6
After elevating the longus colli muscle from the ventral surface of affected vertebral bodies, use Gelpi retractors to hold the muscles apart. Take care to avoid damaging the carotid sheath or esophagus.

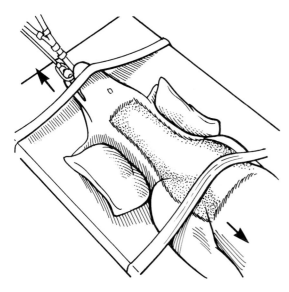

FIG. 34-5
To position the animal for a ventral approach to the cervical vertebrae, place the neck in mild linear traction.

A

Ventral

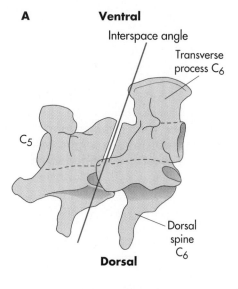

Interspace angle

Transverse process C₆

C₅

Dorsal spine C₆

Dorsal

B

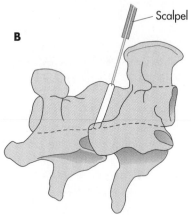

Scalpel

FIG. 34-7
A, Note the slight cranial-to-caudal angle of the cervical vertebral interspaces. **B,** To excise the ventral annulus, the scalpel blade should be inserted at this cranial-to-caudal angle.

venous sinuses, extend the slot no more than one quarter of the length of the vertebra cranially or caudally (see Figs. 34-8 through 34-10).

Gauge the depth of the slot by visualizing three distinct layers of bone while drilling. First, penetrate the hard outer cortical layer of the vertebral body (the white cortical bone exposed when the longus colli muscle is elevated from the vertebral body.) Next, visualize the softer, more hemorrhagic, marrow layer just below the outer cortical layer. This layer is more easily drilled than the outer cortical layer. Drill the outer cortical and marrow layers with 4- to 5-mm diameter carbide burrs. Finally, visualize the 1- to 2-mm thick inner cortical layer of the vertebral body. Once this layer has been reached, drill carefully, using gentle "paintbrush" strokes with a 2- to 3-mm diameter diamond burr. Take care not to break into the spinal canal abruptly. After penetrating the inner cortical layer, use a 3-0 or 4-0 bone curette to enlarge the defect (Fig. 34-11). Carefully curette the dorsal annulus fibrosus and periosteum to expose the dorsal longitudinal ligament. Curette the inner cortical layer of bone to a diameter sufficient to allow removal of the herniated disk but avoid excessive lateral curettage lest laceration of a vertebral venous sinus occurs (see Fig. 34-8). Once exposure is adequate, carefully remove the dorsal longitudinal ligament with fine ophthalmic forceps and a No. 11 scalpel blade, allowing access to the spinal canal (Fig. 34-12). Determine adequate decompression of the spinal cord by visualizing the characteristic bluish hue of dura mater (spinal cord) through the slot (Fig. 34-13). Ensure adequate visualization during manipulation of neural structures. Before closure, irrigate the wound with physiologic saline solution to dislodge any remaining bone fragments from soft tissues. Do not fill the slot with bone graft, fat, or Gelfoam. Appose paired longus colli muscles with simple interrupted sutures. Close subcutaneous tissues and skin routinely.

FIG. 34-8
A, Cross-section of the cervical spine showing vertebral venous sinus and vertebral artery relative to the intervertebral disk and spinal cord; width of the slot is determined by this relationship. **B,** Laminectomized cervical spine showing the shape of vertebral venous sinus and dorsal longitudinal ligament relative to intervertebral spaces; length of the slot is determined by this relationship.

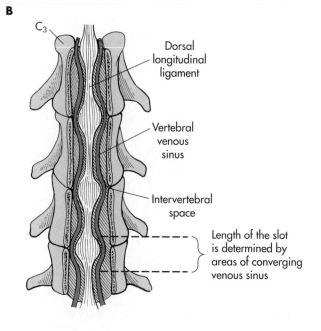

A

Dorsal

C₅

Vertebral venous sinus

Vertebral artery

Width of the slot is determined by location of vertebral venous sinuses at the intervertebral space

B

C₃

Dorsal longitudinal ligament

Vertebral venous sinus

Intervertebral space

Length of the slot is determined by areas of converging venous sinus

Cervical Disk Fenestration

Cervical disk fenestration is performed from intervertebral spaces C2-C3 through C6-C7. It is not indicated for patients with disk material that has herniated into the spinal canal or intervertebral foramen; however, it may benefit patients with diskogenic pain. There is some suggestion that fenestration of alternate disk spaces after ventral slot may decrease recurrence of disk herniation; however, this is controversial. The author does not recommend disk fenestration after ventral slot procedures.

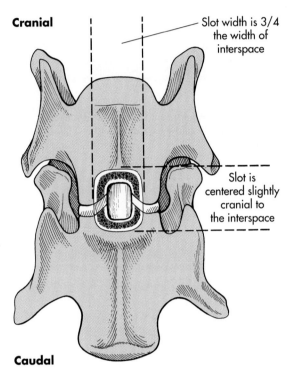

Cranial

Slot width is 3/4 the width of interspace

Slot is centered slightly cranial to the interspace

Caudal

FIG. 34-9
Proper dimensions of a ventral slot, based on length and width of the vertebral body.

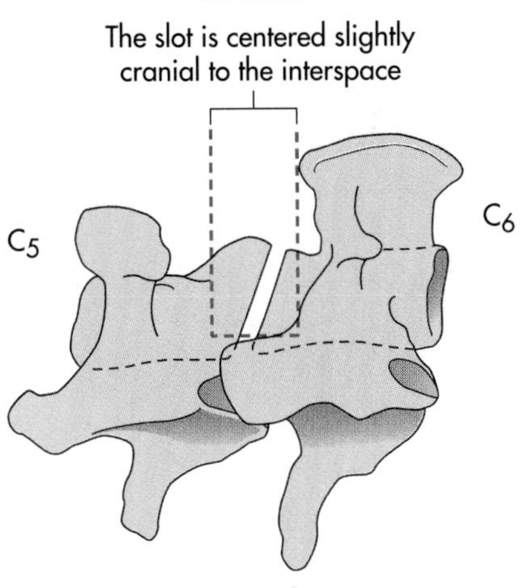

Ventral

The slot is centered slightly cranial to the interspace

C₅   C₆

Dorsal

FIG. 34-10
Cranial and caudal extent of the ventral slot defect, based on caudal-to-cranial angle of the intervertebral space.

Position and prepare the patient for surgery as described above. Make an incision from the thyroid cartilage cranially to the manubrium sterni caudally. Expose each intervertebral space in a similar fashion as the ventral slot; however, separate longus colli muscle only at each intervertebral space. Expose ventral annulus fibrosus with a periosteal elevator. Use a No. 11 scalpel blade to excise a large wedge-shaped piece of ventral annulus fibrosus (Fig. 34-14). Hold the scalpel at the proper cranial-to-caudal angle to facilitate excision of ventral annulus and removal of nucleus pulposus (see Fig. 34-7). Remove nuclear material with an ear loop, tartar scraper, or small bone curette (4-0 or 5-0). Take care to prevent dorsal extrusion of disk fragments into the spinal canal. Close as described above for ventral slot.

Dorsal Cervical Laminectomy and Hemilaminectomy

Dorsal cervical laminectomy is the removal of dorsal lamina from cervical vertebrae to expose the spinal cord (Fig. 34-15). Laminectomy is generally indicated when lesions are located in the dorsal or lateral spinal canal, whereas ventral slot (described above) is generally indicated when the compressive lesion is located in the ventral spinal canal. The specific laminectomy procedure used (i.e., cranial cervical, mid-cervical, caudal cervical) depends on location and etiology of the compressive lesion. Dorsolateral hemilaminectomy and

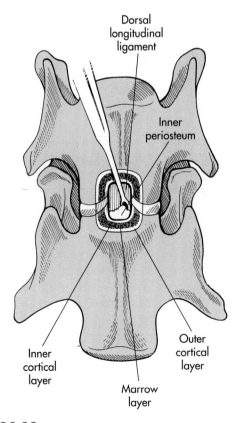

Dorsal longitudinal ligament

Inner periosteum

Inner cortical layer

Marrow layer

Outer cortical layer

FIG. 34-11
The proper depth of the ventral slot defect is determined by identifying outer cortical, medullary, and inner cortical layers of bone; once the inner cortical layer is reached, use a 3-0 or 4-0 curette to expose the dorsal longitudinal ligament.

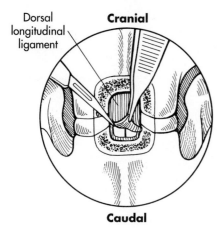

FIG. 34-12
The dorsal longitudinal ligament is grasped with ophthalmic forceps and incised with a No. 11 scalpel blade.

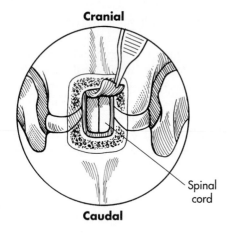

FIG. 34-13
Decompression is complete when the spinal cord is visualized.

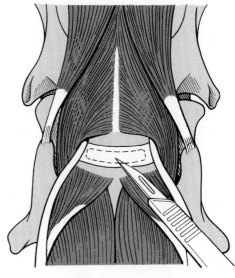

FIG. 34-14
Cut a large rectangular window (fenestration) into the ventral annulus fibrosus to allow exposure and removal of nucleus pulposus.

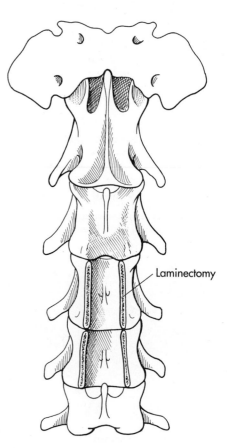

FIG. 34-15
Cervical laminectomy of C4 and C5.

facetectomy is removal of right or left dorsal lamina, a portion of the right or left pedicle, and portions of the articular facet from affected vertebrae (Fig. 34-16).

Dorsal approach to the cranial cervical spine (C1-C2). *Perform cranial cervical laminectomy with the patient in sternal recumbency, head gently flexed in a neutral position, and head and neck supported by a rolled fleece or rigid vacuum type of apparatus (Fig. 34-17). Make a dorsal midline incision from the occipital protuberance to the dorsal spinous process of C4. Expose the median fibrous raphe between paired splenius muscles and dorsal cutaneous branches of the cervical nerves. Use these structures as a guide to perform midline dissection (Fig. 34-18). Divide the splenius muscles over the spinous process of C2 and retract them laterally. Incise paraspinal epaxial muscles on each side of the spinous process of C2 and reflect them from the spine and dorsal laminae with a periosteal elevator. Elevate muscle to the level of C2-C3 articular facets caudally and the ventral aspect of the C1-C2 intervertebral foramina cranially (Fig. 34-19). If a hemilaminectomy is performed, elevate muscle only on the side to be ex-*

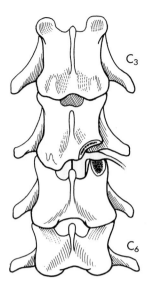

FIG. 34-16
Dorsolateral hemilaminectomy with facetectomy exposing the intervertebral foramen and exiting nerve root.

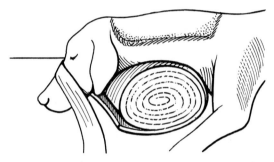

FIG. 34-17
To position an animal for cranial cervical laminectomy, gently flex and support the neck.

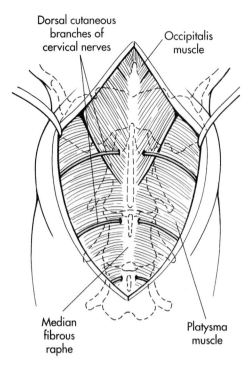

FIG. 34-18
During cervical laminectomy, dissect on the midline of the superficial cervical musculature to expose the median raphe and cutaneous nerves.

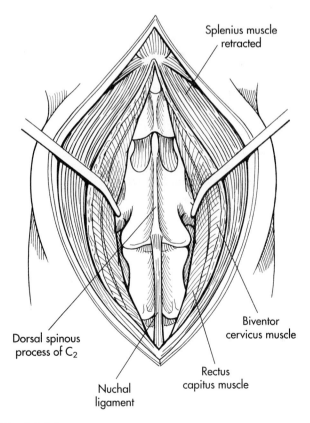

FIG. 34-19
During cranial cervical laminectomy, elevate muscle from the spinous processes and laminae of C1 and C2.

posed. Use self-retaining retractors to facilitate exposure. At the cranial end of the dissection, elevate muscles from the dorsal atlantoaxial ligament; wide elevation of muscles from the dorsal arch of C1 may be performed, depending on needed exposure. Caudally, elevate muscle until the multifidus muscle and nuchal ligament are exposed (see Fig. 34-19). From this point, perform a hemilaminectomy, dorsal laminectomy, or axial laminotomy, as needed (Fig. 34-20). Specific laminectomy techniques are described on p. 1059. Close the surgical wound by suturing muscles to the tendinous raphe in their respective layers. Close subcutaneous tissues and skin routinely.

Dorsal approach to the midcervical spine (C2-C5).
Position the patient in sternal recumbency. Place rolled padding under the neck at the midcervical region. Flex the neck over the padding to elevate the cervical vertebrae and open interarcuate spaces (Fig. 34-21). Position the patient carefully to improve palpation of important anatomic landmarks and enhance visualization of interarcuate ligaments. Make a dorsal midline incision from the occiput to the spinous process of the first thoracic vertebra. Identify

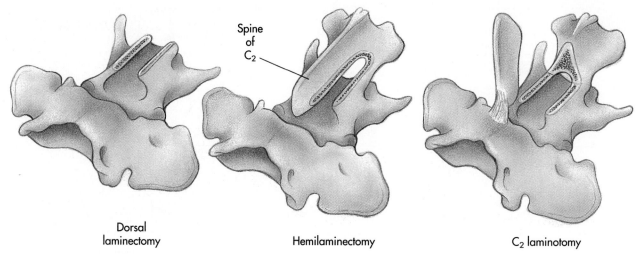

Spine
of
C₂

Dorsal
laminectomy

Hemilaminectomy

C₂ laminotomy

FIG. 34-20
Appearance of a completed C2 dorsal laminectomy, hemilaminectomy, and laminotomy.

the median fibrous raphe and use it as a landmark for midline dissection to the nuchal ligament (Fig. 34-22). Incise along one side of the nuchal ligament and between paired bellies of epaxial muscles. Identify appropriate anatomic landmarks and use a periosteal elevator to remove epaxial muscles from dorsal spinous processes and lamina of affected vertebrae. Dissect to the level of the articular processes; this depth is sufficient to perform deep dorsal laminectomy and avoid the vertebral arteries. Specific laminectomy techniques are described on p. 1059. Close epaxial muscles to the tendinous raphe or nuchal ligament in their respective layers. Close subcutaneous tissue and skin routinely.

Dorsal approach to the caudal cervical spine (C5-T3). Because the scapulae are closely associated with the caudal cervical spine and the vertebral laminae are located deep in epaxial muscles, positioning to enhance exposure is recommended. *Position the patient in sternal recumbency. To encourage elevation of the C6 and C7 dorsal spinous processes and laminae, cradle the neck by gently flexing and elevating it over rolled fleece, sandbags, or a rigid vacuum type of apparatus (Fig. 34-23). Position the front legs against the body to encourage abduction of the scapulae from the midline. Do this either by positioning the legs close to the body with sandbags or by tieing the front legs across the table (see Fig. 34-23). Make a dorsal midline skin incision from the midcervical region to the dorsal spinous process of T3. Locate the fibrous median raphe and continue midline dissection through epaxial muscles. Retract epaxial muscles with self-retaining retractors to enhance exposure of dorsal spinous processes. Palpate the prominent dorsal spinous process of T1 and cranially slanted smaller dorsal spine of C7 (about half of the height of T1) to determine specific anatomic location (see Fig. 34-1). Use a periosteal elevator to expose dorsal spinous processes and laminae of affected vertebrae. Remove dorsal spines of T1 through T3 (as needed) for dorsal laminectomy.* This will have minimal effect on spinal stability as the nuchal ligament is continuous with the supraspinous liga-

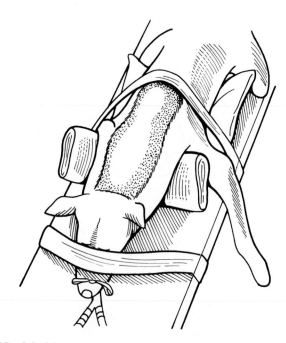

FIG. 34-21
To position an animal for midcervical dorsal laminectomy place the animal in sternal recumbency and flex the neck over padding.

ment. Excise interarcuate ligaments between C6 and T1 (as needed) with a No. 11 scalpel blade to expose the spinal cord. Specific laminectomy techniques are described on p. 1059. Close the surgical wound by suturing epaxial muscles to the tendinous raphe or nuchal ligament in their respective layers. Close subcutaneous tissues and skin routinely.

Dorsolateral approach to the cervical spine. Dorsolateral hemilaminectomy is removal of dorsal spinous processes, the dorsolateral portion of lamina, and dorsal articular facets of affected vertebrae. It is indicated in patients with compressive lesions of the lateral aspect of the spinal canal and intervertebral foramen.

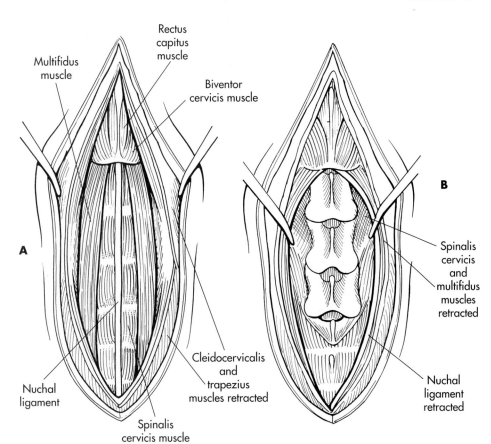

Multifidus muscle

Rectus capitus muscle

Biventor cervicis muscle

A

Nuchal ligament

Spinalis cervicis muscle

Cleidocervicalis and trapezius muscles retracted

B

Spinalis cervicis and multifidus muscles retracted

Nuchal ligament retracted

FIG. 34-22
A, Identify the median fibrous raphe and nuchal ligament during dorsal midcervical laminectomy and use them as landmarks. **B,** Elevate the cervical musculature from dorsal spinous processes and laminae of C3, C4, and C5.

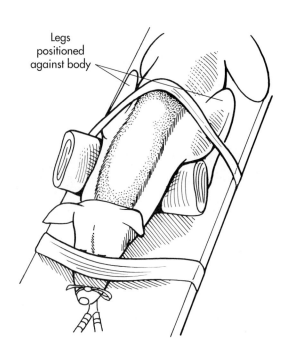

Legs positioned against body

FIG. 34-23
To position an animal for caudal cervical laminectomy, cradle the neck, gently flex it, and elevate it over a rolled fleece, sandbags, or a rigid vacuum type of apparatus. Position the front legs against the body with sandbags or tie them across the table.

Position the patient in sternal recumbency with the head and neck slightly flexed and elevated. Make a dorsal midline skin incision centered over the affected vertebrae. Identify the median fibrous raphe and expose the dorsal spinous processes via midline dissection. Elevate epaxial muscles from the dorsal spinous processes, lamina, and dorsal articular facets of affected vertebrae. Continue dissection and periosteal elevation on the lateral aspect of the articular facet and intervertebral foramen to provide full visualization of the lateral aspect of the vertebral body. Carefully dissect and identify the vertebral artery before examination of the intervertebral foramen. Specific laminectomy techniques are described below. Close epaxial muscles to the tendinous raphe in their respective layers. Close subcutaneous tissues and skin routinely.

☞ **N O T E ·** Performing a dorsolateral hemilaminectomy and facetectomy with rongeurs requires careful dissection and visualization of the lateral aspect of the facet joint.

Laminectomy and laminotomy techniques. Laminectomy is performed with a high-speed pneumatic bone drill, rongeurs, or both. Laminar thickness varies with patient size; larger patients generally have thicker lamina. Vertebral and laminar density varies with age; older animals tend to have denser, more compact bone. Disadvantages of dorsal laminectomy and dorsolateral hemilaminectomy include severe disruption of hard and soft tissues, prolonged operating times, poor visualization of ventral and ventrolateral lesions, and excessive spinal cord manipulation to approach the floor of the spinal canal. It is most efficient to use a high-speed pneumatic drill in conjunction with rongeurs to perform dorsal cervical laminectomy, C2 laminotomy, and dorsolateral hemilaminectomy and facetectomy. First use a high-speed drill with selected carbide and diamond tip burrs to enter the spinal canal. Then use rongeurs to carefully increase exposure by nibbling away bone from the drilled edge.

Remove dorsal spinous processes of affected vertebrae with rongeurs. When using a high-speed drill, identify laminectomy depth by visualizing the white outer cortical layer, the softer, red medullary layer, and the white inner cortical layer. Drill the first two layers using 4- to 5-mm carbide burrs (Fig. 34-24, A). Once the inner cortical layer is reached, use a gentle "paint brush" technique with a 2- to 3-mm diamond tip burr to expose inner periosteum. Gently elevate periosteum and remaining interarcuate ligament with a dental spatula to expose spinal canal and spinal cord (Fig. 34-24, B and C). When performing C2 laminotomy, use a high-speed drill with a 2-mm carbide burr to make fine laminar cuts as necessary to elevate the dorsal spinous process and allow its replacement after exposure of the spinal canal and spinal cord (Fig. 34-25). When performing dorsolateral hemilaminectomy, use a high-speed drill with 4- to 5-mm carbide and 2- to 3-mm diamond burrs to remove lamina and articular facets. Carefully identify

outer cortical, marrow, and inner cortical layers of lamina and articular facets while drilling. Once the inner periosteal layer is reached, use a dental spatula and fine ophthalmic forceps to explore the spinal canal and intervertebral foramen. Identify the vertebral artery located ventral to the intervertebral foramen before manipulating the nerve roots and spinal cord (see Fig. 34-8). When using rongeurs to perform laminectomy procedures, carefully dissect the interarcuate ligament with a No. 15 blade and ophthalmic forceps to expose the intervertebral space and laminar edge. Accentuate the exposed laminar edge by grasping its dorsal spinous process with towel clamps and gently elevating the lamina (Fig. 34-26). Carefully place rongeurs on this edge and remove lamina to expose the spinal canal and spinal cord. Dissect interarcuate ligaments from C6 to T1 to expose the spinal canal and spinal cord. Use of a high-speed drill is recommended.

Cervical Spinal Stabilization

Cervical spinal stabilization is a technique used to repair a cervical fracture/luxation, malformation, malarticulation, or congenital subluxation resulting in spinal instability. Stabilization can be accomplished by various techniques, including pins and methylmethacrylate bone cement, screws and Lubra plate, cross pins, and orthopedic wire. Surgical exposure is performed by either a dorsal or ventral approach as described above. The specific stabilization technique used generally depends on location of the instability (see subsequent sections).

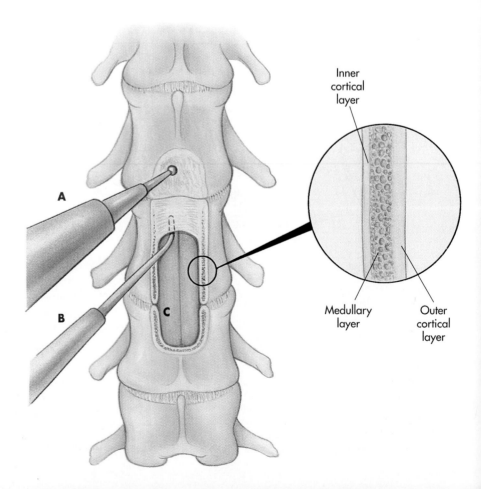

FIG. 34-24
A, Use a pneumatic bone drill to expose outer cortical, medullary, and inner cortical layers of laminar bone. **B,** Elevate periosteum with a dental spatula to gain exposure to the spinal canal. **C,** Expose the spinal cord and nerve roots.

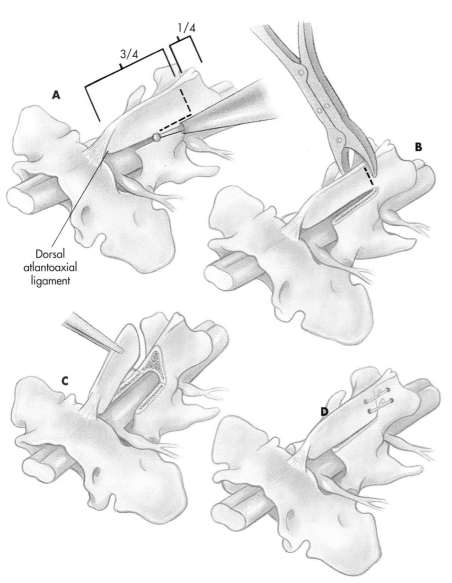

FIG. 34-25
For C2 laminotomy, **A,** measure the dorsal spinous process of C2 to ensure three quarters of its length is removed. Use a high-speed pneumatic drill to make the fine laminar cuts needed to elevate the spinous process of C2. **B,** Use bone cutters to transect the spinous process and laminar bone at predetermined sites. **C,** Retract the spine and lamina of C2 cranially, using the atlantoaxial ligament as a hinge. **D,** Wire the dorsal spinous process and lamina in place after examining the spinal cord.

Dorsal atlantoaxial ligament

HEALING OF THE SPINAL CORD

Three basic categories of change occur following acute injury to the spinal cord: (1) direct morphologic distortion of neuronal tissue, (2) vascular changes, and (3) biochemical and metabolic changes. Controversy exists regarding the relative importance of these closely related categories in the production of functional deficits. Direct morphologic damage of spinal cord tissue (i.e., laceration, compression, stretching) resulting in axonal interruption is felt to be irreversible and untreatable because central axons do not regenerate sufficiently to restore function.

In the case of reversible spinal cord injury, a characteristic series of events occurs during the repair process. Approximately 2 days after injury, a heterogenous population of small cells (most likely of hematogenous origin), including polymorphonuclear, lymphocyte, macrophage, and plasma cells, invade the traumatized tissue. This is essentially an inflammatory response. In a matter of 7 to 20 days, fibroblasts make their appearance and begin laying down scar tissue. A concurrent glial reaction consisting of astrocyte proliferation and expansion of processes occurs. Depending on the extent of spinal cord injury, moderate to extensive fibrosis, nerve fiber degeneration, and multifocal malacia may be seen. Axons that have been severed, compressed, or stretched start to regrow, but will reach the edges of the scar mass and stop. Regeneration of spinal cord axons sufficient to restore function has not been achieved; however, if enough axons remain intact, return to clinically acceptable motor function can be expected.

☞ **N O T E** · The pathophysiology of acute spinal cord injury is probably best viewed as being analogous to that of systemic shock; several complicated processes are involved and at some point an irreversible state may be reached.

SUTURE MATERIALS/SPECIAL INSTRUMENTS

The special instrumentation necessary to perform ventral slot, fenestration, dorsal laminectomy, dorsolateral hemilaminectomy, and spinal stabilization are listed by technique

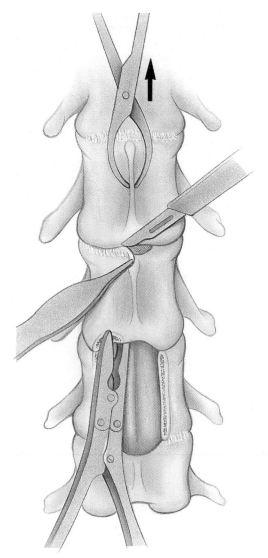

FIG. 34-26
Accentuate the laminar edge by grasping its dorsal spinous process with towel clamps and gently elevating the lamina. Carefully dissect the exposed interarcuate ligament with a No. 15 blade and ophthalmic forceps to reveal the laminar edge. Place rongeurs on this exposed edge and carefully remove the lamina to expose spinal canal and spinal cord.

in Table 34-7. It is important to practice each technique, become familiar with regional anatomy, and learn proper use of special instrumentation before performing these surgeries.

POSTOPERATIVE CARE AND ASSESSMENT

Critical care observation for the first 24 hours postoperatively includes monitoring respiration, administration of analgesics, and observation for gastric dilatation-volvulus and seizure activity (particularly if the patient had preoperative myelography). Blood gas analysis is warranted in animals with ventilatory compromise. Postoperative analgesia is provided by low doses of opioids, thus reducing their respi-

ratory depressant effects. Because postoperative pain can result in vocalizing and swallowing air, periodic abdominal girth measurements should be performed to assess presence of gastric dilatation. Fluids should be administered at maintenance rates and the patient turned every 2 hours until sternal. Corticosteroid administration is generally discontinued postoperatively. If neurologic status deteriorates after surgery, corticosteroids may be given until the cause is determined and corrected. Antibiotic therapy (prophylactic or therapeutic) is determined by criteria listed in Table 34-4.

☞ **NOTE** • Respiratory depression or arrest secondary to cervical spinal cord manipulation has been reported; patients must be carefully monitored for this event.

Ambulatory patients may be discharged 24 to 48 hours after surgery and should be confined for 2 to 3 weeks. They should walk on a harness for 4 to 8 weeks. Nonambulatory patients are treated with frequent hydrotherapy, physiotherapy, elevated padded cage rack, frequent turning, and bladder expression three to four times a day. They should be kept clean and dry to prevent decubital ulcers. Avoid indwelling urinary catheters because they are a frequent cause of urinary tract infection. A supporting cart helps nurse patients to an ambulatory status. Advantages of a cart include unhindered eating, drinking, micturition, and defecation. Additionally, animals with motor function are encouraged to ambulate, and an erect position facilitates physiotherapy. Nonambulatory patients may be discharged when owners are able to care for them. Neurologic exams should be performed at 1, 2, 3, 6, 9, and 12 months postoperatively. Radiographs (of the awake animal) may be performed at 1, 3, 6, 9, and 12 months after surgery.

COMPLICATIONS

Complications associated with ventral slot procedures include instability and collapse of the intervertebral space as a result of creating a slot that is too wide, laceration of a vertebral venous sinus, and iatrogenic spinal cord trauma. Knowledge of anatomic landmarks and proper neurosurgical instrumentation helps avoid such complications. Complications associated with cervical disk fenestration include inadequate removal of nucleus pulposus; dorsal extrusion of disk fragments into the spinal canal, causing neck pain and tetraparesis; diskospondylitis; and continued neck pain after fenestration. Complications associated with dorsal laminectomy include excessive hemorrhage from soft tissue dissection, iatrogenic spinal cord trauma, seroma, and surgical wound infection. Complications associated with dorsolateral hemilaminectomy include nerve root damage and laceration of a vertebral artery.

SPECIAL AGE CONSIDERATIONS

Softer cortical bone of lamina, pedicles, and vertebral bodies of young animals requires less aggressive drilling and rongeuring than the denser, more compact bone of older dogs.

TABLE 34-7

Special Instruments Necessary to Perform Cervical Spinal Surgery

Procedure	Instruments
Special instruments needed for most procedures	High-speed pneumatic or electric drill burrs: carbide and diamond tip, cautery unit (monopolar, bipolar), periosteal elevator/osteotome, suction, hemostatic sponge (Gelfoam), bone wax, dental spatula, dural hook
Ventral slot	Micro suction tip, 3-0 or 4-0 bone curette, vertebral spreaders
Dorsal laminectomy, axial laminotomy, dorsolateral hemilaminectomy, facetectomy	Duck-bill, double-action rongeurs, Lempert rongeurs
Fenestration	Tartar scraper, ear curette, No. 7 Bard-Parker scalpel handle
Spinal stabilization	Steinmann pins, methylmethacrylate bone cement, small fragment reduction forceps, vertebral spreaders

Suggested Reading

Eidelberg E: The pathophysiology of spinal cord injury, *Radiol Clin of N Am,* 15:241, 1977.

Felts JF, Prata RG: Cervical disk disease in the dog: intraforaminal and lateral extrusions, *J Am Anim Hosp Assoc* 19:755, 1983.

Gilpin GN: Evaluation of three techniques of ventral decompression of the cervical spinal cord in the dog, *J Am Vet Med Assoc* 168:325, 1976.

Hurov L: Dorsal decompressive cervical laminectomy in the dog: surgical considerations and clinical cases, *J Am Vet Med Assoc* 15:301, 1979.

Prata RG, Stoll SG: Ventral decompression and fusion for the treatment of cervical disc disease in the dog, *J Am Anim Hosp Assoc* 9:462, 1973.

Rucker NC: Management of spinal cord trauma, *Prog in Vet Neurol* 1:397, 1992.

Swaim SF: Ventral decompression of the cervical spinal cord in the dog, *J Am Vet Med Assoc* 164:491, 1974.

Toombs JP: Cervical intervertebral disk disease in dogs, *Compend Contin Educ Pract Vet* 14:1477, 1992.

Walker TL et al: The use of electric drills as an alternative to pneumatic equipment in spinal surgery, *J Am Anim Hosp Assoc* 17:605, 1981.

SPECIFIC DISEASES

CERVICAL DISK DISEASE

DEFINITIONS

Cervical disk disease is associated with disk degeneration and extrusion causing spinal cord compression and/or nerve root entrapment. **Hansen type I** disk degeneration is characterized by chondroid degeneration of the nucleus pulposus, whereas **Hansen type II** disk degeneration is characterized by fibrinoid degeneration of the nucleus pulposus. **Radiculopathy** is pain associated with nerve root compression. **Myelopathy** is a general term denoting functional disturbances and/or pathological changes in the spinal cord. **Diskogenic pain** is caused by derangement of an intervertebral disk. **Claudication** is a complex of symptoms caused by occlusion of the spinal vasculature.

SYNONYMS

Slipped disk, herniated intervertebral disk, cervical disk extrusion

GENERAL CONSIDERATIONS AND CLINICALLY RELEVANT PATHOPHYSIOLOGY

Intervertebral disk disease is the most common neurologic disorder diagnosed in veterinary patients. Cervical disk disease accounts for approximately 15% of all canine intervertebral disk extrusions (Toombs, 1992). Eighty percent of cervical disk protrusions occur in dachshunds, beagles, and poodles (Seim, Prata, 1982). The most common site of disk extrusion is the C2-C3 intervertebral space; frequency of involvement decreases from C3-C4 to C7-T1.

Disk degeneration is commonly divided into two distinct categories referred to as *Hansen type I* (Fig. 34-27) and *Hansen type II* (Fig. 34-28). Both types of disk degeneration occur in the cervical region; however, Type I extrusions are most common. In animals with cervical disk protrusion, the nucleus pulposus undergoes degenerative changes and loses its ability to absorb shock. Continued degeneration and subsequent protrusion (Hansen type II) or extrusion (Hansen type I) of disk fragments occur spontaneously or secondary to trauma. Location and force of the extrusion or protrusion dictate the degree of neurologic deficits.

DIAGNOSIS
Clinical Presentation

Signalment. Most animals with cervical disk disease have acute neck pain. Middle-age (i.e., 4 to 9 years), chondrodystrophoid breeds (i.e., dachshunds, beagles) are most commonly affected (Seim, Prata, 1982). There is no sex predilection.

History. A stiff, stilted gait, reluctance to move the head and neck, lowered head stance, and muscle spasm of the neck and shoulder muscles are common. Approximately 10% of affected patients are tetraparetic (ambulatory or nonambulatory).

Physical Examination Findings

The location of extruded disk fragments within the spinal canal is the most important factor in determining whether affected animals have pain or tetraparesis. If disk material extrudes in a dorsolateral direction (i.e., between the dorsal longitudinal ligament and vertebral venous sinus), nerve

FIG. 34-27
Hansen type I disk degeneration is characterized by an acute massive extrusion of degenerate nuclear material in the spinal canal.

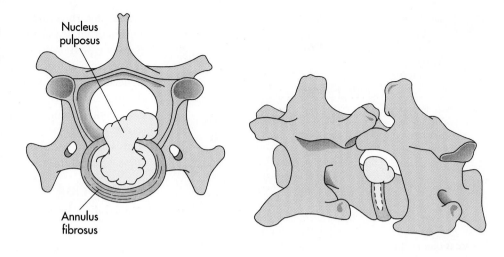

Nucleus pulposus

Annulus fibrosus

FIG. 34-28
Hansen type II disk degeneration is characterized by a slow chronic protrusion of degenerate dorsal annulus fibrosus in the spinal canal.

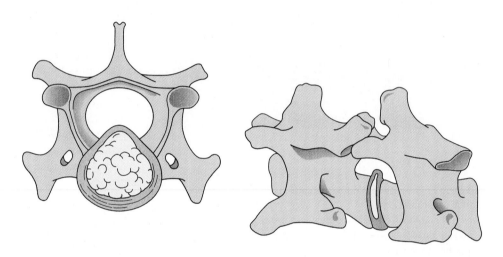

root compression and pain occur (Fig. 34-29). This is the most common location of cervical disk extrusion in dogs. If disk material extrudes directly on the midline (i.e., between fibers of dorsal longitudinal ligament), it causes spinal cord compression and subsequent tetraparesis (Fig. 34-30). These patients may also exhibit neck pain as a result of tethering of nerve roots in the intervertebral foramina. If disk material protrudes against (but not through) the dorsal longitudinal ligament, pain may result from pressure on pain-sensitive fibers of the dorsal annulus fibrosus and dorsal longitudinal ligament (diskogenic pain; Fig. 34-31). Diskogenic pain rarely occurs in dogs.

Occasionally, patients suffer neck pain and front leg lameness (monoparesis) as a result of a dorsolateral disk extrusion in the lower cervical spine (C4-C7) that entraps a nerve root supplying the brachial plexus (see Fig. 33-29). Pressure from disk material on the nerve root causes nerve root ischemia and severe pain and muscle spasm. Pain is often intermittent and generally manifests as a foreleg lameness. Presence of a root signature is helpful in localizing the extruded disk (C4-C7). It is important to carefully evaluate patients with forelimb lameness to exclude cervical disk disease.

☞ **N O T E ·** Dogs with nerve root signatures (forelimb lameness) are often misdiagnosed as having orthopedic rather than neurologic disease. Performing a complete neurologic examination helps distinguish between the two.

Radiography/Ultrasonography

Well-positioned lateral and ventrodorsal survey radiographs of the cervical spine may be diagnostic for cervical disk disease. Classical findings on plain radiographs include a narrowed intervertebral space, collapse of the articular facets, "fogging" of the intervertebral foramen, and/or "trailing" of calcified disk material into the spinal canal (Fig. 34-32). Myelography is indicated if there are no visible narrowed interspaces, no disk material is visible within the spinal canal or intervertebral foramen, a lesion is identified that is not compatible with the neurologic examination, or if precise localization of the disk is necessary to determine the appropriate surgical approach (e.g., ventral slot vs. fenestration, dorsolateral hemilaminectomy vs. ventral slot). Myelography is indicated in 90% to 95% of cervical disk patients. Patients

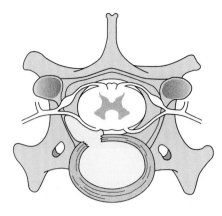

FIG. 34-29
Nerve root entrapment by extruded disk fragments, resulting in radiculopathy.

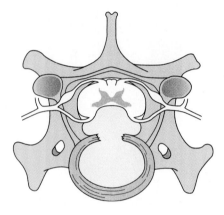

FIG. 34-30
Spinal cord compression by extruded disk fragments, resulting in myelopathy.

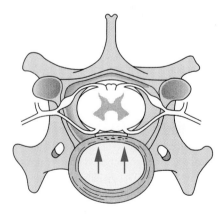

FIG. 34-31
Fibers of the dorsal annulus fibrosus compressed by degenerate nuclear fragments, resulting in diskogenic pain.

with a herniated cervical disk exhibit signs consistent with an extradural mass (Fig. 34-33).

☞ **N O T E** • General anesthesia is necessary to obtain diagnostic radiographs in animals with disk protrusion.

An intraforaminal or lateral disk extrusion is present in some animals with severe neck pain. Intraforaminal disk fragments cannot be seen on plain or contrast ventrodorsal or lateral projections; an oblique cervical radiograph is necessary. To obtain oblique cervical radiographs, the patient is placed in dorsal recumbency, with the entire cervical spine positioned at a 45- to 60-degree angle to the table. The left intervertebral foramina are viewed when the spine is obliqued to the right and vice versa. Fogging of the foramen is diagnostic for intraforaminal disk extrusion (Fig. 34-34).

Laboratory Findings

Patients presenting with cervical disk disease rarely have abnormalities on CBC or biochemical profile. Because most affected patients have severe neck pain, a stress leukogram may be seen. Patients recently treated with corticosteroids may have elevated hepatic enzymes.

DIFFERENTIAL DIAGNOSIS

Presumptive diagnosis of cervical disk disease is based on signalment, careful historical evaluation, physical examination, and neurologic examination. Potential diseases that mimic cervical disk disease include neoplasia, atlantoaxial instability, diskospondylitis, and spinal fracture/luxation. Diagnostic differentials can usually be eliminated by evaluation of physical, hematologic, serum biochemical, cerebrospinal fluid, and radiographic studies. Diagnosis of cervical disk extrusion is confirmed by radiography, myelography, and/or surgery.

MEDICAL MANAGEMENT

Conservative vs. surgical treatment of patients with cervical disk disease is dictated by the patient's history and presenting neurologic signs. A staging system helps determine appropriate therapy (Table 34-8). The most important aspect of conservative management in patients with cervical disk disease is strict cage confinement for 3 to 4 weeks. After this period, 3 to 4 weeks of gradual return to normal activity is recommended. Walks should be restricted to a leash and harness; collars that encircle the neck should be avoided. This duration of forced rest allows resolution of inflammation and facilitates stabilization of the ruptured disk by fibrosis.

Strict confinement and exercise control may or may not be accompanied by administration of antiinflammatories and/or muscle relaxants. It is important to educate the client about potential euphoric effects of antiinflammatory drugs. If strict confinement is not maintained during drug therapy, the patient could potentially worsen because of increased activity leading to further disk extrusion. Antiinflammatory management of patients presenting with *pain alone* may be instituted multiple times without fear of inducing tetraparesis. Moreover, patients treated conservatively that fail to respond may still benefit from surgery. Therefore most patients with mild to moderate neck pain from cervical disk extrusion should be treated conserva-

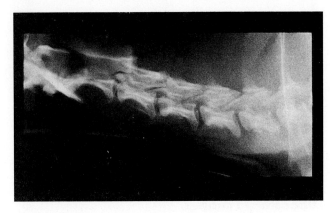

FIG. 34-32
Lateral radiograph of a dog with a C2-C3 herniated intervertebral disk. Notice the "fogged" foramen (herniated disk) and slightly narrowed intervertebral space.

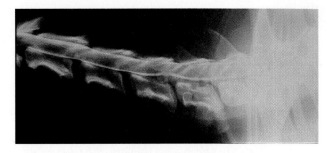

FIG. 34-33
Lateral myelogram of a dog with a C5-C6 herniated intervertebral disk. Notice elevation of contrast column at C5-6 consistent with extradural compression.

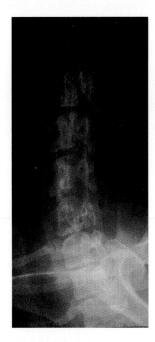

FIG. 34-34
Forty-five- to sixty-degree oblique cervical radiograph showing intraforaminal disk extrusion at C7-T1.

tively before surgical intervention. Commonly used antiinflammatories and muscle relaxants and their dosages are provided in Table 34-9. Antiinflammatory drugs and muscle relaxants can be used independently or in combination. Choosing the proper drug regimen is dictated by the patient's clinical signs and knowing the outcome of therapeutic trials. Recommended corticosteroid dosages vary dramatically among clinicians. Dosages provided in Table 34-9 should be tapered over a 6-day period and followed with serial neurologic examinations. If there is no response, consider repeat corticosteroid therapy, combination therapy, or surgery.

Nonsteroidal antiinflammatory drugs may cause severe gastric irritation and ulceration, particularly if the dosage is above recommended levels, given for extended periods, or given in combination with corticosteroids. **Nonsteroidal antiinflammatory drugs (NSAIDs) should not be used in combination with corticosteroids.** Muscle relaxants are generally unsuccessful when used alone to treat patients with severe neck or back pain; they should be combined with corticosteroids initially. Muscle relaxants can be given in combination with prednisolone, dexamethasone, aspirin, phenylbutazone, or flunixin meglumine. A muscle relaxant can be used alone in patients with mild or moderate neck or back pain, or in those with moderate to severe neck or back pain that are improving but require further treatment. Common clinical presentations and suggested therapeutic regimens are listed in Table 34-10. Knowledge of the potential side effects of commonly used antiinflammatory drugs (or combinations of drugs) is important. A list of common side effects of drugs used to treat patients with cervical disk disease is provided in Table 34-11. **All patients must be placed in strict confinement for 3 to 4 weeks as part of their medical management, especially if drugs are used.**

Patients given antiinflammatory drugs should be monitored carefully for depression, anorexia, abdominal pain, melena, and/or vomiting undigested or digested blood (coffee grounds). If gastrointestinal lesions are suspected, corticosteroids and NSAIDs should be discontinued immediately because gastrointestinal ulceration associated with antiinflammatory medication, spinal cord injury, and stress of hospitalization may be fatal. Drugs listed in Table 34-12 may be used to treat or prevent gastric ulcers.

SURGICAL TREATMENT

The objective of surgery in patients with cervical disk disease is to remove extruded disk fragments from attenuated nerve roots and/or spinal cord. This may result in immediate pain relief and eventual restoration of normal motor function. A ventral slot is most commonly performed for removal of disk material in the cervical region; however, midcervical or caudal cervical hemilaminectomy and facetectomy (see p. 1058) are indicated for removal of disk fragments from the intervertebral foramen. During ventral slot procedures adequate decompression of the spinal cord is achieved when the char-

TABLE 34-8

Staging System to Help Determine Medical vs. Surgical Treatment and Prognosis of Animals with Cervical Disk Disease

Stage	Clinical signs	Radiography	Treatment	Prognosis
I	Single or occasional episodes of mild to moderate neck pain	Radiographs not taken	Conservative	Favorable
		Incidental finding of degenerate disks	Fenestration/ conservative	Favorable
II	First episode of severe neck pain or second episode of mild to moderate neck pain	Radiographs not taken	Conservative	Favorable/guarded
		Extruded disk in canal	Ventral slot	Excellent
III	Uncontrolled neck pain or repeated episodes of neck pain	Extruded disk in canal	Ventral slot	Excellent
		Intraforaminal disk	Dorsolateral hemilaminectomy	Excellent/favorable
IV	Ambulatory tetraparesis* with or without neck pain	Radiographs not taken	Conservative	Guarded
		Extruded disk in canal	Ventral slot	Excellent/favorable
V	Weakly ambulatory tetraparesis† with or without neck pain	Extruded disk in canal	Ventral slot	Excellent/favorable
VI	Nonambulatory tetraparesis‡ with or without neck pain; absence of forelimb sensory deficits	Extruded disk—C2 to C4	Ventral slot	Excellent
		Extruded disk—C4 to C7	Ventral slot	Favorable
VII	Nonambulatory tetraparesis‡ with or without neck pain; forelimb sensory deficits present	Extruded disk in canal	Ventral slot	Guarded

*Ambulatory tetraparesis is hindlimb weakness with a choppy forelimb gait; the patient can rise without assistance and ambulate with evidence of motor weakness.

†Weakly ambulatory tetraparesis is severe tetraparesis; the patient can rise without assistance and take several steps, but tires easily and assumes a recumbent position.

‡Nonambulatory tetraparesis is severe tetraparesis without the ability to ambulate unassisted; voluntary motor movements may or may not be present.

acteristic bluish hue of the dural tube is identified through the slot (Fig. 34-35).

Recurrence of cervical disk extrusion at an alternate intervertebral space is rare; routine fenestration of unaffected disks after ventral slot is unnecessary. Cervical disk fenestration (see p. 1055) may be used to treat patients with neck pain secondary to cervical disk disease. Fenestration relieves pain in some patients, but does not adequately remove compressive disk material from the spinal canal or intervertebral foramen. Patients that undergo fenestration for cervical disk disease exhibit longer morbidity than those treated with ventral decompression (ventral slot). Tetraparesis may occur from overaggressive fenestration.

Preoperative Management

Intravenous fluids and steroids should be given before surgery. In addition to their therapeutic effect, intravenous steroids may protect the spinal cord from the effects of surgical manipulation. The steroid of choice is methylprednisolone sodium succinate (30 mg/kg intravenously).

Anesthesia

Selected anesthetic protocols for animals undergoing cervical spinal cord surgery are provided on p. 1049. The animal's neurologic status and positioning for surgery are important preanesthetic considerations. If the patient is exhibiting motor weakness (e.g., weakly ambulatory or nonambulatory tetraparesis), or will require positioning that may cause respiratory compromise, mechanical ventilatory support should be considered.

Surgical Anatomy

Unique anatomic features of the cervical spine include the following: (1) C1-C2 does not have an intervertebral disk, (2) C6 has a prominent transverse process, (3) C1 has a prominent ventral spinous process, (4) each vertebral body has a characteristic midline ventral ridge, (5) presence of transverse foramen (for vertebral artery and vein) in each cervical vertebra except C7, (6) characteristic cranial-to-caudal slant of each intervertebral space, and (7) location of the vertebral venous sinuses and dorsal longitudinal ligament on the floor of the spinal canal.

Positioning

Patients undergoing a ventral slot or fenestration procedure should be placed in dorsal recumbency with their chest in a V-trough. They must be carefully secured with sandbags or a rigid vacuum type of apparatus to prevent lateral motion. The front legs are taped caudally and a loop of rope is tied around the muzzle, caudal to the maxillary canine teeth. The rope is secured to the table and the front legs are pulled caudally to apply linear traction to the cervical spine (see Fig. 34-5 on p. 1053). Linear traction stabilizes the spine and opens intervertebral spaces and foramina, improving exposure during the ventral slot procedure. An area from cranial to the laryngeal cartilages to caudal to the manubrium sterni should be prepared for surgery (i.e., ventral midline cervical incision). Patients diagnosed with intraforaminal disk extrusion should be positioned in sternal recumbency with the neck elevated, cradled, and gently flexed (see Fig. 34-17 on p. 1057 and Fig. 34-21 on p. 1058).

SURGICAL TECHNIQUE

Perform a ventral slot as described on p. 1051. Once the spinal canal has been reached, remove disk material located on the ventral midline first because removal of laterally located disk material increases the risk of lacerating a venous sinus. A dull, flat dental spatula is best suited for removal of foramenal disk material (Fig. 34-36, A). Bend the dental spatula at a 60-degree angle to facilitate removal of laterally extruded disk material and reduce venous sinus laceration. Gently sweep the spatula along the lateral aspect of the spinal canal (Fig. 34-36, B). Gently tease to loosen disk material from the foramen and encourage fragments to move toward the slot margin where they can either be suctioned using a small suction tip or removed with fine ophthalmic forceps. Take special care when old, calcified disks are encountered because they may be adhered to venous sinus or dura. Carefully tease and manipulate these disks away from the dura with a dental spatula. If severe hemorrhage from a lacerated venous sinus occurs, discontinue manipulation in the spinal canal and consider closing the incision. The technique for controlling venous sinus hemorrhage is discussed in Table 34-1 on p. 1050. *If hemorrhage can be lateralized to one side of the slot, it may be possible to manipulate and remove the disk from the opposite side of the slot, but take care to ensure adequate visualization before manipulation in the spinal canal.*

SUTURE MATERIALS/SPECIAL INSTRUMENTS

Special instrumentation necessary for ventral slot, disk fenestration, and dorsolateral hemilaminectomy is listed in Table 34-7.

POSTOPERATIVE CARE AND ASSESSMENT

Respiration should be monitored and animals should be observed for seizures for 24 hours after surgery. Analgesics should be provided as necessary (Table 34-13) and corticosteroids discontinued immediately postoperatively. Neurologic examination should be performed twice daily. Ambulatory patients are generally discharged by 24 to 48 hours postoperatively. Discharge of nonambulatory patients generally depends on the owner's ability to care for the animal. All patients should be fitted with a harness; neck collars should be avoided. Ambulatory patients should have exercise restricted for 3 to 4 weeks; gradual increase in exercise is allowed over the subsequent 3 to 4 weeks. Stable interbody fusion after ventral slot requires 6 to 8 weeks, after which return to normal activity is recommended. Care of nonambulatory patients is described on p. 1062. Return of neurologic function is difficult to predict postoperatively; it may take 6 to 8 weeks (or longer) for the animal to regain the ability to ambulate.

Significant complications in patients treated surgically for cervical disk disease are uncommon. Possible complications include continued neck pain and/or deteriorating motor status. Treatment of the complication is determined by the cause and surgical treatment used. Successful treatment options are outlined in Table 34-14.

TABLE 34-9

Dosages and Regimens of Drugs Used in Patients with Cervical or Thoracolumbar Disk Disease

Corticosteroids:
Dexamethasone (Azium)

0.2 mg/kg PO or IM BID for 3 days, then SID for 3 days; reevaluate; may repeat treatment once or twice and consider combining with a muscle relaxant; if no response, consider surgery

Prednisolone

0.5 to 1.0 mg/kg PO BID for 3 days, then SID for 3 days; reevaluate; may repeat treatment once or twice; consider combining with a muscle relaxant; if no response, consider surgery

Methylprednisolone (Solu-Medrol)

30 mg/kg IV given once at anesthetic induction; discontinue after 1 dose

Nonsteroidal antiinflammatories:
Aspirin

10 mg/kg PO BID for 7 days; reevaluate; if no response, consider alternative medical therapy or surgery

Phenylbutazone (Butazolidin)

22 mg/kg PO TID (not to exceed 800 mg/day) for 7 days; reevaluate; if no response, consider alternative medical therapy or surgery (not recommended in cats)

Flunixin meglumine (Banamine)

0.5 mg/kg IV, IM, or SC BID for 2 days maximum; reevaluate; if no response, consider alternative medical therapy or surgery

Muscle relaxants:
Methyocarbamol (Robaxin-V)

22 mg/kg PO once as a loading dose, then 11 mg/kg PO TID for 10 days; reevaluate; may repeat treatment once or twice and consider combining with steroids; if no response, consider surgery

Diazepam (Valium)

1.1 mg/kg PO BID (not to exceed 20 mg/day) for 10 days; reevaluate; may repeat once or twice; consider combining with steroids; if no response, consider surgery

PROGNOSIS

Prognosis for patients treated medically or surgically for cervical disk disease depends on neurologic signs, anatomic location of the disk extrusion, and medical or surgical treatment used, but is generally favorable. Clinical factors and probable patient outcomes are outlined in Table 34-8. Ambulatory patients with mild, moderate, or severe neck pain should be pain free or significantly improved by 24 to 48 hours postoperatively. Ambulatory, tetraparetic patients (with or without neck pain) should be pain free 24 to 48 hours postoperatively and motor dysfunction should be resolved by 7 to 10 days. Weakly ambulatory tetraparetic patients (with or without neck pain) should be pain free 24 to 48 hours postoperatively and motor dysfunction should be resolved by 3 to 4 weeks. Nonambulatory tetraparetic

TABLE 34-10

Recommended Medical/Conservative Therapy Based on Clinical Presentation of Dogs with Cervical Disk Disease*

Clinical Presentation	Initial Treatment†	Result	Second Treatment†	Result	Third Treatment†
Mild neck pain; first episode or multiple episodes	Cage rest only	No improvement	Muscle relaxants for 10 days	No improvement	Steroids‡ plus muscle relaxants for 6 days
Moderate neck pain; first episode or multiple episodes	Muscle relaxants for 10 days	No improvement	Steroids‡ plus muscle relaxants for 6 days	No improvement	Repeat second treatment and consider surgery
Severe neck pain; first episode or multiple episodes	Steroids‡ plus muscle relaxants for 6 days	No improvement	Repeat first treatment	No improvement	Consider surgery
Severe neck pain; first episode or multiple episodes	Steroids‡ plus muscle relaxants for 6 days	Slight improvement to moderate or mild neck pain	Muscle relaxants for 10 days	No improvement	Repeat second treatment and consider surgery
Mild, moderate, or severe neck pain and ambulatory tetraparesis	Recommend surgery but consider steroid trial for 1 day	No improvement on steroids	Surgery; ventral slot; preoperative steroids		
Mild, moderate, or severe neck pain and nonambulatory tetraparesis	Surgery; ventral slot; preoperative steroids				
Recurrent mild, moderate, or severe pain; unresponsive to medical management	Surgery; ventral slot; preoperative steroids				

*See Table 34-9 for drug dosages and variations on duration of therapy.
†All patients must be placed in strict confinement for 3 to 4 weeks as part of their medical management, regardless of the drug used or duration of drug therapy.
‡Nonsteroidal antiinflammatory drugs can be substituted for corticosteroids; however, corticosteroids should not be used in combination with nonsteroidal antiinflammatory drugs.

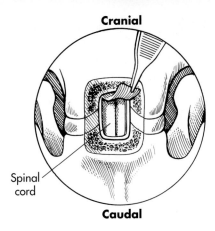

FIG. 34-35
When herniated disk material has been successfully removed, the spinal cord is visible.

TABLE 34-13

Postoperative Analgesics

Oxymorphone (Numorphan)
0.05-0.1 mg/kg IV, IM every 4 hrs (as needed)

Butorphanol (Torbutrol, Torbugesic)
0.2-0.4 mg/kg IV, IM, or SC every 2 to 4 hrs (as needed)

Buprenorphine (Buprenex)
5-15 µg/kg IV, IM every 6 hrs (as needed)

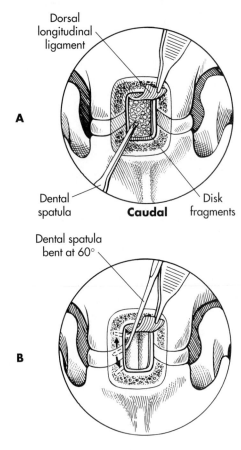

FIG. 34-36
A, Remove ventrally located disk fragments with ophthalmic forceps and a dental spatula. **B,** Remove laterally located (foraminal) disk fragments with a dental spatula bent at 60 degrees; use a sweeping motion to encourage disk removal.

TABLE 34-11

Side Effects of Commonly Used Antiinflammatory Drugs

Drug	Side Effects
Dexamethasone	When used in combination with NSAIDs (i.e., flunixin meglumine), commonly causes gastric ulceration/perforation, colonic ulceration (rare), pancreatitis (rare)
Prednisolone	Same as dexamethasone
Aspirin	Platelet function abnormalities, gastric ulceration/perforation
Phenylbutazone	Bone marrow suppression, gastric ulceration/perforation
Flunixin meglumine	Gastric ulceration, prolonged treatment in combination with steroids commonly causes gastric ulceration/perforation
Methocarbamol	Slight muscle weakness
Diazepam	Central nervous system depression, potential for client abuse

TABLE 34-12

Drugs Used to Treat or Prevent Gastrointestinal Complications of Corticosteroids or NSAIDs

Drug	Dose	Action
Cimetidine (Tagamet)	5-10 mg/kg PO, IV, SC TID to QID	Used to treat ulcers; decreases gastric acid formation by the parietal cell, thus preventing further ulceration by HCl
Ranitidine (Zantac)	2 mg/kg PO, IV, IM, SC BID to TID	Same as cimetidine
Famotidine (Pepcid)	0.5 mg/kg PO SID to BID	Same as cimetidine
Omeprazole (Prilosec)	0.7-1.5 mg/kg PO SID to BID	Used to treat ulcers; blocks proton pump of the parietal cell
Misoprostol (Cytotec)	1-5 µg/kg PO TID	A prostaglandin E analog that is used to prevent NSAID-induced ulcers
Sucralfate (Carafate)	0.5-1.0 g PO TID to QID; give 1 hr after other medications	Used to treat ulcers; gastric and duodenal protectant; acts to coat ulcer; acts as a bandage

TABLE 34-14

Postoperative Complications in Surgical Patients with Cervical Disk Disease

Complication	Surgical Treatment Used	Cause (Based on Radiography)	Course of Action
Continued neck pain	Ventral slot	Slot excessively wide	Neck brace for 2 to 3 weeks; pain control; if no improvement, then cervical stabilization
		Disk material remains	Neck brace for 2 to 3 weeks; pain control; if no improvement, reoperate
		Normal radiographs	Neck brace and treat medically for diskogenic pain
Continued neck pain	Dorsolateral hemilaminectomy	Disk material remains	Neck brace for 2 to 3 weeks; pain control; if no improvement, make oblique radiographs; reoperate if disk present in foramen
Continued neck pain	Fenestration	Disk in canal	Ventral slot, remove disk from canal and foramen
		Disk in foramen	Dorsolateral hemilaminectomy and facetectomy
Deteriorating motor status	Ventral slot	Slot excessively wide	Cervical stabilization
		Disk in canal	Reoperate if disk in spinal canal; if second disk, perform ventral slot
Deteriorating motor status	Dorsolateral hemilaminectomy	Disk pushed into canal	Reoperate to remove disk
Deteriorating motor status	Fenestration	Disk in canal	Ventral slot; remove disk from canal

patients (with or without neck pain) should be pain free 24 to 48 hours postoperatively and motor dysfunction should be resolved by 4 to 6 weeks. Nonambulatory tetraparetic patients have a better prognosis if they do not have foreleg sensory deficits preoperatively, have a C2-C3 or C3-C4 lesion, and regain ambulation within 96 hours postoperatively.

References

Seim HB, Prata RG: Ventral decompression for the treatment of cervical disk diseases in the dog: a review of 54 cases, *J Am Anim Hosp Assoc* 18:233, 1982.

Toombs JP: Cervical intervertebral disk disease in dogs, *Compend Contin Educ Pract Vet* 14:1477, 1992.

Suggested Reading

Bagley RS et al: Cervical vertebral fusion and concurrent intervertebral disc extrusion in four dogs, *Vet Radiol and Ultrasound* 34:336, 1993.

Bagley RS et al: Dysphonia in two dogs with cranial cervical intervertebral disk extrusion, *J Am Anim Hosp Assoc* 29:557, 1993.

Clark DM: An analysis of intraoperative and early postoperative mortality associated with cervical spinal decompressive surgery in the dog, *J Am Anim Hosp Assoc* 22:739, 1986.

Dallman MJ, Paletta P, Bojrab MJ: Characteristics of dogs admitted for treatment of cervical intervertebral disk disease: 105 cases (1972–1982), *J Am Vet Med Assoc* 200:2009, 1992.

Felts JF, Prata RG: Cervical disk disease in the dog: intraforaminal and lateral extrusions, *J Am Anim Hosp Assoc* 19:755, 1983.

Fingeroth JM, Smeak DD: Laminotomy of the axis for surgical access to the cervical spinal cord: a case report, *Vet Surg* 18:123, 1989.

Fry TR et al: Surgical treatment of cervical disc herniations in ambulatory dogs, ventral decompression vs. fenestration: 111 cases (1980–1988), *Prog Vet Neurol* 2:165, 1991.

Gaschen L, Lang J, Haeni H: Intervertebral disc herniation (Schmorl's node) in five dogs, *Vet Radiol and Ultrasound* 36:509, 1995.

Tomlinson J: Tetraparesis following cervical disk fenestration in two dogs, *J Am Vet Med Assoc* 187:76, 1985.

Waters DJ: Nonambulatory tetraparesis secondary to cervical disk disease in the dog, *J Am Anim Hosp Assoc* 25:647, 1989.

WOBBLER SYNDROME

DEFINITIONS

Wobbler syndrome is a disorder of the caudal cervical vertebrae and intervertebral disks (i.e., spondylopathy) that causes spinal cord compression (i.e., myelopathy).

SYNONYMS

Cervical vertebral instability, cervical spondylomyelopathy, cervical malformation-malarticulation, cervical spondylolisthesis, cervical spondylopathy

GENERAL CONSIDERATIONS AND CLINICALLY RELEVANT PATHOPHYSIOLOGY

Wobbler syndrome is a relatively common disease in Doberman pinschers, Great Danes, and other large-breed dogs. The etiology is unknown, but may be nutritional, traumatic, hereditary, or acquired. It is a "syndrome" that probably has multiple etiologies. Wobbler syndrome has been subdivided into five classifications distinguished by the location of the compressive lesion with respect to the spinal canal (Table 34-15). Discussion of the proposed pathophysiology of Wobbler syndrome is divided into each of the proposed disease classifications (i.e., chronic degenerative disk disease, congenital osseous malformations, vertebral tipping, hypertrophied ligamentum flavum/vertebral arch malformations, and "hourglass" compression).

TABLE 34-15

Classification of Wobbler Syndrome

Classification	Age/Breed	Lesion Location	Cause of Compression	General Prognosis
Chronic degenerative disk disease	Adult, male Doberman pinschers	Compresses ventral aspect of spinal cord C5 to C7	Disk degeneration and subsequent hypertrophy of ventral annulus fibrosus	Favorable
Congenital osseous malformation	Young Great Danes and Doberman pinschers	Compresses spinal cord laterally or dorsoventrally C3 to C7	Congenital malformation of vertebral bodies and articular facets	Unfavorable
Vertebral tipping	Adult, male Doberman pinschers	Compresses ventral aspect of spinal cord C5 to C7	Dorsal malposition of the affected vertebral body in the spinal canal	Favorable
Ligamentum flavum/vertebral arch malformation	Young Great Danes	Compresses dorsal aspect of spinal cord C4 to C7	Hypertrophy and hyperplasia of the ligamentum flavum; vertebral arch malformation	Favorable to guarded
Hourglass compression	Young Great Danes	Compresses spinal cord on all sides C2 to C7	Hypertrophy of ligamentum flavum and annulus fibrosus; malformation or degenerative disk disease of articular facets	Guarded

Chronic degenerative disk disease may originate from either vertebral instability (i.e., stress) or primary degeneration of the intervertebral disk (i.e., Hansen type II disk protrusion). The degenerating annulus fibrosus undergoes hypertrophy and/or hyperplasia. Spinal cord compression occurs when the disk space collapses and buckles the redundant annulus fibrosus dorsally (Fig. 34-37, *A*). The dorsal longitudinal ligament (located dorsal to the annulus fibrosus on the floor of the spinal canal) compresses the dura (see Fig. 34-37, *A*). Spinal cord compression in chronic degenerative disk disease is dynamic in that flexion and extension of the neck may vary the degree of spinal cord compression. Generally, dorsal extension of the neck increases spinal cord compression (Fig. 34-37, *B*); ventral flexion (Fig. 34-37, *C*) and linear traction (Fig. 34-37, *D*) decrease compression.

Congenital osseous malformations may occur anywhere along the cervical spine in one or multiple (most common) vertebrae. Malformed vertebrae cause narrowing of the spinal canal as a result of stenosis of the cranial vertebral canal orifice, articular facet deformities, malformation of vertebral pedicles, and/or deformation of vertebral arches (Fig. 34-38). Diets high in calcium exacerbate the malformations in Great Dane puppies. Congenital osseous malformations may be related to disorders of endochondral ossification.

Vertebral tipping is characterized by displacement (tipping) of the craniodorsal surface of the vertebral body (generally C6 or C7) into the spinal canal, causing spinal cord compression (Fig. 34-39). Instability secondary to chronic degenerative disk disease (or vice versa) may be the predisposing factor that allows the vertebral body to become malpositioned.

The compressive lesion in hypertrophied ligamentum flavum/vertebral arch malformations occurs on the dorsal aspect of the spinal cord. Patients with isolated ligamentum flavum abnormalities will probably develop hypertrophy and/or hyperplasia secondary to instability (Fig. 34-40). Vertebral arch malformations may be genetic and/or nutritional in origin. Whatever the cause, the vertebral arch, articular processes, and facets become plump, deformed, and asymmetric. Spinal cord compression is not the result solely of deformation, but of a combination of static deformation and dynamic compression. In dorsal extension, the cranial tip of the deformed vertebral arch of one vertebra is brought closer to the caudodorsal rim of the body of the adjacent cranial vertebra, increasing spinal cord compression (Fig. 34-41, *A*). When the neck is flexed ventrally, the cranial tip of the elongated vertebral arch is retracted, decreasing spinal cord compression (Fig. 34-41, *B*).

Hourglass compression occurs because the spinal cord compression occurs dorsally, ventrally, and laterally (Fig. 34-42). Annulus fibrosus hypertrophy and/or hyperplasia causes ventral spinal cord compression, whereas hypertrophy and/or hyperplasia of the ligamentum flavum produces dorsal spinal cord compression. Degenerative joint disease or malformation/malarticulation of the articular facets causes lateral spinal cord compression. Dynamic hourglass lesions may occur at any level of the cervical spine.

DIAGNOSIS
Clinical Presentation

Signalment. Information concerning sex and breed may assist specific classification of Wobbler syndrome (see Table 34-15). Doberman pinschers and Great Danes account for 80% of the cases. The incidence of chronic degenerative disk disease is twice as likely in males than females. Variation in age of presentation depends on specific classification (see Table 34-15).

History. Affected animals generally become less coordinated over months to years. All four limbs are affected, but

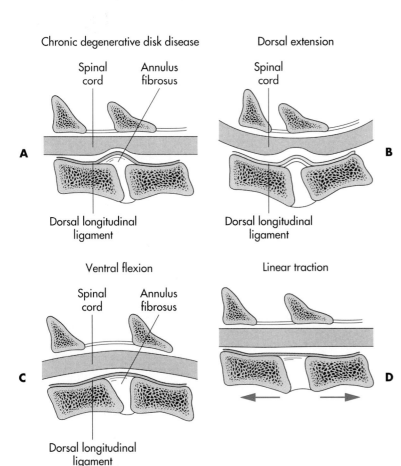

Chronic degenerative disk disease

Dorsal extension

Ventral flexion

Linear traction

FIG. 34-37
A, Chronic degenerative disk disease produces spinal cord compression because of hypertrophy of the annulus fibrosus. **B,** Mechanism by which dorsal extension of the cervical spine increases spinal cord compression in patients with chronic degenerative disk disease. **C,** Ventral flexion of the cervical spine decreases spinal cord compression in patients with chronic degenerative disk disease. **D,** Linear traction of the cervical spine decreases spinal cord compression in patients with chronic degenerative disk disease.

FIG. 34-38
Vertebra with congenital osseous malformation (C7). Notice the malformed facets and deformation of the spinal canal.

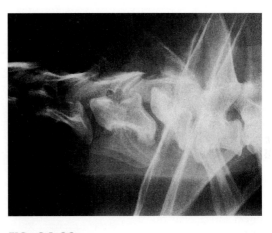

FIG. 34-39
Lateral radiograph of a dog with Wobbler syndrome and C6-C7 vertebral tipping. Notice the cranial dorsal surface of C7 "tipped" into the spinal canal.

signs are generally initiated and more pronounced in the rear legs. Occasionally, an acute exacerbation precipitated by minor trauma may be noted. Approximately 40% of cases have a history of neck pain (Bruecker, Seim, Blass, 1989).

Physical Examination Findings

General physical examination findings are normal in the majority of patients with Wobbler syndrome. Upper motor neuron signs (including a crossed extensor reflex) generally occur in the rear limbs of dogs with chronic disease. A broad-based stance is often noted in the rear legs. Thoracic limb reflex changes are generally mild. A stiff, straight-legged gait and atrophy of the supraspinatus and infraspinatus muscles are common with chronicity. The neck is often carried in ventral flexion because this position produces the least amount of spinal cord compression (see Fig. 34-37, *C*). Dorsal extension of the neck may cause pain and/or accentuate spinal cord compression, with resultant increased motor signs (see Fig. 34-37, *B*). Care should therefore be taken

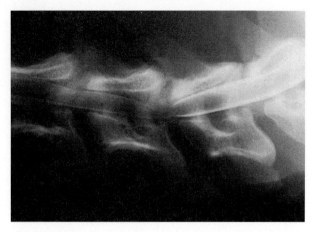

FIG. 34-40
Lateral myelogram of a dog with C5-C6 ligamentum flavum hypertrophy. Notice the ventral deviation of the dorsal contrast column.

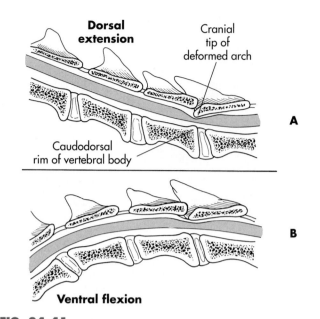

FIG. 34-41
A, Dorsal vertebral arch malformation producing dorsal spinal cord compression. **B,** Ventral flexion causes retraction of the malformed arch, relieving spinal cord compression.

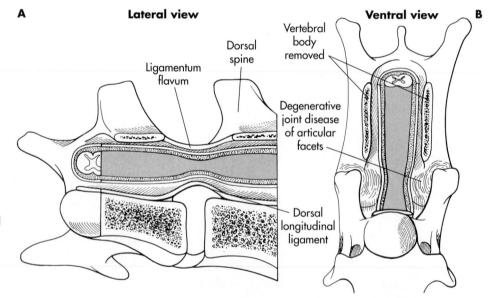

FIG. 34-42
A, Hourglass compression of the ventral spinal cord is caused by redundant dorsal annulus fibrosus; dorsal compression is caused by redundant ligamentum flavum. **B,** Lateral compression is caused by degenerative joint disease or malformation/malarticulation of articular facets.

when manipulating the head and neck. Abnormalities noted on neurologic examination vary and may include pain alone, paraparesis, ambulatory tetraparesis, weakly ambulatory tetraparesis, or nonambulatory tetraparesis. Definitions of each neurologic classification are provided in Table 34-16.

Radiography/Ultrasonography

Plain radiographs of the neck are *not* diagnostic for the affected vertebra, intervertebral space (IVS), or location of the compressive mass within the spinal canal (i.e., dorsal, ventral, and/or lateral). Typical changes on plain radiographs for each classification of Wobbler syndrome are summarized in Table 34-17.

Although plain radiography may help diagnose Wobbler

syndrome, myelography is essential to determine the following: (1) location and number of affected vertebrae and/or intervertebral spaces, (2) location of lesion(s) within the spinal canal (i.e., dorsal, ventral, lateral), (3) degree of spinal cord compression, and (4) occurrence of dynamic compression. Typical myelographic changes expected with each classification of Wobbler syndrome are provided in Table 34-17.

Stress myelography is radiographic imaging of the cervical spine in various stressed positions (i.e., ventral flexion, dorsal extension, and linear traction) during myelography. Stress myelography is essential to diagnose dynamic compressive lesions. Classically, spinal cord compression with chronic degenerative disk disease is worsened with the neck

TABLE 34-16

Neurologic Classification

Neurologic Finding	Definition
Pain	Discomfort on manipulation of the head and neck
Paraparesis	Upper motor neuron deficits and mild-to-moderate motor weakness of the hind limbs; normal thoracic limb function
Ambulatory tetraparesis	Paraparesis with a choppy thoracic limb gait as a result of upper, lower, or upper and lower motor neuron deficits and mild motor weakness
Weakly ambulatory tetraparesis	Severe tetraparesis; patient can still rise without assistance and take several steps, but tires easily and assumes a recumbent position
Nonambulatory tetraparesis	Tetraparesis without the ability to rise or walk

in dorsal extension and improved in ventral flexion and linear traction (see Fig. 34-37, *B* to *D*). Dorsal extension is not recommended in radiographic evaluation of patients with Wobbler syndrome as it may exacerbrate spinal cord compression. A complete myelographic examination, including linear traction, allows formulation of a rational therapeutic approach (Fig. 34-43).

Laboratory Findings

No significant abnormalities are noted in the hemogram or urinalysis of most affected animals. Biochemical analysis may reveal an elevated serum cholesterol in Doberman pinschers with subclinical hypothyroidism. Whether hypothyroidism has an influence on Wobbler syndrome is unclear.

DIFFERENTIAL DIAGNOSIS

Any disorder causing neck pain, paraparesis, or tetraparesis in large-breed dogs (i.e., especially Doberman pinschers and Great Danes) should be considered as differential diagnoses. Diseases that can be mistaken for Wobbler syndrome are listed in Table 34-18. Differentiation is usually possible by signalment, neurologic exam, serum chemistry, cerebral spinal fluid analysis, and radiography/myelography. Diagnosis of Wobbler syndrome is confirmed by plain and stress myelography.

MEDICAL MANAGEMENT

Wobbler syndrome is a chronic, progressive disorder characterized by subtle hindlimb weakness that often progresses to nonambulatory tetraparesis. Medical therapy may cause temporary improvement; however, progression to an unacceptable neurologic status is common. Whether or not a patient is treated conservatively depends on classification of the disorder, degree of neurologic dysfunction, and number of affected vertebrae or intervertebral spaces (Table 34-19).

The most important aspect of conservative management is strict confinement for 3 to 4 weeks. During this period, patients should be fitted with a neck brace. Gradual return to normal activity is recommended over the next 3 to 4 weeks. Walks should be restricted to a leash and harness; neck collars should be avoided. Although this duration of forced rest allows resolution of spinal cord inflammation, the long-term beneficial effect on cervical spinal stabilization, malformations, disk degeneration, and tissue hypertrophy and hyperplasia is unknown.

Strict confinement, use of a neck brace, and exercise control may or may not be accompanied by antiinflammatory therapy. Clients must be educated as to the potential euphoric effects of antiinflammatory drugs. If strict confinement is not maintained during drug therapy, the patient may become too active and have increased paresis as a result of acute spinal cord contusion. Commonly used antiinflammatory drugs and their dosages are listed in Table 34-20. Recommended corticosteroid dosages vary among clinicians. Nonsteroidal antiinflammatory drugs may cause severe gastric irritation and ulceration, particularly if given above recommended doses or for excessive durations or when given in combination with corticosteroids. **Nonsteroidal antiinflammatory drugs should not be used in combination with corticosteroids.** Knowledge of potential side effects of commonly used antiinflammatory drugs (or combinations of drugs) is important (see Table 34-11).

If conservative treatment is successful, spinal cord edema resolves, remyelination occurs, and the animal recovers function. If no improvement is noted by 3 to 4 weeks, or if neurologic deterioration occurs, surgical intervention should be considered.

SURGICAL TREATMENT

The objectives of surgery in patients with Wobbler syndrome are relief of spinal cord compression, cervical spinal stabilization (where necessary), and reversal of neurologic deficits. Although numerous surgical techniques have been described for treatment of Wobbler syndrome, only a few have long-term prognostic merit. The surgical technique of choice is based on classification, clinical presentation, vertebral body or interspace affected, number of lesions present, location of the lesion within the spinal canal, and the presence or absence of a dynamic lesion (Table 34-21). Surgical techniques currently used to treat patients with Wobbler syndrome include ventral slot, ventral stabilization, ventral traction-stabilization, and dorsal laminectomy.

> ☞ **N O T E** • The major disadvantages of ventral slot decompression are difficulty in adequately removing the entire compressive lesion and possible instability caused by the slot.

Techniques that employ decompression and stabilization have improved the outcome of patients with dynamic lesions. Based on pathophysiology of the compressive lesion, techniques using linear traction stretch the annulus fibrosus,

TABLE 34-17

Plain and Myelographic Findings with Wobbler Syndrome

Classification	Plain Film Changes	Myelographic Changes
Chronic degenerative disk disease	Normal; collapse of the intervertebral space; spondylosis; sclerotic endplates; calcified disk; C5 to C7 most often affected	Extradural mass compressing the ventral surface of the spinal cord; lesions are generally dynamic
Congenital osseous malformation	Various osseous malformations; C3 to C7 most often affected	Extradural mass compressing the lateral, ventral, and/or dorsal surface of the spinal cord; lesions are generally static
Vertebral tipping	Tipping of the craniodorsal end of a vertebra into the spinal canal; C6 or C7 most often affected	Normal; extradural mass compressing the ventral aspect of the spinal cord; lesion may be static or dynamic
Ligamentum flavum hypertrophy	Normal; C4 to C7 most often affected	Extradural mass compressing the dorsal surface of the spinal cord (soft tissue); lesions are generally static
Vertebral arch malformation	Normal; sclerosis and malformation of affected laminae; C4 to C7 most often affected	Extradural mass compressing the dorsal surface of the spinal cord (malformed laminae), lesions often have a static and dynamic component
Hourglass compression	Normal; C2 to C7 may be affected	Extradural mass compressing the lateral, ventral, and dorsal surfaces of the spinal cord (soft tissue and osseous); lesions are generally dynamic

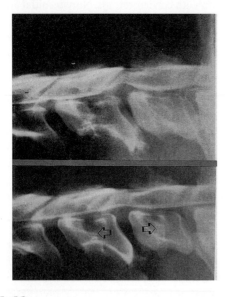

FIG. 34-43
(*Top*) Lateral radiograph of a dog with C6-C7 chronic degenerative disk disease and extradural compression of the spinal cord. (*Bottom*) Linear traction results in spinal cord decompression.

thus relieving spinal cord compression (see Fig. 34-37, *D*). Once the spine is stabilized in traction, the spinal cord remains decompressed and eventually atrophy of the annulus fibrosus occurs, further improving decompression. Several ventral traction-stabilization techniques have been successfully used to treat patients with Wobbler syndrome, particularly those with chronic degenerative disk disease. These include Steinmann pins and methylmethacrylate bone cement, polyvinylidine spinal plates, and Harrington rods. The initial approach for decompression and stabilization is as described

for ventral slot (see p. 1051); however, once the affected IVS is located, the IVS and vertebral bodies cranial and caudal to the affected interspace must be exposed. This increased exposure is necessary for placement of the chosen stabilizing device.

Preoperative Management

The dog is premedicated with intravenous methylprednisolone sodium succinate (30 mg/kg). Intravenous fluids are administered throughout the procedure. Antibiotic therapy is dictated by criteria listed in Table 34-4 on p. 1050.

Anesthesia

Suggested anesthetic protocols for patients with cervical spinal disorders are described on p. 1049. Neurologic status and positioning for surgery are important preanesthetic considerations. If the patient has motor weakness (i.e., weakly ambulatory tetraparetic or nonambulatory tetraparetic), or will require positioning that may cause respiratory compromise (i.e., flexion of the neck, lateral compression of the chest), mechanical ventilatory support should be considered.

Surgical Anatomy

Anatomy of the cervical spine is described on p. 1051 and illustrated in Fig. 34-1 on p. 1052.

Positioning

For a ventral approach, position the animal in dorsal recumbency in a V-trough and carefully secure it to the table to prevent lateral motion. Patients with a dynamic lesion (i.e., chronic degenerative disk disease, hourglass compression, vertebral arch malformation, redundant ligamentum flavum) should be secured to the table with the neck in linear traction. This positioning results in spinal cord decompression. Patients requiring a dorsal approach are placed in sternal recumbency. The use of dynamic positioning is based on patient classification and results of stress myelography. As a general rule, patients requiring dorsal decompression are positioned with the neck elevated and flexed over a rolled fleece or rigid vacuum type of apparatus.

SURGICAL TECHNIQUES
Decompression via a Ventral Slot

Perform a ventral slot as described on p. 1051. Once the spinal canal is reached, carefully remove redundant dorsal annulus fibrosus (i.e., dynamic lesion) or disk material (i.e., static lesion). Remove the ventral midline annulus or disk

---

TABLE 34-18

Differential Diagnoses That Mimic Wobbler Syndrome Using the DAMNIT-V Scheme

Classification	Examples	Diagnostic Differentials/Tools
Degenerative	Cervical disk disease	Static mass on stress myelography
	Bilateral hip dysplasia	Physical exam; neurologic exam; hip radiographs
	Bilateral ruptured cruciate	Physical exam; neurologic exam
Anomalous	Atlantoaxial subluxation	Signalment; plain and stress radiography
Metabolic	Any disorder causing generalized weakness (e.g., Addison's disease)	Neurologic exam; laboratory findings
Nutritional	Nutritional secondary hyperparathyroidism	Dietary history; plain radiography
Neoplastic	Tumors of the cervical spine, spinal cord, or nerve roots	Plain and stress myelography
Immunologic	Polyarthritis	Neurologic exam; laboratory data
	Polymyositis	Neurologic exam; laboratory data
Infectious	Cervical diskospondylitis	Plain radiographs
	Meningitis	CSF analysis
Traumatic	Cervical spinal fracture/luxation	History; plain radiographs
Vascular	Fibrocartilaginous embolism	History; CSF analysis; myelography

---

TABLE 34-19

Conservative vs. Surgical Management for Patients with Wobbler Syndrome

Classification	Clinical Signs*	Number of Lesions	Treatment	Prognosis
Chronic degenerative disk disease, vertebral tipping, hourglass compression	Pain alone	Single or multiple lesions	Conservative	Favorable
			Surgical	Excellent
	Paraparesis	Single or multiple lesions	Conservative	Favorable
			Surgical	Excellent
	Ambulatory tetraparesis	Single lesion	Conservative	Guarded
			Surgical	Favorable
		Multiple lesions	Conservative	Guarded to unfavorable
			Surgical	Favorable to guarded
	Weakly ambulatory tetraparesis	Single lesion	Conservative	Unfavorable to grave
			Surgical	Favorable to guarded
		Multiple lesions	Conservative	Unfavorable to grave
			Surgical	Guarded
	Nonambulatory tetraparesis	Single lesion	Conservative	Grave
			Surgical	Guarded
		Multiple lesions	Conservative	Grave
			Surgical	Guarded to unfavorable
Ligamentum flavum hypertrophy/vertebral arch malformation	Paraparesis	Single or multiple lesions	Conservative	Guarded
			Surgical	Favorable
	Tetraparesis	Single lesion	Surgical	Favorable
		Multiple lesions	Surgical	Guarded
Congenital osseous malformation	Paraparesis	Single lesion (rare)	Conservative	Unfavorable
			Surgical	Favorable
	Tetraparesis	Single lesion (rare)	Surgical	Guarded
	Paraparesis	Multiple lesions	Conservative	Unfavorable
			Surgical	Unfavorable
	Tetraparesis	Multiple lesions	Surgical	Unfavorable to grave

*The definition of each neurologic classification is given in Table 34-16.

TABLE 34-20

Drugs Used in Patients with Wobbler Syndrome

Corticosteroids:
Dexamethasone (Azium)

0.2 mg/kg PO or IM BID for 3 days, then SID for 3 days; reevaluate patient; may repeat treatment once or twice; if no response, consider surgery

Prednisolone

0.5 to 1.0 mg/kg PO BID for 3 days; then SID for 3 days; reevaluate patient; may repeat treatment once or twice; if no response, consider surgery

Methylprednisolone (Solu-Medrol)

30 mg/kg IV given once at anesthetic induction; discontinue after 1 dose

Nonsteroidal antiinflammatories:
Aspirin

10 mg/kg PO BID for 7 days; reevaluate patient; if no response, consider alternative medical therapy or surgery

Phenylbutazone (Butazolidin)

22 mg/kg PO TID (not to exceed 800 mg/day) for 7 days; reevaluate patient; if no response, consider alternative medical therapy or surgery

Flunixin meglumine (Banamine)

0.5 mg/kg IV, IM, or SC BID for 2 days maximum; reevaluate patient; if no response, consider corticosteroid therapy or surgery

material first so as not to lacerate the vertebral venous sinus. Use ophthalmic forceps and a dental spatula to remove laterally located annular or disk fragments. Continue to remove tissue until the bluish hue of the spinal cord is visible, ensuring adequate decompression of the spinal cord. Lavage the surgical wound and close as described for ventral slot (p. 1054).

Stabilization with Pins and Methylmethacrylate

This technique can be used to distract and stabilize up to two affected intervertebral spaces. Advantages of this technique include complete spinal cord decompression without entering the spinal canal and reduced risk of iatrogenic cord trauma. A neck brace is not required postoperatively and a favorable to excellent prognosis can be expected in most ambulatory patients (see Table 34-21).

☞ **N O T E** • This is the author's technique of choice for patients requiring dynamic ventral traction-stabilization.

Perform a ventral slot at the affected IVS(s), to the level of the inner cortical layer (i.e., 75% transdiskal slot) (Fig. 34-44, A). Drill the slot no more than half the width of the vertebral body; slot length is determined by the thickness of

the vertebral endplates. Discontinue burring once the cortical endplate of each vertebral body is removed. Place a modified Gelpi retractor (see below under the discussion of special instruments) in defects burred in the vertebral bodies, cranial and caudal to the affected vertebral bodies (Fig. 34-44, B). Create the defects just large enough to accept the blunted tips of the modified Gelpi retractor. Engage the retractor and distract the affected IVS 2 to 3 mm. Harvest autogenous cancellous bone from the heads of the humeri and place it into the distracted slot. Insert two 7/64- or 1/8-inch Steinmann pins into the ventral surface of the vertebral body cranial to the affected IVS. Insert the pins on the ventral midline of the vertebral body and direct them 30 to 35 degrees dorsolateral, to avoid entering the spinal canal (Fig. 34-45). It is important to engage two cortices with each pin. Cut the pins, leaving approximately 1.5 to 2 cm exposed. Notch the exposed portion of each pin with pin cutters to allow the bone cement to grip the pin and prevent migration. Mix sterile methylmethacrylate bone cement powder with liquid monomer until it reaches a doughy consistency and can be handled without sticking to your surgical gloves. Meticulously mold the cement around each pin; make sure each pin is completely surrounded and covered with bone cement (see Fig. 34-45). Irrigate the bone cement with sterile saline solution for 5 to 10 minutes to dissipate the heat of polymerization. Remove the vertebral spreaders after the cement has hardened. Close the paired longus colli muscles cranial and caudal to the cement mass. Close the remainder of the incision routinely.

Stabilization with Polyvinylidine Spinal Plates

Advantages of this technique over ventral slot decompression alone include adequate spinal cord decompression without entering the spinal canal, reduced risk of iatrogenic spinal cord trauma, and improved recovery. Disadvantages include high incidence of implant failure in patients that do not tolerate a neck brace, need for a donor or bone bank, time necessary for allograft incorporation into an interbody fusion, and inability to provide adequate stabilization in patients with multiple lesions.

Identify the affected IVS and perform a ventral slot as described on p. 1051; however, carry the slot only to the level of the inner cortical layer (i.e., 75% transdiskal slot) (see Fig. 34-44, A). Place the affected IVS in approximately 2- to 3-mm linear traction using modified Gelpi retractors as described for pins and bone cement stabilization (see Fig. 34-44, B). Create the slot configuration to precisely accommodate a full cortical allograft harvested from the distal third of the tibia of a 15- to 20-lb donor. The graft maintains the IVS in linear traction, resulting in spinal cord decompression. Pack the cortical allograft with autogenous cancellous bone harvested from the heads of the humeri before placement in the slot. Once the graft is in place, remove the vertebral spreader. Place the polyvinylidine spinal plate on the ventral surface of the adjacent vertebral

TABLE 34-21

Surgical Techniques for Treatment of Wobbler Syndrome

Classification	Clinical Presentation	Affected Vertebral Body or Interspace	Location of Lesion within Spinal Canal	Dynamic or Static Lesion	Surgical Technique Recommended	Prognosis
Chronic degenerative disk disease/vertebral tipping	Pain alone	C5-C6 or C6-C7	Ventral	Dynamic	Ventral slot or traction-stabilization	Excellent
	Paraparetic	C5-C6 and C6-C7	Ventral	Static	Ventral slot	Excellent
		C5-C6 or C6-C7	Ventral	Dynamic	Ventral slot or traction-stabilization	Excellent to favorable
		C5-C6 and C6-C7	Ventral	Static	Ventral slot +/− stabilization	Excellent to favorable
	Ambulatory tetraparetic	C5-C6 and C6-C7	Ventral	Dynamic	Ventral traction-stabilization	Favorable
		C5-C6 or C6-C7	Ventral	Static	Ventral slot and stabilization	Favorable
		C5-C6 and C6-C7	Ventral	Dynamic	Ventral traction-stabilization	Favorable
		C5-C6 or C6-C7	Ventral	Static	Ventral slot and stabilization	Favorable
	Weakly ambulatory tetraparetic	C5-C6 and C6-C7	Ventral	Dynamic/static	Ventral traction-stabilization	Guarded to favorable
		More than two lesions	Ventral	Dynamic/static	Dorsal laminectomy	Guarded to favorable
		C5-C6 or C6-C7	Ventral	Dynamic	Ventral traction-stabilization	Guarded to favorable
			Ventral	Static	Ventral slot and stabilization	Guarded to favorable
	Nonambulatory tetraparetic	C5-C6 and C6-C7	Ventral	Dynamic/static	Ventral traction-stabilization	Guarded
		More than two lesions	Ventral	Dynamic/static	Dorsal laminectomy	Guarded
		C5-C6 or C6-C7	Ventral	Dynamic	Ventral traction-stabilization	Guarded
			Ventral	Static	Ventral slot and stabilization	Guarded
		C5-C6 or C6-C7	Ventral	Dynamic/static	Ventral traction-stabilization	Guarded to unfavorable
		More than two lesions	Ventral	Dynamic/static	Dorsal laminectomy	Guarded to unfavorable
Congenital osseous malformation	Paraparesis to tetraparesis	Single lesion (rare)	Lateral, ventral, and/or dorsal	Static	Dorsal laminectomy	Favorable
		Multiple lesions	Lateral, ventral, and/or dorsal	Static	Dorsal laminectomy	Unfavorable
Ligamentum flavum hypertrophy	Paraparesis to tetraparesis	Single lesion	Dorsal	Dynamic	Dorsal laminectomy	Favorable
			Dorsal	Static	Ventral traction-stabilization	Favorable
		Multiple lesions	Dorsal	Dynamic/static	Dorsal laminectomy	Guarded
Ventral arch malformation	Paraparesis to tetraparesis	Single lesion	Dorsal	Dynamic	Dorsal laminectomy	Favorable
			Dorsal	Static	Ventral traction-stabilization	Favorable
		Multiple lesions (rare)	Dorsal	Dynamic/static	Dorsal laminectomy	Guarded
Hourglass compression	Paraparesis to tetraparesis	Single lesion	Lateral, ventral, and dorsal	Dynamic	Ventral traction-stabilization	Favorable
			Lateral, ventral, and dorsal	Static	Dorsal laminectomy	Favorable
		Two lesions	Lateral, ventral, and dorsal	Dynamic/static	Ventral traction-stabilization	Guarded
		Multiple lesions	Lateral, ventral, and dorsal	Dynamic/static	Dorsal laminectomy	Guarded

FIG. 34-44
A, To decompress the spinal cord, perform a 75% transdiskal ventral slot at the affected intervertebral space. **B,** Use vertebral spreaders to place the affected intervertebral space in 2- to 3-mm linear traction.

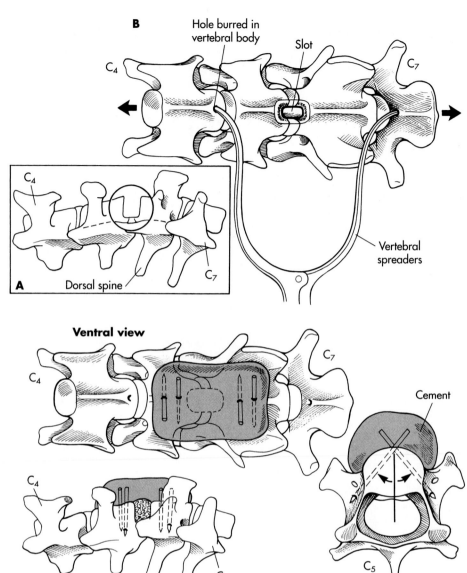

FIG. 34-45
Proper placement of Steinmann pins and bone cement to provide traction and stabilization of the affected intervertebral space.

bodies to secure the bone graft in the slot. Secure the plate with two screws placed in each vertebral body. Drill and tap holes at a 20- to 25-degree angle from the midline to prevent spinal canal penetration (Fig. 34-46). Determine screw length by assessing vertebral body width and depth from cervical spinal radiographs. Place autogenous cancellous bone on the ventral surface of the plate. Suture the paired longus colli muscles over the autogenous cancellous bone to hold it in place. Close the remainder of the incision routinely.

Stabilization with Harrington Spinal Distraction Rods

Harrington spinal distraction rods provide distraction and stabilization in Wobbler patients without the use of a vertebral spreader. Advantages of this technique include adequate spinal cord decompression of two adjacent intervertebral disk spaces without entering the spinal canal, reduced risk of iatrogenic spinal cord trauma, and improved recovery of pa-

tients with two lesions. Disadvantages include inability to distract and stabilize only one IVS, implant cost, and possibility of implant failure in patients that do not tolerate a neck brace.

☞ **NOTE** · This technique is most useful in patients with two adjacent lesions (generally C5-C6 and C6-C7).

Approach the ventral aspect of the affected vertebrae as described for ventral slot on p. 1051. Fenestrate the intervertebral disk spaces of affected vertebrae. Create slots in the vertebral endplates of affected vertebrae with a high-speed burr to precisely accept the tips of the distraction hooks (Fig. 34-47). Turn the centrally placed nuts such that one nut moves toward each end to contact the hooks. Tighten the nuts to distract both hooks and intervertebral disk spaces. Place the IVS in 2 to 3 mm of distraction and

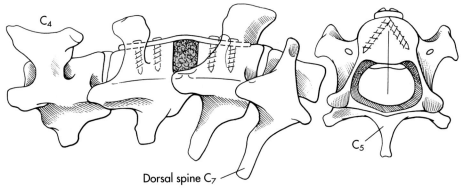

FIG. 34-46
Proper placement of full cortical allograft and polyvinylidine spinal plate to provide traction and stabilization of the affected intervertebral space.

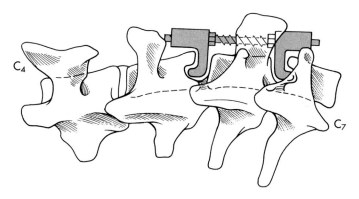

FIG. 34-47
Proper placement of a Harrington rod to provide traction and stabilization of the affected intervertebral space.

crimp the nuts or secure cerclage wire to the bolt adjacent to each nut to prevent loosening. Place cancellous bone in the slotted defects to promote interbody fusion. Approximate longus colli muscles over the cancellous graft and close the remainder of the incision routinely.

Decompression via Dorsal Laminectomy

Identify and expose the dorsal aspect of affected vertebrae as described for dorsal laminectomy on p. 1055. After exposure of the cervical vertebrae, identify affected vertebrae (see the discussion of unique anatomic landmarks of the cervical spine on p. 1051). Remove dorsal spinous processes and laminae with rongeurs and a high-speed surgical burr, respectively. The laminectomy defect may be from three quarters the length of each vertebra to a continuous laminectomy extending from C4 to C7, depending on the extent of the compressive lesion. Limit the width of the laminectomy to the medial aspect of the articular facets of the cranial vertebra (Fig. 34-48). First burr the lamina to the level of the periosteum of the inner cortical layer. Use a dental or iris spatula to carefully penetrate the periosteal layer and enter the spinal canal (see Fig. 34-24 on p. 1060). Use an ophthalmic forceps and No. 11 scalpel blade to gently excise and remove the ligamentum flavum en bloc. If lateral compression exists, use rongeurs to resect the lateral aspects of the vertebral arches to the level of the vertebral artery and vein. Resect hypertrophied joint capsule and ligamentum flavum to achieve lateral decompression of the spinal cord. Place transarticular lag screws for vertebral stabilization if necessary. Drill an appropriate-size hole through the cranial and caudal articular facets, bilaterally. Remove articu-

lar cartilage using a high-speed surgical burr, tap the hole, and place a lag screw. Place cancellous bone around the joints to promote arthrodesis. Place an autogenous fat graft over the laminectomy site to help prevent formation of a fibrous laminectomy membrane that could result in spinal cord compression. Approximate paraspinal muscles and fascia; close remaining tissues routinely.

SUTURE MATERIALS/SPECIAL INSTRUMENTS

See p. 1061 for special surgical instruments for exposure of the cervical spine. Modified Gelpi retractors with blunted ends are useful for distracting affected vertebrae during stabilization procedures and are made by removing the hooked tips of a Gelpi retractor (Fig. 34-49).

POSTOPERATIVE CARE AND ASSESSMENT

Immediate postoperative care includes administration of intravenous fluids and analgesics, monitoring respiration, measurement of abdominal girth every 4 hours for 24 hours (i.e., for gastric dilatation-volvulus), and monitoring for seizures (i.e., particularly if the patient had immediate preoperative myelography). Steroids should be discontinued immediately after surgery and the neck collar replaced with a body harness.

Postoperative use of a neck brace is generally dictated by the technique chosen and patient cooperation. Patients that have ventral traction-stabilization using plastic spinal plates or Harrington rods should wear a neck brace for the first 4 to 6 weeks postoperatively. Neck braces should not be used in

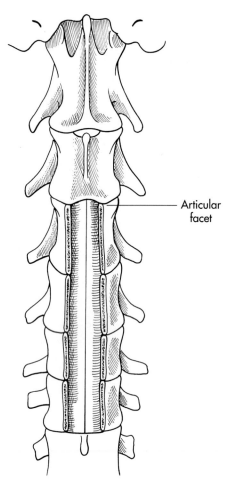

FIG. 34-48
Perform dorsal laminectomy at multiple intervertebral spaces, if necessary, to decompress the spinal cord.

Articular facet

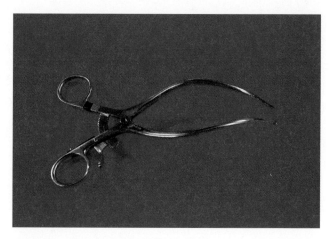

FIG. 34-49
Vertebral spreaders made by cutting the tips off of Gelpi retractors.

patients that do not tolerate them as they may damage the implant while fighting the presence of the neck brace. These patients should be strictly confined to cages.

Postoperative management of ambulatory patients includes strict confinement with harness walks two to three times daily for the first 2 to 3 weeks, then a gradual increase in exercise over the next 6 to 8 weeks. Slippery surfaces should be avoided. Postoperative management of nonambulatory patients includes physiotherapy (passive range-of-motion exercises), hydrotherapy (swimming), and the use of a supporting cart until the dog has regained the ability to walk.

Supporting carts can be constructed from plastic pipe and fabric. Neoprene, nylon, or leather harnesses are useful in weakly ambulatory patients. Special attention to good nursing care of recumbent patients is necessary to avoid decubital ulcers, urinary tract infections, and/or pneumonia. Heavily padded, dry bedding or waterbeds may prevent decubital ulcers.

Patients should be assessed initially by immediate postoperative radiographs to evaluate implants and by neurologic examination 48 hours after surgery. Long-term assessment includes radiographic evaluation at 3, 6, 9, and 12 months postoperatively and neurologic examinations as needed, depending on status (i.e., generally daily until ambulatory, then 1, 2, 3, 6, 9, and 12 months postoperatively).

COMPLICATIONS

Complications may be short-term (e.g., immediate postoperative to 1 month) or long-term (e.g., greater than 1 month) and vary between procedures. Short-term complications and their most likely causes are listed in Table 34-22. The most common long-term complication in patients treated with ventral slot or ventral traction-stabilization for chronic degenerative disk disease, vertebral tipping, or hourglass compression is development of a second compressive lesion at the interspace adjacent to the previously affected interspace. It is presumed that once an IVS is fused, stress at the adjacent interspaces is increased. It is possible that this increased stress encourages development of spinal instability and subsequent spinal cord compression in some patients or that some patients have a predisposition to disk degeneration in the lower cervical spine that encourages a second lesion. Whatever the cause, this phenomenon is referred to as the *domino effect* and has been reported to occur in 25% of patients at 5 to 60 months postoperatively (Fig. 34-50) (Bruecker, Seim, Blass, 1989).

PROGNOSIS

Prognosis for patients treated conservatively is guarded, but also depends on classification, severity of neurologic signs, and number of lesions (see Table 34-19). The prognosis for surgically treated patients is dependent upon disease classification, severity of neurologic deficit, number of lesions, method of therapy available, and quality of aftercare (see Table 34-21).

Reference

Bruecker KA, Seim HB, Blass CE: Caudal cervical spondylomyelopathy: decompression by linear traction and stabilization with Steinmann pins and polymethylmethacrylate, *J Am Anim Hosp Assoc* 25:677, 1989.

TABLE 34-22

Short-Term Postoperative Complications in Wobbler Patients

Classification	Surgical Technique	Short-Term Complication	Cause of Complication
Chronic degenerative disk disease / vertebral tipping / hourglass compression	Steinmann pins and bone cement	Deteriorating neurologic status	Pin in spinal canal; implant failure
		Pin fracture	Insufficient confinement; pin too small
		Pin migration	Unnotched pin; didn't cover pin with cement
		Cement fracture	Never reported
		Implant pulls off vertebrae	Improper angle of pin placement; didn't engage two cortices with pins
	Polyvinylidine spinal plates	Deteriorating neurologic status	Screw in spinal canal; implant failure
		Screw loosening	Insufficient confinement; neck brace not worn
	Harrington rod	Deteriorating neurologic status	Hook in spinal canal; implant failure
		Rod loosens or slips off	Insufficient confinement; neck brace not worn
	Ventral slot	Deteriorating neurologic status	Slot excessively wide; slot caused spinal instability; entire compressive mass not removed; insufficient confinement
	Dorsal laminectomy	Deteriorating neurologic status	Laminectomy caused increased instability; excessive spinal cord manipulation; insufficient confinement
Ligamentum flavum hypertrophy / vertebral arch malformation	Dorsal laminectomy	Deteriorating neurologic status	Laminectomy caused increased instability; excessive spinal cord manipulation; inappropriate articular facet stabilization

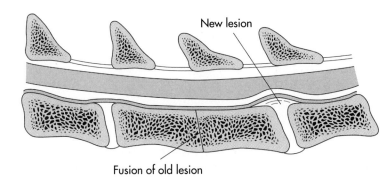

New lesion

Fusion of old lesion

FIG. 34-50
Interbody fusion from a previous traction-stabilization procedure may cause increased stress on the intervertebral spaces cranial and caudal to the fused space. This may result in instability and formation of a second lesion at these stressed spaces.

Suggested Reading

Bruecker KA, Seim HB, Blass CE: Ventral decompression and stabilization using Steinmann pins and polymethylmethacrylate for the treatment of caudal cervical spondylomyelopathy: results of 39 cases, *Vet Surg* 17:1, 1988.

Bruecker KA, Seim HB, Withrow SJ: Clinical evaluation of three surgical methods for treatment of caudal cervical spondylomyelopathy of dogs, *Vet Surg* 18:197, 1989.

Bruecker KA, Seim HB, Withrow SJ: Ventral decompression and lubra-plate stabilization for the treatment of caudal cervical spondylomyelopathy: results of 37 cases, *Vet Surg* 16:84, 1987.

Burke MJ et al: Histochemical study of the annulus fibrosus in normal canine caudal cervical intervertebral discs, *Res Vet Sci* 40:18, 1986.

Dixon BC, Tomlinson JL, Kraus KH: A modified distraction-stabilization technique for canine caudal cervical spondylomyelopathy using an interbody polymethylmethacrylate plug, *Vet Surg* 24:425, 1995.

Dixon BC, Tomlinson JL, Kraus KH: Modified distraction-stabilization technique using an interbody polymethylmethacrylate plug in dogs with caudal cervical spondylomyelopathy, *J Am Vet Med Assoc* 208:61, 1996.

Ellison GW, Seim HB, Clemmons RM: Distracted cervical spinal fusion for management of caudal cervical spondylomyelopathy in large-breed dogs, *J Am Vet Med Assoc* 193:447, 1988.

Goring RL, Beale BS, Faulkner RF: The inverted cone depression technique: a surgical treatment for cervical vertebral instability "Wobbler syndrome" in Doberman pinschers. I. *J Am Anim Hosp Assoc* 27:403, 1991.

Lyman R: Wobbler syndrome: continuous dorsal laminectomy is the procedure of choice, *Prog Vet Neurol* 2:143, 1991.

McKee VM, et al: Vertebral distraction-fusion for cervical spondylopathy using a screw and double washer technique, *J Sm Anim Prac* 31:27, 1990.

Olsson SE: Dynamic compression of the cervical spinal cord, *Acta Vet Scand* 23:65, 1982.

Seim HB: Wobbler syndrome: ventral decompression and stabilization is indicated, *Prog Vet Neurol* 2:143, 1991.

Seim HB: Wobbler syndrome in the Doberman pinscher, *Canine Pract* 19:23, 1994.

Seim HB, Withrow SJ: Pathophysiology and diagnosis of caudal cervical spondylomyelopathy with emphasis on the Doberman pinscher, *J Am Vet Med Assoc* 18:241, 1982.

Trotter EJ et al: Caudal cervical vertebral malformation-malarticulation in Great Danes and Doberman pinschers, *J Am Vet Med Assoc* 168:917, 1976.

Wilson ER, Aron DN, Roberts RE: Observation of a secondary compressive lesion after treatment of caudal cervical spondylomyelopathy in a dog, *J Am Vet Med Assoc* 205:1297, 1994.

ATLANTOAXIAL INSTABILITY

DEFINITIONS

Atlantoaxial instability is an alteration of the dens and/or ligaments that span the multifaceted, diarthrodial atlantoaxial articulation and cause instability, vertebral subluxation, and subsequent spinal cord and nerve root compression.

SYNONYMS

Atlantoaxial subluxation, atlantoaxial luxation

GENERAL CONSIDERATIONS AND CLINICALLY RELEVANT PATHOPHYSIOLOGY

Atlantoaxial instability is probably a congenital and/or developmental problem resulting in an unstable articulation between the first two cervical vertebrae. Laxity may result from fracture, absence, hypoplasia, or malformation of the dens, resulting in a nonfunctional attachment of alar, apical, and/or transverse ligaments (Fig. 34-51, *A*), or improper formation, laxity, or rupture of the alar, apical, transverse, or dorsal atlantoaxial ligaments, resulting in lack of ligamentous support between the atlas and axis (Fig. 34-51, *B*). Trauma may elicit clinical signs in animals with laxity as a result of these causes. Instability predisposes the patient to spinal cord and nerve root compression, often resulting in neck pain and ambulatory to nonambulatory tetraparesis.

DIAGNOSIS
Clinical Presentation

Signalment. Atlantoaxial instability primarily occurs in toy-breed dogs. It has occasionally been reported in large-breed dogs and rarely in cats. It generally (56%) occurs in dogs younger than 1 year of age (McCarthy, Lewis, Hosgood, 1995). Dogs that present with clinical signs at an older age generally have had instability since birth, but recent trauma has caused significant spinal cord and nerve root compression.

History. Progressive tetraparesis and incoordination, often associated with neck pain, are expected. Acute presentations can occur after seemingly minor trauma. Owners may report that the dog dislikes having its head touched.

Physical Examination Findings

General physical examination findings are usually normal. Neurologic examination reveals a dog with motor weakness and UMN signs to the front and hindlegs. Patients present with varying degrees of neck pain. Ventral flexion of the head will often exacerbate neck pain and may worsen the neurologic condition. Care must be exercised during cervical flexion because the dens (if present) can cause spinal cord compression. Forceful flexion must be avoided at all times.

☞ **N O T E** · *Do not* forcefully flex the head of these patients. Flexing the neck may exacerbate neurologic deficits.

Radiography/Ultrasonography

A preliminary lateral radiograph without anesthesia allows diagnosis of atlantoaxial instability with significant subluxation (Fig. 34-52). A flexed lateral view of the anesthetized animal may be necessary to reveal increased laxity and subluxation of C1-C2. The instability is most pronounced dorsally. A gap of 4 to 5 mm between the lamina of C1 and dorsal spine of C2 is diagnostic (see Fig. 34-52). Ventrodorsal and open mouth views may show absence or fractionation of the dens. Because the open mouth view requires flexion of the neck, it is not routinely recommended.

Laboratory Findings

Laboratory findings in patients with atlantoaxial instability are generally normal. Young patients or those previously treated with corticosteroids may have slight elevations in serum alkaline phosphatase activity.

DIFFERENTIAL DIAGNOSIS

Presumptive diagnosis of atlantoaxial instability is made in young, toy-breed dogs with a history of neck pain and acute or progressive, ambulatory or nonambulatory, UMN tetraparesis. Diagnosis of atlantoaxial instability and exclusion of fracture/luxation is confirmed by survey radiography.

MEDICAL MANAGEMENT

Medical treatment consisting of strict confinement for 3 to 4 weeks, a neck brace that maintains the neck and head in extension, and short-term corticosteroids may alleviate symptoms. The neck brace, constructed of padded splint material, such as x-ray film or fiberglass casting material, must be worn during the 3 to 4 weeks of confinement, ensuring maximum scar tissue formation. Corticosteroids (Table 34-23) may be used for 24 to 48 hours. Recurrence is common.

SURGICAL TREATMENT

Surgical correction of atlantoaxial instability is indicated when neurologic dysfunction is mild to severe (i.e., severe neck pain or weakly ambulatory to nonambulatory tetraparesis [with or without neck pain]) or a course of medical therapy has failed. Objectives of surgery include reduction of atlantoaxial subluxation, decompression of spinal cord and nerve roots, and atlantoaxial joint stabilization. Surgical techniques for decompression and stabilization fall into two major categories (i.e., dorsal and ventral).

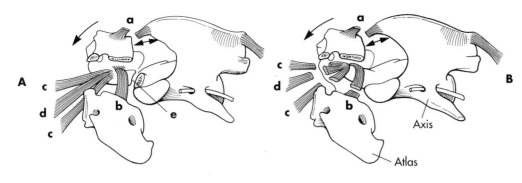

FIG. 34-51
A, Ligamentous structures associated with the atlantoaxial joint. Fracture of the dens and rupture of the atlantoaxial ligament result in instability. (*a*) Dorsal atlantoaxial ligament, (*b*) transverse ligament, (*c*) alar ligaments (paired), (*d*) apical ligament, (*e*) fracture/malformation of the dens. **B,** Rupture of ligamentous supporting structures of the atlantoaxial joint causes atlantoaxial instability. (*a*) Dorsal atlantoaxial ligament, (*b*) transverse ligament, (*c*) paired alar ligaments, (*d*) apical ligament.

TABLE 34-23
Corticosteroid Dosage
Dexamethasone (Azium)
0.2-1.1 mg/kg IM BID

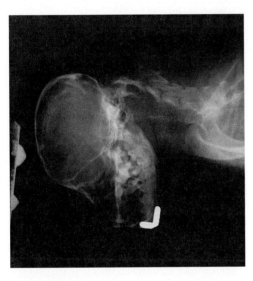

FIG. 34-52
Radiograph of an awake patient with atlantoaxial instability. Notice the increased distance between the dorsal laminae of C1 and dorsal spinous process of C2.

☞ **N O T E** · The author prefers a ventral approach and placement of Kirschner wires and bone cement (see p. 1086).

Preoperative Management

The animal should be given intravenous fluids and steroids before surgery. Steroids are given to protect the spinal cord from the possible effects of surgical manipulation. The steroid of choice is methylprednisolone sodium succinate (30 mg/kg intravenously). Serum glucose concentrations should be assessed before, during (every 30 to 60 minutes), and after surgery in toy breeds. Supplementation with dextrose-containing fluids may be necessary during surgery.

Anesthesia

See p. 1049 for suggested anesthetic protocols for use in dogs with cervical spinal disorders. The patient's neurologic status and positioning for surgery are important preanesthetic considerations. If the patient has motor weakness (e.g., ambulatory tetraparesis, weakly ambulatory tetraparesis, or nonam-

bulatory tetraparesis) or will require positioning that may cause respiratory compromise, mechanical ventilatory support should be considered. Trauma to the cranial cervical spinal cord during reduction of the atlantoaxial instability may cause transient respiratory arrest. Ventilatory support during surgical manipulation of atlantoaxial subluxation is therefore recommended. Care should be taken to avoid hypothermia and these animals should be actively rewarmed after surgery.

☞ **N O T E** · Use extreme care during intubation to avoid excessive neck manipulation in these patients.

Surgical Anatomy

The cervical spine is unique in its variable anatomic configuration from vertebra to vertebra, particularly C1 and C2 (see Figs. 34-1 and 34-3 on p. 1052). Important anatomic variations during surgical repair of atlantoaxial instability are listed in Table 34-24.

Positioning

Patients undergoing a ventral approach are positioned as described for ventral slot procedure on p. 1051 (see Fig. 34-5 on p. 1053). The neck is placed in a slightly extended position and is fixed in mild linear traction. This position reduces the subluxation and decompresses the spinal cord and nerve roots. An area from the intermandibular space to the caudal cervical region, including the heads of the humeri, is aseptically prepared. Patients undergoing a dorsal approach should be positioned in sternal recumbency with the head and neck slightly flexed (see Fig. 34-17 on p.1057). An area from the occiput to the caudal cervical region is aseptically prepared.

TABLE 34-24

Anatomic Variation of the Atlas and Axis Important to Surgical Repair of Atlantoaxial Instability

Vertebrae	Anatomy	Surgical Significance
C1-atlas	Thin dorsal arch (laminae); no dorsal spinous process	Poor implant-holding power dorsally
	No vertebral body, just thin ventral fovea	Poor implant-holding power ventrally
	Ventrolateral diarthrodial joints	Good purchase for implants ventrally; used to evaluate anatomic reduction
	Prominent ventral tubercle	Landmark for surgical localization
	Prominent wings	Moderate implant-holding power dorsally and ventrally
C2-axis	Prominent dorsal spinous process	Moderate implant-holding power dorsally, patient age and size dependent; landmark for surgical localization
	Thin central vertebral body	Poor implant-holding power ventrally
	Prominent cranial articular processes	Good purchase for implants ventrally; used to evaluate anatomic reduction
	Prominent caudal vertebral body	Good ventral purchase for implants
	Dens	May fracture or displace into spinal canal
C1-C2	Bilateral ventrolateral diarthrodial joints	Good purchase for implants ventrally; used to evaluate anatomic reduction
	Dorsal atlantoaxial ligament	Moderate purchase of implants used to replace the ligament

SURGICAL TECHNIQUES
Dorsal Stabilization

The dorsal approach allows reduction of the subluxation and fixation of the dorsal lamina of C1 to the dorsal spine of C2. Bony decompression is provided by hemilaminectomy or reduction of the subluxation. Hemilaminectomy provides dorsal spinal cord decompression, but does not correct the instability or relieve ventral spinal cord compression; in fact, it reduces stability of the fixation. Thus it is not recommended. Rigid immobilization using dorsal lamina of C1 and C2 is often unrewarding. Reduction of the luxation and immobilization of the vertebra, without hemilaminectomy, provide adequate decompression. Dorsal fixation is generally provided by a loop of orthopedic wire, synthetic suture material, or autogenous graft (i.e., nuchal ligament). Regardless of the material chosen, it is passed under the lamina of C1, over the spinal cord, and tied to two holes drilled in the dorsal spine of C2. The fixation relies on fibrous tissue to form a solid union. Frequent postoperative complications with this technique, including breakdown of the suture or bone, tearing out of the suture with minimal strain because the dorsal arch of the atlas and dorsal spinous process of the axis in young toy-breed dogs have the consistency and strength of wet cardboard, and continued micromotion at the atlantoaxial joint, may cause the wire to fatigue and break. Additionally, improper placement of fixation material may result in spinal cord trauma. Inadequate reduction of the subluxation and inappropriate stabilization, especially if used in conjunction with hemilaminectomy, are possible.

Perform a dorsal approach to the cranial cervical spine as described on p. 1056. Periosteally elevate epaxial muscle from the dorsal lamina of the atlas and dorsal spine, lamina, and pedicles of the axis. Carefully incise the atlantoaxial fascia caudal to the arch of the atlas and enter the epidural space. Incise the atlantooccipital fascia cranial to the arch of the atlas and enter the epidural space. Gently thread a loop of 25-gauge orthopedic wire under

the arch of the atlas in a cranial-to-caudal direction. Thread the suture material through this loop of orthopedic wire and gently pull it under the arch of the atlas (Fig. 34-53, A). Drill two holes in the dorsal spinous process of the axis and pass the ends of the suture material through the holes; one from right to left and the other from left to right. Reduce the atlantoaxial joint and tie the suture ends to maintain reduction (Fig. 34-53, B). Close muscle, subcutaneous tissue, and skin routinely.

Ventral Stabilization

The ventral approach allows accurate anatomic reduction for decompression, use of transarticular pins for stability (placed in the most solid portion of the atlas and axis), placement of an autogenous cancellous bone graft to encourage atlantoaxial arthrodesis, and odontoidectomy if indicated (i.e., malformed dens). The technique is easy, fast, safe, and effective and involves the placement of Kirschner wires or screws across the C1-C2 articulation (Fig. 34-53, C). Placement of Kirschner wires is described below. Screws may be used instead of pins, especially in large-breed dogs with traumatic subluxation. The most common complication has been pin migration. This is effectively prevented by applying methylmethacrylate bone cement to the exposed portion of the Kirschner pins. Even though this fixation is not on the tension band side, it provides superior fixation to the dorsal approach.

Approach to the ventral aspect of C1 and C2 is as described for ventral slot on p. 1051. Periosteally elevate longus coli muscles from the ventral aspect of the atlas and axis. Be careful not to cause excessive motion of the atlantoaxial joint during exposure. Identify and open the paired atlantoaxial joints. Dissect the joint capsule from the ventral aspect of the vertebral bodies with a No. 15 scalpel blade to visualize articular cartilage. Use an ASIF small fragment forceps or towel clamp to grasp the midbody of C2 (Fig. 34-54). Place caudal traction on C2 to open the

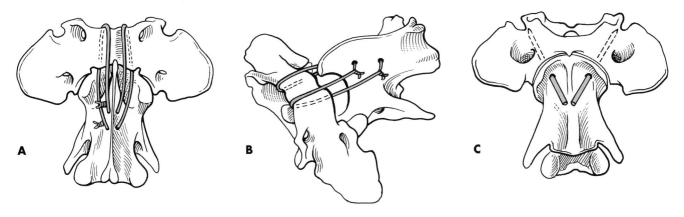

FIG. 34-53
A, For dorsal stabilization of atlantoaxial subluxation, pass wire or suture material under the dorsal arch of C1. **B,** Pass the wire or suture material through holes drilled in the dorsal spine of C2 and secure it. **C,** For ventral stabilization, place Kirschner wires across the atlantoaxial joints.

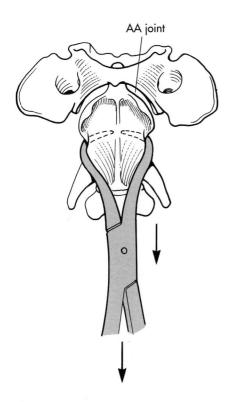

AA joint

FIG. 34-54
Use orthopedic reduction forceps to grasp the body of C2. Use traction and countertraction to reduce the atlantoaxial subluxation.

atlantoaxial joint, enabling safe removal of articular cartilage. Use a bone curette or high-speed pneumatic drill to remove approximately 50% of the articular surface, bilaterally. Expose the head of the humerus, drill a ⅛-in Steinmann pin through the outer cortex, and introduce a size 0 curette to harvest cancellous bone. Transfer the bone graft to the scarified atlantoaxial joints and reduce the subluxation, using the reduction forceps or towel clamps. Select two appropriate-size nonthreaded Kirschner wires

(0.625-in or 0.45-in). Start the first pin close to the midline on the caudoventral body of the axis. Direct the pin medial toward the alar notch on the cranial edge of the atlas, with the point of the pin angled ventrally (Fig. 34-55, A). An air-driven or electric drill facilitates accurate and easy pin placement. Place the second pin through the opposite joint, using similar landmarks. Cut the pins, leaving approximately 5 to 7 mm protruding from the body of C2 and notch or slightly bend the exposed pin. Carefully mold methylmethacrylate bone cement to incorporate both pins (Fig. 34-55, B). Lavage the bone cement with cool saline to dissipate the heat of polymerization. Close muscle, subcutaneous tissue, and skin routinely.

SUTURE MATERIALS/SPECIAL INSTRUMENTS

When using the dorsal approach, braided polyester suture, nonabsorbable monofilament suture, or orthopedic wire are recommended fixation materials. For the ventral approach, methylmethacrylate bone cement is needed to prevent pin migration and small fragment forceps or towel clamps aid in reduction and stabilization during pin placement.

POSTOPERATIVE CARE AND ASSESSMENT

Patients with atlantoaxial instability should be evaluated postoperatively in a similar fashion as patients with other cervical spinal disorders. Because of the anatomic configuration of C1 and C2 in young toy breeds, any form of fixation should be considered marginal. Regardless of whether a dorsal or ventral approach is used, all forms of internal fixation should be supported with a neck brace, and strict cage confinement enforced until radiographic evidence of union.

PROGNOSIS

Generally, prognosis for patients treated medically is unfavorable because of recurrence of clinical signs. Prognosis for patients treated surgically using a dorsal approach is related

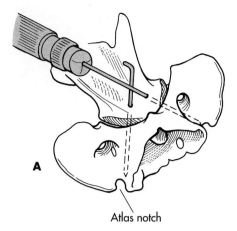

Atlas notch

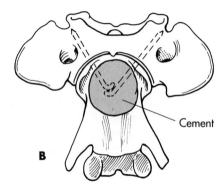

Cement

B

FIG. 34-55
A, Place Kirschner wires in cross-pin fashion; wires are directed toward the alar notch to ensure proper placement.
B, Notch or bend the exposed ends of the Kirschner wires. Mold methylmethacrylate bone cement around both pin ends.

to implant success or failure. If implants fail, prognosis is unfavorable. If implants succeed, prognosis is favorable. Prognosis for patients treated using a ventral approach is favorable to excellent; even patients that present with weakly ambulatory or nonambulatory tetraparesis have favorable return to an ambulatory status.

Reference

McCarthy RJ, Lewis DD, Hosgood G: Atlantoaxial subluxation in dogs, *Compend Cont Educ Pract Vet* 17:215, 1995.

Suggested Reading

Chambers JN, Betts CW, Oliver JE: The use of nonmetallic suture material for stabilization of atlantoaxial subluxation, *J Am Anim Hosp Assoc* 13:602, 1977.

Cook JR, Oliver JE: Atlantoaxial luxation in the dog, *Compend Contin Educ Pract Vet* 3:242, 1981.

Gilmore DR: Nonsurgical management of four cases of atlantoaxial subluxation in the dog, *J Am Anim Hosp Assoc* 20:93, 1984.

Johnson SG, Hulse DA: Odontoid dysplasia with atlantoaxial instability in a dog, *J Am Anim Hosp Assoc* 25:400, 1989.

LeCouteur RA et al: Stabilization of atlantoaxial subluxation in the dog, using the nuchal ligament, *J Am Vet Med Assoc* 177:1011, 1980.

Schultz KS, Waldron DR, Doherty M, et al: Application of ventral pins and polymethylmethacrylate for stabilization of atlantoaxial instability in three dogs, *Vet Surg* 23:426, 1994.

Sorjonen DC, Shires PK: Atlantoaxial instability: a ventral surgical technique for decompression, fixation, and fusion, *Vet Surg* 10:22, 1981.

Stead AC, Anderson AA, Coughlan A: Bone plating to stabilize atlantoaxial subluxation in 23 dogs, *Vet Surg* 30:409, 1991.

Swaim SF, Greene CE: Odontoidectomy in a dog, *J Am Anim Hosp Assoc* 11:663, 1975.

Thomas WB, Sorjonen DC, Simpson ST: Surgical management of atlantoaxial subluxation in 23 dogs, *Vet Surg* 20:409, 1991.

Wheeler SJ: Atlantoaxial subluxation with absence of the dens in rottweiler, *J Sm Anim Prac* 33:90, 1992.

FRACTURES AND LUXATIONS OF THE CERVICAL SPINE

DEFINITIONS

Traumatic or pathologic disruption of osseous and supporting soft-tissue structures of the cervical spine may result in **vertebral fracture** or **luxation** and subsequent spinal cord and nerve root compression.

SYNONYMS

Cervical fracture, cervical dislocation, broken neck

GENERAL CONSIDERATIONS AND CLINICALLY RELEVANT PATHOPHYSIOLOGY

Cervical vertebral fractures and luxations occur less frequently than fractures and luxations of the thoracolumbar spine. The most common cause of cervical fracture/luxation is automobile trauma. Other less frequent causes include dog fights, gunshot injuries, running head first into a solid object, hanging by a leash or collar, and underlying metabolic or neoplastic disorders resulting in bone demineralization (e.g., nutritional secondary hyperparathyroidism, osteosarcoma).

Traumatic spinal fractures/luxations are induced by forces resulting in severe hyperextension, hyperflexion, compression, and/or rotation. They generally occur at or near the junction of a movable (kinetic) and immovable (static) vertebral segment. In the cervical spine, the skull, atlas, and dens and body of the axis form a unit called the *cervicocranium* (Fig. 34-56). The dorsal spinous process of the axis is secured to the lower cervical spine by caudal articular facets, spinalis and semispinalis muscles, and nuchal ligament. This produces a static-kinetic relationship between the cervicocranium and lower cervical spine; the axis (C2) is the point of stress concentration. Traumatic forces applied to the cervical spine therefore culminate at the axis (Fig. 34-57). Failure of supporting structures of the spine to resist such stress results in mechanical discontinuity (i.e., fracture or luxation) with resultant spinal cord and nerve root compression. Proposed areas of the spine with a static-kinetic relationship include craniocervical, cervicothoracic, thoracolumbar, and lumbosacral junctions.

☞ **N O T E ·** The most frequent anatomic location of cervical fracture/luxation is the cranial cervical region with approximately 80% occurring at C1-C2.

Pathologic fractures generally occur when the integrity of bone is compromised because of an underlying disease process. Chronic calcium/phosphorus imbalances, primary and secondary neoplasia (e.g., multiple myeloma, osteosarcoma, metastatic neoplasia), and osteoporosis are examples of systemic disorders that can result in pathologic fracture. The cause of the underlying disorder must be determined and therapy instituted before spinal fracture/luxation repair.

DIAGNOSIS
Clinical Presentation

Signalment. There is no breed or sex predilection. Cervical spinal fractures may occur in any age dog and cat; however, it is most common in patients younger than 5 years of age.

History. Patients with fracture or luxation of the cervical spine typically have a history of trauma. The majority have been hit by an automobile. They may appear to be in pain, hold their neck in a stiff, protected position, and/or present with varying degrees of tetraparesis, depending on the amount of spinal cord contusion/compression. Occasionally, patients may have no significant neurologic deficits on initial presentation; however, deficits may occur several days after injury. Careful physical and neurologic examinations are necessary to detect subtle deficits.

Physical Examination Findings

Animals suspected of suffering from cervical fracture/luxation should be handled with extreme caution. Because trauma is the most common etiology, careful examination of all systems and treatment for shock are important. Patients with no obvious neurologic deficits should undergo a careful cervical spinal examination. Gentle palpation for an area of hyperpathia (i.e., increased sensitivity to pain) can be performed by grasping the ventral aspect of the neck with thumb and fingers and gently squeezing each vertebral body. Discomfort on palpation suggests a lesion and warrants further diagnostics. Careful palpation of the spine may also reveal information as to the type of injury sustained. Crepitus, excessive movement, or anatomic discontinuity of the spine suggests an unstable fracture/luxation. These physical

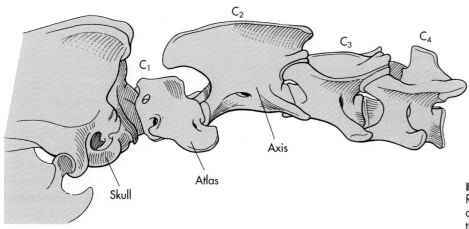

FIG. 34-56
Relationship of the structures (skull, atlas, and dens and body of the axis) that form the cervicocranium.

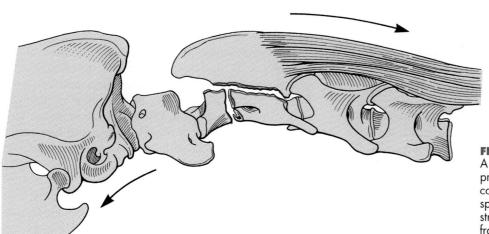

FIG. 34-57
A static-kinetic relationship is produced between the cervicocranium and lower cervical spine; the axis is the point of stress concentration resulting in fracture/luxation.

findings may be an important factor in assessing inherent stability (or instability) of the traumatized spine.

Patients with neurologic deficits should undergo a careful neurologic examination to localize the fracture or luxation and to determine severity of spinal cord and nerve root compression. Characteristic findings of the neurologic examination (UMN or LMN signs to the front limbs, UMN signs to the hind limbs) allow accurate localization of the fracture/luxation. Because the most common location of cervical spinal fracture/luxation is C1-C2, the most likely sign is varying degrees of acute neck pain, with or without upper motor neuron tetraparesis.

Radiography/Ultrasonography

Survey and contrast radiography may be required to accurately diagnose spinal fractures and luxations. Survey radiographs may be taken of conscious or anesthetized animal. Conscious patients may protect the fracture/luxation during positioning; however, an uncooperative patient may cause unpredictable radiographic detail. Survey radiographs of conscious patients should be taken during the initial workup so that spinal injury may be assessed. If surgery is necessary or closer radiographic evaluation is needed, the patient should be anesthetized. Advantages of anesthetizing the patient for radiographs include excellent positioning and quality radiographs. The disadvantage is loss of inherent support and increased instability of the spine during transport and positioning.

☞ **N O T E** · Anesthetized patients with possible neurologic abnormalities should always be handled carefully.

Typical radiographic findings in patients with cervical spinal fracture/luxation include discontinuity of bony structures (i.e., spinous process, lamina, pedicle, vertebral body), malalignment of IVS and/or articular facets, fracture lines in the body and/or spinous processes of involved vertebrae, loss of continuity or malalignment of the spinal canal, or any combination of these (Fig. 34-58). Radiographs of the cervical spine may be difficult to interpret; oblique views are often necessary in addition to standard lateral and ventrodorsal views.

☞ **N O T E** · A complete spinal series of radiographs (i.e., cervical, thoracic, lumbar, and sacral) is needed; 20% of patients with traumatic spinal injury have a spinal fracture/luxation at a second location.

Fractures may be classified as stable or unstable according to radiographic appearance and the force that caused the injury. Forces resulting in laminar and/or pedicle fracture, dorsal spinous process fracture, articular facet fracture, and supraspinous/interspinous ligament rupture (dorsal compartment) are generally considered unstable. Forces resulting in disk rupture, ventral longitudinal ligament rupture, and avulsion fracture of the ventral vertebral body (ventral com-

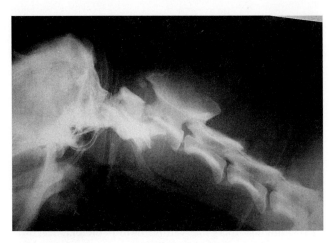

FIG. 34-58
Lateral radiograph of a dog with a C2 fracture. Notice the fracture fragment dorsal to C1 lamina, malalignment of C1-C2 vertebral bodies, and craniodorsal displacement of C2.

partment) are generally considered stable. Forces resulting in a combination of dorsal and ventral compartment injury are generally considered unstable. These are only guidelines; initial neurologic examination, physical examination, and serial neurologic examinations should be undertaken in combination with radiographic appearance to determine ultimate patient management.

☞ **N O T E** · Radiographs only reveal the status of spinal displacement at the time they are taken. It is possible that spinal displacement during the traumatic episode was greater than that seen on radiographs. Evaluating the severity of spinal fracture or luxation radiographically must be done in conjunction with neurologic examination findings.

Myelography may be necessary if there is suspicion of herniated intervertebral disk material (i.e., annulus fibrosus or nucleus pulposus), bone fragments in the spinal canal, no evidence of spinal discontinuity, or when radiographic findings do not correlate with neurologic examination. Myelography is infrequently necessary for definitive diagnosis or surgical planning of patients with cervical fracture/luxation.

Laboratory Findings

Patients with cervical fracture/luxation rarely have abnormalities on CBC and biochemical profile unless the fracture is secondary to a metabolic disorder (e.g., nutritional secondary hyperparathyroidism). Because most patients present with severe neck pain, a stress leukogram may be seen. Patients with a history of trauma or those that have undergone recent treatment with corticosteroids may have elevated concentrations of hepatic enzymes.

DIFFERENTIAL DIAGNOSIS

Presumptive diagnosis of cervical fracture/luxation is based on a young dog presenting with a history of trauma and physical and neurologic examination findings consistent with neck pain and tetraparesis. Other differentials can usually be eliminated by physical, hematologic, serum biochemical, cerebrospinal fluid, and/or radiographic evaluations. Diagnosis of cervical fracture/luxation is confirmed by radiography.

MEDICAL MANAGEMENT

Patient stabilization is the initial objective. Those patients with severe trauma should be treated for shock. The neck should be stabilized with a padded neck brace. Analgesics should be given to control neck pain (see Table 34-13 on p. 1070). Cage confinement should be encouraged. After patient stabilization, physical and neurologic examination should localize the fracture/luxation. Radiographs of the cervical spine are taken while the patient is conscious, for initial assessment. The decision for conservative or surgical management is based on initial neurologic status, radiographic assessment of spinal stability, and serial neurologic examinations.

Stable fractures in patients with strong voluntary motor movements are often managed successfully by conservative means, including strict cage confinement, neck brace, and antiinflammatory agents. Recommended drug treatment regimens are listed in Table 34-25. Serial neurologic examinations should be performed twice daily to determine response to therapy. If the patient does not remain quiet and causes further displacement of the fracture/luxation, is ambulatory but shows severe instability (palpation of a crepitant "click" over the fracture/luxation site while ambulating), remains unacceptably static, or deteriorates neurologically, surgical therapy should be considered. Surgery is also indicated if the fracture/luxation appears unstable, if the patient presents weakly ambulatory or nonambulatory tetraparetic, or if conservative therapy is unsuccessful.

TABLE 34-25

Antiinflammatory Drugs Used with Cervical or Thoracolumbar Fracture/Luxation

Conservative Management:
Dexamethasone (Azium)

0.2-0.5 mg/kg IV at presentation, then 0.2 mg/kg PO BID for 2 days, then SID for 2 days*[†]

Surgical Management:
Methylprednisolone (Solu-Medrol)

30 mg/kg IV given once at anesthetic induction; discontinue after 1 dose

Dexamethasone (Azium)

0.2 mg/kg PO, IM, or IV BID for 1 day, then SID for 1 day*[†] (if steroids are continued after surgery)

*If the patient is improving, discontinue steroids and enforce strict confinement for 3 additional weeks
[†]If signs of gastrointestinal upset or hemorrhage develop, discontinue corticosteroids.

SURGICAL TREATMENT

Objectives of surgery in a patient with traumatic or pathologic cervical spinal fracture/luxation are spinal cord and nerve root decompression and vertebral stabilization. Patients with pathologic fracture must have the cause of the underlying disorder determined and medical therapy instituted before surgical fracture/luxation repair. Once the underlying disorder has been controlled, treatment can be performed as described for traumatic fracture/luxation.

Factors that should be considered when selecting a stabilization technique are location of the fracture/luxation, special anatomic considerations, presence of a compressive lesion within the spinal canal (e.g., osseous fragment, disk material), patient size, patient age, equipment available, and surgeon's experience. The influence that special anatomic considerations and fracture location have on technique selection is outlined in Tables 34-26 and 34-27, respectively. If a compressive lesion is identified within the spinal canal the removal technique is dictated by lesion location (Table 34-27). Ventral lesions are usually removed via ventral slot technique (see p. 1051) and dorsal or dorsolateral lesions via dorsal laminectomy or dorsolateral hemilaminectomy, respectively (see p. 1055). Patient size affects the size and type of implant used to stabilize the fracture/luxation: the larger the patient, the larger the implant. Patient age may influence the surgical technique chosen. Younger animals usually have softer, more cancellous bone, whereas older animals have harder, more compact bone. Implant selection will be based on specific holding power in various regions of the cervical spine. Several equally successful techniques for fracture/luxation stabilization may be chosen, based on availability of specialized equipment or surgeon experience.

☞ **N O T E** · Reduction of the fracture/luxation may be facilitated and maintained by two techniques: (1) by drilling holes in the ventral bodies of the vertebrae cranial and caudal to the fracture/luxation and placing ASIF small fragment reduction forceps in the holes (Fig. 34-59), and (2) by fenestrating adjacent intervertebral disks or drilling holes into adjacent vertebral bodies to accommodate a vertebral distractor to gently distract affected vertebral bodies (see Fig. 34-44, *B* on p. 1080).

C1-C7 body fractures/luxations, traumatic cervical disk extrusions, and atlantoaxial subluxation are generally approached ventrally. The ventral approach to the affected vertebra is performed as described for ventral slot (see p. 1051). Steinmann pins and methylmethacrylate (bone cement) can be used successfully for selected cervical spinal fractures or luxations. Generally, vertebral body subluxation or body fractures occurring from C1-C7 can be adequately stabilized with this technique (see Tables 34-26 and 34-27). Appropriate exposure for pin and bone cement placement generally requires one or two vertebral bodies cranial and caudal to the fracture/luxation to be visible.

TABLE 34-26

Anatomic Variation of Cervical Vertebrae Important for Surgical Repair of Cervical Spinal Fractures/Luxations

Vertebrae	Anatomy	Surgical Significance
C1-Atlas	Thin dorsal arch (laminae); no dorsal spinous process	Poor implant-holding power dorsally
	No vertebral body, just thin ventral fovea	Poor implant-holding power ventrally
	Ventrolateral diarthroidal joints	Good purchase for implants ventrally; used to evaluate anatomic reduction
	Prominent ventral tubercle	Landmark for surgical localization
	Prominent wings	Moderate implant-holding power dorsally and ventrally
C2-Axis	Prominent dorsal spinous process	Moderate implant-holding power dorsally; landmark for surgical localization
	Thin central vertebral body	Poor implant-holding power ventrally
	Prominent cranial articular processes	Good purchase for implants ventrally; used to evaluate anatomic reduction
	Prominent caudal vertebral body	Good purchase for implants ventrally
	Dens	May fracture or displace into spinal canal
C1-C2	Bilateral ventrolateral diarthroidal joints	Good purchase for implants ventrally; used to evaluate anatomic reduction
	Dorsal atlantoaxial ligament	Moderate purchase of implants used to replace the ligament
C3-C7	Small dorsal spinous processes	Poor purchase for implants dorsally
	Prominent articular facets	Good purchase for implants dorsally
	Prominent vertebral bodies	Good purchase for implants ventrally
	Prominent transverse processes of C6	Landmark for surgical localization

☞ **N O T E** · The author strongly recommends using a ventral stabilization technique for C3-C7 fracture/luxations.

In patients with vertebral luxations it is advisable to prepare a ventral slot and pack it with autogenous cancellous bone to encourage interbody fusion. Ventral interbody screw fixation should *not* be used to stabilize vertebral body fracture or luxation because of an unacceptably high incidence of implant failure and vertebral body fracture.

Fractures of the lamina of C1 and dorsal spine and lamina and pedicles of C2 can be approached dorsally as described on p. 1056 and stabilized with orthopedic wire, monofilament or nonabsorbable suture material, or methylmethacrylate to reestablish continuity of displaced fragments (see Fig. 34-53, *A* and *B*). Placement of these various implants is described on p. 1086. Decompressive hemilaminectomy is performed only if bone fragments in the spinal canal cause spinal cord compression. Because laminectomy and hemilaminectomy decrease the stability of an already unstable spine, these procedures should not be routinely performed.

Preoperative Management

Patients should be given intravenous fluids and steroids before surgery; the latter are given to protect the spinal cord from effects of surgical manipulation. The steroid of choice is methylprednisolone sodium succinate (30 mg/kg intravenously). Preoperative prophylactic or therapeutic antimicrobial therapy is dependent on criteria listed in Table 34-4. Patients with open fractures (e.g., gunshot wounds, bite wounds) require antibiotics (see p. xx). Fracture/luxation of

the cervical spine frequently causes laceration of vertebral venous sinuses. Surgical manipulation encourages further hemorrhage. Because venous sinus hemorrhage can be severe and life threatening, blood should be readily available for transfusion.

☞ **N O T E** · Thoracic films should be evaluated in trauma patients for evidence of pneumothorax/pneumomediastinum and/or diaphragmatic herniation.

Anesthesia

Suggested anesthetic protocols for use in animals with cervical spinal disorders are provided on p. 1049. The patient's neurologic status and positioning for surgery are important preanesthetic considerations. Those with motor weakness (i.e., weakly ambulatory or nonambulatory tetraparesis) or those that require special positioning may be predisposed to respiratory compromise. Reduction of cranial cervical fracture/luxations (C1-C3) may also traumatize the cranial cervical spinal cord, causing transient respiratory arrest. Ventilatory support during surgery is therefore recommended.

Surgical Anatomy

The cervical spine has a unique configuration from vertebra to vertebra, particularly C1 and C2 (Fig. 34-60; see also Fig. 34-1 and Fig. 34-3 on p. 1052). Anatomic variations and their surgical significance when considering fracture/luxation repair are listed in Table 34-24.

TABLE 34-27

Summary of Surgical Stabilization Techniques for Cervical Spinal Fractures/Luxations, Depending Upon Fracture Location

Fracture Location	Special Anatomic and Surgical Considerations	Most Reliable Bony Purchase	Approach and Fixation Technique
C1	Respiratory arrest, lack of a vertebral body, thin dorsal arch (laminae)	Dorsal—dorsal arch (laminae) and wings Ventral—diarthroidal joint and wings	Dorsal—wire laminae; screw wings and wire between screws Ventral—pin through joint or wings, with or without bone cement
C1-C2	Respiratory arrest; lack of an intervertebral disk; two lateral diarthroidal joints	Dorsal—dorsal arch of C1; dorsal spinous process of C2 Ventral—diarthroidal joints	Dorsal—wire or suture spine of C2 to arch of C1 Ventral—pins through joint, with or without bone cement; screws through joint
C2	Respiratory arrest; venous sinus hemorrhage; narrow body (dorsal-ventral); thin spinous process	Dorsal—dorsal spinous process Ventral—lateral and caudal aspect of vertebral body	Dorsal—wire dorsal spinous process with or without bone cement Ventral—pins in body or diarthroidal joint and bone cement; ventral body plate
C3-C7	Venous sinus hemorrhage; small dorsal spinous processes	Dorsal—articular facets Ventral—vertebral bodies	Dorsal—screws (large breed) or wires (small breed) through articular facets Ventral—pins in body and bone cement (to span interspace or stabilize body fracture); ventral body plate (plastic or metal); interbody screw

Positioning

Patients undergoing a ventral approach are placed in dorsal recumbency with their chest in a V-trough and carefully secured with sandbags or a rigid vacuum type of apparatus to prevent lateral motion. Front legs are taped caudally and a loop of rope is tied around the muzzle caudal to the maxillary canine teeth. The rope and tape are used to apply traction or counter-traction (based on radiographic evaluation) resulting in complete or partial fracture/luxation reduction and stabilization. An area from the laryngeal cartilages to caudal to the manubrium sterni is prepared for midline cervical incision.

Patients undergoing a dorsal approach should be positioned in sternal recumbency with the head and cervical spine positioned to encourage fracture/luxation reduction and stabilization (see Fig. 34-17 on p. 1057). Cranial cervical, midcervical, and caudal cervical exposures require slight variation in patient position (see Figs. 34-21 and 34-23).

SURGICAL TECHNIQUE
Stabilization with Pins and Methylmethacrylate

The limiting factor of this procedure is the amount of pin purchase in the relatively narrow vertebral bodies of the cranial cervical vertebrae. In patients with a C2 body fracture, pin purchase cranially is established by placing cross pins bilaterally through the atlantoaxial joints (Fig. 34-61), and caudally by placing pins in the caudal aspect of the C2 vertebral body. This fixation is generally adequate

for mid-C2 body fractures. However, if the caudal aspect of the C2 body is fractured, caudal pins are placed in the body of C3.

After fracture/luxation reduction, place two appropriate-sized Steinmann pins at a 20- to 25-degree angle to the midline on the ventral surface of the vertebral bodies cranial and caudal to the fracture/luxation. Drive each pin into the vertebral body to engage two cortices (Fig. 34-62). Cut the pins to protrude 3 to 4 cm from the vertebral body. Notch each pin with a pin cutter and place methylmethacrylate bone cement on the protruding pins, taking care to ensure that each pin is completely surrounded and covered with bone cement. Use cool saline lavage to dissipate the heat of polymerization. Close longus colli muscles cranial and caudal to the bone cement mass. Close sternohyoideus-thyroideus muscle, subcutaneous tissues, and skin routinely.

Stabilization with Ventral Cross Pins

Ventral cross-pin or screw stabilization is performed in patients with C1-C2 luxations or subluxations. The technique is described and illustrated on p. 1086.

Stabilization with Ventral Spinal Plates

Fracture/luxations of C2-C7 may be stabilized by the use of ventral spinal plates. The fracture/luxation is exposed as described for ventral slot; however, the vertebral body cranial and caudal to the fracture/luxation is also exposed.

FIG. 34-59
ASIF small fragment reduction forceps may be used to maintain reduction of a cervical fracture/luxation.

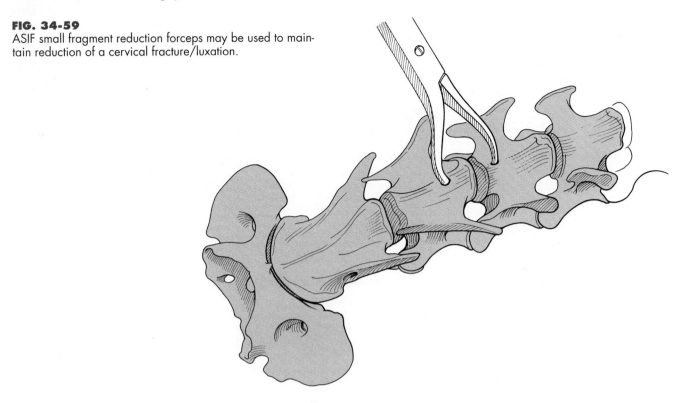

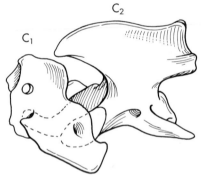

FIG. 34-60
Anatomic configuration of C1 and C2.

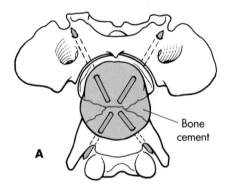

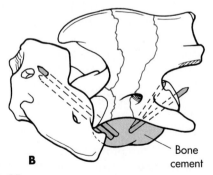

FIG. 34-61
Ventral stabilization of C1 and C2 fracture/luxation using Steinmann pins and methylmethacrylate bone cement in the ventral vertebral bodies. Notice that the pins are placed through the C1-C2 articulation and caudal aspect of the C2 vertebral body.

Reduce the fracture/luxation as described on p. 1091. Fashion an appropriate size plastic or metal plate to the ventral aspect of the vertebral bodies, allowing for two screws cranial and caudal to the fracture/luxation. Determine screw length by evaluating vertebral body size from preoperative radiographs. Drill screw holes 20 to 25 degrees from midline to engage two cortices. Tap the holes and apply the plate across the fracture/luxation (Fig. 34-63). It is impossible to safely engage two cortices unless screws are placed at an angle. Harvest autogenous cancellous bone from the heads of the humeri and place it in the fracture defect. Close longus colli muscles over the plate and graft. Close subcutaneous tissues and skin routinely.

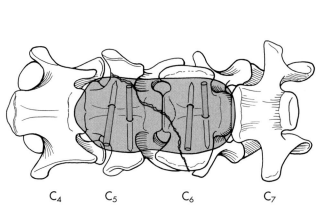

C₄   C₅   C₆   C₇

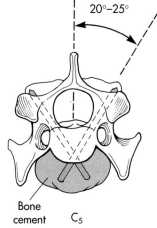

FIG. 34-62
Ventral stabilization of C3 to C7 fracture/luxation using Steinmann pins and methylmethacrylate bone cement in the ventral bodies. Notice that the pins are angled away from the spinal canal.

20°–25°

Bone cement   C₅

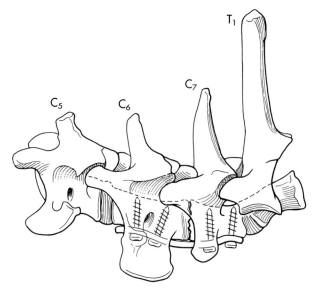

C₅   C₆   C₇   T₁

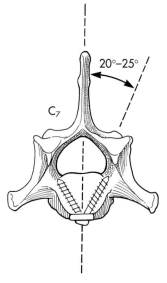

20°–25°

C₇

FIG. 34-63
Ventral stabilization of C3 to C7 fracture/luxation using plastic spinal plates on the ventral vertebral bodies. Notice that the screws are angled away from the spinal canal.

Stabilization Using Articular Facet Screws

Fractures and luxations rarely occur from C3 to C7. As small dorsal spinous processes in this region preclude the use of dorsal spinous process plates, the only dorsal technique for C3-C7 stabilization is articular facet screwing. The spine is approached as described on p. 1055.

Identify the appropriate articular facets of the fractured or luxated vertebrae. Remove the articular surface of each facet with a curette or high-speed pneumatic drill. Reduce the fracture/luxation by grasping the dorsal spinous process cranial and caudal to the fracture/luxation with towel forceps. Bring the articular facets into apposition. Drill and tap appropriate-size holes in each facet. Place one screw in each facet joint in lag screw fashion (Fig. 34-64). Harvest autogenous corticocancellous bone from the dorsal spinous processes of exposed vertebrae. Place the bone graft in and around the stabilized articular facets. Close epaxial muscles, subcutaneous tissues, and skin routinely.

SUTURE MATERIALS/SPECIAL INSTRUMENTS

Careful reduction and stabilization of cervical fractures are facilitated by the use of ASIF small reduction forceps and modified Gelpi retractors.

POSTOPERATIVE CARE AND ASSESSMENT

Patients with cervical spinal fracture/luxation should be evaluated postoperatively in a similar fashion as patients with other cervical spinal disorders. Because of the anatomic configuration of cervical vertebrae, particularly C1 and C2, any form of fixation is marginal at best. It is recommended that all forms of internal fixation be supported with a neck brace and strict cage confinement until radiographic evidence of union.

PROGNOSIS

Prognosis depends on appropriate case management, including assessment of presenting neurologic examination,

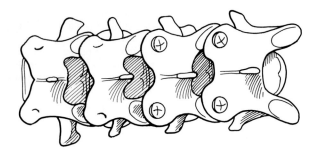

FIG. 34-64
Dorsal stabilization of C3 to C7 fracture/luxation using articular facet screws.

radiographic classification of the fracture/luxation, repair method, and postoperative care. If adequate and early stabilization is performed (conservative or surgical) a favorable prognosis is possible.

Suggested Reading

Blass CE, Waldron DR, van Ee RT: Cervical stabilization in three dogs using Steinmann pins and methacrylate, *J Am Anim Hosp Assoc* 24:61, 1988.

Bruecker KA, Seim HB III: Principles of spinal fracture management, *Sem in Vet Med and Surg* 7:71, 1992.

Reneger WR, Simpson ST, Stoll SG: The use of methylmethacrylate bone cement in cervical spinal stabilization: a case report and discussion, *J Am Anim Hosp Assoc* 16:219, 1980.

Stone EA, Betts CW, Chambers JN: Cervical fractures in the dog: a literature and case review, *J Am Anim Hosp Assoc* 15:463, 1979.

Wong WT, Emms SG: Use of pins and methylmethacrylate in stabilization of spinal fractures and luxations, *J Sm Anim Prac* 33:415, 1992.

NEOPLASIA OF THE CERVICAL VERTEBRAE, SPINAL CORD, AND NERVE ROOTS

DEFINITIONS

Neurofibromas and **neurofibrosarcoma** arise from nerve connective tissue (medullary layer of a nerve fiber). **Schwannomas** are benign tumors of the neurilemma (Schwann cells). **Meningiomas** are slow-growing tumors that arise from arachnoidal tissue. **Astrocytomas** and **ependymomas** arise from spinal cord parenchymal cells.

SYNONYMS

Spinal tumors, spinal cord tumors of the spine, vertebral tumors, nerve root tumors

GENERAL CONSIDERATIONS AND CLINICALLY RELEVANT PATHOPHYSIOLOGY

Tumors may arise from numerous sites in and around the spinal cord. They may be classified as *primary bone, primary spinal cord, primary peripheral nerve root, primary paraspinal soft tissue,* or *metastatic* tumors. It is important to try to classify the tissue of origin because it affects prognosis. Spinal tumors are also classified according to their location relative to the dura (i.e., extradural, intradural-extramedullary, intramedullary; Table 34-28). These locations are usually determined myelographically. The majority of canine cervical vertebral and spinal cord tumors occur extradurally and generally arise from bone (e.g., multiple cartilaginous exostoses, osteosarcoma, fibrosarcoma, multiple myeloma, chondrosarcoma). Tumors may also metastasize to the vertebra, causing spinal cord compression (i.e., hemangiosarcoma, undifferentiated sarcoma, lymphosarcoma). Lymphosarcoma is the most common canine soft-tissue extradural spinal tumor. The majority of canine intradural-extramedullary tumors are nerve sheath tumors (i.e., neurofibroma, neurofibrosarcoma, schwannoma) and meningiomas. Nerve sheath tumors arise from nerve roots, but often cause spinal cord compression because of their close proximity. Meningiomas can arise from any location along the spinal cord, but are generally near the nerve roots. Intramedullary tumors are rare and include astrocytomas and ependymomas. Lymphosarcoma is the most common spinal tumor in cats and generally occurs extradurally. Intradural-extramedullary and intramedullary tumors are rare in cats.

DIAGNOSIS
Clinical Presentation

Signalment. There does not appear to be a sex or breed predilection for cervical vertebral, spinal cord, or nerve root tumors. The majority of patients with cervical spinal tumors are older than 5 years of age; however, benign solitary or multiple cartilaginous exostoses most often occur in patients younger than 1 year of age.

☞ **NOTE •** When considering differentials in patients with neurologic disorders remember that "tumors know no age."

TABLE 34-28

Characteristics of Vertebral, Spinal Cord, and Nerve Root Neoplasia

Extradural:
- 40% of tumors
- Arise from bone and paraspinal tissues
- Prognosis is unfavorable (less than 50-50 chance of improvement)

Intradural-Extramedullary:
- 50% of tumors
- Arise from nerve roots and meninges
- Prognosis is guarded (50-50 chance of getting better)

Intramedullary
- 10% of tumors
- Arise from glial cells
- Prognosis is grave (patient will not get better)

History. The classic history of patients with cervical spinal neoplasia is slowly progressing tetraparesis. However, some patients have an acute onset of neurologic abnormalities preceded by insidious, slowly progressing signs. Careful historical evaluation often reveals that subtle neurologic abnormalities occurred before the acute episode. Historical features may also vary, depending on location of the neoplasm with respect to the dura (i.e., extradural, intradural-extramedullary, or intramedullary).

Physical Examination Findings

Physical and neurologic examination findings associated with vertebral, spinal cord, and nerve root tumors depend on tumor location, degree of spinal cord compression, rate of tumor growth, and associated secondary effects of the tumor. Pain is often associated with cervical spinal tumors, especially if they involve a nerve root (i.e., intradural-extramedullary), cause bone destruction or destruction of adjoining soft tissues, or are extradural. Tumors involving nerve roots of the brachial plexus (spinal cord segments C6-T1) often produce forelimb lameness (i.e., monoparesis), progressing to hemiparesis or tetraparesis. Neurologic examination may reveal UMN signs to the hindlimbs and LMN signs to the forelimbs. Patients with an intramedullary tumor have acute paresis but no pain because there are no sensitive pain fibers within spinal cord parenchyma. The presence of Horner's syndrome (i.e., miosis, ptosis, enophthalmos, and third-eyelid protrusion) localizes the tumor to spinal cord segments C7-T2.

☞ **N O T E** · Diagnosis and lesion localization depends on performance and interpretation of the neurologic examination.

Radiography/Ultrasonography

Survey radiography can be useful in evaluating spinal neoplasia. Osteoproduction and osteolysis from vertebral tumors may be seen on survey radiographs (Figs. 34-65 and 34-66). Some peripheral nerve tumors cause lysis of the intervertebral foramen (Fig. 34-67). Diagnosis of vertebral, spinal cord, and nerve root neoplasms requires myelography. Specific myelographic techniques are described on p. 1044. Myelography identifies the lesion as extradural, intradural-extramedullary, or intramedullary; examples of myelographic abnormalities associated with each classification are described and illustrated on p. 1044-1047. Occasionally, CT scans or MRI may be necessary to accurately determine extent of a vertebral or spinal cord lesion.

Laboratory Findings

Laboratory findings in patients with vertebral and spinal cord neoplasia are generally normal, but may reflect abnormalities caused by a paraneoplastic syndrome. Changes in cerebrospinal fluid are usually noncontributory; however, cell type or evidence of an inflammatory process may suggest neoplasia.

DIFFERENTIAL DIAGNOSIS

A list of differential diagnoses that mimic cervical vertebral and spinal cord neoplasia is provided in Table 34-29. Differential diagnosis of vertebral and spinal cord tumor type is based on location of tumor (i.e., bone, spinal cord, nerve root, or metastasis) and myelographic classification (i.e., extradural, intradural-extramedullary, or intramedullary).

MEDICAL MANAGEMENT

Medical management of cervical spinal tumors is directed at both the primary lesion and secondary effects of the tumor. Corticosteroids are commonly used to decrease peritumoral edema. The steroid of choice is methylprednisolone sodium succinate (Table 34-30). Definitive medical treatment, without surgery, is rarely recommended unless the tumor is inaccessible or the tumor *type* can be more effectively treated with chemotherapy or irradiation alone. Surgical exposure and incisional or excisional biopsy is usually necessary to determine tumor type and plan adjunct therapy.

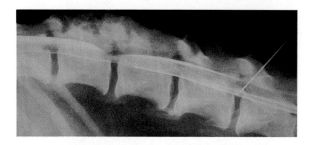

FIG. 34-65
Lateral myelogram of a dog with a tumor of the vertebral body. Notice the osteoproduction involving the dorsal lamina of L2 and L3. Extradural spinal cord compression is evident.

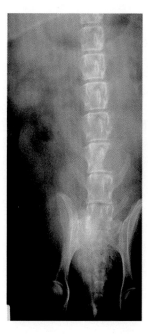

FIG. 34-66
Ventrodorsal radiograph of a dog with a tumor of L5. Notice osteolysis of the lamina, pedicle, vertebral body, and transverse process.

SURGICAL TREATMENT
Preoperative Management

The animal should be given intravenous fluids and steroids before surgery. Steroids are given to protect the spinal cord from the effects of surgical manipulation (see Table 34-20). The steroid of choice is methylprednisolone sodium succinate (30 mg/kg intravenously).

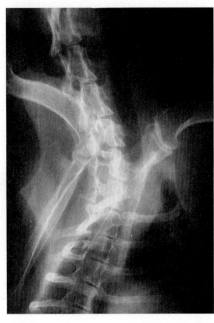

FIG. 34-67
Obliqued (45 to 60 degrees) cervical radiograph of a dog with spinal neoplasia. Notice the enlarged C6-C7 intervertebral foramen.

Anesthesia

See p. 1049 for suggested anesthetic protocols to use in animals with cervical spinal disorders. The patient's neurologic status and positioning for surgery are important preanesthetic considerations. If motor weakness (i.e., ambulatory tetraparesis, weakly ambulatory tetraparesis, or nonambulatory tetraparesis) is present or if positioning may cause respiratory compromise (i.e., sternal recumbency, flexed neck, or lateral chest wall compression), mechanical ventilatory support should be considered.

Surgical Anatomy

The cervical spine has unique and variable anatomic configuration from vertebra to vertebra, particularly C1 and C2 (see p. 1052, Figs. 34-1 and 34-3). Important anatomic variations are described on p. 1051.

Positioning

Generally, patients with cervical vertebral, spinal cord, or nerve root tumors require a dorsal approach because ventral approaches do not provide sufficient exposure for tumor resection. Patients are positioned in sternal recumbency with the head and cervical spine gently flexed. Choice of cranial cervical, midcervical, or caudal cervical laminectomy is based on tumor location and may require slight variation in patient positioning (see Figs. 34-17, 34-21, and 34-23 on pp. 1057, 1058, and 1059, respectively).

SURGICAL TECHNIQUE

Surgical objectives include exposure of the vertebral, spinal cord, or nerve root tumor; wide resection of neoplastic tissue; spinal cord and nerve root decompression; and vertebral stabilization. If wide resection is not possible, biopsy and de-

TABLE 34-29

Differential Diagnoses That Mimic Cervical Vertebral and Spinal Cord Neoplasia Using the DAMNIT-V Scheme

Classification	Examples	Diagnostic Differentials
Degenerative	Cervical disk disease	Plain and contrast radiography
	Wobbler syndrome	History; plain and stress myelography
Anomalous	Atlantoaxial instability	Plain and stress radiography
	Congenital malformation	Plain and stress radiography
Metabolic	Any disorder causing generalized weakness (e.g., Addison's disease)	History; neurologic exam; laboratory findings
Nutritional	Nutritional secondary hyperparathyroidism (may cause pathologic fractures)	Dietary history; plain radiography
Neoplastic	— —	— —
Immunologic	Polyarthritis	Neurologic exam; laboratory data
	Polymyositis	Neurologic exam; laboratory data
Infectious	Cervical diskospondylitis	History; plain and contrast radiographs
	Vertebral osteomyelitis	History; plain and contrast radiographs
	Paraspinal abscess	History; plain and contrast radiographs
	Meningitis	History; CSF analysis
Traumatic	Cervical spinal fracture/luxation	History; plain radiographs
Vascular	Fibrocartilaginous embolism	History; CSF analysis; myelography

TABLE 34-30
Steroid Therapy

Methylprednisolone Sodium Succinate (Solu-Medrol)
30 mg/kg IV, repeated BID if needed; not to exceed 2 doses

compression should be attempted. Definitive diagnosis of tumor type may suggest appropriate adjunct therapy. Patients with tumors of the cranial cervical, midcervical, or caudal cervical vertebrae, spinal cord, or nerve roots are approached via cranial cervical, midcervical, or caudal cervical laminectomy, respectively, as described on p. 1055. Wide laminectomy, laminotomy, facetectomy, and/or foramenotomy are required for adequate exposure of most extradural and intradural-extramedullary tumors. Dorsal laminectomy and durotomy are necessary for exposure and removal of intramedullary tumors. If stabilization is necessary, articular facet screws are placed as described on p. 1095.

SUTURE MATERIALS/SPECIAL INSTRUMENTS

Ultrasonic aspirators use high-frequency ultrasonic vibration to fragment (phacoemulsify) tissue; they reduce dense masses to a nearly liquid state that can be atraumatically aspirated. Ultrasonic aspirators are an invaluable addition to neurosurgical instrumentation, especially in removing neoplastic tissue; however, cost may be prohibitive ($25,000 to $70,000).

POSTOPERATIVE CARE AND ASSESSMENT

Patients with cervical spinal neoplasia should be evaluated postoperatively in a similar fashion as patients with other cervical spinal disorders. Adjunct chemotherapy, irradiation, immunotherapy, or combination therapy is based on results of histopathology and surgical margins.

PROGNOSIS

Prognosis for patients with cervical vertebral, spinal cord, and nerve root tumors depends on tumor type, degree of surgical resection, and sensitivity to adjunct chemotherapy, radiation, immunotherapy, or a combination of any of these factors. Malignant extradural neoplasms usually have an unfavorable prognosis, benign extradural neoplasms have a favorable prognosis, malignant and benign intramedullary neoplasms have an unfavorable-to-grave prognosis, and extradural-intramedullary neoplasms have a guarded prognosis.

Suggested Reading

Bell FW et al: External beam radiation therapy for recurrent intraspinal meningioma in a dog, *J Am Anim Hosp Assoc* 28:318, 1992.

Bichsel P et al: Solitary cartilaginous exostoses associated with spinal cord compression in three large-breed dogs, *J Am Anim Hosp Assoc* 21:619, 1985.

Bradley RL, Withrow SJ, Snyder SP: Nerve sheath tumors in the dog, *J Am Anim Hosp Assoc* 18:915, 1982.

Fingeroth JM, Prata RG, Patnaik AK: Spinal meningiomas in dogs: 13 cases (1972–1987), *J Am Vet Med Assoc* 191:720, 1987.

Gilmore DR: Neoplasia of the cervical spinal cord and vertebrae in the dog, *J Am Anim Hosp Assoc* 19:1009, 1983.

Gilroy BA: Intraocular and cardiopulmonary effects of low-dose mannitol in the dog, *Vet Surg* 15:342, 1986.

Santen DR et al: Thoracolumbar vertebral osteochondroma in a young dog, *J Am Vet Med Assoc* 199:1054, 1991.

Spodnick GJ et al: Prognosis for dogs with appendicular osteosarcoma treated by amputation alone: 162 cases (1978–1988), *J Am Vet Med Assoc* 200:995, 1992.

Troy GC, Hurov LI, King GK: Successful surgical removal of a cervical subdural neurofibrosarcoma, *J Am Anim Hosp Assoc* 15:477, 1979.

CHAPTER 35

Surgery of the Thoracolumbar Spine

GENERAL PRINCIPLES AND TECHNIQUES

DEFINITIONS

Dorsal laminectomy is the removal of the dorsal spinous processes and portions of the lamina, articular facets, and pedicles of affected vertebrae. **Funkquist A** dorsal laminectomy refers to removal of the vertebral lamina, articular facets, and pedicle to a level corresponding to the middle of the dorsoventral diameter of the spinal cord, whereas a **Funkquist B** dorsal laminectomy is removal of the lamina above the dorsal aspect of the spinal cord (articular facets and pedicles are not removed). A **modified dorsal laminectomy** is similar to a Funkquist B procedure; however, the entire caudal articular processes are removed and the laminectomy edges undercut, causing additional exposure of the spinal canal. **Deep dorsal laminectomy** involves removal of dorsal lamina, articular facets, and pedicles to the ventral aspect of the vertebral canal. **Hemilaminectomy** is unilateral removal of lamina, articular facets, and portions of the pedicle of affected vertebrae. **Minihemilaminectomy** or **pediculectomy** is removal of portions of the pedicle at the level of the intervertebral foramen.

PREOPERATIVE CONCERNS

Serial neurologic examinations should be done to determine surgical urgency. Patients with severe neurologic deficits, deterioration, or unacceptably static neurologic examinations may require immediate surgery. Patients with possible unstable spinal fractures or luxations should be immobilized on a rigid platform or placed in a back brace until definitively diagnosed. Spinal surgery generally requires spinal cord and/or nerve root manipulation to treat the underlying disorder (e.g., removal of disk material or neoplasm, fracture stabilization). Preoperative corticosteroid administration may partially protect these structures during surgery; however, steroids may predispose to gastrointestinal ulceration/perforation (see Table 34-11 on p. 1070).

ANESTHETIC CONSIDERATIONS

Anesthetic management for thoracolumbar spinal cord surgery is similar to that described for animals with cervical lesions. A selected anesthetic protocol is given in Table 34-3 p. 1050. Mechanical or intermittent positive-pressure ventilation may help patients with respiratory compromise (e.g., pulmonary hemorrhage).

ANTIBIOTICS

Use of prophylactic or therapeutic antibiotics should be based on criteria provided in Table 34-4 on p. 1050. Cefazolin (Table 35-1) is the antibiotic of choice for neurologic surgery patients because of its low toxicity and excellent *in vitro* activity against common pathogens.

SURGICAL ANATOMY

The vertebral body, lamina, pedicle, dorsal spinous process, transverse processes, accessory processes, and articular facets of each vertebra are unique in anatomic configuration. Figs. 35-1 and 35-2 illustrate the unique anatomy of T11 and L5, respectively. Vertebral venous sinuses run longitudinally on the ventrolateral floor of the spinal canal. The dorsal longitudinal ligament lies directly on the ventral floor of the spinal canal with venous sinuses running on each side (see Fig. 35-17). This is also the location of the intervertebral foramen, its exiting nerve root, and radicular artery. Neurosurgeons should have an appropriate anatomic specimen (in addition to a thorough knowledge of regional anatomy) available for reference.

SURGICAL TECHNIQUES

Patients with surgical disorders of the thoracolumbar spine may be treated by dorsal laminectomy, hemilaminectomy, fenestration, or thoracolumbar spinal stabilization via a dorsal approach. Proper positioning is often critical. Patients with spinal fracture/luxation should be positioned to encourage reduction

---

TABLE 35-1

Perioperative Antibiotic Therapy

Cefazolin (Ancef or Kefzol)

20 mg/kg IV at induction, repeat at 4- to 6-hour intervals for 24 hours

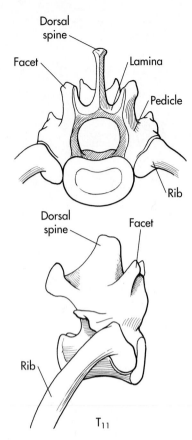

FIG. 35-1
T11 vertebra showing vertebral body, lamina, pedicle, dorsal spinous process, rib, and articular facets.

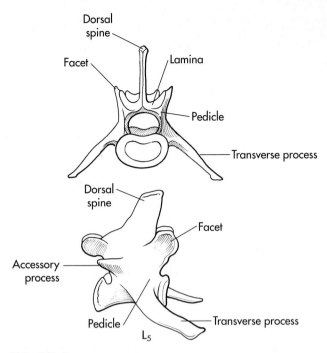

FIG. 35-2
L5 vertebra showing vertebral body, lamina, pedicle, dorsal spinous process, accessory process, transverse process, and articular facet.

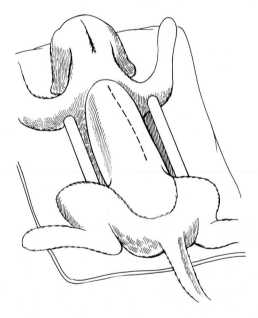

FIG. 35-3
When positioning a dog for dorsal thoracolumbar laminectomy, avoid hyperextending the spine.

of the fracture/luxation and spinal cord decompression. Towels or sandbags placed under the abdomen may divert venous return through vertebral venous sinuses and should be avoided. Avoid hyperextending the spine during positioning (Fig. 35-3). Dorsal laminectomy patients should have their backs gently flexed to open articular facets and interarcuate spaces. For hemilaminectomy, the affected side should be gently rotated dorsally (about 15 degrees) to facilitate lateral exposure of vertebral lamina and articular facets (Fig. 35-4).

Dorsal laminectomy allows entrance to all areas of the thoracolumbar spinal canal and spinal cord (i.e., dorsal, lateral, and ventral). Dorsal decompressive approaches (in order of most commonly to least commonly performed) include modified dorsal, Funkquist A, deep dorsal, and Funkquist B laminectomies. These techniques are indicated for removal of herniated disk fragments, resection of vertebral, spinal cord, and nerve root tumors, and exposure of fracture/luxations.

Modified Dorsal Laminectomy

Modified dorsal laminectomy is indicated for exposure of compressive masses in the ventrolateral and dorsal aspect of the spinal canal (i.e., disk fragments, fracture fragments, vertebral and spinal cord neoplasms). Laminectomy of no more than two consecutive vertebrae should be performed using this technique.

Make an incision over the dorsal midline to include two spinous processes cranial and caudal to the lesion. Use a periosteal elevator or small osteotome to subperiosteally elevate epaxial muscles from dorsal spinous processes, lamina, articular facets, and pedicles of affected vertebrae

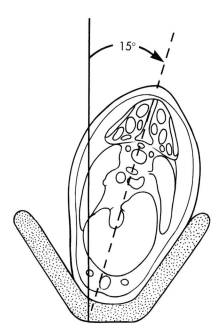

FIG. 35-4
For hemilaminectomy, position the patient with a 15-degree rotation to facilitate lateral exposure of vertebral lamina, pedicle, and articular facets.

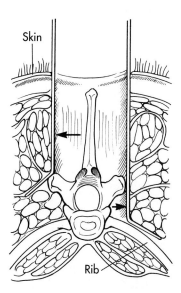

FIG. 35-5
Use a periosteal elevator or small osteotome to subperiosteally elevate epaxial muscles from affected vertebrae.

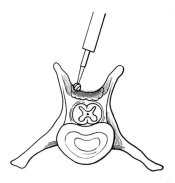

FIG. 35-6
When performing dorsal laminectomy, use a high-speed pneumatic drill to remove the white outer cortical layer of lamina.

(Fig. 35-5). Use Gelpi retractors to facilitate gentle retraction of epaxial musculature during dissection. Control soft-tissue hemorrhage with bipolar cautery. Remove the exposed dorsal spinous processes to the level of the dorsal lamina with large, single-action duckbill rongeurs (see Fig. 8-18). Use a pneumatic air drill to begin burring the outer cortical (white) layer of bone from the lamina of both vertebrae. Remove articular processes of the cranial vertebrae with the drill, working carefully so as much of the cranial articular processes are left intact as possible (Fig. 35-6). Continue drilling the dorsal lamina until the medullary layer of bone is encountered (it is red in appearance, soft, and easily drilled). Carefully burr this layer until the white inner cortical layer is visualized (Fig. 35-7). The inner cortical layer is easily recognized in the midlaminar portion of each vertebral body; however, it becomes more difficult to recognize at the intervertebral space, where bone appears white throughout drilling (Fig. 35-7). Prior to drilling over the intervertebral space, remove the interarcuate ligament (a.k.a., ligamentum flavum, yellow ligament) using sharp dissection with a No. 11 Bard-Parker scalpel blade. Do not use a pneumatic bone drill as it tends to grab soft tissue and force the drill downward toward the spinal canal. Estimate drilling depth at the intervertebral space first by reaching the inner cortical layer at the midlaminar portion of the vertebral body cranial and caudal to the interspace. Drill remaining bone at the intervertebral space to the same level. Once the inner cortical layers of both laminae have been reached, use careful paintbrushlike burring until soft periosteum can be palpated with

a dental spatula. Continue to burr until periosteum is palpable over both vertebrae and the intervertebral space. Use a dental tool and Lempert rongeurs to gently penetrate periosteum, and carefully pry the remaining inner cortical layer away (Fig. 35-7). If necessary, undercut the dorsal laminae to gain additional exposure. Use a 2- to 3-mm diameter carbide or diamond burr to carefully drill away the inner layer of laminar bone (Fig. 35-8). This is the recommended modification, because it provides greater exposure, ensuring atraumatic removal of compressive lesions. If hemorrhage from soft tissue occurs, use suction and bipolar cautery for control. If hemorrhage from bone occurs, apply bone wax to the tip of a periosteal elevator and gently press it on the bleeding surface. Lesions near the vertebral venous sinus should be manipulated with great care. Occasionally, venous sinus hemorrhage is incurred. Proper use of hemostatic agents (e.g., Gelfoam, Surgicel, Avistat) with cottonoid and suction helps control hemorrhage (see

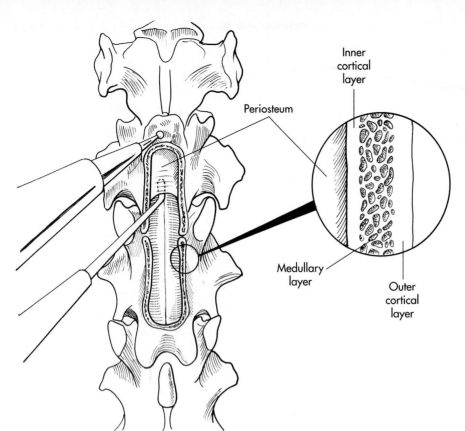

Periosteum

Inner
cortical
layer

Medullary
layer

Outer
cortical
layer

FIG. 35-7
For dorsal laminectomy, carefully drill through outer cortical and medullary layers of bone until the inner cortical layer is reached, then use a paint-brush stroke until periosteum is reached. Three layers of bone are drilled: a thick white outer cortical layer, soft red medullary layer, and a thin white inner cortical layer. Use a dental spatula to penetrate the inner periosteum to expose spinal canal.

Table 34-1 on p. 1050 for technique to control venous sinus hemorrhage). Prior to closure, irrigate the wound with room temperature physiologic saline solution to dislodge any remaining bone fragments from soft tissues. Span the dorsal spinous processes cranial and caudal to the laminectomy site with 20-gauge, stainless steel orthopedic wire (wire is used for cosmetic purposes only). Harvest a piece of subcutaneous fat and place it over the laminectomy site to help prevent dural adhesions. Debride any devitalized muscle and close fascia and epaxial muscles with a simple interrupted pattern over the spanning wire. Close subcutaneous tissues and skin routinely.

Funkquist A Dorsal Laminectomy

Funkquist A dorsal laminectomy provides improved exposure of the lateral aspect of the spinal canal and spinal cord compared to a modified dorsal or Funkquist B laminectomy. This procedure is indicated when compressive masses are located in the dorsal, lateral, or ventrolateral aspect of the spinal canal (i.e., lateral disk extrusions, lateral vertebral, spinal cord, nerve root neoplasms, lateral fracture fragments). Exposure of the spinal canal is limited to two consecutive vertebrae (one intervertebral space). The approach is as described above for modified dorsal laminectomy to the level of laminar and facet exposure.

Remove exposed dorsal lamina and cranial and caudal articular facets with rongeurs or pneumatic drill. Identify outer

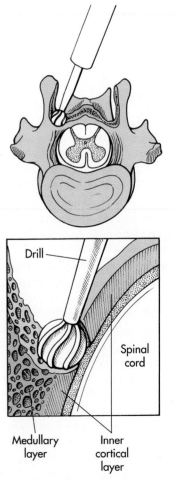

Drill

Spinal
cord

Medullary
layer

Inner
cortical
layer

FIG. 35-8
When performing modified dorsal laminectomy, gain additional lateral exposure by carefully undercutting dorsal lamina and cranial articular facet.

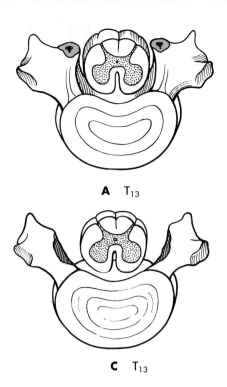

A T₁₃

C T₁₃

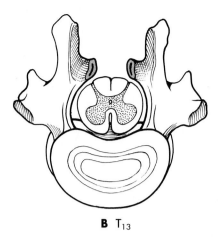

B T₁₃

FIG. 35-9
A, During Funquist type A dorsal laminectomy, remove articular facets and pedicles to expose the dorsal one half of the spinal cord. **B,** During Funquist type B dorsal laminectomy, remove the dorsal lamina, taking care to preserve cranial and caudal articular facets. **C,** Remove the dorsal lamina, cranial and caudal articular facets, and pedicles to the level of the ventral aspect of the spinal canal when performing a deep dorsal laminectomy.

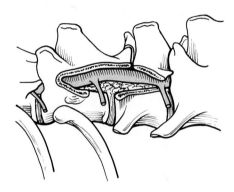

FIG. 35-10
Remove right or left articular facets and pedicles to the level of the ventral floor of the spinal canal during hemilaminectomy.

cortical, medullary, and inner cortical layers of exposed lamina. Enter the spinal canal by carefully penetrating periosteum with a dental spatula or Lempert rongeur. Use double action duckbill and Lempert rongeurs to remove remnants of the lamina, articular facets, and pedicles to a level corresponding to that of a dorsal plane through the middle of the dorsoventral diameter of the spinal cord (Fig. 35-9, A). Carefully explore the dorsal, lateral, and ventrolateral aspect of the spinal canal, spinal cord, and nerve roots. Close as described above for modified dorsal laminectomy.

Funkquist B Dorsal Laminectomy

Funkquist B dorsal laminectomy (Fig. 35-9, B) exposes the dorsal aspect of the spinal canal and spinal cord. It is indicated when compressive masses are located in the dorsal aspect of the spinal canal (i.e., dorsal disk extrusion, dorsal extradural neoplasia, dorsal laminar neoplasia). Laminectomy of up to three consecutive vertebrae can be performed using this technique. The approach is as described above for modified dorsal laminectomy to the level of laminar exposure.

Remove laminar bone with a pneumatic bone drill, taking care to preserve the cranial and caudal articular facets. Identify the outer cortical, medullary, and inner cortical layers as you drill. Remove periosteum from the dorsal lamina with a dental spatula or Lempert rongeurs. Carefully explore the dorsal aspect of the spinal canal and spinal cord. Close as described above for modified dorsal laminectomy.

Deep Dorsal Laminectomy

Deep dorsal laminectomy provides excellent exposure of the dorsal, lateral, and ventral aspects of the spinal canal, spinal cord, and nerve roots. It is indicated when maximal decompression within the limits of one vertebral length is required (e.g., vertebral, spinal cord, or nerve root tumors, and severe disk herniation). This procedure is performed as described for Funkquist A laminectomy to the level of articular facet and pedicle removal.

Carefully rongeur the remaining pedicles to the level of the ventral aspect of the spinal canal (Fig. 35-9, C). Identify vertebral venous sinuses bilaterally and avoid them if possible. Control venous sinus hemorrhage as described in Table 34-1 on p. 1050). Gently manipulate beneath the spinal cord to remove ventrally located masses. Close as described above for modified dorsal laminectomy.

Hemilaminectomy

Hemilaminectomy is indicated when spinal cord is compressed by mass lesions in the lateral, dorsolateral, or ventrolateral spinal canal (e.g., disk extrusion, extradural mass, intradural-extramedullary mass, nerve root tumor, fracture fragment) (Fig. 35-10). Hemilaminectomy is preferable to dorsal laminectomy because it best preserves the structural and mechanical integrity of the spine, is less traumatic, is

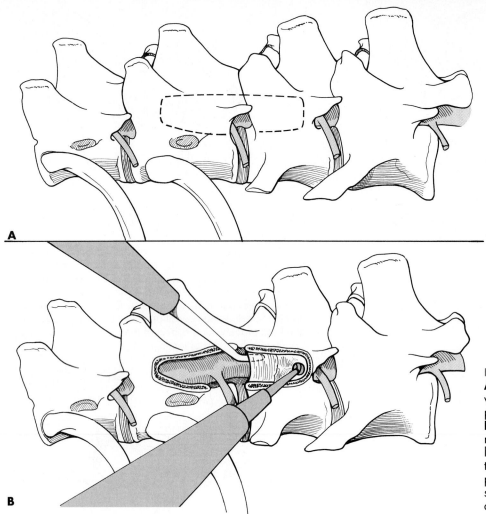

FIG. 35-11
A, During hemilaminectomy, visualize the area of the proposed hemilaminectomy.
B, Drill outer cortical, medullary, and inner cortical layers of lamina and pedicle to the level of the inner periosteum. Use a dental spatula to remove periosteum and enter the spinal canal.

more cosmetic, and reduces the chance of scars causing spinal cord compression. However, the lesion must lateralize myelographically to ensure complete mass removal. Bilateral hemilaminectomy may be performed when the compressive lesion is on both sides of the spinal cord. Unilateral hemilaminectomy can be performed along three consecutive vertebrae without producing clinically significant spinal instability, whereas bilateral hemilaminectomy can be performed along two consecutive vertebrae. Hemilaminectomy may be performed with a high-speed pneumatic drill, high-speed electric drill, or rongeurs.

Make a dorsal midline incision to include two dorsal spinous processes cranial and caudal to the affected intervertebral space or vertebral body. Use a periosteal elevator or small osteotome to elevate epaxial muscles from their attachments on the lateral aspect of the dorsal spinous processes, lamina, articular facet, and pedicle to the level of the accessory process. Use a Gelpi retractor to maintain muscle retraction. Use a drill or rongeur to enter the spinal canal. Regardless of technique used to enter the spinal canal, be careful when manipulating lesions involving the ventral and ventrolateral aspect of the spinal canal, because the vertebral venous sinuses are in close proximity. If venous sinus hemorrhage occurs, control hemorrhage as described in Table 34-1 on

p. 1050. Control soft-tissue hemorrhage with bipolar cautery and hemorrhage from bone with bone wax. Lavage the surgical site with room temperature physiologic saline solution to dislodge any loose bone fragments. Harvest a fat graft from the subcutaneous area and place it over the laminectomy site. Close epaxial muscles to the dorsal midline. Close subcutaneous tissues and skin routinely.

If a drill is used, remove articular processes of the involved intervertebral space with a high-speed drill. Visualize a rectangular area from the base of the dorsal spinous processes dorsally, accessory process ventrally, articular facet of the cranial vertebra, and articular facet of the caudal vertebra (Fig. 35-11, A). Drill the outer cortical bone of this rectangle, beginning cranially and working caudally. Continue to drill through the soft, red, medullary layer to the inner cortical layer. Once the inner cortical layer is reached, use a paint-brush action to expose the soft inner periosteum. Use a dental spatula or Lempert rongeur to carefully enter the spinal canal (Fig. 35-11, B).

If rongeurs are used, remove articular processes of the involved intervertebral space with rongeurs (Fig. 35-12, A). Have an assistant grasp and elevate the dorsal spinous process of the vertebra cranial to the involved intervertebral space with towel forceps (Fig. 35-12, B). This maneuver will open the intervertebral space and facilitate expo-

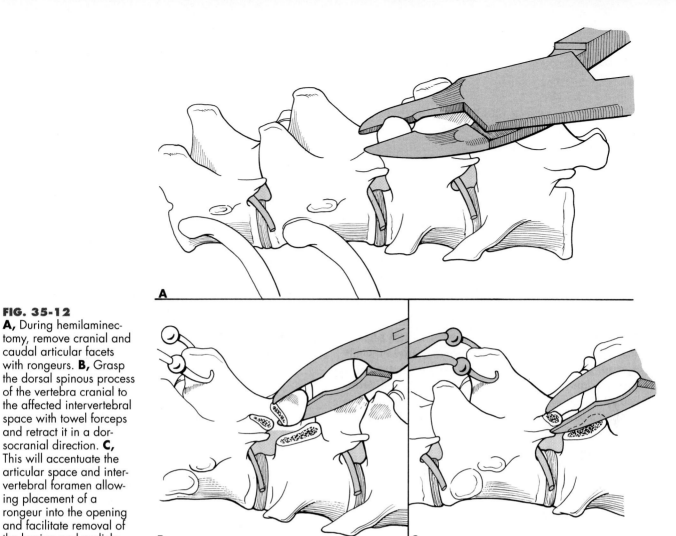

FIG. 35-12
A, During hemilaminectomy, remove cranial and caudal articular facets with rongeurs. **B,** Grasp the dorsal spinous process of the vertebra cranial to the affected intervertebral space with towel forceps and retract it in a dorsocranial direction. **C,** This will accentuate the articular space and intervertebral foramen allowing placement of a rongeur into the opening and facilitate removal of the lamina and pedicle.

sure of the foramen. Place one blade of a Lempert rongeur into the opening and remove a small amount of bone (Fig. 35-12, C). Continue to enlarge the opening cranially and caudally with rongeurs until the laminectomy defect is an appropriate size to allow adequate decompression.

Pediculectomy

Pediculectomy (modified lateral hemilaminectomy) is indicated for lesions confined to the lateral and ventral aspects of the spinal canal (e.g., ventrolateral intervertebral disk extrusion). The initial surgical approach is as described for hemilaminectomy.

Continue epaxial muscle dissection to the level of the caudomedial one fourth of the transverse process at the affected intervertebral space. This allows complete exposure of the intervertebral foramen and associated structures. Using the accessory process as a landmark, drill the slot defect just dorsal and ventral to the accessory process and extend it half the vertebral lengths cranial and caudal. If the radicular artery is encountered, control hemorrhage with bipolar cautery. Determine depth of drilling by identifying outer cortical, medullary, and inner cortical layers. Use caution when drilling the inner cortical layer and removing inner periosteum.

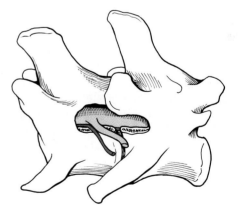

FIG. 35-13
Remove pedicular bone cranial and caudal to the intervertebral foramen during pediculectomy. Cranial and caudal articular facets are preserved.

Identify the spinal nerve from its origin within the spinal canal and its exit from the intervertebral foramen. Retract the nerve with a small blunt hook and remove the remaining portion of the pedicle to extend the defect to the floor of the spinal canal (Fig. 35-13). After removal of disk fragments, harvest a fat graft from the subcutaneous area and place it over the pediculectomy site. Close epaxial muscle, subcutaneous tissues, and skin as described for hemilaminectomy.

HEALING OF THE SPINAL CORD

Healing of the thoracolumbar spinal cord is similar to that described for the cervical spinal cord on p. 1061. The surface plexus of arteries is not as dense in the thoracic spinal cord as in the cervical and lumbar regions. The effect this may have on healing of traumatic lesions is unclear.

SUTURE MATERIALS/SPECIAL INSTRUMENTS

Special instrumentation necessary to perform dorsal laminectomy, fenestration, and spinal stabilization is shown by technique in Table 35-2. It is important to practice each technique, become familiar with regional anatomy, and learn proper use of special instrumentation prior to performing these surgeries.

POSTOPERATIVE CARE AND ASSESSMENT

Immediate postoperative care is determined based on underlying diseases or conditions in Table 35-3. Neurologic status should be determined when the animal has fully recovered from anesthesia, and complete neurologic examinations should be performed daily until discharge. Postoperative care of ambulatory and nonambulatory patients is described in Table 35-4. Ambulatory patients may be discharged 24 to 48 hours postoperatively. Nonambulatory patients require frequent hydrotherapy, physiotherapy, elevated padded cage racks, and bladder expression three to four times a day. Indwelling urinary catheters should be avoided to help reduce urinary tract infections. Keep patients clean and dry to prevent decubital ulcers. A supporting cart helps patients return to an ambulatory status. Advantages of a cart include unhindered eating, drinking, micturition, and defecation. Animals with motor function can be encouraged to ambulate and an erect position facilitates physiotherapy. Nonambulatory patients should remain in the hospital until recovery of bladder function, or until clients can provide appropriate aftercare.

Follow-up neurologic examinations should be performed at 1, 2, 3, 6, 9, and 12 months postoperatively. Spinal radiographs (taken without anesthesia) are recommended at 1, 3, 6, 9, and 12 months postoperatively.

TABLE 35-2

Special Instruments Necessary to Perform Thoracolumbar and Lumbosacral Spinal Surgery

Special instruments needed for most procedures	High-speed pneumatic or electric drill Drill burrs: carbide and diamond tip Cautery unit (monopolar and bipolar) Periosteal elevator/osteotome Suction Hemostatic sponge (Gelfoam) Cottonoid felt sponge Bone wax Dental spatula Dural hook
Dorsal laminectomy, hemilaminectomy, facetectomy, foramenotomy	Duck-bill, double action ronguers Lempert ronguers Microsuction tip Dental spatula Iris spatula Tartar scraper Ophthalmic forceps
Fenestration	Tartar scraper Ear curette No. 7 Bard-Parker scalpel handle 14- to 20-gauge hypodermic needle
Spinal stabilization	Steinmann pins Methylmethacrylate bone cement Plating equipment Dorsal spinous process plates External skeletal fixator

COMPLICATIONS

Potential complications associated with thoracolumbar surgery depend on the type of surgery performed, number of sites operated upon, knowledge of regional anatomy, availability of appropriate neurosurgical instruments, and surgical expertise. Complications associated with dorsal laminectomy, hemilaminectomy, and pediculectomy include iatrogenic spinal cord trauma, seroma, infection, and/or dehiscence. Potential complications associated with fenestration include iatrogenic spinal cord trauma (either from pushing disk into the spinal canal or trauma from inappropriate instrumentation), pneumothorax, scoliosis, ventral abdominal muscle paralysis, diskospondylitis, and recur-

TABLE 35-3

Postoperative Care and Assessment of Patients with Thoracolumbar and Lumbosacral Spinal Disorders

Immediate care (first 24 hours)	Disk	Fx/Lux	Neoplasia
Intravenous fluids	YES	YES	YES
Analgesics (see Table 34-13 on p. 1070)	PRN	PRN	PRN
Corticosteroids	NO	NO	Based on tumor type
Antibiotics	NO	See Table 34-4 on p. 1050	See Table 34-4 on p. 1050
Observe for seizures (particularly if myelogram was performed)	YES	YES	YES
Back brace (T-L only)	NO	Based on postoperative stability	Based on postoperative stability
Neurologic exam	q 24 hrs	q 24 hrs	q 24 hrs

Postoperative Care and Assessment after Thoracolumbar and Lumbosacral Spinal Cord Surgery

Ambulatory Patients
- Strict confinement for 2 to 3 weeks postoperatively
- Physiotherapy for 2 to 3 weeks postoperatively
- Leash walks only for 4 to 8 weeks postoperatively

Nonambulatory patients (perform until ambulatory)
- Physiotherapy
- Hydrotherapy
- Supporting cart
- Padded bedding
- Elevated cage rack
- Bladder expression—TID-QID (avoid urinary catheters)
- Neurologic exams daily

rence of disk herniation. Urinary tract infections may occur secondary to neurologic deficits causing urine stasis. Spinal instability, muscle fibrosis, and/or contracture over the spinal cord may occur if excessive amounts of lamina, articular facets, and pedicles are removed. Guidelines for maximum exposure for each technique are discussed above. Occasionally, inadvertent trauma or resection of a lumbar or thoracic spinal nerve root causes bulging of the abdominal muscle innervated by that nerve. The resulting abnormality may resemble an abdominal hernia in appearance.

SPECIAL AGE CONSIDERATIONS

Care should be taken when performing laminectomy procedures on young dogs as their cortical and cancellous bone is much softer. Less pressure on the drill or rongeur is needed to safely enter the canal.

Suggested Reading

Bartels KE, Creed JE, Yturraspe DJ: Complications associated with the dorsolateral muscle-separation approach for thoracolumbar disk fenestration in the dog, *J Am Vet Med Assoc* 183:1081, 1983.

Bitetto WV, Thacher C: A modified lateral decompressive technique for treatment of canine intervertebral disk disease, *J Am Anim Hosp Assoc* 23:409, 1987.

Caulkins SE, Purinton PT, Oliver JE: Arterial supply to the spinal cord of dogs and cats, *Am J Vet Res* 50:425, 1989.

Flo GL, Brinker WO: Lateral fenestration of thoracolumbar discs, *J Am Anim Hosp Assoc* 11:619, 1975.

Hosgood G: Wound complications following thoracolumbar laminectomy in the dog: a retrospective study of 264 procedures, *J Am Anim Hosp Assoc* 28:47, 1992.

Lubbe AM, Kirberger RM, Verstraete FJM: Pediculectomy for thoracolumbar spinal decompression in the dachshund, *J Am Anim Hosp Assoc* 30:233, 1994.

Seim HB III: Dorsal decompressive laminectomy for T-L disk disease, *Canine Practice* 20:6, 1995.

Shores A: Intervertebral disk syndrome in the dog. III. Thoracolumbar disk surgery, *Compend Contin Educ Pract Vet* 4:24, 1982.

Swain SF: A rongeuring technique for performing thoracolumbar hemilaminectomies, *Vet Med/Small Anim Clin* 71:172, 1976.

Yovich JC, Read R, Eger C: Modified lateral spinal decompression in 61 dogs with thoracolumbar disc protrusion, *J Sm Anim Prac* 35:351, 1994.

Yturraspe DJ, Lumb WV: A dorsolateral muscle-separating approach for thoracolumbar intervertebral disk fenestration in the dog, *J Am Vet Med Assoc* 162:1037, 1973.

SPECIFIC DISEASES

THORACOLUMBAR DISK DISEASE

DEFINITIONS

Thoracolumbar (T-L) disk disease is associated with chondroid degeneration of the nucleus pulposus of intervertebral disks producing extrusion, spinal cord compression, and nerve root entrapment. **Fenestration** is creation of a window or "fenestra" in the lateral or ventral annulus fibrosus to gain access to the nucleus pulposus. **Durotomy** is an incision through dura mater to expose spinal cord parenchyma.

SYNONYMS

Slipped disk, herniated disk, T-L disk disease

GENERAL CONSIDERATIONS AND CLINICALLY RELEVANT PATHOPHYSIOLOGY

Thoracolumbar (T-L) disk disease is the most common cause of small animal neurologic dysfunction. Significant advances have been made in establishing history, signalment, clinical presentation, and radiographic and myelographic findings. However, management methodology is controversial and generally determined by clinical experience, rather than critically analyzed data. Many clinicians recommend early surgical spinal cord decompression and mass removal in most cases. Causes of disk degeneration are unknown, and the pathogenesis of spinal cord changes following compressive injury are unclear. Consequently, therapeutic approaches to spinal cord injury remain unsettled. Pathophysiology and pathogenesis of thoracolumbar disk disease are identical to cervical disk disease discussed on p. 1063 (see Figs. 34-27 and 34-28).

☞ **NOTE** • The most commonly involved sites of T-L disk extrusion are intervertebral disk spaces between T11 and L2; these sites make up approximately 65% to 75% of all disk extrusions.

DIAGNOSIS
Clinical Presentation

Signalment. T-L disk disease primarily occurs in chondrodystrophoid breeds such as dachshunds, Pekingese, beagles, miniature and toy poodles, cocker spaniels, Shih Tzus, Lhasa apsos, and Welsh corgis. Dachshunds have ten times the risk of all other breeds combined. Although disk protrusion occurs in cats, it is rare. Both sexes are equally affected. About 80% of disk problems occur in animals between 3 and 7 years of age (Brown, Helphrey, Prata, 1977).

History. Dogs with T-L disk disease present with various clinical signs. The classic presentation is acute to subacute back pain only, or back pain in addition to varying degrees of paraparesis. Although T-L disk extrusions are variable, many are acute and disruptive. Variables affecting the ultimate severity of spinal cord pathology and subsequent clinical signs are listed in Table 35-5. Acute, rapid extrusions tend to be more deleterious than slow extrusions (i.e., days to weeks). Disk material in the spinal canal may cause inflammation, further exacerbating neural deficits. Onset of clinical signs may occur in minutes or weeks after disk extrusion. Signs may be rapidly progressive, slowly progressive, remain static, or disappear and then later recur. Recurrences are usually caused by further extrusion of the previously affected disk.

Physical Examination Findings

Physical examination findings are usually normal in T-L disk disease patients. Neurologic examination findings vary depending upon the anatomic location of the extrusion, duration of compression, and force of compression at the time of disk extrusion. Varying degrees of back pain and upper motor neuron (UMN) ambulatory or nonambulatory paraparesis are the most common presenting neurologic abnormalities. The origins of pain (i.e., radiculopathy) and paresis (i.e., myelopathy) due to disk extrusion are discussed on p. 1063. Accurate localization of the affected intervertebral space requires careful neurologic examination (see Chapter 33). Severity of spinal cord trauma is assessed by neurologic examination; profound neurologic deficits suggest severe spinal cord insult. Finally, determining the presence or absence of deep pain perception is an important prognostic tool; patients with preservation of deep pain perception generally have a favorable prognosis, while those without deep pain perception have an unfavorable to grave prognosis.

☞ **NOTE ·** It is extremely important that deep pain be properly assessed. A withdrawal reflex does not verify the presence of deep pain. If the animal has deep pain, it should vocalize or otherwise indicate (e.g., dilation of pupils, turning of head, increased heart rate) that the pain was felt.

Radiography/Ultrasonography

Location of an extruded T-L disk is confirmed by radiographic/myelographic examination. Highly collimated

TABLE 35-5
Variables that Affect Neurologic Signs

- Location of extrusion (UMN vs. LMN)
- Acuteness of disk extrusion
- Velocity of disk extrusion
- Mass of material extruded
- Spinal canal diameter to spinal cord diameter ratio

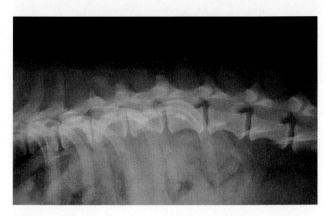

FIG. 35-14
Lateral radiograph of a dog with a T12-T13 herniated intervertebral disks. Notice the wedged intervertebral space, collapsed articular facets, and "fogged" intervertebral foramen.

lateral, ventrodorsal, and oblique projections of the entire T-L spine obtained under general anesthesia are often required. Survey radiographic findings indicative of disk extrusion include narrow or wedged intervertebral space, narrow or "fogged" (i.e., radiodense disk material) intervertebral foramen, collapse of articular facets, and calcified material in the spinal canal. Although survey radiographs may suggest the affected intervertebral space, they are rarely diagnostic (Fig. 35-14).

Myelography is indicated if there are no visible narrowed interspaces, disk material is not visible in the spinal canal or intervertebral foramen, a lesion is found that is incompatible with the neurologic examination, or when precise localization of the disk is necessary (e.g., left versus right side hemilaminectomy, hemilaminectomy versus dorsal laminectomy). Patients with a herniated T-L disk exhibit myelographic signs consistent with an extradural mass (Fig. 35-15). Myelography is described in Chapter 33.

☞ **NOTE ·** The author performs myelograms in nearly 90% of patients with T-L disk extrusions.

Laboratory Findings

CBC and serum biochemical profile abnormalities are rare. Recent corticosteroid therapy may elevate the level of hepatic enzymes in the serum.

DIFFERENTIAL DIAGNOSIS

Presumptive diagnosis of T-L disk disease is based on signalment, history, physical examination, and neurologic exami-

TABLE 35-6

Staging System to Help Determine Medical vs. Surgical Treatment and Prognosis in Animals with Thoracolumbar Disk Disease

Stage	Clinical Signs	Radiography/ Lesion Location	Treatment	Prognosis
I	Single or occasional episodes of mild, moderate, or severe back pain, +/− slight CP* deficits, no motor weakness	Radiographs not taken	Conservative	Favorable
		Incidental finding of degenerate disks	Conservative +/− fenestration	Favorable
II	Second episode or persistent and severe back pain, +/− CP deficits, +/− ambulatory paraparesis†	Radiographs not taken	Conservative +/− fenestration	Favorable/guarded
		Extruded disk in canal	Decompression	Excellent
III	Uncontrolled, severe back pain, +/− CP deficits, +/− ambulatory paraparesis	Extruded disk in canal	Decompression	Excellent
	Weakly ambulatory‡ or nonambulatory§ paraparesis, +/− back pain	Extruded disk in canal	Decompression	Excellent/favorable
IV	Paraplegia,‖ +/− back pain			
	Duration < 48 hrs	Extruded disk in canal	Decompression	Unfavorable
	Duration > 48 hrs	Extruded disk in canal	Conservative or decompression	Unfavorable/grave

*CP, conscious proprioception; †ambulatory paraparesis, patients with hindlimb motor weakness that can rise and ambulate without assistance; ‡weakly ambulatory paraparesis, patients that can rise without assistance, take several steps, tire easily, and assume a sitting or recumbent position; §nonambulatory paraparesis, patients that have lost the ability for unassisted hindlimb ambulation (voluntary motor movements may or may not be present); ‖paraplegia, patients that have complete loss of both motor and sensory function.

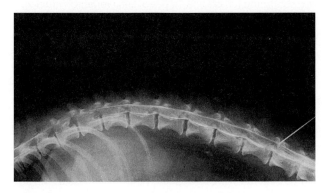

FIG. 35-15
Lateral myelogram of a dog with a T12-T13 herniated intervertebral disk. Notice the severely swollen spinal cord with loss of the contrast column from T11 to L1.

nation. Possible etiologies of spinal disorders are based on history, DAMNIT-V scheme, and myelographic classification given in Chapter 33. The most likely differential diagnoses for extradural masses are intervertebral disk extrusion, fracture/luxation, diskospondylitis, congenital malformation, neoplasia, and vertebral body osteomyelitis. Diagnostic differentials can usually be narrowed by appropriate use of physical examination, hematology, serum chemistry panel, cerebrospinal fluid analysis, and radiography. T-L disk extrusion is confirmed by radiography/myelography and surgery.

Evaluation of history and serial neurologic examinations are needed to formulate appropriate management plans. Establishing onset, course, duration, and severity of motor and sensory impairment helps define prognosis and direct therapy. A staging system may help determine the most appropriate therapy (nonsurgical or surgical) (Table 35-6).

MEDICAL MANAGEMENT

The most important aspect of medical management in **ambulatory patients** is strict cage confinement for 3 to 4 weeks. Next, 3 to 4 weeks of gradual return to normal activity is recommended. Home confinement means discouraging the animal from jumping up and down on furniture, avoiding stairs, confinement to one room when the owner is absent, and restricted leash walks. This forced rest aids resolution of spinal cord and intradiskal inflammation, and facilitates stabilization of the ruptured disk by fibrosis. **Nonambulatory patients** should have easy access to water and food, a soft, dry area to lie down, bladder expression three to four times daily, bowel management, and physiotherapy to maintain muscle mass and joint range of motion. A paraparetic cart may speed recovery by allowing freedom of movement and by improving the patient's attitude.

☞ **NOTE** · The most common mistake made in managing animals with disk extrusions is administration of analgesics or antiinflammatories without appropriate concurrent confinement. Strict cage confinement is mandatory in these patients.

Strict confinement and exercise control are sometimes accompanied by drug therapy. It is important to educate the client regarding the euphoric effects of various medications. If strict confinement is not maintained, excessive activity could cause further disk extrusion with catastrophic neural deficits. Medical management is successful approximately 80% to 90% of the time in patients with just back pain. Commonly used antiinflammatory and muscle relaxant

TABLE 35-7

Recommended Therapy* for Patients with Thoracolumbar Disk Disease Based on Neurologic Signs

Clinical Presentation	Initial Treatment[†]	Result	Second Treatment[†]	Result	Third treatment[†]
Mild to moderate back pain only; first episode or multiple episodes	No drug therapy; cage rest only	No improvement in 5 to 7 days	Muscle relaxant; follow daily	No improvement in 2 to 3 days	Steroids[‡] and muscle relaxant; follow daily
Severe back pain only; first episode or multiple episodes	Muscle relaxant; follow daily	No improvement in 2 to 3 days	Steroids[‡] and muscle relaxant; follow daily	No improvement in 2 to 3 days	Repeat second treatment or consider surgery
+/− Back pain and ambulatory paraparesis	Steroids for 1 day	Improvement	Continue steroids for 6 days	Improvement	Observe
		Static	Steroids 1 day	Improvement	Observe, Consider surgery
		Deterioration	Consider surgery	Deterioration	Consider surgery
+/− Back pain and weakly ambulatory or nonambulatory paraparesis	Recommend early surgery; administer steroids preoperatively				
Recurrent mild, moderate, or severe back pain; unresponsive to medical management	Recommend surgery; administer steroids preoperatively				

*See Table 34-9 on p. 1068 for drug dosages and variations on duration of therapy. [†]All patients are placed in strict confinement for 3 to 4 weeks as part of their medical management regardless of the drug used or duration of drug therapy. [‡]Nonsteroidal antiinflammatory drugs can be substituted for corticosteroids; however, the use of corticosteroids and nonsteroidal antiinflammatory drugs in combination should not be considered.

drugs and their dosages are listed in Table 34-9 on p. 1068. These medications can be used independently or in combination. The choice of drugs is dictated by the patient's clinical signs at presentation and therapeutic trials. Common clinical presentations and suggested therapeutic regimens are listed in Table 35-7. Knowledge of potential side effects of commonly used antiinflammatory drugs is important and are listed in Table 34-11 on p. 1070.

Patients treated with antiinflammatory drugs should be monitored for depression, anorexia, abdominal pain, melena, and vomiting undigested or digested blood (coffee grounds). If gastrointestinal lesions are suspected, antiinflammatory drugs (see Table 34-11) should be discontinued immediately, because ulceration associated with antiinflammatory medication, spinal cord injury, and stress can be catastrophic.

SURGICAL TREATMENT

Surgical treatment objectives for patients with T-L disk disease include gaining access to the spinal canal and removal of disk fragments causing spinal cord and nerve root compression. Surgical treatment is determined by the patient's neurologic status, results of serial neurologic examinations after admission, and response to medical therapy (see Tables 35-6 and 35-7). If presenting signs warrant surgical intervention, or if the patient fails to respond to appropriate medical management, surgery should be considered.

Fenestration has been proposed to eliminate back pain plus prevent further disk extrusion. Because pain is usually due to a combination of nerve root compression and ischemia from extruded disk fragments, fenestration is not the procedure of choice (see Fig. 35-19); removal of extruded disk fragments via laminectomy/pediculectomy is preferred. In rare patients with diskogenic pain (i.e., pressure on the pain-sensitive dorsal longitudinal ligament and dorsal annulus fibrosus), fenestration may alleviate back pain. The role of prophylactic fenestration remains unclear. Because the possibility of multiple disks causing recurrent episodes of back pain is unlikely, laminectomy and mass removal of the single offending disk, rather than prophylactic fenestrations of all disks, are warranted (see Tables 35-6 and 35-7). Decompression in addition to prophylactic fenestration to prevent recurrent disk extrusion at a second site is also controversial. Recurrence of disk extrusion at an adjacent intervertebral space after decompression of the active disk is rare (less than 4.5%); thus prophylactic fenestration is probably not warranted (Brown, Helphrey, Prata, 1977).

It is generally accepted that patients with even mild paraparesis (i.e., motor weakness) should be treated by early decompression and mass removal via dorsal laminectomy, hemilaminectomy, or pediculectomy. Paresis is a strict function of the forces, mechanical deformation, and pressure exerted on the spinal cord. Fenestration does not remove disk material from its extruded location in the spinal canal. The decision to pursue surgical intervention is based on the patient's clinical signs. Generally, the earlier spinal cord decompression is undertaken, the better the chance for complete neural recovery. Patients requiring surgery should be operated within 24 to 48 hours of disk extrusion. Surgery is still a viable option in patients with severe neurologic deficits (i.e., weakly ambulatory or nonambulatory paraparesis) that have been treated medically for 72 to 96 hours before referral; however, they may not recover to a normal neural status (but are often acceptable pets). Patients with several weeks to months of weakly ambulatory or nonambulatory paraparesis may benefit from surgical intervention if there is myelographic evidence of a compressive mass that can be surgically removed. Although the prognosis is unfavorable for complete recovery, the animal may become weakly ambulatory paraparetic with voluntary control of bowel and bladder.

☞ **N O T E** · It is not sufficient to remove lamina, articular facets, and pedicles; laminectomy, hemilaminectomy, or pediculectomy alone without mass removal can be compared with making a hole in the roof of a house to let the water out of the basement. The offending compressive mass lesion (i.e., disk material) must be removed.

Preoperative Management

The animal should be given intravenous fluids and steroids prior to surgery. Intravenous steroids should be given to protect the spinal cord from the effects of surgical manipulation. The steroid of choice is methylprednisolone sodium succinate (30 mg/kg intravenously).

Anesthesia

Suggested anesthetic regimens for dogs with spinal cord injury are given on p. 1050. If the patient requires positioning that may cause respiratory compromise, mechanical ventilatory support should be considered.

Surgical Anatomy

The most common sites for T-L disk extrusion are between T11 and L2. The tough intercapital ligament from T1-2 to T9-10 attaches to each rib head and extends over the dorsal annulus fibrosus (Fig. 35-16), acting as a natural dorsal buttress that helps prevent disk extrusion. The intercapital ligament at T10-11 is smaller than the others; disk herniation may occur at this intervertebral space.

Disk extrusions generally occur at the junction of the vertebral venous sinus and dorsal longitudinal ligament (i.e., area of least resistance) resulting in a ventrolateral location of extruded disk fragments (Fig. 35-17). Disk extrusions may therefore cause varying degrees of nerve root compression and ischemia, spinal cord injury, and venous sinus hemorrhage. Extreme care must be used when manipulating and evacuating disk fragments from the floor of the spinal canal.

Positioning

Patient positioning is dependent upon surgical procedure selected and is described on p. 1101. Generally, patients under-

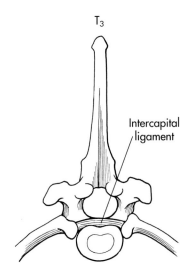

FIG. 35-16
Attachment of the intercapital ligament to each rib head. It spans the dorsal annulus fibrosus.

going dorsal laminectomy, hemilaminectomy, pediculectomy, or dorsolateral fenestration are positioned in sternal recumbency, whereas those undergoing lateral or ventral fenestration are positioned in lateral recumbency.

SURGICAL TECHNIQUE
Spinal Cord Decompression

The most common procedures used to decompress spinal cord and nerve roots (in order of the author's preference) are hemilaminectomy, pediculectomy, modified dorsal laminectomy, Funkquist B laminectomy, Funkquist A laminectomy, and deep dorsal laminectomy. These procedures are described on pp. 1101-1107.

Occasionally, no evidence of extruded disk is seen after entering the canal. Several possibilities exist when this occurs and are listed in Table 35-8, along with a proper course of action for each. Myelotomy, local hypothermia with cool saline, DMSO, naloxone, and thyrotropin releasing hormone are not routinely used in patients with T-L disk extrusions.

Regardless of decompression procedure chosen, enter the spinal canal by carefully lifting off periosteum with a dental spatula, iris spatula, or Lempert rongeur. At this point, disk material, black venous blood ("crankcase oil"), swollen spinal cord, or epidural fat will be visible.

Acute disk protrusions. Acutely extruded disk material may take on various forms. It may be white flecks of disk incorporated in an organized clot, that when incised looks like crankcase oil. This type of disk is often easily suctioned and removal results in full decompression. Extruded material may include portions of the dorsal annulus fibrosus. These fragments are white, firm, and cartilaginous in nature, easy to grasp with ophthalmic forceps, and often can be completely removed as a long continuous strand resulting in full decompression. Occasionally, hard, white chalky disk material is found. Removal is accomplished by continual chipping away at the mass with a dental or iris spatula. Take care to

TABLE 35-8

Course of Action if Disk Material Is not Found at Surgery

Surgical Procedure Performed	Surgical Finding	Course of Action	Result	Second Course of Action
Hemilaminectomy, pediculectomy, dorsal laminectomy	Epidural fat	Correct space? (recount)	Yes	Close; reevaluate: neuro exam, myelogram
			No	Operate correct space
Hemilaminectomy	Swollen cord, no disk	Look for ventral extrusion	Ventral disk identified	Remove disk
			No disk	Perform hemilaminectomy on opposite side
Dorsal laminectomy	Swollen cord, no disk	Look on lateral aspect of canal	Disk identified	Extend dorsal to include pediculectomy
			No disk	Extend laminectomy on one side to floor of spinal canal

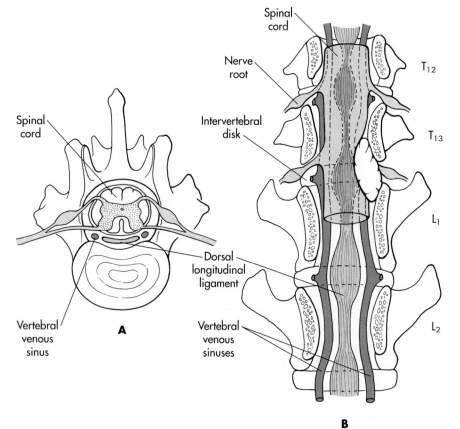

FIG. 35-17
A, Anatomy of thoracolumbar spinal cord and associated ligaments and vessels. Notice the relationship of the vertebral venous sinus and dorsal longitudinal ligament at the level of the intervertebral space and midvertebral body. **B,** Notice the location of extruded disk relative to the nerve root, vertebral venous sinus, and dorsal longitudinal ligament.

protect the spinal cord, nerve root, and venous sinus during dissection, because the majority of disks extrude ventral and lateral (see Fig. 35-17). Mild to moderate shifts of the dural tube back to its normal position following laminectomy and disk removal indicate appropriate decompression.

☞ **NOTE** · If approached within hours or days, acute disk extrusions are generally easily removed with carefully applied suction and manipulation using ophthalmic forceps and dental spatulas.

Chronic disk protrusions. Patients with a chronic history (i.e., months) of medically treated pain and ambulatory paraparesis that finally develop severe motor weakness and require surgery, often have a firm, encapsulated, protruded mass that may be adherent to venous sinus and dura mater (i.e., Hansen type II). Disk removal is difficult due to its hard, encapsulated nature, ventrolateral location (i.e., venous sinus), and adhesions to dura and venous sinus. If venous sinus hemorrhage occurs, control it with hemostatic sponges using the techniques described in Table 34-1.

If the disk can be lateralized, perform a hemilaminectomy, including complete removal of the pedicle. If the disk cannot be lateralized, perform a deep dorsal laminectomy (see p. 1105) and visualize the protruded disk. Remove the entire pedicle to the level of the floor of the spinal canal. Expose the vertebral venous sinus at the level of the affected intervertebral space and transect the sinus, if necessary, to expose the encapsulated disk. Once the disk is adequately exposed, use a No. 11 scalpel blade to incise the disk capsule. Use a dental spatula, iris spatula, and tartar scraper to evacuate the firm disk material. It is rarely necessary to place dural sutures to manipulate the spinal cord and allow adequate visualization and removal of the disk. If the protruded disk is located on the ventral midline and cannot be adequately removed as described above, transect the nerve root at the site of extrusion (permissible only at T3-L3 spinal cord segments). Gently expose the nerve root and radicular vessels and cauterize them with bipolar cautery. As the spinal cord releases, gently roll it off the offending disk for better visualization and less traumatic disk removal. Remove disk material as described above. Do not attempt to reattach the severed nerve root.

Durotomy

Durotomy is rarely indicated. It is not recommended as a therapeutic modality, but may be useful in prognosis. Patients that present with paraplegia (i.e., complete loss of motor function and sensory perception) generally have a poor prognosis. Durotomy to evaluate presence or absence of myelomalacia may be useful in deciding patient outcome.

Carefully tent the dura with fine ophthalmic forceps. Use a gentle longitudinal stroke along the dura with a No. 11 or No. 12 scalpel blade. Penetration of the dura is obviated by the flow of CSF. A 1.5 to 2 cm long incision allows adequate visualization of spinal cord parenchyma. Observe the spinal cord for evidence of central hemorrhagic necrosis, loss of anatomic integrity, and toothpaste-like consistency. These findings are compatible with complete functional loss. Leave the dural incision open. Harvest a subcutaneous fat graft and place it over the laminectomy site.

Disk Fenestration

Three approaches are commonly used to perform disk fenestration: ventral, lateral, and dorsolateral. Advantages and disadvantages of these techniques are listed in Tables 35-9 through 35-11.

Ventral approach. *Place the patient in right lateral recumbency and make a paracostal incision. Enter the abdominal cavity, identify the left kidney, and retract it ventrally. Pack off abdominal viscera caudally with moistened laparotomy pads. Elevate the iliopsoas muscle and locate the short transverse process of L1 for orientation. Digitally depress the aorta and sympathetic trunk to expose the ventral annulus fibrosus of intervertebral disks L1-2 through L5-6 (Fig. 35-18, A). Using a No. 11 scalpel blade or high-speed pneumatic or electric drill, create a*

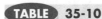

TABLE 35-9

Advantages and Disadvantages of Ventral Fenestration

Advantages
- Avoids the spinal nerve roots
- Minimal hemorrhage

Disadvantages
- Need for a thoracotomy
- Dissection is near major vessels
- Cannot be combined with a decompressive procedure
- Increased risk of pushing disk material into the spinal canal
- Does not provide spinal cord decompression

TABLE 35-10

Advantages and Disadvantages of Lateral Fenestration

Advantages
- Limited muscle dissection
- Minimal hemorrhage
- Does not require abdominal or thoracic surgery
- Can be combined with a hemilaminectomy

Disadvantages
- An assistant is required
- Exposure is difficult in obese animals
- Thoracic disks are difficult to visualize
- Requires dissection near spinal nerves and vessels
- Does not provide spinal cord decompression

TABLE 35-11

Advantages and Disadvantages of Dorsolateral Fenestration

Advantages
- Can be easily combined with a hemilaminectomy procedure

Disadvantages
- Excessive muscle dissection
- Requires dissection near spinal nerves and vessels
- Does not provide spinal cord decompression

window in the ventral annulus. Use a hypodermic needle (14 to 20 gauge), tartar scraper, or curved spatula to remove as much nucleus pulposus as possible. Place the patient through positional changes (i.e., lateral flexion and extension) to encourage evacuation of nuclear material. After all disks have been fenestrated, close abdominal musculature with absorbable suture material. Move the skin incision to the 10th intercostal space and make a thoracotomy incision. Place self-retaining retractors to hold the ribs apart, pack the lungs cranially with moistened laparotomy pads, and dissect parietal pleura from intervertebral disks T9-10 through T13-L1. Avoid aorta, sympa-

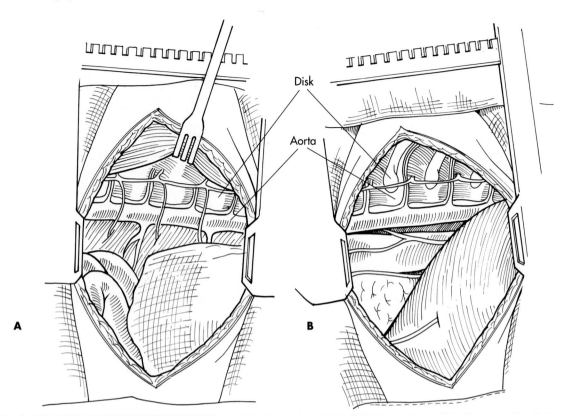

FIG. 35-18
For ventral disk fenestration, perform a, thoracic and, abdominal approach.

thetic trunk, and intercostal vessels (Fig. 35-18, B). Perform disk fenestration as described above. Close the thoracotomy incision routinely.

Lateral approach. This approach is satisfactory for exposing disks T13-L1 through L5-L6. Fenestration of disks T10-11 through T12-13 is more difficult.

Clip and aseptically prepare an area from T6 cranially to the greater trochanter caudally, dorsal spinous processes dorsally to midabdomen ventrally. Place the patient in right lateral recumbency if you are right handed, and left lateral recumbency if you are left handed. Place a 4-inch diameter sand bag or rolled towel under the L2-L6 vertebrae to create an arch effect that helps open the intervertebral spaces. Make a skin incision from the dorsal spine of T9 to the ventral aspect of the ilial wing. Continue the incision through subcutaneous fat, lumbar fascia, a second layer of fat, and to the longissimus dorsi and iliocostalis lumborum muscles. Palpate the short transverse process of L1 for orientation, and with a pair of Kelly forceps, dissect overlying muscle fibers to expose its dorsocranial surface. Identify the lateral annulus fibrosus, located just cranial and slightly ventral to the junction of the transverse process and vertebral body (Fig. 35-19). Use a blunt retractor to expose the lateral surface of the annulus fibrosus; retract muscle fibers dorsally and muscle fibers, spinal nerve, and spinal vessels ventrally. Use a No. 11 scalpel blade to make a window in the lateral aspect of the annulus fibro-

sus. Be careful not to incise dorsal to the junction of the transverse process and vertebral body, as this may result in spinal cord damage. Perform disk fenestration as described for ventral fenestration. To fenestrate disks T10-11 through T12-13, elevate the iliocostalis lumborum muscle off the craniodorsal aspect of the rib to the level of the vertebral body and retract it craniodorsally. Retract the remaining musculature on the cranial aspect of the rib ventrally, exposing the lateral annulus. The thoracic pleura is just ventral to this dissection. Visualization is limited; be careful to stay below the arch of the rib when incising the annulus fibrosus. After all disks have been fenestrated, use positional changes to encourage further evacuation of nuclear material. Close muscle, subcutaneous tissues, and skin routinely.

Dorsolateral approach. *Place the patient in ventral recumbency with the spine gently arched dorsally. Make a dorsal midline skin incision from the dorsal spinous process of T9 to the dorsal spinous process of L6. Continue dissection to the level of the thoracolumbar fascia. Incise the thoracolumbar fascia along the dorsal spinous processes on the side toward the surgeon. Using a periosteal elevator or small osteotome, elevate epaxial muscles from the lateral aspect of the dorsal spinous processes, working in a caudal to cranial direction. Elevate a second level of epaxial muscle from articular facets. Begin by elevating musculature from the caudal aspect of the articular process and progress to the cranial aspect. Use curved scissors to sever muscular attachments close to their tendon of origin to min-*

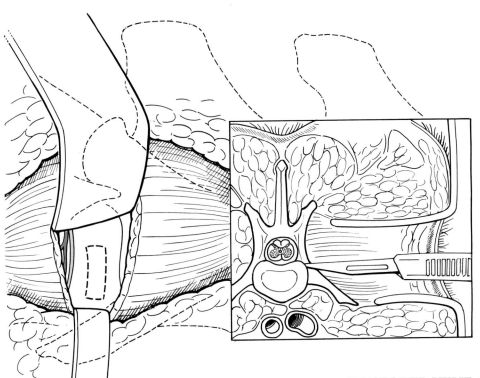

FIG. 35-19
For lateral disk fenestration, perform a lateral epaxial muscle splitting approach.

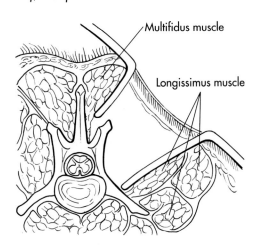

Multifidus muscle

Longissimus muscle

FIG. 35-20
For dorsolateral disk fenestration, perform a dorsolateral epaxial muscle splitting approach.

imize hemorrhage. Place Gelpi retractors to hold muscles apart and improve exposure. Elevate remaining musculature from the dorsal aspect of the transverse processes of lumbar vertebrae and cranial surface of the ribs of thoracic vertebrae. Identify muscular attachments to the accessory process, spinal nerve, and vessels (Fig. 35-20). Retract these structures cranially to expose the lateral surface of the annulus fibrosus. Perform fenestration as described for ventral fenestration. Close muscle, subcutaneous tissues, and skin routinely.

SUTURE MATERIALS/SPECIAL INSTRUMENTS

Special instruments necessary to perform laminectomy and fenestration procedures are listed in Table 35-2.

POSTOPERATIVE CARE AND ASSESSMENT

Patients with T-L disk disease should be evaluated postoperatively in a similar fashion as patients with other T-L spinal disorders (see p. 1109 and Table 35-4). As no inherent or acquired spinal instability is created, physiotherapy is encouraged as soon as the patient has recovered from postoperative discomfort; generally 24 to 48 hours. As the majority of T-L disk patients are small-breed dogs, clients should be instructed in home management and these patients can often be sent home within 72 hours of surgery, even if they are weakly ambulatory or nonambulatory paraparetic.

☞ **NOTE** · If these animals are unable to urinate on their own, express their bladder three to four times daily until voluntary urinations occur. Otherwise the bladder may become atonic.

PROGNOSIS

Prognosis for patients treated medically or surgically for T-L disk disease is generally favorable and is dependent upon neurologic signs and the medical or surgical management selected. Clinical factors and probable patient outcome are outlined in Tables 35-5 and 35-6.

Reference

Brown NO, Helphrey ML, Prata RG: Thoracolumbar disk disease in the dog: a retrospective analysis of 187 cases, *J Am Anim Hosp Assoc* 13:665, 1977.

Suggested Reading

Bauer M et al: Follow-up study of owner attitudes toward home care of paraplegic dogs, *J Am Vet Med Assoc* 200:1809, 1992.

Butterworth SJ, Denny HR: Follow-up study of 100 cases with thoracolumbar disc protrusions treated by lateral fenestration, *J Sm Anim Prac* 32:443, 1991.

Gambardella PC: Dorsal decompressive laminectomy for treatment of thoracolumbar disc disease in dogs: a retrospective study of 98 cases, *Vet Surg* 9:24, 1980.

Gaschen L, Lang J, Haeni H: Intervertebral disc herniation (Schmorl's node) in five dogs, *Vet Radio and Ultrasound* 36:509, 1995.

Henry WB Jr.: Dorsal decompressive laminectomy in the treatment of thoraco-lumbar disc disease, *J Am Anim Hosp Assoc* 11:627, 1975.

Holmberg DL et al: A comparison of manual and power-assisted thoracolumbar disc fenestration in dogs, *Vet Surg* 19:323, 1990.

Horne TR, Powers RD, Swaim SF: Dorsal laminectomy techniques in the dog, *J Am Vet Med Assoc* 171:742, 1977.

Knapp DW et al: A retrospective study of thoracolumbar disk fenestration in dogs using a ventral approach: 160 cases (1976 to 1986), *J Am Anim Hosp Assoc* 26:543, 1990.

Levine SH, Caywood DD: Recurrence of neurological deficits in dogs treated for thoracolumbar disk disease, *J Am Anim Hosp Assoc* 20:889, 1984.

Moore RW, Withrow SJ: Gastrointestinal hemorrhage and pancreatitis associated with intervertebral disk disease in the dog, *J Am Vet Med Assoc* 180:1443, 1982.

Olby NJ, Dyce J, Houlton JEF: Correlation of plain radiographic and lumbar myelographic findings with surgical findings in thoracolumbar disc disease, *J Sm Anim Prac* 35:345, 1994.

Prata RG: Neurosurgical treatment of thoracolumbar disks: the rationale and value of laminectomy with concomitant disk removal, *J Am Anim Hosp Assoc* 17:17, 1981.

Seim HB III: Thoracolumbar disk disease: diagnosis, treatment, and prognosis, *Canine Practice* 20:8, 1995.

Shores A et al: Structural changes in thoracolumbar disks following lateral fenestration, *Vet Surg* 14:117, 1985.

Smith GK, Walter MC: Spinal decompressive procedures and dorsal compartment injuries: comparative biomechanical study in canine cadavers, *Am J Vet Res* 49:266, 1988.

Swaim SF, Vandevelde M: Clinical and histologic evaluation of bilateral hemilaminectomy and deep dorsal laminectomy for extensive spinal cord decompression in the dog, *J Am Vet Med Assoc* 170:407, 1977.

Trevor PB et al: Healing characteristics of free and pedicle fat grafts after dorsal laminectomy and durotomy in dogs, *Vet Surg* 20:282, 1991.

Wagner SD et al: Radiographic and histologic changes after thoracolumbar disc curettage, *Vet Surg* 16:65, 1987.

FRACTURES AND LUXATIONS OF THE THORACOLUMBAR SPINE

DEFINITIONS

Fractures or **luxations of the thoracic or lumbar spine** are caused by traumatic or pathologic disruption of osseous and supporting soft tissue structures, producing spinal cord and nerve root compression.

SYNONYMS

Broken back, spinal fracture, vertebral fracture, vertebral column fracture, dislocated spine

GENERAL CONSIDERATIONS AND CLINICALLY RELEVANT PATHOPHYSIOLOGY

The thoracolumbar spine is the most common site for spinal fractures and luxations. Fractures and luxations occur between T11 and L6 in approximately 50% to 60% of patients with blunt spinal trauma (Selcer, Bubb, Walker, 1991). It appears that the higher incidence of fracture/luxation at certain sites along the vertebral column may not correlate to a difference in muscular or ligamentous attachments, but rather to mobile areas of the vertebral column adjacent to more stable areas of the axial skeleton (such as caudal thoracic and caudal lumbar spine). Fractures of the thoracic spine involving T1 through T9 are relatively uncommon, and when they do occur are generally stable and nondisplaced due to the inherent stability gained by massive epaxial muscle mass, rib attachments, ligamentous support, and intercostal muscle attachments. The most common cause of vertebral fractures is automobile trauma (i.e., approximately 90%) (Selcer, Bubb, Walker, 1991). Other causes include bite wounds, gunshot injuries, and underlying metabolic or neoplastic disorders resulting in bone demineralization (e.g., nutritional secondary hyperparathyroidism, osteosarcoma).

☞ **NOTE** · A complete physical examination should be done. Approximately 40% to 50% of patients with vertebral fractures have associated problems (e.g., pneumothorax, lung contusions, diaphragmatic hernia, urogenital injuries, and other orthopedic injuries) (Selcer, Bubb, Walker, 1991).

Fractures and luxations of the thoracolumbar spine are classified as pathologic or traumatic. Pathologic fractures/luxations generally occur when hereditary or congenital ligamentous instability decreases spinal support (e.g., atlantoaxial instability) or when bone integrity is compromised due to an underlying disease process (e.g., metabolic bone disease, neoplasia). Traumatic fracture/luxations are induced by forces resulting in severe hyperextension, hyperflexion, axial compression, and rotation; often occurring at or near the junction of a mobile and more rigid vertebral segment. Failure of supporting structures of the spine to resist such forces causes mechanical discontinuity with resultant spinal cord and nerve root compression.

☞ **NOTE** · Approximately 20% of patients have a second spinal fracture/luxation (Feeney, Oliver, 1980).

DIAGNOSIS
Clinical Presentation

Signalment. There is no breed or sex predisposition; however, dogs more commonly sustain vertebral fracture/luxation than cats. Vertebral fractures may occur at any age, but are more common in younger animals (i.e., 1 to 2 years of age).

History. Patients with thoracolumbar vertebral fractures typically present because of trauma associated with automobiles. They suffer varying degrees of back pain and paraparesis, depending upon severity of spinal cord and nerve root compression. Occasionally, patients present with subtle neurologic deficits, and careful physical and neurologic examinations are necessary to detect abnormalities.

Physical Examination Findings

Vertebral fracture patients often have concurrent injuries (e.g., pneumothorax, pulmonary contusion, diaphragmatic hernia, and fracture/luxation of the pelvis, ribs, appendicular skeleton, second vertebral fracture). Thorough physical examination is necessary to recognize these injuries before an appropriate course of action can be planned. Extreme care must be taken during physical examination to avoid exacerbating the spinal injury by excessive movement. Patients with profound neurologic deficits should be secured to a rigid platform during examination and preoperative management. Careful palpation of the spine may reveal a depression over its dorsal aspect, a displaced dorsal spinous process caused by rupture of the supraspinous and interspinous ligaments, or fracture of the dorsal spinous processes. If the patient is ambulatory, the back should be palpated for crepitus or excessive movement as the patient moves. These findings also help assess inherent stability or instability of the traumatized spine. A thorough neurologic examination should be performed to locate the fracture, determine the best therapy, and provide prognostic information (i.e., presence or absence of deep pain perception). Specific neurologic examination techniques are discussed in Chapter 33.

Radiography/Ultrasonography

Radiographs are of limited use for evaluating thoracic and lumbar spinal trauma. Survey radiographs may reveal the location of the fracture/luxation and severity of vertebral displacement at the time the radiograph is taken. However, radiographs may not show the maximum displacement at the time of injury; spontaneous reduction of subluxations, luxations, and fractures often occurs prior to radiography. The amount of spinal cord damage may therefore differ in patients with radiographically similar lesions. Radiographs may help determine prognosis when vertebral displacement is severe enough to reduce spinal canal diameter more than 80% in the lateral and ventrodorsal projections; these patients generally have irreversible spinal cord and nerve root compression (Fig. 35-21).

☞ **NOTE** • Neurologic examination findings are more useful than radiographic findings in discerning extent of injury and prognosis. Markedly displaced fractures may be found in ambulatory animals and no discernible radiographic lesion may be evident in animals without deep pain.

Survey radiographs may be taken on the awake or anesthetized patient. Advantages and disadvantages of each are

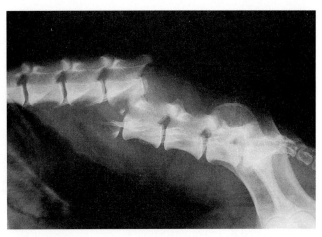

FIG. 35-21
Lateral radiograph of a dog with an L4 fracture. Notice the severe vertebral displacement.

TABLE 35-12
Typical Radiographic Findings with Thoracic and Lumbar Spinal Fracture/Luxation
• Discontinuity of bony structures (i.e., dorsal spinous process, lamina, pedicle, vertebral body)   • Malalignment of intervertebral spaces and/or articular facets   • Fracture lines in the body, lamina, and/or spinous processes of involved vertebrae   • Loss of continuity or malalignment of the spinal canal   • Combination of the above

discussed on p. 1090. Awake lateral and cross-table ventrodorsal projections are recommended. This evaluation, coupled with neurologic examination findings, aids in determining therapy. If surgery is considered, preoperative anesthetized radiographs should be taken for critical evaluation of the vertebral injury (see p. 1042). Because up to 20% have a second spinal fracture/luxation all patients with traumatic spinal injury should have a complete spinal series of radiographs. Typical radiographic findings in patients with thoracic and lumbar spinal fracture/luxation are listed in Table 35-12 (Fig. 35-22, *A* and *B*). A rough idea of spinal stability can be judged by whether the dorsal compartment, ventral compartment, or a combination of dorsal and ventral compartment injury exists (see p. 1090). Myelography may be required if there is a suspicion of herniated intervertebral disk material, bone fragments in the spinal canal, no evidence of vertebral discontinuity, or when radiographic findings do not correlate with neurologic examination (see p. 1042). Typical myelographic findings in patients with thoracic and lumbar spinal fracture/luxation are consistent with an extradural mass and are described and illustrated in Fig. 33-15 on p. 1046.

Laboratory Findings

Patients presenting with just thoracolumbar fracture/luxation generally have stress leukograms and elevated hepatic

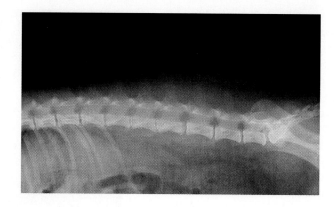

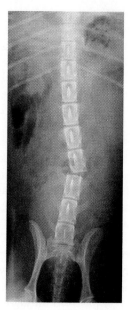

FIG. 35-22
A, Lateral and **B,** ventrodorsal radiographs of a dog with L4-L5 luxation. Notice the accentuated intervertebral space at L4-L5 on the lateral view and lateral vertebral body displacement on the ventrodorsal view.

enzyme levels. However, if concurrent injuries are present, laboratory abnormalities (e.g., elevated BUN and electrolyte abnormalities with uroabdomen, blood gas abnormalities with pneumothorax or pulmonary contusions) may occur.

DIFFERENTIAL DIAGNOSIS

Possible etiology of spinal disorders based on history, DAMNIT-V scheme, and myelographic classification is given in Chapter 33. The most likely differential diagnoses for an extradural mass are intervertebral disk extrusion, fracture/luxation, diskospondylitis, congenital malformation, neoplasia, and vertebral body osteomyelitis. Diagnostic differentials can usually be eliminated by appropriate use of physical, hematologic, serum chemistry, cerebrospinal fluid, and radiographic evaluations. Diagnosis of thoracolumbar fracture/luxation is confirmed by radiography.

Because concurrent injuries are common in patients with thoracolumbar vertebral fracture/luxation, physical examination and patient stabilization, with management of life threatening injuries, is the initial objective. Patients with severe trauma should be treated for shock and the T-L spine stabilized by securing the patient to a rigid platform. After initial stabilization, neurologic examination is performed to localize the fracture/luxation and help determine therapy. Radiographs of the thoracic and lumbar spine should be taken while the patient is conscious for initial assessment. Conservative or surgical management is based on initial neurologic status, serial neurologic examinations, radiographic assessment of spinal stability (i.e., is the fracture stable or unstable) (see Table 35-12), and presence of concurrent injuries.

MEDICAL MANAGEMENT

Medical management includes strict confinement, a back brace, antiinflammatory medication, and serial neurologic examinations (Table 35-13). Ambulatory patients should be restricted to a cage, or a small room or kennel for 2 to 3 weeks. A comfortable, well-padded back brace or body splint constructed from basswood or light-weight, moldable fiberglass supports the spine. Although the efficacy of a back brace may be questioned, it appears useful to counteract excessive ventral and lateral flexion of the torso while the patient is confined. Generally, patients are treated with antiinflammatory drugs. Commonly used antiinflammatory and muscle relaxant drugs and their dosages are listed in Tables 34-9 and 34-25. These medications can be used independently or in combination. Knowledge of potential side effects of commonly used antiinflammatory drugs is important (see Tables 34-11 and 34-12 on p. 1070). Choosing the proper drug regime is dictated by the patient's clinical signs and therapeutic trials. A list of common clinical presentations and suggested medical therapies are listed in Table 35-14.

Neurologic examinations should be performed twice daily for the first week, then daily until the patient is released from the hospital. Nonambulatory patients are treated with strict cage confinement, a back brace, antiinflammatory medications, and serial neurologic examinations. In addition, nonambulatory patients should have easy access to water and food, a soft, dry area to lie down, bladder expression three to four times a day, bowel management, and physiotherapy to maintain muscle mass and joint range of motion. A paraparetic cart is not recommended due to pressure placed on the thoracolumbar spine by the cart's supporting bars.

SURGICAL TREATMENT

Patients that fail to respond to an appropriate course of medical management or present with profound neurologic deficits (see Tables 35-13 and 35-14) are surgical candidates. Objectives of surgical treatment include spinal cord and nerve root decompression and vertebral fracture/luxation stabilization. Decompression is generally provided by fracture/luxation reduction. Laminectomy and mass removal (i.e., disk material, bone fragments) are rarely needed. Stabilization can be provided by multiple procedures; however,

TABLE 35-13 Conservative vs. Surgical Management of Patients with Thoracolumbar Spinal Fracture/Luxations

Initial Neurologic Exam*	Serial Neurologic Exam	Radiographic Assessment	Treatment	Prognosis
Back pain; normal ambulation	Static or improving	Minimal displacement; stable	Conservative	Favorable
	+/− Back pain; ambulatory paraparesis	Moderate or severe displacement; unstable	Improve conservative management Surgically stabilize†	Favorable to guarded Favorable
	+/− Back pain; weakly ambulatory or nonambulatory paraparesis	Minimal, moderate, or severe displacement; unstable	Surgical stabilization†	Favorable to guarded
Back pain; conscious proprioceptive deficits	Static or improving	Minimal to moderate displacement; stable	Conservative	Favorable
	+/− Back pain; ambulatory paraparesis	Moderate to severe displacement; unstable	Improve conservative management Surgically stabilize†	Favorable to guarded Favorable
	+/− Back pain; weakly ambulatory or nonambulatory paraparesis	Minimal, moderate, or severe displacement; unstable	Surgical stabilization†	Favorable to guarded
Back pain; ambulatory paraparesis	Static or improving	Minimal displacement; stable	Conservative	Favorable
	+/− Back pain; weakly ambulatory or nonambulatory paraparesis	Minimal, moderate, or severe displacement; unstable	Surgical stabilization	Favorable to guarded
Back pain; weakly or nonambulatory paraparesis	Improving	No displacement; stable	Conservative	Favorable to guarded
	Static or deteriorating	No displacement; stable; myelogram shows no compressive lesion	Conservative	Favorable to guarded
		Myelogram shows compressive lesion	Surgical decompression-stabilization†	Favorable to guarded
		Minimal, moderate, or severe displacement; unstable	Surgical stabilization†	Favorable to guarded
Back pain; paraplegia	Static	Mild displacement; stable	Paraplegic cart or euthanasia Spinal stabilization and paraplegic cart; or euthanasia	Unfavorable to grave
	Static	Severe displacement; unstable		Unfavorable to grave

*Definition of neurologic status (ambulatory, weakly ambulatory, and nonambulatory paraparesis) is given in Table 35-6 on p. 1111. †Patients retaining even minimal neurologic function deserve the benefits of conservative treatment if surgery is unacceptable to the owner.

TABLE 35-14

Recommended Therapy* for Patients with Thoracolumbar Vertebral Fracture/Luxation Based on Neurologic Signs

Clinical Presentation	Initial Treatment†	Result	Second Treatment†	Result	Third treatment†
Back pain; no paraparesis	No drugs	No improvement	Steroids‡	Improvement	Continue steroids‡
				Deterioration; paraparesis	Consider surgical§ stabilization
Back pain; CP deficits	Steroids‡ for 1 day	Improvement	Continue steroids‡	Improvement	Follow—taper steroids
		Static	Continue steroids‡	No improvement	Consider surgical stabilization
		Deteriorating	Consider surgical stabilization		
Ambulatory paraparesis	Steroids‡ for 1 day	Improvement	Continue steroids‡	Improvement	Follow—taper steroids
		Static	Steroids‡ for 1 more day	Improvement	Follow—taper steroids
				Static or deteriorating	Consider surgical stabilization
		Deteriorating	Consider surgical stabilization		
Weakly ambulatory paraparesis	Recommend early surgery; administer preoperative steroids	Follow radiographically			
Nonambulatory paraparesis	Recommend early surgery; administer preoperative steroids	Follow radiographically			
Paraplegia	See Table 35-13				

*See Table 34-9 on p. 1068 and 34-25 on p. 1091 for drugs, dosages and variations on duration of therapy. †All patients are placed in strict confinement for 3 to 4 weeks, fitted with a back brace, and given a neurologic examination daily as part of their medical management regardless of drug used or duration of drug therapy. ‡Nonsteroidal antiinflammatory drugs can be substituted for corticosteroids, however, the use of corticosteroids and nonsteroidal antiinflammatory drugs in combination should not be considered. §If deep pain perception remains, give the patient the benefit of further conservative therapy if surgery is unacceptable to the owner.

only techniques and various configurations of techniques that have been clinically or biomechanically proven to provide adequate vertebral stabilization are discussed here. These include Steinmann pins and methylmethacrylate (bone cement), vertebral body plates, dorsal spinous process plates, modified segmental spinal fixation, or a combination of the above techniques. Choice of technique is dictated by location of the fracture, size, age, and disposition of the patient, equipment available, and experience of the surgeon.

☞ **N O T E ·** It is important to remember that patients retaining even minimal neurologic function deserve the benefits of conservative treatment if surgery is unacceptable to the owner.

Preoperative Management

The animal should be given intravenous fluids and steroids prior to surgery. Intravenous steroids may be administered to protect the spinal cord from surgical manipulation. The steroid of choice is methylprednisolone sodium succinate (30 mg/kg intravenously).

Anesthesia

Suggested anesthetic regimens for animals undergoing spinal surgery are on p. 1050. If the patient requires positioning that may cause respiratory compromise, mechanical ventilatory support should be considered.

Surgical Anatomy

Anatomy of the thoracolumbar spine is described on p. 1101.

Positioning

Techniques used for surgical stabilization for thoracic and lumbar fracture/luxation require a dorsal approach. Patient positioning is generally sternal recumbency and is described and illustrated in Figs. 35-3 and 35-4.

SURGICAL TECHNIQUE
Steinmann Pins and Bone Cement

This technique provides an effective means of spinal stabilization. It can be performed on any area of the spine (i.e., thoracic, thoracolumbar, lumbar, lumbosacral), in any age or size animal of any disposition, is performed easily, and re-

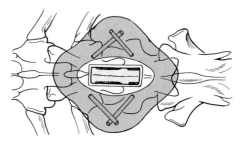

FIG. 35-24
When performing a laminectomy in conjunction with Steinmann pin and methylmethacrylate bone cement stabilization, mold bone cement in the shape of a doughnut to prevent contact of cement and spinal cord.

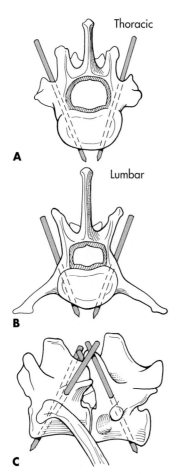

FIG. 35-23
Proper location and direction of in the, **A,** thoratic and **B,** lumbar vertebral bodies. **C,** Lateral view showing proper direction and angle of Steinmann pin placement in two adjacent vertebra.

quires a minimum of special equipment. It does necessitate a thorough knowledge of vertebral anatomy and constant reference to an appropriate anatomic specimen. Dogs weighing less than 15 kg with luxations or fractures close to the endplate can be stabilized with one 20-gm package of methylmethacrylate. Dogs weighing more than 15 kg require two 20-gm packages. Generally, two or three 20-gm packages of methylmethacrylate are required when spanning a vertebral body fracture or when a laminectomy has been performed. Because pin placement is critical and anatomic landmarks vary from vertebra to vertebra, a skeleton should be available for reference during this procedure.

Approach the spine as described for modified dorsal laminectomy (p. 1102). Place towel forceps in the dorsal spinous processes of the vertebrae cranial and caudal to the fracture/luxation; apply traction and countertraction during epaxial muscle elevation from lamina and pedicles. This helps avoid fracture/luxation displacement during dissection. Continue dissection ventrally to the level of the costal fovea of the transverse processes if a thoracic vertebra is involved, or the base of the transverse processes if a lumbar vertebra is involved. If a dorsal laminectomy or

hemilaminectomy is indicated, perform one as described on pp. 1102 and 1105 respectively. Reduce the vertebral fracture/luxation using bone holding forceps or towel clamps applied to the dorsal spinous processes. Facilitate reduction by having two nonsterile assistants apply gentle traction on the head and tail. Maintain reduction of the fracture/luxation with traction on towel clamps, or if a dorsal laminectomy is not performed, place a 0.45-inch Kirschner wire across each articular facet. Use an electric or air driven drill to place Steinmann pins into the vertebral bodies on each side of the fracture/luxation. In the thoracic vertebrae, place pins into the pedicle and drive them into the vertebral body, using the tubercle of the ribs and base of the accessory processes as anatomic landmarks. In the lumbar vertebrae, place pins into the vertebral bodies, using the accessory processes and transverse processes as landmarks. Direct the Steinmann pins cranioventrally and from lateral to medial in the vertebral body cranial to the fracture/luxation, and caudoventrally and from lateral to medial in the vertebral body caudal to the fracture/luxation (Fig. 35-23). Drive each Steinmann pin to exit 2 to 3 mm from the ventral aspect of the vertebral body. Cut the pins 3 to 4 mm below the level of the dorsal spinous processes. Notch each pin at its dorsal aspect with a pin cutter. If a laminectomy was performed, cover the defect with an autogenous fat graft. Thoroughly mix the liquid monomer with polymer powder. Once the methylmethacrylate can be handled without sticking to the surgeon's gloves, pack it around the Steinmann pins making sure it contacts all surfaces of each pin and covers the dorsal aspects. If a dorsal laminectomy or hemilaminectomy has been performed, mold the methylmethacrylate into the shape of a doughnut as it is packed around the Steinmann pins (Fig. 35-24). Take care not to allow methylmethacrylate to contact spinal cord or nerve roots. If a laminectomy was not performed, apply a circular mass of methylmethacrylate, incorporating Steinmann pins, articular facets, lamina, pedicles, and adjacent dorsal spinous process (Fig. 35-25, A). If a fractured vertebral body must be spanned, place pins in the body cranial and caudal to the fractured body (Fig. 35-25, B). Use the same technique as described above. Lavage the methylmethacrylate with cool saline for 5 minutes to dissipate the heat of polymerization. If necessary, excise portions

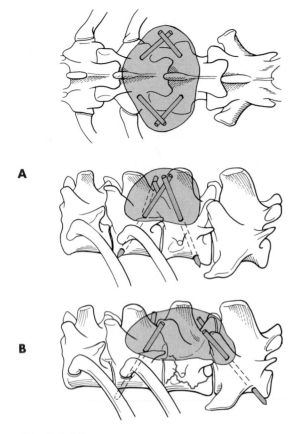

FIG. 35-25
A, If a laminectomy is not performed in conjunction with Steinmann pin and methylmethacrylate bone cement stabilization, mold bone cement around pins, dorsal spinous processes, articular facets, lamina, and pedicles of affected vertebra. **B,** If a vertebral body fracture must be spanned using Steinmann pin and methylmethacrylate bone cement, place pins in the vertebral bodies cranial and caudal to the fractured vertebra.

TABLE 35-15
Advantages and Disadvantages of Dorsolateral Vertebral Body Plating

Advantages
- Can be performed on any age, size, or disposition of patient
- Provides a rigid means of spinal stabilization

Disadvantages
- Need for nerve root resection at the spanned intervertebral space precludes its use below the 4th lumbar vertebra
- Approach to thoracic vertebrae is difficult
- Difficult to ensure the proper drill angle for screw placement
- Requires plating equipment

TABLE 35-16
Advantages and Disadvantages of Dorsal Spinous Process Plating

Advantages
- Provides a secure means of spinal stabilization
- Limited exposure helps retain inherent spinal stability
- Easily performed
- Is compatible with hemilaminectomy

Disadvantages
- Cannot be used in soft bone of younger animals
- Requires a series of three prominent dorsal spinous processes on each side of the fracture/luxation strong enough to support the stresses encountered by an unstable spine
- Not rigid enough to use in hyperactive large-breed dogs
- Cannot be used in patients with small dorsal spinous processes
- Requires specialized equipment

of epaxial muscles adjacent to methylmethacrylate, to facilitate closure. Close lumbodorsal fascia to the dorsal midline with nonabsorbable monofilament suture material in a simple interrupted pattern. Rarely, relief incisions in the lumbodorsal fascia lateral to the methylmethacrylate are necessary to facilitate closure. Close subcutaneous tissues and skin routinely.

Dorsolateral Vertebral Body Plating

This technique provides effective spinal stabilization. It is recommended that an anatomic specimen be available for reference during placement of plates and screws. Advantages and disadvantages of this technique are listed in Table 35-15. Dorsolateral vertebral body plating requires dorsolateral exposure of lamina, pedicles, facet, and transverse process of lumbar vertebrae or lamina, pedicle, facet and rib head of thoracic vertebrae; the approach is as described for hemilaminectomy on p. 1105. Exposure of articular processes of the vertebra to be plated and articular processes of vertebrae cranial and caudal to these is recommended. If the luxation, subluxation, or fracture is close to the intervertebral space,

stabilization of the two adjacent vertebrae is adequate. If a midbody fracture exists, three vertebral bodies are spanned by the plate.

Identify and protect spinal nerve roots encountered cranial and caudal to the fracture/luxation. Using bipolar cautery, carefully cauterize the vessels and nerve root emerging from the intervertebral foramen between the vertebrae to be plated. Carefully sever the vessels and nerve root. If a hemilaminectomy is indicated, perform it now (see p. 1105). Select a bone plate that will allow placement of two screws in each vertebral body cranial and caudal to the affected intervertebral space (luxation, subluxation) or affected vertebral body (fracture). Reduce and stabilize the fracture/luxation by placing towel clamps in the dorsal spinous processes of the vertebrae cranial and caudal to the fracture/luxation to provide a means of traction and countertraction. If a laminectomy is not performed, place a 0.45-inch Kirschner wire through the reduced articular facet to maintain reduction. Lay the plate on the dorsolateral surface of the reduced vertebral body, ventral to the

FIG. 35-26
A, Proper placement of a spinal plate on lumbar vertebrae. Notice that nerve root resection (rhizotomy) is required.
B, For spinal plating of thoracic vertebrae, resect involved ribs to allow placement of the plate against the vertebral bodies. Wire ribs to the dorsal spinous processes after placement of the spinal plate.

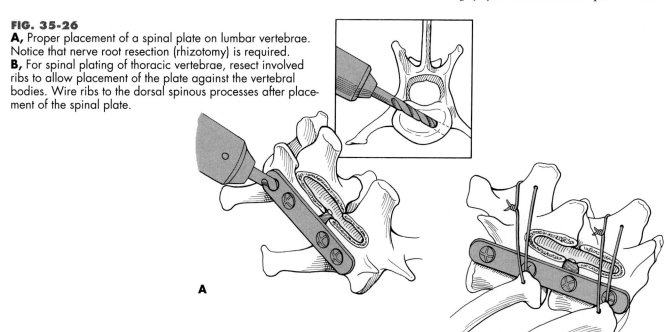

articular facet or laminectomy defect. Drill and tap screw holes to ensure four cortices are engaged cranial and caudal to the involved fracture/luxation. Judge the proper angle for each hole by referring to an anatomic specimen (Fig. 35-26, A). If a laminectomy is performed, use the anatomic location of the spinal cord and spinal canal as reference points to determine proper drill angle. After the hole is drilled, measure the depth with a depth gauge, tap the hole, select an appropriate length screw, and secure the plate to the vertebral body.

For thoracic vertebrae, expose the rib heads of the vertebral bodies to be plated. Use a bone cutting forceps to cut the rib head from its attachment to the vertebral body. Contour the transverse process with rongeurs until the plate lies flat against the vertebral body. Secure the plate as described above. Reattach the severed ribs to the dorsal spinous processes with orthopedic wire (Fig. 35-26, B). Lavage the surgical site with sterile saline solution, harvest an autogenous fat graft and place it over the laminectomy site, appose epaxial muscles with nonabsorbable monofilament suture, and close subcutaneous tissues and skin routinely.

Dorsal Spinous Process Plating

Dorsal spinous process plating using plastic plates provides effective spinal stabilization. Advantages and disadvantages are listed in Table 35-16. Plastic plates are designed to conform to the normal curvature of the spine and come in various sizes. Plate application requires exposure of the dorsal spinous processes and articular facets as described for modified dorsal laminectomy on p. 1102. The technique for reducing and maintaining reduction of the fracture/luxation is as described above.

Make an incision on each side of the dorsal spinous processes, being careful to preserve supraspinous and interspinous ligaments. Elevate epaxial muscles from the dorsal spines and articular facets of at least three vertebrae

cranial and caudal to the fracture/luxation. Do not sever muscle attachments from the lateral aspect of the articular processes. Select two appropriately sized plates and lay them along the space between the dorsal spine and articular facet on each side of the vertebrae (Fig. 35-27, A). Be sure the plates are long enough to grip spinous processes of three vertebrae on each side of the fracture/luxation. Place them such that the roughened surface lies against the dorsal spinous processes. Identify areas of contact that will keep the plates from lying uniformly on the lamina. Remove the plates and use a high-speed air drill to deepen these areas (Fig. 35-27, B). Replace the plates, pass stainless steel bolts through predrilled holes in each plate and between spinous processes, and place washers and nuts on each bolt (see Fig. 35-27, A). Hold the fracture/luxation reduced, and tighten the nuts until plates are in contact between the spinous processes. Lavage the surgical site with sterile saline, debride any devitalized muscle, close epaxial muscles with a nonabsorbable monofilament suture, and close subcutaneous tissues and skin routinely.

Modified Segmental Spinal Fixation

Modified segmental spinal instrumentation provides a simple, versatile, and strong repair of vertebral fracture/luxations. Advantages and disadvantages are listed in Table 35-17. Pin and wire application requires exposure of dorsal spinous processes and articular facets as described for dorsal laminectomy procedures on p. 1101. Number and size of longitudinal and central pins (see below) used are dependent upon size and activity of the patient and relative stability of the fracture/luxation. Generally, large patients with an unstable fracture/luxation, are stabilized with relatively large central pins and a greater number of longitudinal pins (i.e.,

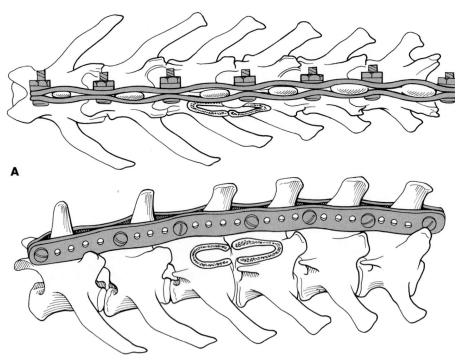

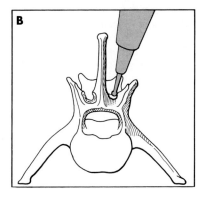

FIG. 35-27
A, Place plastic dorsal spinous process plates on each side of the dorsal spinous processes. Place nuts and bolts through the plates and between spinous processes. **B,** To facilitate uniform plate contact of all dorsal spinous processes spanned by the plate, remove any high points of laminar or articular facet contact by the plates with a high-speed pneumatic drill.

TABLE 35-17
Advantages and Disadvantages of Modified Segmental Spinal Fixation
Advantages
• Can be performed in any area of the spine (i.e., thoracic, thoracolumbar, lumbar, lumbosacral)
• Can be performed in any age, size, or disposition of animal
• Relatively easy to perform
• Requires no special equipment
• Less muscle dissection is required than with Steinmann pins and bone cement or body plating
• Is compatible with dorsal laminectomy procedures
• Provides a strong repair
Disadvantages
• Pin migration and fatigue fracture of orthopedic wire or pins may occur

three to six pins). Moreover, central and longitudinal pin size may be varied and the length of longitudinal pins may be sequentially decreased to achieve a leaf spring effect (Fig. 35-28). If further stiffness is desired, muscular and tendinous attachments lateral to the articular facets are dissected free and a second set of pins is placed in a similar fashion lateral to the facets.

Expose two to three spinous processes and articular facets cranial and caudal to the fracture/luxation, depending upon patient size and activity, and inherent stability of the fracture/luxation. Perform a dorsal laminectomy if indicated, as described on p. 1101. Reduce the fracture/luxation and maintain reduction as previously described above. Drill holes through the bases of articular facets (do not cross the articulation), bases of dorsal spinous processes, and tangentially through the dorsal lamina. Make the holes large enough to accommodate 18- or 20-gauge orthopedic wire. Preplace orthopedic wire through each hole, leaving the ends long enough to wrap around several Steinmann pins. Select two Steinmann pins long enough to include at least two vertebrae cranial and caudal to the affected vertebra (fracture) or intervertebral space (luxation, subluxation), called longitudinal pins. Bend the ends of the longitudinal pins at right angles to extend either into the interspinous space or through holes drilled transversely through the base of the dorsal spinous process. Place longitudinal pins in the space between dorsal spinous processes and articular facets (see Fig. 35-28, A). Place one central pin on each side of the dorsal spinous processes nearest the fracture/luxation. Bend the ends of the central pins to hook around the base of the dorsal spinous processes. Wire the central and longitudinal pins to the base of the articular facets, dorsal lamina, and dorsal spinous processes with the preplaced stands of orthopedic wire (see Fig. 35-28, B). Lavage the surgical site with sterile saline, debride any devitalized muscle, close epaxial muscles with a nonabsorbable monofilament suture, and close subcutaneous tissue and skin routinely.*

SUTURE MATERIALS/SPECIAL INSTRUMENTS

Special instruments necessary are dictated by the stabilization technique chosen. When using methylmethacrylate, an assortment of Steinmann pins of various sizes should be available. Vertebral body plating requires special orthopedic

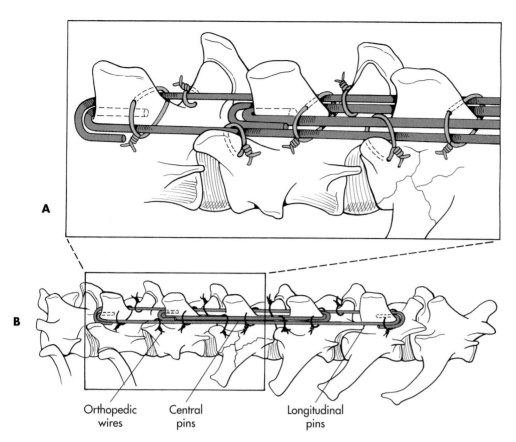

FIG. 35-28
A, Perform modified segmental spinal fixation by wiring central and longitudinal pins to the base of dorsal spinous processes and articular facets. **B,** Place the orthopedic wire through the dorsal spinous process and articular facets.

Orthopedic   Central   Longitudinal
  wires   pins   pins

plating equipment; dorsal spinous process plating requires specially constructed plastic spinal plates; and modified segmental spinal fixation requires assorted Steinmann pins and orthopedic wire.

POSTOPERATIVE CARE AND ASSESSMENT

Patients with thoracic and lumbar fracture/luxation should be evaluated postoperatively in a similar fashion as patients with other T-L spinal disorders (see Table 35-4). See Table 34-13 on p. 1070 for suggested analgesics and dosages.

COMPLICATIONS

Complications associated with use of Steinmann pins and bone cement include iatrogenic injury to the spinal cord or pin migration. Complications associated with vertebral body plating include iatrogenic spinal cord injury, inappropriate screw placement, iatrogenic pneumothorax, or screw and plate migration. Complications associated with dorsal spinal plating include plate slippage and fracture of the dorsal spinous process. Complications associated with modified segmental spinal plating include fatigue fracture of pins or wires or pin migration.

PROGNOSIS

Prognosis for patients treated medically or surgically for thoracic and lumbar fracture/luxation is generally favorable and is dependent upon assessment of apparent neurologic signs and subsequent medical or surgical management chosen.

Clinical factors and probable patient outcome are outlined in Tables 35-13 and 35-14.

References

Feeney DA, Oliver JE: Blunt spinal trauma in the dog and cat: neurologic, radiologic, and therapeutic correlations, *J Am Anim Hosp Assoc* 16:664, 1980.

Selcer RR, Bubb WJ, Walker TL: Management of vertebral column fractures in dogs and cats: 211 cases (1977–1985), *J Am Vet Med Assoc* 198:1965, 1991.

Suggested Reading

Blass CE, Seim HB: Spinal fixation in dogs using Steinmann pins and methylmethacrylate, *Vet Surg* 13:203, 1984.

Bruecker KA, Seim HB III: Principles of spinal fracture management, *Sem Vet Med and Surg* 7:71, 1992.

Carberry CA et al: Nonsurgical management of thoracic and lumbar spinal fractures and fracture/luxations in the dog and cat: a review of 17 cases, *J Am Anim Hosp Assoc* 25:43, 1989.

Dulisch ML, Withrow SJ: The use of plastic plates for fixation of spinal fractures in the dog, *Can Vet J* 20:326, 1979.

Feeney DA, Oliver JE: Blunt spinal trauma in the dog and cat: insight into radiographic lesions, *J Am Anim Hosp Assoc* 16:885, 1980.

Garcia JNP et el: Biomechanical study of canine spinal fracture fixation using pins or bone screws with polymethylmethacrylate, *Vet Surg* 23:322, 1994.

McAnulty JF, Lenehan TM, Maletz LM: Modified segmental spinal instrumentation in repair of spinal fractures and luxations in dogs, *Vet Surg* 15:143, 1986.

Patterson RH, Smith GK: Backsplinting for treatment of thoracic and lumbar fracture/luxation in the dog: principles of application and case series, *Vet Compar Orthop Trauma* 5:179, 1992.

Rouse GP, Miller JI: The use of methylmethacrylate for spinal stabilization, *J Am Anim Hosp Assoc* 11:418. 1975.

Shires PK et al: A biomechanical study of rotational instability in unaltered and surgically altered canine thoracolumbar vertebral motion units, *Prog Vet Neurol* 2:6, 1991.

Swaim SJ: Vertebral body plating for spinal immobilization, *J Am Vet Med Assoc* 158:1683, 1971.

Turner WD: Fractures and fracture-luxations of the lumbar spine: a retrospective study in the dog, *J Am Anim Hosp Assoc* 23:459, 1987.

Waldron DR et al: The rotational stabilizing effect of spinal fixation techniques in an unstable vertebral model, *Prog Vet Neurol* 2:105, 1991.

Walter MC, Smith GK, Newton CD: Canine lumbar spinal internal fixation techniques, *Vet Surg* 15:191, 1986.

Wong WT, Emms SG: Use of pins and methylmethacrylate in stabilization of spinal fractures and luxations, *J Sm Anim Prac* 33:415, 1992.

NEOPLASIA OF THORACOLUMBAR VERTEBRAE, SPINAL CORD, AND NERVE ROOTS

DEFINITIONS

Neoplasms involving the thoracolumbar vertebrae, spinal cord, and nerve roots are similar to those of the cervical region. See p. 1096.

SYNONYMS

Spinal tumors, spinal cord tumors, tumors of the spine, vertebral tumors, nerve root tumors

GENERAL CONSIDERATIONS AND CLINICALLY RELEVANT PATHOPHYSIOLOGY

Tumors of the thoracolumbar vertebrae, spinal cord, and nerve roots are classified by location in and around the spinal cord (i.e., primary bone, primary spinal cord, primary peripheral nerve root, primary paraspinal soft tissue, or metastatic) and by location relative to the dura (i.e., extradural, intradural-extramedullary, or intramedullary). Most canine thoracolumbar vertebral, spinal cord, and nerve root tumors are extradural, generally arising from bone. Tumor types for each location in dogs (i.e., extradural, intradural-extramedullary, intramedullary) are similar to tumor types for cervical vertebrae, spinal cord, and nerve roots (see p. 1096). Lymphosarcoma is the most common spinal tumor in cats and generally occurs extradurally. Intradural-extramedullary and intramedullary tumors in cats are rare. Spinal neoplasia, regardless of location or classification, becomes clinically significant when the enlarging mass compromises neural tissue (i.e., spinal cord or nerve roots) or its invasive growth undermines the vertebra and its supporting structures, leading to pathologic fracture.

DIAGNOSIS
Clinical Presentation

Signalment. There does not appear to be a general sex or breed predilection for patients with thoracolumbar vertebral, spinal cord, or nerve root neoplasia. Most patients are older than 5 years of age. An exception is benign, solitary or multiple cartilaginous exostoses that usually occur in patients younger than 1 year of age.

☞ **N O T E** · When considering differentials in patients with neurologic disorders, remember that "tumors know no age."

History. Historical findings depend on location of the neoplasm relative to the dura. Animals with extradural neoplasia generally present because of acute pain and varying degrees of upper or lower motor neuron paraparesis, while those with intradural-extramedullary neoplasia present with a chronic history (months to years) of dull back pain or hindlimb lameness plus varying degrees of monoparesis or paraparesis. Patients with intramedullary neoplasia present with acute paraparesis (often after a long insidious onset), with or without back pain. Careful historic evaluation often reveals subtle neurologic abnormalities before the acute presenting episode.

Physical Examination Findings

Physical and neurologic examination findings associated with thoracolumbar spinal tumors vary depending upon tumor location (see Fig. 33-9 on p. 1040), degree of spinal cord and nerve root compression, rate of tumor growth, and secondary effects of the tumor (i.e., paraneoplastic syndrome). Some generalizations concerning presenting signs can be made for various classifications of vertebral tumors and are discussed on p. 1096. Patients with tumors involving spinal cord segments T3 to L3 present with varying degrees of back pain and UMN paraparesis, whereas those with tumors involving spinal cord segments L4 to S3 have varying degrees of low back pain and LMN paraparesis (see Chapter 33).

Radiography/Ultrasonography

Abnormal survey radiographs suggesting vertebral, spinal cord, or nerve root neoplasia include osteoproduction, osteolysis, or lysis of the intervertebral foramen (see Figs. 34-65 to 34-67). Diagnosis of most spinal cord and paraspinal vertebral neoplasms requires myelography. Specific myelographic techniques are described in Chapter 33 (see also Figs. 33-13 and 33-14). Myelography classifies neoplasms as extradural, intradural-extramedullary, or intramedullary.

Myelographic abnormalities associated with each classification are illustrated in Figs. 33-15 to 33-17. Occasionally, CT scan or MRI is necessary to accurately determine extent of vertebral, spinal cord, or nerve root involvement.

Laboratory Findings

Laboratory findings are generally normal or reflect paraneoplastic syndromes. Cerebral spinal fluid analysis rarely contributes to a specific diagnosis; however, cell type or evidence of an inflammatory process may support a diagnosis of neoplasia.

DIFFERENTIAL DIAGNOSIS

Differential diagnosis of tumor type is based on location of tumor (i.e., bone, spinal cord, nerve root, or metastasis) and myelographic classification (i.e., extradural, intradural-extramedullary, or intramedullary).

MEDICAL MANAGEMENT

Medical management is directed at the primary lesion and secondary tumor effects. Generally, definitive medical treatment requires surgical exposure and incisional or excisional biopsy to determine tumor type and plan adjunct chemotherapy, irradiation, or combination therapy.

SURGICAL TREATMENT
Preoperative Management

Patients are given intravenous fluids and steroids prior to surgery. Steroids help protect the spinal cord during surgical manipulation. The steroid of choice is methylprednisolone sodium succinate (30 mg/kg intravenously).

Anesthesia

See p. 1101 for suggested anesthetic protocols to use in animals with thoracolumbar spinal disorders.

Surgical Anatomy

Surgical procedures to approach and resect thoracic or lumbar vertebral, spinal cord, and nerve root tumors include dorsal laminectomy and hemilaminectomy, with or without facetectomy and foramenotomy. Each procedure removes various portions of dorsal spinous processes, lamina, pedicles, and articular facets (see p. 1101). Commonly encountered anatomic landmarks of thoracic and lumbar vertebrae are illustrated in Figs. 35-1 and 35-2 on p. 1102.

Positioning

Generally, patients with thoracolumbar vertebral, spinal cord, or nerve root tumors require a dorsal or dorsolateral approach. Patients requiring dorsal laminectomy are positioned with the back gently flexed to open articular facets and interarcuate spaces, facilitating exposure (see Fig. 35-3). Patients requiring hemilaminectomy should have the affected side gently rotated (about 15 degrees) to facilitate dorsolateral exposure of affected vertebrae (see Fig. 35-4).

Surgical Technique

Surgical objectives include exposure of the tumor, wide resection or biopsy of the tumor, spinal cord and nerve root decompression, and occasionally vertebral stabilization. Thoracolumbar vertebral, spinal cord, or nerve root tumors are generally approached via dorsal laminectomy or hemilaminectomy as described on pp. 1101-1105. Wide laminectomy, facetectomy, and foramenotomy are required for adequate exposure of extradural and intradural-extramedullary tumors. Dorsal or hemilaminectomy and durotomy are necessary for exposure and removal of intramedullary tumors. If spinal stabilization is indicated, techniques described for stabilization of thoracic and lumbar spinal fracture/luxations are used (see pp. 1122-1126).

SUTURE MATERIALS/SPECIAL INSTRUMENTS

Ultrasonic aspirators (discussed on p. 1099) are invaluable, especially when removing neoplastic tissue closely associated with, or invading, neural tissues. Other special instruments necessary to perform thoracolumbar dorsal and hemilaminectomy are listed in Table 35-2.

POSTOPERATIVE CARE AND ASSESSMENT

Patients with thoracic and lumbar vertebral, spinal cord, and nerve root neoplasia are evaluated postoperatively just like patients with other thoracolumbar spinal disorders. Adjunct chemotherapy, irradiation, immunotherapy, or combination therapy is based on tumor type and surgical margins. See Table 34-13 on p. 1070 for suggested analgesics and dosages.

PROGNOSIS

Prognosis depends on tumor location (i.e., spine, spinal cord, or nerve root), myelographic classification (i.e., extradural, intradural-extramedullary, or intramedullary), tumor type (i.e., biologic activity), degree of surgical resection, and tumor sensitivity to adjunct therapy. Generally, malignant extradural neoplasms have an unfavorable prognosis, benign extradural neoplasms have a favorable prognosis, malignant and benign intramedullary neoplasms have an unfavorable to grave prognosis, and extradural-intramedullary neoplasms have a guarded to unfavorable prognosis (see Table 34-28, on p. 1096).

Suggested Reading

Bell FW et al: External beam radiation therapy for recurrent intraspinal meningioma in a dog, *J Am Anim Hosp Assoc* 28:318, 1992.

Blass CE et al: Teratomatous medulloepithelioma in the spinal cord of a dog, *J Am Anim Hosp Assoc* 24:51, 1988.

Jeffrey ND, Phillips SM: Surgical treatment of intramedullary spinal cord neoplasia in two dogs, *J Sm Anim Prac* 36:553, 1995.

Lane SB et al: Feline spinal lymphosarcoma: a retrospective evaluation of 23 cats, *J Vet Int Med* 8:99, 1994.

Levy MS et al: Spinal tumors in 37 dogs: clinical outcome and long-term survival *Vet Surg* 24:429, 1995 (abstract).

Moissonnier P, Abbott DP: Canine neuroepithelioma: case report and literature review, *J Am Anim Hosp Assoc* 29:397, 1993.

Nafe LA et al: An enlarged intervertebral foramen associated with an anaplastic sarcoma in a dog, *J Am Anim Hosp Assoc* 19:299, 1983.

Poncelet L et al: Successful removal of an intramedullary spinal paraganglioma from a dog, *J Am Anim Hosp Assoc* 30:213, 1994.

Prata RG, Stoll SG, Zaki FA: Spinal cord compression caused by osteocartilaginous exostoses of the spine in two dogs, *J Am Vet Med Assoc* 166:371, 1975.

Shiroma JT et al: Pathological fracture of an aneurysmal bone cyst in a lumbar vertebra of a dog, *J Am Anim Hosp Assoc* 29:434, 1993.

Spodnick GP et al: Spinal lymphoma in cats: 21 cases (1976–1989), *J Am Vet Med Assoc* 200:373, 1992.

Zaki FA et al: Primary tumors of the spinal cord and meninges in six dogs, *J Am Vet Med Assoc* 166:511, 1975.

CHAPTER 36

Surgery of the Lumbosacral Spine

GENERAL PRINCIPLES AND TECHNIQUES

DEFINITIONS

Dorsal laminectomy of the lumbosacral spine is removal of dorsal spinous processes, lamina, pedicles, and articular facets of L7 and S1, S2, and/or S3. **Hemilaminectomy** is removal of lamina and pedicles on the right or left side. **Facetectomy** is removal of articular facets, either unilaterally (hemilaminectomy) or bilaterally (dorsal laminectomy), to increase exposure to the spinal canal and intervertebral foramen. **Cauda equina** refers to the nerve roots that course through the lumbosacral spinal canal (i.e., L7, S1-3, and Cd 1-5). **Dyesthesia** is the sensation of burning or tingling in areas supplied by entrapped nerve roots.

PREOPERATIVE CONCERNS

Traumatized patients (e.g., victims of automobile accidents) should receive intravenous fluids and be secured to a rigid platform until fractures/luxations are stabilized. Careful physical examination should rule out concurrent trauma to other organ systems (e.g., urinary, cardiopulmonary, associated vertebral or appendicular skeletal fracture/luxations). Surgical urgency is determined by initial and serial neurologic examinations. Generally, patients with acute signs and severe neurologic deficits (e.g., fracture/luxation, acute intervertebral disk extrusion, neoplasia) should have surgery as quickly as possible, while those with chronic signs (e.g., congenital lumbosacral stenosis, diskospondylitis, vertebral osteomyelitis, chronic degenerative disk disease) should be carefully evaluated and staged before medical or surgical treatment. Steroids are generally not administered because their efficacy in nerve root injury is uncertain.

ANESTHETIC CONSIDERATIONS

Suggested anesthetic protocols used in patients with spinal disorders are given on p. 1049.

ANTIBIOTICS

Criteria for use of prophylactic or therapeutic antibiotics are given in Table 34-4 on p. 1050. Selection of an appropriate antibiotic and dose is determined by criteria given in Chapter 10.

SURGICAL ANATOMY

The lumbosacral spine is unique in its anatomic configuration from vertebra to vertebra, particularly L7 and S1. The anatomic variations and surgical significance of each are listed in Table 36-1.

SURGICAL TECHNIQUES

Positioning is critical in patients with lumbosacral disorders. Animals with lumbosacral stenosis (i.e., cauda equina syndrome) should be positioned with the hind legs tucked under the abdomen, thus stretching the interarcuate ligament (also called the ligamentum flavum, yellow ligament) and accentuating the dorsal lumbosacral space (Fig. 36-1). This facilitates exposure for dorsal laminectomy and hemilaminectomy, and may decompress the cauda equina. Patients with lumbosacral fracture/luxation should be positioned to encourage fracture/luxation reduction. Generally, this is accomplished by positioning the patient as illustrated in Fig. 36-1.

Patients with surgical lumbosacral disorders are treated by dorsal laminectomy, hemilaminectomy, facetectomy, or dorsal lumbosacral spinal stabilization. Dorsal laminectomy is most commonly used for decompressing lumbosacral stenosis (i.e., cauda equina syndrome) and exposing and removing herniated disk material, fracture fragments, neoplasms, or paraspinal abscesses at L6-L7 or L7-S1. Unilateral or bilateral facetectomy is performed with laminectomy, if the compressive lesion is located laterally. Hemilaminectomy is most commonly used to expose extradural or intradural-extramedullary lesions involving L6-L7.

Dorsal Laminectomy

Position the patient in sternal recumbency (see Fig. 36-1). Make a dorsal midline incision from the dorsal spinous process of L6 to the first caudal vertebra. Incise the superficial and deep sacral fascia parallel to the skin incision. Using a periosteal elevator or small osteotome, elevate epaxial muscles from their attachments on dorsal spinous processes, lamina, articular facets, pedicles, and accessory processes of L7-S3. Remove the dorsal spinous process of L7 and S1 with rongeurs. Identify the wide interarcuate space of L7-S1; carefully incise and remove

TABLE 36-1

Anatomic Variation of L7 and S1 and Its Surgical Significance

Vertebrae	Anatomy	Surgical Significance
L7	Thick dorsal lamina compared to S1	Has distinct outer cortical, medullary, and inner cortical layers
S1	Thin dorsal lamina compared to L7	Outer cortical, medullary, and inner cortical layers are not distinct
L7-S1 articulation	Most mobile joint in the thoracolumbar spine	Positioning in slight ventral flexion results in significant widening of the interarcuate space during surgery
	Large interarcuate space	Allows limited exposure of the cauda equina prior to laminectomy
	Spinal cord terminates at L5-L6	Only nerve roots course through the L7-S1 spinal canal
	Close association with wings of the ilium	Makes foramenotomy and facetectomy difficult to perform
S1,2,3	Sacral vertebrae are fused	No intervertebral disk spaces; nerve roots exit through separate dorsal and ventral foramina

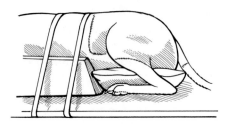

FIG. 36-1
Positioning patients with the hind legs tucked under the abdomen helps accentuate the L7-S1 interarcuate space.

associated soft-tissue structures (i.e., remaining muscle attachments, interarcuate ligament) with a No. 11 scalpel blade. Use a high-speed pneumatic or electric drill to remove the outer cortical and softer medullary layer and identify the inner cortical layer from midbody of L7 to midbody of S2-S3 (Fig. 36-2). The dorsal laminar thickness of L7 and S1 varies greatly; L7 is two to three times thicker than S1. Carefully drill through the inner cortical layer until it becomes soft. Detailed illustrations of each drilled layer are given on p. 1102 and in Fig. 35-7. Penetrate and remove the inner periosteum with a dental or iris spatula until the entire laminectomy site is exposed. Structures present include nerve roots of L7, S1, S2, S3, and caudal nerve roots, vertebral venous sinus, dorsal longitudinal ligament, and dorsal annulus fibrosus. If the L7 or S1 nerve roots appear to be compressed within the foramen or by enlarged facets, perform a facetectomy and/or foramenotomy, respectively, to establish complete nerve root decompression. Using a high-speed drill, remove the cranial articular process of S1 and caudal articular process of L7. Use the drill to approach the intervertebral foramen and Lempert rongeurs to enter the foramen by removing any remaining articular facet. This exposure allows visualization of the intervertebral foramen and exiting L7 nerve root. Lavage the surgical site with warm saline. Harvest a free subcutaneous fat graft and position it over the laminectomy site. Close epaxial muscles with interrupted, monofilament, nonabsorbable suture. Close subcutaneous tissues and skin routinely.

Hemilaminectomy

Hemilaminectomy and facetectomy are indicated for exposure of the lateral aspects of the lumbosacral spinal canal. It is used to remove compressive lesions such as neoplasms, fracture fragments, herniated intervertebral disk material, bulbous articular facets, or paraspinal abscesses.

☞ **N O T E** · Proper technique for controlling venous sinus hemorrhage is discussed in Table 34-1.

Position the patient as for dorsal laminectomy (see Fig. 36-1). Make a dorsal midline skin incision from the dorsal spinous process of L6 to the first caudal vertebra, and continue it through the dorsal sacral fascia. Elevate epaxial muscles from the right or left lateral aspect of the dorsal spinous process, lamina, articular facet, pedicle, and accessory process of the L7-S1 intervertebral space. Visualize the dorsal aspect of the transverse process of L7. Use a high-speed drill to remove lamina, articular facet, and pedicle to the level of the accessory process. Identify outer cortical, medullary, and inner cortical layers while drilling (see p. 1104, Fig. 35-7). Carefully break through the inner periosteal layer with rongeurs and a dental or iris spatula to enter the spinal canal. Identify the vertebral venous sinus located on the floor of the spinal canal. Be careful not to lacerate the sinus while manipulating lesions within the spinal canal. After complete decompression and mass removal, lavage the surgical site with warm saline. Harvest a free subcutaneous fat graft and position it over the laminectomy site. Close epaxial muscles to the dorsal sacral fascia with interrupted, monofilament, nonabsorbable suture. Close subcutaneous tissues and skin routinely.

Spinal Stabilization

Lumbosacral spinal stabilization is a technique that stabilizes a lumbosacral fracture, luxation, or a congenital or acquired stenosis causing spinal instability (see p. 1142). Spinal stabilization can be successfully accomplished by various tech-

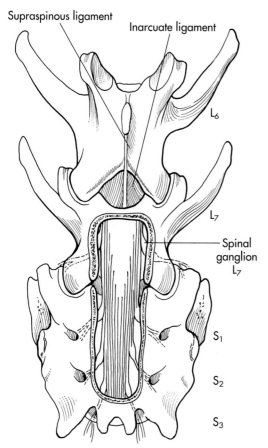

Supraspinous ligament

Inarcuate ligament

L6

L7

Spinal ganglion L7

S1

S2

S3

FIG. 36-2
L7-S1,2 dorsal laminectomy provides exposure of the filum terminale and cauda equina.

niques, including: transilial pins, transilial pins and plastic dorsal spinous process plates, Steinmann pins and methylmethacrylate bone cement, a combination of external skeletal fixation and dorsal spinous process plates, and modified segmental spinal fixation.

HEALING OF THE CAUDA EQUINA

Nerve roots of the cauda equina respond to injury in a similar fashion as peripheral nerves.

Healing of peripheral nerves depends on the extent of injury (i.e., neurotmesis, axonotmesis, or neurapraxia). Neurotmesis occurs if the entire peripheral nerve with all its bundles of fibers is severed or ruptured with a gap between severed nerve ends. Axonotmesis occurs if some axons in the nerve are ruptured but anatomic continuity is maintained. Neurapraxia is an acute transient physiologic dysfunction of a peripheral nerve after trauma; nerve conduction is blocked but degeneration does not occur, and full return of function is expected.

Regrowth of axons is spontaneous, but the time until return of function depends on the extent of injury and the distance from denervated end-organs. Peripheral nerves sustaining mild injury that causes neurapraxia develop transient physiologic dysfunction without anatomic disruption of axons. The nerve regains normal function within 3

months or less (peripheral nerve regeneration occurs at 3 cm per month or approximately 1 mm per day). Peripheral nerves sustaining injury sufficient to cause axonotmesis or neurotmesis undergo immediate degeneration at the site of injury. Degeneration toward the cell body over a distance of two to three nodes of Ranvier generally occurs, and regeneration begins from that site. Nerve processes distal to the injury degenerate completely (i.e., Wallerian degeneration), and after one week a connective tissue framework (i.e., neurilemmal sheath) is left. Within 2 days "sprouting" of the proximal end of the severed axon occurs. Neuron regeneration and return of function depend on several factors. If continuity of the nerve is maintained (i.e., axonotmesis), the distance from injury site to end-organ becomes the most important variable. Little function will be achieved if the distance is more than 25 to 30 cm; the best chance for functional regeneration is a distance of less than 10 to 15 cm. If anatomic nerve continuity is not maintained (i.e., neurotmesis), recovery depends on the distance from the injury to the end-organ, wounding mechanism, time between injury and surgical repair, patient's age and condition, and the surgical technique.

Clean sharp lacerations generally heal better than avulsion, crush, open, or chronic injuries. The earlier a nerve is repaired the better the chance for healing, reinnervation, and normal function of the end-organ. Young, well-nourished, healthy patients usually have faster nerve regeneration. Anatomic alignment of nerve ends and attention to surgical detail ensure that regenerating axons will find their way along the neurilemmal tube to the end-organ, producing functional recovery.

SUTURE MATERIALS/SPECIAL INSTRUMENTS

Special instrumentation necessary to perform dorsal laminectomy, hemilaminectomy, facetectomy, and spinal stabilization is listed by technique in Table 35-2 on p. 1108. It is important to practice each technique, become familiar with regional anatomy, and learn proper use of special instrumentation prior to performing these surgeries.

POSTOPERATIVE CARE AND ASSESSMENT

Critical postoperative care for the first 24 hours typically includes intravenous fluids, analgesics, antibiotics, seizure alert (if workup required a myelogram), and neurologic examinations. Specific care requirements are similar to patients with thoracolumbar spinal disorders. Immediate and long-term postoperative care and assessment for ambulatory and nonambulatory patients are given in Tables 35-3 and 35-4.

COMPLICATIONS

Complications associated with lumbosacral spinal surgery are uncommon. Seroma of the surgical site may occur, but is generally resolved with intermittent or continuous drainage. Bladder function is often impaired, and urinary tract infection commonly occurs. Empty the bladder manually four times daily until normal function returns. If dorsal laminectomy is performed, excessive removal of lamina, articular facets, and pedicles bilaterally could predispose the patient to muscle fibrosis and contracture over the spinal cord, causing spinal cord compression; however, this rarely occurs. Spinal instability has not been observed, even when multilevel exposure is indicated (e.g., L6 to S3). If a spinal stabilization technique is used, complications are generally associated with the specific technique. Patients undergoing hemilaminectomy rarely have significant complications. Iatrogenic nerve root trauma may occur, but nerve roots can tolerate careful surgical manipulation without developing clinically significant neural deficits.

SPECIAL AGE CONSIDERATIONS

Care should be taken when performing laminectomy procedures on young patients, because their cortical and cancellous bone is much softer than in older patients. Less pressure is required when drilling or rongeuring lamina and pedicles in younger patients, and a greater flexibility of the lumbosacral junction allows increased accentuation of the dorsal lumbosacral space during positioning.

Suggested Reading

Evan HE: *Miller's anatomy of the dog,* ed 3, Philadelphia, 1993, WB Saunders.

Koper S, Mucha M: Visualization of the vertebral canal veins in the dog: a radiological method, *Vet Radiol* 18:105, 1975.

Morgan JP, Atiola M, Bailey CS: Vertebral canal and spinal cord mensuration: a comparative study on its effect on lumbosacral myelography in the dachshund and German shepherd dog, *J Am Vet Med Assoc* 191:951, 1987.

Palmer RH, Chambers JN: Canine lumbosacral diseases. Part I. Anatomy, pathophysiology, and clinical presentation, *Comp Contin Educ Pract Vet* 13:61, 1991.

SPECIFIC DISEASES

CAUDA EQUINA SYNDROME

DEFINITIONS

Cauda equina syndrome is a complex of neurologic signs caused by compression of the nerve roots (i.e., cauda equina) coursing through the lumbosacral spinal canal. **Transitional vertebrae** are vertebrae that possess properties of lumbar and sacral vertebrae.

SYNONYMS

Lumbosacral stenosis, cauda equina compression, lumbosacral spondylosis, lumbosacral malformation-malarticulation, lumbosacral instability

GENERAL CONSIDERATIONS AND CLINICALLY RELEVANT PATHOPHYSIOLOGY

Cauda equina syndrome is relatively common and can be categorized as acquired (degenerative) or congenital (developmental). Potential causes are listed in Table 36-2. The respective nerve roots involved are L7, S1-3, and Cd 1-5 (Fig. 36-3).

The cauda equina is the termination or most caudal portion of the spinal cord and adjacent spinal roots. The filum terminale (i.e., caudal end of the spinal cord) in dogs is generally located at L6; however, this depends on the animal's size (the filum terminale in cats and dogs under 7 kg may be L7-S1). Vertebral bodies that contain the cauda equina are L5-L7, S1-S3, and Cd 1-5. Bony and ligamentous boundaries of the cauda equina are: dorsally—lamina, interarcuate ligament, and articular facets; laterally—pedicles; and ventrally—dorsal longitudinal ligament, vertebral venous sinus, dorsal annulus fibrosus, and vertebral body. Congenital or acquired defects causing abnormalities in the skeletal or soft-tissue boundaries may produce cauda equina compression and cauda equina syndrome.

DIAGNOSIS
Clinical Presentation

Signalment. Although there is no breed predilection for congenital cauda equina stenosis, acquired cauda equina syndrome is most commonly diagnosed in large-breed dogs (particularly German shepherds). There is no apparent sex predilection. Most dogs are middle-aged when clinical signs of acquired or congenital cauda equina become apparent; even congenital stenosis often causes clinical signs later in life.

History. Dogs with cauda equina syndrome typically present with a chronic history of back pain and hindlimb lameness, with or without hindlimb weakness. Back pain is due to attenuation of nerve roots, and lameness is either due to pain originating from nerve root entrapment/compression, neurologic deficits secondary to cauda equina com-

TABLE 36-2
Causes of Cauda Equina Syndrome

Acquired

Vertebral fracture or luxation
Diskospondylitis
Vertebral osteomyelitis
Chronic IVD disease
Acute IVD extrusion
Fibrocartilaginous emboli
Neoplasia of the L7-S1 vertebra, surrounding soft tissues, or nerve roots

Congenital

Transitional vertebra
Congenital spinal canal stenosis
Breed influenced spinal canal stenosis
Developmental sacral osteochondrosis

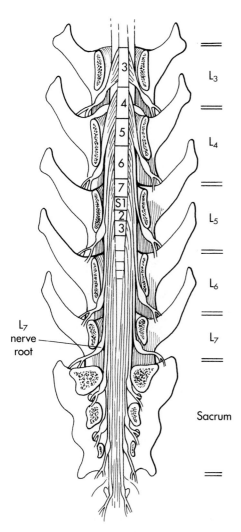

FIG. 36-3
Anatomic relationship of vertebral bodies to spinal cord termination and cauda equina.

pression, or both. The severity of signs depends on location and severity of the lesion. Other historical findings may include scuffing hindlimb toenails, difficulty climbing stairs, a reluctance to jump or sit up on hind legs, urinary or fecal incontinence, abnormal tail carriage, hindlimb muscle atrophy, and excessive chewing on the tail and/or lateral aspect of the hind feet.

Physical Examination Findings

General physical examination findings vary depending upon the cause of cauda equina compression. Patients with fracture/luxation may present with associated life-threatening injuries (e.g., cardiopulmonary, urinary) and signs associated with shock (weak peripheral pulses, tachycardia, prolonged capillary refill time, pale mucous membranes), and/or dyspnea. Patients with infectious causes may have fever and depression; sepsis is unusual. Those with neoplasia may present with systemic signs associated with secondary effects of the tumor (i.e., paraneoplastic syndrome). Animals with congenital stenosis, chronic degenerative disk disease,

or acute disk herniation may have signs that mimic other non-neurologic disorders, including: musculoskeletal disorders (hip dysplasia, chronic stifle instability, polyarthritis); vascular disorders (iliac thrombosis); peripheral neuropathy or myopathy; metabolic disorders causing generalized weakness; primary urogenital tract disease (incontinence, UTI); primary rectal or anal disorders (anal sacculitis, anorectal neoplasia); or distemper radiculopathy.

Neurologic examination findings are related to ischemia and/or compression of nerve roots coursing through the lumbosacral junction (i.e., L7, S1-2, and Cd 1-5). Pain is generally due to nerve root ischemia; paresis is from progressive nerve root ischemia and attenuation. Neurologic signs vary depending on cause and severity of compression, and may be acute or chronic, intermittent or persistent, static or progressive (Table 36-3). The most common neurologic abnormality is lumbosacral hyperpathia (i.e., pain on deep palpation of the lumbosacral junction). Back pain may be accentuated by hyperextension during lumbosacral manipulation. Unilateral or bilateral pelvic limb lameness due to referred pain from attenuation of the L7 and/or S1 nerve root is common. This finding often progresses to loss of conscious proprioception, development of motor weakness, and hind limb atrophy as nerve root ischemia and compression increase. Patellar reflexes may be normal or exaggerated due to loss of antagonism from sciatic innervation (i.e., attenuation of L7, S1-2 nerve roots). This should not be misinterpreted as an UMN sign. Urinary and anal sphincter disturbances may accompany back pain and paraparesis when S2 and S3 nerve roots become compressed. Patients rarely present with sphincter disturbances alone. Initial presenting signs of urinary sphincter disturbance may resemble chronic UTI (e.g., increased urgency, frequent urination). As nerve root compression progresses, urinary incontinence (i.e., dribbling) becomes evident. Generally, clinically apparent anal sphincter dysfunction occurs after urinary sphincter dysfunction, and is manifested by fecal incontinence and anal sphincter hypotonia or atonia on rectal examination. The degree of sphincteric incontinence may be a prognostic indicator; as incontinence increases, the prognosis becomes more unfavorable. Tail carriage or function may be affected as the caudal nerve roots are affected. Abnormalities may include (1) breeds with an erect tail will carry it in a lower position; (2) ability to wag the tail is decreased or absent; (3) tail manipulation results in pain; and (4) loss of tail sensation. Paresthesia and dysesthesia (i.e., burning or tingling sensations in areas supplied by entrapped nerve roots) may occur in the tail, lateral digits, perineum, or genitals and are manifested by the patient's constant licking and chewing of the affected area. Paresthesias and dysesthesias usually occur in the tail and lateral digits.

☞ **N O T E** • Exaggerated patellar reflexes may be a result of loss of antagonism from sciatic innervation (i.e., attenuation of L7, S1-2 nerve roots), not a UMN lesion.

TABLE 36-3

Neurologic Deficits Possible with Cauda Equina Compression

Nerve Involved	Nerve Roots Involved	Neurologic Exam Findings Possible
Cauda equina*	L6, L7, S1-3, Cd1-5	Back pain with or without any of the findings below
Sciatic nerve	L6, L7, S1, +/− S2	Sensory: loss of sensation on lateral digit; licking and chewing of lateral digit; knuckling Motor: decreased withdrawal reflex, especially hock flexion; hindlimb atrophy; motor weakness
Perineal nerve	S1, S2, S3	Sensory: decreased sensation to perineum and caudal thigh; licking perineum
Caudal rectal nerve	S2, S3	Motor: decreased to absent anal sphincter tone on rectal exam
Pelvic nerve	S1, S2, S3	Parasympathetic: loss of bladder control
Pudendal nerve	S1, S2, S3	Motor: varying degrees of urinary incontinence
Caudal nerves	Cd1-5	Sensory: decreased sensation to the tail; pain upon tail manipulation; excessive tail linking Motor: change in tail carriage and tail wag
Femoral nerve†	L4, L5, L6	Sensory: no change expected Motor: patellar reflex appears brisk due to absence of sciatic innervated antagonist muscles

*All neurologic abnormalities involving cauda equina ischemia and/or compression are LMN.
†Although the femoral nerve is not supplied by nerve roots of the cauda equina, when the patellar reflex is performed, it appears brisk (UMN); this is due to loss of antagonist muscles innervated by sciatic nerve and is not a UMN sign.

Radiography/Ultrasonography

Specific imaging techniques used to diagnose cauda equina syndrome vary depending on the cause of cauda equina compression. Patients with fracture/luxation may have survey radiographic findings listed in Table 36-4 (see also Fig. 36-5, p. 1140). Those with neoplasia of the lumbosacral spine, surrounding soft tissue, or nerve roots have survey radiographic and myelographic signs dependent upon tumor location (extradural, intradural-extramedullary, intramedullary; see Fig. 36-11). Patients with infectious cauda equina compression (diskospondylitis, vertebral osteomyelitis) may have osteolysis and/or osteoproduction of the vertebral body, intervertebral space, or both (see Fig. 37-1 on p. 1152).

The process of imaging the lumbosacral spine to diagnose cauda equina compression secondary to chronic degenerative disk disease, intervertebral disk extrusion, or congenital lumbosacral stenosis is often a challenge. Factors influencing the ability to accurately image the L7-S1 junction are listed in Table 36-5. Imaging techniques must be evaluated in light of historical and neurologic examination findings. Commonly performed imaging procedures include survey radiography, stress radiography, myelography, diskography, and epidurography. Results depend on the cause of compression (i.e., chronic degenerative disk disease, intervertebral disk extrusion, or congenital lumbosacral stenosis) and are listed in Table 36-6. Techniques for performing these procedures are discussed and illustrated in Figs. 33-11 to 33-20. Intraosseous venography is technically demanding and results are inconsistent; thus, the technique is not recommended by the author. CT scan and MRI are helpful, but may be cost prohibitive.

Electromyography—particularly of the tail base, pelvic diaphragm, and muscles of sciatic distribution—can reveal spontaneous electrical activity indicative of LMN disease. Electrodiagnostic findings, coupled with typical historical, neurologic, and imaging results may support a diagnosis of cauda equina compression.

Laboratory Findings

Laboratory findings are generally nonspecific. Patients with cauda equina compression secondary to an infection may have leukocytosis, with or without left shift. Patients previously treated with corticosteroids may have a stress leukogram and elevated hepatic enzymes.

DIFFERENTIAL DIAGNOSIS

Differential diagnoses for cauda equina compression include: fracture/luxation; diskospondylitis; vertebral osteomyelitis; fibrocartilaginous emboli; neoplasia of the spine, surrounding soft tissue, or nerve roots; chronic degenerative disk disease; herniated intervertebral disk extrusion; or congenital lumbosacral stenosis. Disorders not associated with the lumbosacral junction that mimic cauda equina syndrome include hip dysplasia, metabolic disorders causing weakness, and degenerative myelopathy. Diagnostic tools include careful historical, physical, and neurologic examinations, laboratory data, multiple imaging procedures, and electrodiagnostics. Surgical exploration may be necessary for a definitive diagnosis.

MEDICAL MANAGEMENT

Medical management of patients with cauda equina compression depends on etiology. The treatment for patients with fracture/luxation is described on p. 1107; for diskospondylitis or vertebral osteomyelitis, p. 1153; and for neoplasia of the spine, surrounding soft tissue, or nerve roots, p. 1148.

TABLE 36-4

Potential Radiographic Findings in Dogs with Cauda Equina Syndrome Associated with Fracture/Luxation

Discontinuity of bony structures (i.e., spinous process, lamina, pedicle, vertebral body)
Malalignment of intervertebral space and/or articular facets
Fracture lines in the vertebral body and/or spinous processes of L7, S1-3
Loss of continuity or malalignment of the spinal canal
Combination of above

TABLE 36-5

Factors Influencing Ability to Accurately Image the L7-S1 Junction

Superimposed density of the wings of the ilium obscuring L7-S1 intervertebral foramen, intervertebral space, and vertebral bodies
Inconsistent termination of the dural sac (i.e., filum terminale)
Exclusively soft-tissue changes not evident on many imaging procedures
Technical difficulty of performing specific imaging procedures (e.g., intraosseous venography, diskography)
Cost of special imaging techniques (e.g., CT scan, MRI)
Inconsistent findings (i.e., false negative results)
Difficulty in interpretation of findings

Medical management of patients with cauda equina compression secondary to chronic degenerative disk disease, intervertebral disk extrusion, and congenital lumbosacral stenosis is based on severity and duration of neurologic signs, as well as serial neurologic examinations (Table 36-7). Medical management consists of strict confinement for 4 to 6 weeks and nonsteroidal antiinflammatory drug (NSAID) therapy (Table 36-8). Steroids are of little benefit to patients with nerve root injury. If nonsteroidal antiinflammatory drug therapy is indicated in the first course of therapy, one of the treatment schedules in Table 36-8 may be tried. Nonsteroidal antiinflammatory drugs may cause serious gastrointestinal side effects; treatment regimes are described in Table 34-12. Potential side effects of aspirin use are platelet function abnormalities and gastric irritation/ulceration. Bone marrow suppression and gastric irritation/ulceration may occur with phenylbutazone. Flunixin meglumine causes gastric irritation/ulceration and prolonged treatment (more than 2 days) may cause gastric ulceration/perforation.

SURGICAL TREATMENT

Surgical objectives include nerve root decompression and vertebral stabilization. Specific surgical procedures for patients with cauda equina compression depend on the etiology. Treatment for patients with fracture/luxation is described on p. 1142, diskospondylitis or vertebral osteomyelitis on p. 1153, and neoplasia of the spine, surrounding soft tissue, or nerve roots on p. 1148. The surgical treatment of patients with cauda equina compression secondary to chronic degenerative disk

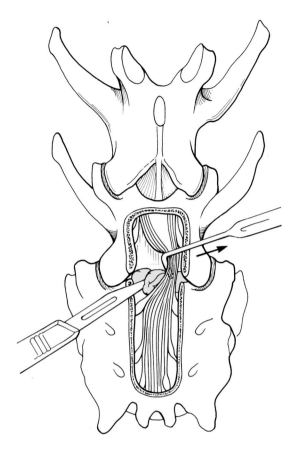

FIG. 36-4
Retract nerve roots laterally with care to facilitate excision of hypertrophied dorsal annulus fibrosus.

disease, intervertebral disk extrusion, and congenital lumbosacral stenosis is based on severity and duration of neurologic signs (see Table 36-7), outcome of medical management (see Table 36-8), results of imaging (see Table 36-6), EMG findings, and serial neurologic examinations (see Table 36-7).

Preoperative Management

Preoperative management of patients with cauda equina compression is similar to that described for patients with other lumbosacral compressive lesions (see p. 1131). Preoperative steroids are not recommended because they do not protect nerve roots.

Anesthesia

Suggested anesthetic protocols for use in patients with lumbosacral spinal disorders are discussed on p. 1049.

Surgical Anatomy

Knowledge of topographic anatomy of the cauda equina and its relationship to lumbar, sacral, and caudal vertebrae will facilitate an understanding of possible neurologic findings in patients with cauda equina compression, as well as the surgical manipulation necessary for decompression (see Fig. 36-3). Dorsal lamina, articular facets and joint capsule, spinal canal diameter, dorsal annulus fibrosus,

Results of Various Imaging Techniques Based on Etiology of Cauda Equina Compression

Imaging Technique	Possible Findings
Chronic degenerative disk disease (DDD)*	
Survey radiographs	Transitional vertebrae[†]; varying degrees of spondylosis[‡]; may be normal
Stress radiographs	Perform flexion and extension; combine with epidurography: *extension:* spinal canal diameter reduces, contrast is obliterated; *flexion:* spinal canal opens, contrast fills previous compression; may be normal
Myelography	Usually normal; extradural compression may be seen if lesion is large and filum terminale reaches far enough caudally; rules out lesion cranial to L6
Diskography	Irregular contrast pattern within the nucleus pulposus; can inject greater than 0.1 ml volume of contrast medium; may be normal (i.e., cannot inject greater than 0.1 ml, smooth contrast pattern)
Epidurography	Contrast flow is stopped or elevated at L7-S1 interspace; combine with stress positioning; may be normal (i.e., contrast flows unobstructed along floor of canal at L7-S1)
Acute intervertebral disk extrusion*	
Survey radiographs	May be normal; may see fogged L7-S1 intervertebral foramen; early spondylosis[‡]
Stress radiographs	Usually normal
Myelography	May be normal; if disk fragments are large and filum terminale extends caudal to L7-S1, may see extradural compression; rules out lesion cranial to L6
Diskography	Extravasation of contrast medium in canal; can inject greater than 0.1 ml volume of contrast medium
Epidurography	Contrast flow is stopped or elevated at L7-S1 interspace
Congenital stenosis	
Survey radiographs	Narrow canal diameter; transitional vertebra[†]; enlarged articular facets; rarely see signs consistent with degenerative disk disease (DDD)
Stress radiographs	Normal early; may see signs consistent with DDD later; combine with epidurography
Myelography	May be normal; may see signs consistent with DDD later if filum terminale extends caudal to L7-S1; rules out lesion cranial to L6
Diskography	Normal early; may see signs consistent with DDD later
Epidurography	Normal early; contrast flow is stopped or elevated at L7-S1 interspace later; combine with stress positioning

*Neurologic examination: interpretation of results of imaging procedures must be performed in light of historical, physical, and neurologic examination findings
[†]Transitional vertebrae are vertebrae that possess properties of two major divisions of the vertebral column. Lumbosacral anomalies include sacralization of L7 (L7 becomes fused [unilaterally or bilaterally] to the sacrum), lumbarization of S1 (S1 becomes a lumbar vertebra and S2 is fused to the sacrum), Cd1 may become fused to S3
[‡]Spondylosis is characterized by any combination of the following survey radiographic signs: collapse of the intervertebral space, sclerosis of vertebral endplates; ventral and lateral proliferation of bony spurs from the vertebral body in an attempt to bridge the intervertebral space (ankylosis), degeneration and collapse of the articular facets

interarcuate ligament, and dorsal longitudinal ligament are all points of anatomy that may play a role in cauda equina compression.

Positioning

Because patients are generally treated via laminectomy, they should be positioned in sternal recumbency with the hind legs tucked under the abdomen to encourage flexion and facilitate exposure of the dorsal lumbosacral intervertebral space (see Fig. 36-1).

SURGICAL TECHNIQUES

Surgical techniques for dorsal laminectomy, hemilaminectomy, facetectomy, and foramenotomy are described on p. 1101.

Patients with Chronic Degenerative Disk Disease

Patients diagnosed with chronic degenerative disk disease require enough exposure of the spinal canal to decompress all attenuated nerve roots. Depending upon neurologic examination findings and results of imaging, adequate decompression involves dorsal laminectomy, with or without foramenotomy and facetectomy. *Perform a dorsal laminectomy on patients with dorsal compression from lamina and interarcuate ligament. Use a No. 11 scalpel blade and ophthalmic forceps to carefully resect the ligament. In patients with lateral compression, perform a facetectomy to decompress the L7 and S1 nerve roots from the bulbous articular facets. In patients requiring further lateral decompression of the L7 nerve root,*

TABLE 36-7

Recommended Therapy* for Patients with Cauda Equina Compression (i.e., Chronic Degenerative Disk Disease, Intervertebral Disk Herniation, Congenital Lumbosacral Stenosis, Lumbosacral Fracture/Luxation, or Diskospondylitis/Vertebral Osteomyelitis†) Based on Clinical Presentation

Initial Treatment§		Result	Second Treatment§	Result	Third Treatment§
Back pain only, with or without paresthesia or dysesthesia					
	Cage rest only	Improvement	Continue cage rest	Improvement	Follow
		Static	NSAIDs‡	Static/deteriorating	Consider surgery
		Deteriorating	Consider surgery¶		
Back pain; mild paraparesis; no urinary incontinence					
	NSAIDs	Improvement	Cage rest/NSAIDs	Improvement	Cage rest/follow
		Static	Continue NSAIDs	Static/deteriorating	Consider surgery
		Deteriorating	Consider surgery		
Back pain; mild paraparesis; early urinary incontinence					
	NSAIDs	Improvement	Cage rest/NSAIDs	Improvement	Cage rest/follow
		Static	Consider surgery		
		Deteriorating	Consider surgery		
Back pain; moderate paraparesis; no urinary incontinence					
	NSAIDs	Improvement	Cage rest/NSAIDs	Improvement	Cage rest/follow
		Static	Consider surgery		
		Deteriorating	Consider surgery		
Back pain; severe paraparesis; no urinary incontinence					
	Consider surgery				
Back pain; moderate or severe paraparesis; urinary incontinence					
	Consider surgery				

*All patients are strictly confined (4 to 6 weeks) as part of their medical management regardless of the drug used or duration of drug therapy.
†Patients suspected of having L7-S1 diskospondylitis or vertebral osteomyelitis should also be treated with antimicrobials (see Tables 34-5 amd 34-6).
‡NSAIDs = nonsteroidal anti-inflammatory drugs; specific drugs, dosages, and duration of therapy are listed in Table 36-8.
§Initial treatment may be the first 24 to 48 hours or 3 to 5 days depending upon results of serial neurologic examinations. Second and third treatments are also dependent upon neurologic status.
¶Regardless of clinical presentation, if a client cannot afford surgery, a course of cage rest and NSAID therapy should be attempted.

perform a foramenotomy to establish complete decompression. Perform unilateral or bilateral facetectomy/foramenotomy based on neurologic exam findings, results of imaging, and surgical findings. Approach nerve root compression from the ventral floor of the spinal canal (i.e., protrusion of dorsal annulus fibrosus) through careful retraction of nerve roots, sharp annular incision, and mass removal (Fig. 36-4). Patients may require all or a variety of the above decompressive techniques. Spinal stabilization is not indicated unless spinal instability is documented (see p. 1142).

Patients with Acute Intervertebral Disk Herniation

In patients with herniated intervertebral disk material, perform a dorsal laminectomy if disk fragments are located on the midline or bilaterally, or a hemilaminectomy if neurologic signs and imaging results lateralize disk fragments to one side. Adequately expose the spinal canal to achieve complete mass removal. Spinal stabilization is generally not indicated unless spinal instability is documented (see p. 1142).

Patients with Congenital Lumbosacral Stenosis

In patients with congenital lumbosacral stenosis, perform a dorsal laminectomy with unilateral or bilateral facetectomy based upon neurologic signs, imaging results, and surgical findings. If stenosis is radiographically or surgically demonstrated extending from L6 to S1, perform a multilevel dorsal laminectomy and bilateral facetectomy from L6 to S1.

TABLE 36-8
Nonsteroidal Antiinflammatory Drugs (NSAID)
Aspirin 10 mg/kg PO, BID for 2 to 3 days*
Phenylbutazone (Butazolidin) 22 mg/kg PO, TID (not to exceed 800 mg/day) for 2 to 3 days*
Flunixin meglumine (Banamine) 0.5-1.0 mg/kg IV, IM, or SC; do not give for more than 2 days
*Reevaluate patient with serial neurologic examinations; if no response, continue the drug or consider alternate NSAID therapy or surgery

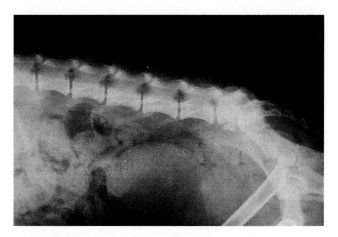

FIG. 36-5
Lateral radiograph of a dog with an L7 fracture. Notice the cranioventral displacement of the sacrum, pelvis, and L7 fracture fragment, which is typical with these fractures.

Remove interarcuate ligaments dorsally and facets laterally to provide complete decompression. Place a free fat graft over the entire laminectomy defect. Spinal stabilization is generally indicated as spinal instability is likely (see p. 1142).

SUTURE MATERIALS/SPECIAL INSTRUMENTS

Special instruments necessary for laminectomy of the lumbosacral junction are similar to those listed in Table 35-2 on p. 1108. It is important to practice each technique, become familiar with regional anatomy, and learn proper use of special instrumentation prior to performing these surgeries.

POSTOPERATIVE CARE AND ASSESSMENT

Critical care observation for the first 24 postoperative hours includes intravenous fluids, analgesics, antibiotics, seizure alert (if the workup required a myelogram), and neurologic examination. A guide to immediate and long-term postoperative care and assessment for ambulatory and nonambulatory patients is given in Tables 35-3 and 35-4 on pp. 1108 and 1109, respectively.

PROGNOSIS

Prognosis for cauda equina compression depends upon the etiology, neurologic deficits on presentation, and treatment regime chosen (i.e., medical or surgical). The prognosis for medically managed patients with mild to moderate back pain, mild lameness, absent or mild paraparesis, and/or no urinary incontinence is favorable to excellent. Medically managed patients with severe back pain, moderate to severe lameness, moderate to severe paraparesis, and/or urinary incontinence is guarded to unfavorable. If patients with mild neurologic deficits show static or deteriorating signs or loss of urinary continence during medical management, early surgical decompression has a better prognosis.

Generally, prognosis for surgically treated patients with acute back pain, mild to moderate lameness, mild to moderate paraparesis, and no urinary incontinence is favorable to excellent. Prognosis for patients with chronic back pain, severe lameness, severe paraparesis, and urinary incontinence is guarded to unfavorable. Regardless of other presenting signs, urinary incontinence implies an unfavorable prognosis if decompression is delayed.

Suggested Reading

Barthez PY, Morgan JP, Lipsitz D: Discography and epidurography for evaluation of the lumbosacral junction in dogs with cauda equina syndrome, *Vet Radiol Ultrasound* 35:152, 1994.

Berzon JL, Dueland R: Cauda equina syndrome: pathophysiology and report of seven cases, *J Am Anim Hosp Assoc* 15:635, 1979.

de Haan JJ, Shelton SB, Ackerman N: Magnetic resonance imaging in the diagnosis of degenerative lumbosacral stenosis in four dogs, *Vet Surg* 22:1, 1993.

Jones JC, Wilson ME, Martels JE: A review of high resolution computed tomography and a proposed technique for regional examination of the canine lumbosacral spine, *Vet Radiol Ultrasound* 35:339, 1994.

Karkkainen M, Punto LU, Tulamo RM: Magnetic resonance imaging of canine degenerative lumbar spine disease, *Vet Radiol Ultrasound* 34:399, 1993.

Koper S, Mucha M: Visualization of the vertebral canal veins in the dog: a radiological method, *Vet Radiol* 18:105, 1975.

McNeel SV, Morgan JP: Intraosseus vertebral venography: a technique for examination of the canine lumbosacral junction, *Vet Radiol* 19:168, 1977.

Morgan JP, Atilola M, Bailey CS: Vertebral canal and spinal cord mensuration: a comparative study of its effect on lumbosacral myelography in the dachshund and German shepherd dog, *J Am Vet Med Assoc* 191:951, 1987.

Morgan JP et al: Lumbosacral transitional vertebrae as a predisposing cause of cauda equina syndrome in German shepherd dogs: 161 cases (1987–1990), *J Am Vet Med Assoc* 202:1877, 1993.

Ness MG: Degenerative lumbosacral stenosis in the dog: a review of 30 cases, *J Sm Anim Pract* 35:185, 1994.

Oliver JE, Selcer RR, Simpson S: Cauda equina compression from lumbosacral malarticulation and malformation in the dog, *J Am Vet Med Assoc* 173:207, 1978.

Palmer RH, Chambers JN: Canine lumbosacral diseases. Part I. Anatomy, pathophysiology, and clinical presentation, *Comp Cont Educ Pract Vet* 13:61, 1991.

Palmer RH, Chambers JN: Canine lumbosacral diseases. Part II. Definitive diagnosis, treatment, and prognosis, *Comp Cont Educ Pract Vet* 13:213, 1991.

Schmid V, Lang J: Measurements on the lumbosacral junction in normal dogs and those with cauda equina compression, *J Sm Anim Pract* 34:437, 1993.

Sisson AF et al: Diagnosis of cauda equina abnormalities by using electromyography, discography, and epidurography in dogs, *J Vet Int Med* 6:253, 1992.

Slocum B, Devine T: L7-S1 fixation-fusion for treatment of cauda equina compression in the dog, *J Am Vet Med Assoc* 188:31, 1986.

Tarvin G, Prata RG: Lumbosacral stenosis in dogs, *J Am Vet Med Assoc* 177:154, 1980.

Watt PR: Degenerative lumbosacral stenosis in 18 dogs, *J Sm Anim Pract* 32:125, 1991.

FRACTURES AND LUXATIONS OF THE LUMBOSACRAL SPINE

DEFINITIONS

Traumatic or pathologic disruption of osseous and supporting soft-tissue structures of the caudal lumbar, sacral, and first caudal vertebrae (i.e., L6, L7, S1-3, Cd1-5) may result in vertebral fracture or luxation and subsequent nerve root compression (i.e., caudal equina).

SYNONYMS

Broken back, caudal lumbar fracture, vertebral fracture

GENERAL CONSIDERATIONS AND CLINICALLY RELEVANT PATHOPHYSIOLOGY

Fractures and luxations of the caudal lumbar vertebra, lumbosacral articulation, sacrum, and caudal vertebrae generally result from direct flexional trauma to the hind quarters. Fractures are usually oblique or short oblique involving the vertebral body of L6 or L7, and may be accompanied by luxation of articular facets. Cranioventral displacement of the caudal segment typically occurs due to muscular forces acting on the sacrum and pelvis, along with the weight of the pelvic mass (Fig. 36-5). Lumbosacral fractures are fairly common due to the static-kinetic relationship of the relatively fixed sacrum to the mobile caudal lumbar and caudal vertebral bodies. The most common cause of fracture/luxation is vehicular trauma. The spinal cord terminates in the body of L6; therefore, neurologic signs are usually associated with trauma to nerve roots of the cauda equina (i.e., L6-7, S1-3, and Cd 1-5) instead of the spinal cord. Due to the ability of nerve roots to resist traumatic injury, substantial displacement of the fracture or luxation may still leave the patient neurologically intact. Conversely, fractures or luxations may occur in which severe displacement of the fracture/luxation segments causes tethering or avulsion of nerve roots, and will occasionally produce trauma to the caudal spinal cord; neurologic deficits in these patients are often profound.

DIAGNOSIS
Clinical Presentation

Signalment. There is no specific age, sex, or breed predilection for canine or feline lumbosacral fracture/luxation. However, dogs are more likely to sustain this injury than cats, and there is a trend of dogs less than 3 years of age being affected more frequently.

History. Nearly 80% to 90% of dogs and cats with lumbosacral fracture/luxation have a history of recent vehicular trauma (Selcer, Bubb, Walker, 1991). Patients generally present with varying degrees of lumbar pain, ambulatory or nonambulatory paraparesis, and decreased anal and tail tone.

Physical Examination Findings

Severe traumatic injury often produces additional injuries (e.g., cardiopulmonary, urinary, diaphragmatic hernia, appendicular skeleton, second vertebral fracture/luxation). A thorough physical examination of each system to identify concurrent injury is necessary. Patients that struggle during physical examination or that have profound neurologic deficits should be secured to a rigid platform to prevent further nerve root trauma until a definitive course of action can be taken.

Lumbosacral fracture/luxation may cause trauma and sustained compression to the cauda equina. The most commonly involved nerve roots are L6-7, S1-3, and Cd1-5. Major nerves associated with these nerve roots include the sciatic nerve (L6, L7, S1, and/or S2), perineal nerve (S1, S2, S3), caudal rectal nerve (S2, S3), pelvic nerve (S1, S2, S3), pudendal nerve (S1, S2, S3), and caudal nerves of the tail (Cd1-5). Because of the regional anatomy innervated by the cauda equina, ischemia and/or compression may produce a wide variety of neurologic signs (see Table 36-3). Although a variety of neurologic deficits may occur, the most common presentation is lumbosacral hyperpathia (i.e., pain on deep palpation of the lumbosacral junction), LMN ambulatory or nonambulatory paraparesis, varying degrees of anal sphincter atonia, and abnormalities in tail carriage and sensation.

Radiography/Ultrasonography

Neurologic examination localizes the lesion to the caudal lumbar and sacral region. Survey radiographs are diagnostic and generally reveal an oblique or short oblique fracture through the vertebral body of L6 or L7, or a luxation or subluxation between L6 and L7 or L7 and S1 (see Fig. 36-5). The caudal vertebral body is characteristically displaced cranioventral to the cranial vertebral body (see Fig. 36-5). Because of the relatively mild neurologic signs that may be seen with marked fracture/luxation displacement on survey radiographs, prognosis is based on neurologic examination findings, not radiologic findings. Moreover, as LMN signs predominate in patients with multiple lesions, neurologic examination may not identify a second thoracolumbar fracture/luxation. A complete series of spinal radiographs is recommended.

☞ **N O T E** · Up to 20% of patients with spinal fracture/luxation have a second fracture/luxation.

Laboratory Findings

Patients presenting with lumbosacral fracture/luxation secondary to severe trauma often have a stress leukogram and elevated hepatic enzymes. If patients sustain concurrent injuries such as uroabdomen, ruptured spleen, or pulmonary contusion, associated laboratory abnormalities may occur. Laboratory findings are usually nonspecific.

DIFFERENTIAL DIAGNOSIS

Fracture/luxation of the lumbosacral spine must be differentiated from other disorders causing cauda equina compression, including congenital lumbosacral stenosis, diskospondylitis, chronic degenerative disk disease, intervertebral disk extrusion, fibrocartilaginous embolism, and neoplasia of the spine, surrounding soft tissue, and nerve roots. Definitive diagnosis is made by analyzing history, neurologic localization, and radiographic results.

MEDICAL MANAGEMENT

Objectives of medical management include immobilization of the spine and patient confinement until fracture/luxation stabilization and union occur. The following conditions are recommended: strict confinement for 4 to 6 weeks in a dry, elevated padded cage; analgesics/nonsteroidal antiinflammatories as needed to control pack pain; urinary bladder expression four times daily; passive physical therapy of the hind legs two to three times daily; and serial neurologic examinations twice daily to assess patient response to therapy.

SURGICAL TREATMENT

Objectives of surgical management are decompression of the cauda equina (i.e., fracture/luxation reduction), followed by adequate spinal stabilization. Infrequently, patients may require dorsal laminectomy for complete decompression (i.e., when bone fragments are present in the spinal canal) or for its prognostic value in evaluating the severity of cauda equina damage. Surgical reduction and stabilization provides immediate relief of back pain, allows freedom of movement, decreases patient morbidity, and protects spinal roots from further trauma. Surgical vs. medical treatment is based on the patient's neurologic status at presentation, response to medical management, and serial neurologic examinations (see Table 36-7). Adequate stabilization of the lumbosacral junction can be provided by (1) transilial pins with Kirschner clamps, bent pins, or bone cement; (2) transilial pins and plastic dorsal spinous process plates; (3) transilial

pin, dorsal spinous process plates, and external skeletal fixation; (4) modified segmental spinal fixation; and (5) Steinmann pins and methylmethacrylate bone cement. Choice of technique is generally dictated by the surgeon's experience and equipment available.

Preoperative Management

Preoperative management of patients with cauda equina compression is similar to that described for any lumbosacral compressive lesion (see p. 1131). If concurrent spinal cord injury is not present, preoperative steroids are not recommended because they do not protect nerve roots. Lumbosacral instability predisposes the patient to further trauma, and care should be taken to support the patient's pelvis during preoperative manipulations.

Anesthesia

Suggested anesthetic regimes for use in patients with lumbosacral spinal disorders are discussed on p. 1049.

Surgical Anatomy

Refer to the description and illustration of topographic anatomy of the cauda equina in Figs. 36-2 and 36-3.

Positioning

The surgical approach for each stabilization technique requires dorsal exposure. Positioning the patient in sternal recumbency with the hind legs tucked under the abdomen encourages flexion of the dorsal lumbosacral region and facilitates fracture reduction and cauda equina decompression (see Fig. 36-1).

SURGICAL TECHNIQUE
L7 Fracture and L7-S1 Luxation

Transilial pins. *Expose dorsal spinous processes and lamina of L6, L7, and the entire median sacral crest as described for dorsal laminectomy on p. 1131. Because of the cranioventral displacement of the sacrum, visualization of the cranial aspect of the sacral crest is obscured by the lamina of L7. L7 laminectomy is not compatible with this technique. Use a periosteal elevator or small osteotome to elevate epaxial muscles and expose the articular processes of L7. Use the tip of a Kelly or Carmalt forceps and carefully place it in the lumbosacral junction. Visually monitor the depth of placement of the forceps to avoid injuring nerve roots. Hook the tip of the forceps under the cranial lamina of the sacrum to act as a lever against the caudal lamina of L7 (Fig. 36-6). Adequate exposure of the lumbosacral junction is facilitated by reducing the fracture/luxation. Prior to attempting reduction, place a bone forceps or towel clamp in the wing of each ilium. Have an unsterile assistant available to provide cranial traction on the patient's head or front legs. Reduce the fracture/luxation by making the simultaneous moves listed in Table 36-9. These manipulations force the sacrum caudodorsally, to reduce the fracture/luxation. Visualize the lumbosacral articular facets; when the articular processes of L7 and S1 are re-apposed,*

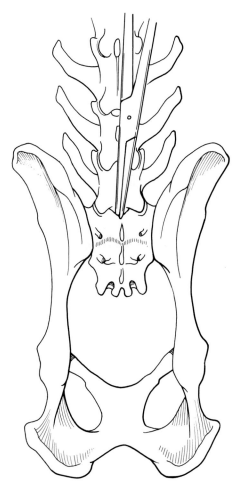

FIG. 36-6
Use of Kelly or Carmalt forceps to aid reduction of an L7 fracture. Hook the tip of the forceps under the cranial lamina of the sacrum and lower the jaws against the caudal lamina of L7.

TABLE 36-9

Manipulation of L7-S1 Fracture/Luxation During Reduction

Grasp the towel clamps or bone forceps on the wings of the ilium and pull caudal and slightly dorsal
Have the assistant place counter traction on the head or front legs
Lever the sacrum against the lamina of L7 while pressing ventrally on L6-7

TABLE 36-10

Selection of Steinmann Pin Size for Transilial Pins

Animal weight	Pin size (inches)
2-5 Kg	7/64
5-10 Kg	3/32
10-20 Kg	1/8
> 20 Kg	3/16

Fractures of the Body of L6 and L7, and Luxation of L7-S1

Transilial pins with dorsal spinous process plates. This technique provides stable fixation by incorporating the caudal lumbar spine to help counteract flexion (i.e., plastic plate) and by using multiple points of fixation to prevent rotational instability (i.e., transilial pins). It is compatible with dorsal laminectomy. *Prepare the dorsum of the back, from the midthoracic region to the base of the tail, for aseptic surgery. Make a dorsal midline skin incision such that three dorsal spinous processes cranial to the fracture/luxation can be exposed, and caudally to a point midway between the tuber ischii. Preserve the interspinous and supraspinous ligaments cranial to the lumbosacral junction by making two parallel lumbosacral fascial incisions on either side of the dorsal spinous processes. Elevate epaxial muscles to the level of the articular facets bilaterally. Carefully expose dorsal spinous processes, lamina, and articular facets of L6, L7, and/or sacrum, depending on location of the fracture. Reduce the fracture/luxation and maintain reduction with transarticular pins as described on p. 1142. Perform a dorsal laminectomy at this time, if indicated (see p. 1131). Select the appropriate size and length of plastic plates and secure them along each side of the dorsal spinous processes as described on p. 1124. Include a minimum of three dorsal spinous processes cranial to the fracture/luxation. Place two transilial Steinmann pins as described on p. 1142 (Fig. 36-8). Be sure to place each pin through predrilled holes in each plastic plate. Prevent pin migration by placing Kirschner clamps on the pin ends, bending the pin ends to 90 degree angles, or notching and covering the pin ends with bone cement as described (see Fig. 36-7). Place a final bolt, washer, and nut through the plates caudal to the transilial pins (see Fig. 36-8). Lavage the*

reduction is anatomic. *Place an 0.062 inch Kirschner wire through each L7-S1 articular facet to maintain fracture/luxation reduction. Next, incise gluteal fascia on the dorsolateral crest of the wings of each ilium, elevate the middle gluteal musculature, and expose the dorsolateral aspect of each ilial crest. Place an appropriate size Steinmann pin (Table 36-10) through the lateral aspect of the ilial wing, across the dorsal lamina of L7, and through the opposite ilial wing. Place a second pin in a similar fashion starting from the opposite side (Fig. 36-7, A). Be sure both pins cross over the dorsal lamina of L7. Prevent pin migration by employing one of the following techniques: 1) bend the ends of each pin at a 90 degree angle (Fig. 36-7, A); 2) connect the pins on each side with double Kirschner clamps of the appropriate size (Fig. 36-7, B); or, 3) notch the pins' ends with a pin cutter and incorporate them with methylmethacrylate bone cement (Fig. 36-7, C). If indicated, remove the interarcuate ligament and perform sacral laminectomy to visualize nerve roots. Lavage the surgical wound with sterile physiologic saline solution, cover the ends of the pins by closing gluteal fascia, and close epaxial muscles by apposing dorsal midline fascia. Close subcutaneous tissue and skin routinely.*

FIG. 36-7
Prevent migration of transilial pins by **A,** bending the ends of each pin at a 90-degree angle; **B,** connecting the pins on each side with a double Kirschner clamp; or **C,** notching the pins' ends with a pin cutter and incorporating them with bone cement.

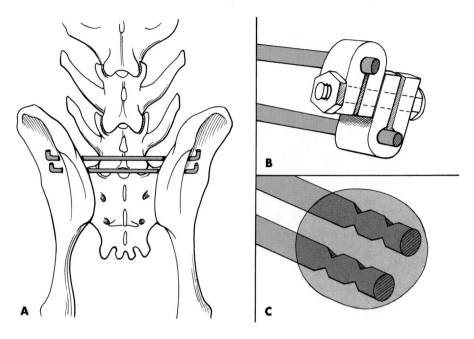

surgical wound and close dorsal lumbar fascia, gluteal fascia, subcutaneous tissue, and skin routinely.

Modified segmental spinal fixation. Modified segmental spinal fixation can be used in patients of all sizes. It does not require deep exposure, is compatible with dorsal laminectomy, simple to perform, versatile (i.e., can be used in combination with other techniques), and results in a stable repair. *Approach the dorsal aspect of the lumbar and lumbosacral spine as described for transilial pins and dorsal spinous process plates on p. 1142. Expose three dorsal spinous processes cranial to the fracture/luxation. Expose, carefully reduce, and maintain fracture/luxation reduction as described for transilial pinning on p. 1142. Perform a dorsal laminectomy at this time, if indicated (see p. 1131). Drill holes in the caudal articular processes and bases of dorsal spinous processes of at least two to three vertebrae cranial to the fracture/luxation. Drill holes in the cranial sacral articular facets to ensure a minimum of two points of fixation per pin in the sacroiliac segment. Preplace 3- to*

4-inch lengths of 18- to 20-gauge stainless steel wire through each hole. Drill two holes transversely through each ilial wing at the level of the dorsal lamina of the sacrum. Bend four appropriate size and length Steinmann pins at a 90-degree angle, remove the points, and pass the pins through the holes drilled in the wings of the ilia. Place the pins alongside the lamina and attach them to the articular facets and dorsal spinous processes using the pre-

Fracture of L6 or L7 Vertebral Bodies and Luxation of L6-L7 or L7-S1

Steinmann pins and methylmethacrylate bone cement. Steinmann pins and methylmethacrylate bone cement can be used in patients of all sizes. This technique requires

exposure of the dorsal surface of the transverse processes of L6 and L7, is compatible with dorsal laminectomy, versatile (i.e., can be used in combination with other techniques), requires constant reference to an anatomic specimen (i.e., spine), and produces a stable repair. Adequately expose the vertebrae cranial and caudal to the fracture or luxation. *Incise muscle attachments to articular facets and periosteally elevate epaxial muscles until the dorsal aspect of the transverse processes of L6 and L7 and dorsal lamina of the sacrum are identi- fied. Reduce the fracture/luxation and maintain reduction as described for transilial pinning on p. 1142. If the frac- ture involves the body of L6, place two pins in the body of L5 and two pins in the body of L7. If an L6-L7 luxation is be- ing repaired, place two pins in the body of L6 and two pins in the body of L7. Place pins and apply bone cement using the technique described on p. 1122. If the fracture involves the vertebral body of L7 or is an L7-S1 luxation, place two pins in the body of L6, two pins in the body of L7, and two pins in the cranial articular process of S1 with penetration through the ilium. If the fracture involves the vertebral body of L7, pin placement in L7 is dictated by the type of fracture present (i.e., avulsion fracture of the endplate, place two pins in L7; transverse fracture, place one or two smaller pins depending on the size of the fracture fragments; com- minuted fracture, no pins should be placed in L7). Insert pins directly into the vertebral bodies of L6 or L7 using the accessory process and transverse process as landmarks. In- sert pins into the center of the cranial articular processes of S1. Drive the pin until it penetrates the gluteal surface of the wing of the ilium. Direct the L6 and L7 pins cranioventral and from lateral to medial, and the S1 pins caudoventral and from lateral to medial. Drive pins to exit 2 to 3 mm from the ventral aspect of the vertebral bodies and wings of the ilia. Cut pins to leave 2 cm protruding and notch the ex-*

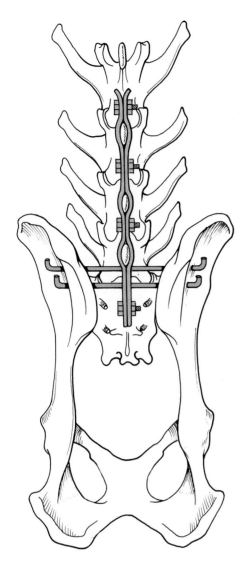

FIG. 36-8
Diagram showing use of transilial pins and plastic dorsal spinous process plates to repair L7-S1 fracture/luxations.

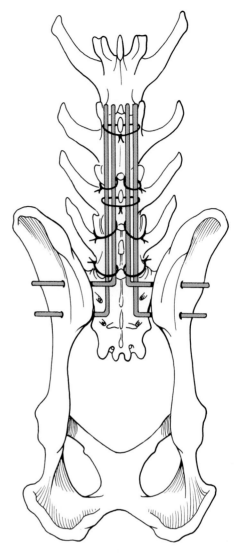

FIG. 36-9
Diagram showing proper pin placement for modified segmental spinal fixation of L6, L7, S1 fracture/luxations.

posed pin heads with a pin cutter. Thoroughly lavage and dry the surgical field (Fig. 36-10). Apply methylmethacrylate bone cement as described on p. 1122 (see also Figs. 35-23 through 35-25). If necessary, excise portions of epaxial muscles adjacent to the methyl methacrylate to facilitate closure. Rarely, relief incisions in the lumbodorsal fascia lateral to the methylmethacrylate are necessary to allow closure of the primary incision. Close subcutaneous tissues and skin routinely.

Transilial pins with dorsal spinous process plates and external skeletal fixation. Transilial pins can be used in patients of all sizes. This technique is compatible with dorsal laminectomy, offers dorsal and ventral compartment fixation, requires minimal special equipment, and results in a stable repair. *Performing a dorsal approach, expose three dorsal spinous processes cranial to the fracture/luxation. Expose dorsal lamina and artic-*

ular facets of affected vertebrae, reduce the fracture/luxation, maintain reduction, and place a dorsal spinous process plate as described on p. 1143. Pull skin and muscle to the center of the incision and percutaneously place a Steinmann pin through skin, muscle, wing of the ilium, holes in the dorsal spinous process plates, opposite ilial wing, and muscle and skin of the opposite side. Place a second Steinmann pin through the vertebral body cranial to the fracture/luxation. Start the pin just caudal to the junction of the transverse process and vertebral body. Pull skin and muscle to the center of the incision and percutaneously insert the pin through skin, epaxial and body wall muscle mass, vertebral body (i.e., just caudal to the junction of the transverse process and vertebral body), and through muscles and skin on the opposite side. Place single clamps on both ends of each Steinmann pin, and attach connecting bars to each side.

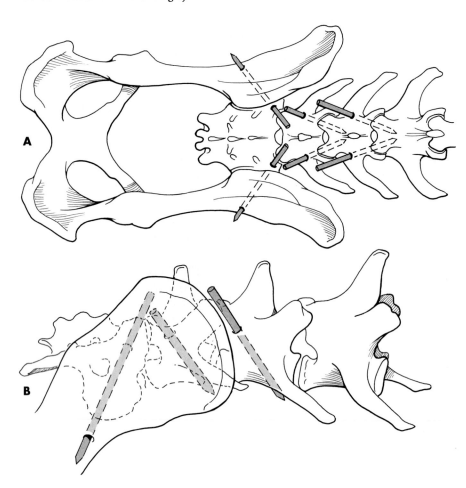

FIG. 36-10
A, Dorsal and **B,** lateral views showing proper pin placement in the ilial wings, articular facets of S1, and vertebral bodies of L6 and L7 when using Steinmann pins and methylmethacrylate bone cement to repair L6, L7, S1 fracture/luxations.

Close dorsal lumbar and sacral fascia, subcutaneous tissues, and skin routinely.

SUTURE MATERIALS/SPECIAL INSTRUMENTS

Depending on the technique chosen, the following special instruments will be needed: plastic dorsal spinous process plates, bone cement, Steinmann pins, skeleton, and Kirschner-Ehmer clamps and connecting bars.

POSTOPERATIVE CARE AND ASSESSMENT

Patients with lumbosacral fracture/luxation should be monitored postoperatively, as are patients with other lumbosacral disorders (i.e., strict confinement, analgesics as needed, short walks using an abdominal sling, frequent urinary bladder evacuation, and daily neurologic examinations). Long–term assessment consists of neurologic examinations and unanesthetized spinal radiographs at 1, 2, 3, 6, 9, and 12 months after surgery.

PROGNOSIS

Prognosis depends on severity of cauda equina compression (i.e., neurologic examination at presentation) and the treatment regimen chosen. Cauda equina nerve roots withstand considerably more trauma than the spinal cord. Patients with 100% lumbosacral spinal canal compromise may retain neurologic function of the hind limbs, anus, urinary bladder, perineum, and tail; their prognosis is favorable. However, patients with profound neurologic deficits (i.e., complete loss of motor function and deep pain perception) should be given a guarded prognosis, regardless of the percentage of spinal canal compromise. As the severity of presenting neurologic deficits increases, early decompression and stabilization allow a more favorable prognosis. If neurologic deterioration during medical management is determined early, immediate surgical intervention produces a more favorable outcome.

☞ **N O T E** · The amount of spinal canal compromise observed on lateral radiographs should *not* be used as a prognostic indicator.

Reference

Selcer RR, Bubb WJ, Walker TL: Management of vertebral column fractures in dogs and cats: 211 cases (1977–1985), *J Am Vet Med Assoc* 198:1965, 1991.

Suggested Reading

Bruecker KA, Seim HB III: Principles of spinal fracture management, *Semin Vet Med Surg* 7:71, 1992.

Dulisch ML, Nichols JB: A surgical technique for management of lower lumbar fractures: case report, *Vet Surg* 2:90, 1981.

Kuntz CA et al: Sacral fractures in dogs: a review of 32 cases, (abstract) *Vet Surg* 22:388, 1993.

Lewis DD et al: Repair of sixth lumbar vertebral fracture-luxations, using transilial pins and plastic spinous-process plates in six dogs, *J Am Vet Med Assoc* 194:538, 1989.

McAnulty JF, Lenehan TM, Maletz LM: Modified segmental spinal instrumentation in repair of spinal fractures and luxations in dogs, *Vet Surg* 15:143, 1986.

Patterson RH, Smith GK: Backsplinting for treatment of thoracic and lumbar fracture/luxation in the dog: principles of application and case series, *Vet Compar Orthop Trauma* 5:179, 1991.

Philips L, Blackmore J: Kirschner-Ehmer device alone to stabilize caudal lumbar fractures in small dogs, *Vet Compar Orthop Trauma* 4:112, 1991.

Shores A et al: Combined Kirschner-Ehmer apparatus and dorsal spinal plate fixation of caudal lumbar fractures in dogs: biomechanical properties, *Am J Vet Res* 49:1979, 1988.

Shores A et al: Combined Kirschner-Ehmer device and dorsal spinal plate fixation technique for caudal lumbar vertebral fractures in dogs, *J Am Vet Med Assoc* 195:335, 1989.

Slocum B, Rudy RL: Fractures of the seventh lumbar vertebra in the dog, *J Am Anim Hosp Assoc* 11:167, 1975.

Ullman SL, Boudrieau RJ: Internal skeletal fixation using a Kirschner apparatus for stabilization of fracture/luxations of the lumbosacral joint in six dogs, *Vet Surg* 22:11, 1993.

Wong WT, Emms SG: Use of pins and methylmethacrylate in stabilization of spinal fractures and luxations, *J Sm Anim Pract* 33:415, 1992.

NEOPLASIA OF THE LUMBOSACRAL SPINE AND NERVE ROOTS

DEFINITIONS

Neoplasms involving the lumbosacral vertebral and nerve roots are similar to those of the cervical and thoracolumbar regions (see pp. 1096 and 1128). Because the spinal cord terminates in the body of L6, primary spinal cord neoplasms are not encountered in the lumbosacral region.

SYNONYMS

Spinal tumors, spinal cord tumors, tumors of the spine, vertebral tumors, nerve root tumors

GENERAL CONSIDERATIONS AND CLINICALLY RELEVANT PATHOPHYSIOLOGY

Tumors of the lumbosacral vertebrae and nerve roots rarely occur. Tumor type, location (i.e., spine, surrounding soft tissue, or nerve root), and classification (i.e., extradural, intradural-extramedullary, or intramedullary) are similar to neoplasms of the cervical, thoracic, and lumbar spine (see pp. 1096). Regardless of tumor type or location, once the encroaching mass becomes large enough to cause cauda equina compression and ischemia, any of the neurologic signs asso-

ciated with cauda equina syndrome or fracture/luxation may occur (see Table 36-3).

DIAGNOSIS
Clinical Presentation

Signalment. There is no sex or breed predilection for patients with tumors of the lumbosacral spine. Generally, patients with spinal tumors are older than 5 years of age. An exception is solitary or multiple cartilaginous exostoses, which usually occur in patients less than 1 year of age.

History. History depends on the specific location of the neoplasm and the degree of cauda equina compression. Patients may present with variable degrees of back pain, with or without LMN ambulatory paraparesis (see Table 36-3). Anal sphincter atonia and urinary incontinence are inconsistent, but occur. Patients with nerve root tumors usually have a chronic history of dull hind leg lameness (i.e., monoparesis from root signature). As the tumor enlarges and compresses more of the cauda equina, paraparesis becomes evident. Patients with vertebral body or surrounding soft-tissue (i.e., extradural) tumors have an acute history of back pain and ambulatory or nonambulatory paraparesis. Careful historical examination may reveal previous (e.g., weeks to months) subtle back pain or hind limb lameness.

Physical Examination Findings

Physical and neurologic examination findings vary depending upon anatomic location of the tumor (i.e., spine, paraspinal soft tissue, nerve root), degree of nerve root compression/ischemia, specific nerve roots involved, and associated secondary effects (e.g., paraneoplastic syndrome). Generally, patients present with any combination of LMN signs associated with cauda equina compression (see Table 36-3). If a single nerve root is involved (e.g., neurofibroma of L7), neurologic examination findings may allow localization of the tumor to that nerve root.

Radiography/Ultrasonography

Radiographic findings suggestive of vertebral neoplasia include vertebral body osteolysis and/or osteoproduction. These findings are generally associated with primary bone tumors (i.e., osteosarcoma, chondrosarcoma, fibrosarcoma). Lysis of an intervertebral foramen suggests a nerve root tumor (i.e., neurofibroma, meningioma) (Fig. 36-11). Diagnosis of lumbosacral neoplasms may require stress radiography, myelography, or epidurography. Specific techniques for performing these procedures are given in Tables 33-8 and 33-9, and Figs. 33-14 through 33-20. Occasionally, CT scan or MRI is needed for a definitive diagnosis. If the neurologic examination accurately localizes the lesion to the lumbosacral space, exploratory laminectomy may provide a definitive diagnosis.

Electromyography, particularly of the tail base, pelvic diaphragm, and muscles of sciatic distribution, can reveal spontaneous electrical activity indicative of LMN disease. Electrodiagnostic findings, plus typical historical,

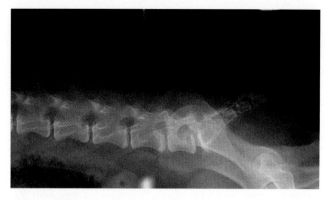

FIG. 36-11
Lateral radiograph of a dog with L7-S1 intervertebral foramen lysis suggestive of nerve root tumor.

neurologic, and imaging results may support a diagnosis of cauda equina compression.

Laboratory Findings

Laboratory findings are generally normal or reflect paraneoplastic syndromes (i.e., hypercalcemia or monoclonal gammopathy). Patients with severe back pain and those treated with corticosteroids may have a stress leukogram.

DIFFERENTIAL DIAGNOSIS

Differential diagnoses for cauda equina compression include: fracture/luxation; diskospondylitis; vertebral osteomyelitis; fibrocartilaginous emboli; neoplasia of the spine, surrounding soft tissue, or nerve roots; chronic degenerative disk disease; herniated intervertebral disk extrusion; or congenital lumbosacral stenosis. Disorders not associated with the lumbosacral junction that may mimic cauda equina compression include hip dysplasia, metabolic disorders that cause generalized weakness, and degenerative myelopathy. Diagnostic tools include careful historical, physical, and neurologic examinations, laboratory data, multiple imaging procedures, and electrodiagnostics. Surgical exploration may be needed for definitive diagnosis.

MEDICAL MANAGEMENT

Medical management is directed at both the primary lesion and secondary effects of the tumor. Corticosteroid therapy is generally not recommended for primary treatment of nerve root injury. However, steroids may be used for their antitumor effects. With most lumbosacral neoplasms, definitive medical treatment requires surgical exposure and incisional or excisional biopsy to determine tumor type and to plan appropriate adjunct chemotherapy, immunotherapy, irradiation, or combination therapy.

SURGICAL TREATMENT

Surgical treatment objectives include the definitive diagnosis of cauda equina compression (i.e., neoplasia, herniated disk, abscess), decompression and mass removal, incisional or excisional biopsy (wide surgical excision is preferred if possi-

ble), tumor staging, and, if necessary, spinal stabilization. If wide surgical excision creates spinal instability, stabilization is performed as described on p. 1142. Definitive histologic diagnosis is used to plan adjunct chemotherapy, immunotherapy, irradiation, or combination therapy.

Preoperative Management

Patients are given intravenous fluids before surgery. Preoperative management of patients with lumbosacral neoplasia is similar to that described for patients with any lumbosacral compressive lesion (see p. 1131). Preoperative steroids are not indicated because they do not protect nerve roots. If lumbosacral instability is suspected, care should be taken to support the pelvis during manipulations.

Anesthesia

Suggested anesthetic regimen for use in patients with lumbosacral spinal disorders are discussed on p. 1049.

Surgical Anatomy

Refer to the description and illustrations of the topographic anatomy of the lumbosacral spinal canal and cauda equina in Figs. 36-2 and 36-3.

Positioning

Exposing neoplasms of the lumbosacral region generally requires a dorsal approach and wide dorsal laminectomy with unilateral or bilateral facetectomy and foramenotomy. If stabilization is needed, a dorsal approach is also recommended. Therefore, position the patient in sternal recumbency with the hind legs tucked under the abdomen to gently flex the lumbosacral junction (see Fig. 36-1). This position facilitates exposure of the dorsal intervertebral space.

SURGICAL TECHNIQUE
Nerve Root Tumors

Tumors involving nerve roots of the cauda equina as they course through the lumbosacral spinal canal are best approached using dorsal laminectomy, facetectomy, and foramenotomy as described on pp. 1131 (Figs. 36-2 and 36-4). It is important to identify the specific nerve root or roots to be resected, and have a knowledge of their effect on the patient's neurologic function (see Table 36-3). Neurologic deficits created by single or multiple nerve root resection may incapacitate the patient to an unacceptable degree. In such cases, biopsy for histopathologic diagnosis and adjunct medical management may be indicated.

☞ **N O T E** · If possible excise the tumor so as to include 2 cm of adjacent normal appearing tissue.

Enter the spinal canal by carefully elevating the inner periosteal layer with a dental or iris spatula and ophthalmic forceps. Remove any remaining epidural fat. Identify cauda equina nerve roots on the floor of the spinal canal. Use a dural hook, dental spatula, or iris spatula to carefully follow the S1 and L7 nerve roots as they course along the floor of the spinal canal. Identify the L7 nerve root as it lies against the caudal aspect of the L7 pedicle, and follow it as it disappears through the L7-S1 intervertebral foramen. Carefully examine each nerve root for evidence of diffuse enlargement or localized bulging. If the lesion is resectable, identify the nerve root involved, carefully cauterize the root cranial to the lesion using bipolar cautery, transect the root with a No. 11 scalpel blade, and carefully elevate the transected portion of the root. Follow the affected nerve root caudal to the lesion and complete the resection as described above. Reexamine the cauda equina to rule out multiple nerve root tumors. Lavage the surgical wound and close tissues routinely.

Tumors Involving the Vertebral Body or Surrounding Soft Tissues

Tumors involving the vertebral body or surrounding soft tissues are best approached via dorsal laminectomy as described in Figs. 36-2 to 36-4. *Perform a dorsal laminectomy to remove affected bone and provide cauda equina decompression. If bony involvement is extensive and nonresectable, use a trephine to biopsy affected bone and perform a dorsal laminectomy to provide cauda equina decompression. If surrounding soft-tissue structures are involved, biopsy representative areas. If neoplastic tissue is cavitated or abscessed, obtain samples for anaerobic and aerobic culture and susceptibility testing. If spinal instability is diagnosed or occurs as a result of decompression, perform spinal stabilization as described on p. 1142.*

SUTURE MATERIALS/SPECIAL INSTRUMENTS

Special instruments necessary for laminectomy and spinal stabilization are listed in Tables 34-7 and 35-2.

POSTOPERATIVE CARE AND ASSESSMENT

Patients with neoplasia of the lumbosacral spine should be monitored postoperatively in a similar fashion as patients with other lumbosacral spinal disorders (see Tables 35-3 and 35-4). In general, strict confinement, analgesics as needed, short walks using an abdominal sling, frequent urinary bladder evacuation, and daily neurologic examinations are indicated. Long-term monitoring and adjunct medical therapy are dependent upon tumor type and surgical margins.

PROGNOSIS

Prognosis depends on tumor type (i.e., biologic activity), surgical margins (i.e., percent of tumor resection), and sensitivity to adjunct therapy (i.e., chemotherapy, immunotherapy, radiation therapy, or combination therapy). Malignant extradural neoplasms tend to have an unfavorable prognosis, benign extradural neoplasms have a favorable prognosis, and extradural-intramedullary neoplasms (i.e., nerve root tumors) have a guarded to unfavorable prognosis.

Suggested Reading

Fingeroth JM, Prata RG, Patnaik AK: Spinal meningiomas in dogs: 13 cases (1972–1987), *J Am Vet Med Assoc* 191:720, 1987.

Lane SB et al: Feline spinal lymphosarcoma: a retrospective evaluation of 23 cats, *J Vet Int Med* 8:99, 1994.

Levy MS et al: Spinal tumors in 37 dogs: clinical outcome and long-term survival, (abstract) *Vet Surg* 24:429, 1995.

CHAPTER 37

Nonsurgical Diseases of the Spine

SPECIFIC DISEASES

DISKOSPONDYLITIS

DEFINITIONS

Diskospondylitis is an infection of the intervertebral disk with concurrent osteomyelitis of adjacent vertebral endplates and vertebral bodies. Infection confined to the vertebral body is referred to as **vertebral osteomyelitis.**

SYNONYMS

Intradiskal osteomyelitis, diskitis, intervertebral disk infection, vertebral spondylitis

GENERAL CONSIDERATIONS AND CLINICALLY RELEVANT PATHOPHYSIOLOGY

Organisms most commonly associated with diskospondylitis are *Staphylococcus aureus* and *Staphylococcus intermedius*. They have been cultured from blood, urine, or both in a significant number of patients with diskospondylitis. Other bacteria and fungi isolated from affected animals are listed in Table 37-1. Infection generally originates in a nonvertebral location (i.e., UTI, pyogenic dermatitis, valvular endocarditis, dental disease) and spreads hematogenously. Vertebral infection usually begins in the endplate, where sludging blood in sinusoidal veins is predisposed to bacterial colonization. Bacteria diffuse through the cartilaginous endplate of the vertebral body to contact the disk, resulting in lysis of the adjacent endplate, disk necrosis, and collapse of the intervertebral space. Rarely, bacteria migrate dorsally and cause epidural abscess formation. Immunosuppressed patients may be predisposed to developing diskospondylitis. Areas of the spine most commonly affected include lumbosacral junction, cervicothoracic junction, thoracolumbar junction, and midthoracic disks. With the exception of the midthoracic spine, each predisposed area is at a static-kinetic junction of the spine (i.e., an area of spinal stability adjacent to an area of relative spinal mobility), encouraging stress concentration. Infrequently, diskospondylitis is caused by foreign body migration or postoperative sequelae to disk fenestration.

Because of the public health hazard, animals with diskospondylitis should be tested for *Brucella canis* infection. People are relatively resistant to infection with *B. canis*, however, and the disease is relatively mild compared with infections caused by other *Brucella*. Symptomatic human patients may experience fever, chills, fatigue, malaise, lymphadenopathy, and/or weight loss.

☞ **N O T E** • Be sure to inform clients of the potential health hazard of keeping *B. canis*–infected pets.

DIAGNOSIS
Clinical Presentation

Signalment. Diskospondylitis usually occurs in large-breed dogs (i.e., 30 to 35 kg or greater), with affected males outnumbering females approximately 2 to 1 (Johnson, Prata, 1983). Large male dogs may have a higher degree of activity and thus place more stress on the spine, presumably predisposing these areas to infection. Some reports suggest that German shepherds are overrepresented. Age at presentation is generally less than 4 years; however, conflicting reports suggest that a significant number of patients may be middle aged or older (i.e., 5 to 9 years) (Gilmore, 1987; Kerwin et al, 1992).

History. The onset of symptoms is generally insidious, but careful historical evaluation may reveal subtle lameness, difficulty jumping, anorexia, depression, and/or weight loss for weeks to months previously. Varying degrees of chronic paraparesis or tetraparesis may occur later; if the condition is acute it may be associated with pathologic fracture, epidural abscess, or the protrusion of infected dorsal annulus fibrosus into the spinal canal.

☞ **N O T E** • The hallmark of patients with diskospondylitis is spinal hyperpathia (i.e., neck or back pain on deep palpation) associated with systemic disease.

TABLE 37-1
Organisms Commonly Cultured from Animals with Diskospondylitis

Bacteria
- *Staphylococcus aureus*
- *Staphylococcus intermedius*
- *Brucella canis*
- *Streptococcus* spp.
- *Escherichia coli*
- *Pasteurella multocida*
- *Actinomyces viscus*
- *Norcardia* spp.
- *Mycobacterium avium*

Fungi
- *Aspergillus* spp.
- *Paecilomyces variotti*
- *Mucor* spp.
- *Fusarium* spp.

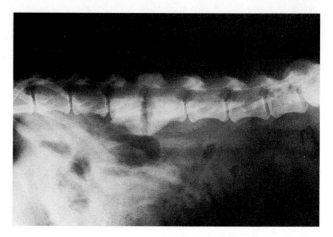

FIG. 37-1
Lateral radiograph of a dog with L3-L4 diskospondylitis. Notice the intradiskal lysis, vertebral endplate lysis, ventral spondylosis, and sclerosis surrounding lytic margins.

Physical Examination Findings

Physical and neurologic examination findings vary, depending on location, severity, and secondary effects of the infection. Patients presented early in the course of the disease may have systemic signs (i.e., depression, weight loss, fever); evidence of spinal involvement includes hyperpathia without paresis. Patients presented later generally have more subtle signs of systemic involvement coupled with profound neurologic signs (i.e., severe, single or multi-level hyperpathia, with varying degrees of paresis caudal to the lesion). Less frequently, patients may have an acute onset of back pain *and* ambulatory or nonambulatory paraparesis or tetraparesis, with or without systemic signs. Diskospondylitis should be considered in any patient with signs of spinal disorder and systemic illness. Specific neurologic signs depend on location of the lesion and are discussed on p. 1039.

Radiography/Ultrasonography

Diagnosis of diskospondylitis is confirmed by survey radiographs. The earliest radiographic signs become evident at 10 to 14 days after initial infection and include lysis of one or both vertebral endplates, followed by collapse of the intervertebral disk space. As the infection progresses, radiographic signs of continued vertebral endplate lysis, proliferative bony changes adjacent to the disk space, sclerotic margins, and ventral osseous proliferation with varying degrees of bridging spondylosis result (Fig. 37-1). Infrequently, and depending upon the offending organisms' continued virulence, vertebral body lysis followed by vertebral body shortening and spinal instability may be seen. The hallmark of diskospondylitis is intradiskal lysis. Patients with spondylosis deformans, an asymptomatic and generally incidental radiographic finding, do not have intradiskal lysis (Fig. 37-2). Bone scintigraphy is helpful in diagnosing early cases of diskospondylitis (i.e., as early as 3 days). Although scintigraphy is extremely sensitive in diagnosing early lesions, false negative results may occur. Myelography is mandatory in

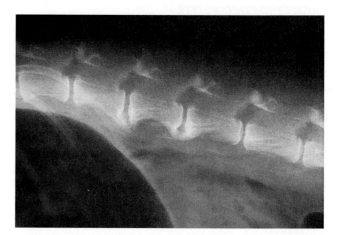

FIG. 37-2
Lateral radiograph of a dog with L2-L3 and L3-L4 spondylosis deformans. Notice the ankylosing spondylitic bridge of mature bone and normal intervertebral space and endplates.

patients requiring surgical intervention. It allows documentation of the presence of an extradural mass, dictates the necessary decompressive technique (i.e., dorsal vs. hemilaminectomy), and may suggest the presence or absence of spinal instability (i.e., stress myelography).

Laboratory Findings

Laboratory abnormalities vary considerably. Generally, a normal or stress leukogram is seen; leukocytosis does not occur unless other systemic abnormalities are present (i.e., UTI, endocarditis, pyoderma, prostatic abscess). The serum biochemical profile is usually normal, unless other systemic abnormalities are present. UTI has been reported in up to 40% of cases; occasionally the same organism is identified in blood and bone cultures (Kornegay, 1993). Blood cultures are positive in 50% to 70% of patients. Cerebrospinal fluid analysis is generally normal but will occasionally show mild protein elevation. A bone culture is generally not performed, but may be done by a percutaneous, fluoroscopically guided needle biopsy (e.g., similar to a bone marrow aspiration biopsy), or by surgical intervention. Culture results are generally unrewarding, but may identify the same organism in urine and blood cultures. Positive *Brucella* titers are occasionally found. The rapid slide test for *Brucella* has many false positive reactions, but few false negatives. Therefore, if the rapid slide test is positive, it should be confirmed with a tube agglutination or agar gel immunodiffusion test.

☞ **N O T E** · Because of the public health risk, perform *Brucella* titers in diskospondylitis patients.

DIFFERENTIAL DIAGNOSIS

Diskospondylitis must be differentiated from spondylosis deformans and spinal neoplasia. Spondylosis and sclerosis are common findings in both spondylosis deformans and diskospondylitis; however, vertebral endplate lysis is only seen with infection (see Fig. 37-2). Similarly, endplate lysis of adjacent or multiple vertebrae is uncommon in spinal neoplasia; lysis is generally associated with the vertebral body, lamina, pedicles, and dorsal spinous processes of a single vertebra (see pp. 1097 and 1148).

MEDICAL MANAGEMENT

Therapy depends on presenting neurologic examination, laboratory data (i.e., urine, blood, and/or bone cultures and *Brucella* titer), and serial neurologic examinations. Generally, patients that present with pain alone or pain and mild paresis, regardless of the number of vertebra affected, are treated with analgesics, antibiotics, and 4 to 6 weeks of strict confinement. Specific antibiotic therapy is based on results of a urine, blood, and/or bone culture and susceptibility testing and *Brucella* titer. Antibiotics chosen should be bactericidal, achieve minimum inhibitory concentrations in bone, and be effective against the causative organism. If cultures and titers are negative, empirical selection of an antibiotic is based on the most likely causative agent (i.e., *Staphylococcus intermedius* or *Staphylococcus aureus*). A β-lactamase resistant antibiotic (e.g., cephradine, clindamycin, cloxacillin) should be used in these patients (Table 37-2). A combination of a tetracycline (i.e., doxycycline, minocycline) plus an aminoglycoside (i.e., streptomycin, gentamicin, amikacin) or fluroguinolone (i.e., enrofloxacin) should be used for diskospondylitis secondary to *B. canis*. Patients should be treated until the *Brucella* titer is negative.

Most patients (i.e., 80% to 90%) respond to an appropriate course of medical management (Johnson, Prata, 1983). Patients unresponsive (i.e., continued hyperpathia without paresis) within 7 to 10 days to medical therapy should be treated with a different antibiotic. If pain persists, a third antibiotic may be attempted, or surgical curettage may be performed to obtain bone samples for culture and susceptibility testing, and to debride intradiskal lesions. Analgesics may be indicated in animals that appear to be in pain. Aspirin (5 to 10 mg/kg TID, PO for 7 days, then as needed up to 3 to 6

TABLE 37-2
Antibiotics for Use in Diskospondylitis*
Amikacin (Amiglyde-V)
10 mg/kg IV, IM, SC, TID
Cephradine (Veslosef)
20 mg/kg PO, TID
Clindamycin (Antirobe)
11 mg/kg PO, BID
Cloxacillin (Cloxapen, Orbenin, Tegopen)
10 mg/kg PO, QID
Doxycycline (Vibramycin)
5 mg/kg PO, BID
Enrofloxacin (Baytril)
5-10 mg/kg PO or IV, BID
Gentamicin (Gentocin)
2 mg/kg IM, BID for 1 week; monitor renal function
Minocycline (Minocin)
10 mg/kg PO, BID
Streptomycin
20 mg/kg BID, IM, for 1 week

*Duration of therapy may be based on one or a combination of the following guidelines:
- Treat for 6 to 8 weeks
- Treat for 2 weeks after resolution of clinical signs
- Treat until radiographic evidence of ankylosing spondylosis
- Treat until *Brucella* titer is negative

weeks) or phenylbutazone (Butazolidin - 22 mg/kg, TID for 7 days, then as needed up to 3 to 6 weeks) are most commonly used. Do not prescribe more than 800 mg of phenylbutazone per day.

SURGICAL TREATMENT

If a medically treated patient shows neurologic deterioration (i.e., paraparesis or tetraparesis) or if a patient presents with an acute onset of spinal hyperpathia and weakly ambulatory or nonambulatory para- or tetraparesis, the following procedures may be performed: myelography, spinal cord decompression, bone samples for culture and susceptibility testing, debridement of intradiskal lesions, and spinal stabilization (if indicated). Myelography should be performed to determine the specific location of the compressive lesion (see p. 1042). Spinal cord decompression may be performed via a dorsal laminectomy or hemilaminectomy; hemilaminectomy is preferred because it creates the least spinal instability. Spinal stabilization is performed if decompression and debridement result in spinal instability, or if instability is documented radiographically (i.e., stress myelography) prior to surgery. Techniques for spinal stabilization are described and illustrated on pp. 1093, 1122, and 1142.

Preoperative Management

See preoperative management for each specific location of the spine affected (i.e., cervical, thoracolumbar, and lumbosacral) on pp. 1049, 1101, and 1131, respectively.

Anesthesia

Suggested anesthetic protocols for spinal surgery are given on p. 1049.

Surgical Anatomy

Anatomic descriptions for each location of the spine affected (i.e., cervical, thoracolumbar, and lumbosacral) are on pp. 1051, 1101, and 1131, respectively.

Positioning

Refer to the surgical procedure chosen for recommendations for appropriate surgical positioning.

Surgical Technique

See surgical technique descriptions for each specific location of the spine affected (i.e., cervical, thoracolumbar, and lumbosacral) on pp. 1051, 1101, and 1131, respectively.

SUTURE MATERIALS/SPECIAL INSTRUMENTS

Avoid using nonabsorbable multifilament sutures (e.g., silk) in infected surgical sites.

POSTOPERATIVE CARE AND ASSESSMENT

After surgery, these patients should be assessed as described on pp. 1062, 1108, and 1133. Antibiotics should be continued for a minimum of 4 to 6 weeks.

PROGNOSIS

Prognosis is dependent upon neurologic examination findings at presentation and the patient's response to initial medical management. Patients with spinal hyperpathia only or spinal hyperpathia plus ambulatory paresis have a favorable to excellent prognosis. Those with spinal hyperpathia and weakly ambulatory paresis, particularly if weakness is a result of spinal pain, have a favorable prognosis. Patients with either of the above neurologic findings that do not respond to an initial course of medication have a guarded to favorable prognosis for responding to either a different antibiotic or surgical bone culture and intradiskal debridement.

Patients with an acute onset of spinal hyperpathia, weakly ambulatory or nonambulatory paraparesis or tetraparesis, evidence of an extradural lesion, and no evidence of spinal instability have a guarded prognosis when treated surgically. If these patients have evidence of spinal instability, the prognosis is guarded to unfavorable.

References

Gilmore DR: Lumbosacral diskospondylitis in 21 dogs, *J Am Anim Hosp Assoc* 23:57, 1987.

Johnson RG, Prata RG: Intradiskal osteomyelitis: a conservative approach, *J Am Anim Hosp Assoc* 19:743, 1983.

Kerwin SC et al: Diskospondylitis associated with *Brucella canis* infection in dogs: 14 cases (1980–1991), *J Am Vet Med Assoc* 201:1253, 1992.

Kornegay JN: Diskospondylitis. In Slatter D, editor: *Textbook of small animal surgery*, ed 2, Philadelphia, 1993, WB Saunders.

Suggested Reading

Dallman MJ et al: Disseminated aspergillosis in a dog with diskospondylitis and neurologic deficits, *J Am Vet Med Assoc* 200:511, 1992.

Kornegay JN, Barber DL: Diskospondylitis in dogs, *J Am Vet Med Assoc* 177:337, 1980.

Lappin MR, Turnwald GH: In Willard MD, Twedt H, Turnwald GH, editors: *Microbiology and infectious diseases in small animal clinical diagnosis by laboratory methods*, ed 2, Philadelphia, 1994, Saunders.

Lobetti RG: Subarachnoid abscess as a complication of diskospondylitis in a dog, *J Sm Anim Pract* 35:480, 1994.

Malik R, Latter M, Love DN: Bacterial discospondylitis in a cat, *J Sm Anim Pract* 31:404, 1990.

McKee VN, Mitten RW, Labuc RH: Surgical treatment of lumbosacral discospondylitis by a distraction-fusion technique, *J Sm Anim Pract* 31:15, 1990.

Smith KR, Kerlin RM, Mitchell G: Diskospondylitis attributable to a gram-positive filamentous bacteria in a dog, *J Am Vet Med Assoc* 205:428, 1994.

Turnwald GH et al: Diskospondylitis in a kennel of dogs: clinicopathologic findings, *J Am Vet Med Assoc* 188:178, 1986.

Watson E, Roberts RE: Discospondylitis in a cat, *Vet Radiol and Ultrasound* 34:397, 1993.

GRANULOMATOUS MENINGOENCEPHALITIS

DEFINITIONS

Granulomatous meningoencephalitis (GME) is an acute, progressive disorder of the central nervous system (CNS), characterized histologically by focal or disseminated perivascular granulomas in the meninges, brain, and spinal cord.

SYNONYMS

GME, inflammatory GME, focal GME, ocular GME, reticulosis, histiocytic encephalitis, neoplastic reticulosis

GENERAL CONSIDERATIONS AND CLINICALLY RELEVANT PATHOPHYSIOLOGY

GME is a neurologic disorder that may affect any portion of the CNS (i.e., meninges, brain, and spinal cord). The lesion is predominant in white matter; however, many dogs have meningeal involvement and occasionally gray matter may be affected. In advanced cases, perivascular lesions extend into the CNS parenchyma and merge with adjacent lesions, forming large coalescent granulomas. The severity of lesions and their regional location (i.e., cerebral, cerebellar, cervical spinal cord, brain stem) are variable. Three forms of the disorder have been described: disseminated, focal, and ocular. History, neurologic examination, laboratory findings, and course of disease may differ depending on the form (Table 37-3). The cause of GME is currently unknown. Suggested hypotheses include a cell-mediated immune response to the sustained presence of an infectious agent; an inflammatory process that may be transformed to a neoplastic one, possibly involving a cell-associated virus; or a genetic predisposition.

TABLE 37-3

Clinical Signs Associated with Various Forms of GME

Form*	Lesion Location†	Clinical Signs‡	Duration of Signs	Prognosis
Disseminated	Lower brain stem Cervical spinal cord Meninges	Acute onset; rapidly progressive; fever may occur early	1 to 8 weeks (25% are dead in 1 week)	Grave; may live 12 to 16 weeks
Focal	Brain stem Cerebral cortex Cerebellum Cervical spinal cord	Insidious onset; signs consistent with a space-occupying mass	3 to 6 months	Unfavorable; may live up to 12 months
Ocular	Ocular nerve	Sudden blindness; anisocoria	3 to 6 months§	Unfavorable; may live 12 to 18 months

*The disseminated and focal forms frequently occur together; the ocular form may occur alone or accompanied by the disseminated or focal forms.
†Although lesions can occur anywhere in the CNS, each form of the disease seems to have a predilection for specific locations. ‡Specific clinical signs are associated with lesion location; see p. 1039 for a description of signs expected in each location. §If the ocular form is present with the disseminated form, duration of signs and prognosis usually follow the disseminated form.

DIAGNOSIS
Clinical Presentation

Signalment. GME occurs in young to middle-aged dogs (i.e., 2 to 6 years); however, occasional reports of dogs as young as 9 months have been described (Thomas, Eger, 1989). Females are more often affected than males. This condition occurs most commonly in toy breeds, particularly poodles and terriers; mixed breeds and larger breeds are affected less frequently. GME is rarely diagnosed in cats.

History. Patients generally present with an acute history of continuous or episodic progression of multifocal neurologic disease that may involve the brain, meninges, and/or cervical spinal cord. Clinical presentation depends on location of lesions and the form of the disease (i.e., disseminated, focal, or ocular) (see Table 37-3).

Physical Examination Findings

Physical and neurologic examination findings are variable and depend on lesion localization and the form of disease present (i.e., disseminated, focal, or ocular) (see Table 37-3). Significant neurologic examination findings include cervical pain evidenced by nuchal rigidity (i.e., suggesting meningeal involvement) or nystagmus, head tilt, blindness, and facial and trigeminal palsy (i.e., suggesting brain stem involvement). Ataxia, paraparesis or tetraparesis, seizures, circling, altered states of consciousness, and behavioral changes are also common. Patients with the disseminated form may present with fever. Animals with the ocular form may have sudden blindness or pupillary abnormalities (i.e., anisocoria, decreased pupillary light reflexes).

Radiography/Ultrasonography

Survey radiographs are normal. Patients that have signs suggesting focal extradural spinal cord lesions (i.e., neck pain and varying degrees of tetraparesis) should have a cerebral spinal fluid (CSF) analysis prior to injecting contrast media into the subarachnoid space. Myelography is generally normal, but occasionally reveals diffuse spinal cord swelling. A CT scan (particularly when contrast-enhanced) may be

helpful in the diagnosis of focal GME. Focal intracranial GME may show contrast enhancement similar to that seen with intracranial neoplasia; enhancement is subjectively less in patients with GME than in patients with focal neoplasia. A presumptive diagnosis of GME is based on signalment, history, progression of clinical signs, CSF analysis, and results of a contrast-enchanced CT scan.

Laboratory Findings

CSF analysis often reveals a mild to marked pleocytosis consisting of lymphocytes, monocytes, and occasional plasma cells. Neutrophils may be seen in up to two thirds of affected animals. They generally make up less than 20% of the total cell count, but occasionally predominate. Protein concentrations are usually mildly to moderately elevated, occasionally without an elevation in cell count. Previous corticosteroid treatment does not appear to dramatically alter CSF cellularity. Techniques for performing cisternal and lumbar taps are described in Chapter 33. Patients with disseminated GME may be neutrophilic.

☞ **N O T E** · CSF obtained from the cistern is preferable to that obtained from a lumbar tap because the medulla and cervical spinal cord are usually more severely affected than the lumbar spinal cord.

DIFFERENTIAL DIAGNOSIS

GME should be suspected in any mature small-breed dog with acute, progressive, multifocal disease involving the brain, meninges, or cervical spinal cord. The differential diagnosis of GME must include other infectious diseases of the brain (i.e., bacterial, viral, fungal, parasitic, rickettsial), extradural cervical spinal disorders (i.e., intervertebral disk extrusion, fracture/luxation, instability, malformation), and primary (i.e., meningioma, glioma, astrocytoma, ependymoma) as well as metastatic neoplasia. Diagnosis is based on history, signalment, onset and progression of clinical signs, CSF analysis, results of imaging techniques, and postmortem examination of CNS tissue. Definitive diagnosis of GME is based on characteristic histopathologic lesions in affected CNS tissue.

MEDICAL MANAGEMENT

Corticosteroids are recommended for treatment of patients with GME. The type of steroid, route of administration, dosage schedule, and duration of therapy depend on initial presenting signs. Patients with moderate to severe clinical signs are initially treated with dexamethasone at 2 mg/kg IV; this dosage is decreased to 0.2 mg/kg daily over 3 to 4 days or until neurologic improvement is noted. The patient is discharged on prednisone (Table 37-4). Variations in the final dosage schedule are dependent upon response to therapy; however, patients should be continued on a maintenance dose indefinitely. If therapy is discontinued, rapid exacerbation of clinical signs often occurs and it may be difficult to achieve a second remission. Patients with mild clinical signs are treated initially with oral prednisone (see Table 37-4). Because of the poor long-term prognosis associated with the use of corticosteroids, alternate therapeutic regimes (antineoplastic drugs, immunosuppressive drugs, radiation therapy) have been tried. At this time, an adequate number of patients have not been treated and followed to determine efficacy. Patients with seizures should be treated with anticonvulsant medications.

SURGICAL TREATMENT

GME is not a surgical disorder.

PROGNOSIS

Prognosis for GME is generally unfavorable to grave (see Table 37-3). Duration of remission with corticosteroid therapy varies with the form of disease: patients with the disseminated form usually do not survive longer than 12 to 16 weeks; those with the focal form may survive for up to 12 months (particularly if the lesion is in the forebrain); patients with purely ocular GME may survive 12 to 18 months. Early diagnosis and aggressive corticosteroid therapy may improve remission time and quality of life.

Reference

Thomas JB, Eger C: Granulomatous meningoencephalomyelitis in 21 dogs, *J Small Anim Pract* 30:287, 1989.

Suggested Reading

Bailey CS, Higgins RJ: Characteristics of cerebrospinal fluid associated with canine granulomatous meningoencephalomyelitis: a retrospective study, *J Am Vet Med Assoc* 188:418, 1986.

Cook JR: Granulomatous meningoencephalomyelitis, *Vet Med Rep* 1:321, 1989.

Cordy DR: Canine granulomatous meningoencephalomyelitis, *Vet Pathol* 16:325, 1979.

Evans SM et al: Radiation therapy of brain masses, *J Vet Int Med* 7:216, 1993.

Plummer SB et al: Computed tomography of primary inflammatory brain disorders in dogs and cats, *Vet Radiol and Ultrasound* 33:307, 1992.

TABLE 37-4
Corticosteroid Therapy of Dogs with GME
Moderate to Severe Clinical Signs   **Dexamethasone**   0.2-2 mg/kg IV
Prednisone   1-2 mg/kg PO BID, for 2 to 3 weeks; taper over a 3- to 4-week period to 2.5 to 5 mg total dose EOD
Mild Clinical Signs   **Prednisone**   1-2 mg/kg PO, BID for 2 to 3 weeks; taper as described above

Sarfaty D, Carrillo JM, Greenlee PG: Differential diagnosis of granulomatous meningoencephalomyelitis, distemper, and suppurative meningoencephalitis in the dog, *J Am Vet Med Assoc* 188:387, 1986.

Speciale J et al: Computed tomography in the diagnosis of focal granulomatous meningoencephalomyelitis: retrospective evaluation of three cases, *J Am Anim Hosp Assoc* 28:327, 1992.

Thomson CE, Kornegay JN, Stevens JB: Analysis of cerebrospinal fluid from the cerebellomedullary and lumbar cisterns of dogs with focal neurologic disease: 145 cases (1985–1987), *J Am Vet Med Assoc* 196:1841, 1990.

DEGENERATIVE MYELOPATHY

DEFINITIONS

Degenerative myelopathy is a neurologic disorder of unknown etiology causing progressive demyelination of long-tract fibers, which begins in the thoracolumbar spinal cord.

SYNONYMS

German shepherd myelopathy

GENERAL CONSIDERATIONS AND CLINICALLY RELEVANT PATHOPHYSIOLOGY

Degenerative myelopathy is a progressive neurologic disorder causing varying degrees of paraparesis. Pathologic findings include loss of myelin in the spinal cord white matter, a process that generally begins in the thoracic region. The cause is currently unknown. Suggested hypotheses include an immune-related disorder in German shepherds, vitamin B deficiency, trauma, vascular disease, and familial neuronal atrophy. Thus far, all suggested etiologies remain unsupported.

DIAGNOSIS
Clinical Presentation

Signalment. Degenerative myelopathy generally occurs in middle-aged to older (i.e., 5 to 7 years) large–breed dogs, particularly German shepherds. There have been rare reports in smaller breeds (e.g., miniature poodles) and cats (Matthews, 1985; Mesfin, Kusewitt, Parker, 1980). There is no sex predilection.

History. Patients usually have a history of slowly progressive hindlimb weakness without back pain; signs may have been present for months. Owners commonly complain that the dog has difficulty rising up on the hind legs or that they hear scuffing or clicking of the hind toenails during ambulation.

Physical Examination Findings

The general physical examination is usually normal. A neurologic examination generally reveals UMN, ambulatory or weakly ambulatory paraparesis without spinal hyperpathia (i.e., back pain). Patients generally have symmetric or asymmetric loss of conscious proprioception (i.e., knuckling, wearing of toenails, stumbling), exaggerated patellar reflexes, and crossed extensor reflexes. Occasionally, patients show LMN (i.e., decreased patellar reflex) and UMN signs. Pain perception and urinary and fecal continence are not lost, even late in the disorder. Thoracic limbs are spared, unless the patient is maintained long enough after complete paraplegia.

Radiography/Ultrasonography

Survey radiographs and myelography are normal in patients with degenerative myelopathy. Myelography is used to eliminate other spinal cord disorders that mimic degenerative myelopathy (e.g., chronic disk protrusion, spinal neoplasia). If a mild disk protrusion is diagnosed on myelography, the degree of spinal cord compression should be correlated with observed neurologic signs before treatment is considered. Patients—particularly German shepherds—may have both diseases coexisting. Surgical treatment of a mild disk protrusion in the face of degenerative myelopathy may not be warranted. MRI may help demonstrate spinal cord lesions.

Laboratory Findings

Laboratory findings are generally normal. Cerebral spinal fluid analysis may show mild increases in protein; however, this finding can be consistent with chronic disk protrusion or spinal neoplasia.

DIFFERENTIAL DIAGNOSIS

The primary differential diagnoses for patients with degenerative myelopathy are chronic disk protrusion (i.e., Hansen type II disk protrusion), spinal neoplasia, and hip dysplasia. Survey radiographs and myelography differentiate chronic` disk protrusion and spinal neoplasia. Because hind leg signs associated with chronic hip dysplasia are caused by joint pain, careful orthopedic and neurologic examination can be used to eliminate this disorder. Some patients show signs of degenerative myelopathy and hip dysplasia. A strong presumptive diagnosis of degenerative myelopathy is based on compatible history and neurologic examination combined with normal survey radiographs and a myelogram. Definitive diagnosis is based on characteristic histopathologic changes in spinal cord parenchyma.

MEDICAL MANAGEMENT

Multiple treatment regimens have been suggested for patients with degenerative myelopathy including corticosteroids, non-steroidal antiinflammatory agents, vitamins (i.e., E and B complex), immune modifiers (i.e., suppressors and stimulants), interferon, and enzyme inhibitors (e.g., aminocaproic acid). Presently, no therapy has consistently been effective. Management of ambulatory and nonambulatory patients with thoracolumbar spinal disorders is described on p. 1108.

SURGICAL TREATMENT

Degenerative myelopathy is not a surgical disorder.

PROGNOSIS

Patients with degenerative myelopathy have an unfavorable prognosis. There is no known medical or surgical treatment that successfully halts the process of demyelination. Progression of this condition to a nonambulatory paraparesis may take months to years, depending upon the patient's neurologic status.

Suggested Reading

Averill DR: Degenerative myelopathy in the aging German shepherd dog: clinical and pathologic findings, *J Am Vet Med Assoc* 162:1045, 1973.

Longhofer SL, Duncan ID, Messing A: A degenerative myelopathy in young German shepherd dogs, *J Sm Anim Pract* 31: 199, 1990.

Matthews NS: Degenerative myelopathy in an adult miniature poodle, *J Am Vet Med Assoc* 186:1213, 1985.

Mesfin GM, Kusewitt D, Parker A: Degenerative myelopathy in a cat, *J Am Vet Med Assoc* 176:62, 1980.

Toenniessen JG, Morin DE: Degenerative myelopathy: a comparative review, *Comp Cont Educ Pract Vet* 17:271, 1995.

SPINAL CORD ISCHEMIA

DEFINITIONS

Fibrocartilaginous embolization (FCE) is the ischemic necrosis of a segment of spinal cord caused by herniation of intervertebral disk material into the spinal cord microvasculature.

SYNONYMS

Necrotizing myelopathy, ischemic myelopathy, embolic myelopathy, vascular episode, fibrocartilaginous infarct

GENERAL CONSIDERATIONS AND CLINICALLY RELEVANT PATHOPHYSIOLOGY

The pathogenesis of canine FCE is poorly understood. Most authors agree that emboli travel to the spinal cord through either arteries or veins. To produce the extent of ischemic myelopathy observed clinically, it is necessary to simultaneously compromise many closely associated small blood vessels. Histopathology usually reveals multiple emboli with staining characteristics much like fibrocartilage found in a degenerating nucleus pulposus. The clinical presence of associated intervertebral disk herniation is variable. Embolization into the ventral spinal artery and its branches as well as vertebral venous sinuses has been demonstrated (Fig. 37-3).

FIG. 37-3
Schematic illustration showing a proposed pathogenesis of a fibrocartilaginous embolism involving extrusion of nuclear material into the vertebral venous sinus or ventral spinal artery and then into small vessels supplying the spinal cord parenchyma.

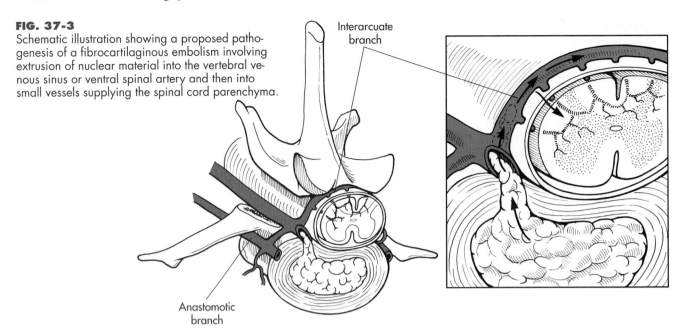

Sudden elevation in central venous pressure, as seen during coughing or vomiting, may be required to propel fibrocartilaginous emboli into the spinal cord's venous drainage. Although other material such as parasites, tissue, metastatic neoplasia, air, fat, foreign bodies, and bacteria could embolize the spinal cord, fibrocartilaginous material is most commonly associated with canine embolic myelopathy.

DIAGNOSIS
Clinical Presentation

Signalment. FCE most commonly affects large non-chondrodystrophoid breeds (e.g., Great Danes, St. Bernards, Labrador retrievers, and German shepherds). The disease is most common in young adults (3 to 7 years); however, it may be seen at almost any age, including dogs as young as 3 months. FCE has also been reported in cats and horses. There is no sex predisposition.

History. Patients typically present with an acute, non-progressive, ambulatory or nonambulatory, tetra-, para-, hemi-, or monoparesis without spinal hyperpathia (i.e., back or neck pain). Frequently, history reveals the dog was running or jumping when clinical dysfunction was detected. In rare instances, there is a history of trauma, but the majority of cases occur acutely without apparent cause. Occasionally, the dog may cry out, as if in pain; however, persistent pain is not a feature.

Physical Examination Findings

Physical examination findings are generally normal. Neurologic examination findings include an acute onset of nonprogressive UMN or LMN, lateralizing, ambulatory or nonambulatory, tetra-, para-, hemi-, or monoparesis, without spinal hyperpathia. Abnormal neurologic findings are consistent with a focal spinal cord lesion anywhere in the five anatomic divisions of the spinal cord (see Fig. 33-9). Typical neurologic signs for each anatomic division are discussed. A

loss of deep pain perception occurs in severe cases of spinal cord ischemia.

Radiography/Ultrasonography

Survey radiographs are generally normal, although mild collapse of an intervertebral space may be seen. If myelography is performed within 12 to 24 hours of the injury, mild spinal cord swelling, suggestive of an intramedullary mass, is seen. If myelography is delayed, spinal cord swelling resolves and a normal study results.

Laboratory Findings

Routine hematologic and serum biochemical analyses are normal. Cerebral spinal fluid analysis is often normal, but may reveal mild protein elevation with normal numbers of leukocytes. Mild xanthochromia (i.e., a yellowish appearance due to hemolyzed blood) sometimes occurs.

DIFFERENTIAL DIAGNOSIS

Fibrocartilaginous embolism must be differentiated from disorders causing acute, focal, asymmetric (i.e., lateralizing signs), nonprogressive paresis without spinal hyperpathia that includes fracture/luxation, intervertebral disk extrusion, and spinal neoplasia. Patients with fracture/luxation generally have persistent back pain; a diagnosis is based on neurologic examination and survey radiographs. Patients with spinal neoplasia present with a variety of clinical and neurologic symptoms; diagnosis is based on myelographic findings compatible with an extradural, intradural-extramedullary, or intramedullary mass (see p. 1044). A presumptive diagnosis of FCE is based on a compatible history and neurologic examination, combined with normal survey spinal radiographs and characteristic myelographic findings (i.e., normal or mild spinal cord swelling). The diagnosis is usually established by eliminating other causes of spinal cord disease; however, a definitive diagnosis is based on histopathologic identification of characteristic fibrocartilaginous emboli and resultant spinal cord infarction.

MEDICAL MANAGEMENT

Therapy depends upon the time of the patient's examination after the onset of clinical signs. Patients presented within 72 hours of the onset of clinical signs should be treated with corticosteroids (Table 37-5), physiotherapy, and confined for 2 to 3 weeks in an elevated cage with dry soft bedding and easy access to food and water. Frequent bladder expressions (i.e., QID) should be induced. Patients presented after 72 hours are treated with supportive care only. Proper treatment of ambulatory and nonambulatory patients is described on pp. 1062 and 1108.

SURGICAL TREATMENT

Fibrocartilaginous embolism is not a surgical disorder.

PROGNOSIS

Prognosis for recovery depends on the site of embolism (i.e., UMN vs. LMN), degree of improvement within 14 days, and the extent of spinal cord damage. Generally, patients with UMN deficits are more likely to recover than patients with LMN deficits. Patients showing improvement within 14 days and those with less extensive spinal cord damage (i.e., based on neurologic examination) are more likely to recover.

TABLE 37-5

Corticosteroid Therapy of Acute FCE

Dexamethasone (Azium)

0.2-0.4 mg/kg PO, TID—then BID for 2 days and SID for 2 days

Suggested Reading

Dyce J, Houlton JEF: Fibrocartilaginous embolism in the dog, *J Sm Anim Pract* 34:332, 1993.

Gilmore DR, deLahunta A: Necrotizing myelopathy secondary to presumed or confirmed fibrocartilaginous embolism in 24 dogs, *J Am Anim Hosp Assoc* 23:373, 1987.

Luttgen PJ: Common degenerative and vascular neurologic disorders in cats and dogs, *Prog Vet Neurol* 1:387, 1990.

Zaki FA, Prata RG: Necrotizing myelopathy secondary to embolization of herniated intervertebral disk material in the dog, *J Am Vet Med Assoc* 169:222, 1976.

Zaki FA, Prata RG, Kay WJ: Necrotizing myelopathy in five Great Danes, *J Am Vet Med Assoc* 165:1080, 1974.

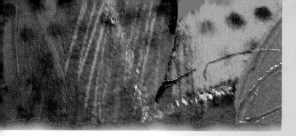

Product Appendix

Abbocatch, Abbott Laboratories, Hospital Products Division, Chicago, Ill.

Achromycin (tetracycline HCl) Lederle Laboratories, Pearl River, N.Y.

Adaptic, Johnson & Johnson, New Brunswick, N.J.

Amiglyde-V (amikacin sulfate), Fort Dodge Laboratories, Inc., Fort Dodge, Iowa

Amoxi-Drops (amoxicillin), SmithKline Beecham Animal Health, Exton, Pa.

Amoxi-Tabs (amoxicillin), SmithKline Beecham Animal Health, Exton, Pa.

Ancef (cefazolin sodium), SmithKline Beecham, Philadelphia, Pa.

Angiocath over-the-needle catheter, Becton Dickinson Vascular Access, Sandy, Utah

Antirobe (clindamycin HCl), The Upjohn Co., Animal Health Division, Kalamazoo, Mich.

Antivenin ([Crotalidae] polyvalent), Fort Dodge Laboratories, Inc., Fort Dodge, Iowa

Aquaphor (cholesterolized anhydrous petrolatum ointment base), Beirsdorf, Inc., Norwalk, Conn.

Argyle thoracic trocar catheter, Sherwood Medical Corp., St. Louis, Mo.

Arquel (meclofenamic acid), Fort Dodge Laboratories, Inc., Fort Dodge, Iowa

Asacol (mesalamine), Procter & Gamble Co., Cincinnati, Ohio

Ascriptin (aspirin, magnesium hydroxide, aluminum hydroxide), Ciba Self-Medication, Inc., Woodbridge, N.J.

Autoclave Tape, 3M Co., St. Paul, Minn.

AutoSuture TA, United States Surgical Corp., AutoSuture Co., Norwalk, Conn.

Avalon Copolymer Flakes, Summit Hill Laboratories, Navesink, N.J.

Azium (dexamethasone), Schering-Plough Animal Health, Union, N.J.

Azulfidine (sulfasalazine), Pharmacia, Inc., Columbus, Ohio

Banamine (flunixin meglumine), Schering-Plough Animal Health, Union, N.J.

Bard Biopty-cut biopsy needle, Bard Urological Division, CR Bard, Inc., Covington, Ga.

Bard Biopty biopsy instrument, Bard Urological Division, CR Bard, Inc., Covington, Ga.

Baytril (enrofloxacin), Miles Agricultural Division, Animal Health Products, Shawnee Mission, Kan.

Biobrane, Winthrop Pharmaceuticals, New York, N.Y.

Biosol (neomycin sulfate), The Upjohn Co., Animal Health Division, Kalamazoo, Mich.

Brethine, Ciba-Geigy Pharmaceuticals, Summit, N.J.

Brevibloc (esmolol HCl), Anaquest, Liberty Corner, N.J.

Bricanyl (terbutaline sulfate), Marion Merrell Dow, Inc., Kansas City, Mo.

Buprenex (buprenorphine), Reckitt & Colman, Richmond, Va.

Butterfly Catheter, Abbott Hospitals, Inc., North Chicago, Ill.

Carafate (sucralfate), Marion Merrell Dow, Inc., Kansas City, Mo.

Cefa-Drops (cefadroxil), Fort Dodge Laboratories, Inc., Fort Dodge, Iowa

Cefadyl (cephapirin sodium), Apothecon, Princeton, N.J.

Cefa-Tabs (cefadroxil), Fort Dodge Laboratories, Inc., Fort Dodge, Iowa

Cefa-Lak (cephapirin sodium), Fort Dodge Laboratories, Inc., Fort Dodge, Iowa

Chloromycetin (chloramphenicol), Parke-Davis, Morris Plains, N.J.

Choledyl SA (oxytriphylline), Parke-Davis, Morris Plains, N.J.

Chronulac (lactulose), Marion Merrell Dow, Inc., Kansas City, Mo.

Clavamox (amoxicillin trihydrate, clavulanate potassium), SmithKline Beeecham Animal Health, Exton, Pa.

Colace (docusate sodium), Bristol-Myers Squibb, Princeton, N.J.

Colyte (polyethylene glycol-electrolyte solution), Reed & Carnrick, Jersey City, N.J.

Conform Stretch Bandages, The Kendall Co., Hospital Products, Boston, Mass.

Cortigel, Savage Laboratories, Melville, N.Y.

Cortosyn, (cosyntropin, mannitol, lyophilized powder), Organon Pharmaceuticals, West Orange, N.J.

Cuprimine (penacillamine), Merck & Co., West Point, Pa.

Cytobin (sodium liothyronine), SmithKline Beecham Animal Health, Exton, Pa.

Cytomel (liothyronine sodium), SmithKline Pharmaceuticals, Philadelphia, Pa.

Cytotec (misoprostol), Searle, Skokie, Ill.

Cytoxan (cyclophosphamide), Bristol-Myers Squibb, Oncology Division, Princeton, N.J.

Debrisan (dextranomer), Johnson & Johnson Medical, Inc., New Brunswick, N.J.

DekNatel Pleur-evac chest drainage system, Sherwood Medical Corp., St. Louis, Mo.

DekNatel thoracic trocar catheter, Baxter Healthcare Corp., Round Lake, Ill.

Denver double-valve peritoneous shunt, Denver Biomaterials, Inc., Denver, Colo.

Depo-Testosterone (testosterone cypionate), The Upjohn Co., Kalamazoo, Mich.

Derma-Clens, SmithKline Beecham Animal Health, Exton, Pa.

Dermaheal, Solvay, Inc., Princeton, N.J.

Dexatrim (phenylpronamolamine HCl), Thompson Medical Co., West Palm Beach, Fla.

Dexon, Davis & Geck, Divison of American Cyanamid Co., Wayne, N.J.

Dibenzyline (phenoxybenzamine HCl), SmithKline Beecham Pharmaceuticals, Philadelphia, Pa.

Didronel (etidronate sodium), Procter & Gamble Pharmaceuticals, Norwich, N.Y.

Dinamap, Critikon, Inc., Tampa, Fla.

Dipentum (olsalazine sodium), Pharmacia, Inc., Columbus, Ohio

Diprivan (propofol), Zeneca Pharmaceuticals, Wilmington, Del.

Dog Bootie, Cold Spot Feeds, Fairbanks, Alaska

Dover red rubber Robinson catheter, Sherwood Medical Corp., St. Louis, Mo.

Dr. Larson's plastic teat tubes, Haver-Lockhart, Shawnee, Kan.

Dulcolax (Bisacodyl), Ciba Consumer Pharmaceuticals, Woodbridge, N.J.

DuoDERM, Conva Tec, A Bristol-Myers Squibb Company, Princeton, N.J.

EEA stapler, Unted States Surgical Corp., Norwalk, Conn.

Elase (fibrinolysin, desoxyribonuclease), Parke-Davis, Morris Plains, N.J.

Elastikon porous adhesive tape, Johnson & Johnson Medical, Inc., New Brunswick, N.J.

Eld feeding tube, Jorgensen Laboratories, Inc., Loveland, Colo.

Enacard (enalapril maleate), Merck Agvet, Iselin, N.J.

Evan's Blue (Direct Blue 53), MCB Manufacturing Chemists, Inc., Cincinnati, Ohio

Feldene (piroxicam), Pfizer U.S. Pharmaceutical Group, New York, N.Y.

Festal II (lipase, amylase, protease), Hoechst-Roussel Pharmaceuticals, Inc., Somerville, N.J.

Flagyl (metranidazole), Searle, Skokie, Ill.

Fluorofil, Mallinckrodt Veterinary, Mundelein, Ill.

Franklin-modified Vim Silverman biopsy needles, V. Mueller, Division of Baxter, McGaw Park, Ill.

Furacin dressing, Norden Laboratories, Inc., Lincoln, Neb.

Garamycin (gentamicin sulfate), Schering Corp., Kenilworth, N.J.

Gelfoam, The Upjohn Co., Kansas City, Mo.

Gentocin (gentamicin sulfate), Schering-Plough Animal Health, Union, N.J.

Geocillin (carbenicillin indanyl sodium), Roerig, New York, N.Y.

GIA stapler, United States Surgical Corp., Norwalk, Conn.

GNC Ca-Mg, General Nutrition Corp., Pittsburgh, Pa.

Golytely, Braintree Laboratories, Inc., Braintree, Mass.

Granulex-V, SmithKline Animal Health, Exton, Pa.

Hemoclip, Solvay Animal Health Inc., Mendota Heights, Mont.

Hemoclip (medium), Edward Weck & Co., Inc., Research Triangle Park, N.C.

Hycodan (hydrocodone), DuPont Pharmaceuticals, Wilmington, Del.

i/d prescription diet, Hills Pet Products, Inc., Topeka, Kan.

ILP stapler, Ethicon, Inc., Somerville, N.J.

Imodium (loperamide), Janssen Pharmaceuticals, Inc., Titusville, N.J.

Imuran (azathioprine), Burroughs Wellcome Co., Research Triangle Park, N.C.

Inderal (propranolol HCl), Wyeth-Ayerst Laboratories, Philadelphia, Pa.

Innovar-Vet (fentanyl, droperidol), Pitman-Moore, Inc., Mundelein, Ill.

Intravent intraoperative tissue expanders, Cox-Uphoff International, Costa Mesa, Calif.

Isovue, Squibb Diagnostic Division, Princeton, N.J.

Isuprel (isoproterenol HCl), Sanofi Winthrop Pharmaceuticals, New York, N.Y.

Jamshidi needle, American Pharmaseal, Valencia, Calif.

Jelco over-the-needle catheter, Critikon, Tampa, Fla.

Kantrim (karamycin sulfate), Fort Dodge Laboratories, Inc., Fort Dodge, Iowa

k/d prescription diet, Hills Pet Products, Inc., Topeka, Kan.

Kefzol (cefazolin sodium), Eli Lilly & Co., Indianapolis, Ind.

Kerlix Rolls, The Kendall Co., Hospital Products, Boston, Mass.

Kling, Johnson & Johnson Medical Inc., New Brunswick, N.J.

K-Y Jelly, Johnson & Johnson Medical Inc., New Brunswick, N.J.

Lanoxin (digoxin), Burroughs Wellcome Co., Research Triangle Park, N.C.

Lasix (furasemide), Hoechst-Roussel Agri-Vet Co., Somerville, N.J.

Leukeran (chlorambucil), Burroughs Wellcome Co., Research Triangle Park, N.C.

Ligaclip, Ethicon, Inc., Somerville, N.J.

Lomotil (diphenoxylate HCl with atropine sulfate), Searle, Skokie, Ill.

Lubafax surgical lubricant, Burroughs Wellcome Co., Research Triangle Park, N.C.

Marlex Mesh, Division of Bard Vascular Systems, Billerica, Mass.

Maxon, Davis & Geck, Division of American Cyanamid Co., Wayne, N.J.

Medrol (methylprednisolone), The Upjohn Co., Kalamazoo, Mich.

Mefoxin (cefoxitin sodium), Merck & Co., West Point, Pa.

Mestinon (pyridostigmine bromide), ICN Pharmaceuticals, Inc., Costa Mesa, Calif.

Metamucil (psyllium), Procter & Gamble Co., Cincinnati, Ohio

Methylene blue injection 1%, Elkins-Sinn, Cherry Hill, N.J.

Michel Clip, V. Mueller, Baxter Healthcare Corp., McGaw Park, Ill.

Michelle trephine, V. Mueller, Baxter Healthcare Corp., McGaw Park, Ill.

Minocin (minocycline HCl), Lederle Laboratories, Pearl River, N.Y.

Morton Lite Salt, Morton Salt Co., Chicago, Ill.

Naprosyn (naproxen), Syntex Laboratories, Palo Alto, Calif.

Nature Made Nutritional Products, Los Angeles, Calif.

Nitropress (nitroprusside sodium), Abbott Laboratories, Abbott Park, Ill.

No. 7 Bard Parker scalpel handle, Becton Dickinson Acute Care, Franklin Lakes, N.J.

No. 11 Bard Parker scalpel blade, Becton Dickinson Acute Care, Franklin Lakes, N.J.

Nolvasan solution, Fort Dodge Laboratories, Inc., Fort Dodge, Iowa

Normosol-R, Sanofi Animal Health, Inc., Overland Park, Kan.

North American Coral Snake Antivenin, Wyeth Laboratories, Inc., Marietta, Pa.

Novafil, Davis & Geck, Division of American Cyanamid Co., Wayne, N.J.

Nu-Gauze, Johnson & Johnson, New Brunswick, N.J.

Numorphan (oxymorphone), DuPont Pharmaceutical, Wilmington, Del.

OK Sterilization Indicators, Propper Manufacturing Co., Inc., Long Island City, N.Y.

Omnipaque (iohexol), Sanofi Winthrop Pharmaceuticals, New York, N.Y.

Orbenin (sodium cloxacillin), SmithKline Beecham Animal Health, Exton, Pa.

Orthoplast splinting material, Johnson & Johnson Medical, Inc., New Brunswick, N.J.

Polydioxanone suture (PDS), Ethicon, Inc., Somerville, N.J.

PLC50 stapler, Ethicon, Inc., Somerville, N.J.

Penrose drains, Davol, Inc., Cranston, R.I.

Pepcid (famotidine), Merck & Co., West Point, Pa.

Periactin (cyproheptadine HCl), Merck & Co., West Point, Pa.

Polytetrafluoroethylene (PTFE), Impra Graft, IMPRA, Inc., Tempe, Az.

Premium CEEA stapler, United States Surgical Corp., Norwalk, Conn.

Preparation-H, Whitehall Laboratories, Inc., New York, N.Y.

Prilosec (omeprazole), Astra Merck, Wayne, Pa.

Primaxin (imipenem-cilastatin), Merck & Co., West Point, Pa.

Pro-Banthine (propantheline bromide), SCS Pharmaceuticals, Chicago, Ill.

Proglycem (diazoxide), Baker Norton Pharmaceuticals, Miami, Fla.

Prolene Mesh, Ethicon, Inc., Somerville, N.J.

Pronestyl (procainamide), Princeton Pharmaceutical Products, New Brunswick, N.J.

Propagest (phenylpropanolamine), Reed & Carnrick, Jersey City, N.J.

Propulsid (cisapride), Janssen Pharmaceuticals, Inc., Titusville, N.J.

Proximate Plus, Ethicon, Inc., Somerville, N.J.

Pulsavac Debridement System, Zimmer, Zimmer Patient Care Division, Dover, Ohio

Q-Tips, Johnson & Johnson Medical, Inc., New Brunswick, N.J.

Radiant Valley Natural Selenium, Perrigo Co., Allegan, Mich.

Radovan Tissue Expander, Mentor Corp., Heyer-Schulte Products Division, Goleta, Calif.

Rapinovet, Mallincrodt Veterinary, Mundelein, Ill.

Regenol (pyridastigmine bromide), Organon, Inc., West Orange, N.J.

Regitine (phentolamine), Ciba-Geigy Pharmaceuticals, Summit, N.J.

Reglan (Metaclopramide HCl), A.H. Robins Co., Inc., Philadelphia, Pa.

Release, Johnson & Johnson Medical, Inc., New Brunswick, N.J.

Renovist (diatrizoate methylglucamine), Bristol-Myers Squibb, Princeton, N.J.

Resco nail shears, Tecla Co., Wallid Lake, Mich.

Rimadyl (nonsteroidal antiinflammatory), Pfizer, New York, N.Y.

Robaxin-V (methocarbanol), A.H. Robins Company, Inc., Philadelphia, Pa.

RU60 stapler, Ethicon, Inc., Somerville, N.J.

Silastic medical grade tubing, Dow Corning Corp., Midland, Mich.

Silastic sheeting #501-3. Dow Corning Corp, Midland, Mich.

Silvadene Cream (silver sulfadiazine), Marion Laboratories, Inc., Kansas City, Mo.

Snyder Hemovac, Zimmer, Inc., Warshaw, Ind.

SoftPaws, Smart Practice, Phoenix, Az.

Soloxine (levothyroxine sodium), Daniels Pharmaceuticals, Inc., St. Petersburg, Fla.

Sovereign feeding tube, Sherwood Medical, St. Louis, Mo.

Specialist cast padding, Johnson & Johnson Medical, Inc., New Brunswick, N.J.

Specialist tubular stockinet, Johnson & Johnson Medical, Inc., New Brunswick, N.J.

Sterrad Chemical Indicator Strip, Johnson & Johnson Medical, Inc., Irvine, Calif.

Stylocath w/L connector, Abbott Laboratories, North Chicago, Ill.

Sublimaze (fentanyl), Janssen Pharmaceutical, Inc., Titusville, N.J.

Supramid, S. Jackson, Inc., Alexandria, Va.

Surgicel, Johnson & Johnson Medical, Inc., Arlington, Tex.

Synthroid (sodium levothyroxine), Boots Pharmaceuticals, Inc., Lincolnshire, Ill.

Tagamet (cimetidine), SmithKline Beecham Pharmaceuticals, Philadelphia, Pa.

Tail Docker/Cutter, Jorgensen Laboratories, Loveland, Colo.

Tapazole (methimazole), Eli Lilly & Co., Indianapolis, Ind.

Tegopen (cloxacillin sodium), Bristol-Myers Squibb, Princeton, N.J.

Tegtmeyer lymph duct cannulator, North American Instrument Co., Hudson Falls, N.Y.

Telfa Pads, The Kendall Co., Hospital Products, Boston, Mass.

Tenormin (atenolol), Zeneca Pharmaceuticals, Wilmington, Del.

Tensilon (edrophonium chloride), Roche Laboratories, Nutley, N.J.

Thoracoabdominal (TA) stapler, United States Surgical Corp., Norwalk, Conn.

Thoraseal III three-bottle underwater chest drainage system, Sherwood Medical Corp, St. Louis, Mo.

Thyro-Tabs (levothyroxine sodium), Vet-A-Mix, Inc., Shenandoah, Iowa

Torbugesic (butorphanol tartrate), Fort Dodge Laboratories, Fort Dodge, Iowa

Torbutrol (butorphanol tartrate), Fort Dodge Laboratories, Fort Dodge, Iowa

Traverse Ointment, Flint Laboratories, Division of Travenol Laboratories, Deerfield, Ill.

Tribrissen (sulfadiazine and trimethoprim), Cooper's Animal Health, Inc., Mundelein, Ill.

Tru-cut biopsy device, Travenol Laboratories, Inc., Deerfield, Ill.

Tru-cut biopsy needle, Travenol Laboratories, Inc, Deerfield, Ill.

Tubegauz, Scholl Manufacturing Co., Inc., Chicago, Ill.

Turnbuckle distraction bars, IMEX Veterinary, Inc., Longview, Tex.

Urecholine (bethanechol chloride), Merck & Co., West Point, Pa.

Valium (diazepam), Roche Animal Health & Nutrition, Nutley, N.J.

Vascular Ties, Sil-Med Corp., Taunton, Mass.

Vasotec (enalapril), Merck & Co., West Point, Pa.

Velosef (cephadrine), Bristol-Myers Squibb, Princeton, N.J.

Vetafil, S. Jackson Company, Alexandria, Va.

Vetbond tissue adhesive, 3M Animal Care Products, 3M Co., St. Paul, Minn.

Vetrap, 3M Animal Care Products, 3M Co., St. Paul, Minn.

Vibramycin (doxycycline), Roerig, New York, N.Y.

Vicryl, Ethicon, Inc., Somerville, N.J.

Vim-Silverman needle, V. Mueller, Division of Baxter, McGaw Park, Ill.

Vivonex, (amino acid enteral nutrition), Sandoz Nutrition, Minneapolis, Minn.

Water Pik, Teledyne Water Pik, Fort Collins, Colo.

w/d prescription diet, Hills Pet Products, Inc., Topeka, Kan.

Westcott style biopsy needle, Manan Medical Products, Northbrook, Ill.

Xeroform, Sherwood Medical, St. Louis, Mo.

Zantac (ranitidine), Glaxo Wellcome, Inc., Research Triangle Park, N.C.

Zefazone (cefmetazole sodium), The Upjohn Co., Animal Health Division, Kalamazoo, Mich.

Zestril (lisinopril), Stuart Pharmaceuticals, Wilmington, Del.

Zyloprim (allopurinol), Burroughs Wellcome, Research Triangle Park, N.C.

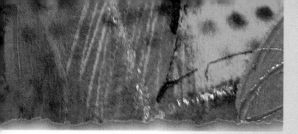

Index

A